HARRISON'S
PRINCIPLES
OF
INTERNAL
MEDICINE

HARRISON'S
PRINCIPLES
OF
INTERNAL
MEDICINE

VOLUME ONE
pages 1 to 1079
SIXTH EDITION

EDITORS

MAXWELL M. WINTROBE

B.A., M.D., B.SC. (Med.), PH.D., D.SC. (Hon.), D.SC. (Hon.), F.A.C.P.

Professor of Internal Medicine; Director, Cardiovascular Research and Training Institute; Director, Laboratory for Study of Hereditary and Metabolic Disorders; University of Utah College of Medicine, Salt Lake City

GEORGE W. THORN

M.D., M.A. (Hon.), LL.D. (Hon.), D.SC. (Hon.), M.D. (Hon.), F.R.C.P.

Hersey Professor of the Theory and Practice of Physic; Samuel A. Levine Professor of Medicine, Harvard Medical School; Physician-in-Chief, Peter Bent Brigham Hospital, Boston

RAYMOND D. ADAMS

B.A., M.A., M.D., M.A. (Hon.), D.M.SC. (Hon.)

Bullard Professor of Neuropathology, Harvard Medical School; Chief of Neurology and Neuropathologist, Massachusetts General Hospital, Boston; Director of Kennedy Laboratories of Massachusetts General Hospital; Co-Director of Eunice Shriver Center, Fernald State School; Associate Physician, University Hospital, Lausanne, Switzerland

IVAN L. BENNETT, JR.

A.B., M.D.

Director, New York University Medical Center, New York

EUGENE BRAUNWALD

A.B., M.D.

Professor and Chairman, Department of Medicine, University of California at San Diego School of Medicine, La Jolla; Chief of Medicine, University Hospital of San Diego County

KURT J. ISSELBACHER

M.D.

Professor of Medicine, Harvard Medical School; Physician and Chief, Gastrointestinal Unit, Massachusetts General Hospital, Boston

ROBERT G. PETERSDORF

A.B., M.D. (Associate Editor)

Professor and Chairman, Department of Medicine, University of Washington School of Medicine; Physician-in-Chief, University of Washington Hospital, Seattle

A BLAKISTON PUBLICATION

McGRAW-HILL BOOK COMPANY

New York · St. Louis · San Francisco · Düsseldorf · London · Mexico · Panama · Sydney · Toronto

HARRISON'S
PRINCIPLES
OF INTERNAL
MEDICINE

Library of Congress Catalog Card Number 76-78960

6 7 8 9 R M R M 9 8 7 6 5

ISBN 07-0 71131-3

FOREIGN LANGUAGE EDITIONS

Portuguese (Fourth Edition)—Editôra Guanabara Koogen, Lta., © 1968
Spanish (Third Edition)—La Prensa Medica Mexicana, © 1965
Italian—Casa Editrice Dr. Francesco Vallardi, Societá Editrice Libraria, Spa., Milan, © 1968
Polish—Panstwowy Zaklad Wydawnictw Lekarskich, expected © 1970
Greek—G. Parissianos Medical and Scientific Books, Athens, expected © 1971

This book was set in Caledonia by The Colonial Press Inc., and printed on permanent paper and bound by Rand McNally and Co. The cover was designed by John Condon; the drawings were done by B. Handelman Associates, Inc. The editors were René Boudreau, Paul K. Schneider, and Diane Drobnis. Eugene Capriotti supervised the production.

NOTICE

Medicine is an ever-changing science. As new research and clinical experience broaden our knowledge, changes in treatment and drug therapy are required. The editors and the publisher of this work have made every effort to ensure that the drug dosage schedules herein are accurate and in accord with the standards accepted at the time of publication. The reader is advised, however, to check the product information sheet included in the package of each drug he plans to administer to be certain that changes have not been made in the recommended dose or in the contraindications for administration. This recommendation is of particular importance in regard to new or infrequently used drugs.

*To all those
who have taught us,
and especially to
our younger colleagues
who continue to
teach and inspire us*

Contributors

AMERICO ABBRUZZESE, M.D.
Clinical Associate in Medicine, Harvard Medical School; Associate in Medicine, Peter Bent Brigham Hospital, Boston.

RAYMOND D. ADAMS, B.A., M.A., M.D., M.A. (HON.), D.M.SC. (HON.)
Bullard Professor of Neuropathology, Harvard Medical School; Chief of Neurology Service and Neuropathologist, Massachusetts General Hospital, Boston.

MENELAOS A. ALIAPOULIOS, M.D., B.S.
Associate in Surgery, Harvard Medical School; Junior Associate in Surgery, Peter Bent Brigham Hospital, Boston.

JAMES C. ALLEN, M.D.
Associate Professor of Medicine and Chief of the Infectious Diseases Unit, State University of New York at Buffalo, School of Medicine, Buffalo, New York.

DAVID H. ALPERS, M.D.
Assistant Professor of Medicine, Washington University School of Medicine; Director, Gastroenterology Division, Department of Internal Medicine, Washington University School of Medicine, St. Louis.

FAYE D. ARUNDELL, M.D.
Clinical Assistant Professor of Dermatology, Stanford University School of Medicine, Stanford, California.

ARTHUR K. ASBURY, M.D.
Associate Professor of Neurology and Associate Director of the Department of Neurology, University of California Medical School at Berkeley, California.

KARL-ERIK ÅSTRÖM, M.D.
Visiting Assistant Professor of Neuropathology, Harvard Medical School; Associate Neuropathologist, Massachusetts General Hospital, Boston.

K. FRANK AUSTEN, M.D.
Professor of Medicine, Harvard Medical School; Physician-in-Chief, Robert Breck Brigham Hospital, Boston.

ROBERT AUSTRIAN, M.D.
John Herr Musser Professor of Research Medicine, University of Pennsylvania School of Medicine, Philadelphia.

HARRY N. BEATY, M.D.
Assistant Professor of Medicine, University of Washington; Head, Division of Infectious Diseases, Harborview Medical Center (King County Hospital), Seattle.

ALBERT R. BEHNKE, B.A., M.D., M.S. (HON.)
Formerly Radiological Medical Director, U.S. Naval Radiological Defense Laboratory, San Francisco.

IVAN L. BENNETT, JR., A.B., M.D.
Director, New York University Medical Center, New York.

DANIEL S. BERNSTEIN, M.D., A.B.
Assistant Professor in Medicine, Harvard Medical School; Senior Associate in Medicine, Peter Bent Brigham Hospital, Boston.

THOMAS C. BITHELL, M.D.
Associate Professor of Internal Medicine and Clinical Pathology, University of Virginia, Charlottesville, Virginia.

DANE R. BOGGS, M.D.
Professor of Medicine; Chief, Hematology Section, Department of Medicine, University of Pittsburgh, Pittsburgh, Pennsylvania.

STUART BONDURANT, M.D.
Robert B. Lamb Professor of Medicine and Chairman, Department of Medicine, Albany Medical College, Albany, New York.

ABRAHAM I. BRAUDE, M.D.
Professor of Medicine; Head, Division of Infectious Diseases, University of California at San Diego School of Medicine, La Jolla.

RALPH W. BRAUER, M.SC., PH.D.
Director, Wrightsville Marine Bio-Medical Laboratory, Wilmington; Professor of Physiology and Pharmacology, Duke University Medical Center, Durham; Visiting Professor of Physiology, University of North Carolina, Chapel Hill.

EUGENE BRAUNWALD, A.B., M.D.
Professor and Chairman, Department of Medicine, University of California at San Diego School of Medicine, La Jolla, California; Chief of Medicine, University Hospital of San Diego County.

THORNTON BROWN, M.D.
Associate Clinical Professor of Orthopedic Surgery, Harvard Medical School; Visiting Orthopedic Surgeon, Massachusetts General Hospital, Boston.

MATTHEW A. BUDD, M.D.
Assistant Professor of Medicine, Harvard Medical School; Associate in Medicine, Beth Israel Hospital, Boston.

GEORGE F. CAHILL, JR., B.S., M.D., M.A. (HON.)
Associate Professor of Medicine and Director, Elliott P. Joslin Research Laboratories, Harvard Medical School; Senior Associate in Medicine, Peter Bent Brigham Hospital, Boston.

EVAN CALKINS, M.D., A.B.
Professor and Chairman, Department of Medicine, State University of New York at Buffalo; Director of Medicine, Edward J. Meyer Memorial Hospital, Buffalo; Attending Physician, Buffalo General Hospital.

CHARLES C. J. CARPENTER, M.D.
Professor of Medicine, Johns Hopkins University School of Medicine; Chief of Medicine, Baltimore City Hospitals, Baltimore.

GEORGE E. CARTWRIGHT, B.A., M.D.
Professor and Head, Department of Medicine, University of Utah College of Medicine, Salt Lake City, Utah.

LEIGHTON E. CLUFF, M.D.
Professor and Chairman, Department of Medicine, University of Florida School of Medicine, Gainesville, Florida.

ROBERT E. COOKE, B.S., M.D.
Given Foundation Professor of Pediatrics and Chairman of

the Department, Johns Hopkins University School of Medicine; Pediatrician-in-Chief, Johns Hopkins Hospital, Baltimore.

LEWIS L. CORIELL, M.A., PH.D., M.D., F.A.A.P.
Professor of Pediatrics, University of Pennsylvania School of Medicine, Philadelphia; Senior Physician, The Children's Hospital, Philadelphia; Director, South Jersey Medical Research Foundation, Camden, New Jersey.

JOHN F. CRIGLER, JR., M.D.
Associate Professor of Pediatrics, Harvard Medical School; Senior Associate in Medicine and Chief, Endocrine Division, Children's Hospital Medical Center, Boston.

EUGENE P. CRONKITE, M.D., D.SC. (HON.)
Chairman, Medical Department, Brookhaven National Laboratory, Upton, New York.

JOSEPH F. DINGMAN, M.D., B.S.
Lecturer in Medicine, Harvard Medical School; Senior Associate in Medicine, Peter Bent Brigham Hospital, Boston.

PHILIP R. DODGE, M.D.
Professor and Chairman of the Department of Pediatrics, Washington University, St. Louis, Missouri.

E. E. EDDLEMAN, JR., B.S., M.D.
Professor of Medicine, University of Alabama Medical College; Associate Chief of Staff for Research and Education, Veterans Administration Hospital, Birmingham.

KENDALL EMERSON, JR., M.D., B.A.
Clinical Professor of Medicine, Harvard Medical School; Physician, Peter Bent Brigham Hospital; Chief of Medicine, Boston Lying-In Hospital, Boston.

KARL ENGELMAN, M.D.
Senior Investigator, Experimental Therapeutics Branch, National Heart and Lung Institute, National Institutes of Health, Bethesda, Maryland.

EDWIN ENGLERT, JR., M.D.
Associate Professor of Medicine and Chairman, Division of Gastroenterology, Department of Internal Medicine, University of Utah Medical Center; Chief, Medical Service, Veterans Administration Hospital, Salt Lake City.

FRANKLIN H. EPSTEIN, M.D.
Professor of Internal Medicine, Yale University School of Medicine, New Haven.

E. HARVEY ESTES, JR., M.D.
Professor and Chairman, Department of Community Medicine, Duke University Medical Center, Durham, North Carolina.

STEFAN S. FAJANS, B.S., M.D.
Professor of Internal Medicine, University of Michigan Medical School, Ann Arbor.

EUGENE M. FARBER, M.D., M.S.
Professor and Executive Head, Department of Dermatology, Stanford University School of Medicine, Stanford, California.

ALVAN R. FEINSTEIN, M.D.
Professor of Medicine and Epidemiology, Yale University School of Medicine, New Haven, Connecticut.

F. ROBERT FEKETY, JR., M.D.
Associate Professor of Medicine; Head, Division of Infectious Diseases, University of Michigan School of Medicine, Ann Arbor.

HARRY A. FELDMAN, A.B., M.D.
Professor and Chairman, Department of Preventive Medicine, State University of New York, Upstate Medical Center at Syracuse, New York.

RICHARD A. FIELD, A.B., M.D.
Professor of Medicine and Director, Division of Endocrinology and Metabolic Diseases, Jefferson Medical College, Philadelphia.

C. MILLER FISHER, M.D.
Associate Clinical Professor of Neurology, Harvard Medical School; Neurologist, Massachusetts General Hospital, Boston.

RUSSELL S. FISHER, M.D., B.S.
Chief Medical Examiner, State of Maryland; Professor of Forensic Pathology, University of Maryland Medical School; Lecturer in Forensic Pathology, Johns Hopkins Medical School; Associate in Public Health Administration, Johns Hopkins School of Hygiene and Public Health, Baltimore.

ALFRED P. FISHMAN, M.D.
Professor of Medicine, Director, Cardiovascular Pulmonary Division, University of Pennsylvania, Philadelphia.

THOMAS B. FITZPATRICK, M.D., PH.D.
Edward Wigglesworth Professor of Dermatology, Harvard Medical School; Chief, Dermatology Service, Massachusetts General Hospital, Boston.

JOHN FOERSTER, M.D.
Assistant Professor of Medicine, University of Manitoba, Winnipeg, Manitoba, Canada.

RICHARD H. FOLLIS, JR., M.D. (DECEASED)
Formerly Armed Forces Institute of Pathology and the Veterans Administration Central Laboratory for Anatomic Pathology and Research, AFIP, Washington, D.C.

EDWARD C. FRANKLIN, M.D.
Professor of Medicine and Head, Division of Rheumatology, New York University School of Medicine, New York.

DONALD S. FREDRICKSON, M.D.
Director of Intramural Research and Chief, Laboratory of Molecular Diseases, National Heart and Lung Institute, National Institutes of Health, Bethesda, Maryland.

LAWRENCE R. FREEDMAN, M.D., B.S.
Associate Professor of Medicine, Yale University School of Medicine, New Haven.

WILLIAM F. FRIEDMAN, M.D.
Assistant Professor of Medicine and Pediatrics; Chief, Divi-

sion of Pediatric Cardiology, University of California at San Diego School of Medicine, La Jolla, California.

ALVIN E. FRIEDMAN-KIEN, M.D.
Associate Professor of Dermatology, New York University School of Medicine, New York.

HARRY W. FRITTS, JR., M.D.
Professor of Medicine, Columbia University, College of Physicians and Surgeons, New York.

GERALD GLICK, M.D.
Associate Professor of
Laboratory of Clinical
College of Medicine,

ROBERT M. GLICKM
Instructor in Medicine
Medicine, Massachuset

JOHN R. GOLDSMIT
Head of Environment
Department of Public

PAUL GOLDHABER
Dean and Professor
School of Dental Me

J. T. GRAYSTON, M
Professor and Chairm
University of Washin

NORTON J. GREEN
Associate Professor
Gastroenterology, Oł
Attending Physician,
cine, Columbus.

SHELDON EDWA
Associate Professor
School of Medicine,

JOHN F. GRIFFIT
Assistant Professor
Medicine, Durham,

T. R. HARRISON,
Professor of Medicine, The Medical College of the
of Alabama, Birmingham, and Distinguished Professor of the University of Alabama.

DONALD H. HARTER, M.D.
Associate Professor of Neurology, Columbia University College of Physicians and Surgeons, New York.

ARTHUR HAUT, A.B., M.D.
Professor of Medicine and Head, Section on Hematology, University of Arkansas School of Medicine, Little Rock, Arkansas.

THOMAS R. HENDRIX, M.D.
Professor of Medicine, Johns Hopkins University School of Medicine, Baltimore.

ALBERT HEYMAN, B.S., M.D.
Professor of Neurology, Duke University School of Medicine, Durham, North Carolina.

ROGER B. HICKLER, M.D.
Lecturer in Medicine, Harvard Medical School; Senior Associate in Medicine, Peter Bent Brigham Hospital; Professor of Medicine, Boston University School of Medicine, Boston; Chief of Medicine, Framingham Union Hospital, Framingham.

FREDERIC L. HOCH, M.D., B.S., M.S.
...sor of Internal Medicine and Associate Professor... Chemistry, Department of Internal Medicine, ...of Michigan Medical Center, Ann Arbor.

...PRICH, M.D.
...Iedicine and Pathology, School of Medicine, ...California, Davis, California.

...HOOK, M.D.
...lholland Professor and Chairman, Department ...University of Virginia School of Medicine, Char-

...HORNICK, M.D.
...essor of Medicine; Head, Division of Infectious ...versity of Maryland School of Medicine, Balti-

...INGBAR, M.D.
...Castle Professor of Medicine, Harvard Medical ...ciate Director, Thorndike Memorial Laboratory, ...Hospital, Boston.

...SELBACHER, M.D.
...Medicine, Harvard Medical School; Physician ...Gastrointestinal Unit, Massachusetts General Hos-

...H B. JACKSON, A.B.
...ssistant Professor in Medicine, University of Mary-...of Medicine, Baltimore.

...W. JARCHO, A.B., M.A., M.D.
...d Head, Department of Neurology; Associate Professor of Medicine, University of Utah College of Medicine, Salt Lake City.

MICHEL JEQUIER, M.D.
Professor of Neurology, University of Lausanne, Switzerland; Chief of Neurology Services, Cantonal Hospital.

CAROL J. JOHNS, M.D.
Assistant Professor of Medicine, Johns Hopkins University School of Medicine, Baltimore.

JOSEPH E. JOHNSON, III, M.D.
Professor of Medicine; Head, Division of Infectious Diseases, University of Florida College of Medicine, Gainesville.

RICHARD L. KAHLER, M.D.
Associate Professor of Medicine, University of California at San Diego School of Medicine; Head, Division of Cardiopulmonary Diseases, Scripps Clinic and Research Foundation, La Jolla, California.

BYRON A. KAKULAS, M.D., M.R.A.C.P., M.C. PATH.
Lecturer in Pathology, Department of Pathology, School of Medicine, Victoria Square, Perth, Western Australia.

JAN KOCH-WESER, M.D.
Assistant Professor of Pharmacology, Harvard Medical School; Assistant Physician, Massachusetts General Hospital, Boston

M. GLENN KOENIG, M.D.
Associate Professor of Medicine; Head, Division of Infectious Diseases, Vanderbilt University School of Medicine, Nashville, Tennessee.

RAYMOND S. KOFF, M.D.
Assistant Professor of Medicine, Boston University School of Medicine; Clinical Investigator, Veterans Administration Hospital, Boston.

VERNON KNIGHT, M.D.
Professor of Medicine and Microbiology, Baylor College of Medicine, Houston, Texas.

JOHN H. KNOWLES, M.D.
General Director and Physician, Massachusetts General Hospital; Professor of Medicine, Harvard Medical School, Boston.

STEPHEN M. KRANE, M.D., A.M. (HON.), A.B.
Associate Professor of Medicine, Harvard Medical School; Physician and Chief, Arthritis Unit, Massachusetts General Hospital, Boston.

CARL KUPFER, M.D.
Director, National Eye Institute, National Institutes of Health, Bethesda, Maryland; formerly Professor and Chairman, Department of Ophthalmology, School of Medicine, University of Washington School of Medicine, Seattle.

DAVID P. LAULER, M.D., B.S.
Assistant Professor of Medicine, Harvard Medical School; Senior Associate in Medicine, Peter Bent Brigham Hospital, Boston.

G. RICHARD LEE, M.D.
Associate Professor of Medicine, College of Medicine, University of Utah, Salt Lake City, Utah.

A. MARTIN LERNER, M.D.
Professor of Medicine; Head, Division of Infectious Diseases, Wayne State University School of Medicine, Detroit, Michigan.

BERNARD LOWN, M.D.
Physician, Peter Bent Brigham Hospital; Associate Professor, Harvard School of Public Health, Boston, Massachusetts.

BERNARD LYTTON, M.B., B.S., F.R.C.S. (ENG.)
Associate Professor and Chief of Urology, Yale University School of Medicine, New Haven.

JANET W. McARTHUR, M.D., A.B., M.S., M.B., D.SC. (HON.)
Associate Clinical Professor of Obstetrics and Gynecology, Harvard Medical School; Associate Physician, Massachusetts General Hospital, Boston.

FRED R. McCRUMB, JR., M.D.
Professor of Medicine, University of Maryland School of Medicine, Baltimore.

VICTOR A. McKUSICK, M.D.
Professor of Medicine and Chief, Division of Medical Genetics, Department of Medicine, Johns Hopkins University School of Medicine, Baltimore, Maryland.

GEORGE V. MANN, M.D.
Associate Professor of Medicine and Associate Professor of Biochemistry, Vanderbilt University School of Medicine; Career Investigator, National Heart and Lung Institute, Nashville, Tennessee.

ALEXANDER MARBLE, M.D., M.A., A.B.
Clinical Professor in Medicine Emeritus, Harvard Medical School; Senior Associate in Medicine Emeritus, Peter Bent Brigham Hospital; Senior Physician, Joslin Clinic and New England Deaconess Hospital; President, Joslin Diabetes Foundation, Inc., Boston.

ALBERT I. MENDELOFF, M.D.
Associate Professor of Medicine, Johns Hopkins University School of Medicine; Physician-in-Chief, Sinai Hospital, Baltimore.

JOHN P. MERRILL, A.B., M.D.
Associate Professor of Medicine, Harvard Medical School; Director, Cardiorenal Section, Peter Bent Brigham Hospital, Boston.

EDWARD S. MILLER, M.D.
Associate Clinical Professor in Medicine, University of Colorado School of Medicine, Denver.

JAY P. MOHR, M.D., MAJ MC
Division of Neuropsychiatry, Walter Reed Army Institute of Research, Washington, D.C.

HUGO W. MOSER, M.D.
Associate Professor of Neurology at the Massachusetts General Hospital, Harvard Medical School; Neurologist, Massachusetts General Hospital; Assistant Superintendent, Fernald School, and Co-Director of Eunice Shriver Laboratories.

KENNETH M. MOSER, M.D.
Associate Professor of Medicine and Director, Pulmonary Disease Division, University of California at San Diego School of Medicine, La Jolla, California.

DON H. NELSON, M.D.
Chief of Medicine, Latter-day Saints Hospital; Professor o Medicine, University of Utah College of Medicine, Salt Lak City.

GEORGE NICHOLS, JR., M.D.
Clinical Professor of Medicine, Harvard Medical School; Senior Associate, Peter Bent Brigham Hospital, Boston.

PHILIP S. NORMAN, M.D.
Associate Professor of Medicine, Johns Hopkins University School of Medicine, Baltimore.

JOHN A. OATES, M.D.
Professor of Medicine and Pharmacology, Vanderbilt University Hospital, Nashville.

E. H. O. PARRY, M.D.
Professor and Chairman, Department of Medicine, Ahmadu Bello University, Zaria, Nigeria.

ROBERT G. PETERSDORF, M.D.
Professor and Chairman, Department of Medicine, University of Washington School of Medicine; Physician-in-Chief, University of Washington Hospital, Seattle.

JAMES J. PLORDE, M.D.
Assistant Professor of Medicine and Preventive Medicine, University of Washington School of Medicine, Seattle.

PETER E. POOL, M.D.
Assistant Professor of Medicine, University of California at San Diego School of Medicine, La Jolla, California.

DAVID C. POSKANZER, M.D., M.P.H.
Associate Professor of Neurology at the Massachusetts General Hospital, Harvard Medical School; Associate Neurologist, Massachusetts General Hospital.

EDWARD P. RADFORD, M.D.
Professor of Environmental Medicine, Johns Hopkins University School of Hygiene and Public Health, Baltimore, Maryland.

CHARLES H. RAMMELKAMP, JR., B.A., M.D., D.SC. (HON.)
Professor of Medicine and Associate Professor of Preventive Medicine, Western Reserve University School of Medicine; Director, Department of Medicine and Research Laboratories, Cleveland Metropolitan General Hospital, Cleveland.

T. J. REEVES, M.D.
Professor and Chairman, Department of Medicine, University of Alabama School of Medicine, Birmingham.

WILLIAM H. RESNIK, M.D.
Clinical Professor of Medicine, Yale University; Consultant Physician, Yale–New Haven Hospital; Consultant Physician, Stamford Hospital, Stamford, Connecticut.

JOHN CHARLES RIBBLE, M.D.
Associate Professor of Pediatrics, Cornell University School of Medicine, New York.

CLAYTON RICH, M.D.
Professor of Medicine and Associate Dean, University of Washington School of Medicine; Chief of Staff, Veterans Administration Hospital, Seattle.

EDWARD P. RICHARDSON, JR., M.D.
Associate Professor of Neuropathology, Harvard Medical School; Neurologist and Neuropathologist, Massachusetts General Hospital, Boston.

EUGENE D. ROBIN, M.D.
Professor of Medicine, University of Pittsburgh Medical School, Pittsburgh, Pennsylvania.

DAVID E. ROGERS, M.D.
Professor Medicine, Dean and Vice President for Medicine, Johns Hopkins School of Medicine; Medical Director, Johns Hopkins Hospital, Baltimore.

EUGENIA ROSEMBERG, M.D.
Director of Research, Medical Research Institute of Worcester, Inc., Worcester, Massachusetts.

JOHN ROSS, JR., M.D.
Professor of Medicine; Chief, Cardiovascular Division, Department of Medicine, University of California at San Diego School of Medicine, La Jolla, California.

RICHARD S. ROSS, M.D.
Professor of Medicine and Director, Cardiovascular Division, Johns Hopkins University School of Medicine; Physician, Johns Hopkins Hospital.

JEAN RUBEIZ, M.D.
Assistant Professor of Neuropathology, American University of Beirut, Lebanon.

DAVID C. SABISTON, JR., M.D.
Professor and Chairman, Department of Surgery, Duke University Medical Center, Durham, North Carolina.

FUAD SABRA, M.D.
Professor of Medicine (Neurology) and Neurologist, Department of Medicine, American University of Beirut, Lebanon.

MARIA Z. SALAM, M.D.
Assistant Clinical Professor of Neurology (Pediatric), Harvard Medical School; Clinical Fellow in Neurology, Massachusetts General Hospital, Boston.

JAY P. SANFORD, M.D.
Professor of Medicine; Head, Division of Infectious Diseases, University of Texas—Southwestern School of Medicine, Dallas.

HERBERT A. SELENKOW, M.D., B.S.
Assistant Professor in Medicine, Harvard Medical School; Senior Associate in Medicine and Director, Thyroid Laboratory, Peter Bent Brigham Hospital, Boston.

ARNOLD M. SELIGMAN, M.D.
Professor of Surgery, Johns Hopkins University School of Medicine; Surgeon-in-Chief, Sinai Hospital, Baltimore.

WALTER H. SHELDON, M.D.
Professor of Pathology, Johns Hopkins University School of Medicine, Baltimore.

CHARLES C. SHEPARD, M.D.
National Communicable Disease Center, Public Health Serv-

ice, U.S. Department of Health, Education and Welfare, Atlanta, Georgia.

LAWRENCE E. SHULMAN, M.D., PH.D.
Associate Professor of Medicine and Director, Connective Tissue Division, Department of Medicine, The Johns Hopkins University School of Medicine, Baltimore.

WILLIAM SILEN, M.D.
Professor of Surgery, Harvard Medical School; Surgeon-in-Chief, Beth Israel Hospital, Boston.

LLOYD H. SMITH, JR., M.D., D.SC. (HON.)
Professor and Chairman, Department of Medicine, University of California, San Francisco Medical Center, San Francisco.

PHILIP J. SNODGRASS, M.D.
Assistant Professor of Medicine, Harvard Medical School; Senior Associate in Medicine, Peter Bent Brigham Hospital, Boston.

EDMUND H. SONNENBLICK, M.D.
Assistant Professor of Medicine, Harvard Medical School; Cardiovascular Division, Department of Medicine, Peter Bent Brigham Hospital, Boston.

WESLEY W. SPINK, B.A., M.D., D.SC. (HON.)
Professor of Medicine, University of Minnesota Hospitals and Medical School, Minneapolis.

EUGENE A. STEAD, JR., B.S., M.D.
Professor of Medicine, Duke University School of Medicine; Durham, North Carolina.

WILLIAM W. STEAD, M.D.
Professor of Medicine, Marquette University School of Medicine, Milwaukee Medical Director, Muirdale Sanatorium, Milwaukee; Chief of Medical Chest Service, Milwaukee County General Hospital, Milwaukee.

JURGEN STEINKE, M.D.
Assistant Professor of Medicine, Harvard Medical School; Senior Associate in Medicine, Peter Bent Brigham Hospital, Boston.

JOHN H. TALBOTT, M.D.
Editor Emeritus, Journal of the American Medical Association, Chicago.

MELVIN L. TAYMOR, M.D., A.B.
Associate Professor of Gynecology, Harvard Medical School; Senior Associate in Surgery, Peter Bent Brigham Hospital, Boston.

LLOYD P. TEPPER, M.D.
Associate Professor of Environmental Health, Department of Environmental Health, University of Cincinnati College of Medicine, Cincinnati, Ohio.

GEORGE W. THORN, M.D., M.A. (HON.), LL.D. (HON.), D.SC. (HON.), M.D. (HON.), F.R.C.P.
Hersey Professor of the Theory and Practice of Physic and Samuel A. Levine Professor of Medicine, Harvard Medical School; Physician-in-Chief, Peter Bent Brigham Hospital, Boston.

WILLIAM A. TISDALE, M.D.
Professor and Chairman, Department of Medicine, University of Vermont College of Medicine, Burlington.

GENNARO M. TISI, M.D.
Assistant Professor of Medicine, University of California at San Diego School of Medicine, La Jolla, California.

ANSGAR TORVIK, M.D.
Assistant Professor of Pathology, Department of Pathology, Ullevaal Hospital, Oslo, Norway.

PHILIP A. TUMULTY, M.D.
Professor of Medicine, Johns Hopkins School of Medicine, Baltimore.

MARVIN TURCK, M.D.
Associate Professor of Medicine, University of Washington School of Medicine; Chief of Medicine, United States Public Health Service Hospital, Seattle.

FRANK H. TYLER, B.A., M.D.
Professor of Medicine, University of Utah College of Medicine, Salt Lake City.

HENRI VANDER EECKEN, H.M., M.D.
Professor of Neurology, Faculty of Medicine, University of Ghent, Ghent, Belgium.

MAURICE VICTOR, M.D.
Professor of Neurology, Western Reserve University School of Medicine; Chief, Neurology Service, Cleveland Metropolitan General Hospital, Cleveland.

ROBERT R. WAGNER, M.D.
Professor and Chairman, Department of Microbiology, University of Virginia School of Medicine, Charlottesville.

HENRY deF. WEBSTER, M.D.
Scientist, National Institute of Neurological Diseases and Stroke, Bethesda, Maryland.

LOUIS WEINSTEIN, M.S., PH.D., M.D.
Professor of Medicine, Tufts University School of Medicine; Lecturer on Infectious Disease, Harvard Medical School; Lecturer in Medicine, Boston University School of Medicine; Chief, Infectious Disease Service, New England Medical Center Hospitals, Boston.

LOUIS G. WELT, M.D.
Alumni Distinguished Professor and Chairman, Department of Medicine, University of North Carolina School of Medicine, Chapel Hill.

JOHN B. WEST, M.D., PH.D.
Professor of Medicine, University of California at San Diego School of Medicine, La Jolla, California.

GORDON H. WILLIAMS, M.D., B.A.
Research Fellow in Medicine, Harvard Medical School; Research Fellow in Medicine, Peter Bent Brigham Hospital, Boston.

MAXWELL M. WINTROBE, B.A., M.D., B.SC. (MED.), PH.D.,
D.SC. (HON. MANIT.), D.SC. (HON. UTAH), F.A.C.P.
Professor of Internal Medicine; Director, Cardiovascular Research and Training Institute, and Director, Laboratory for Study of Hereditary and Metabolic Disorders, University of Utah College of Medicine, Salt Lake City.

SHELDON M. WOLFF, M.D.
Clinical Director and Chief, Laboratory of Clinical Investigation, National Institute of Allergy and Infectious Diseases, National Institutes of Health, Bethesda, Maryland; Clinical Professor of Medicine, Georgetown University School of Medicine, Washington, D.C.

THEODORE E. WOODWARD, M.D.
Professor of Medicine and Head, Department of Medicine, University of Maryland School of Medicine, Baltimore.

GEORGE W. WRIGHT, M.D.
Head of Medical Research, Department of Medicine, St. Luke's Hospital; Associate Clinical Professor of Medicine, Western Reserve University School of Medicine, Cleveland, Ohio.

RICHARD J. WURTMAN, M.D.
Associate Professor of Endocrinology and Metabolism, Department of Nutrition and Food Science, Massachusetts Institute of Technology, Cambridge.

JAMES B. WYNGAARDEN, M.D., F.A.C.P.
Frederic M. Hanes Professor of Medicine and Chairman, Department of Medicine, Duke University Medical Center, Durham.

ROBERT R. YOUNG, M.D.
Assistant Professor of Neurology, Harvard Medical School; Assistant Neurologist (Clinical Neurophysiologist), Massachusetts General Hospital, Boston.

Preface

It often is asked why prefaces are written and whether they are ever read. In his famous preface to *Cromwell,* Victor Hugo pointed out that one seldom inspects the cellar of a house after visiting its salons nor examines the roots of a tree after eating its fruit. Admittedly, the readers of this book will judge it by the substance of its contents and its style, not by the pretexts offered by its editors. It could be added that if the guest has returned several times, then surely he knows that the cellar is well stocked. Why then a preface to a sixth edition?

This preface is intended to indicate the ways in which the present edition maintains or diverges from, as the case may be, the original objectives of this book. By doing this, it will be possible to present the objectives of this textbook of medicine to readers unfamiliar with earlier editions.

When the first group of editors met together twenty-five years ago, they decided to write a textbook of medicine which would conform to the *clinical method* which they had found most useful both as students and as teachers. It was thought that such a book should recapitulate the steps in the process of thinking by which a physician reaches a diagnosis, these being the recording of the patient's symptoms and signs, the consideration of the various disorders that can give rise to them, and the effective utilization of measures which will support and confirm or alter the first impressions and lead ultimately to a firm diagnosis.

The logical first step consistent with this clinical approach is the consideration of the cardinal manifestations of disease. Patients present themselves with symptoms, not diagnoses. Consequently it is basic to good clinical medicine to appreciate the different causes of various manifestations of disease and to understand how they may be produced. This requires an understanding of physiology and of the ways in which deviations from the normal lead to disorders of one kind or another. For this reason material of fundamental biologic importance was incorporated in the first edition of this book and has been regarded as an essential component ever since.

The revolutionary changes in the curricula of many American medical schools, particularly the abbreviation of the standard courses in the sciences basic to clinical medicine and the substitution of shorter "core" courses, has imposed, we believe, additional responsibilities on the modern teacher of clinical medicine and on the modern textbook of medicine. The student who embarks on his clinical training now, although far more sophisticated in many ways than his predecessor of even one generation ago, may not possess as much understanding of the mechanisms of symptoms and disease processes as is required to deal intelligently with clinical problems. This book recognizes the challenge to education posed by such curricula. Clinical biochemistry and pathophysiology form an integral part of this book but, insofar as possible, are considered within the clinical setting.

The interpretation of symptoms usually is most effectively achieved by proceeding from the general to the particular. Symptoms often can be grouped as syndromes. Syndromes are the consequence of a variety of etiologic factors or disease mechanisms and, if these can be recognized and understood, measures to restore the normal physiologic state can be designed and carried out in a logical, systematic fashion. Furthermore, the method of approaching a diagnosis which is based on an analysis of the symptoms, recognition of the syndrome, and consideration of the various disease mechanisms which may have produced it, ensures consideration of the many possible interpretations of the clinical picture which the patient presents. By pursuing such an approach, it is less likely that a disorder which should be considered will be overlooked.

The plan of this book is consistent with this approach. Following a discussion of the editors' general philosophy regarding the approach to the patient (Part One), certain fundamental matters regarding inheritance and growth are discussed (Part Two), such as the inheritance of human disease (Chapter 4), a subject which is assuming greater and greater importance in clinical medicine. Part Three, Cardinal Manifestations of Disease, discusses the mechanisms whereby various symptoms are produced and outlines an approach to the recognition of the diseases of which they may be manifestations.

Discussion of the cardinal manifestations of disease is not limited to a consideration of symptoms and physical signs. With the increasing availability and sensitivity of laboratory methodology and as the result of the introduction of screening procedures for the early detection of disease, an understanding of laboratory data becomes more essential than ever for the effective practice of medicine. Chapters 64, 65, 66, and 67 have been introduced in this edition to meet these needs and to supplement the discussions of laboratory procedures which will be found throughout the book.

Recognition of the importance of altered immune responses as fundamental mechanisms in the pathogenesis of disease has led to the introduction in this edition of Part Four, Disorders Due to Hypersensitivity and Altered Immune Response, where seven chapters are devoted to this important aspect of clinical medicine.

The remainder of the book is concerned with more specific disorders and disease entities. In all these sections, the syndromic approach is emphasized as much as possible, and the reader will find at the beginning of most of the sections, either in the Introduction and/or in the first chapter, a discussion of the approach to the patient having the type of disease considered in that section.

Treatment is discussed in relation to specific disorders or categories of disease (e.g., Chapter 135, Chemotherapy of Infection, Chapter 266, Principles of Drug Therapy in Cardiac Disorders) and is described in terms which are as specific as possible.

A deliberate attempt has been made to avoid long bibliographies. The references at the end of the chapters are limited, for the most part, to reviews and monographs which contain comprehensive bibliographies, together with older works of historical significance.

With the present edition, two of the original editors, Doctors T. H. Harrison and William H. Resnik, have retired, and their places have been taken by Doctors Eugene Braunwald and Kurt J. Isselbacher. The influence of Doctors Harrison and Resnik is clearly evident in this edition and can confidently be predicted to outlast the lives of all the present editors. Their role in the planning of this textbook was profound, and the present editors are deeply indebted to them. But time, like the science of medicine, moves on, and the reader no doubt will detect the influence of the newer editors. Acknowledgement here also is made of the very effective role which Dr. Robert G. Petersdorf has played as an editor, substituting for Dr. Ivan L. Bennett. He has proved to be a very important member of the team.

Once again the editors take pleasure in expressing appreciation to our many colleagues who have so generously responded to editorial suggestions. We continue to be indebted to numerous friends and colleagues for valuable criticisms. Among these are: Dr. Irwin Arias of New York, Doctors K. Frank Austen, Leon Eisenberg and Seymour Kety of Boston, Dr. Gerald Klatskin of New Haven, Dr. Stephen Robinson of Boston, Dr. Rudi Schmid of San Francisco, Doctors John Butler, Lawrence Harker, E. Donnall Thomas, and Frank Parker of Seattle, and Doctors Dean Ashworth, Arthur M. Brown, Edwin Englert, James Freston, Hiroshi Kuida, Richard Levinson, John Moore, Attilio Renezetti, Joseph Thorne, G. Tikoff, and Theophilus Tsagaris of Salt Lake City.

The preparation of the new edition has been ably facilitated by our several secretarial coworkers. We are especially indebted to Mrs. Beatrice A. Fraser, Mrs. Dorothy Starrett, Mrs. Hilda Gardner, and Miss Clo Flahive of Boston, Miss Pat Jaworsky of Baltimore, Miss Jana Maffey and Miss Doris Williams of Seattle, Mrs. Ethel Taggart Christensen of Salt Lake City, and Mrs. Mary Jackson of San Diego.

M.M.W.
G.W.T.
R.D.A.
I.L.B.
E.B.
K.J.I.
R.G.P.

Contents

xvii

HARRISON'S
PRINCIPLES
OF
INTERNAL
MEDICINE

Part One

The Physician and the Patient

Section 1

The Physician and the Patient

1 APPROACH TO THE PATIENT
The Editors

There is no greater opportunity, responsibility, or obligation given a man than that of serving as a physician. In treating the suffering he needs technical skill, scientific knowledge, and human understanding. He who uses these with courage, with humility, and with wisdom will provide a unique service for his fellowman, and will build an enduring edifice of character within himself. The physician should ask of his destiny no more than this; he should be content with no less.

In the practice of medicine the physician employs a discipline which seeks to utilize scientific methods and principles in the solution of its problems, but it is one which, in the end, remains an art. It is an art in the sense that rarely, if ever, can the individual patient be considered the equivalent of an experiment so completely controlled that it is possible to exclude judgment and experience from the interpretation of the patient's reactions. It is an art, too, in the sense that the practicing physician can never be content with the sole aim of endeavoring to clarify the laws of nature; he cannot proceed in his labors with the cool detachment of the scientist whose aim is the winning of the truth, and who, theoretically, is uninterested in the practical outcome of his work. The practicing physician must never forget that his primary and traditional objectives are utilitarian—the prevention and cure of disease and the relief of suffering, whether of body or mind.

THE PATIENT AS A PERSON

The student receives much expert coaching in the methods of physical and laboratory diagnosis, and it is in these areas that he will most easily develop the skills which permit him to be comfortable with the patient. Mastery of the more intangible psychologic aspects of medicine is not so easily acquired, however. The skills essential here depend not simply on instruction but on emotional maturity, manifested by sensitive self-cultivation of the capacity to see deeply and accurately the problems of another human being. The challenge is further magnified by the fact that the examining physician is himself a human instrument, subject to error arising from events in his own biography. The irritability and exasperation of even the kindest and most conscientious physician may sometimes represent not the legitimate protest at the patient's lack of cooperativeness but a basic and not wholly conscious sense of his own insecurity. The successful management of the patient requires emotional maturity on the part of the physician.

Just as the physical growth of each person depends on an adequate and balanced supply of appropriate foodstuffs, so does emotional growth depend on the receipt of proper psychologic nutrients. Although each individual is born with manifold potentialities determined by his genes, the emotional climate in which he grows and develops will shape his eventual character and abilities just as surely as foodstuffs will shape his physique. Invading bacteria influence multitudinous bodily reactions; so also do the emotions possess the capacity to alter behavior, including certain of the biochemical processes of the body.

Any departure from good health carries a potential threat of physical disintegration or crippling disability, and even the most intelligent and best-informed patient should not be considered immune to forebodings just because he refrains from mentioning them. It is especially important that these fears be borne in mind when dealing with the elderly patient, who is rarely unmindful that "the trap is laid" and death is always near.

The attitude of the patient approaching the doctor must always be tinged, for the most part unconsciously, with distaste and dread; his deepest desire will tend to be comfort and relief rather than cure, and his faith and expectation will be directed towards some magical exhibition of these boons. Do not let yourselves believe that however smoothly concealed by education, by reason, and by confidential frankness these strong elements may be, they are ever in any circumstances altogether absent. (Wilfred Trotter)

In the long development of growth from infancy to adult life, there is a progressive change in social relationships, from one of complete dependence on parent, family, and teacher to one of relative independence. At the same time, the process of maturation requires the partial suppression of egocentric drives to the point that the affairs of other members of one's family and social group assume increasing importance. These trends and their modification during life experience affect the development of personality; and deviations in these natural developments prevent satisfactory social adjustment and result in neuroticism.

Illness constitutes a threat not only to the physical integrity of the individual but also to his status in his social group, a fact that is soon learned by every thoughtful physician. Prolonged invalidism during childhood tends inevitably to leave behind an excessive egocentricity, which may become the basis of a lifelong neurosis. In the adult, illness often enforces a return to a posture of dependency, a change usually accompanied by feelings of apprehension and discouragement, sometimes leading to frank anxiety and depression. It is for these reasons that many adults in positions of responsibility express greater concern about the economic and social implications of their illness than about the illness itself. This explains a number of common psychologic defenses which the patient exercises against illness. He may refuse medical aid; or, if he summons the courage to consult a physician, he may minimize or even fail to mention the very symptom about which he is most deeply concerned. On the other hand, there are individuals whose attainment of maturity has been tenuous and uncertain, so that the position of dependency imposed by illness comes as a welcome relief from adult responsibility. They appear to enjoy illness and to resent anything that menaces their state of invalidism. Lesser degrees of this tendency are to be noted among those who consult the physician at the appearance of every new symptom and who are continuously preoccupied with their past illnesses and operations.

It is not easy to keep these simple facts in mind when examining a draped patient in the relatively neutral domain of the hospital ward or even in the private examining room. There are potent obstacles that stand in the way of the physician's making an adequate study of the patient's emotional life. Organic lesions have a way of compelling attention to themselves, and it is less exhausting to limit one's focus to the sphere of physical disease. More time, energy, and experience are necessary to view the patient as an active participant in an enormous moving pageant which includes the personal eccentricities of his forebears, his own fears and patterns of reaction, as well as the hopes for his children's future. It is not enough to know that poverty, insecurity, and perhaps poor vocational and domestic relations are now keeping the patient unhappily depressed, for all too often it is apparent that present socioeconomic (external) factors are not crucial determinants in the contemporary scene. To explain many of the manifestations of illness, it is necessary to view the patient more deeply as an organism with a vast repository of past experiences dating from the earliest days of life, many of which are vaguely remembered, yet have become the foundation of its current system of meeting daily problems. Under the threat of disease, defensive attitudes, which were useful in infancy and childhood but inappropriate in adult life, have a way of reasserting themselves; one of the oldest, the state of readiness for fight or flight (Cannon), may be a precipitating factor in illnesses such as peptic ulcer or hypertension, when called upon too frequently.

The young physician usually finds himself inadequate in his dealings with the patient, for not only does he experience an inevitable sense of insecurity with respect to the patient's problems, but he feels equally uneasy about his newly acquired role of authority and responsibility. Moreover, both he and his older colleague often find it difficult to control their own reactions: disinterest because the patient presents no fascinating problem of organic disease, irritation at his verbosity and lack of clarity and consistency in the recital of the history, annoyance because the patient's illness fails to respond to treatment in the expected manner. The physician can hardly expect to achieve a deep appreciation of the patient's psychologic problems unless he learns to recognize and control his own.

More broadly stated, the physician has a special function in society and should be skilled as a psychologist in human behavior as well as a biologist in human diseases. He brings highly technical knowledge and skills to bear upon the patient's physiologic functioning. He should bring to the suffering patient a quiet humanity, a confidence and security based upon the conviction that all will be done that can be done. The patient must feel that his unique individuality is recognized and appreciated and that his life's problems are meaningful. This is important in patients with well-defined organic disease as well as in the "stress" syndromes largely due to emotional pressures expressed through the body. If we can accept the principle of causality in human behavior, we can, with patience and diligence, learn to fathom some of the patient's motivations even though many of the details very often remain obscure.

Let me see in the sufferer the man alone. . . . Let me be intent upon one thing, O Father of Mercy, to be always merciful to Thy suffering children. (Maimonides)

THE ART OF MEDICINE

Despite the constantly increasing application of scientific methods to the problems of medicine, there remain large areas that are as yet insusceptible of solution by the use of precise methods. To extract the telltale clue from a maze of confusing symptoms, to determine from a mass of conflicting physical signs and laboratory data the ones that are of crucial significance, to know in a borderline case when to initiate and when to refrain from a line of investigation or treatment—the knowledge to accomplish these necessities of medical art is not usually the outcome of laboratory study alone. Involved here are judgments based on "assimilated experience."

Concerning the more personal relations with the patient and the understanding and capacity to peer beyond surface motivations and behavior, no instruction or training can entirely replace an intuitive talent and maturing wisdom. The astute physician will recognize when the casual mention of an apparently trivial complaint is the device for seeking reassurance regarding a feared disorder such as cancer or heart disease. He will at once know or suspect the value of continued probing of the more intimate aspects of the patient's life, and when to overcome a reluctance to discuss them, or to leave them undiscussed, when to express a bright and reassuring prognosis and when and how to utter doubt and caution.

No problem can be more distressing than that presented by the patient with incurable disease, particularly when death is imminent and inevitable. There should be no ironclad, inflexible rule that the patient must be told "everything." Few patients have the courage or faith or stoicism that the advocates of this conviction think they may or should have.

One thing is certain: it is not for you to don the black cap and, assuming the judicial function, take hope away from any patient . . . hope that comes to us all. (William Osler)

The proponents of this principle do not really adhere to their philosophy when they tell the "truth" in such a manner that the kernel of the truth is not conveyed to the patient. How much, for example, is communicated to the patient when the physician says to the patient who has leukemia: "You have more white corpuscles in your blood than is normal, but we found no evidence that any damage has been done." Nor can one conscientiously follow the opposite rule of never telling the patient the truth. How much the patient is to be told will depend on his religious convictions, the wishes of his family, the state of his affairs, and his own desires and character. But even this platitude solves nothing, since it is not merely the recognition of these factors but the physician's wisdom in assessing the relative importance of each that determines how complete a discussion of the facts will best serve the interests of the patient. The younger physician may extract some small measure of consolation from the knowledge that his older and more experienced colleague has no simple and easy formula for meeting the question.

The physician must also be prepared to deal with sentiments commonly experienced at a time of death in the family.

I do not know that I have anything to reproach in my conduct, and certainly nothing in my feelings and intentions towards the dead. But it is a moment when we are apt to think that, if this or that had been done, such event might have been prevented. (Letter to Shelley from Lord Byron on the death of his daughter.)

These words express the feelings of guilt that almost invariably afflict the members of a family when parent or child or spouse has died. The doctor must be prepared to tender what assurance is possible that no fault need be attached to the living.

Somewhat related to this problem is the expiatory attitude of the family when a member becomes gravely or hopelessly ill. The meager resources that may represent the savings of a lifetime of toil may be dissipated in weeks or months in payment for needlessly expensive rooms, private nursing services, and consultations. It is difficult for the physician to oppose these futile gestures too strenuously; they serve more to bring consolation to the family than to assuage the distress of the patient.

Tact, sympathy, and understanding are expected of the physician, for the patient is no mere collection of symptoms, signs, disordered functions, damaged organs, and disturbed emotions. He is human, fearful, and hopeful, seeking relief, help, and reassurance. To the physician, as to the anthropologist, nothing human is strange or repulsive. The misanthrope may become a smart diagnostician of organic disease, but he can scarcely hope to succeed as a physician. The true physician has a Shakespearean breadth of interest in the wise and the foolish, the proud and the humble, the stoic hero and the whining rogue. He cares for people.

CHANGING PATIENT-PHYSICIAN RELATIONSHIPS

The patient-physician relationship described above, a relationship which traditionally has been the goal of all physicians, is in danger of deterioration because of the changing setting in which medicine is increasingly being practiced. In many cases the management of the individual patient requires the active participation of a variety of trained professional personnel—not only physicians, but also nurses, dietitians, biochemists, psychologists and physiatrists, and other paramedical personnel. The patient can benefit greatly from such collaboration, but it is the duty of his physician to guide him through his illness; in order to carry out this increasingly difficult task the physician must have some familiarity with the skills and objectives of his colleagues in the fields allied to medicine. He must also be able to interpret their findings not as isolated phenomena but rather as they contribute to the total clinical picture. In giving his patient an opportunity to receive the full benefits resulting from the important advances which have taken place in the health-related sciences, the physician must retain responsibility for the crucial decisions concerning diagnosis and treatment.

The widening scope of medical practice is altering previously existing physician-patient relationships. An increasing number of patients are being cared for by groups of physicians, by clinics, and by hospitals rather than by the single, independent practitioner. There are many potential advantages in the use of such organized medical groups composed of a number of various specialists, but there are also hazards, both to the patient and the physician. The identity of the physician who is primarily and continuously responsible for each particular patient must be clearly defined. It is this physician who must have an overview of a patient's illnesses and who must maintain familiarity with his reaction to illness, to drugs, and to the problems of daily living. In addition, since a number of physicians may, at any one time, contribute to the care of a particular patient, and since both patients and physicians are increasingly mobile, accurate and detailed record keeping assumes progressively greater importance. It is imperative that the physician promptly commit all relevant data obtained from the clinical and laboratory examinations to his patient's permanent medical record. Only in this way can continuity of patient care be provided.

2 APPROACH TO DISEASE
The Editors

HISTORY

The history of an illness should embody all the facts of medical significance in the life of the patient up to the time he consults the physician; but, of course, his most recent diseases attract the most attention, for these, obviously, are the reason he seeks medical advice. Ideally the narration of symptoms should be in the patient's own words, the principal events being presented in the temporal order in which they occurred. Few patients possess the necessary powers of observation and talent for lucid, coherent description. Usually the help of the physician is needed. He must guide them by questions but at the same time avoid influencing them by inserting his own ideas, especially if the patient is suggestible.

Often it happens that a symptom which has greatly concerned a patient possesses little significance as a medical datum, whereas a seemingly minor complaint may be of importance. Therefore the mind of the physician must be constantly alert to the possibility that any event related by the patient, any symptom however trivial or apparently remote, may be the key to the solution of the medical problem.

An informative history is more than an orderly listing of symptoms. Something always is gained by listening to the patient and noting the way in which he talks about his symptoms. Inflection of voice, facial expression, and attitude may betray important clues as to the meaning of the symptoms to the patient. Thus, listening to this recitation, one discovers not only something about the disease but also something about the patient.

With experience one learns the pitfalls of history taking. What patients relate for the most part are subjective phenomena elusively filtered through minds that vary in their background of past experience. Patients obviously differ widely in their responses to the same stimuli. Their remarks are variably colored by fear of disease, disability, and death and by concern over the consequences of illness to their families. And as if these difficulties were not enough, there are the additional ones created by language barriers, by failing intellectual powers which deprive the subject of accurate recall, or by a disorder of consciousness that makes him unaware of his illness. It is not surprising, then, that even the most careful physician may at times despair of collecting factual data; and often he is forced to proceed with evidence that represents little more than an approximation of the truth.

Viewed in another way, the symptom marks, in the patient's mind, a departure from normal health; in the physician's mind, it initiates a process of inductive and deductive reasoning that culminates in diagnosis. In pondering the various possible explanations of a given symptom or clinical state the physician begins a search for other data, elicited by further questioning of the patient and his family, by physical examination, or by special laboratory tests. The symptoms alone sometimes will provide the most certain clue, as in angina pectoris or epilepsy, where physical findings and laboratory data collected between attacks may give no evidence of the existence of heart or brain disease even when it is manifestly present. In most illnesses, however, the history will not be so decisive, though it may still narrow the number of diagnostic possibilities and guide the subsequent investigation.

It is in the taking of the history that the physician's skill, knowledge, and experience are most clearly in evidence. He has learned from experience how to weigh each given symptom, depending on its nature and the context in which it occurs. He knows when to be incredulous and turn to more reliable sources of information, and he never lets his skepticism blind him to an unusual symptom, a manifestation of some new condition that has previously lain beyond the reach of medical knowledge. Moreover, he knows when to press an interrogation more deeply in a search for further details and when to cast about more broadly, realizing that "disease often tells its secrets in a casual parenthesis." And, finally, he knows how to take advantage of the interview in which the history is gathered to obtain the confidence of his patient and to allay apprehension and fear, the first steps in therapy.

The family history, all too often obtained in a routine, cursory fashion, is a leading tool of clinical genetics and can provide important evidence regarding the nature of the patient's complaints. The use of the family history will be discussed further in Chap. 4, but here it may be pointed out that information regarding symptoms like those of the patient which have occurred in blood relatives, or "run in the family," and knowledge of the ethnic origin of the parents and of consanguinity may be exceedingly helpful. The information must be obtained with tact, however, for patients may be embarrassed by such inquiries. Finally it should be emphasized that the best family history is that which is supported by actual examination of other members of the family. Frequently it is found that some physical deviation from the normal, too subtle to be recognized by a lay person, is quite apparent to the trained observer and that a minor deviation in laboratory data assumes significance when evaluated against a family constellation.

PHYSICAL EXAMINATION

Little need be said about the importance of the physical examination, for early in his training the physician learns that physical signs are the objective and verifiable marks of pathology. The physical sign represents a solid, indisputable fact. However, its significance is enhanced when it confirms a functional or structural change already evidenced by the patient's history. At other times, the physical sign may stand as the only evidence of disease, especially in those cases where the history has been inconsistent and confused or is completely lacking.

If full advantage is to be gotten from the physical examination, it must be performed methodically and thoroughly. Although attention has usually been directed by the history to the offending organ or part of the body, nevertheless the examination must extend to all parts of the body. The patient must be literally scrutinized from top to bottom in an objective search for abnormalities that may yield information concerning present and also future illnesses. Unless the examination procedure is systematic, important parts of it may be forgotten, an error against which even the most skilled clinician must guard. The results of the examination, like the details of the history, should be recorded at the time they are elicited and not hours later when they are subject to the distortions of memory. Many inaccuracies in case study stem from the careless practice of writing or dictating notes long after the examination has terminated.

Skill in physical diagnosis is acquired with experience, but it is not merely technique that determines success in eliciting signs. The detection of a few scattered petechiae or a faint diastolic murmur or a small mass in the abdomen is not a question of keener eyes and ears or more sensitive fingers, but of a mind directed by long experience to be alert to these findings. Skill in physical diagnosis reflects a way of thinking more than a way of doing.

All investigations of the body should be regarded as part of the physical examination. The use of various instruments, such as the ophthalmoscope, sphygmomanometer, galvanometer, microscope, or roentgen tube, are mere extensions of the examination to less accessible structures. Proficiency in their use is part of internal medicine. Tests made on fluids or tissues removed from the patient must be selected carefully; even though the physician may not do the tests, he is responsible for the proper collection of the material and for the interpretation of the results.

INSTRUMENTAL AND LABORATORY EXAMINATIONS

The last century has witnessed the introduction of newer methods of instrumental and laboratory investigation of ever-increasing precision and refinement, and inevitably there has been a drift toward reliance on knowledge gained from these special means of study in the solution of clinical problems. It is essential that one always bear in mind the limitations of these newer methods of examination and their proper use in the practice of medicine. By virtue of their impersonal quality and the complexity of the techniques involved in obtaining them, data secured by instrumental and laboratory methods are frequently surrounded by an aura of authority, without heed to the fact that the data are collected by fallible human beings who are capable of committing

errors of technique, or who may misinterpret the most precise evidence. One must not be misled by the "magic of numbers." Too great emphasis may be placed on minor deviations that may yet lie well within the range of normality. These and other possible errors serve to indicate that laboratory data cannot release the physician from the necessity of careful observation and study of the patient. The wise physician is he who understands the merits and limitations of each source of information, whether it be the history, or the physical examination, or the laboratory investigations. Barring those exigencies that make careful study impracticable or impossible, the history and physical examination should be thorough and painstaking, and the special examinations and laboratory tests should be adequate to furnish what additional information may be necessary. In some cases, it will suffice to use merely the simple tests that should be at the disposal of every practicing physician; in the more obscure cases the full resources of the most advanced teaching hospital may be essential for the successful unraveling of the clinical problem. Moreover, the physician should weigh carefully not only the hazards but also the expense involved in every test that he demands. Every procedure that does not have a specific purpose toward contributing to the management of the patient's illness is a pretentious economic waste resulting from ignorance or callousness or plain charlatanism. Scientific study of a clinical problem does not consist merely of filling a patient's record with endless data. Discrimination in the ordering of laboratory procedures and judgment in appraising the risk and expense of a procedure as against the value of the information to be derived from it are among the criteria by which one estimates the manner in which the art and science of medicine have been fused by the physician.

THE CLINICAL METHOD AND THE SYNDROMIC APPROACH TO DISEASE

The steps described above have as their object the collection of accurate data concerning all the diseases to which human beings are subject, namely, all conditions that "limit life in its powers, enjoyment and duration." But much more is required in making a diagnosis. Each datum must be interpreted in the light of the known facts of anatomy, physiology, and chemistry. The synthesis of these interpretations yields information concerning the affected organ or body system. Further, from the vantage point afforded by such an anatomic diagnosis the physician may then turn to other data, such as the mode of onset and clinical course of the illness, and to the results of laboratory tests, in order to ascertain the nature and degree of physiologic impairment and ultimately the cause of the disease.

All these steps comprise the clinical method, which always proceeds in a series of logical steps. The perceptive student will note certain similarities between the clinical method and the scientific method. Each begins with observational data which suggest a series of hypotheses. These latter are tested in the light of further observations, some clinical, others contrived laboratory procedures. Finally, a conclusion is reached, which in science is called a *theory* and in medicine a *working diagnosis.* The modus operandi of the clinical method, like that of the scientific method, cannot be reduced to a single principle or a type of inductive or deductive reasoning. It involves both analysis and synthesis, the essential parts of cartesian logic. The physician does not start with an open mind any more than does the scientist, but with one prejudiced from knowledge of recent cases; and the patient's first statement directs his thinking in certain channels. He must struggle constantly to avoid the bias occasioned by his own attitude, mood, irritability, and interest.

It is particularly in the study of more difficult patients that one observes most clearly the logical order of the clinical method. Anatomic diagnosis regularly precedes etiologic diagnosis. One seldom succeeds in determining the cause and mechanism of a disease before ascertaining which organ has been involved. An intermediate step is syndromic diagnosis. Most physicians attempt consciously or unconsciously to fit a given problem into one of a series of syndromes. The *syndrome,* in essence, is a group of symptoms and signs of disordered somatic function, related to one another by means of some anatomic, physiologic, or biochemical peculiarity of the organism. It embodies a hypothesis concerning the deranged function of an organ, organ system, or tissue. Congestive heart failure, Cushing's disease, and dementia are examples. In congestive heart failure dyspnea, orthopnea, cyanosis, dependent edema, engorged neck veins, pleural fluid, pulmonary râles, and enlargement of the liver are known to be connected by a single pathophysiologic mechanism—failure of the heart, leading to salt and water retention and high venous pressure. In Cushing's disease the moon facies, hypertension, diabetes, and osteoporosis, are the recognized effects of excess corticosteroids acting on many target organs. In dementia deterioration of memory, incoherence in thinking, faulty judgment, etc., are related through a neuroanatomic and a neurophysiologic principle, i.e., all these disordered intellectual functions are related to slow impairment of the function and destruction of the association areas of the cerebrum.

A syndromic diagnosis usually does not indicate the precise cause of an illness, but it greatly narrows the number of possibilities and, thus, suggests whatever further clinical and laboratory studies are required. The derangements of each organ system in human beings are reducible to a relatively small number of syndromes. Diagnosis is greatly simplified if a given clinical problem conforms neatly to a well-defined syndrome. Then one need only turn to a book for a list of the various diseases that may cause it. The search for the cause of an illness that does not conform to a syndrome is much more difficult, for a seemingly infinite number of diseases may then have to be considered. Nevertheless, the principle remains: the clinical method is an orderly intellectual activity which proceeds almost invariably from symptom to sign, to syndrome, and to disease.

3 CARE OF THE PATIENT
The Editors

Enormous strides have taken place during the past few decades in our knowledge of the mechanisms of disease and in the development of powerful and effective treatment agents. The responsibilities of the physician in his management of the patient have correspondingly grown. When little was known about the pathogenesis of a disorder and when, with rare exceptions, practically all the drugs in the huge pharmacopoeias were virtually placebos, when given in the recommended doses, the therapeutic decisions of the physician were seldom of crucial importance. The scientific physician of the time practiced in an era of therapeutic nihilism. He was aware of the worthlessness of most of the drugs that were available to him, and he displayed his skill as a scientific physician by not tampering mischievously with the natural recuperative powers of the body.

Throw out opium, which the Creator himself seems to prescribe, for we often see the scarlet poppy growing in the cornfields as if it were foreseen that where ever there is hunger to be fed there must also be pain to be soothed; throw out a few specifics which our art did not discover and is hardly needed to apply; throw out wine which is a food and the vapors of which produce the miracle of anesthesia, and I firmly believe that if the whole materia medica, as now used, could be sunk to the bottom of the sea it would be all the better for mankind,—and all the worse for the fishes. (O. W. Holmes, 1860)

The discovery during the past several decades of therapeutic agents capable of exerting decisive influence on the course of disease has made it essential that the physician have some understanding of the disturbed functions induced by disease, of the manner of treatment most likely to exert a beneficial effect, and of the risks involved in the proposed therapeutic plan.

Ideally, treatment should strive for the complete restoration of the patient's health, physical and mental.

But medicine contemplates other subjects besides cure. It aims still to postpone the progress of incurable disease and to put off its evil consequences; and, when, they can no longer be postponed, it seeks to render them more tolerable. (Latham)

These goals, which were hardly attainable at the time of Latham, seldom fail to be achieved with at least some degree of success at the present time. Remedies are available. It is the responsibility of the doctor to use them wisely, with due regard for their action, cost, and potential dangers. Every medical procedure, whether diagnostic or therapeutic, contains within it the potentiality of harm, but it would be impossible to afford the patient all the benefits of modern scientific medicine if every reasonable step in diagnosis and therapy were withheld because of the possible risks. "Reasonable" here implies that the physician has weighed the pros and cons of a procedure and has concluded on rational grounds that it is advisable or essential for the relief of discomfort or the cure or amelioration of disease. When the deleterious effects of the physician's action exceed any advantages that could logically have been anticipated, we are justified in designating these effects as *iatrogenic*. It is necessary only to recall the occasionally dangerous or fatal reactions that followed the use of antibiotics given for a trivial respiratory infection, or the gastric hemorrhage or perforation caused by cortisone administered for a mild arthritis, or the fatal homologous serum jaundice that followed needless transfusions of blood or plasma.

It is equally important to consider the harm physicians may do to patients through ill-considered or unjustified remarks. No matter how placid the patient may seem, he approaches the physician with at least some degree of fear and concern. His anxiety can be enhanced by a too serious demeanor, a flippant remark, or an impressive conference. Many persons have been crippled by a cardiac neurosis because the physician expressed a grave prognosis on the basis of a misinterpreted electrocardiogram. The good physician appreciates the fact that he is always in a position to cause injury by his treatment, by his words, and by his behavior.

It is trite to emphasize that the physician must never become so absorbed in the disease that he forgets the patient who harbors it. Nevertheless, this exhortation cannot be repeated too often. As the science of medicine advances, it is all too easy to become so fascinated by the various manifestations of a malady that one disregards the ailing person: his fears, his concerns about his job and the future of his family, the cost of medical care, the specter of economic insecurity, and similar related problems. Treatment of a patient consists in more than the dispassionate confrontation of a disease. It embodies also the exercise of warmth, compassion, and understanding. In the now famous words of Peabody, "one of the essential qualities of the clinician is interest in humanity, for the secret of the care of the patient is in caring for the patient."

THE GROWING ROLE OF PREVENTIVE MEDICINE

There are few areas of medicine which are less dramatic and less appreciated by the patient and by society, but which are of greater importance to a single individual or to an entire population, than is the intelligent practice of preventive medicine. In this aspect of medical practice, the physician deals with individuals or groups who are not overtly ill or whose complaints may be unrelated to the disease process which he wishes to prevent. The increasing use of the periodic physical examination by large companies, unions, other groups, and single individuals and the ready availability of multiphasic screening tests allow the physician to observe and modify disease processes earlier in their course, even prior to their inception. The finding of an elevated arterial blood pressure, blood sugar, serum uric acid or cholesterol in an asymptomatic person provides an unparalleled opportunity to prevent or retard the development of pathologic changes. The physician may, however, need to exert the full prestige of his position to induce an asymptomatic individual to alter his habits or diet or to follow a therapeutic program throughout the rest of his life. However, the compensation for these efforts, in terms of a patient's increased longevity and well-being, is so great that it fully justifies the effort and attention of every physician.

Part Two

Inheritance and Growth

Section 1

Inheritance and Growth

4 INHERITANCE OF HUMAN DISEASE

Victor A. McKusick

Increasingly in recent years the importance of genetics to medicine has come to be appreciated. The relative importance of those conditions in which genetic factors play a leading role has increased as some other etiologic categories of disease, e.g., infectious and nutritional, have become better understood and better treated.

The mutant gene should be considered an etiologic agent. The variability, yet predictability, of the clinical picture in a genetic disorder in which the etiologic agent, a gene, operates from within is very similar to that of an infectious disease in which the etiologic agent invades from the environment. In studying progressive muscular dystrophy of the pseudohypertrophic type, one is not searching for its cause. The cause, a sex-linked recessive gene, is known. It is the mechanism by which the mutant gene produces the clinical manifestations, and methods for interrupting that mechanism, or compensating for it, that are sought by research in muscular dystrophy.

In addition to those conditions for which a single mutant gene in single or double dose is quite directly responsible, and in addition to those disorders which result from chromosomal aberrations, there are many disorders, including some of the commonest affections of man, e.g., atherosclerosis, hypertension, and certain malformations, in which genetic factors and environmental factors collaborate in a complex manner. For a majority of the diseases of man, causation must not be viewed in the rigid sense of a single etiologic agent—a pattern of thinking engendered by the bacteriologic era of medicine—but rather as a nexus, a network of multiple interacting factors among which the genetic factor or factors are always likely to be important. In coronary artery disease, for example, one cannot say that heredity, high-fat diet, cigarette smoking, particular forms of stress, or any other of many postulated factors is *the* cause. The controversy between genetics and environment, nature and nurture, of an early day has now subsided since it is appreciated that both types of factors are important.

The collaboration of heredity and environment is well illustrated by primaquine sensitivity (glucose 6-phosphate dehydrogenase deficiency) in which hemolytic anemia usually occurs only if the genetically predisposed person is exposed to a chemical of a particular type (Chap. 338); and by suxamethonium (succinylcholine) sensitivity (pseudocholinesterase deficiency) in which the genetically predisposed person suffers no obvious ill effects of his defect unless given the agent mentioned as a muscle relaxant in anesthesia.

An important principle of medical genetics is *heterogeneity.* Many genetic disorders which at first were thought to represent single entities have, on close study, been found to consist of two or more fundamentally distinct entities. There are known, for example, to be two types of X-linked hemophilia (Chap. 346), and the genes for these are at loci rather far apart on the X chromosome. Four or five distinct varieties of hereditary intestinal polyposis can be distinguished on clinical grounds. Several recessively inherited varieties of familial goiter are found to result from separate and distinct biochemical defects.

DEFINITIONS. *Congenital* means "present at birth" and is not synonymous with genetic. Genetic factors may or may not be of importance in the cause of individual congenital malformations. On the other hand, hereditary conditions are not necessarily congenital; at least, clinical manifestations may not appear until much later in life. *Hereditary, genetic,* and *heritable* are roughly synonymous. *Familial* and *heredofamilial* were used previously to designate conditions inherited as recessives, i.e., conditions which often occur in multiple siblings with both parents normal. Since a recessive disorder is as genuinely inherited as a dominant one, these terms have little justification. Possibly the only use for the term *familial* is in connection with disorders with a familial aggregation not yet proved to be genetic in basis.

The word *genotype* refers to the genetic constitution of the individual; *phenotype* refers to the outward expression. The phenotype is, of course, what the physician observes, from which he makes deductions about the genotype. The difference is comparable to that between character and reputation—"genotype" and "character" refer to the true nature of the individual, "phenotype" and "reputation" to the apparent nature. *Karyotype* refers to the chromosomal complement of cells. An *ideogram* is a drawing representing the karyotype.

Abiotrophy is a term introduced by Gowers (1902) to describe the behavior of genetic disorders, such as Huntington's chorea and the spinocerebellar ataxias, in which a system functions normally and may be histologically normal up to a stage more or less late in life. The term refers to an inborn defect which leads to premature deterioration of a particular tissue, organ, or system.

SYNDROMES. As with nongenetic conditions, many hereditary disorders have manifold manifestations, the combination of which is referred to as a *syndrome* ("running together"). Genetic syndromes, excluding those like mongoloid idiocy which are due to a chromosomal aberration, appear to be produced by a single mutant gene which has multiple expressions in the phenotype (so-called "pleiotropism") because the protein, enzymatic or other, which is specified by the gene, has wide implications, at least multiple implications, in the economy of the organism. Genetic linkage—the location on the same chromosome of separate genes for each aspect of the syndrome—cannot account for the syndromal relationships observed in clinical medicine.

The investigation of members of a family with regard to a particular disease trait usually begins from a *proband,* or *propositus* (-a). The proband is the affected person through whom the family is ascertained. The proband is comparable to the *index* case of epidemiologic studies. Often in family studies it is desirable to compare the frequency of a discontinuous trait or the mean level of a biometric trait in the relatives of probands and in the relatives of controls. Data are almost meaningless unless the degree of relationship of the relatives studied is indicated. It means little, for example, to state that 5 percent of the relatives of patients with rheumatoid arthritis have rheumatoid arthritis, but more significance can be attached to the statement that 5 percent of first degree relatives have rheumatoid arthritis. *First degree relatives* are parents, sibs, and offspring; on the average their genetic resemblance to the proband is 0.50, if genetic identity (as in monozygotic twins) is 1.0. *Second degree relatives* are grandparents, aunts and uncles, and grandchildren of the proband; on the average their genetic resemblance to the proband is 0.25.

The aspects of genetics of particular significance to clinical medicine are at least six: (1) cytogenetics, i.e., the study of chromosomes in relation to the phenotype; (2) pedigree patterns, i.e., the behavior in families of single-gene disorders; (3) nature and function of the genetic code; (4) mutation; (5) biochemical aspects of gene action; and (6) the genetics of common disorders (multifactorial inheritance).

CYTOGENETICS IN MAN

It was not until 1956 that the correct chromosome number in man (46) was known and not until 1959 that a microscopically identifiable chromosomal aberration was reported to be the cause of disease in man. These advances were made possible by the introduction of two modifications of technique: (1) the use of colchicine in cell cultures to cause an accumulation of cells in metaphase of mitosis, the stage most favorable for counting the chromosomes; and (2) the use of hypotonic solutions to produce swelling of the nucleus and separation of the chromosomes. The cells studied have been derived from the bone marrow by the usual aspiration technique or from explants of skin or other tissue. Cells grown from the peripheral blood in short-term culture have been particularly useful for family studies and surveys. Use of the mitosis-stimulating properties of phytohemagglutinin is another technique that has facilitated chromosome study. The chromosomes are studied by light microscopy after appropriate fixing and staining (Figs. 4-1 and 4-2).

Mongolism (mongoloid idiocy, Down's syndrome) was found to be characterized by 47 chromosomes, the extra one being one of the smallest autosomes, or nonsex chromosomes (Fig. 4-3). In the *Klinefelter syndrome* it was found that there are 47 chromosomes and a sex chromosome constitution XXY (Fig. 4-4). In the *Turner syndrome* (gonadal aplasia) it was found that there are 45 chromosomes, there being only one sex chromosome, the so-called XO sex chromosome constitution (Fig. 4-5). In both of the latter two cases an abnormality of the sex chromosomes had been suspected because of paradoxic findings on Barr's test of nuclear sex. In the Klinefelter syndrome the subject is ostensibly male but shows the "chromatin-positive" pattern of the normal female; in the Turner syndrome the phenotypic female shows in a majority of cases the "chromatin-negative" pattern of the normal male (Fig. 4-6).

The three conditions above appear to arise through the accident of nondisjunction occurring either during meiosis in one parent (that is, in spermatogenesis or oogenesis) or in the first mitotic cleavage of the zygote. In meiotic nondisjunction both chromosomes of a given pair pass into one cell product rather than separating. Abnormal cells of two types are produced: one with one chromosome too many and one with one chromosome too few. In mongolism the strikingly higher frequency in the offspring of older mothers appears to be due to a higher risk of nondisjunction in older females.

Many other chromosomal aberrations have been discovered. Those which affect the sex chromosomes include XXX, XXXY, XXXXY, XXYY, and XXXX constitutions. Abnormal numbers of X chromosomes are indicated by sex chromatin abnormalities, as indicated in Table 4-1.

The XYY syndrome is of particular significance because the features are, in addition to some degree of mental deficiency, excessive height and behavioral abnormalities leading often to criminality.

Trisomic states (conditions in which, as in mongolism, three chromosomes rather than two of a particular set are present) have been described in which the chromosomes involved are different ones than in mongolism.

Fig. 4-1. The chromosomes of a normal male. On the right are shown the chromosomes of a single somatic cell in the metaphase stage of cell division. The photographic images of the chromosomes have been cut out and arranged according to descending length and varying arm ratio to form the karyotype shown on the left. The sex chromosomes in this normal male are an X, shown with the 6–12 chromosomes, which it resembles, and a Y, shown near chromosomes 21–22, which it resembles.

Table 4-1. CORRELATIONS OF PHENOTYPE, SEX CHROMATIN, AND SEX CHROMOSOMES

	Sex phenotype	Barr bodies (maximum number per cell)	Sex-chromosome constitution
Normal male......	Male		XY
Testicular feminization syndrome	Female (with testes)		XY
Double Y (or XYY) male..........	Male		XYY
Turner syndrome ..	Female		XO
Normal female	Female		XX
Klinefelter syndrome..........	Male		XXY
Klinefelter syndrome..........	Male		XXYY
Triple X syndrome	Female		XXX
Triple X-Y syndrome..........	Male		XXXY
Tetra X syndrome	Female		XXXX
Tetra X-Y syndrome..........	Male		XXXXY
Penta X syndrome.	Female		XXXXX

The only autosomal trisomies that survive after birth have been those involving chromosome 21 (mongolism), 13, or 18. Nonmosaic autosomal monosomy (only one of a given pair of autosomes is present) must be very rare in living children. About one-fifth of spontaneous abortions show a detectable chromosomal abnormality as the probable "cause" of abortion.

Translocation (displacement of part or all of one chromosome onto another) may be balanced (i.e., a full complement of genetic material is present, although in unusual arrangement), or unbalanced (if excess and/or deficiency of genetic material exists). The most frequent form is probably the D-G translocation which can exist in carriers (with the balanced situation) or in mongoloid idiots (with the unbalanced situation).

Deletion (loss of part of a chromosome) also occurs as the basis of congenital syndromes. The most frequent probably is deletion of part of the short arm of chromosome 5 leading to the *cri du chat* syndrome, so called because of the catlike cry of infants with this abnormality; other features are microcephaly, hypertelorism, and mental retardation.

Mosaicism, with a chromosome abnormality present in only a portion of the cells of the individual, is relatively frequent. It arises through an accident in chromosome mechanics in the early embryo and results in an incomplete or mild form of the syndrome observed with the particular chromosomal abnormality in nonmosaic form.

Estimates of the frequency of selected congenital chromosomal errors are given in Table 4-2.

The relationship of demonstrable changes in the chromosomes to neoplastic disease is under active investigation. In many cases of chronic myelocytic leukemia a con-

Fig. 4-2. The chromosomes of a normal female. No Y chromosome is present, and two X chromosomes are present with the 6–12 group.

Fig. 4-3. The chromosomes in mongolism. The chromosomal constitution is that of a normal female except for the presence of an extra chromosome in the set numbered 21.

11

Table 4-2. FREQUENCY OF SELECTED CHROMOSOMAL ABERRATIONS

	A Spontaneous abortions	B Live-born
Sex chromosome abnormalities		
Turner syndrome (all types)......	1/18	1/3,500 "females"
Klinefelter syndrome (all types)......	Probably same as in live-born	1/500 "males"
Extra X chromosomes (females mainly XXX)	Probably same as in live-born	1/1,360 "females"
Autosomal abnormalities		
Trisomy G.........	1/40	1/600
Trisomy 18........	1/200	1/4,500
Trisomy D	1/33	1/14,500
Trisomy 16........	1/33	Almost 0
Triploidy..........	1/22	Almost 0

sistent change in one of the four smallest autosomes has been observed. It appears that deletion, or loss, of part of the long arm of chromosome 21, resulting in the so-called Philadelphia (or Ph[1]) chromosome (Fig. 4-7) may be responsible for most cases of this form of leukemia. Whereas the chromosome aberrations leading to abnormalities of sex, soma, and behavior described above are all congenital, the Philadelphia chromosome (which

Fig. 4-4. *Upper*, a patient with the Klinefelter syndrome. Note the long legs, gynecomastia, and sparse body hair. *Lower*, the chromosomes in the Klinefelter syndrome. The karyotype is abnormal because of the presence of three sex chromosomes (XXY).

is present only in blood cells) arises in postnatal life through chromosome breakage produced by agents such as radiation and, probably, viruses.

THE BEHAVIOR OF GENETIC DISEASE IN FAMILIES

In accordance with the laws of Mendel, many diseases in man occur in families in a characteristic pattern. These are, for the most part, rare conditions and result from "point mutation" in the genetic material, as will be discussed later. The specific pedigree pattern depends on whether the responsible mutant gene is located on one of the autosomal chromosomes or on an X chromosome. It also depends on whether the effects of the gene are evident in single dose, that is, in the heterozygous state, or whether the gene requires double dosage, or the homozygous state, for its expression. According to the type of chromosome bearing the gene in question, a trait is said to be either *autosomal* or *sex-linked*. Depending on whether expression of the gene occurs in the heterozygous state or only in the homozygous state, a trait is said to be either *dominant* or *recessive*, respectively.

Figure 4-8 presents an idealized pedigree pattern of an *autosomal dominant trait*. Within the limits of chance, half the sons and half the daughters of an affected per-

Fig. 4-5. *Upper*, a patient with the Turner syndrome. Note the short stature, broad shieldlike chest with wide intermammary distance, hypoplastic mandible, low-set ears, and webbed neck. Note the scar of the operation for resection of coarctation of the aorta. *Lower*, the chromosomes in the Turner syndrome. Only one sex chromosome, an X, is present.

A

B

Fig. 4-6. *A.* Cell in buccal smear from normal male. No sex chromatin mass is seen in this "chromatin-negative" pattern, which is shown also by most patients with the Turner syndrome. *B.* Cell in buccal smear from normal female, showing a sex chromatin mass adjacent to the nuclear membrane. This "chromatin-positive" pattern is also shown by patients with the Klinefelter syndrome.

son are effected. This follows directly from the fact that the mutant gene is carried by one of a pair of autosomes and that there is a 50 percent chance of the affected parent contributing that chromosome to any given offspring.

As a generalization, dominant traits are less severe than recessive traits. In part an evolutionary or selective reason for this observation can be offered. A dominant mutation which determines a grave disorder that makes reproduction impossible will promptly disappear. On the other hand, even though in the homozygous condition a recessive mutation precludes reproduction, it can gain wide dissemination in heterozygous carriers, if it endows these carriers with a selective advantage.

A biochemical explanation is also possible for the greater severity of recessive traits. One might anticipate a greater derangement when both genes specifying a particular protein, let us say an enzyme, are of mutant type than if only one is mutant.

Another characteristic of dominant characters is wide variability in severity. The degree of severity is referred to as the *expressivity*. Sometimes the expressivity is so much reduced that the presence of the gene cannot be recognized at all, at least by the methods at one's disposal. When this is the case, the trait is said to be *nonpenetrant*. Sometimes in pedigrees of families with a dominant trait, so-called "skipped" generations occur. In the skipped individual, expressivity is so low that the presence of the gene is not recognizable, i.e., the trait is nonpenetrant in that person. The variability results from differences in the environment and in the rest of the genetic make-up, the *genome*. At least in part the variability of dominant traits may be the result of differences in the "normal" allele which accompanies the mutant allele in the heterozygous affected individual. Evidence of the last is provided when one can demonstrate that sib-sib correlations for behavior of the given disease are stronger than the parent-sibling correlations.

Not every person afflicted with an autosomal dominant disorder has an affected parent because a certain proportion have the abnormal gene as a result of fresh mutation occurring in a germ cell of either the father or the mother. The graver the condition, in terms of average interference with reproduction by affected persons, the larger is the proportion of cases which represent new mutation. This follows from the plausible assumption that the frequency of the particular dominant gene is not changing but that an equilibrium exists between addition of new genes to the gene pool through mutation and the loss of genes from the gene pool through failure of reproduction. For a number of dominants, such as achondroplasia and Marfan syndrome, it has been possible to demonstrate paternal age effect. Fathers of sporadic (new mutation) cases are, on the average, 5 to 7 years older than fathers in general. Maternal age effect in some chromosomal aberrations, notably mongolism, is well known; paternal age effect in point mutation is less well known.

Autosomal recessive traits (Fig. 4-9) likewise occur equally often in males and females, as a rule. The affected individuals usually have normal parents, but both parents are heterozygous carriers of the gene in question. Since related individuals are more likely to be heterozygous for the same mutant gene, consanguineous mating, of first cousins, for example, is more likely to result in offspring affected by a recessive trait. Viewed in another way, a greater proportion of the parental matings in families affected by recessive traits are likely to be consanguineous than is true generally. The rarer the recessive trait, the higher is the proportion of consanguineous parental matings.

On the average, among the offspring of two heterozygous parents one-fourth of males and females are expected to be homozygous-affected. One-half will be heterozygous carriers for the trait, and one-fourth will be homozygous for the normal allele.

Affected sibships can usually be ascertained only through the appearance of one or more affected members. Since there is no way to recognize those matings

Fig. 4-7. The chromosomes of bone marrow from a female with chronic myelocytic leukemia. One chromosome 21, marked Ph¹ for Philadelphia chromosome, lacks part of its long arm.

of two appropriately heterozygous parents who are so fortunate as to have no affected children, a collection of sibships containing at least one affected child is a biased sample. More than the expected one-fourth of all children in ascertainable families will be affected. Methods for correcting for the so-called "bias of ascertainment" are available.

If an individual affected by a recessive trait marries a homozygous normal person, none of the children will be affected, but all will be heterozygous carriers. If an individual affected by a recessive trait marries a heterozygous carrier, one-half of the offspring are likely to be

affected. A pedigree pattern superficially resembling that of a dominant trait can result. It was previously thought that two genetic forms of alkaptonuria (Chap. 102) exist —one inherited as an autosomal recessive and one as an autosomal dominant. Closer investigation reveals that the apparently dominant form was the same disease as the clearly recessive one. Because of much inbreeding, homozygous affected individuals frequently mated with heterozygous carriers and a quasi-dominant pedigree pattern resulted.

When two individuals affected by the same recessive

Fig. 4-8. Pedigree pattern of an autosomal dominant trait.

Fig. 4-9. Pedigree pattern of an autosomal recessive trait.

◧ ◑ Male, female, with sickle trait

■ ● Male, female, with sickle-cell anemia

□ ○ Unaffected male, female

Fig. 4-10. Pedigree pattern of an autosomal intermediate trait as illustrated by sickle state.

disease mate, all their offspring are likely to be affected. However, an exception to this generalization occurs if the recessive trait which phenotypically is identical in two parents is in fact determined by genes at different loci. The exception illustrates the genetic axiom: The phenotype is no necessary indication of the genotype. Different genotypes can result in the same phenotype (so-called genetic mimics or genocopies). Or an environmental insult can result in a phenotype indistinguishable from that produced by a mutant gene (a so-called "phenocopy").

Dominant and *recessive* are somewhat arbitrary concepts. When our methods are sufficiently acute, the effect of a recessive gene in heterozygous state can be recognized. Furthermore, a gene which has obvious expression in the heterozygous individual and is therefore considered dominant may have a different effect, quantitatively and even qualitatively, in the homozygous state. The gene for sickle hemoglobin and the states referred to as sickle-cell anemia and sickle-cell trait illustrate the arbitrary nature of the distinction. If sickle-cell anemia is considered as the phenotype, then the condition is recessive, since a homozygous state of the gene is required. The phenotype sickling, however, is dominant since the gene in heterozygous state is expressed. *Intermediate inheritance* is the term sometimes applied to this type of pedigree pattern (Fig. 4-10).

Codominance is the term used for characters which are both expressed in the heterozygote. For example, persons with the blood group AB demonstrate the effects of both the gene for antigen A and the gene for antigen B. Neither is recessive to the other. Similarly the genes for different hemoglobins are both expressed, for example, in the person with both hemoglobin S and hemoglobin C. These examples of codominance again indicate that whether we view the phenotype as recessive or dominant depends largely on the acuteness of our methods for recognizing the products of gene action. This whole discussion illustrates the importance of precise definition of the phenotype. If the particular phenotype occurs only in the homozygote, it is recessive; if it occurs in the heterozygote, it is dominant. Strictly speaking, dominance and recessiveness are attributes of the phenotype, although as a matter of convenience we may speak of dominant or recessive genes.

In traits determined by genes on the X chromosome, either dominance or recessiveness may be observed, just as in autosomal traits. The female with two X chromosomes may be either heterozygous or homozygous for a given mutant gene, and the trait can demonstrate either recessive or dominant behavior. On the other hand, the male with one X chromosome can have only one genetic constitution, namely, *hemizygous*. Regardless of the behavior of the mutant gene in the female, whether recessive or dominant, the mutant gene, if present in the male, is always expressed.

An important characteristic of sex-linked inheritance, both dominant and recessive, is the absence of male-to-male (that is, father-to-son) transmission of the disease. This is a necessary result of the fact that the male contributes his X chromosome to all his daughters but to none of his sons.

Sex-linked (X-linked) recessive inheritance (Fig. 4-11) is illustrated in a classic manner by hemophilia. The pedigree pattern of an autosomal dominant trait is a horizontal one, with affected persons in successive gen-

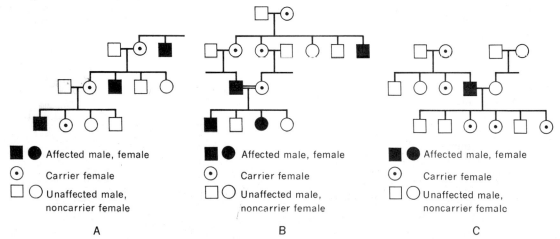

■ ● Affected male, female

⊙ Carrier female

□ ○ Unaffected male, noncarrier female

A

■ ● Affected male, female

⊙ Carrier female

□ ○ Unaffected male, noncarrier female

B

■ ● Affected male, female

⊙ Carrier female

□ ○ Unaffected male, noncarrier female

C

Fig. 4-11. Pedigree patterns of a sex-linked recessive trait. A. Note the "oblique" pattern. B. An affected female can result from the mating of an affected male and a carrier female, as in the case of a consanguineous marriage shown here. C. An affected male mating with a normal, noncarrier female has all normal sons and all carrier daughters.

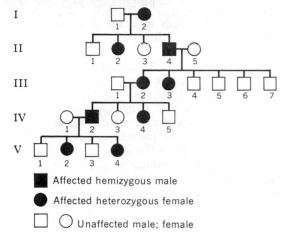

I
II
III
IV
V

■ Affected hemizygous male

● Affected heterozygous female

□ ○ Unaffected male; female

Fig. 4-12. Pedigree pattern of a sex-linked dominant trait.

erations. The pedigree pattern of an autosomal recessive trait tends to be a vertical one, with affected persons confined to a single generation. The pedigree pattern of a sex-linked recessive character tends to be an oblique one because of transmission to the sons of normal carrier sisters of affected males. Bateson compared this pattern to the knight's move in chess. Tracing sex-linked recessive characters through many generations is often difficult because the patronymic of affected persons tends to change with each generation.

To have hemophilia a female must be homozygous for this recessive gene. She must have received a gene for hemophilia from each parent. Such can occur, and has been observed, when a hemophiliac male marries a carrier female (Fig. 4-11B). As with other recessive traits this homozygous state is more likely to result from consanguineous matings. A hemophiliac female may also occur if a carrier mother is impregnated by a mutant sperm from a normal father, or if the phenotypic female has in fact an XO sex chromosome constitution (the Turner syndrome) or an XY constitution (the syndrome of testicular feminization). (In these comments reference is, of course, made to sex-linked recessive hemophilia A and B and not to other hemophilioid states which occur equally frequently in males and females. Also not considered is the rare possibility that unfortunate lyonization, as described below, in a heterozygous female has resulted in a majority of the cells which produce antihemophilic factor having the mutant-bearing X chromosome as the genetically active one.)

A hemophiliac male can have gotten the hemophilia gene *only* from his mother and can transmit it only to his daughters but to none of his sons. *All* daughters of a hemophiliac male are carriers (Fig. 4-11C).

In man one can enumerate more than sixty other diseases inherited as sex-linked recessives, including such significant entities as primaquine sensitivity (Chap. 338), the Duchenne type of progressive muscular dystrophy (Chap. 376), and agammaglobulinemia (Chap. 69). In some, for example, primaquine sensitivity and nephrogenic diabetes insipidus, a partial defect can be dem-

onstrated in the heterozygous female carrier, and one might prefer to call the inheritance sex-linked intermediate. In another condition, choroideremia, hemizygous males, but only the males, have severe impairment of vision, and from this point of view the disease is a sex-linked recessive; but the heterozygous female carriers show striking changes in the fundus oculi on ophthalmoscopy, even though vision is unaffected.

At least one common trait, colorblindness, is inherited as a sex-linked recessive. It is sufficiently frequent (about 8 percent of white males are colorblind) that the occurrence of homozygous colorblind females is no great rarity.

In *sex-linked (X-linked) dominant inheritance* both females and males are affected and both males and females transmit the disorder to their offspring, just as in autosomal dominant inheritance. Superficially the pedigree patterns in the two types of inheritance are similar, but there is a critical difference (Fig. 4-12). In sex-linked dominant inheritance, although the affected female transmits the trait to half her sons and half her daughters, the affected male transmits it to *none* of his sons and to *all* his daughters. Furthermore, in a series of cases females are expected to occur twice as often as males. One of the best studied sex-linked dominant traits is vitamin D–resistant rickets, or hypophosphatemic rickets (Chap. 83). In this condition the hemizygous affected male tends to have more severe clinical involvement than does the heterozygous affected female.

One common trait is inherited as an X-linked dominant: the Xg(a+) blood group. In due course, antisera that directly identify the Xg(a−) blood group will probably be found. These will then be considered co-dominant traits.

Some rare conditions are thought to be inherited as X-linked dominants lethal in the hemizygous male. The characteristics (Fig. 4-13) are (1) occurrence only in females (who are heterozygous for the mutant gene), (2) transmission from affected mother to half her daughters, (3) increased frequency of abortion (male fetus being lost) by affected women. Conditions which appear

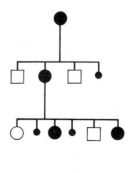

● ○ Affected and unaffected female

□ Unaffected male

⬩ Abortion

Fig. 4-13. Pedigree pattern of a sex-linked dominant trait lethal in the hemizygous male.

to have this mode of inheritance include incontinentia pigmenti, focal dermal hypoplasia, and the orofaciodigital (OFD) syndrome. A male with the last condition was found to be no exception to X-linked dominant, male-lethal inheritance, because in fact he was an instance of XXY Klinefelter syndrome.

Understanding of the behavior of X-linked traits and interpretation of findings in (1) females heterozygous for X-linked genes and (2) persons with an abnormal complement of X chromosomes have been greatly advanced by the *Lyon hypothesis*. There is now good evidence that at an early stage in development one X chromosome of the female becomes relatively inactive genetically (Fig. 4-14). The inactive X chromosome forms the *Barr body*. In each cell it is a random matter whether the X chromosome derived from the mother or that derived from the father is the one that becomes inactive. Once the "decision" is made in a given cell, however, the same X chromosome remains inactive in all descendants of that cell. The adult female is, therefore, a mosaic of two types of cells, those with the mother's X active and those with the father's X active.

The Lyon hypothesis is thought to account for these findings: (1) Heterozygous females tend to vary widely in expression of X-linked recessive genes. As an extreme case, females heterozygous for the hemophilia gene have clinical hemophilia, if most of the pertinent anlage cells destined to produce antihemophilic globulin have the X chromosome with the hemophilia gene active. (2) A mosaic pattern is observed in females heterozygous for

traits such as ocular albinism, an X-linked recessive. The fundi in such females show a mosaic of pigmented and unpigmented areas. (3) Persons with multiple X chromosomes, e.g., the XXX female, have two Barr bodies. All X chromosomes in excess of 1 are inactivated (Table 4-1). These persons have much less drastic abnormalities than would be expected with such excess chromosomal material, if relative inactivation did not occur.

Occurrence of the following types of inheritance in man is uncertain: (1) *holandric (all-male) inheritance*, resulting from the possible location of a gene on the Y chromosome, and (2) *partial sex-linkage*, resulting from the location of a gene on possibly homologous parts of the X and Y chromosomes between which crossing over might occur.

Before leaving sex-linked inheritance, one should note the distribution between sex-linked inheritance and sex-influenced (or sex-limited) autosomal inheritance. Baldness appears to be such a sex-influenced autosomal trait. In man baldness is inherited as an autosomal dominant, but in women for baldness to occur the gene must be in homozygous state, that is, in women baldness behaves like a recessive. In women who develop masculinizing tumors of the ovary, baldness can occur if the genotype is proper. As another example, one can imagine a mutant gene whose sole effect was that of preventing lactation in the female. Even though it were located on an autosomal chromosome, it would not have expression in the male. Idiopathic hemochromatosis (Chap. 107) results from the pathologic effects of excessive accumula-

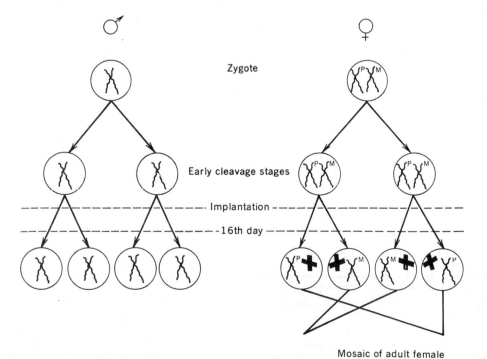

Fig. 4-14. Schematic representation of the phenomenon underlying the Lyon hypothesis. In the normal female, early in embryogenesis (probably soon after implantation) one X chromosome in each cell becomes inactive. Once it has been "decided" whether the maternal (M) or paternal (P) X chromosome will be the inactive one, all descendants of that cell "abide by the decision."

tions of iron within the body, probably as a result of a hereditary defect in the intestinal mechanism regulating iron absorption. Although the inheritance seems to be autosomal dominant, females are rather rarely affected because they have a safety valve on excessive iron accumulation—menstruation and pregnancy.

Note the difficulties in distinguishing sex-linked recessive inheritance from sex-limited autosomal dominant inheritance, if the nature of the disease is such that reproduction of affected males does not occur. The syndrome of testicular feminization (Chap. 97) is an example. The affected individuals are genetic males but, because of endorgan unresponsiveness to androgens, female external genitalia and all the secondary sex characters of the female develop. The affected male does not reproduce and normal females are carriers. The pedigree pattern is precisely that of a sex-linked recessive trait. However, the inheritance can equally well be sex-linked autosomal dominant. In diseases too severe to permit reproduction of affected males—the Pelizaeus-Merzbacher disease (a form of cerebral degeneration), the Duchenne variety of muscular dystrophy (Chap. 376), one variety of gargoylism (Chap. 399)—there is on the basis of pedigree patterns no way to distinguish sex-linked and sex-limited inheritance.

GENETIC COUNSELING. Familiarity with the patterns of disease is useful in diagnosis; if the pedigree pattern is consistent with the mode of inheritance usual for a suspected entity, the diagnosis of that entity is thereby strengthened. Knowing what individuals in a kindred are at risk, one can watch for the earliest signs of hereditary disease.

Furthermore, familiarity with pedigree patterns is essential to genetic counseling. The risk of having an affected child can be stated as 1 in 2 for a person affected by a dominant trait and as 1 in 4 for a couple which has already had a child affected by a recessive disease. For the sister of a male affected by a sex-linked recessive trait the risk of being a carrier is (unless the affected brother represents a new mutation) 1 in 2, of having an affected son one-half of that, or 1 in 4, and the risk of any affected child (considering both sexes) one-half of that, or 1 in 8.

In connection with statements of mendelian risk, it should be made clear to the consultand (person seeking genetic counseling) that the figure is a probability. Parents with one child with cystic fibrosis may take the statement of "1 in 4" to mean that they had their one affected and can now have three children who will be normal. The analogy to tossing coins is useful; with each toss of a true coin the chance of "heads" is 50 percent regardless of the result of earlier tosses. "Chance has no memory."

If a given condition is regularly inherited as a dominant, and if one can be certain that one parent does not have the condition in *forme fruste,* then the risk to later born children is virtually nil. It can be shown that for a rare X-linked recessive disorder of such a nature that the affected males do not reproduce—Duchenne muscular dystrophy is such a condition—about one-third of all cases will be the result of fresh mutation in the X chromosome contributed to the affected male offspring by the mother, and in the other two-thirds of cases the mother will be a heterozygous carrier of the mutation which occurred in an earlier generation. If by chance the carrier female has only one affected son and no affected relative, such as a brother, it is impossible to tell from the pedigree whether she is a carrier or not. Special tests for carrier status for various X-linked disorders have been devised. None is completely discriminatory and probably never can be because of the considerations of the Lyon hypothesis. Screening for heterozygous carriers for X-linked recessives is much more worthwhile than screening for carriers of autosomal recessives. Any X-linked carrier female has a 50 percent chance of having an affected son regardless of the genotype of her husband. An autosomal carrier has a one-fourth chance of having an affected child only if he or she marries another carrier.

Other genetic considerations such as the severity of the disease in question, including its severity in the specific family, must be included in the evaluation. Only the risks should be stated to the persons seeking counsel. The decision as to what action they should follow must be theirs and must take account of factors such as economic status and emotional fortitude. Socially valuable traits partially determined by genetic constitution may be present in the family and outweigh the disadvantage of a mutant gene.

Often the statement of risks is a relief to the persons involved and is not disturbing. For example, a young man with pseudoxanthoma elasticum (Chap. 398), an autosomal recessive trait, was relieved to learn that the likelihood that his children by an unrelated wife would be affected by the severe eye involvement and tendency to hemorrhage is essentially nil. In families affected by a clear-cut, nearly fully penetrant autosomal dominant trait normal persons are sometimes surprised to learn, and considerably relieved, that there is virtually no risk of their offspring being affected.

Genetic counseling in common disorders of multifactor causation presents special problems, which are discussed later.

NATURE AND FUNCTION OF THE GENETIC CODE

The gene is DNA, deoxyribonucleic acid. The function of many genes is to specify the sequence of amino acids that make up a polypeptide chain in a protein, either enzymatic or structural. The code word, or codon, for each amino acid is three-lettered, being spelled in one of four purine or pyrimidine bases: adenine, thymine, guanine, and cytosine (see Table 4-3). The principle of colinearity of the triplet code words in the DNA of the gene and the amino acids in the protein specified by that gene is now well established.

The triplet code for each of twenty specific amino acids is shown in Table 4-3. Messenger RNA (ribonucleic

Table 4-3. THE GENETIC CODE

Second Nucleotide

First nucleotide	A or U	G or C	T or A	C or G	Third nucleotide
A or *U*	**AAA** *UUU* ⎫ **AAG** *UUC* ⎬ Phe **AAT** *UUA* ⎫ **AAC** *UUG* ⎬ Leu	**AGA** *UCU* ⎫ **AGG** *UCC* ⎪ **AGT** *UCA* ⎬ Ser **AGC** *UCG* ⎭	**ATA** *UAU* ⎫ **ATG** *UAC* ⎬ Tyr **ATT** *UAA* ⎫ **ATC** *UAG* ⎬ Stop	**ACA** *UGU* ⎫ **ACG** *UGC* ⎬ Cys **ACT** *UGA* Stop **ACC** *UGG* Trp	A or *U* G or *C* T or *A* C or *G*
G or *C*	**GAA** *CUU* ⎫ **GAG** *CUC* ⎪ **GAT** *CUA* ⎬ Leu **GAC** *CUG* ⎭	**GGA** *CCU* ⎫ **GGG** *CCC* ⎪ **GGT** *CCA* ⎬ Pro **GGC** *CCG* ⎭	**GTA** *CAU* ⎫ **GTG** *CAC* ⎬ His **GTT** *CAA* ⎫ **GTC** *CAG* ⎬ Gln	**GCA** *CGU* ⎫ **GCG** *CGC* ⎪ **GCT** *CGA* ⎬ Arg **GCC** *CGG* ⎭	A or *U* G or *C* T or *A* C or *G*
T or *A*	**TAA** *AUU* ⎫ **TAG** *AUC* ⎬ Ile **TAT** *AUA* ⎭ **TAC** *AUG* Met	**TGA** *ACU* ⎫ **TGG** *ACC* ⎪ **TGT** *ACA* ⎬ Thr **TGC** *ACG* ⎭	**TTA** *AAU* ⎫ **TTG** *AAC* ⎬ Asn **TTT** *AAA* ⎫ **TTC** *AAG* ⎬ Lys	**TCA** *AGU* ⎫ **TCG** *AGC* ⎬ Ser **TCT** *AGA* ⎫ **TCC** *AGG* ⎬ Arg	A or *U* G or *C* T or *A* C or *G*
C or *G*	**CAA** *GUU* ⎫ **CAG** *GUC* ⎪ **CAT** *GUA* ⎬ Val **CAC** *GUG* ⎭	**CGA** *GCU* ⎫ **CGG** *GCC* ⎪ **CGT** *GCA* ⎬ Ala **CGC** *GCG* ⎭	**CTA** *GAU* ⎫ **CTG** *GAC* ⎬ Asp **CTT** *GAA* ⎫ **CTC** *GAG* ⎬ Glu	**CCA** *GGU* ⎫ **CCG** *GGC* ⎪ **CCT** *GGA* ⎬ Gly **CCC** *GGG* ⎭	A or *U* G or *C* T or *A* C or *G*

The DNA codons appear in boldface type; the complementary RNA codons are in italics. A = adenine, C = cytosine, G = guanine, T = thymine, U = uridine (replaces thymine in RNA). In RNA, adenine is complementary to thymine of DNA; uridine is complementary to adenine of DNA; cytosine is complementary to guanine, and vice versa. "Stop" = punctuation. The amino acids are abbreviated as follows:

Ala = alanine	Leu = leucine
Arg = arginine	Lys = lysine
Asn = asparagine	Met = methionine
Asp = aspartic acid	Phe = phenylalanine
Cys = cysteine	Pro = proline
Gln = glutamine	Ser = serine
Glu = glutamic acid	Thr = threonine
Gly = glycine	Trp = tryptophane
His = histidine	Tyr = tyrosine
Ile = isoleucine	Val = valine

acid), in which the nucleotides are complementary to those of DNA so that it is a negative copy of the DNA, conveys the blueprint for amino acid sequence from DNA on a chromosome in the nucleus to the site of protein synthesis on the ribosomes in the cytoplasm (Fig. 4-15). The code dictionary summarized in Table 4-3 was deduced from studies of the messenger RNA code, in which uridine substitutes for thymine. In addition to ribosomal RNA and messenger RNA, a third type, transfer or soluble RNA, is involved in the assemblage of amino acids into polypeptide chains. The process by which RNA is copied from DNA is called *transcription;* the process by which the RNA-DNA blueprint determines the amino acid sequence of a protein is called *translation* (Fig. 4-15).

The limits of the gene have become clearer. As a functional unit, called by Seymour Benzer the *cistron,* the gene is that portion of DNA responsible for specification of a single polypeptide and a *locus* is physically that portion of the linearly arranged genetic material (DNA)

occupied by the cistron or gene. The alternative forms of the gene which occur at the same locus are called *alleles.* For example, the genes for A, B, and O blood types are multiple alleles at one locus. Within a locus there are many mutable sites. Obviously if the gene at a locus is responsible for specifying all the many amino acids in a complex protein, many base pairs are vulnerable to mutation. This much smaller unit is called by Benzer the *muton.* The genetic unit as revealed by recombination is referred to as the *recon.*

The normal process of development occurs by differential gene action; i.e., by activity of some genes but not of others in particular tissues at particular stages. The mechanism controlling differential gene activity, what switches one gene on and another off at a particular stage, is unknown. Dramatic examples of differential gene function are reflected by the shift from synthesis of embryonic hemoglobin to fetal hemoglobin in the first trimester and from fetal hemoglobin to adult hemoglobin in the first months of extrauterine life.

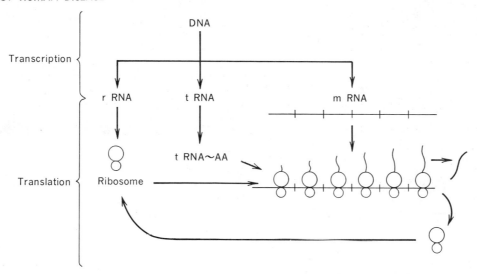

Fig. 4-15. Schema of protein synthesis. (*Courtesy, Dr. Irving M. London*)

MUTATION

This term means change in the genetic material. At least three classes of mutation must be considered. When used without further specification, the term usually refers to "point mutation," that is, change in a single base with substitution of one for another. As seen in Table 4-3, change in DNA from CTT to CAT causes a substitution of valine for glutamic acid in the product protein. This change is the one which occurs in the beta chain of sickle hemoglobin. Similarly, a change from CTT to TTT causes substitution of lysine for glutamic acid, the situation in hemoglobin C. It was first reported that a variant hemoglobin, called Hb I, had lysine (the sixteenth amino acid in the alpha chain) replaced by aspartic acid. Francis Crick insisted, however, that this is not true because change in a single base cannot result in this amino acid substitution. When the matter was re-investigated, it was found that, in fact, glutamic acid is substituted for lysine, a change produced by a single base substitution.

A second class of mutation is that which results in the gross chromosomal abnormalities discussed in the next section. This class includes (1) abnormalities of chromosome number, e.g., missing or supernumerary chromosomes as a result of errors in chromosome segregation during cell division; and (2) abnormalities of chromosome structure, i.e., chromosomal deletions, translocations, inversions, and so on, as a result of chromosome breakage.

A third class of mutation results from nonhomologous pairing and unequal crossing over, as diagrammed in Fig. 4-16. During the meiotic process in gametogenesis, homologous chromosomes pair, but if the matching is not precise, unequal crossing over occurs. The result is either duplication (Fig. 4-16a) of genetic material or deletion. Gene duplication, like the other forms of mutation, has been demonstrably important in evolution. It is

a process by which an organism can experiment with new mutations in one copy of the duplicated gene while retaining an essential function of the original gene. The separate genes that specify the various polypeptide chains of hemoglobin (the beta chain of adult hemoglobin A, the delta chain of adult hemoglobin A_2, the gamma chain of fetal hemoglobin, the epsilon chain of embryonic hemoglobin, and the alpha chain of all four of these hemoglobins) as well as the gene that specifies the single polypeptide chain of myoglobin appear to have evolved from a primordial common ancestral gene through the process of gene duplication and subsequent independent mutation in the separate genes.

Nonhomologous pairing with unequal crossing over also can cause deletion of part of a gene or of part of two contiguous genes. Study of the amino acid sequence in some abnormal hemoglobins suggests that this was the type of mutation responsible, rather than change in a codon which caused a different amino acid to be specified. For example, in hemoglobin Gun Hill five amino acids are missing from the beta chain (amino acids 93 through 97), so that this hemoglobin is only 141 amino acids long rather than 146. Hemoglobin Lepore is another example of mutation due to unequal crossing over. The gene for the beta chain of hemoglobin A and that for the delta chain of hemoglobin A_2 are probably contiguous. In a person with hemoglobin Lepore, the normal beta and delta chains are replaced by a polypeptide chain that has the structure of the delta chain at one end and of the beta chain at the other. As is diagrammed in Fig. 4-16*b*, a fusion gene specifying a hybrid polypeptide chain of this type could have arisen by unequal crossing over.

BIOCHEMICAL ASPECTS OF GENE ACTION

Biochemical genetics has two parts: One, the chemistry of the genetic material (discussed earlier), had its be-

Fig. 4-16. Genetic mutation through nonhomologous pairing and unequal crossing over. *A*. Gene duplication from crossing over between genes. *B*. Creation of a fusion gene through crossing over within a gene, as is thought to have occurred to produce the gene for Lepore hemoglobin.

ginnings with Friedrich Miescher's work on nucleic acid. The second part of biochemical genetics had its origin in the early part of this century, with a physician, Archibald Garrod, and his "inborn errors of metabolism." The disorders he considered were defects in intermediary metabolism resulting from an inherited abnormality of particular enzymes. In its broader implications, biochemical genetics is concerned with the chemical nature of the genetic code and with all the biochemical steps by which that code is translated into an observed characteristic, for example, an inherited disease.

In accordance with the current views, all properties of a protein are a consequence of its amino acid sequence. Probably the proteins specified by genes are not only enzyme proteins but also may be structural proteins, e.g., collagen, or proteins with other functions and properties, such as hemoglobin. The useful concept of "one gene, one enzyme" requires modification to "one gene, one polypeptide," or (see below) "one cistron, one polypeptide."

In the schema outlined earlier, mutation represents a change in the code, that is, a change in the base sequence of DNA. Mutations may be of two types. In "mis-sense" mutations a different amino acid is substituted at a given site in the particular protein, for example, valine for glutamic acid, changing "normal" hemoglobin to sickle hemoglobin. In "non-sense" mutations the change in the base sequence of DNA is such that there is no corresponding amino acid and none of a given protein, e.g., an enzyme, may be found.

The terms borrowed from bacterial genetics, CRM-positive (pronounced "krim-positive") and CRM-negative mutations, correspond to the terms *mis-sense* and *non-sense* mutations, respectively. CRM means cross-reacting material, and in CRM-positive mutations material which

reacts in a normal manner in immunologic tests but is functionally (e.g., enzymatically) ineffective is present. An example of CRM-positive and CRM-negative mutations in man is provided by recessively inherited isolated growth hormone deficiency. Growth hormone is assayed by an immunologic method. Most cases of isolated deficiency have no hormone demonstrable by immunoassay; these are CRM-negative cases. A few have an immunologically demonstrable substance which is apparently ineffective biologically; these are CRM-positive cases.

As stated above, the mutant gene can result in the formation of a different protein or of no protein at all of a given type. If the protein in question is an enzyme, none at all may be formed or an enzyme may be formed which is so impaired in its function that the net effect is the same. In intermediary metabolism such a change can have pathogenetic consequences through any of several mechanisms or through some combination of these. We can represent a hypothetical metabolic process as follows:

$$\text{Gene}_{AB} \qquad \text{Gene}_{BC} \qquad \text{Gene}_{CD}$$
$$\downarrow \qquad\qquad \downarrow \qquad\qquad \downarrow$$
$$\text{Enzyme}_{AB} \qquad \text{Enzyme}_{BC} \qquad \text{Enzyme}_{CD}$$
$$A \longrightarrow B \longrightarrow C \longrightarrow D$$

If a mutant form of gene$_{CD}$ results in no formation of enzyme$_{CD}$ or in the formation of functionally defective enzyme, then the effects may be of several types:

1. The disease characteristic may reflect the deficiency of product D:

$$A \longrightarrow B \longrightarrow C \;\;/\!\!/\!\!\longrightarrow (D)$$

Albinism (Chap. 104) might be cited as an example; melanin is not formed because of a block in tyrosine metabolism. In several forms of genetic cretinism (Chap. 89), thyroid hormone is not formed because of blocks of this type; in the adrenogenital syndrome (Chap. 98), hydrocortisone is not produced.

2. A metabolite just proximal to the block may accumulate in toxic amounts.

$$A \longrightarrow B \longrightarrow \begin{matrix} C \\ C \\ C \end{matrix} \longrightarrow\!\!\!/\!\!\!\!/\longrightarrow (D)$$

An example is alkaptonuria. Homogentisic acid is not metabolized normally. It is excreted in the urine in large amounts. Furthermore its increase in the body in some way leads to a form of degenerative arthritis.

3. If the reactions in questions are reversible, there may be an accumulation of precursors farther back from the site of block.

$$\begin{matrix} A \\ A \\ A \end{matrix} \rightleftharpoons \begin{matrix} B \\ B \end{matrix} \rightleftharpoons C \longrightarrow (D)$$

An example is the accumulation of glycogen in the form of glycogen storage disease (von Gierke's disease) in which the primary defect involves glucose 6-phosphatase (Chap. 111).

Glycogen $\rightleftharpoons$ glucose 1-phosphate $\rightleftharpoons$ glucose 6-phosphate

glucose
6-phosphatase

4. There may be synthesis of products through an accessory pathway which is normally of minor significance.

$$A \longrightarrow B \longrightarrow C \longrightarrow\!\!\!/\!\!\!\!/\longrightarrow (D)$$
$$\downarrow$$
$$X \longrightarrow Y \longrightarrow Z$$

In phenylketonuria, phenylketone products are produced in unusual amounts from phenylalanine, which is not properly metabolized. In hyperoxaluria, an excess production of oxalate may be the result of a defect in the normal metabolism of glyoxylate:

Glycine $\rightleftharpoons$ glyoxylate $\longrightarrow$ formic acid $+ CO_2$

oxalic acid

Undoubtedly these do not exhaust the possible mechanisms of a pathogenetic effect from a mutation in a gene controlling an enzyme.

Metabolic processes are in most instances chains, indeed often networks. A mutation in the genes controlling any of several metabolic steps may lead to the same phenotypic result. Thus, the phenotype is not an indication of the specific genotype. Identical diseases may be produced by mutation of different genes; "genetic mimics," they are called.

A hundred or more disorders have, with varying degrees of reliability, been traced to a deficiency in the activity of a specific enzyme. Almost all behave as recessive traits. Enzyme systems have sufficient margin of safety that the mutant gene must be present in double dose and the deficiency must be complete in order for abnormality to be demonstrable in the phenotype. On the other hand, conditions based on mutation in a gene determining the amino acid sequence of a nonenzymic protein, e.g., hemoglobin, are likely to be dominant in their inheritance pattern. This is because the physical and functional properties of the product protein may be so altered that abnormality occurs even though only about half the product protein is of mutant type. The above principle concerning dominant and recessive inheritance is nicely demonstrated by the methemoglobinemias (Chap. 344), of which dominant and recessive forms exist. The recessive form is due to deficient activity of an enzyme, methemoglobin reductase, of the red cell. The dominant forms have a defect in hemoglobin, these being the several types of hemoglobin M.

The nonenzymic protein which has been subjected to most extensive study is hemoglobin (Chap. 339). Over one hundred mutations in the genes determining the alpha and beta polypeptide chains of hemoglobin have been identified. These mutations have been discovered by finding unitary amino acid changes in variant hemoglobins. Some of the changes involve the same amino acid; e.g., both hemoglobin S and hemoglobin C have a change in the sixth of the 146 amino acids of the beta polypeptide chain. In other variant hemoglobins the change is present in different amino acids of the chain. Understanding of how the particular amino acid substitution alters the function of hemoglobin is steadily increasing.

Another type of process, not strictly enzymatic, by which mutations have pathogenetic effects involves changes in active transport mechanisms in the kidney and elsewhere. Cystinuria (Chap. 102) is an example. Other active transport systems can be cited, such as those involved in the movement of substances such as amino acids across the intestinal mucosa, of substances like bilirubin into and out of the liver cell, and of electrolytes across the muscle cell membrane. All these mechanisms are vulnerable to the effects of mutation in the determinant genes, and diseases for which such mutation is probably responsible can be cited.

Structural genes, i.e., those specifying the amino acid sequence of proteins have for the most part been discussed to this point. "A pile of bricks is not a house," however. Other genes have a controlling role, ensuring an orderly interplay of the structural genes in development and in the adult organism. Mutation can occur also in these controlling genes with resultant disease. The evidence is coming mainly from the study of microorganisms; although a number of disorders of man are suspected to result from mutation in controlling genes, critical evidence is not easily assembled.

The complex machinery of protein synthesis, of which the framework is DNA-RNA-ribosomes, has become more clearly understood in recent years. Of potential therapeutic importance is the demonstration that intermediate steps in protein synthesis can be modified by various measures. It is possible, for example, that although a warped

Fig. 4-17. Schematic representation of the spectrum of disease in regard to the relative importance of genetics (G) and exogenous (E) factors in etiology and pathogenesis.

and enzymatically weak protein is formed in a given disorder, the amount synthesized can be increased by some means and the disease abolished or ameliorated.

The Genetics of Common Disorders

All disease is in some degree genetic and in some degree environmental in etiology and pathogenesis. As to the relative importance of endogenous and exogenous factors, disease can be thought of as falling on a spectrum (Fig. 4-17). Near the genetic end (G) are simply inherited disorders such as phenylketonuria and galactosemia, but these are not at the extreme end because exogenous factors, diet in these specific examples, can importantly modify the phenotype. Near the environmental end (E) are infectious diseases but again not at the extreme end because twin and other studies indicate a significant role of genotype in susceptibility.

In the analysis of disorders affecting all systems, two classes of disorders, with regard to the role of genetic factors, are evident: (1) rare, simply inherited disorders (near the G end of the spectrum); (2) common disorders in which genetic factors play some role. Examples in the gastrointestinal system are familial polyposis of the colon and peptic ulcer; in the cardiovascular system, hereditary hemorrhagic telangiectasia and coronary artery disease; in the connective tissue system, Marfan's syndrome, lupus erythematosus; in the eye, retinitis pigmentosa and glaucoma.

The common disorders are, for the most part, multifactorial in causation. The etiology is a nexus in which

environmental and genetic factors collaborate in a complex way in determining the disease.

Questions asked in connection with common disease are mainly two: How significant are genetic factors in etiology? By what mechanism does the mutant gene contribute to the pathogenesis?

Methods for evaluating the role of genetic factors in common diseases are mainly six:

1. *Family studies.* If genetic factors are important, a familial aggregation for the disorder should be demonstrable. Familial aggregation can have other than a genetic basis; thus, evidence from family studies is per se not critical.

2. *Twin studies.* Monozygotic twins, because of genetic identity, should show a higher concordance rate (i.e., "both affected") than dizygotic twins show, if genetic factors are significantly involved.

3. *Interracial comparisons.* Races have different frequencies of many genes. If genetic factors are important in etiology, the frequency of common diseases may vary from race to race. A difficulty in interpretation of racial data is the uncertainty of environmental comparability. Races are social as well as biologic entities.

4. *Component analysis.* Whenever a factor is shown to be an important element of the etiologic nexus, its genetics can be studied by family studies, twin studies, racial comparisons, and animal homologies. Lipid metabolism in atherosclerosis is an example.

5. *Blood group and disease association.* A simply inherited trait such as a specific blood group can, in some instances, be shown to occur more frequently with a given common disease than would be expected by chance. Some physiologic peculiarity of the person with that blood group seems to predispose him slightly but definitely to the disorder. The best example is the association between blood group O and peptic ulcer (Chap. 5). Another is the association of non-O and venous thromboembolic disease. Demonstration of association is evidence of a genetic factor in the disorder. Failure to demonstrate association does not exclude the importance of genetic factors.

6. *Animal homologies.* If one has available in animals a disorder seemingly identical to a common disease of man, then one may be able to do breeding experiments and extensive biochemical and physiologic investigations that will throw light on the two questions stated above.

The collaboration of multiple genes appears to be involved in determining stature; i.e., stature is a polygenic trait. Environmental factors, such as nutrition and chronic infectious disease, also influence stature; thus, stature is a multifactorial trait, to use the more general term. When the stature of a large group of persons is plotted, the distribution curve is a "normal," bell-shaped Gaussian

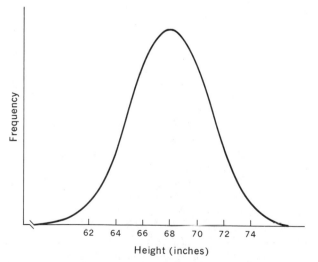

Fig. 4-18. Distribution curve for stature in the southeastern part of England. The mean is 68 in., and the standard deviation 2.6 in. *(Drawn from data analyzed by Cedric O. Carter)*

Fig. 4-19. Distribution curves for blood pressure. Normal blood pressure increases with age and is somewhat different in males and females; hence the separate plots. Note that all show positive skew, i.e., a tail at the end of the curve for higher pressures. [Bøe, et al., Acta med. scandin. 157: (suppl. 321), 1957].

one (Fig. 4-18). This suggests that the multiple genes involved in determining a person's height interact in an additive manner. By way of contrast, the distribution curve for blood pressure is "skewed" (Fig. 4-19), suggesting that the multiple genes determining level of blood pressure interact in a multiplicative manner. This conclusion is supported by the fact that if a logarithmic scale is used for blood pressure, the curve is "normalized" (Fig. 4-20). As a corollary to the view that blood pressure is a polygenic trait, essential hypertension is interpreted as the condition present in those persons whose particular assemblage of genes determines a level of blood pressure at the upper end of the distribution curve. What one calls essential hypertension and what one calls normotension are largely arbitrary decisions.

That a rather small number of genes can produce a continuous distribution is indicated by the example shown in Figure 4-21. Stature is assumed to be deter-

mined by two genetic loci on different chromosomes, each with three alleles in frequencies such that an allele (called "−") which decreases stature by 2 in., one (called "0") which determines the average stature of 68 in., and one (called "+") which increases stature by 2 in. have a relative frequency of 1:2:1. Five classes of gametes produced by each sex have the following frequencies (derived from Table 4-4): −−, $\frac{1}{16}$; −0, $\frac{1}{4}$; 00, $\frac{6}{16}$; +0, $\frac{1}{4}$; ++$\frac{1}{16}$. Zygotes formed from random union of gametes in these proportions have four stature genes (two at each of the two loci), and the possible combinations of +, 0, and − alleles found among the zygotes are nine in number. The relative frequencies of these are derived from Table 4-5 and plotted in Figure 4-21. A satisfactory approximation to a normal distribution is obtained, particularly when environmental influences blur the separation of groups. This example illustrates that even in conditions, like essential hyperten-

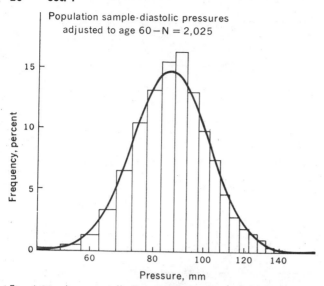

Population sample-diastolic pressures
adjusted to age 60—N = 2,025

Fig. 4-20. An essentially "normal" curve results when adjustment for age and sex differences are made and a logarithmic blood pressure scale is used. (*Courtesy of J. A. Fraser Roberts*)

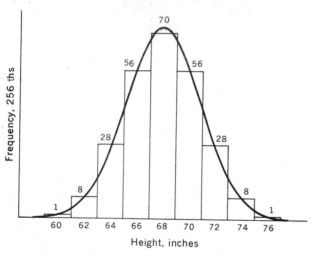

Fig. 4-21. Distribution curve for stature assuming that only two loci, each with three alleles, determine this characteristic. A small number of genes combined with environmental influence can result in a continuous distribution. (*Example from Cedric O. Carter*)

Table 4-4. PROPORTIONS OF EXPECTED
TYPES OF GAMETES

		Chromosome 1		
		Allele − 1/4	Allele 0 1/2	Allele + 1/4
Chromosome 2	Allele − 1/4	1/16 − −	1/8 − 0	1/16 − +
	Allele 0 1/2	1/8 0 −	1/4 0 0	1/8 0 +
	Allele + 1/4	1/16 + −	1/8 + 0	1/16 + +

Table 4-5. PROPORTIONS OF EXPECTED
TYPES OF ZYGOTES

		Male gametes				
		− − 1/16	− 0 1/4	0 0 6/16	0 + 1/4	+ + 1/16
Female gametes	− − 1/16	60 in. 1/256	62 in. 4/256	64 in. 6/256	66 in. 1/64	68 in. 1/256
	− 0 1/4	62 in. 4/256	64 in. 1/16	66 in. 6/64	68 in. 1/16	70 in. 1/64
	0 0 6/16	64 in. 6/256	66 in. 6/64	68 in. 36/256	70 in. 6/64	72 in. 6/256
	0 + 1/4	66 in. 1/64	68 in. 1/16	70 in. 6/64	72 in. 1/16	74 in. 4/256
	+ + 1/16	68 in. 1/256	70 in. 1/64	72 in. 6/256	74 in. 4/256	76 in. 1/256

sion, which appear to be polygenic, it is worthwhile to search for single-gene determined biochemical and physiologic mechanisms.

REFERENCES

Carter, C. O.: "Human Heredity," Baltimore, Penguin Books, Inc., 1962.

Court Brown, W. M.: "Human Population Cytogenetics," Amsterdam, North-Holland Publishing Company, 1967.

Harris, H.: Molecular Basis of Hereditary Disease, Brit. Med. J., 1:135–141, 1968.

Jink, H. et al.: Venous Thromboembolic Disease and ABO Blood Type, Lancet, 1:539–542, 1969.

McKusick, V. A.: "Human Genetics," 2d ed., Englewood Cliffs, N.J., Prentice-Hall, Inc., 1969.

——: "Mendelian Inheritance in Man. Catalogs of Autosomal Dominant, Autosomal Recessive and X-linked Phenotypes," 2d ed., Baltimore, The Johns Hopkins Press, 1968.

Perutz, M. F., and H. Lehmann: Molecular Pathology of Human Hemoglobin, Nature, 219:902–909, 1968.

Roberts, J. A. F.: "Introduction to Medical Genetics," 4th ed., London, Oxford University Press, 1967.

Rowley, J. D.: Cytogenetics in Clinical Medicine, J.A.M.A., 207:914–919, 1969.

Stanbury, J. B., J. B. Wyngaarden, and D. S. Fredrickson (Eds.): "The Metabolic Basis of Inherited Disease," 2d ed., New York, McGraw-Hill Book Company, 1966.

5 BLOOD GROUPS

J. Foerster and M. M. Wintrobe

Blood groups represent systems of antigenic determinants found on the surface of red cells. These antigens are inherited according to simple mendelian laws and are thought to be the products of allelic or closely linked genes. The major systems of antigens (e.g., ABO and Rh) are inherited independently of each other.

Blood groups are identified by means of specific antibodies occurring in serum, either "naturally," or after immunization with foreign red cells or soluble blood group substances. Chemical characterization of blood group antigens has lagged far behind serologic and genetic studies, and so far only the ABO and Lewis systems have lent themselves to extensive biochemical analysis. The study of the latter systems has been greatly facilitated by the discovery that the antigens in question occur not only as surface components of cells, but are also found in water-soluble form in the tissue fluids and secretions of most people.

THE ABO SYSTEM

The ABO antigens are inherited as simple mendelian characters, the blood group of an individual depending on the presence of two out of the three allelic genes: A, B, and O. The possible genotypic and corresponding phenotypic combinations are listed in Table 5-1. Anti-

Table 5-1. THE ABO BLOOD GROUPS

Phenotype (group)	Genotype	Agglutinogens on red cells	Isoagglutinins in serum
0	OO	none	anti-A anti-B
A	AA AO	A	anti-B
B	BB BO	B	anti-A
AB	AB	A and B	none

SOURCE: M. M. Wintrobe, "Clinical Hematology," 6th ed., Philadelphia Lea & Febiger, 1967.

bodies reacting with a particular blood group substance in this system are regularly found in the serum when the corresponding antigen is absent from the red cells. These antibodies were originally thought to occur "naturally," but are now known to arise early in life as a result of exposure to ABO-like polysaccharides occurring ubiquitously in food and other exogenous sources.

In addition to antibodies against A and B antigens, reagents are known which react preferentially with O cells. The antigen defined by these reagents is known as H-substance. Its synthesis is thought to be under the control of an allelic pair of genes, *Hh*, which is inherited independently of the ABO system. Thus the *H* gene in single or double dose gives rise to the H character, and the rare *h* allele, when present in double dose, results in its absence. The H-active material is probably in turn a precursor substance which under the influence of *A* and *B* genes is converted into A and B active substances respectively, thereby accounting for the presence of large quantities of H substance in O individuals.

The capacity to secrete A-, B-, or H-substances into tissue fluids and secretions is controlled by a pair of allelic genes *Sese*. *Se* is considered dominant over *se*, and only homozygous *sese* individuals therefore are nonsecretors of A-, B-, and/or H-substances.

The Lewis system is closely related to the ABO system, although the two allelic genes, *Le* and *le*, which define this system, are inherited independently of the *ABO*, *Hh*, and *Sese* genes. In single or double dose *Le* gives rise to Le^a specific structures; *le* in double dose results in their absence. Le^b specificity, once thought to arise from the activity of an allele of the *Le* gene, is now considered to be an interaction product of *H* and *Le* genes. Most nonsecretors of A, B or H-substances still secrete the Le^a substance, and the secretion of Le^a is therefore considered *not* to be under the control of the *Sese* genes.

The chemical composition of *secreted* ABH and Lewis substances is remarkably similar. They are composed of a carbohydrate moiety which constitutes about 85 percent of the molecule and an amino acid moiety which makes up the remaining 15 percent. The peptide residues are always composed of the same 15 amino acids, and 4 of these, threonine, serine, proline and alanine, make up two-thirds of all the amino acids present. The peptides appear to have structural functions only and are thought to form a firm, spiny backbone to which a large number of relatively short oligosaccharide chains, constituting the blood group substances, are attached at intervals. The carbohydrate moiety of all the ABH and Lewis substances is qualitatively similar in composition. Each contains a methyl-pentose, L-fucose; a hexose, D-galactose; two amino sugars, N-acetyl-D-glucosamine and N-acetyl-D-galactosamine; and a 9-carbon sugar, N-acetyl neuraminic acid. One of these sugars appears to be immunodominant in each of the blood group substances studied.

Cellular blood group substances are much more difficult to isolate, but both A and B active materials have been obtained in water-soluble form. In contrast to the blood group substances found in secretions, these cell-derived extracts are glycolipids. Nevertheless it appears that the oligosaccharide chains which confer blood group specificity on the glycolipid blood group substances of red cells as well as the glycoprotein substances found in secretions are identical, thereby accounting for the similarities in the specificity of antigenic determinants on red cells and on secretions.

The complicated interrelationship between A, B, H, and Lewis substances was clarified considerably when it was recognized that the gene systems controlling these four expressions appear to act sequentially on a common glycoprotein precursor substance. Genetic control presumably comes about through the formation of specific glycosyl transferase enzymes or through some mechanism controlling their function. A simplified version of such a proposed scheme is illustrated in Figure 5-1.

Two precursor chains are recognized on the basis of a $1 \rightarrow 3$ (type I) or $1 \rightarrow 4$ (type II) linkage of the terminal galactosyl unit to the subterminal N-acetyl-

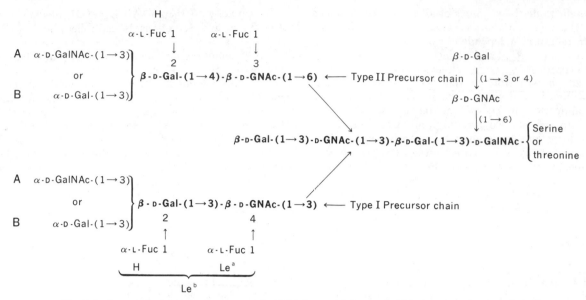

Fig. 5-1. *Proposed composite structure of A, B, H, Le^a and Le^b specific blood group substances linked to serine or threonine spines of the polypeptide backbone. Gal refers to galactose; Fuc to fucose; GNAc to N-acetylglucosamine; GalNAc to N-acetylgalactosamine. The numerical notations (e.g., 1 → 4) refer to the respective carbon positions at which linkage occurs. The precursor substance is identified by **Bold Type**; the determinants characteristic of a given blood group substance are in light type and are identified by their appropriate symbols, namely A, B, H, Le^a, and Le^b. The structure shown is a composite which includes all determinants. In individual blood group substances certain residues will be missing; e.g., H, Le^a, and Le^b specific blood group substances lack A and B specific determinants, and Le^a substance also lacks the H specific determinant. See text and references for details. (After K. O. Lloyd, et al., Biochemistry 7:2976, 1968).*

galactosamine residue. The latter precursor chain has cross-reactivity with antisera to type XIV pneumococcal polysaccharide.

The transferase controlled by the H gene is thought to add L-fucose in α-linkage to the carbon 2 position of either chain to form an H-active structure. The enzyme controlled by the *Le* gene, also a fucosyl transferase, adds L-fucose in α-linkage to the 4 position of the subterminal N-acetylglucosamine unit in chains of type I only, as chains of type II already are substituted at this position. The resultant structure has Le^a specificity. When both *H* and *Le* genes are present, two fucosyl units are added to adjacent sugars on chains of type I, resulting in a structure which, on the basis of inhibition experiments, is thought to be that of the Le^b determinant.

The presence of the fucosyl unit conferring H specificity to the precursor substance is considered to be essential for the functioning of the transferases controlled by the *A* and *B* genes. Thus N-acetyl-D-galactosamine added in α-linkage to carbon 3 of the terminal galactosyl unit confers A-specificity to the H-active precursor substance, whereas addition of D-galactose in identical linkage results in B specificity. The addition of these terminal nonreducing sugars effectively masks the serologic reactivity of the H-active groupings, and the Le^a-active determinants are similarly masked by the substitutions controlled by the *A*, *B*, and *H* genes. The *Se* gene does not bring about structural changes but simply controls the expression of the *ABH* genes for the blood group substances in secretion.

In the case of A substance, differences in the degree of expression of the antigen are well known. Indeed, a spectrum of A exists, extending from the strong A$_1$ to the weak A$_x$ antigen, reflecting a large series of determinant alleles. These differences in A likely represent genetically determined variations in the ability to bind a specific antibody, although the alternate possibility of differences in the number of binding sites per red cell cannot be excluded with certainty. Incomplete expression of blood group antigens also has been noted in rare instances of diseases, such as acute leukemia.

THE Rh SYSTEM

In 1940 Landsteiner and Wiener made the surprising discovery that the sera of rabbits and guinea pigs immunized with the red cells of Rhesus monkeys agglutinated not only the donor erythrocytes but also those of most Caucasian New Yorkers. Those individuals whose red cells were agglutinated by these sera were termed *Rh-positive*, the others, *Rh-negative*. It was subsequently discovered that heterologous antirhesus antibodies do not actually react with red cell antigens presently known to be part of the Rh system, but rather, they react with another antigen (LW) shared by both rhesus and human cells. The original observation did, however, stimulate immediate inquiry into the nature of unexplained intragroup transfusion reactions and incompatibilities between mother and child which result in erythroblastosis fetalis (Chap. 338); and it was found that most of these reactions could be accounted for by antibodies resembling those described by Landsteiner and Wiener.

From this modest beginning has evolved the most complex of human blood group systems, presently characterized by approximately 30 different serologic specificities and an almost unlimited number of complex alleles. Undoubtedly much of the present confusion surrounding this system is related to the fact that chemical definition of these antigens has lagged far behind serologic and genetic studies.

Two systems of nomenclature describing this complex system need to be considered. According to Fisher, the inheritance of Rh antigens is determined by three pairs of closely linked allelic genes. Thus each parent would contribute a set of three Rh genes, C or c, D or d, E or e, each defining a single antigen. A person might therefore inherit CDe from one parent and cde from another, to mention only the two most commonly observed genotypes. This theory also assumes that crossover of linked genes can take place, thereby accounting for the maintenance of the rarer combinations by occasional crossing over from the common heterozygotes. Wiener, on the other hand, postulates a single gene to accommodate a large number of alleles. An equally important part of Wiener's theory implies the existence of several families

of antibodies directed against the same Rh determinant (*agglutinogen*), but each having specificity for different aspects of its structure. These structural aspects defined by a given serologic specificity have been termed *blood factors*. According to this scheme, which is outlined in Table 5-2, a given antigenic determinant (agglutinogen) may be recognized by antibodies of heterogeneous specificities directed against any one of its constituent "blood factors." Thus, for example, the presence of the antigenic determinant rh, which is the product of gene r, may be inferred from serologic reactions which are specific for its constituent blood factors hr', hr", and hr. Unfortunately the structure of complex antigens, and particularly its mode of synthesis, cannot be derived exclusively from an analysis of agglutination reactions. Confirmation of these assumptions will therefore have to await the structural definition of the antigenic determinants in question.

Other Blood Group Systems

The inheritance of M, N, or MN blood group substances appears to be associated with two allelic genes L^m and L^n. Indeed, it seems likely that the synthesis of MN antigens is similar to that of the ABO system, being the result of sequential, gene-controlled changes in a common precursor substance. This is suggested by the association of both M and N activities with the same macromolecule, by the presence of N activity in M preparations derived from cells of the genotype MM, and the exposure of common specificities in M and N preparations by the removal of N-acetylneuraminic acid. It appears likely that N substance is a precursor of M substance. The chemical nature of M and N substances has been investigated extensively, and it has been shown that carbohydrate units with terminal nonreducing acetylneuraminic acid residues are important constituents of their determinant structures.

The Ss antigens are related to M and N in much the same way as C and c are related to D and d, probably existing as closely linked loci on the same chromosome. Many other antigens such as Hu, He, and Mi are now also known to belong to the MnSs system.

The P blood group system appears to be determined by the three alleles P^1, P^2, and the very rare gene, p, which in double dose results in the absence of P_1 and P_2 antigens. Another determinant, P^k also seems to be associated with the P system but is genetically independent of the P^1, P^2 genes. It has been postulated that the P^k determinant, like the Bombay specificity of the ABO system, results from the absence of a very frequent gene dominant in character. The Tj^a antigen is also known to be part of the P system. Thus, naturally occurring anti-Tj^a antibodies are found in the sera of all pp individuals and react with red cells of P_1, P_2, and P^k phenotype. If anti-Tj^a sera are absorbed with P_2 cells, anti-P_1 activity is left behind, confirming the specificity of these reactions. The clinical importance of the P blood group system derives from the fact that antibodies regularly occur

Table 5-2. WIENER'S GENE DESIGNATIONS, CORRESPONDING AGGLUTINOGENS AND BLOOD FACTORS, AND FISHER-RACE NOTATIONS

Genes		Frequency among Caucasoids, %	Corresponding agglutinogens	Blood factors present
Wiener	Fisher Race			
r	cde	38.0	rh	hr',hr",hr
r'	Cde	0.6	rh'	rh',hr"
r'^w	C^wde	0.005	rh'^{w}	rh',rh^w,hr"
r''	cdE	0.5	rh"	rh",hr'
r^y	CdE	0.01	rh^y	rh',rh"
R^o	cDe	2.7	Rh$_0$	Rh$_0$,hr',hr",hr
R^1	CDe	41.0	Rh$_1$	Rh$_0$,rh',hr"
R^{1w}	C^wDe	2.0	Rh$_1^w$	Rh$_0$,rh',rh^w,hr"
R^2	cDE	15.0	Rh$_2$	Rh$_0$,rh",hr'
R^z	CDE	0.2	Rh$_z$	Rh$_0$,rh',rh"

NOTE: Wiener, in his publications, uses italics for gene symbols and for genotypes, regular type for agglutinogens and phenotypes and boldface type for symbols for blood factors and for the corresponding antibodies used to detect the blood factors in question. Further, to distinguish the symbols for genotypes and phenotypes, the letter "h" is omitted and only superscripts are used in gene symbols.

SOURCE: M. M. Wintrobe, "Clinical Hematology," 6th ed., Philadelphia, Lea and Febiger, 1967.

in the serum of individuals who lack the corresponding P antigen. Thus, in addition to the anti-P + P_1 + P^k (= anti-Tj^a) antibody found in the sera of pp individuals, anti-P_1 antibody is found in P_2 subjects and anti-P (= anti-P_1 + anti-P_2) antibody occurs in the serum of P^k individuals.

Many other blood group systems have been described (Table 5-3), some of which possess clinical or anthropologic importance because of their high incidence in the population (e.g., Tj^a, Vel, k), difficulties associated with their detection in the laboratory (Kidd), or peculiarities in ethnic distribution (Diego). So-called "private

Table 5-3. BLOOD GROUPS

Name of system	Antigens of major clinical importance	Other identified antigens
ABO, Hh, LEWIS .	A, B, Le^a	H, Le^b
Rh..............	D	D^u
	C, c	C^u, C^w, C^x
	E, e	E^u, E^w
MNSs...........	S	M, N, s, M_1, M_2, M^g, Mi^a, Vw, Hu, He, U
P................	....	P_1, P_2, P^k, Tj^a
Kell.............	K	k, Kp^a, Kp^b, Js^a, Js^b, K^u, K^w
Duffy...........	Fy^a	Fy^b
Kidd............	Jk^a	Jk^b
Lutheran.......	....	Lu^a, Lu^b
Ii..............	....	I, i
Diego..........	....	Di^a, Di^b

antigens" (e.g., By, Sw^a, Levay) are of little or no clinical significance, except in the families in which they exist.

CLINICAL SIGNIFICANCE OF BLOOD GROUPS

BLOOD TRANSFUSION REACTIONS. These are of great variety (Table 342-1). Those related to blood group incompatibility are among the most serious. The blood groups A, B, and D (Rh) are involved in by far the greatest majority, perhaps 95 percent of all cases. This is because anti-A and anti-B antibodies occur "naturally," and D is, like A and B, a good antigen to which antibodies are produced readily. The first encounter with ABO incompatible blood may result in a hemolytic transfusion reaction; the first exposure of an Rh-negative person to Rh-positive blood will not, because of the lack of natural (or preformed) antibodies. Such a transfusion may, however, sensitize the individual to the Rh antigens in question, and the resultant antibodies may then lead to a hemolytic transfusion reaction on subsequent exposure to similarly incompatible cells. The Kell system (Kk) also is important because many K-negative persons can be sensitized to K by transfusion. The same holds true for E and c, but the danger is smaller. The remaining blood groups are of comparatively minor clinical im-

portance, although most transfusions are potentially sensitizing. Scarcity of sera and the labor involved make it impractical to type routinely for all the known antigens, but the use of a sensitive cross-match test together with the Coombs test for "incomplete" antibodies is a helpful and essential safeguard.

Blood group incompatibility is responsible for at least one disease, erythroblastosis fetalis (Chap. 338). In addition, the anti-red cell antibodies of some other acquired hemolytic anemias have specificity for blood group antigens, most commonly those belonging to the Rh system. This includes many cases of idiopathic autoimmune hemolytic anemia and certain instances of drug-induced hemolytic anemia, most notably those seen in association with alpha-methyl-dopa therapy.

ABO antigens are also known to act as potent transplantation antigens in man. It has been found, for instance, that graft recipients pretreated with incompatible ABO antigens will reject subsequent skin allografts in a markedly accelerated manner from donors incompatible for the same ABO antigens, whereas skin grafts from ABO-compatible individuals are accorded survival times characteristic of first grafts in nonsensitized individuals. It seems clear, therefore, that matching techniques for organ transplantation must take cognizance of ABO incompatibilities between donor and recipient.

The association of blood groups with certain diseases is a well-documented phenomenon. Thus, gastric carcinoma and pernicious anemia are particularly common in individuals with blood group A, and there is an even closer association between blood group O and duodenal ulceration, especially in nonsecretors. The reasons underlying these correlations are not understood.

MEDICOLEGAL AND ANTHROPOLOGIC IMPORTANCE. The usefulness of serologic examinations in medicolegal and anthropologic work is readily apparent. It has been calculated that, with the ABO system and the two subgroups of A, the MNSs blood groups, P, the Rh system, Lutheran, Lewis, and Kell, the total number of possible different combinations of serologic recognizable phenotypes is 23,616, and the number of genotypes is 972,000. Because of technical and other difficulties, the P, Lewis, Kell, Duffy, and Kidd systems are not recommended for use in problems of parentage or identity, but even without them, when blood of the mother, the child, and the alleged father is available, it is possible to exonerate 51 percent of all men of Western European origin who are wrongfully accused of paternity.

Of additional medicolegal importance is the fact that the antigens A, B, and H are present in the secretions of most individuals and can readily be extracted with aqueous solutions from tissues and organs, especially salivary glands and gastric mucosa. High concentrations of blood group substances can also be found in secretions such as saliva, gastric juice, and semen. As a consequence it is possible to apply blood grouping to the examination of dried stains of these secretions as well as to saline extracts of muscle tissue.

In human genetics and anthropology the blood groups are of the utmost value for a number of reasons. The first is that they are sharply distinguishable "all-or-none" characteristics which do not grade into each other. Then again, they are simple, genetically speaking, and are inherited in a known way according to mendelian principles. Furthermore, they owe nothing to environment in their inheritance, nor are they subject to variations because of natural selection, as is the case, for example, with skin color. Hence, the blood groups are especially fitted to throw light on the moderately remote as well as the recent origins of mankind. Wide differences in frequency in different races have been observed. Consequently the blood groups provide valuable anthropometric measurements.

Considerable and interesting data are being accumulated concerning the ethnologic distribution of the blood groups. Thus the incidence of B has been found highest in certain parts of Asia and declines in all directions from central Asia except for a subsidiary high center in Africa. In the Old World the lowest figures have been found in the Scandinavian countries, and in Australia the gene seems to have been absent until very recent times. A similar complete absence has been found in the living aborigines of North America as well as in the Basques. Group O reaches levels of practically 100 percent among certain Indian tribes in the United States. In the aborigines of America the gene for N is relatively rare, while in those of Australia it is very common. The factor P is much commoner in the blood of American Negroes than in that of American whites. The Rh-negative gene (*cde*) has been found in 13 to 17 percent of modern inhabitants of Europe and in white inhabitants of America. In the Basques it reaches very high levels (28.8 percent); in contrast, in a study of Eskimo only 1 out of 2,522 was found to be Rh-negative.

REFERENCES

Lloyd, K. O., E. A. Kabat, and E. Licerio: Immunochemical Studies on Blood Groups, XXXVIII, Biochemistry, 7:2976, 1968.

Mollison, P. L.: "Blood Transfusion in Clinical Medicine," 4th ed., Philadelphia, F. A. Davis Company, 1967.

Race, R. R., and Ruth Sanger: "Blood Groups in Man," 5th ed., Philadelphia, F. A. Davis Company, 1968.

Watkins, W. M.: "Blood Group Substances," Science, 152: 172, 1966.

Wintrobe, M. M.: "Clinical Hematology," 6th ed., Philadelphia, Lea & Febiger, 1967.

6 GROWTH AND DEVELOPMENT
Robert E. Cooke

The phrase "growth and development" has acquired a variety of vague meanings, ranging from changes in height to changes in emotional capacity. In this chapter, growth is defined as an increase in size with time, with particular emphasis on accretion of new protoplasm (largely protein and water) as opposed to changes in volume or weight such as might occur with edema. Development is defined as an increase with time in numbers of functions or in complexity of function, with biologic or behavioral aspects, or both, implied in that function.

Growth, as defined here, has two components—increase in cell number and increase in cell size. At various periods in life after conception, particularly early in gestation, increase in cell number may be primarily responsible for growth. During fetal life between 40 and 50 successive divisions take place, with an increase from one cell to 12×10^{12} cells at the time of birth. From birth to adulthood another four divisions occur. Early growth thereby occurs in a geometric progression. Subsequently there is a greater tendency for arithmetic accretion of protein. Numerous attempts have been made to develop equations describing growth. In general an S-shaped curve best fits the data.

In recent years more precise measurement of cell size has been possible by chemical analysis rather than by microscopic observations, including counts of mitotic activity. It has been determined that 6.2 to 7 $\mu\mu g$ of DNA characterize most diploid cells. In the absence of polyploidy, measurement of total DNA content of one or more tissues establishes cell number. Protein and DNA analyses on similar samples make possible the calculation of cell size, since the water and protein contents of the body bear a straight-line relationship.

Liver nuclei demonstrate polyploidy under a variety of conditions, and the number and size of these cells cannot be determined readily by these simple analyses; actual counts of nuclei and chromosomes are necessary. Available data indicate that one tissue may differ markedly from another in respect to cell multiplication at various stages of growth. Muscle tends to approximate overall growth changes because it represents at least 40 percent of the total lean body mass. Furthermore, cell multiplication may occur in spurts rather than as a continuous process. Likewise, growth as determined by changes in cell size varies markedly from one tissue to another and from one period of life to another.

The assessment of the growth rate of one tissue or another, or of the whole individual, must be related to the particular biologic age of the individual—i.e., the extent of maturation. In the human being, there is great variation in the onset of adolescence. The peak growth rate in height, for example, may occur anywhere over a 5-year period in chronologic age.

Development, as defined in this chapter, though far more difficult to quantify, also proceeds sporadically and in a nonlinear fashion. The appearance of marked increases in activity of certain enzymes—e.g., tyrosin hydroxylase—corresponds to certain biologic stages but may also exhibit considerable variability in time of peak activity. Likewise, the development of behavioral characteristics, when expressed in terms of norms, proceeds along a fairly smooth curve. However, the individual infant or child exhibits marked variability in rate of progress from one month or year to the next. For example, most infants show a fairly regular sequence of developmental milestones, but it is not unusual to see delays, then spurts; e.g., creeping may be delayed but walking accelerated.

CONTROL OF GROWTH AND DEVELOPMENT

Both phenomena obviously represent the interplay of genetic and environmental factors. Growth rates within a family show much less variability than when compared with those of the general population. Tall parents in general have tall children. However, in a process as complex as growth, many genes are involved, with rates of synthesis of many proteins being controlled by independently segregating genetic loci. It is not surprising, then, that physical size of a population has a normal Gaussian distribution. Environmental factors modify genetic expression considerably, however. Occasional monozygotic twins may differ markedly in size at birth, probably because of circulatory abnormalities. Geneticists some years ago predicted that the average height of the population would decrease because short persons were reproducing at a more rapid rate than the tall. Yet average height may actually be increasing because of environmental factors (possibly nutritional). At least greater growth rates are seen in the first 20 years of life now than in the previous generation.

A clearer understanding of the genetic control of development has come from the demonstration of various molecular forms of cell enzymes. Lactic dehydrogenase (LDH), for example, has been shown to be a variety rather than a single molecular species, with differing electrophoretic mobilities, amino acid sequences, and polypeptide groupings. The distribution of particular isozymes differs from one organ or tissue to another. Particular isozymes are present in varying amounts from one period in life to another. A variety of LDH appears in the testis in the human being and in several animal species only at sexual maturation. The mechanisms for turning genetic action on and off at a particular stage in the development of the individual remain unknown.

Exactly the same principles that apply to control of physical growth and maturation apply to behavioral development. The past tendency to attribute intelligence solely to genetic factors and the present tendency to disregard genetic factors in establishing relative limits for intellectual development are both contrary to the facts.

Gesell and others believed that behavior unfolded in an immutable manner, uninfluenced by experience and determined entirely by the innate potential of the individual. This hypothesis was supported by the fact that normative data collected on large numbers of infants and children indicated a fairly regular pattern for the appearance of a large number of items of behavior indicating cognitive and affective maturation.

Early experience, however, has been shown to alter behavioral development substantially. It has been shown that the longer the exposure to an underprivileged home the greater the fall in intellectual quotient. Children with inferior family and environmental histories, when placed in adoptive homes before the age of two years, despite obviously low IQ scores in the true parents and average but not superior IQ scores in the foster parents, had normal intelligence levels at five years, seven years, and thirteen years of age.

Studies of the intellectual development of twins reared in somewhat different environments show a greater correspondence in comparison with other children in the population but less than twins reared together.

The work of Hebb, Harlow, Riesen, and Piaget has reemphasized the influence of learning experiences on subsequent learning ability. Intelligent behavior results from the acquisition of and exploitation of many programs or schemata for solving problems. The initiative for searching for such programs is dependent on motivation—the genesis of which seems obscure but related in part to previous success or failure.

OPTIMAL GROWTH AND DEVELOPMENT

The possible relationship of longevity to rate of growth raises the issue that the maximal rate of growth may not necessarily be optimal. Much of the experimental data indicate that rate of growth in experimental animals and to an extent in human beings may be influenced by diet. Restriction of intake during gestation and prior to weaning may permanently slow growth despite free access to food thereafter. Increased longevity seemed to be associated with the limited food intake. Only one experiment has been designed to show that aging is probably associated with dietary factors rather than being directly related to accelerated rate of growth. The administration of growth hormone to animals previously subjected to dietary restriction restored growth rate to normal without shortening longevity. Diet, likewise, alters rate of maturation of certain tissues in a manner similar to the aging process. Concentrations of alkaline phosphatase, ATPase, and catalase and histidase increase with age in the rat liver.

The manipulation of diet can produce enzyme patterns in the younger rat comparable to those of a much older animal. Although changes in cell structure, water content, and the like may be responsible for some of these effects, the fact that changes in enzyme activity are in opposite directions lends significance to the findings.

Maximum behavioral development may or may not be optimal, just as with physical growth. Most of the evidence, however, indicates that superior intellectual performance is correlated with good emotional adjustment. Studies of the social success and accomplishments of gifted children negate the lay impression that "genius is tainted with madness." The more favorable environments of such children may be in part responsible for such adjustments. The fact that man has the longest ontogenetic preparatory period permitting opportunities for social training makes possible significant improvement of behavioral development providing the necessary condition for each child can be determined.

MEASUREMENT

The recording of changes in physical size and shape with age is important and a fairly reliable indicator of health. Many systems have been developed to facilitate comparisons with normal children of the same age, body build, weight, and height. The determination of prenatal growth and of premature birth in the past has been assessed primarily in terms of weight; gestational age, although necessarily inaccurate, is being utilized more frequently because of the relatively frequent occurrence of intrauterine growth disturbances. A combination of the two would seem desirable.

The prediction of adult size from measurements during childhood is reasonably accurate, particularly if height and bone age are measured and if parental size is also appreciated. Height at three years shows a better correlation with height at maturity than at any other age. The correlation of childhood measurements with adult height were: birth, 0.77; one year, 0.67; two years, 0.75; and at five years, 0.79. One formula for prediction is that of Weech:

$$H_m = 0.545 \, H_2 + 0.544 \, A + 14.84 \text{ in.} \quad \text{(boys)}$$
$$H_m = 0.545 \, H_2 + 0.544 \, A + 10.09 \text{ in.} \quad \text{(girls)}$$

where H_m = height at maturity
H_2 = height at two years
A = average of parents' height

The standard deviation of difference in actual over predicted height is about 1 in.

The assessment of physical development is rapidly being improved. Such determinations as bone age, EEG, enzyme levels, and steroid excretion patterns indicate changes in function and serve to establish biologic age, particularly in the newborn period and at adolescence, when profound functional changes occur.

By the application of multivariate equations utilizing as data measurements of body size, body weight, body water, body chloride, creatinine excretion, cell number, etc., biologic age may be predicted with great precision (± 6 to 9 months in a child). Such predictions permit appropriate estimation of the degree of growth failure in relation to change in chronologic and biologic age. Growth failure can be thought of as loss of months or years of growth rather than centimeters or kilograms, thereby permitting better appreciation of the possibilities for and extent of "catch-up" growth.

For the investigator such calculations permit a better understanding of physiologic function in the maturing infant or child so that physiologic function may be properly compared from one child to the next. Unfortunately, accurate prediction of biologic age in the fetus and premature and in the aged is not yet feasible.

The measurement of intellectual development is now being criticized excessively—by modern psychologists especially. The evidence is irrefutable that there is a high correlation between test scores at ages four years and fourteen and school performance, although exceptions occur. Developmental quotients at one year correlate poorly with intelligence quotients in later childhood. However, low developmental scores at six, nine, and twelve months predict serious abnormality in later life with remarkable accuracy.

The major criticism of IQ predictions arises from the attempts of some investigators to attribute intelligence solely to genetic factors. The Gaussian distribution of intelligence test scores has been used as an argument for the genetic basis of intelligence. Unquestionably, there are multiple genetic factors with phenotypic manifestations far removed from primary gene action and, therefore, subject to great environmental alteration. The environmental factors probably have their greatest impact in the first 4 years of life, but, unfortunately, they have not been well characterized. Terms such as "cultural deprivation" and "inadequate stimulation" are used to describe the early environments of many children who later do poorly in school and in employment. The details of such experience that hinder or promote intellectual development in the human infant and child require much elaboration.

ABERRATIONS IN GROWTH AND DEVELOPMENT

Specific disturbances in physical growth and biologic development as well as behavioral development are discussed in other sections of this text. Retarded growth and slow intellectual development far exceed acceleration in frequency. The causes are multiple, and in no way can the terms "growth retardation" or "mental retardation" be considered as an adequate diagnosis. The etiology or pathophysiology leading to retardation must be searched for, even though at present the majority of cases cannot adequately be explained.

If the pathogenetic factor in growth can be ascertained and corrected, remarkable acceleration or catch-up growth may occur. In some cases of congenital heart disease, for example, surgical correction of the defect may lead to an increase in height age of several years occurring in several months. If excessive delay in correction occurs, eventual stature may be stunted.

Experience with correction of defects causing mental retardation is exceedingly limited. However, there are a few examples of young children reared in bizarre circumstances who seemed to have exhibited catch-up development when the biologic and behavioral environment was improved.

REFERENCES

Bloom, B. S.: "Stability and Change in Human Characteristics," New York, John Wiley & Sons, Inc., 1964.

Cheek, D. B.: Human Growth: Body Composition, Cell Growth, Energy, and Intelligence. Philadelphia, Lea & Febiger, 1968.

Riesen, A. H.: Effects of Early Deprivation of Photic Stimulation, pp. 61–85 in S. F. Osler, and R. E. Cooke, "The Biosocial Basis of Mental Retardation," Baltimore, The Johns Hopkins Press, 1965.

Skeels, H. M.: Adult Status of Children with Contrasting Early Life Experiences. A Follow-up study. Monogr. Soc. Res. Child. Develop., 31:1–56, 1966.

Zinkham, W. H., A. Blanco, and L. J. Clowry, Jr.: An Unusual Isozyme of Lactate Dehydrogenase in Mature Testes: Localization, Ontogeny, and Kinetic Properties, Ann. N.Y. Acad. Sci., 121:571–588, 1964.

7   THE DEVELOPMENT OF PERSONALITY

Raymond D. Adams

The term *personality* encompasses all the physical and psychologic traits that characterize man—that distinguish him from all other individuals in his universe.

The notion that every person is a complex of physical peculiarities, determined by inheritance, is accepted as a fundamental datum of biology. One has but to look at resemblances between parent and child to find ample confirmation of it. Only the extent of human variation occasions surprise. Just as no two people are identical, not even monozygotic twins, so too, do they differ in body chemistry or any other quality that one might choose to measure. These qualities, together with certain inherited predilections to disease, explain why any one person may have an unpredictable reaction to a pathogenic agent when a whole population is exposed. Strictly speaking, normal man is an abstraction, just as is a typical case of disease.

But it is in other seemingly nonphysical attributes that man displays the greatest variety of subtle differences. Here reference is made to a patient's variable place on a scale of physical and mental energy, in capacity for effective work, in intellectual power which makes him susceptible to different degrees of training and education, in sensitivity, temperament, and emotional responsivity, in aggressiveness or passivity, in character, and in adaptability to stress. The composite of these qualities and the life experiences which have helped shape them form the basis of the personality structure of man.

The justification for a chapter on this subject in a book which essays to present the principles of internal medicine stems from the fact that major and minor departures from the usual trends in personality development become common sources of medical complaint later in life when they interfere with somatic function, happiness, and effective adaptation in society. As such they fall under the purview of the physician; and if they are sufficiently grave, they demand the attention of the psychiatrist. The recognition of these disorders requires a knowledge of the bases of normal personality development as a frame of reference. The rules and principles underlying these abnormal deviations—the manner in which heritable traits of personality and unfortunate life experiences combine to account for their appearance—comprise psychopathology. These principles have emerged largely from observations of man as a social animal and have been more studied by social than medical scientists; but in the final analysis, personality attributes are as biologic as the reflexes, instincts, emotions, and drives from which they are derived.

THE ROOTS OF SOCIAL BEHAVIOR

Social behavior, like neurologic and psychologic functions in general, depends to a great extent on the development and maturation of the brain, and these are functions of genetic factors and environmental influence. No other organ in the body undergoes such an amazing number of changes from early embryonal to adult life, which explains the unfolding of an infinite array of human behavior, abilities, and mental capacities. The most rapid changes in the brain occur before birth, and they are the least understood because they take place in the remote recesses of the womb, where they are relatively inaccessible to the eye of the physician and scientist. But, unlike all other animals, man then proceeds through a long period of postnatal development. No other creature is more helpless at birth, possibly because the relatively small size of the female pelvic outlet in our species precludes large size and degree of fetal development of the brain. The weight of the brain at different ages reflects this; the ratio of brain weight in adulthood to birth is 3.5 to 4.0 in man and only 2.2 in the chimpanzee. The difference is qualitative as well as quantitative. Whereas the neocortex in general increases fourfold from birth to maturity, the motor areas for hand, tongue, and larynx (the parts subserving manual dexterity and speech) and the suprasensory areas of parietal lobe (concerned with symbolization and thinking) expand proportionately more. The time required for postnatal development provides another dimension, being longer for man than for any other mammal. This extended period of development, so essential to the unfolding of vast human potential, carries with it a liability—an unusually long period of possible exposure to the action of environmental influences that are beyond the control of the individual himself. In a purely evolutionary sense the whole structure of human social organization into family units has as its primary purpose to protect the child in this period while enabling him to realize his full potential through training and education.

Limitations of space allow no more than a few glimpses of the nervous substructure of the prodigious repertoire of behavioral sequences of development. The histologic studies of Conel trace the enlargement of cortical neurones as their dendritic plexuses are elaborated and synaptic surfaces expanded. The observations of Flechsig (verified by Langworthy, Yakovlev, and others) reveal the sequential changes in myelination of the axones of nerve cells in different parts of the brain, which have been shown to proceed in a time-linked orderly fashion. Minkowski, Hooker, Gesell, André-Thomas are other names, famous for their cataloguing of the changing patterns of motility, sensation, and instinctual and emotional drives in early life and their relationship to stages of anatomic development. Reassuring to adults is the finding of Kaes and Rose that brain development continues on into adult years.

The most advanced phases of man's behavior, called *social* because they involve human interaction for their emergence, must be viewed as a continuation of these basic reflex and instinctual patterns. Their progressive elaboration is reinforced by the adaptive processes and the attendant emotions which they engender. Pleasure accompanies behavior demanded by evolution (e.g., the sexual act, so necessary for reproduction), and anxiety and fear guard the organism against conditions leading to maladaptation. But here we begin to see the workings of another principle—that biologic evolution merges with but is finally superseded by cultural evolution. The latter is uniquely human. Man is the only animal with the capacity to change his environment in a systematic fashion. Only he can anticipate the future and plan for it; and, of the advanced primates, man is the only one capable of symbolization and communication by words. It is through language that he becomes capable of thinking through the consequences of an action before attempting it, of abstracting from the concrete to the general, and of perceiving relationships between elements without the necessity of actual manipulation of those elements. Also, language is the agency whereby the experiences of the past generation are transmitted to the next. Thus man builds continuously on his cultural heritage. The growth of our knowledge has become exponential.

THE DEVELOPMENT OF INDIVIDUAL COMPONENTS OF PERSONALITY

As William James once remarked, "The baby, upon entering this world, assailed by sensations from eyes, ears, nose, skin and entrails, all at once, must feel it as one blooming, buzzing confusion." And the ways our complex nervous system brings these to order during development and maturation are nothing short of miraculous.

At the time of birth the human organism is 9 calendar months along his life cycle, and already some degree of individuality has been stamped on him, for no two infants look alike, even though many of the physical characteristics do not become definite until later, being somehow obscured by the delicacy of immaturity. One baby manifestly differs from others in vigor of movement, amount of sleep required, degree of irritability, and strength of instinctual demands. With respect to patterns of behavior, however, at birth he is still virtually a pulp.

Then commences the unfolding of a vast sequence of maturational changes that will transform him from a helpless vegetative state dominated by incretory and excretory activities, with limited capacity to perceive or react to the world about, to a confident, vigorous, intelligent, self-disciplined adult. From the standpoint of postural control, at the age of six months he sits, at twelve to fifteen months he walks, at two years he runs, at six years he may be acquiring the rudiments of athletic prowess or musical skill. In the area of perception he proceeds from the stage of fleeting interest in lights and movement, to which he makes sketchy, wavering ocular responses, to fine discrimination of color, size, and form. At the time of birth he grasps an object reflexly, with eyes wandering or vacantly transfixed, while by six years of age he expertly scans a figure prior to reproducing its form with a crayon. At birth there is only the cry, lacking all modulation and social meaning and marking the lowest level of language; in 2 years it is converted into articulate sounds, intelligible to others as words and already uttered in short sentences, and in 6 years these words take the form of complex syntactic speech by which the child can interrogate adults or inquire in a primitive way about causality. In personality structure, by the age of six he is aware of his identity as a person, occupying a finite part of space, separable from the physical world about, capable of self-assertion and of controlling the behavior of others in ways that foreshadow what he will later be like as an adult.

Each major item in this emergence of an individual from a reflex-dominated organism to one capable of independent decision is age-linked, and the work of André-Thomas and Arnold Gesell and their students have provided us with catalogues of some of the principal postnatal steps. These have been put to the service of neurologic medicine because they faithfully reflect the healthy function of the nervous system at different stages of growth and development. Deviations from normal sensory, motor, reflex, emotional, and social adaptive functions acquire pathologic significance only if they depart from an average standard. The child's neurologic status may thus be expressed as a developmental quotient (DQ). Gesell conceives this trajectory of developmental sequence essentially as an effluorescence of genetically determined events, whereas Piaget looks upon it as a biologic adaptation, a continuous creative interaction between the organism and its environment.

INTELLIGENCE AND COGNITION. Piaget, one of the most critical developmental psychologists of our time, divides the development of intelligence, one of the principal components of personality, into three major periods: *sensorimotor* (birth to two years), *concrete operations* (two to twelve years), and *formal operations* (twelve years through adult life). The sensorimotor period is one in which the congenital sensorimotor schemata and reflex patterns become differentiated from inchoate general behavior, to emerge later as the elementary processes of intelligence. The period of concrete operations is divided into a preconceptual phase (from two to four years) during which symbols are constructed; the intuitive phase (four to seven years) when concepts of space, causality, and time are acquired; and the logical phase (seven to twelve years) in which thought becomes differentiated from perception and action, permitting the classifying, ordering, and numbering of sensory data. The period of formal operations is one of systematization and recombination of the concrete operations, in the course of which the logical steps of abstract thought are mastered.

Facility in the acquisition of these more complex components of cognition is believed also to be determined by genetic factors. Individuals vary widely in their levels of achievement. Binet and many of the so-called "psychometrists" who followed him deduced this fact after devising tests and measuring these functions in a large population. Thus arose the idea of a human trait called *native intelligence,* defined as capacity for purposive behavior and ability to reason and to solve problems; they also found this capacity to be age-linked and expressible as an intelligence quotient (IQ). But their results were obviously contaminated with the effects of verbal skill, education, and scholastic achievement. Moreover, in educable children further statistical analyses of intelligence showed it to be relatively constant from one period to another but to consist not of a single, universal trait but of an aggregate of special abilities. Verbal skill, arithmetic ability, concept of space, speed of learning and memorizing, all essential components of types of intelligent behavior, were found to correlate only roughly with capacity for abstract thought and creativity. The role of intervening experience in the steps of maturation of cognitive function has been emphasized. In fact, it is the richness, complexity, and diversity of stimulation in a favorable social environment that results in the complete functional organization of mind. This is only another way of rephrasing Gesell's idea that "the primary elements in the child's disposition, capacities, and traits are determined largely by heredity but achieved through maturation which requires interaction with environment."

The time course of the cognitive functions of learning, remembering, perceiving, organization of sensory data, solving problems, and pursuing intellectual tasks is of interest. All are well developed by school age. The scheduling of formal education at six years is thus decided by an observed level of nervous organization which allows attentive interest, persistence of effort, the acquisition of written word and number symbols, and tolerance of separation from the family unit. Interestingly, the wide range of differences between individuals, varying from imbecility to genius, becomes increasingly evident as formal education proceeds. Also, many special defects of perception, speech, memory, etc. not earlier manifest in the simple play of the small child, become apparent at this stage when he is forced to compete with others of his age group. Without educational opportunity the natively intelligent mind never realizes its full potentiality.

EMOTIONAL DEVELOPMENT. Much of the child's individuality is undoubtedly attained through the stresses of human relations, which condition and habituate him. It is here that the extensive and pervasive interpenetration of the environment, which completes the patterns of organic growth, becomes apparent. The Freudian formulation of instinctual and emotional development, the most systematic and complete theory yet devised, conceives of emotional development as a series of predictable modifications of the sexual instinct. The latter is defined not merely as the impulse to sexual gratification but more broadly as desire for the pleasure and satisfaction with which such activities are endowed. The energy of sexual impulse, called *libido,* is traced in this scheme back to the earliest sensory pleasures attendant upon the activities of the oral and genital parts of the body. Successively the sexuality of the child expands to include many of the activities of the mother and other members of the same and finally the opposite sex. Powerful repressive forces are exerted upon the sexual impulse by social custom but always with the risk of the energy of sexual drive being displaced to other systems of thought or activities which may then motivate behavior in unexpected ways. Personality development is regarded essentially as a process of sexual maturation, the final purpose of which is to assure procreation and the establishment of the individual as an integral part of a new family. Perversions, arrests, or regressions of this process are thought to be the source of psychopathic and neurotic behavior. This hormic, or motivational, aspect of behavior and the dependence of it on the formation of sexual bonds between infant and mother, family members, and others is confirmed by the studies of monkeys by Harlow. The baby monkey, if deprived of the warmth of social contact with other animals of its kind, grows up to be totally inadequate as a sexual partner, parent, or member of monkey society.

There are many who believe the Freudian emphasis on sexuality takes far too restricted a view of the human personality. While it is true that the tie to the mother can be conceived as a derivative of the nursing act, body contact with mother soon becomes less important than touch, smell, sight, and sound, as a determinative factor in the infant's behavior as he becomes involved in the complex activities of daily care. Perceptual and cognitive maturation enable the infant to relate many initially disconnected and separate experiences to the person who provides them and, thereby, to distinguish the mother from other persons in the environment. Soon many others, such as siblings, father, teacher, etc., begin to figure in special nonsexual ways in his life.

In the formation of the personality, especially the part concerned with feeling and emotional sensitivity, basic temperament and other qualities play a part. Some children by nature tend from the beginning to be happy, cheerful, and unconcerned about immediate frustrations, and others are irritable and difficult. By the third month of postnatal life Thomas and his associates were able to recognize individual differences in activity-passivity, regularity-irregularity, intensity of action, approach-withdrawal, adaptive-unadaptive, high-low threshold of response to stimulation, positive-negative mood, high-low selectivity, and high-low distractability. Ratings at this age were found to correlate well with others made at two years of age and reasonably well with the results of a third examination at five years. Many of these characteristics are presumably genetic but are influenced by the spirit of the environment provided by parents. But, as Cross and his associates have shown, the initial characterstics of the infant also influence parental reaction, just as their behavior influences his.

The more common traits such as the tendency to worry about health and other problems, to be anxious or serene, timid or bold; the power of instinctual drive and need of satisfaction, the sympathy one has for others, the sensitivity to criticism and degree of disorganization resulting from adverse circumstances are presumably traceable to some of the more basic instincts and emotions.

SOCIAL ADAPTATION. Early life requires a long succession of human interactions, first to parents, then to family, other children, and finally to a widening circle of individuals in the classroom, commercial world, and community at large. Capacity to cooperate, to subjugate one's own egocentric needs to those of the group, to lead or be led, appear as modes of response. Qualities of temperament and emotionality such as aggression, passivity, tendency to anxiety, depression, and elation usually are felt and most clearly expressed in relation to individuals in the social environment.

The basis of these social reactions is less clear than that of cognitive qualities of mind and of temperament. The frequency of aggressive behavior in children, for example, is often used as an argument for an innate aggressive instinct. In actuality this is a derived mode of reaction, and such interpretation is an instance of a widespread tendency to explain infantile behavior by a priori assignment of adult motives, assumed on the basis of spurious analogies. In the normal child, aggression usually originates in innate curiosity or takes the form of a defense reaction or a response to frustration and failure, for all of which aggressiveness is a suitable mediator. Its greater frequency in the abnormal child may be correlated with defects in the organism, as in the case of brain injury, and also with resultant distortions in its environment which give rise to faulty identification models. Moreover, the frequency of display of aggressive behavior is a function of the culture in which the child is reared. While encouraged in our culture, where it is recognized as a desirable manifestation of energetic and vigorous action, becoming unacceptable only if assaultive and violent, it may not at all be condoned in other cultures. The capacity for aggression is indeed inherent in the impulse life of man, as it is in all animals, but its frequency of evocation and display are conditioned by other determinants.

The greatest demands and the greatest frustrations in social development are likely to occur during late childhood and adolescence. The child's difficulty is apt to become manifest in his inability to adjust to the exigencies of the classroom. The adolescent is faced with an even greater diversity of environmental challenges. Half emancipated from family ties, he must seek the recognition and respect of his peers. To do this he needs a field for the full exploitations of his power of abstract thought; and for the first time he becomes concerned with what he is and what he will be. In his search for personal identity he becomes more critical of parents and turns increasingly to larger social groups for his sense of belonging. If his relations with his parents have been soundly constructed and if the parents meet his doubts and criticisms with sympathetic understanding, this temporary unsettling of his primary family position leads to a resynthesis of his relations with them on a firm and lasting basis. The development of adult sexual characteristics and the further evolution of psychosexual impulses cause him to experience a bewildering array of new physical sensations. These sensations lead to an upsurge of interest in physical sex and psychologic sensitization to new aspects of interpersonal relationships along this line. The developing ability for abstract conceptualization provides the foundation for advanced education, for scientific study and creativity, and for increasing concern about the basic meanings and values of human existence.

These types of social development continue as long as life continues. As social roles change, as intellectual and physical capacities first advance and later recede, new challenges demand new adaptations. The success of these is enhanced always if started from a solid base of accomplishment in a secure work role, from a position as a stable member of a family unit, and from an acceptable view and philosophy of one's place in life. Conditions which thwart the healthy development of proper attitudes toward health, family, work, and religion often become the sources of maladjustment in later life.

PSYCHOPATHOLOGIC TRENDS AND THEIR SOURCES

The physician faced with countless human problems, no two of which are ever alike, searches among this bewildering kaleidoscope of developmental events for tendencies which indicate the action of pathogenic agencies and the beginnings of social maladjustment. If identified, attempts are made to modify them and to prevent or control, by appropriate measures, their consequences. The assumption that this is possible is the main premise of the entire mental health movement in the United States. The following disturbances should alert the physician to the possibility of psychopathologic deviation:

1. *Sense deprivation and insufficiency of stimulation.* In the earliest period of life sense deprivation appears to be a factor that impairs perceptual development. An animal reared in darkness for several months has been shown to fail to acquire all the natural visual perceptions and visuomotor reactions when later put in light. A human example of this is amblyopia exanopsia, where ocular imbalance has prevented one eye from accommodating and being stimulated in binocular vision. The wandering eye fails to develop as an effective organ despite the integrity of the refractive media, retina, and nervous connections with the brain. Another example is the deaf child who remains mute, or if he speaks, is unable to learn to modulate his own voice in a pleasing fashion. It is doubtful, however, if sensory deprivation has many other effects on man. Human environment is such a busy, noisy, dazzling place that it is hard to imagine sensory deprivation occurring under most conditions of daily life even in the most impoverished circumstances. However, transient derangements in mentation may occur when disease imposes complete quiet in a darkened room or a respirator. Extreme degrees of sensory deprivation, lasting many hours, may disorganize perceptual processes to a degree where illusions and hallucinations may supervene, often with panic. Such depri-

vation psychoses become increasingly frequent in the brain-damaged child and the elderly person, presumably because their adaptive powers are weakened by inadequacy of cerebral mechanisms.

Potentially significant degrees of insufficient stimulation should be suspected in orphans and in families where the mother is absent much of the time or is disturbed by psychiatric illness. Corrective measures involve increased adult contact.

2. *Emotional deprivation.* Emotional deprivation in early life, so clearly pathogenic in the lives of young animals, has been postulated as a cause of mental retardation and neurosis in man. Bowlby's monograph summarizes the literature on this subject and concludes that early separation from mother has persistent and irreversible effects manifest in both intelligence and personality. The work of Goldfarb provides some further documentation of this fact. In comparing two groups of orphaned children (one of which had spent the first 3 years in an orphanage before being placed in a foster home, the second group put immediately in a foster home), he found lower IQ, poorer school performance, and more sociopathic traits in the first group. Skeels and Scogel had earlier observed that orphans given over to the care of affectionate foster mothers early in life raised their IQs from 64 to 91, while the control group had IQs that fell from 86 to 60. However, the fault of all such studies is the difficulty in being sure that the experimental and control groups are comparable and that the psychologic tests, which require a certain degree of activity, maturity, and motivation on the part of the child, are sufficiently accurate in early life and therefore comparable from one time to another. Bowlby's original monograph, which presents well the deleterious effects of maternal neglect, puts too much stress on their irreversibility. Children left alone for long periods during the first year prove to be relatively inactive and disinterested in their environments, but when moved to a more stimulating atmosphere they usually catch up with their more fortunate colleagues. Here it is a mistake to assume that maternal deprivation constitutes a major factor in the causation of definite and permanent mental retardation. Lesser degrees of diminished intellectual stimulation during childhood, lack of encouragement to study, to learn, to excel in school, unquestionably impair intellectual achievement and increase the rate of school failure and drop-out. But these effects are better understood in terms of poor examples being set for emulation, lack of opportunity to acquire self-discipline, lack of satisfying goals, etc.

Children placed early in foster homes and orphanages and those of the lowest social and economic groups are more likely to be subject to the effects of impoverished emotional environment and inadequate motivation. And, these are often the very ones whose innate capacity for adaptation is most limited.

3. *Deprivation of discipline, parental overindulgence and failure of emancipation from family.* Whether unintelligent, thoughtless, cold parents can induce abnormal character in a child is a moot point. The possibility

that the child is exhibiting the same inherited traits as the parent cannot be excluded. There is no doubt that the child needs guidance and help in making the transition from a state of helplessness and total dependence to one of independence and capability of effective interaction with its social environment. Certain demanding and difficult items of behavior must be taught by reward and at times punishment in order to keep the behavior within the bounds of acceptability. A vacillating, incomprehensible discipline confuses the child and may result in either epsiodes of violent and assaultive behavior or withdrawal. Many early behavior problems seem traceable to a period of excessive parental dependence. In fact one of the great dangers of any prolonged childhood illness is its tendency to strengthen unduly the ties to parents and to inculcate unnatural concern about health. Lack of firm, intelligent, parental discipline will interfere with adaptive processes in the well endowed as well as the retarded child.

Here the physician must guard against undue criticism of the practices of child rearing. It is easy to find fault with parental care because few parents are well instructed in such matters before having children; and the child may be born when the parents themselves are having problems. The possibility that the parents' behavior may also be conditioned by that of the child must not be overlooked. A jittery, overly active, unhappy baby may cause the frustrated parent to lose patience and neglect him, thus creating a vicious circle. The child with a developmental or other disease, not able to comprehend a complex world, not able to understand the language of the parent, often withdraws from human contact, preferring to deal with simpler objects in the physical world. He often appears out of contact with people and is uncritically labeled *autistic.* Intelligent correction involves helping the parents understand the normal reactions of the growing child and helping the child satisfy his physical and emotional needs in ways that are acceptable to society.

4. *Specific deficits in cerebral function.* Every blemish, every physical abnormality becomes a cross to bear during the formative years, when the child or adolescent seeks tribe approval, but it is the restricted cerebral deficit that dislocates him most consistently. The child with the developmental speech disorder (stammer, stutter, dyslexia, or word deafness) not only stands apart, but the training and education to which his intelligence entitles him are blocked. If forced in his school work beyond the capabilities of his language mechanism, he becomes rebellious and aggressive or gives up completely and withdraws; and not infrequently all social development, which at this age is so completely centered in the classroom, is thwarted. Sometimes the fault is only a delay in language development, which will later correct itself as the mysterious process of cerebral dominance is strengthened.

This latter type of disturbance emphasizes another notable aspect of child development—its unevenness and irregularity. Just as no two humans are ready to walk at the same age, so too are they different with respect to the time of acquisition and stable functioning of language mechanisms and other complex behavioral sequences. The total language repertoire covers a span of 15 to 20 years and is matched in length only by such activities as learning to use numerical symbols, to think, and to reason. Presumably these language and other functions depend on maturation of parts of the brain, and delay often is genetically determined (90 percent of stutterers are males) but exercise and guidance are also necessary for their full development. The tendency among psychiatrists in recent years has been to seek out and attempt to treat the patient's reaction to the frustration caused by these deficits rather than to apply methods of teaching which assist in language development.

Medical action involves the discovery and assessment of the native capacities of the child and helping him to improve them by training and to make a healthy adjustment to any inadequacies thereof.

THE ORIGINS OF PSYCHOPATHY, NEUROSIS, AND PSYCHOSIS

Lack of socialization, of coming to understand the actions, feelings, and needs of other members of one's social group, inability to perceive one's own personality deficits, and extremes of egocentricity, which stand as the central issues in the development of psychoneurosis, are evident by the time adolescence is reached. Indeed, *neurosis* is definable in such terms, and *psychosis* signifies but a more global disorganization of mental function and behavior but again expressed to a maximum degree in disordered social relationships. In later life, the neurotic person habitually attempts to preserve his selfish ways in each newly formed social circle. Being socially unacceptable on this account, conflict situations arise which engender anxiety and depression. The complete detachment of the autistic child, the amorality of the constitutional psychopath, the major deviations of temperament and mood of the hereditary manic-depressive, the characteristic difficulty in thinking and affective relationship of the schizophrenic patient have also declared themselves by the end of childhood and early adolescence. And, now one confronts the key problem: To what extent do neurosis, psychopathy, and psychosis have their roots in the early thwarting or perversion of the natural processes of personality development, and to what degree are they determined by genetic factors?

The answers to these questions cannot be given with finality. Experienced clinicians tend to believe that genetic factors are actually more important than environmental. The discovery that unusually tall males with severe acne vulgaris and aggressive psychopathic behavior have two Y chromosomes is an example of a newly discovered genetic relationship. And then, too, there is the fact that deliberate alteration of the social environment has so far never been shown to prevent a major psychiatric disease, although admittedly the wise counseling of parents has been helpful in the management of children with behavior problems. Children identified as high-risk individuals because of early tru-

ancy, conflict with the law, and general social maladjustment, if transferred to a more stable and helpful environment, have, as a group, not turned out better than others who were left alone. Admittedly such investigations are open to many criticisms, and it is for this reason that the mental hygienists have been supported in the United States, even though evidence that their methods are effective is still lacking.

There are other considerations than the development of frank neurosis or psychosis for there are countless unhappy, maladjusted individuals who cannot be included among the psychologically ill. It is with reference to these conditions that one looks for early psychopathologic trends. Adolescent turmoil often seems to stem from unhealthy parent-child relationships, which have engendered excessive dependence or hostility. The result may be either a failure of emancipation or a rejection of family ties and a lasting sense of isolation. Similarly, sexual deviations of adolescent and adult life are often ascribed to lack of early education. The ambivalence of Western society, which evinces interest in sex but then imposes sanctions on its expression, contributes to the problem. Too little is known about the early conditioning that inculcates the traits of masculinity and femininity. Certainly hormonal control plays but a minor part. The basis of homosexuality or sexual perversions is not known. Ignorance of sex and impoverishment of human relations account later for many sexual misadventures.

The sensitivity of the adolescent to the good opinion of his peers renders him psychologically vulnerable to any minor variation in his own physique and to pernicious influences in his social environment. If in addition he should be endowed with limited intellectual and physical capacity, the grounds for persistent and indomitable feelings of inferiority are laid, especially if he is forced to compete in situations which result in repeated failure. The individualization of education and vocational training for such adolescents is essential, both to permit the talented individual to exploit his abilities and to direct the youngster with specific limitations into activities that constructively develop his personality.

It is during the period of late childhood and adolescence, when the psychologic structure is least stable, that transient symptoms, many resembling the psychopathologic states of adult life, are most frequent. Great caution must be exercised lest such temporary maladaptive patterns be misinterpreted. While some of these behavioral disorders represent the early signs of schizophrenia and manic-depressive psychosis, diseases that usually become manifest for the first time around puberty, many of them have a way of disappearing as adult years are reached. One can only surmise that the turbulence of the adolescent period came to be controlled rather late.

CONCLUSION

The internist no less than the psychiatrist must learn to think of his patient in dynamic terms as an organism with a history, with a set of sentiments, attitudes, opinions, and expectations, and with a profound dependence on the forces of his social environment. Assessment of the patient must be as much in terms of his abilities and his disabilities, as in terms of what he is, was, and will be. Clinical diagnosis and treatment are most effective when based on a conception of man that recognizes both the existence of mental diseases and at the same time stresses personality as a series of forces continuously emerging and never fully complete. Developmental disturbances, if global and severe, are usually due to a general structural abnormality of the brain or the effects of disease, whereas maturational delays, related often to inherited predisposition in interaction with social environment and tending to derange nervous function in specific ways (autism, delayed speech and dyslexia, dyscalculia, and uncontrollable or dysinhibited behavior) are not. These latter will be considered further in Chap. 29. The most subtle aberrations in social adjustment, expressed as psychoneurosis and psychosis, will receive separate analysis in Section 10.

REFERENCE

Eisenberg, L.: Normal child development, chap. 38.2 in "Comprehensive Textbook of Psychiatry," A. M. Freedman and H. I. Kaplan (Eds.), Baltimore, Williams and Wilkins Company, 1967.

8 THE AGING PATIENT

The Editors

The clinical phenomena presented under Cardinal Manifestations of Disease depend on pathologic derangements of biologic processes. Only when considered with reference to a time scale in the human life cycle called aging do such biological processes, or morbid derangements thereof, acquire full significance in medicine.

Aging includes the acquired changes which need time for their development and also involutional changes which are as much a part of mammalian life as the autumnal decline of the leaves of deciduous trees. Accumulations of lipofuscins in cells, of cholesterol in the arteries or gall bladder, and of chalk in the cartilages, all require time; hence, they are more advanced in the aged than in the young. Certain changes such as those in the subdeltoid tendon sheath or about the vertebral bodies occur from stress, and the oftener the stress is repeated, the more marked the changes. Hence old persons show more change than younger ones. Involution probably also plays a part in altering the composition of the tissue in all these cases, but age and repeated exposure to a noxious influence are also necessary to evoke clinical evidence of impaired function.

Aging, then, may be defined as the sum of the losses of function and structure of the callosities, scars, and nodular hyperplasias due to "wear and tear" and to involution. Wear and tear includes trauma; infection; overstimulation by emotional, dietary, or other abuses; dietary inadequacies; exposure to inclement weather; or exhausting exertion. Involution may be defined as the physiologic changes in cellular activity leading to the al-

tered structure and functional capacity characteristic of all senescent members of any species. The age at which, in any tissue, involution becomes manifest may show racial as well as familial patterns, varying by years or even decades.

THE MEASURE OF GROWTH AND AGING

The natural length of life is an integral characteristic, built, in some mysterious way, into the organism. The rat is old at 2 years; the rhesus monkey survives for 20 to 25 years; the Galapagos tortoise lives to be 100 years old. Man, like the African elephant, may expect to live for 70 to 75 years. The duration of animal and human life correlates roughly with the size of the brain. Despite all the publicity about medical science lengthening man's life, the change has been only a statistical change brought about by controlling infant mortality and infectious disease. Thereby, more people are enabled to reach the upper limit of life expectancy, but this limit has not been extended. In fact, since Biblical times, when man was said to be allotted three score and ten years, the span of human life has not appreciably lengthened. The clock inevitably runs down for the average person before the seventy-fifth year, and it seems to make little difference whether he lives in a luxurious urban villa or a primitive hut. Only the exceptionally endowed person lives beyond this age.

The disease to which man ultimately succumbs, whether cancer, coronary occlusion, or some other malady, does not greatly alter his predetermined life span. If he were fortunate enough to avoid such conditions, his life would not be lengthened much beyond 10 years. Interestingly, delay in growth by undernutrition early in life has been shown in animals to delay aging and the vulnerability to disease in their senescence. Whether overnutrition has the opposite effect is not known. It also has been observed that whole body irradiation hastens aging and increases susceptibility to disease and death.

To the biologist and physician, death is not the main consideration. What is more meaningful are indices of *vitality*, of resistance to disease, of organ efficiency. In point of fact *senescence* is defined in such terms, i.e., the decline of vitality, the progressive lowering of biologic efficiency, the diminution of the capacity of the organism to maintain itself as an efficient machine. Early loss of certain functions is called *involution;* unexpected, premature decay of any given tissue or cell population has been termed *abiotrophy* (Chap. 4).

The composite of overt bodily changes due to senescence, such as the cessation of bodily growth, wrinkling of the skin, grayness of the hair, loss of teeth, involution of the sexual organs, loss of acuity of the senses, bent posture, weakening of muscular power and coordination, rigidity of the mind, conservative views, and forgetfulness, are known to every observant human. When considered one by one, it is evident that waning vitality or senescence has different times of onset and rates of progress in different organ systems. Measurements of visual and auditory acuity are said to reach their maximum at the age of ten years, and resistance to infection, at fifteen years, whereas intellectual power reaches its peak at twenty-one, and muscular power and coordination at twenty-five. According to Shock, between the ages of thirty and seventy-five, maximum oxygen uptake during exercise decreases 60 percent and maximum ventilation volume, 47 percent. Vital capacity decreases 44 percent, and cardiac output at rest, 30 percent. Kidney plasma flow is reduced 50 percent, glomerular filtration rate 31 percent, and the number of glomeruli in the kidneys, 44 percent. Both adrenal and gonadal activity decrease, basal metabolic rate is reduced 16 percent and the body water content, 18 percent, but the speed of return of blood acidity to equilibrium after exercise declines 83 percent. Brain weight decreases 10 percent, blood flow to the brain, 20 percent, the number of taste buds, 64 percent, the number of fibers in nerves, 37 percent and nerve conduction velocity, 10 percent. It is important, therefore, in the evaluation of the condition of a patient to discriminate between the effects of age and of disease. Diagnostic criteria should be age-linked and cannot be related directly to functional values based on a normal population of young medical students. Likewise, in therapy it is essential to adjust drug dosages to functions which decrease with age, especially cerebral and renal function.

Details concerning changes with age in special organs and tissues will be found in the appropriate sections, viz. nervous system (Chap. 352), skeletal muscles (Chap. 373), kidneys (Chap. 298), and skin and supporting tissues (Chap. 400). From time to time various organs and tissues have been singled out as special targets of the aging process. It is not true, however, that men are "as old as their arteries." Men may die of coronary atherosclerosis before they are old enough to vote; these arteries are diseased, not old. Men are as old as their skins, their scalps, their cerebral cortices, and all their other tissues.

THE CELLULAR BASIS OF AGING

Many mechanisms are presumed to underlie the effects of age on the cellular constituents of various organ systems. Investigative efforts have been directed along a number of lines, viz., (1) the decline in the functional efficiency and finally the deterioration and death of highly specialized, nondividing cells, such as the muscle fiber, neuron, etc.; (2) the failure of the process of mitosis in tissues composed of dividing cells; (3) the accumulation of somatic cell mutations; (4) the progressive alteration of the structural protein, collagen, which constitutes about a third of the body protein; (5) alterations in immune responsiveness and the development of autoimmunologic reactions.

Thus, nerve and muscle cells which cease to divide early and must last the lifetime of the organism are known to have a variable life span. If accidentally destroyed by disease, they are never replaced. Even in the absence of disease, there is a steady outfall which begins about the end of the period of growth and maturation and continues at an accelerated pace into the se-

nium. Functional deficits in organs such as the brain are in large measure to be ascribed to cell loss. Fortunately each organ is endowed with a generous safety factor, a protective excess of cells that must be exhausted before symptoms appear. The extent to which cells begin to falter functionally before their final disintegration is unknown but, in red corpuscles at least, decreasing quantities of certain enzymes have been recorded.

The cytologic events leading to death of nondividing cells are but little understood. In man as well as animals accumulation of lipofuscin in the cytoplasm of these cells is so constant a phenomenon that it can be used as the most reliable cytologic index of age. Called *wear and tear pigment, lipochrome,* or *lipofuscin,* these yellow granules form in the cytoplasm of nerve and muscle cells, being derived in all probability from lysosomes or, possibly, mitochondria. Simultaneous with their formation, the cell diminishes in volume presumably due to loss of other cytoplasmic components such as Nissl bodies (the main cytoplasmic RNA in nerve cells) and mitochondria. Also, the nucleus becomes smaller with infolding of nuclear membrane and alteration of nucleolus. Histochemical stains reveal a depletion of oxidative as well as phosphorylative enzymes. All of these changes have been verified in tissue culture.

Again, alterations occur in the capacity for cell growth and multiplication. Contrary to the original experiments of Alexis Carrel, which showed that cells removed from the animal body and properly sustained and nourished in tissue culture could continue to live and divide forever, Hayflick and his colleagues found that each fibroblast is destined to divide only a certain number of times. Fibroblasts from a human infant divide about 50 times; those of a twenty-year-old, about 30 times; and those from an eighty-year-old person, about 20. Towards the end of the life cycle of the cell, chromosomal aberrations and peculiarities of cell division begin to appear. Only if a special neoplastic type of change takes place with the cells becoming "mixoploid" (50 to 350 chromosomes per cell, many of which are abnormally formed), do cells attain the immortality postulated by Carrel. Male (XY) and female (XX) cells behave alike, whether grown singly or together. Probably leukocytes and liver cells also possess a genetically determined limitation for mitosis.

Hayflick sees the diminishing capacity of cells in vitro to divide as an intrinsic property of the cells themselves, a deterioration of the "genetic program that orchestrates the development of cells." Perhaps with the passage of time the DNA of the dividing cell becomes clouded with an ever-increasing number of copying errors. Depletion with age of certain enzymes involved in the transcription of DNA for the synthesis of proteins may occur. In all events these studies trace the secret of aging in dividing cells back to some obscure degeneration of inherited information-containing molecules in the cell nucleus which provide the final control of cell division. Whether cells in vivo behave differently from cells in tissue culture is not known.

It is important to appreciate that once the fibers of

collagen are laid down, they are not renewed. Labeled constituents of collagen show no "turnover." Aging collagen contracts more strongly when heated (tensile strength and elasticity increase) possibly due to the formation of more H bonds along the sides of the collagen strands between tropo-collagen molecules. The amino acids of aging collagen, particularly hydroxyproline, become less soluble. A diminishing amount of extractable elastin also runs parallel to age, but the change is less marked than in collagen. Chemical analyses have shown the aspartic and glutamic acid components of elastic tissue and amide nitrogen content to increase with age, whereas glycine, proline, and valine decrease.

Little is known regarding the reasons for the cellular changes which occur with age.

It is well recognized that certain diseases are found more frequently in persons of advancing age than in younger ones. Certain types of tumors, vascular diseases of the heart and brain, infections, especially pulmonary ones, and fractures of the hip are well known examples. The reasons, insofar as they are understood, can be best outlined in the various sections which deal with these disorders.

REFERENCES

Birren, J. E.: Human Ageing, a Biological and Behavioral Study, U.S.P.H.S. Publication 986, 1963.

Bourne, G. H., et al.: "Structural Aspects of Aging, "New York, Hafner Publishing Co., 1961.

"Ciba Foundation Colloquia on Ageing," vol. 1. "General Aspects," Boston, Little, Brown and Company, 1955.

Hayflick, L.: Human Cells and Aging, Sci. Am., 218:32, 1968.

Korenchevsky, V., and G. H. Bourne: "Physiological and Pathological Aging," New York, Harper Publishing Company, 1961.

Shock, N. W.: The Physiology of Aging, Sci. Am., 206:100, 1962.

Strehler, B. L.: The Biology of Aging, Am. Instit. Biol. Sci., Publication 6, 1960.

Verzar, F.: The Aging of Collagen, Sci. Am., 208:104, 1963.

Part Three

Cardinal Manifestations and Approach to Disease

Section 1

Pain

9 GENERAL CONSIDERATIONS

Raymond D. Adams and William M. Resnik

Pain, it has been said, is one of "Nature's earliest signs of morbidity." Few will deny that it stands preeminent among all the sensory experiences by which man judges the existence of disease within himself. There are relatively few maladies that do not have their painful phases, and in many of them pain is a characteristic without which diagnosis must always be in doubt. It seems appropriate, therefore, to begin a section on the cardinal manifestations of disease with a discussion of the more general aspects of pain.

The painful experiences of the sick pose manifold problems for the practitioner of medicine, and the student should know something of these problems in order to prepare himself properly for the task ahead. He must be ready to diagnose disease in patients who have felt only the first rumblings of discomfort, before other symptoms and signs of disease have appeared. To cope effectively with problems of this type requires a sound knowledge of the sensory supply of the viscera and a familiarity with the typical symptoms of many diseases. He will be consulted by some patients who seek treatment for pains that appear to have no obvious structural basis, and further inquiry will disclose that worry, fear, and other troubled emotional states may have aggrandized relatively minor aches and pains. To understand problems of this type requires insight into the psychologic factors which influence behavior and a knowledge of psychiatric disease. Next, he must manage the "difficult pain cases," in which no amount of investigation will bring to light either medical disease or psychiatric illness, and it is here that he will sense the need of a sound and assured clinical approach to the pain problem. Finally, he must care for the patients with intractable pain, often from an established and incurable disease, who demand relief either by drug or the "less moderate means of surgery." The possibilities of the latter require a comprehension of the anatomic pathways of pain.

END ORGANS, AFFERENT TRACTS, AND NUCLEI OF TERMINATION OF PAIN PATHWAYS

Pain is now regarded by most physiologists and psychologists as a sensation which depends on its own specific sensory apparatus. The receptors in the skin and deep structures are fine, freely branching nerve endings, which form an intricate network. A single primary pain neurone, with its cell body in the posterior root ganglion, subdivides into many small peripheral branches to supply an area of skin of at least several square millimeters. The cutaneous area of each neurone overlaps with those of other neurones, so that every spot of skin is within the domain of from two to four sensory neurones. These free nerve endings are also found in many of the other specialized sensory receptors in the skin, such as the Krause end-bulbs, the Ruffinian plumes, and Pacinian corpuscles, which may account for the extremes of hot, cold, and pressure sensation becoming painful. However, the whole subject of specific nerve endings for each modality of sensation has been reinvestigated. It appears now that free nerve endings themselves may serve as receptors for other types of sensation. They are the only end organ in the cornea where touch, temperature, and pain are felt.

The sensory nerve fibers for pain course through somatic and visceral nerves, where they are mixed with motor fibers, and they enter the spinal cord and brain stem through the posterior roots and the cranial nerves, respectively. The fibers are of two sizes, one very small, 2 to 4 μ in diameter, with a slow conducting velocity, the other somewhat larger, 6 to 8 μ, with more rapid transmission rates. As the posterior root fibers enter the spinal cord to terminate in the posterior horn of the spinal cord, they divide into two groups. A lateral unmyelinated bundle of thin fibers turns into the substantia gelatinosa where it synapses with (1) many small neurones, whose axons connect with the secondary ascending main neurones in the same and adjacent segments, and (2) more directly, with the large secondary pain neurones themselves. The axons of these small neurones compose

43

the tract of Lissauer. The medial myelinated division synapses with the large secondary sensory neurones in the substantia gelatinosa and the posterior horn of gray matter before ascending in the posterior column. The axones of the secondary sensory neurones ascend for two to three segments and cross through the anterior commissure to take their place as the anterolateral spinothalamic tract. Other pain fibers presumably ascend on the same and opposite side through a chain of short neurones which reside in the gray matter. Some of the nerve cells in the posterior horns send their axones to the central gray matter and to anterior horn cells of the same segment and adjacent segments and subserve such reflex functions as the flexor reflex, of which

Babinski's sign is but a part. The anterolateral spinothalamic tract continues upward to the posterolateral nucleus of the thalamus. This tract lies in the anterior part of the lateral and the anterior funiculi of the spinal cord and passes through the retroolivary part of the medulla and the dorsolateral parts of the pons and midbrain (Fig. 9-1, see also Fig. 9-2). The most superficial fibers are those from the opposite foot and leg and the successively deeper ones from the trunk, arm, neck, and face. Before reaching the thalamus, collateral branches are given off to other segmental structures, such as the reticular formation of the brain stem and the hypothalamus. In addition there appears to be a great diminution in the number of fibers as one pursues the tract upward, which means that many of the ascending fibers are terminating in structures located in the brain stem. The thalamic termination of the spinothalamic tracts along with the secondary trigeminothalamic tracts synapse with the third sensory neurones, which project to the cortex in the parietal lobes. Physiologists are not agreed, however, as to the cortical terminus, for electrical stimulation of the cortex in the conscious human being does not produce a painful sensation but only a tingling as a rule, nor do parietal lobe lesions cause central pain except in rare instances Nearly all pain fibers from the periphery cross to the contralateral half of spinal cord, brain stem, and thalamus, but a few are believed to ascend ipsilaterally, at least for a considerable distance. This point is still being studied.

The pain-sensitive structures in the viscera and integuments of the body, the mechanisms of their excitation, and the peripheral nervous pathways are now fairly well established. The skin and mucous membranes are sensitive to pain, as are also many of the mesodermal tissues. As a means of quick orientation it should be remembered that the facial structures and anterior cranium are the field of the trigeminal nerves; the back of head, second cervical; the neck, third cervical; epaulet area, fourth cervical; deltoid area, fifth cervical; the thumb, sixth cervical; the index finger, seventh cervical; middle finger, eighth cervical; the little finger, first thoracic; the nipple segment, fifth thoracic; the umbilicus, tenth thoracic; the groin, first lumbar; the medial side of knee, third lumbar; the great toe, fifth lumbar; the little toe, first sacral; the back of thigh, second sacral; and genitosacral areas, third, fourth, and fifth sacrals (Figs. 25-1 and 25-2). The first to fourth thoracic nerves are the important dermatomes for the intrathoracic viscera, and the sixth, seventh, and eighth thoracic segments for the upper abdominal organs (see Figs. 25-1 and 25-2). The student should memorize these facts just as he has the multiplication table.

The stimuli that are effective in arousing the sensation of pain vary to some degree for each tissue. The very existence of pain impulses arising from viscera was debated until it was demonstrated that the adequate stimuli for pain originating in the heart or digestive tract, for example, are different from those which cause pain in the skin. The latter is sensitive to pricking, cutting, and burning, whereas these same forms of stimulation give rise to no distress when applied to the stomach or intestine.

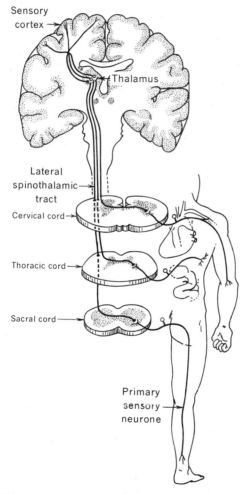

Sensory cortex

Thalamus

Lateral spinothalamic tract

Cervical cord

Thoracic cord

Sacral cord

Primary sensory neurone

Fig. 9-1. Diagram of pain pathways. Stimuli acting on free nerve endings in the skin, muscles, blood vessels, and viscera give rise to sensory impulses, which are transmitted along the primary sensory neurones into the posterior horn of the spinal cord. The secondary sensory neurones cross to the opposite side of the spinal cord almost immediately, within one or two segments, and combine to form the lateral spinothalamic tract, which terminates in the posterolateral nucleus of the thalamus. The third sensory neurone conveys the impulse from the thalamus to the cortex of the postcentral convolution. Visceral pain fibers, although they pass through the sympathetic ganglions en route to the spinal cord, do not differ from other somatic pain fibers.

Pain in the gastrointestinal tract is produced by local trauma of an engorged or inflamed mucosa, distension or spasm of smooth muscle, and traction upon the mesenteric attachment. Severe pain may be induced in voluntary muscles by ischemia, the basis for the condition known as *intermittent claudication*, and also by the injection of water or irritating solutions. Also, prolonged contraction of muscles is a source of pain. Joints are insensitive to pricking, cutting, or cautery, but the synovial membrane responds to hypertonic saline solution and inflammation. Ischemia, the only proved cause of pain in the heart muscle, is responsible for the pain of angina pectoris and myocardial infarction. Arteries give rise to pain when punctured with a needle, when induced to pulsate excessively, as in migraine, and in certain diseases affecting their walls, such as temporal arteritis. Distortion of cranial vessels by traction, displacement, or distension is a common cause of headache.

PHYSIOLOGY AND PSYCHOLOGY OF PAIN

SUPERFICIAL PAIN. There are distinct differences in the characteristics of pain arising in the skin and that originating in the viscera. The effective stimulus for pain in the skin and superficial structures may be mechanical, thermal, chemical, or electrical. At their lowest levels these stimuli may evoke sensations of touch, pressure, warmth, or cold. Only when they reach a certain intensity, usually approaching tissue destruction, does pain develop, and the resulting experience is thereafter a mixed one, combining pain with the original sensation. Wolff points out that the threshold for burning pain with a thermal stimulus is approximately two thousand times the threshold for warmth. Tissue damage is believed to be a common effect of all pain stimuli, a fact from which our concept of the fundamental biologic or self preservation value of pain derives much of its plausibility.

The threshold for the perception of pain is defined as the lowest intensity of stimulus which is recognized as pain. It is approximately the same in all persons. The pain threshold is lowered by inflammation of the peripheral nerve endings and is raised by local anesthetics (such as procaine), lesions of the peripheral and cerebral nervous system, centrally acting analgesic drugs, and distraction or suggestion. Neurotic patients in general have the same pain threshold as normal subjects, but their reaction may be excessive or abnormal. The threshold in the frontal-lobotomized patient is undiminished, but he no longer reacts to his pain. The intensity of the pain stimulus bears a roughly quantitative relationship to the reported degree of sensory experience. The ratio between the two is expressed by the Weber-Fechner law, which states that when a series of progressively increasing stimuli is applied, in order for minimal sensory differences to be perceived, the new stimulus must be increased by a constant fraction of the previously effective one.

Pain arising in the skin has a pricking or burning quality and is localized with a high degree of precision. Pricking pain has a more rapid rate of conductivity than burning pain, being transmitted by the larger pain fibers.

Together they constitute the "double response" of Lewis. A painful stimulus to the toe produces first a pricking pain and about 2 sec later a burning pain. Ischemia of the nerve subserving an area of skin, produced by application of a tourniquet, abolishes pricking pain before burning pain.

In the skin, localization of the pain stimulus is achieved by the simultaneous stimulation of multiple overlapping sensory neurones. Analgesia results from the interruption of all sensory neurones, and hypalgesia from the interruption of a few leaving others intact.

DEEP (INCLUDING VISCERAL) PAIN. The existence of visceral pain was long disputed, but it is now generally accepted that pain arising in the viscera does occur, provided that the stimuli are adequate. There is sound evidence that pain from viscera and deep skeletal structures is mediated through a common sensory apparatus and that the character and behavior of both are essentially the same. Hence, when we discuss visceral pain, the same principles will apply to deep skeletal pain. The pain is recognized by the patient as being "deep," i.e., deep to the skin; it is dull and aching in quality (although occasionally burning, as in the heartburn of esophageal disorders and rarely in anginal pain); the double response is absent; the pain is poorly localized and its borders are only vaguely delineated. It is probable that the high threshold and poor localization of deep pain are related, in part at least, to the relatively sparsely occurring sensory endings in the deep structures, in contrast to the closely distributed and overlapping terminals in the skin where pain threshold is low and accurately localized. Probably the most important characteristics are its relatively crude segmental localization beneath the surface of the body and its frequent reference to certain areas of the body. The simplest explanation for these latter phenomena is that suggested by Lewis:

If we suppose that certain tissues are represented in great detail in the sensorium, we can also understand that pain arising in these tissues may be localized with accuracy. But in other tissues having only a massive cerebral representation, localization may be expected to be less accurate. Segmental reference of deep pain may mean no more than that, centrally, the deep tissues supplied by a given cord segment have a general but little detailed representation. Thus, the impulses received whether these are derived from a viscus or from a deep somatic tissue, would tend to awaken very similar sensory impressions, and to be localized over a general sphere having no precise margins. And it may be regarded as natural enough that the general reference should be to regions that are relatively superficial, regions from which we are habitually receiving sensory impressions, and which are endowed with some positional sense.

The above concept implies that when pain originates in a viscus or deep skeletal tissue, the sensorium recognizes and localizes the pain as arising not in the exact region wherein it occurs but roughly in any or all structures innervated by cord segments subserving the affected viscus or deep somatic tissue. The pain appears to be projected toward the body surfaces supplied by these seg-

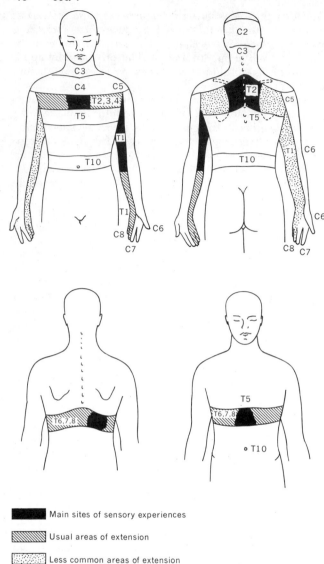

■ Main sites of sensory experiences

▨ Usual areas of extension

░ Less common areas of extension

Fig. 9-2. Radiation and sites of reference of cardiac pain (*upper*); gallbladder pain (*lower*).

ments. For example, the sensory fibers from the heart terminate in the first through the fourth thoracic cord segments (possibly in some cases the fifth thoracic); and pain arising in the heart as the result of ischemia is not localized specifically in the region of the heart or in the precise region of the injured myocardium but in those superficial and deep structures whose sensory nerves also end in the first through the fourth thoracic spinal segments (see Fig. 9-2, showing theoretic distribution of heart pain in the first through fourth thoracic segments). Unfortunately, from the standpoint of diagnosis, the same cord segments receive fibers from the aorta, pulmonary artery, esophagus, and skeletal structures, which explains why pain arising in them may resemble that of myocardial infarction.

Referred Pain. All that has been said about segmental localization of deep pain applies also to referred pain, a term used in clinical medicine to indicate the appearance of pain in a location of the body some distance from the viscus in which the pain originates. According to the hypothesis of Lewis and Kellgren, presented above, the referred pain is an integral part of the phenomenon of visceral pain. Thus, with cardiac pain in which sensory impulses enter mainly the left half of the first through fourth thoracic cord segments, the reference of pain to the arms is explained by the anatomic fact that the first thoracic segment supplies the inner surface of the arm as well as the thorax and heart. Thus it is just as natural for heart pain to appear in the characteristic location in the left arm as it is in the anterior midchest.

This view of visceral and referred pain has an understandable basis in neuroanatomy, for as was said, the thin, slowly conducting pain fibers terminate on small inhibitory neurones in the substantia gelatinosa, whose axones course into several adjacent segments. It is the activation of these neurones that induces a presynaptic depolarization of both large and small pain afferents, raising their threshold of excitation differentially. The unevenness of their inhibitory effects within any given segment might explain why, in the total area bounded by the first through fourth thoracic myotomes, heart pain should so commonly appear only in the anterior midline. It also explains why visceral pain may sometimes overflow into territories completely unrelated to the known innervation of the involved viscus, for example, the appearance of anginal pain in the jaws. Clinical experience teaches us that spread of pain beyond the limits that are "normal" is due in some cases at least to an unusual intensity of pain; thus an anginal pain that is ordinarily confined to the midsternal region (second through fourth thoracic nerves) may spread to the neck and shoulders (third through seventh cervical nerves). In other cases, extension of pain outside the normal boundaries may be due to coexistent lesions in structures with innervation not too distant from the cord segments primarily involved in the cardiac pain. Thus an anginal pain may be localized high in the epigastrium (seventh and eighth thoracic nerves) when peptic ulcer or gallbladder disease is also present. This may be because of summation of stimuli reaching the affected cord segments. It would explain why visceral pains overflowing into neighboring cord segments beyond the limits that are normal for the viscus tend preferentially to wander into higher rather than lower segments. (The inhibitory connections are more numerous in the cephalad structures which have a more abundant representation in consciousness than in caudad ones.)

Deep Skeletal Pain. Since there is sound experimental evidence for the view that visceral pain and deep skeletal pain are mediated through a common deep sensory system, it is not surprising that their characteristics should be similar and that on occasion differentiation between the two may be extremely difficult. Thus a small tear or injury in a lumbar muscle or ligament innervated by the twelfth thoracic or first lumbar nerve may give rise to a pain whose quality and localization, including radiation into the groin and scrotum, are indistinguishable from those of pain caused by renal colic. A similar injury in the right upper rectus muscle may cause a pain that mimics closely the pain of gallbladder colic; and a lesion in a muscle or ligament deep in the chest wall may cause pain with radiation to the left arm, identical in localization with that of angina. Under these circumstances, differentiation of somatic from visceral pain must be made on grounds other than the location and reference of pain.

HYPERESTHESIA, HYPERALGESIA, HYPERPATHIA, AND INVOLUNTARY SPASMS

In the past it has been customary to use the first two of these terms to designate a lowering of the threshold to touch and pain stimuli and the third for a state of pain with a normal or raised threshold but overreaction. The latter may even occur with anesthesia, as in *anesthesia dolorosa*. Any real distinction between these states is ephemeral. Probably only with inflammation is the pain threshold consistently lowered. What is most characteristic of all chronically painful states, and these frequently implicate nerves or central neural structures, is that the part is unusually sensitive to all stimuli, even those which normally do not evoke pain, and the elicited pain is unnatural, radiant, outlasts the initiating stimulus, and is modifiable by fatigue, emotion, etc. One sees listed here many of the characteristics of causalgia, spinal cord pain, phantom pain, zoster neuralgia, thalamic pain, and the like. The explanation currently offered for these states is that at the peripheral as well as central level the system of pain fibres is in equilibrium with other sensory fibers. A kind of inhibition is exerted on the pain system at all times by the small neurones in the substantia gelatinosa, to speak now only of the peripheral nervous system. Since the largest afferent fibers suppress most actively this inhibitory neuronal system, nerve injury, which destroys some of the larger sensory fibers (as happens in herpes zoster and also represents one phase of nerve regeneration after injury) permits overresponse of secondary sensory neurones. According to Melzack and Wall, the small neurones of the substantia gelatinosa constitute a kind of "gate control system," which modulates input. The large, low threshold fibers in a peripheral nerve most effectively activate the gateway cells. This explains the common experience of relieving pain by rubbing, vibration, etc.

Unlike other sensory experiences, pain tends to cause involuntary spasms in the skeletal muscles supplied by the same or adjacent segments of the spinal cord, e.g., spasm of the right upper rectus muscle with a gallstone impacted in the cystic duct or of the pectoral muscles in myocardial infarction.

Pain sensation may be induced by stimulation of the receptors or by irritation of peripheral nerves or roots, and in certain areas of the body it may be abolished by diseases which affect the peripheral or cerebral nervous system or by a surgical procedure which may accomplish the same result. Pain in a circumscribed region may be terminated by section of the nerve which supplies that region (neurotomy) or the spinal roots (posterior rhizotomy); pain in a limb or one side of the trunk may be interrupted by section of the anterolateral spinothalamic tract (lateral spinal tractotomy in the spinal cord or lateral medullary tractotomy in the medulla).

PERCEPTION OF PAIN. The arrival of pain impulses at the thalamocortical level of the nervous system is attended by conscious awareness of the pain stimulus. Clinical study has not informed us of the exact localization of the nervous apparatus for this mental process. It is not entirely abolished by a total hemispherectomy including the thalamus on one side. It is often said that impulses reaching the thalamus create awareness of the attributes of sensation and that the parietal cortex is necessary for the appreciation of the intensity and localization of the sensation. This seems an oversimplification. Probably a close and harmonious relationship between thalamus and cortex must exist in order for a sensory experience to be complete. The traditional separation of sensation (in this instance awareness of pain) and perception (awareness of the painful stimulus) has been abandoned in favor of the view that sensation, perception, and the various conscious and unconscious responses to a pain stimulus comprise an indivisible process.

Although similar to other sensory or perceptive phenomena in certain respects, such as predictable response to given intensity of stimulus, pain differs in other ways. One of its most remarkable characteristics is the strong feeling tone, or affect, with which it is endowed, nearly always one of unpleasantness. Furthermore, pain does not appear to be subject to negative adaptation. Most stimuli, if applied continuously, soon cease to be effective, whereas pain may persist as long as the stimulus is operative and, by establishing a central excitatory state, may even outlast the stimulus.

Stereotaxic surgery by Sweet and Mark on the thalamus in cases of intractable pain permits dissection of the anatomy of the pain experience. Lesions in the terminus of the lateral spinothalamic tract in the postcrolateral nucleus abolish pain and temperature sensation in the contralateral side of the body while leaving the patient with all his misery or affect of pain. Lesions in the centrum medianum abolish the painful state without altering pain and temperature sensation. Thus, at this level there must be a balance of inhibitory and facilitatory sensory systems, and one cannot understand intractable pain in terms simply of excitation of chains of neurones.

PSYCHOLOGIC ASPECTS OF PAIN. A discussion of this problem could hardly be complete without some reference to the influence of emotional states or to the importance of racial, cultural, and religious factors on the pain response, especially the overt expressions. It is common knowledge that some individuals, by virtue of training, habit, or phlegmatic character, are relatively stoical and that others are excessively responsive to pain. Rarely one encounters individuals who are totally incapable of experiencing pain throughout their lifetime, not from any lack of sensory endings or peripheral sensory apparatus but from some peculiarity of central reception.

Lastly, it is important to keep in mind the devastating effects of chronic pain. As Ambroise Paré is alleged to have said, "There is nothing that abateth so much the strength as paine." Continuous pain can be observed to have an adverse effect on the entire nervous system. There is increased irritability, fatigue, troubled sleep, poor appetite, and loss of emotional stability. Courageous men are reduced to a whimpering, pitiable state that may arouse only the scorn of a healthy person. They are irrational about illness and may make unreasonable demands of family and physician. This state, which may be termed *pain shock*, once established, requires delicate but firm management. Of course the effect of narcotic drugs often complicates the picture.

CLINICAL APPROACH TO THE PATIENT WITH PAIN AS THE PREDOMINANT SYMPTOM

One of the most frequent errors is to think of pains always in terms of the severe intractable pains of disease, overlooking the fact that there are thousands of other pains which are part of the daily sensory experience of otherwise healthy individuals. To mention but a few, there is the momentary, hard pain over an eye, in the temporal region, or in the ear or jaw, which strikes with alarming suddenness; the more persistent ache which arises in some fleshy part such as the shoulder, neck, thigh, or calf; the darting pain in an arm or leg; the fleeting precordial discomfort that arouses momentarily the thought of heart disease; the breath-taking catch in the side; the cluster of abdominal pains with their associated intestinal rumblings; and the brief discomfort upon movement of a joint. These *normal pains*, as they should be called, occur at all ages, tending to be brief and to depart as obscurely as they come. They acquire medical significance only when elicited by the inquiring physician or when presented as a complaint by the worried patient; and of course they must always be distinguished from the *abnormal pains* of disease.

When pain by its intensity, duration, and the circumstance of its occurrence appears to be abnormal or constitutes one of the principal symptoms of disease, an attempt should be made by careful analysis of it to reach a tentative decision as to its cause and the mechanism of its production. This can usually be accomplished by a very thorough interrogation of the patient in which he is encouraged to relate as accurately as possible the main characteristics of the pain. This is followed by a physical examination and not infrequently by special laboratory tests, of which there has been much refinement in recent years.

LOCATION OF PAIN. When the pain is caused by a superficial lesion, the cause and effect are usually so obvious that no problem is posed. It is the deep lesion, whether involving somatic or visceral structures, that causes trouble, and here exact localization becomes especially important. We have already seen that pain originating from such tissues no longer is sensed as coming from them but is instead roughly segmental, i.e., within the territory of the cord segments innervating the structure. The identification of the segments involved is of value, for it sets the limit on the diagnostic possibilities

that must be considered, i.e., to those structures having a corresponding innervation. Thus an epigastric or subxiphoid pain or one in the opposite region in the back obliges one to search for its cause in all those structures innervated by the sixth through eighth thoracic cord segments, i.e., the esophagus, stomach, duodenum, pancreas, biliary tract, the upper retroperitoneal structures, as well as the deep somatic tissues in this region. Also one must consider the possibility that a lesion in a viscus innervated by spinal segments above or below the sixth through eighth thoracic cord segments may at times be the source of pain that has spread outside its normal boundaries and involved the epigastrium (Fig. 9-2).

PROVOKING AND RELIEVING FACTORS. These factors are of greater value than quality of pain in providing important data concerning its mechanism. Pain related to breathing, swallowing, and defecation focuses attention on the respiratory apparatus, the esophagus, and the lower bowel, respectively. A pain coming on a few minutes after the beginning of general bodily movement and relieved within a few minutes by rest indicates ischemia as the probable cause. Pain occurring several hours after meals and relieved by food or alkali suggests the irritative effect of acid on the raw lining of the stomach or duodenum. Pain that is brought on or relieved by certain movements or postures of parts of the body is usually due to the activity of diseased skeletal structures (bones, muscles, ligaments). Pain that is enhanced by cough, sneeze, and strain is usually radicular in origin or arises in ligamentous structures. Pain that is increased or altered by cutaneous stimuli is due to disease in sensory tracts in the peripheral or central nervous system. These are a few examples illustrating the paramount importance of determining with the greatest possible accuracy the factors that influence the appearance or relief of pain.

QUALITY AND TIME-INTENSITY CHARACTERISTICS OF THE PAIN. These features are of importance. However, too much stress should not be laid on the adjectives that the patient uses to describe his pain. His choice of words will depend, in part at least, on his vocabulary and on what he imagines is taking place. "Crushing" or "squeezing" are commonly employed to describe an anginal pain, and this implication of pressure does have some significance, since the pain may depend on an associated involuntary contraction of the pectoral muscles. Another patient with the same disease, however, may describe the pain as "exploding" or "burning." Far more important than the adjective used is the information that the pain is steady and does not fluctuate. Similarly, the ulcer pain is frequently designated as "gnawing"; but again, the deep, steady quality is more important than the word used to denote it. Gallbladder colic and renal colic are misnomers, if by colic is meant a "paroxysmal abdominal pain due to spasm, obstruction or distension of any of the hollow viscera." *In both these disorders, the pain is steady.* The aching quality of all deep pains is usually characteristic, but there are in addition several other informative attributes. A true colicky pain, one that is rhythmic and cramping, suggests an obstructive lesion in a hollow viscus. If the patient is a woman and has had children, it is a good idea to ask whether her "cramp" resembles the pains she had during childbirth. A pain that is steady and varies little or not at all from moment to moment means that the stimulus to pain is steady and unwavering, as in angina pectoris and peptic ulcer. Thus a pain in the anterior midsternal region whose intensity fluctuates appreciably within the space of a minute or two is not due to angina, even though the history may appear to suggest a relation to exertion. Similarly, a high epigastric pain appearing several hours after a meal and even apparently relieved by food is not caused by an ulcer if the pain fluctuates perceptibly within seconds or a few minutes. The stimulus to ulcer pain does not quickly vary in intensity. A throbbing pain indicates that an arterial pulsation is giving rise to painful stimuli. Sharp, transitory pain is caused by disease of nerve roots or ganglions, as exemplified by tic douloureux or tabes, or by some disorder in a somatic tissue such as a tear of a muscle or ligament; and often there is a background of dull, aching pain. Particularly noteworthy here is the abrupt intensification of the dull ache of root pain by cough, sneeze, or strain which momentarily increases the intraspinal pressure and stretches or alters the position of the root.

MODE OF ONSET OF THE PAIN. This factor is also important. A pain reaching its full intensity almost immediately after its appearance suggests a rupture of tissue. The pain of a dissecting aortic aneurysm often develops in this manner. In fact, the suddenness and the severity of the pain, reaching a peak of intensity within seconds or minutes, sometimes provides the first clue differentiating this type of chest pain from that caused by myocardial infarction. A similarly rapid accession of pain may occur with the rupture of a peptic ulcer.

DURATION OF THE PAIN. This is another important attribute. Anginal pain rarely lasts less than 2 or 3 min or more than 10 or 15 min. Ulcer pain may continue for an hour or more, unless terminated by the ingestion of food or alkali or a tumbler of water.

SEVERITY OF PAIN. In any given disease, the severity of pain is subject to wide variation, and also patients differ in their tolerance to it. Therefore one cannot judge the gravity of an illness by the intensity of the pain. As a rule, pains that completely interrupt work and pleasurable activity, require opiates for relief, enforce bed rest, and awaken the patient from sound sleep are to be taken more seriously than those which have the opposite characteristics.

TIME OF OCCURRENCE. An accurate determination must be made of the time of occurrence. The relationship of ulcer pain to the preceding meal has already been described. Postural aches come after prolonged activity and disappear with rest, whereas arthritic pains are usually most severe during the first movements after prolonged inactivity. The mechanism for this latter phenomenon is not known; nor do we understand why painful lesions of the bone, such as those caused by metastatic cancer, are likely to be most disturbing during the night. It is possible that the occurrence or aggravation of such pains is due to enhanced awareness of painful stimuli at a time when the mind is not distracted by other stimuli; or it may be that the pains are now more easily evoked by unconscious movements made during sleep when protective reflexes are in abeyance.

It should be obvious from these remarks that the full significance of a pain is usually not revealed by any one single characteristic. It is only by combining all these data that one can determine its anatomic site and its mechanism. In general, *the most important and revealing clues are obtained from the answers to the questions: What brings on the pain? What relieves it?* Pain is a subjective manifestation, not a state to be observed or measured. The accuracy of our data depends on the skill with which we frame our questions and on the powers of observation and memory of the person answering them.

Finally the diagnostic value of measures which *reproduce* and *relieve the pain* should be stressed. Not only are they important for diagnosis, but they convince the patient that the physician understands and can control the mechanism of his pain and the illness behind it. Climbing several flights of stairs under the physician's supervision may settle the question of the presence or absence of angina pectoris. An injection of procaine into a tender area in the chest wall or some other skeletal structure with complete disappearance of the pain may establish a skeletal origin and exclude the possibility of visceral disease. Reproducing the distress sometimes caused by aerophagia merely by distending the esophagus or stomach with air, or reproducing the vague but sometimes alarming sensation of pressure in the chest caused by unconscious hyperventilation by having the patient hyperventilate are other examples of how the principle of the reproduction of pain may be usefully employed.

A systematic interrogation of the patient will not lead to accurate diagnosis in every instance, but the habit of searching for the identifying characteristics of pain will enable the physician to increase his skill in this difficult field. Furthermore, after becoming familiar with the customary responses to these questions, he becomes more alert to the anxious, the hysterical, or the depressed patient who while complaining of pain seems incapable of describing any of its details, or unwilling to do so. Instead, there is preoccupation with theories of what is wrong or with the treatments or mistreatments already given. Finally, there will always be cases that defy solution, when the physician can proceed only by repeatedly reexamining the patient, explaining the need for continued observation, and enlisting his aid and forbearance during this trying period. Asking the patient to tolerate a certain amount of pain without the use of powerful analgesics is usually effective, particularly when the possibility of drug addiction is explained to him.

INTRACTABLE PAINS

In the relatively rare circumstances when all manner of investigation has failed to throw light on the cause and mechanism of the pain, demands for pain-relieving surgery may become increasingly insistent. The physician may in desperation turn to measures which are more dangerous than the disease. Here the commonest source of error is to operate unnecessarily on the hysterical patient (see Chap. 370), only to discover too late that each operative procedure leaves a new pain, often at a higher level than the first. Depressive psychosis may masquerade as a painful state, and electric shock therapy may dramatically terminate the illness. Sometimes a half dozen or more operations are unsuccessfully performed on a single patient. The safest rule to follow in these cases is not to use opiates continuously or to recommend operation for the relief of pain unless a reasonable diagnosis has been made. For the pains of metastatic cancer, the thalamic pain of vascular disease of the brain, and other incurable diseases, the relative advantages of the controlled use of opiates versus lateral spinothalamic tractomy or frontal lobotomy must be carefully weighed in each patient. The age of the patient, life expectancy, and mental state are all of importance in selecting the treatment procedure. Too often today an operation on the spinal cord or brain is chosen in preference to narcotics and the controlled use of drugs. Forgotten is the fact that many patients with cancer were formerly kept relatively comfortable and active by the judicious use of morphine and its analogues and were never subjected to costly operations or deprived of any of those qualities of mind and character which are so treasured by their families.

Superficial pain arising in integumentary structures rarely presents a problem in therapy. Acetylsalicylic acid, 0.30 to 0.60 Gm orally every 4 hr, usually suffices. Acetophenetidin may be added. These two drugs are a particularly effective combination when one element of pain is integumentary. Commercial proprietary preparations of these drugs containing caffeine or amphetamine such as A.S.A., Empirin compound, or Edrisal are available in most pharmacies. The caffeine or amphetamine is particularly useful if there is central nervous system depression. When this type of pain is not effectively controlled by nonnarcotic analgesics, codeine should be given. Usually the addition of small amounts (8 to 30 mg) of codeine phosphate to the standard dose of acetylsalicylic acid and acetophenetidin is effective. A preparation containing codeine phosphate 8 to 30 mg, acetylsalicylic acid 0.23 Gm, acetophenetidin 0.16 Gm, and caffeine 0.032 Gm is commercially available (Empirin compound with codeine phosphate). Codeine, 30 to 45 mg every 3 hr, gives maximal analgesia with minimal side effects. Adequate rest and relief of muscle tension should also be encouraged. The application of heat, especially moist heat, is usually beneficial. Occasionally, cold applications are preferred; but with the exception of cooling packs applied to an inflamed, burning skin or to a causalgia, cold is more likely to aggravate than to soothe the painful condition.

Occasionally integumental and deep pains of skeletal structures are of such severity as to require more powerful narcotic analgesics, such as meperidine hydrochloride (Demerol) in doses of 50 to 100 mg orally or intramuscularly, methadone hydrochloride 5 to 10 mg orally or subcutaneously, or dihydromorphine hydrochloride (Dilaudid) 1.0 to 2.0 mg orally or subcutaneously. These drugs are most useful in conditions when sedation is not required. When pain is unusually severe and some degree of euphoria is desired, morphine is the ideal drug. It should be given in doses of 8.0 to 15.0 mg orally or subcutaneously. Frequently a dose as small as 4.0 to 6.0 mg will relieve pain without causing undesirable nausea and vomiting. If the original dose is too small, a second dose of the same or slightly larger size can be given in 2 hr. This divided dose is less likely to induce nausea and vomiting than the larger single dose, because the stimulating effect of the first dose is insufficient to produce these symptoms and the depressant effect which follows reduces the sensitivity of the vomiting mechanism or renders it refractory to the second dose. Since all these narcotic analgesics are, for the most part, detoxified by the liver, they either should not be used or should be given in only half the usual dosage in cases of liver disease, myxedema, adrenal insufficiency, and other states in which the metabolic rate is reduced. Morphine and related narcotic analgesics tend to cause pruritus and therefore should be used with care in patients with skin irritability. The possibility of initiating addiction in susceptible individuals must be carefully evaluated in every instance.

If the patient exhibits mental tension, insomnia, and restlessness, a sedative drug such as phenobarbital or sodium amytal may be given with the analgesic agents. Sedative medication, especially the quick-acting barbiturates, should not be used alone for the control of pain, because they sometimes cause excitement and confusion under these circumstances.

Visceral pain originating in the stomach, gallbladder, intestines, or heart is usually very poorly controlled by the nonnarcotic analgesics. Various combinations of acetylsalicylic acid and acetophenetidin usually prove to be ineffective unless given with sedatives. The narcotic analgesics are the agents of choice, but of course they should never be given until the physician is certain that the relief of the pain will not mask the state of his patient. If sedation is not desirable, and if constipation is a troublesome problem, the newer synthetic analgesics, meperidine in doses of 50 to 100 mg orally or intramuscularly or methadone 5 to 10 mg by mouth or subcutaneously every 4 to 6 hr, are recommended. Like morphine, these drugs are habit-forming, but they do not share with morphine the properties of strong analgesia, sedation, and euphoria. Patients with severe visceral pain who are also anxious or fearful and unable to relax or sleep should be given morphine sulfate in doses of 8 to 15 mg subcutaneously. The well-known spasmogenic effects of morphine are partially counteracted by atropine sulfate, 0.3 to 0.4 mg. Aminophylline, 0.5 Gm intravenously, overcomes much of this undesirable spastic action; a rectal suppository of 0.5 Gm, although less effective, may be substituted.

Intractable pain due to incurable diseases such as metastatic carcinoma is one of the most difficult of therapeutic problems. As a rule, one resorts to narcotic drugs because of their strong analgesic action, and habituation is accepted as the lesser of two evils. An alternative is "pain-relieving surgery." Section of peripheral nerves, the lateral spinothalamic tracts in the spinal cord (cordotomy) or the lateral part of the medulla, stereotaxic thalamotomy, and lobotomy are relatively safe procedures which have advantages in certain cases over the continuous use of opiates.

REFERENCES

Cohen, H.: The Mechanism of Visceral Pain, Trans. Med. Soc. London, 64:35, 1944.

Feindel, W. H., G. Weddell, and D. C. Sinclair: Pain Sensibility in Deep Somatic Structures, J. Neurol., Neurosurg. Psychiat., 11:113, 1948.

Hardy, J. D., H. G. Wolff, and H. Goodell: "Pain Sensations and Reactions," Baltimore, The Williams & Wilkins Company, 1952.

Lewis, T.: "Pain," New York, The Macmillan Company, 1942.

Ryle, J. A.: "The Natural History of Disease," London, Oxford University Press, 1936.

White, J. C., and W. H. Sweet: "Pain, Its Mechanisms and Neurosurgical Control," Springfield, Ill., Charles C Thomas, Publisher, 1955.

10 HEADACHE
John F. Griffith and Raymond D. Adams

The term *headache* should encompass all aches and pains located in the head, but in common language its application is restricted to unpleasant sensations in the region of the cranial vault. Facial, pharyngeal, and cervical pain are put aside as something different and are discussed here in Chaps. 13 and 355.

Headache, along with fatigue, hunger, and thirst, represents man's most frequent discomforts. Medically speaking, its significance is often abstruse, for it may stand as a symptomatic expression of disease or of some minor tension or fatigue, incident to the affairs of the day. Fortunately, in most instances it reflects the latter, and only exceptionally does it warn of serious disease seated in intracranial structures. But, it is this dual significance, the one benign, the other potentially malignant, that keeps the physician on the alert. Systematic approach to the headache problem necessitates a broad knowledge of the medical and surgical diseases of which it is a symptom and a clinical methodology which leaves none of the common and treatable causes unexplored.

GENERAL CONSIDERATIONS

In the introductory chapter on pain reference was made to the necessity, when dealing with any painful state, of determining its quality, location, duration, and time course and conditions which produce, exacerbate, or relieve it. When headache is considered in these terms, a certain amount of useful information is obtained by careful history, but perhaps less than one might expect.

Unfortunately, physical examination of the head itself is seldom useful.

As to quality of cephalic pain, the patient is rarely helpful in his description. In fact persistent questioning on that point occasions surprise, for the patient usually assumes that the word *headache* should have conveyed enough information to the examiner about the nature of the discomfort. Most headaches are dull, deeply located, and of aching character, a pain recognizable as of the type that usually arises from structures deep to the skin. Seldom is there reported the superficial burning, smarting, or stinging type of pain localized to the skin. When asked to analogize the sensation to another sensory experience, the patient may make some allusion to tightness, pressure, or bursting feeling, terms which then give clue to a muscular tension or psychologic state.

Queries about the intensity of the pain are seldom of much value since they reflect more the patient's attitude toward the condition and his customary way of reporting things that happen to him than the true severity. As usual, the bluff, hearty person tends to minimize his discomfort, whereas the neurotic may dramatize it. Degree of incapacity is a better index. A severe migraine attack seldom allows performance of the day's work. The pain which awakens the patient from sleep at night, or prevents sleep, is also more likely to have a demonstrable organic basis. As a rule, the most intense cranial pains are those which accompany subarachnoid hemorrhage and meningitis, which have grave implications, or migraine and paroxysmal nocturnal orbitotemporal ("cluster") headaches, which are benign.

Data regarding *location* of the headache are apt to be more informative. If the source is in deep structures (extracranial, subdermal, or intracranial), as is usually the case, the correspondence with the site of the pain is fairly precise. Inflammation of an extracranial artery causes pain well localized to the site of the vessel. Lesions of paranasal sinuses, teeth, eyes, and upper cervical vertebrae induce less sharply localized pain but one that is still referred in a regional distribution that is fairly constant. Intracranial lesions in the posterior fossa cause pain in the occipital-nuchal region, homolateral if the lesion is one-sided. Supratentorial lesions induce frontotemporal pains, again homolateral to the lesion if it is on one side. But localization can also be very uninformative or misleading. Ear pain, for example, seldom means disease in the ear, and eye pain may be referred from parts as remote as the occiput or cervical spine.

Duration and *time-intensity curve* of headaches in both the attack itself and the life-profile are most useful. Of course, the headache of bacterial meningitis or subarachnoid hemorrhage occurs usually in single attacks over a period of days. Single, brief, momentary (1 to 2 sec) pains in the cranium are presently uninterpretable and are significant only because they indicate no serious underlying disease. Migraine of the classic type has its onset in the early morning hours or daytime, reaches its peak of severity in a half hour or so, and lasts, unless treated, for several hours up to 1 to 2 days, often terminated by sleep. In the life history a frequency of more than a single attack every few weeks is exceptional. In contrast to this is the nightly occurrence (1 to 2 hr after onset of sleep) over a period of several weeks to months of the rapidly peaking, nonthrobbing orbital or supraorbital pain of cluster headache, which tends to dissipate within an hour. The headache of intracranial tumor characteristically can occur at any time of day or night, interrupt sleep, vary in intensity, and last a few minutes to hours, only to recur later in the day. The life profile is one of increasing frequency and intensity over a period of months. Tension headache, once commenced, may persist continuously for weeks or months, though waxing and waning from hour to hour.

Headache that bears a more or less constant relationship to certain biologic events and also to physical environmental changes may prove to be informative. Premenstrual headaches most typically relate to premenstrual tension during the period of oliguria and edema formation; they usually vanish after the first day of vaginal bleeding. The headaches of cervical arthritis are most typically intense after a period of inactivity, and the first stiff movements are both difficult and painful. Hypertensive headaches, like those of cerebral tumor, tend to occur on waking in the morning, but, as with all vascular headaches, excitement and tension may provoke them. Headache from infection of nasal sinuses may appear, with clocklike regularity, upon awakening and in mid-morning, and is characteristically worsened by stooping. Eye-strain headaches naturally follow prolonged use of the eyes, as in reading, peering for a long time against glaring headlights in traffic, or in watching cinema. Atmospheric cold may evoke pain in the so-called "fibrositic" or "nodular" headache or when the underlying condition is arthritic or neuralgic. Anger, excitement, or irritation may initiate common migraine in certain disposed individuals; this is more typical of common migraine than of the classic type.

PAIN-SENSITIVE STRUCTURES AND MECHANISMS OF HEADACHE

Understanding of headache has been greatly augmented by the observations of surgeons during operations on man. These operations inform us that the following cranial structures are sensitive to mechanical stimulation: (1) skin, subcutaneous tissue, muscles, arteries, and periosteum of skull; (2) delicate structures of eye, ear, and nasal cavity; (3) intracranial venous sinuses and their tributary veins; (4) parts of the dura at the base of the brain and the arteries within the dura mater and pia-arachnoid; (5) the trigeminal, glossopharyngeal vagus, and first three cervical nerves. The bony skull, much of the pia-arachnoid and dura, and the parenchyma of the brain lack sensitivity. Interestingly, pain is practically the only sensation produced by stimulation of the listed structures.

The pathways whereby sensory stimuli, whatever their source, are conveyed to the central nervous system are the trigeminal nerves for structures in the anterior two-thirds of the skull and the glossopharyngeal, vagus, and first three cervical nerves for those in the posterior third. The central connections through spinal cord and brainstem to thalamus are comparable to those already depicted in Chap. 9.

The pain of intracranial disease is referred, by a mechanism already discussed, to some part of the cranium lying within the areas supplied by the aforementioned nerves (V, IX, X, C-I, II, III). There may be an associated local tenderness of the scalp at the site of reference. Dental or jaw pain may also have cranial reference. The pain of disease in other parts of the body is not referred to the head, although it may initiate headache by other means.

By analysis of several types of headache, Wolfe and his colleagues have demonstrated that most "spontaneous" cranial pains can be traced to the operation of one or more of the following mechanisms:

1. distension, traction, and dilatation of the intracranial or extracranial arteries
2. traction or displacement of large intracranial veins or the dural envelope in which they lie
3. compression, traction, or inflammation of sensory cranial and spinal nerves
4. voluntary or involuntary spasm and possibly interstitial inflammation of cranial and cervical muscles

More specifically, the intracranial mass lesions only cause headache if in a position to deform, displace, or exert traction on vessels and dural structures at the base of the brain, and this may happen long before intracranial pressure rises. In fact the artificial induction of high intraspinal and intracranial pressure by the subarachnoid or intraventricular injection of sterile saline does not result in headache. Some have interpreted this to mean raised intracranial pressure does not cause headache, a conclusion which is called into question by the demonstrable relief of headache by lumbar puncture and lowering the cerebrospinal fluid (CSF) pressure in some patients. Actually, most patients with high intracranial pressure complain of recurrent bioccipital and bifrontal headache, probably due to traction on vessels or dura. As to localization, the pains follow the patterns mentioned above; those deflecting the falx or pressing on superior longitudinal or straight sinuses induce pain behind or above the eye; if the lateral part of the lateral sinus is involved, the pain is felt in the ear. Displacement of tentorium elicits pain felt in the supraorbital region.

Dilatation of the temporal arteries with stretching of surrounding sensitive structures is believed to be the mechanism of most of the pain of migraine. Extracranial, temporal, and occipital arteries, when involved in a peculiar giant-cell arteritis (cranial or "temporal" arteritis), a disease which afflicts individuals over fifty years of age, always give rise to headache of dull aching and throbbing type, at first localized and then more diffuse. Characteristically it is severe and persistent over a period of weeks or months. The offending artery, strangely, is not always tender to pressure, yet section of it, as in biopsy, relieves the pain. Evolving atherosclerotic thrombosis of internal carotid, anterior, and middle cerebral arteries is sometimes accompanied by pain in the forehead or temple; with vertebral artery thrombosis, the pain is postauricular, and basilar artery thrombosis causes pain to be projected to the occiput and sometimes the forehead.

In *infection or blockage of paranasal sinuses,* accompanied usually by pain over the antrum or in the forehead (from the ethmoid and sphenoid sinuses the pain localizes around the eyes on one or both sides or in the vertex or other part of the cranium, especially in disease of the sphenoid sinuses), the mechanism involves changes in pressure and irritation of pain-sensitive sinus walls. Usually it is associated with tenderness of the skin in the same distribution. The pain may have two remarkable properties: (1) When throbbing, it may be abolished by compressing the carotid artery on the same side. (2) It tends to recur and subside at the same hours, i.e., on awakening, with gradual disappearance when the person is upright, and coming again in the late morning hours. The time relations are believed to yield information concerning the mechanism; morning pain is ascribed to the sinuses filling at night, and its relief on arising, from emptying after the erect posture has been assumed. Stooping intensifies the pain by pressure change, as does blowing the nose sometimes; and amphetamine (inhalant), which reduces swelling and congestion, tends to relieve the pain. Some believe that the highly sensitive orifice of the sinus is the source, but more probably, the pain arises in the sensitive mucous membrane of the sinus. However, it may persist after all purulent secretions have disappeared, due probably to a mechanism of blockage of the orifice by boggy membranes and a vacuum or suction effect on the sinus wall (*vacuum sinus headaches*). The condition is relieved when aeration is restored. During air flights both earache and sinus headache tend to occur on descent, when the relative pressure in the blocked viscus falls.

Headache of ocular origin, located as a rule in the orbit, forehead, or temple, is of steady, aching type and tends to follow prolonged use of the eyes in close work. Ocular muscle imbalance is believed to be the mechanism. There is experimental evidence to show that the main faults are hypermetropia and astigmatism (not myopia), which result in sustained contraction of extraocular as well as frontal, temporal, and even occipital muscles. Correction of the refractive error abolishes the headache. Traction on the extraocular muscles during eye surgery and on the iris will evoke pain. Another mechanism is involved in the raised intraocular pressure seen in acute glaucoma or iridocyclitis, which causes steady, aching pain in the region of the eye. When intense, it may radiate throughout the distribution of the ophthalmic division of the trigeminal nerve. As for ocular pain in general, it is important that the eyes should always be refracted, but eyestrain is probably not as frequent as one would expect from the wholesale dispensing of spectacles.

The mechanism of *headaches accompanying disease of ligaments, muscles, and apophyseal joints* in the upper spine, which are referred to occiput and nape of neck on the same side, can be in part reproduced by the injection of hypertonic saline into these structures. Such pains are especially frequent in late life with rheumatoid and hypertrophic arthritis and tend also to occur after whiplash injuries to the neck. If the pain is arthritic in origin, the first movements after being still for some hours are both stiff and painful. In fact, evocation of pain by active and passive motion of the spine should indicate traumatic or other disease to movable parts. The pain of myofibrositis, evidenced by tender nodules near the cranial insertion of cervical and other muscles, is more obscure. There are no pathologic data as to the nature of these vaguely palpable lesions, and it is uncertain whether the pain actually arises in them. They may represent only the deep tenderness felt in the region of referred pain or the involuntary secondary protective spasm of muscles. Characteristically, the pain is steady (nonthrobbing) and spreads from one to both sides of the head. Exposure to cold or draft may precipitate it. While severe at times, it seldom prevents sleep. Massage of muscles and heat have unpredictable effects and relieve the pain in some cases.

The *headache of meningeal irritation* (infection or hemorrhage), which is of acute onset, severe, generalized, deep-seated and constant, and especially intense at the base of the skull and associated with stiffness of neck on bending forward, has been ascribed by some authorities to increased intracranial pressure. Indeed the withdrawal of CSF may afford some relief. But, dilatation and congestion of inflamed meningeal vessels must also be a factor. It seems more probable, therefore, that the pain is due to the chemical irritation of nerve endings in the meninges. The mechanism of the pain, therefore, is probably identical with that occurring in acute inflammatory conditions elsewhere.

Lumbar puncture headache, which is characterized by a steady occipital-nuchal but also frontal pain coming on a few minutes after arising from a recumbent position and relieved within a few minutes by lying down, has as its cause a persistent leakage of CSF into the lumbar tissues through the needle site. The CSF pressure is low (often 0 in lateral decubitus position), and the injection of sterile isotonic saline intrathecally relieves it. The headache is usually increased by compression of the jugular veins and is unaffected by digital obliteration of one carotid artery. It seems probable that in the upright position a low intraspinal and negative intracranial pressure exerts traction on dural attachments and dural sinuses by caudal displacement of the brain. Understandably, then, headache following cisternal puncture is rare. As soon as the leakage of CSF stops and CSF pressure is gradually restored (usually from a few days up to a week or so), the headache disappears. "Spontaneous" low-pressure headache may follow a sneeze or strain, due presumably to rupture of the spinal arachnoid along a nerve root.

The mechanism of the throbbing or steady headache which accompanies febrile illnesses (acute tonsillitis, typhoid fever, malaria, and sandfly fever), located in frontal or occipital regions or generalized, is probably vascular. It is much like histamine headache in being relieved on one side by carotid artery compression and on both sides by jugular vein compression or the subarachnoid injection of saline. It is increased by shaking the head. It seems probable that the meningeal vessels pulsate unduly and stretch pain-sensitive structures around the base of the brain. In certain cases, however, the pain may be lessened by compression of temporal arteries, and in these cases a component of the headache seems to be derived from the walls of extracranial arteries, as in migraine.

PRINCIPLE VARIETIES OF HEADACHE

Innumerable diseases are associated with headache through the operation of some of the aforementioned mechanisms. Usually there is no difficulty in diagnosing the headache of glaucoma, purulent sinusitis, bacterial meningitis, and brain tumor, and a fuller account of these special headaches will be found where these diseases are described in later sections of the book. It is when headache is chronic, recurrent, and unattended by other important signs of disease that the physician faces one of his most difficult medical problems.

The following types of headache should then be considered:

MIGRAINE. There are two identifiable, closely related syndromes, one called *classic* or *typical,* the other, *common* or *atypical.* Positive family history in 80 percent of cases, onset in childhood or adolescence, and early neurologic symptoms such as homonymous hemianopia, paresthesias, aphasia, hemiparesis (present only in classic form), unilateral throbbing pain, sensitivity to light and sound, nausea and sometimes vomiting, and relief by ergotamine are listed as the identifying characteristics of both groups. When all are present diagnosis is easy, but with only one or two there may be uncertainty. Common migraine is more likely to give trouble, especially if the age of onset is later and the attacks are not preceded by neurologic signs, occur with greater frequency, and have less predictable response to ergotamine than classic migraine. Also, if the headache is more clearly provoked by psychologically stressful situations, the possibility of psychiatric illness introduces itself more immediately. Special difficulties are also raised by unusual neurologic manifestations (see Chap. 358).

CLUSTER HEADACHE. This headache is also called *paroxysmal nocturnal cephalalgia, migrainous neuralgia,* and *histamine headache* (Horton). It is characterized by male predominance, uniformly constant, unilateral orbital localization, and onset within 2 or 3 hr after falling asleep (it is infrequent during the waking hours). The pain is usually intense, with lacrimation, blocked nostril then rhinorrhea, and sometimes flush, miosis, ptosis, and edema of cheek, all lasting approximately an hour. It tends to recur nightly for several weeks or a few months (hence the term *cluster*), followed by complete freedom for years. The pain of a given attack may leave as rapidly as it began. Clusters may recur over the years, being possibly more likely in times of stress, prolonged strain, overwork, and with upsetting emotional experiences.

Rarely, the condition may continue for 6, 7, or 8 years. The picture is so characteristic that it cannot be confused with any other disease, though to those unfamiliar with it the possibility of a carotid aneurysm, hemangioma, brain tumor, or sinusitis may be suggested. Appropriate x-rays and carotid arteriography will always exclude such conditions but usually are unnecessary. In the differential diagnosis orbital (nasociliary, supraorbital, Sluder's sphenopalatine) neuralgias must also be considered (see Chap. 355).

In the life history profile the clusters of headache may last for weeks. The clusters may be single or recur two or three times, with years of freedom in between, during which such precipitating factors as alcohol are no longer effective. Often the pain involves the same orbit in each cluster.

The relationship of the cluster headache to migraine remains conjectural. A portion of the cases have a background of migraine, which led to the earlier postulation of migrainous neuralgia, but the majority do not. The family history of migraine, or of cluster headache, is less frequent than in migraine.

TENSION HEADACHE AND VARIOUS OTHER CRANIAL PAINS WITH PSYCHIATRIC DISEASE. The headache is usually bilateral, often with diffuse extension over the top of the cranium. Occipital-nuchal localization is also common. Although described as pain, close questioning may uncover other sensations, viz., fullness, tightness, pressure (as if the head is surrounded by a band or in a vise), on which a nonthrobbing aching pain is engrafted. The onset of a given attack is more gradual than in migraine and not infrequently is added to a pressure ache which lasts unremittingly for weeks or months. In fact, this is the only type of headache that exhibits the peculiarity of being absolutely continuous day and night for long periods of time. Although sleep may be possible, whenever the patient awakens, the headache is present; and the common analgesic remedies have no beneficial effect unless the pain is intense and of aching type.

As to mechanism, the ascription of it to sustained muscle activity, shown by the electromyogram, is only a partial explanation. The continuous pressing quality of milder cephalic sensations at times when the patient is relaxed hardly seems to be attributable to physiologic stimulation and suggests instead that the condition is maintained by focused attention on the head (occasioned by worry and fear of intracranial disease. Moreover, it must be remembered that all types of headache in their late stages may give rise to muscle tension. In contrast to the migrainous patient, whose profile of headache is periodic and lifelong, with tendency to lessen in late adult years, tension headache occurs more often in middle age and usually coincides with anxiety and depression in the trying times of life. Many premenstrual headaches are of this type, and there is an increased incidence of this type of tension headache at menopause.

Psychologic studies of groups of patients with tension headaches have revealed prominent symptoms of anxiety, hypochondriasis, and to a lesser extent, depression. When psychiatric syndromes are searched for headache, it is evident that the majority of patients with anxiety neurosis and other syndromes (hysteria, obsessive-compulsive neurosis, schizophrenia) in which anxiety is a prominent symptom, exhibit this type of headache. With endogenous and reactive depressions it is less frequent, though the incidence is increased in the late-life involutional and hypochondriacal states (see Chap. 369). Migraine and traumatic headaches may be complicated by tension headache.

Other odd cephalic pains, e.g., boring pains, "clavus hystericus," may occur in hysteria and raise perplexing problems in diagnosis. Their bizarre character, persistence in the face of every known therapy, absence of other signs of disease, and the presence of the stigmata of the hysterical personality, provide the basis for correct diagnosis (see Chap. 369).

HEADACHE OF ANGIOMA AND ANEURYSM. Many authorities have declared that a vascular malformation may give rise to periodic hemicranial pain of a type that is indistinguishable from migraine except for its constancy of location (invariably on the same side) in all attacks. The temporal profile of any given attack shows the onset to be sudden or very acute, with the pain reaching a peak within minutes. Neurologic disturbances such as unilateral numbness, weakness, or aphasia tend to occur after the onset of the headache and to outlast it. Should hemorrhage occur, the headache is often extremely severe and localizes more towards the occiput and neck, lasting many days in association with stiff neck. A cranial or cervical bruit and, of course, blood in CSF, establish the diagnosis but it may require verification by arteriography. Other clinicians have denied the relationship of a migrainelike syndrome to angioma or aneurysm, and indeed, entirely adequate statistical data proving or disproving it are wanting. Even appropriate response to ergotamine is not conclusive and may be obtained in angiomatous headaches. Of course, vascular lesions may exist for long periods of time without headache, or the latter may develop many years after other manifestations, such as epilepsy and hemiplegia (see Chap. 351).

TRAUMATIC HEADACHE. Severe, chronic, continuous or intermittent headaches appear as the cardinal symptom of two posttraumatic syndromes, separable in each instance from the headache that immediately follows head injury (i.e., that of scalp laceration and contusion with sanguinous CSF and increased intracranial pressure). The latter lasts several days or a week or two.

The Headache of Chronic Subdural Hematoma. Headache and dizziness of fluctuating severity, followed by drowsiness, stupor, coma, and hemiparesis are the usual manifestations of chronic subdural hematoma. The head injury may have been minor and forgotten by patient and family. The headaches are deep-seated, steady, unilateral or generalized, and respond to the usual analgesic drugs. The typical attack profile of the headache and other symptoms is one of increasing frequency and severity over several weeks or months. Diagnosis is now established by arteriography (see Chap. 358).

Headache of Posttraumatic Nervous Instability. Here, headache is a prominent feature of a complex syndrome comprised of giddiness, fatigability, insomnia, nervousness, trembling, irritability, inability to concentrate, and tearfulness. The pain displays many variations from one day to another and also a highly individualized pattern of localization. Often it centers on the site of injury, where there is also tenderness. Reference to throbbing pain as well as pressure is obtained. Particular importance is attached to its persistence, intensification by mental and physical effort, stooping, noise, bright light, and confusion. The patient looks and acts much like a person in an agitated depression, and indeed, many neurologists believe such a state to be a posttraumatic neurosis or depression. The severity and duration of the headache bear no relation to the magnitude of the injury; some of the worst cases have had minor injuries without loss of consciousness, and major injuries may leave no headache in their wake. Unsettled litigation surely prolongs the discomfort and disability. The observation that histamine may reproduce some of the more severe headaches has suggested to some a vascular origin. Cephalic tenderness and aching pain sharply localized to the scar of the scalp laceration represent in all probability a different problem, raising the question of a traumatic neuralgia. With whiplash injuries to the neck, unilateral retroauricular or occipital pain suggest traumatism of the corresponding nerves (see Chaps. 13 and 358).

HEADACHES OF BRAIN TUMOR. Headache is the outstanding symptom of cerebral tumor. Unfortunately, the quality of the pain has no specific feature. It tends to be deep-seated, nonthrobbing (or throbbing), and aching or bursting. Attacks last a few minutes to an hour or more and occur once or many times during the day. Activity and frequent change in the position of the head may provoke pain, while rest in bed diminishes its frequency. Nocturnal awakening because of pain, although typical, is by no means diagnostic (see above). Unexpected forceful (projectile) vomiting may punctuate the illness in its later stages. As the tumor grows, the pain becomes more frequent, severe, and sometimes is nearly continuous terminally. But there are exceptions, some headaches being mild and tolerable, others as agonizing as that of the headache of bacterial meningitis and subarachnoid hemorrhage. If unilateral, the headache is homolateral to the tumor 9 out of 10 times. Supratentorial tumors are felt anterior to the interauricular circumference of the skull; posterior fossa tumors behind this line. Bifrontal and bioccipital headache, coming on after unilateral headaches, signify the development of increased intracranial pressure.

APPROACH TO THE PATIENT WITH HEADACHE

Obviously very different possibilities are raised by a patient who presents himself for the first time in his life with severe headache and another one who has had recurrent headache over a period of years. The chances of uncovering the cause in the first instance are much greater than the latter, and some of the underlying conditions (meningitis, subarachnoid hemorrhage, epidural hematoma, glaucoma, and purulent sinusitis) are more serious.

In searching for the cause of recurrent headache one should investigate the status of cardiovascular and renal systems by blood pressure and urine examination, eyes (fundoscopic, intraocular pressure, and refraction), the sinuses by transillumination and x-rays, the cranial arteries by palpation (and biopsy), the cervical spine by effect of passive movement and x-rays, and the nervous system by neurologic examination and psychic function by mental status.

Hypertension is, of course, frequent in the general population and is always difficult to prove as a cause of recurrent headaches. Minor elevations of blood pressure may be a result rather than the cause of nervous tension. No doubt severe hypertension with diastolic blood pressures of over 110 mm Hg are regularly associated with headache, and measures which reduce blood pressure can be shown to relieve the headache. But it is the moderate hypertensive when subject to numerous and severe headaches who gives concern. If headache is severe and frequent, there is usually an underlying anxiety or tension state or a common migraine syndrome that is exacerbated by blood vessel disease. The mechanism of the puzzling hypertensive phenomenon of occipital pain, present on awakening in the morning and wearing off during the day, is uncertain.

The adolescent with daily frontal headaches represents a special type of problem. Often their relationship to eyestrain is unclear, and refraction of the eyes and new eyeglasses do not relieve the condition. Anxiety or tension is probably a factor in such cases, but it is difficult to be certain of a causal relationship. Some of the most persistent and inexplicable headaches, which have led to a survey by a battery of diagnostic procedures for tumor, have proven in the end to be depression.

Equally puzzling is the somber, tense adult whose primary complaint is headache, or the migrainous person who in late life or at menopause begins to have daily headaches. Here it becomes important to assess mental status along the lines suggested in Chaps. 18, 30 and 369, looking for evidences of anxiety, depression, and hypochondriasis. The quality and persistence of the headache are suggestive of the possibility of psychiatric illness. Sometimes, a direct question as to the patient's idea of what is the matter may elicit suspicion and fear of brain tumor.

The most worrisome type of patient, in our experience, is the one who has only headache of increasing frequency and severity over a period of months or a year or so. Usually it becomes necessary to resort to a complete neurologic survey, including careful inspection of optic discs and x-rays of skull, electroencephalogram, lumbar puncture, and radioactive-isotope scanning to rule out brain tumor, abscess, or subdural hematoma.

Every elderly person with severe headache of some few days or weeks duration should be considered as a possible case of cranial arteritis. Increased sedimentation rate, fever, and anemia may be conjoined, but only in a minority of cases, unfortunately. The finding of a thickened temporal artery is important, and arterial biopsy establishes the diagnosis and often relieves the pain.

TREATMENT

The most important steps in the treatment of headache are those measures which uncover and remove the underlying disease or functional disturbance.

For the common everyday headache due to fatigue, stuffy atmosphere, or excessive use of alcohol and tobacco, it is simple enough to advise avoidance of the offending activity or agent, and symptomatic therapy in the form of acetylsalicylic acid, 0.6 Gm (in the form of aspirin or Anacin) will suffice. Some patients who invariably have headache when constipated and hypochondriacs who not infrequently suffer incapacitating headache, fatigue, and depression whenever bowel elimination does not meet their expectation, are not easily helped. Certainly, simple explanation, an anti-constipation regimen, and drugs which counteract depression (see Ch. 369) are preferable to the continuous use of analgesics. Premenstrual headache, if troublesome, can usually be helped by the use of a diuretic compound for the week preceding the menstrual period and a mixture of mild analgesic and tranquilizing medications (acetylsalicylic acid, 0.6 Gm and phenobarbital, 30 mg). If the headaches are severe and incapacitating, they should be treated as common migraine (see Chap. 367).

Hypertensive headaches respond to agents which lower blood pressure and relieve muscle tension. Chlorothiazide (Diuril), 250 to 500 mg twice a day, and methyldopa (Aldomet), 250 to 500 mg per day, when combined with a small amount of phenobarbital, 15 mg t.i.d., have given the best results. Meprobamate, 200 mg t.i.d., or chlordiazepoxide HCl (Librium), 5 mg t.i.d., may be administered in place of phenobarbital. For the morning occipital ache a capsule containing sodium nitrite, 30 mg, caffeine sodium benzoate, 0.5 Gm, and acetophenetidine, 0.6 Gm, has been useful. A simplified version is to supply the caffeine in a cup of strong black coffee and to give with it acetylsalicylic acid.

The muscle tension headaches respond best to massage, relaxation, and to a combination of drugs which relieve anxiety (phenobarbital, amobarbital, meprobamate, and chlordiazepoxide HCl) and pain [acetylsalicylic acid, propoxyphene HCl (Darvon) or Percodan]. Stronger analgesic medication may be needed (codeine or meperidine HCl). Psychotherapy is usually not beneficial in this group of patients.

Recurrent vascular headaches (common migraine) and classic migraine should be treated according to the plan outlined in Chap. 367.

The headache of the syndrome of posttraumatic nervous instability requires supportive psychotherapy in the form of reassurance and frequent explanation of its benign and transient nature, a program of increasing physical activity, and drugs which allay anxiety and depression. Tender scars from scalp laceration may be novocainized repeatedly (subcutaneous injection of 5 ml of 1% procaine) with some degree of success. Settlement of litigation as soon as possible works to the patient's advantage.

Heat, massage, salicylates, and indomethacin (Indocin) or phenylbutazone (Butazolidine) usually effect some improvement in those arthritic diseases of the cervical spine which are associated with cervicocranial pain (see Chap. 13).

Corticosteroid therapy is indicated in cranial arteritis to prevent disastrous blindness by occlusion of the ophthalmic arteries and in certain cases of rheumatoid arthritis. The headaches of cranial tumor often respond surprisingly well to large doses of methylprednisolone acetate and like compounds.

In conclusion, it is well to mention the importance of general hygenic measures. Young physicians in particular are apt to seek a specific therapy for each headache syndrome and give little thought to the general health of the patient. We have observed that most of the recurrent and chronic headaches are likely to be more severe and disabling whenever the patient becomes nervous, sick, and tired. A well-rounded diet, adequate rest, a reasonable amount of physical exercise, and a balanced view of the sources of daily anxieties and how to cope with them should be the goal of all therapeutic programs.

REFERENCES

Wolff, H. G.: "Headache and Other Pain," Fair Lawn, N.J., Oxford University Press, 1947.

Friedman, A. P.: "Research and Clinical Studies in Headache," Baltimore: The Wilkins & Wilkins Company, 1967.

Vinken, P. J. and G. W. Bruyn: "Handbook of Clinical Neurology," vol. 5, "Headache and Cranial Neuralgias," Amsterdam North Holland Publishing Company, 1968.

11 PAIN IN THE CHEST

T. R. Harrison, W. M. Resnik, T. J. Reeves, and E. Braunwald

The common problem in patients who complain of chest pain involves the distinction of trivial disorders from coronary disease, which is attended by the threat of sudden death. There is little parallelism between the severity of the pain and the gravity of its cause. An incorrect positive diagnosis of a hazardous condition such as angina pectoris is likely to have harmful psychologic and economic consequences. In no field of medicine is accurate diagnosis more important or, at times, more difficult.

The apparently bizarre radiation of pain arising in the thoracic viscera can usually be explained in terms of the known facts concerning nerve supply. These have been considered in Chap. 9. One occasionally sees a patient with extension of pain to a location which cannot be logically explained. In most instances, such an individual will be found to have more than one disorder capable of causing pain in the chest. The presence of the second and often silent condition may affect the radiation of the pain produced by the primary disorder. Thus, when the pain of angina pectoris extends to the back, the patient may be found to have also a significant degree of spinal arthritis. Similarly, the radiation of anginal pain to the abdomen commonly occurs in individuals who have some upper abdominal disorder, such as a hiatus hernia, disease of the gallbladder, pancreatitis, or peptic ulcer. When such instances are excluded, there is only an occasional patient who presents a distribution of pain which cannot be logically explained in terms of the known facts about nerve supply.

The common tendency to assume that the presence of an objective abnormality, such as a hiatus hernia or right bundle branch block, necessarily means that an atypical chest pain arises in the stomach or the heart is to be strongly condemned. Such an assumption is justified only if a careful history indicates that the behavior of the pain is entirely compatible with the site of origin which is suggested by the objective finding.

THE LEFT-ARM MYTH. There is a long tradition, widely accepted by physicians and laymen, that pain in the left arm, especially when appearing in conjunction with chest pain, has a unique and ominous significance as being almost certain evidence of the presence of ischemic heart disease. This is a myth that has neither theoretic nor clinical foundation. From a theoretic standpoint, any disorder involving the deep afferent fibers of the upper thoracic region should be capable of causing pain in the chest, the left arm, both areas, or neither area. Hence a pain of trivial significance arising in skeletal tissues innervated by upper (first to fourth) thoracic nerves would be expected to produce left-arm-area pain. These expectations are exactly in accord with clinical observation. Thus, almost any condition which is capable of causing pain in the chest may induce radiation to the left arm. Such localization is common not only in patients with coronary disease but also in those with numerous other types of chest pain. Although pain due to myocardial ischemia most frequently is substernal and radiates down the ulnar aspect of the left arm (Chap. 271) and is pressing and constricting in nature, the location, radiation, and quality of pain are of less diagnostic significance than is the behavior of the pain, in terms of the conditions which induce it and relieve it.

The majority of individuals also believe that cardiac pain is situated in the region of the left breast and therefore left inframammary pain is one of the common symptoms that brings the patient to seek medical advice. It differs radically from the pain due to myocardial hypoxia, i.e., angina pectoris, in that it is usually a long-lasting, dull ache, occasionally accentuated by sharp stabs. It has no relationship to exertion and may be accompanied by tenderness over the precordium.

Chest pain which occurs after the patient sits down

and upon completion of activity usually is not angina pectoris.

Only the more important or more common conditions listed will be considered in the text.

PAIN DUE TO OXYGEN DEFICIENCY OF THE MYOCARDIUM

PHYSIOLOGIC CONSIDERATIONS OF THE CORONARY CIRCULATION. Pain due to myocardial ischemia occurs when the oxygen supply to the heart is deficient in relation to the oxygen need. The oxygen consumption of this organ is closely related to the physiologic effort made during contraction. It is dependent primarily on three factors: (1) the frequency of cardiac contraction, (2) the tension developed by the myocardium and, (3) the contractile state of the myocardium. When cardiac contractility, arterial pressure, and heart rate remain constant, an elevation of stroke volume produces an efficient type of response because it leads to an increase in the external work of the heart (i.e., in the product of cardiac output and arterial pressure) with little accompanying augmentation of myocardial oxygen requirements. Thus, a rise in flow load causes less increment in myocardial oxygen consumption than does a comparable increase in cardiac work per minute brought about by elevation either of pressure or of heart rate. However, the net effects of these hemodynamic variables depend not on oxygen need alone but rather on the balance between the demand and the supply of oxygen. The heart is always active and the coronary venous blood is normally much more desaturated than that from other areas of the body. Thus the removal of more oxygen from each unit of blood, which is one of the adjustments commonly utilized by exercising skeletal muscle, is already employed in the heart of an individual in the basal state. Therefore, this organ has only one effective means of obtaining the additional oxygen required for greater contractile activity and this is by increase in the coronary blood flow.

It follows, from hydrodynamic considerations, that the flow of blood through the coronary arteries is directly proportional to the pressure gradient between the aorta and the ventricular myocardium during systole and the ventricular cavity during diastole but is proportional to the fourth power of the radius of the coronary arteries. Thus, a relatively slight alteration in coronary diameter will produce a large change in coronary flow, provided that other factors remain constant. In the normal heart, coronary blood flow occurs primarily during diastole, when it is unopposed by myocardial constriction of the coronary vessels. Coronary flow is regulated primarily by myocardial oxygen needs, probably through the release of vasodilator metabolites. Although changes in coronary flow occur with activation of autonomic nerves to the coronary vessels, these alterations result primarily from the effects of these nervous stimuli on myocardial contraction and therefore on the heart's oxygen consumption.

The coronary dilatation which normally occurs during exercise, is impaired in patients with fixed coronary narrowing due to coronary arteriosclerosis. Thus, physical exertion, or any condition which increased heart rate, arterial pressure, or myocardial contractility tends to precipitate anginal attacks by increasing myocardial oxygen needs in the face of impaired oxygen delivery. Bradycardia usually has the opposite effects, and this apparently explains the rarity of angina in patients with complete heart block, even when this disorder is associated with coronary disease.

CAUSES OF MYOCARDIAL HYPOXIA. By far the most frequent underlying cause is organic narrowing of the coronary arteries secondary to coronary atherosclerosis. Less frequently, narrowing of the coronary orifices due to syphilitic aortitis or to distortion by a dissecting aneurysm may be responsible. A drug, such as ergot, which causes constriction of the coronary arteries, may occasionally induce anginal attacks in the absence of organic disease. There is no evidence that vasoconstriction or increased cardiac contractile activity (rise in heart rate or blood pressure, or increase in contractility due to liberation of catecholamines or adrenergic activity) due to emotion can precipitate angina unless there is also structural narrowing of the coronary vessels.

Aside from conditions which narrow the lumen of the coronary arteries, the only other frequent causes of myocardial hypoxia are disorders, such as aortic stenosis, which cause a marked disproportion between the perfusion pressure and the ventricular work. Under such conditions the systolic rise in left ventricular pressure is not, as in hypertensive states, balanced by a corresponding elevation of aortic perfusion pressure, and most of the coronary flow occurs during diastole. Therefore, an increase in heart rate is especially harmful because it shortens diastole more than systole and thereby decreases the total available perfusion time per minute.

Patients with marked right ventricular hypertension may have exertional pain which is, in most respects, identical with that of the common type of angina. It is likely that this discomfort results from relative ischemia of the right ventricle brought about by the increased oxygen needs and by the elevated intramural resistance, with sharp reduction of the normally large systolic perfusion of this chamber.

In persons with *syphilitic aortitis,* angina is not uncommon and the relative roles of aortic insufficiency and of coronary ostial narrowing are difficult to assess. However, the latter factor is absent in patient with rheumatic aortic insufficiency, in whom angina occurs less frequently than in patients with luetic disease. However, angina is frequent and severe in patients with rheumatic aortic regurgitation and stenosis.

The importance of tachycardia, decline in blood pressure, or diminution in arterial oxygen content will be apparent from the above discussion. However, these are precipitating and aggravating factors rather than underlying causes of angina.

THE EFFECTS OF MYOCARDIAL HYPOXIA. The most common of these is anginal pain, which is considered in some detail in Chap. 271. It is usually described as a heavy pressure or squeezing and occurs particularly on walking, especially after meals, on cold days against a wind or uphill. When anginal pain is induced by walking, it forces the patient to stop or reduce his speed. It occurs with anger, excitement, and other emotional states. The exact mechanism of the pain stimulus is still unknown. The evidence that oxygen deficiency is in some way responsible appears to be overwhelming, but the precise mechanism of its action has not been established.

As a rule, myocardial infarction is associated with a pain similar in quality and distribution to that of angina but of great intensity and longer duration. The pain of myocardial infarction is not relieved by rest or by coronary dilator drugs. Occasionally, it is minimal or even completely absent. In such instances, it is possible that preexisting longstanding myocardial ischemia has damaged the nerve fibers which would otherwise conduct the pain impulses.

A second effect of myocardial ischemia is often seen in the electrocardiogram. Most persons with angina have normal tracings between attacks, and the record may even remain normal during the episode of pain. However, in many instances, depression of the S-T segments appears in leads I, II, AVL, or in those from the left precordium during exertion. The finding of deep, ischemic type of S-T segment depressions during an attack of pain with a return to normal after the pain subsides strongly suggests that the pain is anginal in origin. There is strong experimental evidence that such depressions, as well as the elevations which are usually seen in patients with infarction and are observed in a few patients during anginal attacks, are related to alterations in ionic balance (Chap. 260). It appears that the net effect of very severe ischemia is to produce S-T segment elevations, while less marked ischemia has the reverse effect. The value and limitation of electrocardiographic changes occuring after exercise in the diagnosis of angina pectoris are discussed in Chap. 271.

A third effect of myocardial hypoxia is alteration in contraction. It has been shown that the left ventricular end-diastolic pressure may rise during anginal attacks, particularly if they are prolonged. This indicates transient depression of left ventricular function, which is presumably induced by the decreased contractility of the ischemic areas. On auscultation a fourth heart sound is also frequently heard during the anginal episode.

The beneficial effect of nitrites was originally ascribed by Lauder Brunton to reduction in tension in the arteries and thus, presumably, in the heart. Subsequent studies in animals pointed toward absolute increase in coronary flow. However, direct measurements in man suggest that the increase in coronary flow is relative and that the beneficial effects of these agents are dependent on a reduction in the oxygen requirements of the heart.

Another characteristic effect of myocardial hypoxia is liability to sudden death. This may never occur, despite hundreds of anginal episodes. However, it may supervene early in the disease and even in the first attack. When the conducting system is involved, the patient may die from atrioventricular block, with standstill of the ventricle.

However, the usual mechanism is probably ventricular fibrillation, which can often be seen to occur in animals following ligation of a coronary artery.

PAIN DUE TO IRRITATION OF SERIOUS MEMBRANES OR JOINTS

PERICARDITIS. Experimental studies made on man indicate that the visceral and the internal surface of the parietal pericardium are ordinarily insensitive to pain, although when the latter is sufficiently inflamed, painful stimuli may originate from it. The most highly sensitive region is the lower part of the external surface of the parietal layer, and the pain associated with inflammation of the remaining part usually arises in the adjacent pleura. These observations explain why noninfectious pericarditis (that associated with uremia and with myocardial infarction) with relatively mild inflammation is usually painless or accompanied rarely with very mild pain, whereas infectious pericarditis, being nearly always more intense and spreading to the neighboring pleura, is usually associated with typical pleuritic pain (i e, aggravated by breathing, coughing, etc.). Since the central part of the diaphragm receives its sensory supply from the phrenic nerve, which arises from the third to fifth cervical segments of the spinal cord, pain arising from the lower parietal pericardium and central tendon of the diaphragm is felt characteristically at the tip of the shoulder, the adjoining trapezius ridge, and the neck. Involvement of the more lateral part of the diaphragmatic pleura, supplied by branches from the intercostal nerves (sixth to ninth thoracic), causes pain not only in the anterior chest but also in the upper abdomen and corresponding region of the back, thus sometimes simulating the pain of acute cholecystitis or pancreatitis.

Pericarditis causes three distinct types of pain. By far the commonest is the pleuritic pain, related to respiratory movements and always aggravated by cough or deep inspiration, sometimes brought on by swallowing, because the esophagus lies just beyond the posterior portion of the heart, sometimes by change of bodily position. It is sharper, more left-sided, is frequently referred to the neck or flank, and lasts longer than angina pectoris. This type of pain is due to the pleuritic component of the pleuropericarditis so commonly present in the infectious forms. The next commonest pericardial pain is the steady, crushing substernal pain identical with that of acute myocardial infarction; if the pleuritic component is absent, differentiation on the basis of the pain alone is impossible. The mechanism of this steady substernal pain is not certain, but it is probable that it arises from the highly inflamed inner parietal surface of the pericardium or from the irritated afferent cardiac nerve fibers lying in the periadventitial layers of the superficial coronaries. The third type of pain, one that a priori should appear to be the most common and characteristic, is actually quite uncommon. This pain is synchronous with the heartbeat and is felt at the left border of the heart and left shoulder. Rarely, all three types may be present simultaneously.

The painful syndromes which may follow operations on the heart ("post commissurotomy syndrome"), myocardial infarction, or trauma to the heart are discussed in later chapters (Chaps. 270 through 272). Such pains often but not always arise in the pericardium.

Pleural pain is very common and may be identical with that of pericarditis. However, its sharp superficial quality and its aggravation by each breath readily distinguishes it from the deep dull steady unwavering pain of myocardial ischemia.

The pain resulting from *pulmonary embolism* may resemble that of acute myocardial infarction and in massive embolism it is located substernally. In patients with smaller emboli the pain is located more laterally and is pleuritic in nature. The pain of mediastinitis or of mediastinal emphysema (Chap. 293) usually resembles that of pleuritis but is more likely to be maximal in the substernal region, and the associated feeling of constriction may cause confusion with myocardial infarction. The pain due to *acute dissection of the aorta* is usually extremely severe. It is localized to the center of the chest, lasts for hours, and requires unusually large amounts of analgesics for relief. It often radiates into the back but is not aggravated by changes in position or respiration.

The *costochondral and chondrosternal articulations* are the commonest sites of anterior chest pain. Objective signs in the form of swelling (Tietze's syndrome), redness, and heat are very rare, but sharply localized tenderness is common. The pain may be "neuritic," i.e., darting and lasting for only a few seconds, or a dull ache enduring for hours or days. An associated feeling of tightness due to muscle spasm (see below) is frequent. When the discomfort endures for a few days only, a story of minor trauma or of some unaccustomed physical effort can be obtained. The chronic variety of this discomfort is common in persons with arthritis of the spine and also in patients with ischemic heart disease, but in many instances no associated disorder is found. It should be emphasized that *pressure on the chondrosternal and costochondral junctions is an essential part of the examination of every patient with chest pain.* A large percentage of patients with this disorder, and especially those who also have minor and innocent T-wave alterations (Chap. 260), are erroneously labeled as having coronary disease. The dire consequences of such a mistake have already been emphasized.

Pain secondary to *subacromial bursitis* and *arthritis of the shoulder and spine* may be precipitated by exercise of the local area but not by general exertion. It may be brought out by passive movement of the involved area as well as by coughing.

PAIN DUE TO TISSUE DISRUPTION

Rupture or tear of a structure may give rise to pain that sets in abruptly and reaches its peak of intensity almost instantly. Such a story would, therefore, arouse the suspicion of dissecting aneurysm, pneumothorax, mediastinal emphysema, a cervical disk syndrome, or rupture of the esophagus. However, the patient may be too ill to recall the precise circumstances, or the pain may be atypical and increase gradually in severity. Likewise, other and more benign conditions, such as a slipped costal cartilage or an intercostal muscle cramp, may produce pain with an abrupt onset.

PAIN DUE TO INCREASED MUSCLE TENSION

This is of two varieties, depending on whether the discomfort arises in skeletal or smooth muscle. The former is very frequent, and the usual causes are discussed later in some detail. A very rare type is *intercostal cramp*, which, except for the location, is identical with the common night cramp in the calves. Here, again, the coexistence of insignificant variations in the electrocardiogram *often* leads to the tragedy of a false positive diagnosis of ischemic heart disease.

It is likely that increased tension in visceral musculature is responsible for the chest pain associated with some esophageal disorders, the splenic flexure syndrome, aerophagia, and diverticulum of the stomach. There is uncertainty whether the same mechanism or pinching of nerve fibers causes the discomfort of hiatal hernia, a disorder that can mimic the pain of myocardial ischemia exactly as regards location, quality, and intensity but not as regards precipitating and alleviating factors.

CLINICAL ASPECTS OF SOME OF THE COMMONER CAUSES OF CHEST PAIN

Some of the features of pericarditis have already been described, and those of the more serious causes of chest pain such as myocardial ischemia (angina pectoris and infarction), dissecting aneurysm, and disorders of the pleura, esophagus, stomach, duodenum, and pancreas are considered in the appropriate chapters dealing with these problems. Here, we are concerned with the discussion of those causes which are not considered in more detail elsewhere.

PAIN ARISING IN THE CHEST WALL OR UPPER EXTREMITY. This may develop as a result of muscle or ligament strains brought on by unaccustomed exercise and felt in the costochondral or chondrosternal junctions or in the chest wall muscles. We mention the upper extremities and especially the left because of the deeply ingrained legend that pain in the left arm has a specific significance in indicting the heart. Other causes are *osteoarthritis* of the dorsal or thoracic spine and displaced *cervical discs.* Pain in the left upper extremity and precordium may be due to compression of portions of the brachial plexus by a cervical rib or by spasm and shortening of the anterior muscle secondary to high fixation of the ribs and sternum. Finally, pains in the upper extremity (shoulder-hand syndrome) and in the pectoral muscles may, through unknown mechanisms, occur in patients with ischemic heart disease.

Skeletal pains in the chest wall or shoulder girdles or arms are usually recognized quite easily. Localized tenderness of the affected area is usually present, and the pain is sometimes clearly related to movements involving the painful locus. Thus deep breathing, turning or twisting of the chest, and movements of the shoulder girdle and arm will elicit and duplicate the pain of which the patient complains. The pain may be very brief, lasting only a few seconds, or dull and aching and enduring for hours. The duration is, therefore, likely to be either longer or shorter than untreated anginal pain, which usually lasts for only a few minutes.

These skeletal pains often have a sharp or sticking quality. In addition, there is frequently a feeling of tightness which is probably due to associated spasm of intercostal or pectoral muscles. This may produce the "morning stiffness" seen in so many skeletal disorders. The discomfort is unaffected by nitroglycerin but often abolished by infiltration of the painful areas with procaine (Novocain).

When chest wall pain is of recent origin and follows some unusual activity involving the pectoral muscles, it presents no problem in diagnosis. However, *long-standing skeletal pain is frequent in persons who also have angina pectoris.* This association is sometimes coincidental, because both disorders are very common. In other instances, it seems that the coronary disease is responsible for the chest wall pain, the exact mechanism being uncertain but similar to that responsible for the well-known shoulder-hand syndrome. This coexistence of the two different types of chest pain in the same patient is a frequent cause of a confusing history because in the patient's mind the anginal needle may be hidden in the skeletal haystack. Thus every middle-aged or elderly patient who has long-standing anterior chest wall pain merits careful study.

Detailed questioning will sometimes reveal that what was originally thought by the patient to be a single type of discomfort actually comprises two different pains which, though similar in quality and area, differ as regards duration and initiating factors. When the history is inconclusive, the postexertional electrocardiogram may furnish decisive information. However, both false positive and false negative tracings may be obtained, according to whether they are interpreted loosely or critically (Chap. 271). It may thus be necessary to study the pain itself and to learn by direct observations whether exercise alone or postprandial exertion, or even postprandial effort undertaken holding an ice cube, is capable of producing it. Repeated tests may be required, the effects of preceding placebos, as compared to nitroglycerin, on the amount of exertion required to induce the pain being compared. *The confusion created by the presence of innocent skeletal pain impairs the reliability of the history and is probably the commonest cause of errors—both positive and negative—in the diagnosis of angina pectoris.*

Emotional disorders are also common causes of chest wall pain. Usually, the discomfort is experienced as a sense of "tightness," sometimes called "aching," and occasionally it may be sufficiently severe as to be designated a pain of considerable magnitude. Since the discomfort has almost always the additional quality of tightness or constriction and, furthermore, since it is often localized across the sternum, although it may be felt in other areas of the anterior chest, it is not surprising that this type of pain is frequently confused with that of myocardial ischemia. Ordinarily, it lasts for a half hour or more and may persist for a day or less with slow fluctuation of intensity. The association with fatigue or emotional strain is usually clear, although it may not be recognized by the patient until called to his attention. The pain probably develops through unconscious and prolonged increase of muscle tone (as in frowning in the face, or as can be quickly produced in the hand by tightly clinching the fist), often enhanced by an accompanying hyperventilation (by causing a contraction of the chest wall muscles similar to the painful tetany of the extremities). When the hyperventilation and/or the associated adrenergic effect due to anxiety also causes innocent changes in the T waves and S-T segments, the confusion with coronary disease is strengthened. However, the long duration of the pain, the lack of any relation to exertion but association rather with fatigue or tension, and the usual periodic occurrence on successive days without any limitation of capacity for exercise usually make the differentiation from ischemic pain quite clear.

As compared to these two causes (the chest wall muscle and ligament strains and the contraction of the pectoral muscles due to reflex influences, fatigue, or tension) the various other conditions that may cause skeletal discomfort are uncommon and readily recognized after appropriate observation: spinal arthritis, herpes zoster, anterior scalene and hyperabduction syndromes, malignant disease of the ribs, etc.

The several *abdominal disorders* which may at times mimic anginal pain may usually be suspected from the history, which ordinarily will indicate some relationship to swallowing, eating, belching, the expulsion of flatus, etc. Pain resulting from gastric or duodenal ulcer is epigastric or substernal, commences about 1 to 1½ hr after meals and is usually promptly relieved by antacids or milk. Occasionally, as in some patients with hiatal hernia, the gastrointestinal x-ray will be of crucial significance. Rarely, it may be necessary to inflate the stomach or the splenic flexure with air, in order to satisfy both the doctor and the patient that one of these organs is responsible for a tight pain in the lower chest. Roentgenographic examination is also often helpful in differentiating biliary, gastrointestinal, aortic, pulmonary, and skeletal disease pain from angina pectoris. It should be emphasized again that the demonstration of the presence of a coexistent abdominal disorder such as hiatal hernia does not constitute proof that the chest pain of which the patient complains is due to this. Such disorders are frequently asymptomatic and are not at all uncommon in patients who also have angina pectoris.

APPROACH TO THE PATIENT WITH PAIN IN THE CHEST

Most individuals with this complaint will fall into one of two general groups. The first consists of persons with prolonged and often severe pain without obvious initiating factors. Such persons will frequently be gravely ill. The problem is that of differentiating such serious conditions as myocardial infarction, dissecting aneurysm, and pulmonary embolism from each other and from less grave causes. In some such instances, the careful history will provide significant clues, while objective evidence of crucial importance will appear within the subsequent 2 or 3 days. Thus, when the initial examinations are not decisive, a watch and wait policy, with repeated electrocardiograms coupled with measurements of the transaminase, sedimentation rate, etc., will commonly provide the correct answer.

The second group of patients comprises those who have brief episodes of pain, with otherwise apparently excellent health. Here, the resting electrocardiogram will rarely supply decisive information, but records taken after exercise will often reveal characteristic changes (Chap. 271). However, in many instances it is the study of the subjective phenomenon, i.e., of the pain itself, that will lead to the diagnosis. Of the several methods of investigation which are available for such patients, three are of cardinal importance.

A detailed and *meticulous history* of the behavior of the pain is the most important method. The location, radiation, quality, intensity, and, especially, duration of the episodes are important. Even more so is the story of the aggravating and alleviating factors. Thus a history of sharp aggravation by breathing, coughing, or other resporatory movements will usually point toward the pleura, pericardium (because of the associated pleuropericarditis), or mediastinum as the site, although chest wall pain is likewise affected by respiratory motions. Similarly, a pain which regularly appears on rapid walking and vanishes within a few minutes upon standing still will usually mean angina pectoris, although here, once again, a similar story will rarely be obtained from patients with skeletal disorders.

When the history is inconclusive, the *study of the patient at the time of the spontaneous episode* will often supply crucial information. Thus the electrocardiogram, which may be normal both at rest and after exercise in the absence of pain, will occasionally demonstrate striking changes when recorded during an anginal episode. Similarly, x-ray of the esophagus or of the stomach may show no evidence of cardiospasm or of hiatal hernia except when the observation is made during the pain.

The third method of study represents the *attempt to produce and alleviate the pain at will*. This procedure is necessary only when doubt exists following the history or when needed for psychotherapeutic purposes. Thus the demonstration that a localized pain, which can be reproduced by pressure on the chest, is completely relieved by local infiltration with procaine will often be of conclusive importance in convincing the patient that the heart is not the site. The discomfort due to distension of the stomach or of the splenic flexure with air is frequently mistaken by the patient, and occasionally by the physician, for pain of cardiac origin. The simple demonstration, by passing a tube to the appropriate area and inflating with air, that the pain can be exactly reproduced may be not only of diagnostic but also of psychotherapeutic value. However, the demonstration that such procedures will reproduce the patient's pain may be misleading in persons who have angina in addition to another disorder. It may, therefore, be necessary to study also the effect of exercise on the pain and on the electrocardiogram.

When, as is not rarely the case, the history is atypical, the correct diagnosis of angina pectoris will often depend in large measure on the response to nitroglycerin. Here, a number of pitfalls should be avoided. If the patient has previously had the drug, careful questioning may be necessary to avoid errors. Thus disappearance after its sublingual administration does not necessarily prove that there is a cause and effect relationship. It is necessary to be certain that the pain vanishes more rapidly (usually within 5 min) and more completely when the drug is used than when it is not employed. A false negative impression concerning the effect of nitroglycerin may be the result of the use of a deteriorated preparation which has been exposed to light. It is thus necessary to be sure that the dosage used is sufficient to induce a pharmacologic effect in the form of a slight flush or a mild pounding headache. In doubtful instances, repeated exercise tests, with and without preceding administration of nitroglycerin, are necessary. The demonstration that the time required for a given exercise to produce pain is consistently and considerably longer when it is undertaken within a few minutes after a sublingual nitroglycerin pill than after a placebo may, in some instances, represent the sole method for accurate recognition of angina pectoris. A completely negative response to such repeated tests constitutes almost conclusive evidence against angina.

SUMMARY

The location of a pain in the chest has little diagnostic import. The concept that radiation from the anterior chest to the left arm necessarily indicates coronary disease as a cause is an old wives' tale. The several thoracic viscera and the chest wall have nerve fibers which pass by a final common pathway to the pain-receptive areas of the brain. One can no more identify the cause of the pain by its location alone than one can hear the ring of a telephone and know the city from which the call originated. Differences in the quality and duration of pain may be of diagnostic value. However, the most important aspect of the history in the diagnosis of *brief and recurrent chest pain is the relationship to various precipitating and alleviating factors*. The observation of the effect of exercise on the electrocardiogram and on the pain is often conclusive. In many instances the study of the effect of nitroglycerin on the amount of exercise required to produce pain is crucial.

In the spontaneously arising pains of long duration, as in myocardial infarction, dissecting aneurysm, pulmonary embolism, acute pericarditis, gallbladder colic, incarcerated hiatal hernia, acute pancreatitis, in all of which the pain may be identical in location, severity, character, and sites of reference, it is often the corollary data, clinical and laboratory, that finally determine the diagnosis.

Reproducing and alleviating the discomfort is not only sometimes of value in establishing the diagnosis but of immense psychologic benefit to the patient when he learns that an apparently mysterious and disturbing disorder can be mimicked and relieved at will.

When, as will occasionally occur, the thorough examination leaves one in doubt, observation over a period of time will often clarify the question, at least to the extent of establishing or excluding the more serious causes of the pain. Under such circumstances the patient should be advised to follow the same exertional and dietary regime which one would advise in any healthy middle-aged person, because this is essentially the same as that advised for a person with minimal myocardial ischemia. At the same time, fear can be alleviated by the reassurance that this regime is aimed not at treatment of an existing condition but at preventing future vascular disease.

REFERENCES

Braunwald, E.: The Determinants of Myocardial Oxygen Consumption, The Physiologist, 12:65, 1969.

Burch, G. E., J. M. Phillips, and N. P. De Pasquale: Cardiac Causalgia, Am. Heart J., 76:725, 1968.

Capps, J. A.: Pain from the Pleura and Pericardium, Assoc. Research Nervous and Mental Disease, Proc. (1942) 23: 263, 1943.

Friedberg, C. K.: Angina Pectoris—Diagnosis, Differential Diagnosis, Prognosis and Treatment, Chap. 19 in "Diseases of the Heart," 3d ed., pp. 734–769, Philadelphia, W. B. Saunders Company, 1966.

Hurst, J. W., and R. B. Logue: Symptoms Due to Heart Disease, Chap. 3 in "The Heart," 1st ed., pp. 47–53, New York, McGraw-Hill Book Company, 1966.

Keefer, C. S., and W. H. Resnik: Angina Pectoris: A Syndrome Caused by Anoxemia of the Myocardium, Arch. Intern. Med., 41:769, 1928.

Keele, K. D.: Pain Complaint Threshold in Relation to Pain of Cardiac Infarction, Brit. Med. J. (Lancet), 1:670, 1968.

Pain and Its Clinical Management, Med. Clinics N. Am., 52: 1–228, 1968.

Prinzmetal, M., and R. A. Massumi: Anterior Chest Wall Syndrome: Chest Pain Resembling Pain of Cardiac Origin, J.A.M.A., 159:177, 1955.

Wehrmacher, William H.: "Pain in the Chest," Springfield, Ill., Charles C Thomas, Publisher, 1964.

Wood, P.: The Chief Symptoms of Heart Disease, Chap. 1 in "Diseases of the Heart and Circulation," 3d ed., pp. 1–25, Philadelphia, J. B. Lippincott Company, 1968.

12 ABDOMINAL PAIN
William Silen

The correct interpretation of acute abdominal pain is one of the most challenging demands made of any physician. Since proper therapy often requires urgent action, the luxury of the leisurely approach suitable for the study of other conditions is frequently denied. Few other clinical situations demand greater experience and judgment, because the most catastrophic of events may be forecast by the subtlest of symptoms and signs. Nowhere in medicine is a meticulously executed detailed history and physical examination of greater importance. The etiologic classification in Table 12-1, although not complete, forms a useful frame of reference for the evaluation of patients with abdominal pain.

The diagnosis of "acute or surgical abdomen" so often heard in emergency wards is not an acceptable one because of its often misleading and erroneous connotation. The most obvious of "acute abdomens" may not require operative intervention, and the mildest of abdominal pains may herald the onset of an urgently correctible lesion. Any patient with abdominal pain of recent onset requires early and thorough evaluation with specific attempts at accurate diagnosis.

SOME MECHANISMS OF PAIN ORIGINATING IN THE ABDOMEN

INFLAMMATION OF THE PARIETAL PERITONEUM. The pain of parietal peritoneal inflammation is steady and aching in character and is located directly over the inflamed area, its exact reference being possible because it is transmitted by overlapping somatic nerves supplying the parietal peritoneum. The intensity of the pain is dependent upon the type and amount of foreign substance to which the peritoneal surfaces are exposed in a given period of time. For example, the sudden release into the peritoneal cavity of a small quantity of *sterile* acid gastric juice causes much more pain than the same amount of grossly contaminated neutral fecal material. Enzymatically active pancreatic juice incites more pain and inflammation than does the same amount of sterile bile containing no potent enzymes. Blood and urine are often so bland as to go undetected if exposure of the peritoneum has not been sudden and massive. In the case of bacterial contamination, such as in pelvic inflammatory disease, the pain is frequently of low intensity early in the illness until bacterial multiplication has caused the elaboration of irritating substances.

So important is the rate at which the irritating material is applied to the peritoneum that a perforated peptic ulcer may be associated with entirely different clinical pictures

Table 12-1. SOME IMPORTANT CAUSES OF ABDOMINAL PAIN

I. Pain originating in the abdomen
   A. Parietal peritoneal inflammation
      1. Bacterial contamination, e.g., perforated appendix, pelvic inflammatory disease.
      2. Chemical irritation, e.g., perforated ulcer, pancreatitis, mittelschmerz
   B. Mechanical obstruction of hollow viscera
      1. Obstruction of the small or large intestine
      2. Obstruction of the biliary tree
      3. Obstruction of the ureter
   C. Vascular disturbances
      1. Embolism or thrombosis
      2. Vascular rupture
      3. Pressure or torsional occlusion
      4. Sickle-cell anemia
   D. Abdominal wall
      1. Distortion or traction of mesentery
      2. Trauma or infection of muscles
      3. Distension of visceral surfaces, e.g., hepatic or renal capsules
II. Pain referred from extraabdominal sources
   A. Thorax—e.g., pneumonia, referred pain from coronary occlusion
   B. Spine—e.g., radiculitis from arthritis
   C. Genitalia—e.g., torsion of the testicle
III. Metabolic causes
   A. Exogenous
      1. Black widow spider bite
      2. Lead poisoning and others
   B. Endogenous
      1. Uremia
      2. Diabetic coma
      3. Porphyria
      4. Allergic factors (C'1 esterase deficiency)
IV. Neurogenic causes
   A. Organic
      1. Tabes dorsalis
      2. Herpes zoster
      3. Causalgia and others
   B. Functional

dependent only upon the rapidity with which the gastric juice enters the peritoneal cavity. *The pain of peritoneal inflammation is invariably accentuated by pressure or changes in tension of the peritoneum,* whether produced by palpation or by movement as in coughing or sneezing. Consequently, the patient with peritonitis lies quietly in bed preferring to avoid motion in contrast to the individual with colic who may writhe incessantly.

The intensity of the tonic muscle spasm accompanying peritoneal inflammation is dependent upon the location of the inflammatory process, the rate at which it develops, and the integrity of the nervous system. Spasm over a perforated retrocecal appendix or perforated ulcer into the lesser peritoneal sac may be minimal or absent because of the protective effect of overlying viscera. As in pain of peritoneal inflammation, a slowly developing process often greatly attentuates the degree of muscle spasm. Catastrophic abdominal emergencies such as a perforated ulcer have been repeatedly associated with minimal or occasionally no detectable pain or muscle spasm in obtunded, seriously ill debilitated elderly patients or in psychotic patients.

OBSTRUCTION OF HOLLOW VISCERA. The pain of obstruction of hollow abdominal viscera is classically described as intermittent, or colicky. Yet, the lack of a truly cramping character should not be misleading, because distension of a hollow viscus may produce steady pain with only very occasional exacerbations. Although not nearly as well localized as the pain of parietal peritoneal inflammation, some useful generalities can be made concerning the distribution of the pain caused by the obstruction of hollow intraabdominal viscera.

The colicky pain associated with obstruction of the small intestine is usually periumbilical or supraumbilical and is poorly localized. As the intestine becomes progressively dilated with loss of muscular tone, the colicky nature of the pain may become less apparent. With superimposed strangulating obstruction, pain may be felt in the lower lumbar region if the obstructing mechanism causes severe traction on the root of the mesentery. Pain arising in the colon is usually perceived in the region involved by the pathologic process.

Sudden distension of the biliary tree produces a steady rather than colicky type of pain, and hence the term "biliary colic" is misleading. Acute distension of the gallbladder usually causes pain in the right upper quadrant with radiation to the right posterior thorax or to the tip of the right scapula, and distension of the common bile duct is often associated with pain in the epigastrium radiating to the upper lumbar region. Considerable variation is common, however, so that differentiation between these may be impossible. The typical subscapular pain of lumbar radiation is frequently absent. Gradual dilatation of the biliary tree as in carcinoma of the head of the pancreas may cause no pain or only a mild aching sensation in the epigastrium or right upper quadrant. The pain of distension of the pancreatic ducts is similar to that described for distension of the common bile duct but in addition is very frequently accentuated by recumbency and relieved by the upright position.

Obstruction of the urinary bladder results in dull suprapubic pain, usually low in intensity. Restlessness without specific complaint of pain may be the only sign of a distended bladder in an obtunded patient. In contrast, acute obstruction of the intravesicular portion of the ureter is characterized by severe suprapubic and flank pain which radiates to the penis, scrotum, or inner aspect of the upper thigh. Obstruction of the ureteropelvic junction is felt as pain in the costovertebral angle, whereas obstruction of the remainder of the ureter is associated with flank pain, which often extends into the corresponding side of the abdomen.

VASCULAR DISTURBANCES. A frequent misconception, despite abundant experience to the contrary, is that pain associated with intraabdominal vascular disturbances is sudden and catastrophic in nature. The pain of embolism or thrombosis of the superior mesenteric artery, or that of impending rupture of an abdominal aortic aneurysm certainly may be severe and diffuse. Yet just as frequently, the patient with occlusion of the superior mesenteric artery has only mild continuous diffuse pain for 2 or 3 days before vascular collapse or findings of peritoneal inflammation are present. The early, seemingly insignificant discomfort is caused by hyperperistalsis rather than peritoneal inflammation. Indeed, absence of tenderness and rigidity in the presence of continuous diffuse pain in a patient likely to have vascular disease is quite characteristic of occlusion of the superior mesenteric artery. Abdominal pain with radiation to the sacral region, flank, or genitalia should always signal the possible presence of a rupturing abdominal aortic aneurysm. This pain may persist over a period of several days before rupture and collapse occur.

ABDOMINAL WALL. Pain arising from the abdominal wall is usually constant and aching. Movement and pressure accentuate the discomfort and muscle spasm. In the case of hematoma of the rectus sheath, now most frequently encountered in association with anticoagulant therapy, a mass may be present in the lower quadrants of the abdomen. Simultaneous involvement of muscles in other parts of the body usually serves to differentiate myositis of the abdominal wall from an intraabdominal process which might cause pain in the same region.

REFERRED PAIN FROM EXTRAABDOMINAL SOURCES AND FROM ABDOMEN TO OTHER AREAS

Pain referred to the abdomen from the thorax, spine, or genitalia may prove a vexing problem in differential diagnosis, because diseases of the upper abdominal cavity such as acute cholecystitis, perforated ulcer, or subphrenic abscesses are frequently associated with intrathoracic complications. A most important, yet often forgotten, dictum is that the possibility of intrathoracic disease must be considered in every patient with abdominal pain, especially if the pain is in the upper abdomen. Systematic questioning and examination directed towards detecting the presence or absence of myocardial or pulmonary infarction, pneumonia, pericarditis, or esophageal disease, the intrathoracic diseases which most often masquerade as abdominal emergencies, will often provide sufficient clues to establish the proper diagnosis. Diaphragmatic pleuritis resulting from pneumonia or pulmonary infarction may cause pain in the right upper quadrant and pain in the supraclavicular area, the latter radiation to be sharply distinguished from the referred subscapular pain caused by acute distension of the extrahepatic biliary tree. The ultimate decision as to the origin of abdominal pain may require deliberate and planned observation over a period of several hours, during which time repeated questioning and examination will provide the proper explanation.

Referred pain of thoracic origin is often accompanied by splinting of the involved hemithorax with respiratory lag and decrease in excursion more marked than that seen in the presence of intraabdominal disease. In addition, apparent abdominal muscle spasm caused by referred pain will diminish during the inspiratory phase of respiration, whereas it is persistent throughout both respiratory phases if it is of abdominal origin. Palpation over the area of referred pain in the abdomen also does not usually accentuate the pain and in many instances actually seems to relieve it. The frequent coexistence of thoracic and abdominal disease may be misleading and confusing, so that differentiation might be difficult or impossible. For example, the patient with known biliary tract disease often has epigastric pain during myocardial infarction, or biliary colic may be referred to the precordium or left shoulder in a patient who has suffered previously from angina pectoris. The explanation for the radiation of pain to a previously diseased area has not been elucidated.

Referred pain from the spine, which usually involves compression or irritation of nerve roots, is characteristically intensified by certain motions such as cough, sneeze, or strain and is associated with hyperesthesia over the involved dermatomes. Pain referred to the abdomen from the testicles or seminal vesicles is generally accentuated by the slightest pressure on either of these organs. The abdominal discomfort is of dull aching character and is poorly localized.

METABOLIC ABDOMINAL CRISES

Pain of metabolic origin may simulate almost any other type of intraabdominal disease. Here several mechanisms may be at work. In certain instances such as hyperparathyroidism, the metabolic disease itself may produce an intraabdominal process such as pancreatitis. Primary hyperlipemia may also be accompanied by severe pancreatitis, which can lead to unnecessary laparotomy unless recognized. C'1 esterase deficiency associated with angioneurotic edema is also often associated with episodes of severe abdominal pain. Whenever the cause of abdominal pain is obscure, a metabolic origin must always be considered. Abdominal pain is the hallmark of familial Mediterranean fever (Chap. 256).

The problem of differential diagnosis is often not readily resolved. The pain of porphyria and lead colic usually are difficult to distinguish from that of intestinal obstruction, because severe hyperperistalsis is a prominent feature of both. The pain of uremia or diabetes is nonspecific, and the pain and tenderness frequently shift in location and intensity. Diabetic acidosis may be precipitated by acute appendicitis or intestinal obstruction, so that if prompt resolution of the abdominal pain does not result from correction of the metabolic abnormalities, an underlying organic problem should be suspected. Black widow spider bites produce intense pain and rigidity of the abdominal muscles and of the back, an area infrequently involved in disease of intraabdominal origin.

NEUROGENIC CAUSES

Causalgic pain may occur in diseases which injure nerves of sensory type. It has a burning character and is usually limited to the distribution of a given peripheral nerve. Normal stimuli such as touch or change in temperature are transformed into, and may precipitate, this type of pain, which is also frequently present in a patient at rest. A helpful finding is the demonstration that cutaneous pain spots are irregularly spaced, and this may be the only indication of the presence of causalgic pain. Even though the pain may be precipitated by gentle palpation, rigidity of the abdominal muscles is absent, and the respirations are not disturbed. Distension of the abdomen is uncommon, and the pain has no relationship to the intake of food.

Pain arising from spinal nerves or roots may be caused by herpes zoster, impingement by arthritis, tumors, herniated nucleus pulposus, diabetes, or syphilis, comes and goes suddenly, and is of a lancinating type. Again it is not associated with food intake, abdominal distension, or changes in respiration. Severe muscle spasm, as in the gastric crises of tabes dorsalis, is common but is either relieved or is not accentuated by abdominal palpation. The pain is made worse by movement of the spine and is usually confined to a few dermatome segments. Hyperesthesia is very common.

Psychogenic pain conforms to none of the aforementioned patterns of disease. Here the mechanism is hard to define, and the most common problem is the hysterical adolescent or young woman who frequently loses an appendix and other organs because of abdominal pain. Ovulation or some other natural event that causes brief mild abdominal discomfort may be maximized as an abdominal catastrophe.

Psychogenic pain varies enormously in type and location but usually has no relation to meals. It is often at its onset markedly accentuated during the night. Nausea and vomiting are rarely observed, although occasionally the patient reports these symptoms. Spasm is seldom induced in the abdominal musculature and if present does not persist, especially if the attention of the patient can be distracted. Persistent localized tenderness is rare, and, if found, the muscle spasm in the area is inconsistent and often absent. Restriction of the depth of respiration is the most common respiratory abnormality, but this occurs in the absence of thoracic splinting or change in the respiratory rate.

APPROACH TO THE PATIENT WITH ABDOMINAL PAIN

There are few abdominal conditions which require such urgent operative intervention that an orderly approach need be abandoned, no matter how ill the patient. Only those patients with exsanguinating hemorrhage must be rushed to the operating room immediately, but in such instances only a few minutes are required to assess the critical nature of the problem. Under these circumstances, all obstacles must be swept aside, adequate access for intravenous fluid replacement obtained, and the operation begun. Many patients of this type have expired in the radiology department or the emergency room while awaiting such unnecessary examinations as electrocardiograms or films of the abdomen. *There are no contraindications to operation when massive hemor-*

rhage is present. Although exceedingly important, this situation fortunately is relatively rare.

Nothing will supplant an orderly painstakingly *detailed history*, which is far more valuable than any laboratory or roentgenologic examination. This kind of history is laborious and time-consuming, making it not especially popular even though a reasonably accurate diagnosis can be made on the basis of the history alone in the majority of cases. The *chronological sequence of events* in the patient's history is often more important than emphasis on the location of pain. If the examiner is sufficiently open-minded and unhurried, asks the proper questions, and listens, the patient will often himself provide the diagnosis. Careful attention should be paid to the extraabdominal regions which may be responsible for abdominal pain. An accurate menstrual history in a female patient is essential. Narcotics or analgesics should be withheld until a definitive diagnosis or a definitive plan has been formulated, because these agents often make it more difficult to secure and to interpret the history and physical findings.

In the examination, simple critical inspection of the patient, for example of his facies, position in bed, and respiratory activity, may provide valuable clues. The amount of information to be gleaned is directly proportional to the *gentleness* and thoroughness of the examiner. Once a patient with peritoneal inflammation has been examined in a brusque manner, accurate assessment by the next examiner becomes almost impossible. For example, eliciting rebound tenderness by sudden release of a deeply palpating hand in a patient with suspected peritonitis is cruel and unnecessary. The same information can be obtained by gentle percussion of the abdomen (rebound tenderness on a miniature scale), a maneuver which can be far more precise and localizing. Asking the patient to cough will elicit true rebound tenderness without the need for placing a hand on the abdomen. Furthermore, the brusque demonstration of rebound tenderness will startle and induce protective spasm in a nervous or worried patient in whom true rebound tenderness is not present. A palpable gallbladder will be missed if palpation is so brusque that voluntary muscle spasm becomes superimposed upon involuntary muscular rigidity.

As in history taking, there is no substitute for sufficient time spent in the examination. It is important to remember that abdominal signs may be minimal but nevertheless exceptionally meaningful if carefully assessed with consistent symptomatology. Signs may be virtually or actually totally absent in cases of pelvic peritonitis, so that careful *pelvic and rectal examination are mandatory in every patient with abdominal pain.* The presence of tenderness on pelvic or rectal examination in the absence of other abdominal signs must not lead the examiner to exclude such important operative indications as perforated appendicitis, diverticulitis, twisted ovarian cyst, and many others.

Much attention has been paid to the presence or absence of peristaltic sounds, their quality and frequency. Auscultation of the abdomen is probably one of the least rewarding aspects of the physical examination of a patient with abdominal pain. Severe catastrophes, such as strangulating small-bowel obstruction or perforated appendicitis, may occur in the presence of normal peristalsis. Conversely, when the proximal intestine above an obstruction becomes markedly distended and edematous, peristaltic sounds may lose the characteristics of borborygmi and become weak or absent even when peritonitis is not present. It is usually the severe chemical peritonitis of sudden onset which is associated with the truly silent abdomen. Assessment of the patient's state of hydration is important. The hematocrit and urinalysis permit an accurate estimate of the severity of dehydration, so that adequate replacement can be carried out.

Laboratory examinations may be of enormous value in the assessment of the patient with abdominal pain, yet with but a few exceptions they rarely establish a diagnosis. Leukocytosis should never be the single deciding factor as to whether or not operation is indicated. A white blood cell count greater than 20,000 may be observed with perforation of a viscus, but pancreatitis, acute cholecystitis, pelvic inflammatory disease, and intestinal infarction may be associated with marked leukocytosis. A normal white blood cell count is by no means rare in cases of perforation of abdominal viscera. The diagnosis of anemia may be more helpful than the white blood cell count, especially when combined with the history.

The urinalysis is also of great value in indicating to some degree the state of hydration or to rule out severe renal disease, diabetes, or porphyria. Determination of the blood urea nitrogen, blood sugar, and serum bilirubin may also be helpful. The serum amylase determination is overrated, since in carefully controlled series where the determination has been done within the first 72 hours, the amylase was less than 200 Somogyi units in one-third of the cases, between 200 and 500 in another one-third, and greater than 500 in one-third. Since many diseases other than pancreatitis, e.g., perforated ulcer, strangulating bowel obstruction, and acute cholecystitis, may be associated with very marked increase in the serum amylase, great care must be exercised in denying an operation to a patient solely on the basis of an elevated serum amylase level. The determination of the output of urinary amylase is probably more accurate than the estimation of the serum amylase in the diagnosis of pancreatitis.

Abdominal paracentesis has proved to be a safe and effective diagnostic maneuver in patients with acute abdominal pain. It is of special value in patients with blunt trauma to the abdomen where evaluation of the abdomen may be difficult because of other multiple injuries to the spine, pelvis, or ribs and where blood in the peritoneal cavity produces only a very mild peritoneal reaction. The gallbladder is the only organ which may continue to seep fluid following accidental perforation, so that the region of this organ must be assiduously avoided. Determination of the pH of the aspirated fluid to ascertain the site of a perforation is misleading, because even highly acid gastric juice is rapidly buffered by peritoneal exudate.

Plain and upright or lateral decubitus x-rays of the abdomen may be of the greatest value. They are usually unnecessary in patients with acute appendicitis or strangulated external hernias. However, in intestinal obstruction, perforated ulcer, and a variety of other conditions, films may be diagnostic. During a search for free air, the patient should be kept in the decubitus or upright position for at least 10 min before the appropriate film is taken lest a small pneumoperitoneum be missed. In rare instances, barium or water-soluble medium examination of the upper gastrointestinal tract may demonstrate partial intestinal obstruction which may elude diagnosis by other means. If there is any question of obstruction of the colon, oral administration of barium sulfate should be avoided. On the other hand, barium enema is of inestimable value in cases of colonic obstruction and should be used with greater frequency where the possibility of perforation does not exist.

Sometimes, even under the best of circumstances with all available auxiliary aids and with the greatest of clinical skill, a definitive diagnosis cannot be established when a patient is evaluated initially. Nevertheless, despite lack of a clear anatomic diagnosis it may be abundantly clear to an experienced and thoughtful physician and surgeon on clinical grounds alone that operation is indicated. Should that decision be questionable, watchful waiting with repeated questioning and examination will often elucidate the true nature of the illness and indicate the proper course of action.

REFERENCES

Cope, Z.: "The Early Diagnosis of the Acute Abdomen," 10th ed., Fair Lawn, N.J., Oxford University Press, 1953.

Fitz, R. H.: Perforating Inflammation of the Vermiform Appendix: With Special Reference to Its Early Diagnosis and Treatment, Trans. Assoc. Am. Physicians, 1:107, 1886.

Glenn, F.: Pain in Biliary Tract Disease, Surg. Gynecol. Obstet., 122:495, 1966.

Holman, E.: The Art of Abdominal Percussion in the Presence of Inflammation, Surg. Gynecol. Obstet., 93:775, 1951.

Lewis, T.: "Pain," New York, The Macmillan Company, 1942.

—— and J. H. Kellgren: Observation Relating to Referred Pain, Visceromotor Reflexes and Other Related Phenomena, Clin. Sci., 4:47, 1939.

Silen, W., M. F. Hein, and L. Goldman: Strangulation Obstruction of the Small Intestine, Arch. Surg., 85:121, 1962.

13 PAIN IN THE BACK AND NECK

Thornton Brown, Michel Jequier, and Raymond Adams

The following remarks concern mainly the lower back, since it is most frequently the site of disabling pain. The lower spine and pelvis, with their many muscular and tendinous attachments, are relatively inaccessible to palpation and also to inspection, even through the medium of x-ray. For want of reliable physical signs and laboratory tests, it is often necessary to depend on the patient's description of his pain, which may not be altogether accurate, and his behavior during the execution of certain maneuvers. Seasoned clinicians, for these reasons, come to appreciate the need of a systematic clinical approach, the description of which will be one of the main purposes of this chapter.

ANATOMY AND PHYSIOLOGY OF THE LOWER BACK

The spine is roughly divisible into two parts: an anterior column of articulated vertebral bodies and intervertebral disks held together by the anterior and posterior longitudinal ligaments and annulus fibrosus which together constitute the supporting pillar of the body; and a posterior segment consisting of pedicles and laminas, fused to form the walls of the spinal canal, which provides protection for the spinal cord.

The stability of the spine depends on two types of supporting structures, the ligamentous (passive) and muscular (active). Active muscular support and movement are contributed by the erector spinae, abdominal, glutei maximus, psoas, and hamstring muscles.

The vertebral and paravertebral structures derive their innervation from the recurrent branches of the spinal nerves. Pain endings and fibers have been demonstrated in the ligaments, muscles, periosteum of bone, outer layers of annulus fibrosus, and synovium of the articular facets. The sensory fibers from these structures and the sacroiliac and lumbosacral joints join to form the sinovertebral nerves which pass via the recurrent branches of the spinal nerves of the first sacral and the fifth to first lumbar vertebras into the gray matter of the corresponding segments of the spinal cord. Efferent fibers emerge from these segments and extend to the muscles through the same nerves. The sympathetic nerves contribute only to the innervation of blood vessels and appear to play no part in voluntary and reflex movement, though they do contain sensory fibers.

The parts of the back that possess the greatest freedom of movement and hence are most frequently subject to injury, are the lumbar and cervical. The majority of their movements are reflex and are the basis of posture.

GENERAL CLINICAL CONSIDERATIONS

TYPES OF LOW BACK PAIN. Of the several symptoms of disease of the spine (pain, stiffness or limitation of movement, and deformity), pain is of foremost importance by virtue of its frequency and its disabling effects. Four types of pain may be differentiated: local, referred, radicular, and that arising from secondary (protective) muscular spasm. One must identify these several types of pain by the patient's description, and here reliance is placed mainly on the character, location, and the conditions which modify them. The mechanism

of the several types of pain has already been described in Chap. 9.

Local pain is caused by any pathologic process which impinges upon or irritates sensory endings. Involvement of structures which contain no sensory endings is painless. The substance of the vertebral body may be destroyed by tumor, for example, without evocation of pain, whereas lesions of periosteum, synovial membranes, muscles, annulus fibrosus, and ligaments are often exquisitely painful. Although painful states are often accompanied by swelling of the affected tissues, this is not apparent if a deep structure of the back is the site of disease. Local pain is steady, sometimes intermittent, of the aching type, and rather diffuse but is always felt in or near the affected part of the spine. Often there is involuntary splinting of the spine segments by paravertebral muscles, and certain movements or postures which alter the position of the injured tissues aggravate or relieve the pain. Firm pressure upon superficial structures in the region of the involved structure usually evokes tenderness which is of aid in identifying the site of the abnormality.

Referred pain is of two types, that projected from the spine into regions lying within the area of the lumbar and upper sacral dermatomes and that projected from the pelvic and abdominal viscera to the spine. Pain due to diseases of the upper lumbar spine is usually referred to the anterior aspects of the thighs and legs; and that from the lower lumbar spine is referred to the gluteal regions, posterior thighs, and calves. Pain of this type tends also to be deep, of aching quality, and rather diffuse. In general the referred pain parallels in intensity the local pain in the back. In other words, maneuvers which alter local pain have a similar effect on referred pain, though not with such precision and immediacy as in "root pain." Pain from visceral disease usually is felt within the abdomen or flanks and may be modified by the state of activity of the viscera. Its character and temporal relationships are those of the particular visceral structure involved, and posture and movement of the back have relatively little effect, either on the local pain or that referred to the back.

Radicular, or "root," *pain* has some of the characteristics of referred pain but differs in its greater intensity, distal radiation, circumscription to the territory of a root, and the factors which excite it. The mechanism is distortion, stretching, irritation, or compression of a spinal root, most often central to the intervertebral foramen. The pain is sharp, often quite intense, and nearly always radiates from a central position near the spine to some part of the lower extremity. It is usually superimposed on the dull ache of referred pain. Cough, sneeze, and strain characteristically evoke this sharp radiating pain, though these maneuvers may also jar or move the spine and enhance local pain. Any motion which stretches the nerve, i.e., forward bending with the knees extended or "straight-leg raising," excites radicular pain; and jugular vein compression, which raises intraspinal pressure and may cause a shift in the position of the root, has a similar effect. The fourth and fifth lumbar and first sacral roots, which form the sciatic nerve, if involved in disease, cause pain which extends mainly down the posterior aspects of thigh, the postero- and anterolateral aspects of the leg, and into the foot, in the distribution of this nerve —so-called "sciatica." Tingling, paresthesias, and numbness or sensory impairment of the skin, soreness of the skin, and tenderness along the nerve usually accompany radicular pain. Also reflex loss, weakness, atrophy, fascicular twitching, and often stasis edema may occur if motor fibers are involved in the anterior roots.

Pain resulting from muscular spasm is usually mentioned in relation to local pain, but it deserves separate consideration. As stated above, muscle spasm is associated with most conditions which result in local pain. Muscles in a state of persistent tension give rise to a dull ache, which Smith-Petersen called "secondary pain." One can feel the tautness of the erector spinae and gluteal muscles and demonstrate by palpation that the pain is localized to them.

Other pains often of undetermined origin are sometimes described by patients with chronic disease of the lower back. In the legs drawing, pulling, cramping sensations (without involuntary muscle spasm), tearing, throbbing, or jabbing pains, feelings of burning or coldness are difficult to interpret and, like paresthesias and numbness, should always suggest the possibility of nerve or root disease.

Since it is often difficult to obtain physical or laboratory confirmation of painful disease of the lower spine, the importance of an accurate history and description of symptoms cannot be overemphasized. Frequently the most important lead comes from the knowledge of the mode of onset and circumstances which initiated the pain. Inasmuch as many painful affections of the back are the result of injury incurred during work or in an accident, the possibility of exaggeration or prolongation of pain for personal reasons, or even hysteria or malingering, must always be kept in mind.

THE EXAMINATION OF THE LOWER BACK. *Inspection* of the spine, buttocks, and legs when standing erect, walking, stooping, and squatting is of value. The patient's resting posture should be noted because faulty posture predisposes to pain in the lumbosacral and sacroiliac regions. With sciatica the lumbar spine is often scoliotic, with the convexity toward the normal side, though the converse may occur. Also, a slight flexion or flattening of the lumbar lordosis is common with acute painful states. The presence of a definite kyphosis usually signifies deformity of one of the vertebral bodies, e.g., fracture. Spasm of paravertebral muscles on one or both sides is often obvious during inspection. One may also notice a hypotonia of the gluteus maximus on the affected side with drooping of the gluteal fold.

The next step in the examination is observation of the spine, hips, and legs during certain motions. During the procedure it is well to remember that no advantage accrues from trying to find out how much the patient can be hurt. Instead, it is much more important to deter-

mine when and under what conditions the pain commences. One looks for limitation of the natural motions of the patient as he disrobes and while he is standing, sitting, and reclining. When standing, the motion of forward bending normally produces flattening and reversal of the lumbar lordotic curve and exaggeration of the dorsal curve. With lesions of the lumbosacral region which involve the posterior ligaments, articular facets, or erector spinae and with ruptured lumbar discs the patient attempts to avoid stretching these structures. As a consequence, the erectores spinae remain taut and prevent motion in the lumbar spine. Forward bending then occurs at the hips and at the lumbar-thoracic junction. With disease of the lumbosacral joints and spinal roots, the patient bends in such a way as to avoid tensing the hamstring muscles and putting undue leverage upon the pelvis. In unilateral "sciatica," with its increased curvature toward the side of the lesion, lumbar and lumbosacral motions are splinted and bending is mainly at the hips; at a certain point the knee on the affected side is flexed to relieve hamstring spasm and tilting of the pelvis, and to slacken the roots and sciatic nerve.

Lateral bending is usually less instructive than forward bending. However, in unilateral ligamentous or muscular strain, bending to the opposite side aggravates the pain by stretching the damaged tissues. Moreover, in lateral disc lesions, bending of the spine toward the side from which the trunk lists is restricted.

In diseases of the lower spine, flexion while sitting can normally be performed easily, even to the point of bringing the knees in contact with the chest. The reason for this is that knee flexion relaxes the hamstring muscles and relieves stretch of the sciatic nerve. The lumbar and lumbosacral joints and the normal curve of the spine need not be altered under these conditions. On the other hand, if the knees are extended, the same impedance of movement noted during forward bending, while standing with the legs straight, is observed.

The study of motions in the reclining position yields the same information as those in the standing and sitting positions, with the difference that there is less pressure on the discs. Passive lumbar flexion is like active forward bending in the standing position. With lumbosacral lesions and sciatica, it causes little pain and is not limited as long as the hamstrings and sciatic nerve are relaxed (knee flexed). With lumbosacral and lumbar spine disease (e.g., arthritis), passive flexion of the hips is free, whereas flexion of the lumbar spine is impeded and painful. Passive straight-leg raising (possibly up to 90° except in those who are congenitally stiff), like forward bending in the standing posture with the legs straight, places the sciatic nerve and its roots, also the hamstrings, under tension, thereby producing pain. It also rotates the pelvis, thus causing lumbar joint pain. Consequently, in diseases of the lumbosacral joints and of the lumbosacral roots, this movement is limited on the affected side and, to a lesser extent, the opposite side. Lasegue's sign (pain and limitation of movement during elevation of the leg when the knee is extended) is but a variation of this test, as are Goldthwait's sign (limited extension at the knee after the thigh has been flexed on the trunk), Lewin's sign (snapping back of the knee into flexion when released), and Bragaard's sign of pain in the opposite leg during straight-leg raising. The evoked pain is always referred to the diseased side, no matter which leg is flexed. In disease of the lumbosacral joints there may also be slight limitation of straight-leg raising, though rarely to the degree seen in disease of the lumbosacral roots.

The motion of hyperextension is best performed with the patient standing or lying prone. If the condition causing back pain is acute, it may be difficult to extend the spine in the standing position. A patient with lumbosacral strain can usually extend or hyperextend the spine without aggravation of pain. If involved in an active inflammatory or other acute process, however, vertical pressure upon these joints will increase the pain. Also, if there is ligamentous strain, no enhancement of pain occurs because the posterior segments of the spine are relaxed during extension. The converse is true if there is strain of extensor muscles, for hyperextension places the muscular attachments to the periosteum under tension. Although disease of articular facets may limit ex-

tension, little or no pain is produced. In lumbar disc disease (except in the acute phase of the illness), extension of the spine is usually tolerated well, though in some patients with a displaced disc fragment situated posterolaterally, pain is evoked by extension rather than flexion. A reversed Lasegue's sign (limitation in the hyperextension of straight leg while in prone position) suggests spinal nerve involvement at the midlumbar level or a lesion of the lumbosacral joint.

Palpation and percussion of the spine are the last steps in the examination. The approach must always be gentle since rough percussion of the designated area of pain only confuses the physician and antagonizes the patient. It is preferable to palpate first those regions which are the least likely to evoke pain. At all times the examiner should know what structures are being palpated (see Fig. 13-1). Localized tenderness is seldom pronounced in disease of the spine because the involved structures are so deep that they rarely give rise to surface tenderness. Mild superficial and poorly localized tenderness signifies only a disease process within the affected segment of the body, i.e., dermatome.

Tenderness over the costovertebral angle often indicates genitourinary disease, adrenal disease (Rogoff's sign), or an injury to the transverse processes of the first or second lumbar vertebra [Fig. 13-1 (1)]. Hypersensitivity on palpation of the transverse processes of the other lumbar vertebras as well as the overlying erector spinae muscles may signify fracture of the transverse process or a strain of muscle attachments.

Upon palpation of the spinous processes and interspinous ligaments any deviation in the anteroposterior or lateral plane must be particularly noted. Such a deviation usually indicates spondylolisthesis. Tenderness of the interspinous ligaments is indicative of disc lesions [Fig. 13-1 (2)].

Tenderness in the region of the articular facets between the fifth lumbar and first sacral vertebras is consistent with a lumbosacral disc disease [Fig. 13-1 (3)]. It is also not infrequent in rheumatoid arthritis.

Rectal and pelvic examination constitute an essential part of the diagnostic study of all cases of low back pain and sciatica.

Upon completion of the examination of the back a search for motor, reflex, and sensory changes (see Syndrome of Ruptured Disc, below), particularly in the lower extremities, should be made.

SPECIAL LABORATORY PROCEDURES. Laboratory tests often aid in diagnosis. Depending on the circumstances, these may include measurement of the serum proteins, phosphatases (alkaline and acid), calcium, phosphorus, uric acid, serum electrophoresis (myeloma proteins), tuberculin, agglutination for Brucella, sedimentation rate, and rheumatoid factor. X-rays should be taken in every case of low back pain and sciatica in the anteriorposterior, lateral, and oblique planes of the lumbar spine (looking for abnormal mobility with disc disease) and at times, the thoracic spine. Stereoscopic or laminographic films may provide further information if the regular x-rays show abnormalities. In many cases of low

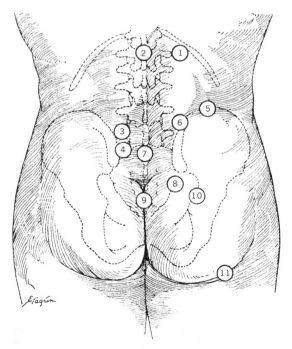

Fig. 13-1. (1) Costovertebral angle. (2) Spinous process and interspinous ligament. (3) Region of articular fifth lumbar to first sacral facet. (4) Dorsum of sacrum. (5) Region of iliac crest. (6) Iliolumbar angle. (7) Spinous processes of fifth lumbar to first sacral vertebras (tenderness = faulty posture or occasionally spina bifida occulta). (8) Region between posterior superior and posterior inferior spines. Sacroiliac ligaments (tenderness = sacroiliac sprain; often tender with fifth lumbar to first sacral disk). (9) Sacrococcygeal junction (tenderness = sacrococcygeal injury, i.e., sprain or fracture). (10) Region of sacrosciatic notch (tenderness = fourth to fifth lumbar disk rupture and sacroiliac sprain). (11) Sciatic nerve trunk (tenderness = ruptured lumbar disk or sciatic nerve lesion).

back pain with neurologic manifestations, examination of the spinal canal with a contrast medium (myelogram) is necessary. This study can be combined with tests of dynamics of the cerebrospinal fluid, and a sample of the fluid should always be removed for cytologic and chemical examination prior to the installation of the contrast medium (Pantopaque, Myodil, or air). Injection and removal of Pantopaque require special skill and should not be attempted without previous experience with the procedure. If done properly, the procedure is harmless. Injection of contrast medium directly into the intervertebral disc (discograms) has recently become popular but is still controversial. The technique of this procedure is more complicated than that of myelographic examination, and the risk of damage to nerve roots or the introduction of infection is not inconsiderable. In the authors' opinion, the results do not warrant the risk involved.

PRINCIPAL CONDITIONS WHICH GIVE RISE TO DISABLING PAIN IN THE LOWER BACK

CONGENITAL ANOMALIES OF THE LUMBAR SPINE

Anatomic variations of the spine are not at all infrequent, and although not of themselves the source of pain and functional derangement, they may be of importance because they dispose to strain by permitting excessive mobility or the adoption of abnormal postures.

There may be a lack of fusion of the laminas of the neural arch—a spina bifida—of one or several of the lumbar vertebras, or of the sacrum. Hypertrichosis or hyperpigmentation in the sacral area may betray the condition, but it may remain entirely occult until disclosed by x-ray. The anomaly induces pain only when accompanied by malformation of vertebral joints or stretching and distortion of nerve roots.

Spondylolysis, another important anomaly, consists of a bony defect in the pars interarticularis, which is replaced by cartilage, permitting a forward displacement of the vertebral body, pedicles, superior articular processes, leaving the laminae, inferior articular processes and spinous processes behind (spondylolisthesis). Although of congenital origin, the first symptoms of disordered function (low back pain radiating to the thighs, tightness of back muscles, and signs of involvement of spinal roots—paresthesias and sensory loss, muscle weakness, and reflex impairment) may not appear until later in life and are often precipitated by an injury.

Articular facets of the vertebras may be set in an unusual plane, either oblique or frontal, rather than the sagittal one as in the normal lumbar spine; there may also be an abnormality of the number of mobile lumbar vertebras (either six or four). The lowest vertebra may be asymmetric in its relation to the sacrum. Although these abnormalities have been blamed for chronic low back pain, large surveys suggest that they bear no relationship to it.

TRAUMATIC AFFLICTIONS OF THE LOWER BACK

Trauma constitutes the most frequent cause of low back pain.

In severe acute injuries, the examining physician must be careful to avoid further damage. In tests of motility, all movements must be kept to a minimum until an approximate diagnosis has been made and adequate measures have been instituted for the proper care of the patient. If the patient complains of pain in his back and cannot move his legs, his spine may have been fractured. His neck should not be flexed nor should he be allowed to sit up. (See Chap. 356 for further discussion of spinal cord injury.)

SPRAINS AND STRAINS. The terms *strain* and *sprain* are used loosely by most physicians. It is probably impossible to differentiate between them. Here we shall use only the word strain. Strain should designate a minor injury which does not produce gross structural damage. The abnormal mechanical force may be acute, as in heavy lifting, or mild and persistent, due to maintenance of an abnormal posture. The latter is often occupational. Rest and relaxation promptly alleviate the discomfort, attesting to the lack of major structural change. What formerly was regarded as sacroiliac strain or sprain is now known to be due to discogenic disease in most instances. This is caused by lifting heavy objects with the spine in a position of imperfect mechanical balance, as when lifting and turning at the same time. Sudden unexpected motion is particularly dangerous.

The diagnosis of lumbosacral and sacroiliac strains with injury of the various structures of the lower back depends upon the description of the injury, the localization of the pain by the patient, the finding of localized tenderness, and the augmentation of pain when tension is exerted on the involved structures by the appropriate maneuvers. The prompt alleviation of the pain by rest and relaxation indicates the existence of a strain. The role of recovery depends on the degree of damage, pre-existing disc disease, etc. It may, however, be relieved by local infiltration of an anesthetic agent, a finding which is also helpful in diagnosis.

Sacroiliac strain, once so popular as an explanation of unilateral back pain, is now highly controversial. Because of their irregular surfaces, the sacroiliac bones are interlocked, and joint movement is minimal and is further restricted by strong sacroiliac ligaments. Only violent injury could derange this well-protected and stable joint. Multiple pregnancies close together may be another cause. When the joint is injured, the principal symptom is a localized ache which is made worse by compression of the pelvis. It must be remembered that involvement of a spinal nerve root (fifth lumbar or first sacral) associated with injury to the disk is the more common cause of pain and local tenderness in the area of the sacroiliac joint.

VERTEBRAL FRACTURES. Fractures of the lumbar vertebral body are usually the result of flexion injuries. This is most likely to occur in falls from a height; often the calcaneus is also fractured. Nearly always there is localized tenderness over the fractured vertebra. Spasm of the lower lumbar muscles, limitation of movements of the lumbar spine, and the x-ray appearance of the damaged portion of the lumbar spine (with or without neurologic abnormalities) are the basis of clinical diagnosis. The pain is usually immediate, though occasionally it may be delayed for days, and some patients are found to have had crushed fractures of the vertebral body without being able to recall any traumatic episode.

Fractured transverse processes, which are almost always associated with tearing of the paravertebral muscles, are diagnosed by the finding of deep tenderness at the site of the injury, local muscle spasm on one side, and limitation of all movements which stretch the lumbar muscles. Radiologic evidence provides the final confirmation.

PROTRUSION OF LUMBAR INTERVERTEBRAL DISCS. This condition is now recognized as the major cause of severe and chronic or recurrent low back and leg pain. It is most likely to occur between the fifth lumbar and first sacral vertebras and, with lessening frequency, between the fourth to fifth lumbar, the third to fourth lumbar, the second to third lumbar, and the first to second lumbar vertebras. Almost nonexistent in the thoracic spine, it is next most frequent at the sixth to seventh and fifth to sixth cervical vertebras. The cause is usually a flexion injury, but in a considerable proportion of cases no trauma is recalled. Degeneration of the posterior longitudinal ligaments and the annulus fibrosus, which occurs in most adults of middle and advanced years, may have taken place silently or have been manifested by mild, recurrent lumbar ache. A sneeze, lurch, or other trivial movement may then cause the nucleus pulposus to extrude through the frayed ligament.

The fully developed syndrome of ruptured intervertebral disc consists of backache, abnormal posture, and limitation of motion of the spine (particularly flexion). Nerve root involvement is indicated by radicular pain, sensory disturbances (paresthesias, hyper- and hyposensitivity in dermatome pattern), motor abnormalities (weakness and atrophy, coarse twitching and fasciculation, and muscle spasms), and impairment of tendon reflexes. Since herniation of the intervertebral lumbar discs most often occurs between the fourth and fifth lumbar vertebras and the fifth lumbar and first sacral vertebras with irritation and compression of the fifth lumbar and first sacral roots, respectively, it is important to recognize the clinical characteristics of lesions of these two roots. *Lesions of the fifth lumbar root* produce pain in the region of the hip, groin, posterolateral thigh, lateral calf to the external malleolus, dorsal surface of the foot, and the first or second and third toes. Paresthesias may be in the entire territory or only the distal parts of these territories. The tenderness is in the lateral gluteal region and near the head of the fibula. Weakness, if present, involves the extensor of the big toe and of the foot. Either the knee or ankle reflex may be diminished, but these reflexes are usually unchanged. Walking on the heels may be more uncomfortable than walking on the toes. In *lesions of the first sacral root* the pain is felt in

the midgluteal region, posterior thigh, posterior calf to the heel, and the plantar surface of the foot and fourth and fifth toes. Tenderness is most pronounced over the midgluteal region (sacroiliac joint), posterior thigh, and calf. Paresthesias and sensory loss are mainly in the lower leg and outer toes, and weakness, if present, involves the flexor muscles of the foot and toes, abductors of the toes, and hamstring muscles. The ankle reflex is diminished to absent in the majority of cases. Walking on the toes is more uncomfortable than on the heels. With lesions of either root there may be limitation of straight-leg raising during the acute, painful stages.

Low back pain may also be caused by degeneration of the intervertebral disc, without frank extrusion of fragment of disc tissue. Or the herniation may occur into the adjacent vertebral body, giving rise to Schmorl's nodules. In such cases there are no signs of nerve root involvement though the back pain may be referred to the leg.

The rarer *lesions of the fourth and third lumbar roots* give rise to pain in the anterior part of the thigh and knee, with corresponding sensory loss. The knee-jerk is diminished or abolished. An inverted Lasegue sign is positive when the third lumbar root is affected.

The syndrome is usually unilateral. Only with massive derangements of the discs do bilateral symptoms and signs occur, and these may then be associated with paralysis of the sphincters. The pain may be mild or severe. All or part of the above syndrome may be present. There may be back pain with little or no leg pain; rarely leg pain may be experienced without pain in the back. The rupture of multiple lumbar or lumbar and cervical discs is not infrequent, attesting to a basic disorder of the entire disc including the annulus fibrosus.

When all components of the syndrome are present, the diagnosis is easy; when only one part is present, particularly backache, it may be difficult, especially if there has been no accident. Since similar symptoms may occur without demonstrable disc rupture, other diagnostic procedures are required. Plain x-rays usually show no abnormality or at most a narrowing of the intervertebral space or traction spurs, which is indicative of disc degeneration; hence one must resort to Pantopaque myelography. This will reveal in most cases an indentation of the lumbar subarachnoid space or deformity of the root sleeve. Unfortunately, a small ruptured disc may not show, especially at the L-5 S-1 level. The electromyogram is helpful in showing denervation of leg muscles (see Chap. 390). The protein of the cerebrospinal fluid is elevated in some instances.

Tumor of the spinal canal, epidural or intradural, may produce a syndrome similar to that of ruptured disc (see Chap. 356).

ARTHRITIS

Arthritis will be discussed more fully elsewhere. It need only be mentioned that osteoarthritis is much more frequent than rheumatoid and that the latter may take two forms, one in which the spinal involvement is but a part of a generalized arthritis, often with other signs of "connective tissue disease" and the other limited almost exclusively to the spine, sacroiliac joints, and hips (rheumatoid spondylitis or Marie-Strümpell arthritis) (Chap. 390). An extreme form of osteoarthritis in the cervical region, sometimes leading to spinal cord or nerve compression, is called spondylosis (see Chap. 356).

Rheumatoid spondylitis, which often begins with involvement of the sacroiliac joints, induces continuous aching pain and stiffness in the back or in the buttocks and thigh. Fatigue and other systemic manifestations are usually present. Expansion of the chest is limited when the thoracic spine is involved. However, the disease rarely reaches an advanced degree without pain. Acute painful exacerbations are probably due to involvement of the apophyseal joints. The pain is centered in the spine and is worse on movement, especially after the patient has been inactive. Pain during the night or in the early morning hours is another common feature. It may be partially relieved by activity and is often aggravated by seasonal and barometric changes. The effect of salicylates, which usually alleviate the pain to some degree, may be taken as another diagnostic feature. Signs of root involvement may coexist.

Ankylosing spondylitis, a disease closely related to rheumatoid arthritis of the spine, is an important cause of low back pain. The majority of its victims are men, usually in their twenties (onset may be to fifty years). The initial complaint of recurrent low-back pain and stiffness, with or without recurrent sciatic pain, or more vague symptoms (tired back, soreness, aching, or "catches in the back") may precede demonstrable x-ray changes by several years. It differs from rheumatoid spondylitis, which is more frequent in women, affects usually the upper spine (especially cervical), and extends to the whole back; only a third of patients with ankylosing spondylitis develop arthritic changes in the shoulders, hips, knees, and ankles. The aortic valve may become involved, giving rise to insufficiency (spondylitic heart disease). The sedimentation rate is usually elevated, but constitutional symptoms are rare. Recurrent iritis and uveitis are present in approximately 25 percent of patients. X-rays show the sacroiliac and apophyseal joints to be blurred and anterior and lateral spinal ligaments calcified. A therapeutic response to phenylbutazone (Butazolidine) or indomethacin (Indocin) and exercises is also quite characteristic (see Chap. 386). Discogenic disease also figures in the differential diagnosis.

In *osteoarthritis,* by contrast, pain in the spine may or may not be accompanied by the motor, reflex, or sensory changes of root involvement. The pain in the spine is of the same type as in rheumatoid spondylitis and is also accompanied by a sense of stiffness and limitation of movement. It differs slightly in being more clearly aggravated by motion, more readily relieved by rest, and less pronounced at night. Fatigue and systemic symptoms are notably absent. The severity of the pain is not clearly related to the degree of the process as seen in the x-ray. X-ray evidence of the disease in the spine is found in a majority of individuals beyond the age of

fifty as is clicking in the neck on head movement. The presence of such changes should not be accepted as establishing an arthritic source of a severe and progressive pain, since it may be due to a more serious unrelated condition, such as a neoplasm.

Injury may exacerbate the pain of both rheumatoid and osteoarthritis. (See Chap. 390 for further discussion of spondylitis.)

OTHER DESTRUCTIVE DISEASES

INFECTIOUS, NEOPLASTIC AND METABOLIC DISEASES.
Metastatic carcinoma (breast, bronchus, prostate, thyroid, hypernephroma, stomach, uterus), multiple myeloma, and lymphoma are the common tumors which involve the spine; tuberculosis and pyogenic osteomyelitis are the most frequent infections, though brucellosis, typhoid fever, actinomycosis, and blastomycosis are known to occur.

Special mention should be made of the spinal *epidural abscess* (usually staphylococcal), which necessitates urgent surgical treatment. The symptoms are a localized pain, spontaneous as well as on percussion and palpation, often with radicular radiation, and a rapidly developing flaccid paraplegia appearing in a febrile patient.

Destructive lesions of any type may develop silently, i.e., without any pain, as long as they are limited to the osseous tissue. Upon spreading to the periosteum or to the adjacent spinous structures, however, they become the source of much pain of both local and referred type, and often one or more spinal roots are implicated as well, with the typical radicular type being added to the clinical picture. A "spontaneous" fracture may initiate pain. Pain caused by neoplasms of the spine tends to be of aching character and more or less steady, though occasionally waxing and waning. It is especially severe at night, seeming to be only slightly benefited by rest; yet activity during the day also worsens the pain. As the disease progresses, the pain increases in duration and severity. It may then be of a throbbing character. The most important physical finding, which should lead one to suspect a destructive lesion, is an intensification of the pain by jarring the spine, by percussing the spinous processes gently with the fist or a reflex hammer, or by exerting a steady pressure upon these parts. Axial compression (downward pressure exerted on the head or dropping on the heels from the toe position) may also serve to intensify the pain. Nocturnal pain, spinal ache, and percussion sensitivity are also characteristic of Pott's disease and osteomyelitis. The establishment of the cause of the pain is often delayed because the first x-rays may not disclose the lesion. (Nearly a cubic centimeter of bone must be destroyed in a vertebral body before it is visible in an x-ray.) If these are negative, they should be repeated after an interval of a few weeks. Other laboratory data, such as white blood count and smear, sedimentation rate, and electrophoresis of serum proteins, and acid and alkaline phosphatase in the serum are helpful.

In so-called "metabolic bone diseases" (osteoporosis

of either the postmenopausal or senile type or osteo-malacia) a considerable degree of loss of bone substance may occur without any symptoms whatsoever. Many such patients do, however, complain of aching in the lumbar or thoracic area. This is most likely to occur following an injury, sometimes of trivial degree, which leads to collapse or wedging of a vertebra. Certain movements greatly enhance the pain, and certain positions relieve it. One or more spinal roots may then be involved. Paget's disease of the spine is nearly always painless. It may lead to compression of the spinal cord. The recognition of these bone disorders is discussed in some detail elsewhere (Chaps. 356 and 381).

REFERRED PAIN FROM VISCERAL DISEASE

The pain of disease of the pelvic, abdominal, or thoracic viscera is often felt in the region of the spine; i.e., it is referred to the more posterior parts of the spinal segment which innervates the diseased organ. Occasionally back pain may be the first and only sign. The general rule is that pelvic diseases are referred to the sacral region, lower abdominal disease to the lumbar region (centering around the second to fourth lumbar vertebras), and upper abdominal diseases to the lower thoracic spine (eighth thoracic to the first and second lumbar vertebras). Characteristically there are no local signs, no stiffness of the back, and motion is of full range without augmentation of the pain. However, some positions, e.g., flexion of the lumbar spine in the lateral recumbent position, may be more comfortable than others.

LOW THORACIC AND UPPER LUMBAR PAIN IN AB-DOMINAL DISEASE. Peptic ulceration or tumor of the wall of the stomach and of the duodenum most typically induces pain in the epigastrium (see Chaps. 11, 12, and 314); but if the posterior wall is involved, and particularly if there is retroperitoneal extension, the pain may be felt in the region of the spine. Usually the pain is central in location or is more intense on one side. If very intense, it may seem to encircle the body. It tends to retain the characteristics of pain from the affected organ; e.g., if due to peptic ulceration, it is relieved by food and soda and appears about 2 hr after a meal.

Diseases of the pancreas (peptic ulceration with extension to the pancreas, cholecystitis with pancreatitis, tumor) are apt to cause pain in the back, being more to the right of the spine if the head of the pancreas is involved and to the left if the body and tail are implicated.

Diseases of retroperitoneal structures, e.g., lymphomas, sarcomas, and carcinomas, may evoke pain in this part of the spine with some tendency toward radiation to the lower abdomen, groins, and anterior thighs. A secondary tumor of the ileopsoas region on one side often produces a unilateral lumbar ache with radiation toward the groin and labia or testicle; there may also be signs of involvement of the upper lumbar spinal roots. An aneurysm of the abdominal aorta may induce a pain which is localized to this region of the spine but may be felt higher or lower, depending on the location of the lesion.

The sudden appearance of obscure lumbar pain in a patient receiving anticoagulants should arouse the suspicion of retroperitoneal bleeding.

LUMBAR PAIN WITH LOWER ABDOMINAL DISEASES. Inflammatory diseases of segments of the colon (colitis, diverticulitis) or tumor of the colon cause pain which may be felt in the lower abdomen between the umbilicus and pubis, or in the midlumbar region, or in both places. If very intense, the pain may have a beltlike distribution around the body. A lesion in the tranverse colon or first part of the descending colon may be central or left-sided, and its level of reference to the back is to the second to third lumbar vertebras. If the sigmoid colon is implicated, the pain is lower, in the upper sacral region and anteriorly in the midline suprapubic region or left lower quadrant of the abdomen.

SACRAL PAIN IN PELVIC (UROLOGIC AND GYNECO-LOGIC) DISEASES. Although gynecologic disorders may manifest themselves by back pain, the pelvis is seldom the site of a disease which causes obscure low back pain. For the most part the diagnosis of painful pelvic lesions is not difficult, for a thorough palpation of structures by abdominal, vaginal, and rectal examination may be supplemented by methods (sigmoidoscopy, barium enema, pyelography) which adequately visualize all these parts.

Menstrual pain itself may be felt in the sacral region. It is rather poorly localized, tends to radiate down the legs, and is of a crampy nature. The most important source of chronic back pain from the pelvic organs, however, is the uterosacral ligaments. Endometriosis or carcinoma of the uterus (body or cervix) may invade these structures, while malposition of the uterus may pull on them. The pain is localized centrally in the sacrum below the lumbosacral joint but may be more on one side. In endometriosis the pain begins during the premenstrual phase and often continues until it merges with menstrual pain. Malposition of the uterus (retroversion, descensus, and prolapse) characteristically leads to sacral pain, especially after the patient has been standing for several hours. Postural adjustments may also evoke pain here when a fibroma of the uterus pulls on the uterosacral ligaments. Carcinomatous pain due to implication of nerve plexuses is continuous and becomes progressively more severe; it tends to be more intense at night. The primary lesion may be inconspicuous, being overlooked upon pelvic examination. Papanicolaou smears and a pyelogram are the most useful diagnostic procedures. X-ray therapy of these tumors may produce sacral pain consequent to swelling and necrosis of tissue, the so-called "radiation phlegmon of the pelvis." Low back pain with radiation into one or both thighs is a common phenomenon during the last weeks of pregnancy.

Chronic prostatitis, evidenced by prostatic discharge, frequency of urination, and slight reduction in sexual potency, may be attended by a nagging sacral ache; it may be mainly on one side, with radiation into one leg if the seminal vesicle is involved on that side. Carcinoma of the prostate with metastases to the lower spine is another cause of sacral or lumbar pain. It may be present without urinary frequency or burning. Spinal nerves may be infiltrated by tumor cells, or the spinal cord itself may be compressed if the epidural space is invaded. The diagnosis is established by rectal examination, x-rays of the spine, and measurement of acid phosphatase (particularly the prostatic phosphatase fraction). Lesions of the bladder and testes are usually not accompanied by back pain. When the kidney is the site of disease, the pain is ipsilateral, being felt in the flank or lumbar region.

Visceral derangements of whatever type may intensify the pain of arthritis, and the presence of arthritis may alter the distribution of visceral pain. With disease of the spine in the lumbosacral region, for example, distension of the ampulla of the sigmoid by feces or a bout of colitis may aggravate the arthritic pain. In patients with arthritis of the cervical or thoracic spine, the pain of myocardial ischemia may radiate to the back.

OBSCURE TYPES OF LOW BACK PAIN AND THE QUESTION OF PSYCHIATRIC DISEASE

The practicing physician is consulted by many individuals who complain of low back pain of obscure origin. A safe rule is to assume that all of them have some type of primary or secondary disease of the spine and its supporting structures or of the abdominal or pelvic viscera. If the pain is of acute onset and short duration, it may be due to only a minor trauma, a so-called "fibrositis," or some form of articular disease. If it is recurrent, the possibility of a ruptured disc causing an instability of the spine must be considered. If it is severe and progressive, neoplasia, a tuberculous infection, and rheumatoid spondylitis should be kept in mind. Adolescent girls and boys are subject to an obscure form of epiphyseal disease of the spine (Scheuermann's disease) which may cause low back pain upon exercise over a period of 2 to 3 years.

POSTURAL BACK PAIN. Many slender asthenic individuals and some fat middle-aged individuals have discomfort in the back. Their backs ache much of the time, and the pain interferes with effective work. The physical examination is negative except for slack musculature and poor posture. The pain is diffuse in the mid or low back and characteristically is relieved by bed rest and induced by the maintenance of a particular posture over a period of time. Pain in the neck and between the shoulder blades is a common complaint among thin, tense, active women and seems to be related to taut trapezius muscles.

PSYCHIATRIC ILLNESS. Low back pain may be encountered in compensation hysteria and malingering, in anxiety or neurocirculatory asthenia (formerly called neurasthenia), in depression and hypochondriasis, and in many nervous individuals whose symptoms and complaints do not fall within any category of psychiatric illness.

Again it is probably correct to assume that pain in the back in such patients usually signifies disease of the spine and adjacent structures, and this should always be carefully looked for. However, the pain may be exaggerated, prolonged, or woven into a pattern of invalidism or disability because of coexistent or secondary psychologic factors. This is especially true when there is the possibility of personal gain (notably compensation). The patients seeking compensation for protracted low back pain without obvious structural disease tend, after a time, to become suspicious, hostile toward the medical profession or anyone who might question the authenticity of their illness, and uncooperative. One notes in them a tendency to describe their pain poorly and to prefer, instead, to discuss the degree of their disability and their mistreatment in the hands of the medical profession. These features and a negative examination of the back should lead one to suspect a psychologic factor. A few patients, usually frank malingerers, adopt the most bizarre attitudes, such as being unable to straighten up or walking with the trunk flexed at almost a right angle (camptocormia) (see Chap. 370).

The depressed and hypochondriac patient represents a troublesome problem, and a common error is to minimize the importance of anxiety and depression or to ascribe them to worry over the illness and its social effects. The more common and minor back ailments, e.g., those due to osteoarthritis and postural ache, are enhanced and rendered intolerable by the irritable moodiness and self-concern. Such patients are often subjected to surgical procedures, which prove ineffective. The disability seems excessive for the degree of spinal malfunction, and misery and despair are the prevailing features of the syndrome. One of the most reliable diagnostic measures is the response to drugs which alleviate the depression (see Chap. 371).

PAIN IN THE NECK AND SHOULDER

This topic has been discussed to some extent in the chapter on thoracic pain, and further references will be found under Pain in the Extremities.

It is useful to distinguish here three major categories of painful disease—those of the spine, cervical plexus, and shoulder. Although the pains in these three regions of the body may overlap, the patient himself usually can indicate the site of the origin. Pain arising from the cervical spine is nearly always felt in the spine (though it may be projected to the shoulder and arm), is evoked or enhanced by certain movements or positions of the neck, and is accompanied by tenderness and limitations of motions of the neck. Similarly, pain of brachial plexus origin is experienced in and around the shoulder or between the shoulders, is induced by the performance of certain tasks with the arm and by certain positions, and is associated with tenderness of structures above the clavicle. There may be a palpable abnormality above the clavicle (aneurysms of subclavian artery, tumor, cervical rib). The combination of circulatory symptoms and signs referable to the lower part of the brachial plexus, manifested in the hand by obliteration of pulse when the patient takes and holds a full breath with the head tilted back or turned (Adson's test), unilateral Raynaud's phenomenon, trophic changes in the fingers, and sensory loss over the ulnar side of the hand with or without interosseous atrophy, complete the clinical picture. X-rays showing a cervical rib or deformed thoracic outlet or superior sulcus tumor of the lung (Pancoast syndrome) offer confirmation of the diagnosis. Pain, localized to the shoulder region, influenced by motion, and associated with tenderness and limitation of motions (extension, abduction, external and internal rotation), points to tendinitis with calcium deposition of the rotator cuff of muscles surrounding the shoulder joint. Often the term *bursitis* has been used loosely to designate this tendinitis, capsulitis, or muscular tear. Spine, plexus, and shoulder pain all may radiate into the arm or hand, but sensory, motor, and reflex changes always indicate involvement of nerve roots (in disease of the spine), plexus, or nerves.

Osteoarthritis of the cervical spine may cause pains which radiate into the back of the head, shoulders, and arms on one or both sides of the thorax. Coincident involvement of nerve roots is manifested by paresthesias, sensory loss, weakness, or tendon reflex change. Should bony ridges form in the spinal canal (spondylosis), the spinal cord may be compressed, with resulting weakness and atrophy and sometimes sensory disturbances in the arms and spastic weakness and ataxia with loss of vibratory and position sense in the legs. A Pantopaque cervical myelogram reveals the degree of encroachment on the spinal canal and the level at which the spinal cord is affected. The authors have experienced the greatest difficulty in distinguishing spondylosis with or without disc rupture and spinal cord compression from primary neurologic diseases (syringomyelia, amyotrophic lateral sclerosis, or tumor) with an unrelated osteoarthritis of the cervical spine, particularly at the fifth to sixth and sixth to seventh cervical vertebras, where the disc spaces are often narrowed in the adult. A combination of nervous tension with osteoarthritis of the cervical spine or a painful injury to ligaments and muscles after an accident in which the neck is forcibly extended and flexed (e.g., whiplash injury to spine) are extremely vexatious clinical syndromes. If the pain is persistent and limited to the neck, the problem will sometimes prove to have been due to disruption of a disc, but it is often complicated by psychologic factors.

One of the commonest causes of neck, shoulder, and arm pain is disc herniation in the lower cervical region. As with rupture of the lumbar discs, the syndrome includes the aforementioned disorder of spinal function and evidence of neural involvement. It develops after a trauma which may be major or minor (sudden hyperextension of the neck, diving, forceful manipulations, chiropractic treatment, etc.). Virtually every patient exhibits an abnormality in full motion of the neck (limitation and pain). Hyperextension is the movement that most consistently aggravates the pain. With laterally situated disc lesions between the fifth to sixth cervical vertebras, the symptoms and signs are referred to the sixth cervical roots, i.e., pain felt at the trapezius ridge,

tip of the shoulder, anterior upper arm, radial forearm, and often in the thumb; paresthesias and sensory impairment or hypersensitivity in the same regions; tenderness in the area above the spine of the scapula and in the supraclavicular and biceps regions; weakness in flexion of the forearm; diminished to absent biceps and supinator reflexes (triceps retained or exaggerated). With sixth to seventh cervical disc disease and involvement of the seventh cervical root, the pain is in the region of the shoulder blade, pectoral region and medial axilla, posterolateral upper arm, dorsal forearm and elbow, index and middle fingers, or all the fingers; tenderness is most pronounced over the medial aspect of the shoulder blade opposite the third to fourth thoracic spinous processes, in the supraclavicular area and triceps region; paresthesias and sensory loss are most pronounced in the second and third fingers or tips of all the fingers; weakness is in extension of the forearm (occasionally wristdrop is present) and in the hand grip; the triceps reflex is diminished to absent, and the biceps and supinator reflexes are preserved. Cough, sneeze, and downward pressure on the head in the hyperextension position exacerbate pain, and traction (even manual) tends to relieve it.

Unlike lumbar discs, the cervical ones, if large and centrally situated, may result in compression of the spinal cord (central disc, all of the cord; paracentral disc, part of the cord, i.e., Brown-Sequard syndrome). The central disc is often nearly painless, and the cord syndrome may simulate a degenerative disease (amyotrophic lateral sclerosis, combined system disease). A common error is to fail to think of a ruptured disc in the cervical region in patients with obscure symptoms in the legs. The diagnosis of ruptured cervical disc should be confirmed by the same laboratory procedures that were mentioned under lumbar disc.

Metastases in the cervical spine may be very painful, but the problem is not different from that of secondary deposits of tumor in other parts of the spine.

Shoulder injuries (rotator cuff), subacromial or subdeltoid bursitis, the frozen shoulder (periarthritis or capsulitis), tendinitis, and arthritis may develop in patients who are otherwise well, but these conditions are also frequent in hemiplegics or in individuals suffering from coronary heart disease. The pain is often severe and extends toward the neck and down the arm into the hand. The dorsum of the latter may tingle without other signs of nerve involvement. Vasomotor changes also may occur in the hand (shoulder-hand syndrome), and after a time, osteoporosis and atrophy of cutaneous and subcutaneous structures occur (Sudeck's atrophy or Sudeck-Leriche syndrome). These conditions fall more within the province of orthopedics than of medicine and will not be discussed in detail. The physician, however, must know that they can be prevented by proper exercises.

The carpal tunnel syndrome, with paresthesias and numbness in palmar distribution of the median nerve and aching pain which extends up into the forearm, may be mistaken for disease of the shoulder or neck.

MANAGEMENT OF BACK PAIN

A muscular strain is always benign in character, and one may expect full recovery in 2 to 4 weeks. Ligamentous strains, if severe, may last longer, from 6 to 12 weeks. The underlying principle of therapy in both is immobilization in a recumbent position that relaxes and removes pressure from the injured structure. Usually lying on the side with knees and hips flexed is the favored position. If the erector spinae are strained, the optimal position is hyperextension; the same is true of strains of the posterior and sacroiliac ligaments. This position is best maintained by having the patient lie with a small pillow or blanket under the lumbar spine or lie face down. During the acute phase of any injury of this type, application of cold, in the form of an ice bag or cold water bottle (ethyl chloride spray of the skin is said to give dramatic relief at times), is indicated. It reduces the circulation and consequently the swelling. After the third or fourth day, heat is desirable to improve the circulation and to relax protective muscle spasm. Analgesic medication should be given liberally during the first few days [codeine, 30 mg and aspirin, 0.6 Gm, meperidine (Demerol) 50 mg, or morphine 10 to 15 mg]. When ready for ambulation, after some days in bed, the patient may need protection of the injured part, preferably adhesive strapping, in cases of muscle strain, or a belt or brace. Plaster casts should be avoided. Ambulatory treatment is supplemented by corrective exercises designed to strengthen trunk muscles, especially the abdominal, overcome faulty position, and to increase the mobility of the spinal joints. Only if these measures prove inadequate and the patient is partially disabled over long periods of time by an unstable, painful lower back (recurrent lumbosacral backache) should operative intervention be considered.

In the treatment of an acute rupture of a lumbar or cervical disc, complete bed rest is essential and strong analgesic medication is required. Traction is of little value in lumbar disc disease, and it is best to permit the patient to find the most comfortable position. Later, traction, if of any value, keeps the patient confined to bed. In contrast, traction is of great help in rupture of cervical discs. Often the pain subsides after 2 to 3 weeks in bed, and the patient may remain free of pain upon resuming normal activities. He may suffer some minor recurrence of the pain but be able to carry on his usual activities, and eventually he will recover. There is always danger of relapse. To prevent this, mild muscle-strengthening exercises of the spine after the pain has subsided (see Fig. 13-2) and avoidance of activities which favor spine injury (see Fig. 13-3) are recommended. If the pain does not subside after a trial of prolonged bed rest (several weeks) and the myelogram demonstrates a large disc, an operative removal, preferably without spine fusion, should be undertaken. The final decision as to the time and necessity of surgery depends on the duration and gravity of the pain and the neurologic disorder.

For the many patients with back pain who do not fall

Fig. 13-2. Front of postural instruction sheet. Patient is instructed as follows:

Exercises should be taken on a padded floor. Exercise 3 should be omitted unless otherwise instructed. Start exercises by doing each one ——— times morning and evening, increasing the series one a day until you are doing each one ——— times morning and evening. Exercises are essential in obtaining a proper muscular balance, but a correct posture is acquired only through conscious effort.

Remember—
1. When standing or walking, toe straight ahead and take most of your weight on heels.
2. Try to form a crease across the upper abdomen by holding the chest up and forward and elevating the front of the pelvis.
3. Avoid high heels as much as possible.
4. Sit with the buttocks "tucked under" so that the hollow in the low back is eradicated.
5. When possible, elevate the knees higher than the hips while sitting. This is especially important when driving (driver's seat forward) or riding as a passenger in an automobile.
6. Sleep on your back with knees propped up or on your side with one or both knees drawn up. Bed should be firm.
7. Do not lift loads in front of you above the waist line.
8. Never bend backward.
9. Do not bend forward with knees straight. Always "squat."
10. Avoid standing as much as possible.
Learn to Live 24 Hours a Day without a Hollow in the Lower Part of Your Back

into any one of the above categories, simple measures are beneficial. For the adolescent with a suspicion of epiphyseal disease, restricted activity (avoidance of vigorous sports) for a few months or years and a supporting garment help. Muscle-strengthening exercises and a physical conditioning program are indicated for postural backache (see Fig. 13-2). Spine fusion should be reserved only for the exceptional patient with disabling and persistent pains.

Spondylosis of the cervical spine, if painful, is helped by bed rest and traction; if signs of spinal cord involvement are present, a collar to limit movement may halt the progression and even lead to improvement. Decompressive laminectomy with sectioning of denticulate ligaments is reserved for severe instances of the disease with advancing neurologic symptoms. The shoulder-hand syndrome may benefit from stellate ganglion blocks or ganglionectomy, but the basic treatment is physiotherapy,

Correct	Incorrect	Correct	Incorrect

Fig. 13-3. Reverse side of postural instruction sheet showing correct and incorrect methods of lifting, sitting, and sleeping.

with surgical procedures being used only as measures of last resort.

14 PAIN IN THE EXTREMITIES
Eugene A. Stead, Jr.

Pain in the extremities comes from disturbances within the tissues of the extremities or from irritation at any level of the sensory nerve paths serving the extremity, or it is referred from deep somatic or visceral structures.

DISTURBANCES WITHIN THE TISSUES

Any lesion causing inflammation, swelling, ischemia, or destruction of pain-sensitive tissues of the extremity may cause pain. Burns, frostbite, and chemical injuries are painful. Arthritis, cellulitis, abscesses, osteomyelitis and hematomas, tumors, Paget's disease, and bone changes with hyperparathyroidism cause varying degrees of pain. Degeneration of nerves and trauma to nerve trunks are painful. Damage to nerves or to muscles from ischemia is painful.

IRRITATION OF SENSORY NERVES

Involvement of the nerves at any point in their course from the extremity to the spinal cord may cause pain in the extremity. The pain of cervical rib, ruptured intervertebral disk, spinal cord tumor, and tabes dorsalis falls into this group. Central pain from involvement of the

spinothalamic tract and thalamus is occasionally seen (see Chap. 9).

PAIN REFERRED FROM DEEP STRUCTURES

The pain of angina pectoris and myocardial infarction frequently radiates to the inner surfaces of the arms. Pain from the hip may be referred to the knee. Pain from the deep muscles of the back or from the vertebras may be the source of pain referred to the extremity.

CAUSES OF PAIN IN THE EXTREMITIES

PAIN FROM TRAUMA, INFLAMMATION, AND SWELLING. The immediate response to trauma is due to mechanical stimulation of nerve endings. Pain persisting after the injury may result from chemical stimuli produced by the injured tissues. Lewis has described the reactions in skin made hyperalgesic by injury. Needle pricks too light to awaken pain in uninjured skin will arouse a response in a traumatized area. Pain is easily induced by friction or warming, and often by cooling. Distension of the skin by direct stretching or by venous congestion causes pain. If injured skin is rubbed, pain is felt immediately; this subsides and is followed in about 15 sec by a second pain which lasts a minute or more. If the circulation to the part is obstructed, the initial pain is unaltered, but the second pain rises to a greater intensity and persists until approximately 1 min after the circulation is restored. The first pain comes from direct stimulation of sensory nerves, the second from a relatively stable pain-giving substance released into, and held within, the tissue space. The chemical nature of this substance is not known. Skin made hyperalgesic by injury, regardless of the mechanism of the injury, will respond to heat and congestion with burning pain. If this reaction occurs diffusely in the skin of the extremities without obvious cause, the burning pain from warmth and congestion is called *erythromelalgia*.

The injury to the skin caused by heat is well recognized. That prolonged cold will cause tissue damage in many ways comparable to burns is less commonly realized. Prolonged immersion of the feet or prolonged exposure to cold with the feet in wet boots will cause severe tissue damage to the point of gangrene, even though actual freezing does not occur. Freezing, of course, causes tissue damage and may produce gangrene. Fibrosis and ischemic neuritis are common after any form of injury from cold and may cause persistent tenderness and pain.

In bacterial infections, the mechanical factor of rapidly forming edema increases local tissue pressure and causes pain in skin already made hyperalgesic by chemical factors associated with injury. Congestion aggravates the pain, and elevation of the part alleviates it. Less rapid edema formation usually does not cause pain, because the tissues stretch gradually. Patients with cardiac edema complain of heaviness of the legs and occasionally of diffuse tenderness. Edema associated with varicose veins may cause a sense of fullness and dull ache. In acute thrombophlebitis, pain may arise from the involved veins.

It may be aggravated by ischemia secondary to sympathetic vasoconstriction resulting from the sensory stimuli from the inflamed veins. Tumor masses may cause pressure on bone or peripheral nerves.

Arthritis is a common cause of pain in the extremities. When the process is *acute,* as in pyogenic arthritis, gout, and many cases of rheumatic fever, pain is likely to be severe at rest and intensified by the slightest movement. The other signs of inflammation—swelling, redness, and warmth—are pronounced.

In chronic arthritis of the degenerative type, which is especially common in the knees (Chap. 387), pain is usually present only on motion, although there may be minimal discomfort at rest because of local spasm of muscles. Heat and redness are lacking, and swelling may be present or absent. In elderly women with arthritis of the distal interphalangeal joints (Heberden's nodes), pain may be lacking despite striking deformity.

Rheumatoid arthritis (Chap. 386), which is often most pronounced in the hands, is characterized by marked fluctuations in the intensity of the inflammation, and hence of the pain. Prolonged periods of freedom from symptoms other than slight stiffness in the morning and minimal swelling alternate with exacerbations of mild to severe aching, associated with swelling and heat and lasting a few hours to many weeks.

Pain arising in the bones of the extremities is likely to be severe, throbbing, worse at night, and associated with pronounced localized tenderness. Trauma, osteomyelitis, neoplasms, metabolic diseases of bone (Chap. 381), and pulmonary osteoarthropathy are the most important causes.

The syndrome of sore, painful shoulder with superficial and deep areas of exquisite tenderness is common. It frequently begins as wryneck and at times occurs in a number of persons closely associated with one another. Marked spasm prevents abduction of the arm at the shoulder. The entire upper extremity may feel numb and queer. There is no fever. Biopsy of the skin and muscles shows apparently normal tissues. Light freezing of the skin with ethyl chloride or procainization of the superficial and deep tender areas frequently gives dramatic relief of pain, relief which may be permanent. The mechanism of pain production in this syndrome is not known.

PAIN FROM ISCHEMIA, THROMBOSIS, EMBOLISM, AND ARTERITIS. Interference with blood supply may result from obliterative arterial disease or embolus or from arteriolar spasm secondary to stimulation of sensory receptors or nerves. It may be aggravated in polycythemia by the adverse effect of increased viscosity of the blood. The pain may be produced by the action on sensory nerve endings of metabolites accumulating in the muscles or by changes in the nerves themselves.

The sensations produced by ischemia to the extremity are familiar to all. When the blood supply is occluded, the part gradually becomes numb and paralyzed and we say the part has "gone to sleep." If the part is not moved, pain does not develop. The sensation at the end of the fingers becomes dulled in about 12 to 15 min. At that time, light pressure on the fingers may hurt, and stroking the finger tips causes an unpleasant sensation. Later, pain is dulled, and much later, analgesia develops. On release of the arterial occlusion, unpleasant tingling occurs, particularly in the fingers. This tingling is not the result of the inrush of blood into the fingers, because it occurs if blood is released only into the proximal part of the extremity. It results from changes in the main nerves of the arm during recovery. Stroking the fingers accentuates it. The paresthesias produced by the injury and recovery of the nerve from ischemia are similar to those produced by chronic disease processes involving the peripheral nerves or nerve roots.

If the extremity is exercised while the circulation is completely occluded, a continuous diffuse aching pain develops in the muscles because the sensory nerves are stimulated by the formation of stable metabolites. The pain is present during and between contractions. It is frequently described as a cramp, but the muscles are flaccid. If the contractions are continued, the muscles become tender. On release of the tourniquet, the pain disappears in a few seconds, probably as the result of the carrying away of readily diffusible metabolites.

If the brachial artery at the elbow or the femoral artery at the inguinal ligament is occluded by digital pressure for ½ hr, instead of by application of a cuff, much less change in the circulation occurs, because collateral circulation is not stopped. Loss of sensation does not occur, and on release of the occlusion, the reactive hyperemia is much less intense than with the cuff.

In occlusive vascular disease of the vessels of the legs, a common symptom is pain with tenderness of the muscles which is relieved by rest. It is called *intermittent claudication,* and it represents in the muscles of the extremities the same changes which occur in the heart with angina pectoris. The resting muscle is receiving an adequate supply of blood for normal metabolism. When muscle metabolism is increased by exercise and occlusive vascular disease prevents increase of the blood supply, metabolites accumulate in the muscles and stimulate the sensory nerve endings. The nature of the chemical substances has not been determined. The more severe the circulatory impairment, the less exercise is required to produce the pain and the more slowly the pain disappears on rest.

In occlusive vascular disease, the nerves themselves may become ischemic and cause severe and persistent pain. This pain, in certain instances, is aggravated by dependency because of stimuli resulting from congestion. In addition to Buerger's disease and arteriosclerosis, ischemic neuritis is a prominent symptom in small-vessel involvement of the type seen in periarteritis nodosa.

Embolus or thrombus in the brachial or femoral vessels frequently produces sufficient circulatory impairment to cause pain. The pain in thrombosis is indistinguishable from the pain of embolism. The pains do not occur at the site of occlusion but in the muscles and tissues distal to it. The time of onset of the pain will depend on the temperature of the part, the amount of activity, and the amount of associated vasospasm. If the part is warm and still, the limb may become numb before the muscle pain is produced. Heat applied to a limb with poor circulation may cause gangrene from (1) increased metabolism of tissue without corresponding increase in blood supply or (2) lack of cooling effect of the blood. When heat above body temperature is applied to the skin, the blood normally acts as a cooling system; in the presence of arterial occlusion, local heating causes an immediate rise in temperature of the part. If the part is exercised, the muscle pain occurs early. Twenty-four hours after an embolus has lodged, the vessel wall may be tender because of periarterial inflammation. Occlusion of small blood vessels does not cause pain unless ischemia of muscle or nerve is produced.

Normal skin hurts when warmed after severe exposure to cold. This is a response to direct injury from the cold. The white, cold fingers in Raynaud's phenomenon may be painful. In scleroderma the thickening of the connective tissue combined with spasm of the digital arteries may result in painful ulceration of the fingers and eventual loss of the terminal phalanges.

The pain from ischemia or infection is frequently altered or absent in patients with diabetes because of associated peripheral neuropathy. Whenever a painful-looking lesion of the extremity is treated casually by the patient, neuropathy should be suspected. Tabes dorsalis, leprosy, senile cortical atrophy, and syringomyelia should be considered.

The circulation to the extremities can be greatly modified by overactivity of the sympathetic nervous system. In many instances of injury, inflammation, or thrombophlebitis, sensory stimuli arising in the extremity may produce intense reflex vasoconstriction, and the resulting ischemia may cause diffuse pain. Relief of the vasoconstriction by paravertebral procaine block of the appropriate sympathetic ganglions may cause striking relief of pain. Similarly, sensory impulses arising from ischemic areas after arterial occlusion by an embolus or thrombus may stimulate sympathetic nervous system activity and reflex spasm. Paravetrebral block will relieve the spasm of collateral vessels, and if circulation improves sufficiently, pain will disappear.

PAIN FROM NEUROPATHY, NEURITIS, GANGLIONITIS, AND PRESSURE ON NERVES OR NERVE ROOTS. Involvement of the peripheral nerves frequently causes unpleasant sensations in the extremities. In diabetic neuropathy, numbness may be accompanied by diffuse pains through both lower extremities. Any combination of sensory loss and pain may occur in peripheral nerve damage from infection, poisons, or mechanical factors such as trauma or pressure. Spinal cord tumors and slipped intervertebral disks are common causes of nerve root pain. Inflammation of the dorsal root ganglions results in the syndrome of herpes zoster. The redness and blistering is attributed to antidromic vasodilatation from stimulation of the sensory nerves. Impulses arising in sensory nerves or ganglions and passing peripherally to the sensory end organs are called *antidromic*. Involvement of the dorsal root ganglions, dorsal roots, and adjacent spinal cord produces the lightning pains in the extremities typical of tabes dorsalis. Paralysis from pressure in the axilla may be caused by crutches or by sleeping with the arm thrown over the back of a chair. The latter usually occurs in alcoholic stupor and is called "Saturday night paralysis."

PAIN FROM IMMOBILIZATION, SPASM, AND CRAMPS. Prolonged immobilization of a part results in stiffness of muscles and joints. The muscles tighten and splint the joint, and motion is prevented. An attempt to move the part produces pain. Local infiltration with procaine will frequently allow a great improvement in motility, which may be permanent. Similar spasm occurs after trauma. A painful sprain of the ankle which prevents walking may be relieved in a few minutes by procainization. Even in acute arthritis part of the pain may be secondary to spasm and may respond to curare or procaine, which relax the muscle. In acute poliomyelitis, nonparalyzed muscles may be sore and contracted. Application of hot packs gives relief.

Muscles placed in unusual positions may go into intense contraction and cause severe pain. Cramps in the foot or leg occurring at night are common. They are relieved by forcefully extending the joint so as to stretch the cramped muscles. In nocturnal cramps, pain occurs so quickly that simple ischemia would seem unlikely. They differ from the cramps of arterial disease in that the pain is not brought on by exercise. Painful muscle cramps occur in tetany and in chloride deficiency. Whether the pain of tetany is caused by ischemia from the prolonged contraction or related to damage because of the intensity of the contraction is not known.

Unaccustomed, strenuous exercise causes aching, tender muscles, tendons, and joints. The pain results from low-grade injury to the muscles from repetitive maximal contractions.

GLOMUS TUMOR. Tumor of the glomus, the specialized arteriovenous anastomosis of the skin, produces unusual vasomotor phenomena and radiating pain. It is characteristically a small (a few millimeters in diameter), extremely painful, purplish nodule either in the skin of the extremity or under the nail. Pain is caused by contact or change of temperature and may spread to involve the entire extremity. Why these tumors are so painful is not clear. While most observers have noted an unusually rich nerve supply, others have not found it.

PAIN FROM CAUSALGIA. Pain in the extremity associated with signs of local circulatory dysfunction is seen in nerve injuries after amputations and in persons with coronary arterial disease with or without myocardial infarction. It occurs in the hand-shoulder syndrome. The above conditions have one thing in common: local injury sets up a reaction which at first appears to be the result of sensory stimuli from the injured part. Later changes occur in the peripheral nerves, spinal cord, or central nervous system so that the process continues after the injury has apparently healed.

Classic Causalgia. Injury to any nerve, more commonly the medial or sciatic nerve, may give rise after a few days or weeks to a burning pain. The gross injury to the nerve may have been severe or trivial. The pain will be caused by light friction; deep pressure is less painful.

Heat usually provokes the pain. The skin becomes smooth and glossy and is frequently wet with sweat. It has a red or purplish tint. The temperature of the involved part is usually said to be increased. The pain is frequently relieved by sympathectomy. Causalgic pain may result from the activation of sensory fibers by sympathetic impulses. If injury links the two systems so that leakage of efferent sympathetic impulses into the sensory nerves can occur, most of the clinical phenomena of causalgia, including the relief by sympathetic block, can be explained.

The initiating mechanisms of causalgia are unknown. Several theories have been advanced: (1) The sensitivity of the skin may result from vasodilator substances released by repeated centrifugal impulses arising in the injured area. It is known that stimulation of the paralyzed end of a cut cutaneous nerve results in vasodilatation which may be accompanied by itching and burning pain. (2) The sensitivity of the skin may result from a lack of inhibition of pain and thermal neurones due to loss of large sensory fibers (see Chaps. 9 and 25).

Regardless of the local mechanism, it appears that other mechanisms central to the extremity are capable of continuing the process once the causalgia has been present for some time. At this stage, dorsal root section or sections of the spinothalamic tract may not modify the pain. Chain reactions within the short interconnecting nerves in the spinal cord have been postulated. Paravertebral block or sympathectomy should be done early before these central changes occur and before the patient becomes a drug addict. Because the patient's complaints are so bizarre and because the original injury may be mild, causalgia is frequently mistaken for a compensation neurosis.

Phantom Limb Pain. After amputation of a limb, the patient may complain of pain which he localizes in the removed part. At times this may be caused by a neuroma of the cut nerves or by the faulty construction of the stump. The stump may show vasomotor changes. In most instances, therapy directed toward the stump does not relieve the pain; at times, paravertebral block of the sympathetic ganglions does. The clinical observations suggest that, as in causalgia, pain may begin locally but that changes may take place in the central nervous system which are responsible for its continuation.

Hand-Shoulder Syndrome. Myocardial infarction is frequently complicated by persistent shoulder pain with marked limitation of motion. At times, swelling of the hand and wrist and contraction of the palmar fascia are present. The elbow is not involved. Atrophy of skin and osteoporosis may follow. Similar disturbances in shoulder and hand function have occurred in association with trauma, hemiplegia, herpes zoster, and cervical osteo-arthritis. This syndrome may occur without recognized associated diseases. The exact mechanism of this fairly common syndrome is unknown.

APPROACH TO THE PATIENT

A careful history will usually yield important clues. The pain may be felt in the region of the knee when the disease is in the hip or in the foot when the knee is the seat of the disorder. Pain on first arising in the morning, particularly when associated with stiffness, suggests a disturbance of joints or muscles. When the bone is affected, there is commonly nocturnal aggravation. Pain of throbbing character usually arises in tense tissues with free blood supply, and hence suggests bone as the source. Sharp shooting pain of brief duration, brought on by coughing or sneezing, is common with disorders of the vertebral column or of the posterior nerve roots. Relief of discomfort by elevation suggests venous obstruction; relief by dependency suggests an arterial lesion. Pain ascribed to walking may actually be due to standing and may have its source in the lumbar spine or feet. Pain due to ischemia of muscles is characteristically induced by walking, with latency of onset and of offset. Disorders of joints are likely to be accompanied by pain on local movement, the duration of the discomfort paralleling that of the movement.

The history having suggested the responsible structure, the suspicion is confirmed or disproved by the physical findings and the appropriate special procedures. Since these are mentioned in the later chapters dealing with the disorders of the various systems of the body, they need not be cited here. However, it should be emphasized that x-ray examination, while often invaluable in the case of long-standing disease of the bones, may be entirely negative in the presence of serious skeletal disorders of recent origin. This is especially important in regard to acute osteomyelitis and to the earlier stages of metastatic neoplasms of bone.

REFERENCES

Allen, E. V., N. W. Barker, and E. A. Hines, Jr.: "Peripheral Vascular Diseases," Philadelphia, W. B. Saunders Company, 1946.

Doupe, J. C., C. H. Cullen, and G. Q. Chance: Post-traumatic Pain and the Causalgic Syndrome, J. Neurol., Neurosurg. Psychiat., 7:33, 1944.

Lewis, Thomas: "Pain," New York, The Macmillan Company, 1942.

——: "Vascular Disorders of the Limbs," New York, The Macmillan Company, 1946.

Section 2

Alterations in Body Temperature

15 DISTURBANCES OF HEAT REGULATION

Ivan L. Bennett, Jr. and
Robert G. Petersdorf

In health, the body temperature of man is maintained within a narrow range despite extremes in environmental conditions and physical activity. To a lesser but nonetheless remarkable extent, this is true of other mammals as well. An almost invariable accompaniment of systemic illness is a disturbance in temperature regulation, very often an abnormal elevation, or *fever*. In fact, fever is such a sensitive and reliable indicator of the presence of disease that thermometry is probably the commonest clinical procedure in use.

Even in the absence of a frank febrile response, interference with heat regulation by disease is evident. This may take the form of flushing, pallor, sweating, and abnormal sensations of cold or warmth, or it may consist of erratic fluctuations of body temperature within normal limits when a patient is at bed rest.

CONTROL OF BODY TEMPERATURE

The principal source of body heat is the combustion of foods. The greatest amount of heat is generated in the liver and the voluntary muscles. Heat production by muscle is of particular importance because the quantity can be varied according to the need. In most circumstances this variation consists of small increases and decreases in the number of nerve impulses to the muscles, causing unapparent tensing or relaxing. When, however, there is a strong stimulus for heat production, muscle activity may increase to the point of shivering, or even to a generalized rigor.

Heat is lost from the body in several ways. Small amounts are used in warming food or drink and in the evaporation of moisture from the respiratory tract. Most heat is lost from the surface of the body, by *convection* (transfer of heat to a fluid medium, i.e., ambient air), *radiation* (the exchange of electromagnetic energy between the body and the radiant environment) and *evaporation* (passage of water from liquid to gaseous state). Evaporation is particularly important when the ambient temperature exceeds that of the body, when it becomes the major source of heat loss.

The principal method of regulating heat loss is by varying the volume of blood flowing to the surface of the body. A rich circulation in the skin and subcutaneous tissues carries heat to the surface, where it can escape. In addition, sweating increases heat loss by providing water to be vaporized. The sweat, or eccrine, glands are under the control of the sympathetic nerves which in this instance mediate cholinergic stimuli. Heat loss by sweating may be tremendous because as much as 1 liter of sweat per hour may be elaborated.

When the need is for conservation of warmth, adrenergic autonomic stimuli cause a sharp reduction in the blood flow to the surface. This causes vasoconstriction and transforms the skin and subcutaneous tissue into layers of insulation.

The control of body temperature, integrating the various physical and chemical processes for heat production or loss, is a function of cerebral centers located in the hypothalamus. A high decerebrate animal displays a normal temperature if the hypothalamus is left intact. On the other hand, an animal whose brainstem has been sectioned loses ability to control body temperature, which consequently tends to vary with the environment, a condition referred to as *poikilothermia*. Although the centers in the anterior hypothalamus were generally thought to be responsible for heat loss and those in the posterior hypothalamus to control heat conservation, this separation may be an oversimplification. In fact, a new area anterior to the hypothalamus may have important integrating functions in temperature control.

It is probable that the cerebral temperature-regulating centers are affected by more than one kind of stimulus. Experiments on animals show that variation in the temperature of the blood flowing through the brain can cause activation of the appropriate counteracting feedback mechanisms, either for heat loss or for heat production. There is evidence that these centers also may be stimulated by sensory impulses, e.g., the flushing and sweating which may occur after ingestion of highly seasoned food. Furthermore, cutaneous stimuli may exert considerable feedback control on the temperature-regulating mechanisms. Physiologic variations in endocrine function may affect the body temperature; for example, the mean body temperature of women is higher during the second half of the menstrual cycle than it is between the onset of menstruation and the time of ovulation. The sensations of intense heat followed by diaphoresis that characterize the vasomotor instability experienced by some women at the menopause are undoubtedly a result of endocrine imbalance.

A basic problem on which information is needed is why the normal body temperature of warm-blooded animals is in the neighborhood of 98 to 103°F. Animals or human beings whose cervical cords have been severed maintain about the same body temperature, although fluctuations tend to be greater because of lack of neural control. There may be some intrinsic chemical regulating mechanism in the tissues.

Sweating, so important in man, is supplanted by panting and radiation from the body surface in many animals. In the rabbit, for example, the surface of the large ears is of great importance in dissipating heat.

Diseases of many types derange temperature regulation and fever is the result in many animals, but notable exceptions exist. The laboratory mouse responds to most "pyrogenic" stimuli with a profound drop in body temperature, and the rat gives variable responses, sometimes showing an elevation of temperature and sometimes showing a hypothermic response to disease. Furthermore, when mice or rats are maintained at high ambient temperatures, their response to materials known to be pyrogenic in man is no longer irregular but is constantly febrile. This is a striking demonstration of the influence of environment and other factors upon the outward expression of the derangement in body temperature control which occurs in disease.

NORMAL BODY TEMPERATURE

It is not practical to designate an exact upper level of normal body temperature because there are small differences among normal persons. There are rare individuals whose temperatures are always elevated slightly above accepted "normal" levels, and there is considerable variation in temperature in a given case. In general, however, it is safe to regard an oral temperature above 98.6°F in a person who has been lying in bed as an indication of disease. An oral temperature above 99.2°F in a person who has been engaged in moderate activity has the same significance. The temperature may be as low as 96.5°F in healthy individuals. Rectal temperature is usually 0.5 to 1.0°F higher than oral temperature. In very hot weather the body temperature may be elevated by 0.5° or perhaps even 1.0°F.

There is a distinct diurnal variation in body temperature in healthy man. Oral readings of 97°F are relatively common on arising in the morning. Body temperature rises steadily through the day, reaches a peak of 99°F or greater between 6 P.M. and 10 P.M., and then drops slowly to reach a minimum at 2 A.M. to 4 A.M. Although it might be postulated that this diurnal variation is dependent upon increasing activity during the day and rest at night, the pattern is not reversed in individuals who work at night and sleep during the day for long periods of time.

The febrile patterns of most human diseases also tend to follow this normal diurnal pattern. Fevers tend to be higher, to "spike," in the evening, and many patients with febrile disease have relatively normal temperatures in the early morning hours.

Severe or prolonged exercise or very hot baths can produce a transient elevation in body temperature, which is quickly compensated for by increased dissipation for the skin and lungs. Such elevations are not properly classified as fevers. Body temperature is somewhat labile in young children, and transient elevations after relatively slight exertion in warm weather are frequently observed in this group.

DISORDERED THERMOREGULATION

All fevers are accompanied by an *increase in heat production,* and abrupt rises after shaking chills may involve as much as a 600 percent increase for a short time. Elevation of body temperature itself increases metabolic activity about 7 percent for each degree Fahrenheit. There is no question, however, about the major importance of *decrease in heat loss* in fevers of any duration. Abrupt rises after severe exertion in healthy individuals are compensated for within a few minutes, but in illness the compensatory mechanism fails and the elevation is sustained. When it is considered that a 10 percent decrease in heat loss will result in a body temperature of 106°F within a few hours, the cardinal role of defective heat loss in fever is more easily appreciated. DuBois has pointed out the existence of a "safety valve" in human adults. When hyperthermia reaches dangerous levels, the mechanisms for heat loss are suddenly activated; consequently, oral temperatures above 106°F are rare in man. While the operation of this cutoff can be spoken of as analogous to the action of a thermostat, there is no evidence to support the existence of any physiologic equivalent of a "thermostat" in the regulation of body temperature; the analogy should not be substituted for a frank admission of ignorance of the basic mechanisms involved.

Deviations of 5°F from the normal body temperature of 98.6°F do not interfere appreciably with most bodily functions. Convulsions are common at temperatures higher than 106°F, and irreversible brain damage, presumably due to protein denaturation (impairment of normal enzymic functions) is common when temperatures of 108°F are reached. Conversely, when temperatures are lowered to 91°F, loss of consciousness occurs, at 86°F poikilothermia sets in, and between 83 and 84°F ventricular fibrillation supervenes.

The systemic symptoms accompanying deviations in temperature are poorly understood. For example at temperatures of 102°F many patients have malaise, drowsiness, weakness, and generalized aches and pains. Many others, however, feel entirely well. Why some individuals are able to tolerate fever so well, while others become markedly ill remains an enigma. Perhaps the inciting stimulus rather than fever per se is the major determinant of systemic complaints.

DISEASES OF THE NERVOUS SYSTEM. Disease of the regulatory centers in the hypothalamus may affect body temperature. Cases have been observed in which there was destruction of the centers controlling heat-conserving mechanisms, with resulting hypothermia. More commonly, cerebral lesions are manifested by hyperthermia; this may occur with tumors, infections, degenerative diseases, or vascular accidents. It is not uncommon in cerebral apoplexy for the temperature to rise to 105 to 107°F during the last few hours before death.

Heat stroke ("sunstroke") is an interesting example of fever due to interference with the controlling mechanism. Here the central mechanisms for cooling seem suddenly to fail and the patient ceases to sweat, despite the fact that his temperature is rising. Some of the highest temperatures ever observed in human beings (112 to 113°F) have been in cases of heat stroke. A temperature higher than 114°F is not compatible with life.

INCREASED HEAT PRODUCTION. Patients with thyrotoxicosis frequently have an elevation in temperature 1 to 2°F above the normal range. This is ascribable to the increased amount of heat produced by an increase in the activity and rate of the metabolic processes. Dinitrophenol, a drug which was formerly used for weight reduction in obese persons, causes elevation of temperature; this too seems to be caused by an increased metabolic activity, produced by some mechanism outside the thyroid.

IMPAIRMENT OF HEAT LOSS. Patients with congestive heart failure often have an elevation of body temperature, between 0.5 and 1.5°F. Perhaps this elevation is caused by impairment of heat dissipation as a result of diminished cardiac output, decline in cutaneous blood flow (with increasing insulation of the central temperature core), the insulating effect of edema, and the increased heat production incident to the muscular activity of dyspnea. On the other hand, patients with congestive heart failure are likely to have other causes of fever, such as venous thrombosis, pulmonary embolism and infarction, myocardial infarction, rheumatic fever, and urinary tract infection. However, since slight fever is so regularly present even in the absence of such complications, the circulatory disturbance may be responsible.

Patients with skin disorders such as ichthyosis or congenital absence of sweat glands may have fever in a warm environment because of inability to lose heat from the surface of the body. Similarly, individuals taking drugs which impair sweating [atropine, propantheline (Pro-Banthine)] may have fever in warm weather.

HYPOTHERMIA. From the clinical standpoint, reduction of body temperature is of far less frequency and importance than is elevation. Daily variation of temperature within the "subnormal" range, i.e., 97 to 98.6°F, is observed in nearly all healthy individuals. The temperature range may be somewhat lower than normal, i.e., 96 to 97.5°F, in patients with myxedema and during the first day or so after critical fall in temperature associated with infectious disease. Oral temperatures below 96°F are rarely encountered, as there is apparently a potent countering mechanism which opposes falls below that level. This barrier may, of course, be broken through exposure to extreme cold. Furthermore, when cerebral function has been impaired, as by alcohol or large doses of sedative drugs, less severe chilling can result in a fall in body temperature. An example of this is the hypo-

thermic temperatures found in vagrants who are found in unheated rooms, railroad yards, and other exposed places after alcoholic debaucheries. The lowered body temperature in shock may be due to impaired cerebral regulation or to inability to produce adequate heat.

One condition in which profound hypothermia may develop is myxedema with coma (Chap. 89). Body temperature in such a patient may gradually sink to 80 to 85°F. Attending personnel may fail to recognize this because the clinical thermometer registers only as low as it has been shaken; hence a series of falsely high readings in the range of 95 to 97°F may be recorded.

REFERENCES

Brengelman, G., and A. C. Brown: Temperature Regulation, pp. 1050–1069 in "Physiology and Biophysics," T. C. Ruch and H. D. Patton (eds.), Philadelphia, W. B. Saunders Company, 1965.

Dubois, E. F.: "Fever and the Regulation of Body Temperature," Springfield, Ill., Charles C Thomas, Publisher, 1948.

Pickering, G. W.: Regulation of Body Temperature in Health and Disease (Lancet), 1:1 and 59, 1958.

16 CHILLS AND FEVER
Ivan L. Bennett, Jr. and Robert G. Petersdorf

In view of the extensive knowledge of physiologic mechanisms controlling body temperature mentioned in the previous chapter, it is surprising that so little is known about the ways in which diseases upset thermoregulation.

Some bacteria, particularly gram-negative species, produce endotoxins which are pyrogenic (Chap. 134, 144), and a few viruses also cause fever when injected into man or animals. Many microorganisms, however, possess no demonstrable pyrogenic toxin, and of course, fever accompanies diseases which do not involve invasion of the body by any known parasite. Omitting disorders which involve cerebral thermoregulatory centers directly, febrile diseases may be grouped as follows: (1) All *infections*, whether caused by bacteria, rickettsias, viruses, or more complex parasites, may cause fever. (2) *Mechanical trauma*, as in crushing injuries, frequently gives rise to fever lasting 1 or 2 days. Not infrequently, however, complicating infection sets in. (3) Most *neoplastic diseases* are associated with fever. In most patients, fever in patients with cancer is related to obstruction or infection produced by the tumor. In some neoplasms, however, particularly cancers of the liver, stomach, and pancreas, fever may be due to the tumor per se, particularly following metastasis to the liver. Hypernephroma can produce hectic fever with daily chills. In lymphosarcoma or Hodgkin's disease, fever may be one of the prominent early manifestations. (4) Many *hematopoietic disorders* are characterized by pyrexia, examples being acute hemolytic episodes and the leukemias. (5) *Vascular accidents* of any magnitude nearly always cause fever, examples being myocardial, pulmonary, and cerebral infarctions. (6) *Diseases due to immune mechanisms* are almost always febrile. These include the collagen diseases, drug fevers, and serum sickness. (7) Certain *acute metabolic disorders,* such as gout, porphyria, and thyroid crisis, sometimes are associated with fever.

PATHOGENESIS OF FEVER

Several hypotheses have been offered to explain disturbed temperature regulation in disease. Some investigators have attributed fever to shifts in body water which interfere with heat production and heat loss. It is true that newborn infants may become febrile when fluid intake is inadequate and that the temperature elevation subsides promptly when fluid is administered. In adults, there are occasional instances of fever associated with extracellular fluid deficit when the ambient temperature is above 90°F. On the other hand, "dehydration" is not ordinarily associated with fever in adults, and the clinical practice of attributing fever to this cause is to be deprecated.

Some have attempted to account for fever on the basis of alterations in endocrine function, with particular reference to the thyroid and adrenals. There is little clinical or experimental evidence to support this idea. Temperature regulation is normal in Addison's disease and in Cushing's syndrome. Body temperature is slightly above normal in thyrotoxicosis and a little low in myxedema, but these differences are entirely in keeping with the metabolic rate and there is no real evidence of impaired thermoregulation in either disease.

There was a renewal of interest in a role of the endocrines in the pathogenesis of fever with the finding that abnormalities of etiocholanolone metabolism exist in some patients with "periodic" fever (Chap. 256). Although administration of progesterone and some of its congeners and of etiocholanolone results in fever in man, there is no evidence that specific steroid fevers (notably etiocholanolone fever) exist.

The common factor in febrile diseases whether or not they are infectious in origin is *tissue injury.* The hypothesis which best fits clinical and experimental observations is that fever results from disturbance of cerebral thermoregulation brought about by a product or products of tissue injury. It has been shown experimentally that inflammatory exudates cause fever when injected intravenously into normal animals, and similar results have been obtained in human subjects. Probably the major source of pyrogenic material is the polymorphonuclear leukocyte, although other cells may also release fever-producing substances.

While considering the pathogenesis of fever, the sequence of events which follows intravenous injection of killed bacteria or of purified bacterial endotoxin is relevant. Figure 16-1 shows a typical human response to injection of typhoid vaccine. Body temperature does not begin to rise until about an hour after injection of the

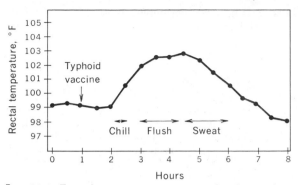

Fig. 16-1. Typical temperature response of a human being to intravenous injection of a comparatively large dose of typhoid vaccine—100,000,000 organisms.

pyrogen. During this interval, the patient notes no discomfort and his appearance is unchanged. Then, rather suddenly, there is malaise, he complains of cold, and within minutes he is burrowing down into the bedclothes, asking for more blankets. He begins to shiver and is soon having a shaking chill which lasts 10 to 20 min. During this time, the skin is pale and cold but rectal temperature rises steeply. After subsidence of the rigor, the patient gradually feels warmer, skin circulation increases, and within 2 hr he is flushed and complains of feeling feverish. After another hour, profuse sweating begins and body temperature begins to return toward normal.

ENDOGENOUS PYROGEN. The pathophysiologic counterpart of these clinical events has been worked out to a large extent in experimental animals. Following its injection, endotoxin is removed rapidly from the bloodstream by the fixed phagocytes of the reticuloendothelial system. At the same time there is, in most species, a profound leukopenia, and these cells are marginated along blood vessel walls. During this period, they appear to be activated to release a fever-producing substance into the circulation. This humoral factor, which has been called *endogenous pyrogen,* is presumably the substance which acts on the thermoregulatory centers to produce fever. Endogenous pyrogen has been found in the bloodstream of animals given endotoxin, antigens (in previously sensitized animals) antigen-antibody complexes, and those with experimental pneumococcal, streptococcal, staphylococcal, and viral infections. Biologically, endogenous pyrogen behaves similarly to sterile inflammatory exudates. It is a low-molecular-weight protein, which is heat-labile and probably basic and may be closely related to lysozomal enzymes. Its biochemical structure has not been worked out, but there is suggestive evidence that it exists in cells in an inactive precursor form. Whether endogenous pyrogen is the sole mediator of fever, or whether some of the agents which incite its release—such as endotoxin—can activate the thermoregulatory centers directly is unknown.

ACCOMPANIMENTS OF FEVER

The perception of fever by patients varies enormously. Some individuals can tell with considerable accuracy whether their body temperatures are elevated, apparently by sensations of warmth in the skin. Others, notably patients with tuberculosis, may be wholly unaware of body temperatures as high as 103°F. Often, also, patients may pay no attention to fever because of other unpleasant symptoms such as headache (Chap. 10) and pleuritic pain.

Pain in the back, generalized myalgias, and arthralgia without arthritis are common in fever. Whether these symptoms reflect the presence of an infectious agent or are merely a nonspecific accompaniment of pyrexia is not clear.

Abrupt onset of fever with a *chill* or *rigor* is characteristic of some diseases and, in the absence of antipyretic drugs, rare in others. Athough repeated rigors suggest pyogenic infection with bacteremia, a similar pattern of fever may occur in noninfectious diseases such as lymphoma and hypernephroma. It is important to differentiate a true chill which is accompanied by teeth chattering or bed shaking from the chilly sensation which occurs in almost all fevers, particularly those in viral infections. In some instances, however, a true rigor occurs in viremia.

Herpes labialis, so-called "fever blister," results from activation of the herpes simplex virus by elevated temperature and occurs frequently in patients undergoing artificial fever therapy. For reasons which are obscure, fever blisters are common in pneumococcal infections, streptococcosis, malaria, meningococcemia, and rickettsioses but are rare in mycoplasma pneumonia, tuberculosis, brucellosis, smallpox, and typhoid.

Delirium can result from elevation of body temperature and is particularly common in patients with alcoholism or cerebral arteriosclerosis.

Convulsions are not infrequent in febrile children, especially those with a family history of epilepsy, although febrile convulsions do not, in general, reflect serious cerebral disease.

CLINICAL IMPORTANCE OF FEVER

The clinical thermometer was one of the first instruments of precision to be introduced into the practice of medicine. Its objectivity and simplicity make it an immensely valuable aid to physical diagnosis. Nowadays we are so accustomed to graphic temperature charts in hospitals and the ready availability of the clinical thermometer for use in the home that we scarcely realize our great dependence upon them. Determination of the body temperature assists in estimating the severity of an illness, its course and duration, and the effect of therapy, or even in deciding whether a person has an organic illness.

A question frequently asked is whether fever is beneficial. There are a few infections of man in which pyrexia appears definitely to be beneficial to the host, examples being neurosyphilis, some gonococcal infections, and chronic brucellosis. Certain other diseases, such as uveitis and rheumatoid arthritis, sometimes improve after fever therapy. In experimental animals some pneumococcal and cryptococcal infections have been influenced in favor of the host animal by raising the body temperature. Aged and debilitated patients with infection may exhibit little or no fever, and this is generally interpreted as a bad prognostic sign. In the great majority of infectious diseases, however, there is no reason to believe that pyrexia accelerates phagocytosis, antibody formation, or other defense mechanisms.

Fever has its detrimental aspects. The greater velocity of all metabolic processes accentuates weight loss and nitrogen wastage. The work and the rate of the heart are increased. Sweating aggravates loss of fluid and salt. There may be discomfort due to headache, photophobia, general malaise, or unpleasant sensation of warmth. The rigors and profuse sweats of hectic fevers are particularly unpleasant for the patient.

In elderly individuals with overt or potential cardiac or cerebral vascular disease, fever may be particularly deleterious.

MANAGEMENT OF FEVER. Since fever ordinarily does little harm and imposes no great discomfort, antipyretic drugs are rarely necessary and may obscure the effect of a specific therapeutic agent and of the natural course of the disease. There are situations, however, in which lowering of the body temperature is of vital importance: heat stroke, postoperative hyperthermia, delirium due to high pyrexia, and shock associated with fever and heart failure. Under these circumstances, sponging the body surface with cool saline or the application of cool compresses to the skin and forehead may be employed. There is no advantage to sponging with alcohol which, because of its pungent odor, makes some patients ill. When high internal temperature is combined with cutaneous vasoconstriction, as in heat stroke or postoperative hyperthermia, the cooling measures should be combined with massage of the skin in order to bring blood to the surface, where it may be cooled. Immediate immersion in a tub of ice water should be considered a lifesaving emergency procedure in patients with heat stroke if the internal body temperature is in excess of 108°F. Cooling blankets which can be set at hypothermic temperatures are a highly effective means for external cooling and have supplanted immersion into ice in most instances.

If antipyretic drugs, such as aspirin (0.3 to 0.6 Gm), are employed to bring about a fall in temperature, the ill effects of the unpleasant diaphoresis, sometimes associated with an alarming fall in blood pressure and the subsequent return of fever, occasionally accompanied by a chill, can be mitigated by enforcing a liberal fluid intake and by administering the drug regularly and frequently at 2- or 3-hr intervals.

The discomfort of a rigor can be alleviated in many patients by the intravenous injection of calcium gluconate. This procedure will stop the shivering and chilliness but has no influence on the ultimate height of the fever. Severe disruptive rigors sometimes need to be abolished with morphine sulfate (10 to 15 mg subcutaneously).

DIAGNOSTIC SIGNIFICANCE OF FEVER

Illnesses of unknown etiology in which fever is a prominent or the only manifestation are frequent. Fever is not an indication of any particular type of disease; it is merely a reaction to injury comparable to alterations in leukocyte count or increased erythrocyte sedimentation rate. In approaching patients with fever, two cardinal diagnostic principles must be kept in mind: (1) Most of the time fever is a manifestation of a common disease, and fever associated with a pulmonary infiltrate is much more likely due to pneumococcal than to pneumocystics pneumonia. (2) The diagnosis of febrile illnesses must occur in the context of the epidemiologic setting. For example, an acute 7-day febrile illness in a soldier in Vietnam is probably due to malaria, scrub typhus, or leptospirosis; in a college student in the United States it may represent infectious mononucleosis or some other viral infection, and in an octogenarian following prostatectomy it is probably an indication of urinary tract infection, wound infection, pulmonary infarction, or aspiration pneumonia. When fever becomes prolonged (2 to 3 weeks) and assumes a central feature in the patient's illness, it is defined as fever of unknown origin, or FUO. The more important probabilities to be considered in dealing with a patient with FUO are discussed below.

FEBRILE ILLNESSES OF SHORT DURATION

Acute febrile illnesses of less than 2 weeks' duration are a common occurrence in medical practice. In many instances they run their courses, progressing to complete recovery, and a precise diagnosis is not made. In most instances, however, it is safe to assume that the illness is of infectious origin. Although short febrile illnesses can be noninfectious, i.e. allergic fevers due to drugs or serums, thromboembolic disease, hemolytic crises, or gout, they are decidedly in the minority.

Most undiagnosed acute febrile infectious diseases are probably viral, since diagnostic methods for bacterial infection are better, and they are rapidly brought under control by the chemotherapeutic agents in common use. It is not practical to carry out tests needed to identify all the known viruses, and furthermore, there must be a considerable number of as yet unidentified viruses pathogenic for man.

The following characteristics, while not restricted solely to acute infections, are highly suggestive that infection is present:
1. Abrupt onset
2. High fever, i.e., 102 to 105°F, with or without chills
3. Respiratory symptoms—sore throat, coryza, cough
4. Severe malaise, with muscle or joint pain, photophobia, pain on movement of the eyes, headache
5. Nausea, vomiting, or diarrhea
6. Acute enlargement of lymph nodes or spleen
7. Meningeal signs, with or without spinal fluid pleocytosis
8. Leukocyte count above 12,000 or below 5,000 per cu mm

None of the symptoms or signs listed is encountered only in infection. Many of these features could be seen in acute myeloblastic leukemia or disseminated lupus erythematosus. Nevertheless, in a given instance of acute febrile illness with some or all of the manifestations listed, the probabilities strongly favor infection, and the patient can be given reasonable reassurance that he will probably recover in a week or two, regardless of a precise diagnosis.

It is desirable of course, to establish an accurate diagnosis, and whatever steps are practicable in the circumstances to establish the cause should be taken. Cultures of the throat, blood, urine, or feces should be obtained *before* institution of antibacterial chemotherapy. Skin and/or serologic tests should be carried out when indicated.

PROLONGED FEBRILE ILLNESSES

Some of the knottiest problems in the field of internal medicine are found in cases of prolonged fever in which the diagnosis remains obscure for weeks or even months. Eventually, however, the true nature of the illness usually reveals itself, since a disease which causes injury sufficient to evoke temperature elevations of 101°F or higher for several weeks does not often subside without leaving some clue as to its nature.

The elucidation of problems of this sort calls for skillful application of all diagnostic methods—careful history, thorough physical examination, and the considered application of good laboratory examinations.

It is obviously not possible or practical in this section to mention all the known entities which may cause prolonged febrile disease, or even to give an adequate discussion of the differential diagnosis of the more frequent ones. Additional details about the manifestations and differential diagnosis of the entities mentioned will be found elsewhere.

INFECTIOUS DISEASES

The infections occupy a less prominent position among the causes of prolonged fever now than formerly, because of the common practice of administering antibiotic drugs to any patient in whom fever persists for more than a few days. Consequently, many infections are at present being eradicated by more or less "blind" therapy, without their nature or location being determined accurately. Nevertheless, patients with infection comprise the greatest percentage in any group of patients with FUO. Furthermore, certain infections do not respond to the usual antibiotic therapy. In general, this does not apply to virus diseases because they tend to run their courses more or less acutely and do not often cause continued illness lasting many weeks or months, irrespective of chemotherapy.

TUBERCULOSIS. (Chap. 174.) This disease proves to be responsible for puzzling febrile disease with surprising frequency, despite the facts that there is a fairly effective therapy and that the simple procedure of chest x-ray is usually sufficient for diagnosis of the commonest clinical form. The drugs given as therapeutic trials may not include those with tuberculostatic activity such as streptomycin or isoniazid. Extrapulmonary forms of tuberculosis may not be easily located, e.g., disease of the bones, deep lymph nodes, genital or urinary organs. Furthermore, the pulmonary lesions of miliary tuberculosis may not be detectable by x-ray until very late in the course of the disease. In considering the possibility of tuberculous infection, the skin test may be of great assistance, since negative reaction to a properly executed skin test rules out the possibility of tuberculosis except in rare instances of overwhelming disease. A positive skin reaction, on the other hand, does not prove that tuberculosis is causing the patient's illness, but in its presence tuberculosis must be kept in mind as a possibility until another cause for the fever is found.

BACTERIAL ENDOCARDITIS. (Chap. 137.) In the classical subacute form of the disease, a heart murmur is nearly always present; therefore, absence of murmur largely eliminated this disease from consideration. The correct diagnosis is likely to be missed in middle-aged or elderly patients, in whom a heart murmur may not be given much weight. For example, an elderly patient with subacute bacterial endocarditis may first present following the occurrence of a cerebral embolus and may be regarded as having had a hemorrhage or thrombosis because of arteriosclerosis. The best clinical practice is to culture the blood of *every* patient who has fever and a heart murmur. Bacterial endocarditis without cardiac murmurs is seen most frequently in intravenous drug users who develop infection on the tricuspid valve, and every such individual who presents with fever should be assumed to have endocarditis until proved otherwise. In addition, antibiotics mask SBE because these drugs often render blood cultures negative until the drugs have been excreted or metabolized. For this reason, patients suspected of having SBE who have received antimicrobials, should have blood cultures taken for several days after administration of the drugs is discontinued.

BRUCELLOSIS. (Chap. 154.) This infection is most unlikely in an American city dweller but has to be considered in farmers, veterinarians, or slaughterhouse workers. Arthralgia and myalgia are common, but actual redness and swelling of joints are rare in this disease. Peripheral leukocytosis is seldom seen in brucellosis. In active febrile disease the blood culture and bone marrow culture frequently are positive, and specific agglutinins are *nearly always* present in the serum.

SALMONELLA INFECTION. (Chaps. 149 and 150.) Although typhoid fever is subject to great variability and may cause fever for several weeks, it should not often be a cause of prolonged fever of obscure origin, since cultures of feces or blood will be positive, and the specific antibodies are detected in the agglutination reaction. Other salmonella organisms may, however, cause prolonged febrile illness, and these may present greater diagnostic difficulty. Routine serologic tests may not be helpful, and antibiotics, including chloramphenicol (Chloromycetin), may not be effective. Repeated culture of the blood or of bone marrow may yield the causative organism. There may eventually be localization of infection in a joint or the pleural cavity from which the etiologic agent can be obtained.

PYOGENIC INFECTION. (Chap. 136.) Chemotherapy often does not succeed in eradicating localized pyogenic infection, and in certain locations inflammation may be relatively asymptomatic. These infections include osteomyelitis of the vertebrae or pelvic bones, subdiaphragmatic, hepatic, perinephric, renal cortical, retropharyngeal, and mediastinal abscesses, cholangitis, bronchiectasis, and pelvic inflammatory disease. The right upper quadrant, pericolonic, periappendiceal, and pelvic regions are particularly prone to sequestration of abscesses. X-ray studies are often helpful, but many times exploratory surgery must be performed to achieve both diagnosis and cure.

AMEBIASIS. (Chap. 240.) Amebic colitis usually evokes symptoms pointing to disease of the colon. Hepatic involvement, on the other hand, may not give a distinctive clinical picture, and prolonged fever may be the principal manifestation. Some assistance may be obtained from a history of dysentery, or from tenderness or enlargement of the liver and elevation of the right leaf of the diaphragm. The complement fixation test has little diagnostic value. Therapeutic trial of an antiamebic drug, such as chloroquine or emetine, which acts on the hepatic form of amebiasis, may be justified.

HISTOPLASMOSIS. (Chap. 188.) This infection is prevalent in the region of the Mississippi Valley of the United States, although in most individuals it is not clinically recognizable. The disease may, however, be manifested as a chronic febrile illness, with localizing manifestations pointing to many organ systems. Fever, leukopenia, anemia, hepatomegaly, and splenomegaly in a person who has resided in a geographic area where histoplasmosis occurs should suggest the possibility. The skin reaction to histoplasmin is often positive but may be negative in disseminated histoplasmosis, which is the form most likely to cause prolonged pyrexia. The complement fixation reaction, on the other hand, is nearly always positive in disseminated disease. The organisms may be demonstrated in biopsy of involved tissue or in bone marrow.

COCCIDIOIDOMYCOSIS. (Chap. 187.) This disease needs to be considered in persons who have traveled through, or resided in, the southwest part of the United States. Clinical manifestations are like those of the various forms of tuberculosis. The coccidioidin skin test and serologic reaction to this antigen are positive.

SCHISTOSOMIASIS. (Chap. 250.) Persons who have lived in the Caribbean islands, in Africa, or in the Far East may have prolonged febrile illness associated with this infestation. Diarrhea, bladder symptoms, cough, hepatosplenomegaly, and anemia are suggestive. Diagnosis is made by finding the ova in feces or urine or in rectal or hepatic biopsy. Salmonella infection, including bacteremia, is common in schistosomiasis and may be responsible for fever.

COLLAGEN DISEASES

Under this term is included a broad spectrum of diseases in which there are histologic evidences of disorders

of collagen and the blood vessels. Some of these diseases are particularly important causes of prolonged febrile illness.

DISSEMINATED LUPUS ERYTHEMATOSUS. (Chap. 392.) This disease is by no means rare, being encountered with greater frequency in American hospitals than typhoid fever. The possibility should receive special consideration in a young woman with fever, polyarthritis, low or low-normal leukocyte count, anemia, pulmonary infiltrations or pleural involvement, and hematuria and other evidence of acute nephritis. Behavioral abnormalities, orbital edema, and salivary gland swelling are less common features. The diagnosis can be made with confidence in patients who develop the full clinical picture, or by demonstration of LE cells or a rise in titer of antinuclear factor. The diseases likely to be confused with disseminated lupus erythematosus are rheumatic fever and rheumatoid arthritis.

PERIARTERITIS NODOSA. (Chap. 391.) Features which particularly point to this syndrome are febrile illness in a male of any age, with leukocytosis, eosinophilia, anemia, asthma, peripheral neuritis, arthritis or muscle pain, hypertension, and evidence of renal involvement. Lesions in medium-sized arteries can give rise to the clinical pictures of myocardial infarction, mesenteric embolism, and peripheral vascular disease. There may be a variety of cutaneous eruptions. The only conclusive method of diagnosis is biopsy of a muscle or a skin lesion or of other tissue excised at operation.

RHEUMATOID ARTHRITIS. (Chap. 386.) In its earlier stages there may not be characteristic swelling and deformity of joints but only vague pains in muscles and joints, together with fever, slight anemia, and malaise. Differentiation from rheumatic fever and from disseminated lupus erythematosus may be difficult. Sometimes the diagnosis cannot be made until the more characteristic picture of the disease develops, or the latex test becomes unequivocally positive.

RHEUMATIC FEVER. (Chap. 269.) Fever, with or without muscle and joint pains, may persist for weeks and months at a time. A history of preceding attacks or of an upper respiratory infection before onset of the systemic illness, the presence of a heart murmur, relative tachycardia, and arrythmias or conduction defects are suggestive findings. Significant elevation of the antistreptolysin O titer is present in 80 percent of cases, and other acute phase reactants (antihyaluronidase, antistreptokinase) in the remainder. It may be difficult to differentiate active rheumatic fever with carditis from SLE, rheumatoid disease, bacterial endocarditis, and *atrial myxoma*. This intracardiac tumor may present with fever, arthralgias, peripheral embolic phenomena, and heart murmurs. Cardiac angiography is diagnostic. It is particularly important to consider myxoma in the differential diagnosis because it can be removed completely by open-heart surgical techniques.

HENOCH–SCHÖNLEIN, OR ALLERGIC, PURPURA. (Chap. 245.) There may be fever, joint pains, and evidences of renal and pulmonary involvement. The results of the capillary fragility test and platelet count are normal. Differentiation from lupus erythematosus, rheumatic fever, and acute glomerulonephritis may be difficult. Diagnosis will depend on the finding of hemorrhagic occurrences, usually in the intestinal lumen or in joints.

NEOPLASTIC DISEASES

Fever is a common manifestation of cancer but a very rare accompaniment of benign tumors. In patients in the age range where cancer is common, unexplained fever should always suggest the possibility of neoplasm.

CARCINOMAS AND SARCOMAS. Certain malignant processes seem especially likely to cause fever. Notable are sarcomas involving bone or lymphoid tissue, hypernephroma, carcinoma of the pancreas or stomach, and metastatic cancer of the liver. Occasionally the clinical picture is strongly suggestive of pyogenic infection, with hectic fever, chills, sweats, and marked leukocytosis; and patients have been subjected to laparotomy with preoperative diagnoses such as empyema of the gallbladder, localized peritonitis, or liver abscess.

HODGKIN'S DISEASE. Fever may be the principal symptom and only objective finding early in the course of Hodgkin's disease, especially when the principal involvement is in the abdominal viscera or retroperitoneal regions. Cases with splenomegaly and vague abdominal distress have been confused with typhoid fever. Pel-Ebstein fever is seen in a minority of cases of Hodgkin's disease. The diagnosis of this disorder is made by biopsy.

HEMATOPOIETIC DISEASES

Disorders of blood formation or blood destruction are frequently associated with fever.

LEUKEMIAS. It is not uncommon for acute leukemia to be mistaken for acute infection at the onset. The acute leukemias are nearly always accompanied by fever, sometimes as high as 105°F. The correct diagnosis will be suggested by rapid development of anemia and characteristic changes in peripheral blood and bone marrow. Chronic leukemia, particularly lymphatic, may be characterized by low-grade fever, but because of the typical changes in circulating leukocytes, is not often a diagnostic problem. Both acute and chronic leukemias may be accompanied by infection, which may be responsible for the fever, and before it is assumed that fever in a patient with leukemia is due to the blood dyscrasia, infection must be ruled out by appropriate tests and cultures.

HEMOLYTIC EPISODES. Most of the hemolytic diseases are characterized by bouts of fever. Acute crises of hemolysis may give rise to shaking chills and marked elevations of temperature. The difficulty sometimes encountered in differentiating sickle-cell disease from acute rheumatic fever is well known. The presence of these hemolytic disorders is suggested by the more rapid development of anemia than occurs in other febrile illnesses and by the usual accompaniment of reticulocytosis and jaundice.

Fever is not characteristic of severe anemia due to external blood loss or of the anemia of uremia.

VASCULAR DISEASE

Reference has already been made to the fever of collagen diseases, all of which are accompanied by vascular lesions. In addition, certain other diseases of the blood vessels, not always regarded as being in the same category as the collagen diseases, may cause chronic illness.

TEMPORAL, OR CRANIAL, ARTERITIS. (Chap. 394.) This is a disease of old people, featured by severe aching pain in the temporal area, headache, muscle and joint pains, fever, and leukocytosis. There may be accompanying visual defects or blindness due to involvement of the retinal artery. The temporal or occipital arteries may be inflamed and tender. Diagnosis is not difficult if the superficial arteries are carefully palpated and temporal artery biopsy is performed.

THROMBOEMBOLIC DISEASE. In migratory thrombophlebitis, segments of large veins become inflamed and thrombosed. There is usually local pain and swelling, but sometimes the lesions are cryptic. Symptomless thrombosis of deep calf or pelvic veins may cause prolonged febrile illness as a result of repeated small pulmonary emboli. These emboli may not be manifested by pleuritic pain or hemoptysis, but cough, dyspnea, or vague thoracic discomfort is likely to be present. Careful examination of the legs and repeated examination of the lungs should reveal the diagnosis. Sometimes these patients present with a nephrotic syndrome due to renal vein thrombosis.

MISCELLANEOUS

SARCOIDOSIS. Ordinarily, fever is not characteristic of sarcoidosis, but it is prominent in a minority of cases, especially those characterized by arthralgia, hilar lymphadenopathy, and cutaneous lesions resembling erythema nodosum, or in those with extensive hepatic lesions. Diagnosis is suggested by lymphoid enlargement, ocular lesions, and hyperglobulinemia and is clinched by biopsy of skin, lymph nodes, or liver.

REGIONAL ENTERITIS. Inflammatory lesions of the large and small bowel rarely present as FUO's but an occasional individual who has only fever, abdominal pain, and subtle changes in bowel habits, will be found to have regional enteritis.

DRUG FEVER. (Chap. 73.) This is an important cause of cryptic fever, and a careful history of drug intake should be taken in every patient with unexplained fever. Fever due to allergy to one of the antibiotics may become superimposed on the fever of the infection for which the drug was given, resulting in a very confusing picture. Often fever is due to common drugs including sulfonamides, arsenicals, iodides, thiouracils, barbiturates, and laxatives especially those containing phenolphthalein. Any questions of drug fever can be resolved rapidly by discontinuing all medication. The diagnosis can be further substantiated by giving a test dose of the drug after fever has subsided, but this may result in a very unpleasant or even dangerous reaction.

FAMILIAL MEDITERRANEAN FEVER. (Chap. 256.)

MALINGERING. Rarely, a patient will produce purposeful elevations in temperature. Many methods have been employed to cause the thermometer to register higher than the true temperature. If malingering is suspected, all that is necessary to prove it is to repeat the temperature determination immediately after a high reading has been obtained, with someone remaining at the bedside while the thermometer is in place.

PROLONGED LOW-GRADE TEMPERATURE ELEVATIONS

Not infrequently a patient, while not appearing acutely ill, has been subject to elevation of body temperature above the "normal" level, i.e., his temperature has been in the range of 99.0 to 100.5°F. Prolonged low-grade fever may be a manifestation of serious illness, or it may be a matter of no real consequence. Possibly there are some individuals whose "normal" temperatures are in this range. However, there is no certain way of identifying such individuals. The possibilities to be considered in such cases vary considerably according to the age groups concerned.

In children temperature regulation may be somewhat erratic even up to the age of twelve years. Children may therefore have slight temperature elevations when excited or after exercise. A mother may note that her child's skin feels hot when he has been playing and may find his temperature slightly above normal. Reexamination on subsequent days may reveal the same elevation from time to time. This poses the question whether the "fever" is an indication of disease or of imperfect thermoregulation. If the physical examination reveals no abnormality, if the appetite is good and the child is gaining weight, and if there is no anemia or urinary abnormality, it is fairly safe to advise the parent to cease taking temperatures and forget about "fever." Real harm can be done by restricting the activity of an otherwise healthy child because of misinterpretation of the significance of low-grade fever.

In young adults chronic low-grade temperature elevation cannot easily be imputed to imperfect thermoregulation. Here tuberculosis, brucellosis, rheumatic fever or other collagen disease, as well as many of the conditions mentioned in the preceding section have to be considered. A special problem encountered in females of this age group is *habitual hyperthermia,* and every experienced physician has encountered examples of the syndrome. The patient may have temperatures of 99.0 to 100.5°F regularly or intermittently for years and also usually has a variety of complaints characteristic of psychoneurosis, such as fatigability, insomnia, bowel distress, vague aches, and headache. Prolonged careful study and observation fail to reveal evidence of organic disease. Unfortunately, many of these people go from doctor to doctor and are subjected to a variety of unpleasant, expensive, and even harmful tests, treatments, and operations. The diagnosis of this syndrome can be made with reasonable certainty after a suitable period of observation and study, and if the patient can be convinced of its validity, a real service will have been rendered.

In a patient past middle age even low-grade fever should always be regarded as a probable indication of organic disease. The possibilities to be considered in this age group are the same as those discussed above in the section Prolonged Febrile Illnesses.

RELAPSING AND RECURRENT FEVERS

Occasionally patients are encountered who have recurrent bouts of high fever at more or less regular intervals. The following are among the diseases which have to be considered:

MALARIA. (Chap. 241.) The disease had vanished from the United States almost completely, but Vietnam war veterans constitute an important and sizable reservoir of this infection, as do other persons recently arrived from foreign countries. It is most unusual, however, for malaria to recur after a symptom-free interval of 1 year or more. Seizures recur at 2- or 3-day intervals, or more irregularly in falciparum infections, depending on the maturation cycle of the parasite. Diagnosis depends on demonstration of the parasites in the blood.

RELAPSING FEVER. (Chap. 182.) This disease occurs in the southwest part of the United States, as far east as Texas, and in many other parts of the world. The recurrences are related to some cycle in the development of the parasites. Diagnosis is by demonstration of the spirochetal organisms in stained films of the blood.

RAT-BITE FEVER. (Chaps. 162 and 183.) Two etiologic agents—Spirillum minus and Streptobacillus moniliformis can be transmitted by the bite of a rat. Both may cause an illness characterized by periodic exacerbations of fever. The clue as to the diagnosis depends on obtaining a history of rat bite 1 to 10 weeks previous to the onset of symptoms. The cause can be established by appropriate laboratory procedures.

PYOGENIC INFECTION. In rare instances, localized pyogenic infections give rise to periodic bouts of fever separated by afebrile and relatively symptom-free intervals. The so-called "Charcot's intermittent biliary fever," cholangitis with biliary obstruction due to stones, is an example. The febrile attacks are sometimes associated with slight jaundice. There should be a history suggestive of cholelithiasis, and during the attacks tenderness can be elicited in the right upper quadrant. Urinary tract infection, with episodes of ureteral obstruction due to small stones or inspissated pus, can also cause recurrent fever.

HODGKIN'S DISEASE. In perhaps 5 to 10 percent of cases, there is seen at some time during the course of the disease the so-called "Pel-Ebstein fever"—bouts of fever lasting 3 to 10 days, separated by afebrile and asymptomatic periods of 3 to 10 days. These cycles may be repeated regularly over a period of several months. In rare instances this periodicity of the fever has been sufficiently striking to suggest the correct diagnosis before lymphadenopathy or splenomegaly became evident.

DIAGNOSTIC PROCEDURES

When faced with so large a number of possibilities, it is obvious that no single plan can be outlined for the systematic study of every problem in unexplained fever. In any given patient, the history, physical examination, and most importantly, the epidemiologic setting must determine the diagnostic approach. If the features suggest the presence of infectious disease, the main dependence will be upon bacteriologic and immunologic methods, whereas in an obscure febrile disorder in a person in the "cancer age group" the best chance of early diagnosis may lie in x-ray studies and biopsy.

Careful elicitation of the patient's past history and the chronologic development of his symptoms may provide important leads. Places of recent residence, contact with domestic or wild animals and birds, preceding acute infectious diseases such as diarrheal illness or boils, contact with persons with tuberculosis, may provide clues to infection. Localizing symptoms may give a clue to an organ system affected by neoplasm or infection.

In the physical examination, careful search is made for skin lesions and for petechial hemorrhages in the ocular fundi, conjunctivas, nail beds, and skin. The lymph nodes are carefully palpated, with special attention to the retroclavicular, axillary, and epitrochlear areas. The finding of a heart murmur may be important. Detection of an abdominal mass may be the first lead to diagnosis of neoplastic disease. Palpable enlargement of the spleen suggests infection, leukemia, or lymphoma and points away from a diagnosis of cancer. Enlargement of the liver and spleen suggests lymphoma, leukemia, chronic infection, or cirrhosis. A large liver without palpable spleen points to liver abscess or metastatic cancer. The rectum and the female pelvic organs may reveal masses or abscesses and the testicles, teratoma, or tuberculosis. Useful laboratory examinations include cultures of blood, bone marrow, urine, or other body fluids; examination of blood smears for parasites or for evidence of hematologic disorder; tests for hemolysins, LE cells, serologic studies, and antinuclear antibodies. Among x-ray examinations, chest films, which may need to be repeated at intervals, are most useful. Intravenous pyelograms may provide useful clues to disease of kidneys, ureters, or retroperitoneal regions. Lymphangiograms are helpful in the diagnosis of retroperitoneal cancer, abdominal aortograms in renal tumors, abscesses, cysts or pancreatic masses, and cardiac angiograms in atrial myxomas. Gastrointestinal x-rays are of little aid except in regional enteritis. On the other hand, liver scan is the single most useful test in the diagnosis of disease in the right upper quadrant. Lung scans may reveal pulmonary emboli.

Biopsy often is the best means of definitive diagnosis. Bone marrow aspiration may be helpful, not only for the histology of the marrow but also for occasional demonstration of other disease processes such as metastatic carcinoma or granulomas and for culture. Needle biopsy of the liver is a very useful procedure and can be done with reasonable safety. It may be helpful not only with primary or metastatic disease of the liver, but also because the liver may reveal existence of other diseases such as histoplasmosis, schistosomiasis, brucellosis, tuberculosis, sarcoidosis, or lymphoma. Lymph node biopsy is helpful in diagnosis of many diseases, including the lymphomas, metastatic cancer, tuberculosis, and mycotic infections. However, inguinal nodes are notoriously unsatisfactory for biopsy and are too frequently chosen because of their easy accessibility. Axillary, cervical, and supraclavicular nodes are much more likely to yield helpful information, and the node excised need not necessarily be large. Muscle biopsy may be of assistance in the recognition of dermatomyositis, periarteritis nodosa, sarcoidosis, and trichinosis.

Exploratory laparotomy has been advocated as the most definitive diagnostic maneuver in FUO, but is valuable only when other investigations, including history, physical examination, x-rays, and laboratory data, point to the abdomen as a likely source of disease. Blind exploration of the abdomen simply because the diagnosis is obscure is to be deprecated.

THERAPEUTIC TRIALS

It is common practice to give a trial of antibiotic therapy to patients with unidentified febrile disorders. Occasionally this kind of marksmanship is effective, but in general, "blind" therapy does more harm than good.

Undesirable features include drug toxicity, superinfection due to resistant pathogenic bacteria, and interference with accurate diagnosis by cultural methods. Furthermore, a coincidental fall in temperature not due to therapy is likely to be interpreted as response to treatment, with the conclusion that an infectious disease is present. If therapeutic trials are instituted, they should be as specific as possible. Examples are: isoniazid and streptomycin or PAS for tuberculosis; aspirin for rheumatic fever; chloroquine and/or emetine for hepatic amebiasis; penicillin and streptomycin for enterococcal endocarditis, and chloramphenicol for salmonella bacteremia. Shotgun broad-spectrum therapy is contraindicated because it is unlikely to yield useful information and is more likely to be toxic. Similarly, cortisone or ACTH are nonspecific. These drugs have an antipyretic effect and produce euphoria in many individuals, but the apparent improvement induced by these agents tells little about the nature of the underlying disease.

REFERENCES

Atkins, E.: Pathogenesis of Fever, Physiol. Rev., 40:580, 1969.

Geraci, J. E., L. A. Weed, and D. R. Nichols: Fever of Obscure Origin—The Value of Abnormal Exploration in Diagnosis, J.A.M.A., 169:1306, 1959.

Petersdorf, R. G.: The Physiology, Pathogenesis and Diagnosis of Fever, Med. Times, 96:50, 1968.

——, and P. B. Beeson: Fever of Unexplained Origin: Report of 100 Cases, Medicine, 40:1, 1961.

——, and I. L. Bennett, Jr.: Factitious Fever, Ann. Intern. Med., 46:1039, 1957.

Section 3

Alterations in Nervous Function

17 GENERAL CONSIDERATIONS
Raymond D. Adams

The symptoms and signs of nervous disease, which comprise the subject material of this section, are probably the most frequent and the most complex in all of medicine. Naturally, they interest students of neurology and psychiatry, but they are so often found in patients who do not have classifiable diseases of the nervous system that they inevitably become the concern of every physician.

A lucid exposition of the diverse and complex manifestations of nervous disease is difficult, and a certain bias, which will be apparent at once to specialists in this field, is almost unavoidable. The method chosen here is somewhat unconventional and requires a few

words of explanation. The aim has been to bring together all the expressions of disordered nervous function. They are described in some detail, and the most generally accepted explanations from anatomy, biochemistry, physiology, and psychology are offered. No distinction is drawn between relatively simple phenomena, such as motor and sensory paralysis, which are usually based on an easily demonstrated structural change, and the most complex ones, such as anxiety, depression, or paranoia, to which at present no gross or microscopic pathologic changes can be assigned.

An attempt has been made, wherever indicated, to present both the neurologic and the psychologic conceptions of the more complex cerebral phenomena, but the emphasis is on the neurologic because it is more understandable to physicians and surgeons, since the approach is the same as that to all other medical diseases.

NEUROLOGIC (MEDICAL) AND PSYCHOLOGIC CONCEPTIONS OF NERVOUS DISEASE

An understanding of these two conceptions of nervous disease is necessary in order to appreciate current trends in neurology and psychiatry. At the very beginning of this brief exposition of methodology and clinical approach, it should be stated that the terms *neurologic* and *psychologic* do not denote the respective activities of neurologists and psychiatrists. Neurologic means the concepts of medicine applied to the study of nervous disease. They may be and are used by physicians, psychiatrists, and neurologists. Psychologic comprises another set of ideas, largely nonmedical and used by many psychiatrists as well as by neurologists and other physicians. In other words, the conception, the method, or the subject matter does not strictly pertain to any one discipline.

The *neurologic conception* starts with the assumption that all the phenomena of nervous disease are related to a pathologic process within the nervous system. This process may be obvious, like a cerebral infarct or tumor; or it may be impossible to see even with an ordinary light microscope, like the encephalopathy of delirium tremens. In all instances the pathologic process is the result of some physical or chemical change, and the visible lesion may represent only its most advanced and often irreversible stage. The symptoms and clinical signs of nervous disease are the expressions of the activity of the pathologically altered nervous system. These clinical manifestations vary widely and include, on the one hand, the relatively simple, easily elicited, stereotyped objective signs, such as motor paralysis or ataxia, and on the other, the most complex, difficult to evoke, highly individualized, subjective signs, such as hallucination, delusion, or obsessive thought. This is perhaps the most difficult idea for the student to grasp—that there is no necessary difference between "physical" and "mental" or "organic" and "functional" symptoms. To the neurologist, as to other physicians, all these symptoms have their objective as well as their "conscious" or subjective aspects, and the prominence of one or the other should not change our way of looking at them. In either the paralyzed or the delirious patient, something of normal behavior has been lost as a consequence of nervous disease (negative or deficit symptoms), and often something new in his behavior has emerged, presumably because of the unbalanced or unrestrained action of the undamaged parts of the brain (positive symptoms). Some symptoms, like the dementia of general paresis, are understandable largely through the structural alteration of the brain, and the clinical picture is a combination of deficits of function and the activity of intact parts of it. The patient still exhibits behavior and thinking and still responds to his environment. No doubt previous personality structure, educational level, etc., modify the clinical state. Other symptoms, such as a paranoid idea, though believed to be based on a neuropathologic process, are more difficult to analyze, for we cannot easily identify the primary defect nor trace its effects in the patient's reaction. Such symptoms and reactions become more comprehensible when viewed against the background of all previous life experiences, to some of which they may be related. The previous life experiences thus become part of the present illness, but though possibly explaining the content of the nervous symptom and its mode of evolution, they do not explain its occurrence. The neurologic examination becomes merely a device which permits one to sample systematically the activities of the altered nervous system at one moment, and special techniques, particularly refined psychologic methods, may be needed to supplement it. Also, special laboratory procedures, such as biochemical tests of the blood, the electroencephalogram (EEG), the examination of the cerebrospinal fluid, and x-rays, yield additional objective data that cannot be obtained by simple clinical observation. Pathologic study provides the final confirmation of the location and character of the disease. The goal of the neurologic method, or of neuropathology (the laboratory study of nervous disease), is to define the essential pathologic processes underlying disease and to determine their cause and mechanism. A complete theory of a nervous disease should embrace all aspects of it, the anatomic, pathologic, biochemical, and physiologic, as well as psychologic. The method is that of the medical sciences and of medicine itself.

The *psychologic conception of disease* rests on many of the same assumptions as the neurologic concept. For example, it is assumed that in many patients psychologic difficulties are caused by structural changes at the molecular, chemical, or tissue level. They may be due to a genetic or developmental defect, and a lesion may be visualized. But another aspect is emphasized, that the nervous disorder, like the content of the mind, is determined within broad limits by previous life experiences. Certain features of personality, the degree of emotional maturity, and the capacity to adjust adequately to a social situation, which are thought to depend to a considerable extent on learned patterns of reaction, are the sources of pathology. More particularly, aberrations of mental function are regarded as immature and unstable reactions to environmental circumstances, derived, it is believed, from personality inadequacy or traceable to unfortunate experiences in early life. Some of these experiences are easily remembered, i.e., "conscious," others are forgotten, i.e., "unconscious," and can be recalled with difficulty and sometimes only through the free-association method of psychoanalysis. In either case the principal method of approach is to review the patient's autobiography and determine the relationship of the present symptoms to past experiences. The symptoms and signs of mental disease, whether the grandiose delusion of the general paretic or the phobia of a neurotic person, are regarded as responses to a number of stimulus situations acting upon individuals who differ from normal mainly in that they have learned to think and to react emotionally in an abnormal manner. Since their symptoms are often traced to psychic conflicts that have arisen in their personal life, they are in this sense psychogenic. By interview and frank discussion, the physician endeavors to demonstrate these relationships to the patient and thereby to assist him to adjust to them satisfactorily. The ultimate aim of the psychologic study of disease or of psychopathology, which is the scientific study of the psychologic origins of symptoms, is to discover abnormal mental processes and to find their psychologic cause and mechanism. Examples of some of the established mechanisms are conflict, projection, repression, conditioning, and arrest of libido. It is held, particularly by some of the more narrowly trained psychoanalysts, that all psychologic theories of mental disorder must be couched in psychologic terms and that anatomic, biochemical, physiologic, and pathologic terms have no place in such a formulation. In general, the method is that of psychology, and the conception is in line with rationalistic philosophy.

The authors would suggest that each method and each conception of disease has its place in medicine. However, the two methods operate at entirely different levels. In the *diagnosis* of nervous disease the physician's first responsibility is to record accurately all the symptoms and signs obtained in a single examination or a series of them. Here the method is that of any of the medical disciplines. A purely psychologic approach is not of great diagnostic value because eliciting the patient's biography and finding psychologic explanations for his symptoms is a time-consuming procedure and commits one prematurely to a formula of the present illness that may be totally erroneous. In the strict interpretation of nervous disorders both the neurologic and psychologic conceptions come into play; the symptom(s) which appear indicate, upon neurologic analysis, which part of the nervous system has been damaged, but the precise form the symptom takes, especially in complex behavioral derangements, will be divulged by the psychologic study of the premorbid and morbid personality. In *therapy* and in the *management* of many diseases, including those for which there is no known treatment, a detailed knowledge of the patient's personality and his general reactions are, on the other hand, quite indispensable. Success in all fields of medicine depends on the ability to deal with the patient as a troubled individual. Here the psychologic method is of practical value, and the neurologic one often has relatively less to offer. This is a province of medicine where trained psychiatrists may function with great skill. In *theorizing* about disease and in doing *medical research,* however, the neurologic method and concept provide the soundest approach, for they embrace all the methods of medicine and the medical sciences, anatomic, physiologic, biochemical, and neuropathologic, as well as psychologic. Here the psychologic method has limited application, and though it yields useful data about the evolution of symptoms and their content or form, it will probably never explain completely *a disease of the nervous system.*

All that has been said applies to nervous diseases, and thus, from the very beginning, we are confronted by one of the crucial problems of neurology—that of defining a nervous disease. Failure to do this has resulted in great confusion and has been an obstacle to research. The authors propose to define nervous disease as one *in which there is a lesion in the nervous tissue or in which reasonable evidence of an anatomic abnormality or a consistent physical or biochemical disturbance obtains.* This should be distinguished from an abnormal psychologic reaction, which is defined as *a disorder of behavior caused by maladjustment in social relations.* Worry over the loss of a job or the ill health of a child, with all its potential visceral reverberations, would not be classified as a disease. These and countless other daily problems are better looked upon as natural psychologic and physiologic reactions to social problems and dealt with at a psychologic level. A persistent anxiety state without obvious cause in a previously healthy young housewife, on the other hand, would be viewed differently. Most psychiatrists would consider it a reaction to some unconscious conflict, whereas many neurologists might consider it an unexplained socially evoked disorder as mysterious as was hyperthyroidism a century ago. We suggest that anyone who essays to investigate it should do so with a completely open mind and be prepared to review critically any apparently satisfactory explanation, whether psychologic or neurologic. Mania, depression, paranoia, and the several varieties of schizophrenia, which are the major problems of psychiatry, have, unfortunately, an uncertain status. Many experienced psychiatrists would probably agree that they are diseases, rather than deviate ways of living or abnormal psychologic reactions, and that the more comprehensive methods of medicine and the medical sciences offer a more promising approach than does psychology. To the neurologist the major deficiencies in the study of these latter disorders of the nervous system in the past few years have been the relative overemphasis on psychopathology and the neglect of neuropathology, using this term in its broadest sense.

NEUROLOGY AND PSYCHIATRY

All the former has been said to explain the different ways in which neurologists and psychiatrists conceptualize the problems of nervous disease. Actually, the fields of neurology and psychiatry are broad and touch every medical and surgical specialty. Both are concerned with disturbances of behavior, conduct, thinking, and emotional control due to diseases of the brain. In addition, neurology includes as its subject matter many diseases of the nervous system that do not alter the mind, and psychiatry is occupied with countless problems of adjustment in daily life, which are sources of much unhappiness and disability and yet cannot be defined as nervous diseases.

Certain major manifestations of mental illness and of neurologic disease, those most likely to be encountered by general practitioners and internists, will be discussed in the first half of this book, and an attempt will be made to explain them in terms of current anatomic, physiologic, and psychologic theory. A comprehensive account of the major psychiatric and neurologic diseases will be presented in the second half of this book in their appropriate place, with diseases of the nervous system. A systematic discussion of normal personality development will be found in Part 2, Chap. 7. Neurologic disorders will be discussed in sequence, ranging from the most frequent and general symptoms and signs to the most specific.

THE IMPORTANCE OF PSYCHOLOGIC MEDICINE

The magnitude of the field of psychologic medicine can hardly be overestimated, and emphasis on the neurologic method is not intended to depreciate the importance of the psychologic approach. Every physician would agree that illness invariably creates problems for the patient and his family. Some, such as the temporary loss of employment or interruption of normal activities, are relatively minor. Others, such as fear of disability or death, may be so overwhelming as to demand the most thoughtful treatment. The need to understand the patient and his reactions must be taken into account in every medical procedure, even in history taking, where the reliability and validity of symptoms must be evaluated against the background of the patient's personality and his cultural environment. The group of illnesses called the *psychoneuroses* or *neuroses* are known to manifest a wide variety of symptoms that may be confused with those of medical disease.

Of even greater significance is a second large category of diseases of unknown origin (peptic ulcer, mucous colitis, ulcerative colitis, bronchial asthma, atopic dermatitis, urticaria, angioneurotic edema, hay fever, Raynaud's disease, hypertension, hyperthyroidism, amenorrhea and other disturbances of menstruation, enuresis, dysuria, rheumatoid and other forms of arthritis, headache, syncope, and epilepsy) in which a stressful personal problem appears often to be associated with the initial development, exacerbation, or prolongation of symptoms. Three lines of evidence tend to set these *psychosomatic diseases* apart from all others. (1) A large series of observations, made by Cannon, Wolff, Mittelman, Wolf, Cobb, Finesinger, White, Jones, and others, have established the fact that the function of the offending organ is excited and possibly deranged by strong emotions and assuaged by tranquility and feelings of security. (2) A careful analysis of the biographies of patients with these diseases has shown what is believed to be an inordinately high incidence of resentment, hostility, dependence or independence, suppressed emotionality, and inability to communicate matters of emotional concern or to differentiate between reality and subjective falsification (cf., studies of Lindemann, Dunbar, French, and Alexander). (Studies of personality promised at first to show a special group of personality traits to be operating in each disease, but subsequent inquiry indicates that this is not the case.) (3) A search through the biographic data of patients with these diseases has shown relationship between exacerbations of symptoms and the occurrence of frustrating or disturbing incidents; and unsuccessful medical therapy has seemed to result when these emotional factors were neglected.

In the field of psychosomatic disease, despite intensive investigation by psychiatrists in the last 30 years, the reports of which make up an enormous literature, very few facts have been established. Surely it can be said that, like the psychoneuroses, they are "part disturbances" of the personality. But they differ from the psychoneuroses in that (1) they have different symptoms; (2) as a rule they last longer; (3) they have in most instances a known and demonstrable pathologic basis and often a known cause, e.g., allergy in asthma and atopic dermatitis; (4) treatment has been concerned more directly with the relief of symptoms and has tended to be directed by different groups of specialists; (5) the incidence of frank psychoneuroses in this group of patients is no greater than in the population at large, and these psychosomatic disorders are not more frequent in neurotic individuals. No complete proof has thus far been adduced that psychic factors are the primary cause of any of these psychosomatic diseases any more than they are the cause of angina pectoris or exophthalmic goiter. Moreover, the concepts formed about these diseases in recent years, although educationally useful, have not been of great theoretical value. There is no evidence that the therapeutic results obtained by a thoughtful understanding physician, unsophisticated in psychologic theory, are less good than those of the most experienced psychiatrists.

The basic fault in this field of psychologic medicine, as it was in the "somatic medicine" that flourished before and after the First World War, is that one aspect is stressed with too little reference to the other. As pointed out by Wolff in his scholarly exposition of the mind-body relationship, the logical fallacy of such ideas as "psychogenic," "psychosomatic," and "emotional causes of disease" is that they imply a mind acting in opposition to a body.

A third group of illnesses that fall more clearly in the borderland between medicine, neurology, and psychiatry might be termed the *functional overlays of organic disease*. Here under the stress of disease, usually one that is frightening or painful and disabling, an illness of definite organic type becomes complicated by psychologic symptoms which have no direct (causal) relationship to it. At least two patterns of reaction can be discerned: (1) a type of hysterical conversion (cf. Chap. 370) in which some physical symptom such as paralysis, sensory loss, tremor, vomiting, or loss of equilibrium are added to the signs of organic (sometimes neurologic) disease. Inquiry may show that the patient may have exhibited some positive evidence of emotional instability or immaturity in the past, but often this is unclear. The domestic situation may give some clue as to the reason for persistent invalidism. (2) Affective reactions of anxiety or depression (cf. Chaps. 18 and 369), the latter being more frequent and masquerading under the guise of fatigue, insomnia, apathy, and disinterest or suspiciousness. These seem to bear no certain relationship to the nature of the illness, although the fatigue-exhaustion syndrome has been especially frequent after infectious hepatitis, influenza, brucellosis, and Icelandic disease. Again, previous temperament and personality may provide some hint of a natural tendency to anxiety and depression. The separation of the psychologic disturbance from the organic disease assumes importance because the treatment of the two, especially the psychologic one, requires special methods.

An ancient approach to this broad area of psychologic medicine, first suggested by Claude Bernard and ably espoused by Adolph Meyer, regards man as a psychobiologic unit functioning in relationship to his physical and his uniquely social environment. Disease is conceived of as representing a faulty or inadequate adaptation of the organism to the environment. Sometimes the maladaptation can be traced to a single agent in the environment, such as the tubercle bacillus, without which the disease tuberculosis could not develop. In other instances, as in a recurrent infection, the condition is much more complex, indicating a primary physical defect in the individual, such as an agammaglobulinemia. Again, exhaustion from a prolonged stressful situation or malnutrition may have rendered the patient susceptible to the infectious agent. Seldom even in straightforward disease, such as tuberculosis or delirium tremens, can one reduce the problem to a single physical or psychic factor. Hence, it is proposed that a rigid and narrow physical or psychologic approach must be supplanted by this broader, more biologic one, which attempts to weigh each of several factors that make up the equation of disease. At present this is difficult, for all the factors in many diseases, particularly in psychoneurotic and psychosomatic ones, have not been isolated and studied. Until such time as new facts are obtained, the physician must cope with a huge population of patients, as many as 50 percent, who suffer from obscure ailments and diseases, and he is forced to employ inadequate methods of diagnosis and treatment. Fortunately, most of these illnesses are benign and of relatively minor importance, and time and kindly reassurance will alleviate them; some of them represent psychoneuroses that are not disabling. The physician and student must acquire a sensitivity to psychologic problems without becoming so mindful of them that every illness is reduced to a naive psychologic formula. Above all, an open mind should be adopted, one that will permit critical review of all hypotheses in this field and acceptance of only those based on the valid data of controlled clinical observation and scientific experiment.

REFERENCES

Carter, A. B.: The Functional Overlay, Brit. Med. J. (Lancet) 2:1196, 1967.

Cobb, S.: "Emotions and Clinical Medicine," New York, W. W. Norton & Company, Inc., 1950.

Finesinger, J. E.: Psychiatric Components in Medical Disease: Psychosomatic Medicine, New Engl. J. Med., 227:578, 1942.

Masserman, J. H.: "Behavior and Neurosis: An Experimental Psychoanalytic Approach to Psychobiologic Principles," Chicago, The University of Chicago Press, 1943.

Wolf, S., and H. G. Wolff: "Human Gastric Function: An Experimental Study of a Man and His Stomach," Fair Lawn, N.J., Oxford University Press, 1947.

18 NERVOUSNESS, ANXIETY, AND DEPRESSION

Raymond D. Adams

Upon close questioning the majority of patients who enter a physician's office or a hospital will admit to being nervous, anxious, or depressed. Evidently the natural human reactions to the prospect of real or imaginary disease or to the stresses of contemporary social environment are being experienced. If they stand in clear relationship to a stressful situation, e.g., anxiety over pressing economic reverses or grief over the death of a loved one, these states may be accepted as normal, and they become the basis of medical consultation only when excessively intense and uncontrollable or when accompanying derangements of visceral function are excessive. The problem increases in complexity when similar symptoms occur in individuals who are not undergoing immediately stressful or depressing experiences; and any threatening situation, if it exists, is either unknown to the conscious mind of the patient or has been at least partly suppressed. The relationship between social stimulus and the prevailing alteration of mood can then be discovered only by gentle probings by the psychologically sophisticated physician. Once the connection is established and the problem dealt with realistically, the symptoms become understandable and often disappear.

There is still another broad category of nervousness, anxiety, and depression, the significance of which we cannot fully comprehend. These are states in which the individual suffers profound and prolonged anxiety and depression without obvious explanation. Delving into the unconscious mind fails to reveal a plausible psychogenesis. In many such instances a genetic factor appears to operate, and the principal features of the illness and its natural cause are so stereotyped as to indicate a fundamental derangement of the emotional apparatus of the nervous system. These latter states we would categorize as diseases even though they do not possess an established mechanism or pathology.

The problem confronting every physician is to recognize these nervous disorders in all their variations and to decide whether they constitute the nervous reactions of a normal person, a pathologic reaction the psychologic antecedents of which are veiled in the obscurities of the unconscious mind, or a grave occult disease of the nervous system demanding the attention of specialists in psychologic medicine.

In this chapter the cardinal features of these conditions will be described along with current views of their psychologic and physiologic origins; and lines of inquiry that might help determine their significance will be suggested.

NERVOUSNESS

By this rather vague term the lay person usually refers to a state of restlessness and overactivity, tension, uneasy apprehension, or hyperexcitability. But it may also mean other things, such as thoughts of suicide, fear of killing one's child or spouse, a distressing hallucination or paranoid idea, or frank hysterical behavior. Careful questioning as to its exact nature is always necessary.

In its usual signification, a period of nervousness may represent no more than one of the variations to which many otherwise normal individuals are subject. For example, adolescence rarely passes without its period of turmoil as the young person attempts to emancipate himself from his family and to adjust to school work and the opposite sex (cf. Chap. 7). In the female the menses are accompanied by increased tension and moodiness, and of course, the menopause is another critical period. Some individuals claim they have been nervous in all their social relations throughout life, and one should then suspect a psychoneurosis or psychosis even though adjustment to school, family, and work seems to have been adequate. Others come to the physician because of a recent development of nervousness; in this instance one must consider a variety of conditions such as psychoneurosis, psychosis, endocrine disease (e.g., hyperthyroidism), a drug reaction (corticosteroid therapy), or withdrawal reaction from a drug (alcoholic or barbiturate delirium). Some patients complain of nervousness that attends the development of a medical disease; it would appear then to be secondary, i.e., occasioned by fear of disability, dependency, or death.

Nervousness even in its simplest form is reflected in many important activities of the human organism. When it is present, there is often a mild somberness of mood and increased tendency to tears and anger (emotionality). Fatigue that bears no proper relationship to sleep and rest is frequent; and sleep is often troubled, as are eating and drinking habits. The patient subject to headaches often reports these symptoms to have increased in frequency and intensity. All these, then, along with sweating, awareness of cardiac action, queer sensations in the head or giddiness, upset stomach, and frequency of micturition, indicate that the nervous state is inducing some of the same visceral changes that occur with anxiety. Thus, it would appear that nervousness and anxiety constitute a graded series of reactions, anxiety being usually a more intense and protracted nervousness; the underlying cause and mechanisms appear to be essentially the same for both conditions (see p. 369).

THE ANXIETY STATE

Anxiety is "the fundamental phenomenon and central problem of neurosis . . . a nodal point, linking up all kinds of most important questions, a riddle of which the solution must cast a flood of light upon our whole mental life." (Freud) From the viewpoint of the social historian, anxiety is said to be "the most prominent mental characteristic of Occidental civilization." (Willoughby) In these varied contexts anxiety has a broad meaning, more or less equivalent to social and psychologic unrest. In more general psychologic terms it has been defined as "an emotional state arising when a continuing strong desire seems likely to miss its goal." (McDougall)

The more strictly medical meaning of the word *anxiety*, and the one used in this chapter, designates a state characterized by a subjective feeling of fear and uneasy anticipation (apprehension), usually with a definite topical content and associated with the physiologic accompaniments of fear, i.e., breathlessness, choking sensation, palpitation, restlessness, increased muscular tension, tightness in the chest, giddiness, trembling, sweating, flushing, and broken sleep. By topical content is meant the idea, the person, or the object about which the person is anxious. The several vasomotor, visceral, and chemical changes that underlie many of the symptoms and signs are mediated through the autonomic nervous system, particularly the sympathetic part of it, and involve the thyroid and adrenal glands.

Forms of Anxiety

Anxiety manifests itself in acute episodes, lasting a few minutes, or as a protracted state continuing for weeks, months, or even years. In the acute attacks, called *anxiety attacks* or *panics*, breathlessness, palpitation, choking, sweating, and trembling accompany an intense fear of dying, losing one's reason, or committing a horrid crime. In states of chronic anxiety, nervousness, restlessness, irritability, excitability, fatigue, pressure or tension headaches, and insomnia again are the major symptoms, but they tend to be milder and less frightening but by no means less disabling. Discrete anxiety attacks and protracted states of anxiety are not mutually exclusive, though they often occur separately. Episodic anxiety occurring in attacks, without any major disorder of mood or of thinking, is usually classified as an *anxiety neurosis;* the prolonged state of anxiety is called *neurocirculatory asthenia*. These two conditions will be discussed in greater detail in Chap. 369. Anxiety symptoms are a prominent feature in the syndrome of posttraumatic nervous instability (cf. Chap. 358).

Physiologic and Psychologic Basis

The cause, mechanism, and biologic meaning of anxiety have been the subjects of much speculation. The psychologist has come to regard anxiety as anticipatory behavior, i.e., a state of uneasiness concerning something which may or will happen in the future. It is believed to be based on an inherited instinctual pattern (fear); and the occurrence of this emotional state in situations that would not be expected to provoke it could be an example of a conditioned or learned response.

The only well-systematized psychologic theory is that put forth by psychoanalysts, who look upon anxiety as a response to a situation which in some manner threatens the security of the individual. Anxiety is a response to danger, the topical content of which lies in the unconscious mind. It is pointed out that the somatic symptoms of anxiety are similar to those of fear. The postulated danger is internal rather than external; a primitive drive that is not compatible with current social practices has been aroused and can be satisfied only at risk to the individual.

Most psychiatrists accept this theory and believe that psychotherapeutic interviews will disclose the anxiety-provoking stimulus of which the patient is himself unaware. Once insight is gained into the psychodynamic mechanism, the anxiety symptoms are said to subside.

A search for evidences of visceral disease in patients with anxiety has thus far been unrewarding. A reduced capacity for physical work and strong effort has suggested the possibility of a defect in aerobic metabolism, as evidenced by increased oxygen consumption and an excessive rise in blood lactate. Moreover, such patients seem unable to tolerate the physiologic and biochemical effects of work as well as does the average person. Whether these differences are of primary significance or are due merely to lack of training and poor physical condition has not been settled.

A number of endocrinologic studies have been done and have yielded interesting data. The urinary excretion of epinephrine has been found elevated in some individuals; in others, an increase in the urinary excretion of norepinephrine has been noted; in still a third group, normal values for both epinephrine and norepinephrine were obtained. Elmadjian and his associates have observed that aldosterone excretion in patients with anxiety neurosis is two or three times that of normal control subjects. This work has been in part corroborated by Venning, who demonstrated an increase in aldosterone excretion in medical students experiencing fear and anxiety while preparing for examination. The interpretation of these observations is not certain, but it is becoming increasingly evident that prolonged and diffuse anxiety is a pattern of behavior determined by a biochemical abnormality of certain parts of the brain.

Diagnosis of Anxiety

Clinical diagnosis of the anxiety state depends upon recognition of (1) the implicit or subjective disturbance, i.e., the uneasiness and apprehension, and (2) the subjective and more objective vasomotor or visceral changes. The presence of diffuse or more or less circumscribed attacks of autonomic or thyroid and adrenal excitation, *without psychic counterpart,* does not establish the diagnosis of anxiety. Similar autonomic and endocrine discharges may occur with thyrotoxicosis, pheochromocytoma, corticosteroid therapy (usually in large doses), hypoglycemia, and menopause. Penfield has described them also as a manifestation of tumors of the third ventricle (diencephalic autonomic epilepsy), and they have occasionally occurred as a prelude (aura) to a frank convulsive state. When the psychic components of anxiety are fully described by a patient who admits to having visceral manifestations, one must consider as diagnostic possibilities anxiety neurosis, depression, hysteria, psychasthenia,

schizophrenia, or a drug or endocrine psychosis. The differential diagnosis of the anxiety state will be discussed more fully in Chap. 369. The data obtained by history and physical examination, if analyzed carefully, usually permit distinction between pure derangements of autonomic nervous and endocrine systems and true anxiety. One of the commonest sources of error is to mistake an anxious depression for an anxiety neurosis.

DEPRESSION

There are few individuals who do not experience periods of discouragement and despair, and these become manifestly more frequent as modern society increases in complexity, demanding ever greater inhibition of one's impulses and greater conformity to a group. As with anxiety, depression of mood that is appropriate to a given situation in life seldom becomes the basis of medical complaint. The patient then seeks help only when he cannot overcome or control his grief or unhappiness. But, there are numerous instances where he does not fully recognize its cause, and in this respect, the symptoms are viewed as indicative of disease for which help is sought. Thus, depression, like anxiety, may be either a normal reaction or a pathologic state, and the distinction may require searching analysis of the medical data by a discerning physician.

Information about depressions, like knowledge of all psychiatric syndromes, is gained from three sources: the history obtained from the patient; the history obtained from the family or a friend in close contact with the patient; and the findings on examination.

The majority of patients who suffer from depression give a history of "not feeling well," of being "low in spirits," "blue," "glum," "unhappy," or 'morbid." They are vaguely aware that their emotional reactions have changed; activities that were formerly pleasant are no longer so. But it often happens that these patients do not perceive their unhappiness and instead complain of being nervous, worried, fatigued, or unable to think with accustomed efficiency. Pain of obscure origin may be the predominant topic of their conversation, as may any other symptom common in adult life, e.g., tinnitus, dry mouth, burning tongue, arthritis, constipation, pruritus. Multiplicity and persistence of complaint has led to many of these persons being classed as hypochondriacs; and indeed, the most typical examples of excessive preoccupation with symptoms in middle-aged and elderly persons are found in depressed individuals. Since these associated symptoms are so frequent and are often a misleading feature of depression, they will be presented in further detail.

LASSITUDE, FATIGUE, LACK OF ENERGY, POOR APPETITE. A decrease in energy output is a common symptom. The patient complains of being continuously without energy and of tiring out of proportion to the amount of work done. The appetite is usually poor; the patient derives no real enjoyment from eating and may comment, "I only eat to live," "I only eat because I have to." Weight loss is common and probably due to decreased food intake; and the majority of severely depressed patients are constipated. Exceptionally, there is weight gain because of continued food intake and reduced activity. Sexual desire also wanes; complete loss of libido is common.

LOSS OF INTEREST AND INCAPACITY FOR ENJOYMENT. These are noted by both the patient and his family. When formerly the patient found pleasure in his work and was quite capable of doing it well, even the simplest tasks now demand great effort. He feels that he lacks his former efficiency in work and often ascribes this to forgetfulness. However, when one questions his employer, one learns that there has been no impairment of memory or judgment but only a lack of the usual interest in and enthusiasm for work. Also, when the patient's memory is systematically tested, the deficit in memory of which he complains appears as a difficulty in concentration rather than a true memory deficit. This lack of interest and enthusiasm extends also to other activities. Absorbing recreational pursuits now give no pleasure. Cherished friendships are abandoned simply because it is too much of an effort to see people. Irritability is also frequent, and patients who formerly were quite placid and imperturbable find themselves easily irritated by trivial happenings. The noises of children playing about the house are intolerable. However, if the patient is overcritical or harsh with them, he feels guilty and reproaches himself.

WORRY AND DIFFUSE CONCERN. These symptoms are prominent in most cases of depression. Patients find themselves worrying about things that have not happened or feeling apprehensive and fearful about the outcome of some ordinary activity. Incidents that occurred years before may be the objects of concern. For example, the patient may become very much upset and unhappy and may cry about the death of a relative that occurred many years before. He is assailed by pessimistic thoughts and by feelings of inadequacy and unworthiness and is often preoccupied with the possibility of suicide.

INSOMNIA. Almost always present, insomnia manifests itself in several ways. The patient may find it difficult to fall asleep; or he may fall asleep quickly but soon awaken and be unable to return to sleep. Some patients state that they do not awaken during the night but their sleep is restless and unsatisfactory. Usually, when unable to sleep, they cannot remain quietly in bed. Plagued by pessimistic thoughts, they arise, walk about the house, smoke a cigarette, get something to eat, and resort to various measures to induce sleep. Bad dreams or nightmares are common. Occasionally there is excessive sleep, and the patient finds relief from his worries in slumber.

A closely related complaint is that of not feeling rested upon awakening in the morning. Patients frequently state, "I feel more tired upon awakening than I did before I went to sleep." A diurnal variation in mood swing is characteristic. In most patients all symptoms are worse in the morning and improve as the day progresses. Occasionally the reverse is true, and the symptoms are worst in the afternoon or evening.

ANXIETY. A large proportion of depressed patients experience anxiety. There may be anxiety attacks in which the patient becomes tense and apprehensive, perspires freely, and experiences palpitation and labored respiration. These symptoms may occur in discrete attacks or may continue in milder form over a long period of time. There may be crying spells in association with attacks of tenseness and palpitation for reasons not apparent to the patient or to an observer.

NERVOUSNESS. This is another common symptom. Very often depressed patients and psychoneurotic patients state that nervousness is their chief complaint. They may mean by this term a vague, ineffable psychologic state or a feeling of uneasy expectancy or of impending doom, the precise nature of which is uncertain. Again, nervousness may mean tenseness, inner tremulousness, or a diffuse uneasiness. Depressed patients also use "nervousness" to mean a feeling of sadness, with outbreaks of spontaneous weeping.

PAIN. Though it is not generally appreciated, pain may occasionally be one of the earliest, if not the first, manifestations of depression, occurring before other obvious depressive symptoms appear. The pain is often described as "tearing," "pulling," "twisting," "burning," or "clamping" and may be localized or migratory. In one patient it appeared first in the right external auditory canal and then successively in the right chest and shoulder, the left pudendal region, and both lower extremities, starting in the left instep and radiating upward to the left groin, then in the right instep radiating to the right groin. The pain is usually constant from the time of onset. There may be fluctuations in severity, however, with exacerbations which the patient associates with fatigue and emotional disturbances.

The family, in relating the story of the illness, usually can do more than just verify many of the patient's symptoms. They can give a clearer idea of the degree of worry, the extent of disability, the depth of the alteration of emotional reaction, and the distressing effect of the patient's disturbed behavior on others. Moreover, they are often helpful in documenting the time of onset of the illness, the natural fluctuations, and the response to therapy.

SIGNS OF DEPRESSION. Before considering the objective signs on examination, it should be pointed out that the chief abnormalities occur in three domains of psychic function: emotion, ideation, and psychomotor activity. Abnormalities in these three spheres are designated by some psychiatrists as the cardinal signs or "unit symptoms" of the disorder.

The *facial expression* is often plaintive, troubled, pained, or anguished. The patient's attitude and manner betray the prevailing mood of depression, discouragement, and despondency. In other words, the affective response, which is the outward expression of feeling, is consistent with the depressed mood. The patient's eyes during the course of the interview may become tearful, or he may cry openly. At times the immobility of the face will mimic the facies of parkinsonism.

The stream of speech, from which the ideational content is determined, is slow. At times the patient is mute and speaks neither spontaneously nor in response to questions. Again, he may speak very slowly with a long period between his spontaneous utterances, or there may be a long delay between the questions asked by the examiner and the answers given by the patient. The retardation is present regardless of the topic of conversation and is not restricted to certain subjects as it is in the case of emotional blocking (selective retardation) seen in other psychiatric illnesses. At times the flow of speech is accelerated rather than retarded, but still the topical content tends to be restricted to a few subjects, such as the patient's symptoms and his personal problems.

The *motor activity may be decreased* in varying degrees, from slow and deliberate movement even to total cessation as in stupor. Frequently the patient will sit for hours in one place without moving; the slightest movement appears to require great effort. Again, motor activity may be increased to the point of restlessness and agitation, the patient pacing the floor, wringing his hands, and loudly bemoaning his fate.

The *content of speech* varies and is largely conditioned by the past experiences of the patient. Conversation is replete with pessimistic thoughts and fears of cancer or other serious diseases. Expressions of self-depreciation, self-accusation, feelings of unworthiness, inferiority, guilt, a belief that life is not worthwhile, and suicidal preoccupation less often enter the conversation. Although systematized ideas of persecution are not common in depression, the patient often believes he is not liked by his relatives or friends. The patient's reaction to these ideas is usually one of agreement, since he himself feels unworthy and sees no reason for people wanting him around or enjoying his company. In severe depressions some of the ideas expressed by the patient are bizarre and assume the form of somatic and nihilistic delusions. Various parts of the body are said to be "rotting"; there have been "no normal bowel movements for weeks or months"; "all my blood is dried up"; "I am half dead," etc. In severe depressions auditory, visual, tactile, or olfactory hallucinations occur, and as a rule their salient features are consistent with the depressed mood.

Personal and abstract judgment is often pessimistically tinged by the depressed mood. The patient evaluates his illness as a hopeless one and his business as destined for certain failure. His outlook toward the future is pessimistic and hopeless. Insight may be entirely lacking. The patient may insist that he is suffering from malignancy or some incurable disease despite repeated reassurance to the contrary. However, some patients do realize that they are depressed and that their feelings are for the most part determined by this depression.

ETIOLOGY AND MECHANISM. Psychiatrists are not in complete agreement concerning the cause of the depressive syndrome. There are two schools of thought, one of which contends that the depressive reaction has its genesis in hereditary factors, the other, based largely on psychoanalytic theory, considers it to be a psychogenic disturbance brought about by the inability of a rigid personality to adjust its instinctual drives to the demands of the environment. The latter theory, while

interesting, has not been substantiated and has not resulted in the development of effective psychotherapeutic measures. Rauwolfia compounds and other agents used to treat nervousness and anxiety may induce a depressive mood, a fact of considerable theoretical importance (cf., Chap. 371).

CLINICAL SIGNIFICANCE. All these symptoms and signs comprise a clinical syndrome of importance because of its frequency and gravity. Errors in diagnosis in our best hospitals are numerous and at times serious. Large numbers of such patients tend to accumulate in the various medical clinics, taking up the time of the medical staff that attempts to give them symptomatic therapy. Here the serious consequences of misdiagnosis lie mainly in the fact that the patient does not receive the appropriate treatment for his depression (see Chap. 371). When anxiety symptoms are prominent, an incorrect diagnosis of anxiety neurosis may be made. This mistake, or the false attribution of depression to some environmental circumstance, may obscure the fact that the illness is in reality an endogenous psychosis, and the patient may unexpectedly commit suicide even while receiving psychotherapy. Again, despondency or depression due to unfortunate life circumstances may be misdiagnosed as an endogenous depression and treated by the more drastic methods of electroshock or powerful antidepressant drugs rather than by supportive therapy.

Depression may occur intermittently in conjunction with all the psychoneuroses and persistently in manic-depressive psychosis and in association with medical and neurologic diseases. Chronic infection, endocrine disorders (hyperparathyroidism, hypothyroidism, or Addison's disease), or neoplasia may at times produce chronic fatigue that is difficult to distinguish from depression.

The most important point to be remembered is that if a patient presents any one of the above symptoms, it is incumbent upon the physician to take a complete history and to examine the mental status in some detail in an effort to determine the existence of a depressive state. Once it is established, since it is but one cardinal manifestation of several psychiatric illnesses, the physician must then undertake a differential diagnosis along the lines suggested in Chap. 369.

TREATMENT OF ANXIETY AND DEPRESSION. See Chap. 369 and 371.

SELF-CONSCIOUSNESS AND PARANOID TENDENCIES

Although the most frequent patterns of abnormal nervous reaction have been described, this chapter would not be complete without brief reference to states of self-consciousness and distrust of others as sources of medical complaint. Not a few adolescents and young adults are assailed by doubts of their adequacy to adapt to social situations. They are timid, shy, unable to think of anything to say ("tongue-tied"), and their embarrassment may be so obvious that others make fun of them. This state may often be traced to simple inexperience, a lack of opportunity to be in social groups, and is corrected in time by further contact with people their own age. A few painful social experiences in the past may have conditioned them to react with panic and fear to a social group. Always the more severe and persistent forms of this so-called "inferiority complex," with a tendency to be overly concerned about and to misinterpret the thoughts and actions of others, should raise the question of a malevolent schizoid trend. Admittedly this is exceptional, however, and not a few individuals, whose nervous reactions are not wholly classifiable, go through life tortured by doubts of their own social competence without ever gaining complete control of themselves and without ever a sign of schizophrenia. They are called *introverted* or *neurotic.* Whether they later become subjects of paranoid reactions and depressions is still a matter of conjecture.

19 LASSITUDE AND ASTHENIA
Raymond D. Adams

The term *weakness* is used by patients to describe a variety of subjective complaints which vary in their import and prognostic significance. Most subjective disorders embraced by this term will be found, on careful questioning, to fall within the following classification:

I. Lassitude, fatigue, lack of energy, listlesssess, and languor. These terms, while not synonymous, shade into each other; all refer to weariness and a loss of that sense of well-being typically found in persons who are healthy in body and mind. Symptoms of this type are present in a large majority of all patients and have little diagnostic specificity. For the sake of brevity this group of complaints will be considered together under Lassitude and Fatigue.
II. Weakness, loss of muscular strength, and asthenia. These may be either persistent or episodic.
   A. Persistent weakness: This may be (1) restricted to certain muscles or groups of muscles (paresis, palsy, paralysis) or (2) general, involving the entire musculature, in which instance the term *asthenia* or *myasthenia* is used. Paralysis is discussed in Chap. 21. The generalized type of weakness will be considered below under Asthenia. It is far less common than lassitude and more likely to indicate serious disease.
   B. Recurrent weakness: Many patients complain of "attacks of weakness," and careful questioning reveals that a diminished sense of alertness, a feeling of lightheadedness, or a sensation of faintness is the actual symptoms. These complaints are subjectively different from lassitude and asthenia, and the causes are likewise different; such recurrent attacks of weakness are discussed in Chap. 20.

It should be restated that the unqualified term weakness is so vague as to be almost useless and that a sound clinical approach to this problem entails, as the initial step, an analysis of what the patient himself means when he uses this and similar terms.

LASSITUDE AND FATIGUE (Lack of Energy, Languor, Listlessness, Weariness, and Neurasthenia)

Of all symptoms these are among the most frequent and at the same time the most abstruse, More than half of all patients make direct complaint of this group of symptoms or admit their presence when questioned. During the Second World War they figured so prominently in military medicine that the term *combat fatigue* was applied to all acute psychiatric illnesses on the battlefield. Therefore, it behooves every student of medicine to learn as much as possible about these symptoms and their physiologic and psychologic antecedents.

Lassitude or fatigue most commonly refers to a feeling of weariness or tiredness. Patients who complain of this symptom have a more or less characteristic way of describing it. They speak of being "all in," "without pep," having "no ambition," "no interest," or "being fed up." They are inclined to lie down. On close analysis there is a difficulty in initiating activity, and also in sustaining it.

This condition is the familiar aftermath of prolonged labor or great physical exertion, and under such circumstances it is accepted as a physiologic reaction. When, however, the same symptoms or similar ones appear in no relation to such antecedents, they are recognized as being unnatural, and the patient rightly suspects some recently acquired disease.

The physician's first task then is to determine whether his patient is merely suffering from the physical and mental effects of overwork without realizing it. Overworked and overwrought people are everywhere observable in our society. Their actions are both instructive and pathetic. They seem to be impelled by notions of duty and refuse to think of themselves. Or, as is often the case, some personal inadequacy prevents them from deriving pleasure from any activity except their work, in which they indulge as a defense mechanism. Such individuals often experience a variety of symptoms such as weariness, irritability, nervousness, and sleeplessness. The behavior of these individuals and their varied symptomatology are best understood by referring to psychologic studies of the effect of fatigue on normal individuals.

THE EFFECT OF FATIGUE ON THE NORMAL PERSON

According to the most authoritative sources, fatigue has several effects, some explicit, others implicit. These are (1) a series of physiologic changes in many organs of the body, (2) an overt disorder of behavior in the form of reduced output of work, known as *work decrement,* and (3) an expression of dissatisfaction and a subjective feeling of tiredness or weariness in association with a variety of psychologic changes.

Fatigue indicates the presence of changes in the physiologic balance of the body. Continuous muscular work results in depletion of muscle glycogen and accumulation of lactic acid and probably other metabolites which reduce the contractility and the recovery of active muscle. It is said that the injection of blood of a fatigued animal into a rested one will produce the overt manifestations of fatigue in the latter. During fatigue states muscle action is tremulous, and movements become clumsy and cannot be sustained for long without increasing effort. The rate of breathing increases; the pulse quickens; the blood pressure rises and the pulse pressure widens; and the white blood count and the metabolic rate are increased. These reactions bear out the hypothesis that fatigue is in part a manifestation of altered metabolism.

The decreased capacity for work or productivity which is the direct consequence of fatigue has been investigated by industrial psychologists. Their findings show clearly the importance of the motivational factor on work output, whether it be in the operation of an ergograph or the performance of heavy manual labor. Also it appears that there are individual differences in the energy potential of human beings, just as there are differences in physique and temperament. Some people are strong and vigorous from birth, whereas others are weak and lacking in energy.

The subjective feelings of fatigue have been carefully recorded. Aside from weariness the tired person complains of nervousness, restlessness, inability to deal effectively with complex problems, and a tendency to be upset by trivialities. The number and quality of his associations in tests of mental functions are reduced. Behavior tends to be less rational than normal, and the capacity to deliberate and to reach judgments is impaired. The worker physically exhausted after a long, hard day is unable to perform adequately his duties as head of a household, and the example of the tired businessman who becomes the proverbial tyrant of the family circle is well known. A disinclination to try and the appearance of ideas of inferiority are other characteristics of the fatigued mind.

Instances of fatigue and lassitude resulting from overwork are not difficult to recognize. A description of the patient's daily routine will usually suffice; and if he can be persuaded to live at a more reasonable pace, his symptoms promptly subside. Errors in diagnosis are usually in the direction of ascribing fatigue to overwork, chronic infection, or anemia when it actually reflects a psychoneurosis or depression.

FATIGUE AS A MANIFESTATION OF PSYCHIATRIC DISORDER. The great majority of patients who enter a hospital because of unexplained chronic fatigue and lassitude have been found to have some type of psychiatric illness. In former times the term *neurasthenia* was applied to this group of patients, but since fatigue rarely exists as an isolated phenomenon, the current practice is to label such cases according to the total clinical picture. The usual associated symptoms are nervousness, anxiety, irritability, depression, insomnia, palpitation, headaches, breathlessness, inability to concentrate, sexual disorders, and disturbances of appetite. In one series of cases of severe fatigue in a general hospital, 75 percent were diagnosed as anxiety neurosis or tension state. Depression and "psychosomatic disease" accounted for another 10 percent,

and the remainder had miscellaneous illnesses with hysterical, obsessive, or phobic symptoms.

Several features are common to the psychiatric group. The fatigue is frequently worse in the morning. The patient often desires to lie down but finds himself unable to sleep when he does. The feeling of fatigue relates more to some activities than to others; at times certain affairs are prosecuted with great vigor; while even the thought of other activities completely exhausts the patient. A careful inquiry into the circumstances under which the fatigue first occurred or recurs often reveals a specific relationship to certain events. Instances of an acute episode of fatigue coming on during an unpleasant emotional experience, in connection with a grief reaction, or after a surgical operation have been noted. And, finally, the feeling of tiredness extends to mental as well as physical activities. The individual's capacity for sustained mental effort, as in solving problems or carrying on a difficult conversation, is impaired.

Depressing emotion, whether grief from bereavement or a phase of manic-depressive or involutional psychosis, has its characteristic effect on the impulse life and energy of the individual. The initiation of activity is difficult, and the capacity for work is reduced. Lassitude and fatigue are a more prominent feature in many mild depressive illnesses than is the depression of mood. Patients typically complain that everything they do, whether mental or physical, requires great effort, and all their accustomed activities no longer give the usual satisfaction and enjoyment. Sleep is poor, with a tendency to early morning waking. Such individuals are at their worst in the morning, both in spirit and in energy output, and tend to improve as the day wears on. It is difficult to decide whether their fatigue is a primary effect of disease or is secondary to lack of interest.

Many physicians may question whether all patients with chronic fatigue as seen in everyday practice deviate far enough from normal to justify a diagnosis of psychoneurosis or depressive psychosis. Some people because of circumstances beyond their control have no purpose in life and much idle time. They become bored with the monotony of their daily routine. Such conditions are conducive to fatigue, just as optimism or enthusiasm for a new enterprise dispels fatigue. There are other patients who, as far as one can tell, were reasonably healthy and well-adjusted until they met some adversity which aroused fear and worry. They then develop a state which may be classified as simple nervousness or reactive anxiety with the usual lassitude and fatigue, sleeplessness, and difficulty in concentration. Reactions such as these are understandable to everyone who has had "stage fright" or "buck fever." The sense of physical weakness, the utter incapacity to act, the sudden transformation of a normally well-ordered mind into intellectual chaos, and the exhaustion which follows the episode are indelible experiences in the minds of most of us.

PSYCHOLOGIC THEORIES. The significance of lassitude and fatigue in these different life situations and psychiatric illnesses has been the subject of much speculation. Physiologists have remarked on the enervating effect of strong emotion and have argued that a simple prolongation of the emotional experience would provide a rational explanation for all the symptoms of chronic anxiety. This, however, only takes the explanation one step further back and does not account for the patient's being emotionally aroused at a time when there is no explicit stimulus to emotion.

The dynamic schools of psychiatry, particularly the psychoanalytic, have postulated that chronic fatigue, like the anxiety from which it derives, is a danger signal that something is wrong; some activity or attitude has been persisted in too intensely or too long. The purpose of fatigue may be regarded as self-preservation, not merely as a protection against physical injury but also to preserve the individual's self-esteem, his concept of himself. Another hypothesis is that the fatigue is the result of the exhaustion of one's store of energy by the demands of repression. The characteristic situation in which the fatigued patient finds himself is said to be one in which effective behavior is of a type forbidden by the patient's own idea of what is permissible to him as a member of society. Fatigue then is not a negative quality, a lack of energy, but an unconscious desire for inactivity. A reciprocal relationship is believed to exist between fatigue and anxiety. Both are believed to be protective devices, but anxiety is the more imperative. It calls the individual to take some positive action to extricate himself from a predicament, whereas fatigue calls for inactivity. Both fatigue and anxiety operate blindly. The individual does not perceive what it is that must be done or stopped. All this happens at an unconscious level.

Other psychiatrists are not satisfied with the psychoanalytic hypothesis, especially for cases of lifelong weakness and fatigability. They point out that individuals differ basically in energy potential. Certain persons, it is believed, seem endowed with a limited store of energy. The physiologic or psychologic basis for this deficiency is unknown. Eugene Kahn regards it as a constitutional inadequacy and states that at present it cannot be decided whether this is inborn or acquired. Under the heading "Psychopath Weak in Impulse," he describes the individual who has an evident physical inferiority. He is a weakling; his vitality is low. He is unusually susceptible to disease and requires longer to convalesce than the average. Such a person may spend half his life recuperating from illnesses that would not bother a normal person. Vigorous games tire him, and his performance is usually so poor that he takes no interest in sports. Unless born in favorable economic circumstances he earns a meager livelihood. He seeks and accepts subordinate positions and usually cannot establish an independent social position of his own. He gives the impression of weakness of will, dullness, or nervousness, though many such individuals possess an average or superior intellectual endowment. His success is limited by lack of drive and industry. Sexual impulse is also weak, and he may find marriage impossible. He requires medical attention throughout life and, whenever subjected to any unusual stress, is apt to break down and complain of nervousness, lassitude, insomnia, and many other vague symptoms. The physical inferiority and lack of sexual impulse bring to mind that dwarfs of endocrine origin often show this same deficiency in impulse life, as do also the majority of patients with mental retardation. This weakness in impulse is found in the chronic invalid seen in everyday practice.

It is perfectly obvious that these various psychologic theories are not mutually exclusive. Undoubtedly there are certain individuals whose impulse to activity is weak throughout life, and this deficiency probably is largely, if not exclusively, determined by genetic factors. It is equally clear that boredom, lack of interest, depression of mood, and strong emotion, regardless of the conditions under which they arise, are usually accompanied by fatigue and lassitude. The more chronic varieties of fatigue are probably in most instances related to psychiatric illnesses, and here the proposition that fatigue, like anxiety, is part of a psychologic defense mechanism seems most applicable.

LASSITUDE AND FATIGUE IN CHRONIC INFECTION, ENDOCRINE, AND OTHER MEDICAL DISEASES. Chronic infection is another cause of chronic fatigue, though a much less frequent one. Everyone has at some time or other sensed the abrupt onset of extreme enervation, a tired ache in all the muscles of the body as an acute infection develops, or the listlessness that accompanies an afternoon fever. In chronic infections symptoms of lassitude, fatigue, mental depression, and vague aches and pains are of course more persistent and may even obscure those of the underlying illness. Also, there is often a period of easy fatigability, irritability, and inability to work effectively after a protracted febrile illness. Some diseases, e.g., influenza, brucellosis, and hepatitis, are more likely to be followed by these convalescent symptoms than others. If symptoms of this type are prolonged, it is often difficult, if not impossible, to decide whether they are due to the disease in question or to the presence of chronic anxiety or depression. In many chronic diseases such as infectious hepatitis and brucellosis, neurotic symptoms are often added to those of the original disease, but it is more likely that the primary fatigue state has a biochemical basis.

Metabolic and *endocrine disturbances* (see Chaps. 86 and 373) of various types may produce lassitude or fatigue. The symptom is likely to be extremely marked and to be associated with true muscular weakness. In Addison's disease and Simmonds's disease it dominates the clinical picture. Aldosterone deficiency is another established cause of chronic fatigability (cf. Chap. 92). In persons with hypothyroidism with or without frank myxedema, lassitude is usually pronounced. It is also present in many patients with hyperthyroidism, although often less troublesome than the associated nervousness. Uncontrolled diabetes may be accompanied by excessive fatigability. Hyperparathyroidism, Cushing's disease, and hypogonadism are other instances of endocrine disease in which lassitude may be prominent (see appropriate chapters).

Any type of nutritional deficiency may, when severe, cause lassitude, and in the early stages of the disease this may be the only complaint. Weight loss and the dietary history may be the only objective clues as to the nature of the illness. Most patients who have had a myocardial infarct are left with a sense of fatigue.

Amongst the neurologic diseases in which fatigability is a prominent symptom should be mentioned posttraumatic nervous instability, Parkinson's syndrome, multiple sclerosis, and postapoplectic states. The fatigue in Parkinson's disease may be present for months or years before the neurologic symptoms are recognized. It probably depends on a subjective awareness of the early stages of the motor deficit (akinesia). The majority of patients who have recovered from a stroke complain of persistent fatigue. Relapse in multiple sclerosis may be preceded by inexplicable fatigability, and fever and exposure to environmental heat, even for a brief period, exhaust the patient's energy.

DIFFERENTIAL DIAGNOSIS. Since a large variety of physical and emotional disorders may be accompanied by lassitude, the following discussion is limited to causes likely to be obscure.

When chronic fatigue and lassitude are the presenting symptoms, the commonest cause is a psychoneurosis or depressive psychosis. The basis of diagnosis is the nature of the symptoms and its pervasive effect on both mental and physical function, the associated psychiatric symptoms, usually of anxiety or depression, and the absence of signs of somatic disease. However, since psychic and somatic disorders frequently coexist, it is wise to search for organic disease before concluding that the illness is entirely psychogenic. The clinical examination should be thorough and prompt; unnecessary prolongation of the procedure may aggravate an anxiety state, if present. A careful inquiry should be made for situational factors in the patient's life which could possibly be related to the psychiatric symptoms. If found, measures should be taken to assist the patient to understand how these factors are affecting him. If reassurance that no somatic disease is present and discussion of the patient's problems do not afford relief, a psychiatric consultation is desirable. If the diagnosis is obscure, psychiatric appraisal should be part of the initial examination. Common errors are to mistake a depressive illness in which the leading symptom is chronic fatigue for a psychoneurosis; to fail to recognize the basic energy lack in an "asthenic psychopath" and to attempt to treat him as an individual with a chronic somatic disease or a recently acquired neurotic illness; and to misjudge the relative importance of psychic and somatic factors in a chronic medical disease.

Obscure infections and surgical operations may cause symptoms which closely resemble those of psychoneurosis. Indeed, individuals who have suffered from all three conditions report that the "nuclear" emotional state is similar. As a rule, aches and pains, weight loss, and low-grade fever are more prominent in chronic infection, and anxiety is in the foreground of the neurotic illness. In the United States tuberculosis, subacute bacterial endocarditis, chronic brucellosis, chronic pyelonephritis, subacute infectious hepatitis, or certain parasitic infections such as malaria and hookworm should be considered as a cause

of an illness of this type. The status of chronic brucellosis has been especially difficult to evaluate. Unfortunately there is no reliable method (other than blood culture, which is rarely positive in chronic cases) of diagnosing this condition.

Anemia (Chap. 61), when moderate to severe, and regardless of the type, should be accepted as a cause of lassitude. The severity of the symptom is more likely to parallel the hemoglobin level of the blood than the number of erythrocytes. It is the author's impression that mild grades of anemia are usually asymptomatic and that lassitude is ascribed to anemia much too often. *Nutritional deficiency*, combined with anemia, is one of the most frequent causes of lassitude and fatigability in many parts of the world.

The diagnosis of the fatigue and lassitude which accompany endocrine diseases may be difficult. These conditions are relatively rare in comparison to the psychiatric diseases which cause chronic fatigue. One of the most helpful points to keep in mind is that many of these patients are actually experiencing some degree of asthenia as well as fatigue. Details as to the most reliable methods of diagnosis of these rare diseases will be found in later chapters of the book.

Almost any type of chronic *exogenous* or *endogenous intoxication* is likely to be associated with lassitude, which, however, is only rarely the chief complaint. Among the commoner examples are alcoholism, bromism, prolonged ingestion of barbiturates, morphine addiction, and uremia. In these the clue to diagnosis is usually provided by the more troublesome complaints. In patients with acute infections, malignant tumors, and almost any other type of serious disease, other symptoms are in the foreground and are much more likely to be of diagnostic value than is the associated lassitude itself.

Lassitude of sudden onset is likely to be due to (1) an acute infection, (2) a disturbance of fluid balance, especially one producing extracellular fluid deficit, or (3) rapidly developing circulatory failure of either peripheral or cardiac origin. In these various disorders, discussed in detail in later chapters, the subjective manifestation—lassitude—is likely to be accompanied by outspoken objective phenomena, i.e., fever, tachycardia.

GENERALIZED MUSCLE WEAKNESS AND ASTHENIA

As can be judged from the foregoing remarks, the evaluation of lassitude and fatigue involves distinctions between a number of psychiatric and medical diseases; in contrast, the presence of weakness and myasthenia turns one to a rather different class of neurologic diseases which involve nerve and muscle. The symptomatic state of weakness, clearly differentiated from fatigability, is relatively infrequent.

True neural weakness and myasthenia are probably never due to psychologic disorders. Weakness does not attain significant degree in states of anemia, chronic infection, or nutritional depletion, except through the intermediation of some disorder of the neuromuscular apparatus such as a polyneuropathy. This is not to say that the chronically ill and debilitated patient is as strong as a normal healthy individual. Clearly maximal power of contraction and muscle volume are lessened, but the degree of change falls below the threshold of the methods ordinarily used in the examining room and sick bed. In such states the patient's complaints are more likely to center on other aspects of his medical disease, such as lassitude and pain, rather than loss of muscular power.

The proper determination of muscular weakness depends on two lines of inquiry: (1) a history of reduced efficiency in the performance of accustomed duties; (2) actual reduction by clinical tests of *peak power* (maximal single contractions) and endurance of some or all the major groups of muscles. It conducted systematically from head to foot, as outlined in Chap. 373, one may ascertain, by reference to one's idea of normal muscular power for age and sex, whether all the muscles or a given group of them fall below standard. Further, weakness having been demonstrated, the next step is to determine whether there is rapid weakening with continued activity, evinced by tests of sustained contraction of the affected muscles and rapid recovery with rest, as in myasthenia gravis. A series (30 to 60) of maximal contractions of the muscles of a limb, with and without a tourniquet which occludes arterial circulation, will help decide whether the special impairment of contraction that occurs in the biochemical contracture syndromes (cf. Chaps. 377 and 378) or the carpopedal spasms of tetany are present.

Diseases of the peripheral nervous system are among the best-known causes of weakness, and the additional indications of their presence are muscular atrophy, loss of tendon reflexes, and disturbances of sensation, usually in a distal pattern. If all these findings are present, there is no difficulty in distinguishing this class of disease from the myopathies, where the weak muscles may be large (pseudohypertrophic) or small (atrophic) and where reflexes diminish in proportion to the loss of muscular power. A polyneuropathy can further be separated on clinical grounds alone from the true myasthenic states, where failing neuromuscular conduction results in rapid weakening of contraction without associated atrophy, loss of tendon reflexes, or sensory changes. But it is the mild subclinical polyneuropathies that give trouble. In states of chronic renal and hepatic failure one usually finds some degree of weakness, and at autopsy it is found to be based on slight degrees of peripheral nerve degeneration and focal denervation atrophy. Diabetes mellitus, chronic nutritional deficiency, and carcinomatosis are also frequently associated with mild degrees of weakness and atrophy due to a polyneuropathy. In old age a similar picture of motor unit denervation appears in the weak, thin muscles and is due presumably to a degeneration of anterior horn cells and their axones.

Polymyopathies and the myasthenic states are the other principal causes of muscular weakness, either persistent or periodic. Muscular dystrophy in its early stages may occasion only slight weakness in certain muscle groups, and polymyositis has almost identical effects. The former is characteristically familial and its temporal course is slow; the latter has a rapid evolution (in terms of a few weeks) and often is associated with dermatitis (dermatomyositis) and disease of connective tissues or carcinoma. Large doses of corticosteroids given over a period of months or Cushing's disease cause weakness of proximal limb muscles due to segmental degeneration of muscle fibers. In hyperthyroidism and hypothyroidism there are characteristic disturbances of muscle function and size which will be described fully in Chap. 378. Hyperparathyroidism and Addison's disease cause a persistent mild generalized weakness due to some obscure disturbance in the muscle fiber and in adrenal deficiency states, especially in aldosterone deficiency, changes in sodium and potassium levels may interfere with the contraction of the muscle fibers. Many of these and other subtle diseases of muscle can be distinguished by referring to the time course of the disturbance of muscle function and the topography of the muscular affection (cf. Chap. 373).

Not all muscular weakness is due to disease of peripheral nerve or muscle. Central motor disturbances such as early Parkinson's disease or a phenothiazine dyskinesia may induce slowness of muscle action and slight diminution in power without altering the tendon reflexes.

In conclusion, it should be emphasized again that the distinction between lassitude and weakness is of primary importance, for the diseases which underlie these two states are very different. It is usually only in the early stages of a disease causing weakness when one is likely to make mistakes, for as the weakness progresses to frank paresis or paralysis the problem is one which obviously can be analyzed only along the lines described in Chap. 21. Admittedly, the separation of lassitude and weakness is not a sharp one; the former symptom often shades into the latter. Some patients with obvious weakness also complain of fatigue, but very few patients complaining of lassitude are really found to be weak, even though they may use this term to describe their feelings. The elicitation of weakness requires the testing of muscular efficiency. The analysis of fatigue and lassitude requires probing into the psychiatric state as well as the search for medical and neurologic diseases.

The considerations mentioned will lead to an accurate evaluation of the cause of weakness in many patients. Even so, there will remain a group of subjects (unfortunately, not rare) in whom the most exhaustive investigation fails to uncover the cause. In some such individuals time will furnish the answer, but in others recovery will eventually occur without the cause being known.

REFERENCES

Adams, R. D., D. Denny-Brown, and C. M. Pearson: "Diseases of Muscle: a Study of Pathology," 2d ed., New York, Paul B. Hoeber, Inc., 1962.

Walton, J. N.: "Diseases of Voluntary Muscle," 2d ed., Boston, Little, Brown and Company, 1969.

20 FAINTNESS, SYNCOPE, AND EPISODIC WEAKNESS

Raymond D. Adams and
T. R. Harrison

Episodic faintness, lightheadedness or giddiness, and reduced alertness are frequent and vexatious symptoms. The patient may refer to these symptoms as "weak spells" when he actually means loss of vigor, weakness of limbs, or impaired alertness. Any difference between faintness and syncope appears to be only quantitative. Since syncope, though less common, is more definite, it will be considered in greater detail. Those types of episodic weakness, such as myasthenia gravis and familial periodic paralysis, which are associated with striking reduction of muscular strength but not with impairment of consciousness, are discussed in other chapters. Epilepsy, which is also associated with episodic unconsciousness, differs from syncope in most other respects. It is discussed in Chap. 28.

CARDINAL FEATURES OF SYNCOPE

The term *syncope* literally means a "cutting short," "cessation," or "pause," and it is synonymous with swoon or faint. Syncope comprises a generalized weakness of muscles, with inability to stand upright and impairment of consciousness. Abrupt onset, brief duration, and complete recovery within a few minutes are other distinguishing features. Faintness, in contrast, refers to lack of strength, with a sensation of impending faint; it is an incomplete faint. Both faintness and syncope vary somewhat according to their mechanism, but both conform roughly to the following pattern.

The syncopal attack develops rapidly, but it is doubtful whether consciousness is ever terminated with the absolute suddenness of an epileptic seizure. At the beginning of the attack, the patient is nearly always in the upright position, either sitting or standing (the Stokes-Adams attack [cf. Chap. 265] is exceptional in this respect). Usually the warning of the impending faint is a sense of "feeling badly." The patient is assailed by giddiness, the floor seems to move, and surrounding objects begin to sway. His senses become confused, he yawns or gapes, there are spots before his eyes, or vision may dim, and his ears may ring. Nausea and sometimes actual vomiting accompany these symptoms. If the patient can lie down promptly, the attack may be averted without complete loss of consciousness. If he cannot, there is "loss of senses" and falling to the ground. What is most noticeable, even at the beginning of the attack, is a striking pallor or ashen-gray color of the face, and very often the face and body are bathed in cold perspiration. As a rule, the deliberate onset enables the patient to lie down or at least protect himself as he slumps. A hurtful fall is exceptional.

The depth and duration of the unconsciousness vary. Sometimes the patient is not completely oblivious of his surroundings. His senses are confused, but he may still be able to hear the voices or see the blurred outlines of people around him. Again, unconsciousness may be profound, and there may be complete lack of awareness and of capacity to respond. The patient may remain in this state for seconds to minutes or even as long as half an hour.

Shortly after the beginning of unconsciousness, convulsive movements occur in some instances. These usually consist of several clonic jerks of the arms and twitchings of the face. Rarely is there a generalized tonic-clonic convulsion. Usually the person who has fainted lies motionless, with skeletal muscles completely relaxed. Sphincter control is usually maintained. The pulse is feeble or cannot be felt; the blood pressure is low, and breathing is almost imperceptible. The reduction in vital functions, the striking pallor, and unconsciousness simulate death.

Once the patient is in a horizontal position, perhaps from having fallen, gravitation no longer hinders the flow of blood to the brain. The strength of the pulse improves, and color begins to return to the face. Breathing becomes quicker and deeper. Then the eyelids flutter, and consciousness is quickly regained. There is from this moment onward a correct perception of the environment. The patient is nevertheless keenly aware of physical weakness; and if he rises too soon, another faint may be precipitated. Headache and drowsiness, which, with mental confusion, are the usual sequelae of a convulsion, do not follow a syncopal attack.

CLASSIFICATION OF CAUSES OF RECURRENT WEAKNESS, FAINTNESS, AND DISTURBANCES OF CONSCIOUSNESS

The following list is based on established or assumed physiologic mechanisms. Some of the disorders frequently cause episodic weakness but rarely syncope. A few are especially apt to cause syncope associated with convulsive twitchings. These features are indicated in accompanying parentheses. Unless this specific notation is made, it may be assumed that the disorder in question is likely to cause faintness (when mild) and syncope (when severe).

I. Circulatory (deficient *quantity* of blood to the brain—common causes of either faintness or syncope)
  A. Peripheral
    1. Psychogenic (vasovagal-vasodepressor) syncope
    2. Postural hypotension
    3. Increased intrathoracic pressure, e.g., tussive syncope
    4. Other causes of peripheral circulatory failure Diseases of autonomic and peripheral nervous system (Chap. 36)
  B. Cardiac (acute cardiac failure, see Chap. 264)
    1. Alterations in rate or rhythm
      a. Bradycardia (sinus, AV block)
      b. Neurogenic (reflex bradycardia) Hypersensitive carotid sinus, vagovagal attacks
      c. Ectopic tachycardias (Chap. 265) (especially ventricular tachycardia and fibrillation)

2. Acute myocardial injury (especially infarction, see Chap. 271)
3. Mechanical hindrance
   a. Aortic stenosis
   b. Chronic pulmonary hypertension
   c. Disorders of pulmonary vessels, e.g., embolism
II. Other causes of weakness and episodic disturbances of consciousness
   A. Chemical (defective *quality* of blood to the brain)
      1. Hyperventilation (faintness common, syncope seldom occurs)
      2. Hypoglycemia (episodic weakness common, faintness occasional, syncope rare)
   B. Cerebral
      1. Cerebrovascular disturbances (cerebral ischemic attacks, see Chap. 357)
      2. Emotional disturbances, anxiety attacks, and hysterical seizures (see Chaps. 369 and 370)

This list of conditions which cause weakness, faintness, and disturbances of consciousness is deceptively long and involved. Close study, however, reveals that the commoner types of faint are reducible to a few simple mechanisms. In order not to obscure the central problem of fainting by too many details, only a few of the commoner varieties likely to be encountered in clinical practice are discussed below.

COMMON TYPES OF SYNCOPE

VASOVAGAL, VASODEPRESSOR (PSYCHOGENIC) SYNCOPE. This is the ordinary faint, and the description already given applies most perfectly to this form of it. The loss of consciousness usually takes place when the systolic pressure falls to 70 mm Hg or below. The pulse is weak or imperceptible, and its rate may be either slowed or slightly increased. Sudden vasodilatation, particularly of intramuscular vessels, is responsible for the fall in blood pressure and the inadequate cerebral circulation. It has been thought to represent a response to an emotional or physical stimulus which would ordinarily call for immediate strenuous physical activity. In the absence of such activity, there is sudden pooling of blood in the muscles, with inadequate venous return, decline in cerebral blood flow, and loss of consciousness. These considerations explain the rarity of vasovagal syncope in the recumbent position or during active muscular exercise, which increases the venous return. However, this explanation is somewhat speculative, and there are surprisingly few studies of this type of syncope.

Vasovagal or vasodepressor faints occur (1) in normal health as a consequence of a strong emotional experience or in conditions that favor vasodilatation, e.g., hot, crowded rooms, especially if the person is tired, hungry, or ill; (2) in anxiety states and neurocirculatory asthenia; (3) during pain; (4) after injury to tissues as a consequence of some combination of shock, pain, and psychologic factors.

POSTURAL HYPOTENSION WITH SYNCOPE. This type of syncope affects persons who have a chronic defect in, or a variable instability of, vasomotor reflexes. The character of the syncopal attack differs little from that of the vasovagal or vasodepressor type. The effect of posture is the cardinal feature of it. Sudden arising from a recumbent position or standing still is the condition under which it usually occurs.

Nature has provided man with several mechanisms by which his circulation adjusts to the upright posture. The pooling of blood in the lower parts of the body is prevented by (1) pressor reflexes which induce constriction of peripheral arteries and arterioles; (2) reflex acceleration of the heart by means of aortic and carotid reflexes; (3) improvement of venous return to the heart by activity of the muscles of the limbs and by increased rate of respiration. A normal individual placed on a tilt table to relax his muscles and tilted upright has a slightly diminished cardiac output, and blood accumulates in the legs to a slight degree. This is followed by a slight transitory fall in systolic blood pressure and then, within a few seconds, by a compensatory rise. Some normal individuals, if tilted on a table, will faint. In them it has been found that at first the blood pressure falls slightly and then stabilizes at a *lower* level. Shortly thereafter these compensatory reflexes suddenly fail, and the blood pressure falls precipitously. This also happens in some of the conditions listed below. In others, e.g., after surgical sympathectomy in diseases of the sympathetic nervous system and in the unusual condition or chronic orthostatic hypotension, the blood pressure never stabilizes after tilting but falls steadily to a level at which cerebral circulation cannot be maintained.

Postural syncope tends to occur under the following conditions: (1) in otherwise normal individuals who for some unknown reason have defective postural reflexes; (2) rarely, as part of a syndrome which comprises chronic orthostatic hypertension, symptoms of peripheral preganglionic autonomic and extrapyramidal disorder; (3) after prolonged illness with recumbency, especially in elderly individuals with flabby muscles; (4) after a sympathectomy that abolishes vasopressor reflexes; (5) in diabetic and other neuropathies, tabes dorsalis, and diseases of the nervous system which cause flabby, weak muscles and paralysis of vasopressor reflexes; (6) in persons with varicose veins because of pooling of blood in the abnormal venous channels; (7) in patients receiving antihypertensive and certain sedative and antidepressive drugs.

In some cases of *chronic orthostatic hypotension*, there is degeneration of preganglionic autonomic neurones with anhidrosis and other symptoms of sympathetic and parasympathetic paralysis (sphincteric disturbances, impotence, lack of tears, lack of saliva, pupillary paralysis) and extrapyramidal disorder (tremor, ataxia, rigidity). The hypotension differs from that already described in that the systolic and diastolic blood pressures fall rapidly as soon as the patient assumes an upright position, but there is no compensatory tachycardia, pallor, sweating, nausea, or other symptoms. The loss of consciousness is usually abrupt and may be attended by confusion. Recumbency restores the circulation of the brain, with a prompt return to consciousness. The pooling of blood in the abdomen and legs does not excite vasoconstriction of peripheral vessels. This is apparently because of the abnormality in the autonomic nervous system. There is also evidence that patients with this type of postural hypotension are deficient in release of norepinephrine and epinephrine. Repeated attacks may result in mental confusion, slurred speech, and other neurologic signs.

Micturition syncope, a condition usually seen in the elderly when they arise from bed at night to urinate, is probably a form of postural syncope. It has been suggested, however, that vasomotor reflexes from the bladder itself play a contributory part.

SYNCOPE OF CARDIAC ORIGIN (CARDIAC SYNCOPE). The occurrence of fainting in patients with a permanently slow pulse was first described by Morgagni and subsequently by Adams and by Stokes. It is today known as the Stokes-Adams syndrome. The heart rate is usually less than 40, and the electrocardiogram shows a transient or permanent atrioventricular block. Rarely, this may be present only during the attack. Usually without more than a momentary sense of weakness, the patient suddenly loses consciousness. This may occur at any time of the day or night, regardless of the position of the body. When the patient is upright, the unconsciousness will develop after a more brief period of asystole than with the recumbent position. According to Engel, 4 to 8 sec of asystole produce coma in the erect position, and 12 to 15 sec are required in recumbency. If cardiac standstill is more than 12 sec, the patient turns pale, falls unconscious, and may exhibit a few clonic jerks. The blood pressure falls rapidly during the period of asystole. With the resumption of the heartbeat, the face and neck become flushed. Longer periods of asystole, up to 5 min, result in coma, ashen-gray pallor giving way to cyanosis, stertorous breathing, fixed pupils, incontinence, and bilateral Babinski signs. Prolonged confusion and neurologic signs due to the relative ischemia of parts of the brain supplied by narrowed, arteriosclerotic arteries may persist in some patients, and permanent impairment of mental function is not unknown. Cardiac faints of this type may recur several times a day. Occasionally the heart block is transitory, and the electrocardiogram taken later shows only evidence of myocardial disease. Another form is that in which the heart block is reflex and due to irritation of the vagus nerves. Examples of this phenomenon have been observed with esophageal diverticula, mediastinal tumors, carotid sinus disease, glossopharyngeal neuralgia, and pleural and pulmonary irritation. However, reflex bradycardia is more commonly of the sinoatrial type than of the atrioventricular type.

Aortic stenosis and, less often, insufficiency dispose to fainting attacks. In rare instances it is due to heart block, but the more frequent mechanism appears to be diversion of blood from the brain to the exercising muscles in a patient who is unable to increase his cardiac output because of the mechanical hindrance. A characteristic clinical feature is that the faint occurs during or immediately after exertion. There may be an initial pallor, weakness,

or lightheadedness, or no warning whatsoever. Unconsciousness may last as long as half an hour and convulsions sometimes occur.

Closely related, and probably also a form of *effort syncope,* is that which occurs in some 20 percent of patients with *primary pulmonary hypertension.* Here exercise leads to dizziness, epigastric distress, and faintness followed by nausea, vomiting, and abdominal cramps. The attacks last from a few seconds to several minutes. Effort syncope in the absence of signs of aortic stenosis should lead to a search for the diagnostic evidence of dilatation of the pulmonary artery, accentuation of pulmonary second sound, or right ventricular hypertrophy. Again the cause of the faint seems to be an impaired cardiac output.

Paroxysmal atrial and ventricular tachycardia cause unconsciousness by interfering with cardiac filling and output. Bigeminal rhythm (Chap. 265) may rarely have the same effect. Most patients who faint because of paroxysmal ectopic tachycardia are aware of the preliminary rapid heart action. Otherwise, the syncopal attack does not differ from the aforementioned types.

A cardiac faint, sometimes fatal, may occur in patients with disease of the coronary arteries. No explanation for death is found at autopsy. Such faints, as well as those occurring during myocardial infarction, may be due to ventricular tachycardia, ventricular fibrillation, heart block, or rarely, to severe pain alone.

CAROTID SINUS SYNCOPE. The carotid sinus is normally sensitive to stretch and gives rise to sensory impulses carried via the intercarotid nerve of Hering (branch of the glossopharyngeal nerve) to the medulla oblongata. Massage of one or both carotid sinuses, particularly in elderly persons, cause a reflex slowing of the heart or even heart block, a fall of blood pressure without cardiac slowing, or an interference with the circulation of the ipsilateral cerebral hemisphere.

Syncope due to carotid sinus sensitivity may be initiated by turning of the head to one side, by a tight collar, or as in a few reported cases, by shaving over the region of the sinus. The absence of such stimuli is of no aid in diagnosis, since spontaneous attacks may occur. The attack nearly always begins when the patient is in an upright position, usually when he is standing. The onset is sudden, often with falling. Clonic convulsive movements are not infrequent in the vagal and depressor type of carotid sinus syncope. Unilateral paresthesias or convulsions have been reported in the central type. The period of unconsciousness seldom lasts longer than a few minutes. The sensorium is immediately clear when consciousness is regained. The majority of the reported cases have been in males.

In a patient displaying faintness on compression of one carotid sinus, it is important to distinguish between the benign disorder, hypersensitivity of one carotid sinus, and a much more serious condition, atheromatous narrowing of the opposite carotid or of the basilar artery (see Chap. 357).

Other forms of vasovagal syncope have been described. Exceptionally intense pain of visceral origin may inhibit cardiac action through vagal stimulation. We have observed instances of cardiac standstill during an attack of gallbladder colic, for example. The patient had been treated for epilepsy for several years despite her statements that pain always preceded loss of consciousness. Weiss has cited other examples, such as esophageal or mediastinal lesions, bronchoscopy, needling of body cavities, etc. Vagal and glossopharyngeal neuralgia are known to occasionally induce a reflex type of fainting. Again the sequence is always pain then syncope—in this instance the pain is localized to the base of the tongue, pharynx or larynx, tonsillar area, and ear. It may be triggered by pressure at these sites. Section of the ninth or tenth cranial nerve relieves the condition. It has been suggested that the cardiovascular effects are attributable to excitation of the dorsal motor nucleus of the vagus via collateral fibers from the nucleus of the tractus solitarius. The rare vertiginous faint which accompanies intense vertigo from labyrinthine or vestibular disease may be another example of reflex vagal stimulation.

TUSSIVE SYNCOPE ("LARYNGEAL VERTIGO"). This condition is rare, but it should be mentioned because it illustrates another mechanism of fainting—that resulting from a paroxysm of coughing. The few patients that the authors have observed have been men with chronic bronchitis. After hard coughing the patient suddenly becomes weak and loses consciousness momentarily. The unconsciousness that results from breath holding in infants is probably similar. Not all the underlying physiologic changes are known. It is said that the intrathoracic pressure becomes elevated and interferes with the venous return to the heart. The Valsalva maneuver of trying to exhale against a closed glottis is believed to produce an identical effect. Episodes of faintness and lightheadedness are not infrequent in pertussis and chronic laryngitis. Exceptionally, some other strong activity, such as laughing, straining at stool, running upstairs, or lifting, may produce a similar syndrome. *Breath-holding* spells of infancy and childhood are probably another example of the Valsalva phenomenon of straining with closed glottis, leading to diminished cardiac filling and reduced output (see Chap. 365).

SYNCOPE ASSOCIATED WITH CEREBROVASCULAR DISEASE. This is infrequent, and when it occurs, there is usually partial or complete occlusion of the large arteries in the neck. The best examples are found in the "aortic arch syndrome" (pulseless disease) where the innominate and common carotid and vertebral arteries have become narrowed. Physical activity, then, may critically reduce blood flow to the upper brainstem, causing abrupt loss of consciousness (cf. Chap. 357). Stenosis or occlusion of vertebral arteries and the "vertebral steal syndrome" is another example. Fainting is said also to occur occasionally in patients with congenital anomalies of the upper cervical spine (Klippel-Feil syndrome) or cervical spondylitis where the vertebral arteries are compromised. Head turning may then cause piercing neck pain, nausea, vomiting, vertigo, visual scotomas, and finally unconsciousness. If one carotid artery is occluded, heavy massage or pressure on the other may cause loss of consciousness, a kind of carotid syncope.

Pathophysiology of Syncope

In the final analysis the loss of consciousness in these different types of syncope must be caused by a change in the nervous elements in those parts of the brain which subserve consciousness. Syncope resembles epilepsy in this respect; yet there is an important difference. In epilepsy, whether major or minor, the arrest in mental function is almost instantaneous and, as revealed by the electroencephalogram, is accompanied by a paroxysm of activity in certain groups of cerebral neurones. Syncope, on the other hand, is not so sudden. The difference relates to the essential pathophysiology—a sudden spread of an electric discharge in epilepsy, and the more gradual failure of cerebral circulation in syncope.

During syncopal attacks, measurements of cerebral circulation (Schmidt-Kety and Gibbs's methods) demonstrate a significant degree of reduction in cerebral blood flow and of cerebral oxygen utilization (cerebral metabolism). Cerebral vascular resistance is decreased. The electroencephalogram reveals high-voltage slow waves, 2 to 5 per sec, coincident with the loss of consciousness. If the ischemia lasts only a few minutes, there are no lasting effects on the brain. If it persists for a longer time, it may result in necrosis of the border zones between the major cerebral and cerebellar arteries.

Conditions Often Associated with Episodic Weakness and Faintness but Not with Syncope

ANXIETY ATTACKS AND THE HYPERVENTILATION SYNDROME. This condition is discussed in detail in Chaps. 18 and 366, and it is necessary here only to state that this disorder is one of the commonest causes of recurrent faintness without actual loss of consciousness, the symptoms *are not relieved by recumbency*, and the diagnosis depends in large measure on reproducing the symptoms by hyperventilation. Two mechanisms are involved in the attacks: the loss of carbon dioxide as the result of hyperventilation and the release of epinephrine. Both mechanisms are said to be initiated by anxiety or allied emotional disturbances. Hyperventilation results in hypocapnia, alkalosis, increased cerebrovascular resistance, and decreased cerebral blood flow.

Of aid in diagnosis, as well as in therapy, is the demonstration to the patient of many of the symptoms of anxiety attack by voluntary hyperventilation for a period of 2 to 3 min and the cautious, slow, intravenous injection, during a period of several minutes, of 0.01 to 0.1 mg epinephrine. However, it must be admitted that the initial symptoms of the attack are not usually reproduced and that in some cases such measures are entirely without demonstrable effect.

HYPOGLYCEMIA. Another frequent cause of obscure episodic weakness is spontaneous hypoglycemia. When severe, the condition is likely to be due to a serious disease, such as a tumor of the islets of Langerhans or advanced adrenal, pituitary, or hepatic disease, in which instances there may be a confusion or even a loss of consciousness. When mild, as is usually the case, hypoglycemia is of the reactive type (Chap. 96) and occurs 2 to 5 hr after eating. The fasting blood glucose is normal. The diagnosis depends largely upon the history and the reproduction by the injection of insulin of a symptom complex exactly similar to that occurring in the spontaneous attacks.

ACUTE INTERNAL HEMORRHAGE. This condition, usually within the gastrointestinal tract, is an occasional cause of syncope. Peptic ulcer is the commonest source of the hemorrhage. When pain is absent, as it often is, and when there is no hematemesis, the cause of the weakness, faintness, or even unconsciousness may remain obscure until the passage of a black stool.

CEREBRAL ISCHEMIC ATTACKS. The attacks which occur in some patients with arteriosclerotic narrowing or occlusion of the major arteries of the brain are all of identical pattern, and indicate a temporary focal deficit in cerebral function. The main symptoms vary from patient to patient and include dim vision, hemiparesis, numbness of one side of the body, dizziness, and thick speech, and to those may be added an impairment of consciousness. The mechanism of this vascular syndrome has not been fully elucidated. Some physicians hold that localized vasospasm is responsible; other ascribe the attacks to small focal vascular lesions. The author's own investigations suggest some other mechanism than either of these. The condition is discussed in Chap. 357.

HYSTERICAL FAINTING. Hysterical fainting, which is rather frequent, usually occurs under dramatic circumstances. These are described in Chap. 370. The attack is unattended by any outward display of anxiety. The evident lack of change in pulse and blood pressure or color of the skin and mucous membranes distinguishes it from the vasodepressor faint induced by a shocking emotional experience. The diagnosis is based on the bizarre nature of the attack in a person who exhibits the general personality and behavior characteristics of hysteria.

Differential Diagnosis

OF SYNCOPE FROM OTHER TRANSISTORY NERVOUS DISORDERS. More typical varieties of syncope must be distinguished from other disturbances of cerebral function, the most frequent of which is akinetic or some other form of epilepsy (see Chap. 28). The epileptic attack may occur day or night, regardless of the position of the patient; syncope rarely appears when the patient is recumbent, the only common exception being the Stokes-Adams attack. The patient's color does not usually change in epilepsy; pallor is an early and invariable finding in all types of syncope, except chronic orthostatic hypotension and hysteria, and it precedes unconsciousness. Epilepsy is more sudden in onset, and if an aura is present, it rarely lasts longer than a few seconds before consciousness is abolished. The onset of syncope is usually more deliberate.

Injury from falling is frequent in epilepsy and rare in syncope for the reason that only in the former are protective reflexes instantaneously abolished. Tonic-convulsive movements with upturning eyes are frequent in epilepsy in contrast to syncope, though the same cannot be said of clonic movements of the arms. The period of unconsciousness tends to be longer in epilepsy than in syncope. Urinary incontinence is frequent in epilepsy and rare in syncope, but since it may be observed occasionally in syncope, it cannot be used as a means of excluding this condition. The return of consciousness is prompt in syncope and slow in epilepsy. Mental confusion, headache, and drowsiness are the common sequelae of epilepsy, whereas physical weakness with clear sensorium characterizes the postsyncopal state. Repeated spells of unconsciousness in a young person at a rate of several per day or month are much more suggestive of epilepsy than syncope. It should be emphasized that no one of these points will absolutely differentiate epilepsy from syncope, but taken as a group and supplemented by electroencephalograms (see Chap. 21), they provide a means of distinguishing the two conditions.

OF THE DIFFERENT TYPES OF SYNCOPE. Differentiation of the several conditions that diminish cerebral blood flow is discussed in some detail in Chap. 26, and only a few points need to be repeated here.

When faintness is related to reduced cerebral blood flow resulting directly from a disorder of cardiac function, there is likely to be a combination of pallor and cyanosis, pronounced dyspnea, and distension of the veins. When, on the other hand, the peripheral circulation is at fault, pallor is usually striking but not accompanied by cyanosis or respiratory disturbances, and the veins are collapsed. When the primary disturbance lies in the cerebral circulation, the face is likely to be florid and the breathing slow and stertorous. During the attack a heart rate faster than 150 per min indicates an ectopic cardiac rhythm, while a striking bradycardia (rate less than 40) suggests the presence of complete heart block. In a patient with faintness or syncope attended by bradycardia, one has to distinguish between the neurogenic reflex and the myogenic (Stokes-Adams) types. Occasionally, electrocardiographic tracings will be needed, but as a rule, the Stokes-Adams seizures can be recognized by their longer duration, by the greater constancy of the heart rate, by the presence of audible sounds synchronous with atrial contraction, and by marked variation in intensity of the first sound, despite the regular rhythm (Chap. 265). Clinical diagnosis may at times be difficult or impossible.

The color of the skin, the character of the breathing, the appearance of the veins, and the rate of the heart are therefore valuable data in diagnosis *if the patient is seen during the attack.* Unfortunately, the physician does not have the opportunity to see most of the patients during their "spells" of weakness. Hence he must obtain the proper clues from the patient's story. It is therefore of primary importance that the physician be familiar with the *circumstances* and the *precipitating* and *alleviating* factors in a given episode of weakness or fainting.

The following points are also helpful in the differential diagnosis of syncope:

Type of Onset. When the attack begins with relative suddenness, i.e., over the period of a few seconds, carotid sinus syncope or postural hypotension is likely. When the symptoms develop gradually during a period of several minutes, hyperventilation or hypoglycemia (spontaneous or induced by insulin) is to be considered. Onset of syncope during or immediately after exertion suggests aortic stenosis and, in elderly subjects, postural hypotension. Exertional syncope is likewise occasionally seen in persons with aortic insufficiency.

Position at Onset of Attack. Attacks due to hypoglycemia, hyperventilation, hypertensive encephalopathy, or heart block are likely to be independent of posture. Faintness associated with a decline in blood pressure (including carotid sinus attacks) and with ectopic tachycardia usually occurs only while in the sitting or standing position, whereas faintness resulting from orthostatic hypotension or orthostatic tachycardia is apt to set in shortly after change from the recumbent to the standing position.

Associated Symptoms. The associated symptoms during an attack are important, for palpitation is likely to be present when the attack is due to anxiety or hyperventilation, to ectopic tachycardia, or to hypoglycemia. Numbness and tingling in the hands and face are frequent accompaniments of hyperventilation. Irregular jerking movements and generalized spasms without loss of consciousness or change in the electroencephalogram are typical of the hysterical faint. Genuine convulsions during the attack, although characteristic of epilepsy, may occasionally occur with heart block and with hypertensive encephalopathy.

Duration of Attack. When the duration of the seizure is very brief, i.e., a few seconds to a few minutes, one thinks particularly of carotid sinus syncope or one of the several forms of postural hypotension. A duration of more than a few minutes but less than an hour particularly suggests hypoglycemia or hyperventilation.

SPECIAL METHODS OF EXAMINATION

In many patients who complain of recurrent weakness or syncope but do not have a spontaneous attack while under the observation of the physician, an attempt to *reproduce* attacks is of great assistance in diagnosis. In order to avoid the effects of suggestion, rigid controls must be adopted. Thus, if one wishes to determine whether the attacks in a given subject are hypoglycemic in type and may be reproduced by insulin injection, it is necessary to control the observations by injecting other drugs such as atropine, nitroglycerin, or histamine which evoke subjective symptoms of a different type. When properly controlled, the insulin test is of great value in the diagnosis of spontaneous hypoglycemia. Without such controls the procedure is useless.

When hyperventilation is accompanied by faintness, the pattern of symptoms can be reproduced readily by having the subject breathe rapidly and deeply for 2 or 3 min. This test is often of therapeutic value also because the underlying anxiety tends to be lessened when the patient learns that he can produce and alleviate the symptoms at will simply by controlling his breathing.

Among other conditions in which the diagnosis is commonly clarified by reproducing the attacks are carotid sinus hypersensitivity (massage of one or the other carotid sinus), orthostatic hypotension, and orthostatic tachycardia (observations of pulse rate, blood pressure, and symptoms in the recumbent and standing positions), and tussive syncope by Valsalva maneuver. In all such instances one should remember that the *crucial point is not whether symptoms are produced* (the procedures mentioned frequently induce symptoms in healthy persons) but whether the exact pattern of symptoms that occurs in the spontaneous attacks is reproduced in the artificial seizures.

Multiple mechanisms of syncope frequently coexist. Combinations of hypoglycemia, hyperventilation, and postural hypotension, or any two of them, are frequent. In order to reproduce exactly the spontaneous symptoms, it may be necessary to have the patient stand and hyperventilate at a time when the blood sugar has been reduced by insulin administration. When tremor, palpitation, and fright are present in the spontaneous attacks, it may be necessary to carry out these procedures in association with the administration of epinephrine. There is great psychotherapeutic value to the patient in knowing that the physician can turn his "spells" on and off at will and, therefore, is not guessing about their cause and significance.

Lastly, the electroencephalogram is helpful in diagnosis. In the interval between epileptic seizures it may show some degree of abnormality in 40 to 80 percent of cases. In the interval between syncopal attacks it should be normal.

TREATMENT

Fainting in most instances is due to a relatively innocent cause. In dealing with patients who have fainted the physician should think first of those causes of fainting that constitute a therapeutic emergency. Among them are massive internal hemorrhage and myocardial infarction, which may be painless. In an elderly person a sudden faint, without obvious cause, should arouse the suspicion of complete heart block, even though all findings are negative when the physician sees the patient.

If the patient is seen during the preliminary stages of fainting or after he has lost consciousness, one should make sure that he is in a position which permits maximal cerebral blood flow, i.e., with head lowered between the knees, if sitting, or lying supine. All tight clothing and other constrictions should be loosened and the head turned so that the tongue does not fall back into the throat, blocking the airway. Peripheral irritation, such as sprinkling or dashing cold water on the face and neck or the application of cold towels, is helpful. If the temperature is subnormal, the body should be covered with a warm blanket. If available, aromatic spirit of ammonia may be given cautiously by inhalation. One should be prepared for a possible emesis. Nothing should be given by mouth until the patient has regained consciousness. Then ½ tsp aromatic spirit of ammonia in a half glass of cold water, or a sip of brandy or whiskey, may be given. The patient should not be permitted to rise until his sense of physical weakness has passed, and he should be watched carefully for a few minutes after rising.

As a rule, the physician sees the patient after the faint has occurred, and he is asked to explain why it happened and how it can be prevented in the future. The prevention of fainting depends on the mechanisms involved. In the usual vasovagal faint of adolescents, which tends to occur in periods of emotional excitement, fatigue, hunger, etc., it is enough to advise the patient to avoid such circumstances. If the patient is sickly, measures to improve general health and circulatory efficiency are useful. In postural hypotension the patient should be cautioned against arising suddenly from bed. Instead, he should first exercise his legs for a few seconds, then sit on the edge of the bed and make sure he is not lightheaded or dizzy before he starts to walk. He should sleep with the headposts of the bed elevated on wooden blocks 8 to 12 in. high. A snug elastic abdominal binder and elastic stockings are often helpful. Drugs of the ephedrine group (ephedrine sulfate, 8 to 16 mg) may be useful if they do not cause insomnia. If there are no contraindications, a high intake of sodium chloride, which expands the extracellular fluid volume, may be beneficial.

In the syndrome of chronic orthostatic hypotension special corticosteroid preparations (Florinef acetate tablets, 2 to 4 mg per day in divided doses) have given relief in some cases. Binding of the legs (G suit) and sleeping with head and shoulders elevated are helpful.

The treatment of carotid sinus syncope involves first of all instructing the patient in measures that minimize the hazards of a fall (see below). Loose collars should be worn, and the patient should learn to turn the whole body, rather than the head alone, when looking to one side. Atropine or the ephedrine group of drugs should be used, respectively, in patients with pronounced bradycardia or hypotension during the attacks. Radiation or surgical denervation of the carotid sinus has apparently yielded favorable results in some patients, but it is rarely necessary. Once the possibility has been excluded that the attacks are due to a narrowing of major cerebral arteries, emphatic reassurance is essential for such patients, the majority of whom are under the mistaken impression that strokes or cardiac disease are responsible for the episodes.

The treatment of the various cardiac arrhythmias which may induce syncope is discussed in Chap. 265. The treatment of hypoglycemia will be found in Chap. 96 and of the hyperventilation syndrome and hysterical fainting in Chaps. 366 and 370.

The chief hazard of a faint in most elderly persons is not the underlying disease but rather fracture or other trauma due to the fall. Therefore, patients subject to recurrent syncope should cover the bathroom floor and bathtub with rubber mats and should have as much of their home carpeted as is feasible. Especially important is the floor space between the bed and the bathroom, because faints are common in elderly persons when walking from bed to toilet. Outdoor walking should be on soft ground rather than hard surfaces, when possible, and the patient should avoid standing still, which is more likely than walking to induce an attack.

A number of the topics considered in this chapter are discussed elsewhere in this book. The mechanisms of the circulatory disorders which may cause syncope are considered in Chap. 36. Epilepsy as a cause of recurrent unconsciousness is discussed in Chap. 28. The hyperventilation syndrome is considered in Chap. 366.

REFERENCES

Engel, G. L.: "Fainting," Springfield, Ill., Charles C Thomas, Publisher, 1950.

Gowers, W. R.: "The Borderland of Epilepsy," London, J. A. Churchill, 1907.

21 MOTOR PARALYSIS
Raymond D. Adams

The motor system may undergo dissolution in several ways during the course of nervous disease. In diffuse progressive disorders of the cerebrum there may be disintegration first of the highest, most complex nervous organizations, including learned patterns of volitional movement, and then of more elementary ones. Thus, concepts or memories of specialized, learned movement patterns may be lost while less complicated semivolitional or automatic movements are retained. Later there may be a paralysis of all voluntary movements without change in or with exaggeration of reflexes, as decortication proceeds. In lesions of basal ganglia and cerebellum, volitional movements and normal postures are altered by the presence of abnormal movements (tremor, chorea, athetosis), abnormal postures (dystonia), or incoordination (ataxia). In lesions of the brainstem all volitional movements are abolished on one or both sides of the body with release of certain obligatory postural states (decerebrate) and with normal or enhanced spinal reflexes. In lesions of the spinal cord paralysis of voluntary movement may occur with either increase or abolition of reflex activity. In lesions of peripheral nerves and skeletal muscles all movements, learned, instinctual, automatic, postural, and reflex, are lost, since this is the final common pathway.

These and other impairments of motor function may be somewhat arbitrarily subdivided into (1) paralysis due to affection of lower motor neurones, (2) paralysis due to disorder of upper motor neurones, (3) abnormalities of coordination (ataxia) due to lesions in cerebellum, (4) abnormalities of movement and posture due to disease of extrapyramidal motor system, (5) apraxic or nonparalytic disturbances of purposive movement due to involvement of cerebrum. The first two types of motor disorder and the cerebral disorders of movement will be discussed briefly in the following pages; cerebellar ataxia and extrapyramidal motor abnormalities will be considered in Chap. 22.

DEFINITIONS. The term *paralysis* is derived from two Greek words, *para*, beside, and *lysis,* a loosening. In medicine it has come to refer to an abolition of function, either sensory or motor. When applied to voluntary muscles, paralysis means loss of contraction due to interruption of some part of the motor pathway from the cerebrum to the muscle fiber. Lesser degrees of paralysis are sometimes spoken of as *paresis*, but in everyday medical parlance motor paralysis usually stands for either partial or complete loss of function. The word *plegia* comes from the Greek word meaning stroke; and the word *palsy,* from an old French word, has the same meaning as paralysis. All these words are used interchangeably in medical practice, though it is preferable to use paresis for slight and paralysis or plegia for severe loss of motor function.

Paralysis Due to Disease of the Lower Motor Neurones

Some of the essential facts concerning the anatomy and physiology of this system of motor nerve cells are well known. A few of them deserve brief comment because they explain important clinical phenomena.

Each motor nerve cell through the extensive arborization of the terminal part of its fiber comes into contact with 100 to 200 or more muscle fibers; altogether they constitute "the motor unit." All the variations in force, range, and type of movement are determined by differences in the number and size of motor units called into activity and the frequency of their action. Feeble movements involve only a few small motor units; powerful movements recruit many more units of increasing size. When a motor neurone becomes diseased, as in progressive muscular atrophy, it may manifest increased irritability, and all the muscle fibers that it controls may discharge sporadically in isolation from other units. The result of the contraction of one or several such units is a visible twitch, or *fasciculation,* which can be recorded in the electromyogram as a large diphasic or multiphasic action potential. If the motor neurone is destroyed, all the muscle fibers to which it is attached undergo a profound atrophy, namely, denervation atrophy. For some unknown reason the individual denervated muscle fibers now begin to be sensitive to circulating acetylcholine and contract spontaneously, though they can no longer do so in response to a nerve impulse or as a part of a motor unit. This isolated activity of individual muscle fibers is called *fibrillation* and is so fine that it cannot be seen through the intact skin but can be recorded only as

a repetitive short-duration spike potential in the electromyogram (see Chap. 374).

The motor nerve fibers of each ventral root intermingle as the roots join to form plexuses, and although the innervation of the muscles is roughly metameric, or according to segments of the spinal cord, each large muscle comes to be supplied by two or more roots. For this reason the distribution of paralysis due to disease of the anterior horn cells or anterior roots differs from that which follows a lesion of a peripheral nerve.

All motor activity, even of the most elementary reflex type, requires the cooperation of several muscles. The analysis of a relatively simple movement, such as clenching the fist, affords some idea of the complexity of the underlying neural arrangements. In this act the primary movement is a contraction of the flexor muscles of the fingers, the flexor digitorum sublimis and profundus, the flexor pollicis longus and brevis, and the abductor pollicis brevis. In the terminology of Beevor, these muscles act as *agonists* or *prime movers* in this act. In order that flexion may be smooth and forceful the extensor muscles (antagonists) must relax at the same rate as the flexors contract. The muscles which flex the fingers also flex the wrist; and since it is desired that only the fingers flex, the muscles which extend the wrist must be brought into play to prevent its flexion. The action of the wrist extensors is *synergic*, and these muscles are called *synergists* in this particular act. Lastly the wrist, elbow, and shoulder must be stabilized by appropriate flexor and extensor muscles, which serve as *fixators*. The coordination of agonists, antagonists, synergists, and fixators involves reciprocal innervation and is managed by segmental spinal reflexes under the guidance of proprioceptive sensory stimuli. Only the agonist movement in a voluntary act is believed to be initiated at a cortical level.

If all or practically all peripheral motor nerves supplying a muscle are destroyed, both voluntary and reflex movements are abolished. The muscle becomes soft and yields excessively to passive stretching, a condition known as *flaccidity*. Muscle tone—the slight resistance that normal relaxed muscle offers to passive movement—is reduced (hypotonia or atonia). The denervated muscles undergo extreme atrophy, usually being reduced to 20 or 30 percent of their original bulk within 3 months. The reaction of the muscle to sudden stretch, as by tapping its tendon, is lost. And, finally, it may be demonstrated that the muscle will no longer respond to electric stimuli of short duration, i.e., faradic stimuli, but still does respond to currents of long duration, i.e., to galvanic stimuli. This alteration of electric response is known as *Erb's reaction of degeneration*. If only a part of the motor units in the muscles are affected, partial paralysis or paresis will ensue. The atrophy will be less, the tendon reflexes weakened instead of lost, and the reaction of degeneration may not be obtained. Quantitative testing by determination of strength-duration curves is a means of showing partial denervation, but electromyographic evidence of fibrillations and fasciculations may also be obtained.

The tonus of muscle and the tendon reflexes are now

known to depend on the muscle spindles and the afferent fibers to which they give origin and on the small anterior horn cells whose axones terminate on the small muscle fibers within the spindles. These small spinal motor neurones are called *gamma neurones* in contrast to the large *alpha neurones.* A tap on a tendon, by stretching the spindle muscle fibers, activates afferent neurones which transmit impulses to alpha motor neurones. The result is the familiar brief muscle contraction or tendon reflex. The spindle muscle fibers are then relaxed (unloaded), which terminates the reflex. Thus the setting of the spindle fibers and the state of excitability of the gamma neurones (normally inhibited by the corticospinal fibers and other supranuclear neurones) determine the level of activity of the tendon reflexes and the responsiveness of muscle to stretch. Other mechanisms of inhibitory nature, involving Golgi tendon organs, are brought into play in more powerful stretching of muscle.

Lower motor neurone paralysis is the direct result of physiologic arrest or destruction of anterior horn cells or their axones in anterior roots and nerves. The signs and symptoms vary according to the location of the lesion. Probably the most important question for clinical purposes is whether sensory changes coexist. The combination of flaccid, areflexic paralysis and sensory changes usually indicates involvement of mixed motor and sensory nerves or affection of both anterior and posterior roots. If sensory changes are absent, the lesion must be situated in the gray matter of the spinal cord, in the anterior roots, in a purely motor branch of a peripheral nerve, or in motor axones alone. The distinction between nuclear

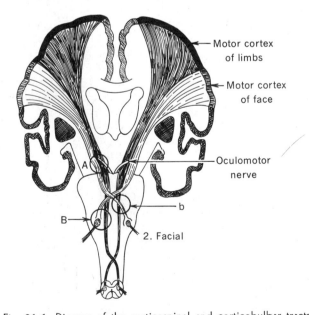

Fig. 21-1. Diagram of the corticospinal and corticobulbar tracts. Lesion at (*A*) produces ipsilateral oculomotor palsy and contralateral paralysis involving face, arm, and leg. Lesion at (*B*) causes ipsilateral facial paralysis of peripheral type and contralateral paralysis of arm and leg. Lesion at (*b*) results in ipsilateral facial weakness of upper motor neurone of central type and contralateral paralysis of arm and leg. (*Bergmann and Staeheln: "Krankheiten des Nervensystems," Berlin, Springer-Verlag, 1939.*)

(spinal) and anterior root (radicular) lesions may at times be impossible to make. The presence of spasticity in muscles weakened by a spinal lesion points to the integrity of the segments below the level of the lesion.

Paralysis Due to Disease of the Upper Motor Neurones

Several anatomic and physiologic facts concerning the upper motor neurones are worthy of note. It was formerly believed that the corticospinal tract originated from the large motor cell of Betz in the fifth layer of the precentral convolution. However, there are only about 25,000 to 30,000 Betz cells, whereas the pyramidal tract at the level of the medulla contains approximately 1 million axones. This tract must, therefore, contain many fibers that arise not from the giant Betz cells of the motor cortex (area 4 of Brodmann) but rather from the smaller Betz cells of area 4 and the cells of the adjacent precentral area 6) and postcentral cortex (areas 1, 2, 3, 5, 7). Numerous research workers have questioned the premotor, motor, and parietal cortical origin of all the fibers of the pyramid. Some are said to arise in other parts of the cerebrum or basal ganglia, and Brodal and his associates believe that some ascend from spinal cord. The most critical degeneration studies of van Crevel, however, have shown that when areas 4, 6, 1, 2, 3, 5, and 7 are removed in the cat, if one waits several months, all will be found degenerated and none can be traced to other parts of the cerebral cortex. The pyramidal tract is the only long fiber connection between the cerebrum and the spinal cord. At the level of the internal capsule these corticospinal fibers are intermingled with many others destined to end in the globus pallidus, substantia pallidus, substantia nigra, and reticular substance and with others ascending from the thalamus. The fibers to the cranial nerve nuclei become separated at about the level of the midbrain and cross the midline to the contralateral cranial nerve nuclei (Fig. 21-1). These fibers form the corticomesencephalic, corticopontine, and corticobulbar tracts. The decussation of the pyramidal tract at the lower end of the medulla is variable in different individuals. A small number of fibers, 10 to 20 percent, do not cross but descend ipsilaterally as the uncrossed pyramidal tract. Exceptionally, all of them cross; rarely, none. The termination of the corticospinal tract is in relation to nerve cells in the intermediate zone of gray matter, and not more than 10 to 15 percent establish direct synaptic connection with anterior horn cells. These new facts derived from degeneration studies must of necessity modify current views of the anatomy of the pyramidal tract and suggest new interpretations.

The motor area of the cerebral cortex is difficult to define. It includes that part of the precentral convolution which contains Betz cells, but as already mentioned, it probably extends anteriorly into area 6 and posteriorly into the anterior parietal lobe, where it overlaps the sensory areas. Physiologically it is defined as the region of electrically excitable cortex from which isolated movements can be evoked by stimuli of minimal intensity. The muscle groups of the contralateral face, arm, trunk, and leg are represented in the motor cortex, those of the face being at the lower end of the precentral convolution and those of the leg in the paracentral lobule on the medial surface of the cerebral hemisphere. These motor points are not fixed but vary somewhat with the conditions of previous stimulation. The parts of the body capable of the most delicate movements have, in general, the largest cortical representation.

Table 21-1. DIFFERENCES BETWEEN PARALYSIS OF UPPER AND LOWER NEURONE TYPES

Upper, supranuclear motor paralysis	*Lower, spinomuscular, or infranuclear paralysis*
Muscle groups affected diffusely, never individual muscles	Individual muscles may be affected
Atrophy slight and due to disuse	Atrophy pronounced, 70 to 80 percent of total bulk
Spasticity with hyperactivity of the tendon reflexes	Flaccidity and hypotonia of affected muscles with loss of tendon reflexes
Babinski sign	Plantar reflex, if present, is of normal flexor type
Fascicular twitches not produced	Fascicular twitches may be present
Normal reactions to galvanic and faradic current	Loss of faradic reaction, retention of galvanic action (reaction of degeneration)

Area 6, the premotor area, is also electrically excitable but requires more intense stimuli to evoke movements, and the movements produced are more complex than those evoked from area 4. Very strong stimuli elicit movements from a wide area of premotor frontal and parietal cortex, and the same movements may be obtained from several points. From this it may be assumed that one of the functions of the motor cortex is to synthesize simple movements into an infinite variety of finely graded, highly differentiated patterns.

Upper motor neurone paralysis may be due to lesions in the cerebral cortex, subcortical white matter, internal capsule, brainstem, or spinal cord. The distribution of the paralysis varies with the locale of the lesion, but there are also other typical features. Paralysis due to a lesion of the upper motor neurones always involves a group of muscles, never individual muscles, and if any movement is possible, the proper relationships between antagonist, synergists, and fixators are always preserved. The paralysis never involves all the muscles on one side of the body, even in the hemiplegia resulting from a complete lesion of the corticospinal tract. Movements that are invariably bilateral, such as those of the eyes, jaw, pharynx, larynx, neck, thorax, and abdomen, are little if at all affected. The hand and arm muscles suffer most severely, the leg muscles next, and of the cranial musculature only the muscles of the lower face and tongue are involved to any significant degree. Broadbent was the first to call attention to this distribution of

paralysis, and this predilection of certain muscles to paralysis with pyramidal tract disease is referred to as *Broadbent's law.* Paralysis of pyramidal type is rarely complete for any long period of time, and in this respect it differs from the total and absolute paralysis due to a lesion of the lower motor neurones. The paralyzed arm may suddenly move during yawning or stretching, and various other reflex activities can be elicited at all times. However, acute disorders may abolish function in parts of the nervous system distant from the site of the lesion. For example, a sudden lesion of the pyramidal tract in the cervical spinal cord may not only cause paralysis of voluntary movements but also abolish all of the spinal reflexes. This is known as *spinal shock.* It usually lasts but a few days or weeks and is replaced by spasticity of the paralyzed muscles. This phenomenon of *spasticity* is another characteristic of lesions of the upper motor neurones and is due to a release of spinal reflex mechanisms or the release of a "normal component in movement from its natural competitor" (Denny-Brown). Spasticity does not appear immediately after the onset of a sudden lesion but develops gradually over several weeks. In exceptional cases the paralyzed limbs remain flaccid. The spasticity affects some muscle groups more than others. The arm is usually held in a flexed position, and any attempts to extend it encounter resistance, which is maximal at the beginning and then yields (clasp-knife phenomenon). The leg is maintained in an extended position, and passive flexion is resisted. If the limbs are moved to a new position, either flexion or extension, that position is maintained (shortening and lengthening reaction). If patients have suffered paresis due to a lesion of the pyramidal tract, they not infrequently display associated movements upon attempting to carry out a voluntary movement with the weak limb. Attempts to flex the arm may result in involuntary pronation (the pronation phenomenon); or when the hemiplegic leg is flexed, the foot may automatically dorsiflex and evert (Strümpell's tibialis phenomenon). When the patient is asked to make alternating movements with the paretic limb, the healthy limb may mimic these movements (i.e., *mirror movements*).

Table 21-1, modified from Stewart, shows the main differences between paralyses of the lower and those of the upper motor neurones.

APRAXIC OR NONPARALYTIC DISORDERS OF MOTOR FUNCTION

Aside from upper and lower motor neurone paralysis with cerebral lesions there may be loss of purposive movement without paralysis. This is called *apraxia* and may be explained as follows. Many simple actions are acquired by learning or practice. These depend on the formation of movement patterns, particularly those which involve manufacture, i.e., the use of tools and instruments as well as gestures. Once established, they are remembered and may be reproduced under the proper circumstances. Any purposive act may be conceived as occurring in several stages. First, the idea of an act

must be aroused in the mind of the patient by an appropriate stimulus situation, perhaps by a spoken command
to do something. This idea or concept is then translated
into action by excitation of patterns of premotor or motor
cortical neurones in proper sequence, which are transmitted to lower centers by the corticospinal tracts. These
latter initiate particular movements of individual muscle
groups but also modify or suppress the subcortical mechanisms that control the basic attitudes and postures of the
body. In right-handed and most left-handed individuals
the neural mechanisms for the formulation of an idea of
an act (motor schema or image) in response to a spoken
command or a verbal stimulus and its reproduction are
believed to be centered in the posterior and inferior part
of the left parietal lobe, near the angular gyrus; these
areas, near the language mechanism, are connected with
the left premotor regions for the control of the right hand
and with the motor areas of the right cerebral hemisphere
through the corpus callosum for the control of the left
side.

A failure to execute certain acts in the correct context
while retaining the individual movements upon which
such acts depend is the main feature of *apraxia*. The
most adequate clinical test of motor deficits of this type
is to observe a series of self-initiated actions such as
using a comb, a razor, a toothbrush, or a common tool,
or gesturing, i.e., waving goodbye, saluting, shaking the
fist as though angry, or blowing a kiss. These may be
called forth by a command or a request to imitate the
examiner. Of course, failure to follow a spoken or written
request may be due to aphasia that prevents understanding of what is asked, or an agnosia may prevent
recognition of the tool or object to be used. But aside
from these sources of difficulty there remains a peculiar
motor deficit in which the patient appears to understand
but has lost his memory of how to perform a given act,
especially if called upon for it in an unnatural setting.
He is said then to have *ideational apraxia*. Or he may
have the idea of what he wants to do or what others
command him to do but cannot translate the idea of
the sequence of movements into a precise well-executed
act. This is called *ideomotor apraxia*. The failure is evident both after spoken command and in requests to imitate the gestures of the examiner. Sometimes these two
conditions may be dissociated; the patient, while not
aphasic, cannot execute a spoken command but can still
imitate the act if it is called forth by gesture. Finally
there is a disorder of movement sequences which consists of an inexplicable ineptitude in the use of a part of
the body for all actions. This is called *motor* or *kinetic
apraxia*. Apraxia may be limited to only one group of
muscles, such as tongue or lips as in Broca's aphasia (see
Chap. 29). Confused or demented patients may fail entirely to understand what the examiner requests and be
unable to perform many self-initiated actions. They have
ideational apraxia. If this deficit can be singled out, it
reflects a specific loss of certain learned patterns of
movement (a "specific amnesia" so to speak, analogous
to the amnesia of words in aphasia). The added element
of mental confusion tends usually to obscure the disorder.

Thus, ideational apraxia is most often manifest in diffuse or bilateral cerebral lesions; ideomotor apraxia
means major hemisphere parietal disease, and the effect
is bilateral; left-sided ideomotor apraxia indicates a lesion
in the corpus callosum and adjacent white matter of one
or other hemisphere; motor (kinetic) apraxia signifies a
lesion in the premotor cortex opposite to the affected
hand.

The latter lesions (of areas 6 and 8) which leave the
more posterior part of the motor and the sensory cortex
intact have an added feature in that many voluntary
movements, while retained, are slow and awkward. Moreover, grasping and sucking reflexes are manifest. The
tendon reflexes are lively, and the plantar reflexes are
flexor. In some cases in which basal ganglia are also
involved voluntary contractions of hand and foot may
persist unduly on tactile stimulation of the palmar and
plantar surfaces, so that the patient is unable to release
his grip or dorsiflex his foot (*tonic innervation*) voluntarily even after the stimulus is removed. In lesions of
the parietal lobe a whole series of aversion or avoidance
reactions to sensory stimuli become manifest. For a more
complete discussion of the several types of apraxia, see
Chap. 30.

Examination Scheme for Motor Paralysis and Apraxia

The first step is to inspect the paralyzed limb, taking
note first of its posture and of the presence or absence
of muscle atrophy, hypertrophy, and fascicular twitchings. The patient is then called upon to move each muscle
group, and the power and facility of movement are
graded and recorded. The range of passive movement
is then determined by moving all the joints. This provides information concerning alterations of muscle tone,
i.e., hypotonia, spasticity, and rigidity. Dislocations, disease of joints, and ankyloses may also be revealed by
these same maneuvers. Muscle bulk is then inspected.
Slight atrophy may be due to disuse from any cause, i.e.,
pain, fixation as the result of a cast, or any type of paralysis. A pronounced atrophy usually occurs only with
denervation of several weeks' or months' standing.

The tendon reflexes are then tested. The usual routine
is to try to elicit the jaw jerk (increased in pseudobulbar
palsy) and the supinator, biceps, triceps, quadriceps, and
Achilles tendon reflexes. Two cutaneous reflexes are then
tested, the abdominal and the plantar reflexes. (The
extensor plantar reflex is Babinski's sign.)

If there is no evidence of upper or lower motor neurone disease, but certain acts are nonetheless imperfectly
performed, one should look for a disorder of postural
sensibility or of cerebellar coordination or rigidity with
abnormality of posture and movement due to disease of
the basal ganglions (cf. Chap. 22). In the absence of
these disorders, the possibility of an apraxic disorder can
be investigated by watching the patient's own movements and those called forth by specific command and
gesture.

Hysterical paralysis may pose problems. Usually it is

easily distinguished from chronic lower motor neurone disease by the areflexia and severe atrophy that are so characteristic of the latter condition. Diagnostic difficulty arises only in certain acute cases of upper motor neurone disease that lack all the usual changes in reflexes and muscle tone. In hysterical paralysis one arm or one leg or all one side of the body may be affected. The hysterical gait is sometimes diagnostic in itself (see Chap. 23). Often there is loss of sensation in the paralyzed parts and sometimes loss of sight in the eye, of hearing in the ear, and of smell in the nostril on the paralyzed side, a group of sensory changes that is never seen in organic brain disease. The patient should be asked to move the affected limbs; as he does so, the movement is seen to be slow and jerky, often with contraction of both agonist and antagonist muscles simultaneously or intermittently. Hoover's sign and Babinski's combined leg flexion test are helpful in distinguishing hysterical from organic hemiplegia. To elicit Hoover's sign, the patient, lying on his back, is asked to raise one leg from the bed against resistance; in a normal individual the back of the heel of the contralateral leg is pressed firmly down, and the same is true when the patient with organic hemiplegia attempts to lift the paralyzed leg. The hysteric exerts little force with the good leg or will contract it more strongly under these circumstances than as a primary willed action. To carry out Babinski's combined leg flexion test, a patient with an organic hemiplegia is asked to sit up without using his arms; when he does so, the paralyzed or weak leg flexes at the hip, and the heel is lifted from the bed while the heel of the sound leg is pressed into the bed. This sign is absent in hysterical hemiplegia.

DIFFERENTIAL DIAGNOSIS OF PARALYSIS

The diagnostic consideration of paralysis may be simplified by the following subdivisions, which relate to the location and distribution of weakness.

1. *Monoplegia* refers to weakness or paralysis of all the muscles in one limb, whether leg or arm. It should not be applied to paralysis of isolated muscles or groups of muscles supplied by a single nerve or motor root.

2. *Hemiplegia* is the commonest distribution of paralysis—loss of strength in arm, leg, and sometimes face on one side of the body.

3. *Paraplegia* indicates weakness or paralysis of both legs. It is most commonly found in spinal cord disease.

4. *Quadriplegia* indicates weakness of all four extremities. It may result from lesions involving peripheral nerves, gray matter of the spinal cord, or corticospinal tracts bilaterally in the cervical cord, upper brainstem, or cerebrum. *Diplegia* is a special form of quadriplegia in which the legs are affected more than the arms.

5. *Isolated paralyses* refer to weakness localized to one or more muscle groups.

MONOPLEGIA

The physical examination of patients who complain of weakness of one extremity often discloses an unnoticed weakness in another limb, and the condition is actually hemiplegia or paraplegia. Or instead of weakness of all the muscles in a limb, only isolated groups are found to be affected. Ataxia, sensory disturbances, or pain in an extremity will often be interpreted by the patient as weakness, as will the mechanical limitation resulting from arthritis or the rigidity of parkinsonism.

In general, the presence or absence of atrophy of muscles in a monoplegic limb can be of diagnostic help.

PARALYSIS WITHOUT MUSCULAR ATROPHY. Long-continued disuse of a limb may lead to atrophy, but this is usually not so marked as in diseases that denervate muscles; the tendon reflexes are normal, and the response of the muscles to electric stimulation and electromyogram are unaltered.

The most frequent cause of monoplegia without muscular wasting is a lesion of the cerebral cortex. Only occasionally does it occur in diseases which interrupt the corticospinal tract at the level of the internal capsule, brainstem, or spinal cord. A vascular lesion (thrombosis or embolus) is commonest, but of course, a tumor or abscess may have the same effect. Multiple sclerosis and spinal cord tumor, early in their course, may cause weakness of one extremity, usually the leg. As indicated above, weakness due to damage to the corticospinal system is usually accompanied by spasticity, increased reflexes, and an extensor plantar reflex (Babinski's sign), and the electric reactions and electromyogram are normal. However, acute diseases that destroy the motor tracts in the spinal cord may at first (for several days) reduce the tendon reflexes and cause hypotonia (the condition known as *spinal shock*). This does not occur in partial or slowly evolving lesions and occurs only to minimal degree in lesions of brainstem and cerebrum. In acute diseases affecting the lower motor neurones the tendon reflexes are always reduced or abolished, but atrophy may not appear for several weeks. Hence one must take into account the mode of onset and the duration of the disease in evaluating the tendon reflexes, muscle tone, and degree of atrophy before reaching an anatomic diagnosis.

PARALYSIS WITH MUSCULAR ATROPHY. This condition is more frequent than paralysis without muscular atrophy. In addition to the paralysis and reduced or abolished tendon reflexes, there may be visible fasciculations. If completely paralyzed, the muscles exhibit an electric reaction of degeneration and the electromyogram shows reduced numbers of motor units (often of large size), fasciculations at rest, and fibrillations. The lesion may be in the spinal cord, spinal roots, or peripheral nerves. Its location can usually be decided by the distribution of the palsied muscles (whether the pattern is one of nerve, spinal root, or spinal cord involvement), by the associated neurologic symptoms and signs, and by special tests (cerebrospinal fluid examination, x-ray of spine, and myelogram).

Brachial atrophic monoplegia is relatively rare, and when present, it should suggest in an infant a brachial plexus trauma, in a child poliomyelitis, in an adult poliomyelitis, syringomyelia, amyotrophic lateral sclerosis, or brachial plexus lesions. Crural monoplegia is more frequent and may be caused by any lesion of thoracic or lumbar cord, i.e., trauma, tumor, myelitis, multiple sclerosis, etc. It should be noted that multiple sclerosis almost never causes atrophy and that ruptured intervertebral disk and the many varieties of neuritis rarely paralyze all or most of the muscles of a limb. Muscle dystrophy may begin in one limb, but by the time the patient is seen the typical more or less symmetric pattern of proximal limb and trunk involvement is evident. A unilateral retroperitoneal tumor may paralyze the leg by implicating the lumbosacral plexus.

HEMIPLEGIA

This is the most frequent distribution of paralysis in man. With rare exceptions (a few unusual cases of poliomyelitis or motor system disease) this pattern of paralysis is due to involvement of the corticospinal tract.

LOCATION OF LESION PRODUCING HEMIPLEGIA. The site or level of the lesion, i.e., cerebral, capsular, brain stem, or spinal cord, can usually be deduced from the associated neurologic findings. Diseases localized in the cerebral cortex, cerebral white matter (corona radiata), and internal capsule usually evoke weakness or paralysis of the face, arm, and leg on the opposite side. The occurrence of convulsive seizures or the presence of a defect in speech (aphasia), a cortical type of sensory loss (astereognosis, loss of two-point discrimination, etc.), anosognosia, or defects in the visual fields suggest a cortical or subcortical location.

Damage to the corticospinal tract in the upper portion of the brain stem (see Fig. 21-1) may cause paralysis of the face, arm, and leg on the opposite side. The lesion in such cases is localized by the presence of a paralysis of the muscles supplied by the oculomotor nerve on the same side as the lesion (Weber's syndrome) or other neurologic findings. With low pontine lesions a unilateral abducens or facial palsy is combined with a contralateral weakness or paralysis of the arm and leg (Millard-Gubler syndrome). Lesions of the lowermost part of the brain stem, i.e., in the medulla, affect the tongue and sometimes the pharynx and larynx on one side and arm and leg on the other side. These "crossed paralyses," so common in brainstem diseases, are described in Chap. 355.

Rarely, a homolateral hemiplegia may be caused by a lesion in the lateral column of the cervical spinal cord. At this level, however, the pathologic process often induces bilateral signs, with resulting quadriparesis or quadriplegia. If one side of the spinal cord is extensively damaged, the homolateral paralysis is combined with a loss of vibratory and position sense on the same side and a contralateral loss of pain and temperature (Brown-Séquard syndrome).

Muscle atrophy of minor degree often follows lesions of the corticospinal system but never reaches the proportions seen in diseases of the lower motor neurones. The atrophy is due to disuse. When the motor cortex and adjacent parts of the parietal lobe are damaged in infancy or childhood, the normal development of the muscles and the skeletal system in the affected limbs is retarded. The palsied limbs and even the trunk on one side are small.

This does not occur if the paralysis begins after the greater part of skeletal growth is attained (after puberty). In the hemiplegia due to spinal cord injury muscles at the level of the lesion atrophy as a result of damage to anterior horn cells or ventral roots.

CAUSES OF HEMIPLEGIA. In this condition vascular diseases of the cerebrum and brainstem exceed all others in frequency. Trauma (brain contusion, epidural and subdural hemorrhage) ranks second, and other diseases such as brain tumor, brain abscess and encephalitis, demyelinative diseases, complications of meningitis, tuberculosis, and syphilis are of decreasing order of importance. Most of these diseases can be diagnosed by the mode of evolution and the conjoined clinical and laboratory data presented in the chapters on neurologic diseases. For further discussion see Chap. 357.

PARAPLEGIA

Paralysis of both lower extremities may occur in diseases of the spinal cord and the spinal roots or of the peripheral nerves. If onset is acute, it may be difficult to distinguish spinal from neural paralysis, for in any acute myelopathy spinal shock may result in abolition of reflexes and flaccidity. As a rule in acute spinal cord diseases with involvement of corticospinal tracts, the paralysis affects all muscles below a given level; and often, if the white matter is extensively damaged, sensory loss below a particular level (loss of pain and temperature with lateral spinothalamic tracts and loss of vibratory and position sense with posterior columns) is conjoined. Also, in bilateral disease of the spinal cord, the bladder and bowel sphincters are paralyzed. Alterations of cerebrospinal fluid (dynamic block, increase in protein or cells) are frequent. In peripheral nerve diseases both sensory and motor loss tend to involve the distal muscles of the legs more than the proximal ones (an exception is acute idiopathic polyneuritis), and the sphincters are often spared or only briefly deranged in function. Sensory loss, if present, is more likely to consist in distal impairment of touch, vibration, and position sense, with pain and temperature spared in many instances. The cerebrospinal fluid protein may be normal or elevated.

For clinical purposes it is helpful to consider separately the acute and the chronic paraplegias and to divide the chronic ones into two groups, those which occur in infancy and those which begin in adult life.

Acute paraplegia, beginning at any age, is relatively infrequent. Fracture dislocation of the spine with traumatic necrosis of the spinal cord, spontaneous hematomyelia with bleeding from a vascular malformation (angioma, telangiectasis), thrombosis of a spinal artery with infarction (myelomalacia), and dissecting aortic aneurysm or atherosclerotic occlusion of nutrient spinal arteries arising from the aorta with resulting infarction (myelomalacia) are the commonest varieties of sudden paraplegia (or quadriplegia, if the cervical cord is involved). Postinfectious or postvaccinal myelitis, acute demyelinative myelitis (Devic's disease if the optic nerves are affected), necrotizing myelitis, and epidural abscess or tumor with spinal cord compression tend to develop somewhat more slowly, over a period of hours or days, or they may have a subacute onset. Poliomyelitis and acute idiopathic polyneuritis, the former a purely motor disorder with meningitis, the latter predominantly motor but often with minimal sensory disturbances (paresthesias or objectively demonstrated impairment), must be distinguished from the other acute myelopathies and from one another.

In pediatric practice, delay in starting to walk and difficulty in walking are common problems. These conditions may be associated with a systemic disease such as rickets or may indicate mental deficiency or, more commonly, some muscular or neurologic disease. Congenital cerebral disease accounts for a majority of cases of infantile diplegia (weakness predominant in the legs, with the arms minimally affected). Present at birth or manifest in the first months of life, it may appear to progress; but actually it is stationary and only becomes apparent as the motor system develops. Later there may seem to be slow improvement as a result of the normal maturation processes of childhood. Congenital malformation of the spinal cord or birth injury of the spinal cord are other possibilities. Friedreich's ataxia and familial paraplegia, progressive muscular dystrophy, and the chronic varieties of polyneuritis tend to appear later during childhood and adolescence and are slowly progressive.

In adult life multiple sclerosis, subacute combined degeneration, spinal cord tumor, ruptured cervical disk and cervical spondylosis, syphilitic meningomyelitis, chronic epidural infections (fungous and other granulomatous diseases), Erb's spastic paraplegia and motor system disease, and syringomyelia represent the most frequently encountered forms of spinal paraplegia. (See Chap. 356 for discussion of these spinal cord diseases.) The several varieties of polyneuritis and polymyositis must be considered in their differential diagnosis, for they, too, may cause paraparesis.

QUADRIPLEGIA

All that has been written about the common causes of paraplegia applies to quadriplegia. The lesion is usually in the cervical rather than the thoracic or lumbar segments of the spinal cord. If it is situated in the low cervical segments and involves the anterior half of the spinal cord, as in occlusion of the anterior spinal artery, the arm paralysis may be flaccid and areflexic and the leg paralysis spastic (anterior spinal syndrome). There are only a few points of difference between the common paraplegic and quadriplegic syndromes. In infants, aside from developmental abnormalities and anoxia of birth, an inherited cerebral disease (Schilder's disease, metachromatic leukoencephalopathy, lipid storage disease) may be responsible for a quadriparesis or quadriplegia. Congenital forms of muscular dystrophy may be recognized soon after birth and also infantile muscular atrophy (Hoffmann-Werdnig disease).

In adults repeated cerebral vascular accidents may lead to bilateral hemiplegia, usually accompanied by pseudobulbar palsy.

ISOLATED PARALYSIS

Paralysis of isolated muscle groups usually indicates a lesion of one or more peripheral nerves. The diagnosis of a lesion of an individual peripheral nerve is made on the presence of weakness or paralysis of the muscle or group of muscles and impairment or loss of sensation in the distribution of the nerve in question. Complete transection or severe injury to a peripheral nerve is usually followed by atrophy of the muscles it innervates and by loss of their tendon reflexes. Trophic changes in the skin, nails, and subcutaneous tissue may also occur.

Knowledge of the muscular and sensory function of each individual nerve is needed for a satisfactory diagnosis. Since lesions of the peripheral nerves are relatively uncommon in civil life, it is not practical for the general physician to keep all these facts in his memory, and a textbook of anatomy or Chap. 354, the Section on mononeuropathies, should be consulted. It is, however, of considerable importance to decide whether the lesion is a temporary one of conduction only (neuropraxia) or whether there has been a pathologic dissolution of continuity, requiring nerve regeneration for recovery. Electromyography may be of value here.

All the diseases mentioned in the differential diagnosis of monoplegia, hemiplegia, paraplegia, and quadriplegia will be discussed in the chapters on neurologic diseases.

MUSCULAR PARALYSIS AND SPASM UNATTENDED BY VISIBLE CHANGE IN NERVE OR MUSCLE

A discussion of motor paralysis would not be complete without some reference to a group of diseases that appear to have no basis in visible structural change in motor nerve cells, nerve fibers, motor end-plates, and muscular fibers. This group is comprised of myasthenia gravis, myotonia congenita (Thomsen's disease), familial periodic paralysis, disorders of potassium, sodium, calcium, and magnesium metabolism, tetany, tetanus, botulinus poisoning, black widow spider bite, and the thyroid myopathies. In these diseases, each of which possesses a fairly distinctive clinical picture, the abnormality is purely biochemical, and even if the patient survives for a long time, no visible microscopic changes develop. An understanding of these diseases requires knowledge of the processes involved in nerve and muscle excitation and in the contraction of muscle. They will be discussed in Chaps. 377 and 378.

22 TREMOR, CHORIA, ATHETOSIS, ATAXIA AND OTHER ABNORMALITIES OF MOVEMENT AND POSTURE

Raymond D. Adams

In this chapter are discussed the automatic, static, and less modifiable postural activities of the human nervous system. These are believed, on good evidence, to be an expression of the activity of the *older motor system*, meaning, according to S. A. K. Wilson, who introduced this term, the extrapyramidal motor structures in the basal ganglions and brainstem.

In health, the activities of both the old (extrapyramidal) and the new (pyramidal) motor system are blended. The static postural activities of the former are indispensable to voluntary, or willed, movement of the latter.

This close association of the pyramidal and extrapyramidal systems is shown by human disease. Lesions of the pyramidal tract result not only in paralysis of volitional movements of the contralateral half of the body but in the appearance of a fixed posture or attitude in which the arm is maintained in flexion and the leg in extension (predilection type of Wernicke-Mann or hemiplegic dystonia of Denny-Brown). Similarly, decerebration from a lesion in the upper pons or midbrain releases another posture in which all four extremities are extended and the cervical and thoracolumbar spine dorsiflexed. In these released action patterns one has evidence of extrapyramidal postural and righting reflexes which are mediated through bulbospinal and other brainstem structures.

The student may be dismayed to read in current articles trenchant criticism of the validity of the concept of the pyramidal tract and division of motor system into pyramidal and extrapyramidal. Extremists claim the pyramidal tract may be severed in animals and even in men without lasting motor deficits. But it must be remembered that this tract is such a puny thing in most mammals, even in small monkeys, that it can hardly be compared to that of man, and there has yet to be a pathologically proven example in man of complete interruption of this tract with preserved voluntary motor function.

If an oversimplification may be permitted for clarity of exposition, the extrapyramidal motor system may be subdivided into two parts: (1) the striato-pallidonigral and (2) the cerebellar. Disease in either of these parts will result in disturbances of movement and posture without significant paralysis. These two major systems and the symptoms that result when they are diseased are reviewed on the following pages.

THE BASAL GANGLIA: PHARMACOLOGY AND PATHOLOGICAL ANATOMY

As an anatomic entity the basal ganglia have no precise limitation. The list of basal structures originally thought to have some part in motor function, such as the caudate and lenticular nuclei and amygdaloid body, has been greatly expanded by physiologists to include the field of Forel and zona incerta, subthalamic nucleus of Luys, substantia nigra, red nucleus, dentate nucleus of cerebellum, and the reticular formation of the brainstem. The anatomic connections between these structures and other parts of the brain, such as with the cerebral cortex and afferent sensory systems, are too intricate to present

in a textbook of medicine. The reader must refer to a neuroanatomy textbook.

Perhaps the principal new anatomic idea to emerge in recent years is the central position that the *ventrolateral nucleus of the thalamus* plays in the ascending limb of circuits which involve the cortex-pons-cerebellum-dentate nucleus-*thalamus*-cortex, and the cortex-striatum-subthalamic nucleus and substantia nigra-*thalamus*-cortex. Indeed it would seem that all the extrapyramidal motor systems at this level of the nervous system are funneled through the ventrolateral nucleus up to the motor cortex and pyramidal system. Descending pathways to the spinal cord are disputed; probably there are polysynaptic descending systems of fibers through the reticular formation of pons and medulla. It is noteworthy that some of the descending and ascending systems from and to the cortex pass through the internal capsule, hence lesions here and in the cerebral white matter may simultaneously involve both pyramidal and extrapyramidal systems.

A second and most exciting development of recent years has been in the biochemistry and pharmacology of the basal ganglia. In man the substantia nigra, putamen, and caudatum are rich in norepinephrine. Precursors of this substance are shown in the following metabolic pathway:

L—phenylalanine
    hydroxylase
L—Tyrosine
    oxidase
L—Dopa (3–4 hydroxyphenylalanine)—Dopaquinone—Indolquinone—melanin
    decarboxylase
L—Dopamine—homoprotocatechuric acid—homovanillic acid
    oxidase
L—Norepinephrine
    methylase
L—Epinephrine

Dopa is seen to be a step not only in the metabolism of norepinephrine but also of melanin. The former is an important intercellular transmitter substance; the latter is contained in the pigmented neurones of substantia nigra and other brainstem nuclei which degenerate in Parkinson's disease.

This new field of neuropharmacology opened up when it was discovered that prolonged use of tranquilizer medication such as reserpine and chlorpromazine induced Parkinson's syndrome and many other disorders of the extrapyramidal system such as athetosis and other dyskinesias of neck and spinal musculature. Some of these disorders have been permanent, persisting for months and years after the drugs were discontinued; usually they are transitory. Interestingly, reserpine depletes the striatum (putamen and caudate nuclei) of its norepinephrine unless iproniazid is given beforehand or at the same time. The quantity of dopa in the striatum and substantia nigra is diminished in Parkinson's disease. It can be replenished by giving dopa orally or intravenously, with concomitant reduction in extrapyramidal symptomatology.

Some of the most significant facts about clinicopathologic relationships in man are to be found in the writings of a number of famous neurologists. In 1912 S. A. K. Wilson delineated the syndrome of chronic lenticular degeneration, and at about the same time Van Woerkem observed a disturbance of cerebral function in other forms of liver disease. In 1920 Oskar and Cecile Vogt described a number of other motor disturbances associated with lesions limited to the striatum. Lewy was one of the first to describe the pathology of paralysis agitans, and Tretiakoff (in postencephalitic forms) and Hassler (in paralysis agitans) subsequently established the localization of at least part of the lesions in the substantia nigra. The thorough studies of Huntington's chorea by Bielschowsky in 1919 related the choreoathetosis to lesions in the caudate nucleus and putamen. A long series of observations, the most recent ones being those of J. Purdon Martin, have demonstrated the relationship between hemiballismus and lesions in the subthalamic nucleus of Luys.

Unfortunately, many of the classic cases leave much to be desired. In some instances the disease process was of diffuse type, and many other parts of the brain were affected, as in Wilson's hepatolenticular degeneration. Also, lack of quantitative neuropathologic methods hampered progress in the field. Even now the topography of the pathologic findings in several of these diseases (e.g., dystonia musculorum deformans) has not been fully determined.

Table 22-1 presents clinicopathologic correlations accepted by many neurologists; however, there is still much uncertainty as to finer details.

The symptoms that lend themselves best to clinical analysis are akinesia, rigidity, chorea, athetosis, dystonia, and tremor.

AKINESIA

When analyzed along classic neurologic lines, into primary functional deficits and secondary release effects, akinesia stands as the negative or deficit symptom of extrapyramidal disease. By the term *akinesia* one refers to the disinclination of the patient to use an affected part of the body, to engage it freely in all the natural actions of the body. Paralysis, the negative symptom of pyramidal disease, is different in that there is diminution of strength in the part and it cannot be used effectively in the desired movement. In this respect, too, it is unlike apraxia, where movements are lost because of a lesion which erases the memory of the motor schema which combines sequence of movements to form an intended action. The parkinsonian patient exhibits the phenomenon of akinesia most clearly in his extreme underactivity. He sits motionless for long times. In looking to the side he moves his eyes not his head. In arising from a chair he fails to make all the little adjustments needed (putting feet back, putting hands on arms of chair, etc.). Yet he is not weak (paretic) or apraxic. Formerly, akinesia was attributed to rigidity, which could reasonably hamper all movements, but now that stereotaxic surgery can abolish both tremor and rigidity it becomes clear that the motor deficit or akinesia is still there. Strictly interpreted it would appear that, apart from their contribution to the maintenance of postures, the basal ganglia must provide something essential to the performance of the large variety of semiautomatic actions that make up the full repertoire of natural human mobility.

A point of interest is whether akinesia is an invariable manifestation of all extrapyramidal diseases, without which there could be no secondary release effects such as flexion dystonia, athetosis, chorea, and rigidity. The question has no clear answer. While seemingly true of Huntington's and Sydenham's chorea, double athetosis, and Parkinson's disease, one cannot be sure of the existence of either akinesia or paralysis in hemiballismus.

ALTERATIONS OF MUSCLE TONE (SPASTICITY, RIGIDITY, HYPOTONIA)

Already it has been pointed out that muscle tone (the small resistance to muscle stretch offered by healthy muscle) is enhanced in the many conditions that cause a paralysis of voluntary movement by interrupting the corticospinal tract. The special distribution of the increased tone, i.e., greater in antigravity muscles (extensors of leg and flexors of the arm in man), the sudden augmentation of tone with gradual yielding upon quick movement (the

Table 22-1. CLINICOPATHOLOGIC CORRELATIONS

Symptoms	Principal location of morbid anatomy
Unilateral plastic rigidity with static tremor (Parkinson's syndrome)	Contralateral substantia nigra plus (?) other structures
Unilateral hemiballismus and hemichorea	Contralateral subthalamic nucleus of Luys, prerubral area, and Forel's fields
Chronic chorea of Huntington's type	Caudate nucleus, putamen, pallidum (?), and, in some cases, corpus Luysi
Athetosis and dystonia	Contralateral putamen
Cerebellar ataxia, i.e., intention tremor, slowness in starting and stopping alternating, voluntary movements, hypotonia, rebound phenomenon	Homolateral cerebellar hemisphere or middle and inferior cerebellar peduncles, superior brachium conjunctivum (ipsilateral if below, contralateral if above the decussation)
Decerebrate rigidity, i.e., opisthotonos, extension of arms and legs, modification of these postures by turning of head and neck (increased extensor and decreased flexor tone on side toward which head is turned)	Lesion usually bilateral in tegmentum involving red nuclei or structures between red nuclei and vestibular nuclei. Rarely above tentorium in subthalamus
Palatal and facial myoclonus (rhythmic)	Lesion in the central tegmental tract, inferior olivary nucleus, and olivodentate connections.
Diffuse myoclonus	? cerebellar cortex, ? thalami

lengthening reaction or clasp-knife phenomenon), and the absence of resistance upon slow movement, its disappearance in relaxed muscle with "electromyographic silence," and exaggerated tendon reflexes are the identifying characteristics of this spasticity. This type of hypertonus is believed in some instances to be due to hyperactivity of the small gamma motor neurones, resulting in increase in the sensitivity of the spindle muscle fibers to stretch; in other instances it seems clearly related to excessive activity of the larger alpha motor neurones. The "gamma spasticity" is abolished by procaine injection of the motor nerve, which paralyzes the small gamma motor and sensory fibers, leaving the larger ones intact, without weakening the willed contractions of the muscle, whereas the "alpha spasticity" is not affected.

In the state known as *rigidity* the muscles are continuously or intermittently firm, tense, and prominent; and the resistance to passive movement is intense and even, like that noted in bending a lead pipe or in stretching a strand of toffee. Although present in all muscle groups, both flexor and extensor, on the whole, it tends to be more prominent in those which maintain a flexed posture, i.e., flexor muscles of trunk and limbs. It appears to be somewhat greater in the large muscle groups, but this may be merely a question of muscle mass. Certainly the smaller muscles of the face and tongue and even those of the larynx are often affected. The tendon reflexes are not enhanced. Nevertheless, like "gamma spasticity," this rigidity is said to be abolished by procaine, and Foerster had earlier demonstrated that it is eradicated by posterior root section. In the electromyographic tracing, motor unit activity is more continuous than in spasticity, persisting even after relaxation.

A special type of rigidity, first noted by Negro in 1901, is the *cogwheel phenomenon*. When the hypertonic muscle is passively stretched, the resistance may be rhythmically jerky, as though the resistance of the limb were controlled by a ratchet. A number of different explanations of this phenomenon have been suggested. Wilson postulated it might be due to a minor form of the lengthening-shortening reaction, but a more likely explanation is an associated static tremor that is masked by rigidity during an attitude of repose but emerges faintly during manipulation.

Rigidity is prominent in extrapyramidal diseases such as paralysis agitans, postencephalitic Parkinson's syndrome, and some cases of athetosis and cerebral palsy.

The *tension hypertonus of athetosis* differs from both spasticity and rigidity. Strictly speaking, it takes two forms, one which occurs during the involuntary athetotic movement, and another which appears in the absence of any involuntary motion. Clinically these forms of hypertonus are variable from one moment to the next and are paradoxic in that they sometimes disappear during a rapid passive movement or when the limb is passively shaken. The tendon reflexes may be normal or brisk. The lengthening and shortening reactions are absent. This form of variable hypertonus is found in cases of double athetosis and choreoathetosis and in some cases of dystonia musculorum deformans. Usually in Sydenham's and

Huntington's chorea a state of hypotonia prevails, sometimes as strikingly as in sensory polyneuropathies and lower motor neurone paralyses.

INVOLUNTARY MOVEMENTS

CHOREA. Derived from the Greek word meaning "dance," chorea refers to widespread arrhythmic movements of a forcible, rapid, jerky type. These movements are involuntary and are noted for their irregularity, variability, relative speed, and brief duration. They are quite elaborate and of variable distribution. In some respects they resemble a voluntary movement in their complexity, yet they are never combined into a coordinated act. The patient may, however, incorporate them into a deliberate movement, as if to make them less noticeable. When superimposed on voluntary movements, they may take on a grotesque and exaggerated character. Grimacing and peculiar respiratory sounds may be other expressions of the movement disorder. Usually they are discrete, but if very numerous, they may flow into one another; the resultant picture then resembles athetosis. They may be limited to a limb or to an arm and leg on one side (hemichorea), or they may involve all parts of the body. Normal volitional movements are, of course, possible, for there is no paralysis, but they too may be excessively quick and poorly sustained. The limbs are often unusually slack or hypotonic. A choreic movement may be superimposed on a tendon reflex, giving rise to the "hung-up reflex." The tendon reflexes tend to be pendular from the associated hypotonia; when the knee jerk is elicited with the patient sitting, the leg swings back and forth four or five times, like a pendulum, rather than one or two times as in a normal person.

Chorea appears in typical form in Sydenham's chorea and was noted also in the acute stages of epidemic encephalitis lethargica. It is a feature also of Huntington's chorea (chronic chorea), where the movements tend more typically to be choreoathetotic. Vascular lesions in the subthalamus, particularly those in and near the subthalamic nucleus of Luys, may result in wild flinging movements of the opposite arm and leg (hemiballismus). As these subside, they become almost indistinguishable from chorea.

ATHETOSIS. This term is from a Greek word meaning "unfixed" or "changeable." The condition is characterized by an inability to sustain the fingers and toes, tongue, or any other group of muscles in any one position. The maintained posture is interrupted by continuous, slow, sinuous, purposeless movements. These are most pronounced in the digits and the hands but often involve the tongue, throat, and face. One can detect as basic patterns of movement an extension and pronation and flexion and supination of the arm, and alternating flexion and extension of the fingers. They may be unilateral, especially in children who have suffered a hemiplegia at some previous date (posthemiplegic athetosis). The movements are slower than those of chorea, but in many cases gradations between the two (choreoathetosis) are seen. Most athetotic patients exhibit variable degrees of motor deficit due in some instances to associated pyramidal tract disease. Discrete individual movements of the tongue, lips, and hand are often impossible, and attempts to perform such voluntary movements result in a contraction of all the muscles in the limb (an *intention spasm*). Variable degrees of rigidity are generally associated, and these may account for the slower quality of athetosis, in contrast to chorea. It must be admitted, however, that in some cases it is almost impossible to distinguish between chorea and athetosis.

Athetosis or choreoathetosis of all four limbs is a cardinal feature of a curious state known as *double athetosis*, which begins in childhood. Athetosis appearing in the first months of life usually represents a congenital or postnatal condition such as hypoxia, kernicterus, or birth injury. Postmortem examination in some of the cases has disclosed a peculiar pathologic change of probable hypoxic etiology, a status marmoratus in the striatum; in others there has been a loss of medullated fibers, a status dysmyelinisatus, in the same regions.

TORSION SPASM OR DYSTONIA. Torsion spasm is closely allied to athetosis, differing only in that the larger axial (trunk, girdle muscles) rather than appendicular ones are involved. It results in bizarre, grotesque movements and positions of the body. The word *dystonia* has been given to these movements but, unfortunately, is also applied to any fixed posture which may be the end result of a disease of the motor system. Thus Denny-Brown speaks of hemiplegic dystonia, the flexion dystonia of parkinsonism, extensor dystonia with retraction of head and arching or twisting of back. If the latter meaning is given, it would be better to speak of athetosis of the trunk as torsion spasms or phasic dystonia, in contrast to fixed dystonia. The former, like athetosis, may show remarkable fluctuations, sometimes the whole musculature of the body may be thrown into spasm by an effort to move an arm or to speak. If mild, the torsion spasm may be limited to the lumbar or cervical muscles or those of one limb and may cease when the body is at rest.

Torsion spasm may be seen in the condition of double athetosis after hypoxic damage to the brain, in kernicterus, and rarely, in Wilson's hepatolenticular degeneration. It is most characteristic of the syndrome designated *dystonia musculorum deformans* but also occurs in other conditions such as the postphenothiazine dyskinesias and Hallevorden-Spatz disease (Chap. 364).

Chorea, athetosis, and torsoin spasm are all closely related. The movements are elaborate and depend for their expression on cortical mechanisms. Paralytic lesions involving the pyramidal tract abolish the involuntary movements. The hypotonia in chorea and some cases of athetosis, the pendular reflexes, and some degree of interference with the natural movements are also reminiscent of the syndrome that follows disease of the cerebellum. Lacking, however, are intention tremor and true incoordination or ataxia.

MYOCLONUS. This term refers to several different motor disorders, some localized, others diffuse. Like chorea, the myoclonic movement is involuntary and arrhythmic, but it is much faster than chorea, being concluded in a few hundred milliseconds. Variations in degree are noteworthy; it may consist of no more than a flick of a single muscle or part of a muscle, but the larger movements always betray its nature, involving as they do a group of muscles. Thus myoclonus can be distinguished from fasciculation. Sensory relationships are another prominent attribute. Flickering light, a series of loud sounds, or abrupt contact with some part of the body may regularly initiate a jerk, sometimes as a direct sensorimotor effect, again through the mechanism of startle. One special variety is evoked by willed movement, presumably through a proprioceptive mechanism. Hence, one may speak of action or intention myoclonus, auditory or visual myoclonus. A series of intense stimuli may recruit a series of myoclonic jerks into a full-blown seizure, as happens often in the familial myoclonic epilepsy syndrome of Unverricht-Lundborg. The pathology of the latter is usually a lipid storage disease or an amyloid nerve cell inclusion.

Familial types of myoclonus may persist in almost pure form or in association with mild ataxia over a period of many years. In the child and adult, herpes simplex encephalitis may present as a confusional state and dementia with myoclonus. In the elderly adult diffuse myoclonus is a prominent symptom in Jakob-Creutzfeld's disease. Intention myoclonus is often a sequela to anoxic encephalopathy. Postsomnolescent myoclonus jerks of arms for 20 to 30 min after a night's sleep is reported by some patients with idiopathic epilepsy. In all these diseases the pathologic changes are so widespread that anatomic localization is impossible. The least degrees of it are seemingly related to diseases of thalamus and cerebellum. Indeed cerebellar incoordination and intention tremor are combined with diffuse myoclonus of action or intention type in several of the aforementioned diseases i.e. lipidoses, and Lafora body type of myoclonus.

The term *myoclonus* unfortunately has also been assigned to a rather different motor phenomenon—that of repetitious, rhythmic clonus of some part of the "branchial cleft" or craniocervical musculature. An example is "nystagmus of the palate" (rhythmic contractions at the rate of 10 to 50 or more per min of soft palate, pharyngeal muscles, vocal cords, facial muscles, and diaphragm). The lesions producing this state, which we would prefer to designate as a form of continuous *bulbar, facial,* or *diaphragmatic clonus,* have been situated in all instances in the central tegmental tract, inferior olivary nucleus, or olivocerebellar tract. Vascular lesions, tumors, and encephalitic processes have all been causative.

The main fault with our concept of myoclonus is that it covers too many motor disorders. When movements are grouped according to their brevity or involuntary nature, one must include the normal dormescent start or jerk of a limb as one falls asleep, and the motor components of a natural startle reaction. The obligatory Moro response also falls within the group, as well as the form of epilepsy known as infantile, or salaam, spasms and the falling spells of the petit mal triad. Metrazol injections cause myoclonus of limbs, which has shown to depend on a lower brainstem (medullary reticular) mechanism.

Another problem arises on the clinical side in distinguishing diffuse myoclonus from other abrupt involuntary movements such as tremors, chorea, and restricted forms of epilepsy (epilepsia partialis continua). Speed of movement, lack of rhythmicity, and relationships to sensory stimulation prove to be the most reliable identifying features of the larger group of myoclonic disorders. There is an advantage in trying to separate the arrhythmic diffuse from the rhythmic restricted form in that each stands as a diagnostic attribute of a whole category of nervous diseases.

TREMOR. This consists of a more or less regular rhythmic oscillation of a part of the body around a fixed point, involving alternate contractions of agonist and antagonist muscles. The rate is usually 3 to 6 beats per sec, but faster frequencies do occur; in any one individual the rate is fairly constant in all affected parts, regardless of the size of the muscle or of the part of the body. Tremors usually involve the distal part of the limbs, the head, tongue, or jaw, and rarely the trunk.

There are many different types of tremor, and only a few are recognized as bearing any meaningful relationship to disease of the extrapyramidal motor system; but since tremors have not been discussed elsewhere, all the different types will be considered here.

Tremors can be classified in several ways. They may be subdivided according to their distribution, amplitude, regularity, and relationship to volitional movement. The following tremors should be familiar to every physician:

Static (Parkinsonian) Tremor. This is a coarse, rhythmic tremor, with an average rate of 4 to 5 beats per sec, most often localized in one or both hands, and occasionally, in the jaw or tongue. Its most characteristic feature is that it occurs when the limb is in an attitude of repose, and willed movement at least temporarily suppresses it. If the tremulous limb is completely relaxed, the tremor usually disappears, but the average patient rarely achieves this state. In some cases the tremor is constant; in others it varies from time to time and with the progress of the disease extends from one group of muscles to another. In paralysis agitans the tremor tends to be rather gentle and more or less limited to the distal muscles, whereas in postencephalitic parkinsonism and hepatolenticular degeneration it often has a wider range and involves proximal muscles. In many cases there is a variable degree of rigidity of plastic type. The tremor interferes with voluntary movements surprisingly little; it is not uncommon to see a patient who has been trembling violently raise a full glass of water to his lips and drain the contents without spilling a drop. The handwriting of these patients is often small and cramped (micrographia). The gait may be of a festinating type (see Chap. 23, Disturbances of Gait). It is the combination of static tremor, slowness of movement, rigidity, and flexed postures without true paralysis that constitutes Parkinson's syndrome (also called amyostatic syndrome).

The exact pathologic anatomy of static tremor is unknown. In paralysis agitans and postencephalitic Parkinson's syndrome, the visible lesions are predominantly in the substantia nigra. In hepatocerebral degeneration, where this syndrome is mixed with cerebellar ataxia, the lesions are more diffuse. A similar tremor, without rigidity, slowness of movement, flexed postures, or masked facies, is seen in senile individuals. Unlike Parkinson's disease, it does not progress.

Action Tremor. This term refers to a tremor present when the limbs are actively maintained in a certain position, as when outstretched, and throughout voluntary movement. It may increase slightly as the action of the limbs becomes more precise, but it never approaches the degree of augmentation in fine movement of intention tremor. It is easily made to disappear when the limbs are relaxed. Probably the *action tremor* is but an exaggeration of normal or physiologic tremor, which ranges from 6 to 8 per sec, being slower in childhood and old age. More particularly, in adults the tremor is of small excursion, has a frequency of 8 per sec, and is somewhat irregular. The tremor involves the outstretched hand, head, and less often, the lips and tongue, and it interferes little with voluntary movements such as handwriting and speech. This type of tremor is seen in numerous medical, neurologic, and psychiatric diseases and is therefore more difficult to interpret than static tremor. When occurring as the only neurologic abnormality in several members of a family, it is known as *familial* or *hereditary tremor*. Familial tremor may begin in childhood, but usually comes on later and persists throughout adult life. Being worse when the patient is under observation, it becomes a source of embarrassment because it suggests to the onlooker that the patient is nervous. A curious fact about familial tremors is that one or two drinks of an alcoholic beverage may abolish them, and they may become worse after the effects of the alcohol have worn off. Similar tremors are seen in delirious states, such as delirium tremens, in the chronic alcoholic patient as an isolated symptom ("the morning shakes"), and in general paretics. An action tremor, usually more rapid than the above, is also characteristic of hyperthyroidism and other toxic states, and a similar tremor is frequently observed in patients suffering intense anxiety. In fact it can be reproduced by injections of epinephrine. Severe action tremor may also accompany certain diseases of the basal ganglia, including parkinsonism.

Intention Tremor. The word *intention* is ambiguous in this context because the tremor itself is not intentional. The term means, instead, that the tremor requires for its full expression the performance of an exacting, precise, willed movement. The term *ataxic tremor* has been suggested because it is always combined with cerebellar ataxia. The tremor is absent when the limbs are inactive and during the first part of a voluntary movement, but as the action continues and greater precision of movement is demanded (e.g., in touching a target such as the patient's nose or the examiner's finger), a jerky, more or less rhythmic interruption of forward progression, with side-to-side oscillation, appears. It continues for a fraction of a second or so after the act is completed. The tremor may seriously interfere with the patient's performance of skilled acts. Sometimes the head is involved (titubation). This type of tremor invariably indicates disease of the cerebellum and of its connections. When the disease is very severe, every movement, even the lifting of a limb, results in a wide-ranging tremor of such violence as to throw the patient off balance. This latter state is occasionally seen in multiple sclerosis, Wilson's disease, and vascular lesions of midbrain and subthalamus.

Hysterical Tremor. Hysterical tremors may simulate any of the aforementioned varieties and are difficult to diagnose. One notable feature is that they usually do not correspond to any of the better known types of organic tremor. Most often they are restricted to a limb and are seldom as regular as the static tremors of paralysis agitans. If the affected limb is restrained by the examiner, the tremor may move to another part of the body. It persists during movement and at rest and is less subject to the modifying influences of posture and willed movement than are organic tremors. This manifestation of hysteria is exceedingly rare.

OTHER INVOLUNTARY MOVEMENTS. There are other abnormalities of movement, about which only a few words can be said. They vary from simple irritative phenomena to complex psychologically related phenomena, such as compulsions.

Spasmodic Torticollis. This is an intermittent or continuous spasm of sternomastoid, trapezius, and other neck muscles, usually more pronounced on one side, with turning or tipping of the head. It is involuntary and cannot be inhibited and thereby differs from habit spasm or tic. This condition should be considered a form of dystonia. It is worse when the patient sits, stands, or walks, and usually contactual stimulation of the chin or of the back of the head partially alleviates the muscle imbalance. Psychiatric treatment is ineffectual. In severe cases muscle sectioning, neurectomy, section of the anterior cervical roots, or cryothalamotomy have given favorable results.

Other Craniocervical Spasms. Blepharaclonus (inability to keep open the eyes), lingual spasms, "spastic" dysphonia, facial spasms, and cervicothoracic spasms are all special varieties of involuntary movement, appearing usually in late middle life and the senium. Facial, cervical, and thoracic spasms have occurred with striking frequency during phenothiazid medication. Transiency, or nonprogressivity, unresponsiveness to psychotherapy, and uncertain amelioration by all pharmacologic agents characterize most of them. Exceptionally, these drug-induced dyskinesias, as they are called (actually athetosis), persist for months or years after the medication is discontinued.

Tics and Habit Spasms. Many individuals throughout life are prone to habitual movements, such as sniffing, clearing the throat, protruding the chin, or blinking, whenever they become tense. The patient admits that the movements are voluntary and that he feels compelled to make them in order to relieve tension; they can be inhibited for a time by an effort of will but reappear when attention is diverted. In certain cases they become so ingrained that the person is unaware of them and unable to control them. Children between five and ten years of age are especially liable to habit spasms. The movements are often purposive coordinated acts which normally serve the organism; it is only their incessant repetition when uncalled for that constitutes a habit. Stereotypy is their main identifying feature. Multiple convulsive tics (*Gilles de la Tourette's disease*) is a more severe form of the same condition. In children it is best to ignore the habit spasm and at the same time to arrange for more rest and a calmer environment. In adults relief of nervous tension by tranquilizing drugs and psychotherapy is helpful, but the disposition to tic formation persists.

Writer's cramp and other so-called "occupational spasms" should be mentioned here if only to indicate their unclassifiable status. Usually a middle-aged man or woman begins to observe upon attempting to write that all the muscles of thumb and fingers either go into a spasm or are in some way inhibited. Usually it is the spasm that interferes, and it may be painful and spread into the forearm or even the shoulder. Sometimes the spasm fragments into a tremor which interferes with the execution of fluid, cursive movements. Although limited to writing, exceptionally it may involve other equally demanding motor acts. At all other times and in the execution of grosser movements the hand is normal. Psychogenesis has been claimed, but careful clinical analysis will disprove it. Many patients learn to write in new ways or to use the other hand though that, too, may be involved. Hypnosis is usually without effect. Liversedge has stated that about half of the patients can be helped by a deconditioning procedure that delivers an electric shock whenever the spasm occurs. His results have not been verified by others. Aside from the spasm there is no other neurologic abnormality.

EXTRAPYRAMIDAL MOTOR DISTURBANCES DUE PRIMARILY TO DISEASES OF THE CEREBELLUM

Isolated lesions in the midline flocculonodular lobe result in grave disturbances of equilibrium. Often the symptoms are exhibited only when the patient attempts to stand and walk. He sways, staggers, titubates, and reels (see under Cerebellar Gait, Chap. 23). There may be no disturbance in coordination and no intention tremor of the limbs. A midline tumor of the cerebellum, such as medulloblastoma, usually produces this syndrome.

Extensive lesions of one cerebellar hemisphere, especially the anterior lobe, cause disturbances of coordination in volitional movements of the ipsilateral arm and leg. This is known as *ataxia*. The movements are characterized by an inappropriate range, rate, and strength of each of the various components of the motor act and by an improper sequence of those components. Electromyographic analysis has shown that ataxia is manifested as a decomposition of movement consisting of abnormal duration and sequences of bursts of contraction and relaxation of agonists and antagonists of a joint, usually a large joint (Carrera and Mettler). This incoordination is also called *asynergia*. The defects are particularly noticeable in acts that require rapid alternation of movements. Slowness in acceleration and deceleration, which is almost invariably present, impedes the performance (dysdiadochokinesis). The direction of purposive movement is frequently inaccurate. Owing to delay in arresting a movement, the patient may overshoot his mark. The antagonist muscles do not come into play at the proper time, possibly because of the hypotonia that is almost always present. This may be demonstrated by having the patient flex his arm against a resistance that is suddenly released. The patient with cerebellar disease will sometimes strike his face because he fails to check the flexion movement (Holmes rebound phenomenon). In movements requiring accurate direction, as the limb approaches its destination it may stop short and then advance by a more or less rhythmic series of jerks and oscillations (intention tremor). In addition to hypotonia, there may be, in acute cerebellar lesions, some slight weakness. Bilateral lesions of the cerebellar hemispheres and midline flocculonodular lobe lead to such a severe disturbance in all movements that the patient may be unable to stand or walk or use his limbs effectively. In addition, there are ocular and speech disturbances, namely, nystagmus, skew deviation of the eyes, and dysarthria. Lesions of the cerebellar peduncles have the same effect as extensive hemispheral lesions. This syndrome due to involvement of one cerebellar hemisphere may be observed in a tumor or abscess or in vascular lesions of the brainstem and cerebellar peduncles. The ataxia tends to be bilateral and symmetric in primary atrophy or degeneration of the cerebellum.

SOME GENERAL FEATURES OF ALL EXTRAPYRAMIDAL MOTOR DISTURBANCES

From the above discussion of many special types of motor disorder the reader must not think that they always appear in pure form. Various combinations occur in diseases. For example, Wilson's disease usually presents with a Parkinson-like picture of tremor, rigidity, slowness of movement, and flexion dystonia of trunk, but exceptionally there is athetosis, tonic innervation, phasic dystonia, and action myoclonus. Hallevorden-Spatz disease may take the form of universal rigidity and flexion dystonia or choreoathetosis. Occasionally the degeneration of Huntington's chorea leads to rigidity rather than choreoathetosis. Pyramidal and various of these extrapyramidal disorders may be associated in patients with cerebral diplegia. Nonetheless certain combinations tend to occur with greater or lesser frequency in certain diseases, as will be pointed out in Chaps. 361, 363, and 364. The benign restricted or localized spasms and twitches are the most obscure disorders with reference to both their pathologic anatomy or physiology.

In broad terms all the extrapyramidal disorders should be viewed in terms of the primary deficit (negative symptom) and the new phenomena (movements, abnormal postures, tremors, etc.) which have appeared. These latter (positive symptoms) are presently ascribed to release from or disequilibrium of the undamaged parts of the nervous system. The clearest negative effect is usually evidenced as an akinesia or disinclination to use the affected muscles. The difficulty in rapid sequences of movement stands as another negative effect both in diseases of basal ganglia and cerebellum. In fact this latter symptom, presenting as a clumsiness, may be the only fault manifest in certain maladroit children. Stress and nervous tension characteristically worsens both the motor deficiency and the abnormal movements in all of these extrapyramidal syndromes, just as relaxation helps the motor performance. All the movement disorders are abolished in sleep.

One of the most remarkable discoveries of recent years, to be credited largely to the pioneering efforts of neurosurgeons (Meyer, Cooper) has been the abolition of tremors, rigidity, and involuntary movements of the limbs by a surgical lesion in the medial segment of the globus pallidus or the ventrolateral nucleus of the thalamus. The effects are contralateral. Usually the lesion has been made by the injection first of procaine (Novocain) and then either alcohol, cooling and freezing (Cooper), or electrocoagulation (White and Sweet and Leksell). The operation has been successful in temporarily alleviating tremor or rigidity (or both) on one side. The procedure is successful in approximately 80 percent of cases of paralysis agitans, and the postural abnormality in dystonia musculorum deformans and double athetosis has responded somewhat less consistently. The operations have been perfected to the point where the mortality rate is less than 1 percent, and the risk of hemiplegia or some other sequel is less than 10 percent. Of course, as the disease progresses, the beneficial effects are lost. The therapeutic procedure indicates that the pallidum and ventrolateral nucleus, probably through their connections with the cerebral cortex (motor cortex and its pyramidal pathway), are essential for the expression of these extrapyramidal syndromes. The indications for these surgical procedures are discussed in Chap. 364.

EXAMINATION AND DIFFERENTIAL DIAGNOSIS

In Chap. 21 the methods of examining the motor system were described at some length, so only a few additional remarks concerning extrapyramidal disorders need be made here. These abnormalities are best demonstrated by seeing the patient in action. If he complains of a limp after walking a distance or of difficulty in climbing stairs, he should be observed under these conditions. Tests of rate, regularity, and coordination of voluntary movement must be sufficiently varied and demanding of the patient's motor coordination to bring out the defect. The physician must cultivate the habit of accurately observing and describing abnormalities of movement and must not be content merely to give the condition a name or to force it into some category such as chorea or tic or myoclonus. The main postures of the body in all common acts should be noted. Aside from the assessment of muscle power and of gait, the usual test applied to the upper limb is to ask the patient to touch the examiner's fingertip and then the tip of his own nose repeatedly (*finger-to-nose test*). In testing the leg the patient is asked to place his heel on one knee and then to run it down his shin and back to the knee (*heel-to-knee-to-shin test*). Finer movements of the hand may be tested by having the patient successively touch each finger to his thumb or pat his thigh rapidly or by having him use tools or handle objects. The performance of rapidly alternating movements such as pronation and supination or opening and closing the hands are valuable tests.

The fully developed extrapyramidal motor syndromes can be recognized without difficulty once the physician has become familiar with the typical pictures. The mental picture of Parkinson's syndrome, with its slowness of movement, poverty of facial expression, and static tremor and rigidity, should be fixed in mind. Similarly, the gross distortions and postural abnormalities of dystonia, whether widespread in trunk muscles or involving only neck muscles, as in spasmodic torticollis, once seen should thereafter be familiar. Athetosis, with its instability of postures and ceaseless movements of fingers and hands; intention spasm; chorea, with its more rapid and complicated movements; and the abrupt movements of myoclonus that flit over the body are other standard syndromes. Characteristic of all is the presence of a mild defect in the voluntary use of the affected parts.

The clinical differences between pyramidal and extrapyramidal disorders are summarized in Table 22-2.

Table 22-2. CLINICAL DIFFERENCES BETWEEN PYRAMIDAL AND EXTRAPYRAMIDAL SYNDROMES

	Pyramidal	Extrapyramidal
Character of rigidity	Clasp-knife effect	Plastic, equal throughout passive movement or intermittent (cogwheel rigidity)
Distribution of rigidity	Flexors of arms, extensors of legs	Flexors of all four limbs and trunk
Shortening and lengthening reaction	Present	Absent
Involuntary movements	Absent	Presence of tremors, chorea, athetosis, dystonia
Tendon reflexes	Increased	Normal or slightly increased
Babinski's sign	Present	Absent
Paralysis of voluntary movement	Present	Absent or slight

Early or mild forms of these conditions, like all medical diseases, may offer special difficulties in diagnosis. Cases of paralysis agitans, seen before the appearance of tremor, are often overlooked. The patient may complain of being nervous and restless or may have experienced an indescribable stiffness and aching in certain parts of the body.

Because of the absence of weakness or of reflex changes, the case may be considered psychogenic or rheumatic. It is well to remember that Parkinson's syndrome often begins in a hemiplegic distribution, and for this reason the illness may be misdiagnosed as cerebral thrombosis. A slight masking of the face, a suggestion of a limp, blepharoclonus (uninhibited blinking of eyes when the bridge of the nose is tapped), a mild rigidity, failure of an arm to swing naturally in walking, or loss of certain movements of cooperation will help in diagnosis at this time. Every case presenting the syndrome of Parkinson or other abnormality of movement and posture in adolescence or early adult life should be surveyed for hepatolenticular degeneration by tests of liver function and split-lamp examination for corneal pigmentation (Kayser-Fleischer ring); if facilities are available, urinary aminonitrogen excretion and copper excretion should be determined.

Mild or early chorea is often mistaken for simple nervousness. If one sits for a time and watches the patient, the diagnosis will often become evident. There are cases, nonetheless, in which it is impossible to distinguish simple nervousness from early Sydenham's chorea, especially in children, and there is no laboratory test upon which one can depend. The first postural manifestation of dystonia may suggest hysteria, and it is only later, when the fixity of the postural abnormality, the lack of the usual psychologic picture of hysteria, and the relentlessly progressive character of the illness become evident, that accurate diagnosis is reached. Another common error is to assume that a bedfast patient who has complained of dizziness, staggering, and headaches and exhibits no other neurologic abnormality is suffering from hysteria. The flocculonodular cerebellar syndrome is demonstrable only when the patient attempts to stand and walk.

REFERENCES

Carrera, R. M. E., and F. A. Mettler: Function of the Primate Brachium Conjunctivum and Related Structures, J. Comp. Neurol., 102:151, 1955.

Denny-Brown, D.: Diseases of the Basal Ganglia and Subthalamic Nuclei," Fair Lawn, N.J., Oxford University Press, 1945.

Martin, J. Purdon, and Ian R. McCaul: Acute Hemiballismus Treated by Ventrolateral Thalamolysis, Brain, 82:104, 1959.

23 VERTIGO AND DISORDERS OF EQUILIBRIUM AND GAIT

Maurice Victor and
Raymond D. Adams

The terms to describe sensations of unbalance are often rather ambiguous, and the patient must be carefully questioned. He often uses *dizziness* to indicate not only a sense of rotation but also vague sensory experiences such as unsteadiness, insecurity, weakness, faintness, and light-headedness. Blurring of vision and even petit mal epilepsy may be referred to as dizzy spells. *Giddiness* has almost the same significance, with perhaps more implication of altered consciousness and swaying sensation. *Vertigo* literally means "sense of turning" either of one's body or of the surroundings, a definition which, with a few important qualifications to be mentioned below, is used throughout this chapter. *Equilibrium* refers simply to a state of balance or equipoise in which opposing forces, such as gravity and postural reflexes, exactly counteract each other.

Disorders of equilibrium are suitably considered in connection with dizziness and vertigo because of their frequent conjunction (vertiginous ataxia). Other disorders of equilibrium quite independent of vertigo, e.g., those due to a loss of joint and muscle sense (sensory ataxia) or cerebellar disease (cerebellar ataxia) are also considered briefy in this chapter.

ANATOMIC, PHYSIOLOGIC, AND PSYCHOLOGIC CONSIDERATIONS

Several mechanisms are responsible for the maintenance of a balanced posture and make us aware of the body's position in relation to its surroundings—afferent impulses from the eyes, labyrinths, muscles, and joints relay information about the position of the body in space. In response to these impulses the organism is capable of making fine and rapid postural adjustments to maintain equilibrium, most of which do not demand volitional control. The most important of the afferent impulses are the following:

1. Impulses from the retina and possibly proprioceptive impulses from the ocular muscles, which activate reflexes that influence the position of head and neck.

2. Impulses from the labyrinths, which are highly specialized spatial proprioceptors, whose primary function is to register changes in direction of motion (either acceleration or deceleration) and in the position of the body. The semicircular canals respond to movement and angular momentum, and the otoliths—the sense organs of the utricle and saccule—are mainly concerned with orienting the organism in reference to gravity.

3. Impulses from the proprioceptors of the joints and muscles, which regulate reflex, postural, and voluntary movement. Those from the neck are of special importance in relating the position of the head to the rest of the body.

The cerebellum, the vestibular nuclei, the red nuclei, and other brainstem ganglionic centers are the most important central structures concerned with regulating posture.

Important psychologic phenomena are also involved in the maintenance of equilibrium, namely, those which deal with the relationship between ourselves and the external world. We learn to perceive that portion of space occupied by our body and construct from sensory data a set of integrated sensory experiences called by some neurologists, *the body schema*. The space around our body,

i.e., the external world, is then said to be represented by another schema. Those two schemata are neither static nor independent: they are constantly being modified and adapted to one another; their interdependence is ascribed to the fact that the various sense organs which supply the information on which the two schemata are based are usually simultaneously activated by any movement of our bodies. By a process of learning we see objects as having motion or being still, when we are either moving or stationary. Motion of an object in space is always relative. At times, especially when our own sensory experience is incomplete, we mistake movement of our surroundings for movements of our own body as, for example, the illusion of movement which is experienced in a stationary train when a neighboring train is moving. Hence, in this frame of reference, orientation of the body in space is possible only by the maintenance of an orderly relationship between the body schema and the schema of the external world. As a corollary, disorientation in space or disequilibrium occurs when this relationship is upset.

On clinical grounds, disorders of equilibrium may be divided into three groups: (1) true vertigo; (2) pseudovertigo, or giddiness; and (3) abnormalities of equilibrium without either vertigo or giddiness.

VERTIGO

CHARACTERISTICS. In disorders in which vertigo is a leading symptom, the patient's history assumes special importance in diagnosis, for this symptom may be accompanied by no objective signs. The diagnosis of vertigo is an easy matter when the patient reports that objects in his environment spun around, or his body was turning, or his head was spinning. Very often, however, he is not so explicit. He may state that there was a feeling of to-and-fro or up-and-down movement of the body, usually the head; or he may relate that the floor or walls seemed to undulate or sank or rose up toward him or that he was pulled strongly to one side or to the ground, as though drawn by a strong magnet. This feeling of impulsion is particularly characteristic of vertigo. With milder degrees of vertigo, the patient may have difficulty in describing his symptoms. It may help to ask him whether his present symptoms are similar to the feeling of movement one experiences when coming to a halt after being rapidly rotated. Or, it may be necessary to induce vertigo by rotating the patient rapidly in one direction and have him compare it to his symptoms.

The symptoms of vertigo are usually paroxysmal and of short duration, but at times they may linger for weeks or even months. The chronic state may or may not follow an acute attack; in this latter instance the patient complains of a continuous state of imbalance, of swaying, or a vague sense of movement in the environment.

All but the mildest forms of vertigo are accompanied by varying degrees of nausea and vomiting, nystagmus, headache, and ataxia, as well as by the need to avoid movement of the head. When the attack is at its height, the slightest movement of the head may aggravate the sense of whirling or rotation and of nausea; after the acute symptoms have subsided, vertigo may be evoked only by movement of the head. One form of paroxysmal vertigo (the positional vertigo of Barany) depends entirely on changes in position of the head (see Chap. 355, Diseases of Cranial Nerves).

Stance and gait are almost invariably affected during an attack of vertigo. In exceptionally severe attacks the patient may without warning be thrown to the ground and only then experience vertigo, nausea, and vomiting. Some patients may be so ataxic that they are unable to sit or to stand. In less severe cases the patient may feel unsteady in walking, tending to veer to one side. This type of gait disturbance, which depends on an abnormality of labyrinthine or vestibular function, may be called *vertiginous ataxia*. It is noteworthy that in these circumstances the coordination of individual movements of the limbs is not impaired—a point of difference from most instances of cerebellar disease.

Headache is often associated with vertigo. Loss of consciousness as part of a vertiginous attack rarely occurs and usually signifies another category of disorder, such as syncope or seizure.

DISTINCTION BETWEEN TRUE AND FALSE VERTIGO. It is important to distinguish clearly between true vertigo and a second group of symptoms which do not have the same significance, i.e., *pseudovertigo*. The latter symptoms may be described as a feeling of uncertainty, lightheadedness, or a swimming sensation; or the patient may feel as though he is going to fall or is walking on air. These sensory phenomena are particularly common in psychoneurotic states and in introspective individuals with an overawareness of various body parts. Other peculiar aberrations, for example, a feeling of lengthening of the legs or a sensation as if the ground were receding, may be remarked upon. A feeling of light-headedness is frequently brought about by hyperventilation, and similar symptoms occur in patients with anemia, hypertension, and pulmonary disease, particularly emphysema. In anemia, mild hypoxia is the probable mechanism, and ischemia is probably the cause in emphysematous patients, in whom an attack of coughing may lead to dizziness or even fainting, owing to impaired venous return to the heart (tussive syncope). The dizziness that so often accompanies hypertension is more difficult to evaluate. In some cases it may be due to associated nervousness; in others, it may depend upon transient changes in the intracranial vasculature. *Postural* dizziness is a closely related complaint. Individuals in poor physical condition and many elderly persons, especially if they have cerebrovascular disease, are troubled upon arising from a recumbent or sitting position or after stopping by a momentary giddiness or a swaying type of dizziness with dimming of vision or spots before the eyes. These symptoms last only for several seconds or a minute, during which time the patient may find it necessary to stand still or to steady himself by holding on to a nearby object. There need be no fall in brachial blood pressure at the time of symptom production. The condition may be due to a momentary failure of reflex vasoconstriction in over-

coming the "pooling" effect of gravity upon the circulating blood. This type of dizziness may occur in normal individuals on arising and is more pronounced after a hot bath; it is a frequent complaint in patients convalescing from debilitating illness. A mild syncopal reaction of any type may give rise to similar symptoms and may be described by the patient as "dizziness."

In practice it is not difficult to separate these symptoms from true vertigo; there is not the feeling of rotation nor of impulsion so characteristic of the latter. In addition, the ancillary symptoms of true vertigo, including varying degrees of nausea, vomiting, headache, ataxia, and the need to keep the head immobile, do not occur.

NEUROLOGIC SIGNIFICANCE. A disorder of any of the following structures may give rise to vertigo.

1. Cerebral cortex
2. Ocular muscles
3. Cerebellum
4. Labyrinthine-vestibular apparatus
5. Brainstem

Vertigo may constitute the aura of an epileptic seizure, indicating a cerebrocortical origin. This usually occurs with lesions of the temporal lobe, mainly on the lateral aspect of the middle and posterior portions or at the parietotemporal junction. The patients experience a sensation of movement, either of their body away from the side of stimulation or of the environment in the opposite direction. This type of vertigo lasts for only a few moments before being submerged in the seizure activity. Vertiginous seizures may occur very rarely as a reflex phenomenon, the result of vestibular (e.g., caloric) stimulation.

Ocular disturbances may give rise to vertigo and may even be accompanied by unsteadiness; this occurs most frequently at the outset of an ocular muscle paralysis when the patient looks in the direction of action of the paralyzed muscle. The vertigo is apparently due to a faulty projection of the visual field, the patient being presented with two conflicting images. Some people experience a type of giddiness or uncertainty when wearing bifocal lenses for the first time. The necessity of adapting to an unusual visual environment, as in looking down from a height, may result in a similar sensation. These types of vertigo are usually mild and transient and of relatively little clinical significance.

Whether *lesions of the cerebellum* can produce vertigo seems to depend on what portion of this structure is involved. Thus vertigo may be absent despite large lesions of the cerebellar hemispheres but present if the vestibulocerebellar connections are damaged.

For all practical purposes the problem of vertigo resolves itself into deciding whether this symptom has its origin in the labyrinth, in the vestibular division of the eighth cranial nerve, or in the vestibular nuclei and their immediate connections with other structures in the brainstem. A number of features, especially the form of the attack and the associated symptoms, help to make this decision.

Vertigo of labyrinthine origin (aural vertigo) tends to occur in paroxysmal attacks. It has an abrupt onset, is maximal at the beginning, and subsides in a matter of minutes or in an hour or two. Similarly, the nausea, vomiting, pallor, immobility, and ataxia associated with the attack are short-lived. The accompanying nystagmus tends also to be transient and characteristically is rather fine, rotatory, and most pronounced when the eyes are turned away from the offending labyrinth. Occasionally, vertigo of labyrinthine origin may take a more chronic form. However, it seldom continues for more than a few days or weeks, the central mechanisms apparently compensating for the peripheral lesion. Labyrinthine vertigo is frequently associated with deafness and tinnitus, since the pathologic process in the inner ear encroaches on the cochlear apparatus. Labyrinthine vertigo may accompany an ear infection (labyrinthitis) or occur as a cardinal symptom of Ménière's disease, vestibular neuronitis, or Barany's positional vertigo.

Vertigo of acoustic nerve origin, associated as a rule with an acoustic neuroma, is usually mild and intermittent (lasting weeks or months) but it has all the main elements of true vertigo (sense of turning, impulsion, preferred posture, etc.). It may be the initial symptom but more often occurs an interval of time (months or years) after the associated impairment of hearing. Once established, coarse horizontal nystagmus to the side of the tumor and finer nystagmus to the opposite side are demonstrable. Impaired caloric responses and high frequency deafness (without recruitment) confirm the eighth nerve affection. Involvement of adjacent cranial nerves (VII, V, X) and cerebellum (ipsilateral ataxia), the late signs of a cerebellopontine angle mass, facilitates diagnosis.

Vertigo of brainstem origin usually lasts longer than aural vertigo and may disorganize the patient's equilibrium for several weeks or even longer. In these cases, auditory function is usually spared, since vestibular and cochlear fibers become separated soon after entering the brainstem. It is a fairly reliable clinical rule that the combination of auditory and vestibular symptoms occurs only in diseases that involve the inner ear or eighth cranial nerve. Nystagmus which accompanies central lesions tends to be coarse and protracted, is more marked on lateral gaze to one side than the other, and may have a vertical component, particularly on upward gaze. Vertical nystagmus nearly always indicates disease of the brainstem. A demyelinative lesion may affect vestibular connections, and this diagnosis should always be considered when a young person has a severe and protracted attack of vertigo without auditory symptoms. Vascular and neoplastic lesions may also give rise to vertigo through involvement of the vestibular nuclei and their immediate connections. In addition, there may be signs of interference with other segmental mechanisms of the lower brainstem or the long sensory and motor tracts that pass through it. These features clearly exclude a labyrinthine or vestibular nerve localization.

Diagnosis

When the patient's complaint is dizziness, it is first necessary to obtain a clear description of the symptoms.

The element of rotation or a similar sensation, the sense of impulsion, and the accompanying nausea and vomiting, nystagmus, headache, and ataxia usually distinguish the case of true vertigo from one of giddiness. The latter has no element of rotation or impulsion, and the ancillary manifestations are absent. Although fearful of falling or swooning, the patient can nonetheless walk without difficulty if forced to do so. Smothering and choking feelings, palpitation, trembling, sweating, and a sense of fear or apprehension complete the usual clinical picture of neurotic dizziness. Frequently in cases of recurrent aural vertigo, i.e., *Ménière's syndrome*, symptoms of anxiety and depression may be added to the total clinical picture, which adds to the difficulty of interpretation (see Chap. 355).

If the physician is uncertain whether the patient has true vertigo, it is sometimes helpful to induce these sensations in order that the patient may compare them with his usual attacks. This can be done by having the patient breathe deeply for 3 minutes (which causes giddiness in most persons), stoop over for a minute and then straighten up (postural giddiness), and while standing, turn rapidly in one direction 10 times in order to provoke vertigo. If the patient fails to distinguish these sensations, his history is probably inaccurate and he should be asked to take careful note of his sensations during his next spontaneous attack.

In some cases the attack may be so abrupt and severe that the patient falls immediately to the ground without loss of consciousness. Here the diagnosis of vertigo may be clarified by nausea, vomiting, and dizziness, which almost invariably follow such a fall. If the vertigo has been very mild in degree, it is helpful to elicit a history of disinclination to walk during the attack, a tendency to list to one side, discomfort in sitting or riding in a vehicle, and a preference for maintaining one position fixedly.

A neurologic examination, including tests of ocular movements and nystagmus, cranial nerve function, gait, and coordination of limbs, should be carried out on all patients with dizziness as the presenting complaint. The eardrums should be inspected and hearing tested by the methods indicated in Chap. 24. Vestibular function should also be tested. This is commonly done by irrigating the ear with 5 ml ice water for a period of 30 sec, the head being tilted forward 30° from the body axis, since in this position the horizontal canal is brought into a vertical position. The normal labyrinthine responses consist of falling to the side of the vestibular lesion, past-pointing to that side, and rotary nystagmus on gaze to the opposite side. The nystagmus begins about 20 sec after the irrigation and persists for 90 to 120 sec. The duration of these periods is variable, however, and comparison of the affected and normal labyrinths is more important.

Attempts to reproduce the dizziness should include observation of the patient when his body position is suddenly changed from sitting to recumbency with the neck hyperextended and the head turned first to the right and on the next trial to the left. In Barany's positional vertigo, within 5 to 10 sec after becoming recumbent with the offending ear down, the eyes are seen to jerk in a coarse horizontal nystagmus and the patient feels dizzy. This lasts 10 to 15 sec and the direction of the dizziness is reversed upon returning to a sitting position.

DISTURBANCES OF EQUILIBRIUM (GAIT)

Probably no aspect of equilibrium is more interesting or affords greater opportunity for diagnosis than the analysis of the patient's gait.

The normal gait seldom attracts attention. The body is erect, the head straight, and the arms hang loosely and gracefully at the sides, each moving rhythmically forward with the opposite leg. The feet are slightly everted, and the steps are of moderate length and approximately equal, the internal malleoli of the tibias almost touching one another. With each step there is coordinated flexion of hip and knee and dorsiflexion of foot and a barely perceptible elevation of the hip so that the foot clears the ground. The heel strikes the ground first, and inspection of shoes will show that this part is most subject to wear. In the erect posture, the muscles of greatest importance in maintaining equilibrium are the erector spinae and the extensors of the hips and knees.

When analyzed in greater detail, the requirements for locomotion in an upright, bipedal position can be reduced to the following elements: (1) antigravity support of the body; (2) stepping; (3) an adequate degree of equilibrium; and (4) a means of propulsion. The support of the body is provided by the antigravity reflexes which maintain firm extension of knees, hips, and back muscles, but modifiable by position of head and neck. These reflexes depend on the integrity of the spinal cord and lower parts of the brainstem (pontine transection leads to exaggeration of these antigravity reflexes—decerebrate rigidity). Stepping, the second element, is a basic movement pattern, present at birth, and integrated at the midbrain level. Its appropriate stimulus is contact of the sole with a flat surface and inclination of the body forward and alternately from side-to-side. Equilibrium involves the preservation of balance at right angles to the direction of movement. The center of gravity during the continuously unstable equilibrium which prevails in walking must shift from side to side within narrow limits as the weight is borne first on one foot then the other. Propulsion is provided by leaning forward and slightly to one side and permitting the body to fall a certain distance before being checked by the support of the leg. Here both forward and alternating lateral movements must occur. But in running, where at one moment both feet are off the ground, a forward drive or thrust by the hind leg is also needed. Locomotion may fail in the course of neurologic diseases when one or more of these mechanical principles is prevented from operating, as we shall see.

There are many individual variations of gait, and it is a commonplace observation that the sound of an individual's footsteps, notably his pace and heaviness of tread, may identify him. The manner of walking and the carriage of the body may even provide clues to character, personality, and occupation. Furthermore, the gaits of men and women differ, the steps of women being quicker and shorter and the movement of their trunk and hips more graceful and delicate. Certain female characteristics of gait, if observed in the male, immediately impart an impression of femininity; or male characteristics in the female, one of masculinity.

Since normal body posture and locomotion require visual information (we see where we are going and pick our steps), labyrinthine function, and proprioception, it is of interest to note the effect of deficits in these senses on normal function. A blind man or a normal one who is blindfolded may walk very well. He moves cautiously, to avoid collision with objects, and on smooth pavement shortens his step slightly; with the shortening there is less rocking of the body and he seems unnaturally stiff. A man without labyrinthine function (as happens after prolonged streptomycin therapy) shows a slight unsteadiness in walking and he cannot descend stairs without holding onto a banister. Running is also difficult. Characteristically, he has great difficulty in focusing on a stationary object when he is moving, so that he cannot drive a car. Proof that he is dependent on visual cues comes from his performance blindfolded where he is seen to be unsteady and to stagger to some extent, but usually he does not fall. A loss of proprioception, as in a complete lesion in the posterior columns of the spinal cord in the high cervical region, abolishes for a long time the capacity for independent locomotion. After years of training the patient will still have difficulty in starting to walk and in propelling himself forward. As Purdon Martin has illustrated, he holds his hands in front of his body, bends body and head forward, walks with a wide base with irregular uneven steps but does rock his body. If he loses his balance, he shows no reactions to protect his equilibrium. If he falls, he cannot arise without help, and he cannot get up from a chair. He is unable to crawl or to get into an "all-fours" posture. When standing, if blindfolded, he immediately falls. Thus the postural reactions are demonstrably more dependent on proprioceptive than on visual or labyrinthine information.

When confronted with a disorder of gait, the examiner must observe the patient's natural stance and the attitude and dominant positions of the legs, trunk, and arms. It is good practice to watch the patient as he walks into the examining room, because he is apt to walk more naturally then than during special tests. He should be asked to stand with his feet together, head erect, with eyes first open and then closed. Swaying due to nervousness may be overcome by asking that he touch the tip of his nose with the finger of first one hand and then the other. Next the patient should be asked to walk forward and backward, with his eyes first open and then closed. Any tendency to reel to one side, as in cerebellar disease, can be checked by having him walk around a chair. When the affected side is toward the chair, the patient tends to walk into it; and when it is away from the chair, he veers outward in ever-widening circles. More delicate tests of gait are walking a straight line heel to toe or having the patient arise quickly from a chair and walk briskly and then stop or turn suddenly. If all these tests are successfully executed, it may be assumed that any difficulty in locomotion is not due to disease of the proprioceptive mechanisms or cerebellum. Detailed neurologic examination is then necessary in order to determine which of the many other possible diseases is responsible for the patient's disorder of gait.

The following abnormal gaits are so distinctive that with a little practice they can be recognized at a glance.

CEREBELLAR GAIT. The main features of this gait are *wide base* (separation of legs), *unsteadiness, irregularity,* and *lateral reeling*. Steps are uncertain, some are shorter and others longer than intended, and the patient may lurch to one side or the other. The unsteadiness is more prominent on quickly arising from a chair and walking, on stopping suddenly while walking, or on turning abruptly. If the ataxia is severe, the patient cannot stand without assistance. If lesser in degree, standing with feet together and head erect, with eyes either opened or closed, may be difficult. In its mildest form the ataxia is best demonstrated by having the patient walk a line heel to toe. After two or three steps he loses his balance and must step to one side to avoid falling. Romberg's sign, i.e., marked swaying or falling with the eyes closed but not with the eyes open, is not a feature of cerebellar disease. Compensation may be effected by shortening the step and shuffling, i.e., keeping both feet simultaneously on the ground. The defect in the cerebellar gait is not in antigravity support, steppage, or propulsion but in the coordination of proprioceptive, labyrinthine, and visual information in reflex coordination of movements. The abnormality of gait may or may not be accompanied by other signs of cerebellar incoordination and intention tremor of the arms and legs. The presence of the latter signs depends on involvement of the cerebellar hemispheres as distinct from anterior and midline structures; if the lesion is unilateral, they are always on the same side.

Cerebellar gait is most commonly seen in multiple sclerosis, cerebellar hemorrhage, medulloblastoma of the cerebellar vermis, and the cerebellar degenerations. In certain forms of cerebellar degeneration (e.g., the type associated with chronic alcoholism) the disease process reaches a plateau and then remains stable for many years, and the gait disorder, in these circumstances, becomes altered to some extent. The base is wide and the steps are still short, but more regular; the trunk is inclined slightly forward, the arms are held away from the sides, and the gait assumes a somewhat rhythmic quality. In this way the patient can walk for long distances, but he lacks the capacity to make the necessary postural adjustments in response to sudden changes in his position. In this respect, among others, cerebellar ataxia differs from that due to drunkenness (see below).

GAIT OF SENSORY ATAXIA. This gait is due to an impairment of proprioception resulting from interruption of afferent nerve fibers in the peripheral nerves, posterior roots, posterior columns of the spinal cords, or medial lemnisci; it may also be produced occasionally by a lesion of both parietal lobes. Whatever the location of the lesion, the patient is deprived of knowledge of the position of his limbs. The principal features of the resulting

gait disorder are the *uncertainty*, the *irregularity*, and the *stamp* of the feet. Hunt characterized this type of gait very well when he said that the ataxic patient is recognized by "his stamp and stick." When the ataxia is of moderate severity, there is great difficulty in standing and walking, and in advanced cases there is a complete failure of locomotion, although muscular power is retained. The legs are kept far apart to correct the instability, and the patient carefully watches the ground and his legs. As he steps out, the legs are flung abruptly forward and outward, often lifted higher than necessary. The steps are of variable length, and many are attended by an audible stamp as the foot is banged down on the floor. The body is held in a slightly flexed position, and the weight may be supported on the cane that the severely ataxic patient so often carries. The incoordination is greatly exaggerated when the patient is deprived of visual cues, as in walking in the dark. Most patients, when asked to stand with feet together and eyes closed, show greatly increased swaying or actual falling (Romberg's sign). It has been said that a lame man whose shoes are not worn in any one place is probably suffering from sensory ataxia. There is invariably a loss of vibratory and position sense in the feet and legs. Gaits of this type are observed in tabes dorsalis, Friedreich's ataxia, subacute combined degeneration, syphilitic meningomyelitis, chronic polyneuritis, and those cases of multiple sclerosis in which posterior column disease predominates.

HEMIPLEGIC AND PARAPLEGIC (SPASTIC) GAIT. In hemiplegia the leg is held stiffly and does not flex freely and gracefully at the knee and hip. It tends to rotate outward and describes a semicircle, first away from and then toward the trunk (circumduction). The foot scrapes along the floor, and the toe and outer side of the sole of the shoe are worn. One can diagnose the hemiplegic gait by hearing the slow rhythmic scuff of the foot along the floor. The other muscles of the body on the affected side are weak and stiff to a variable degree, particularly the arm, which is carried in a flexed position and does not swing naturally. This type of gait disorder is most frequently associated with vascular disease of the brain.

The spastic paraplegic gait is entirely different from the gait of sensory ataxia, though the two may be combined. Each leg is advanced slowly and stiffly with restricted motion at the knee and hip. The patient looks as though he were wading in water. The legs are extended or slightly bent at the knees and may be strongly adducted at the hips, tending almost to cross ("scissors" gait). The steps are regular and short. Movements of the legs are slow, and the patient may be able to advance only with great effort. An easy way to remember the main features of the hemiplegic and paraplegic gait is by the letter S, which begins each of its descriptive adjectives—spastic, slow, scuffing. The defect is in the stepping mechanism and in propulsion, not in support or equilibrium. Cerebral spastic diplegia, multiple sclerosis, syringomyelia, spinal syphilis, combined system disease, spinal cord compression, and familial spinal spastic ataxia are the common causes of spastic paraparesis.

FESTINATING GAIT. This term comes from the Latin

festinatio, haste, and is appropriate for the gait disorder of both paralysis agitans and postencephalitic Parkinson's syndrome. *Rigidity* and *shuffling,* in addition to *festination,* are the cardinal features of this gait. When they are joined to the typical tremors, rigidity, and slowness of movement, there can be little doubt as to the diagnosis.

The general attitude of the patient is one of flexion; rigidity and immobility of the body are other conspicuous features. There is a paucity of the automatic movements made in sitting, standing, and walking; the head does not turn in looking to one side, the arms are seldom folded, and the legs are rarely crossed. The arms are held stiffly as though in preparation for writing, and the facial expression is unblinking and masklike.

In walking, the trunk is bent forward and the arms are carried ahead of the body and do not swing. The legs are stiff and bent at the knees and hips. The steps are short and the feet barely clear the ground as the patient shuffles along. Once forward or backward locomotion is started, the upper part of the body advances ahead of the lower part, as though the patient were chasing his center of gravity. His steps become more and more rapid, and he may fall if not assisted. This is the festination, and it may occur when the patient is walking forward or backward, taking the form of either propulsion or retropulsion. The defect is in rocking the body from side to side so as to clear the floor and in moving the legs quickly enough to catch the center of gravity in forward propulsion. Other unusual gaits are sometimes observed in the postencephalitic patient. For example, he may be unable to take his first step forward because he cannot lift one foot, or until he hops or takes one step backward; or walking may be initiated by a series of short steps that give way to a more normal gait; occasionally such a patient may run better than he walks.

ATHETOTIC, DYSTONIC, AND CHOREIC GAITS. These are less common than the preceding gait disorders. The athetotic patient is rigid, and his body often assumes the most grotesque postures. One arm may be held aloft and the other one behind the body with wrist and fingers alternately undergoing slow flexion, extension, and rotation. The head may be inclined in one direction, the lips alternately retract and then purse, and the tongue intermittently protrudes from the mouth. The legs advance slowly and awkwardly. Sometimes the foot is plantar flexed at the ankle, and the weight is carried on the toes; or it may be dorsiflexed or inverted. This type of gait is typical of congenital athetosis.

In dystonia musculorum deformans the first symptom may be a limp due to inversion or plantar flexion of the foot or a distortion of the pelvis. The patient stands with one leg rigidly extended or one shoulder elevated. The trunk may be in a position of exaggerated lordosis and the hips are partly flexed, with a tilting forward of the pelvis. Because of the muscle spasms that deform the body in this manner, the patient may have to walk with knees flexed. The gait may seem normal as the first steps are taken, but as the patient walks, one or both legs become flexed, giving rise to the "dromedary" gait. In the more advanced stages walking becomes impossible owing to torsion of the trunk or the continuous flexion of one leg.

In *chorea* the gait is often bizarre. As the patient stands or walks there is a continuous play of irregular "choreic" movements affecting the face, neck, and hands, and in the advanced stages, the large proximal joints and trunk. The positions of the trunk and upper parts of the body vary with each step. There are jerks of the head, grimacing, squirming, twisting movements of the trunk and limbs, and peculiar respiratory noises. The general features of these conditions are described more fully in Chap. 364.

STEPPAGE, DROP-FOOT, OR EQUINE GAIT. This is caused by paralysis of the pretibial and peroneal muscles. The legs must be lifted abnormally high in order for the feet to clear the ground. There is a slapping noise as the foot strokes the floor. The anterior and lateral border of the sole of the shoe becomes worn. The steps are regular and even; otherwise, walking is not remarkable. The steppage gait may be unilateral or bilateral and occurs in diseases that affect the peripheral nerves of the legs or motor neurones in the spinal cord, such as poliomyelitis, progressive muscular atrophy, and Charcot-Marie-Tooth disease (peroneal muscular atrophy). It may also be observed in patients with peripheral types of muscular dystrophy.

WADDLING GAIT. This gait is characteristic of progressive muscular dystrophy. The attitude of the body may be straight, but more often the lumbar lordosis is accentuated. The steps are regular but a little uncertain. With each step there is an exaggerated elevation of the hip, and once the weight is on this hip, it yields to an abnormal degree so that the upper trunk then inclines to that side. This alternation of lateral trunk movements results in the rolling gait, or *waddle,* a term suggested by Oppenheim. The gluteal musculature is weak and inefficient, although leg muscles may appear well developed. Muscular contractures leading to an equinovarus position of the foot may complicate childhood cases, so that the waddle is combined with circumduction of the legs and "walking on the toes."

STAGGERING OR DRUNKEN GAIT. This is characteristic of alcoholic and barbiturate intoxication. The drunken patient totters, reels, tips forward and then backward, threatening each moment to lose his balance and fall. Control over trunk and legs is greatly impaired. The steps are irregular and uncertain. The patient appears stupefied and indifferent to the quality of his performance, but under certain circumstances he can momentarily correct his defect.

The frequently used adjectives *drunken* and *reeling* do not describe aptly the gait of cerebellar disease, except, perhaps, the most acute and severe cases. The intoxicated patient reels in many different directions, unlike the patient with cerebellar disease, and no effort is made to correct the reeling by watching the legs or the ground, as in cerebellar or sensory ataxia. In the drunken patient, despite a wide diversity of excursions of all parts of the body, balance may be exquisitely maintained. In contrast, the patient with cerebellar disease has great difficulty in maintaining his balance if he sways or lurches too far to one side.

HYSTERICAL GAIT. This may take any one of several forms—monoplegic, paraplegic, or hemiplegic. The monoplegic or hemiplegic patient does not lift the foot from the floor while walking; instead, he drags it as a useless member or pushes it ahead of him as though it were a skate. The characteristic circumduction is absent in hysterical hemiplegia, and the typical hemiplegic posture, hyperactive tendon reflexes, and Babinski's signs are missing. The hysterical paraplegic cannot very well drag both legs, and usually he depends on a crutch or remains helpless in bed; the muscles may be rigid with contractures or flaccid. The gait may be quite dramatic. Some patients look as though they were walking on stilts, and others lurch wildly in all directions, actually demonstrating by their gyrations the most remarkable ability to make rapid postural adjustments.

Astasia-abasia, in which the patient, though unable to either stand or walk, retains normal use of his legs while in bed, is nearly always hysterical. When such a patient is placed on his feet, he takes a few normal steps and then becomes unable to advance his feet; he lurches wildly and crumples to the floor if not assisted.

FRONTAL LOBE ATAXIA. Equilibrium and the capacity to stand and walk may be severely disturbed by diseases that affect the frontal lobes, particularly their medial parts. Although this disorder of gait is sometimes spoken of as an ataxia, or as an *apraxia* since the difficulty in walking cannot be accounted for by weakness or loss of sensation alone, it is probably neither. It most likely represents a loss of integration at the cortical and basal ganglionic level of the essential elements of stance and locomotion which were acquired in infancy and are often lost in senility.

The patient assumes a posture of slight flexion, with the feet placed farther apart then normal. He advances slowly, with small, shuffling hesitant steps. At times the patient halts, unable to advance without great effort, although he does much better with a little assistance. Turning is accomplished by a series of tiny, uncertain steps which are made with one foot, the other being planted on the floor as a pivot. The initiation of walking becomes progressively more difficult, and in advanced cases the patient may be unable to take a step or even to stand, and he falls backward.

Some patients are able to make complex movements with their legs, such as drawing imaginary figures, at a time when their gait is seriously impaired. In most cases, however, all movements of the legs are slow and awkward, and the limbs, when passively moved, offer variable resistance (Gegenhalten). An inability to turn in bed is highly characteristic, and may eventually become complete. These motor disabilities are usually associated with dementia, but there need be no parallelism in the evolution of these disorders. Grasping, groping, hyperactive tendon reflexes, and Babinski signs may or may not be present. The end result in many cases is a "cerebral paraplegia in flexion" (Yakovlev), in which the patient lies curled up in bed, immobile and mute, his limbs fixed by contractures in an attitude of flexion. If one frontal lobe is affected, awkwardness of movement appears in the opposite arm and leg, simulating cerebellar ataxia at times except for the absence of intention tremor, pendular reflexes, Holmes's rebound sign, etc.

SENILE GAIT. Elderly persons often complain of difficulty in walking, and examination may disclose no abnormality other than the slightly flexed posture of the senile and short uncertain steps, *marche à petits pas*. Speed, balance, and all the graceful, adaptive movements are lost. The exact nature of this gait disorder is not understood. It may represent no special neurologic defect, but only a general defensive reaction to all forms of defective locomotion. Or, it may represent an early or mild form of frontal lobe ataxia (see above).

REFERENCES

Altmann, F.: Diagnostic Significance of Vertigo. *In* The Vestibular System and Its Diseases. Wolfson, R. J., Ed. University of Pennsylvania Press, Philadelphia, 1966, pp. 353–374.

Citron, L., and Hallpike, C. S.: Observations Upon the Mechanism of Positional Nystagmus of the So-Called "Benign Paroxysmal Type," J. Laryngol. & Otol., 70:253, 1956.

Martin, J. P.: The Basal Ganglia and Locomotion. Ann. Roy. Coll. Med., 32:219, 1963.

Symonds, C.: The Significance of Vertigo in Neurological Diagnosis. J. Laryngol. & Otol., 66:295, 1952.

24 COMMON DISTURBANCES OF VISION, OCULAR MOVEMENT, AND HEARING

*Maurice Victor
and Raymond D. Adams*

Disturbances of vision and hearing, perhaps more properly considered under diseases of cranial nerves, present so many special problems that they will be dealt with in a separate chapter.

DISORDERS OF VISION

Here the most frequent complaint is blurred, impaired, or distorted vision, and less often, diplopia, ocular pain, irritation of eyes, or inability to keep the eyelids open. It is to be noted that patients do not always distinguish between mild diplopia and a true impairment or diminution of vision in one or both eyes; either condition may be described as blurring or dimming, and there may also be surprising inaccuracy in stating whether one or both eyes are affected. In late childhood and adolescence increasing difficulty in focusing eyes and in seeing clearly usually can be traced to developing myopia, though one must rule out ocular or suprasellar tumors. In the middle years (forty-five to fifty) presbyopia, an almost invariable accompaniment of age, is the usual explanation of this phenomenon; and still later in life glaucoma and cataract are the most frequent causes.

Episodic blindness in one or both eyes merits separate consideration. When it is bilateral and the blind spots are bordered by bright lines and then followed by unilateral headache and nausea, classic migraine is almost invariably the diagnosis. Episodic blindness limited to one eye, lasting a few minutes only but usually recurring (amblyopia fugax), indicates atherosclerosis of the carotid artery with impending thrombosis. Obscurations of vision of minutes' duration attend increased intracranial pressure and papilledema; they often herald permanent blindness and secondary optic atrophy.

Distortions of vision take several forms. The perceived objects may appear too small (micropsia), too large (macropsia), or they may seem to be askew. Such phenomena always suggest a lesion of the temporal lobes. The latter may also be accompanied by complex visual hallucinations (of landscapes, of people, etc.), which actually represent a sensory seizure (see Chap. 28).

ANATOMIC AND PHYSIOLOGIC CONSIDERATIONS

The first neuronal elements in the visual pathway are the rod and cone cells situated in the deepest layer of the retina. The cones are responsible for sharp vision and color discrimination, and they alone are present in the fovea. The rods, which are more sensitive to low intensities of light, predominate in the rest of the retina. Visual impulses are transmitted through the second system of neurones, the bipolar cells, to the ganglion cells, the axones of which form the optic nerve after first perforating the sclera at the optic disk, which has a sievelike structure, the *lamina cribrosa*. The absence of visual end organs at this point accounts for the blind spot in the field of vision. The optic nerve is actually a part of the central nervous system, with glial cells between its fibers but no Schwann cells as in the other cranial and spinal nerves.

The optic nerves extend from the disk to the optic chiasm, where their fibers undergo partial decussation (Fig. 24-1). The rearranged optic fibers continue as the optic tract, which partially encircles the cerebral peduncles and synapses with cells in the lateral geniculate body. From these cells arises the fourth system of neurones, the final visual pathway, comprising the geniculocalcarine tract. These fibers lie close to the wall of the temporal horn of the lateral ventricle. The upper ones take a direct course posteriorly, the lower ones loop forward over the temporal horn of the lateral ventricle into the temporal lobe (Meyer's loop) before they pass posteriorly and join the upper fibers on their way to the calcarine cortex.

The types of visual field defect resulting from lesions in different parts of the visual pathways are shown in Fig. 24-1. A prechiasmal lesion causes either a scotoma (an island of impaired vision within the visual field) or a cut in the peripheral part of the visual field. A small scotoma in the macular part of the visual field may seri-

Fig. 24-1. Diagram showing the effects on the fields of vision produced by lesions at various points along the optic pathway. A, complete blindness in left eye; B, bitemporal hemianopsia; C, nasal hemianopsia of left eye; D, right homonymous hemianopsia; E and F, right upper and lower quadrant hemianopsias; G, right homonymous hemianopsia with preservation of central vision. (Homans: "A Textbook of Surgery," Springfield, Ill., Charles C Thomas, Publisher, 1945.)

ously impair visual acuity. Demyelinative, toxic (methyl alcohol, quinine, and certain of the phenothiazine tranquilizing drugs), nutritional (so-called "tobacco-alcohol" amblyopia), and vascular diseases are the usual causes of scotomas. The toxic states are characterized by symmetrical bilateral scotomas and the nutritional disorders by more or less symmetrical central or centrocecal ones (involving both the fixation point and the blind spot). These scotomas are predominantly in the distribution of the papillomacular bundle, but it is not certain whether the primary effect is on the nerve fibers or the ganglion cells. Vascular lesions, taking the form of hemorrhages or microinfarcts (cytoid bodies) in the retina or infarcts in the optic nerve, cause unilateral scotomas. Demyelinative diseases give rise to unilateral or asymmetric bilateral scotomas. If the lesion is near the optic disk, there may be swelling of the optic nerve head, i.e., papillitis, which can usually be distinguished from papilledema by the marked impairment of vision it produces.

Another common defect encountered on visual field examination is concentric constriction. This may be due to papilledema, in which case it is usually accompanied by an enlargement of the blind spot. A concentric constriction of the visual field, at first unilateral and later bilateral, and pallor of the optic disks (optic atrophy) should suggest chronic syphilitic optic neuritis. Glaucoma is another cause of this type of field defect. Tubular vision, i.e., constriction of the visual field to the same degree regardless of the distance of the visual test stimulus from the eye, is a sign of hysteria. In organic disease, e.g., chorioretinitis, the area of the constricted visual field enlarges as the distance between the patient and the stimulus increases.

Hemianopsia means blindness in one-half the visual field. *Bitemporal hemianopsia*, indicating a lesion of the decussating fibers of the optic chiasm, is due to tumor of the pituitary gland or of the infundibulum or third ventricle, to meningioma of the diaphragm of the sella, or occasionally, to a large suprasellar aneurysm of the circle of Willis. *Homonymous hemianopsia* (a loss of vision in corresponding halves of the visual fields) indicates a lesion of the visual pathway behind the chiasm and, if *complete*, gives no more information than that. *Incomplete homonymous hemianopsia* has more localizing value: if the field defects in the two eyes are similar (*congruous*), the lesion is likely to be in the calcarine cortex; if *incongruous*, the visual fibers in the parietal or temporal lobe are more likely to be implicated. Since the fibers from the peripheral lower quadrants of the retina extend for a variable distance into the temporal lobe, lesions of this lobe may be accompanied by a homonymous upper quadrantic field defect. Parietal lobe lesions may affect the lower quadrants more than the upper.

If the entire optic tract or calcarine cortex on one side is destroyed, there is complete homonymous hemianopsia, including half the field that represents the macula. Incomplete lesions of the optic tract and radiation usually spare central (macular) vision. It must be kept in mind that apparent macular sparing is frequently due to imperfect fixation of gaze. A lesion of the tip of one occipital lobe produces central homonymous hemianopsia because half the macular fibers of both eyes terminate there. Lesions of both occipital poles result in bilateral central scotomas; and if all the calcarine cortex on each side is completely destroyed, there is complete "cortical" blindness. Altitudinal or horizontal hemianopsias are more often due to lesions of the occipital lobes below or above the calcarine cortex than of optic chiasm.

In addition to blindness, i.e., "visual anesthesia," there is another category of visual impairment, which consists of a defect of visual perception, i.e., *visual agnosia*. The patient can see but cannot recognize objects unless he hears, smells, tastes, or palpates them. The failure of visual recognition of words is called *alexia*. The ability to recognize visually presented objects and words depends not only upon the integrity of the visual pathways and primary visual areas of the cerebral cortex (area 17 of Brodmann) but also upon those cortical areas which lie just anterior to the cerebral cortex in the *dominant* hemisphere (areas 18 and 19 of the occipital lobe and the angular gyrus). Visual-object agnosia and alexia result from lesions of these latter areas or from a lesion of the left calcarine cortex combined with one which interrupts the fibers crossing from the right occipital lobe. These subjects are discussed further in Chaps. 25 and 30.

The optic nerves also contain the afferent fibers for the pupillary reflexes. These fibers leave the optic tract and terminate in the superior colliculi. A lesion of the optic nerve or tracts may abolish the pupillary light reflex; the pupil is dilated and unreactive. Cerebral lesions, on the other hand, leave the pupillary light reflex unaltered. The lack of direct reflex in the blind eye and of consensual reflex in the sound one means that the afferent limb of the reflex arc (optic nerve) is the site of the lesion. A lack of direct light reflex with retention of the consensual reflex places the lesion in the efferent limb of the reflex arc (the homolateral oculomotor nucleus or nerve). Loss of light reflex without visual impairment or ocular palsy (Argyll Robertson pupillary phenomenon) is thought to be due to a lesion in the superior colliculi or periaqueductal region (see below).

Amaurosis refers to blindness from any cause. *Amblyopia* refers to an impairment or loss of vision which is not due to an error of refraction or some other disease of the eye. Hemeralopia and Nyctalopia mean poor twilight or night vision and are associated with vitamin A deficiency and pigmentary degeneration of the retina.

Hereditary diseases account for a significant proportion of cases of congenital or childhood amblyopia. These take the form of anophthalmia, bulbar atrophy (Norrie's disease), hypoplasia of optic nerves, retinitis pigmentosa, often combined with other conditions such as dwarfism polydactyly and gonadal deficiency (Lorain-Moon-Biedl disease), polyneuropathy and deafness (Refsum's disease), vestibulo-cerebellar ataxia and mental deficiency (Hallgren's disease) or mental deficiency alone. Pigmentary degeneration and optic atrophy are also common causes in adult years; some of the former are drug induced.

DIPLOPIA AND STRABISMUS AND DISORDERS OF THE THIRD, FOURTH, AND SIXTH NERVES

Strabismus (squint) refers to an ocular imbalance that results in improper alignment of the two eyes. It may be due to paralysis of an eye muscle; the ocular deviation results from the unrestrained activity of the opposing muscle. It may be due to inequality of tone in the muscles that hold the two eyes in a central position. The former is called *paralytic strabismus* and is primarily a neurologic problem; the latter is *nonparalytic strabismus* (referred to as *concomitant* strabismus if the squinting eye has a full range of movement) and is an ophthalmologic problem. Any type of ocular imbalance causes diplopia for the reason that images then fall on disparate or noncorresponding parts of the two retinas. After a time, however, the patient learns to suppress the image of one eye. This almost invariably happens early in concomitant strabismus of congenital nature, and the individual grows up with a diminished visual acuity in that eye (*amblyopia ex anopsia*).

The oculomotor, trochlear, and abducens nerves innervate the extrinsic and intrinsic musculature of the eye. A knowledge of their origin and anatomic relationships is essential to an understanding of the various paralytic ocular syndromes. The oculomotor nucleus consists of several groups of nerve cells ventral to the aqueduct of Sylvius, at the level of the superior colliculi. The nerve cells that innervate the iris and ciliary body are situated anteriorly in the so-called "Edinger-Westphal nucleus." Below this nucleus are the cells for the superior rectus, inferior oblique, internal rectus, and inferior rectus, in that order from above downward. Convergence is under the control of the medial groups of cells, the nucleus of Perlia. The cells of origin of the trochlear nerves are just inferior to those of the oculomotor nerves. The sixth nerve arises at a considerably lower level, from a paired group of cells in the floor of the fourth ventricle at the level of the lower pons. The intrapontine portion of the facial nerve loops around the sixth nerve nucleus before it turns anterolaterally to make its exit; a lesion in this locality usually causes a homolateral paralysis of both lateral rectus and facial muscles.

All three nerves, after leaving the brainstem, course anteriorly and pass through the cavernous sinus, where they come into close proximity with the ophthalmic division of the fifth nerve, and together they enter the orbit through the superior orbital fissure. The oculomotor nerve supplies all the extrinsic ocular muscles except two—the superior oblique and the external rectus—which are innervated by the trochlear and abducens nerves, respectively. The voluntary part of the levator palpebrae muscle is also supplied by the oculomotor nerve, the involuntary part being under the control of autonomic fibers which also supply the sphincter pupillae and the ciliary muscles (muscles of accommodation).

Although all the extraocular muscles probably participate in every movement of the eyes, particular muscles move the eyes in certain fields. The lateral rectus rotates the eye outward; the medial rectus, inward. The function of the vertical recti and the obliques varies according to the position of the eye. When the eye is turned outward, the elevators and depressors of the eye are the superior and inferior recti; when the eye is turned inward, they are the inferior and superior obliques, respectively. In contrast, torsion of the eyeball is effected by the oblique muscles when the eye is turned outward, and by the recti when it is turned inward.

Accurate binocular vision is achieved by the associated action of the ocular muscles, which allows a visual stimulus to fall on exactly corresponding parts of the two retinas. Conjugate movement of the eyes is controlled by centers in the cerebral cortex and brainstem. Area 8 in the frontal lobe is the center for voluntary conjugate movements of the eyes to the opposite side. In addition, there is a center in the occipital lobe concerned with contralateral following movements. Fibers from these centers pass to the opposite sides of the brainstem, where they connect with lower centers for conjugate move-

ments: those for the right lateral gaze are thought to be in the proximity of the right abducens nucleus; those for the left lateral gaze are near the left abducens. Simultaneous innervation of one internal rectus and the other external rectus during lateral gaze is a function of the medial longitudinal fasciculus. The arrangements of nerve cells and fibers for vertical gaze and convergence are situated in the pretectal areas and paramedian zones of the midbrain tegmentum.

OCULAR MUSCLE AND GAZE PALSIES

There are three types of paralysis of extraocular muscles: (1) paralysis of isolated ocular muscles, (2) paralysis of conjugate movements (gaze), and (3) syndromes of mixed gaze and ocular muscle paralysis.

Characteristic clinical disturbances result from single lesions of the third, fourth, or sixth cranial nerves. A complete third nerve lesion causes ptosis (since the levator palpebrae is supplied mainly by the third nerve), an inability to rotate the eye upward, downward, or inward, a divergent strabismus due to unopposed action of the lateral rectus muscle, a dilated nonreactive pupil (iridoplegia), and paralysis of accommodation (cycloplegia). When only the muscles of the iris and ciliary body are paralyzed, the condition is termed *internal ophthalmoplegia*. Fourth nerve lesions result in an extorsion of the eye and a weakness of downward gaze, so that patients commonly complain of special difficulty in going downstairs. Head tilting, to the opposite shoulder, is especially characteristic of fourth nerve lesions. This maneuver causes a compensatory intorsion of the lower eye, enabling the patient to obtain binocular vision. Lesions of the sixth nerve result in paralysis of abduction and a convergent strabismus owing to the unopposed action of the internal rectus muscles. With incomplete sixth nerve palsies, turning the head toward the side of the paretic muscle may overcome diplopia. The foregoing signs may occur with various degrees of completeness, depending on the severity and site of the lesion or lesions.

Ocular palsies may be central, i.e., due to a lesion of the nucleus or the intramedullary portion of the cranial nerve, or peripheral. Ophthalmoplegia due to a lesion in the brainstem is usually accompanied by involvement of other cranial nerves or long tracts. Peripheral lesions, which may or may not be solitary, have a great variety of causes; the most common are aneurysm of the circle of Willis, tumors of the base of the brain, carcinomatosis of the meninges, herpes zoster, and syphilitic meningitis. The third-nerve palsy that occurs with diabetes is probably due to infarction of the third nerve, and the prognosis for recovery in such cases, as with other nonprogressive diseases of the peripheral nerve, is usually excellent. The points of difference between lesions within and outside of the brainstem are tabulated in Table 24-1, and the various intramedullary and extramedullary cranial nerve syndromes are described in Tables 355-1 and 355-2. See also diagrams in Ch. 357.

When the ocular palsy is slight, there may be no obvious squint or defect in ocular movement; yet the patient experiences diplopia. Study of the relative posi-

Table 24-1. COMPARISON OF LESIONS WITHIN AND OUTSIDE
THE BRAIN STEM

Effect	Lesions within the brain stem	Lesions external to the brain stem
Involvement of multiple contiguous nerves	±	+
Involvement of sensorimotor tracts	+, often "alternating" or crossed sensory or motor palsies	±
Disturbance of consciousness	+	0 (+ late)
Evidence of other segmental disturbances of the brain stem such as decerebrate rigidity, tonic neck reflexes, pseudobulbar palsy	+	0 (+ late)
X-ray evidence of erosion of cranial bones or enlargement of foramens	0	+

tions of the images of the two eyes then becomes the most accurate way of determining which muscle is involved. The image seen by the affected eye is usually less distinct, but the most reliable way of distinguishing the two images is by the red glass test. *A red glass is placed in front of the patient's right eye.* He is then asked to look at a flashlight, held at a distance of a meter, to turn his eyes in various segments of his visual fields, and to state the position of the red and white images. The relative positions of the two images are plotted as indicated in Fig. 24-2.

Three rules aid in the analysis of ocular movements by the red glass test. (1) The direction in which the distance between the images is at a maximum is the direction of action of the paretic muscle. For example, if the greatest separation is in looking to the right, either the right abductor or the left adductor muscle is weak. (2) The image projected farther to the side belongs to the paretic eye. If the patient looks to the right and the red image is farther to the right, then the right abducens muscle is weak. If the white image is to the right of the red, then the left internal rectus muscle is weak. (3) In testing vertical movements, again the image of the eye with the paretic muscle is the one projected most peripherally in the direction of eye movement. One ignores lateral separation at this time. It must be remembered that there are two elevator and two depressor muscles. The responsible muscle may be either one of the obliques or vertical recti muscles. For example, if the maximum separation of images occurs on looking downward and to the left, and the white image is projected farther down than the red, the paretic muscle is the left inferior rectus. If the maximum separation occurs on looking down and to the right, and the white image is lower than the red, the paretic muscle is the left superior oblique. Separation of images on looking up and to the right or left will simi-

larly distinguish paresis of the inferior oblique and superior rectus muscles.

Monocular diplopia may occur and is related to diseases of the lens and refractive media of the eye. Also, paresis of accommodation may produce diplopia for near vision; its cause is unknown.

PARALYSIS OF CONJUGATE MOVEMENT (GAZE). The term *conjugate gaze,* or *conjugate movement,* refers to the simultaneous movement of the two eyes in the same direction. An acute lesion in one frontal lobe may cause paralysis of contralateral gaze. The eyes turn toward the side of the lesion. The ocular disorder is temporary (several days' duration). In bilateral frontal lesions the patient may be unable to turn his eyes voluntarily (oculomotor apraxia) in any direction—up, down, or to the side—but retains fixation and following movements, which are believed to be occipital lobe functions. Gaze paralysis of cerebral origin is not attended by strabismus or diplopia. The usual causes are vascular occlusion with infarction, hemorrhage, and abscess or tumor of the frontal lobe. With certain extrapyramidal disorders, e.g., postencephalitic parkinsonism or Huntington's chorea, ocular movements may be limited in all directions, especially upward. Lesions of the superior colliculus and tegmentum, near the posterior commissure, interfere with voluntary reflex upward gaze, and often movements of convergence as well as the pupillary light reflexes are abolished (Parinaud's syndrome). There also exists a pontine center for conjugate lateral gaze, probably in the vicinity of the abducens nuclei. A lesion here causes ipsilateral gaze palsy, with the eyes turning to the opposite side. Vertical and lateral gaze palsies are combined in the supranuclear ophthalmoplegia syndrome of Steele-Richardson. The palsy tends to last longer than with cerebral lesions and is frequently accompanied by other signs of pontine disease. Fully developed forms of gaze paralysis are readily discerned, but lesser degrees may be overlooked unless one pays special attention to the predominant position of the eyes and tests the ability to sustain conjugate movement.

In skew deviation, a poorly understood disorder of gaze, the eyes diverge, one looking down, the other up. The deviation is constant in all fields of gaze. It may occur with any lesion of the posterior fossa but particularly one in the brainstem. The lesion is on the side of the lower eye.

MIXED GAZE AND OCULAR PARALYSES. These are always a sign of intrapontine or mesencephalic disease. With a lesion of the lower pons in or near the sixth-nerve nucleus, there is a homolateral paralysis of the lateral rectus muscle and a failure of adduction of the opposite eye, i.e., a combined paralysis of the sixth nerve and of conjugate lateral gaze. Lesions of the medial longitudinal fasciculi interfere with lateral conjugate gaze in another way. On looking to the right, the left eye fails to adduct; on looking to the left, the right eye fails to adduct. The abducting eye shows nystagmus. This condition is referred to as *internuclear ophthalmoplegia* and should always be suspected when only adduction of the eyes is affected. If the lesion is in the lower part of the medial longitudinal fasciculi, convergence is intact; if the lesion is in the higher part, i.e., near the oculomotor nuclei, convergence may be lost (anterior internuclear ophthalmoplegia).

NYSTAGMUS. This refers to involuntary rhythmic movements of the eyes; it is of two types, oscillating (pendular) and rhythmic (jerk). In jerk nystagmus, the movements are distinctly faster in one direction than the other; in pendular nystagmus, the oscillations are roughly equal in rate for the two directions, although on conjugate lateral gaze, the pendular type may resemble the jerk type, with the fast component to the side of the gaze.

In testing for nystagmus, the eyes should first be examined in the central position and then during upward, downward, and lateral movements. If nystagmus is monocular (as described below), each eye should be tested separately, with the other one covered. Labyrinthine nystagmus is most obvious when visual fixation is prevented by shielding the eyes; brainstem and cerebellar nystagmus are brought out best by having the patient fixate on a finger. Labyrinthine nystagmus may vary with the position of the head; hence these various tests should be performed with the head in several different positions. In particular, the postural nystagmus of Bárány is evoked by hyperextension of the neck, with the patient in the supine position. Optokinetic nystagmus should be tested by asking the patient to look at a rotating cylinder on which several stripes have been painted or a striped cloth moved across the field of vision.

A few irregular jerks are observed in many normal individuals when the eyes are turned far to the side. These so-called "nystagmoid movements" are probably similar to the tremulousness of a muscle that is contracted maximally. Occasionally a fine rhythmic nystagmus can be obtained in extreme lateral gaze, but if it is bilateral and disappears as the eyes move a few degrees toward the midline, it usually has no clinical significance.

Pendular nystagmus is found in a variety of conditions in which central vision is lost early in life, such as albinism and in various other diseases of the retina and refractive mediums. The syndrome of miners' nystagmus, formerly a common cause of industrial disability, occurs after many years of work in comparative darkness. The oscillations of the eyes are very rapid, increase on upward gaze, and are often associated with vertigo, head tremor, and intolerance of light. *Spasmus nutans* is a specific type of pendular nystagmus of infancy and is accompanied by head nodding and occasionally by wry positions of the neck. The prognosis is good; most infants recover within a few months.

Jerk nystagmus is the commoner type. It may be lateral or vertical, particularly on ocular movement in these planes, or it may be rotary. By custom, the direction of the nystagmus is named according to the direction of the fast component. There are several varieties of jerk nystagmus. When one is watching a moving object—e.g., the passing landscape from a train window or a rotating drum with vertical stripes—a rhythmic jerk nystagmus, *optokinetic nystagmus*, normally appears. The slow phase is a result of visual fixation; the quick phase is compensa-

Fig. 24-2. Diplopia fields with individual muscle paralyses. The dark glass is in front of the right eye, and the fields are projected as the patient sees the images. *A.* Paralysis of right external rectus. Characteristic: right eye does not move to the right. Field: horizontal homonymous diplopia increasing on looking to the right. *B.* Paralysis of right internal rectus. Characteristic: right eye does not move to the left. Field: horizontal crossed diplopia increasing on looking to the left. *C.* Paralysis of right inferior rectus. Characteristic: right eye does not move downward when eyes are turned to the right. Field: vertical diplopia (image of right eye lowermost) increasing on looking to the right and down. *D.* Paralysis of right superior rectus. Characteristic: right eye does not move upward when eyes are turned to the right. Field: vertical diplopia (image of right eye uppermost) increasing on looking to the right and up. *E.* Paralysis of right superior oblique. Characteristic: right eye does not move downward when eyes are turned to the left. Field: vertical diplopia (image of right eye lowermost) increasing on looking to left and down. *F.* Paralysis of right inferior oblique. Characteristic: right eye does not move upward when eyes are turned to the left. Field: vertical diplopia (image of right eye uppermost) increasing on looking to left and up. (Cogan: "Neurology of the Ocular Muscles," 2d ed., Springfield, Ill., Charles C Thomas, Publisher, 1956.)

tory. With unilateral cerebral lesions, particularly in the parieto-occipital region, there is loss of optokinetic nystagmus when the moving stimulus, e.g., the drum, moves toward the side of the lesion.

Aside from optokinetic nystagmus, lateral and vertical nystagmus are most frequently due to barbiturate intoxication. Jerk nystagmus may signify disease of the labyrinthine-vestibular apparatus. Labyrinthine stimulation or irritation produces a nystagmus with the fast phase to the opposite side. The slow component reflects the effect of impulses derived from the semicircular canals, and the fast component is a corrective movement. Vestibular-labyrinthine nystagmus may be horizontal, vertical, or most characteristically, rotary. Vertigo, nausea, vomiting, and staggering are the usual accompaniments (see Chap. 23). Brainstem lesions often cause a coarse unidirectional nystagmus, which may be horizontal or vertical; the latter is usually brought out on upward gaze and rarely on downward gaze. The presence of vertical nystagmus is pathognomonic of disease in the tegmentum of the brainstem. Vertigo is inconstant, and signs of disease of other nuclear structures and tracts in the brainstem are frequent. Jerk nystagmus of this type is frequent in demyelinative or vascular disease, in tumors, and syringobulbia. Cerebellopontine angle tumors cause a coarse bilateral horizontal nystagmus, with the fast component to the side of the lesion. Nystagmus probably does not occur with cerebellar disease unless the fastigial nuclei and their connections with the vestibular nuclei are involved. The nystagmus that occurs only in the abducting eye and is said to be a pathognomonic sign of multiple sclerosis probably represents an incompletely developed form of internuclear ophthalmoplegia. The movement of the adducting eye (which does not show nystagmus) is impaired.

Convergence nystagmus is a rhythmic oscillation in which a slow abduction of the eyes in respect of each other is followed by a quick movement of adduction. It is usually accompanied by other types of nystagmus and by one or more features of Parinaud's syndrome. Occasionally there is also a jerky retraction movement of the eyes (*nystagmus retractorius*) or eyelids or a maintained spasm of convergence, best brought out on attempted elevation of the eyes to command. These unusual phenomena all point to a lesion of the upper midbrain tegmentum and are usually manifestations of vascular disease or of pinealoma.

Seesaw nystagmus, one eye moving up, the other down, is occasionally observed in conjunction with bitemporal hemianopia. Its mechanism is unknown.

Oscillopsia refers to illusory movement of the environment, in which objects seem to move back and forth, to jerk or to wiggle. It may or may not occur with turning of the eyes and consequent displacement of the image on the retina, and is said to be characteristic of the nystagmus of multiple sclerosis.

ALTERATIONS OF PUPILS

Pupil size is determined by the balance of innervation between the dilator and constrictor fibers. The pupillo-dilator fibers arise in the posterior part of the hypothalamus, descend in the lateral tegmentum of the midbrain, pons, medulla, and cervical spinal cord to the eighth cervical and first thoracic segments, where they synapse with the lateral horn cells. The latter give rise to preganglionic fibers that synapse in the superior cervical ganglion; the postganglionic fibers course along the internal carotid artery and traverse the cavernous sinus to join the first division of the trigeminal nerve, finally reaching the eyes as the long ciliary nerves. The pupillo-constrictor fibers arise in the nucleus of Edinger-Westphal, join the oculomotor nerve, and synapse in the ciliary ganglion with the postganglionic neurones that innervate the iris and ciliary body.

The pupils are usually equal in size, though if the eyes are turned to one side, the pupil of the abducting eye dilates slightly. Pupil size varies with light intensity; as one pupil constricts under a bright light (direct reflex), the other unexposed pupil does likewise (consensual reflex). Pupillary constriction is also part of the act of convergence and accommodation for near objects.

Interruption of the sympathetic fibers either centrally, between the hypothalamus and their point of exit from the spinal cord, or peripherally, in the neck or along the carotid artery, results in miosis and ptosis (due to paralysis of the levator palpebrae), with loss of sweating of the face, and occasionally enophthalmos (Bernard-Horner syndrome). Stimulation or irritation of the pupillodilator fibers has the opposite effect, i.e., lid retraction, slight proptosis, and dilatation of the pupil. The ciliospinal pupillary reflex, evoked by pinching the neck, is effected through these efferent sympathetic fibers. Abnormal dilatation of the pupils (mydriasis), often with loss of pupillary light reflexes, may result from midbrain lesions and is a frequent finding in cases of deep coma. Extreme constriction of the pupils (miosis) is commonly observed with pontine lesions, presumably because of bilateral interruption of the pupilodilator fibers.

The functional integrity of the sympathetic and parasympathetic nerve endings in the iris may be determined by the use of certain drugs. Atropine and homatropine dilate the pupils by paralyzing the parasympathetic nerve endings, while physostigmine and pilocarpine constrict them, the former by inhibiting cholinesterase activity at the neuromuscular junction and the latter by direct stimulation of the sphincter muscle of the iris. Cocaine dilates the pupils by stimulating the sympathetic nerve endings. Morphine acts centrally to constrict the pupils.

In chronic syphilitic meningitis and other forms of late syphilis, particularly tabes dorsalis, the pupils are usually small, irregular, and unequal; they do not dilate properly in response to mydriatic drugs and fail to react to light, although they do constrict on accommodation. This is known as the *Argyll Robertson pupil*. The exact locality of the lesion is not certain; it is generally believed to be in the tectum of the midbrain proximal to the oculomotor nuclei, where the descending pupillodilator fibers are in close proximity to the light-reflex fibers. The possibility of a partial third-nerve lesion or a lesion of the ciliary ganglion has not been excluded. A dissociation of the light reflex from the accommodation-convergence reaction is sometimes observed with other midbrain lesions, e.g., pinealoma, multiple sclerosis, and diabetes mellitus; in these diseases miosis, irregularity of pupils, and failure to respond to a mydriatic are not constantly present. Another interesting pupillary abnormality is the myotonic reaction, sometimes referred to as *Adie's pupil.* The patient may complain of blurring of vision or may have suddenly noticed that one pupil is larger than the other. The reaction to light and convergence are absent if tested in the customary manner, although the size of the pupil will change slowly on prolonged stimulation. Once contracted or dilated, the pupils remain in that state for some minutes. The affected pupil reacts promptly to the usual mydriatic and miotic drugs but is unusually sensitive to a 2.5 percent solution of Mecholyl, a strength that will not affect a normal pupil. The myotonic pupil usually appears during the third or fourth decade and may be associated with absence of knee jerks, and hence be mistaken for tabes dorsalis.

DISTURBANCES OF HEARING

Tinnitus and *deafness* are frequent symptoms and always indicate disease of the ear or of the auditory nerve and its central connections.

Tinnitus, or ringing in the ears, is a purely subjective phenomenon and may also be reported as a buzzing, whistling, hissing, or roaring sound. It is a very common symptom in adults and may be of no significance, as, for example, the hissing sound due to wax in the external auditory canal or a blocked eustachian tube. On the other hand, it is regularly associated with disease of the eighth nerve, inner ear, or ossicles; severe and prolonged tinnitus in the presence of normal hearing is very rare. If tinnitus is localized to one ear and is described as having a tonal character, such as ringing or a bell-like tone, and particularly if the recruitment phenomenon (see below) is present, it is probably cochlear in origin. Noises described as rushing water or escaping steam point more to disease of the nerve or even the brainstem. Clicking sounds are caused by intermittent contraction of the tensor tympani. A pulsating tinnitus synchronous with the pulse may be related to an intracranial vascular malformation; however, this symptom must be carefully judged, since introspective individuals often report hearing their pulse when lying with one ear on a pillow. Certain drugs such as salicylates and quinine produce tinnitus and transient deafness. Nervous individuals are less tolerant of tinnitus than are more stable persons; depressed or anxious patients may demand relief from tinnitus that has existed for years.

Examination of hearing should always begin with inspection of the external auditory canal and the tympanic membrane. A watch or whispered words are suitable means of testing hearing at the bedside, the opposite ear being closed by the finger. If there is any suspicion of deafness or a complaint of tinnitus or vertigo, or if the patient is a child with a speech defect, then hearing must be tested further. This can be done with the use of tuning forks of different frequencies, but the most accurate results are obtained by the use of an electric audiometer and the construction of an audiogram, which reveals the entire range of hearing at a glance. An auditory recruitment test may also be helpful: the difference in hearing between the two ears is estimated, and the loudness of the stimulus delivered to each ear is then increased by regular increments. In nonrecruiting deafness (characteristic of a nerve trunk lesion) the original difference in hearing persists in comparisons above threshold. In recruiting deafness (as occurs in Ménière's disease) the more defective ear gains in loudness and finally is equal to the better one.

Deafness is of two types: (1) nerve deafness, due to interruption of cochlear fibers, and (2) conduction deafness, due to disease of the middle ear (or occlusion of the external auditory canal or eustachian tube). In differentiating these two types, the tuning fork tests are of value. When the vibrating fork is held several inches from the ear (the test for air conduction), sound waves can be appreciated only as they are transmitted through the middle ear and will be reduced with disease in this location. When the fork is applied to the skull (test for bone conduction), the sound waves are conveyed directly to the cochlea, without the intervention of the middle ear apparatus, and will therefore not be reduced when the disease is confined to the middle ear. With affection of the cochlea or eighth nerve, both air and bone conduction will be reduced or lost. Normally air conduction is better than bone conduction. These principles form the basis for several tests of auditory function.

In *Weber's test*, the vibrating fork is applied to the forehead in the midline. In middle ear deafness the sound is localized in the affected ear, in nerve deafness, in the normal ear. In *Rinné's test* the fork is applied to the mastoid process, the other ear being closed by the observer's finger. At the moment the sound ceases the fork is held at the auditory meatus. In middle ear deafness the sound cannot be heard by air conduction after bone conduction has ceased (abnormal or negative Rinné test). In nerve deafness the reverse is true (normal or positive Rinné test), although both air and bone conduction may be quantitatively decreased. In *Schwabach's test,* the patient's bone conduction is compared with that of a normal observer. In general, high-pitched tones are lost in nerve deafness and low-pitched ones in middle ear deafness, but there are frequent exceptions to this rule.

The common causes of middle ear deafness are otitis media, otosclerosis, and rupture of the eardrum. Nerve deafness has many causes. The internal ear may be aplastic from birth (hereditary deaf-mutism), or it may be damaged by rubella in the pregnant mother. Acute purulent meningitis or chronic infection spreading from the middle ear are common causes of nerve deafness in childhood. The auditory nerve may be involved by tumors of the cerebellopontine angle or by syphilis. Deafness may also result from a demyelinative plaque in the brainstem. A series of genetically determined syndromes which feature a neural type of deafness, some congenital, others progressive, have recently come to light. The most interesting of these are: hereditary deafness with nephritis (Alport's disease); hereditary deafness with goitre (Pendred's disease); hereditary heart disease with deafness

(Jervell and Lang-Nielsen disease); hereditary deafness with renal disease and digital anomalies; hereditary deafness with various combinations of mental retardation, retinitis pigmentosa and polyneuropathy as in Hallgren's disease, Alstrom's disease, Refsum's disease; hereditary deafness with skin abnormalities such as albinism, lentigines, piebaldness, white forelock (Waardenburg's disease), onchydystrophy and pegged teeth, atopic dermatitis, anhydrosis; hereditary deafness with muscular dystrophy. Of the types of conduction deafness hereditary otosclerosis is the most frequent (causes 50 percent of deafness in adulthood); other types are observed with cranial, ear, jaw, and other congenital anomalies (Treacher-Collins disease, Engelman's diaphyseal dysplasia etc.). Hysterical deafness may be difficult to distinguish from organic disease. In the case of bilateral deafness, the distinction can be made by observing a blink (cochleoorbicular reflex) or an alteration in skin sweating (psychogalvanic skin reflex) in response to a loud sound. Unilateral hysterical deafness may be detected by an audiometer, with both ears connected, or by whispering into the bell of a stethoscope attached to the patient's ears, closing first one and then the other tube without the patient's knowledge.

REFERENCES

Cogan, D.: Brain Lesions and Eye Movements in Man. Chap. 17 in "The Oculomotor System," M. Bender (Ed.), p. 417, New York, Harper & Row Publishers, Incorporated, 1964.

Pasik, P., and T. Pasik: Oculomotor Functions in Monkeys with Lesions of the Cerebrum and Superior Colliculi, Chap. 3 in "The Oculomotor System," M. Bender (Ed.), p. 40, New York, Harper & Row Publishers, Incorporated, 1964.

Konigsmark, B. W.: Hereditary Deafness in Man, Publication of Dept. of Otology, Johns Hopkins University, 1969.

25 DISORDERS OF SENSATION

Maurice Victor and Raymond D. Adams

Loss or perversion of somatic sensation not infrequently represents the principal manifestation of disease of the nervous system. The logic of this is clear enough, since the major anatomic pathways of the sensory system are distinct from those of the motor system and may be selectively disturbed by disease. An understanding of these sensory disorders depends on a knowledge of applied anatomy, physiology, and the use of special tests designed to indicate the nature of the disordered function and its locality.

Ideally, one should be familiar with the sensory organs in the skin and deep structures, the distribution of the peripheral nerves and the spinal roots, and the pathways by which the sensory impulses are conveyed through the spinal cord and brainstem to the thalamus and parietal lobe cortex. These topics were introduced in Chap. 9,

General Considerations of Pain. Unfortunately, space does not permit a detailed review here of the anatomy of the sensory system nor of its physiology. The interested reader may turn to the references at the end of the chapter. Nor is a final statement on the physiology of the sensory system possible, because our notions about the physiology of receptors and pain are in a state of constant revision. But, the generally accepted views about the cutaneous distribution of sensory spinal roots and peripheral nerves can be obtained from Figs. 25-1 and 25-2.

Disorders of the somatic sensory apparatus pose special problems for the patient. He is confronted with derangements of sensation which may be unlike anything he had previously experienced, and he has few words in his vocabulary to describe what he feels. He may say that a limb feels "numb" and "dead" when in fact he means weakness or paralysis and not a sensory disturbance. Observant individuals may discover a loss of sensation, for example, inability to feel discomfort on touching an object hot enough to blister the skin or unawareness of articles of clothing and other objects in contact with the skin. Or the disease may induce a new and unnatural series of sensory experiences, which are as often a source of complaint as loss of sensation. If nerves, spinal roots,

Fig. 25-1. Distribution of the sensory spinal roots on the surface of the body. (Holmes: "Introduction to Clinical Neurology," Edinburgh, E. & S. Livingstone, Ltd., 1946.)

Fig. 25-2. The cutaneous fields of peripheral nerves. (*Haymaker and Woodhall: "Peripheral Nerve Injuries," Philadelphia, W. B. Saunders Company, 1945.*)

or spinal tracts are only partially interrupted, a touch may arouse tingling or pricking (Novocaine feeling), meaning presumably that at least some of the remaining touch and pain fibers are functional but acting abnormally. Similarly, burning and pain may represent over activity of surviving thermal and pain fibers (causalgia). The lesion may be in the peripheral nerve, the lateral spinothalamic tract in the spinal cord or brainstem, or the thalamus. Hyperesthesia or hyperpathia are frequent. Tightness and drawing and pulling sensations, a feeling of a band or girdle around the limb or trunk, are common, with partial involvement of pressure fibers. These abnormal sensations are called *paresthesias,* or *dysesthesias,* if they are unpleasant; and their character and distribution inform us of the anatomy of the lesion involving the sensory system.

EXAMINATION OF SENSATION

The examination of sensation is the most difficult part of the neurologic examination. For one thing, test procedures are relatively crude and inadequate, and at times no objective sensory loss can be demonstrated despite symptoms that clearly indicate the presence of such a

deficit. Also, a response to a sensory stimulus is difficult to evaluate objectively, and the examiner's conclusions depend on the patient's interpretations of sensory experiences. This, in turn, depends on his general awareness, responsiveness, and desire to cooperate, as well as his intelligence, level of education, and the degree of suggestibility and fatigue. At times, children and relatively uneducated persons are better witnesses than more sophisticated individuals who are likely to analyze their feelings too minutely.

The detail in which sensation is tested will be governed by the clinical situation. If the patient has no sensory complaints, it is sufficient to examine vibration and position sense in the fingers and toes, to test the appreciation of pain over the face, trunk, and extremities, and to determine whether the sensory findings are the same in symmetric parts of the body. A rough survey of this sort may detect sensory defects of which the patient is unaware. On the other hand, more thorough testing is in order if the patient has complaints referable to the sensory system, or if there is localized atrophy or weakness, ataxia, trophic changes of joints, or painless ulcers.

A few other general principles should be mentioned.

One should not press the sensory examination in the presence of fatigue, for an inattentive patient is a poor witness. When first dealing with a patient, sensory testing is of necessity preceded by a history and often by a general examination; under these circumstances it is best to aim for a quick orientation regarding the whole sensory system and to return to the details when the patient is rested. The examiner must also avoid suggesting symptoms to the patient. After having explained in the simplest terms what is required, he should interpose as few questions and remarks as possible. Consequently, the patient must not be asked, "Do you feel that?" each time he is touched but simply told to say "yes" or "sharp" every time he has been touched or feels pain. The patient should not be permitted to see the part under examination. For short tests it is sufficient that he close his eyes; during more detailed testing it is preferable to screen his eyes from the part being examined. Finally, the findings of the sensory examination should be accurately recorded on a chart.

Sensation is frequently classified as *superficial* (cutaneous, exteroceptive) and *deep* (proprioceptive); the former comprises the modalities of light touch, pain, and temperature; the latter includes the sense of position, passive motion, vibration, and deep pain.

SENSE OF TOUCH. This is usually tested with a wisp of cotton. The patient is first acquainted with the nature of the stimulus by applying it to a normal part of the body. Then he is asked to say "yes" each time various other parts are touched. A patient simulating sensory loss may say "no" in response to a tactile stimulus. Cornified areas of skin, such as the soles and palms, will require a heavier stimulus than normal, and the hair-clad parts a lighter one because of the numerous nerve endings around the follicle. The patient is more sensitive to a moving stimulus of any kind than a stationary one. The application of the examiner's or preferably the patient's finger tips is a useful method of mapping out an area of tactile loss, as Trotter originally showed.

More precise testing is possible by using a von Frey hair. By this method, a stimulus of constant strength can be applied, and the threshold for touch sensation determined.

SENSE OF PAIN. This is most efficiently estimated by pinprick, although it can be evoked by a great diversity of noxious stimuli. The patient must understand that he is to report the degree of sharpness of the pin and not simply the feeling of contact or pressure of the point or even a special sensation due to penetration of the skin. If the pinpricks are applied rapidly, their effects may be summated and excessive pain may result; therefore, they should be delivered not too rapidly, about 1 per sec, and not over the same spot.

It is almost impossible, using an ordinary pin or needle, to apply each stimulus with equal intensity. This difficulty can be largely overcome by the use of an algesimeter, which enables one not only to give constant stimuli but also to grade their intensity and determine threshold values. Even when the pinpricks are of equal intensity, an isolated stimulus may be reported as excessively sharp, apparently because of direct contact with a pain spot.

If an area of diminished or absent sensation is encountered, its boundaries should be demarcated to determine whether it has a segmental or peripheral nerve distribution or whether sensation is lost below a certain level. Such areas are best delineated by proceeding from the region of impaired sensation toward the normal, and the changes may be confirmed by dragging a pin lightly over the skin.

DEEP PRESSURE SENSE. One can estimate this sense simply by pinching or pressing deeply on the tendons and muscles; no special virtue is attached to the traditional and somewhat sadistic use of the testicle for this test. Pain can often be elicited by heavy pressure even when superficial sensation is diminished; conversely, in some diseases, such as tabetic neurosyphilis, the loss of deep pressure sense may be more prominent.

THERMAL SENSE. The proper evaluation of this form of sensation requires attention to certain details of procedure. One may fail consistently to evoke a sensation of hot or cold, if small test objects are used. The perception of thermal stimuli are relatively delayed, especially if the test objects are applied only lightly and momentarily against the skin. At a temperature below 10°C or above 50°C, sensations of cold or warmth become confused with pain. As the temperature of the test object approaches that of the skin, the patient's response will be modified by the temperature of the skin itself.

The following procedure for testing thermal sensation is therefore suggested. The areas of skin to be tested should be exposed for some time before the examination. The test objects should be large, preferably Erlenmeyer flasks containing hot and cold water. Thermometers, which extend into the water through the flask stoppers, indicate the temperature of the water at the moment of testing. At first, extreme degrees of heat and cold (e.g., 10 and 45°C) may be employed to delineate roughly an area of thermal sensory disturbance; the patient will report that the flask feels "less hot" or "less cold" over such an area than over a normal part. If areas of impaired sensation are found, the borders may be accurately determined by moving the flask along the skin from the insensitive to the normal region. The qualitative change should then be quantitated as far as possible by estimating the *differences in temperature* which the patient is able to recognize. The patient is asked to report whether one stimulus is *warmer or colder* than another and whether a given stimulus is warm or cold, since the cooler of the two may be interpreted as warm. The range of temperature difference between the two flasks is gradually narrowed by mixing their contents. A normal person is capable of detecting a difference of 1° when the temperature of the flasks is in the range of 28 to 32°C. In the warm range he should readily recognize differences between 35 and 40°C and in the cold range, between 10 and 20°C. In many older persons and in others with poor peripheral circulation (especially in cold weather), the responses may be modified in an otherwise normal patient.

The sensation of heat or cold depends not only on the temperature of the stimulus but also on the duration of the stimulus and the area over which it is applied. This principle may be employed to detect slight degrees of sensory impairment; the patient may be able to distinguish small differences in temperature when the bottom of the flask is applied for 3 sec but unable to do so if only the side of the flask is applied for 1 sec. Throughout the test procedure, especially when small temperature differences are involved, the area of sensory disturbance should be continually checked against perception in normal parts.

POSTURAL SENSE AND THE APPRECIATION OF PASSIVE MOVEMENT. These modalities are usually lost together, although in any particular case one may be disproportionately affected.

Abnormalities of postural sensation may be revealed in several ways. When the patient extends his arms in front of him and closes his eyes, the affected arm will wander from its original position; if the fingers are spread apart, they may undergo a series of slow-changing postures ("piano-playing" movements, or *pseudoathetosis*). In attempting to touch the tip of the nose with his index finger, the patient may miss the target repeatedly.

The lack of position sense in the legs may be demonstrated by displacing the limb from its original position and asking the patient to point to his large toe. If postural sensation is defective in both legs, the patient will be unable to maintain his balance with feet together and eyes closed (Romberg's sign). This sign should be interpreted with caution. Even a normal person in the Romberg position will sway slightly more with his eyes closed than open. A patient with lack of balance due to motor disorders or cerebellar disease will also sway more if his visual cues are removed. Only if there is a marked discrepancy between the state of balance with eyes open and closed can one confidently state that the patient shows Romberg's sign, i.e., loss of proprioceptive sensation. Mild degrees of unsteadiness in nervous or suggestible patients may be overcome by diverting their attention, e.g., by having them alternately touch the index finger of each hand to their nose while standing with their eyes closed.

The appreciation of passive movement is first tested in the fingers and toes, and the defect, when present, is reflected maximally in these parts. It is important to grasp the digit firmly at the sides opposite the plane of movement; otherwise the pressure applied by the examiner in displacing the digit may allow the patient to identify the direction of movement. This applies to the testing of the more proximal segments of the limb as well. The patient should be instructed to report each movement as "up" or "down" in relation to the previous stationary position. It is useful to demonstrate the test with a large and easily identified movement, but once the idea is clear to the patient, the smallest detectable changes in position should be tested. The range of movement normally appreciated in the digits is said to be as little as 1°. Clinically, however, defective appreciation of passive movement is judged by comparison with a normal limb or,

if bilaterally defective, on the basis of what the examiner has through experience learned to regard as normal. Slight impairment may be disclosed by a slow response or, if the digit is displaced very slowly, by a relative unawareness that movements have occurred; or after the digit has been displaced in the same direction several times, the patient may misjudge the first movement in the opposite direction; or after the examiner has moved the toe, the patient may make a number of small voluntary movements of the toe, in an apparent attempt to determine its position or the direction of movement.

THE SENSE OF VIBRATION. This is a composite sensation comprising touch and rapid alterations of deep pressure sense. Its conduction depends on both cutaneous and deep afferent fibers, which ascend in the dorsal columns of the cord. It is therefore rarely affected by lesions of single nerves but will be disturbed in cases of polyneuritis and disease of the dorsal columns, medial lemniscus, and thalamus. For this reason, vibration and position sense are usually lost together, although one of them (usually vibration sense) may be affected disproportionately. With advancing age, vibration sense may be diminished at the toes and ankles.

Vibration sense is tested by placing a tuning fork with a low rate of vibration (128 d.v.) over the bony prominences. The examiner must make sure that the patient responds to the vibration and not simply to the pressure of the fork. Although there are mechanical devices to quantitate vibration sense, it is sufficient for clinical purposes to compare the point tested with a normal part of the patient or of the examiner. A 256-d.v. fork can be used for finer testing. The level of vibration-sense loss due to spinal lesions can be estimated by placing the fork over successive vertebral spines.

DISCRIMINATIVE SENSORY FUNCTIONS. Damage to the sensory cortex or to the sensory projections from thalamus to cortex results in a special type of disturbance that affects mainly the patient's ability to make sensory discriminations. Lesions in these structures may disturb postural sense but leave the so-called "primary modalities" (touch, pain, temperature, and vibration sense) relatively little affected. In such a situation, or if a cerebral lesion is suspected on other grounds, discriminative function should be tested further by the following tests.

Two-point Discrimination. The ability to distinguish two points from one is tested by using a compass, the points of which should be blunt and applied simultaneously and painlessly. The distance at which such a stimulus can be recognized as double varies greatly; 1 mm at the tip of the tongue, 3 to 6 mm at the finger tips, 1.5 to 2 cm on the palms and soles, 3 cm on the dorsa of the hands and feet, and 4 to 7 cm on the body surface. It is characteristic of the patient with a lesion of the sensory cortex to mistake two points for one, although occasionally the opposite occurs.

Cutaneous Localization and Number Writing. The ability to localize cutaneous stimuli is tested by touching various parts of the patient's body and asking him to point to the part touched or to the corresponding part on the examiner's limb. Recognition of *number writing*, or of the direction of lines drawn on the skin, also depends on localization of tactile stimuli.

Appreciation of Texture, Size, and Shape. Appreciation of *texture* depends mainly on cutaneous impressions, but the recognition of *shape and size* of objects is based on impressions from deeper receptors as well. The lack of recognition of shape and form, therefore, though frequently found with cortical lesions, may also be present with lesions of the spinal cord and brainstem due to interruption of tracts transmitting postural and tactile sensation. Such a sensory defect, called *stereoanesthesia,* should be distinguished from *astereognosis,* which connotes an inability to identify an object by palpation, the primary sense data being intact. The latter defect is essentially a tactile agnosia and is associated with lesions lying posterior to the postcentral gyrus in the dominant hemisphere. In practice, a pure astereognosis is rarely encountered, and the term is employed where the impairment of tactile and joint sense is of insufficient severity to account for the defect in recognition.

Extinction of Sensory Stimuli and Sensory Inattention. In response to bilateral simultaneous testing of symmetric parts, the patient may acknowledge only the stimulus on the sound side, or he may improperly localize the stimulus on the affected side, whereas stimuli applied to each side separately are properly appreciated. This phenomenon of *extinction* or cortical *inattention* is characteristic of parietal lobe lesions, the symptomatology of which is considered in Chap. 31.

A few other terms require definition, since they may be encountered in reading about sensation. Most of them are pedantic, and it is recommended that the simplest terms possible be used. *Anesthesia* refers to a loss and *hypesthesia* to a diminution of all forms of sensation. Loss or impairment of specific cutaneous sensations is indicated by an appropriate prefix or suffix, e.g., *thermoanesthesia* or *thermohypesthesia, analgesia* (loss of pain) or *hypalgesia, tactile anesthesia* (loss of sense of touch), and *pallanesthesia* (loss of vibratory sense). The term *hyperesthesia* requires special mention; although it implies a heightened receptiveness of the nervous system, careful testing will usually demonstrate an underlying sensory defect, i.e., an elevated threshold to tactile, painful, or thermal stimuli; once the stimulus is perceived, however, it may have a severely painful or unpleasant quality (*hyperpathia*).

SENSORY SYNDROMES

SENSORY CHANGES DUE TO INTERRUPTION OF A SINGLE PERIPHERAL NERVE

These changes will vary with the composition of the nerve involved, depending on whether it is predominantly muscular, cutaneous, or mixed. Since proprioceptive fibers run for at least a portion of their course with the muscular (mainly motor) nerves, and cutaneous sensibility is carried in sensory nerves, each of these sensory systems may be affected separately. In lesions of cutaneous nerves, it is said that the area of tactile anesthesia is more extensive than the one for pain due to greater overlapping of pain fibers.

Because of overlap from adjacent nerves, the area of sensory loss following division of a cutaneous nerve is always less than its anatomic distribution. If a large area of skin is involved, the sensory defect characteristically consists of a central portion, in which all forms of cutaneous sensation are lost, surrounded by a zone of partial loss, which becomes less marked as one proceeds from the center to the periphery. The sense of deep pressure and passive movement is intact because it is carried by muscular nerves. Along the margin of the hypesthetic zone the skin becomes excessively sensitive. A light contact may be felt as a smarting, mildly painful sensation. According to Weddell, this is due to collateral regeneration from surrounding healthy nerves into the denervated region (see Chap. 9).

In lesions involving the brachial and lumbosacral plexuses, the sensory disturbance is no longer confined to the territory of a single nerve and is accompanied by muscle weakness and reflex change.

SENSORY CHANGES DUE TO MULTIPLE NERVE INVOLVEMENT (POLYNEUROPATHY)

In most instances of polyneuropathy the sensory changes are accompanied by varying degrees of motor and reflex loss. Usually the sensory impairment is symmetric, with notable exceptions in some instances of diabetic and periarteritic neuropathy. Since the longest and largest fibers are most affected, the sensory loss is most severe over the feet and legs and less severe over the hands. The abdomen, thorax, and face are spared except in the most severe cases. The sensory loss usually involves all the modalities, and although it is manifestly difficult to equate the impairment of pain, touch, temperature, vibration, and position sense, one of these may seemingly be impaired out of proportion to the others. One cannot accurately predict, from the patient's symptoms, which mode of sensation will be disproportionately affected. The term *glove-and-stocking anesthesia* is frequently employed to describe the sensory loss of polyneuropathy and draws attention to the predominantly distal pattern of involvement. It is an inaccurate term insofar as the border between normal and impaired sensation is not sharp; the sensory loss shades off gradually, and the transition to normal sensation occurs over a variable vertical extent of the limb. In hysteria, by contrast, the border between normal and absent sensation is usually sharp.

SENSORY CHANGES DUE TO INVOLVEMENT OF MULTIPLE SPINAL NERVE ROOTS

Because of considerable overlap from adjacent roots, division of a single sensory root does not produce complete loss of sensation in any area of skin. Compression of a single sensory cervical or lumbar root (in herniated intervertebral disks, for example) causes varying degrees of impairment of cutaneous sensation, however. When two or more roots have been completely divided, a segmental zone of sensory loss can be found in which reduction of pain perception is greater in extent than touch. Surrounding the area of complete loss is a narrow zone of partial loss, in which a raised threshold accompanied by overreaction (*hyperesthesia*) may or may not be demonstrated. The presence of muscle paralysis, atrophy, and reflex loss indicates involvement of ventral roots as well.

THE TABETIC SYNDROME. This results from damage to the large proprioceptive fibers of the posterior lumbosacral roots. It is usually caused by neurosyphilis, less often by diabetic or other types of neuropathy. Numbness or paresthesias and lightning pains are frequent complaints, and areflexia, atonicity of the bladder, abnormalities of gait (Chap. 23), and hypotonia without muscle weakness are found on examination. The sensory loss may consist only of loss of vibration and position sense in the lower extremities, but in severe cases, loss or impairment of superficial or deep pain sense or of touch may be added. The feet and legs are most affected, much less often the arms and trunk.

COMPLETE SPINAL SENSORY SYNDROMES. In a complete transverse lesion of the spinal cord, all forms of sensation are abolished below a level that corresponds with the lesion. There may be a narrow zone of "hyperesthesia" at the upper margin of the anesthetic zone. It is important to remember that during the evolution of such a lesion there may be a discrepancy between the level of the lesion and that of the sensory loss, the latter ascending as the lesion progresses. This can be understood if one conceives of a lesion evolving from the periphery to the center of the cord, affecting first the outermost fibers carrying pain and temperature sensation from the legs. Conversely, a lesion advancing from the center of the cord may affect these modalities in the reverse order.

PARTIAL SPINAL SENSORY SYNDROMES. Hemisection of the Spinal Cord (Brown-Séquard Syndrome). In rare instances disease is confined to one side of the spinal cord; pain and heat sensation are affected on the opposite side, and proprioceptive sensation, on the same side as the lesion. The loss of pain and temperature sensation begins two or three segments below the lesion. An associated motor paralysis on the side of the lesion completes the syndrome. Tactile sensation is not involved, since the fibers from one side of the body are distributed in tracts (posterior columns and anterior spinothalamic) on both sides of the cord.

LESIONS OF THE CENTRAL GRAY MATTER (SYRINGO-MYELIC SYNDROME). Since fibers conducting pain and temperature cross the cord in the anterior commissure, a lesion in this location will characteristically abolish these modalities on one or both sides but will spare tactile sensation. The commonest cause of such a lesion is syringomyelia, less often, tumor and hemorrhage. This type of dissociated sensory loss usually occurs in a segmental distribution, and since the lesion frequently involves other parts of the gray matter, varying degrees of segmental amyotrophy and reflex loss may be added. If the lesion has spread to the white matter, corticospinal and posterior column signs will be present as well.

POSTERIOR COLUMN SYNDROME. There is loss of vibratory and position sense below the lesion, but the sense of pain, temperature, and touch are affected relatively little or not at all. This lesion may be difficult to distinguish from an affection of large fibers in sensory roots (tabetic syndrome). In some diseases vibratory sensation may be involved predominantly whereas in others position sense is more affected. It should be stressed that an interruption of proprioceptive fibers may interfere with discriminative sensory function, such as two-point discrimination and recognition of size, shape, and weight, and that impairment of this function may occur with posterior column disease alone. Paresthesias in the form of tingling and "pins-and-needles" sensations or girdle sensations are a common complaint with posterior column disease, and pain stimuli may also produce unpleasant sensations.

THE ANTERIOR SPINAL ARTERY SYNDROME. With occlusion of the anterior spinal artery or other destructive lesions that predominantly affect the ventral portion of the cord, there is a relative or absolute sparing of proprioceptive sensation and loss of pain and temperature sensation below the level of the lesion. Since the corticospinal tracts and the ventral gray matter also fall within the area of distribution of the anterior spinal artery, paralysis of motor function forms a prominent part of this syndrome.

DISTURBANCES OF SENSATION DUE TO LESIONS OF THE BRAINSTEM. A characteristic feature of lesions of the medulla and lower pons is that in many instances the sensory disturbance is crossed, i.e., there is loss of pain and temperature sensation of one side of the face and of the opposite side of the body. This is accounted for by involvement of the trigeminal tract or nucleus and the lateral spinothalamic tract on one side of the brainstem. In the upper pons and midbrain, where the spinothalamic tracts and the medial lemniscus become confluent, an appropriately placed lesion may cause a loss of all superficial and deep sensation over the contralateral side of the body. Cranial nerve palsies, cerebellar ataxia, or motor paralysis are often associated, as indicated in Chaps. 355 and 357.

SENSORY LOSS DUE TO A LESION OF THE THALAMUS (SYNDROME OF DEJÉRINE-ROUSSY)

Involvement of the nucleus ventralis posterolateralis of the thalamus, usually due to a vascular lesion or tumor, causes loss or diminution of all forms of sensation on the opposite side of the body. Position sense is affected more frequently than any other sensory function, and deep sensory loss is usually, but not always, more profound than cutaneous loss. There may be spontaneous pain or discomfort ("thalamic pain"), sometimes of the most torturing and disabling type, on the affected side, and any form of stimulus may have a diffuse, unpleasant, lingering quality. Emotional disturbance also aggravates the painful state. This overresponse is usually associated with an elevated threshold; i.e., a stronger stimulus is necessary to produce a sensation, in spite of the greater discomfort experienced by the patient once the sensation had been evoked. The thalamic pain syndrome may occasionally accompany lesions of the white matter of the parietal lobe.

SENSORY LOSS DUE TO LESIONS IN THE PARIETAL LOBE

There is a disturbance mainly of discriminative sensory functions on the opposite side of the body, particularly the face, arm, and leg. Loss of position sense, impaired ability to localize touch and pain stimuli, elevation of two-point threshold, a general inattentiveness to sensory stimuli on one side of the body, and astereognosis (if the lesion is in the dominant hemisphere) are the most prominent findings. It is generally taught that the primary modalities of sensation (pain and temperature, touch and vibratory sense) are not affected by lesions which are confined to the cerebral cortex, but this statement requires modification. In acute, deep parietal lesions the primary modalities may be abolished, and as was said, it may be followed by the "thalamic pain syndrome," but usually the impairment takes a different form from that due to thalamic lesions. Thus, with cortical lesions, one examination may disclose no sensory abnormalities, whereas the patient's responses may be inconstant and irregular on the next examination. This type of response is often attributed to hysteria. Other features of parietal lobe symptomatology and the differences between dominant and nondominant parietal lobe syndromes will be considered in Chap. 30.

SENSORY LOSS DUE TO SUGGESTION AND HYSTERIA

The possibility of suggesting sensory loss to a patient has already been mentioned. In fact, hysterical patients almost never complain spontaneously of cutaneous sensory loss, although they may use the term *numbness* to indicate a paralysis of a limb. Complete hemianesthesia, often with reduced hearing, sight, smell, and taste, as well as impaired vibration sense over only half the skull, is a common finding in hysteria. Anesthesia of one entire limb or a sharply defined sensory loss over part of a limb, not conforming to the distribution of root or cutaneous nerve, is also frequently observed. Postural sensation is rarely affected. The diagnosis of hysterical hemianesthesia is best made by eliciting the other relevant symptoms of hysteria or, if this is not possible, by noting the discrepancies between this type of sensory loss and that which occurs as part of the usual sensory syndromes.

REFERENCES

Holmes, Gordon: "Introduction to Clinical Neurology," 2d ed., chaps. 8 and 9, Baltimore, The Williams & Wilkins Company, 1952.

Kibler, R. F., and P. W. Nathan: A Note on Warm and Cold Spots, Neurology, 10:874, 1960.

Mayo Clinic: "Clinical Examinations in Neurology," 2d ed., Philadelphia, W. B. Saunders Company, 1963.

Oppenheimer, D. R., E. Palmer, and G. Weddell: Nerve Endings in the Conjunctiva, J. Anat., 92:322, 1958.

Melzack, R., and P. Wall: Pain Mechanisms: A New Theory. Science, 150:971, 1965.

Mountcastle, V. B.: Central Nervous Mechanisms in Sensation. Chaps. 61, 62, and 63 in Medical Physiology, V. B.

Mountcastle (Ed.), 12th ed., vol. 2, pp. 1345–1464, St. Louis, The C. V. Mosby Company, 1968.

26 COMA AND RELATED DISTURBANCES OF CONSCIOUSNESS

Raymond D. Adams

The practitioner of medicine is frequently called upon to treat patients whose principal abnormality is an impairment of consciousness, which varies from inattentiveness and simple confusion to coma. In large municipal hospitals it is estimated that as many as 3 percent of total admissions are due to diseases that have caused coma, and although this figure seems high, it serves to emphasize the importance of this class of neurologic diseases and the necessity for every student of medicine to acquire a theoretic as well as a practical knowledge of them.

The terms *consciousness, confusion, stupor, unconsciousness,* and *coma* have been endowed with so many different meanings that it is almost impossible to avoid ambiguity in their usage. They are not strictly medical terms, but literary, philosophic, and psychologic ones as well. The word *consciousness* is the most difficult of all. William James once remarked that everyone knew what consciousness was until he attempted to define it. To the psychologist consciousness denotes a state of awareness of one's self and one's environment. Knowledge of one's self, of course, includes all "feelings, attitudes and emotions, impulses, volitions, and the active or striving aspects of conduct" (English)—in short, an awareness of all one's own mental functioning, particularly the cognitive processes. These can be judged only by the patient's verbal account of his introspections and, indirectly, by his actions. Physicians, being practical men for the most part, have learned to place greater confidence in their observations of the patient's general behavior and his reactions to overt stimuli than in what he says. For this reason when they employ the term *consciousness,* they usually do so in its commonest and simplest signification, namely, a state of awareness of the environment. This narrow definition has another advantage in that the word *unconsciousness* is its exact opposite—a state of unawareness of environment or a suspension of those mental activities by which man is made aware of his environment. To add to the ambiguity, psychoanalysts have given the word *unconscious* a still different meaning; for them it stands for repository of impulses and memories of previous experiences that cannot be immediately recalled to the conscious mind.

DESCRIPTION OF STATES OF NORMAL AND IMPAIRED CONSCIOUSNESS

The following definitions, while admittedly unacceptable to most psychologists, are of service to medicine, and they will provide the student with a convenient terminology for describing the mental states of his patients.

NORMAL CONSCIOUSNESS. This is the condition of the normal individual when fully awake, in which he is responsive to psychologic stimuli and "indicates by his behavior and speech that he has the same awareness of himself and his environment as ourselves." This normal state may fluctuate during the course of the day from keen alertness or deep concentration with a marked constriction of the field of attention to general inattentiveness and drowsiness.

SLEEP. Sleep is a state of physical and mental inactivity from which the patient may be aroused to normal consciousness. A person in sleep gives little evidence of being aware of himself or his environment, and in this respect he is unconscious. Yet he differs from a comatose patient in that he may still respond to unaccustomed stimuli and at times is capable of some mental activity in the form of dreams, which leave their traces in memory. And, of course, he can be recalled to a state of normal consciousness when stimulated.

INATTENTIVE, CONFUSIONAL, AND CLOUDY STATES OF CONSCIOUSNESS. In these conditions the patient does not take into account all elements of his immediate environment. Like delirium, these states always imply an element of sensorial clouding or imperceptiveness. The term *confusional* lacks precision, for often it signifies an inability to think with customary speed and coherence. Here the difficulty is in defining thinking.

An inattentive, severely confused person is usually unable to do more than carry out a few simple commands. His capacity for speech may be limited to a few words or phrases, or he may be voluble. He is unaware of much that goes on around him and does not grasp his immediate situation. A moderately confused individual can carry on a simple conversation for short periods of time, but his thinking is slow and incoherent, and he is unable to stay with one topic. Often he is disoriented in time and place. In mild degrees of confusion the disorder may be so slight that it is overlooked unless the examiner is searching in his analysis of the patient's behavior and conversation. The patient may even be roughly oriented as to time and place and able to speak freely on almost any subject. Only occasional irrelevant remarks betray an incoherence of thinking. Patients with mild or moderately severe confusion may be subjected to psychologic testing. The degree of confusion often varies from one time of day to another and tends to be least pronounced in the early morning. Severe confusion or stupor may resemble semicoma during periods when the patient is drowsy or asleep. Many events that happen to the confused patient leave no trace in his memory; in fact, capacity to recall later events that transpired in any given period is one of the most delicate tests of mental clarity. However, careful analysis will show the defect to be one of inadequate registration and fixation of items rather than a fault in retentive memory.

Some neurologists regard *delirium* as a state of confusion with excitement and hyperactivity, and in some medical writings the terms *delirium* and *confused-cloudy*

states are used interchangeably. It is undoubtedly true that the delirious patient is nearly always confused. However, the vivid hallucinations which characterize delirious states, the relative inaccessibility of the patient to other events than those to which he is reacting at any one moment, his extreme agitation and tremulousness, and the tendency to convulse suggest a cerebral disorder of a somewhat different type. The clearest evidence of the relationship of inattention, confusion, stupor, and coma is that the patient may pass through all these states as he becomes comatose or emerges from coma. The author has not observed any such relationship between coma and delirium. These distinctions are drawn with greater clarity in Chap. 30.

At times a patient with certain types of aphasia, especially jargon aphasia, may create the impression of confusion, but close observation will reveal that the disorder is confined to the sphere of language and that behavior is otherwise natural.

STUPOR. In stupor mental and physical activity are reduced to a minimum. Although inaccessible to many stimuli, the patient opens his eyes, looks at the examiner, and does not appear to be unconscious. Response to spoken commands is either absent or slow and inadequate. As a rule tendon or plantar reflexes are not altered. On the other hand, tremulousness of movement, coarse twitching of muscles, restless or stereotyped motor activity, and grasping and sucking reflexes are not infrequent, depending on the way in which disease affects the nervous system. In psychiatry the term *stupor* means a state in which impressions of the external world are normally received, but activity is suspended or marked by negativisim, e.g., catatonic schizophrenia.

COMA. The patient who appears to be asleep and is at the same time incapable of sensing or responding adequately to either external stimuli or inner needs is in a state of coma. Coma may vary in degree, and in its deepest stages no reaction of any kind is obtainable. Corneal, pupillary, pharyngeal, tendon, and plantar reflexes are all absent. With lesser degrees of it pupillary reflexes and ocular movements and other brainstem reflexes are preserved, and there may or may not be extensor rigidity of the limbs and opisthotonos, signs which, as Sherrington showed, indicate decerebration. Respirations are often slow or rapid and may be periodic, i.e., Cheyne-Stokes breathing. In still lighter stages, referred to as *semicoma*, most of the above reflexes can be elicited, and the plantar reflexes may be either flexor or extensor (Babinski's sign). Moreover, pricking or pinching the skin, shaking and shouting at the patient, or an uncomfortable distension of the bladder may cause the patient to stir or moan and his respirations to quicken.

THE ELECTROENCEPHALOGRAM AND DISTURBANCES OF CONSCIOUSNESS

One of the most delicate confirmations of the fact that these states of altered consciousness are expressions of neurophysiologic changes is the electroencephalogram. In the normal waking state the electrical potentials of the cortical neurones are integrated into regular waves of two frequency ranges, from 8 to 15 (alpha rhythm) and 16 to 25 (beta rhythm). These wave forms are established by adolescence, but certain individual differences in general pattern and dominance of alpha waves are maintained throughout adult life. With sleep these cortical potentials slow down and amplitude (voltage) of the individual waves increases. At one stage in light sleep characteristic bursts of 14 to 16 per sec waves appear, the so-called "sleep spindles," and in deep sleep all the waves of normal frequency and amplitude are replaced by slow ones of high voltage (1¼ to 3 per sec). Similarly, some alteration in brain waves occurs in all disturbances of consciousness except the milder degrees of confusion. This alteration usually consists of a disorganization of the electroencephalographic pattern, which shows random, slow waves of high voltage in stages of confusion; more regular, slow, 2 to 3 per sec waves of high voltage in stupor and semicoma; and slow waves or even suppression of all organized electrical activity (isoelectric state) in the deep coma of hypoxia and ischemia, the so-called "brain death syndrome" (see Chap. 363). The electroencephalograms of deep sleep and light coma resemble one another. However, not all diseases that cause confusion and coma have the same effect on the electroencephalogram. Some, such as barbiturate intoxication, may cause an increase in frequency and amplitude of the brain waves. In epilepsy the disturbance of consciousness is usually attended by paroxysms of "spikes" (fast waves of high amplitude) or by the characteristic alternating slow waves and spikes of petit mal. Other diseases, such as hepatic coma, characteristically cause a slowing in frequency and an increasing amplitude of "brain waves" and special triphasic waves. Whether all metabolic diseases of the brain induce similar changes in the electroencephalogram has not been determined. Probably there are differences between them, some of which may be significant (see Chap. 353).

MORBID ANATOMY AND PHYSIOLOGY OF COMA

In recent times there has been some clarification and amplification of earlier neuropathologic observations that the smallest lesions associated with protracted coma are always to be found in the midbrain and thalamus. The essence of more recent neurophysiologic studies, to be found in the writings of Bremer, of Morison and Dempsey, and of Moruzzi and Magoun, is that an ascending series of destructive lesions of spinal cord, medulla, pons, and cerebellum have no effect on the state of consciousness until the level of midbrain and diencephalon (thalamus) is reached. High brainstem transections invariably induce states of prolonged unresponsiveness, whereas stimulation of the upper brainstem reticular formation causes a drowsy or sleeping animal to suddenly become alert and his EEG to change correspondingly. As anesthetic agents abolish consciousness, they are found to suppress the activity of the upper reticular activating system, without interfering, at least at certain levels, with the transmission of specific sensory impulses.

Anatomic studies show the reticular activating system of the upper brainstem to receive collaterals from the specific sensory pathways and to project, not just to the sensory cortex of the parietal lobe, as do the thalamic relay nuclei for somatic sensation, but to the whole of the cerebral cortex. The latter has corticofugal connections which feed back nerve impulses to the reticular formation. Sensory stimulation, it would seem, then, has the double effect of conveying to the brain information about the outside world but also of providing some of the energy for activating those parts of the nervous system on which consciousness depends.

These new data are in line with the older ideas of Herbert Spencer and Hughlings Jackson—that the diencephalon and cerebral cortex always function together as a unit and represent the highest levels of integrative nervous activity, called by Penfield *centrencephalic*. While anatomic details have yet to be worked out and the precise physiology of the reticular activating system leaves much to be desired, being more complicated than this simple formulation would suggest, nevertheless, as a working idea it will make some of the following neuropathologic observations more comprehensible.

The study of a large series of human cases in which coma has preceded death by several days will bring to light two major types of lesion. In the first group a macroscopically visible lesion such as a tumor, abscess, intracerebral, subarachnoid, subdural, or epidural hemorrhage, massive infarct, or meningitis is demonstrable; usually the lesion involves a portion only of the cortex and white matter, leaving much of the cerebrum intact. Rarely, it is located in the thalamus or midbrain, which would make the coma understandable. But in the other instances the coma will always be related to a temporal lobe–tentorial herniation with compression, ischemia, and secondary hemorrhage in the midbrain and lower thalamus or with downward displacement of the brainstem. A detailed clinical record will show the coma to have coincided with these secondary displacements and herniations. Exceptionally, a widespread bilateral damage to the cortex and subcortical white matter will be found—the result of bilateral infarcts or hemorrhages, viral encephalitis, hypoxia, or ischemia—without thalamic or midbrain lesions. In the second group (and this is larger than the first) with no visible lesion seen by the naked eye, often no abnormality is divulged by any technique of pathology. The lesion, here caused by a metabolic or toxic state, is subcellular or molecular. In some instances the grossly normal brain will reveal a demonstrable cellular change under the light microscope which may be characteristic, e.g., hepatic coma. Usually the microscopic lesions are too diffuse for clinico-anatomic correlation. Thus, pathologic changes are compatible with physiologic deductions that the state of prolonged coma correlates with lesions of all parts of the cortical-diencephalic systems of neurones, but it is only in the upper brainstem where they may be small and discrete.

MECHANISMS WHEREBY CONSCIOUSNESS IS DISTURBED IN DISEASE

Knowledge of diseases of the nervous system is so limited that it is not possible to identify all the different mechanisms by means of which consciousness is disturbed. Already several ways in which the mesencephalic-diencephalic-cortical systems are deranged have been identified; there are probably many others.

In a number of disease processes there is direct interference with the metabolic activities of the nerve cells in the cerebral cortex and the central cerebral nuclear masses of the brain. Hypoxia, hypoglycemia, hyper- and hypoosmolar states, acidosis, alkalosis, hyper- and hypokalemia, hyperammonemia, and deficiencies of thiamine, nicotinic acid, vitamin B_{12}, pantothenic acid, and pyridoxine are well-known examples. The intimate details of these underlying biochemical changes have not yet been fully elucidated, but methods are becoming available for their study. The rate of cerebral blood flow can now be determined in human beings with considerable accuracy (Schmidt-Kety method) by measuring the rate of diffusion of inert gases such as N_2O or krypton into the brain, namely, the time required for the gas to reach the same degree of concentration in the jugular venous blood as in arterial blood after a 10-min inhalation of the gas. The normal value of cerebral blood flow (CBF) is 700 to 800 ml per min. The cerebral metabolic rate (CMR — oxygen consumption per minute) can be determined at the same time by measuring the oxygen difference between arterial and jugular blood and multiplying this difference by the rate of cerebral blood flow. Glucose and other nutrients and metabolites can be measured as they enter and leave the brain. Microchemical tests can be done on brain tissues and cerebrospinal fluid (CSF). Normally the brain consumes 3.3 ml O_2 per 100 Gm brain per minute. The relevant point for our discussion is that cerebral metabolism or blood flow are reduced in all the metabolic disorders leading to coma. Oxygen values of below 2.0 ml per 100 Gm are incompatible with an alert state. In hypoglycemia the cerebral blood flow is normal or above normal, whereas the cerebral metabolic rate is diminished, owing to deficiency of substrate. In thiamine and vitamin B_{12} deficiency the cerebral blood flow is normal or slightly diminished, and the cerebral metabolic rate is diminished, presumably because of insufficiency of coenzymes. Extremes of body temperature, either hyperthermia (temperature over 106°F) or hypothermia (temperature below 97°F), probably induce coma by exerting a nonspecific effect on the metabolic activity of neurones.

Diabetic acidosis, uremia, hepatic coma, and the coma of systemic infections are examples of endogenous intoxications. The identity of the toxic agents is not entirely known. In diabetes acetone bodies (acetoacetic acid, β-hydroxybutyric acid, and acetone) are present in high concentration, and in uremia there is probably accumulation of dialyzable toxin, perhaps phenolic derivatives of the aromatic amino acids. In both conditions "dehydration" and serum acidosis may also play an important role. In many cases of hepatic coma, elevation of blood NH_3 to levels five to six times normal has been found. Lactic acidemia and other organic acids may affect the brain by lowering its pH to less than 7.3. The mode of action of bacterial toxins is unknown. In all these conditions the cerebral metabolic rate tends to be reduced, whereas cerebral blood flow remains normal. In water intoxication the membrane excitability of nerve cells is altered by hyponatremia and changes in intracellular K levels.

Drugs such as barbiturates, bromides, dilantin, alcohol, glutethimide and phenothiazines induce coma by their direct suppressive effect on the neurones of the cerebrum and diencephalon. Others such as methyl alcohol, ethylene glycol, and paraldehyde result in metabolic acidosis. Many additional pharmacologic agents have no direct action on the nervous system but lead to coma through the mechanism of circulatory collapse and inadequate cerebral circulation. In toxic and metabolic diseases, although the patient usually approaches coma through a state of drowsiness, confusion, and stupor, and the reverse sequence occurs as he emerges from it, each disease has its special effects manifesting itself by a characteristic clinical picture. This means that the mechanism and topography of the lesion will be different.

A critical decline in blood pressure, usually to a systolic level below 70 mm Hg, affects neural structures by causing a decrease in cerebral blood flow and, secondarily, a diminution in cerebral metabolic rate. If decline in blood pressure is episodic, the corresponding clinical picture is syncope (see Chap. 20). Here the clinical picture is one of physical weakness usually preceding and following the loss of consciousness, the whole process being acute and promptly reversible.

The sudden, violent, and excessive discharge of *epilepsy* is another mechanism. Usually a Jacksonian convulsion has little effect on consciousness until it spreads from one side of the body to the other. Coma immediately ensues, presumably because the spreading of the seizure discharge to central neuronal structures paralyzes their function. Other types of seizure in which consciousness is interrupted from the very beginning are believed to originate in the diencephalon.

Concussion exemplifies still another special pathophysiologic mechanism. In "blunt" head injury it has been shown that there is an enormous increase in intracranial pressure of the order of 200 to 700 lb per sq in., lasting a few thousandths of a second. Either the vibration set up in the skull and transmitted to the brain or this sudden high intracranial pressure is believed to be the basis of the abrupt paralysis of the nervous system that follows head injury. That the increased pressure itself may be the main factor has been suggested by experiments in which raising the intraventricular pressure to a level approaching diastolic blood pressure has abolished all vital functions.

As was pointed out above, large, destructive, and space-consuming lesions of the brain, such as hemorrhage, tumor, or abscess, interfere with consciousness in two ways. One is by direct destruction of the midbrain and diencephalon; the other, far more frequent, is by producing herniation of the medial part of the temporal lobe through the opening of the tentorium and crushing the upper brain against the opposite free edge of the tentorium. Here the mechanism is again mechanical and probably circulatory.

CLINICAL APPROACH TO THE COMATOSE PATIENT

Coma is not an independent disease entity but is always a symptomatic expression of disease. Sometimes the underlying disease is perfectly obvious, as when a healthy individual is struck on the head and rendered unconscious. All too often, however, the patient is brought to the hospital in a state of coma, and little or no information about him is immediately available. The physician must then subject the clinical problem to careful scrutiny from many directions. To do this efficiently, he must have a broad knowledge of disease and a methodical approach to the problem that leaves none of the common and treatable causes of coma unexplored.

It should be pointed out that when the comatose patient is seen for the first time, simple therapeutic measures take precedence over diagnostic procedures. A quick survey should make sure that the comatose patient has a clear airway and is not in shock (circulatory collapse) or, if trauma has occurred, that he is not bleeding from a wound. In patients who have suffered a head injury there may be a fracture of the cervical vertebrae, and therefore one must be cautious about moving the head and neck lest the spinal cord be inadvertently crushed. There must be an immediate inquiry as to the previous health of the patient: whether the patient had suffered a head injury or had been seen in a convulsion, and the circumstances in which he was found. The persons who accompany the comatose patient to the hospital should not be permitted to leave until they have been questioned.

DIAGNOSIS. The temperature, pulse, respiratory rate, and blood pressure are of aid in diagnosis. Fever suggests a severe systemic infection such as pneumonia, bacterial meningitis, or a brain lesion that has disturbed the temperature-regulating centers. An excessively high body temperature, 107 to 110°F, associated with dry skin should arouse the suspicion of heat stroke. Hypothermia is frequently observed in alcoholic or barbiturate intoxication, extracellular fluid deficit, peripheral circulatory failure or myxedema. Slow breathing points to morphine, barbiturate intoxication, or hypothyroidism, whereas deep, rapid breathing suggests pneumonia but may occur in diabetic or uremic acidosis (Kussmaul's respiration) or with intracranial diseases as a central neurogenic hyperpnea. The rapid breathing of pneumonia is often accompanied by an expiratory grunt, cyanosis, and fever. Diseases that elevate the intracranial pressure or damage the brain, especially the brainstem, often cause slow, irregular, or periodic (Cheyne-Stokes) breathing. The pulse rate is less helpful, but if exceptionally slow, it should suggest heart block or, if combined with periodic breathing and hypertension, an increase in intracranial pressure. A tachycardia of 160 or above calls attention to the possibility of an ectopic cardiac rhythm with insufficiency of cerebral circulation. Marked hypertension occurs in patients with cerebral hemorrhage and hypertensive encephalopathy and, at times, those with increased intracranial pressure; whereas hypotension is the usual finding in the coma of diabetes, alcohol or barbiturate intoxication, or internal hemorrhage, myocardial infarction, dissecting aortic aneurysm, gram-negative bacillary septicemia, and Addison's disease.

Inspection of the skin may also yield valuable information. Cyanosis of the lips and nail beds means inadequate oxygenation. Cherry-red coloration indicates carbon monoxide poisoning. Multiple bruises, and in particular a bruise or boggy area in the scalp, favor cranial trauma. Bleeding from an ear or nose or orbital hemorrhage also raises the possibility of trauma. Puffiness and hyperemia of face and conjunctivas and telangiectasia are the usual stigmas of alcoholism; marked pallor suggests internal hemorrhage. The presence of a maculo-hemorrhagic rash indicates the possibility of meningococcal infection, staphylococcus endocarditis, typhus, or Rocky Mountain spotted fever. Pellagra may be diagnosed from the typical skin lesions on face and hands. The face may be myxedematous. In pituitary hypoadrenalism the skin is sallow. Excessive sweating suggests hypoglycemia or shock, and dry skin, diabetic acidosis and uremia. Skin turgor is reduced in dehydration. Hemorrhagic blisters will have formed over pressure points if the patient has been motionless for a time.

The odor of the breath may provide clues to the nature of a disease causing coma. The odor of alcohol is easily recognized (Vodka is odorless). The spoiled-fruit odor of diabetic coma, the uriniferous odor of uremia, and the musty fetor of hepatic coma are distinctive enough to be identified by physicians who possess a keen sense of smell.

The next step in the physical examination should give special attention to the status of the nervous system. Although the examination is limited in many ways, careful observation of the stuporous or comatose patient may yield considerable information concerning the function of different parts of the nervous system. One of the most helpful procedures is to sit at the patient's bedside for 5 to 10 min and observe what he does. The predominant postures of the body, the position of the head and eyes, the rate, depth, and rhythm of respiration, and the pulse should be noted. The state of responsiveness should then be estimated by noting the patient's reaction when his name is called and his capacity to execute a simple command or to respond to painful stimuli. The most effective painful stimuli are supraorbital pressure, sternoid pressure, or pinching the side of the neck or inner parts of the upper arms or thighs. By grading these stimuli, one may titrate the response, so to speak, and evaluate both the degree of coma and changes from hour to hour in the course of the disease. Vocalization may persist in stupor and light coma and is the first response to be lost. Deft avoidance movements of parts stimulated, and grimacing are preserved in light coma and substantiate the integrity of corticomedullary and corticospinal tracts.

Usually it is possible to determine whether or not the coma is accompanied by meningeal irritation or focal disease in the cerebrum or brainstem. With meningeal irritation from either bacterial meningitis or subarachnoid hemorrhage, there is resistance to active and passive flexion of the neck but not to extension, turning, or tipping the head. Resistance to movement of the neck in all directions indicates disease of the cervical spine or is part of generalized rigidity. In infants, bulging of the anterior fontanel is at times a more reliable sign of meningeal irritation than stiff neck. A temporal lobe or cerebellar pressure cone or decerebrate rigidity may also limit passive flexion of the neck and may be confused with meningeal irritation.

Evidence of disease of a cerebral hemisphere, diencephalon, midbrain, pons, or medulla can be obtained even though the patient is comatose by noting the residual movement, prevailing postures of the body, respiratory rhythm and frequency, and status of cranial nerves. This is of more than passing importance because severe and persistent derangements of these functions are frequent with mass lesions of the brain and rare in metabolic disorders (except in terminal stages). A hemiplegia, in most instances, reflects a contralateral hemispheral lesion and is revealed by lack of restless movements, grasp reflex, and avoidance movements. The paralyzed limbs are slack and remain in uncomfortable positions. If lifted from the bed, they "fall flail." The cheek puffs out in expiration on the paralyzed side, and the eyes are often turned away from the paralysis (toward the lesion). Painful stimuli may provoke a moan or grimace on one side and not the other, reflecting a hemianesthesia. A homonymous hemianopsia in a stuporous patient is revealed by attraction of eyes to visual stimuli presented on one side and not the other.

Of the various tests of brainstem function those which have been most useful are: pattern of breathing, pupillary size and reactivity, and ocular movement and oculovestibular reflexes. As to patterns of abnormal breathing in progressive lesions which reduce the state of consciousness from confusion and inattention to stupor and coma, the earliest abnormality with cerebral lesions is the appearance of posthyperventilation apnea (period of apnea after 5 to 10 deep breaths). Its presence indicates bifrontal disease, wherein lies the mechanism, according to Plum, for activating rhythmic breathing when CO_2 is reduced. In coma due to massive cerebral lesions the rate of respiration increases slightly, and as it progresses an irregularity appears which gives way to the waxing-waning Cheyne-Stokes respiration (CSR). This means that the centers in the midbrain now isolated from the cerebrum are rendered more sensitive than usual to CO_2 (hyperventilation drive); and by intermittently reducing plasma CO_2 to low levels a temporary apnea follows. With midbrain–upper pontine lesions a state of *central neurogenic hyperpnea* (CNH) rather like

Kussmaul breathing, supervenes. Here respirations are increased in rate (up to 100 per min) and in depth, to the extent that respiratory alkalosis may result. The reflex mechanisms for respiratory control in the lower brainstem have in this instance been released, and the threshold of respiratory activation is low. This respiratory drive continues despite low arterial CO_2 tensions and elevated pH. Oxygen therapy (unlike the hyperventilation of pneumonia, pulmonary congestion, etc.) does not modify the pattern. Low pontine-level lesions sometimes cause *apneustic breathing* (where there is a pause of 2 to 3 seconds after full inspiration) or other abnormal patterns, such as short cycle clusters (3 to 4) of respiration without waxing or waning followed by a pause (Biot respirations) or respiration alternans in which a few breaths are omitted from time to time. With lesions of medulla the rhythm of breathing is chaotic, being irregularly interrupted, the breath varying in rate and depth. This has been called "ataxia of breathing," not a very appropriate term. The latter progresses to apnea, as may also CSR or CNR; in fact, respiratory arrest is the mode of death of most patients with serious central nervous disease. As Plum and Fisher both point out, when certain supratentorial brain lesions progress to the point where the temporal lobe and cerebellum herniates, one may observe a succession of respiratory patterns (CSR—CNP—Biot breathing to ataxic breathing) indicating extension of the functional disorder from upper to lower brainstem.

With midbrain lesions the pupils dilate to 4 to 5 mm and become unreactive to light; and with severe destruction of the tissue at this level (anoxic pannecrosis), they will finally dilate widely and not respond. Pontine tegmental lesions cause miotic pupils with only slight reaction to strong light. Thus, the preservation of pupillary light reflexes indicates integrity of the pupillary dilatation and constrictive mechanisms in midbrain. Ciliospinal pupillary dilatation is also lost in brainstem lesions (see Chap. 24). Unilateral Horner's syndrome (miosis, ptosis, exophthalmos, and reduced sweating) may be observed homolateral to a predominantly one-sided lower brainstem lesion, usually medullary. The pupillary reactions are of great importance because drug intoxications and metabolic disorders which cause coma leave the pupils unaffected. Exceptions are glutethimide (Doriden) and deep ether anesthesia where the pupils may be of medium size or slightly enlarged and unreactive for several hours; opiates (heroin and morphine) which cause pinpoint pupils with light reflex so small that it can be seen only with a magnifying glass; and atropine poisoning where the pupils are widely dilated and fixed.

Ocular movements are altered in a variety of ways. In light coma from metabolic abnormalities the eyes rove from side to side in random fashion like the slow eye movements of light sleep. They disappear as brainstem function becomes depressed. Oculocephalic reflexes (doll's eye movements), elicited by briskly turning or tilting the head, with eyes moving conjugately in the opposite direction, are exaggerated. They are not present in the normal person and if elicitable, evidence is obtained of the integrity of the tegmental structures of midbrain and pons which integrate ocular movements, and of the third, fourth, and fifth cranial nerves. Irrigation of each ear with 30 to 100 ml ice water (or just cold water if not completely comatose) will normally cause nystagmus away from the stimulated side (see Chap. 24). In comatose patients in whom the fast corrective "cortical" phase of nystagmus is lost the eyes are deflected to the side irrigated with cold water or away from the side irrigated with hot water. The position is held for 2 to 3 min. These oculovestibular reflexes are also lost in brainstem lesions. If only one eye abducts and the other fails to adduct in the lateral conjugate movement, there is indication of interruption of the medial longitudinal fasciculus (on the side of adductor paralysis). Irrigating both ears with ice water with head extended to 60° will sometimes induce vertical conjugate movements. An abducens palsy (sixth nerve) is reflected by a turning in of the eye due to unopposed action of internal rectus muscle, and oculomotor palsy results in abduction from unopposed action of abducens muscle. The eyes may be held conjugately to one side at all times in a coma—away from the side of the paralysis with large cerebral lesions (looks at the lesion) and toward the side of the paralysis with unilateral pontine lesions (looks away from the lesion). And, during a one-sided seizure the eyes jerk toward the convulsing side of face, arm, and leg (opposite to the irritative focus). The eyes may be turned down and inward (looking at nose) in thalamic and upper midbrain lesion (Parinaud's syndrome, see Chap. 24). Retractory and convergence nystagmus and ocular bobbing [brisk downward movements of both eyes with slow elevation to the original position (two-to-three times a minute)] occur with lesions in midbrain tegmentum and lower pons respectively. The major brainstem structural lesions, including temporal lobe herniation, abolish most, if not all, conjugate ocular movements when producing coma, whereas metabolic disorders do not. Of the intoxications, barbiturates and diphenylhydantoin (Dilantin) are the only common drugs which affect ocular movements, but they leave pupillary reactions intact.

As to the meaning of prevailing postures and movements in the comatose patient it may be said that restless, grasping, picking movements of one arm or arm and leg or all four extremities signify that the corticospinal tract(s) is intact; variable resistance to passive movement (paratonic rigidity) and strong grasping or complex avoidance movements have the same signification and if bilateral, the coma usually is not deep. Focal seizures require intact corticospinal motor system and are seldom seen with massive destruction of a cerebral hemisphere. Often these elaborate forms of semivoluntary movement are present on the "good side" in patients with extensive disease in one hemisphere and probably represent some type of disequilibrium of cortical and subcortical movement patterns. Definite choreic, athetotic, or even hemiballismic movements indicate disorder of subthalamic and basal ganglionic structures, just as they do in the alert patient. *Decerebrate rigidity* with jaw clenched, neck retracted, arms and legs stiffly extended and internally rotated appears in the condition of diencephalic-midbrain

suppression of temporal lobe pressure cone, with hemorrhages and infarction of upper pons and midbrain and with certain metabolic disorders such as hypoglycemia and hypoxia. Occasionally the mechanism of the decerebrate posture is unclear, as with certain bilateral subacute encephalitic, demyelinative and infarctive cerebral lesions. *Decorticate rigidity*, with arm or arms in flexion and adduction and leg(s) extension, signifies higher lesions in cerebral white matter, internal capsules, and thalamus. *Diagonal postures*, opposite arms and legs flexed and extended, probably mean supratentorial lesions; extended arms and flexed legs are probably fragments of decerebrate postures and point to midpontine lesions. *Abolition of all postures and movements* indicates acute bilateral corticospinal interruption, profound coma, and low pontine-medullary lesions involving reticular facilitatory (extrapyramidal) mechanisms.

Lower brainstem reflexes are seldom helpful in the analysis of coma. Only in the most profound metabolic comas and intoxications and in the hypoxemic pannecrosis of the entire brain (brain-death syndrome) are coughing, swallowing, and spontaneous respirations all abolished. Further, the tendon and plantar reflexes give little indication of what is happening. Tendon reflexes may be preserved until late and may be normal or slightly reduced on the hemiplegic side. The plantar reflexes may be absent or extensor. Only in deep coma or in states of decerebrate rigidity will a cerebral hemiplegia not be detected by flaccidity and motionless arm and leg.

A history of headache before or at the onset of coma, recurrent vomiting, and papilledema affords the best clues to increased intracranial pressure. This can be confirmed by lumbar puncture, which is usually safe unless there is a herniation of the temporal lobe through the tentorium or of the cerebellum through the foramen magnum. In the latter instance the cerebrospinal fluid pressure may not reflect intracranial pressure. Papilledema may develop within 12 to 24 hr in brain trauma and brain hemorrhage but, if pronounced, usually signifies brain tumor or abscess, viz., a lesion of longer duration. Multiple retinal or large subhyaloid hemorrhages are usually associated with ruptured saccular aneurysm or hemorrhage from an angioma. Papilledema, with widespread retinal exudates, hemorrhages, and arteriolar changes, is an almost invariable accompaniment of hypertensive encephalopathy. In patients with evidence of increased intracranial pressure, lumbar puncture, although admittedly dangerous because it may promote further herniation, is nevertheless necessary in some instances. See Chaps. 24 and 401 for further discussion of retinal changes.

LABORATORY PROCEDURES. Unless the diagnosis is established at once by history and physical examination, it is necessary to carry out a number of laboratory procedures. If poisoning is suspected, the gastric contents must be aspirated and saved for later chemical analysis. A catheter is passed into the urinary bladder, and a specimen of urine is obtained for determination of specific gravity, sugar, acetone, and albumin content. Urine of low specific gravity and high protein content is nearly always found in uremia, but proteinuria may also occur for 2 or 3 days after a subarachnoid hemorrhage or with fever. Urine of high specific gravity, glycosuria, and acetonuria are almost invariable in diabetic coma; but glycosuria and hyperglycemia may result from a massive cerebral lesion. If bromide or barbiturate intoxication is suspected, it can be verified by special tests for these substances. A blood count is made, and in malarial districts a blood smear is examined for malarial parasites. Neutrophilic leukocytosis occurs in bacterial infections and also with brain hemorrhage and softening. Venous blood should be examined for glucose, nonprotein nitrogen, CO_2, sodium bicarbonate, pH, NH_3, sodium, potassium, chlorides, and Ca. The cerebrospinal fluid must be drawn, and the pressure, presence of blood, white cell count, and results of Pandy's test should be recorded. Bloody cerebrospinal fluid occurs in cerebral contusion, subarachnoid hemorrhage, brain hemorrhage, and occasionally with hemorrhagic infarcts due to thrombophlebitis or arterial embolism. If there is pleocytosis, a stained smear of the sediment should be searched for bacteria, and a rough quantitative sugar determination should be done. The standard cerebrospinal fluid formula in bacterial meningitis is elevated pressure, high white cell count (5,000/20,000), elevated protein, and subnormal sugar values. The fluid should be saved for quantitative tests for sugar and protein, and a bacterial culture and Wassermann reaction should be performed. If the pressure is suspected of being elevated, a number 22 needle should be used. A very high pressure must be slowly reduced by removal of 10 to 15 ml over a period of 15 to 20 min, and urea, mannitol, or other hypertonic solutions should be given intravenously. Also, a corticosteroid may be given to reduce brain swelling over a longer period of time. Jugular compression tests are obviously contraindicated. X-rays of the skull should be obtained as soon as possible after these procedures, preferably on the way from the emergency ward to the hospital room.

CLASSIFICATION OF COMA AND DIFFERENTIAL DIAGNOSIS

The demonstration of focal brain disease or meningeal irritation, with cerebrospinal fluid abnormality, helps in differential diagnosis. The diseases that frequently cause coma can be conveniently divided into three classes, as follows:

Classification of Coma

I. Diseases that cause no focal or lateralizing neurologic signs or alteration of the cellular content of the cerebrospinal fluid
   A. Intoxications (alcohol, barbiturates, opiates, etc.) (Chaps. 118, 119 and 120)
   B. Metabolic disturbances (diabetic acidosis, uremia, Addisonian crises, hepatic coma, hypoglycemia, hypoxia (Chap. 363)
   C. Severe systemic infections (pneumonia, typhoid fever, malaria, Waterhouse-Friderichsen syndrome)
   D. Circulatory collapse (shock) from any cause, and cardiac decompensation in the aged (Chap. 20)
   E. Epilepsy (Chaps. 28 and 368)
   F. Hypertensive encephalopathy and eclampsia (Chap. 357)
   G. Hyperthermia or hypothermia
   H. Concussion (Chap. 358)
II. Diseases that cause meningeal irritation, with either blood or an excess of white cells in the cerebrospinal fluid, usually without focal or lateralizing signs
   A. Subarachnoid hemorrhage from ruptured aneurysm, occasionally trauma (Chap. 357)
   B. Acute bacterial meningitis (Chap. 360)
   C. Some forms of virus encephalitis (Chap. 361)
   D. Acute hemorrhagic leukoencephalitis (Chap. 362)
III. Diseases that cause focal or lateralizing neurologic signs, with or without changes in the cerebrospinal fluid
   A. Brain hemorrhage (Chap. 357)
   B. Brain softening due to thrombosis or embolism (Chap. 357)
   C. *Brain abscess* (Chap. 360)
   D. Epidural and subdural hemorrhage and brain contusion (Chap. 358)
   E. Brain tumor (Chap. 359)
   F. Miscellaneous, i.e., thrombophlebitis, some forms of virus encephalomyelitis (Chap. 361)

With the clinical tests outlined above clearly in mind one can usually ascertain whether a patient with coma falls in one of the above categories. Concerning the group of comas without focal, lateralizing, or meningeal signs, which includes most of the secondary metabolic diseases of the brain, intoxications (both exogenous and endogenous), concussion, and postseizure states, it should be pointed out that a previous neurologic disease may have left residue which confuse the clinical picture. An earlier hemiparesis from vascular disease or trauma may reveal itself in an alcoholic or hepatic coma, uremia, or hyperglycemic encephalopathy. Also, in hypertensive encephalopathy, transitory focal signs may sometimes be present. And occasionally, for no understandable reason one leg may seem to move less or one plantar reflex be extensor in a metabolic coma. In actuality, the diagnosis of postepileptic coma or concussion depends on observation of the precipitating event or indirect evidence thereof; usually the diagnosis is not too long obscure, for another fit may occur and recovery of consciousness, once the seizures cease, is usually prompt. The final determination of the exact toxic or metabolic disorder requires the synthesis of a variety of clinical and laboratory data, which will be described in other parts of the book.

With respect to the comas of group II the signs of meningeal irritation (head retraction, stiffness of neck or forward bending, Kernig and Brudzinski leg flexion signs) are usually elicitable in both bacterial meningitis and subarachnoid hemorrhage. However, if the coma becomes deep, stiff neck may disappear or be absent from the beginning. Here diagnosis is established by CSF examination. In the coma of bacterial meningitis, unless it is associated with brain swelling and cerebellar herniation, the CSF pressure is not exceptionally high (usually less than 400 mm); if the pressure is high, as death approaches there are signs of compression of the medulla with fixed, dilated pupils, arrest of respiration, and fall in arterial blood pressure. Patients in coma from ruptured aneurysms also have high CSF pressure and often a massive hemispheral and ventricular extension of the hemorrhage.

In patients with group III type of coma it is the inequality of sensory-motor disturbances in the two arms and legs and the aforementioned changes in respiratory pattern, pupillary and ocular reflexes, and the remaining postural states that provide clues to serious structural lesions in the segmental brainstem apparatus. As the latter become prominent, they may obscure earlier signs of cerebral disease. It is noteworthy that bilateral cerebral infarction or hemorrhage or traumatic necrosis and hemorrhage may resemble the comatose state of metabolic and toxic diseases, since brainstem mechanisms may be preserved; contrariwise, hepatic, hypoglycemic, and hypoxic coma will sometimes look like the coma of brainstem lesion by causing decerebrate postures. Usually, however, the CSF pressure is elevated and the fluid sanguineous in massive cerebral hemorrhage. Unilateral infarction due to anterior, middle, or posterior cerebral artery occlusion seldom produces more than a stupor or light coma; if bilateral, however, coma may be profound. Evidence of brainstem displacement and temporal lobe herniation is manifested by increased or altered ventilation (CSR, CNH), bilateral Babinski signs, dilated pupil on the side of the lesion, decerebrate postures, dilated pupils, and loss of full ocular movements. The coma itself gives no clue as to the nature of the original mass lesion. The terminal pattern of a descending gradient of diencephalic, mesencephalic, pontomedullary paralysis of nervous paralysis is identical in all. Differential diagnosis must depend on the other data.

An error which must be cautioned against is the diagnosis of irreversible coma (brain-death syndrome) on the basis of complete abolition of all brainstem and cerebral activity and isoelectric (flat) EEG if there is hypothermia or evidence of intoxication. Only with hypoxia and cerebral ischemia can this diagnosis be made securely.

Diagnosis has as its prime purpose the direction of therapy, and it matters little to the patient whether or not we diagnose a disease for which we have no treatment. The treatable forms of coma are drug intoxications, toxemia from systemic infections, epidural and subdural hematoma, brain abscess, bacterial and tuberculous meningitis, diabetic acidosis, and hypoglycemia.

RELATIVE INCIDENCE OF DISEASES THAT CAUSE COMA

There have been only a few attempts to determine the relative incidence of diseases that lead to coma. A report from the Boston City Hospital (Solomon and Aring) includes the largest series of clinical cases but was heavily skewed by the large local problem of chronic alcoholics, which made up 60 percent of all admissions in coma. Trauma (13 percent), cerebral vascular disease (10 percent), poisonings (3 percent), epilepsy (2.4 percent),

diabetes, bacterial meningitis, pneumonia, uremia, and eclampsia followed in that order. In the series of fatal cases studied at the Cook County Hospital (Holcomb), accuracy of clinical diagnosis was not more than 50 percent and did not improve with increasing length of survival (in half the fatal cases the patient died in the first 24 hr and in two-thirds, within 48 hr). Again, trauma, cerebrovascular disease, meningitis, and alcoholism accounted for the majority of cases. In a series of 386 cases of coma of uncertain etiology Plum and Posner observed that approximately 40 percent turned out to be metabolic, 25 percent, drug intoxications, and the remainder to be neurologic disease of supra- or infra-tentorial structures. Diagnostic accuracy was much greater in this recent series than in that of Holcomb.

Of course, figures like these do not provide information concerning coma caused by multiple factors. For example, a patient with a cerebral vascular lesion, old or recent, and diabetes mellitus may lapse into coma during an insulin reaction at a time when there is still sugar in the urine. Only by appreciating the interplay of these several common factors is one likely to reach the correct diagnosis.

The differential diagnosis of diseases that cause focal or lateralizing signs and meningitis will be taken up under the discussions of traumatic, neoplastic, vascular, and infective diseases of the brain.

CARE OF THE COMATOSE PATIENT

Impaired states of consciousness, regardless of their cause, are often fatal because they not only represent an advanced stage of many diseases but also add their own characteristic burden to the primary disease. The main objective of therapy is, of course, to find the cause of the coma, according to the procedures already outlined, and to remove it. It often happens, however, that the disease process is one for which there is no specific therapy; or as in hypoxia or hypoglycemia, the disease process may already have expended itself before the patient comes to the attention of the physician. Again, the problem may be infinitely complex, for the disturbance may be attributable not to a single cause but rather to several possible factors acting in unison, no one of which could account for the total clinical picture. In lieu of direct therapy, supportive measures must be used, and, indeed, it may be said that the patient's chances of surviving the original disease often depend in large measure on their effectiveness.

The physician must give attention to every vital function in the insensate patient. The following is a brief outline of the more important procedures. In order for them to be carried out successfully a well-coordinated team of nurses under constant guidance of a physician is needed.

1. If the patient is in shock, this takes precedence over all other abnormalities. The treatment of shock is discussed in Chap. 36.

2. Shallow and irregular respirations and cyanosis require the establishment of a clear airway and oxygen.

The patient should be placed in a lateral position so that secretions and vomitus do not enter the tracheobronchial tree. Pharyngeal reflexes are usually suppressed, and therefore an endotracheal tube can be inserted without difficulty. Stagnant secretions should be removed with a suction apparatus as soon as they accumulate, since they will lead to atelectasis and bronchopneumonia. Oxygen can be administered by mask in a 100 percent concentration for 6 to 12 hr, alternating with 50 percent concentration for 4 hr. The depth of respiration can be increased by the use of 5 to 10 percent carbon dioxide for periods of 3 to 5 min every hour. Atropine should not be given; edema of the lungs and fluid in the tracheobronchial passages are not glandular secretions. Furthermore, atropine thickens this fluid and also may disturb temperature regulation of the body. Aminophylline is helpful in controlling Cheyne-Stokes breathing. Respiratory paralysis dictates the use of a positive-pressure respirator or electrophrenic stimulator, but in the author's experience neither has been effective in comatose states in which there is disorganization of respiratory centers.

3. The temperature-regulating mechanisms may be disturbed, and extreme hypothermia, hyperthermia, or an unrecognized poikilothermia may occur. In hyperthermia, removal of blankets and use of alcohol sponges and cooling solutions are indicated.

4. The bladder should not be permitted to become distended. If the patient does not void, a retention catheter should be inserted. If more than 500 ml urine is found in the bladder, decompression must be carried out slowly over a period of hours. Urine excretion should be kept between 500 and 1,000 ml per day. The patient should not be permitted to lie in a wet or soiled bed.

5. Diseases of the central nervous system may upset the control of water, glucose, and salt. The unconscious patient can no longer adjust his intake of food and fluids by hunger and thirst. Salt-losing and salt-retaining syndromes have both been described with brain disease. Water intoxication and severe hyponatremia may of themselves prove fatal. The maintenance of water and electrolytes will be discussed in Chap. 88. If coma is prolonged, the insertion of a stomach tube will ease the problem of feeding the patient and maintaining fluid and electrolyte balance.

6. One should not attempt to forestall the development of bronchopneumonia by the prophylactic use of penicillin and streptomycin or some other broad-spectrum antibiotics; instead, appropriate ones should be administered when the infection occurs. The legs should be examined each day for signs of phlebothrombosis.

7. If the patient is capable of moving, suitable restraints should be used to prevent a possible fall out of bed.

8. Convulsions should be controlled by measures outlined in Chap. 368.

REFERENCES

Fisher, C. M.: Neurological Examination of the Comatose Patient, Acta Neurol. Scand., 1969.

Holcomb, B.: Causes and Diagnosis of Various Forms of Coma, J.A.M.A., 77:2112, 1921.

Plum, E., and J. Posner: "Diagnosis of Stupor and Coma," Philadelphia, F. A. Davis Company, 1966.

Solomon, P., and C. D. Aring: The Causes of Coma in Patients Entering a General Hospital, Am. J. Med. Sci., 188:805, 1938.

27 SLEEP AND ITS ABNORMALITIES
Raymond D. Adams

Sleep, that familiar yet inexplicable condition of repose in which consciousness is in abeyance, is obviously not abnormal; yet there is no absurdity in considering it in connection with abnormal phenomena. There are no doubt irregularities of sleep which approach serious extremes, just as there are unnatural forms of waking.

Inasmuch as sleep is an elementary phenomenon of life and an indispensable phase of man's existence, everyone has had much personal experience of sleep, or the lack of it, and has observed others in sleep. It requires no special knowledge of medicine, therefore, to know something about this condition or to appreciate its importance to health and well-being. Nearly all the great writers of the past have expressed their views on the psychologic and physical benefits of sleep, but probably none with more feeling than Sterne, who has Tristram Shandy remark: "'Tis the refuge of the unfortunate—the enfranchisement of the prisoner—the downy lap of the hopeless, the weary, the broken-hearted; of all the soft, delicious functions of nature this is the chiefest; what a happiness it is to man, when anxieties and passions of the day are over. . . ."

Physicians are often sought by individuals who suffer an illness caused by or accompanied by some derangement of sleep. Most often the problem is one of sleeplessness, but sometimes it concerns peculiar phenomena occurring in connection with sleep.

NORMAL SLEEP

The natural physiologic changes discoverable in sleeping man can be summarized as follows: temperature falls less than 1° but skin temperature rises, only to fall sharply on awakening; BMR reduced 10 to 15 percent; pulse rate slows 10 beats or so; blood pressure falls 10 to 30 mm Hg; sweating increased; gastric, salivary, and lacrimal secretions reduced; intestinal action continues and sphincters are closed; volume of urine diminished; pupils contracted and eyes diverged and turned up; musculature becomes atonic and tendon jerks depressed or absent; Babinski sign present in some persons; breathing deepens and slows, becoming Cheyne-Stokes in some elderly persons; EEG at first shows interruption of alpha rhythm and appearance of slow waves, then sleep spindles of 15 to 18 c per sec and finally delta waves of 2 to 3 c per sec.

More detailed analysis of sleep behavior in recent years has shown that typical slow (EEG) sleep pattern becomes interrupted for brief periods by fast cortical activity. The record looks more like that of an alert person but he remains inactive, his cervical muscles are atonic, and there are at this time rapid eye movements. It is in this period of so-called "paradoxical sleep" (PS) that all dreaming occurs. Paradoxical sleep always bears a certain relationship to slow sleep (SS); it invariably follows it and makes up about 25 percent of the total sleep period. From this discovery it must be argued that sleep behavior is not a unitary function but involves neural organization at more than one level of the nervous system.

Theories as to the anatomic substratum of sleep are numerous. Most of the older ideas about the existence of a sleep center, located somewhere in the walls of the third ventricle, have largely been replaced by a dynamic conception of arousal systems in the reticular activating areas of the upper brainstem and of inhibitory systems from cortex and other regions. Decorticate man, like animals, exhibits natural cycles of sleeping and waking, but paradoxical sleep disappears only when lesions occur in the pontine tegmentum. However, at any level to expect that one nucleus would be responsible for either alertness or sleep would be a gross simplification, for some neurones (e.g., cerebral cortex) are shown to be active during sleep and others not.

The means whereby these systems of neurones are suppressed during sleep is the other great unsolved problem. Over the years fatigue products, acidosis, toxins, and hormones have all had their advocates. Pieron was the first to show that a substance which he called hypnotoxin appears in the CSF of fatigued dogs and when injected into the ventricles of control animals, induces true sleep. And now Monnier has obtained a substance in the dialysate of the blood of sleeping animals that will cause an alert animal to fall asleep. The nature of this substance is unknown. Barbiturates and like soporific drugs act on the upper reticular activating system; tranquilizing drugs which are conducive of sleep by quieting anxiety have their main effects on the hippocampus and cerebral cortex.

Man's sleep pattern is based on daylight living. He learns to adapt all of his activities to the variations in the length of the day. This is a tedious process of conditioning, as every parent knows who struggles to get children off to bed. Temperature, pulse, blood pressure, metabolic rate, amount of physical activity, efficiency of nervous function are all adjusted to wake-sleep pattern. People vary in their capacity to adapt to sudden alteration of their circadian rhythm, with all its biologic nuances, as when moving abruptly to another part of the world, or taking on night work.

The sleep requirement per day and the relative amounts of slow and paradoxical sleep change steadily during the early years of life. The infant sleeps most of the time and gradually, as sleep lessens, adjusts its awake pattern to daylight. Paradoxical sleep at first predominates and then diminishes to 25 percent. By puberty the need of sleep is reduced to 10 to 11 hr, and the adult seldom sleeps more than 7 to 8, the woman needing about an hour more than the man. Slow sleep normally varies in depth; one usually plunges into the deepest sleep within the first hour of going to bed, and as various measurements have shown, sleep lightens after 3 to 4 hours, again becoming somewhat deeper after 5 to 6 hours. Exceptionally, especially in those who work best in the afternoon and night, the deepest sleep comes later in the night and awakening in the morning is difficult. During light sleep many small restless movements are made, often activated by sensory stimuli; each person has his own repertory of them. Kleitman has found that the normal person makes 30 to 60 movements in 8 hr sleep, the duration of movement averaging 8 to 10 secs for a total of about 5 min per night. The febrile patient sleeps with less movement than the normal one.

THE EFFECTS OF LOSS OF SLEEP

Of the conditions making for human efficiency, sleep is one of the most important. Sleep is absolutely essential to normal body metabolism. Experimental animals deprived of sleep will die within a few days, no matter how well they are fed, watered, and housed.

Despite the many studies of the effect of sleeplessness on human beings and animals, we still do not know as much as we should about it. Experiments on human beings have taken the form of enforced abstention from sleep for several days, with tests administered before, and after. One group of psychologists succeeded in keeping their subjects going in a state of apparent wakefulness for more than 200 hr. The surprising result was that on tests such as tapping, aiming at targets, reading letters, and calculation there was no failure of performance even after the loss of two nights' sleep. The sleepless subjects did fail, however, in tasks requiring sustained attention. They could do as well as they normally would on short tests, but on longer ones of the same degree of difficulty they became slow and inaccurate. Another characteristic was sluggishness of attention in shifting from one task or one test item to another. It was difficult for the subjects to redirect their activity; once started on a given line, they could hardly be diverted from it. After 3 days, they could no longer read. Whatever their achievement on the tests, all subjects reported numerous symptoms, such as burning eyes, headache, dazed feeling, nervousness, emotional instability, loss of motor power and coordination, slurred speech, drooping eyelids, and distressing visual hallucinations. In general deportment they were alternately irritable and silly, tending to laugh at anything said to them. There was a progressive decrease in the alpha waves in the EEG.

The reason for the relatively good test performance in the face of these bodily sensations is the ability of the normal individual to compensate. He can "shake himself out of it" and apply himself with an effort that overcomes his deficiencies. The extra effort put forth to remain oriented to the task cannot be maintained without cost. The energy consumed during an arithmetic test, as measured by the metabolic rate, is about three times greater in persons who have lost sleep.

Another surprising finding was that the subjects recovered on less than 35 percent of the sleep that had been lost. Furthermore, the first 8 to 12 hr of sleep is predominantly of the slow type, with very little paradoxical sleep. In other words, the amount of sleep required after the experiment is not equal to the number of hours that they were kept awake. Probably the explanation is that the subjects were not fully awake at all times, and in the latter part of the experiment they may have been half asleep.

A corollary of this hypothesis is that persons who sleep for long periods do not necessarily obtain the maximum benefits from sleep. Sleep may be sound and restful or light and fitful. In sound sleep the psychogalvanic test of skin resistance of the palm is raised, and in poor sleep it remains the same as in the waking state. It has also been found that only in sound sleep does the blood pressure fall. From these fragmentary studies it must be concluded that the value of sleep to the metabolism of the human organism is a function of its depth multiplied by its length, and that long hours spent in bed are no substitute for sound sleep.

Dreaming has been found by Aserinsky and Kleitman to occur always during the period of paradoxical sleep when the electroencephalogram reveals fast waves. This has been shown by awakening the patient when this brain wave pattern appears. Most subjects, if left alone, will awaken without remembering that they have dreamed. Jouvet finds that "paradoxical state" or "dream state" depends on a pontine mechanism.

DERANGEMENTS OF SLEEP

INSOMNIA. The word *insomnia* signifies want of sleep and is used popularly to indicate any interference with the duration or depth of sleep. As every physician knows from practical experience, this is not a disease, but a symptom of many diseases, which differ widely in their nature and gravity. It is associated equally with trivial ailments and with conditions which jeopardize life. The persistence and severity of insomnia are no guide to the diagnosis of the condition on which it depends.

Since insomnia is often a symptom of a minor illness, there is a tendency for the physician to make light of it. Yet few common conditions cause more misery and discomfort to the patient. When deprived of the nightly restoration of his energies, he grows weary and his whole mental and physical vigor is impaired. He seems to exhaust his fund of reserve force. His tolerance of pain, noise, and the countless irritations of everyday life is reduced. This, in turn, reflects itself in his psychologic reaction to all the ordinary symptoms of disease. Also, the capacity for effective work is intimately related to the ability to sleep. In fact, sound sleep is one of the most reliable measures of sound health.

Once there was a tendency to formulate elaborate classifications of insomnia according to the nature of the diseases in each of the different organ systems of the body.

This approach has little to offer because, in the final analysis, the factors operating in all these diseases are relatively few. Most instances of unyielding insomnia are due to (1) the presence of pain and discomfort or (2) anxiety (with muscular tension) and other nervous disorders.

Several types of sensory disorder may cause abnormal wakefulness. The pain of spine and root or peripheral nerve disease may be particularly troublesome at night, and the same is true of abdominal discomfort in a number of gastrointestinal diseases, such as pancreatic carcinoma. Tired, aching, restless legs, which has been described as the "restless leg syndrome" (*anxietas tibialis*) may regularly delay the onset of natural sleep. Excessive fatigue may give rise to many abnormal muscular sensations of a similar nature. *Acroparesthesias,* that peculiar nocturnal tingling numbness of the hands which is so common in women, may awaken the patient nightly, as does also cluster headache, which nearly always occurs 2 to 3 hr after falling asleep.

Insomnia is a frequent complaint of patients suffering from psychiatric disease. Its simplest form is that of a reactive nervous state in which domestic and business worries keep the patient in a turmoil. Also, vigorous mental activity late at night or excitement which leaves the muscles tense counteracts drowsiness and sleep. Under these circumstances there is difficulty in falling asleep and a tendency to sleep late in the morning. Sleeplessness is also commonly recorded in the histories of patients suffering from psychoneuroses and psychoses. In a valuable study of the character of sleep in psychiatric patients Muncie concludes that illnesses in which anxiety and fear are prominent symptoms usually result in difficulty in falling asleep and light, fitful, or intermittent sleep. Also, disturbing dreams, so common in such conditions, may awaken the patient, and he may even try to stay awake in order to avoid them. The sleep pattern is altered, but quality and quantity are little if at all diminished. In contrast, the depressive illnesses, particularly manic-depressive or involutional depression, cause either light sleep in the early part of the night or early morning waking and inability to return to sleep. Quantity of sleep is reduced and nocturnal motility increased, according to the study of Hinton. If anxiety is combined with depression, both the above patterns are observed. In states of mania all types of sleep disorder are known to occur. The sleep rhythm may be totally deranged in acute confusional states and delirium. In the latter the patient may only doze for short periods both day and night. The total amount and depth of sleep in a 24-hr period is reduced. Frightening hallucinations may prevent sleep. The senile and arteriosclerotic patient tends to catnap during the day and then refuse to go to bed at night; his nocturnal sleep is intermittent, and the total amount may be either increased or decreased.

Finally, there are patients who are convinced of the absolute necessity of obtaining sleep of a certain ideal quantity or quality. These are the "sleep pedants" and the "sleep hypochondriacs" of Laudenheimer. They become obsessed with the importance of sleep. Every night they are in a panic lest they remain awake; they cannot sleep because of their anxiety over it. Often they claim to be sleepless the night through, when in fact they are seen fast asleep on more than one occasion. They demonstrate the truth of William McDougall's statement that "peace of mind is an essential preliminary to sleep." Especially interesting is that group for whom insomnia becomes the excuse for all inadequacies and failures in adjustment to the everyday problems of living. Such individuals, although they want to sleep, worry about the loss, and their mental agitation actually opposes sleep.

Whatever the cause may be, the physician should always be on his guard when listening to reports of the amount of sleep lost by victims of insomnia, because they are usually exaggerated. Every individual who has lain awake at night will recall how much longer the time seemed than it actually was. This is an example of an illusion in the perception of unfilled time.

DISTURBANCES IN THE TRANSITIONAL PERIOD OF SLEEP (SOMNOLESCENT STARTS, SENSORY PAROXYSMS, CIRCADIAN RHYTHM, AND NOCTURNAL PARALYSIS).

As sleep comes on, it would appear that certain nervous centers may be excited to a burst of insubordinate activity. The result is a sudden start that rouses the incipient sleeper. It may involve one or both legs or the trunk, less often, the arms. If the start occurs repeatedly during the process of falling asleep and is a nightly event, it may become a matter of great concern to the patient. These starts are more apt to occur in individuals in whom the sleep process develops slowly, and it has been observed that they are especially frequent in tense, nervous persons. It is probable that some relationship exists between these nocturnal starts and the sudden isolated jerk of a leg, or arm and leg, which may occur in healthy, fully conscious individuals. It does not appear to be related to epilepsy despite certain superificial resemblances. Disturbances of this nature may be the stimulus for night terrors. These somnolescent starts must be distinguished from flexor spasms of the legs, which occur in individuals who have suffered disease of the pyramidal tracts and from a rare condition known as nocturnal myoclonus in which the legs are involved in brusque flexion or extension movements of such force as to awaken the patient.

Sensory centers may be disturbed in a similar way either as an isolated phenomenon or in association with phenomena that induce motion. As the patient drops off to sleep he may be roused by a sensation that darts through his body. Such sensory symptoms are often in the domain of one of the special senses, especially hearing. A sudden clang or crashing sound disturbs commencing sleep. Sometimes a sudden flash of light occurs as sleep is coming on. A sensation of being lifted and dashed to earth or of being turned is probably a similar sensory paroxysm involving the labyrinthine mechanism.

Curious paralytic phenomena, so distressing to a patient as to cause him to seek medical advice, may also occur in the transition from the sleeping to the waking state. Sometimes in an otherwise healthy individual a state supervenes in the morning in which, although awake, conscious, and fully oriented, he is unable to innervate a single muscle. He lies as though still asleep with eyes closed and is all the while engaged in a struggle for movement. He has the impression that if he could move a single muscle, the spell would instantly vanish and he would regain full power. It has been reported that the slightest cutaneous stimulus such as the touch of a hand may abolish the paralysis. Such attacks are usually transient and of no special significance. They have also been reported to occur during the development of sleep. They may be related to narcolepsy.

NIGHTMARES AND NIGHT TERRORS.

Awakening in a state of terror has happened to nearly everyone. Children and nervous adults are especially prone to it. Fevers dispose to it, and it has been said that any upsetting condition of the body, such as a disturbance of digestion, may have a similar effect. Bad dreams, stimulated directly by recent memory of blood-curdling television programs before going to bed, may account for night terrors in children. Some psychologists have drawn a distinction between the nightmare which is merely a terrifying dream and that in which there are visual hallucinations and motor activity. Considering the predominantly visual nature of dreams, it is doubtful if such a separation is valid. Probably any difference is only one of degree.

A night terror is probably always connected with an alarming dream. The victim sits up or jumps out of bed, shouts, or rushes frantically from his room. He is at first unconscious of his surroundings, but usually the intensity of emotional disturbance and the physical activity awaken him. The following morning he may have only a hazy recollection of the experience.

Such phenomena are of little significance as isolated events in childhood but must be distinguished from nocturnal epilepsy. They seldom persist beyond adolescence. If they occur with excessive frequency and continue very long, a relationship to other disturbances, such as psychoneurosis, usually exists.

SOMNAMBULISM AND SLEEP AUTOMATISM.

Examples of sleep-walking come to the attention of the practicing physician not infrequently. This condition likewise occurs more often in children than in adults. After being asleep for a time, the patient arises from his bed and walks about the house. He may turn on a light or perform some other familiar act. There is no outward sign of emotion; the eyes are open, and the sleeper is guided by vision, thus avoiding familiar objects. The sight of an unfamiliar object may awaken him. If spoken to, he makes no response; if told to return to bed, he may do so but more often must be led back to it. Sometimes he will mutter strange phrases or sentences over and over. The following morning he usually has no memory of the episode.

Most psychiatrists hold that these are dissociated mental states similar to the hysterical trance and fugue, except that they begin during sleep. Undoubtedly this is true, and sleep walking may be accepted as evidence of a nervous disorder, probably of the psychoneurotic variety. There are nonetheless examples of this in adults who have no other signs of mental illness. One can only regard such a case as an isolated disorder of sleep-waking mechanism. It is probably allied to talking in one's sleep, though the two conditions seldom occur together.

Half-waking somnambulism, or sleep automatism, is a state in which an adult patient, half-roused from sleep, goes through a fairly complex routine such as going to a window, opening it, and looking out, but afterward recalling only a part of the episode. The patient may injure himself during sleepwalking.

NOCTURNAL EPILEPSY. Paroxysmal abnormalities of the brain waves of the type seen in epilepsy tend to occur in epileptic patients during or shortly after the onset of sleep. This characteristic electroencephalographic pattern has been found so frequently in the epileptic patient that the practice of artificially inducing sleep in order to obtain confirmation of epilepsy has been adopted in many laboratories. Of course, it has long been known that epilepsy occurs during sleep.

The sleeping epileptic patient attracts attention to his condition by a cry, violent motor activity, or labored breathing. As in the diurnal seizure, after the tonic-clonic phase, he becomes quiet and falls into a state resembling sleep but from which he cannot be aroused. His appearance depends on the phase of the seizure he happens to be in when first observed. Seizures of this type may occur at any time during the night, and some patients may have all their seizures at night. If the seizure during the night is unobserved, the only indication of it may be disheveled bedclothes, a few drops of blood on the pillow, wet bed linen from urinary incontinence, a bitten tongue, or sore muscles. In some children the occurrence of a seizure is betrayed only by incoherent behavior or a headache, the common aftermath of a convulsive disorder that was unnoticed. Rarely, a patient may die in an epileptic seizure during sleep, presumably from being smothered by bedclothes, aspirating vomitus, or for some more obscure reason.

Other less well-defined types of seizure occur at night. The patient may arise as though in a night terror and perform complex acts. He may be excited and overactive and, if restrained, become combative. After some minutes he is subdued and returns to sleep. The following morning he disclaims all memory of the episode. Probably this does not represent a psychomotor seizure but is instead a night terror. An electroencephalographic study may be helpful in such cases.

Nocturnal jerks of the legs, also called *nocturnal myoclonus*, is another troublesome symptom because it interferes with sleep night after night. Only recently has it been classified as a myoclonic form of epilepsy. It is unaccompanied by all other epileptic manifestations. Anticonvulsant drugs are said to control the condition, though in two cases the author has had better success with an occasional dose of Pantopon. It differs from the restless leg syndrome in that involuntary movements occur.

Epilepsy may occur in conjunction with both night terrors and somnambulism, and the question then arises whether the latter is in the nature of postepileptic automatism. Usually, no such relationship is established.

PROLONGED STATES OF SLEEP AND REVERSAL OF SLEEP-WAKING RHYTHM. Encephalitis lethargica, or "epidemic encephalitis," that remarkable illness which appeared on the medical horizon during the great pandemic influenza following the First World War, has provided some of the most dramatic instances of prolonged somnolence. In fact, protracted sleep lasting days to weeks was such a prominent symptom that the disease was called "sleeping sickness." The patient appeared to be in a state of continuous sleep, or "somnosis," and remained awake only while stimulated. Although the infective agent was never isolated, the pathologic anatomy was fully divulged by many excellent studies, all of which demonstrated a destruction of neurones in the midbrain, subthalamus, and hypothalamus. Patients surviving the acute phases of the illness often had difficulty in reestablishing the normal sleep-waking rhythm. As the somnolence disappeared, some patients exhibited a reversal of sleep rhythm, tending to sleep by day and stay awake at night and Parkinson's syndrome (Chap. 361).

Hypersomnia also occurs in trypanosomiasis, the common cause of sleeping sickness in Africa, and with a variety of diseases localized to the floor and walls of the third ventricle. Small tumors in the posterior hypothalamus and midbrain have been associated with arterial hypotension, diabetes insipidus, and somnolence lasting many weeks. Such patients can be aroused, but if left alone, they immediately fall asleep. Tumors of the brain, in general, show a tendency to cause drowsiness and increased amounts of sleep, but those of the diencephalon more so than any others (e.g., than posterior fossa ones). Traumatic brain lesions and other diseases have been found to produce similar clinical pictures.

NARCOLEPSY AND CATAPLEXY. The term *narcolepsy* has been used rather loosely. According to most authorities, it should refer to peculiar brief recurrent attacks of sleep and not to prolonged or continuous sleep. *Cataplexy* is a sudden brief loss of muscular power evoked by strong emotion, usually laughter. Although a few of the reported cases are doubtless examples of hysteria, there is unquestionably a well-defined clinical entity which bears no relationship to neurosis or any other known psychiatric condition. This will be discussed further in Chap. 366.

SLEEP PALSIES AND ACROPARESTHESIAS. Curious and at times distressing paresthetic disturbances develop during sleep. Everyone is familiar with the phenomenon of an arm or leg falling asleep. The immobility of the limbs and the maintenance of uncomfortable postures without being aware of them permits pressure to be applied to exposed nerves. The ulnar, radial, and peroneal nerves are quite superficial in places; pressure of the nerve against an underlying bone may interfere with intraneural circulation of the compressed segment. If this lasts for half an hour or longer, a sensory and motor paralysis sometimes referred to as *sleep palsy* may develop. This condition usually lasts only a few hours or days, but if the compression is prolonged, the nerve may be severely damaged so that functional recovery awaits regeneration. Unusually deep sleep, as in alcoholic intoxication, or anesthesia renders the patient especially liable to sleep palsies merely because he does not heed the discomfort of an unnatural posture.

Acroparesthesias are frequent in adult women and are not unknown to men. The patient will say that after being asleep for a few hours she is awakened by an intense numbness, tingling, prickling, a feeling of "pins and needles" in her fingers and hands. There are also aching, burning pains or tightness and other unpleasant sensations. At first there is a suspicion of having slept on the arm, but the usual bilaterality and the occurrence regardless of the position of the arms dispel this notion. Usually the paresthesias are in the distribution of the median nerves. Vigorous rubbing of the hands restores normal sensation, and the paresthesias subside within a few minutes, only to return later or upon first awakening in the morning. The condition never occurs during the daytime unless the patient is lying down or sitting with the arms and hands in one position. It may be unilateral but is more often bilateral. It never occurs in the feet. When acroparesthesias are frequent, the hands may at all times feel swollen, stiff, clumsy, slightly numb, and sometimes distressingly painful. Careful examination discloses little or no objective sensory loss, though in some cases touch and pain sensation have been slightly altered in parts supplied by the median nerves. Slight atrophy and weakness of the abductor pollicis brevis and opponens pollicis have been noted, and in a few cases it has been marked (carpal tunnel syndrome). The use of the hands for heavy manual work during the day seems to aggravate the condition, and a holiday or a period of hospitalization may relieve it. It often occurs in young housewives with a new baby or in factory workers who perform a routine skill. Recently it has been demonstrated that there is a compression of the median nerves in the carpal tunnel of the wrist by thickened carpal ligaments, tenosynovitis, bony overgrowth (as in acromegaly), or amyloid deposit (multiple myeloma). The injection of 50 mg hydrocortisone beneath the carpal ligament and the use of Diuril or one of its analogs has given immediate relief in a respectable number of cases. The section of the carpal ligament has nearly always cured recalcitrant cases.

DIAGNOSIS OF DISORDERS OF SLEEP

The diagnosis of the cause of insomnia may be troublesome. The difficulty is usually not with the severe case of insomnia as much as with the chronic one. A common source of error is failure to recognize an underlying psychiatric illness such as anxiety neurosis or depressive psychosis. This failure can be avoided only by having the main symptoms of these illnesses clearly in mind and making particular inquiry concerning them in every case.

Somnolescent starts, somnolescent sensory paroxysms, and night terrors may all be confused with nocturnal epilepsy, but actually the only real problem here is to distinguish between night terrors and epilepsy. This may at times be difficult, if not impossible. The occurrence of other types of seizures, especially if they occur during the daytime, the lack of any display of terrifying emotion,

and the presence of urinary incontinence and tongue biting all indicate epilepsy. Often electroencephalographic confirmation can be obtained.

In the diagnosis of diseases that cause protracted somnolence, a thorough neurologic study, with x-rays of skull, electroencephalogram, and lumbar puncture, must be employed. Diabetes insipidus, signs of pituitary insufficiency, blindness in parts of visual fields, ophthalmoplegia, and sometimes extrapyramidal motor disturbances are helpful in that they indicate disease in areas adjacent to the posterior hypothalamus and midbrain. But, probably the most frequent cause of excess drowsiness is that due to medication which acts either directly on the diencephalon or alters some component of blood, e.g., Na or K, and thereby affects the nervous system.

Sleep palsies must be distinguished from other diseases affecting the peripheral nerves. The onset during sleep, maximal functional disturbance immediately afterward, and steady improvement are the main characteristics. A delay in the appearance of muscular atrophy may be perplexing unless it is remembered that it takes 2 to 3 months for denervation atrophy to develop fully. The syndrome of acroparesthesias is often mistaken for ruptured cervical disk, anterior scalene and cervical rib syndrome, peripheral neuritis, multiple sclerosis, or psychoneurosis. The nocturnal incidence, the localization to the fingers and hands in the median nerve distribution, and the lack of other neurologic signs are diagnostic. A tourniquet around the arm just above the elbow may reproduce the acroparesthetic syndrome.

TREATMENT

In general, there are three varieties of wakefulness. For best management, treatment should be based on the type exhibited by the patient. In younger patients the most frequently observed type of insomnia is the inability to fall asleep. These individuals have become more and more tense during the day and are unable to relax. This type of insomnia usually lasts from 1 to 3 hr, and then the individual sinks into an exhausted, deep sleep which continues through the night. For these patients a quick-acting, fairly rapidly destroyed hypnotic such as secobarbital (Seconal), 0.1 Gm given 15 to 20 min before going to bed, is useful.

The second group consists of patients who are able to go to sleep but who awaken in 2 or 3 hr and lose sleep in the middle of the night. They awaken during the period when sleep normally lightens and some are alternately awake and asleep all the rest of the night. Often these are sick persons with a debilitating or painful illness which generates more pain and restlessness as muscles relax and leave painful areas unsplinted. In others, fever, sweats, dyspnea, or other distressful symptoms develop and demand attention. Frequently, these patients secure relief from pentobarbital (Nembutal), 0.1 Gm given at bedtime. For cardiac patients who have Cheyne-Stokes respiration or moderate orthopnea, a rectal suppository of aminophylline, 0.5 Gm given at bedtime, will frequently relieve the respiratory distress and promote sleep. When pain is a factor in insomnia, acetylsalicylic acid 0.3 to 0.6 Gm, should be given with the sedative. Occasionally, codeine phosphate, 30 mg, may be required when pain is severe.

The third group of insomnia patients consists of those who go to sleep promptly and sleep well most of the night, only to awaken too early in the morning. Most of these individuals are older persons who turn night into day. They go to bed and get up earlier and earlier so that soon they are sleeping during the day and are alert during the night. Into this category also fall those individuals who are under great tension, worry, or anxiety or are overworked and exhausted. These people sink into bed and sleep through sheer exhaustion, but around 4 or 5 A.M. they awake with their worries and are unable to get back to sleep. Most of these patients are benefited by barbital, 0.3 Gm given with fruit juice or milk at bedtime. For debilitated patients the compressed tablets of insoluble material should be crushed to ensure proper absorption or sodium barbital should be substituted. Chloral hydrate, 1.0 Gm given with fruit juice at bedtime, is also effective and may be substituted for barbital if desired.

Patients with serious mental agitation, delirium, or excitement who require prompt, easily controlled, relatively safe sedation should receive whiskey, 30 to 60 ml by mouth, or paraldehyde, 15 to 30 ml by mouth in iced fruit juice, or the same dose of the latter by rectum but diluted with 200 ml physiologic saline solution or 120 ml olive oil. For frankly delirious patients 25 to 50 mg of chlorpromazine (t.i.d.) has been a most helpful medication. Generally, it is wise to avoid barbiturates with highly agitated patients, since occasionally they may precipitate serious mental confusion, excitement, or even manic tendencies. Chloral hydrate, 1.0 to 2.0 Gm by mouth, is also useful in the management of these individuals and frequently proves more satisfactory than the barbiturates.

A word of caution about oversedation is wise in any discussion of sedative drugs. All too frequently they are abused in that they are given when not needed, the dosage is too great, or the wrong preparation is used. These drugs are a common source of constipation, lead to fatigue and lack of energy and strength, and interfere with the patient's recovery from his illness.

When large dosages of quicker-acting barbiturates, 0.4 to 0.6 Gm daily, are given for more than a few weeks, there is real danger of habituation, which once developed, is pernicious in character. Withdrawal, unless accomplished skillfully and in graded steps, may cause serious mental disturbance or precipitate convulsions. The chronic insomniac who has no other symptoms should not be permitted to use sedative drugs as a crutch on which to limp through life. The solution of this problem is rarely to be found in medication. One should search out and correct the underlying difficulty using medication only as a temporary helpful tool. A good book, pleasure in staying awake, and belief that the human organism will always get as much sleep as needed are helpful.

Barbiturate sedatives may be of value in treating night terrors, and if their differentiation from nocturnal epilepsy is impossible, a trial on diphenylhydantoin sodium (Dilantin Sodium) and phenobarbital is indicated. (See Chap. 368 for further information concerning anticonvulsant medication.)

REFERENCES

Kleitman, N.: "Sleep and Wakefulness," Chicago, The University of Chicago Press, 1934.

Kremer, M., R. W. Gilliatt, J. S. R. Golding, and T. G. Wilson: Acroparesthesiae in the Carpel-tunnel Syndrome. Brit. Med. J. (Lancet), II:590, 1953.

Miller, H. R.: "Central Autonomic Regulations in Health and Disease," p. 260, New York, Grune & Stratton, Inc., 1942.

Muncie, W.: "Psychobiology and Psychiatry," p. 104, St. Louis, The C. V. Mosby Company, 1939.

28 RECURRENT CONVULSIONS
Raymond D. Adams

The magnitude of the problem of epilepsy and its importance in our society can hardly be overstated. The statistics of Lennox and Lennox show that at least 1,000,000 persons in the United States are or have been subject to seizures. After apoplexy, epilepsy is the most frequent neurologic disorder. Therefore, the physician must know something of the nature and etiology of this common condition and of the mechanism whereby symptoms are produced.

Epilepsy is an intermittent disorder of the nervous system due presumably to a sudden, excessive, disorderly discharge of cerebral neurones. This was the postulation of Hughlings Jackson, the eminent British neurologist of the nineteenth century, and modern electrophysiology offers no evidence to the contrary. This discharge results in an almost instantaneous disturbance of sensation, loss of consciousness, convulsive movements, or some combination thereof. A terminologic difficulty arises from the diversity of the clinical manifestations. It seems improper to call a condition a convulsion when only an alteration of sensation or of consciousness takes place. The word *seizure* is preferable as a generic term and also lends itself to qualification. Motor or convulsive seizure is therefore not tautologic, and one may speak also of sensory seizures. The word *epilepsy*, which in times past meant the "falling evil," has many unpleasant connotations, and although it is a useful medical term, probably it is best avoided in open discussions until the general public becomes more enlightened.

Epilepsy may begin at any age. It may occur once in the lifetime of an individual or several times a day. Sometimes it is an obvious symptom of a brain disease that also manifests itself in other ways, and at times it is the solitary expression of deranged cerebral function in an individual who otherwise maintains perfect health. The latter is the more frequent circumstance and explains why the convulsive state has for so long been looked upon as a disease entity. However, it is illogical to suppose that a convulsion occurring by itself represents a disease, whereas one occurring in combination with other symptoms is only a manifestation of a disease. The convulsive state must always be looked upon as symptomatic. Use of such epithets as "genuine" or "essential" or "idiopathic" merely point to obscure causation and the more benign nature of the disease.

THE COMMON TYPES OF CONVULSIVE DISORDERS

In a statistical survey of nearly 2,000 patients it was reported that 51 percent of all epileptic patients had had *generalized convulsions;* 8 percent, minor seizures referred to as *petit mal;* 1 percent, *psychic* or *psychomotor seizures;* and the remaining 40 percent, two or even all three types, the most prominent form being psychomotor. Thus psychomotor epilepsy is almost as frequent as grand mal. Although the total number of seizures that had a focal onset was not determined, these data give some notion of the principal forms of the convulsive state in the majority of patients.

THE GENERALIZED CONVULSION (GRAND MAL, MAJOR EPILEPSY)

The term *convulsion* is most applicable to this form of seizure. The patient may sense its possible approach by any of several subjective sensations. For some hours he may feel apathetic, depressed, irritable, or the opposite —unusually alert or even ecstatic. Flatulence, constipation, and headache are other prodromal symptoms, and myoclonic twitches, i.e., sudden movements that affect one or another limb or the trunk, may precede the convulsion by some hours. In approximately half the cases there is some type of sensation or movement of one part of the body before the loss of consciousness or the generalized convulsion. This is called the *aura,* and as will be explained later, it provides the most reliable clue to the location of the underlying disease. The most frequent aura is an epigastric sensation, a sinking or gripping feeling, a strangulation or palpitation. A tingling numbness of the fingers or lips or some other part of the body, a flashing light or panorama, and disagreeable taste or odor are other well-known sensory auras. Clonic twitches, tonic contraction of the muscles of a limb, and turning of the head and eyes are somatic motor auras that at first take the form of focal epilepsy and end in a generalized seizure. They may spread from one part of the body to another in an orderly, predictable sequence. Usually, by the time all one side of the body is affected there is a loss of consciousness. The aura, though truly a warning of the oncoming seizure, is actually the first part of the seizure and not a prodrome. It seldom lasts more than a few seconds.

The generalized convulsion, or *fit,* as it is often called, begins with a sudden loss of consciousness and falling to the ground. The whole musculature is seized in a violent spasm. The contraction of the diaphragm and chest muscles produces a characteristic cry. The eyes turn up or to one side, the face is contorted, the jaw is set, often with biting of the tongue and oozing of saliva or blood from the lips, and the limbs may assume any of several positions. With continued spasm of the respiratory muscles, breathing is impossible, and the color of the skin and mucous membranes becomes dusky or cyanotic. After a fraction of a minute the rigid or tonic state of the muscles gives way to a series of clonic jerking movements. Air begins to enter the lungs in short convulsive gasps, and a bloody froth, a mixture of saliva and blood from a bitten tongue or cheek, forms on the lips. The arms, legs, face, and head jerk violently. After a minute or two the movements become slower, then irregular, and finally cease. The patient then lies relaxed, breathing rather deeply and sweating profusely. There may have been loss of control of urine and occasionally of feces. The state is now one of deep coma, and even the most intense pain evokes no response. Plantar reflexes are often extensor. One or both pupils may not react. After a few minutes the patient stirs and then opens his eyes. His first remarks or questions usually betray mental confusion. For the next several minutes or even hours there is a tendency toward incoherence of thought and drowsiness. Often the patient falls into a deep sleep. Headache is another frequent postseizure or postictal symptom. The patient himself is completely unaware of what has happened or at most remembers only the aura. He may come to his senses in a hospital or other strange place, and his only way of telling that something has happened is by the hiatus in his memory, his disheveled appearance, the bitten tongue, and a soreness of the vigorously exercised muscles. Injury may be sustained during the fall and as a consequence of violent muscular contraction; one or several vertebras may be crushed. Periorbital subcutaneous hemorrhages may reflect the violence of the exertion during the seizures.

Convulsions of this type ordinarily come singly or in groups of two or three and may occur when the patient is awake or asleep. About 5 to 8 percent of patients at some time have a series of seizures without regaining consciousness between times. This is known as *status epilepticus* and demands urgent treatment. Instead of the whole sequence of changes described above, only one part of the seizure may occur; for example, there may be only the aura without loss of consciousness, or the entire spell may consist of a brief loss of consciousness and momentary spasm of the limbs. Anticonvulsive medication abbreviates the seizure.

PETIT MAL (MINOR EPILEPSY, SMALL ILLNESS, L'ABSENCE)

In contrast to the generalized seizure, these attacks are so brief that they are often overlooked. In fact, many patients may have them for years before their true nature is recognized.

The attack comes without warning and consists of sudden loss of consciousness. The person is motionless, and a staring expression of the face and failure to speak or to respond to commands are the only signs of abnormality.

In contrast to grand mal, motor disturbances are conspicuously absent, and at most only a few flickering contractions of the eyelids and facial muscles and jerking of the arms at a rate of three contractions per second are seen. The patient does not fall, as a rule, and he may continue such complex acts as walking or even riding a bicycle during an attack. After 2 to 15 sec or more, consciousness is regained abruptly and fully, and the patient promptly resumes whatever action he was performing before the seizure. To the patient there is only a blank place, an "absence," in his stream of consciousness.

Closely related to petit mal are the *akinetic seizures,* in which the patient suddenly loses consciousness and falls motionless to the ground, and the myoclonic seizure, which consists of a sudden violent contraction of some part of or all the body, often followed by a lapse of posture with falling and loss of consciousness of a few seconds' duration (*generalized myoclonus*). Because of frequent association with petit mal and the similarity of the electroencephalographic pattern, Lennox groups petit mal, the akinetic seizure, and myoclonic seizure into a single entity called the *petit mal triad.*

Episodes of this type are much more frequent in childhood and adolescence. Another characteristic is their great frequency. As many as several hundred may occur in one day. Although benign, they may, if frequent, derange the mental processes so that the patient does poorly in school. Rarely, a series of them in close succession will interrupt consciousness for a longer period of time. This is known as *petit mal status. Pyknolepsy* is an almost obsolete term for frequent petit mal during childhood, terminating at puberty. When present as the only type of seizure during childhood, petit mal may give way to or be combined with grand mal, in a majority of cases by the age of sixteen years.

PSYCHOMOTOR EPILEPSY (EPILEPTIC EQUIVALENTS, PSYCHIC VARIANTS, EPILEPTIC MANIA OR DELIRIUM

This differs in several ways from the two types of seizure discussed above. (1) The aura, if it occurs, is often a complex hallucination or perceptual illusion. There may be an unpleasant smell or taste or the revival of a complicated visual scene involving people, dwellings, etc., usually taken from past experiences and resembling a dream. Furthermore, the patient's perception of what is seen and heard and his relationship to the outside world are altered. Objects appear to be far away or unreal (*jamais vu*); or strange objects or persons may seem familiar (*déjà vu phenomenon*). Hughlings Jackson applied the term *dreamy state* to these psychic disturbances. (2) Instead of losing all control of his thoughts and actions, the patient behaves as though he were partially conscious during the attack. He may get up and walk about, unbutton or remove his clothes, attempt to speak, or even continue such habitual acts as driving a car. If he is asked a specific question or given a command, it is evident that he is out of contact with the examiner and does not understand. When restrained, he may resist with great energy and at times can be violent. This type of behavior is said to be *automatic,* presumably because the patient behaves like an automaton. (3) Convulsive movements, when present, are likely to consist of chewing, smacking and licking of the lips, and less often, tonic spasms of the limbs or turning of the head and eyes to one side.

In any given case one or several of these phenomena may be observed. In the series studied by Lennox and Lennox, which numbered 414 cases, 43 percent of patients displayed some of these motor or psychomotor phenomena; 32 percent, the automatic state; and 25 percent, the psychic changes. Because of the concurrence of these three symptom complexes, they have referred to the whole group as the *psychomotor triad.* These types of seizure vary in frequency and duration. Some are very brief, lasting only for seconds, and others continue for hours or days. This calls to mind that the duration of the seizure is an unsatisfactory criterion for classification. Two-thirds of the patients have generalized convulsions at some time in their lives.

In addition to these three major types, the clinicians of the nineteenth century recognized many other special forms of epilepsy, some of which were given descriptive names. The term *tonic seizure* referred to tonic muscle contractions, to the exclusion of phasic qualities. *Epilepsia partialis continua* specified a regular repetitive clonic contraction of one group of muscles, not progressing to a generalized seizure. The terms *focal motor* or *focal sensory epilepsy* were applied to a tonic or clonic movement or a sensation restricted to one portion of the body. *Myoclonic epilepsy* referred to a syndrome of epilepsy and isolated twitches of a muscle or group of muscles, the latter being *myoclonus* (see Chap. 22). Random, arrhythmic myoclonus in a sense might be designated as *epilepsia partialis discontinua et disseminata*. It is usually caused by a more or less diffuse disease of the cerebral and cerebellar cortex and possibly of other parts of the nervous system, such as the thalamus.

In childhood a number of other forms of epilepsy occur, related presumably to the immaturity of the child's nervous system. The seizures of the newborn (*neonatal epilepsy*) are fragmentary and brief. Infantile or salam spasms, i.e., brief flexion of neck and limbs, are peculiar to the age period of six months to three to four years. *Febrile seizures* appear only in the age period of eighteen months to six years. Photic reflex epilepsy is induced by flickering light in childhood and adolescence Chap 365.

It is obvious that the traditional division of seizures into three main general types leaves much to be desired. Whereas petit mal is a more or less homogeneous type, grand mal may represent a phase of generalization of the seizure discharge, regardless of its origin or the initial symptoms of the seizure. Psychomotor epilepsy, as will be evident upon further analysis, is not a uniform syndrome but encompasses a diversity of clinical phenomena. Moreover, careful study of the first symptoms of the seizure and the use of the electroencephalogram have given us a new means of subdividing seizures according to other more significant attributes.

Common Focal Seizure Patterns

The seizure pattern provides information that not only is of great value in determining the topography of the disease causing the convulsive disorder but affords a new basis of classification that will serve until the etiology is discovered. The most definite focal seizure patterns are listed below. They are so helpful in the localization of cerebral lesions that every student of medicine should be familiar with them. These types of epilepsy are often termed *focal* because they can be traced to a circumscript lesion in one part of the brain.

MOTOR SEIZURES (GENERALIZED, CONTRAVERSIVE, FOCAL MOTOR, AND JACKSONIAN SEIZURES)

A lesion in one or other frontal lobe may give rise to a generalized or major convulsive seizure of the type described above, without introductory sensory aura. In some cases there is a turning movement of the head and eyes to one side, simultaneous with loss of consciousness, and in others there are no turning movements. It has been postulated that in both types of seizure, the one with and the one without contraversive movements, the discharge from the frontal lobe spreads rapidly into an integrating center such as the thalamus, with immediate loss of consciousness. In cases with head and eye turning, the discharge is believed to reach area 8 (area for contralateral turning of head and eyes), although it has been found that contralateral turning of the head and eyes can be induced in the experimental animal by stimulation of temporal or occipital as well as of the premotor cortex.

Do most cases of generalized motor seizures (grand mal) of idiopathic type have a frontal focus? Unfortunately, this question cannot be answered at the moment. Such a focus has been found in only a small number of such cases, and these may not be representative of the whole group.

The characteristics of the *Jacksonian motor seizure* are well known. It begins usually with a twitching of the fingers of one hand, the face on one side, or one foot. The movements are clonic and rhythmic; their speed varies. They may occur in bursts, or paroxysms. The disorder then spreads or marches from the part first affected to other muscles on the same side of the body—from the face to the neck, hand, forearm, arm, trunk, and leg; if the first movement is in the foot, the order is reversed. The high incidence of onset in the lips, fingers, and toes probably is related to the greater cortical representation of these parts of the body. The disease process or focus of excitation is usually the Rolandic cortex, area 4 (Fig. 31-1) on the opposite side; in a few cases it has been found in the post-Rolandic convolution. Lesions confined to the premotor cortex (area 6) are said to induce contractions of an arm, face, neck, or all of one side of the body. Perspiration and piloerection, sometimes of the parts of the body involved in a focal motor seizure, suggest that these autonomic functions have cortical representation in the Rolandic area. Some neurologists distinguish focal motor and Jacksonian motor seizures by the absence of a characteristic march in the former, but both have essentially the same localizing significance.

Another type of focal motor epilepsy, the previously mentioned *epilepsia partialis continua*, consists of rhythmic clonic movements of one group of muscles, usually in the face, arm, or leg. These may continue for a variable period of time, minutes to weeks or months. The seizure usually does not march to other parts of the body. Its localizing value has not been settled. Some cases have a lesion in the opposite sensorimotor areas of the cerebral cortex.

SOMATIC, VISUAL, AND OTHER SENSORY SEIZURES

Somatic sensory seizures, either focal or "marching" to other parts of the body on one side, nearly always indicate a parietal lobe lesion. The usual sensory disorder is described as a numbness or a tingling or "pins-and-needles" feeling. Other variations are sensations of crawling (formication), buzzing, electricity, or vibration. Pain and thermal sensations are infrequent. The onset is in the lips, fingers, and toes in the majority of cases, and the spread to adjacent parts of the body follows a pattern determined by sensory arrangements in the postcentral (post-Rolandic) convolution of the parietal lobe. In Kristiansen and Penfield's series the seizure focus was found in the postcentral convolution in 24 of 55 cases; it was central, either pre- or post-Rolandic, in 18, and precentral in 7 cases. One may conclude that this type of sensory phenomenon always indicates a focus in or near the post-Rolandic convolution of the opposite cerebral hemisphere; if localized in the head, the locus is in the lowest part of the convolution, near the Sylvian fissure; if in the foot or leg, the upper part near the superior sagittal sinus is involved.

Visual seizures are also of localizing significance. Lesions in or near the striate cortex of the occipital lobe usually produce a sensation of lights, of darkness, or of color. According to Gowers, red is the most frequent color, followed by blue, green, and yellow. The patient may tell of seeing stars or moving lights in the visual field on the side opposite the lesion. Sometimes they appear to be straight ahead of the patient. Often, if they occur on only one side of the visual field, he believes only one eye to be affected, the one opposite the lesion, probably because the average person is unaware that he has two corresponding visual fields. It is curious that a seizure arising in one occipital lobe may cause momentary blindness in both eyes. It has been noted that seizures in the lateral surface of the occipital lobes (Brodmann's areas 18 and 19) are more likely to cause twinkling or pulsating lights. Complex visual hallucinations are usually due to a focus in the posterior part of the temporal lobe, near its junction with the parietal, and they may be associated with auditory hallucinations. Often the visual images, either those of the hallucination or of objects seen, are distorted and seem too small (*micropsia*) or unnaturally arranged.

Auditory hallucinations are rather infrequent as an initial manifestation of a seizure. Occasionally a patient with a focus in the superior temporal convolution on one side will report a buzzing or a roaring in his ears. A human voice sometimes repeating recognizable words has been noted a few times in patients with lesions in the more posterior part of the dominant temporal lobe.

Vertiginous sensations of a type suggesting vestibular stimulation may be the first symptom of a seizure. The lesion is usually localized in the superior posterior temporal region or at the junction between parietal and temporal lobes. Foerster is said to have evoked a sensation of vertigo by stimulating the parietal lobe, and in one of Penfield's cases the lesion was there. Occasionally with a temporal focus vertigo is followed by an auditory sensation. Giddiness is also a frequent prelude to a seizure, but this has so many different meanings that it is of little diagnostic import.

Olfactory hallucinations are often associated with disease of the inferior and medial parts of the temporal lobe, usually in the region of the hippocampal convolution or the uncus (hence the term *uncinate seizures*, after Jackson). Usually the smell is exteriorized, i.e., projected to someplace in the environment, and is of a disagreeable nature. Gustatory hallucinations have also been recorded in proven cases of temporal lobe disease. Sensations of thirst and salivation may be associated. Stimulation of the upper surface of the temporal lobe in the depths of the Sylvian fissure during neurosurgical operations has reproduced peculiar sensations of taste.

Visceral sensations arising in the thorax, epigastrium, and abdomen are among the most frequent of the auras. They are described as a vague, indefinable feeling, a sinking sensation in the pit of the stomach, and a weakness in the epigastrium or substernal area that rises to the throat and head. In several such cases the seizure discharge has been localized to the upper bank of the Sylvian fissure, but in a few cases lesions were in the upper intermediate or medial frontal areas near the cingulate gyrus. Palpitation and acceleration of pulse at the beginning of the attack have also been related to a temporal lobe focus.

PSYCHIC PHENOMENA

The studies of many neurologists have served to establish the close relationship between psychic changes and the temporal lobe. Disease of either temporal lobe may be accompanied by seizures that have many of the characteristics outlined under Psychomotor Epilepsy. In addition to olfactory and gustatory hallucinations, there are often others of more complex visual and auditory type with feelings of unreality, and partial or complete interruption of consciousness may be observed. Compulsive thought or action may recur in a fixed pattern during each seizure. Automatic behavior or even frank psychoses of many different types, lasting for hours or days, may be induced by seizure discharges or electrical stimulation of the temporal lobe. Masticatory movements are also frequent.

LOSS OF CONSCIOUSNESS

A lapse of consciousness is the initial event in petit mal, which is believed now to represent a disorder of the diencephalon, the so-called "centrencephalic epilepsy." Lesions in the prefrontal regions have been observed to abolish consciousness at the very beginning of the seizure, presumably through the effects on the diencephalon and midbrain structures.

The various motor, sensory, or psychic phenomena may be combined in many different sequences. These presumably indicate the spread of a seizure discharge from one cortical area to another. A flash of light followed by tingling of one side of the body suggests that the epileptic discharge began in the occipital lobe and extended to the somatic sensory areas in the parietal lobe. A smell of something burning, followed by chewing and smacking movements, and then loss of speech would be interpreted as a spread of the seizure discharge from the region of the uncus to the upper parts of the temporal and the inferior frontal lobe. A focal motor seizure followed by a tonic contraction of one side of the body and then turning of the head and eyes contralaterally would indicate a successive involvement of the motor, premotor, and contraversive cortical field for head and eyes. Little is known about the factors that facilitate or inhibit the spread of seizure discharges from one part of the brain to another.

THE EVOCATION OF SEIZURES (Reflex Epilepsy)

For a long time it has been known that seizures could be evoked in susceptible individuals by a physiologic or psychologic stimulus. Approximately 1 in every 15 patients will have remarked that their seizures occur under special circumstances, such as being exposed to flickering light, passing from darkness to light or the reverse, being startled by a loud noise, hearing a series of monotonous sounds or music, touching, rubbing, or hurting a particular part of the body, making certain movements, i.e., eating, reading, carrying out some complex mental task, or being subjected to fright or other strong emotion. The evoked seizure may be focal (beginning often in the part of the body that has been stimulated) or generalized and may take the form of one or a series of myoclonic jerks, a petit mal, or a grand mal. In a few instances *reflex epilepsy*, as it is called, has been due to a focal cerebral disease, such as a tumor, but more often its cause cannot be ascertained. W. Watson has discovered a strong tendency to familial incidence in a variety of myoclonic jerking elicited by photic stimulation (photic epilepsy), and some patients in whom this phenomenon had been noted were unaware of ever having had a seizure. Also of interest in these cases of evoked seizure has been the phenomenon of willfully averting the seizure by undertaking some mental task, e.g., thinking about some distracting subject or counting, or by initiating some physical activity.

Patients of this type suggest to us that epilepsy is a

natural state, a physiologic event resulting from excitation and subsequent inhibition of an injured part of the cerebrum.

PATHOPHYSIOLOGY AND BIOCHEMISTRY OF EPILEPSY

From what has been said about epilepsy it is obvious that a satisfactory theory must account for the following clinical and pathologic data. (1) The majority of demonstrable epileptogenic lesions are situated in or near the cerebral cortex, which suggests that some property of the six-layered neural organization of this structure disposes to this condition. (2) The lesions of any given disease may or may not give rise to epilepsy; some peculiarity of the lesion must, therefore, determine this phenomenon. (3) The epileptic focus, once present, is known to become active, i.e., to discharge, only on occasion, or at least the electrical discharge which attends it only then becomes detectable in the electroencephalogram or expresses itself as an overt seizure. (4) Several events, some of physiologic or psychologic nature and others biochemical, are potent in activating the seizure focus or facilitating its spread. The former include photic and other sensory stimuli; the latter, such agents as pentylenetetrazol (Metrazol), picrotoxin, acetylcholine, excessive hydration, and alkalosis. (5) The seizure discharges upon reaching a certain intensity spread along preformed pathways from their site of origin to other cortical areas and to the diencephalon and brainstem. (6) Some inhibitory process counteracts and ultimately terminates the seizure discharge. (7) In many cases in human beings no cortical lesion has been demonstrated by current neuropathologic methods, and in this group there may be a genetic factor. The evidence on this latter point is not altogether convincing. Certainly, epilepsy and paroxysmal disturbances in the electroencephalogram have been observed in a large series of identical twins. However, the incidence of convulsions among blood relatives of epileptic patients is only two or three times that in the public at large, and a specific genetic pattern has never been established.

Investigations of epilepsy have centered on human cases of focal epilepsy and on experimentally induced focal epileptic lesions in the mammalian cortex. In both man and animal the neurophysiologic analogue to the convulsive seizure in human beings has been identified as a burst of high voltage spike waves, followed by repetitive, self-sustained discharge of electrical activity akin to posttetanic potentiation. This posttetanic potentiation is found so consistently in or near epileptic foci as to be accepted by many as the electrical sign of the epileptic lesion. The afterdischarge, once started, continues at a regular frequency of 10 to 14 per sec. Within a short time (seconds to minutes), the intervals between spikes increase; they tend then to be grouped, and their voltage rises. When the pauses between bursts reach 1/2 sec or more, the afterdischarge ceases altogether and the area of cortex becomes electrically inactive and inexcitable. The basis of the potentiation of the spike discharge is

little understood. Once started, its continuation involves a recycling or feedback process. Cessation indicates a rivalry between two opposing processes, the initial one excitatory, the final one inhibitory. A possible physiologic basis of these two processes has been demonstrated by Eccles at the spinal level. Each motor anterior horn cell, when activated, stimulates through a collateral branch another cell, the Renshaw cell, which is inhibitory in its action and imposes this inhibition on the anterior horn itself. Phillips has noted a similar arrangement between the Betz cells in the cerebral cortex and other interneurones that inhibit the Betz cells. Thus, both anterior horn cells and Betz cells can initiate excitation in another cell via their main axone, which in turn inhibits their own activity. Moreover, on the afferent side of neurone activation each sensory cell from the end organ to the cerebral cortex is monitored by a central descending inhibitory system. And, deafferentation itself is shown to increase the excitability of motor neurones.

The histologic changes in the seizure focus in man and experimental animals have been singularly difficult to interpret. In man epileptogenic foci are found not in gliotic scars but in neighboring intact regions of the brain. Whether the latter contain full populations of nerve cells with all their natural excitatory and inhibitory cortical mechanisms cannot be easily evaluated under the microscope. Golgi preparations are said to show a diminished number of dendritic arborizations and smaller synaptic surface of neurones.

A convulsive seizure could be conceived, therefore, either as an excessive excitation resulting from narrowly focused afferent stimulation on the injured cerebral cortex or as a deficiency of suppressive influences from either the afferent neurones or the special inhibitory neurones of the cortex. Strychnine, one of the most potent agents for discharging neurones and producing seizures, does not facilitate the excitatory postsynaptic potential of motor neurones but, rather, diminishes their inhibitory postsynaptic potentials. Solutions of strychnine, by themselves too weak to have any effect on the cortex, condition it in such a fashion that sensory stimuli conveyed to it will discharge the altered neurones and thus produce convulsive activity. This state of affairs resembles that which prevails in epileptic patients, where a silent, subliminal epileptic focus is discharged by a particular type of sensory stimulus and is restored to its quiescent state by inhibitory neurones.

Since electrical activity is believed to depend on chemical changes (flux of Na, K, Ca, Mg), it is rather to be expected that the effects of these ions would be studied in epilepsy. Hypocalcemia, hyponatremia, and hypokalemia, as well as hypoxia and alkalosis, for example, do increase the seizure tendency, but it is unclear as to whether they play a part in naturally occurring seizures. Also, a search has been made for special excitatory and inhibitory substances in the brain. Acetylcholine is known to be an effective convulsive agent when applied to the animal cortex, and cholinesterase inhibitors, such as isopropylfluorophosphate, likewise produce seizures. Cortical lesions in epileptic patients have been found to contain an increased amount of acetylcholinesterase and in a test tube are unable to "bind" acetylcholine. After a seizure there are increased amounts of acetylcholine in human cerebrospinal fluid. Barbiturates and diphenylhydantoin (Dilantin) are said to act as anticonvulsants because they enhance the acetylcholine-binding power of the cerebral cortex.

With respect to inhibitory substances Florey found that cerebral and spinal cord tissue contain an agent identified as gamma aminobutyric acid (GABA), which if applied to the cortex, blocks excitation of the superficial layer and augments inhibition—an action opposite to that of strychnine. It is formed from glutamic acid, and one of the coenzymes which catalyzes its synthesis is pyridoxine (vitamin B_6), lack of which is known to produce seizures in animals and man. Metrazol and picrotoxin are said to act by preventing the inhibitory effect of GABA. The action of GABA as an intrinsic anticonvulsant has not been fully explored. Given intravenously, it is said to protect animals against chemically induced seizures; others have not confirmed this effect.

A number of metabolic changes have been measured during a generalized convulsion. Presumably they are secondary. Oxygen utilization by the cerebral cortex increases, and of course, the violent generalized motor activity and arrest of respiration produce a hypoxia. CO_2 production in the convulsant brain is increased, and there is a relative acidosis. In the postseizure period cerebral vessels are dilated, and the oxygen content of the cerebral tissue increases. Hypoxic encephalopathy may occasionally complicate a prolonged motor seizure or status epilepticus and give rise to a postepileptic encephalopathy (neuronal loss in some cortical layers, hippocampus, and cerebellum).

Although high-amplitude activity of a group of neurones represents the "functional unit of epilepsy," it is the spread of this electrical potential to other parts of the nervous system that characterizes the whole convulsive seizure both clinically and electroencephalographically. The spread of these discharges proceeds along preformed pathways, i.e., via the uncinate fibers to adjacent cortical fields, via the corpus callosum to corresponding parts of the contralateral cerebral hemisphere, or along corticothalamic and thalamocortical pathways to the diencephalon and reticular formation. Some of the metabolic factors listed above may facilitate this spread. Little is known about agents that interfere with the spread of the seizure discharge. Acting on the assumption that the spread of seizure discharge is responsible for many of the undesirable features of the seizure, the corpus callosum has been sectioned in animals and human beings, and although the results were not conclusive, the seizures usually remained unilateral. The anticonvulsant activity of phenobarbital and diphenylhydantoin is believed to be mainly in preventing the spread of seizure discharges rather than in suppressing the epileptic focus.

Certain occurrences in the seizure, such as the cry, the motor activity, and the sensory experience, may be regarded as the direct manifestations of the seizure discharge in the brain. From the more general neurophysiologic point of view, they are excitatory. Others, like the lapse of consciousness of petit mal, are inhibitory. Electrical stimulation of the brain through the intact skull, as in electroshock convulsions for the treatment of depression or by the application of electrodes on the surface of the brain, is observed to produce the same changes. This initial outburst lasts for only a brief period of time and is often followed by a total or subtotal paralysis or inhibition of cerebral function. Similarly a focal motor seizure, for example, may result in suppression of activity in motor areas and a temporary paralysis of the involved muscles (Todd's postepileptic or exhaustion paralysis). The loss of consciousness that follows a generalized motor seizure, in contradistinction to that of petit mal, is probably due to a postexcitatory paralysis of either diencephalic or midbrain structures. Vital functions may also be arrested, but usually for only a few seconds. In rare instances, however, death may occur owing to a cessation of respiration, derangement of cardiac action, or some unknown cause. The automatic behavior so characteristic of psychomotor epilepsy appears in some instances to be a direct stimulatory effect in the temporal lobe and in others is a postexcitatory, inhibitory, or paralytic effect.

The electroencephalogram provides a delicate proof of Hughlings Jackson's theory of epilepsy—that it is an excessive, disorderly discharge of cortical neurones. At the onset of the focal seizure this is registered in or near the focus as a series of spikes or sharp waves interrupting the normal alpha and beta waves. The clinical spread of the seizure has its electroencephalographic equivalent in the extension of the abnormal electrical waves; and with generalization of the seizure (grand mal) the entire electroencephalographic recording surface of the brain exhibits spikes of high voltage. Petit mal is accompanied by a characteristic cold wave–spike complex occurring simultaneously in all cortical leads and presumably taking origin from a diencephalic focus. At first there was thought to be a characteristic electroencephalographic picture for psychomotor epilepsy, but further studies have not confirmed this. The postseizure state, sometimes called *postictal disturbance of cerebral function*, also has its electroencephalographic correlate in random generalized slow waves; with recovery the electroencephalogram returns to normal. If the electroencephalographic tracing is obtained during the interval between seizures, it is abnormal to some degree in approximately 40 percent of fully conscious and 75 percent of sleeping patients.

The electroencephalographic changes are discussed in Chap. 353.

DISEASES CAUSING SYMPTOMATIC EPILEPSY

In the list of diseases of the nervous system with which every physician must be familiar, a few stand apart by reason of their tendency to produce recurrent convulsions. The seizures are said to be symptomatic in contrast to the large majority of cases in which epilepsy is idiopathic. The physician must distinguish by the usual clinical and laboratory methods the different diseases that may cause, accompany, or precipitate convulsions.

DISEASES LOCALIZED IN THE CEREBRAL HEMISPHERES

Almost any type of cerebral lesion may cause seizures; on the other hand, no cerebral lesion is invariably accompanied by them. In patients with cerebral lesions the seizures are usually focal, leading in most instances to a generalized convulsion of grand mal type; less commonly they are of the petit mal type.

CEREBRAL TUMORS. They give rise to seizures in 35 to 60 percent of cases; in approximately 10 percent of all cases of tumor the seizure is the initial symptom. The nearer the tumor is to the excitable motor cortex, the greater is the likelihood of seizures. Tumors of the cerebellum and brainstem are seldom associated with any of the types of seizures described above, but they may cause episodes of decerebrate rigidity, i.e., opisthotonos and extension of all four extremities, sometimes called *tonic cerebellar fits.*

CEREBRAL TRAUMA. Trauma may cause seizures immediately after the injury, i.e., within hours or days, or after an interval of several months or years. In the former case seizures are rare; in the latter they vary in incidence, being more frequent in the severer grades of head injury. Uncomplicated concussion results in epilepsy in only about 0.5 percent of cases, which is about the expected frequency in the population at large, whereas with penetrating injuries, the incidence rises to approximately 20 percent and some figures have been as high as 40 percent. The average interval between the head injury and the first seizure is about 9 months, with a range of 6 months to 2 years or longer. The frequency of seizures varies from patient to patient; as years pass they tend to become less frequent.

CEREBROVASCULAR DISEASES. Although seizures occur at the time of the hemorrhage or infarction in a small percentage of cases, it has been said that vascular disease is rarely responsible for recurrent convulsions. This is true of atherosclerotic thrombosis and lacunar state and all types of brainstem infarction. Recently, however, analysis of our own material showed that cases of vascular disease of the cerebral cortex, particularly of embolic infarction, resulted in recurrent convulsions in about 20 percent of cases, a frequency nearly as high as in traumatic disease of the cerebral cortex. Hypertensive encephalopathy is often attended by convulsions. Venous thrombosis and infarction are a notable cause of focal epilepsy, and the same is true of vascular lesions in infancy and childhood, which may be either arterial or venous in nature. Seizures are also a frequent manifestation of vascular malformations.

CEREBRAL INFECTIONS. All types of cerebral infection may lead to epilepsy. Brain abscess is accompanied by seizures in about 50 percent of cases, and they often continue after the abscess has been drained or removed surgically. The seizures that accompany viral encephalitis, dementia paralytica, and other inflammatory diseases of the brain are related to cortical lesions. Inclusion-body encephalitis and subacute sclerosing encephalitis give rise to arrhythmic myoclonus, which is often combined with progressive dementia. In diseases that do not involve the cerebral cortex, such as encephalitis lethargica, there is little or no disposition to epilepsy.

DEGENERATIVE DISEASES. All types of degenerative diseases, if they affect the cerebral cortex, may be associated with recurrent seizures. Lipid-storage diseases and Jakob-Creutzfeldt disease tend usually to cause myoclonic dementia. Tuberous sclerosis is almost invariably accompanied by seizures. They occur but are infrequent in Alzheimer's disease and Pick's disease. About 3 percent of multiple sclerosis patients have convulsions in some phase of their illness.

CONGENITAL MALDEVELOPMENT OF THE BRAIN. This is frequently associated with epilepsy, which may be part of the syndrome of mental retardation, spastic diplegia, and other disturbances of motor function. The seizures usually develop in the first weeks or months of life. Special types of infantile and childhood seizures are discussed later in Chap. 365.

METABOLIC DISEASES

Conditions that disturb the metabolism of the brain may induce recurrent seizures. With hypoxia of whatever cause the damage to the cerebral cortex is associated with a series of seizures that begin within a few hours and continue intermittently for a variable period of time, usually a few days. Many of the surviving patients are not subject to epilepsy, but a small group develops intention myoclonus. Pyridoxine deficiency, phenylketonuria, and argininosuccinic aciduria are associated with seizures beginning in early life and continuing for the lifetime of the patient. Cerebral edema, resulting from excess ingestion of water or large infusions of glucose and water, may be attended by one or several generalized convulsions followed by headache and mental confusion. Uremia is accompanied by muscular twitching and, occasionally, by one or more terminal convulsions. Low blood calcium due to rickets or hypoparathyroidism often results in both tetany and seizures. Hypoglycemia, as from an overdose of insulin or an insulin-secreting islet cell tumor, often induces seizures, but they invariably follow an initial period of mental confusion, stupor, or coma. The usual history is for the attack to begin several hours after a meal or following a period of fasting. Seizures occur frequently in alcoholic patients and in those who have become addicted to barbiturates during the period of withdrawal.

DRUG INTOXICATION. The classic examples of direct seizure evocation by drugs are camphor, Metrazol, and picrotoxin. Withdrawal from barbiturates and alcohol in addicted individuals also gives rise to generalized convulsions.

APPROACH TO THE CLINICAL PROBLEM OF RECURRENT SEIZURES

A history of recurrent attacks of loss of consciousness or awareness associated with abnormal movements or confusion is usually sufficient to establish a diagnosis of epilepsy. With such patients a very thorough history, a complete physical and neurologic examination, testing of the visual fields, and laboratory studies, including x-ray examination of the skull and an electroencephalogram, should be done. The results of these essential procedures will determine to which of the categories in the above classification the case belongs and whether it should be labeled idiopathic epilepsy.

The history should be particularly searching in regard to epilepsy in the family history and occurrence of head trauma or infections in the past; and careful description of the disease itself, including prodromata, aura, manifestations during the seizure and the postictal period, must be obtained. Seizures in other members of the family favor the diagnosis of idiopathic epilepsy. Signs of pulmonary or ear infection or of congenital heart disease with a right-to-left shunt should suggest, in a patient with recently acquired seizures, the possibility of a brain abscess. The presence of a heart murmur and fever or of atrial fibrillation favor embolism. Head trauma of a serious nature, followed by seizures at an interval of several weeks to 2 years, indicates that an injury may have given rise to convulsions. A regularly recurring aura, especially of a focal nature, may indicate the presence of a localized lesion in the brain. Similarly, a focal convulsive movement at the onset of the seizure probably indicates a localized cerebral lesion. A transient monoplegia or hemiplegia (Todd's paralysis) in the postictal period also has considerable significance in localizing a lesion. In fact, its presence may provide the best clue to a focal brain lesion. A history of other neurologic symptoms such as headache, localized paralysis, or mental changes often indicates the need for special diagnostic studies.

A general physical examination may provide clues to the legion of conditions associated with epilepsy. The presence of protuberances over the skull may suggest an underlying pathologic condition. Vascular nevi over the body, especially over the face and in the retina, may be associated with vascular abnormalities within the skull. Small tumors, often pedunculated, distributed over the body surface bring to mind the diagnosis of von Recklinghausen's disease and, when associated with seizures, may indicate an intracranial glioma or neurofibroma. White spots over the trunk and limbs and sebaceous adenomas of the face point to the diagnosis of tuberous sclerosis. Smallness of an arm or leg points to a congenital defect of brain. Cranial nerve disturbances are also helpful in diagnosis; thus, a sixth-nerve paralysis is often associated with increased intracranial pressure. Localized weakness, differences in reflexes, or the presence of abnormal reflexes, such as Babinski's response, all have potential localizing value.

The question of what laboratory procedures should be done in cases of epilepsy can be answered only on the basis of the clinical findings. With generalized convulsions simple blood chemistries are among the first things to do. The determination of blood glucose helps orient the examiner in instances of hypoglycemia and hyperglycemia; the calcium level provides the main clue to hypocalcemia, the blood urea nitrogen (BUN) to kidney disease, and sodium and potassium levels to multiple metabolic disturbances including dilutional hyponatremia. X-rays of the skull should be taken in all cases. Significant findings related to increased intracranial pressure include erosion of the clinoid processes and, in infants and children, separation of the sutures. Hyperostoses, erosions of the skull, abnormal vascular markings, and intracranial calcifications are other findings of importance that may appear in skull x-rays. Because of the frequency of cerebral metastases from primary carcinoma of the lung, chest films should be made in all patients suspected of having intracranial neoplasm.

Lumbar puncture can be of considerable value in elucidating the causes of epilepsy. If the history, neurologic examination, or skull x-rays show any abnormality, especially if it suggests a focal lesion in the brain, then a lumbar puncture is mandatory. Of special importance are determination of the pressure, cell count, total protein, and serologic tests. Increased pressure points to an expanding intracranial lesion. An abnormal cell count often indicates an infectious process. An elevation in total protein (greater than 100 mg per 100 ml) favors the diagnosis of a tumor. If the pressure is normal, but other symptoms or signs point to a recently acquired, localized brain lesion, an arteriogram or pneumoencephalogram may be needed. If, in addition to localizing signs, the patient shows signs of increased intracranial pressure, whether by papilledema or high cerebrospinal fluid pressure, then a ventriculogram may be preferred to a pneumoencephalogram, although arteriography is now used more frequently than air visualization because of its greater safety. The visualization of the cerebral hemisphere by these procedures may be of particular help to the neurosurgeon in localizing the lesion and in planning a surgical approach to it.

The electroencephalogram, although now routinely employed in the definitive diagnosis of cases with epilepsy, is not absolutely conclusive, since it may be normal in some patients, particularly if the seizures are relatively infrequent, or abnormal in diseases that do not cause epilepsy. The test is of particular value in diagnosing petit mal, for here clinical or subclinical attacks are apt to be frequent enough to register during the electroencephalographic test. Abnormal electrical waves may manifest themselves in other types of epilepsy as well, and the electroencephalogram may be abnormal during the interseizure period, demonstrating either focal or generalized abnormalities of cortical activity. Activation of the electroencephalogram by photic stimulation, drug-induced sleep, or Metrazol injection is now standard procedure in many laboratories.

The type of clinical study in any given case is dictated to some extent by the age of the patient. Up until early adulthood the plan should be outlined as below. Most patients in this age group turn out to have idiopathic epilepsy. With increasing age, the incidence of idiopathic epilepsy becomes less and symptomatic epilepsy increases. Thus the appearance of convulsions for the first time at a period past middle age should be presumptive evidence of brain tumor until every effort has been made to rule it out.

The most frequent causes of recurrent convulsions in different age groups are presented in Table 28-1.

Table 28-1. CAUSES OF RECURRENT CONVULSION IN DIFFERENT AGE GROUPS

Age of onset, yr.	Probable cause
Infancy, 0–2	Congenital maldevelopment, birth injury; metabolic (hypocalcemia, hypoglycemia), B$_6$ deficiency, phenylketonuria
Childhood, 2–10	Birth injury, trauma, infections, thrombosis of cerebral arteries or veins, beginning of idiopathic epilepsy
Adolescence, 10–18 ...	Idiopathic epilepsy, trauma, congenital defects
Early adulthood, 18–35	Trauma, neoplasm, idiopathic epilepsy, alcoholism, drug addiction
Middle age, 35–60	Neoplasm, trauma, vascular disease, alcoholism, drug addiction
Late life, over 60	Vascular disease, degeneration, tumor

DIFFERENTIAL DIAGNOSIS

The clinical differences between a seizure and a syncopal attack were presented in Chap. 20 and need not be repeated here. It must be emphasized once again that there is no single criterion for distinguishing between them. The author has erred in calling akinetic seizures simple faints and in mistaking cardiac or carotid sinus faints for seizures. Petit mal may be difficult to identify because of the brevity of attacks. One helpful maneuver is to have the patient count for 5 to 10 min. If he is having petit mal, he will blink or stare, pause in counting, or skip one or two numbers. Psychomotor seizures are the most difficult of all to diagnose. These attacks are so variable in character and so likely to induce minor disturbances in conduct rather than obvious interruptions of consciousness that they may be diagnosed as temper tantrums, hysteria, psychopathic behavior, or acute psychosis.

A special problem in diagnosis is offered by states of mental dullness and confusion. Epileptic patients as seen in hospital and office practice usually show no mental deterioration, regardless of the type of seizure. Therefore, the appearance of dementia, confusion, or some other derangement of mental function should suggest the possibility of recurrent subclinical seizures not controlled by medication, drug intoxication, postseizure psychosis, or a brain disease that has caused both dementia and seizures. To distinguish these clinical states may require careful observation, along the lines suggested in Chap. 30, and electroencephalography.

REFERENCES

Lennox, W., and M. Lennox: "Epilepsy," Boston, Little, Brown & Company, 1960.
Penfield, W., and H. Jasper: "Epilepsy and the Functional Anatomy of the Brain," Boston, Little, Brown & Company, 1954.

29 AFFECTIONS OF SPEECH
Raymond D. Adams and Jay P. Mohr

Language or speech functions are of fundamental significance to man, in both his social intercourse and his private intellectual life; and when they are disordered as a consequence of developmental anomaly or disease of the brain, the resultant physiologic loss exceeds all others in gravity—even blindness, deafness, and lameness.

The physician is concerned with all derangements of language function, including those of reading and writing, because they are the source of much unhappiness and disability and are almost invariably manifestations of disease of the brain. Furthermore, language is the means whereby the patient communicates his complaints and his feelings to his physician and, at the same time, the medium for that interpersonal transaction between physician and patient which we call psychotherapy. Thus, any disease process that interferes with speech or the understanding of spoken words touches the very core of the patient-physician relationship. Finally, the clinical study of language disorders serves to illuminate the abstruse relationship between psychologic functions and the anatomy and physiology of the cerebrum. Language mechanisms fall halfway between the well-localized sensorimotor functions and the complex mental functions, such as imagination and thinking, which cannot be localized.

GENERAL CONSIDERATIONS

It has often been remarked that man's commanding position in the world rests on the possession of two faculties: (1) the ability to employ verbal symbols as a "background for his own ideation" and as a means of transmitting his thoughts to others of his kind; and (2) the remarkable facility of his hands. One curious and provocative fact is that the evolution of both speech and manual dexterity occurs in relationship to neurophysiologic pathways located in one cerebral hemisphere. This is a departure from nearly all other localizable neurophysiologic patterns, which are organized according to a bilateral and symmetric plan. The dominance of one cerebral hemisphere, usually the left, emerges with speech and the preference for the right hand, especially in writing; and a lack of development or loss of cerebral dominance as a result of disease disturbs both these traits.

There is abundant evidence that higher animals are able to communicate with each other by vocalization and gestures. However, the content of their communications is their feeling tone at the moment. This *emotional language*, as it is called, was studied by Charles Darwin, who noted that it underwent increasing differentiation in the animal kingdom. Similar instinctual patterns of emotional expression are observed in man. In fact, they are the earliest type of speech to appear (in infancy) and may have been the first to develop in primitive man. Moreover, the language we use to express joy, anger, and fear is retained even after destructive lesions of the dominant cerebral hemisphere; i.e., the neural arrangements that subserve emotional expression are bilateral and symmetric and do not even depend exclusively on the cerebrum. The experiments of Cannon and Bard have amply demonstrated that emotional expression is possible in animals after the removal of both cerebral hemispheres, provided the diencephalon, and particularly the hypothalamus and lower parts of the neuraxis, remain undamaged. In the human infant emotional expression is well developed at a time when the cerebral cortex is still immature.

Propositional, or symbolic, speech differs from emotional speech in several ways. Instead of communicating feeling, it transmits ideas from one person to another and requires in its development the substitution of a series of sounds or marks for objects or concepts. This type of speech is not found in animals nor in the human infant. It is not instinctive but learned and is therefore subject to all the modifying influences of social and cultural environments. However, the learning process becomes possible only after the nervous system has reached a certain degree of maturity. The units of propositional language, i.e., words and phrases, have acquired symbolic value and have become the medium of our thought processes. Facility in symbolic language, which is acquired over a period of 15 to 20 years, depends on both maturation of the nervous system and education.

THE DEVELOPMENT OF LANGUAGE

The acquisition of symbolic language by the infant and child has been observed methodically by a number of eminent scientists, and their findings provide a basis for understanding the various derangements of speech.

First, there is the *babbling* and *lalling stage* during which the infant of a few weeks of age emits a variety of sounds in combinations of vowel and labial or nasoguttural consonants. This predominantly motor speech activity is no doubt stimulated and reinforced by auditory sensations, which become linked to the kinesthetic ones arising from the speech musculature. It is not clear whether the capacity to hear and understand the spoken word precedes or follows the first motor speech. Possibly it varies from one infant to another, but certainly both speaking and auditory perception of words develop very early in life. Soon babbling merges with *echo speech*, in which the infant repeats parrotlike whatever he hears. Thereafter, auditory, visual, and kinesthetic sensations are gradually combined, and a sound comes to stand for or symbolize an object. Nouns are learned first, then verbs and other parts of speech. Single words and groups of words are used meaningfully in thinking and talking. They form propositions, which, according to Hughlings Jackson, are the very essence of speech. By the age of eighteen to twenty-four months the average infant can construct a phrase; in the months and years that follow,

he learns to speak in full sentences. A six-year-old child has a speaking vocabulary of several thousand words and an even larger understanding vocabulary. To learn the name of an object requires the formation of a link between the visual perceptive (association) regions of occipital lobes and the auditory perceptive region in the left temporal lobe, probably by way of the angular gyrus. In order to learn to say a name it is necessary to have a link between the auditory perceptive region (Wernicke) and the center for motor patterns of speech (Broca).

The child is now ready for the next stage, reading. This involves the association of graphic visual symbols with the auditory and kinesthetic images of words that have already been acquired. Usually the written word is learned by associating it with the spoken word rather than the seen object. It is held that the angular gyrus and contiguous parieto-occipital areas are critically involved in the establishment of these cross-modal associations. Writing is learned soon after reading, and word auditory-visual symbols now must become linked to cursive movements of the hand. Only those destined to become literate learn to read and write; and to be a complete master of the art of writing is an attainment of only a few select members of our society.

Language development appears to proceed in an orderly manner, but there are individual variations in the actual time at which each successive stage is reached and, to a limited extent, in the order of the different stages. Maturational delays are frequent. The pattern appears to be set by the neurologic equipment of the individual at any given age. Psychologic factors are of minor importance, at least in the beginning. There is, therefore, good reason why educators have found it unprofitable to teach reading and writing before the sixth year.

Anthropologists have suggested that the individual merely recapitulates the language development of his race. It is supposed that gestures and the utterance of simple meaningful sounds first occurred in primitive man as a differentiation of emotional speech. Gradually these movements and sounds became the conventional signs and verbal symbols of concrete objects, then of the abstract qualities of objects. Signs and spoken language were the first means of human communication; graphic records appeared much later. The American Indian, for instance, never attained a written language. Writing began as pictorial representation, and only much later were alphabets devised. The reading and writing of words and propositions have been relatively recent developments.

The increasing importance of language in contemporary society may be overlooked unless we reflect on the proportion of man's time devoted to purely verbal pursuits. *External speech*, by which we mean the expression of thoughts by spoken and written words and reception of the thoughts of others, is an almost continuous activity when human beings are gathered together; and *internal speech*, or the formation in our minds of unuttered words, is the "coin of mental commerce." It goes on even during a state of preoccupation, when a man is apt to think in words and may, in doing so, subconsciously utter words.

THE ANATOMY OF THE LANGUAGE FUNCTIONS

The conventional teaching is that there are three language areas, situated, in most individuals, in the left cerebral hemisphere (Fig. 31-1). Two are receptive and one executive. The two receptive areas are closely related and embrace what may be referred to as the central language zone. One, subserving auditory language reception, is situated in the posterior part of the first and second temporal convolutions (areas 41 and 42) near the primary auditory receptive area in Heschl's convolutions; the other, subserving visuolexic functions, occupies the angular convolution (area 39) in the inferior parietal lobule adjacent to the primary visual receptive areas. The intervening areas between these auditory and visual language "centers," the inferior temporal region (area 37), and the supramarginal convolution, are also part of this central language zone and are involved in language formulation. The executive area, situated at the posterior end of the third frontal convolution (referred to as Broca's area, or area 44) is for motor aspects of speech. Of dubious significance as a unique "writing center" is the foot of the second frontal convolution above Broca's area. These sensory and motor areas are connected by the arcuate bundle of nerve fibers which passes through the isthmus of the temporal lobe, and other connections may traverse the external capsule of the lenticular nucleus (subcortical white matter of the insula). From Broca's area there are fiber connections with the lower Rolandic cortex which in turn innervates the speech apparatus. These language areas are also connected with the thalamus and to corresponding areas in the minor cerebral hemisphere through the corpus callosum and anterior commissure.

There has been much difference of opinion concerning these cortical areas, and objection has been made to calling them centers, for they do not represent histologically circumscribed structures of constant function and fixed localization. Actually there is relatively little information concerning their anatomy and physiology. A competent neuroanatomist could not distinguish under the microscope some of these cortical speech areas from other parts of the cerebral cortex. Crude electrical stimulation of the parts of the cortex concerned with speech while the patient is alert and talking (during craniotomy under local anesthesia) causes only an arrest of speech. Knowledge of the location of speech functions has come almost exclusively from the study of human beings who have succumbed to focal brain diseases. From the available information it seems almost certain that the whole language mechanism is not divisible into a number of parts, each depending on a certain fixed group of neurones. Instead, speech must be regarded as a sensorimotor process roughly localized in the opercular or peri-Sylvian region of the left cerebral hemisphere, and the more complex elaborations of speech probably depend on the entire cerebrum.

Carl Wernicke, more than any other person, must be credited with the anatomic-psychologic scheme upon which contemporary ideas of *aphasia* rest. Paul Broca, of Paris, had made the fundamental observation that a lesion of the posterior part of the left inferior frontal convolution deprived a man of speech. But Wernicke's original study showed that a lesion in the posterior part of the left superior temporal convolution, near the termination of the acoustic pathway, would result not in loss of speech but in distorted words (paraphasia, i.e., interchange of words of similar sound or meaning, neologisms, and sometimes unintelligible jargon), a failure to comprehend what is said and written, an inability to repeat what is said, and an inability to communicate by writing. The rapid, fluent paraphasic quality of the speech he ascribed to a loss of the internal correction of the activities of the motor speech area of Broca by the receptive language zone. The occurrence of *alexia* with lesions in the auditory language field he explained as a consequence of the fact that one learns to read by associating written symbols with previously learned auditory ones. Similarly, *agraphia* would be expected because one learns to write by linking visual word symbols with kinesthetic ones for hand movement.

In collaboration with his pupils, Wernicke proposed a classification of language disorders, dividing them into three groups according to whether the disorder was (1) of the central receptive or the motor mechanisms of language, (2) of their connections with one another, or (3) of the afferent visual and auditory pathways by which the language mechanism was activated or of the efferent motor pathway by which its executive function was carried out through lower centers. The anatomy of the primary receptive and executive language disorders was said to be *cortical* (localized in the superior temporal and inferior frontal respectively); the anatomy of the lesion which separated the primary receptive zones from frontal motor zones was predicted to be transcortical (perhaps in insula and external capsule); and that which interrupted afferent and efferent pathways was subcortical. The latter were noted to be of two types: (1) motor in the form of *pure word muteness* and (2) sensory in the form of *pure word deafness*. Later Dejerine added a third, (3) *pure word blindness*.

Wernicke and his students established location of the lesions, so they believed, for the cortical and subcortical types of aphasia but those of the transcortical and conduction disorders were inconsistent, being sometimes insular and sometimes in the cortex more posteriorly, i.e., in the posterior Sylvian arc, (the cortex of posterior-superior temporal and inferior parietal lobes).

The verification of Wernicke's scheme by Liepmann, Lichtheim, and other of his pupils required many years of work and the development of systematic clinical and pathologic methods of study. Once the scheme was presented, it came immediately under sharp attack from many quarters. The anatomy of it struck several critics as being too neat, and for the more dynamically oriented workers it gave too little attention to the psychologic aspects of language. Pierre Marie, Henry Head, von Monakow, Arnold Pick, and Kurt Goldstein subsequently offered other ways of subdividing language function, again based on the manner in which speech deteriorated in disease. However, when they sought to correlate clinical and anatomic data, they always came back to an anatomic plan which differed little from that of Wernicke and his colleagues.

Most contemporary students of aphasia, while appreciative of the fundamental importance of Wernicke's contributions, find the division into cortical, subcortical, and transcortical (or conduction) disorders somewhat misleading, for the lesions never respect these anatomic boundaries; and to use these terms, as did Wernicke, to refer to mechanisms that involved predominantly cortical, subcortical, or transcortical organizations of neurones or their connections postulates a kind of physiologic organization, the existence of which is known only by inference. The word *conduction disorder* is especially confusing for it could apply to sensory pathways for the activation of the language mechanism as well as to efferent pathways for the execution of speech and to connections with the medial temporal regions concerned with learning and memory. Furthermore, the idea of subdividing the language mechanism into strictly sensory and motor parts with identifiable anatomic connections with one another can only impress the modern student as a somewhat outdated notion of neurophysiology. Not even the sensorimotor cortex for voluntary hand movements works that way.

Early and recent work on aphasia indicates that human language depends in some way upon the integrity of an anatomic region situated between the primary input zones of the temporal and occipital lobes and the output zone in the inferior frontal lobe of the dominant hemisphere. This places the mechanism in close connection with the cortical sensory association and cross-modal elaboration areas of the superior temporal and inferior parietal lobes, with the corresponding parts of the opposite cerebral hemisphere through the corpus callosum, with medial parts of the temporal lobes (learning-memory mechanisms) and with the diencephalon. The acquisition of language appears to involve, in part, the establishment of specific, item-by-item, cross-modal, verbally-mediated associations. But quite unknown at present is how these verbal relations are organized into a mechanism of extraordinary complexity—one that can be activated (controlled) by a variety of visual and auditory stimuli, that permits variable arrangements of words into an infinite number of sequences with unimaginable speed and efficiency and makes endless combinations of them available for our thinking and problem solving and for communicating our ideas through speech and writing.

From the available clinical and pathologic data it may be concluded that the locus of the anatomic lesion is more significant than the extent of brain damage. Localization of the lesion is in most instances predictable from the clinical symptomatology, but there are variations. For example, patients with lesions of Broca's area (area 44) do not always suffer the same degree of disturbance of speech. This lack of consistency in the anatomy of any given speech disorder has engaged the attention of many students of aphasia, and several different hypotheses have been proposed to explain it. The "classic" one has been that the net effect of any lesion depends not only on locus and extent of lesion but on the degree of cerebral dominance. If cerebral dominance is poorly established, a left-sided lesion has less effect on speech than if dominance is strong. Unfortunately, handedness and cerebral dominance are not recorded in many of the 1,500 cases collected by Henschen from the world's medical literature. Another factor which imparts an element of unpredictability to the anatomy of speech is that no two individuals acquire language in the same way; some depend more on auditory sense, others on visual. Lastly, clinical analyses of speech disorders may fail to identify a biologically meaningful functional deficit. We may then be trying to correlate a phenomenon of secondary importance to the anatomy of the lesion.

CEREBRAL DOMINANCE AND ITS RELATIONSHIP TO SPEECH AND HANDEDNESS

The functional supremacy of one cerebral hemisphere is so crucial to language function that it must be considered in greater detail. There are three ways of determining that the left side of the brain is dominant: (1) the loss of speech when disease occurs in certain parts of the left hemisphere and its preservation in diseases involving the right hemisphere; (2) the greater facility in the use of the right hand, foot, and eye; (3) the arrest of speech immediately after the injection of amobarbital (Amytal Sodium) or some other drug in the left internal carotid artery. Only (2) and (3) are of use in deciding the cerebral dominance of a living and healthy patient. Unfortunately, the Amytal Sodium or Wada test does not reproduce the syndrome of major hemisphere inactivation. There is only mutism followed by a brief period of groping for names. Presumably it gives information about the localization of motor output areas rather than of sensory ones.

Of the general population approximately 90 to 95 percent are right-handed; the remainder prefer the left hand. A person is said to be right-handed if he chooses the right hand for intricate complex acts and is more skillful with it. The preference is more complete in some than others. Most individuals are neither completely right-handed nor completely left-handed but favor one hand for more complicated tasks. Orton refers to this as *intergrading*. The manner in which dextrality and sinistrality are acquired is of interest. Most infants and small children are ambidextrous in their first actions. Writing may be carried out with either hand at first, and "mirror writing" at this early stage is frequent. Between the ages of two and six years one hand and one foot are selected for throwing and kicking a ball, sawing a board, cutting bread, etc. By middle childhood there is usually no doubt as to the dominant side. The reason for hand preference is still controversial. There is strong evidence of a hereditary factor, but the mode of inheritance is uncertain. Learning is also a factor; for many children are shifted at an early age from left to right (shifted sinistrals) because it is a handicap to be left-handed in a right-handed world. Many right-handed persons sight with the right eye, and it has been said that eye preference determines hand preference. Even if true, this still does not account for eye dominance. It is noteworthy that handedness develops simultaneously with language, and the most that can be said at the present is that speech localization and the preference for one eye, one hand, and one foot are all manifestations of some fundamental and inherited tendency not yet defined. Anatomic difference between the dominant and the minor cerebral hemispheres is uncertain except that the occipital horn of the left lateral ventricle is usually larger than the right, and the left sulcus lunatus more prominent. No consistent differences in the electroencephalogram between the two hemispheres have been found.

Left-handedness may result from disease of the left cerebral hemisphere in early life, and this probably accounts for its higher incidence among the feeble-minded and brain-injured. Presumably the neural mechanisms for language then become centered in the right cerebral hemisphere. Handedness and cerebral dominance may fail to develop in some individuals, and this is particularly true in certain families. Developmental defects in speech and reading, stuttering, "mirror writing," and general clumsiness are much more frequent in these families.

Differences in degree of cerebral dominance do unquestionably account for some of the inconsistency in the cerebral localization of speech in different individuals. In studies of groups of left-handed individuals who suffer cerebral derangements of speech it has been noted that approximately 75 percent of them have had lesions in the left cerebral hemisphere. Further, in those aphasias due to the right cerebral lesions, the patient is always left-handed, and the speech disorder tends to be less severe and enduring. The latter may take the form of an expressive disturbance rather than alexia or amnestic aphasia; and visuoconstructive troubles are prominent, as are also faults in calculation and recognition of one's neurologic deficits (anosognosia).

The functional capacities of the minor hemisphere in speech are not fully documented by careful anatomic studies. Always there is some uncertainty as to whether any residual function after lesions of the major hemisphere is due to recovery of parts of its language zones or to the activity solely of the minor hemisphere. Reasonably well established are the following more or less verbal functions of the minor hemisphere: motor responses of mimicry, social anticipation (smiling, handshaking, modesty reactions) and self care (washing and feeding), avoidance behavior to noxious stimuli and capability of training in performances of cross-matching visually presented simple words with pictures.

TYPES OF LANGUAGE DISORDER ENCOUNTERED IN MEDICINE

These can be divided into four categories:

1. Disturbances of speech that occur with diseases affecting the higher nervous integrations, namely, delirium and dementia. Speech is seldom lost in these conditions but is instead merely deranged as part of a general impairment of intellectual functions. These conditions will not be discussed further here (see Chap. 31). *Palilalia* and *echolalia*, in which the patient repeats, parrotlike, the syllables and words which he hears, are special abnormalities usually observed in states of dementia generally with conjoined extrapyramidal signs.

2. The loss or disturbance of speech due to a cerebral lesion that does not deprive a man of his reason or paralyze other motor or sensory functions. This condition has been termed *aphasia;* milder degrees of it have been called *dysphasia.*

3. A defect in articulation with intact mental functions and normal comprehension and memory of words. This is a pure motor disorder of the muscles of articulation and may be due to flaccid or spastic paralysis, rigidity, repetitive spasms (stuttering), or ataxia. The term *anarthria* or *dysarthria* has been applied to some of these conditions.

4. Loss of voice due to a disease of the larynx or its innervation, with resulting *aphonia* or *dysphonia.* Articulation and internal language are unaffected.

In the practice of medicine the most frequent and troublesome disorders of speech are aphasia, stuttering, dysarthria, and aphonia.

Types of Aphasia

Systematic examination will usually make it possible to decide whether the patient has a *global aphasia* (with loss of all or nearly all speech functions; a motor aphasia (*Broca's aphasia*), sometimes called verbal or executive aphasia; *Wernicke's aphasia,* a receptive or sensory aphasia predominantly auditory and visual in type; or *dissociative speech syndromes:* of the central language area from the motor area, of the motor speech area from lower centers, of auditory verbal aphasia (word deafness), of alexia (inability to read), and of amnestic aphasia. Writing is disturbed to some extent in the majority of cases of aphasia and is rarely disturbed alone.

GLOBAL OR TOTAL APHASIA. Global or total aphasia is due to a lesion that destroys a large part of the speech areas of the major cerebral hemisphere. It is an affection of all input and output zones that are concerned with receiving sensory stimuli for speech as well as for expression. Usually it is due to occlusion of the left internal carotid or middle cerebral artery, but it may be caused by a massive hemorrhage (hypertensive or traumatic), an infiltrative tumor, or other lesion. The middle cerebral artery nourishes all the speech areas, and nearly all the aphasic disorders due to vascular occlusion are caused by involvement of this artery or its branches. Left hemispherectomy for glioma or epilepsy has had a similar effect on all speech functions.

Most of the patients with global aphasia are speechless or can say at most a few words; they cannot read or write and can understand only a few simple spoken words and phrases. Related signs include right hemiplegia, hemianesthesia, and homonymous hemianopia. The state of consciousness may vary from full alertness to semicoma. The patient may participate in common gestures of greeting, show modesty and avoidance reactions, and engage in self-help activities. Improvement depends on the nature and extent of the disease and whether or not the right cerebral hemisphere had previously engaged in language formulation and expression. With the passage of time some degree of understanding of spoken speech may be evident and a few words of speech may return. However, if the left hemisphere was strongly dominant, there will usually be little or no recovery, which casts doubt on the popular notion that the right hemisphere can take over speech function.

WERNICKE'S APHASIA. The syndrome has two components. The first is an impairment in phonemic hearing, which reflects the proximity of the lesion to the primary auditory cortex of Heschl's transverse gyri and involvement of auditory association areas, separating them from the angular gyrus. The second is a general impairment of language-dependent behavior, which may reflect the major role the auditory region plays in the regulation of language.

The defect in auditory functions is manifested by an impairment of repetition of spoken words and the matching of two sequences from a series of identical auditory stimuli or rhythms. Repetition is confined to short words or words of which the components are widely separated in phonemic composition. A few simple commands may still be executed but not complex ones. The patient gestures freely, talks volubly, and appears unaware of his deficit. The errors of word formation are in the nature of paraphasia, and take the form of substitution of words or jargon sounds similar in sound to the correct response (literal paraphasia) or the substitution of words of similar meaning for one another (verbal paraphasia). When severely disorganized, the speech may be reduced to an incomprehensible gibberish or jargon.

The general impairment of language-dependent behavior may be more or less disassociated from the deficits in phonemic hearing, and may occasionally appear in more isolated form. Certain neurologists have referred to this as "central aphasia." Although all the sensory and motor apparatus required in the activation and expression of language behavior appears intact, the patient is unable to understand what is said to him, to read aloud or for comprehension, to speak in properly constructed sentences, or to communicate by writing. Vocal speech is marred by paraphasias, as indicated above, and also by impairments in the construction of phrases in spontaneous speech. The patient is unable to name from sight or touch items whose names he can repeat from dictation. He is unable to write from dictation words he can copy from sight or even from touch. The copying performance is slow and laborious and conforms to the exact contours of the model (including the examiner's handwriting style) in a "servile" fashion. He is unable to cross-match words from dictation to sight, yet he can match a word to itself by sight alone and can repeat the word from dictation. Overall, performance is impaired on those tasks which require previous experience to indicate a relationship between two formally dissimilar stimuli (e.g., the sound of the word "cat" and printing the letters of the word "cat"). But preserved are those performances which can be accomplished by indicating or producing a response which is formally identical to that given (e.g., copying from sight the word "cat").

With the passage of time, the impairment in phonemic hearing may improve and with it, the apparent understanding of words. Of the several speech faults, repetition of spoken language, especially of unfamiliar words, is most likely to remain impaired. Extreme variability of performance is frequently striking. When testing is conducted in single steps with pauses between trials, a surprising degree of intact performance may be noted, but any increase in rate and variation of material presented results in failure. A common error is to interpret flaws in verbal production as a primary expressive aphasia, but in actuality, there is no abnormality of the articulatory-phonetic performance as there is in verbal output disorders of purely motor type. This is the reason we prefer to avoid the term *expressive aphasia,* i.e., it includes more than just motor output disorders.

As a rule, the lesion involves the posterior Sylvian region (temporal and parietal) and is usually caused by an embolic occlusion of the lower division of the left middle cerebral artery. Subcortical slit hemorrhage in the temporoparietal region, and involvement of the temporal isthmus and adjacent white matter by tumor, abscess, or extension from putaminal or thalamic hemorrhage may have similar effects.

The posterior Sylvian region, comprising posterior superior temporal, opercular supramarginal, and posterior insular gyri, appears to encompass a variety of language functions, since seemingly minor changes in size and locale of lesion are associated with important changes in syndromes in a spectrum of Wernicke's aphasia, conduction aphasia, pure word deafness, as well as a number of variants of these syndromes. The interesting theoretic problem raised by the consideration of general impairment in language-dependent behavior is whether or not the deficits observed represent disturbance of a unitary language function in the posterior Sylvian region or, instead, a series of sensorimotor activities of which the required anatomic pathways happen to be crowded together in a small region of the brain. In view of the multiple ways in which language deteriorates in disease, the latter hypothesis seems more likely.

MOTOR SPEECH DISORDERS (BROCA'S APHASIA). Although the nature of Broca's aphasia remains somewhat in doubt we have chosen to apply the term, as have others, to a primary deficit in motor speech production. Uncertainty relates always to the degree to which it may be combined with impairment in language-dependent behavior. In our experience there is a wide range of variation in the motor deficit, from the mildest cortical type of dysarthria with entirely intact "inner language" to a complete loss of all means of communication through lingual, phonetic, and manual action. Since the muscles that can no longer be used in speech still function in other acts, the term *motor (kinetic)*, or *ideomotor, apraxia* seems applicable to certain components of the deficit.

In the fully developed syndrome the patient will have lost all power of expressing himself by spoken words. No longer can he speak spontaneously in conversation, read aloud, or repeat words he hears. If any words remain accessible to him, they will be "yes" or "no" and perhaps a few other habitual expressions. One at first suspects the lingual and phonetory apparatus of being paralyzed until it is observed that the patient has no difficulty chewing, swallowing, clearing his throat, licking his lips, and even vocalizing without words. Often the lower part of the face is weak on the opposite (right) side and occasionally the arm and leg as well. The tongue may deviate away from the lesion, i.e., to the right. For a time, despite good preservation of auditory comprehension and ability to read, commands to purse the lips properly, to lick the lips, to blow, smack, and make other purposeful movements are poorly executed, which means that the ideomotor apraxia has extended to other acts. Imitation of the examiner's actions are better performed, and self-initiated actions are normal. The patient may repeat his few remaining words over and over again, as if compelled to do so. The words of well-known songs may be sung, and others are uttered as expletives, when the patient is angered or excited, making the point that he is "speechless" but not "wordless." Usually, the patient recognizes his ineptitude and own mistakes. Failing in attempts to correct them he may exhibit signs of exasperation or despair.

Most patients with Broca's aphasia have as much trouble writing as speaking. Should their right hand be paralyzed, they cannot print with their left one; and if manual mobility is spared, they do not succeed in writing out their replies to questions or in indicating their needs. Writing to dictation is impossible but letters and words can still be copied.

Comprehension of spoken and written language, while normal under many conditions of testing may break down when novel material is rapidly presented, varying with the degree of associated central aphasia.

Broca's aphasia due to vascular lesions (the common ones) usually regresses in time, and as words return, the patient's utterances are noted to be slow, laborious, slurred, and many of the small words (articles, prepositions, conjunctions) are omitted, giving the speech an agrammatic character (*agrammatism*). There is loss also of all the natural accent, word emphasis, and melody of language (*dysprosody*), and the coordination of respiration and speaking are faulty.

The rate of clearing, in fact the natural course of the

neurologic syndrome, varies with the nature of the causative lesion. An embolus in the upper main division (Rolandic) of the middle cerebral artery causes the most abrupt onset and rapid regression (sometimes hours or days). Because of the distribution of this artery there is frequently an associated right-sided faciobrachial paresis and a *left*-sided brachial apraxia. Atherosclerotic thrombosis, tumor, subcortical hypertensive hemorrhage, traumatic hemorrhage, etc., may also declare themselves in this way if they should involve the premotor cortex which lies in the posterior part of the left inferior frontal convolution (area 44 of Broca).

Pure word mutism also causes the patient to be wordless but leaves his inner speech intact. Since this is anatomically more in the nature of a dissociation of the motor cortex for speech from lower centers, we shall describe it with the dissociative syndromes.

DISSOCIATIVE SPEECH SYNDROMES

These are characterized by an impairment in the activation of executive functions of the language mechanism by the interruption of major afferent connections or of major efferent (motor) connections with lower centers, and it also includes separation of the more strictly receptive parts of language from the purely motor ones, i.e., a break in sensorimotor integration. The patient generally appears to be normal except for the specific deficit, sensory or motor, i.e., his behavior with respect to language-dependent tasks and his utilization of words in thinking (inner speech) are normal.

ISOLATION OF BROCA AND WERNICKE AREAS. Here, a lesion (usually hypoxia and ischemia with water-shed infarction) isolates the auditory and motor speech mechanisms separating them from the rest of the brain. The patient exhibits a defect in auditory and visual word comprehension and lacks useful speech. Presumably information from the rest of the brain cannot be transferred to Wernicke's area for conversion into verbal form. Speech is fluent, rapid and paraphrasic. There is dysnomia. Spoken phrases are repeated, parrot-like, unlike the Wernicke aphasic syndrome.

CONDUCTION DISORDER WITH SEPARATION OF CENTRAL LANGUAGE AREA FROM MOTOR SPEECH AREA. Here the principal abnormality consists of paraphasia in self-initiated speech and in repeating what is heard. In contrast, the articulatory-phonetic process is normal and the patient has no difficulty in comprehending what he hears and sees. He is alert and aware of his deficit. One of the best ways of eliciting the defect is to have the patient repeat nonsense syllables. Careful analysis of the disturbance shows that in the formation of words the mistakes are of a type seen in literal paraphasia, that is to say that words of somewhat similar structure (phonemic similarity) but different meaning are interchanged. Often it can be shown that the oral, pharyngeal, lingual musculature is not correctly controlled to produce the word intended, yet there is no element of dysarthria or dysprosody. The disorder becomes more apparent when the rate of presentation of auditory material is increased and as the uttered words become more polysyllabic. Since nouns are the longest words in the sentence, one may gain an inaccurate impression that they are specifically affected.

The lesion in autopsied cases is superficial in the cortex and subcortical white matter and is located in the upper bank of the Sylvian fissure involving the supramarginal gyrus of inferior parietal lobule and occasionally the posterior part of the superior temporal region. It presumably interrupts fiber systems in the insula. The usual cause is an embolus in a branch (ascending parietal or posterior temporal) of the middle cerebral artery. Deeper, larger lesions in position to interrupt the arcuate fasciculus connecting the temporal and frontal lobes are likely to involve other pathways as well, giving rise to a more extensive speech deficit (central aphasia or Wernicke's aphasia and dysnomia). These latter types of aphasia, as they regress, may resolve into conduction aphasia. More anterior insular lesions usually include some degree of Broca's aphasia.

PURE WORD DEAFNESS. This syndrome is characterized by impaired auditory comprehension and inability to repeat what is said or to write to dictation. Inner speech, manifested by facile and correct use of words in thinking and discussing problems, correctly phrased self-initiated utterances, correct writing, reading, and copying are all intact. The patient may declare that he cannot hear, but shouting does not help him, sometimes to his surprise. By audiometric testing no hearing defect is found. Ordinary sounds can be distinguished. Sometimes the patient thinks he has heard a question or statement when he has not; he acts on a combination of visual cues and distorted sounds and then proceeds to give an irrelevant answer. If his listener looks incredulous he reacts by being more insistent. When the patient is able to describe his auditory experience, he says that words are a jumble of noises. Often the syndrome is not pure and elements of paraphasia enter, which helps in distinguishing the condition from true deafness.

In most instances the lesion has been bilateral in the superior temporal gyrus, in position to separate the primary auditory cortex in the transverse gyrus of Heschl from the secondary and tertiary association areas of the superior-posterior part of temporal lobe. The few unilateral lesions have been in the major (dominant) hemisphere. Requirements of smallness and superficiality of lesion in cortex and subcortical white matter are best fulfilled by a small embolic occlusion of a branch of the lower division of the middle cerebral artery. More extensive lesions lead to Wernicke's aphasia.

PURE WORD BLINDNESS. In this state a literate person loses the ability to read, to copy, and often to name colors. He can no longer name or point on dictated command to visual letter stimuli or the words of which they are composed. However, understanding spoken language, repetition, writing to dictation, and conversation are all intact. Often the subject makes no complaint about his difficulty; it is discovered almost by accident. In tests he reads a single letter at a time (this may be seen in otherwise normal patients who have bilateral hemianopia with only central vision remaining) but commonly he utters letter-name responses that seem to have little connection with the presented letters. The response may be corrected and the defect obscured if other visual cues are available, such as the bottle on which the words Coca-Cola appear. Associated with this there may be impaired naming of common colors when presented in isolation, and impaired naming of unseen objects which the subject touches. When the dominant hemisphere is involved, as it usually is in such cases, there may be a right homonymous hemianopia, an amnestic defect (see Chap. 30), and a hemisensory defect on the right due to involvement of the left occipital lobe, the left fornix and its decussation, and the left thalamus, respectively, a combination which nearly always signifies thrombosis or embolism of the left posterior cerebral artery.

The anatomy of the lesions is usually such as to destroy the left visual striate cortex and association areas 18 and 19 as well as the connections of the right visual cortex and association areas to the left angular gyrus. This disconnection usually occurs in the splenium of the corpus callosum. Less often the lesion may be confined to the left occipital lobe and the deep central white matter of the parietal lobe, cutting through the right occipital–left parietal connection. In this case the right homonymous hemianopia may be absent. With purely left cerebral lesions a primary or secondary tumor or, rarely, multifocal leucoencephalopathy or trauma may be the underlying disease. The associated disturbances of color naming are not dependent on a lesion of the corpus callosum. In large lesions of the left parietaloccipital region alexia may be combined with right-left confusion, acalculia, and difficulty in naming of fingers and other parts of the body (Gerstmann's syndrome) (see Chap. 31).

PURE WORD MUTENESS (SUBCORTICAL MOTOR APHASIA). The patient will have lost all capacity to speak, while retaining perfectly the ability to write, to think with words, to understand spoken words, and to read. Although usually paretic, the lips, tongue, pharynx, and larynx show none of the apraxic disturbance seen in Broca's aphasia. With recovery or in milder degrees of the disorder, vocal utterances are dysarthric due to paresis and are extremely slow, with inadequate volume and intonation.

The causative lesion, usually vascular, is located in the motor cortex, separating it from the premotor, or is located beneath both Broca's convolution and the motor cortex, separating them from subcortical motor centers.

AMNESTIC–DYSNOMIC APHASIA. This may be a relatively early or an isolated manifestation of nervous disease. The patient loses the ability to name objects. Partial degrees of it are associated with pauses in speech, groping for a word, the substitution of another word. When shown a series of uncommon objects, the patient may tell of their use instead of giving their names. The difficulty applies not only to objects seen but to the names of things heard or felt, but such tests are more difficult to employ.

Recall of the names for letters, digits, and other printed verbal material is almost invariably preserved. That the deficit is principally one of naming is shown by the fact that the patient makes correct use of the object and is usually able to point to it when asked to do so. As a rule, he will choose the correct name from a series shown him or given to him verbally. There is a tendency among patients to explain failure as one of forgetfulness, which indicates their partial unawareness of the defect.

The causative lesion is usually deep in the temporal lobe, in position, probably, to interrupt connections of sensory speech areas with the hippocampal-parahippocampal regions concerned with learning and memory. Mass lesions, such as a tumor or an otogenic abscess, are the most frequent, and as they enlarge, an upper contralateral quadrantic visual field defect, or Wernicke's aphasia, is produced. Occasionally, dysnomia appears with diseases which occlude the temporal branches of the posterior cerebral artery. Alzheimer's disease and senile dementia may begin or present early a phase in which there is a dysnomic or amnestic type of aphasia. Usually, however, by the time the patient's difficulty is recognized, other disorders of speech have been added, as well as indifference, apathy, and abulia.

APPROACH TO THE CLINICAL PROBLEM OF APHASIA

In investigating a case of aphasia it is first necessary to inquire into the patient's native language, his handedness, and his previous education. Many naturally left-handed children are trained to use their right hand for writing; therefore, in determining this point we must ask which hand is used for throwing a ball, threading a needle, or using a spoon or common tools such as hammer, saw, or bread knife. One should quickly ascertain whether the patient has other signs of a gross cerebral lesion such as hemiplegia, facial weakness, homonymous hemianopia, or cortical sensory loss. When hemiplegia, hemianesthesia, and homonymous hemianopia are present, the aphasic disorder is usually of global type. Such a constellation of signs is but rarely coincident with pure central aphasia, Wernicke's aphasia, or one of the dissociative syndromes. Dyspraxia of limbs and speech musculature, in response to spoken commands or visual mimicry, is generally associated with Broca's aphasia and sometimes central aphasia. Bilateral or unilateral homonymous hemianopia without motor weakness tends often to be linked to pure word blindness (alexia or dyslexia) or to amnestic-dysnomic aphasia. Bilateral hemiplegias are associated not infrequently with pure word muteness. Multiple small embolic vascular lesions, causing a variety of focal cerebral signs, are the lesions most likely to be accompanied by Wernicke's aphasia, alexia, or pure word deafness.

It is important before the beginning of the examination to determine whether the patient is alert and mentally clear or suffering from confusion, because this may interfere with accurate assessment of language. One must also avoid the effects of fatigue as far as possible by making the interview short. Explanation of the purpose of the tests, sympathy, and encouragement are often necessary to assure full cooperation.

Many elaborate examination schemes have been devised for testing the language functions; (see monographs of Weisenberg and McBride, Goldstein, and Schuell); some of them lead to refinements that are of little physiologic or clinical significance. The following procedure will yield sufficient data for diagnosis in most cases.

1. In ordinary conversation does the patient spontaneously utter intelligible words in proper sequence and well-constructed phrases and sentences? The fluency of speech, the extent of vocabulary, the grammatic construction of sentences, the accuracy of word usage, and clarity of enunciation should all be observed and examples incorporated into the record of the interview. Wrong choice of words, misplacement of words or syllables, omission of essential words, and use of disjointed phrases may be slight in degree and take the form of either literal or verbal paraphasia; if severe, they may result in an unintelligible jabbering or jargon. Can the patient repeat or copy what he hears or reads?

2. Can the patient understand what he hears? If he is unable to speak, give him a series of commands of increasing complexity. Ask him to close his eyes, open his mouth, hold up his left hand, place the index finger of the left hand to the right ear, etc. Often the patient will execute the first one or two simple commands correctly and will fail on all others, sometimes repeating the first act over and over (perseveration). Auditory comprehension may be difficult to assess in conversation because of many visual cues that are unwittingly transmitted by the examiner. The most dependable proof of intact repetition is the ability to repeat complex and unusual words and phrases given without gesture and out of context of previous conversation.

3. Can the patient read? Written questions or commands should be present and the responses observed. If motor speech is absent, the patient can be asked to select correct words for objects shown or words spoken by pointing to the corresponding words in a list. Recognition of similarity and dissimilarity between groups of words on the list may be tested by having him point successively to those words designating vegetables, flowers, inanimate objects, etc. If writing is intact, tests of copying or transcribing from print to script or vice versa will indicate whether he can see a word without knowing its meaning.

4. Can the patient write spontaneously? If his right hand is paralyzed, he should be encouraged to try with his left. It must also be determined whether or not he can write from dictation and can copy words or sentences. Transcription from print to script and vice versa should also be tested.

5. If he is able to speak, can he name common objects shown visually, such as a penny, button, pencil, fountain pen, handkerchief, the various parts of a wrist watch, safety pin, key, flashlight, matches? If not, does he recognize the correct name when he hears it? Are gestures appropriate?

Nonfluency distinguishes the anterior or frontal group of aphasias; fluency with failure of comprehension and repetition characterizes the posterior group of aphasias.

Disorders in the Development of Language in Children

A close parallelism exists between the symptoms observed in adults who have suffered a loss in language functions as a result of brain injury and those seen during the development of language skills. This reminds us that there may be faulty development of language and of cerebral dominance. It has been found that a high percentage of these patients have a strong family background of speech disorders and that strong preference for the right or the left hand is not present. Males are affected much more frequently than females (ratios as high as 10:1).

Developmental disorders of language and congenital deafness are far more frequent than aphasia. These include developmental alexia (special reading disability), developmental word deafness, developmental motor aphasia (motor speech delay), and developmental apraxia (abnormal clumsiness of the limbs). The development of language, instead of proceeding in the manner outlined in the early part of this chapter, is arrested or delayed. Disorders of this type are probably due to slowness in the normal processes of maturation rather than an acquired or developmental disease. These conditions are often misunderstood by parents, teachers, and physicians. Sometimes the unfortunate child is judged to be feebleminded or lazy. Another frequent error is to assume the condition is due to psychologic factors, since nervousness, stubbornness, poor sleep, headaches, etc., are frequently associated.

CONGENITAL WORD DEAFNESS. If an individual is born deaf, he can learn to talk only after special training; he is "deaf and dumb." Should deafness develop within the first few years of life, after speech has been acquired, the child gradually loses speech but can be retaught by the lip-reading method. His speech is harsh, poorly modulated, and unpleasant, and he is apt to make many peculiar throat noises of a snorting or grunting kind. Such patients may be bright and alert and also clever at pantomime and gesturing. They are inattentive to household noises and do not appear to understand what is said to them. The deafness can be demonstrated at an early age by careful observation of the child's responses to sounds, but it cannot be accurately tested before the age of three or four years. The psychogalvanic reflex technique for testing reaction to sounds and tests of the labyrinths, which are frequently unresponsive in deaf-mutes, may be helpful. In contrast, the idiot or moron is stupid in all his actions and talks little because he has nothing to say. Developmental word deafness may be difficult to distinguish from true deafness. Usually the parents have noted that the word-deaf child responds to loud noises and music, though obviously this does not assure perfect hearing, particularly for high tones. The word-deaf child

does not understand what is said, and there is delay and distortion of speech. These children are alert, active, and inquisitive and may chatter incessantly. They adopt a language of their own design, and attentive parents come to understand it. This peculiar type of speech is known as *idioglossia*. It is also observed in children who have marked difficulty in the articulation of certain consonants. They learn to lip-read very quickly and are clever at acting out their own ideas.

CONGENITAL WORD BLINDNESS (ALEXIA). In this unusual condition the patient has good eyesight and is able to see the word but not to grasp its meaning. There is no loss of the ability to recognize the meaning of objects, pictures, and diagrams. Usually with assiduous training, the patient, who is otherwise bright and intelligent, can learn to read individual letters and a few simple words. Spelling is impossible. Often the patient cannot write anything of his own composition but can copy skillfully. Lesser degrees of congenital alexia are commoner than the severe forms and pose serious problems in the classroom. Some 10 percent of school children have some degree of this disability. The problem is a complex one, for difficulty in learning to read well is unquestionably influenced by the teaching techniques used in the school. Only a few of the severely handicapped children have a right homonymous hemianopia or a right-sided sensory loss; most of them show no other abnormality. The majority have no other signs. The important genetic study of Hallgren shows that the condition is inherited as an autosomal dominant trait and is unrelated to psychologic factors; speech delay, articulatory abnormalities, and difficulty in reading digits may be associated. Also, there is a statistically higher incidence of left handedness.

ABNORMALITIES OF ARTICULATION AND PHONATION (LISPING, DYSLALIA). A number of odd varieties of deficient articulation may come to the notice of the physician. One is *lisping,* in which the s sound is replaced by *th*; e.g., "thister" for "sister." Another condition, called *lallation* or *dyslalia,* a common speech disorder observed in early childhood, is characterized by multiple substitutions or omissions of consonants. In severe forms, speech may be almost unintelligible. These children are unaware that their speech differs from that of other persons and are distressed at not being understood. Milder degrees consist of the failure to pronounce only one or two consonants. For example, there may be imperfect enunciation of the sound r so that it sounds like w. "Running a race" becomes "wunning a wace." The nature of this disorder is not known. It has been suggested that the development of language in some children is so rapid that there is a partial failure of both perceptive and imitative speech. The patient usually recovers spontaneously from this disorder or responds promptly to speech therapy, which is best carried out at about the age of five years. These abnormalities are more frequent among feebleminded than normal children, and mental defect should always be suspected if numerous consonants are mispronounced and the condition persists beyond the age of twelve or thirteen years. The speech disorder resulting from *cleft palate* is easily recognized. Many of these patients also have a harelip, and the two abnormalities together interfere with suckling and later in life with the enunciation of labial and guttural consonants. The voice has an unpleasant nasality and often, if the defect is severe, there is an audible escape of air through the nose.

STAMMERING AND STUTTERING AND CLUTTERED SPEECH. Stammering and stuttering are difficult to classify. In some respects they belong to the developmental disorders, but they differ from them in being largely centered in articulation. They consist of a spasm of the muscles of articulation when an attempt is made to speak. The spasm may be tonic and result in a complete block of speech, sometimes called *stammering,* or a repetitive spasm that leads to repeated utterance of the first syllable, i.e., a stutter, or the words may come out in rapid clusters, all poorly enunciated. Certain syllables offer greater difficulty than others. The patient falters on an initial consonant or syllable, which he repeats over and over again before he finally succeeds in enunciating the rest of the word, e.g., p-p-paper, b-b-b-boy. The severity of the stutter is increased by excitement, as in speaking before strangers or a group of people. The spasms may overflow into other muscle groups not directly concerned with speech. Males are affected three times as often as females. The time of onset may be when the child first begins to talk, i.e., at two or three years of age, or between the ages of six and eight years. These latter are the two critical periods of language development. Many of these children also have some degree of reading and writing disability. Slowness in developing hand preference or enforced change from left- to right-handedness are noted in many cases. If mild, the condition tends to develop or to be present only during periods of emotional distress; and it usually disappears spontaneously during adolescent or early adult years. If severe, it persists all through life, regardless of treatment, but tends to improve as the patient grows older.

The essential character of stuttering is difficult to define. There is no detectable paralysis or incoordination of speech musculature, which seems to function normally in other commonplace acts and when the patient is alone and relaxed or singing. Stuttering differs from apraxia in that the muscles, when called upon to perform the specific act, go into voluntary spasm; but since the spasm does not occur during other movements in which these muscles are involved, it differs from the intention (tension) spasm of athetosis. It appears to represent a special category of movement disorder and is much like writer's cramp, another motor disorder of unknown etiology.

Everyone who has studied stuttering and stammering has been impressed with the high incidence of similar disabilities in other members of the same family, sometimes going back several generations. This and the preponderance in males suggest a sex-linked characteristic, but the inheritance does not follow a simple pattern.

Many of the patients, probably as a natural result of this impediment to free social intercourse, become increasingly fearful of speaking and have feelings of inferiority after a few years. By the time adolescence and adulthood are reached, emotional factors are so prominent that many physicians have mistaken stuttering for neurosis. Usually there is little or no evidence of any personality deviation before the onset of stuttering, and psychotherapy by competent psychiatrists, though unquestionably helpful in relieving emotional tension and assisting a satisfactory adjustment to the condition, has not significantly modified the underlying defect. Occasionally, stuttering will develop during adult life as a consequence of brain disease.

Emphasis on maturational delay in the language disorders of children is relative. Tumors, vascular lesions of the dominant hemisphere may abolish speech as in the adult, but the effects (especially before the 6th or 7th years) are always transitory.

Disorders of Articulation and Phonation

The third group of speech abnormalities is that of the disorders of articulation. In simple dysarthria there is no abnormality of the cortical centers. The dysarthric patient is able to understand perfectly what he hears, and if literate, he reads and has no difficulty in writing, even though unable to utter a single intelligible word. This is the strict meaning of being inarticulate.

The act of speaking is a highly coordinated sequence of contractions of the larynx, pharynx, palate, tongue, lips, and respiratory musculature. These are innervated by the hypoglossal, vagal, facial, and phrenic nerves. The nuclei of these nerves are controlled through the corticobulbar tracts by both motor cortices. As with all movements, there is also an extrapyramidal influence from the cerebellum and basal ganglions. A current of air is produced by expiration, and the force of it is finely regulated and coordinated with the activity of other muscles engaged in speech. *Phonation,* or the production of vocal sounds, is a function of the larynx. Changes in the size and shape of the glottis and in the length and tension of the vocal cords are effected by the action of the laryngeal muscles. Vibrations are set up and transmitted to the column of air passing over the vocal cords. Sounds thus formed are modified as they pass through the nasopharynx and mouth, which act as resonators. Articulation consists of contractions of the tongue, lips, pharynx, and palate, which interrupt or alter the vocal sounds. Vowels are of laryngeal origin, as are some consonants; but the latter are formed for the most part during articulation. For instance, the consonants *m, b,* and *p* are labial, *l* and *t* are lingual and *nk* and *ng* are nasoguttural.

Defective articulation and phonation are best observed by listening to the patient during ordinary conversation or while reading aloud from a newspaper or a book. Test phrases or the rapid repetition of lingual, labial, and guttural consonants may bring out the particular abnormality. Disorders of phonation call for an examination of the apparatus of voice. The movements of the vocal cords should be inspected with the aid of a hand mirror, or, even better, a laryngoscope, and those of the tongue, palate, and pharynx by direct observation.

Defects in articulation may be subdivided into several

types: paralytic dysarthria, spastic and rigid dysarthria, and ataxic dysarthria.

PARETIC DYSARTHRIA. This is due to a neural or bulbar (medullary) paralysis of the articulatory muscles (lower motor neurone paralysis). Bulbar poliomyelitis and "progressive bulbar palsy" are examples of diseases that may produce partial or complete anarthria. In the latter the shriveled tongue lies inert on the floor of the mouth, and the lips are relaxed and tremulous. Saliva constantly collects in the mouth because of dysphagia, and drooling is troublesome. Speech becomes less and less distinct. There is special difficulty in the correct utterance of vibratives, such as *r*; and as the paralysis becomes more complete, lingual and labial consonants are finally not pronounced at all. Lesser degrees of this abnormality are observed in myasthenia gravis. Bilateral paralysis of the palate, which may occur with diphtheria, poliomyelitis, or involvement of the tenth cranial nerve by tumor, produces a disorder of articulation similar to that of the cleft palate. The voice has a nasal quality, since the posterior nares are not closed during phonation, and certain consonants, such as *n*, *b*, and *k*, are altered. The abnormality is sometimes less pronounced in recumbency and increased when the head is thrown forward. Bilateral paralysis of the lips interferes with enunciation of labial consonants; *p* and *b* are slurred and sound more like *f* and *v*.

SPASTIC AND RIGID DYSARTHRIA. These are more frequent than the paralytic variety. Diseases that involve the corticobulbar tracts, usually vascular disease or motor system disease, result in the syndrome of pseudobulbar palsy. The patient may have had a minor stroke some time in the past affecting the corticobulbar fibers on one side; but since the bulbar muscles are probably represented in both motor cortices, there is no impairment in speech or swallowing from a unilateral lesion. If another stroke occurs involving the other corticobulbar tract and possibly the corticospinal tract at the pontine, midbrain, or capsular level, the patient immediately becomes anarthric or dysarthric and dysphagic. Unlike bulbar paralysis due to lower motor neurone involvement, there is no atrophy or fasciculation of the paralyzed muscles, the jaw jerk is exaggerated, the palatal reflexes are retained, emotional control is poor (pathologic laughter and crying), and sometimes breathing becomes periodic (Cheyne-Stokes). The patient may be anarthric and aphonic for a time, but as he improves, or in mild degrees of the same condition, speech is thick and indistinct, much like that of partial bulbar paralysis.

In paralysis agitans, or postencephalitic Parkinson's syndrome, one observes an extrapyramidal disturbance of articulation. The patient speaks slowly and articulates poorly, slurring over many syllables and trailing off the end of sentences. The voice is low-pitched, monotonous, and lacking inflection. The words are pronounced hastily. In advanced cases speech is almost unintelligible; only whispering may be possible at this stage. It may happen that the patient finds it impossible to talk while walking but can speak if he sits or lies down.

In chorea and myoclonus, speech may also be severely affected, and the defect is distinguished from the speech of pseudobulbar palsy or paralysis agitans by the interruptions of the abnormal movements. Grimacing and other characteristic motor signs must be depended upon for diagnosis. Pyramidal and extrapyramidal disturbances of speech may be combined in generalized cerebral diseases such as general paresis, in which slurred speech is one of the cardinal signs.

In many cases of capsular hemiplegia or partially recovered Broca's aphasia the patient is left with a dysarthria that may be difficult to distinguish from a pure articulatory defect. Careful testing of other language functions, especially writing, may bring out the aphasic quality.

ATAXIC DYSARTHRIA. This is characteristic of acute and chronic cerebellar lesions. It may be observed in multiple sclerosis, Friedreich's ataxia, cerebellar atrophy, and heat stroke. The principal speech abnormality is slowness; imprecise enunciation, monotony, and unnatural separation of the syllables of words (scanning) are other features. Coordination of speech and respiration are poor. There may not be enough breath to utter certain words, and others may be ejaculated explosively. *Scanning dysarthria* is distinctive, but in some cases, especially if there is some possibility of spastic weakness of the tongue from corticobulbar tract involvement, it is impossible to predict the anatomy of disease from analysis of speech alone. Myoclonic jerks involving the speech musculature may be superimposed on cerebellar ataxia in a number of diseases.

Aphonia and Dysphonia

Finally, a few points should be made concerning the fourth group of language disorders, i.e., disturbances of voice. In adolescence and early adult life there may be a persistence of the unstable "change of voice" normally seen in boys soon after puberty. As though by habit, the patient speaks part of the time in a falsetto voice. This can usually be overcome by training.

Paresis of the respiratory movements, as in poliomyelitis and acute infectious polyneuritis, may affect voice because insufficient air is provided for phonation and speech. Also, disturbances in the rhythm of respiration may interfere with the fluency of speech. This is particularly noticeable in so-called "extrapyramidal diseases," and one may note that the patient tries to talk upon inspiration. Reduced volume of speech due to limited excursion of the breathing muscles is another common feature; the patient is unable to speak above a whisper or to shout.

Paresis of both vocal cords causes complete aphonia. There is no voice, and the patient can speak only in whispers. Since the vocal cords normally separate during inspiration, their failure to do so when paralyzed may result in an inspiratory stridor. If one vocal cord is paralyzed, the voice becomes hoarse, low-pitched, and rasping.

Another curious condition about which little is known is *spastic dysphonia*. The authors have seen several cases, middle-aged or elderly men and women, otherwise healthy, who gradually lost the ability to speak quietly and fluently. Any effort to speak resulted in contraction of all the speech musculature so that the patient's voice was strained and phonation was labored. This is apparently a neurologic disorder of undetermined kind. The patients are not neurotic, and psychotherapy has been ineffective. This condition differs from the stridor caused by spasm of the laryngeal muscles in tetany.

Instability or changeableness of voice, a common problem for adolescent boys, may persist into adult life. Its basis is not known. Voice training has been helpful in many patients.

DIAGNOSIS

Speech is such a complex act that it has not been possible to present all its facets. Nothing, for example, has been said here about speech changes during various psychiatric illnesses. This does not mean that the psychiatric syndromes are unimportant, for there is no doubt that hysterical aphonia, the various tics that interrupt the speech of tense individuals, and the altered rate, fluency, and content of speech in the psychoses pose formidable problems.

In diagnosing disorders of speech the physician must attempt in every case to decide first whether the problem is one of aphasia, dysarthria, or dysphonia. The examination procedure outlined above will, if carried out systematically, permit this first and important step to be made.

If the patient is aphasic, it should be determined whether his aphasia is of global, central, Wernicke, or Broca type or whether it is a restricted disorder of motor function, a pure alexia, or word deafness. The differential diagnosis has already been given and also the significance of associated neurologic signs. Identification of the type of aphasia is of localizing value and it may provide an important lead as to the underlying brain disease.

The general physician is frequently called upon to examine children who show some disorder of speech or delay in language development. From the above remarks it will be seen that these disorders fall into several broad categories, of which stuttering, delay in onset of speech, dyslalia, partial or complete deafness, word deafness, cleft palate, lisping, and word blindness are the most frequent. When faced with problems of this type, the physician must ask several questions. *Is the child partially or completely deaf? Does he have a more generalized mental or neuromuscular defect—is he feebleminded or suffering from an infantile hemiplegia or spastic diplegia? Does he stammer, stutter, or show dyslalia?* In attempting to answer these questions, the parents' account of the child's development and his behavior at home is most helpful. Failure to respond to noise of any kind suggests deafness. An interest in sounds and music but not in stories or conversation, together with slow development of understanding and use of speech are indicative of high-tone deafness or word deafness (auditory verbal agnosia). Delayed onset of suckling, head control, sitting, standing, walking, etc., necessitate neurologic examina-

tion; one should look particularly for spastic weakness or rigidity of the limbs and poor motor control of the tongue, as well as mental retardation. The latter can be assessed at an early age by intelligence tests, such as the performance part of the Stanford-Binet test. If the child is otherwise normal, recitation of a nursery rhyme will disclose a stammering, stuttering, lallation of cleft palate speech.

Disturbances of articulation point to involvement of a different set of neural structures, such as the motor cortices, the corticobulbar pathways, the seventh, ninth, and tenth nuclei, the brainstem, and extrapyramidal nuclei and tracts. Often it is necessary to use other neurologic findings to decide which of these are implicated in any given case. The important distinction between the pseudobulbar or supranuclear palsies and the bulbar palsies is grasped only with difficulty by the average student. The information obtained by localizing these two major types of dysarthria is extremely helpful in differential diagnosis.

Dysphonia should lead to an investigation of laryngeal disease either primary or secondary to an abnormality of innervation.

TREATMENT

The sudden loss of speech would be expected to cause great apprehension, but except for almost pure motor defects, most patients show remarkably little concern. It appears that the very lesion that deprives them of speech also causes at least a partial loss of insight into their own disability. This reaches almost a ludicrous extreme in some cases of Wernicke's aphasia, in which the patient becomes indignant when others cannot understand his jargon. Nonetheless, as improvement occurs, many patient do become discouraged. Reassurance and a positive program of speech rehabilitation are the best ways of helping the patient at this stage.

The contemporary methods of training and reeducation in overcoming an aphasic defect have never been critically evaluated. Most aphasic difficulty is due to vascular disease of the brain, and nearly always this is accompanied by some degree of spontaneous improvement in the days, weeks, and months that follow the stroke. Sometimes recovery is complete within hours or days; at times not more than a few words are regained after a year or two of assiduous speech training. Nevertheless, it is the opinion of many experts in the field that speech training is worthwhile.

One must decide for each patient whether speech training is needed and when it should be started. As a rule, therapy is not advisable in the first few days of an aphasic illness, because one does not know how lasting it will be. Also, if the patient suffers a severe global aphasia and can neither speak nor understand spoken and written words, the speech therapist is helpless. Under such circumstances, one does well to wait a few weeks until some one of the language functions has begun to return. Then the physician may begin to encourage and help the patient to use the function to a maximum degree. In milder aphasic disorders the patient may be sent to the speech therapist as soon as the illness has stabilized.

The methods of speech training are specialized, and it is advisable to call in a person who has been trained in this field. However, inasmuch as the benefit is largely psychologic, an interested member of the family or a schoolteacher can be used if a speech therapist is not available in the community.

The language problems of children are serious and demand skillful diagnosis and treatment. Often, excellent results are obtained. Most of the well-organized urban school systems have remedial reading teachers who will take over the problem once it has been evaluated medically. The emotional problems that often accompany the developmental disturbances of language and of cerebral dominance must be dealt with gently and firmly.

The physician should by wise counseling help the patient understand the nature of this problem and try to avoid some of the secondary and emotional problems that the speech disorder creates. Prolonged psychotherapy helps with the emotional problems but has not, in the author's experience, corrected the underlying speech defect. Fortunately, the natural course of mild stuttering is toward improvement during adolescence, and many patients recover spontaneously by adult life. In severe cases a lifelong problem must be faced, and none of the present methods of therapy, including psychoanalysis, has corrected the defect.

There is no special treatment for the dysarthric disturbance of speech.

REFERENCES

Alajouanine, T.: Verbal Realization in Aphasia, Brain, 79: 1–29, 1956.

Brain, R.: Aphasia, Apraxia, Agnosia, chap. 83 in "Neurology, S. A. K. Wilson and N. Bruce (Eds.), 2d ed., vol. 3, Baltimore, The Williams & Wilkins Company, 1955.

Geschwind, N.: Disconnection Syndromes in Animals and Man. Brain, 88:237–294, 585–644, 1965.

Hallgren, B.: Specific Dyslexia. Supp. 65 of Acta Psychiat. Neurol., 1950.

Nielsen, J. M.: "Agnosia, Apraxia, Aphasia: Their Value in Cerebral Localization," 2d ed., New York, Hafner Publishing Company, Inc., 1962.

Orton, S. T.: "Reading, Writing and Speech Problems in Children," New York, W. W. Norton & Company, Inc., 1937.

30 DELIRIUM AND OTHER CONFUSIONAL STATES AND KORSAKOFF'S AMNESTIC SYNDROME

Raymond D. Adams and Maurice Victor

Every physician sooner or later discovers through clinical experience the need for special competence in assessing the mental faculties of his patients. He must be able to observe with detachment and complete objectivity their character, intelligence, mood, memory, judgment, and other attributes of personality in much the same fashion as he observes the nutritional state and the color of the mucous membranes. The systematic examination of these affective and cognitive functions permits him to reach certain conclusions regarding mental status, and these are also of value in understanding the patient and his illness. Without the data obtained from the study of the mental status, errors will be made in evaluating the reliability of the patient's history, in diagnosing the neurologic or psychiatric disease from which he suffers, and in conducting any proposed therapeutic program.

Perhaps the content of this chapter will be more clearly understood if we repeat a few of the introductory remarks of Chap. 17. The main thesis of the neurologic physician is that mental and physical functions of the nervous system are simply two aspects of the same neural process. The mind is no more or less than the self-regulating, goal-seeking activities, the same ones that are manifest in all mammalian life. It is only because of the prodigious complexity of man's brain, his high capacity for memory of past experiences, his imagination, and power of reasoning, his capacity to make conscious choice and to reflect on the working of his own psychic processes that the illusion of separation of mind and body was created. Biologists and psychologists have reached the modern monistic view by placing all protoplasmic activities of the nervous system (growth, development, behavior, and mental function) in a continuum and noting the inherent purposiveness and creativity common to all of them. The physician is persuaded of its truth by his daily experiences with disease, in which every known aberration of behavior, intellect, and personality appear as expressions of diseases of the cerebrum.

In this chapter we are concerned with common disturbances of sensorium and intellection that have not been previously discussed and which stand as cardinal manifestations of certain cerebral diseases. The most frequent of these are confusion, disturbances of memory, and abnormalities of thinking or reasoning.

DEFINITION OF TERMS

The following nomenclature, though tentative, is useful and will be employed throughout this textbook:

Confusion, as stated in Chap. 26, is a term that has two meanings. The commonest refers to a general reduction in alertness, attentiveness, and perception of environmental stimuli, an inability to take notice of, i.e., to register all elements of, a situation within a short period of time. Often there are misinterpretations of stimuli, and hallucinations and drowsiness may be prominent. The other usage designates slowness and inefficiency in thinking, often with failure in subsequent recall. Thus, in the first sense confusion is aligned with disorders of consciousness, attention, and perception, and as was pointed out in Chap. 26, it may represent one stage on the way to coma or emergence therefrom. The term *delirium* is often used to specify a disorder of consciousness, perception, and attention, but it connotes in addition excessive alertness, sleeplessness, and frenzied excitement. Mental activity may be interrupted by the abrupt intrusion of hallucinations, which are frequent. We believe that confusion and delirium represent essentially different types of cerebral disorder. In many textbooks of psychiatry, however, confusion and delirium are grouped together and called toxic-exhaustive psychosis or "organic reaction type," indicating their postulated cause and pathologic basis. Confusion as an impairment of thinking, on the other hand, is related to derangements of intellect, i.e., dementia.

The term *amnesia* means loss of the ability to form memories despite an alert state of mind. It presupposes an ability to grasp the problem, to use language normally, and to maintain adequate motivation. The failure is mainly one of retention, recall, and reproduction, and it should be distinguished from states of drowsiness and confusion, where the learned material seems never to have been adequately assimilated. *Dementia* means loss of reason or, more particularly, a deterioration of intellect. Implied in the word is the idea of a gradual enfeeblement of mental powers in a person who formerly possessed a normal mind. *Amentia*, by contrast, indicates a congenital feeblemindedness.

OBSERVABLE ASPECTS OF BEHAVIOR AND THEIR RELATION TO CONFUSION, DELIRIUM, AMNESIA, AND DEMENTIA

In the strict sense the intellectual, emotional, volitional, and behavioral activities of the human organism are so complex and varied that one may question the possibility of using derangements of them as reliable guides to cerebral disease. Certainly they have not the same reliability and ease of anatomic and physiologic interpretation as sensory and motor paralysis or aphasia. Yet one observes certain of these higher cerebral disturbances recurring with such regularity in certain diseases as to be useful in clinical medicine; and some of them gain in specificity because they are often combined in certain ways to form syndromes, which are essentially what states of confusion, delirium, amnesia, and dementia are. Of course, we do not always know the value of certain elements of these syndromes, i.e., which are of primary or secondary importance.

The components of mentation and behavior that lend themselves to bedside examination are (1) the processes of sensation and perception; (2) the capacity for memorizing; (3) the ability to think, reason, and form logical conclusions; (4) temperament, mood, and emotion; (5) initiative, impulse, and drive; (6) insight. Of these (1), (2), and (3) may be grouped as cognitive, (4) as affective, and (5) as conative or volitional. Insight includes essentially all introspective observations made by the patient concerning his own normal or disordered functioning. Each component of behavior and intellection has its objective side, expressed in the manifest ef-

fects of certain stimulus conditions on the patient and his behavioral responses, and its subjective side, expressed in what the patient says he thinks and feels.

Disturbances of Perception

Perception, i.e., the processes involved in acquiring through the senses a knowledge of the "world about" or of one's own body, involves many things aside from the simple sensory process of being aware of the attributes of a stimulus; it includes the selective focusing and maintaining of attention, elimination of all extraneous stimuli, and recognition of the stimulus by knowing its relationship to personal remembered experience. One must appreciate that the perception of an object undergoes predictable types of derangements in disease. Most often there is a reduction in the number of perceptions in a given unit of time and failure to properly synthesize them and relate them to the ongoing activities of the mind. Or there may be apparent inattentiveness, fluctuations of attention, distractibility (pertinent and irrelevant stimuli now having equal value), inability to persist in an assigned task, and in the reporting and reacting to only a small part of a complex of stimuli. Qualitative changes also appear, mainly in the form of sensory distortions and misinterpretation and misidentification of objects and persons (illusions); and these, at least in part, form the basis of hallucinatory experience in which the patient reports and reacts to stimuli not present in his environment. The loss of ability to perceive simultaneously all elements of a large complex of stimuli is sometimes explained as a "failure of subjective reorganization." Major disturbances in the perceptual sphere, sometimes called "clouding of the sensorium," occur most often in confusional states and deliria, but quantitative deficiency may become evident in the advanced stages of amentia and dementia.

Disturbances of Memory

Memory, i.e., the retention of learned experiences, is involved in all mental activities. It may be arbitrarily subdivided into several parts, namely, (1) registration, which includes all that was mentioned under perception; (2) mnemonic integration and retention; (3) recall; and (4) reproduction. As was stated above, in disturbances of perception and attention there may be a complete failure of learning and memory for the reason that the material to be learned was never assimilated. In Korsakoff's amnestic syndrome newly presented material appears to be temporarily registered but cannot be retained for more than a few minutes, and there is nearly always an associated defect in the recall and reproduction of memories formed before the onset of the illness (retrograde amnesia). Dislocation of events in time and the fabrication of stories, called *confabulation*, constitutes a third feature of the syndrome. Sound retention with failure of recall is at times a normal state; but when it is severe and extends to all events over a given period of time, it is usually due to hysteria or malingering. Proof that the processes of registration and recall are intact under these circumstances comes from hypnosis and suggestion, by means of which the lost items are fully recalled and reproduced. In Korsakoff's amnestic state the patient fails on all tests of learning and recent memory and his behavior accords with his deficiencies of information. Since memory is involved to some extent in all mental processes, it becomes the most testable component of mentation and behavior.

Disturbances of Thinking

Thinking, which is central to so many important intellectual activities, remains one of the most elusive of all mental operations. If by thinking we mean selective ordering of symbols for problem solving and capacity to reason and form sound judgments (the usual definition), obviously the working units of most complex experiences of this type are words and numbers. The activity of substituting word and number symbols for the objects for which they stand (symbolization) is a fundamental part of the process. These symbols are formed into ideas or concepts, and the arrangement of new and remembered ideas into certain orders or relationships, according to the rules of logic, constitute another intricate part of thought, presently beyond the scope of analysis. In a general way one may examine thinking for speed and efficiency, ideational content, coherence and logical relationships of ideas, quantity and quality of associations to a given idea, and propriety of the feeling and behavior engendered by an idea.

Information concerning the thought processes and associative functions is best obtained by analyzing the patient's spontaneous verbal productions and by engaging him in conversation. If he is taciturn or mute, one may then have to depend on his responses to direct questions or upon written material, i.e., letters, etc. One notes the prevailing trends of the patient's thoughts, whether his ideas are reasonable or precise and coherent or vague, circumstantial, tangential, and irrelevant, and whether his thought processes are shallow and completely fragmented. Disorders of thought are frequent in deliria, and in degenerative and other types of cerebral disease. The organization of thought may be disrupted with fragmentation, repetition, and perseveration. This is spoken of as incoherence and marks many confusional delirious states. The patient may be excessively critical, rationalizing, and hairsplitting; this is a type of thinking often manifest in depressive psychoses. Derangements of thinking may also take the form of a virtual flight of ideas. The patient moves nimbly from one idea to another, and his associations are numerous and loosely linked. This is a common feature in hypomanic or manic states. The opposite condition, poverty of ideas (the more frequent condition), is characteristic both of depression, where it is combined with gloomy thoughts, and of dementing diseases, where it is part of a general reduction in all intellectual activity. Thinking may be distorted in such a way that the patient fails to check his ideas against reality. When a false belief is maintained in spite of normally convincing contradictory evidence, the patient is said to have a delusion. Delusion is common to many illnesses, particularly manic-depressive and schizophrenic states. Ideas may seem to have been implanted in the patient's mind by some outside agency such as radio, television, or atomic energy. These reflect the passivity feelings characteristic of manic-depressive and schizophrenic psychoses. Other distortions of logical thought, such as gaps or condensations of logical associations, are typical of schizophrenia, of which they constitute a diagnostic feature.

Disturbances of Emotion, Mood, and Affect

The emotional life of the patient is expressed in a variety of ways, and there are several points to be made about it. In the first place, rather marked individual differences in basic temperament are to be observed in the normal population; some persons are throughout their life cheerful, gregarious, optimistic, and free from worry, whereas others are just the opposite. In fact, the unusually volatile, cyclothymic person is believed to be liable to manic-depressive psychosis and the suspicious, withdrawn, introverted person to schizophrenia and paranoia. Strong, persistent emotional states such as fear and anxiety may occur as reactions to life situations and may be accompanied by derangements of visceral function. If excessive and disproportionate to the stimulus, they have medical significance; they are usually manifestations of an anxiety neurosis or depression. Variations in the degree of responsiveness to emotional stimuli are also frequent and, when excessive and persistent, are important. In depression all stimuli tend to enhance the somber mood of unhappiness. Emotional response that is excessively labile, variable from moment to moment, and poorly controlled or uninhibited is a condition common to many diseases of the cerebrum, particularly those involving the corticopontine and corticobulbar pathways. It may constitute a part of the syndrome of pseudobulbar palsy. All emotional expression may be lacking, as in apathetic states or severe depressions, or the patient may be a victim of every trivial problem in daily life; i.e., he cannot control his worries. Finally, the emotional response may be inappropriate to the stimulus, e.g., a depressing thought is amusing and attended by a smile, as in schizophrenia.

Since there are relatively few overt manifestations of temperament, mood, and other emotional experiences described above, the physician must evaluate these states by the appearance of the patient and by verbalized accounts of his feelings. For these purposes it is convenient to divide emotionality into mood and feeling or affect. By mood is meant the prevailing emotional state of the individual without reference to the stimuli impinging upon him, i.e., his immediate environmental circumstances. It may be pleasant and cheerful or melancholic. The language, e.g., the adjectives used, and the facial expressions, attitudes, postures, and speed of movement most reliably betray the patient's mood.

By contrast, feelings or affects are said to be emotional experiences evoked by environmental stimuli. According to some psychiatrists, feeling is the subjective component and affect, the overt manifestation. Others apply either word to the subjective state. The difference between mood as a prevailing emotional state and feeling and affect as emotional reactions to stimuli may seem rather tenuous, but these distinctions are considered valuable by psychiatrists.

Impulse, that basic biologic urge, driving force, or purpose, by which every organism is directed to reach its full potentialities, appears to be another extremely important and observable but neglected dimension of behavior. Again, one notes wide normal variations from one person to another in strength of impulse to action and thought, and these individual differences are present throughout life. One of the most conspicuous pathologic deviations is an apparent constitutional weakness in impulse in certain neurotic individuals. Moreover, with many types of cerebral disease, particularly those which involve the posterior orbital parts of the frontal lobes, a reduction in impulse is coupled with an indifference or lack of concern about the consequences of actions. In such cases all other measurable aspects of psychic function may be normal. Extreme degrees of lack of impulse, or abulia, take the form of mutism and immobility, called *akinetic mutism*. Psychomotor retardation is a lesser degree of the same state and is also a feature of depression, in which instance mood alternation and extreme fatigability are conjoined, or of cerebral disease.

Lastly, insight, the state of being fully aware of the nature and degree of one's deficits, becomes manifestly impaired or abolished in relation to all types of cerebral disease that cause disorders of behavior. Rarely does the patient with any of the aforementioned states seek advice or help for his illness. Instead, his family usually brings him to the physician. Thus, it appears that the diseases which produce all these abnormalities not only evoke observable changes in behavior but also alter or reduce the capacity of the patient to make accurate introspections of his own psychic function. This fact stands as one of the most incontrovertible proofs that the cerebrum is the organ both of behavior and of all inner psychic experiences; that is to say, behavior and mind are but two inseparable aspects of the function of the nervous system.

COMMON SYNDROMES

This entire group of acute confusional states is characterized principally by clouding of consciousness with prominent disorders of attention and perception that interfere with clarity of thinking and the formation of memories. One syndrome, here called *hyperkinetic delirium*, includes overactivity, sleeplessness, tremulousness, and hallucinations. Convulsions often precede the delirium. In a variant of this syndrome, here called *hypokinetic delirium*, drowsiness, and reduced awareness and responsiveness are the principal abnormalities, and perceptual disorder and degree of activity are less important. A second syndrome is a confusional state in which there

is manifest reduction in alertness, attentiveness, and sensorial registration. A third syndrome consists of a confusional state occurring in a patient with some other cerebral disease. The latter disposes him to the acute psychosis which we have chosen to designate as a *beclouded dementia*. These illnesses tend to develop acutely, to have multiple causes, and to terminate within a relatively short period of time (days to weeks) leaving the patient without residual damage. These two syndromes will be described separately.

Delirium

CLINICAL FEATURES. These are most perfectly depicted in the alcoholic patient. The symptoms usually develop over a period of 2 or 3 days. The first indications of the approaching attack are difficulty in concentrating, restless irritability, tremulousness, insomnia, and poor appetite. One or several generalized convulsions are the initial major symptom in 30 percent of the cases. The patient's rest becomes troubled by unpleasant and terrifying dreams. There may be momentary disorientation or an occasional irrational remark.

These initial symptoms rapidly give way to a clinical picture that, in severe cases, is one of the most colorful and dramatic in medicine. The state of consciousness becomes altered; it is clouded in that the patient is inattentive and unable to perceive all elements of his situation— as though he were in a twilight state. He talks incessantly and incoherently and looks distressed or perplexed; his expression is in keeping with his vague notions of being annoyed or pursued by someone who seeks to injure him. From his manner and from the content of his speech it is evident that he misinterprets the meaning of ordinary objects and sounds around him and has vivid visual, auditory, and tactile hallucinations, often of a most unpleasant type. At first he can be brought momentarily into touch with reality and may in fact answer questions correctly; but almost at once he relapses into his preoccupied, confused state, gives wrong answers, and is unable to think coherently. The clouding of sensorium is revealed by his inability to repeat or reverse series of digits or to do serial additions or subtractions. As a rule he is disoriented. Before long he is unable to shake off his hallucinations even for a second and does not recognize his family or his physician. Tremor and restless movements are usually present and may be violent. The countenance is flushed, and the conjunctivas are injected; the pulse is rapid and soft, and the temperature may be raised. There is much sweating, and the urine is scanty and of high specific gravity.

The symptoms abate, either suddenly or gradually, after 2 or 3 days, although in exceptional cases they may persist for several weeks. The most certain indication of the end of the attack is the occurrence of sound sleep and of lucid intervals of increasing length. Recovery is usually complete.

Delirium is subject to all degrees of variability, not only from patient to patient but in the same patient from day to day and hour to hour. The entire syndrome may be observed in one patient and only one or two symptoms in another. In its mildest form, as so often occurs in febrile diseases, it consists of an occasional wandering of the mind and incoherence of expression interrupted by periods of lucidity. This form, lacking motor and autonomic overactivity, is sometimes referred to as a *quiet delirium* (here, *hypokinetic delirium*) and is difficult to distinguish from other confusional states. The more severe form of active delirium and tremulousness, best exemplified by delirium tremens, is characterized by a great excess of motor activity, severe insomnia, and marked confusion, which may progress to a "muttering stupor" and/or coma, which in about 10 percent of patients ends fatally.

MORBID ANATOMY AND PATHOPHYSIOLOGY. The brains of patients who have died in delirium tremens usually show no pathologic changes of significance. A number of diseases, however, may cause delirium and also give rise to focal lesions in the brain, such as focal embolic encephalitis, viral encephalitis, Wernicke's disease, or trauma. The topography of these lesions is of particular interest. They tend to be localized in certain parts of the brain, particularly in the midbrain and subthalamus and in the temporal lobes, where they involve the reticular activating and limbic systems.

Penfield's studies of the human cortex during surgical exploration clearly indicate the importance of the temporal lobe in producing visual, auditory, and olfactory hallucinations. With subthalamic and midbrain lesions, there may occur visual hallucinations of a pleasurable type accompanied by good insight, namely, the peduncular hallucinosis of Lhermitte.

The electroencephalogram in delirium shows nonfocal slow activity in the 5 to 7 per sec range, a state that rapidly returns to normal as the delirium clears. However, in other cases only activity in the fast beta frequency is seen, and in milder degrees of delirium there is usually no abnormality at all.

An analysis of the several conditions conducive to delirium suggests at least three different physiologic mechanisms. In alcoholism and barbiturate intoxication the clinical manifestations appear after the withdrawal of drugs known to have a strong inhibitory effect on certain areas of the central nervous system. Presumably their release and overactivity are then the basis of delirium. In this respect it is interesting to note that delirium tremens is made up of symptoms which are the antithesis of alcoholic intoxication. In the case of bacterial infections and poisoning by certain drugs, such as atropine and scopolamine, the delirious state probably results from the direct action of the toxin or chemical on these same parts of the brain. Thirdly, destructive lesions such as acute inclusion body encephalitis of the temporal lobes cause delirium by disturbing the function of certain areas.

Psychophysiologic mechanisms have also been postulated. It has long been suggested that some individuals are much more liable to delirium than others. There is much reason to doubt this hypothesis, for it has been shown that all of a group of randomly selected persons would develop delirium if the causative mechanisms were strongly operative. This is to be expected, for any healthy

person under certain circumstances may experience phenomena akin to those found in delirium. Thus after repeated auditory and visual stimulation the same impressions may continue to be perceived even though the stimuli are no longer present. Moreover, it has been shown that a healthy individual can be induced to hallucinate by placing him in an environment as free as possible of sensory stimulation. A relation between delirium and dream states has been postulated because in both there is a loss of appreciation of time, a richness of visual imagery, indifference to inconsistencies and "defective reality testing." Moreover, patients may refer to some of these delirious symptoms as a "bad dream," and normal persons may hallucinate in the so-called "hypnagogic state," the short period between sleeping and waking. In general, however, formulations in the field of dynamic psychology seem more reasonably to account for the topical content of delirium than to explain its occurrence. Wolff and Curran, having observed the same content in repeated attacks of delirium due to different causes, concluded that the content depends more on age, sex, intellectual endowment, occupation, personality traits, and past experience of the patient than on the cause or mechanism of the delirium.

The main difficulty in understanding delirium arises from the fact that it has not been possible from clinical studies to ascertain which of the many symptoms have physiologic significance. What is the basis of this altered consciousness, this sensorial alteration, the lack of harmony between actual sensory impressions of the present and memory of those in the past? Obviously, there is something missing from total behavior, something that leaves the patient at the mercy of certain sensory stimuli and unable to attend to others, yet at the same time incapable of discriminating between sense impression and fantasy. There appears to be some lack of inhibition of sensory processes, which may also be the basis of the sleep disturbance (insomnia) and the convulsive tendency.

Acute Confusional State Associated with Reduced Mental Alertness and Responsiveness (Includes Primary Mental Confusion and Hypokinetic Delirium)

CLINICAL FEATURES. Here a conjunction of two syndromes is necessary because at a practical level they may be impossible to distinguish from one another. In the most typical examples all mental functions are reduced to some degree, but alertness, attentiveness, and the ability to grasp all elements of the immediate situation suffer most. In its mildest form the patient may pass for normal, and only failure to recollect and reproduce happenings of the past few hours or days reveals the inadequacy of mental function. The more obviously confused patient spends much of his time in idleness, but what he does do may be inappropriate and annoying to others. Only the more automatic acts and verbal responses are properly performed, but these may permit the examiner to obtain from the patient a number of relevant and accurate replies to questions about age, occupation, and residence. Reactions are slow and indecisive, and it is difficult for the patient to sustain a conversation. He may doze during the interview and is observed to sleep more hours each day than is natural or the same number at more irregular intervals. Responses tend to be rather abrupt, brief, and mechanical. Perceptual difficulties are frequent, and voices, common objects, and the actions of other persons are frequently misinterpreted. Often one cannot discern whether the patient hears voices and sees things that do not exist, i.e., whether he is actively hallucinating, or is merely misinterpreting stimuli in the environment. Inadequate perception and forgetfulness results in a constant state of bewilderment. Failing to recognize his surroundings and having lost all sense of time, he repeats the same question and makes the same remarks over and over again.

As the confusion deepens, conversation becomes more difficult, and at a certain stage the patient no longer notices or responds to much of what is going on around him. Replies to questions may be a single word or a short phrase spoken in a soft tremulous voice or whisper. The patient may be mute. Irritability may or may not be present. It was to this profound impairment of all cognitive functions that Bonhoeffer, a German authority on delirium, gave the name *amentia*. Some patients are extremely suspicious; in fact, a paranoid trend may be the most pronounced and troublesome feature of the illness.

In its most advanced stages confusion gives way to stupor and finally to coma. As the patient improves, he may pass again through the stage of stupor and confusion in the reverse order. All this informs us that at least one category of confusion is but a manifestation of the same disease processes that in their severest form cause coma.

In some instances the mental aberration never exceeds that of confusion with stupor; in others, with more than the usual degree of irritability and restlessness, one cannot fail to notice the striking resemblance to delirium. It is to this latter state that we attach the term *hypokinetic delirium* with all the implications, anatomic and physiologic, described under hyperkinetic delirium. In both there is a clouding of consciousness, impairment of attention, slowness, and disordered perception and association of ideas. The point is that if tremor, vivid hallucinations, vigilant excited attitude, insomnia, and the low convulsive threshold are inconspicuous, the differentiation is nearly impossible. The same diagnostic difficulty arises when a delirium is complicated by an illness that superimposes stupor (e.g., delirium tremens with pneumonia). Actually, typical cases showing one or the other of these two syndromes are easily distinguished. Difficulty in distinguishing these two states is the reason that many writers such as Romano and Engel and Lipowski insist on there being but one disordered mechanism, the manifestations of which they call *delirium*. The present writers would disagree, for they believe several pathogenetic mechanisms of different types and involving different parts of the brain to be included in this category of acute, reversible cerebral disease.

(See Chaps. 118 and 120 for discussions of some of the diseases which cause delirious states.)

MORBID ANATOMY AND PATHOPHYSIOLOGY. All that has been said on this subject in Chap. 26 is applicable to at least one subgroup of the confusional states. In the others no consistent pathologic change has been found. The electroencephalogram is of interest because it is almost invariably abnormal in more severe forms of this syndrome, in contrast to delirium, where the changes are relatively minor. High-voltage slow waves in the 2 to 3 per sec (delta) range or the 5 to 7 per sec (theta) range are the usual finding.

Senile and Other Dementing Brain Diseases Complicated by Medical Diseases (Beclouded Dementia)

Many elderly patients who enter the hospital with medical or surgical illness are mentally confused. Presumably the liability to this state is determined by preexisting brain disease, in this instance senile dementia, which may or may not have been obvious to the family before the onset of the complicating illness. Other cerebral diseases (vascular, neoplastic, demyelinative) may have the same effect of increasing the patient's liability to delirium.

All the clinical features of hypokinetic delirium or confusion described in the previous sections may be present. The severity may vary greatly. The confusion may be reflected only in the patient's inability to relate sequentially the history of his illness, or it may be so severe that he is virtually *non compos mentis*.

Although almost any complicating illness may bring out this confusion, it is particularly frequent with infectious disease, especially in those cases which resist the effects of antibiotic medication; with posttraumatic and postoperative states, notably after concussive brain injuries and removal of cataracts (in which case the confusion is probably related to being temporarily deprived of vision); and with congestive heart failure, chronic respiratory disease, and severe anemia, especially pernicious anemia. Often it is difficult to determine which of several possible factors is responsible for the confusion in this heterogeneous group of illnesses. There may be more than one factor. A cardiac patient with a confusional psychosis may be febrile, have marginally reduced cerebral blood flow, be intoxicated by one or more drugs, or be in electrolyte imbalance. The same is true of postoperative confusional states, where a number of factors such as fever, infection, dehydration, and drug intoxication may be incriminated. The presence of alcoholism may further complicate the matter.

When he recovers from the medical or surgical illness, the patient usually returns to his premorbid state, though his shortcomings, now drawn to the attention of the family and physician, may be more obvious than before.

Coincidental Development of Acute Schizophrenic or Manic-depressive Psychosis during a Medical or Surgical Illness

A certain proportion of psychoses of the schizophrenic or manic-depressive type first become manifest during an acute medical illness or following an operation or parturition. A causal relationship between the two is usually sought but cannot be established. Usually the psychosis began long before but was not recognized. The diagnosis of the psychiatric illness must proceed along the lines suggested in Chaps. 371 and 372. Close observation will usually reveal a clear sensorium and relatively intact memory, which permits differentiation from the acute confusional states.

KORSAKOFF'S AMNESTIC SYNDROMES AND THE RESIDUAL MENTAL STATES FOLLOWING DELIRIUM AND CONFUSION

The majority of patients suffering from the delirious confused states recover completely after a few days or weeks. Afterwards one can detect no evidence of damage to the nervous system. In contrast, in cases of beclouded dementia, as the sensorial disturbance subsides, the patient is left with the same mental weakness that existed before the onset of the confusional state. Sometimes the dementia seems more pronounced afterward, and the family will later remark that the patient's mind failed at the time of the acute illness. However, one has the impression that they merely became aware of the insidiously developing dementia at this time.

There is another group of cases, by no means small or insignificant, in which the acutely delirious or confused patient is left with a severe deficit. The inattentiveness, hallucinations, and sleep disorder disappear. The patient is alert, easily engaged in conversation, and quite proper in his general deportment. Nevertheless, he is incompetent to look after himself. A careful evaluation of his mental status will reveal a severe memory deficit of the type found in Korsakoff's psychosis. The distinguishing feature of this latter illness is not memory loss alone but the disproportionate affection of memory in relation to the patient's alertness and the integrity of other faculties. It is further characterized by the inability to learn new facts and, in its early stages, by confabulation. This state, once fully developed, may be permanent, though often there is some improvement in learning capacity and memory as the months pass. It represents a special type of dementia.

The clinical features of Korsakoff's psychosis are presented in detail in Chap. 363. Although frequently observed in patients who suffer from alcoholism and malnutrition, the same clinical picture may occur with other diseases, such as ruptured saccular aneurysm and subarachnoid hemorrhage, tuberculous meningitis, and tumors in the walls of the third ventricle.

OTHER BEHAVIORAL DISORDERS ASSOCIATED WITH CEREBRAL DISEASE

When one attempts to categorize all the patients with relatively acute or subacute disorders of mentation and behavior under the section headings above, there are still a considerable number that remain difficult to classify. They present themselves as an almost infinite variety of syndromes in which the following abnormalities of function may occur: reduced or increased levels of speech, thought and action; disorientation as to time and place; idleness and lack of interest; loss of spontaneity and sense of humor; muteness and hypokinesia, resistiveness and negativism; hostility, lack of observance of social custom, use of abusive and vulgar language; inexplicable fright, euphoria, and lack of proper concern; complaint of visual distortion, of excess sensitivity to sounds; distortions of smell and taste; inability to find the names of objects, to follow a conversation, to think coherently; sexual indiscretion, lack of modesty, and other signs of disinhibition; seizures; disturbances of sleep. Obviously these many symptoms do not all have the same basic significance and the majority possess only relative localizing value. They may be associated with definite hemiparesis, hemihypesthesia, frank aphasia, or homonymous hemianopia, but even without these lateralizing signs they point to the existence of cerebral disease.

Syndromes comprising these elements may be observed in subacute inclusion body encephalitis, Behcet's meningoencephalitis, adult toxoplasmosis, infectious mononucleosis, acute or subacute demyelinative diseases (acute or subacute recurrent multiple sclerosis), granulomatous and other forms of angiitis, gliomatosis cerebri, carcinomatosis with encephalopathy of multifocal type, multiple tumor metastases, acute and subacute bacterial endocarditis, and thrombopenia with small vessel thrombosis (Moschcowitz's disease). A fuller account of some of these cerebral symptoms will be found in descriptions of these diseases.

Classification of Deliria or Acute Confusional States and Korsakoff's Amnestic Syndrome

The syndrome itself and its main clinical relationships are the only satisfactory basis for classification until such time as the actual cause and pathophysiology are discovered. The tendency in the past to subdivide the syndromes according to their most prominent symptom or degree of severity, e.g., "picking delirium," "microptic delirium," "acute delirious mania," "muttering delirium," has no fundamental value.

I. Hyperkinetic Delirium
   A. In a medical or surgical illness (no focal or lateralizing neurologic signs; cerebrospinal fluid usually clear)
      1. Typhoid fever
      2. Pneumonia
      3. Septicemia, particularly erysipelas and other streptococcal infections

4. Rheumatic fever
5. Thyrotoxicosis and ACTH intoxication (rare)
6. Postoperative and posttraumatic states

B. In neurologic disease that causes focal or lateralizing signs or changes in the cerebrospinal fluid
   1. Vascular, neoplastic, or other diseases, particularly those involving the temporal lobes and upper brainstem
   2. Cerebral contusion and laceration (traumatic delirium)
   3. Acute purulent and tuberculous meningitis
   4. Subarachnoid hemorrhage
   5. Encephalitis due to viral causes and to unknown causes, e.g., infectious mononucleosis

C. The abstinence states (after drug intoxications), exogenous intoxications and postconvulsive states; signs of other medical, surgical, and neurologic illnesses absent or coincidental
   1. Alcoholism (delirium tremens), barbiturates, chlordiazepoxide, glutethimide
   2. Drug intoxications: camphor, caffeine, ergot, bromides, scopolamine, atropine, amphetamine
   3. Postconvulsive delirium

II. Hypokinetic Delirium and Non-Delirious Confusional States Associated with Psychomotor Underactivity

A. Associated with a medical or surgical disease (no focal lateralizing neurologic signs; cerebrospinal fluid clear)
   1. Metabolic disorders: hepatic stupor, uremia, hypoxia, hypercapnia, hypoglycemia, porphyria
   2. Infective fevers, especially typhoid
   3. Congestive heart failure
   4. Postoperative, posttraumatic, and puerperal psychoses

B. Associated with drug intoxication (no focal or lateralizing signs; cerebrospinal fluid clear): opiates, barbiturates, bromides, Artane, etc.

C. Associated with diseases of the nervous system (the focal or lateralizing neurologic signs and cerebrospinal fluid changes of these conditions are commoner than in delirium)
   1. Cerebral vascular disease, tumor, abscess
   2. Subdural hematoma
   3. Meningitis
   4. Encephalitis
   5. Preexisting neurologic disease (e.g., senile dementia) complicated by a medical or surgical disease

D. Beclouded dementia, i.e., senile brain disease in combination with infective fevers, drug reactions, heart failure, etc.

III. Korsakoff's amnestic syndrome

A. Deficiency of thiamine
   1. Alcoholic disorders with peculiar dietary habits, gastrointestinal diseases, etc.

B. Subarachnoid hemorrhage from ruptured aneurysms

C. Tumors and infective granulomas in walls of the third ventricle

D. Bilateral post-cerebral artery occlusion

E. Inclusion-body encephalitis

With reference to the differential diagnosis acute delirious confusional states, one must also have a secure approach because such illnesses are observed almost daily on the medical and surgical wards of a general hospital. Occurring as they do during an infective fever, in the course of another illness such as cardiac failure, or following an injury, operation, or the excessive use of alcohol, they never fail to create grave problems for the physician, the nursing personnel, and the family. The physician often has to diagnose without the advantage of a lucid history, and his program of treatment may constantly be threatened by the patient's agitation, sleeplessness, and uncooperative attitude. The nursing personnel are often sorely taxed by the necessity of providing a satisfactory environment for the convalescence of the patient and, at the same time, maintaining a tranquil atmosphere for the other patients on the ward. And the family is appalled by the sudden specter of insanity and all it entails.

Under such circumstances, it is a great temptation to rid oneself of the clinical problem by transferring the patient to a psychiatric hospital. This, in the author's opinion, is an unwise action, for it may result in the inexpert management of the underlying medical disease and may even jeopardize the patient's life. It is far better for the physician to assume full responsibility for the care of such patients and to familiarize himself with management of this group of nervous disorders.

The first step in diagnosis is to recognize that the patient is confused. This is obvious in most cases, but, as pointed out above, the mildest form of confusion, particularly when some other acute alteration of personality is prominent, may be overlooked. In these mild forms a careful analysis of the patient's thinking as he gives the history of his illness and the details of his personal life will usually reveal an incoherence. Digit span and serial subtraction of 7s from 100 are useful bedside tests of the patient's capacity for sustained mental activity. Memory of recent events is one of the most delicate tests of adequate mental function and may be accomplished by having the patient relate all the details of his entry to the hospital, laboratory tests, etc.

Once it is established that the patient is confused, the differential diagnosis must be made between delirium, simple or primary mental confusion, a beclouded dementia, and Korsakoff's psychosis. This can be done usually by careful attention to the patient's degree of alertness and wakefulness, his capacity to solve new problems, his memory, accuracy of perception, and hallucinations. The presence of Korsakoff's psychosis may not become evident until the patient's general state improves. The distinction between confusional states and dementia is also difficult at times. It has been said that the patient with the acute confusional psychosis has a clouded sensorium, i.e., he is inattentive, and inclined to inaccurate perceptions and hallucinations, whereas the patient with dementia has a clear sensorium. However, it is the authors' impression that many severely demented patients are as beclouded as those with confusional psychoses, and that the two conditions are at times indistinguishable, except for their different time courses. All this suggests that the parts of the nervous system affected may be the same in both conditions. When the physician is faced with this problem, the history of the mode of onset becomes of great value. The confusional psychosis has an acute or subacute onset and is usually reversible, whereas dementia is always chronic and tends to be more or less irreversible.

Once a case has been classified as delirium, primary mental confusion, or Korsakoff's psychosis, it is important to determine its clinical associations. A thorough medical and neurologic examination and often a lumbar puncture should be done. The other medical and neurologic findings are of great value in indicating the underlying disease to be treated, and they also give information concerning prognosis. In the neurologic examination, particular attention should be given to language functions, visual fields and visual-spatial discriminations, cortical sensory functions, and calculation and other test performances that require normal functioning of the temporal, parietal, and occipital lobes. Confusional states are frequent with diseases of these parts of the brain. Moreover, some of the signs of the latter are often mistaken for a confusional psychosis.

Schizophrenia and manic-depressive psychosis can usually be separated from the confusional stress by the presence of a clear sensorium and good memory.

The treatment is directed to eradicating or controlling the underlying disease process.

CARE OF THE DELIRIOUS AND CONFUSED PATIENT

The primary therapeutic effort in treating the delirious and confused patient in a general hospital is to control the underlying medical disease. Delirum seldom lasts more than a few days, and if the patient can be kept on a medical ward, the social stigma that attaches to incarceration in a mental institution is avoided. In the author's experience only a few delirious patients are so agitated and noisy as to annoy others, and should this happen, many general hospitals now have some facilities for isolating the mentally disturbed patient. Delirium of this severity is rare in infectious diseases but is, of course, not infrequent in alcoholism (delirium tremens), drug intoxication, and other medical diseases.

Important objectives are to quiet the patient and protect him against injury. A private nurse, an attendant, or a member of the family should be with the patient at all times, if this can be arranged. Depending on how active and vigorous he is, a locked room, screened windows that cannot be opened by the patient, and a low bed or mattress on the floor should be arranged. It is often better to let the patient walk about the room than to tie him into bed, which may excite or frighten him so that he struggles to the point of complete exhaustion and collapse. If he is less active, the patient can usually be kept in bed by leather wrist restraints, a restraining sheet, or a net thrown over the bed. Unless contraindicated by the primary disease, the patient should be permitted to sit up or walk about the room part of the day.

All drugs that could possibly be responsible for delirium—particularly opiates, barbiturates, bromides, atro-pine, hyoscine, cortisone, adrenocorticortropic hormone (ACTH), and salicylates in large doses—should be discontinued (unless withdrawal effects are believed to underlie the illness). Paraldehyde and chloral hydrate are the only sedatives that can be trusted under these circumstances. Paraldehyde, which is preferred, may be given orally or rectally in doses of 10 to 12 ml. For oral administration, mixing it with fruit juices makes it more palatable, though alcoholic patients will take it in any form and seem to enjoy it. Chlorpromazine, chlordiazepoxide, and diazepam are often extremely effective if given in full doses, and should be continued until natural sleep is restored. One must be cautious in attempting to suppress agitation completely. To accomplish this may require very large doses of drugs, and vital functions may be dangerously impaired. The purpose of sedation is to assure rest and sleep so that the patient does not exhaust himself. Continuous warm baths or warm packs are also effective in quieting the delirious patient, but very few general hospitals have proper facilities for this valuable method of treatment.

A fluid intake and output chart should be kept, and any fluid and electrolyte deficit should be corrected according to the methods outlined in Chap. 296. The pulse and blood pressure should be recorded at intervals of 2 hr in anticipation of circulatory collapse. Transfusions of whole blood and vasopressor drugs may be lifesaving.

Finally, the physician should be aware of many small therapeutic measures that may allay fear and suspicion and reduce the tendency to hallucinations. The room should be kept well lighted, and if possible, the patient should not be moved from one room to another. Every procedure should be explained in detail, even such simple ones as the taking of blood pressure or temperature. The presence of a member of the family may enable the patient to maintain contact with reality.

It may be some consolation and also a source of professional satisfaction to remember that most delirious patients tend to recover if they are placed in good hygienic surroundings and competently nursed. The family should be reassured on this point. They must also understand that the abnormal behavior and irrational actions of the patient are not wilful but rather are symptomatic of a brain disease.

See also Chapter 31 for care of demented patient.

REFERENCES

Bonhoeffer, K.: Die Psychosen in Gefolge von akuten Infektionen, etc. in "Handbach der Psychiatrie," G. L. Aschaffenburg (Ed.), Spez. Teil 3, pp. 1–60, Leipzig, 1912.

Lipowski, Z. J.: Delirium, Clouding of Consciousness and confusion. *J. Nervous Mental Dis.*, 145:227, 1967.

Romani, J., and G. L. Engel: Physiologic and Psychologic Considerations of Delirium, Med. Clinics N. Am. 28:629, 1944.

Whitty, C. W. M., and O. L. Zangwill (Eds), "Amnesia," London, Butterworth & Co. (Publishers), Ltd., 1966.

Wolff, H. G., and D. Curran: Nature of Delirium and Allied States, Arch. Neurol. Psychiat., 33:1175–1935.

31 | DERANGEMENTS OF INTELLECT AND BEHAVIOR INCLUDING DEMENTIA AND OTHER CEREBRAL DEFECT SYNDROMES

*Raymond D. Adams and
Maurice Victor*

Increasingly, as the number of elderly adults in our population rises, the internist is consulted because an otherwise healthy individual begins to lose his capacity to function effectively as head of a family or as a worker. This may have several significations—indicating the beginning of a brain tumor, the formation of a chronic subdural hematoma, or the development of a chronic drug intoxication, a chronic meningoencephalitis (syphilis), degenerative cerebral disease, a chronic low-pressure hydrocephalus, a degenerative brain disease, or a depressive psychosis. In former times when there was little that could be done about any of these clinical states no great premium was attached to diagnosis. But modern medicine now offers the means of treating several of these conditions and in some instances of restoring the patient to normal health and effectiveness. Early recognition of the underlying pathologic process improves chances of recovery. For this reason and because of the frequency of these problems every practicing physician stands a chance of becoming involved.

The following information will be helpful in understanding the nature of some of these clinical problems.

THE CLINICAL SYNDROME OF DEMENTIA

In current neurologic parlance the term *dementia* usually denotes a clinical state comprised of failing memory and loss of other intellectual functions due to chronic progressive degenerative disease of the brain. It may or may not be associated with signs of disease in one or more of the motor, sensory, or speech areas of the cerebrum. The chronicity of the process is ordinarily emphasized, but the illogic of setting apart any one constellation of cerebral symptoms on the basis of their speed of onset or duration is obvious. We would like to propose that the state of dementia be regarded as a generic syndrome of multiple causation and mechanism, and that a degeneration of neurones is only one of the causes.

The earliest signs of dementia may be so subtle as to escape the notice of even the most discerning physician. Often an observant relative of the patient or an employer is the first to become aware of a certain lack of initiative, irritability, loss of interest, and inability to perform up to the usual standard. Later there is distractibility, inability to think with accustomed clarity, reduced general comprehension, perseveration in speech, action, and thought, and defective memory, especially for recent events. Frequently a change in mood becomes apparent, deviating more often toward depression than elation. The direction of this deviation is said to depend on the previous personality of the patient rather than upon the character of the disease. Excessive lability of mood may also be observed, i.e., an easy fluctuation from laughter to tears on slight provocation. Moral and ethical standards are lost, early in some cases and late in others. Paranoid ideas and delusions may develop. As a rule, the patient has little or no realization of these changes in himself; he lacks insight. As the condition progresses, there is loss of almost all intellectual faculties, with mental retardation and extreme incoherence and irrationality. Mutism, unresponsiveness, dysarthria, aphasia, and sphincteric incontinence may be added to the clinical picture. In a late stage a secondary physical deterioration also takes place. Food intake, which may be increased in the beginning of the illness, is in the end usually limited, with resulting emaciation. Any febrile illness or metabolic upset induces stupor or coma, indicating the precarious state of cerebral compensation. Finally the patient remains in bed most of the time and dies of pneumonia or some other intercurrent infection. This whole process may evolve over a period of months or years, usually the latter.

Many of these alterations of behavior are the direct result of disease of the nervous system; expressed in another way, the symptoms are the primary manifestations of neurologic disease; others are secondary, they are reactions to the catastrophe of losing one's mind. For example, the dement is said to seek solitude to hide his affliction and may thus appear asocial or apathetic. Again, excessive orderliness may be an attempt to compensate for failing memory; apprehension, gloom, or irritability may express general dissatisfaction with a necessarily restricted life. It would appear that even in a state of fairly advanced deterioration, the patient is still capable of reacting to his illness and to the individuals who care for him.

Attempts to relate loss of memory and failing intellectual function to lesions in certain parts of the brain have been eminently unsuccessful. Two types of difficulty have obstructed progress in this field. (1) There is the problem of defining, analyzing, and determining the significance of the so-called "intellectual" functions. (2) The morbid anatomy of these diseases is so diffuse and complex that it cannot be fully localized and quantitated.

In the most careful analyses of the intellectual functions, certain general and certain specific factors have been isolated. The general factors are not localized at the moment to any one area of the brain, whereas the specific ones do have at least a regional localization in the cerebrum. Spearman, Thurstone, and others have been able to single out a number of specific factors such as verbal capacity, ability to appreciate spatial relationships, ability to learn and to reason inductively and deductively, facility in the use of numbers and in numerical calculation, and retentive memory. All these qualities are tested in standard intelligence and achievement tests. Memory correlates poorly with all the other factors and seems to be an independent item. There is an intercorrelation between all the other factors. In other words, a person who performs well in tests of verbal capacity tends to do well on tests of spatial orientation, numerical relationships, learning, and reasoning. Some general factor, ?G factor of Spearman, is being measured by each test and determines in part the level of performance. In addition, there are special aptitudes or factors (S. factors of Spearman) that account for individual superiorities' or (in disease) inferiorities in one or another test.

Morbid Anatomy and Pathologic Physiology of Dementia

In dementia the memory impairment, which is a constant feature, may occur with extensive disease in any part of the cerebrum. Yet it is interesting to note that the function of certain parts of the diencephalon and of the hippocampi may be more fundamental to retentive memory than the rest of the cortex, and as will be pointed out below, it may be certain of the corticothalamic connections that are particularly concerned with this function. Failure in tests of verbal function (the most advanced degree of which is aphasia) is closely associated with disease of the dominant cerebral hemisphere, and particularly the speech areas in the frontal, temporal, and parietal lobes and insula. Loss of capacity for arithmetic, reading, and numerical calculation (acalculia) is related to lesions in the posterior part of the left (dominant) cerebral hemisphere. Impairment in drawing or constructing simple and complex figures with blocks, sticks, picture arrangements, etc., as shown by tests of visual construction is most pronounced in right (nondominant) parietal lobe lesions, as will be pointed out below. Thus, the clinical picture resulting from cerebral disease depends in part on the extent of the lesion, i.e., the amount of cerebral tissue destroyed, and on the specific locality of the lesion.

Dementia is related usually to obvious structural disease of the cerebrum and the diencephalon. Knowledge of the detailed anatomy of the diencephalic nuclei and their connections with one another and with the various parts of the cerebral cortex is so limited that it has thus far been impossible to define either the topography of many of the diseases with which we are concerned or the nature of the lesion. In some diseases, such as Alzheimer's and Pick's presenile or senile dementia, the main process appears to be a degeneration and loss of nerve cells in the association areas, with secondary changes in the cerebral white matter. In others, such as Huntington's chorea, Jakob-Creutzfeldt pseudosclerosis, and the cerebrobasal ganglionic and cerebrocerebellar degenerations, loss of neurones in the cerebral cortex is accompanied by a similar degeneration of neurones in the putamen and caudate nuclei and the cerebellum, respectively. Arteriosclerotic vascular disease results in multiple foci of infarction all through the thalami, basal ganglions, brainstem, and cerebrum and, in the latter, in the motor, sensory, or visual projection areas as well as in the association areas. Severe trauma may cause contusions of cerebral convolutions and degeneration of the central white matter (Strich), which result in protracted stupor, coma, or dementia (rare). Most diseases that produce dementia are quite extensive, and the frontal lobes are affected more often than other parts of the cerebrum.

Other mechanisms than the destruction of brain tissue may operate in some cases. Chronic increased intracranial pressure or chronic hydrocephalus (with large ventricles the pressure may not exceed 180 mm), regardless of cause, is often associated with a general impairment of mental function. There the factor of compression of tracts in the cerebral white matter is the main factor. The compression of one or both cerebral hemispheres by chronic subdural hematomas may cause a widespread disturbance of cortical function. A diffuse inflammatory process is at least in part the basis for dementia in syphilis and in neurotropic virus infections such as "inclusion body encephalitis." Presumably there is loss of neurones and also inflammatory derangement of the function of others. Lastly, several of the toxic and metabolic diseases discussed in Chap. 26 may interfere with nervous function over a long period of time and create a clinical picture similar to, if not identical with, that of dementia. One must suppose that the altered biochemical environment has affected the excitability of the neurones.

(The details of all the diseases which cause dementia will be found in Chaps. 363 and 364.)

Bedside Classification of Dementing Diseases of the Brain

The conventional classification of dementing diseases of the brain is usually according to etiology, if known, or pathology. Another more practical approach, which follows logically from the method by which the whole subject has been presented in this book, is to subdivide the diseases into three categories on the basis of the associated clinical and laboratory signs of medical disease and the accompanying neurologic signs. Once the physician has determined that the patient suffers a dementing illness, he must then decide, from the medical, neurologic, and laboratory data, into which category the case fits. This classification may at first seem somewhat artificial. However, it is likely to be more useful to the student or physician not conversant with the many diseases that cause dementia than a classification based on pathology.

CLASSIFICATION

I. Diseases in which dementia is usually associated with clinical and laboratory signs of other medical disease
   A. Hypothyroidism
   B. Cushing's disease
   C. Nutritional deficiency states such as pellagra, Wernicke's disease and Korsakoff's syndrome, pernicious anemia, and subacute degeneration of spinal cord and brain
   D. Neurosyphilis: general paresis and meningovascular syphilis
   E. Hepatolenticular degeneration
   F. Cerebral arteriosclerosis (coronary disease, pseudobulbar symptoms)
   G. Bromidism
II. Diseases in which dementia is associated with other neurologic signs but not with other obvious medical disease
   A. Invariably associated with other neurologic signs
      1. Huntington's chorea (choreoathetosis)

2. Schilder's disease and related demyelinative diseases (spastic weakness, pseudobulbar palsy, blindness, deafness)
3. Amaurotic family idiocy and other lipid-storage diseases (myoclonic seizures, blindness, spasticity, cerebellar ataxia)
4. Myoclonic epilepsy (diffuse myoclonus, generalized seizures, cerebellar ataxia)
5. Jakob-Creutzfeldt disease (diffuse myoclonus)
6. Cerebrocerebellar degeneration (cerebellar ataxia)
7. Cerebral-basal ganglia degeneration (apraxia-rigidity)
8. Dementia with spastic paraplegia (spastic legs)
   B. Often associated with other neurologic signs
1. Cerebral arteriosclerosis
2. Brain tumor
3. Brain trauma, such as cerebral contusion, mid-brain hemorrhage, chronic subdural hematoma
III. Diseases in which dementia is usually the only evidence of neurologic or medical disease
   A. Alzheimer's disease and senile dementia
   B. Pick's disease
   C. Marchiafava-Bignami disease (sometimes with frontal lobe signs)
   D. Some cases of brain tumor of frontal lobes and corpus callosum
   E. Low-pressure hydrocephalus

Many of these diseases are discussed more fully in other sections of this book. The special features of the dementia that accompanies arteriosclerotic, senile, syphilitic, traumatic, nutritional, and degenerative diseases are discussed in the appropriate chapters.

Differential Diagnosis

The first difficulty in dealing with this class of patients is to make sure of deterioration of intellect and personality change. It may be necessary to examine the patient several times before one is confident of the clinical findings.

There is always a tendency to assume that mental function is normal if patients complain only of nervousness, fatigue, insomnia, or vague somatic symptoms and to label the patients psychoneurotic. *This will be avoided if one keeps in mind that psychoneuroses rarely begin in middle or late adult life.* A practical rule is to assume that all mental illnesses beginning during this period are due either to structural disease of the brain or to depressive psychosis.

A mild dysphasia must not be mistaken for dementia. The aphasic patient appears uncertain of himself, and his speech may be incoherent. Furthermore, he may be anxious and depressed over his ineptitude. Careful attention to the patient's language performance will lead to the correct diagnosis in most instances. Further observation will disclose the fact that the patient's behavior, except for speech, is within normal limits.

The depressed patient presents another type of problem. He may remark that his mental function is poor or that he is forgetful and cannot concentrate. Scrutiny of his remarks will show, however, that he actually remembers all the details of his illness and that no qualitative change in mental ability has taken place. His difficulty is either a lack of energy and interest or an anxiety that prevents the focusing of attention on anything except his own problems. Even during mental tests his performance may be impaired by his emotions, in much the same way as that of the worried student during his examinations. This condition of emotional blocking is called *experiential confusion.* When the patient is calmed by reassurance, his mental function is normal, a proof that intellectual deterioration has not occurred. The hypomanic patient fails in tests of intellectual function because of his restlessness and distractibility. It is helpful to remember that the demented patient rarely has sufficient insight to complain of mental deterioration; and if he admits to poor memory, he seldom realizes the degree of his disability. The physician must never rely on the patient's statements as to the efficiency of mental function and must always evaluate a poor performance on tests in the light of the emotional state and motivation at the time the test is given.

The neurologic syndrome associated with metabolic or endocrine disorders, i.e., ACTH therapy, hyperthyroidism, Cushing's disease, Addison's disease, or the postpartum state may be difficult to diagnose because of the wide variety of clinical pictures that may be shown. As will be stated in Chap. 372, some patients appear to be suffering from a dementia, others from an acute confusional psychosis; or if mood change or negativism predominate, a manic-depressive psychosis or schizophrenia is suggested. In these conditions some degree of clouding of sensorium and impairment of intellectual function can usually be recognized, and these findings alone should be enough to exclude schizophrenia and manic-depressive psychosis. It is well to remember that acute onset of mental symptoms always suggests confusional psychosis or delirium. Inasmuch as many of these conditions are completely reversible, they must be distinguished from dementia.

Once it is decided that the patient suffers from a dementing disease, the next step is to determine by careful physical examination whether there are other neurologic signs or indications of a particular medical disease. This enables the physician to place the case in one of the three categories in the bedside classification. X-rays of skull, electroencephalogram, lumbar puncture and pneumoencephalogram should be carried out in most cases. Usually these procedures necessitate admission to a hospital. The final step is to determine by the total clinical picture which disease within any one category the patient has. Table 372-1 and 2 shows the major points in differential diagnosis.

SPECIAL SYNDROMES CAUSED BY DISEASES OF PARTS OF THE CEREBRUM

Symptoms and signs of disease of one part of the cerebrum may occur singly or in combination with dementia, and they provide important information about the location of a disease process and at times about its nature. This is an appropriate place, therefore, to review briefly the known effects of disease of different parts of the cerebrum. Agnosia, apraxia, and aphasia will be only mentioned, since they are treated more extensively in Chaps. 25, 29, and 357.

FRONTAL LOBES. In Fig. 31-1, it may be seen that the frontal lobes lie anterior to the central, or Rolandic, sulcus and superior to the Sylvian fissure. They consist of several functionally different parts, which are conventionally designated in the neurologic literature by numbers (according to a scheme devised by Brodmann) and by letters (in the scheme of von Economo and Koskinas).

The posterior parts, areas 4 and 6 of Brodmann, are specifically related to motor function. Voluntary movement in man depends on the integrity of these areas, and lesions in them produce spastic paralysis of the contralateral face, arm, and leg. This is discussed in Chap. 21, Motor Paralysis. Lesions limited more or less to the premotor areas (area 6) are accompanied by prominent grasp and sucking reflexes. Lesions in areas 8 and 24 of Brodmann interfere with the mechanism concerned with turning the head and eyes contralaterally. Lesions in areas 44 and 45 of the major hemisphere abolish or reduce verbalization, deglutition, and chewing. Lesions in area 44 of the dominant cerebral hemisphere, usually the left one, have often resulted in loss of verbal expression, the aphasia of Broca. Lesions in the medial limbic or piriform cortex (areas 23 and 24), wherein lie the mechanisms controlling respiration, circulation, and micturition have relatively unclear clinical effects.

The remainder of the frontal lobes (areas 9, 10, 11, 12, and 13 of Brodmann), sometimes called the *prefrontal areas*, have less specific and measurable functions. The following groups of symptoms have been observed in patients with diseases limited to one or both frontal lobes or to the central white matter and anterior part of the corpus callosum by which they are joined.

1. Change of personality, usually expressed as lack of concern over the consequences of any action, which may take the form of a childish excitement (moria of Jastrowitz), an inappropriate joking and punning (*witzelsucht* of Oppenheim), or an instability and superficiality of emotion, or irritability.

2. Slight impairment of intelligence, usually described as lack of concentration, vacillation of attention, inability to carry out planned activity, difficulty in changing from one activity to another, loss of recent memory, or lack of initiative and spontaneity.

3. Motor abnormalities such as decomposition of gait and upright stance, trunk ataxia of Bruns, abnormal postures, reflex grasping or sucking, incontinence of sphincters, and akinetic mutism.

The most pronounced changes have been observed in cases with bilateral disease of frontal lobes, and there has been much doubt as to the effect of a lesion involving only one frontal lobe. Nevertheless, the most careful psychologic tests on patients with lesions of either frontal lobe demonstrate a slight elevation of mood with increased talkativeness and tendency to joke, a lack of tact, inability to adapt to a new situation, and loss of initiative.

Several careful studies of lobotomized patients have

Fig. 31-1. Diagram to show cortical areas, numbered according to the scheme of Brodmann. The speech areas are in black, the three main ones being 39, 41, and 45. The zone marked by vertical stripes in the superior frontal convolution is the secondary motor area which, like Broca's area 45, if stimulated causes vocal arrest. (*Redrawn from "Handbuch der Inneren Medizin," Berlin, Springer-Verlag, 1939.*)

now been published. Of course, very few of these patients were normal before the operation, so that base-line measurements of mental ability were not always obtainable. However, some patients of normal intellect have received this treatment for severe neurosis or intractable pain. They are said to have shown little or no loss of ability in their performance on intelligence tests, depending on the extent of the procedure; and if worry, fears, compulsions, and suffering from pain were incapacitating, the loss of these traits resulted in test scores actually higher than before the operation. However, careful examination usually will disclose a slight lowering of general intelligence, a decrease in drive or energy, a definite change of personality in the form of shallow emotional life, a lack of tact, and inability to direct and sustain activity toward future goals. Also there is a diminution of traits related to neuroticism, such as suggestibility, rigidity of character, self-criticism, and introversion.

The function of the frontal lobes cannot be determined simply by the study of human beings who have suffered injury or disease of this part of the brain. Symptoms from lesions of a part of the nervous system are not identical with the functions of that part. The symptoms of frontal lobe deficit must depend both on a loss of certain parts of the cerebrum and on the functional activity of the remaining portions of the nervous system. There is no doubt that the human mind is changed by disease of the frontal lobes, but it is difficult to say in what way it is changed. Intelligence, emotional feeling and expression, memory, visual fixation, postural control, regulation of respiration and blood pressure—all are intact in animals and human beings without frontal lobes. Perhaps at present it is best to regard the frontal lobes as that part of the brain which orients the individual, with all his percepts and concepts formed from past life experiences, toward action that is projected into the future.

TEMPORAL LOBES. The boundaries of the temporal lobes may be seen in Fig. 31-1. The Sylvian fissure separates the superior surface of each temporal lobe from the frontal and anterior parts of the parietal lobes. There is no definite anatomic boundary between the temporal and occipital lobes either inferiorly or laterally or between temporal and parietal lobes. The temporal lobe includes the superior, middle, and inferior temporal, fusiform, and hippocampal convolutions and the transverse convolutions of Heschl, which is the auditory receptive area present on the superior surface within the Sylvian fissure. The hippocampal convolution was once believed to be related indirectly to the olfactory bulb, but now it is known that lesions here do not cause anosmia. The fibers from the homolateral lower quadrant of each retina course through the central white matter en route to the occipital lobes, and lesions that interrupt them characteristically produce a contralateral homonymous upper quadrant defect of visual fields. Hearing and labyrinthine function, also localized in the temporal lobes, are bilaterally represented, which accounts for the fact that unless both temporal lobes are affected, there is no demonstrable loss of hearing. Loss of equilibrium has not been observed with temporal lobe lesions. Extensive disease in the superior and middle convolutions of the left temporal lobe in right-handed individuals results in Wernicke's aphasia. This syndrome, discussed in Chap. 29, Affections of Speech, consists of jargon aphasia and inability to read, to write, or to understand the meaning of spoken words. Probably the basic defect in all these is the loss of memory for words.

Between the auditory and olfactory projection areas there is a large expanse of temporal lobe which has no assignable function. This is the temporal association area. Patients with tumors and vascular lesions of this part of the brain have been examined on numerous occasions, but usually the full extent of the disease has not been determined, even by pneumoencephalography, arteriography, or isotopic scanning procedures. Cases of temporal lobectomy for tumor have provided more valuable material, but again it has seldom been possible to be certain that other parts of the brain were not involved. The most careful psychologic studies have shown a difference between cases involving loss of the dominant and the nondominant temporal lobe. With lesions of the dominant side there is impairment in learning verbal material presented aloud; with nondominant lesions there is a similar failure in tests with visually presented material. In addition, about 20 percent of both right and left lobectomy patients have shown a syndrome similar to that described

for the prefrontal parts of the brain; but more significant is the fact that in the other cases little or no defect in personality was exhibited. The study of cases of uncinate epilepsy, with the characteristic dreamy state, olfactory or gustatory hallucinations, and masticatory movements, suggests that all these functions are organized through the temporal lobes. Similarly, stimulation of the posterior parts of the temporal lobes of epileptic patients during surgical procedures has brought to light the interesting fact that complex memories and visual and auditory images, some with strong emotional content, can be aroused in fully conscious human beings. Recent studies of the effect of stimulation of the amygdaloid nucleus, which is in the anterior and medial part of the temporal lobe, have shed additional light on this subject. Symptoms may be evoked not unlike some of those of schizophrenic patients. Complex emotional experiences that have occurred previously may be revived. There are remarkable autonomic effects. Blood pressure rises, pulse increases, respirations are increased in frequency and depth, and the patient looks frightened. These effects have been discussed in Chap. 28, Recurrent Convulsions. Ablation of these nuclei has eliminated uncontrollable rage reactions in psychotic patients. Excision of the hippocampal and adjacent convolutions bilaterally has been carried out recently, with a disastrous loss of ability to learn new experiences or to establish new memories (Korsakoff's psychosis). All this suggests the important role of the temporal lobes in auditory and visual perception and imagery, in learning and memory, and in the emotional life of the individual.

Bilateral ablation of temporal lobes, so far studied only in monkeys, produces an animal that displays a curious tendency to react to every visual stimulus without seeming to recognize it (psychic blindness) and to examine every object in its environment by oral and manual contact. Placidity, with lack of the usual emotional response to stimuli, was another prominent feature.

To summarize, in man the temporal lobe syndromes include the following:

I. Effects of unilateral disease of the dominant temporal lobe
   A. Quadrantic homonymous anopia
   B. Wernicke's aphasia
   C. Impairment in verbal tests of material presented through the auditory sense
   D. Dysnomia or amnestic aphasia
II. Effects of unilateral disease of nondominant temporal lobe
   A. Quadrantic homonymous anopia
   B. Impairment of mental function with inability to judge spatial relationship in some cases
   C. Impairment in nonverbal tests of visually presented material

PARIETAL LOBES. This part of the human nervous system is the subject of one of the most interesting discussions of cerebral function that has occurred in this century: its role in the formation of the body image or body schema.

It has long been known that the postcentral convolution is the terminus of somatic sensory pathways from the opposite half of the body. It has also been learned that destructive lesions here do not abolish cutaneous sensation but instead cause mainly a defect in sensory discrimination with variable impairment of sensation. In other words, pain, touch, and thermal and vibratory sensation are largely retained, whereas stereognosis, sense of position, distinction between single and double contacts (two-point threshold), and the localization of sensory stimuli are lost. There is also the phenomenon of extinction, viz., if both sides of the body are touched simultaneously, only the stimulus on the normal side is perceived. This type of sensory disturbance, sometimes called *cortical sensory defect,* is discussed in Chap. 25, Disorders of Sensation. Later it was noted that extensive lesions deep in the white matter of the parietal lobes produce a contralateral homonymous hemianopia, and lesions in the angular gyrus of the dominant hemisphere result in an inability to read.

More recent investigations have centered about the function of the parietal lobes in perception of position in space and of the relationship of the various parts of the body to one another. Since the time of Babinski it has been known that patients with a large lesion of the minor parietal lobe are often unaware of their hemiplegia and hemianesthesia. Babinski called this condition *anosognosia.* Related psychologic disorders are lack of recognition of the left arm and leg when seen or felt by the other hand, neglect of the left side of the body in dressing, an imperception of external space on the left side, and constructional apraxia, an inability to perform the movements of constructing simple figures. *Agnosia* and *apraxia* are discussed in Chaps. 21 and 25.

Another frequent constellation of symptoms, usually referred to as *Gerstmann's syndrome,* occurs with lesions of the dominant parietal lobe. This consists of inability to write (agraphia), inability to calculate (acalculia), failure to distinguish right from left, and loss of recognition of various parts of the body. An ideomotor apraxia may or may not be conjoined.

The effects of disease of the parietal lobes differ according to whether the dominant (left hemisphere in a right-handed person) or nondominant lobe is involved. These may be tabulated as follows:

I. Effect of unilateral disease of parietal lobe, right or left
   A. Cortical sensory syndrome and sensory extinction (or total hemianesthesia with large acute lesions of white matter)
   B. Mild hemiparesis, unilateral muscular atrophy in children
   C. Homonymous hemianopia or visual inattention, and sometimes neglect of one-half of external space
   D. Abolition of opticokinetic nystagmus to one side
II. Effects of unilateral disease of dominant parietal lobe (left hemisphere in right-handed patients), additional phenomena
   A. Disorders of language (especially alexia)
   B. Gerstmann's syndrome
   C. Bimanual astereognosis (tactile agnosia)
   D. Bilateral apraxia of ideomotor type
III. Effects of unilateral disease of minor parietal lobe (right

hemisphere in right-handed patients), additional phenomena
   A. Anosognosia
   B. Neglect of left side of body
   C. Neglect of visual space to the left of the midline

In all these lesions, if the disease is sufficiently extensive, there may be a reduction in the capacity to think clearly, inattentiveness, and impairment of memory.

It is impossible at this time to present a formula of parietal lobe function in general. It does seem reasonably certain that both the parietal and occipital lobes participate in sensory functions, especially in those which provide consciousness of one's surroundings, of the relationship of objects in the environment to one another, and of the position of the body in space. In this respect, as C. M. Fisher has suggested, the parietal lobe may be regarded as a suprasensory mechanism for transmodal (intersensory) relationships, particularly tactile and visual, which are the basis of our concepts of space.

OCCIPITAL LOBES. The occipital lobes are the terminus of the visual pathways and are essential for visual sensation and perception. Lesions in one occipital lobe result in homonymous defects in the contralateral visual fields. Bilateral lesions cause cortical blindness, a state of blindness without change in optic fundi or pupillary reflexes. If areas 18 and 19 of Brodmann are affected (Fig. 31-1), there is loss of visual recognition, with retention of some degree of visual acuity, a state termed *visual agnosia,* or *mind blindness.* In the classic form of this blindness an individual with intact mental powers is unable to recognize objects, even though by tests of visual acuity and perimetry he appears to see sufficiently well to do so. Psychologists have demonstrated several special types of visual agnosia. In the simultagnosia of Wolpert, the patient, though able to see the individual parts of a picture, is unable to gather the meaning of the whole. Similarly, in prosopagnosia the patient is unable to recognize a human face even though he sees all the individual details of it. Alexia, or inability to read, and visual spatial agnosia, or inability to recognize actual or abstract space, with resulting disorientation, are other special types of agnosia. Often the patient with bilateral lesions of the occipital lobes (cerebral cortical blindness) is unaware of his visual difficulty, i.e., has an agnosia for it. This state is known as *Anton's syndrome.* In *Holmes' syndrome* visual disorientation may be combined with a homonymous hemianopia. Left occipital lobe lesions in combination with a lesion of splenium of corpus callosum causes alexia without agraphia (see Chap. 29).

This whole problem of both visual and tactile agnosia has recently been reexamined. In most of the reported cases tests of primary visual sensation or visual acuity have been inadequate. By controlling the time factor in visual perception and the adaptation time, and by testing the simultaneous perception of multiple points in the visual field, it is possible to show that the visual function is more often impaired than was at first suspected. The division of the visual process into sensation and perception becomes highly artificial.

Visual function is discussed further in Chap. 24.

CORPUS CALLOSUM. A congenital defect or extensive lesion of the corpus callosum disconnects the dominant cerebral hemisphere which controls speech, praxis, and handedness, from the nondominant. The patient speaks, reads, understands spoken words and writes correctly with the right hand. He uses the right hand skillfully. In contrast the left hand is maladroit; and attempts at writing with the left hand result in an aphasic performance. He can read correctly in the right visual field but not in the left. Objects are identified and named by tactile examination with the right hand but not the left. Verbal commands are performed with the right hand but not the left (apraxia). In bifrontal and corpus callosum lesions (tumor, anterior cerebral infarct, Marchiafava-Bignami disease) a corpus callosum syndrome is combined with bilateral grasp reflexes, abulia, and psychomotor impairment.

DIAGNOSIS OF FOCAL CEREBRAL DISEASE. In summarizing the special effects of disease of different parts of the cerebral hemispheres, several points should be made. Extensive lesions in one or both frontal lobes often encroach on motor areas and, in doing so, cause a weakness of muscle groups on the opposite side of the body. This is especially noticeable in the face and is sometimes more pronounced during emotional expression than on voluntary movement. It may affect the arm and leg as well. In some instances the weakness may be rather slight, and a slowness and stiffness of movement with grasp reflex, slightly increased tendon reflexes, and Babinski's sign on the contralateral side are observed. A rather "absentminded" type of urinary and fecal incontinence is also frequent. Motor aphasia—an inability to speak—indicates involvement of the inferior frontal convolution of the dominant frontal lobe. Anosmia and blindness are neighborhood symptoms, resulting from extension of a lesion on the orbital surfaces of the frontal lobes to the olfactory bulbs and optic nerves.

An upper quadrantic homonymous anopia is the most reliable sign of disease of either the right or left temporal lobes; this localization should always be considered if dementia and this visual disturbance are conjoined. Uncinate or psychic seizures also establish a temporal lobe lesion but do not indicate the laterality. Bizarre disturbances of thinking and affect, often indistinguishable from schizophrenia, may follow temporal lobe seizures. In lesions of the dominant temporal lobe, Wernicke's aphasia is the most characteristic feature.

Cortical sensory deficit is the common neurologic abnormality in disease of either parietal lobe and is often combined with hemiplegia. With left-sided lesions in the inferior parietal lobule there is alexia and a contralateral homonymous hemianopia. Gerstmann's syndrome localizes a lesion in the more posterior parts of the parietal and the lateral occipital lobes of the dominant hemisphere. The curious disturbances of body awareness or body scheme and of parts of the body to the left of the midline are usually found with lesions of the nondominant parietal lobe. Focal seizures arising in the parietal lobe usually consist of a focal or Jacksonian sensory disturbance.

Occipital lesions are distinguished by the almost exclusive affection of visual functions, a circumstance that rarely occurs in pure form with temporal or parietal lesions. The affection may take the form of homonymous hemianopia or of one of the more complex disorders of visual recognition.

In the syndrome of dementia the components of which vary from one disease to another, one may discern the effects of impaired functioning of the several lobes of the brain, and their defects are maximized, always, by bilaterality of lesion and involvement of corpus callosum. Some of these components, such as amnesia, calculation difficulty, reduced verbal function, altered visual spatial relationships, have localizing value even when present in slight degree. In combination they inform the examiner of the diffuse topography of the cortical lesions. Others such as impairment of capacity to think and reason, reduced impulsivity, altered emotionality have little value in localization.

THE APPROACH TO THE CLINICAL PROBLEM OF CONFUSION AND DEMENTIA

The physician presented with a patient suffering from a diffuse or focal cerebral disease must adopt an examination technique designed to expose fully the intellectual defect. Abnormalities of posture, movement, sensation, and reflexes cannot be relied upon for the full demonstration of the neurologic deficit, for it must be remembered that the association areas of the brain may be severely damaged without demonstrable neurologic signs of this type.

Three categories of data are required for the recognition and differential diagnosis of dementing brain disease:

1. A reliable history of illness
2. Findings on mental examination, i.e., so-called "mental status," as well as on the rest of the neurologic examination.
3. Special laboratory procedures, lumbar puncture, x-rays of the skull, electroencephalogram, and sometimes pneumoencephalogram.

The history should always be supplemented by information obtained from a person other than the patient, because through lack of insight he is often unaware of his illness; indeed, he may be ignorant even of his chief complaint. Special inquiry should be made about the patient's general behavior, capacity for work, personal habits, and such faculties as memory and judgment.

This performance of an examination of the mental status must be systematic. At a minimum it should include the following:

I. Insight (patient's replies to questions about his chief symptoms): What is your difficulty? Are you ill? When did your illness begin?

II. Orientation (knowledge of personal identity and present situation):

Person: What is your name? What is your occupation? Where do you live? Are you married?

Place: What is the name of the place where you are now? How did you get here? What floor is it on? Where is the bathroom? What are you doing now?

Time: What is the date today? What time of day is it? What meals have you had? When was the last holiday?

III. Memory:

Remote: Tell me the names of your children and their birth dates. When were you married? What was your mother's maiden name? What was the name of your first school teacher?

Recent past: Tell me about your recent illness (compare with previous statements). What did you have for breakfast today? What is my name or the nurse's name? When did you see me for the first time. What were the headlines in the newspaper today? Give the patient a simple story orally or written and ask him to retell it after 3 to 5 min.

Retention: Repeat these numbers after me (give series of 3,4,5,6,7,8 digits at speed of 1 per second). Now when I give a series of numbers, repeat them in reverse order.

Visual span: Show the patient a picture of several objects and then ask him to name what he has seen and to note any inaccuracies.

IV. General information: Ask about names of presidents, well-known historic dates, the names of large rivers, of large cities, etc.

V. Capacity for sustained mental activity:

Calculation: Test ability to add, subtract, multiply, and divide. Subtraction of serial 7s from 100 is a good test of calculation as well as of attention.

Abstract thinking: See if the patient can detect similarities and differences between classes of objects, or explain a proverb or a fable.

VI. General behavior: Attitudes, general bearing, stream of thought, attentiveness, mood, manner of dress, etc.

VII. Special tests of localized cerebral functions: grasping, sucking, aphasia battery, praxis with both hands, cortical sensory function, drawing of clock face, map of U.S.A., or Europe, floor plan of house, etc.

In order to enlist the patient's full cooperation, the physician must prepare him for questions of this type. Otherwise, the first reaction will be one of embarrassment or anger because of the implication that his mind is not sound. It should be pointed out to the patient that some individuals are rather forgetful and that it is necessary to ask specific questions in order to form some impression about their degree of nervousness when being examined. Reassurance that these are not tests of intelligence or of sanity is helpful.

A more formal and reliable method of examining the mental capacity of adults is the Wechsler-Bellevue test. This can be given by a psychologist or by the physician if he has carefully read the instructions for administering and scoring the test. The *Mental Examiners' Handbook*, by F. L. Wells and J. Ruesch, published by the Psychological Corporation, is helpful to those not familiar with this type of examination. Tests of retention of verbal material and the recall of a series of learned digits or of visually presented objects are of value in estimating the degree of deterioration. In the Wechsler-Bellevue test the discrepancy between the vocabulary, picture completion, information, and object assembly tests as a group (these correlate well with premorbid intelligence and are relatively insensitive to dementing brain disease) and arithmetic, block design, digit span, and digit-symbol tests provide an index of deterioration.

Although the form of confusion or dementia does not indicate a particular disease, certain combinations of symptoms and neurologic signs are more or less characteristic and may aid in diagnosis. The mode of onset, the clinical course, the associated neurologic signs, and the accessory laboratory data constitute the basis of differential diagnosis. It must be admitted, however, that some of the rarer types of "degenerative" brain disease are at present recognized only by pathologic examination. The correct diagnosis of treatable forms of senile (over sixty years of age) or presenile (forty to sixty years) dementias, such as general paresis, subdural hematoma, brain tumor, bromide or other chronic drug intoxication, normal pressure hydrocephalus, pellagra and related deficiency states, and hypothyroidism, is of greater practical importance than the diagnosis of the untreatable ones.

MANAGEMENT OF THE DEMENTED PATIENT. Dementia is a clinical state of the most serious nature, and usually it is worthwhile to admit the patient to the hospital for a period of observation. The physician then has an opportunity to see him several times in a new and fairly constant hospital environment, and certain special procedures such as x-rays of the skull, lumbar puncture, analysis of blood for drugs, basal metabolic rate, an electroencephalogram, and often a pneumoencephalogram can be carried out at this time. The management of the demented patient in the hospital may be relatively simple if he is quiet and cooperative. If the disorder of mental function is severe, a nurse, attendant, or member of the family must stay with him at all times. Provision must be made for adequate food and fluid intake and control of infection, using the same measures outlined for the delirious patient.

Once it is established that the patient has an untreatable dementing brain disease, a responsible member of the family should be apprised of the medical facts. The patient should be told that he has a nervous condition for which he is to be given rest and treatment. Nothing is accomplished by telling him more. The family should be given the prognosis, if the diagnosis is sufficiently certain for this to be done. If the dementia is slight and circumstances are suitable, the patient may remain at home, continuing activities of which he is capable. He should be spared responsibility and guarded against injury that might result from imprudent action. If he is still at work, plans for occupational retirement should be carried out. In more advanced stages of the disease mental and physical enfeeblement become pronounced and institutional care should be advised. Seizures should be treated symptomatically. Nerve tonics, vitamins, and hormones are of no value in checking the course of the illness or in regenerating decayed tissue. They may, however, offer some support to the patient and family. Sometimes stimulants in the form of dextroamphetamine, caffeine and nicotinic acid cause transitory improvement in mental function. Undesirable restlessness, nocturnal wandering,

belligerency or anxiety may be reduced by some of the tranquilizing drugs (see Chap. 121).

Section 4
Alterations in Circulatory and Respiratory Function

32 DYSPNEA
Harry W. Fritts, Jr.

While resting quietly a normal man breathes with effortless ease. His rhythm is leisurely and somewhat irregular; his frequency is usually below 16 breaths per minute; and if he is of average size, his tidal volume is less than 600 ml. To generate this flow of air he expends a very small amount of energy. Indeed, Otis, Fenn, and Rahn have estimated that the calories needed for 24 hr of quiet breathing are fewer than those contained in an ordinary bar of candy. Translated into more precise terms, this indicates that the respiratory muscles of a resting man utilize less than 2 percent of the total energy consumed by the body. It is, therefore, not surprising that quiet breathing is a largely subconscious process.

Even when exercise lifts breathing to the conscious level the normal man does not find the sensation unpleasant. He may complain of breathlessness as he approaches the point of exhaustion, but his discomfort is ameliorated by a feeling of exhilaration or accomplishment. If, however, airflow is artificially impeded, or if ventilatory motion is restricted by strapping his chest and abdomen, awareness of breathing becomes a sensation of distress. Such distress has been characterized by the word *dyspnea*, derived from the Greek roots *dys* (hard) and *pnoe* (breathing). Thus, in its broadest context *dyspnea* denotes an unpleasant awareness of breathing, ranging in intensity from mild discomfort to agony.

Although *dyspnea* has never been a precise term, its current meaning is ambiguous because the word is used in two different ways. On the one hand physicians remark, "The patient complained of dyspnea," while on the other they say, "The patient appeared dyspneic." In the first instance the physician substitutes the noun *dyspnea* for the words used by the patient to describe his symptoms; in the second he employs the adjective *dyspneic* to describe an observed abnormality in the breathing pattern of the patient. Though the choice of definitions is a matter of personal preference, ambiguity can be minimized by using *dyspnea* to denote the overall subject of uncomfortable breathing, by using the words of the patient to describe his symptoms, and by employing precise terms to characterize the breathing pattern, e.g., "a rapid rate with small tidal volumes." This approach has the advantage of separating signs from

symptoms, an important distinction because the two are often poorly correlated. Some patients with seemingly normal ventilatory patterns complain bitterly of distress, while others with obviously abnormal frequencies and tidal volumes deny symptoms. As stressed by Gaensler, the patient's account of his discomfort involves many factors, including intelligence, ability to articulate sensations, and threshold for sensory stimuli.

Quantification

Like pain, respiratory discomfort cannot be measured directly, although a number of indices have been devised to predict when discomfort will appear. Three of the most popular have been the Breathing Reserve, the Walking Ventilation, and the Dyspnea Index. All three relate the minute volume of ventilation (MVV) to the maximum breathing capacity (MBC), and all provide information about the fraction of the capacity actually being utilized. For instance the Breathing Reserve, calculated as the difference between the MBC and the MVV, represents the amount of the capacity still available to the person. This amount is customarily expressed as a percentage of the MBC by the following simple formula:

$$\% = \frac{MBC - MVV}{MBC} \times 100$$

Although there is considerable individual variability, most people are asymptomatic when the calculated index is above 70 percent, and most are aware of their breathing when the index is below this level. Accordingly, an average normal man, having an MBC of 150 liters per min, would begin to be breathless only after his MVV exceeded 50 liters per min, a rate of air movement adequate for heavy exercise. In contrast a patient with advanced emphysema, having an MBC of only 50 liters per min, would have discomfort when his MVV reached 15 liters per min, a rate of air movement only slightly greater than that maintained at rest. These calculations shed light on the severe handicap imposed by a disease like emphysema.

Conditions Associated With Respiratory Distress

The foregoing considerations suggest that the relation between the actual ventilation and the maximal capacity to move air is one of the determinants of breathlessness. It therefore follows that stimuli which increase ventilation or disorders which reduce capacity will tend to make discomfort appear. Among stimuli known to be associated with increased ventilation are arterial hypoxemia, arterial hypercapnea, arterial acidemia, muscular exercise, fever, hypermetabolism, systemic hypotension, and an elevated pressure in the great veins and chambers of the right side of the heart. Among disorders known to reduce ventilatory capacity are weakened respiratory muscles, an abnormal chest wall, a low total lung volume, a stiffened lung, and an increased resistance to airflow. All these factors are obvious sources of respiratory discomfort; other influences are less easily understood. For instance, normal man will experience discomfort if he breathes into an apparatus which forces him to maintain a small tidal volume, yet he can obtain relief by taking occasional deep breaths. Also, paralyzing the respiratory muscles with curare can lead to discomfort, even though the alveolar ventilation is adequately maintained by a mechanical respirator.

These observations have led to the view that uncomfortable breathing is related not only to the absolute values of ventilation and capacity, but to a variety of other influences. One is any condition which augments the energy required for a particular level of ventilation. Another is any factor which causes the patient to utilize either a frequency or a tidal volume which is not his normal one.

MECHANISMS OF DYSPNEA

The respiratory center, a complex array of cells in the pons and medulla, is particularly sensitive to changes in carbon dioxide tension and hydrogen ion concentration in the blood and cerebrospinal fluid. The carotid and aortic chemereceptors respond principally to the blood oxygen tension; other receptors in the aortic arch and carotid arteries are sensitive to blood pressure. These peripheral elements transmit impulses centrally through the glossopharyngeal and vagus nerves.

Information about the position and motion of the thorax and lungs travels centrally through several pathways. The intercostal nerves transmit information about the muscles and joints of the chest wall; the phrenic nerves subserve the same function for the muscle of the diaphragm. In addition, the vagi carry impulses from intrapulmonary receptors which signal the state of expansion of the lungs. These impulses, constituting the sensory arm of the Hering-Breuer reflex, provide a means of regulating the respiratory cycle, because inflation tends to limit inspiration and to initiate the expiration of air. Though highly developed in animals, this reflex appears to be relatively weak in normal man.

Despite this detailed knowledge of normal respiration, the precise mechanism producing the sensation of breathlessness remains an enigma. Popular theories have stressed an overloaded respiratory center, fatigue of the respiratory muscles, excessive energy expenditures, and stimulation of intrapulmonary receptors. These re-

ceptors are thought to respond to conditions which increase the stiffness of the lung, and therefore to play a role in the breathlessness occurring in conditions such as pulmonary vascular congestion, pulmonary edema, atelectasis, or diffuse granulomatous disease.

A number of studies have focused attention on the neural circuits regulating the behavior of the respiratory muscles. Campbell has postulated that sensory elements, particularly muscle spindles, play a central role in comparing the tension in the muscle to the degree of stretch. According to him, respiratory discomfort can arise when the tension is inappropriately large for a particular muscle length. Though the exact role of this mechanism has not been determined, there is little doubt that impulses from the respiratory muscles can play an important part in the origin of respiratory discomfort.

Finally, breathlessness often may represent the operation of several mechanisms, rather than the effect of any single one.

DIFFERENTIAL DIAGNOSIS

The separation of an abnormal breathing pattern from respiratory symptoms is an important first step in the approach to the patient. At times, bizarre patterns may be unassociated with distress. One example is the Kussmaul breathing seen in diabetic acidosis. The patient's minute ventilation may be greatly increased, yet he will be unaware of this augmentation. Similarly, many patients with Cheyne-Stokes respiration are oblivious of the change in their breathing pattern. Quite often patients with anemia overventilate, particularly during exercise, but complain chiefly of weakness or tiredness. As a general rule, these diseases produce changes in other organ systems which overshadow the effect on respiration.

Those patients who have breathlessness as a principal symptom usually have one of the following conditions: (1) obstructive disease of the lung, (2) interstitial and alveolar disease of the lung, (3) disease of the chest wall or respiratory muscles, (4) disorders of the heart and circulation, or (5) anxiety neurosis or hysteria. Since each of these conditions is discussed in detail in Part 8, Sec. 3, the ensuing paragraphs stress those points in the evaluation of the patient which will help distinguish one of the conditions from the others.

OBSTRUCTIVE DISEASE OF THE LUNG. (See Chap. 283.) Among the diseases causing acute airway obstruction are asthma, bronchiolitis, and croup. In each, a careful history and a detailed physical examination almost always will establish the diagnosis. In contrast, chronic airway obstruction may be more difficult to recognize, because of the wide variety of signs and symptoms which accompany it. Usually, patients with chronic airway obstruction give a history of shortness of breath for many months. At first breathlessness occurs only with heavy exercise; later with moderate activity; and finally at rest. Characteristically, breathlessness is associated with chronic cough, productive of variable amounts of sputum. Frequent respiratory infections accentuate the cough, quantity of sputum, and breathlessness. The patient may complain of becoming short of breath at night, and he may say that relief comes from bringing up large volumes of secretions. Such a story usually, though not always, permits chronic airway obstruction to be distinguished from the orthopnea or the paroxysmal nocturnal dyspnea that occurs with heart failure. Finally, some patients give a history of wheezing.

The physical examination is especially important; signs of airway obstruction include prolongation of expiration, utilization of the muscles of the neck to lift the anterior part of the upper thorax, retraction of the soft tissues of the thorax during inspiration, and retraction of the lower rib margins as inspiration begins. Often better felt than seen, retraction usually denotes either a low position of the diaphragm or an abnormally low intrapleural pressure, both of which are characteristic of obstructive disease. Other signs include expiratory wheezes and, if the disease is advanced, evidence of right-sided heart failure. Contrary to the popular view, an increased anteroposterior diameter of the chest is one of the less-valuable signs of obstructive lung disease.

Roentgenograms of the chest may be misleading. For instance the leaves of the diaphragm may be low and flat, or they may be at normal levels and rounded. In the latter case their slow rise during a forced expiration will be visible only by fluoroscopy. If the chest is long and narrow, estimating the size of the heart is hazardous, so that even with right ventricular enlargement the transverse cardiac diameter may be normal.

One of the useful bedside tests is to have the patient make a forceful expiration. Prolongation may be plainly evident. If it is not, demonstration that he is unable to blow out a match with his mouth held widely open confirms his failure to achieve a high rate of expiratory flow. When this happens, the MBC will usually be markedly reduced.

Finally, a high hematocrit may reflect chronic arterial hypoxemia and a high venous bicarbonate an elevated tension of carbon dioxide in the blood. Whether or not these changes are present, an analysis of arterial blood is very important.

INTERSTITIAL AND ALVEOLAR DISEASE OF THE LUNG. (See also Chap. 284.) This category embraces a large number of diseases, ranging from acute pneumonia to chronic disorders such as tuberculosis, sarcoid, carcinoma, pneumoconiosis, and idiopathic fibrosis of the lung. The history varies with the etiology, and the signs elicited by physical examination also will depend on the nature and stage of the disease. In almost all these diseases roentgenograms will be abnormal. In the chronic disorders the patient characteristically overventilates at rest and even more while active.

Pulmonary function tests show modest reductions in MBC and vital capacity, and increased stiffness of the lung is often present. Although the oxygen saturation may be low at rest and may fall further with exercise, the carbon dioxide tension is seldom elevated. Indeed, until the late stages of these diseases, the carbon dioxide tension is usually low.

DISEASES OF THE CHEST WALL OR RESPIRATORY MUSCLES. The three most common disorders of the bony thorax causing breathlessness are fractured ribs, kyphoscoliosis, and arthritis of the spine. All interfere with the motion of the thorax and consequently impair ventilation. In each instance the history, physical examination, and standard roentgenograms will permit the diagnosis to be made.

By way of contrast, diagnosing weakness of the respiratory muscles is more difficult. Primary myopathies are uncommon, but almost any debilitating illness, including those associated with prolonged bed rest, can cause the skeletal muscles to atrophy from disuse. When this happens, breathlessness will disappear as the patient regains his general strength.

HEART FAILURE. (See also Chap. 264.) Deciding whether breathlessness originates from disease of the lungs or of the heart often presents a problem. Though a chronic cough usually signifies pulmonary disease, cough as well as wheezing may occur in heart failure. Though breathlessness at night may have a pulmonary origin, acute attacks which awaken the patient and cause him to sit upright are most often caused by heart disease. The important clues, which come from associated symptoms and signs of cardiac dysfunction, include cardiomegaly, hypertension, valvular lesions, or angina. Rales may signify either pulmonary infection or cardiac decompensation, and their diagnostic value is limited. Also, breathlessness of cardiac or pulmonary origin may occur in the absence of rales. In a similar way, the value of roentgenograms is often limited because either pulmonary congestion or pulmonary infection can produce shadows in the lungs.

Tests of pulmonary function usually show some reduction in both the vital capacity and the maximum breathing capacity, and in some instances changes in the mechanical properties of the lungs. Except in the presence of intracardiac shunts, the arterial saturation in nonpulmonary heart disease is almost always above 90 percent, and the carbon dioxide tension is low.

One of the conditions most difficult to distinguish in the differential diagnoses is pulmonary emboli. Right-sided heart failure in the absence of signs of intrinsic lung disease should suggest the possibility of multiple small emboli, but often diagnosis is uncertain without angiography or lung scanning. While the arterial tension of oxygen may be subnormal, the carbon dioxide tension is seldom elevated, an important point of distinction between cor pulmonale secondary to emboli and that caused by obstructive pulmonary disease.

NEUROSIS. Several clues may suggest that breathlessness is associated with psychiatric illness. The most important is the patient's tendency to hyperventilate and occasionally to inspire deeply and expire audibly without relation to exercise. He feels as if he is being smothered, when in fact he is hyperventilating. The breathing pattern is frequently strange, with irregularities in both frequency and tidal volume. At other times the pattern is one of maintained hyperventilation, to the point where the patient complains of tingling in the extremities, or even a sensation of faintness. Watching the patient breathe during sleep is a valuable diagnostic procedure. If the abnormal breathing pattern disappears, psychogenic causes should be suspected. Similarly, observing the patient when he does not know he is being watched is helpful, because the respiratory pattern may be completely different when he is alone.

CONCLUSIONS

The detailed mechanisms of respiratory distress are largely unknown, even though a large number of conditions associated with breathlessness are well characterized. The history, physical examination, roentgenograms, standard laboratory tests, and, where indicated, special tests of respiratory and cardiac function usually will lead to the diagnosis. However, there will remain a group of patients with no measurable abnormalities who appear to have genuine respiratory distress. In these persons careful follow-up during the course of illness will usually reveal concrete signs.

REFERENCES

Campbell, E. J. M.: The Relationship of the Sensation of Breathlessness to the Act of Breathing, pp. 55–63 in "Breathlessness," Oxford, Blackwell Scientific Publications, Ltd., 1966.

Comroe, J.: Some Theories of the Mechanism of Dyspnoea, pp. 1–7 in "Breathlessness," Oxford, Blackwell Scientific Publications, Ltd., 1966.

Cournand, A., D. W. Richards, R. A. Bader, M. E. Bader, and A. P. Fishman: The Oxygen Cost of Breathing, Trans. Assoc. Am. Physicians, 67:162, 1954.

Euler, C. von: The Control of Respiratory Movement, pp. 19–32 in "Breathlessness," Oxford, Blackwell Scientific Publications, Ltd., 1966.

Gaensler, E. A.: "Dyspnea: Diagnostic and Therapeutic Implications," in "Disease a Month," Chicago, The Year Book Medical Publishers, Inc., May, 1961.

——, and G. W. Wright: Evaluation of Respiratory Impairment, Arch. Environ. Health, 12:146, 1966.

Guz, A., M. I. M. Noble, J. G. Widdicombe, D. Trenchard, W. W. Mushin, and A. R. Makey: The Role of Vagal and Glossopharyngeal Afferent Nerves in Respiratory Sensation, Control of Breathing and Arterial Pressure Regulation in Conscious Man, Clin. Sci., 30:161, 1966.

Otis, A. B., W. O. Fenn, and H. Rahn: Mechanics of Breathing, J. Appl. Physiol., 2:592, 1950.

Richards, D. W., Jr.: The Nature of Cardiac and Pulmonary Dyspnea, Circulation, 7:15, 1953.

Sears, T. A.: The Respiratory Motoneurone: Integration at Spinal Segmental Level, pp. 33–45 in "Breathlessness," Oxford, Blackwell Scientific Publications, Ltd., 1966.

Widdicombe, J. G.: Respiratory Reflexes, pp. 585–630 in "Handbook of Physiology," sec. 3, vol. 1, Respiration," American Physiology Society, 1964. Washington, D.C.

Wright, G. W., and B. V. Branscomb: The Origin of the Sensations of Dyspnea, Trans. Clin. & Climatol. Assoc., 66:116, 1954.

33 CYANOSIS, HYPOXIA, AND POLYCYTHEMIA

*T. R. Harrison, M. M. Wintrobe,
R. L. Kahler, and E. Braunwald*

CYANOSIS

The term *cyanosis* is used to describe the clinical sign of a bluish color of the skin and mucous membranes resulting from an increased amount of reduced hemoglobin, or of hemoglobin derivatives, in the small blood vessels of those areas. Hence it is to be distinguished from *argyria*, in which the deposition of silver salts causes a bluish discoloration of the skin. In the latter condition there is a metallic tint and the blue color persists despite pressure, whereas the truly cyanotic skin becomes pale when sufficient pressure is exerted to express the blood from the vessels.

Cyanosis is usually most marked in the lips, nail beds, ears, and malar eminences. In the last region the line of distinction between true cyanosis and the ruddy color which is commonly seen in robust elderly subjects cannot always be clearly drawn. Furthermore, the "red cyanosis" of polycythemia vera (Chap. 343) must be distinguished from the true cyanosis discussed here. A cherry-colored flush, rather than cyanosis, is caused by carboxyhemoglobin (Chap. 116).

Certain modifying factors influence the degree of cyanosis. These include the thickness of the epidermis, the quality of cutaneous pigment, and the color of the blood plasma, as well as the state of the cutaneous capillaries. The accurate clinical detection of the presence and degree of cyanosis is difficult, as proved by oximetric studies. Some observers can reliably detect central cyanosis when the arterial saturation has fallen to 85 percent; others may not detect it until the saturation has reached 75 percent.

The *fundamental mechanism of cyanosis* consists of an increase in the amount of reduced hemoglobin in the vessels of the skin. This may be brought about either by an increase in the amount of venous blood in the skin as the result of dilatation of the venules and venous ends of the capillaries, or by a decrease in the oxygen saturation in the capillary blood.

As a general rule, cyanosis becomes apparent when the mean capillary concentration of reduced hemoglobin exceeds 5 Gm per 100 ml. It is the absolute rather than the relative amount of reduced hemoglobin which is important in producing cyanosis. Thus, in a patient with severe anemia the relative amount of reduced hemoglobin in the venous blood may be very large when considered in relation to the total hemoglobin. However, since the latter is markedly lowered, the absolute amount of reduced hemoglobin may still be small, and therefore patients with severe anemia and marked arterial desaturation do not display cyanosis. Conversely, the higher the total hemoglobin content, the greater the tendency toward cyanosis; thus, patients with marked polycythemia tend to be cyanotic at higher levels of arterial oxygen saturation than patients with normal hematocrit values. Likewise, local passive congestion, which causes an increase in the total amount of hemoglobin in the vessels in a given area, may cause cyanosis even though the average percentage saturation is not altered.

Cyanosis also is observed when nonfunctional hemoglobin is present in the blood, as little as 1.5 Gm per ml methemoglobin or 0.5 Gm sulfhemoglobin being sufficient to produce cyanosis (Chap. 344).

True cyanosis may be subdivided into two general categories: central and peripheral. In the central type, there is arterial blood unsaturation or an abnormal hemoglobin derivative, and the mucous membranes and skin are both affected. Peripheral cyanosis is generally due to a slowing of blood flow to an area because of vasoconstriction resulting from cold exposure, shock, congestive failure, and peripheral vascular disease; often, in these conditions, the mucous membrane of the oral cavity or those beneath the tongue may be spared. Clinical differentiation between central and peripheral cyanosis may not always be simple, and in conditions such as cardiogenic shock with pulmonary edema there may be a mixture of both types.

Differential Diagnosis

CENTRAL CYANOSIS. Decreased arterial oxygen saturation results from a low oxygen tension in the arterial blood. This may be brought about when there is a corresponding decline in the tension of oxygen in the inspired air without sufficient compensatory alveolar hyperventilation to maintain alveolar oxygen tension. Cyanosis does not occur in a significant degree in an ascent to an altitude of 8,000 ft but is marked in a further ascent to 16,000 ft. The reason for this becomes clear on studying the S shape of the oxygen dissociation

Table 33-1. CAUSES OF CYANOSIS

I. Central cyanosis
  A. Decreased arterial oxygen saturation
    1. Decreased atmospheric pressure—high altitude
    2. Impaired pulmonary function
      a. Alveolar hypoventilation
      b. Uneven relationships between pulmonary ventilation and perfusion
      c. Impaired oxygen diffusion
    3. Anatomic shunts
      a. Certain types of congenital heart disease
      b. Pulmonary arteriovenous fistulas
      c. Multiple small intrapulmonary shunts
  B. Hemoglobin abnormalities
    1. Methemoglobinemia—hereditary, acquired
    2. Sulfhemoglobinemia—acquired
    3. Carboxyhemoglobinemia (not true cyanosis)
  C. Polycythemia (not true cyanosis)
II. Peripheral cyanosis
  A. Reduced cardiac output
  B. Cold exposure
  C. Redistribution of blood flow from extremities
  D. Arterial obstruction
  E. Venous obstruction

curve (Fig. 33-1). At 8,000 ft the tension of oxygen in the inspired air is about 120 mm Hg, the alveolar tension is approximately 80 mm Hg, and the hemoglobin is nearly completely saturated. However, at 16,000 ft the oxygen tensions in atmospheric air and alveolar air are about 85 and 50 mm Hg, respectively, and the oxygen dissociation curve shows that the arterial blood is only about 75 percent saturated. This leaves 25 percent of the hemoglobin in the reduced form, an amount likely to be associated with cyanosis in the absence of anemia.

Impaired pulmonary function, through alveolar hypoventilation, perfusion of unventilated or poorly ventilated areas of lung, or an increase in the barriers to diffusion through which the gas must pass to reach hemoglobin, is common cause of central cyanosis. This may occur acutely, as in extensive pneumonia or in pulmonary edema, or with chronic pulmonary diseases (e.g., emphysema). In the last situation clubbing of the fingers and polycythemia are generally present. However, in many types of chronic pulmonary disease with fibrosis and obliteration of the capillary vascular bed, cyanosis does not occur because there is no significant volume of circulation through unaerated portions.

A less-common, but important, cause of decreased arterial oxygen saturation is shunting of systemic venous blood into the arterial circuit. Certain types of congenital heart disease are associated with cyanosis (Chap. 268). Since blood normally flows from a high- to a low-pressure region, in order for a cardiac defect to result in a right-to-left shunt it must ordinarily be combined with an obstructive lesion distal to the defect or with elevated pulmonary vascular resistance. The commonest congenital cardiac lesion associated with cyanosis is the combination of ventricular septal defect and pulmonary outflow tract obstruction (tetralogy of Fallot). The more severe the obstruction, the greater the degree of right-to-left shunting and resultant cyanosis. The mechanisms for the elevated pulmonary vascular resistance which may produce cyanosis in the presence of intra- and extracardiac communications without pulmonic stenosis are discussed elsewhere (Chap. 268). In patients with patent ductus arteriosus, pulmonary hypertension, and right-to-left shunt, differential cyanosis results; i.e., cyanosis occurs in the lower extremities but not in the upper extremities.

Pulmonary arteriovenous fistulas may be congenital or acquired, solitary or multiple, microscopic or massive. The degree of cyanosis produced by these fistulas depends upon their size and number. They occur with some frequency in hereditary hemorrhagic telangiectasia (Chap. 347). Arterial oxygen unsaturation also occurs in some patients with cirrhosis, although it is uncommon in this condition. A number of factors may explain this observation; pulmonary arteriovenous fistulas or portal vein–pulmonary vein anastomoses have been demonstrated in some patients.

In patients with central cyanosis due to arterial oxygen unsaturation, the severity of cyanosis increases with exercise. With increased extraction of oxygen from the blood by the exercising muscles, the venous blood returning to the right side of the heart is more un-saturated than at rest, and shunting of this blood or its passage into lungs incapable of normal oxygenation intensifies the cyanosis. Also, since the systemic vascular resistance normally decreases with exercise, passage of right ventricular blood into the systemic circuit is made easier by exercise in patients with congenital heart disease and communications between the two sides of the heart.

Arterial blood unsaturation is ascertained by subjecting an arterial blood sample to Van Slyke analysis for determining oxygen content and capacity or by directly determining the hemoglobin saturation by oximetric or spectrophotometric techniques. A much more sensitive measurement, especially when the saturation is near normal, is the measurement of arterial blood oxygen tension (P_{O_2}) by means of an oxygen electrode.

Cyanosis is produced by small amounts of circulating methemoglobin and by even smaller amounts of sulfhemoglobin (Chap. 344). Although they are uncommon causes of cyanosis, these abnormal hemoglobin pigments should be sought by spectroscopic analysis when cyanosis is not readily explained by malfunction of the circulatory or respiratory systems. Generally, clubbing does not occur with them, but there may be minimal polycythemia.

PERIPHERAL CYANOSIS. Probably the most common cause of peripheral cyanosis is that due to generalized vasoconstriction resulting from exposure to cold air or water. This is clearly a normal response to the stimulus and is transient.

When the cardiac output is low, as in severe congestive heart failure or shock, cutaneous vasoconstriction occurs as a compensatory mechanism, so that blood is diverted to more vital areas (kidneys, central nervous system, heart), and intense cyanosis associated with cool extremities may result. Even though the arterial blood may be normally saturated, the reduced volume flow through the skin and the reduced oxygen tension at the venous end of the capillary result in cyanosis.

Acute arterial obstruction to an extremity generally results in pallor and coldness, but there may be associated slight cyanosis. If there is venous obstruction, the extremity is usually congested and markedly cyanotic, and there is true stagnation of blood flow. Stasis of a lesser degree resulting from increased blood viscosity probably contributes to the cyanosis in some patients with polycythemia vera.

Certain features are important in arriving at the proper cause of cyanosis.

1. The history, particularly the duration (cyanosis present since birth is usually due to congenital heart disease); possible exposure to drugs or chemicals which may produce abnormal types of hemoglobin.

2. Clinical differentiation of central as opposed to peripheral cyanosis. Objective evidence by physical or radiographic examination of disorders of the respiratory or cardiovascular systems.

3. The presence or absence of clubbing of the fingers. (Clubbing without cyanosis is frequent in patients with

Fig. 33-1. Relationship between oxygen tension and oxygen saturation of the hemoglobin of the blood. The heavy line is for blood at pH 7.44. The curves to the right and left are for bloods of pH 7.24 and 7.64, respectively, and indicate quantitatively the magnitude of the Bohr effect for hydrogen ion concentration changes of these magnitudes.

During vigorous muscular effort the increase in acidity of the blood causes the dissociation curve to shift to the right, raises the tissue oxygen tension for any given degree of saturation of the hemoglobin, and thus makes oxygen more available to the muscles. On the other hand, any condition, such as high altitude, which causes respiratory alkalosis moves the dissociation curve to the left. This facilitates oxygen uptake in the lungs by increasing the oxygen saturation at a given level of alveolar oxygen tension.

Beneath the abscissas are plotted the calculated arteriovenous oxygen differences, upon the presumption of the right-heart venous oxygen content normally being 5 vol percent less than the arterial content, and with constant cardiac output in the following states: N = normal person, arterial oxygen content 20 vol percent; AA = same person suffering from arterial hypoxia sufficient to lower the arterial oxygen content to 14.6 vol percent (= 73 percent saturation), but with oxygen consumption unaltered; MA = same person with 100 percent increase in oxygen consumption; AN = anemic patient, arterial oxygen content 10 vol percent, with arterial saturation and oxygen consumption same as in normal person. The heavy dots indicate the mean oxygen tension in each instance.

subacute bacterial endocarditis and in association with nonspecific ulcerative colitis, and it may occasionally occur in healthy persons or as an occupational effect.) Slight cyanosis of the lips and cheeks, without clubbing of the fingers, is common in well-compensated patients with mitral stenosis and is probably due to minimal arterial hypoxia resulting from fibrotic changes in the lungs secondary to long-standing congestion combined with reduction of cardiac output. The combination of cyanosis and clubbing is frequent in many patients with certain types of congenital cardiac disease and is seen occasionally in persons with advanced pulmonary disease or pulmonary arteriovenous shunts. On the other hand, cyanosis due to acquired cardiac disease, to acute hypoxia, or to acute disorders of the lungs is not associated with clubbed fingers.

4. Determination of arterial blood oxygen tension or oxygen saturation. Spectroscopic and other examinations of the blood for abnormal types of hemoglobin.

It is clear from the previous discussion that cyanosis is a clinical sign intimately related to hypoxia, i.e., a reduction in the oxygen concentration or tension in the body. The term *hypoxia* is preferable to the less-precise expression *anoxia*, which refers to the total absence of oxygen, a state incompatible with life.

HYPOXIA

The fundamental purpose of the cardiorespiratory system is to make possible delivery of oxygen (and sub-

Table 33-2. CAUSES OF HYPOXIA

I. Decreased oxygen delivery to the tissues
   A. Generalized hypoxia
      1. Arterial hypoxia
         a. Low atmospheric oxygen tension
         b. Diminished oxygenation in the lungs
         c. Systemic venous-to-arterial shunts
      2. Anemic hypoxia
         a. Diminished hemoglobin concentration
         b. Altered hemoglobin
      3. Circulatory hypoxia (ischemia, stagnation)
   B. Specific organ hypoxia
      1. Reflex
      2. Organic
II. Increased oxygen requirements
   A. Thyrotoxicosis
   B. Exercise
III. Improper oxygen utilization

strates) to the cells and to remove carbon dioxide (and other metabolic products) from them. Proper maintenance of this function depends on an intact cardiovascular and respiratory system and a supply of air containing adequate oxygen.

When hypoxia occurs as the result of a decline in oxygen tension in the inspired air, respiration is stimulated, alveolar ventilation increases, and the carbon dioxide tension in the alveoli and in the arterial blood falls. This respiratory alkalosis causes a leftward shift in the oxygen dissociation curve (Fig. 33-1) and enables a given alveolar oxygen tension to cause a greater degree of oxygen uptake by the hemoglobin (Bohr's effect.) Thus, at an alveolar oxygen pressure of 55 mm Hg, a rise in pH from 7.44 to 7.64 will cause the arterial saturation to increase from 80 to nearly 90 percent.

However, when hypoxia results from interference with the passage of air into the lungs or from the perfusion of poorly ventilated alveoli, carbon dioxide tension usually remains normal or even rises; and the oxygen dissociation curve tends to remain unchanged or move to the right. Under these conditions the percentage saturation of the hemoglobin in the arterial blood at a given level of alveolar oxygen tension does not rise and may even fall. Thus arterial hypoxia and cyanosis are likely to be more marked in proportion to the degree of depression of alveolar oxygen tension when such depression results from pulmonary disease than when the depression occurs as the result of a decline in the partial pressure of oxygen in the inspired air.

The respiratory mechanisms may be considerably impaired without the development of a significant degree of arterial hypoxia. This is because the properties of hemoglobin are such that its dissociation curve is practically flat above 100 mm Hg of oxygen tension, and almost flat to about 80 mm Hg. When the tension of oxygen in the alveoli falls below the point at which the slope of the dissociation curve tends to become more nearly vertical, a rapid decline in the amount of oxygen in the arterial blood occurs.

If the flow of blood through the tissues and the oxygen consumption of the tissues remain constant, then the amount of oxygen extracted in the tissues as the blood passes through the capillaries will also remain constant. Therefore, if the oxygen content of arterial blood is reduced, the venous blood emerging from the capillary will have less oxygen by an amount corresponding to the initial abnormal reduction in the arterial blood.

The clinical features of arterial hypoxia depend on how rapidly it develops. Barcroft pointed out that when hypoxia develops rapidly, the picture resembles drunkenness; when it develops slowly, it simulates fatigue. In either case cyanosis is likely to be striking. When the arterial hypoxia is of long duration, clubbing of the fingers usually appears.

Anemic Hypoxia. This includes various states, one of which is associated with anemia and others in which there is a partial conversion to non-oxygen-carrying derivative pigments (Chap. 344). Any decrease in hemoglobin concentration is attended by a corresponding decline in the oxygen-carrying power. Under such conditions the P_{O_2} in the arterial blood remains normal, but the absolute amount of oxygen transported per unit volume of blood is diminished. As the anemic blood passes through the capillaries, and the usual amount of oxygen is removed from it, the P_{O_2} in the venous blood declines to a greater degree than would normally be the case.

Carbon monoxide intoxication (Chap. 116) is accompanied by the equivalent of anemic hypoxia in that the hemoglobin which is combined with the carbon monoxide (carboxyhemoglobin) is unavailable for oxygen transport. But, in addition to this, the presence of carboxyhemoglobin increases the affinity of normal hemoglobin for oxygen at low levels of P_{O_2} (i.e., shifts the lower portion of the dissociation curve of hemoglobin to the left), so that the oxygen can be unloaded only at lower tensions. By such formation of carboxyhemoglobin a given degree of reduction in oxygen-carrying power produces a far greater degree of tissue hypoxia than the equivalent reduction in hemoglobin due to simple anemia.

The P_{O_2} in the venous blood is decreased in both anemic hypoxia and arterial hypoxia. However, the P_{O_2} in the arterial blood is not reduced in anemic hypoxia, and the decrease in mean capillary and in tissue P_{O_2} is less than in arterial hypoxia with similar levels of venous P_{O_2}. Patients with anemia of moderate severity do not exhibit any manifestations of oxygen deficiency while at rest but are likely to display such symptoms on exertion. With severe anemia, symptoms of hypoxia may be present even at rest.

Circulatory Hypoxia. Even though the blood is normal as regards quantity and kind of pigment and is normally saturated with oxygen, and even though the oxygen consumption of the tissues remains normal, reduced P_{O_2} at the venous end of the capillary necessarily occurs if the volume of blood through the tissues (oxygen delivery) is reduced. The clinical pictures which occur when circulatory hypoxia is generalized, as a result of circulatory failure, are discussed in detail in Chap. 264.

Specific Organ Hypoxia. Decreased circulation to a specific organ may be due to organic arterial or venous obstruction or may occur as a reflex phenomenon. The latter may occur when vasoconstriction to, for instance, the limbs, results from an attempt to maintain adequate perfusion to more vital organs, as in severe congestive heart failure. When organic disease of the arteries develops, ischemic hypoxia results, with accompanying pallor. Venous obstruction results in congestion, and the term stagnant hypoxia is applicable.

Increased Oxygen Requirements. Even if oxygen diffusion into arterial blood is unhampered and the hemoglobin is qualitatively and quantitatively normal, the P_{O_2} in venous blood (hence, mean capillary tension) may be reduced if the oxygen consumption of the tissues is elevated without a corresponding increase in volume flow per unit of time. Such a situation may be encountered in febrile states and in thyrotoxicosis. Under such conditions the circulation may be considered deficient relative to the metabolic requirements. Thus, this type of metabolic hypoxia is comparable to circulatory hypoxia, in that in both conditions the volume flow of blood is decreased relative to the needs of the tissues, the difference being that in one case the primary defect is the volume flow of blood and in the other the primary defect is an increased oxygen need by the tissues.

Ordinarily, the clinical picture of patients with hypoxia due to an elevated basal metabolic rate is quite different from that of other types of hypoxia; the skin is warm and flushed, owing to increased cutaneous blood flow which dissipates the excessive heat produced, and cyanosis is absent in these patients.

Exercise is a classic example of increased tissue oxygen requirements. The increased demands are normally met by several mechanisms: (1) by increasing the cardiac output and thus increasing oxygen delivery to the tissues; (2) by preferentially directing the blood to the exercising muscles and away from resting muscles (by changing vascular resistance in various beds, in some areas by direct effects, in others by reflex effects); (3) by increasing oxygen extraction from the delivered blood and widening the arteriovenous oxygen differences. If the capacity of these mechanisms is exceeded, then hypoxia, especially of the exercising muscles, will result.

Improper Oxygen Utilization. The administration of cyanide (Chap. 116) (and several other similarly acting poisons) leads to a paradoxic state in which the tissues are unable to utilize oxygen and the venous blood, in consequence, tends to have a high oxygen tension. This is a type of metabolic disturbance in which the defect is not in the supply of oxygen to the tissues, but in the capacity of the tissues to utilize oxygen. The number of mechanisms transferring electrons to oxygen is limited. It is only by a defect in one or more of these mechanisms, or by failure of preceding oxidations to provide electrons for them, that diminution in oxygen utilization can occur. Thus, cyanide paralyzes the electron-transfer function of cytochrome oxidase so that it cannot pass electrons to oxygen, whereas reduction of tissue temperature slows the rates of metabolic reactions that produce such electrons. Diphtheria toxin is believed to inhibit the synthesis of one of the cytochromes and thus interfere with oxygen consumption and energy production by the cells involved.

Effects of Hypoxia

The symptoms of local oxygen deficiency depend on the tissues affected and are, therefore, protean in nature; they will not be discussed here. When hypoxia is general, all parts of the body may suffer some impairment of function, but those parts which are most sensitive to the effects of hypoxia give rise to symptoms which dominate the clinical picture. The *changes in the central nervous system* are especially important, and here the higher centers are most sensitive. Acute hypoxia, therefore, produces impaired judgment, motor incoordination, and a clinical picture closely resembling that of acute alcoholism. When hypoxia is long-standing, the symptoms consist of fatigue, drowsiness, apathy, inattentiveness, and delayed reaction time, simulating manifestations of severe fatigue. As hypoxia becomes more severe, the centers of the brainstem are affected and death usually results from respiratory failure. The gasping reflex, being a primitive mechanism, persists to the last. Measurements of cerebral blood flow indicate that with reduction of arterial oxygen tension, cerebrovascular resistance decreases and cerebral blood flow increases. This mechanism tends to minimize the cerebral hypoxia. On the other hand, reduction of arterial P_{O_2}, when accompanied by diminution of P_{CO_2}, increases cerebrovascular resistance, and volume flow per unit of time is decreased. It would appear, therefore, that when hypoxia is associated with increased ventilation and hypocapnia, it is enhanced, at least in the higher levels of the central nervous system, by a reduction in volume flow of blood per unit of time. Compared with the brain, the phylogenetically older spinal cord and peripheral nerves are relatively insensitive to hypoxia, and symptoms due to disturbance of these structures usually do not appear. There is evidence that hypoxia causes constriction of pulmonary arteries. This has the advantage of shunting blood away from poorly ventilated areas toward better-ventilated portions of the lung. However, it has the disadvantage of causing increased pulmonary vascular resistance and an increased burden on the right ventricle.

Some of the *metabolic effects of severe acute hypoxia* are well known in regard to the liver and muscles. In these structures the breakdown of the primary foodstuff, carbohydrate, normally proceeds anaerobically (i.e., without oxidation) to the stage of formation of pyruvic acid. The further oxidation of pyruvate requires the availability of oxygen, and when this is deficient, the breakdown is impaired and increasing proportions of pyruvate become reduced to lactic acid, which cannot be further broken down anaerobically (Chap. 75). Hence, there is an increase in the blood lactate, with decrease in bicarbonate and a corresponding acidosis. Since the total energy obtained from foodstuff breakdown is greatly reduced under these circumstances, the amount of energy available for continuing resynthesis of energy-rich phosphate compounds becomes inadequate. As the breakdown of the latter substances is the immediate source of energy driving the myriad of anabolic reactions which take place in tissues, such deficiency of energy-rich phosphate compounds produces a complex disturbance of cellular function. Whether or not the more subtle effects of mild hypoxia upon, for example, the central nervous system are mediated through lesser degrees of such disordered metabolism remains to be demonstrated.

Most of the useful respiratory response to hypoxia originates in special chemosensitive cells in the carotid and aortic bodies, although the respiratory center is also stimulated directly by oxygen lack. The peripheral chemoreceptors are extremely rugged and continue to function after other tissues have been damaged by hypoxemia. The chemoreceptors are stimulated by a reduction in their oxygen supply below their needs either by lowered arterial P_{O_2} or by lowered blood flow to them.

The acute effects of hypoxia on the *reaction of the blood* are complicated, because two different antagonistic influences are at work. If respiration is stimulated by hypoxia, the resulting increase in ventilation, with loss of carbon dioxide, tends to make the blood more alkaline. On the other hand, the diffusion of additional quantities of lactic acid from the tissues into the blood tends to make the blood more acid. In either case the total amount of bicarbonate, and hence the carbon dioxide–combining power, tends to be diminished. With mild hypoxia there is likely to be respiratory alkalosis; severe hypoxia is attended by metabolic acidosis (see Chap. 297).

The heart, although relatively sensitive to hypoxia as compared with most of the structures of the body, is less sensitive than the nervous system. Consequently, in the absence of severe coronary artery disease, serious manifestations of cardiac impairment do not commonly occur when there is generalized hypoxia, and the manifestations arising in the nervous system dominate the picture. It is known that diminished oxygen tension in any tissue results in local vasodilatation. In generalized hypoxia diffuse vasodilatation results in an elevation of total cardiac output. In patients with preexisting heart disease, particularly coronary artery disease, the combination of hypoxia and the peripheral tissues' requirements for an increase of cardiac output may precipitate congestive heart failure. In prolonged or severe hypoxia hepatic and renal function may also be impaired.

One of the important mechanisms of compensation for prolonged hypoxia is an increase in the amount of hemoglobin in the blood. This is due not to direct stimulation of the bone marrow but to the effect of an erythropoiesis-stimulating factor (erythropoietin). The kidney is the chief site of production or activation of erythropoietin, which then acts upon the stem cells. Assayable levels of erythropietin are increased by hypoxia, and its production has been found to be regulated by the balance between tissue oxygen supply and demand.

POLYCYTHEMIA

The term *polycythemia* signifies an increase above the normal in the number of red corpuscles in the circulating blood. This increase is usually, though not always, accompanied by a corresponding increase in the quantity of hemoglobin and in the volume of packed red corpuscles. The increase may or may not be associated with an increase in the total quantity of red blood cells in the body. It is important to distinguish between *absolute* polycythemia (an increase in the total red corpuscle mass) and *relative* polycythemia, which occurs when, through loss of blood plasma, the concentration of the red corpuscles becomes greater than normal in the circulating blood. This may be the consequence of abnormally lowered fluid intake or of marked loss of body fluids, such as occurs in persistent vomiting, severe diarrhea, copious sweating, or acidosis (Chap. 297). Loss of electrolytes from the extracellular compartment, when not accompanied by corresponding loss of water, leads to a decline of osmolar concentration in the extracellular fluid. The resulting shift of water into the tissue cells may produce relative polycythemia, sometimes of high grade. In certain types of peripheral circulatory failure there is a loss of plasma into the interstitial fluid, again resulting in relative polycythemia. Such a shift takes place largely in the periphery, with the result that the polycythemia may be more marked in capillary blood than in that from central blood vessels.

Because the term *polycythemia* is used loosely to refer to all varieties of increase in the number of red corpuscles, the terms *erythrocytosis* and *erythremia* are preferred in referring to two forms of absolute polycythemia. *Erythrocytosis* denotes absolute polycythemia which occurs in response to some known stimulus; *erythremia* (polycythemia rubra vera) refers to the disease of unknown etiology, which is discussed elsewhere (Chap. 343).

Erythrocytosis develops as a consequence of a variety of factors and represents a physiologic response to conditions of hypoxia. As noted above, sojourn at high altitudes leads to defective saturation of arterial blood with

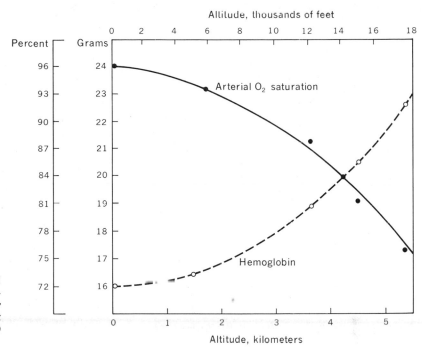

Fig. 33-2. Relationship between mean arterial oxygen saturation (percent) and the mean hemoglobin content (Gm per 100 ml) in healthy male residents at various altitudes. (*Hurtado et al.; courtesy, Archives of Internal Medicine.*)

oxygen and stimulates the production of more red corpuscles. There is evidence that oxygen saturation rather than oxygen tension is the more important determinant of the erythropoietic response to chronic hypoxia (Fig. 33-2). Immediately on ascent to a high altitude, symptoms such as fatigue, dizziness, headache, nausea, vomiting, ringing in the ears, and prostration may appear. In most persons adaptation soon occurs, with the development of polycythemia and other compensatory adjustments. However, a disorder may set in insidiously a few years later, or even as long as 20 years after continued residence at high altitudes, leading to the development of a condition known as *chronic mountain sickness* or *seroche* (*Monge's disease*). Two forms have been described, an emphysematous type in which dyspnea is prominent and bronchitis is common; and an erythremic type in which prominent manifestations are a florid color which turns to cyanosis on mild exertion, mental torpor, fatigue, and headache. Those affected are usually in the fourth to sixth decades. Return to sea level promptly relieves the symptoms. Brisket disease of cattle, a disorder of young calves grazing at high altitudes in Utah and Colorado, which is characterized by pulmonary hypertension and subsquent right-sided heart failure, is not a true counterpart of Monge's disease, since it is not associated with sustained oxygen unsaturation or polycythemia.

Any chronic pulmonary disease which alters ventilation-perfusion relationships or seriously impairs gas diffusion may produce chronic hypoxemia and lead to erythrocytosis. *Emphysema* is the commonest of the chronic pulmonary conditions which is associated with erythrocytosis. Pulmonary arteriovenous fistulas or cavernous hemangioma of the lung may lead to impaired saturation of arterial blood with oxygen, with the conse-

quent development of erythrocytosis and of a clinical picture resembling closely that of certain types of congenital heart disease. The increased blood viscosity secondary to the polycythemia (Fig. 33-3) results in an elevation of pulmonary arterial pressure and, combined with the elevation of pulmonary vascular resistance resulting from hypoxia, the increased viscosity further elevates right ventricular pressure and contributes to the development or intensification of cor pulmonale. Although phlebotomy may be attempted in patients with chronic pulmonary disease with hematocrit values of 50 to 60 percent or more, its value is limited since the diminished blood viscosity is offset by a decrease in oxygen transport.

The mechanical conditions present in very obese individuals may cause primary alveolar hypoventilation and result in arterial unsaturation, erythrocytosis, hypercapnea, and somnolence (Chap. 284). Because certain of these patients resemble the fat, sleepy, red-faced boy of Dickens' *The Pickwick Papers*, the condition has been termed the *Pickwickian syndrome*. This syndrome is observed less commonly in nonobese individuals, and the specific cause is unclear. Decreased sensitivity of the respiratory center to CO_2 may play a role. The increased oxygen cost of breathing found in obese individuals is a contributing factor.

The partial shunting of blood from the pulmonary circuit, such as occurs in congenital heart disease, causes the most striking erythrocytosis resulting from abnormalities in the heart or lungs. Erythrocyte counts as high as 13 million, per cu mm, which are possible only when the red corpuscles are smaller than normal, have been observed in such cases, with volumes of packed red blood cells even as high as 86 ml per 100 ml of blood. As the polycythemia develops, there is a progressive rise in blood viscosity (Fig. 33-3), with the sharpest increase beginning when

Fig. 33-3. Correlation of hematocrit value with specific viscosity of the blood. (*Rudolph et al.; courtesy, Pediatrics.*)

the volume of packed red blood cells reaches 65 to 70 percent. Cautious phlebotomy is sometimes performed in severely symptomatic patients with extremely high hematocrit levels, but it should not be continued if there is no symptomatic improvement. The commonest defect producing such polycythemia is pulmonary stenosis associated with a right-to-left shunt that allows venous blood to enter the systemic arterial tree without transversing the lungs. Other conditions include transposition of the great arteries, tricuspid atresia, persistent truncus arteriosus, and other less-common anomalies, discussed in Chap. 268. Although erythrocytosis does not usually occur in patients with acquired heart disease, it may occasionally be seen in persons with mitral stenosis.

The excessive use of coal-tar derivatives and other forms of chronic poisoning (Chap. 116), by producing abnormal hemoglobin pigments such as methemoglobin and sulfhemoglobin (Chap. 344), also may cause erythrocytosis. Another chemical agent, cobalt, has produced erythrocytosis in experimental animals, but the mechanism is obscure. Carriers of certain abnormal hemoglobins which have a high oxygen affinity, such as $Hb_{Chesapeake}$ (Chap. 339), are slightly polycythemic.

Erythrocytosis is found in Cushing's syndrome and can be produced by the administration of large amounts of adrenocortical steroids. Especially intriguing are the instances of polycythemia observed in association with various tumors. These have been chiefly of two varieties, *infratentorial* and *renal*. The tumors in the posterior fossa of the skull have usually been vascular (hemangioblastomas). The renal tumors have included hypernephroma, adenoma, and sarcoma. Other tumors that have been associated with polycythemia include *uterine myoma* and

hepatic carcinoma. Polycythemia also has been reported in association with polycystic disease of the kidneys and hydronephrosis. However, only a small proportion (0.3 to 2.6 percent) of the various renal disorders mentioned above have been associated with polycythemia. Plasma erythropoietin levels have been found elevated in a number, though not all, of the cases so studied. Erythropoiesis-stimulating activity has been demonstrated in tumor extracts and in renal cyst fluid, and polycythemia has disappeared after the associated tumor was removed.

The term *stress erythrocytosis* has been applied to the polycythemia seen occasionally in very active, hard-working persons in a state of anxiety, who appear florid but who have none of the characteristic signs of erythremia— no splenomegaly nor leukocytosis with immature cells in the blood. In such individuals the total red blood cell mass is normal and the plasma volume is below normal.

In essence, then, erythrocytosis is known to develop in the presence of:

1. Defective saturation of arterial blood with oxygen, resulting from (*a*) decreased atmospheric pressure and (*b*) impaired pulmonary ventilation

2. Congenital disorders that permit right-to-left shunts

3. Defect in circulating blood pigment

4. Polycythemia produced by the adrenocortical secretions

5. Humoral mechanisms of less well-defined nature which may play a role, as suggested by the cases of polycythemia associated with a variety of tumors, malignant and benign, and with certain renal disorders mentioned above

It is clear, however, that some instances of erythrocytosis cannot be explained by these long-recognized mechanisms.

The differential diagnosis of polycythemia is discussed in the chapter on erythremia (Chap. 343).

REFERENCES

Bakshi, S. P., J. L. Fahey, and L. E. Pierce: Sausage Cyanosis—Acquired Methemoglobeinemic Nitrite Poisoning, New Engl. J. Med., 277:1072, 1967.

Barcroft, J.: "The Respiratory Functions of the Blood," London, Cambridge University Press, 1925.

Burwell, C. S., E. D. Robin, R. D. Whaley, and A. G. Bickelmann: Extreme Obesity Associated with Alveolar Hypoventilation: A Pickwickian Syndrome, Am. J. Med., 21:811, 1956.

Comroe, J. H., Jr.: "Physiology of Respiration," 1st ed., Chicago, The Year Book Medical Publishers, Inc., 1965.

——, R. E. Forster, A. B. Dubois, W. A. Briscoe, and E. Carlsen: "The Lung—Clinical Physiology and Pulmonary Function Tests," 2d ed., Chicago, The Year Book Medical Publishers, Inc., 1962.

Donati, R. M., R. D. Lange, and N. I. Gallagher: Nephrogenic Erythrocytosis, Arch. Intern. Med., 112:960, 1963.

——, J. M. McCarthy, R. D. Lange, and N. I. Gallagher: Erythrocytosis and Neoplastic Tumors, Ann. Intern. Med., 58:47, 1963.

Edwards, M. J., M. J. Novy, C. Waters, and J. Metcalfe:

Improved Oxygen Release: An Adaptation of Mature Red Cells to Hypoxia, J. Clin. Invest., 47:1851, 1968.

Gordon, A. S., G. W. Cooper, and E. D. Zanjani: The Kidney and Erythropoiesis, Seminars Hematol., 4:337, 1967.

Hurtado, A.: Some Clinical Aspects of Life at High Altitudes, Ann. Intern. Med., 53:247, 1960.

Jacobson, L. O., C. W. Gurney, and E. Goldwasser: The Control of Erythropoiesis, pp. 297–327, in "Advances in Internal Medicine," W. Dock and I. Snapper (Eds.), vol. 10, Chicago, The Year Book Medical Publishers, Inc., 1960.

Lundsgaard, C., and D. D. Van Slyke: Cyanosis, Medicine, 2:1, 1923.

Murray, J. F.: Classification of Polycythemic Disorders with Comments on the Diagnostic Value of Arterial Blood Oxygen Analysis, Ann. Intern. Med., 64:892, 1966.

Rudolph, A. M., A. S. Nadas, and W. H. Borges: Hematologic Adjustments to Cyanotic Congenital Heart Disease, Pediatrics, 11:454, 1953.

Weil, J. V., G. Jamieson, D. W. Brown, and R. F. Grover: The Red Cell Mass—Arterial Oxygen Relationship in Normal Man, J. Clin. Invest., 47:1627, 1968.

Wintrobe, M. M.: "Clinical Hematology," 6th ed., Philadelphia, Lea & Febiger, 1967.

34 EDEMA
Louis G. Welt

Edema is defined as an increase in the extravascular component of the extracellular fluid volume. It may be localized or have a generalized distribution depending on the primary lesion. It is recognized by the clinician in its gross generalized form by puffiness of the face (which is most readily apparent in the periorbital areas) and by the persistence of an indentation of the skin following pressure. This is known as *"pitting" edema*. In its more subtle form it may be detected by the fact that the rim of the bell of the stethoscope leaves an indentation on the skin of the chest that lasts a few minutes. One of the first symptoms a patient may note is the ring on a finger fitting more snugly than in the past. Lastly, it should be cautioned that the volume of the interstitial space may increase by several liters before edema is recognized by the patients from the symptoms or by the physician through physical examination. *Ascites* and *hydrothorax* refer to accumulation of excess fluid in the peritoneal and pleural cavities, respectively. *Anasarca*, or "dropsy," refers to gross generalized edema.

PATHOGENESIS

A more detailed discussion of the volume and distribution of body fluids is presented in Chap. 296. About one-third of the total body water is confined to the extracellular space. This compartment, in turn, is composed of the plasma volume and the interstitial space. Under ordinary circumstances the plasma volume represents about 25 percent of the extracellular space, and the remainder is in the interstitium. The forces that regulate the disposition of fluid between these two components of the extracellular compartment are frequently referred to as the *Starling forces*, owing to the masterful description presented by that noted physiologist.

In general terms, two forces tend to promote a movement of fluid from the vascular to the extravascular space, and these forces are the *hydrostatic pressure within the vascular system* and the *colloid osmotic pressure* in the interstitial fluid. In contrast, the factors which promote a movement of fluid into the vascular compartment are the *colloid oncotic pressure* contributed by the plasma proteins, and the *hydrostatic pressure within the interstitial fluid*, referred to as the *tissue tension*. These forces are balanced so that there is a large movement of water and diffusible solutes from the vascular space at the arteriolar end of the microcirculation and back into the vascular compartment at the venous end.[1] In addition, fluid is returned from the interstitial space into the vascular system by way of the lymphatics, and unless these channels are obstructed, lymph flow tends to increase if there is a tendency toward a net movement of fluid from the vascular compartment to the interstitium. In this fashion, all these forces are usually balanced so that a given steady state exists with respect to the size of the two compartments, and yet a large exchange between them is permitted. However, should any one of these factors be altered significantly, one can see how there may be a net movement of fluid from one component of the extracellular space to the other.

An increase in pressure in the vessels of the microcirculation may readily result from an increase in venous pressure due to local obstructive phenomena in the venous drainage, or to congestive heart failure, or to the simple expansion of the vascular volume by the administration of large volumes of fluid at a rate in excess of the ability of the kidneys to excrete these excesses. The colloid oncotic pressure of the plasma may be reduced owing to any of the factors that may induce hypoalbuminemia, such as malnutrition, liver disease, and loss of protein into the urine or into the gastrointestinal tract, or to a severe catabolic state.

Damage to the capillary endothelium increases the permeability of these vessels, which permits the transfer to the interstitial compartment of a fluid containing more protein than usual. Injury to the capillary walls may be the result of chemical, bacterial, thermal, or mechanical agents. Increased capillary permeability may also be a consequence of a hypersensitivity reaction. Lastly, damage to the capillary endothelium is presumably responsible for inflammatory edema, which is easily recognized by the presence of other signs of inflammation—redness, heat, and tenderness.

In any attempts to formulate a hypothesis concerning the pathophysiology involved in edematous states, it is exceedingly important to discriminate between the pri-

---

[1] There is no final resolution of the argument whether the exchange of fluid and solutes occurs between capillary endothelial cells or through the cells themselves.

mary events, which account for the maldistribution of fluid between the two components of the extracellular space, and the predictable secondary consequences, which include the retention of salt and water. There are instances in which an abnormal retention of salt and water may, in fact, be the *primary* disturbance. In these circumstances the edema is a secondary manifestation of the generalized increase in volume of the extracellular fluid. These special instances are usually related to those conditions characterized by an acute reduction in renal function (such as acute tubular necrosis or acute glomerulonephritis) and other disorders characterized by the primary production of excess mineralocorticoid or inappropriate secretion of the antidiuretic hormone.

These latter circumstances aside, one can create a hypothesis which is admittedly at least incomplete but within which one can begin to understand the concatenation of events in a variety of edematous states and perceive many of the features common in the pathophysiology of each. The basic premise is that the primary disorder concerns one or more alterations in the Starling forces such that there is a net movement of fluid from the vascular system into the interstitium or from the arterial compartment of the vascular space into the chambers of the heart or into the venous circulation itself. In either event, a diminished arterial volume may be anticipated to have certain consequences that lead to retention of salt and water. If retention of an increment of salt and water repairs the volume deficit, the stimuli to retain salt and water should be dissipated and a new steady state achieved. If, on the other hand, retention of salt and water does not repair the volume deficit because the increased volume of fluid cannot be sustained in the appropriate component of the vascular bed, the stimuli are not dissipated and the retention of salt and water continues. The sequence of events can be explored in a variety of circumstances.

Obstruction of Venous and Lymphatic Drainage to a Limb

The simplest condition to examine may be the consequences of lymphatic and venous obstruction to a limb. This must increase the hydrostatic pressure in the microcirculation so that more fluid is transferred from the circulation than can be reabsorbed at the venous end; furthermore, the alternate route, the lymphatic channels, are stipulated to be obstructed as well. This event must of necessity cause an increased volume of interstitial fluid in the limb at the expense of the plasma volume. The diminished plasma volume has a variety of consequences:

RENAL HEMODYNAMIC CHANGES. The diminished volume of plasma can be expected to reduce the perfusion of the kidney and decrease the glomerular filtration rate. Since one of the most important influences regulating the excretion of salt (and water) may be the filtered load itself, this would promote the excretion of lesser quantities of salt and smaller volumes of water. Other consequences

of a hemodynamic nature are presumably conditioned by alterations in plasma volume. For reasons that are as yet unclear, it seems quite well established that an influence of "volume" on the rate of excretion of salt functions independently of its filtered load and independently of mineralocorticoid secretion. The nature of this regulatory mechanism is unknown, but a direct correlation occurs between alterations in volume and alterations in the excretion of salt. The phenomenon may be related to the character and distribution of blood flow to the kidney, but there are other alternatives. In any event, a diminished plasma volume can readily diminish the excretion of salt owing to alterations in renal hemodynamic parameters.

HUMORAL FACTORS. Ample evidence reveals that a diminished volume of plasma in some fashion promotes an increased secretion of aldosterone. This is due to an increase in an aldosterone-stimulating agent, which is dependent on the presence of intact kidneys and may well be angiotensin. This, in turn, may be increased in the plasma owing to some influence on the renal circulation related to alterations in flow or pressure, or to the chemical composition of intraluminal fluid that may stimulate the release of renin from the juxtaglomerular apparatus. In turn, the renin reacts with renin substrate to form angiotensin I, and the latter is converted enzymatically to angiotensin II, which stimulates the secretion of aldosterone. Whatever the precise sequence of events, a diminished plasma volume promotes increased secretion of this mineralocorticoid which implements the renal tubular reabsorption of sodium.

The influence of alterations in plasma volume or the excretion of sodium salts was mentioned in relation to possible alterations in renal hemodynamics. There are data that suggest the possibility that the increase in volume of some component(s) of the extracellular space promotes the secretion of a "natriuretic" hormone, also referred to as a *third factor*, or *volume effect*. The unambiguous demonstration of such a hormone, its site(s) of secretion, and its characterization are yet to be presented.

The retention of sodium owing to the hemodynamic and humoral factors alluded to above may, in turn, be accompanied directly by an increased reabsorption of water. If not, then the primary retention of sodium thus dictates some increase in the effective osmolality of body fluids, promotes thirst and the acquisition of water, and promotes the secretion of antidiuretic hormone, which then implements the retention of water.

In the context of the disorder under discussion, the volume of the extracellular fluid (about 140 mM sodium per liter of water) is increased. This increment tends to accumulate in the interstitium of the limb in which venous and lymphatic drainage are obstructed until the tissue tension is great enough to counterbalance the primary alteration in the Starling forces, at which time no further fluid will accumulate in that limb. At this point the additional accumulation of fluid will repair the deficit in plasma volume, and the stimuli to retain more salt and water are dissipated. The net effect is an increase in the volume of interstitial fluid in a local area, and the secondary responses repair the plasma volume deficit incurred by the primary event.

This same sequence may be translated easily to many other edematous states.

Nephrotic Syndrome

The primary alteration in this disorder is a diminished colloid oncotic pressure due to exorbitant loss of protein into the urine. This should promote a net movement of fluid into the interstitium and initiate the sequence of events described above. However, so long as the hypoalbuminemia is severe, the increment of fluid cannot be restrained within the vascular compartment, and hence the stimuli to retain salt and water are not abated.

Cirrhosis

Measurements of blood volume in cirrhosis of the liver are commonly increased when the disorder is accompanied by a fairly large system of dilated venous radicles. Nevertheless, the arterial volume is quite likely diminished in size. If the primary event in the formation of ascites is due to obstruction of the lymphatic drainage of the liver as well as obstruction of the portal venous system, it is likely that the enlarged venous system has promoted a deficit in the arterial component. Once again, the sequence of events already described will come into play, and salt and water will be retained. So long as the venous bed continues to enlarge and the collection of fluid in the peritoneal cavity increases, the deficit in volume of the arterial side of the circulation is not repaired and the stimuli persist to retain salt and water. In addition, considerable data suggest that there are arteriovenous shunts in this disorder. One consequence of these shunts is a reduced renal blood flow despite an increase in cardiac output. In this fashion the alterations due to renal hemodynamic factors are fortified.

Although the diseased liver admittedly may not inactivate aldosterone and antidiuretic hormone in a competent fashion, it is unlikely that this plays a significant role in salt and water retention. Some suggest that this difficulty in inactivation permits the development of higher levels of these humoral agents, which may amplify the responses in terms of salt and water retention. This seems unlikely since, in the first place, a tendency to diminished inactivation of these hormones might be expected to retard their rates of secretion; furthermore, it is apparent that if one provides a mechanism for the loculated ascitic fluid to reach the interstitium of the abdominal wall by the use of a prosthetic device, there is an immediate diuresis of salt and water. This is presumably because if the ascitic fluid reaches the interstitial space elsewhere, it can be reabsorbed into the circulation and this, in turn, will repair the volume deficit and dissipate the stimuli responsible for the retention of salt and water. Unfortunately, these devices are soon obstructed by scar tissue and hence have not been a practical form of therapy. Nevertheless, this experience emphasizes that deficient inactivation of these hormones by the diseased liver plays no important role in implementing the edematous state.

Congestive Heart Failure

In this disorder it is postulated that the defective systolic emptying of the chambers of the heart promotes an accumulation of blood in the heart and venous circulation at the expense of the arterial volume, and the oft-repeated sequence of events is initiated. In many instances of mild heart failure a small increment of volume may be achieved, which may repair the volume deficit and establish a new steady state. This may result because up to a point an increase in the volume of blood within the chambers of the heart appears to promote a more forceful contraction and may thereby increase the volume ejected in systole. However, if the cardiac disorder is more severe, retention of fluid cannot repair the arterial volume deficit. The increment accumulates in the venous circulation, and the increase in hydrostatic pressure therein promotes the formation of edema in the lungs as well as elsewhere. The pulmonary edema impairs gas exchange and may induce hypoxia, which embarasses cardiac function still further. The volume of blood within the chambers of the heart becomes ever larger and reaches a point where this increase affects systolic emptying adversely, thus worsening the heart failure.

Cylic Edema

There is a syndrome characterized by periodic episodes of edema without obvious cause. It has been observed most commonly (but not exclusively) in women, and there appears to be some relationship to the menstrual cycle. The fact that most cases are seen in women may be due, in part at least, to the unfortunate cosmetic consequences of facial edema which is more likely to disturb women than men. Another feature of this disorder is fairly constant, large, diurnal alterations in weight so that the patient may weigh several pounds more in the evening than in the morning after having been in the upright posture most of the day.

No one knows whether all these patients represent a single type of disorder with varying degrees of intensity. A large diurnal weight change suggests the possibility that patients may well have increased capillary permeability in general, which is emphasized daily by the upright posture and the consequent increased hydrostatic pressure in the vessels. The episodes of more frankly sustained edema may be the result of a further increase in capillary permeability due to some other influence. If, in fact, it truly occurs more commonly in women and is correlated with the menstrual cycle, there may be some hormonal influence on the permeability of vessels which permits the loss of plasma volume into the interstitial space and the sequence of events secondary to a contraction in plasma volume. An occasional patient has been reported in whom

Fig. 34-1. Sequence of events leading to the formation and the retention of salt and water.

the loss of plasma volume was so striking as to induce peripheral vascular collapse; and in one instance, at least, this was so severe as to cause death.

This general formulation is represented graphically in Fig. 34-1. As mentioned earlier, this is certainly incomplete, and the amplification presented in this discussion may well have serious defects of omission and error. Allusion has been made to some of the unknown areas. One more which deserves further comment concerns the precise role of the mineralocorticoid hormone in these problems. Although increased quantities of aldosterone have been demonstrated to be secreted in these various edematous states, it must be emphasized that augmented levels of aldosterone (or other mineralocorticoids) do not always promote the accumulation of edema, as witnessed by the lack of striking fluid retention in most instances of primary aldosteronism. Furthermore, although normal subjects will retain some salt and water under the influence of a potent mineralocorticoid such as deoxycorticosterone acetate or 9-alpha-fluorohydrocortisone, this accumulation appears to be self-terminative despite continued exposure to the steroid and to salt and water. It is probable that the failure of normal subjects to accumulate fluid indefinitely reflects an increase in glomerular filtration rate, other hemodynamic influences, and the effect of the increase in volume which promotes an increased excretion of salt independent of the filtered load of sodium. The role of aldosterone in the accumulation of fluid in these edematous states discussed above may be

more effective because these patients are unable to repair the crucial deficit in volume.

Throughout this discussion it has been assumed that the retention of sodium salts is primary to water retention. This is attested to by (1) the usual failure to accumulate edema if sodium is not available in the diet and (2) the successful use of pharmacologic agents and other measures that promote the excretion of sodium in the urine. In most circumstances the mechanisms responsible for maintaining a normal effective osmolality in the body fluids continue to operate efficiently so that sodium retention promotes thirst and secretion of the antidiuretic hormone, which, in turn, lead to the ingestion and retention of approximately 1 liter of water for each 140 mM sodium retained. Similarly, measures which promote the loss of sodium into the urine are accompanied by antithetical responses leading to the net loss of an equivalent volume of water from the body.

DIFFERENTIAL DIAGNOSIS

Despite numerous inconsistencies encountered in the explanation for the various factors and mechanisms concerned in edema formation, the primary cause can usually be determined. As a rule, localized edema can be readily differentiated from generalized edema. The great majority of patients with noninflammatory generalized edema of significant degree suffer from cardiac, renal, hepatic, or nutritional disorders. Consequently, the differential diagnosis of generalized edema should be directed toward implicating or excluding these several conditions. The considerations listed below should suffice to differentiate the common causes of edema.

Localized Edema

Edema originating from inflammation or hypersensitivity is usually readily identified; allusion has been made to characteristics of this type of edema. Localized edema due to venous or lymphatic obstruction (thrombophlebitis, chronic lymphangitis, resection of regional lymph nodes, filariasis, etc.) may demonstrate in a local area all the characteristics of edema occurring from generalized retention of salt and water. It should be reemphasized that lymph edema is peculiarly intractable because restriction of lymphatic flow results in increased protein concentration in interstitial fluid, a circumstance which severely impedes removal of retained fluid.

Edema of Heart Failure

Evidence of heart disease as manifested by cardiac enlargement, diastolic murmurs, and gallop rhythm plus evidences of cardiac failure, such as dyspnea, basilar rales, diminished vital capacity, prolonged circulation time, venous distension, increased venous pressure, and hepatomegaly, usually provides abundant evidence of the pathogenesis of edema resulting from heart failure.

Edema of the Nephrotic Syndrome

The classic triad—massive proteinuria, hypoproteinemia, and hypercholesterolemia is usually present. This syndrome may occur during the course of a variety of kidney diseases, which include glomerulonephritis, diabetic glomerulosclerosis, amyloid infiltration, renal vein thrombosis, diffuse connective tissue diseases, and hypersensitivity reactions. A history of previous renal disease may or may not be elicited; more commonly, it is not.

Edema of Acute Glomerulonephritis

The edema occurring during the acute phases of glomerulonephritis is characteristically associated with hematuria, proteinuria, and hypertension. Some evidence supports the view that the fluid retention is due to increased capillary permeability; but probably in most instances the edema in this disease results from primary retention of sodium and water by the kidneys owing to acute renal insufficiency and the consequent development of a congested state. However, discrimination between congestive heart failure and a congested state in acute renal insufficiency is often difficult. The congested state differs from congestive heart failure since it is characterized by a normal or increased cardiac output, normal or diminished circulation time, a reduction in the packed cell volume, a normal arteriovenous oxygen difference, and failure to respond to a digitalis preparation. Patients commonly have severe evidence of pulmonary congestion on chest x-ray before cardiac enlargement is significant, and these patients frequently lie supine in bed with no tachypnea. If one cannot discriminate between the congested state and congestive heart failure, use of a cardiac glycoside is more prudent but especial care should be taken to avoid digitalis intoxication.

Edema of Cirrhosis

Ascites plus evidence of hepatic disease (collateral venous channels, hepatomegaly, spider angiomas, and jaundice) characterize edema of hepatic origin. The ascites is frequently extremely refractory to treatment; the lack of therapeutic response can be ascribed to the fact that intraabdominal fluid collects as a result of a combination of obstruction of hepatic lymphatic drainage, portal hypertension, hypoalbuminemia, and relatively high protein content of the ascitic fluid. The latter may be due to escape of a protein-containing fluid through the lymphatic vessels of the liver capsule or through the portal vessels, the lymphatic drainage of which is impeded. Edema may also occur in other parts of the body in patients with cirrhosis as a result of hypoalbuminemia. Furthermore, the sizable accumulation of ascitic fluid may be expected to increase intraabdominal pressure and impede venous return from the lower extremities; hence, it tends to promote accumulation of edema in these limbs as well.

Edema of Nutritional Origin

An inadequate diet over a prolonged period may produce hypoproteinemia and edema. In some instances of extreme malnutrition the degree of transudation appears to be disproportionately great for the degree of serum protein deficit observed. Coexisting beriberi heart disease may augment edema of this origin. In the latter condition, increased cardiac output and blood flow, in addition to those factors usually present in heart failure and capillary dilatation, may further favor edema formation. More striking edema is commonly observed when these famished subjects are provided with an adequate diet. The mechanism is not clear, but the ingestion of more food may increase the quantity of salt taken, which is retained along with water. The edema may be more apparent than under other circumstances, because the subcutaneous tissue is so depleted of fat that modest collections of edema may be more obvious than they would be in an obese subject.

GENERAL DIFFERENTIAL CRITERIA

Aside from the criteria already mentioned, certain other points may help elicit the cause of edema.

The distribution of edema is an important guide to the cause. Thus, edema of one leg or of one or both arms is usually the result of vascular or lymphatic obstruction. Edema resulting from hypoproteinemia characteristically is generalized, but it is especially evident in the eyelids and face and tends to be most pronounced in the morning because of the recumbent posture assumed during the night. Edema associated with heart failure, on the other hand, tends to be more extensive in the legs and to be accentuated in the evening, a feature also determined largely by posture. In the rare types of cardiac disease, such as tricuspid stenosis and constrictive pericarditis, in which orthopnea may be absent and the patient may prefer the recumbent posture, the factor of gravity may be equalized and facial edema observed. Less common causes of facial edema include trichinosis, allergic reactions, and myxedema. Unilateral edema occasionally results from cerebral lesions affecting the vasomotor fibers on one side of the body; paralysis also reduces lymphatic and venous drainage on the affected side.

The color, thickness, and sensitivity of the skin are important. Local tenderness and increase in temperature suggest inflammation. Local cyanosis may signify a venous obstruction. Generalized but usually slight cyanosis commonly indicates congestive heart failure. In individuals who have had repeated episodes of prolonged edema, the skin over the involved area may be thickened, hard, and often red.

The venous pressure is of great importance in evaluating edema. Elevation of this measurement in an isolated part of the body usually reflects venous obstruction. Generalized elevation of venous pressure is almost pathognomonic of congestive heart failure, although it may be present in the congestive state that accompanies acute renal insufficiency. Ordinarily significant increase in venous pressure can be recognized by the level at which cervical veins collapse; in doubtful cases and for accurate recording, the venous pressure should be measured.

Determination of the concentration of serum proteins, and especially of serum albumin, clearly differentiates those patients in whom edema is due entirely or in part to diminished intravascular colloid osmotic pressure. The presence of proteinuria affords useful clues. The complete absence of protein in the urine is evidence against (but does not exclude) either cardiac or renal disease as a cause of edema. In a patient with edema without proteinuria, the presence of a palpable liver constitutes strong evidence that hepatic disease may be the cause of the edema. Slight to moderate proteinuria is the rule in patients with heart failure, whereas persistent massive proteinuria usually reflects the presence of the nephrotic syndrome. Since the liver may be palpable in subjects with heart failure or hepatic disease, the presence of proteinuria in a patient who does not have a palpable liver suggests the possibility of the nephrotic syndrome. Aside from the points mentioned, which bear directly on the question of the type of edema, much valuable information can be obtained from other features of the examination. Some of these are the presence or absence of heart disease, the character of the urinary sediment, the dietary history, and a history of alcoholism.

It should be emphasized that edema may originate from a variety of abnormal states; it is not, therefore, necessarily a consequence of only one of the disorders enumerated above. For example, in a diabetic patient, edema may be the result of hypoalbuminemia associated with the nephrotic syndrome with intercapillary glomerulosclerosis, increased venous pressure associated with congestive heart failure due to atherosclerotic and hypertensive heart disease, and the anemia consequent to uremia.

SUMMARY

Edema limited to a local area suggests either obstruction or local capillary damage. The obstruction may be lymphatic, venous, or both, and the local capillary damage may be due either to inflammation or to allergy. Significant generalized edema may occur before it can be appreciated clinically. It appears first in tissues that are expansible and may be demonstrable only by pressure against a bony eminence such as the tibia. The presence of generalized edema requires investigation especially for evidence of cardiac, renal, or hepatic disease and occasionally for manifestations of nutritional deficiency.

The primary factors promoting transfer of fluid from the intravascular to the extravascular compartment of the extracellular fluid space are reasonably clear. The secondary factors that induce salt and water retention include a variety of hemodynamic humoral mechanisms, the nature of which, although clarified by recent investigations, can still not be formulated by any single hypothesis with confidence.

REFERENCES

deWardener, H. E., I. H. Mills, W. F. Clapham, and C. J. Hoyter: Studies on the Effluent Mechanism of the Sodium Diuresis Which Follows the Administration of Intravenous Saline in the Dog, Clin. Sci., 21:249, 1961.

Starling, E. H.: The Fluids of the Body, in "The Herter Lectures," New York, W. T. Keener and Co., 1909.

Welt, L. G.: Water Balance in Health and Disease, chap. 6 in "Diseases of Metabolism," 5th ed., G. G. Duncan (Ed.), Philadelphia, W. B. Saunders Company, 1964.

35   PALPITATION
William H. Resnik and Eugene Braunwald

Palpitation is a disagreeable subjective phenomenon which may be defined as an awareness of the beating of the heart. Palpitation is not pathognomonic of any particular group of disorders; even when it occurs as a more or less prominent complaint, the diagnosis of the underlying disease is made largely on the basis of other associated symptoms and data, rather than from an analysis of the palpitation alone. Nevertheless, palpitation is frequently of considerable importance in the minds of patients. The clear association of the symptom with the function of the heart and the fear that it may represent heart disease account for the patient's apprehension about it. Concern is all the more pronounced in patients who know or who have been told that they may have heart disease; to them palpitation may seem to be an omen of impending disaster. Since the resulting anxiety may be associated with increased activity of the autonomic nervous system, with consequent alteration of the cardiac rate and rhythm and the vigor of contraction, the patient's awareness of these changes may then lead to a vicious cycle.

Palpitation may be described by the patient in various terms, such as "pounding," "fluttering," "flopping," and "skipping," and in most cases it will be obvious that the complaint is of a sensation of disturbed heartbeat. Not infrequently, the patient complains of throbbing in the neck or upper part of the abdomen, when under similar circumstances most persons would refer the palpitation to the precordium.

In the various conditions discussed below, palpitation may be the chief source of the patient's discomfort and the outstanding complaint. It must not be inferred, however, that in all these disorders palpitation is always a symptom of great magnitude, even from the patient's standpoint.

The wide variability in the sensitivity to alterations in cardiac activity among different individuals must be appreciated. Some patients seem to be unaware of the most serious tachycardias; others are seriously troubled by an occasional extrasystole.

PATHOGENESIS OF PALPITATION

Under ordinary circumstances the rhythmic heartbeat is imperceptible to the healthy individual of average or placid temperament. Palpitation may be experienced by normal persons who have engaged in strenuous physical effort or have been strongly aroused emotionally. This type of palpitation is physiologic and represents the normal awareness of an overactive heart—i.e., a heart that is beating at a rapid rate and at the same time expelling more than the usual amount of blood with each beat. Since palpitation due to overactivity of the heart may occur also in certain pathologic states, e.g., severe anemia or thyrotoxicosis, it is commonly assumed that it is the overactivity *per se* or the associated increased stroke output that is responsible for the symptom. However, overactivity of the heart is generally associated with several other alterations in cardiac function, including acceleration of heart rate, steeper gradient of development of intraventricular pressure during the period of isometric contraction, and increased intensity of the heart sounds, especially of the first sound.

When palpitation is heavy and regular, it is usually caused by an augmented stroke volume, and it should raise the question of a variety of hyperkinetic circulatory states (anemia, arteriovenous fistula, thyrotoxicosis, and the so-called idiopathic hyperkinetic heart syndrome), aortic or mitral regurgitation, and atrial or ventricular septal defect. But unusual movements of the heart within the thorax are also frequently the mechanism of palpitation. Thus, the ectopic beat and/or the compensatory pause may be appreciated, since both are associated with alterations in cardiac motion.

IMPORTANT CAUSES OF PALPITATION

It is impracticable to enumerate all the circumstances under which palpitation may occur. Hence, only those disorders will be mentioned in which palpitation may be a prominent symptom.

PALPITATION DUE TO DISORDERS OF THE MECHANISM OF THE HEARTBEAT. Extrasystoles. The symptoms are fairly consistent, and in most cases the diagnosis will be suggested by the patient's story. The premature contraction and the post-premature beat are often described as a "flopping" or as if "the heart turns over." The pause following the premature contraction may be felt as an actual cessation of the heartbeat, in contrast with the complete unawareness of pauses of similar duration when the heart beats normally or when atrial fibrillation with a slow ventricular rate occurs. The patient's apprehensions seem to magnify the duration of the interval and sometimes may make him wonder if the heart will ever resume its beat. The first ventricular contraction succeeding the pause may be felt as an unusually vigorous beat and will be described as "pounding" or "thudding." Any one or all of these different symptoms initiated by the premature contraction may be experienced by the patient.

Usually the identification of the extrasystole as the cause of palpitation is a simple matter. When extrasystoles are numerous, clinical differentiation from atrial fibrillation can be made by any procedure that will bring about a definite increase in the ventricular rate; at increasingly rapid heart rates, the extrasystoles usually diminish in frequency and then disappear, whereas the irregularity of atrial fibrillation increases. Heart block, with dropped beats, is the only other common arrhythmia with which the premature contraction is likely to be confused; here, simple auscultation will reveal the absence of the premature beat prior to the pause.

The Ectopic Tachycardias. These conditions, which are considered in some detail in Chap. 265, are other common and medically more important causes of palpitation. Strangely, ventricular tachycardia, one of the most serious arrhythmias, rarely is manifested as palpitation; and this may be related to the abnormal sequence, and hence impaired coordination and vigor, of ventricular contraction.

If the patient is seen between attacks, the diagnosis of ectopic tachycardia and its type will have to depend on the history, but of course the precise diagnosis can be made only when an electrocardiogram and observations on the effect of carotid sinus pressure are made during the episode. The mode of onset and offset gives the most important lead. Determining this mode may prove difficult, for in many cases of rapid heart action, it is not impossible to ascertain with certainty whether there was an actual sudden onset or whether there was a preceding period of anxiety followed by the rapid, but not abrupt, development of sinus tachycardia. It is usually even more difficult to ascertain the exact characteristics of the off-set of the tachycardia.

PALPITATION DEPENDENT ON ORGANIC OR FUNCTIONAL DISTURBANCE ORIGINATING OUTSIDE THE CIRCULATORY SYSTEM. Once again, only the more important and common conditions, particularly those which may not be readily recognized, will be mentioned.

Thyrotoxicosis. In its fully developed form, thyrotoxicosis will usually be evident and offers little difficulty in the way of diagnosis. It is particularly likely to be overlooked in the presence of myocardial failure. The suspicion that thyrotoxicosis is present may be aroused by the detection of any one of its characteristic features, and the diagnosis will be confirmed by the procedures mentioned in Chap. 89.

Anemia. When mild, anemia may cause palpitation during exertion; when severe, it causes palpitation at rest. In some patients the coloring of the skin may not reveal the cause of the symptom, but appropriate studies of the blood will clarify the situation.

Fever. Palpitation may be present in acute infections, particularly in the early stages; but here the symptom is merely an insignificant phenomenon in the midst of other obviously more important ones. Palpitation may be a prominent symptom in an individual suffering from one of the chronic and sometimes more obscure febrile illnesses, such as incipient tuberculosis, chronic brucellosis, subacute bacterial endocarditis, or acute rheumatic fever with carditis and relatively few or no joint manifestations. Carditis in acute rheumatic fever and subacute bacterial endocarditis cannot of course be considered causes of palpitation originating outside the heart. They are considered in this group because the presenting symptoms, including palpitation, are often only those of an infection without localizing symptoms that direct suspicion to the heart. The problem is to determine that the cause of the palpitation is an infectious illness and to carry out the usual procedures to reveal the type of infection.

Hypoglycemia. Palpitation is often a prominent feature of this condition and appears to be related to release of epinephrine. The diagnosis is confirmed by appropriate blood sugar estimations and by prompt relief of all symptoms on the administration of glucose in one form or another (Chap. 96).

Aerophagia. Many patients who complain of "gas" and belching also complain of palpitation, possibly due in some cases to an associated anxiety state. This type of palpitation is readily recognized by the history of relief through eructation.

Tumors of the Adrenal Medulla (Pheochromocytomas). Such tumors may give rise to recurrent attacks, including paroxysms of hypertension and palpitation which are identical to those seen following the injection of epinephrine or norepinephrine. This type of tumor is a rather uncommon cause of palpitation and is mentioned chiefly because cure may be effected by surgical removal (Chap. 93). A similar syndrome may be produced when monoamine oxidase (MAO)-inhibitor drugs are taken concurrently with sympathomimetic drugs, such as ephedrine or amphetamine.

Drugs. The relationship between the development of palpitation and the use of tobacco, coffee, tea, alcohol, epinephrine, ephedrine, aminophylline, atropine, or thyroid extract is obvious.

PALPITATION AS A MANIFESTATION OF THE ANXIETY STATE. Persons who are healthy physically and well adjusted emotionally may have palpitation under certain circumstances. Thus, during or immediately after vigorous physical exertion or during sudden emotional tension, palpitation is common and is usually associated with outspoken tachycardia. Occasionally a healthy person may be conscious of his heartbeat when he is lying on the left side, but this type of palpitation is clearly due to the better transmission of the heart sounds to the ear when he is in that position. Lifting the head from the pillow will bring about a striking diminution or immediate disappearance of the symptom.

In some patients, palpitation may be one of the outstanding manifestations of a transitory episode of acute anxiety which may never recur, i.e., after this one episode or between infrequent bouts of increased nervous tension, the patient may experience no palpitation. In other persons the palpitation may, with other symptoms, represent prolonged anxiety neurosis or anxious depressions or a lifelong disorder indicative of disturbed autonomic function. The latter condition has been called neurocirculatory asthenia (see Chap. 369). Whether these illnesses are simply an expression of a chronic, deep-seated anxiety state superimposed on a normal autonomic nervous system or whether they depend on a constitutional or inherited autonomic instability is not yet entirely clear. At any rate, the clinical significance of this differentiation between the transitory and the enduring forms is that the former is often dissipated by firm reassurance from the physician, whereas the latter is usually resistant even to the most thorough and expert psychiatric care. In the latter case, the patient must be treated with most carefully planned psychologic support and tranquilizing medications. This chronic form of palpitation is known by various names, such as *Da Costa's syndrome, soldier's heart, effort syndrome, irritable heart, neurocirculatory asthenia,* and *functional cardiovascular disease.* Aside from palpitation, the chief symptoms are those of an anxiety state.

Physical examination usually reveals the typical findings of the hyperkinetic syndrome. These include a left parasternal lift, a precordial or apical systolic murmur, a wide pulse pressure, and a rapidly rising pulse. Electrocardiograms may display minor depressions of the S-T junction and inversion of T waves and so occasionally lead to a mistaken diagnosis of coronary disease; this is particularly likely to occur when these findings are associated with complaints by the patients of an aching feeling of substernal tightness, commonly present in emotional stress. The presence of any kind of organic disease is one of the commonest causes of the underlying anxiety which frequently produces this functional syndrome.

The diagnosis of this type of anxiety state depends on

Table 35-1. ITEMS TO BE COVERED IN HISTORY

Does the palpitation occur:	*If so, suspect:*
As isolated "jumps" or "skips"?.....................................	Extrasystoles
In attacks, known to be of abrupt beginning, with a heart rate of 120 beats/min or over, of regular or irregular rhythm?	Paroxysmal rapid heart action
Independent of exercise or excitement adequate to account for the symptom?	Atrial fibrillation, atrial flutter, thyrotoxicosis, anemia, febrile states, hypoglycemia, anxiety state
In attacks developing rapidly though not absolutely abruptly, unrelated to exertion or excitement?..	Hemorrhage, hypoglycemia, tumor of the adrenal medulla
In conjunction with the taking of drugs?............................	Tobacco, coffee, tea, alcohol, epinephrine, ephedrine, aminophylline, atropine, thyroid extract, monoamine oxidase inhibitors
On standing?...	Postural hypotension
In middle-aged women, in conjunction with flushes and sweats?..........	Menopausal syndrome
When the rate is known to be normal and the rhythm regular?...........	Anxiety state

the presence of the findings mentioned above. Even when a patient presents undoubted objective evidence of structural cardiac disease, a superimposed anxiety state should be considered responsible for the symptoms when the clinical picture is that which has been described. Normal values for vital capacity and for circulation time make it extremely improbable that the dyspnea that accompanies this type of palpitation is due to organic cardiac disease. It is noteworthy that an anxiety state, in contrast to heart disease, causes a sighing type of dyspnea. Also pain localized to the region of the apex, lasting for hours or days, and accompanied by hyperesthesia is due usually to an anxiety state, not to structural cardiac disease. Palpitation associated with organic cardiac disease is nearly always accompanied by arrhythmia or by marked tachycardia, whereas the symptom may exist with regular rhythm and with a heart rate of 80 beats per min or less in patients with the anxiety state. Giddiness due to this syndrome can usually be reproduced by hyperventilation (Chap. 20) or by change from the recumbent to the erect posture.

The treatment of the anxiety cardiac syndrome depends on removal of the cause. In many instances a thorough examination of the heart and a statement that it is normal will suffice. Instructions to take more rather than less physical exercise will reinforce these statements. Frequently, the demonstration that the physician can reproduce not only the palpitation but many other symptoms of the anxiety state merely by the subcutaneous injection of 0.5 to 1.0 ml 1:1,000 epinephrine serves to convince the patient that his symptoms are not the result of some mysterious disorder but are rather the effect of a well-understood physiologic mechanism. This is especially true when the initial anxiety has been mainly the result of fear of heart disease. When the anxiety state is a manifestation of chronic anxiety neurosis or depressive psychosis, the symptoms are more likely to persist.

Management of patients with palpitation and the anxiety cardiac syndrome is facilitated by a clear understanding on the physician's part of the mechanisms of the symptoms. The palpitation is probably related to release of epinephrine and to the lower perception threshold. The pain probably arises in the intercostal tissues as a result of the pounding of the heart. The hyperventilation with its ensuing train of symptoms (Chap. 20) is analogous to sighing. It is possible that the entire syndrome is related to decline of the normal inhibitory effect of the cerebral cortex on those hypothalamic centers which normally control the sympathetic system ("cortical-hypothalamic imbalance"). Explanation of these physiologic mechanisms to the patient and reassurance that they are not indicative of serious disease is one of the most important therapeutic steps.

The commonest causes for palpitation have been enumerated and briefly discussed. Because this symptom occurs in such a wide variety of disorders which have no common or closely related underlying disturbance of structure or function, it is impossible to follow closely any predetermined plan of study in elucidating the significance of the symptom. The exact procedure will vary, of course, with the circumstances under which the patient is seen. Table 35-1 summarizes the main points of information that will be ascertained in the history. These questions and others formulated according to circumstances of the individual case will serve to suggest the additional lines of inquiry that may be necessary for analysis and appraisal of palpitation.

One point merits special emphasis. As a rule palpitation produces anxiety and fear out of all proportion to its seriousness. When the cause has been accurately determined and its significance explained to the patient, his concern is often ameliorated and may disappear entirely.

REFERENCES

Cohen, M. E., and P. D. White: Life Stress and Bodily Disease, vol. 29, chap. 56, in "Research Publications of the Association for Research in Nervous & Mental Disease," Baltimore, The Williams & Wilkins Company, 1950.

Kjellberg, S. R., V. Rudhe, and T. Sjöstrand: The Effect of Adrenaline on the Contraction of the Human Heart under Normal Circulatory Conditions, Acta Physiol. Scand., 24:333, 1952.

Siecke, H., and H. E. Essex: Relation of the Difference in Pressure across the Mitral Valve to the Amplitude of the First Heart Sound in Dogs with Atrioventricular Block, Am. J. Physiol., 192:135, 1958.

Wood, P.: "Diseases of the Heart and Circulation," 3d ed., pp. 17 and 18, Philadelphia, J. B. Lippincott Company, 1968.

Yu, P. N., B. J. B. Yim, and C. A. Stanfield: Hyperventilation Syndrome. Changes in the Electrocardiogram, Blood Gases, and Electrolytes during Voluntary Hyperventilation; Possible Mechanisms and Clinical Implications, A.M.A. Arch. Intern. Med., 103:902, 1959.

36 HYPOTENSION AND THE SHOCK SYNDROME

Karl Engelman and
Eugene Braunwald

HYPOTENSION

The differential diagnosis of hypotensive states and the development of a rational plan of therapy require understanding of the normal regulation of arterial pressure.

CONTROL OF ARTERIAL PRESSURE. Arterial pressure must be maintained at levels sufficient to permit adequate perfusion of the extensive capillary networks in the systemic vascular bed. The level of pressure in the central arterial bed is in a large measure dependent on two factors—the volume of blood ejected by the left ventricle per unit of time, i.e., the cardiac output, and the resistance to blood flow offered by the vessels in the peripheral vascular bed. The resistance of a blood vessel, in turn, varies inversely as the fourth power of its radius, and at any given level of cardiac output arterial pressure is therefore largely dependent upon the degree of constriction of the smooth muscle in the walls of the arterioles. Though resistance to flow also varies with the viscosity of the fluid and the length of the vessels, alterations in these factors are ordinarily of only secondary importance.

Cardiac output is controlled largely by factors which regulate ventricular end-diastolic volume, the level of myocardial contractility, and heart rate (Chap. 263). The autonomic nervous system plays a major role in the maintenance of arterial pressure by its influences on the cardiac output and on the degree of constriction of the resistance (arterioles) and capacitance (venules and veins) vessels. The afferent limbs of the autonomic reflex arcs regulating arterial pressure arise in stretch receptors in the aortic arch and the carotid sinuses. Impulses are transmitted along afferent fibers in the glossopharyngeal and vagus nerves to extensive central autonomic connections in the medulla. Synapses connect not only the sympathetic and parasympathetic nuclei and efferent arcs, but also the cerebral cortex and hypothalamic nuclei which control hormonal secretion via the pituitary gland.

A rapid reduction of arterial pressure diminishes the stimulation of baroreceptors, which in turn evokes an activation of sympathetic outflow and inhibition of parasympathetic activity. As a result, the vascular smooth muscles in arterioles and veins constrict, while heart rate and myocardial contractility are augmented. In addition, adrenal medullary secretion is increased, as are the output of antidiuretic hormone (ADH), adrenocorticotrophic hormone (ACTH), and aldosterone; all of these effects act to restore the arterial pressure to control levels. Opposite changes occur if arterial pressure is raised acutely. Thus, the operation of the baroreceptor system normally serves to buffer the body from a variety of influences which would otherwise produce marked alterations in arterial pressure.

MEASUREMENT OF ARTERIAL PRESSURE. Arterial pressure is determined clinically with a pneumatic cuff; ordinarily, this indirect method provides slight underestimation of the true arterial pressure. Considerable error may be introduced if proper precautions are not taken in determining blood pressure by this method. The arterial pressure may be significantly underestimated if the air in the cuff is released too rapidly, especially in the presence of bradycardia or an irregular rhythm, or if inadequate inflation of the cuff does not result in complete vascular occlusion. This indirect method is most accurate when, in normal-sized adults, cuffs 12 to 14 cm in width are employed. However, when a cuff of this size is used on children or adults with unusually thin arms, blood pres-

Table 36-1. RANGE OF NORMAL BLOOD PRESSURES

Age, years	Systolic blood pressure, mean ± 2 SD, mmHg	Diastolic blood pressure, mean ± 2 SD, mmHg
Newborn	80 ± 16*	46 ± 16*
1......	96 ± 30	66 ± 25
2......	99 ± 25	64 ± 25
4......	99 ± 20	65 ± 20
6......	100 ± 15	56 ± 8
8......	105 ± 16	57 ± 9
10......	111 ± 17	58 ± 10
13......	118 ± 19	60 ± 10

Age	Male	Female	Male	Female
20–24....	123 ± 18†	116 ± 18†	76 ± 14†	72 ± 12†
25–29....	125 ± 17	117 ± 15	78 ± 11	74 ± 12
30–34....	126 ± 17	120 ± 18	79 ± 13	75 ± 14
35–39....	127 ± 18	124 ± 19	80 ± 13	78 ± 13
40–44....	129 ± 19	127 ± 23	81 ± 12	80 ± 14
45–49....	130 ± 22	131 ± 25	82 ± 13	82 ± 15
50–54....	135 ± 25	137 ± 27	83 ± 14	84 ± 16
55–59....	138 ± 25	139 ± 28	84 ± 14	84 ± 16
60–64....	142 ± 27	144 ± 29	85 ± 16	85 ± 17

* (Newborn to 13 years). Includes both males and females. From R. J. Haggerty, M. W. Maroney, and A. S. Nadas: Essential Hypertension in Infancy and Childhood, A.M.A. J. Dis. Child., 92:535, 1956.

† (20 to 64 years). From A. M. Master, C. I. Garfield, and M. B. Walters, Normal Blood Pressure and Hypertension, Philadelphia, Lea & Febiger, 1952.

sure may be seriously underestimated, or conversely, it may be overestimated when employed on an arm or thigh greater than 20 cm in girth. Marked vasoconstriction resulting in severely attenuated limb blood flow and/or marked reductions in pulse pressure may also result in serious underestimation of arterial pressure by the auscultatory method. Direct intraarterial recordings may reveal a normal or even an elevated pressure, while the absence of Korotkoff sounds makes the pressure unobtainable by the indirect methods.

THE "NORMAL" BLOOD PRESSURE. The "normal" blood pressure has been difficult to define. Traditional statistical approaches define normality on the basis of values included within two standard deviations of the mean of pressures obtained in a large population of healthy individuals. Analysis of blood pressures obtained from a study of 74,000 presumably healthy, working adults, aged twenty to sixty-four years, revealed that in both sexes the levels of systolic and diastolic pressures rise gradually but progressively with age (Table 36-1). There is little variation in the distribution of pressures at the lower end of the scale over the entire age span, but all curves are skewed to the right for the older subjects. This distribution reflects the increased incidence of hypertension with aging. Chronic hypotension, however, occurs only rarely.

ACUTE HYPOTENSION AND SHOCK

Not commonly, physicians are called upon to treat patients who acutely develop severe hypotension or shock. These two terms are not synonymous; although shock is usually associated with hypotension, a previously hypertensive patient may be in shock despite an arterial pressure within normal limits, and hypotension may occur in the absence of shock. *Shock* may be defined as a state in which there is widespread, serious reduction of tissue perfusion which, if prolonged, leads to generalized impairment of cellular function.

The most common clinical causes of shock are listed in Table 36-2. Since maintenance of arterial pressure is dependent on cardiac output and peripheral vasomotor tone, marked reductions in either of these variables without a compensatory elevation of the other results in systemic hypotension. Reduction of cardiac output due to hypovolemia or acute myocardial infarction is among the most frequently encountered and easily categorized causes of shock. Failure of neurogenic mechanisms resulting in decreased vasoconstrictor impulses is another well defined category; in many patients, particularly in the late stages of shock, multiple factors play a role in the development of circulatory failure.

Hypovolemia has been studied much more extensively than any other cause of shock; the mechanism of development is usually readily evident and well understood, and therapy, i.e., restoration of blood volume, is both simple and effective if applied before irreversible tissue damage occurs. Whether the primary insult is the external loss of blood, plasma, or water and salt or the internal sequestration of these fluids in a hollow viscus or body cavity, the general effect is similar, i.e., reduced venous return

and decreased cardiac output. For purposes of a general discussion of shock, hemorrhagic hypovolemia will be used as the model, but the general physiologic consequences of the various etiologies of reduced tissue perfusion are similar.

Table 36-2. ETIOLOGIC FACTORS IN SHOCK

I. Hypovolemia
    A. External Fluid Losses
        1. Hemorrhage
        2. Gastrointestinal
          a. Vomiting (pyloric stenosis, intestinal obstruction)
          b. Diarrhea
        3. Renal
          a. Diabetes mellitus
          b. Diabetes insipidis
          c. Excessive use of diuretics
        4. Cutaneous
          a. Burns
          b. Exudative lesions
          c. Perspiration and insensible water loss without replacement
    B. Internal sequestration
        1. Fractures
        2. Ascites (peritonitis, pancreatitis, cirrhosis)
        3. Intestinal obstruction
        4. Hemothorax
        5. Hemoperitoneum
II. Cardiogenic
    A. Myocardial infarction
    B. Arrhythmia (paroxysmal tachycardia or fibrillation, severe bradycardia)
III. Obstruction to blood flow
    A. Pulmonary embolus
    B. Tension pneumothorax
    C. Cardiac tamponade
    D. Dissecting aortic aneurysm
    E. Intracardiac (ball-valve thrombus, atrial myxoma)
IV. Neuropathic
    A. Drug induced
        1. Anesthesia
        2. Ganglion-blocking or other antihypertensive drugs
        3. "Ingestion" (barbiturates, glutethimide, phenothiazines)
    B. Spinal cord injury
    C. Orthostatic hypotension (primary autonomic insufficiency, peripheral neuropathies)
V. Other
    A. Infection
        1. Gram-negative septicemia (endotoxin)
        2. Other septicemias
    B. Anaphylaxis
    C. Endocrine failure (Addison's Disease, myxedema)
    D. Anoxia

Depending upon the severity and rate of development of hypovolemia, the shock syndrome may develop abruptly or evolve gradually. If the precipitating factors progress unabated, the endogenous defense mechanisms, while initially competent to maintain adequate circulation, eventually are extended beyond their capacity for compensation. The development of the shock syndrome may be thought to evolve through several stages which merge with one another:

1. The period in which the blood volume deficit is relatively minor and in which the patient may be asymptomatic. In a previously healthy individual compensation for an acute blood loss of as much as 10 percent of the normal blood volume (as with venesection of 500 ml blood from a donor) is achieved acutely by constriction of the arteriolar bed and an augmentation of heart rate and myocardial contractility. Other responses with more gradual effects include the increased secretion of antidiuretic hormone and aldosterone, which results in salt and water retention and the redistribution of fluid into the intravascular compartment. Arterial pressure is maintained and cardiac output is normal, or only slightly reduced, primarily as a consequence of selective reductions of blood flow to the skin, kidney, and muscle beds.

2. With a reduction of blood volume of 15 to 25 percent, cardiac output falls markedly, and despite intense arteriolar constriction in most vascular beds, arterial pressure declines. Generalized venoconstriction occurs, increasing the fraction of the total blood volume in the central circulation and tending to sustain venous return. With this massive reflex adrenergic discharge there is tachycardia, intense cutaneous vasoconstriction, pallor, diaphoresis, piloerection, oliguria, apprehension, and restlessness.

3. Once the patient has achieved this state of maximal mobilization of compensatory mechanisms, small additional losses of blood result in rapid deterioration of the circulation, with life-threatening reductions of cardiac output, blood pressure, and tissue perfusion. The duration of this shock state, the severity of tissue anoxia, and the age and underlying physical state of the patient are of primary importance in determining the ultimate outcome. If tissue perfusion is restored rapidly, recovery may be expected. However, if shock persists, the severe vasoconstriction may itself become a complicating factor and by reducing tissue perfusion even further may initiate a vicious cycle leading to an irreversible state due to widespread cellular injury. Anoxia, hypercapnia, and acidosis result from hypoperfusion of tissues; these metabolic derangements ultimately result in failure of the energy-requiring active transport systems of cell membranes. The integrity of the cells is compromised, and potassium ions, intracellular enzymes, peptides, and other vasoactive compounds are released into the circulation. Of special importance during prolonged profound shock is stasis of the microcirculation of the bowel and breakdown of the mucosal barrier, which leads to the entry of bacteria and bacterial toxins into the bloodstream. Because many of these substances are potent vasodilators, there may be widespread inhibition of vasoconstrictor tone, which depresses arterial pressure despite intense sympathetic activity. Blood flow to the brain and heart is further reduced, and infarction of these vital organs usually leads to death.

Just as cardiac output may fall to dangerous or even fatal levels due to actual fluid losses or sequestration with diminished venous return, cardiac failure or intrathoracic obstruction to blood flow may have a similar effect. Furthermore, even in the presence of a normal blood volume and cardiac function, "vasomotor collapse" due to drug-induced or neuropathic failure of sympathetic vasomotor activity can result in shock due to reduction of peripheral resistance and the pooling of blood in the venous bed. Finally, a complex form of shock may result from infection, especially gram-negative bacteremia with endotoxin release, from anaphylaxis, anoxia, and endocrine disorders which affect myocardial function, fluid and electrolyte balance, vasomotor tone, and general tissue metabolic processes.

Treatment of the patient with shock should be directed toward the rapid restoration of cardiac output and tissue perfusion. General supportive measures must be undertaken immediately, sometimes even before the etiology of the shock state has been identified. Whether shock results from decreased cardiac output due to a primary reduction in intravascular volume or a reduction of "effective blood volume" with pooling of blood in certain vascular beds, the most effective means of restoring adequate circulation is by the rapid infusion of volume-expanding fluids (whole blood, plasma, plasma substitutes, or isotonic electrolyte solutions). However, when shock is secondary to, or is accompanied by, cardiac failure with increased central venous pressure, the infusion of volume-expanding fluids may result in pulmonary edema. Here attention must be directed toward restoring cardiac function with cardiotonic drugs such as the digitalis glycosides and isoproterenol, and an attempt should be made to support arterial pressure at levels sufficient to maintain the coronary perfusion pressure (Chap. 271). Arrhythmias, which may also contribute to the low cardiac output, should be corrected (Chap. 265).

The appearance of the external jugular veins may be helpful in differentiating between shock with high or low central venous pressure. However, a catheter inserted into the superior vena cava is the best means for continuously monitoring venous pressure and is of considerable value in guiding therapy; such a catheter should be inserted in patients with shock whenever possible. Serial measurements of venous pressure, urine flow rate, heart rate, and the clinical and mental state of the patient often provide more important indices of the efficacy of therapy than arterial pressure changes.

There is considerable debate concerning the efficacy of vasocontrictor drugs in shock. In patients with severe peripheral constriction these agents are often ineffective and may actually reduce the already lowered tissue perfusion. However, these drugs are usually helpful in patients with inadequate vasoconstrictor responses. The use of alpha adrenergic blocking agents or massive doses of adrenal glucocorticoids in shock secondary to gram-negative septicemia with endotoxin release is also a matter of considerable controversy and cannot yet be considered a routine procedure.

CHRONIC HYPOTENSION

Although many patients have been treated for chronic "low blood pressure," most of these individuals, with systolic pressures in the range of 90 to 110 mm Hg, are normal and may actually have a greater life expectancy than their cohorts with higher pressures. Patients with true chronic hypotension may complain of lethargy, weakness, easy fatigability, and dizziness or faintness, especially if arterial pressure is lowered further when the erect position is assumed. These symptoms are presumably due to a decrease in perfusion of the brain, heart, skeletal muscle, and other organs.

Although arterial pressure is usually normal or even slightly elevated in patients with congestive heart failure, chronic hypotension occasionally results from severe reductions of the cardiac output, particularly in patients with stenotic valvular lesions and in patients with chronic constrictive pericarditis. The major endocrine causes of chronic hypotension are associated with deficient gluco- and mineralocorticoid secretion and resultant reductions of the intravascular and interstitial fluid volume. Hypotension is usually more pronounced in patients with primary adrenocortical insufficiency than in those with hypopituitarism because secretion of the salt-retaining adrenocortical hormone, aldosterone, is partially preserved in pituitary insufficiency (Chap. 87).

Malnutrition, cachexia, chronic bed rest, and a variety of neurologic disorders may result in chronic hypotension, especially in the standing position. Interference with the neural pathways anywhere between the vasomotor center and the efferent sympathetic nerve endings on the blood vessels or heart may prevent the vasoconstriction and increase in cardiac output which occur as a normal response to a reduction in arterial pressure. Multiple sclerosis, amyotrophic lateral sclerosis, syringomyelia, syphilitic or diabetic tabes dorsalis, peripheral neuropathies, spinal cord section, diabetic neuropathy, extensive lumbodorsal sympathectomy, and the administration of drugs interfering with nerve transmission in the sympathetic nervous system are all associated with orthostatic hypotension. In addition, idiopathic orthostatic hypotension (primary autonomic insufficiency), a rare condition in which there is degeneration of central and/or peripheral autonomic nervous structures, may result in such severe orthostatic hypotension that syncope or seizures occur when the patient arises from recumbency. This condition is progressive and characterized by ascending anhydrosis and loss of hair, decreased BMR, reduced norepinephrine production, deficient secretion of lacrimal and salivary glands, ileus, bladder atony, and absence of tachycardia on standing despite the marked reduction of blood pressure.

Specific therapy is not available for most of the neurologic causes of orthostatic hypotension, and treatment with sympathomimetic drugs has not proved effective over prolonged periods. However, the expansion of extracellular volume, which may be achieved with a high (10 to 20 Gm per day) salt diet and/or the potent synthetic salt-retaining steroid, 9-α-fluorohydrocortisone (0.1 to 0.5 mg per day) may be helpful. Tight, full-length, elastic supportive hose to reduce orthostatic pooling of blood in the legs may also arterial pressure, and in the

most severe cases pressurized aviator suits may be necessary to permit ambulation.

REFERENCES

Beecher, H. K., F. A. Simeone, C. A. Burnett, S. L. Shapiro, E. F. Sullivan, and T. B. Mallory: The Internal State of the Severely Wounded Man on Entry to the Most Forward Hospital. *Surgery* 22:672, 1947.

Master, A. M., C. I. Garfield, and M. B. Walters: Normal Blood Pressure and Hypertension, Philadelphia, Lea and Febiger, 1952.

Weil, M. H., and H. Shubin: Diagnosis and Treatment of Shock, Baltimore, The Williams & Wilkins Company, 1967.

37 ELEVATION OF ARTERIAL PRESSURE

Karl Engelman and Eugene Braunwald

Patients with elevations of arterial pressure are usually asymptomatic, and the blood pressure abnormality often arouses attention only incidentally during military, life insurance, or other periodic physical examination. Because hypertension results in secondary organ damage and a reduced life span, it should be evaluated fully and, when appropriate, treated.

DIAGNOSIS OF HYPERTENSION. Often, however, the first question is whether patients with a moderately elevated routine blood pressure recording are truly hypertensive. It is well established that anxiety, discomfort, physical activity, or other stress can acutely and transiently raise arterial pressure. Most individuals have a higher pressure when initially examined than after several measurements made in the course of a single visit; in order to establish the diagnosis of hypertension it is necessary to document in the course of several examinations that arterial pressure remains elevated. Patients with transient or "labile" hypertension may not require treatment, but should be reexamined periodically, since over the course of time such individuals often develop sustained hypertension.

Systolic hypertension in the presence of a normal or reduced diastolic pressure is rarely considered to be responsible for organ damage, but usually reflects other pathologic processes. It is most commonly seen in elderly patients with decreased compliance of the aortic wall. In patients with severe bradycardia, thyrotoxicosis, severe anemia, fever, aortic valvular insufficiency, arteriovenous shunts or fistulas, and the hyperkinetic heart syndrome, systolic hypertension is due to an elevated stroke volume, often accompanied by a rapid diastolic runoff.

Patients with true systemic hypertension have an increased mean arterial pressure with elevations of both systolic and diastolic pressures. Regardless of the primary etiology, the hemodynamic abnormality in most of these patients is increased vascular resistance, especially at the level of the smaller muscular arteries and arterioles, though a small number of patients may also have an increased cardiac output, particularly in the early stages of the illness. In a small fraction of patients, hypertension is associated with hypervolemia or increased blood viscosity secondary to polycythemia.

ETIOLOGY OF HYPERTENSION

A specific etiology for the increase in peripheral resistance which is responsible for the elevated arterial pressure cannot be defined for at least 90 percent of patients with hypertensive disease. Numerous experimental studies have sought to define the role of a variety of components ultimately responsible for idiopathic, or so-called "essential," hypertension. Evidence for the role played by abnormal psychologic stimuli comes from the finding that chronically stressed animals may become hypertensive, and that sedatives and tranquilizers are helpful in the treatment of many hypertensive patients. Another neurogenic mechanism, the resetting of the sensitivity of the baroreceptors, occurs in hypertensive dogs so that they appear to recognize elevated arterial pressures as normal. The importance of salt intake is suggested by studies showing that rats can be made hypertensive when given excessive dietary salt, and epidemiologic studies have also suggested this as a factor of possible etiologic significance in man; other studies have indicated that increased water and sodium in the walls of arterioles may result in increased peripheral resistance.

It appears that all of the above-mentioned factors play some role in patients with essential hypertension, which might be best regarded as a multifactorial disease related to abnormalities of the regulatory mechanisms normally concerned with the homeostatic control of arterial pressure. Page has described a "mosaic pattern" of how the complex interrelationships of central and sympathetic nervous influences, vascular defects, water and electrolyte metabolism, and cardiac activity can combine to produce the hypertensive state. In addition, hereditary and racial factors seem to play significant roles in the development of hypertension, since this disease is often found in families and is especially prevalent and virulent among certain ethnic groups, such as the American Negro population.

More specific etiologic relationships have been established for a smaller group of patients with systemic hypertension (Table 37-1). Primary renal diseases associated with the development of serious hypertension (as distinguished from renal damage secondary to hypertension) have been recognized for years, although in many cases the exact mechanism of blood pressure elevation is unknown. Hypertension may develop suddenly during the course of acute glomerulonephritis and it is usually a prominent feature in the late stages of renal damage due to chronic glomerulonephritis (Chap. 304) or pyelonephritis (Chap. 303). Polycystic renal disease, renal infarction, or partial occlusion of the renal artery due to congenital or acquired vascular defects are also

Table 37-1. CLASSIFICATION OF ARTERIAL HYPERTENSION

I. Systolic hypertension with wide pulse pressure
   A. Decreased compliance of aorta (arteriosclerosis)
   B. Increased stroke volume or cardiac output
      1. Arteriovenous fistula
      2. Thyrotoxicosis
      3. Hyperkinetic heart disease
      4. Fever
      5. Psychogenic
      6. Aortic valvular insufficiency
      7. Patent ductus arteriosus
II. Systolic and diastolic hypertension (increased peripheral vascular resistance)
   A. Renal
      1. Chronic pyelonephritis
      2. Acute and chronic glomerulonephritis
      3. Polycystic renal disease
      4. Renovascular stenosis or renal infarction
      5. Most other severe renal disease (arteriolar nephrosclerosis, diabetic nephropathy, etc.)
   B. Endocrine
      1. Acromegaly
      2. Adrenocortical hyperfunction
         a. Cushing's disease and syndrome
         b. Primary hyperaldosteronism
         c. Congenital or hereditary adrenogenital syndromes ($17\text{-}\alpha$-hydroxylase and $11\text{-}\beta$-hydroxylase defects)
      3. Pheochromocytoma
   C. Neurogenic
      1. Psychogenic
      2. "Diencephalic syndrome"
      3. Familial dysautonomia (Riley-Day)
      4. Poliomyelitis (bulbar)
      5. Polyneuritis (acute porphyria, lead poisoning)
      6. Increased intracranial pressure (acute)
      7. Spinal cord section
   D. Miscellaneous
      1. Coarctation of aorta
      2. Increased intravascular volume (excessive transfusion)
      3. Polyarteritis nodosa
   E. Unknown etiology
      1. Essential hypertension ($>90\%$ of all cases of hypertension)
      2. Toxemia of pregnancy
      3. Acute intermittent porphyria

implicated as etiologic factors, the latter having been clearly related to activation of the renin-angiotensin-aldosterone pressor system.

The most clearly defined etiologic relationships in the development of hypertension are found among the endocrine disorders. Adrenocortical hormones have also been implicated in the hypertensive syndromes associated with tumors or hyperplasia of the anterior pituitary (Cushing's Syndrome, primary hyperaldosteronism, Chap. 92), as well as with various congenital or hereditary enzyme defects (hypertensive adrenogenital syndromes). Secretion of excessive qualities of the pressor catecholamines, norepinephrine and epinephrine, associated with pheochromocytomas, i.e., chromaffin cell tumors arising from the adrenal medulla or sympathetic ganglia, are also commonly associated with hypertension (Chap. 93). Patients with acromegaly (Chap. 87) may have hypertension, but the mechanism of their blood pressure elevation is less clear. The presence of these endocrinopathies is usually readily recognizable and distinguishable from essential hypertension by their distinctive clinical and biochemical features.

EFFECTS OF HYPERTENSION

Following an asymptomatic latent period, clinical manifestations which reflect the underlying pathologic sequelae of the hypertensive state usually become apparent. Cardiac, renal, and central nervous system effects due to accelerated vascular damage are most prominent, and if unaltered by therapy, they often ultimately result in symptomatic illness and death.

EFFECTS ON HEART. Cardiac compensation for the excessive work load imposed by increased systemic pressure is at first sustained by the presence of left ventricular hypertrophy. Ultimately, the function of this chamber deteriorates, it dilates, and the symptoms and signs of heart failure appear (Chap. 264). Angina pectoris may also occur due to accelerated coronary arterial disease and/or increased myocardial oxygen requirements as a consequence of the increased myocardial mass which exceeds the capacity of the coronary circulation. On physical examination the heart is enlarged and has prominent left ventricular impulse. The sound of aortic closure is accentuated, and there may be a faint murmur of aortic insufficiency. Presystolic (atrial) gallop sounds appear frequently in hypertensive heart disease and a protodiastolic (ventricular), or summation, gallop rhythm may be present. Electrocardiographic changes of left ventricular hypertrophy are common, while evidence of ischemia or infarction may be observed late in the disease. The majority of deaths due to hypertension result from myocardial infarction or congestive heart failure.

NEUROLOGIC EFFECTS. The neurologic effects of long-standing hypertension can be divided into retinal and central nervous system changes. Because the retina is the only tissue in which the arteries and arterioles can be examined directly, repeated ophthalmoscopic examination provides the opportunity to observe the progress of the vascular effects of hypertension. The Keith-Wagener-Barker classification of the retinal changes in hypertension (Table 37-2) has provided a simple and excellent means for serial evaluation of the hypertensive patient. Table 37-2 includes both the criteria for grouping the retinal findings of hypertension and the secondary arteriolosclerotic changes. Increasing severity of hypertension is associated with focal spasm and progressive general narrowing of the arterioles, as well as the appearance of hemorrhages, exudates and papilledema. These retinal lesions often produce scotomata, blurred vision, and even blindness, especially in the presence of papilledema or hemorrhages of the macular area. Hypertensive lesions may develop acutely, and if therapy results in significant reduction of blood pressure, may show rapid resolution. Rarely, these lesions resolve without therapy. In contrast,

Table 37-2. CLASSIFICATION OF HYPERTENSIVE AND ARTERIOLARSCLEROTIC RETINOPATHY

| Degree | Hypertension | | | | | Arteriolarsclerosis | |
| | Arterioles | | Hemor-rhages | Exudates | Papilledema | Arteriolar light reflex | AV crossing‡ defects |
	General narrowing A/V ratio*	Focal spasm†					
Normal	3/4	1/1	0	0	0	Fine yellow line, red blood column	0
Grade I	1/2	1/1	0	0	0	Broadened yellow line, red blood column	Mild depression of vein
Grade II	1/3	2/3	0	0	0	Broad yellow line, "copper wire," blood column not visible	Depression or humping of vein
Grade III	1/4	1/3	+	+	0	Broad white line, "silver wire," blood column not visible	*a)* Right-angle deviation, tapering and disappearance of vein under arteriole *b)* Distal dilatation of vein
Grade IV	Fine, fibrous cords	Obliteration of distal flow	+	+	+	Fibrous cords, blood column not visible	Same as grade III

* This is the ratio of arteriolar/venous diameters.
† This is the ratio of diameters of region of spasm to proximal arteriole.
‡ Arteriolar length and tortuosity increases with severity.

retinal arteriolosclerosis is a degenerative process resulting from endothelial and muscular proliferation, and it accurately reflects similar changes in other organs. Sclerotic changes do not develop as rapidly as hypertensive lesions nor do they regress appreciably with therapy. As a consequence of increased wall thickness and rigidity, sclerotic arterioles distort and compress the veins as they cross within their common fibrous sheath, and the reflected light streak from the arterioles is changed by the increased opacity of the vessel wall.

Central-nervous-system dysfunction also occurs frequently in patients with hypertension. Occipital headaches, most often in the morning, are among the most prominent early symptoms of hypertension. Dizziness, lightheadedness, vertigo, tinnitus, and dimmed vision or syncope may also be observed, but the more serious manifestations are due to vascular occlusion or hemorrhage. With severe long-standing hypertension, patients develop multiple focal or large vascular infarcts or hemorrhages which result in destruction of brain tissue. The focal changes may be manifested as personality or memory deficits, but the larger lesions which produce major strokes are responsible for up to 10 to 15 percent of deaths occurring secondary to hypertension.

RENAL EFFECTS. Vascular damage in hypertension also affects the kidneys. Arteriolosclerotic lesions of the afferent and efferent arterioles and the glomerular capillary tufts are the most common renal vascular lesions and result in decreased glomerular filtration rate and tubular dysfunction. Proteinuria and microscopic hematuria occur due to glomerular lesions, and approximately 10 percent of the deaths secondary to hypertension result from renal failure. Blood loss in hypertension occurs not only from renal lesions, but epistaxis, hemoptysis, and metrorrhagia also occur more frequently in these patients.

MALIGNANT HYPERTENSION. Although these complications of hypertension are serious and are often eventually fatal after many years of the disease, a small fraction, variously estimated as between 1 and 5 percent, of patients with essential hypertension enter an accelerated phase which usually results in rapid death. This "malignant" phase of hypertension is associated with very high levels of arterial pressure and characteristic rapidly progressive necrosis of the walls of small arteries and arterioles with concentric collagenous endothelial thickening leading to diminution or occlusion of the vascular lumen. These lesions of arteriolonecrosis result in massive proteinuria, hematuria and rapidly progressive uremia, grade IV retinopathy with papilledema, and cerebral edema with increased intracranial pressure, mental confusion, and seizures. These manifestations progress rapidly over a period of days to weeks and if therapy is not effective, death occurs from uremia or an intracranial vascular accident.

As a consequence of the pathologic changes secondary to the elevated arterial pressure, treatment of patients with systemic hypertension is directed toward lowering pressure in an attempt to halt or reverse the progressive organ damage. In certain instances specific therapy or cure of the primary etiologic factor can be achieved by repair of a stenotic renal artery lesion or coarctation of the aorta, or by removal or functional suppression of a humor which secretes pressor substances. However, because of the unknown etiology of the hypertension in the majority of patients, therapy is directed primarily toward the major physiologic abnormality, i.e., it is designed to lower systemic vascular resistance. Because the sympathetic nervous system plays such an important role in the maintenance of peripheral resistance, many effective antihypertensive drugs act by interfering with the vasoconstrictor impulses mediated by this system (Chap. 276). Although arterial pressure can be reduced in the majority of patients, hypertension is a chronic disease, and a therapeutic program must usually be maintained for the duration of the patient's life.

REFERENCES

Combined Staff Conference: Recent Advances in Hypertension, *Am. J. Med.*, 39:616, 1965.

Freis, E. D.: Hemodynamics of Hypertension, *Physiol. Rev.* 40:27, 1960.

Page, I. H., and J. W. McCubbin: The Physiology of Arterial Hypertension, p. 2163, in W. F. Hamilton (Ed.), "Handbook of Physiology," vol. 3, Washington, D.C., The American Physiological Society, 1965.

Scheie, H. G.: Evaluation of Ophthalmoscopic Changes of Hypertension and Arteriolarsclerosis, A.M.A. Arch. Ophthalmol. 49:117, 1953.

38 COUGH AND HEMOPTYSIS
George W. Wright

COUGH

It is estimated that as much as 100 ml secretion is produced daily by the tracheobronchial mucosa. During the night, especially in older persons whose swallowing reflex is less competent, an added amount of secretion trickles into the trachea from the supralaryngeal region The accumulating secretions are moved, in part directly via the ciliary escalator and in part by the cough mechanism, to the pharynx, where the material is then swallowed or expectorated. In some persons, the volume and character of the secretions are such that the entire quantity can be moved by ciliary action alone, but when the secretions are unusually voluminous or difficult to move, the force of coughing is required to maintain clear air passages Under ordinary circumstances cough is considered to be an integral part of the "normal" act of tracheobronchial cleansing.

Cough, with or without the expulsion of secretions, may be a manifestation of disease. In a manner similar to other "clinical manifestations" which are in reality simply altered patterns of normal function, as for example increased frequency of urination or inappropriate breathlessness, sudden changes in cough pattern may be alarming, but gradual changes tend to be ignored by both patient and physician. A more precise delineation of the normal cough and sputum pattern would improve its clinical usefulness. With the increasing awareness that chronic bronchitis in its severe form is one of the common causes of serious morbidity, quantitative and qualitative cough and sputum patterns have been more extensively studied. The pattern indicative of disease has been more sharply defined, but there is still no agreement as to what is "normal." In a population thought to be healthy and having no experience of cigarette smoking, 23 percent admitted to a daily cough with phlegm, swallowed or expectorated, occurring the first thing in the morning only. Thus, a brief period of cough upon arising from sleep would seem acceptable as a normal pattern for clearing the air passages, even if associated with some phlegm. In contrast, cough, with or without phlegm, occurring *throughout* the day should require sufficient medical examination to exclude abnormal causes.

Like sneezing, cough may be a reflex mechanism. It can be invoked or, to some degree, inhibited voluntarily. It is initiated by stimulation of the mucosa or deeper structures in the larynx, trachea, and major bronchi. The nerve pathways involved are the glossopharyngeal and vagus. Direct stimulation of these nerves or their sensory endings in such places as the external ear, neck, and esophagus may also produce cough. Accumulation of mucus on the surface or inflammation, drying, cooling, and chemical stimulation of the mucosa will initiate this reflex, prompting a desire to cough. Changes in the intramural tension of the bronchi by contraction of smooth muscle or effects of gravity invoked by changes in posture may also play a role in initiating the cough reflex.

MECHANISM OF COUGH. The mechanical train of events leading to the expulsive action of a cough is complex. Combined pressure and cinefluorographic studies suggest the following mechanism. After an inspiration, the laryngeal end of the air tubes is firmly closed, and intrathoracic pressure is raised by an expiratory effort. A sudden release of the closed glottis creates a high gradient of pressure between the intrabronchial gas and that in the pharynx. Rates of air flow as high as 600 liters per minute may occur momentarily. It is believed that this high rate of flow moves secretions along the wall of the tubes. At almost the same moment, as the intratracheal pressure rapidly falls, a bronchial transmural pressure gradient is set up because the intrapulmonary air distal to the smaller bronchi is trapped against a higher resistance in the smaller tubes. This momentarily high transmural pressure produces a transient narrowing, if not complete closure, of the lumen of the trachea and major bronchi. These two events, namely narrowing of the lumen and augmented velocity of air flow, push the foreign material toward the oral pharynx in the same manner that a pea is expelled better from a closely fitting tube than from a loosely fitting one. Expulsion of mucus can occur without preliminary closure of the glottis, as for example through a tracheostomy. Cough is, however, not as effective in the tracheotomized person or in one whose respiratory muscles are weakened.

CAUSES OF COUGH. By far the commonest source of bronchial irritation associated with an abnormal cough pattern is that induced by cigarette smoking. Wynder, Lemon, and Mantel, in a study of the epidemiology of persistent cough, demonstrated that 45 percent of their population who smoked from 1 to 10 cigarettes per day and 70 percent of those who smoked more than 21 cigarettes per day had persistent cough. Expectoration of phlegm occurred in 90 percent of those with persistent cough. To what extent cough is directly related to chemical irritation or to hypersecretion has not been determined, but it can be assumed that both play a role. It is apparent from these observations that the use of cough and phlegm as a meaningful early sign of serious underlying lung disease other than chronic bronchitis is of limited value in those who smoke a pack or more of cigarettes daily. Nevertheless, no person with a chronic cough should ever be dismissed lightly as having a "cigarette cough" even though this is often the case.

In most instances of a rather abrupt change in the cough pattern, as for example that associated with the common cold, pneumonia, or pulmonary embolism and infarction, there are other signs and symptoms sufficiently alarming to bring the patient to a physician. Other diseases which begin less abruptly may have as their sole initial symptom an alteration in the cough pattern, and it is in these situations that particular care must be taken to find the cause of a persistently altered cough pattern. Subtle changes in the cough pattern may be due to tuberculosis, fungus infections, tumors, bronchiectasis, sarcoidosis, and many other diseases. Thorough use of roentgenographic and sputum study techniques as well as bronchoscopy must be resorted to under these conditions.

The great importance of cough and sputum as manifestations of chronic bronchitis are discussed in Chap. 283. Cough occurs in emphysema, where the cough mechanism tends to be ineffective and a low-grade chronic bronchitis often develops.

Cough, for the most part not associated with hypersecretion, may occur in diseases of the heart. Pressure of enlarged chambers and vessels on the vagus nerve may play a role in such coughs. Far more common, however, is the peculiar recurring single cough, at times little more than a "clearing of the throat," which is quite characteristic of mild pulmonary edema. In frank pulmonary edema cough is usually more severe.

As a rule, cough has a protective purpose, but it can also be harmful. Distal bronchial secretions tend to be spread peripherally during cough and may spread disease within the lung. Trauma to the tracheobronchial wall or larynx may lead to bleeding or play a role in the development of infection. The muscular effort involved in coughing is relatively great and may aggravate heart failure in patients who have passive congestion of the lungs.

Ribs may be fractured as the result of cough, and this is a not uncommon cause of severe chest pain. Muscle soreness likewise develops in chronic prolonged cough. The pain induced by these two mechanisms often presents a difficulty in differential diagnosis. During a prolonged paroxysm of cough, the persistent high intra-thoracic pressure may so impede venous return that cardiac output falls and cerebral ischemia occurs. This form of "cough" syncope may be associated with fainting and convulsions. It is most common in the elderly with cerebral arteriosclerosis. Such attacks developing in a person operating a mechanical device may lead to disastrous consequences. Cough may also be harmful in a public-health sense because of its potential for spreading infection.

HEMOPTYSIS

Bleeding from the lungs and major air passages is an important and fairly common medical problem. It is, of course, necessary to ascertain that the blood is actually coming from the tracheobronchial tree and not from the gastrointestinal tract or the nasopharynx. Blood which comes from the lungs is usually bright red, frothy in appearance, and mixed with phlegm. That from the stomach tends to be dark red or brown and mixed with food particles. Blood from actively bleeding gums or nasopharynx is virtually always bright red and as a rule is not frothy. In contrast to the retching and vomiting associated with hematemesis and the clearing of the throat or blowing of the nose associated with nasopharyngeal bleeding, the blood which comes from the lung is almost always associated with coughing or with the sensation that something has come into the back of the throat which requires throat clearing. Vomiting often causes coughing and vice versa, but the sequence of these events helps to determine the source of the blood.

In view of the extraordinary vascularity of the lung, it is remarkable that hemoptysis is not more common. It seems likely that some capillary bleeding may occur periodically within the lungs and may never be brought up to the pharynx, but instead be reabsorbed at its point of origin. Pneumonia, chronic passive congestion of the lungs, and pulmonary infarction frequently are associated with frank hemoptysis. However, emphysema, a disease characterized by actual destruction of the most distal pulmonary vascular components, is associated with hemoptysis only infrequently.

CAUSES OF HEMOPTYSIS. The most common causes of hemoptysis are infections, neoplasms, and cardiovascular disorders, but include many other more uncommon causes such as arteriovenous aneurysm, foreign body, parasites, and broncholith. Thoracic trauma, with or without rib fracture, may also produce hemoptysis. Several studies of the etiology of hemoptysis have been made in large groups of patients. The frequency of the various causes differs according to the source, i.e., whether the study is of a population survey, a general hospital, or a surgical clinic. In some groups the cause remains undetermined in as many as 45 percent of cases even after thorough and prolonged search, while in others, only approximately 10 percent of cases is undiagnosed. In general hospitals, hemoptysis is caused by neoplasms in 5 percent, lower respiratory tract infection in 35 percent, tuberculosis in

10 percent, and cardiovascular disease in 10 percent of patients; the remaining 40 percent are undiagnosed. In more limited populations—especially those related to surgical clinics—the proportions are strikingly different, with neoplasm and lower respiratory tract infection accounting for 75 percent of cases and only 7 or 8 percent remaining undiagnosed.

It is not known with certainty whether or not hard coughing alone can lead to hemoptysis. Chronic bronchitis is the cause of most episodes of severe prolonged cough not associated with disorders such as neoplasms or abscess. In view of the altered mucosa in bronchitis, it is not surprising that bleeding or hemoptysis would occur. In some populations chronic bronchitis probably is the underlying etiology of most episodes of mild hemoptysis.

The sputum in bacterial pneumonia nearly always contains blood at some stage in the course of the disease. In the virus pneumonias bleeding is not nearly so common or profuse. In most pneumonias the sputum seldom resembles pure blood but is mixed with mucopurulent material.

In the early stages of pulmonary tuberculosis hemoptysis may be minor but is often persistent. In the more extensive cavitary forms of the disease a large vessel may erode, producing massive or, rarely, even fatal hemorrhage. Because the blood from a tuberculous cavity may be heavily contaminated with organisms, hemoptysis may be associated with an extensive spread of the disease to other parts of the lung via the bronchial system.

It is estimated that hemoptysis occurs on one or more occasion in virtually all patients with bronchiectasis, and in many this is the most frightening aspect of the disease. Chronic inflammation and erosion of the mucosa in the bronchiectatic area presumably causes the bleeding. Hemoptysis is so common and recurrent in bronchiectasis that patients learn to ignore it.

Lung tumors often first manifest their presence by hemoptysis. Bronchial carcinoma should be suspected as the cause of hemoptysis in any patient with a history of smoking a pack or more of cigarettes daily for 20 or more years. At least 50 percent of bronchial neoplasms lead to hemoptysis. With adenoma of the bronchus bleeding may be very profuse.

Pulmonary infarction is one of the commonest causes of hemoptysis occurring in patients hospitalized for reasons other than lung infection. Pulmonary embolism without infarction is less likely to produce hemoptysis. Pulmonary infarction should be suspected as the cause of hemoptysis (1) whenever there is associated pleural pain without clear evidence of pneumonia, (2) in all patients with congestive heart failure, (3) in the postoperative and posttraumatic states, (4) in all bedridden patients, (5) whenever there are signs of phlebothrombosis, and (6) in patients who have transient elevations of serum bilirubin and lactic dehydrogenase with a normal value for serum transaminase.

Pulmonary vascular congestion secondary to heart disease is a common cause of hemoptysis. This is particularly true in mitral stenosis (Chap. 270) but is less common with other causes of congestive failure. Rarely, hemoptysis occurs in patients with systemic arterial hypertension, presumably due to a rupture of a submucosal artery.

Hemoptysis also occurs in the purpuras and leukemias and has been reported in association with anticoagulant therapy. That it does not occur more commonly when clotting is compromised suggests that spontaneous intermittent small-vessel bleeding in the lung parenchyma may in fact be rather uncommon.

REFERENCES

Committee on Etiology of Chronic Bronchitis, Medical Research Council: Definition and Classification of Chronic Bronchitis, Brit. Med. J. (Lancet), 1:775, 1965.

Committee on Therapy, American Thoracic Society: The Management of Hemoptysis, Am. Rev. Resp. Dis., 93: 471, 1966.

Loudon, R. G., and L. C. Brown: Cough Frequency in Patients with Respiratory Disease, Am. Rev. Resp. Dis., 96:1137, 1967.

——, and G. B. Shaw: Mechanics of Cough in Normal Subjects and in Patients with Obstructive Respiratory Disease, Am. Rev. Resp. Dis., 96:666, 1967.

Salem, H., and D. M. Aviado: Antitussive Drugs, Am. J. Med. Sci., 247:585, 1964.

Wynder, E. L., F. R. Lemon, and N. Mantel: Epidemiology of Persistent Cough, Am. Rev. Resp. Dis., 91:679, 1965.

Section 5

Alterations in Gastrointestinal Function

39 ORAL MANIFESTATIONS OF DISEASE

Paul Goldhaber

DISTURBANCES OF THE TEETH AND DENTAL TISSUES

DEVELOPMENTAL DISTURBANCES. Since tooth structure, unlike bone, does not undergo physiologic remodeling, developmental disturbances severe enough to cause obvious alterations in the morphologic features or integrity of the teeth provide relatively permanent evidence that a systemic disturbance has acted during that particular phase of tooth development.

The most common type of defect is *enamel hypoplasia*, which results from an aberration in enamel formation due to disturbance of those ameloblasts actively secreting enamel matrix. The defects range from deep pits or grooves extending horizontally around the surface of the crown to defective or completely absent incisal edges or occlusal surfaces. The teeth most frequently affected are the permanent central incisors, cuspids, and first molars, the crowns of which develop during the first year of life. The systemic factors most frequently thought to be involved are serious gastrointestinal disturbances and deficiencies of calcium, phosphorus, or vitamins A and B.

Mottled enamel is a form of hypoplasia due to excessive fluoride ingestion. It consists of white spotting of the enamel or, in more severe forms, of pitting, brownish staining, and brittleness. It should be noted that these effects occur at levels of fluoride significantly higher than that recommended for the artificial fluoridation of drinking water in order to prevent dental caries.

Amelogenesis imperfecta is a hereditary condition in which enamel is absent or is thin, brown, and easily fractured. *Dentinogenesis imperfecta*, also hereditary and usually associated with *osteogenesis imperfecta*, affects the dentin rather than the enamel, giving the teeth a characteristic translucence. Because the union between the dentin and enamel is defective, the latter chips easily, exposing the underlying dentin, which rapidly wears down or fractures.

Congenital syphilis may give rise to characteristic "screwdriver" upper central incisors with notched incisal edges (Hutchinson's incisors) and first molars with rough, pitted occlusal surfaces (mulberry molars).

Complete or partial *anodontia* may occur in *hereditary ectodermal dysplasia*, a syndrome characterized by partial or complete absence of sweat glands, defective or absent sebaceous glands, hair follicles, and other ectodermal structures. When some teeth are present, they are usually cone-shaped.

Intrinsic *staining* of the teeth may be due to a number of factors. Erythroblastosis fetalis may give rise to green, brown, or blue coloration due to the deposition of blood pigment in the enamel and dentin of the developing teeth. In teeth which develop after birth, when hemolysis has ceased, the stain does not develop. A yellow-brown discoloration may be caused by the administration of *tetracycline* to infants or to women in the last trimester of pregnancy In cases of *congenital porphyria*, porphyrins are incorporated in the developing teeth, giving rise to a reddish-brown coloration which fluoresces red in ultraviolet light.

ODONTOGENIC TUMORS. The odontogenic tumors are neoplasms derived primarily from the tissues involved in odontogenesis. The *ameloblastoma,* an example of an ectodermally derived tumor, is the most aggressive tumor in the group and may occur at any age. Most frequently, it occurs in the molar-ramus area, originating as a central lesion of bone which gradually grows and expands the bone. Although the tumor may recur following resection, the prognosis is favorable, since the tumor is slow-growing and rarely, if ever, metastasizes. The *odontomas* are mixed tumors derived from both ectoderm and mesoderm which usually form a slow-growing mass composed of numerous structures having a morphologic resemblance to miniature teeth.

DENTAL CARIES, PULPAL AND PERIAPICAL INFECTION, AND SEQUELAE. Dental caries, the principal cause of tooth loss up to the fourth decade of life, is characterized by a bacteria-induced progressive destruction of the mineral and organic components of the outer enamel and underlying dentin. Numerous long-term public health studies have clearly shown that the artificial fluoridation of drinking water supplies to a level of 1 part per million leads to a 50 to 75 percent reduction in the occurrence of dental caries in permanent teeth of children, presumably due to an alteration of the developing enamel crystals during tooth formation which makes them more resistant to acid dissolution.

If the carious lesion progresses unchecked, there is eventual infection of the dental pulp, giving rise to an *acute pulpitis.* During the early stages of pulpitis moderately severe pain may result from thermal changes, particularly cold drinks. It is noteworthy that toothache in persons flying at high altitudes (aerodontalgia) occasionally occurs in persons having early pulpal inflammation or recently filled teeth. The cause of this phenomenon is not known, but in some instances the pain appears to be related to the sinuses rather than the teeth. As more of the pulp becomes involved because of advanced caries, heat or reclining may stimulate the onset of even more severe and continuous pain. At this stage, damage to the pulp is irreversible, and treatment consists either of extraction or thorough removal of the remaining contents of the pulp chamber and root canals followed by sterilization and filling with an inert material (root canal therapy).

If the pulpitis is not treated, infection may spread beyond the apex of the tooth into the periodontal ligament, giving rise to pain on chewing or percussion. The most common manifestation of periapical disease is the *periapical granuloma,* a localized mass of chronic granulation tissue which slowly expands at the expense of the surrounding alveolar bone. The *chronic periapical granuloma* may present the above symptoms or may be asymptomatic. If allowed to persist untreated the periapical granuloma may give rise to a *periapical cyst* or a *periapical abscess*—all three lesions appearing as radiolucent areas on roentgenograms. The acute periapical abscess may extend into the surrounding bone marrow, resulting in an *osteomyelitis.* More frequently, the abscess perforates the cortical plate and, following the path of least resistance, spreads through various tissue spaces, giving rise to cellulitis and bacteremia, or discharges into the oral cavity, into the maxillary sinus, or through the skin.

The symptomatology produced by cellulitis depends on which tissue space is affected. For example, *Ludwig's angina* originates from an infected mandibular molar, involves the submaxillary space, and subsequently extends into the sublingual and submental spaces. Clinically, this is manifested by swelling of the floor of the mouth, elevation of the tongue, and difficulty in swallowing and breathing. With continued swelling, there may be edema of the glottis, necessitating an emergency tracheotomy. Spread of the infection to the parapharyngeal spaces may lead to cavernous sinus thrombosis.

PERIODONTAL DISEASE

After the third decade chronic destructive periodontal disease (*periodontitis*) is responsible for the loss of more teeth than dental caries. It begins as a marginal inflammation of the gingivae (gingivitis), which slowly spreads to involve the underlying alveolar bone and periodontal ligament. As the disease progresses, the alveolar bone is resorbed, resulting in loss of periodontal ligament fiber attachment from the tooth to the bone. The separation of the soft tissue from the tooth surface results in "pocket" formation, the inner aspect of which bleeds readily on probing or spontaneously during chewing. Frank pus sometimes exudes from under the gingival margin, accounting for the use of the now outmoded term "pyorrhea." With continued loss of alveolar bone the involved teeth become mobile. As the periodontal pockets deepen, the pocket orifice may become occluded, leading to the formation of a *periodontal abscess.* The prognosis for teeth with advanced bone loss, extreme mobility, and recurrent abscess formation is usually poor or hopeless, and the usual treatment is extraction.

The most important local etiologic factors associated with this disease are thought to be *poor oral hygiene,* resulting in the accumulation of grossly visible adherent masses of bacteria (*bacterial plaque*), calculus (mineralized bacterial plaque), and food impaction. The margins of overextended fillings also play a role as local irritating factors. Occlusal trauma, particularly due to grinding and clenching habits, may be involved. Therapy is aimed at elimination of these factors and the development of a local environment which can be maintained in health by good oral hygiene.

Systemic factors are thought to modify the response of the host to the local factors, but their nature is more obscure. In some instances, however, there are characteristic alterations in the gingiva in response to a number of specific systemic conditions. For example, during *pregnancy* the gingiva may become edematous and friable with a raspberry-like appearance of the interdental papillae. Occasionally, a tumorlike mass may develop in an interdental area (Plate 5-1); this usually regresses following parturition. The use of the anticonvulsant drug *diphenylhydantoin sodium* (Dilantin) frequently results in fibrous hyperplasia of the gingiva which may actually cover the teeth, interfere with mastication, and cause a serious esthetic problem (Plate 5-2). A similar clinical picture, although usually more generalized and extensive, occurs in *idiopathic familial fibromatosis*. The latter condition appears to be hereditary in nature.

A relatively common gingival disease, found predominantly in young adults in college or the armed forces, is *acute necrotizing ulcerative gingivitis* (Vincent's infection; trench mouth) (Plate 5-3). This disease is characterized by tender or painful gingivae, bleeding on pressure, and the pathognomonic sign of papillary or marginal gingival necrosis and ulceration. Clinical evidence suggests that the etiology of this disease has a psychosomatic component. Unlike *acute herpetic gingivostomatitis*, (Plate 5-4), with which this disease is most frequently confused, in patients with acute necrotizing ulcerative gingivitis fever or malaise rarely develop, and patients respond rapidly to penicillin or broad-spectrum antibiotics.

With regard to the *systemic effects of oral disease* it should be noted that both infected periapical lesions and periodontal disease provide potential sources of infection which may spread to other sites. Transient bacteremias have been demonstrated after simple massage of inflamed gingivae, as well as during tooth extraction. The frequent association of tooth extraction with the subsequent occurrence of subacute bacterial endocarditis has led to the prophylactic use of antibiotics in dental patients with a history of rheumatic fever or other evidence of valvular disease.

DISEASES OF THE JAWS

DEVELOPMENTAL DEFECTS. The most serious and common developmental disturbance of the jaws is *cleft palate* (approximately 1 per 1,000 births), which ordinarily presents as a large continuous defect in the midline of the hard and soft palates connecting the nasal and oral cavities and leads to difficulties in eating, drinking, and speech. In mild cases only the soft palate is involved. In more severe cases, the defect may extend anteriorly and follow the line of fusion to the left or right between the premaxilla and the maxilla, producing, in addition, a cleft of the alveolar ridge between the lateral incisor and cuspid, and a cleft lip (*harelip*). A cleft of the lip may occur without a cleft palate. The former is usually repaired surgically before the patient is one month old. Surgery for cleft palate is ordinarily delayed until the patient is about 1½ years old in order to avoid injury to the growth centers in the maxilla. An obturator may be used to close the defect if the cleft is too large.

GENERALIZED SKELETAL DISTURBANCES. There are many systemic bone diseases which may affect the mandible or maxilla. In *Paget's disease* involvement of the jaw occurs relatively late. It is interesting to note that the classic history of the patient needing to buy hats of larger size has its counterpart in the oral cavity, for patients with dentures may need to have them remade periodically because of progressive enlargement of the jaw, usually the maxilla. *Monostotic fibrous dysplasia* of the jaws develops as a painless swelling of the outer plate of bone

leading to malocclusion due to the displacement of the developing tooth germs. The chief complaints of patients with *eosinophilic granuloma, Letterer-Siwe disease,* or *Hand-Schüller-Christian disease* may include sore mouth, tooth mobility, and malodorous breath. When the involved teeth are extracted, the sockets heal with difficulty.

ENDOCRINE DISTURBANCES. The jaws are most severely affected by endocrine diseases which occur during the period of growth and development. In *cretinism* the jaws are small, and eruption and shedding of the primary teeth are delayed. The effects are less severe in *juvenile myxedema*. The oral manifestation of *adult myxedema* is thickening of the lips and tongue. *Hyperthyroidism* in children leads to premature shedding of the deciduous teeth and accelerated eruption of the permanent teeth. In pituitary dwarfs the small jaws cannot accommodate the teeth, giving rise to malocclusion. In *gigantism* the teeth erupt earlier but are widely spaced because of the large size of the mandible and maxilla, which have a normal relationship. In *acromegaly*, accelerated growth of the mandibular condyle leads to a downward and forward elongation of the mandible with resultant prognathism. The tongue enlarges, and often lateral indentations develop from pressure against the teeth. The first sign of *hyperparathyroidism* may be a giant-cell tumor of the jaw, which may appear radiographically as a cystic area in the maxilla or mandible. These cystlike lesions must be differentiated from periapical cysts due to pulpal infection and from fissural cysts, such as median palatine, nasopalatine, and globulomaxillary cysts, which arise from epithelial cells trapped during the fusion of various developing bones. Other radiographic changes, such as loss of lamina dura and alveolar bone resorption, coupled with loosening of teeth are often related to concomitant advanced periodontal disease rather than to hyperparathyroidism per se (see Chap. 90).

DISEASES OF THE ORAL MUCOSA AND TONGUE

HEMATOLOGIC DISTURBANCES. Oral manifestations are common in both the acute and chronic forms of all types of leukemia, particularly *monocytic leukemia*. They consist of local gingival bleeding, enlargement, and necrosis. Petechiae and ulceration of the oral mucosa may also be evident. Extensive ulcerations of the gingivae, buccal mucosa, lips, soft palate, pharynx, and tonsils may also occur in *agranulocytosis*. In thrombocytopenic states multiple petechiae, ecchymoses, and bleeding gingivae may be observed. The mucous membranes of the oral cavity, including the papillae of the tongue, are atrophic in the *Plummer-Vinson* syndrome (see Chaps. 40, 313). As a result, the tongue is red, smooth, and sore, and there is difficulty in swallowing. Of interest is the finding that the atrophic mucous membranes had a predisposition toward the development of oral carcinoma. The oral symptoms in *pernicious anemia* are similar (see Chap. 337).

VITAMIN DEFICIENCIES. *The oral effects of deficiency of the B group of vitamins* involve the soft tissues primarily, giving rise to reddening and ulceration of the oral

Table 39-1. PIGMENTED LESIONS OF THE ORAL MUCOSA

Condition	Usual location	Clinical features	Course
Black hairy tongue	Dorsum of tongue	Elongation of filiform papillae of tongue, which take on a brown to black coloration.	Long-lasting but may disappear spontaneously.
Heavy metal pigmentation (bismuth, mercury, lead)	Gingival margin	Thin blue-black pigmented line along gingival margin due to prior treatment for syphilis with bismuth or mercury or from accidental absorption of lead.	Long-lasting.
Amalgam tattoo	Gingiva and mucobuccal fold	Small blue-black pigmented areas associated with embedded amalgam particles in soft tissues; these will show up on radiographs as radiopaque particles.	Remains indefinitely.
Fordyce's disease................	Buccal and labial mucosa	Aggregation of numerous, small yellowish spots just beneath mucosal surface; no subjective symptoms.	Remains without apparent change indefinitely.
Addison's disease................	Any area in mouth but mostly on buccal mucosa	Blotches or spots of bluish-black to dark-brown pigmentation occur early in the disease accompanied by diffuse pigmentation of skin; other symptoms of adrenal insufficiency.	Condition controlled by steroid therapy.
Peutz-Jeher syndrome	Any area in mouth	Dark-brown spots on lips, buccal mucosa, and palate with characteristic distribution of pigment around lips, nose, eyes, and on hands; concomitant intestinal polyposis.	Lesions remain indefinitely.
Malignant melanoma	Any area in mouth	The tumor may appear as a raised, painless, brown-black lesion or may be amelanotic; it may be ulcerated and infected.	Early metastasis leads to death.

mucosa and tongue, swelling and burning of the tongue, and fissuring at the corners of the lips (*angular cheilosis*). Severe vitamin C deficiency (*scurvy*) is manifested by petechiae in the oral mucosa; swollen, ulcerated, bleeding gingivae; and loosening of teeth.

PIGMENTATIONS (See Table 39-1). The spread of irregular spots or blotches of brown pigment throughout the oral mucosa, primarily the buccal mucosa, may be the first sign of *Addison's disease*. The pigmentation associated with the *Peutz-Jegher* syndrome is readily differentiated because of its history, characteristic distribution around the lips, eyes, and nostrils, as well as its intraoral distribution. Both *lead poisoning* and *bismuth poisoning* may be manifested by a dark line along the gingival margin, particularly in individuals who have poor oral hygiene. Bismuth poisoning may also demonstrate pigmented patches elsewhere in the oral mucosa.

INFECTIONS. See Tables 39-2 and 39-3 and Chap. 136.

DERMATOLOGIC DISEASES. See Tables 39-2 and 39-3 and Chap. 400.

TONGUE ALTERATIONS. See Table 39-4.

MALODOROUS BREATH. A distinctly unpleasant odor of the breath (halitosis) may emanate from any patient with *infections of the upper respiratory tract*, especially in bronchiectasis and lung abscess. Halitosis may occur with oral sepsis as in *stomatitis, gingivitis*, or extensive *caries*. Some persons who smoke excessively may have halitosis. Occasionally otherwise normal persons will exhibit halitosis without obvious cause. A *fishy odor* of the breath is found in patients with hepatic failure, an *ammoniacal or urinary odor* is found in azotemia, and a *sweet, fruity* odor is typical of diabetic acidosis.

DISEASES OF THE SALIVARY GLANDS

Conditions affecting the salivary glands include mumps parotitis (Chap. 231), Mikulicz's disease (Chap. 386), and Sjögren's syndrome (Chap. 386). Inflammation of the salivary glands (*sialadenitis*) is usually associated with the presence of a salivary stone (*sialolithiasis*) in the duct of one of the major salivary glands. The classic history of pain and swelling of the gland around mealtimes is due to the partial blockage of salivary flow by the stone. Localization of the stone may be accomplished by palpation or by roentgenograms with or without the use of an intraductal injection of radiopaque material (*sialography*).

Xerostomia, or dryness of the mouth, is due to salivary gland dysfunction and may be temporary or permanent. Among the factors which cause temporary dyness are emotional factors (such as fear), infection of the glands, and administration of drugs, such as atropine or antihistamines. Radiation to the area may produce a more permanent xerostomia due to atrophy of the glands. A similar dryness may occur in Sjögren's syndrome.

Table 39-2. VESICULAR, BULLOUS, OR ULCERATIVE LESIONS OF THE ORAL MUCOSA

Condition	Usual location	Clinical features	Course
Viral diseases:			
Acute herpetic gingivostomatitis (herpes simplex)	Lip and oral mucosa	Presence of labial vesicles which rupture and crust, and intraoral vesicles which quickly ulcerate; extremely painful to pressure; acute gingivitis, fever, malaise, foul odor, and cervical lymphadenopathy; occurs primarily in infants and children.	Heals spontaneously in 10–14 days, unless secondarily infected.
Recurrent herpes labialis	Mucocutaneous junction of lip	Eruption of groups of vesicles which may coalesce, then rupture and crust; painful to pressure or spicy foods.	Lasts about 1 week, but condition may be prolonged if secondary infection occurs.
Herpangina (Coxsackie A; also possibly Coxsackie B and ECHO viruses)	Oral mucosa, pharynx, tongue	Sudden onset of fever, sore throat and oropharyngeal vesicles usually in children under 4 years, summer months; diffuse pharyngeal injection and vesicles (1–2 mm), grayish white surrounded by red areola; vesicles enlarge and ulcerate.	Incubation period 2–9 days; fever for 1–4 days; recovery uneventful.
Foot, hand, and mouth disease (Coxsackie A-16)	Oral mucosa, pharynx, palms, and soles	Fever, malaise, headache with oropharyngeal vesicles which become painful, shallow ulcers.	Incubation period 2–18 days; lesions heal spontaneously in 2–4 weeks.
Bacterial or fungous diseases:			
Acute necrotizing ulcerative gingivitis ("trench mouth," Vincent's infection)	Gingiva	Painful, bleeding gingiva characterized by necrosis and ulceration of gingival papillae and margins plus lymphadenopathy and foul odor.	Continued destruction of tissue followed by remission, but may recur.
Primary syphilis (chancre)	Lesion appears where organism enters body; may occur on lips, tongue, or tonsillar area	Small papule develops rapidly into a large, painless ulcer with indurated border; unilateral lymphadenopathy occurs; chancre and lymph nodes contain spirochetes; serologic tests positive by 3d to 4th weeks.	Healing of chancre occurs in 1–2 months, followed by secondary syphilis in 6–8 weeks.
Secondary syphilis	Oral mucosa frequently involved with mucous patches, primarily on palate but also at commissures of mouth	Maculopapular lesions of oral mucosa, about 5–10 mm in diameter with central ulceration covered by grayish membrane; eruptions occur on various mucosal surfaces and skin accompanied by fever, malaise, and sore throat.	Lesions may persist from several weeks to a year.
Tertiary syphilis	Palate and tongue	Gummatous infiltration of palate or tongue followed by ulceration and fibrosis; atrophy of tongue papillae may produce characteristic bald tongue and glossitis.	Gumma may destroy palate, causing complete perforation.
Tuberculosis	Tongue, tonsillar area, soft palate	A solitary, irregular ulcer covered by a persistent exudate; ulcer has an undermined, indurated border.	Lesion may persist.
Histoplasmosis	Any area in mouth, particularly tongue, gingiva, or palate	Numerous small nodules which may ulcerate; hoarseness and dysphagia may occur because of lesions in larynx, usually associated with fever and malaise.	May be fatal.

Table 39-2. VESICULAR, BULLOUS, OR ULCERATIVE LESIONS OF THE ORAL MUCOSA (*continued*)

Condition	Usual location	Clinical features	Course
Dermatologic diseases:			
Mucous membrane pemphigoid..	Primarily mucous membranes of the oral cavity, but may also involve the eyes, urethra, vagina, and rectum	Painful, grayish-white collapsed vesicles or bullae with peripheral erythematous zone; gingival lesions desquamate, leaving ulcerated area.	Protracted course with remissions and exacerbations; involvement of different sites occurs slowly; corticosteroids may control severe cases.
Erythema multiforme..........	Primarily the oral mucosa and skin of hands and feet	Intraoral ruptured bullae surrounded by an inflammatory area; lips may show hemorrhagic crusts; the "iris" or "target" lesion on the skin is pathognomonic; patient may have severe signs of toxicity.	Onset very rapid; condition may last 1–2 weeks; may be fatal.
Pemphigus vulgaris...........	Oral mucosa and skin	Ruptured bullae and ulcerated oral areas; mostly in older adults.	With repeated recurrence of bullae toxicity may lead to cachexia, infection and death within 2 years.
Neoplastic diseases:			
Squamous cell carcinoma	Any area in mouth, most commonly on lower lip, tongue, and floor of mouth	Ulcer with elevated, indurated border; failure to heal, pain not prominent; lesions tend to arise in areas of leukoplakia or in smooth or atrophic tongue.	Invades and destroys underlying tissues or may metastasize to regional lymph nodes.
Acute leukemia	Gingiva	Gingival swelling and superficial ulcerations followed by hyperplasia of gingiva with extensive necrosis and hemorrhage; deep ulcers may occur elsewhere on the mucosa complicated by secondary infection.	Fatal.
Lymphosarcoma	Gingiva, palate, tongue, and tonsillar area	Elevated, ulcerated area which may proliferate rapidly, giving the appearance of a traumatic inflammatory lesion; swelling of regional lymph nodes.	Fatal.
Other Conditions:			
Recurrent aphthous stomatitis ..	Any place on oral mucosa	Single or clusters of painful ulcers found anywhere on mucosa with surrounding erythematous border; lesions may be 10–15 mm in diameter.	Lesions heal in 1–2 weeks but may recur monthly or several times a year.
Traumatic ulcers	Any place on oral mucosa; dentures frequently responsible for ulcers in vestibule	Localized, discrete ulcerated lesion with red border; produced by accidental biting of mucosa, penetration by a foreign object, or chronic irritation by a denture.	Lesion usually heals in 7–10 days when irritant is removed, unless secondarily infected.

ORAL CANCER

Oral cancer constitutes more than 5 percent of all human cancers. *Squamous cell carcinoma* is the most common malignant oral tumor, accounting for approximately 90 to 95 percent of all oral malignant tumors. Of interest is the fact that most of these tumors occur on the lips, primarily the lower lip, rather than intraorally (Plate 5-6). About half of the intraoral tumors involve the tongue, primarily the posterior two-thirds and the lateral borders. The major etiologic factor in lip cancer appears to be exposure to intense sunlight. Predisposing factors for intraoral carcinoma include tobacco (usually in the form of cigar or pipe smoking, or snuff placed in the mucobuccal fold), excessive consumption of alcohol, syphilitic glossitis, and the atrophic mucosa of the Plummer-Vinson syndrome. There is some evidence to suggest that liver disease, particularly cirrhosis, is also important in some types of intraoral carcinoma. Although numerous instances of carcinoma of the tongue adjacent to a sharp tooth or dental appliance have been reported, animal studies with chronic irritation per se, as well as epidemiologic studies, cast doubt on this apparent rela-

Table 39-3. WHITE LESIONS OF ORAL MUCOSA

Condition	Usual location	Clinical features	Course
Pachyderma oris	Any area in mouth	Elevated white lesion due to hyperkeratosis and thickening of the oral epithelium secondary to chronic irritation.	Removal of irritant leads to healing in 2–3 weeks.
Leukoplakia	Any area in mouth	White patch or raised plaque with sharply defined borders; in more severe cases the lesion is indurated and rough, and may be fissured and eroded; pain not present in early lesions.	Carcinoma frequently arises in the more severe type of lesion.
Lichen planus (Plate 5-5)	Any area in mouth but most often on buccal mucosa	Varied appearance of lesion due to arrangement of grayish-white papules which coalesce to make up the pattern; a reticular network is most common; oral lesions may precede skin lesions.	May disappear spontaneously.
Moniliasis (thrush)	Any area in mouth	Creamy white curdlike patches which reveal a raw, bleeding surface when scraped; found in sick infants, debilitated elderly patients, or patients receiving high doses of corticosteroids or broad-spectrum antibiotics.	Responds favorably to antifungal therapy after correction of predisposing causes.
Chemical burns	Any area in mouth	White slough due to necrosis of epithelium and underlying connective tissue caused by contact with agents (e.g., aspirin) applied locally or the use of undiluted sodium perborate or hydrogen peroxide as a mouthwash; removal of slough leaves a raw, painful surface.	Lesion heals in several weeks if not secondarily infected.

tionship. The most common *precancerous lesion* in the oral cavity is *leukoplakia,* which is a whitish patch on the mucosa that histologically shows alterations that include hyperkeratosis, acanthosis, and dyskeratosis. *All chronic ulcerative lesions which fail to heal within 1 to 2 weeks should be considered potentially malignant* and must be biopsied in order to make the definitive diagnosis. It is noteworthy that in their early stages intraoral epidermoid carcinomas are rarely painful, in contrast to similar-appearing inflammatory lesions.

The prognosis for patients with carcinoma of the lip is usually good, since these malignant tumors are noted sooner and apparently metastasize later. On the other hand, patients with carcinoma of the tongue have a poorer prognosis, particularly as the location of the tumor occurs more posteriorly on the tongue. Intraoral carcinomas may spread by direct invasion to the underlying bone. Involvement of nerves, such as the inferior alveolar nerve or mental nerve, may result in numbness or paresthesia of the lower lip on the ipsilateral side. Depending on the site of origin of the intraoral carcinoma, metastases usually spread to the submaxillary or cervical lymph nodes.

NEUROLOGIC DISTURBANCES

A number of neurologic disturbances have a direct effect on oral and paraoral structures. *Trigeminal neu-*

ralgia (tic douloureux) is an example of a syndrome involving the trigeminal nerve. It is characterized by extremely severe, unilateral, lancinating pain of the face occurring spontaneously or set off by pressure on a "trigger zone" on the face. Facial palsy is a unilateral disturbance of the motor branch of the facial nerve due to either trauma, surgical sectioning, or tumor involvement. When it is of acute onset and unknown cause, possibly a localized infection in the nerve, it is called *Bell's palsy.* It may be due to cranial herpes zoster in some instances. The condition is manifested by drooping of the corner of the mouth, inability to close the eye on the same side, and difficulty in speech and eating. In mild cases the symptoms may disappear spontaneously within a month. Alternations in taste sensation in the anterior two-thirds of the tongue due to disturbance of the sensory component of the facial nerve occurs in some cases and indicates a more central location of the lesion in the nerve.

The pain associated with the *glossopharyngeal neuralgia syndrome* is similar in type and intensity to that found in trigeminal neuralgia, being set off by a trigger zone in the pharynx and affecting the posterior region of the tongue, pharynx, soft palate, and ear. Disturbance of the hypoglossal nerve leads to dysfunction of the tongue musculature and atrophy. Bilateral nerve involvement prevents protrusion of the tongue, whereas unilateral involvement leads to deviation of the protruded tongue toward the affected side.

Table 39-4. ALTERATIONS OF THE TONGUE

Type of change	Clinical features
Alterations in size or morphology:	
Macroglossia..............	Enlarged tongue which may be part of a syndrome found in developmental conditions such as Down's syndrome; may be due to tumor (hemangioma or lymphangioma), metabolic disease (such as primary amyloidosis), or endocrine disturbance (such as acromegaly or cretinism).
Fissured ("scrotal") tongue...	Dorsal surface and sides of tongue covered by painless shallow or deep fissures which may collect debris and become irritated.
Median rhomboid glossitis....	Congenital abnormality of tongue with ovoid, denuded area in the median posterior portion of the tongue.
Alterations in color:	
"Geographic" tongue ("wandering rash").......	Asymptomatic inflammatory condition of the tongue, with rapid loss and regrowth of filiform papillae, leading to appearance of denuded red patches "wandering" across the surface of the tongue.
Hairy tongue..............	Elongation of filiform papillae of the medial dorsal surface area due to failure of keratin layer of the papillae to desquamate normally; brownish-black coloration may be due to staining by tobacco, food, or chromogenic organisms.
"Strawberry" and "raspberry" tongue.................	Appearance of tongue during scarlet fever due to the hypertrophy of fungiform papillae plus changes in the filiform papillae.
"Bald" tongue.............	Complete atrophy of papillae which may occur in pernicious anemia, severe iron deficiency anemia, pellagra, or syphilis; may be accompanied by painful, burning sensations.

DISTURBANCES OF THE TEMPOROMANDIBULAR JOINT

Pain in the area of the temporomandibular joint frequently causes the patient to seek therapy. It may be due to posterior displacement of the condyle in the fossa leading to displacement of the meniscus and chronic trauma. *Dislocation of the condyle anteriorly* beyond the articular eminence due to sudden stretching or tearing of the capsular ligament may result in a locking of the mandible in an open position. Reduction of the dislocated jaw may be accomplished by a downward and posterior pressure applied bilaterally intraorally to the buccal surfaces of the mandible in the region of the angle of the jaw. Padding of the thumbs is essential to avoid injury due to the sudden closure of the mandible as it snaps back into position. Condylar fracture should be suspected in patients with pain and swelling in the condylar area and a history of recent facial trauma. In *osteoarthritis* the clinical signs and symptoms may be minimal despite extensive changes in the condyle. Temporomandibular joint involvement occurs less frequently in *rheumatoid arthritis*. When affected the joints are swollen and painful, leading to limitation of movement, particularly on arising in the morning. In children the disease may lead to malocclusion. *Ankylosis* of the joint may occur eventually, necessitating a condylectomy.

The myofascial pain syndrome, the most common disorder of the temporomandibular joint, is characterized by facial pain and mandibular dysfunction. The pain is often localized in the ear or jaw and may extend to the neck and shoulder. The mandibular dysfunction is manifested by limitation of movement, particularly an inability to open to the fullest extent. It is thought that such patients are predisposed to the syndrome because of increased musculature tension and hyperexcitable reflexes related to emotional tension. The precipitating factor appears to be the stretching of an abnormal focus of pain which initiates a self-sustaining pain-spasm-pain cycle. Treatment of the pain-dysfunction syndrome involves the use of drugs to relieve the pain, lessen cortical excitability, and relax the muscles. Local anesthetics are used intramuscularly in the region of the trigger zone or as superficial sprays in an attempt to break the pain-spasm-pain cycle.

REFERENCES

Bhaskar, S. N.: "Synopsis of Oral Pathology," St. Louis, The C. V. Mosby Company, 1965.

Gorlin, R. J., and J. J. Pindborg: "Syndromes of the Head and Neck," New York, McGraw-Hill Book Company, 1964.

Jacobson, F. L. (Ed.): Symposium on Oral Diagnosis and Treatment Planning, Dent. Clinics N. Am., 1963.

McCarthy, P., and G. Shklar: "Diseases of the Oral Mucosa," New York, McGraw-Hill Book Company, 1964.

Maccomb, W. S., and G. H. Fletcher: "Cancer of the Head and Neck," Baltimore, The Williams & Wilkins Company, 1967.

Mitchell, D. F. (Ed.): Symposium on Oral Medicine, Dent. Clinics N. Am., 1968.

Shafer, W. G., M. K. Hine, and B. M. Levy: "A Textbook of Oral Pathology," Philadelphia, W. B. Saunders Company, 1966.

40 DYSPHAGIA
Thomas R. Hendrix

Dysphagia, or difficulty in swallowing, is a most relia-ble symptom and indicates the presence of disease or motor dysfunction. Dysphagia should never be dismissed as an emotional disturbance or be confused with globus hystericus, which is the term used to indicate the sensa-tion of a lump or tightness in the throat independent of swallowing.

The most characteristic manifestation of dysphagia is the sensation of food "sticking" somewhere in its passage to the stomach, usually at the level of the obstructing lesion but sometimes referred to the suprasternal notch, even though the obstruction may be at the lower end of the esophagus. Pain may accompany dysphagia, especially if esophageal spasm is induced by the peristaltic waves attempting to force the bolus through the obstruction. If the pain is mild, it tends to be localized to the site of obstruction; if more severe, it radiates more widely, into the base of the neck, angles of the jaw, arms, epigastrium, or back. Sometimes pain, in a sense, may even cause dysphagia, as when the throat is so sore that swallowing is difficult. For further details regarding these symptoms, see Chap. 313.

Normal swallowing is a complex function dependent upon coordination of voluntary muscular structures of the oropharynx, striated muscles protecting the larynx and respiratory passages, as well as relaxation of the esophag-eal sphincters and the peristaltic wave itself; hence dysphagia may occur as a consequence of derangement or incoordination of any of the elements of the swallowing act as well as narrowing of the lumen by inflammatory stricture or tumor.

For clinical purposes it is useful to separate dysphagia into that of oropharyngeal or esophageal origin, because symptoms, etiology, and treatment are usually different.

OROPHARYNGEAL DYSPHAGIA. Symptoms associated with dysphagia caused by disorders of oropharyngeal structures include aspiration with swallowing, regurgita-tion of fluid into the nose, pharyngeal pain with swallow-ing, and inability of the tongue to move the bolus into the pharynx. Dilatation and atony of pyriform sinuses and pharynx and retention of contrast media in the val-leculae are characteristic radiographic findings in patients with pharyngeal dysfunction. In addition, aspiration of contrast medium into the trachea or regurgitation into the nasopharynx and apparent obstruction at the upper esophageal sphincter (cricopharyngeus) may be found.

Neuromuscular disorders are the most common causes of oropharyngeal dysphagia. Examples of these disorders are cerebral vascular accidents which cause pseudobulbar palsy (see Chap. 21) or bulbar palsy, poliomyelitis, motor system disease, diphtheritic polyneuritis, myasthenia gravis, myotonic dystrophies and restricted muscular dys-trophies (oculopharyngeal and laryngoesophageal), and dermatomyositis. Ulcerative lesions such as pharyngitis, Vincent's angina, monilia stomatitis, viral infections with herpetic lesions, and retropharyngeal abscess interfere by causing pain and thereby inhibiting the initiation of deglu-

tition. Plummer-Vinson syndrome (Paterson-Kelly syn-drome, or sideropenic dysphagia), may also be listed here, since the difficulty in swallowing in this disorder resembles that due to a neuromuscular disorder, although pain may be an additional disturbing feature. Limited pathologic studies have shown both epithelial and muscle atrophy. It is clear that the dysphagia is not due to the character-istic web, or mucosal fold, of the anterior aspect of the cricopharyngeal area, because the web often persists long after the symptoms have been relieved by iron replace-ment.

Oropharyngeal dysphagia may be caused by narrowing of the lumen of the pharynx or upper esophagus by tumor, granulomatous disease, Zenker's diverticulum, or an enlarged thyroid.

ESOPHAGEAL DYSPHAGIA. Symptoms indicating that the cause of dysphagia is to be found in the esophagus range from retrosternal fullness with swallowing to failure of the bolus to pass through the esophagus associated with pain relieved only by regurgitation of the offending bolus. Barium swallows in patients with dysphagia of esophageal origin show segmental narrowing of the eso-phageal lumen, failure of peristalsis, or both. Abnormali-ties of peristalsis may be characterized more precisely by intraluminal manometric studies.

Mechanical narrowing of the esophageal lumen is most frequently caused by carcinoma either of squamous type, arising from the esophagus itself, or adenocarcinoma of the cardia extending up into the esophagus. Rarely, be-nign tumors may reach sufficient size to cause dysphagia. Inflammatory strictures most commonly result from reflux esophagitis but are also caused by ingestion of corrosive substances, such as lye, or by trauma from foreign bodies or instrumentation. In addition, a lower esophageal ring may produce dysphagia by obstructing the esophageal lumen. Extrinsic pressure from aneurysms, vascular anomalies, mediastinal tumors, or paraesophageal dia-phragmatic hernias may compress the esophageal lumen sufficiently to cause dysphagia. Finally, the motility dis-turbances associated with diffuse esophageal spasm, cardiospasm, and esophageal reflux may be the basis of dysphagia. Although esophageal peristalsis is absent in the majority of patients with scleroderma, dysphagia does not become a prominent symptom until reflux esophagitis has led to an inflammatory stricture.

DIFFERENTIAL DIAGNOSIS. Determination of the basic mechanism responsible for dysphagia is usually a simple matter, but identification of the exact disorder responsible for it may be quite difficult. For example, cancer of the esophagus sometimes presents with a sudden rather than gradual onset, and the x-ray may have a smooth, sym-metrical appearance such as is more commonly seen with benign stricture or cardiospasm; even esophagoscopy may be inconclusive, and biopsy may yield deceptive results if the tissue shows only inflammatory reaction and does not include neoplastic cells. Similarly, neuromuscular disorders and disturbances of esophageal motility inter-fering with swallowing may be difficult to classify.

Certain symptoms associated with dysphagia, however, have diagnostic value. Hiccups, together with difficulty in swallowing, suggest a lesion at the terminal portion of the esophagus, such as carcinoma, achalasia, or hiatal hernia. Dysphagia followed after an interval of some duration by hoarseness usually means extension of a malignant growth beyond the walls of the esophagus and the involvement of a recurrent laryngeal nerve. When the hoarseness comes first and the dysphagia later, the primary lesion is almost always in the larynx. This combination of laryngeal and pharyngeal symptoms may also occur in polymyositis or dermatomyositis or with any disease causing bilateral involvement of vagus nerves or nuclei (poliomyelitis and polyneuritis). In motor system disease, the most common cause of a mixture of bulbar and pseudobulbar palsy, dysphagia is usually combined with dysphonia and dysarthria; the jaw jerk is hyperactive and the tongue atrophic. Dysphagia and unilateral wheezing virtually always indicate a mediastinal mass involving the esophagus and a main or large bronchus. Coughing with each swallow of food or drink means a fistulous communication between the esophagus and the trachea. Coughing occurring sometime after swallowing may be due to regurgitation of food, most common in achalasia and Zenker's diverticulum.

DIAGNOSTIC PROCEDURES. Examination of the mouth and pharynx should disclose those lesions the effect of which is to impede the transfer of food from the mouth to the esophagus, because of either pain or mechanical interference. When lesions of the hypopharynx (e.g., *chronic abscess secondary to tuberculosis of the spine*) or of the larynx (e.g., *tuberculosis* or *carcinoma*) are suspected, examination with a mirror is necessary.

The most important diagnostic technique in the evaluation of dysphagia is a barium swallow. It usually makes it possible to determine whether dysphagia is caused by mechanical obstruction or esophageal motor abnormality. Absence of esophageal peristalsis can best be demonstrated by barium swallows with the patient in Trendelenburg's position. If there is no peristalsis, barium will remain in the esophagus until the patient is tilted upright. Since the muscular action of the pharynx is so rapid, it is useful when studying disorders of the pharynx and upper esophagus to record barium swallows cineradiographically. Projection of the film at slow speed permits detection and analysis of abnormalities of pharyngeal function.

If barium swallow shows a lesion within the esophagus or a narrowing of the lumen, esophagoscopy is the most direct method for establishing the nature of the lesion. In addition to inspecting the lesion, biopsies should be taken to differentiate inflammatory from neoplastic lesions. A malignant stricture is not ruled out with certainty, however, if the biopsy shows only normal tissue or chronic inflammation, because tumors invading the esophagus from the cardia often spread beneath the mucosa and may be missed by a superficial biopsy. In such circumstances repeat biopsies or exfoliative cytology would be necessary. Cytologic studies by experienced personnel are very accurate in the diagnosis of esophageal cancer.

Motor abnormalities of the pharynx and esophagus may be suspected by viewing the movement of a swallowed radiopaque bolus by fluoroscopy, but to characterize these abnormalities definitely the motor response of pharynx and esophagus to swallowing must be studied by recording intraluminal pressure from several points simultaneously. Records are best obtained by use of a train of water-filled, perfused catheters connected to external pressure transducers or strain gages. Examination of manometric records of swallows will demonstrate whether the wave is normally propagated over the length of the esophagus, whether the pressure generated by the peristaltic wave is normal and sufficient to propel the bolus, and, finally, whether sphincter relaxation is complete, of adequate duration, and properly coordinated with the peristaltic wave. Combining manometric with cineradiographic techniques has added greatly to our understanding of pharyngoesophageal function.

REFERENCES

Davenport, H. W.: "Physiology of the Digestive Tract," 2d. ed., Chicago, The Year Book Medical Publishers, Inc., 1966.

Ingelfinger, F. J.: The Physiologic Background of Heartburn, Esophagitis, and Cardiospasm, Arch. Intern. Med., 105: 770, 1960.

Siegel, C. I., and T. R. Hendrix: The Clinical Value of Esophageal Motor Studies, Postgrad. Med., 29:505, 1961.

Stevens, M. B., et al.: Aperistalsis of the Esophagus in Patients with Connective-tissue Disorders and Raynaud's Phenomenon, New Engl. J. Med., 270:1218, 1964.

Winans, C. S., and L. D. Harris: Quantitation of Lower Esophageal Sphincter Competence, Gastroenterology, 52: 773, 1966.

Wynder, E. L., and J. H. Fryer: Etiologic Considerations of Plummer-Vinson (Paterson-Kelly) Syndrome, Ann. Intern. Med., 49:1106, 1958.

41 INDIGESTION
Kurt J. Isselbacher and Matthew A. Budd

"Indigestion" is a term frequently used by patients to describe a multitude of symptoms generally appreciated as distress associated with the intake of food. The term is thus nonspecific and may have a different meaning for the patient and the physician. In approaching the patient with indigestion it is important for the physician first to elicit a good description of this complaint. To some patients indigestion refers to a feeling that digestion has not proceeded naturally. There is a sense of abdominal fullness, pressure, or actual pain. Others may use the term to describe heartburn, belching, distension, or flatulence. These complaints will be considered in this chapter. Discussed elsewhere are the closely related but distinct symptoms of dysphagia, nausea and vomiting, and anorexia (Chaps. 40 and 42).

Indigestion may occur as a result of disease of the gastrointestinal tract or in association with pathologic states in other organ systems. As a result of systematic clinical and laboratory study, a definable pathophysiologic process often can be shown to be responsible for the symptoms in a given case of indigestion. Frequently, however, clear etiologic explanations for the patient's complaints of indigestion are not established. Such cases are often designated as "functional indigestion," with a strong implication that psychosomatic factors underlie the complaints. Although it is clear that psychic factors may lead to symptoms of indigestion, the designation of "functional indigestion" is rarely if ever a satisfactory explanation, serving only to rephrase the patient's symptomatology. A psychogenic cause should not be assumed until organic causes of indigestion have been thoroughly excluded.

After having ascertained the patient's definition of indigestion, it is also important to determine (1) the location and duration of the discomfort, (2) the temporal relation of the symptoms to the ingestion of food, and (3) the possible relation of the symptoms to the ingestion of specific types of food (e.g., fatty foods, milk).

PAIN PATTERNS

True visceral abdominal pain as seen in indigestion is mediated over visceral afferent nerves which accompany the abdominal sympathetic pathways (see Chap. 12). Visceral pain is generally described as dull and aching in nature (with a diffuse midline localization) or as fullness or pressure. The location of the discomfort corresponds generally to the segmental level of the affected organ. Abdominal visceral pain can be produced experimentally by artificially increasing pressure in a hollow viscus. Usually this type of pain is the result of distension or exaggerated muscular contraction of a viscus, and it is noteworthy that inflammation lowers the threshold to such stimuli.

The visceral pain of indigestion should be distinguished from the sharp, lateralized, and localized pain patterns seen in many acute abdominal processes involving the peritoneum. In contrast to true visceral pain, this pain is mediated over cerebrospinal afferent nerves. Again it is of a dull, aching type whether from inflammation of the viscera or of peritoneal surfaces.

In view of the diffuse nature of true visceral abdominal pain, the main clue comes from the segmental level of the viscus; in any given segmental region there is no way of determining which of several viscera are the source of it (Table 41-1). The following rules, already given in Chap. 9, are useful: *Substernal pain* of gastrointestinal origin usually arises from disorders in the esophagus or cardia of the stomach. Because pain in this area is frequently of cardiac origin, heart disease must be considered carefully and excluded. *Epigastric pain* is generally of gastric, duodenal, biliary, or pancreatic origin. As the pathologic process in the biliary tract and pancreas becomes more intense, as, for example, in inflammatory states, the pain lateralizes and localizes, e.g., biliary pain to the right upper quadrant and tip of the right scapula and pancreatic pain to the epigastrium, left upper quadrant, and back. *Periumbilical pain* is generally associated

Table 41-1. DISTRIBUTION OF VISCERAL PAIN AND EXAMPLES OF DISORDERS FREQUENTLY INVOLVING THE SPECIFIC ORGAN

Organ	Location of referred pain	Frequent disorders
Esophagus.........	Substernum, epigastrium	Peptic esophagitis, hiatus hernia stricture, carcinoma
Stomach..........	Epigastrium	Gastritis, peptic ulcer, carcinoma
Duodenum (first and second portion...	Epigastrium	Peptic ulcer
Duodenum (third portion, jejunum and ileum).......	Periumbilical	Regional enteritis, lymphona, gastroenteritis (infectious), intestinal obstruction
Gallbladder........	Epigastrium, right upper quadrant, right side of back	Cholelithiasis, cholecystitis
Pancreas..........	Epigastrium, left side of back	Pancreatitis, pancreatic carcinoma
Liver.............	Right upper quadrant	Passive congestion of liver, hepatitis, cirrhosis
Colon.............	Below umbilicus	Ulcerative colitis, carcinoma, partial obstruction

with small-bowel disease. *Pain below the umbilicus* is often of appendiceal, large-bowel, or pelvic origin.

TEMPORAL RELATIONSHIPS OF PAIN AND INDIGESTION

The establishment of the temporal patterns of a patient's complaints often provides useful diagnostic information. First, it is important to ascertain whether the symptoms are *constant* (continually present over extended periods of time), as may occur, for example, with an infiltrating gastric carcinoma, or *intermittent* as in acute gastritis following an alcoholic binge or in association with the use of certain drugs. Symptoms are occasionally *seasonal;* this can occur in peptic ulcer disease where in some patients symptoms may be more prominent in the spring and autumn.

Another important and often diagnostic feature is the relation of pain or indigestion to ingestion of food. This relationship is especially significant or helpful if symptoms occur either during or minutes after the meal or if they occur several hours (4 or more) after eating. *Early postprandial symptoms* may reflect esophageal disease, because they may be associated with disordered swallowing function. In such instances, the distress or other symptoms of indigestion often are experienced substernally. Early postprandial complaints occur also in gastric disorders such as acute gastritis or carcinoma. *Late post-*

prandial indigestion, i.e., that occurring several hours after eating, may reflect failure of the stomach to empty adequately as in pyloric stenosis or gastric atony. It may also be a symptom of duodenal ulcer, in which case it classically occurs several hours after the meal, when the ulcerated mucosa is exposed to acid secretions of the stomach unbuffered by food. Conversely, the relief of pain following food ingestion is also seen in patients with peptic ulcer and is presumably due to the neutralization of the acid by the ingested food. Late postprandial indigestion also may result from the impaired digestive and absorptive processes, as in pancreatic insufficiency. Pain occurring *nocturnally* and with *recumbency* may be seen in patients with hiatus hernia and carcinoma of the pancreas.

FOOD INTOLERANCE

There are a number of situations in which specific foods or types of foods appear to be related to indigestion. Careful documentation of this relationship is sometimes of great help in arriving at an etiologic diagnosis.

Some foods may be poorly tolerated because of their consistency. For example, patients with esophageal stricture or carcinoma may tolerate liquids well, but the ingestion of solids may be associated with discomfort, especially substernal distress (see Chap. 313). Certain foods may be tolerated poorly because the intestinal tract cannot assimilate them adequately. This may occur following the ingestion of fatty foods in patients with pancreatic or biliary tract disease.

Individuals may lack a specific enzyme required for assimilation of a certain nutrient. As an example, patients may lack or have a deficiency of the mucosal enzyme lactase, which catalyzes the hydrolysis of lactose. When lactase deficiency exists on a congenital or acquired basis (e.g., in sprue, ulcerative colitis) (Chap. 316), the ingestion of milk (where the carbohydrate is lactose) results in distension, flatulence, and diarrhea.

There are a number of other conditions or disorders in which specific foods are poorly tolerated. Foods may be poorly tolerated because they initiate *allergic reactions* or exert a deleterious or *toxic effect* on the intestinal tract of susceptible individuals (e.g., gluten in patients with nontropical sprue). Finally certain substances may lead to systemic effects because of biochemical defects which render them particularly hazardous. Examples of this are galactose intolerance in galactosemia (Chap. 112), and branched-chain amino acid intolerance in maple syrup (urine) disease (Chap. 102).

The above mechanisms do not explain the majority of clinical situations in which indigestion is associated with the eating of specific foods. For example, a history of fatty-food intolerance or an inability to eat cabbage, cucumbers, or spicy foods is commonly obtained from patients with indigestion. However, the mechanisms underlying the production of symptoms in these circumstances is still unclear.

ADDITIONAL SYNDROMES COMMONLY DESCRIBED AS INDIGESTION

GASEOUSNESS, FLATULENCE, AEROPHAGIA. There are a number of common clinical syndromes which may be described by the patient as "indigestion" and which appear to be related to the presence of increased quantities of gas in the intestinal tract. The major portion of intraluminal gas represents swallowed air, with a variable quantity produced within the intestinal lumen itself. A degree of air swallowing, or *aerophagia,* is present in normal individuals and can be observed by the radiologist at fluoroscopy. Under certain circumstances, such as chronic anxiety, poor eating habits, or actual intestinal disease itself, aerophagia may increase in magnitude and lead to symptoms in its own right.

Early postprandial fullness and pressure, relieved by eructation and accompanied by a large amount of air seen on x-ray in the gastric fundus, is often referred to as the *magenblase* (i.e., gastric bubble) *syndrome.* Acute gastric distension by swallowed air can occasionally produce sharp pains which may mimic angina pectoris. This sequence of events may be especially perplexing in older patients with coronary artery disease, because it is well recognized that true angina pectoris may itself be precipitated by the ingestion of a large meal. Fatty meals delay gastric emptying and hence the passage of swallowed air down the intestine. This relationship may explain, in part, the prolonged sense of fullness and eructations experienced by many individuals after a fatty meal.

Swallowed air that is not eructated passes on in the intestinal tract and may either produce diffuse abdominal distension or become trapped in the splenic flexure of the colon. Distension of this segment of the colon produces a sensation of left upper quadrant fullness and pressure with radiation to the left side of the chest. This is known as the *splenic flexure syndrome.* Patients will often describe relief of pain with defecation or with the expulsion of flatus. Diagnosis may be made by demonstrating, on physical examination, a note of increased tympany in the extreme left lateral portion of the upper abdomen or by the visualization of large amounts of air in the splenic flexure of the colon by radiography.

A second major source of intestinal gas is that produced within the lumen by fermentative action of bacteria on carbohydrates and proteins. Increased amounts of intraluminal gas production due to this mechanism have been demonstrated in conditions associated with abnormal bacterial colonization of the small intestine and in patients with carbohydrate malabsorption.

Increased gas production has also been shown to occur following the ingestion of certain foods (e.g., the legumes) which contain significant quantities of nonabsorbable sugars. As in the case of swallowed air, increased amounts of intraluminally produced gas can produce symptoms by causing distension, pain, increased motility (with diarrhea), or flatulence.

HEARTBURN. Heartburn, or pyrosis, is a sensation of warmth or burning located substernally or high in the epigastrium. Experimental studies in human beings have shown that esophageal distension or increased motor activity is associated in most subjects with a feeling of fullness and burning in this area.

Heartburn may occur with organic disease of the intestinal tract and is usually associated with gastroesophageal reflux. This is frequently the case in hiatus hernia. In this setting, heartburn occurs after a large meal or with stooping or bending. Esophageal reflux of acid contents at these times leads to symptoms by either the production of abnormal motor activity or direct mucosal irritation (i.e., esophagitis). Heartburn may also be seen in the absense of a demonstrable anatomic or motor pathologic condition, in which case it is frequently accompanied by aerophagia and for lack of other explanation is often attributed to psychologic factors.

INDIGESTION DUE TO DISEASE OUTSIDE THE INTESTINAL TRACT

A multitude of extraintestinal disease processes may result in indigestion by mechanisms which are poorly understood. Indigestion may be the presenting complaint, for example, in congestive heart failure, uremia, pulmonary tuberculosis, and neoplastic disease. Under these circumstances the symptoms of indigestion may present with no unique features to suggest that they are in fact due to some other systemic disease process.

DIAGNOSTIC APPROACH TO THE PATIENT WITH INDIGESTION

Indigestion represents a challenging and difficult diagnostic problem because of the nonspecific nature of its manifestations. The evaluation of indigestion must include initially a thorough medical work-up, with ultimate confirmation or exclusion of pathophysiologic derangements by the appropriate diagnostic procedures.

A careful history should include an assessment of the patient's general medical health, including the possibility of diseases in extraintestinal organ systems which may produce indigestion. Careful evaluation of psychologic factors is crucial, because they often play an etiologic or contributory role in the patient's problem. Of particular importance is the presence of anxiety, depressive reactions, and hysteria (Chaps. 369 and 370). Evaluation of the patient's intestinal problem must include an assessment of his nutritional status, changes in weight, and appetite.

A clear and detailed description of the specific symptoms should be obtained, particularly the patient's definition of the term "indigestion." The nature of the pain or its frequency and time of occurrence, its relationship to meals, and the special circumstances which lead to its exacerbation or relief should be elicited. Associated intestinal symptoms such as nausea and vomiting, abnormal bowel habits, steatorrhea, diarrhea, and melena should also be sought. Physical examination rarely establishes

the specific diagnosis, but it may be useful in detecting disease in other organ systems (for example, congestive heart failure) which can affect intestinal physiology.

X-ray examination of the alimentary tract is crucial to the evaluation of the patient with indigestion. This may involve examination of the esophagus, stomach, small intestine, colon, and biliary tract. Esophagoscopy, gastroscopy or sigmoidoscopy also may be helpful or necessary. Stools should be examined for appearance, occult blood, fat, and muscle fibers. As stated above, careful attempts must be made to exclude nonintestinal disease, especially cardiac disease.

Unfortunately, even after completion of careful diagnostic studies many cases of indigestion will turn out to have no clear explanation. Some of these are psychogenic and may respond to appropriate psychiatric measures. Others represent physiologic derangements which are undetectable by currently available diagnostic methods. Still others represent actual disease processes in early stages which may be diagnosable by conventional methods at a later date. The ultimate evaluation of indigestion requires, therefore, the utmost in sensitivity, diligence, and patience on the part of the examining physician.

REFERENCES

Calloway, D. H.: Respiratory Hydrogen and Methane as Affected by Consumption of Gas Forming Foods, Gastroenterology, 51:383, 1966.
Coghill, N. F.: Dyspepsia, Brit. Med. J., 4:97, 1967.
Jones, C. M.: Digestive Tract Pain, New York, The Macmillan Company, 1938.
Levitt, M. D., and F. J. Ingelfinger: Hydrogen and Methane Production in Man, Ann. N.Y. Acad. Sci., 150:75, 1968.
Pollock, J. H.: "Gaseous Digestive Conditions," Springfield, Ill., Charles C Thomas, Publisher, 1958.
Smith, L. A.: Pattern of Pain in Diagnosis of Upper Abdominal Disorders, J.A.M.A., 156:1568, 1954.

42 ANOREXIA, NAUSEA, AND VOMITING

Kurt J. Isselbacher and Matthew A. Budd

Energy balance in man represents a sensitive coordination and balance between food intake on one hand and work, heat production, and stored energy on the other. Physiologically this balance involves two related phases: a short-term set of mechanisms responsive to the daily changes in energy requirements and long-term mechanisms responsible for the regulation of metabolic reserves and body composition. Energy regulation involves a complex array of neural and chemical stimuli, as yet incompletely understood, which appear to be integrated, at the hypothalamic level, into two centers: a lateral hypothalamic one which initiates feeding and is referred to as the "feeding center" and a medial center resulting in the sensation of satiety and cessation of feeding after a meal has been taken.

Hyperorexia refers to the ingestion of food in excess of metabolic needs and may occur for a variety of neurologic, endocrinologic, and psychologic reasons. *Bulimia* is an extreme form of hyperorexia in which the patient's hunger recurs shortly after eating, resulting in the consumption of frequent large meals throughout the day and night. Such behavior is seen with hypothalamic lesions or in mentally disturbed persons. *Parorexia* describes an appetite for unusual foods and is not strictly concerned with the hunger mechanism. Such behavior may characterize diseases producing metabolic derangements (e.g., Addison's disease) or may be seen in the mentally disturbed.

ANOREXIA

Anorexia, or loss of the desire to eat, is a prominent symptom in a wide variety of intestinal and extraintestinal disorders. It must be clearly differentiated from satiety and from specific food intolerance. Anorexia occurs in many disorders and as a result *by itself is of little specific diagnostic value*. The mechanisms whereby hunger and appetite are modified in various disease states are poorly understood.

Anorexia is commonly seen in diseases of the gastrointestinal tract and liver. For example, it may precede the appearance of jaundice in hepatitis, or it may be a prominent symptom in gastric carcinoma. In the setting of intestinal disease, anorexia should be clearly differentiated from *sitophobia*, or fear of eating because of subsequent or associated discomfort. In such circumstances, appetite may persist, but the ingestion of food is curtailed nonetheless. Sitophobia may be seen, for example, in regional enteritis (especially with partial obstruction) or in patients with gastric ulcer following partial or total gastrectomy.

Anorexia may also be a prominent feature of severe extraintestinal diseases. For example, anorexia may be profound in severe congestive heart failure and contribute significantly to the cachexia in these patients. It may be a major symptom in patients with uremia, pulmonary failure, and various endocrinopathies (e.g., hyperparathyroidism (Addison's disease, and panhypopituitarism). While a frequent accompaniment of organic disease, it is often seen with psychogenic disturbances, such as anxiety or depression.

ANOREXIA NERVOSA

This disease may assume such severe proportions as to be life-threatening. Anorexia nervosa, as the syndrome is called because of present-day attribution to psychogenic factors, is characterized initially by voluntary and marked reduction in the intake of food, leading to malnutrition. Severe caloric restriction in these patients may result in weight loss amounting to as much as 50 percent of the normal body weight and profound deficiencies of essential vitamins and minerals. Death from starvation may result. The disease is seen predominantly in women, although men are also affected occasionally. It generally occurs in early adulthood but can be seen even earlier.

The major clinical feature of anorexia nervosa is profound weight loss in a person with no other signs of demonstrable organic illness. Some patients relate that they experience severe hunger which they consciously curb in the beginning of the illness in order to lose weight. Others complain of a profound loss of appetite. Once anorexia becomes severe, peculiar habits in connection with food may be seen, the main purpose of which is to limit food ingestion which causes distress. Patients may hide or surreptitiously dispose of food; alternatively they may induce emesis or catharsis by a variety of methods. Patients with anorexia nervosa generally demonstrate strength and tolerance for physical activity which is remarkably great in light of their impaired nutritional state. This contrasts with certain endocrine or neoplastic diseases which cause marked weight loss. Only as the degree of malnutrition becomes extreme does weakness become pronounced.

Anorexia nervosa may be a manifestation of a variety of mental disorders and psychiatric diseases. Most often it occurs in adolescents with excessive concern about obesity and physical appearance. These are the most difficult problems of all, and it is to this group that the term anorexia nervosa applies. Occasionally it may be a prominent symptom in hysteria, as a somatic abnormality, and obsessive patients may adhere to ritualistic diets in pursuit of slimness. The severely depressed patient may lose his interest in food, and the psychotic individual may develop delusions about the dangers of eating.

Clinical examination of the patient with anorexia nervosa reveals emaciation, often of extreme degree. There may be signs of vitamin deficiencies as well as caloric undernutrition. The blood pressure, basal metabolic rate, and body temperature may be subnormal. There is neither increased skin pigmentation nor abnormalities in hair distribution; specifically, there is no loss of pubic axillary hair. Mental status surveys usually elicit none of the typical features of hysteria, obsessive-compulsive or phobic neuroses, or depression.

Laboratory tests are of value primarily to aid in the exclusion of systemic diseases which might account for extreme weight loss, such as carcinomatosis, diabetes mellitus, and intestinal malabsorption. However, when the underlying organic disease is subtle and not readily diagnosed by history, physical examination, or laboratory tests, the patient may be prematurely and hence incorrectly labeled as having anorexia nervosa. This is frequently the case in regional enteritis, especially that occurring in childhood and adolescence. It is obviously essential to explore fully all possibilities of underlying organic disease before making a diagnosis of anorexia nervosa.

In the differential diagnosis, anorexia nervosa must be distinguished from panhypopituitarism. There is, however, only a superficial resemblance between these two conditions. While amenorrhea may occur in both diseases, in anorexia nervosa hair distribution, breast tissue, as well as thyroid and adrenal function remain normal until the terminal stages of the disease. In addition, strength and tolerance for exercise are much greater in anorexia nervosa than in panhypopituitarism.

In extreme cases of anorexia nervosa, it may be necessary to give nutriments by nasogastric tube or parenterally in order to sustain life. However, since anorexia nervosa often is accompanied by psychologic conflicts, optimal management includes resolution of the patient's peculiar ideas about food. In some patients a period of anorexia nervosa will terminate spontaneously, even in the absence of psychotherapy. However, in these individuals basic conflicts remain unresolved, and a relapse or other evidence of maladjustment is likely to occur at a later date.

NAUSEA AND VOMITING

Nausea and vomiting may occur independently of one another, but generally they are so closely allied that they can conveniently be considered together. *Nausea* denotes the feeling of the imminent desire to vomit, usually referred to the throat or epigastrium. *Vomiting* refers to the forceful oral expulsion of intestinal contents, while *retching* denotes the labored rhythmic respiratory activity that frequently precedes emesis. Extremely forceful *projectile vomiting* is a special form of vomiting which has significance because it connotes the presence of increased intracranial pressure.

Nausea often precedes or accompanies vomiting. It is usually associated with diminished functional activity of the stomach and alterations of the motility of the duodenum and small intestine. Accompanying severe nausea there is often evidence of altered autonomic (especially parasympathetic) activity: pallor of the skin, increased perspiration, salivation, and the occasional association of hypotension and bradycardia (vasovagal syndrome). Anorexia is also often present.

Following a period of nausea and a brief interval of retching, a sequence of involuntary visceral and somatic motor events occurs resulting in emesis. The stomach plays a relatively passive role in the vomiting process, the major ejection force being provided by the abdominal musculature. With relaxation of the gastric fundus and gastroesophageal sphincter, a sharp increase in intraabdominal pressure is brought about by forceful contraction of the diaphragm and abdominal wall. This, together with concomitant annular contraction of the gastric pylorus, results in the expulsion of gastric contents into the esophagus. Increased intrathoracic pressure results in the further movement of esophageal contents into the mouth. Reversal of the normal direction of esophageal peristalsis may play a role in this process. Reflex elevation of the soft palate during the vomiting act prevents the entry of the material into the nasopharynx, whereas reflex closure of the glottis and inhibition of respiration helps to prevent pulmonary aspiration.

Repeated emesis may have deleterious effects in a number of different ways. The process of vomiting itself may lead to traumatic rupture or tearing in the region of the cardioesophageal junction resulting in massive hematemesis, the so-called Mallory-Weiss syndrome. Prolonged vomiting may lead to dehydration and the loss of gastric secretions (especially hydrochloric acid) to metabolic alkalosis with hypokalemia. Finally, in states of central nervous system depression (coma, etc.), gastric contents may be aspirated into the lungs with a resulting aspiration pneumonitis.

VOMITING MECHANISM. The act of vomiting is under the control of two functionally distinct medullary centers: the *vomiting center* and the *chemoreceptor trigger zone*. The vomiting center controls and integrates the actual act of emesis. It receives afferent stimuli from the intestinal tract and other parts of the body, from higher cortical centers, especially the labyrinthine apparatus, and from the chemoreceptor trigger zone. The important efferent pathways in vomiting are the phrenic nerves (to the diaphragm), the spinal nerves (to the abdominal musculature), and visceral efferent nerves (to the stomach and esophagus).

The chemoreceptor trigger zone is also located in the medulla but by itself is incapable of mediating the act of vomiting. Activation of this zone results in efferent impulses to the medullary vomiting center, which in turn initiates the act of emesis. The chemoreceptor trigger zone can be activated by many stimuli including drugs such as apomorphine, cardiac glycosides, and ergot alkaloids. Certain of the phenothiazine derivatives appear to antagonize the effects of the above-mentioned drugs on the chemoreceptor trigger zone.

CLINICAL CLASSIFICATION. Nausea and vomiting are common manifestations or organic and functional disorders. The precise mechanisms triggering vomiting in the various clinical states are poorly understood, making classification of mechanisms difficult. The categories mentioned below serve to illustrate some of the many disorders which can be accompanied by nausea and vomiting.

Acute Abdominal Emergencies. Many of the disorders in this category which lead to the "surgical abdomen" are associated with nausea and vomiting. Notably, vomiting may be seen with inflammation of a viscus as in acute appendicitis or acute cholecystitis, obstruction of the intestine, or acute peritonitis (see Chap. 12).

Chronic Indigestion. In many of the disorders falling in this category (see Chap. 41) nausea and vomiting may be prominent. Emesis may be either spontaneous or self-induced and may lead to relief of symptoms, as, for example, in uncomplicated peptic ulcer. Nausea and vomiting may accompany the distension and pain seen in the aerophagic syndromes. Often in patients with chronic indigestion, nausea and vomiting may be provoked by specific foods (e.g., fatty foods) for reasons that are poorly understood.

Acute Infectious Disease. Acute systemic infections with fever, especially in young children, are frequently accompanied by vomiting and often severe diarrhea. The mechanism whereby infections remote from the gastrointestinal tract produce these manifestations is unclear. Viral, bacterial, and parasitic infections of the intestinal tract may be associated with severe nausea and vomiting, often with diarrhea. Severe nausea and vomiting may be prominent in viral hepatitis, even before the appearance of jaundice.

Disorders of the Nervous System. Central nervous system disorders which lead to increased intracranial pressure may be accompanied by vomiting, often projectile. Brain swelling due to inflammation, anorexia, acute hydrocephalus, neoplasms, etc., may thus be complicated by vomiting. Disorders of the labyrinthine apparatus and its central connections which underlie vertigo may be accompanied by vomiting with nausea and retching. Acute labyrinthitis and Ménière's disease are examples of such disturbances. Migraine headaches, tabetic crises, and acute meningitis are additional examples of disorders of the nervous system which can lead to vomiting. In the reactive phase of hypotension with syncope, there may be nausea and vomiting.

Diseases of the Heart. Severe nausea and vomiting may be present in acute myocardial infarction, especially of the posterior wall of the heart. Nausea and vomiting may also be seen in congestive heart failure, perhaps related to congestion of the liver. The possibility that these symptoms may be due to drugs (e.g., opiates or digitalis) should always be borne in mind in patients with cardiac disease.

Metabolic and Endocrine Disorders. Nausea and vomiting commonly accompany several endocrinologic disorders, including diabetic acidosis and adrenal insufficiency, especially adrenal crises. The morning sickness of early pregnancy is another instance of nausea and vomiting possibly related to hormonal changes.

Drugs and Chemicals. The side effects of many drugs and chemicals include nausea and vomiting. In some instances this is due to gastric irritation which stimulates the medullary vomiting center.

Psychogenic Vomiting. This term is applied to the vomiting which may occur as part of any emotional upset on a transitory basis or more persistently as part of a psychic disturbance. Close observation will usually disclose the condition to be one of regurgitation rather than of vomiting, and weight loss may not correspond at all to patients' description of the frequency and severity of vomiting. As discussed earlier in this chapter, anorexia nervosa is an emotional disturbance which may be associated not only with anorexia but also with vomiting. Often patients with emotional disorders and vomiting maintain a relatively normal state of nutrition, because a relatively small amount of the ingested food is vomited.

DIFFERENTIAL DIAGNOSIS. Vomiting should be distinguished from *regurgitation*, which refers to the expulsion of food in the absence of nausea and without the abdominal diaphragmatic muscular contraction which is a part of vomiting. Regurgitation of esophageal contents may occur with esophageal stricture or diverticula. Regurgitation of gastric contents is generally seen with gastroesophageal sphincter incompetence, especially with hiatus hernia or in association with peptic ulcer usually when pylorospasm supervenes.

The temporal relationships of vomiting to eating may be of help diagnostically. Vomiting which occurs predominantly in the morning is often seen early in pregnancy and in uremia. Alcoholic gastritis is commonly accompanied by early morning emesis, the so-called "dry heaves." Vomiting which occurs shortly after eating may suggest pylorospasm or gastritis. On the other hand, vomiting which occurs 4 to 6 hours or longer after eating and involves the elimination of large quantities of undigested food often indicates gastric retention (as in diabetic gastric atony or pyloric obstruction).

The character of the vomitus offers clues to the diagnosis. If the vomitus contains free hydrochloric acid, the obstruction may be due to an ulcer; absence of free hydrochloric is more compatible with gastric malignancy. A feculent or putrid odor reflects the results of bacterial action on the intestinal contents. Such vomiting may be seen with low-intestinal obstruction, peritonitis, or gastrocolic fistula. Bile is commonly present in gastric contents whenever vomiting is prolonged. It has no significance unless constantly present in large quantities, when it may signify an obstructive lesion below the ampulla of Vater. The presence of blood in the gastric contents usually denotes bleeding from the esophagus, stomach, or duodenum.

REFERENCES

Anand, B. K.: Nervous Regulation of Food Intake, Physiol. Rev., 41:677, 1961.

Bliss, E. L., and C. H. H. Branch: "Anorexia Nervosa," New York, Hoeber Medical Division, Harper & Row, Publishers, Incorporated, 1960.

Borison, H. L., and S. C. Wang: Physiology and Pharmacology of Vomiting, Pharmacol. Rev., 5:19, 1953.

Mayer, J.: General Characteristics of the Regulation of Food Intake, chap. I, in "Alimentary Canal," vol. I, Washington, D.C., American Physiological Society, 1967.

43 CONSTIPATION, DIARRHEA, AND DISTURBANCES OF ANORECTAL FUNCTION

Albert I. Mendeloff

NORMAL COLONIC FUNCTION

MOTOR AND ABSORPTIVE FUNCTIONS. When one considers that a north-woods lumberjack may consume several kilograms of foodstuffs per day, furnishing him nearly 6000 Cal, and yet produce a stool which weighs only 100 to 200 Gm, of which nearly three-quarters is water, the efficiency of the gut becomes clearly evident. Just as slight changes in renal function may result in the excretion of abnormal amounts of urine, so relatively minor deviations in the absorption of water, in intestinal tone, in propulsive motility, or in rectal sensitivity may result in dramatic changes in the caliber and consistency of the stools.

On a normal mixed diet the stomach is nearly empty several hours after food is ingested. By the time the head of the food column reaches the ileocecal valve, 99 percent of the carbohydrate, 99 percent of the protein, and 97 percent of the fats have been broken down into absorbable form and entered the portal venules and the lacteals.

When the intestinal bolus reaches the terminal ileum, it proceeds very sluggishly unless the stomach empties; the so-called "gastroileal reflex" causes the ileum to empty into the cecum by a rapid series of small squirts. The ileocecal valve can probably function as a true sphincter, slowing down the entry of ileal contents into the cecum, but it also serves to prevent reflux, at least of gas, from cecum into ileum. The ileal volume reaching the cecum daily is about 600 ml, a slurry thoroughly churned in the right colon by segmental contractions of the haustra. Every now and then a coordinated wave involving a short length of colon pushes the soggy mass along into the next area; reflexes brought on by eating activate an occasional massive contraction; this empties a sizable area of right and transverse colon of its contents, which then are packed into the left colon. Defecatory reflexes originate from the rectal walls, which normally are approximated around a small lumen empty of feces; when sigmoid contraction distends the rectal musculature, the defecatory reflex center in the sacral cord causes an increase in intraabdominal pressure through descent of the diaphragm, closure of the glottis, contraction of the abdominal wall musculature, and tensing of the pelvic floor. The later descent of the pelvic floor and the inhibition of tone of the external anal sphincter complete the skeletal muscular phase of defecation. Central nervous system impulses simultaneously engage sacral parasympathetic nerves to contract the smooth muscle of the pelvic colon. However, if the external sphincter is voluntarily contracted, the sigmoid colon relaxes, and the fecal mass slips back up into the rectosigmoid.

INNERVATION. The colon and rectum are supplied with both sympathetic and parasympathetic nerves carrying both sensory and motor fibers. Sympathetic elements from the lower six thoracic segments travel to the right colon via the superior mesenteric plexus; the left colon receives sympathetic fibers originating in the lumbar segments of the cord gathered into the inferior mesenteric plexus, branches of which follow the inferior mesenteric artery. The rectum receives sympathetic innervation from the hypogastric or presacral nerve. Parasympathetic cholinergic fibers to the right colon are assumed to be part of the vagus, passing through the celiac plexus. The left colon and rectum receive all their parasympathetic innervation via the nervi erigentes, originating in the sacral nerves and joining the sympathetic fibers in the pelvic plexuses, from which some accompany the inferior mesenteric artery. The anus and external anal sphincter are supplied by the inferior hemorrhoidal branch of the internal pudendal nerve and by the perineal branches of the fourth sacral nerves, which nerves also innervate the levatores ani. Sensory nerves from the skin and mucous membrane of the anal canal are plentiful and go to the sacral cord.

The functional significance of the sympathetic supply to the lower bowel is unclear. Careful studies in man following dorsolumbar sympathectomy have failed to reveal any consistent dysfunction of colon or rectum. Attempts to relieve colon pain syndromes by presacral neurectomy have been unavailing. The parasympathetic cholinergic innervation of the colon seems to be of sole importance in the motor and secretory functions of that organ; cholinergic drugs correspondingly activate such functions and result, when large enough dosages are employed, in watery diarrhea, cramps, and pain.

The mechanism of defecation has been previously described, and the important contribution of the abdominal musculature, the levatores ani, and the external anal sphincter noted. The internal anal sphincter, a smooth muscle, relaxes when the rectum is distended and seems to help allow gas to escape without full defecatory movements. Sensory innervation of the anal canal permits the brain to discriminate as to whether rectal contents are liquid, gaseous, or solid.

CONTINENCE AND INCONTINENCE

The defecation reflex depends upon the presence of a neuroreceptor system beginning in the smooth muscle of the upper rectum. When its tension reaches a threshold, this musculature contracts, joining and augmenting an entire complex of abdominal wall contraction, internal anal sphincter relaxation, and opening of the external anal sphincter. The reflex is believed to be further augmented by the anal sensation of feces passing though the anal canal, and perhaps also by associated reflexes like that of micturition. The central representation of defecation lies, in experimental animals, in the medulla near the vomiting center, and it may be transiently disturbed in many vascular insults to the brain. Voluntary inhibition of defecation, described earlier, is mediated through rapid relaxation of the abdominal musculature and the contraction of the external anal sphincter.

This sequence of events can take place in persons whose sacral cord has been destroyed—i.e., all its elements can function in the absence of an intact peripheral nerve supply—but the strength of such a denervated contraction is weak, and evacuation is generally incomplete unless laxation, usually by enema, reenforces the reflex. Cord transection abolishes the cerebral appreciation of the urge to defecate. Thus disease or trauma to the higher spinal cord and the brain can produce in the function of colon and rectum the same range of disturbances of function as occur in the bladder (see Chap. 49). The colon may become hypotonic, the external sphincter ineffective, and the defecatory reflexes dulled; the levatores ani are often weak and the abdominal musculature unable to produce and sustain effective pressure increases.

The inability to appreciate anal sensation, whether due to central disease, peripheral neuritis of sacral nerves, or surgical interruption of anal innervation, as in treatment of hemorrhoids and perirectal abscess, may also weaken the responses and is often particularly troublesome when the stool is semisolid or liquid. The "sensing" of the consistency of rectal contents by anal receptors has been demonstrated only recently; it provides some explanation for the unpleasant fact that many surgical repairs of the anorectal area look anatomically excellent but the patient is incontinent of any fecal material other than a hard dry stool.

Sudden interruption of function of the central nervous system, as by cerebral vascular accident, interferes with this whole defecatory complex at many levels, and usually results in fecal incontinence of some degree. The dysfunction is maximal at the onset of the process and generally returns toward normal over a period of weeks. In most forms of neurologic disease resulting in incontinence, the reflex may be satisfactorily activated by rectal distension, most practically produced by a combination of aperients and enemas, which results in a mass movement in the more proximal bowel, augmenting the reflex evacuation from the rectum. As sensation from the anal area returns, the passage of stool through the anus reenforces the reflex. Since the bowel is filled infrequently, and irrigation techniques are generally effective and not dangerous, fecal incontinence in such patients is usually much less troublesome than is urinary incontinence. Fecal impactions may be prevented by regularly administered enemas, control of diet, use of drugs, and regular exercises for strengthening the voluntary anal muscles.

DISORDERED BOWEL FUNCTION

SYMPTOMS. Exaggerations of the motor components of normal gastrointestinal activity constitute the most important early symptoms of gastrointestinal diseases. In the small intestine rapid propulsive motility may be associated with dyssynergy, the combination giving rise to cramping contractions. Because of the rather imprecise character of man's system for the detection and recognition of the sources of visceral pain, these cramps are usually projected to the midline—if they originate in the duodenum, to the epigastrium; if from the jejunum, to the umbilicus; if from the lower ileum, to the area just below the umbilicus. In the colon, dyssynergic activity is rarely projected to the midline but usually is lateralized along the general course of the offending organ. Since the colon is large, festooning the abdomen, and full of fluid and partially compressible gas, contractions in one or another area of the bowl may force the contents back toward the cecum; a simultaneous dyssynergic contraction anywhere else in the colonic wall may trap gas in the area intervening, distending a relaxed but otherwise innocent portion of the bowel so that discomfort is referred to the distended site, often in the splenic or hepatic flexure. Excessive gas results entirely from air swallowed with food or drink or from such "tics" as sighing or forced belching. Sharp, unpleasant contractions in the left lower quadrant associated with straining at stool and partially relieved by defecation, are called *tenesmus*. A sensation of urgent need to defecate—*rectal urgency*—is an extremely distressing symptom associated with irritability of the rectum. Sharp pain in the anal area is made worse by defecation and is usually associated with

an inflammatory response in the skin of the anus—*anal pain*.

After establishing the presence or absence of these deviations, the physician must find out whether or not eating or defecation exacerbates or relieves them, whether the patient tries to mitigate the discomfort by moving about or by lying still, or by holding the abdominal wall immobilized with his hands or against the mattress. Although the general topography of the area of distress may localize findings to large or small intestines, relief by defecation is a feature of disturbance of the left colon, as exacerbation by eating is a feature of malfunction of the small intestine or right colon. Restlessness occurs with colic; peritoneal irritation tends to immobilize the patient. All these disturbances originate as increases in the tone of the bowel wall, and pressure relationships between adjacent segments of intestine determine not only the tension exerted against the wall but also the speed and character of the flow of the fluid contents along the lumen. As increased tension may compress the vessels nourishing the gut wall, so disease or contraction of the nourishing vasculature may deprive the wall of its ability to contract, to absorb, or to secrete. Unabsorbed residue or unduly large volumes of secretions attract more fluid into the lumen, further distending the gut; if large volumes of swallowed air cannot be passed quickly along the small bowel to the cecum, as is usual, the movements of the air-fluid mixture in the small intestine become loud enough to be noticed by the patient; such *borborygmi* are heard normally in the colon. Sudden changes in volume of the abdomen—*distension*—occur when the intraluminal volume of small or large bowel increases, because of paralysis of neuromuscular elements, abnormal handling of gas, or mechanical obstruction behind which muscular contractile activity is greatly increased. Bowel sounds may be absent if the wall is paralyzed, faint if the injury is submaximal, or increased if a viable area is forced to raise its intraluminal pressure in order to drive fluid past an obstructed segment. Sudden changes in pain reference occurring during the course of an illness usually indicate that the peritoneal surfaces have become involved, with more accurate cerebral localization of the underlying disturbance, and perhaps with associated development of spasm or guarding of the overlying musculature.

DIARRHEA AND CONSTIPATION. *Diarrhea* and *constipation* are terms given to alterations in the normal pattern of human defecation habits. There is no standard definition by which patients or physicians may classify strictly the deviation from normal; the range of variation in bowel habits among apparently healthy persons is extraordinarily wide, so that the deviation must, in the last analysis, be compared with each patient's own previous habit pattern rather than with that characterizing the mean, the median, or the mode of the population. Such comparisons involve so many associated functions that it will suffice for the purposes of this discussion to define diarrhea as the frequent passage of unformed stools, and constipation as an undue delay in the evacuation of feces. It is the task of the physician to understand enough of the normal and disturbed physiology of digestion, absorption, and propulsive motility that he may ask pointed questions of the patient which serve to define more precisely the locus, the nature, and, the severity of the disturbance. Since the gastrointestinal tract is a primitive organ upon which all manner of stimuli, from hunger to fear, rage, fever, and fatigue, from grossly infected or chemically toxic ingesta to the most subtly allergenic refined foods, exert effects that disturb function, this task is rarely simple.

ACUTE DIARRHEA. Acute disturbances of bowel function are relatively common and usually manifest themselves as diarrhea. The sudden onset of loose stools in a previously healthy person commonly is due to an active infection, and much less often to the ingestion of preformed toxins, poisonous chemicals or drugs, or to acute radiation sickness. When the patient is first seen, the history will usually point toward the source of the trouble: the eating of a particular meal or food in company with others who have also become similarly ill within 24 hr of eating the suspected food is *prima facie* evidence that a preformed toxin has been ingested; diarrhea developing in a number of patients within 28 to 72 hr after a common meal should make one suspect a salmonella infection. The presence of fever, malaise, muscle aching, and profound epigastric or periumbilical discomfort with severe anorexia suggests an inflammatory disease of the small intestine. The stools are characteristically watery, often accompanied by the explosive passage of gas; there is no rectal urgency or tenesmus and little hypogastric cramping. On physical examination one finds a generally tender abdomen without guarding, and one hears "whooshing" peristaltic sounds. A variant of the syndrome consists only of severe periumbilical pain and vomiting. The hemogram usually is within normal limits. Such an entity is commonly produced by infection with a virus, of which a number of species have been identified. The disease is called *viral gastroenteritis,* runs an acute course for 2 to 3 days, then gradually subsides.

The stool in viral gastroenteritis never contains recognizable exudate—it is singularly free of inflammatory cells, blood, or fibrin. Culture of the stool is usually nonproductive. By contrast, inflammatory diseases of the colon almost always result in leukocytic exudate and fibrin in the feces; stools may give cultures positive for organisms of the genus *Salmonella* or *Shigella* or may on microscopic examination show motile forms and/or cysts of various parasites, the most important of which in the United States is *Endamoeba histolytica.* Colonic infections usually are accompanied by hypogastric cramping, tenesmus, and rectal urgency. The patient may not have true anorexia but may be afraid to eat because eating stimulates the urge to defecate. There is usually fever and leukocytosis.

The physician must remember that an acute diarrhea may be the presenting symptoms of any type of systemic infection or of a hitherto-silent chronic gastrointestinal disease, of which the most well-defined are regional enteritis and ulcerative colitis; the latter may occasionally begin with fulminant dysentery, the former more often presenting as a tender mass in the right lower quadrant with mild diarrhea. Generalized cramping and diarrhea may follow use of a parasympathomimetic drug. Tenesmus, urgency, and left-sided hypogastric tenderness and cramping are classic symptoms of diverticulitis; the stool may contain pus, blood, or both, usually with much mucus. A fecal impaction may make a patient have rectal urgency, ask for a bedpan or visit the toilet often, but expel only a little watery exudate or nothing. Short-circuiting operations on the intestine and stomach usually result in at least mild diarrhea for months after the operation.

Differential diagnosis of these varied entities is made by history, physical examination, gross and microscopic appearance of the stools, appropriate bacteriologic studies, and proctoscopy. It is important to see the excreta put out by the patient, not just to rely on his description or on that of a third party. Toilets are not distinguished for satisfactory lighting nor upset patients for careful observation, and even trained personnel seldom display a curiosity sufficient to overcome the unpleasantness of a stool held close enough for accurate appraisal. Since fluid and electrolyte losses in diarrhea may be so great as to be life-threatening, the patient is given supportive care until studies indicate specific treatment. If no definitive etiologic agent can be identified, barium enema and upper gastrointestinal x-rays should be carried out. Upper gastrointestinal films may be very misleading when the barium meal is fed within the first few days of an acute enteritis or colitis and should be reserved for a time when the whole disease has become more quiescent.

CHRONIC DIARRHEA. A history of bouts of loose stools extending over a period of months or years, usually intermittent in character, calls for painstaking investigation. One particularly wants to know the circumstances of the first such bout—did it follow an acute infection, an operation, an emotional upset of severe degree? The number of days or weeks lost by the patient from his daily occupation on account of the illness, changes in weight and strength, and the appearance of the patient give important leads as to the nature and severity of the underlying disease. By the time the patient sees a physician the presenting symptoms may not be diarrhea but rather those of serious malnutrition, since any long-continued illness of this type may interfere with appetite as well as with the absorptive and digestive functions of the gastrointestinal tract. Associated signs and symptoms may reveal that the diarrhea and malnutrition are due to a generalized disorder which may involve the intestines functionally or structurally—hyperthyroidism, tuberculosis, lymphosarcoma, to name a few. More often, no such disorder will be found, and the physician must consider another, more specifically gastrointestinal disease.

A long history of intermittent diarrhea unaccompanied by fever, weight loss, blood in the stools, or significant loss of working capacity suggests a disturbance of emotional or, less commonly, of allergic origin, and associated symptoms should be elicited (Chaps. 18 and 72). A detailed dietary history is important in such cases, in order to establish the adequacy of the nutrient intake and to allow the patient a chance to ventilate his ideas on the relationship of food and eating to his symptoms. In such disordered functional states, the patient usually has a fairly formed stool on arising in the morning but then has one or two loose stools within the next hour. A similar pattern may occur after the evening meal. The stool caliber is usually small, and there may be mild discomfort, relieved by defecation, in the left lower quadrant of the abdomen. Such a triad of symptoms makes up the diarrheal component of the "irritable colon" syndrome, an extremely common disorder in anxious, nervous people, in which the symptoms result from exaggeration of normal colonic function.

When the history suggests that the diarrheal episodes have been characterized by blood in the stools, or by fever, malaise, anorexia, and weight loss in addition, one suspects a chronic inflammatory process involving either small bowel or colon or both. Regional enteritis may attack any portion of the intestine, producing an encroachment on the lumen and episodes of partial obstruction, ulcerations of the mucous membrane, or local abscesses and fistulas of the abdominal or anal skin, of the bladder, or of other loops of bowel. On proctoscopic examination the rectum is found to be uninvolved, and the stools show little microscopic exudate, although they are often positive for occult blood, gross bleeding being infrequently encountered. Tuberculosis and lymphosarcoma of the intestine can give similar symptoms and may be impossible to differentiate, although usually the roentgenologic appearances are dissimilar. The involvement may be primarily colonic, the most important disease entity being ulcerative colitis, whether idiopathic or due to amebic infestation, venereal lymphogranuloma, or chronic bacillary dysentery. Here the feces show pus cells and red cells when the disease is active, and proctoscopy is usually diagnostic. Stool cultures and examinations for parasites on numerous occasions are important aspects of the medical investigation.

When the patient presents with diarrhea of more than a few months' duration, without fever, blood in the stools, or cramping pain, but with weight loss, weakness, and symptoms of nutritional deficiency diseases (Chaps. 316 and 334), one focuses attention on the small intestine. In children celiac disease and cystic fibrosis of the pancreas are the important disorders to be differentiated; in older patients the same distinction between an absorptive defect and a digestive disorder must still be made in order to distinguish idiopathic steatorrhea from chronic pancreatitis. Whereas the stools in disease of the left colon are loose, often contain exudate on microscopic examination, and weigh less than 200 Gm per 24 hr, the stools associated with malabsorption are bulky, free of exudate, and weigh more than 300 Gm per 24 hr. Such a 24-hr collection, impounded in a collecting vessel, often has a shiny appearance and a foul odor which are almost diagnostic. See Chap. 316 for differential diagnosis of malabsorption.

A history of progressive disease characterized by arthritis, abdominal pain, diarrhea, and weight loss in middle-aged men suggests the diagnosis of Whipple's disease. Lymphosarcomas of low degrees of malignancy may produce malabsorption syndromes by blockage of lymphatic channels from the small bowel; areas of gut with poor motility may become "blind loops" and harbor large numbers of bacteria, which deconjugate bile salts and utilize nutrients needed by the host. The presenting symptoms of such pathologic disturbances may be diarrhea and macrocytic anemia, or watery diarrhea with or without increased fat content. Surgical revisions of the bowel, multiple jejunal diverticulosis, regional enteritis, and mesenteric vascular insufficiency may result in such conditions. Rarer causes of diarrhea are the enormous hypersecretion of gastric juice due to endocrine tumors, and the cramping diarrhea associated with high circulating levels of serotonin (see Chap. 105).

Special techniques are often needed to define clearly all these abnormalities. Duodenal intubation and analysis of digestive juices for pancreatic enzymes is a procedure of considerable importance in ruling out primary disease of the pancreas. Nevertheless, the aid of the skilled radiologist is probably more useful than any test in interpreting all but the earliest manifestations of these syndromes. Pancreatic calcification, fistulas, distortions of the duodenal loop, diffuse granulomatous diseases of the small bowel, diverticula, polyps, ulcerated areas, stenosis, and obstruction—all these can be identified by modern radiologic techniques, which provide in addition baseline data for evaluating the natural history of the disease and response to therapy.

CONSTIPATION. Whereas diarrhea may be a dangerous symptom per se, with its accompaniment of dehydration and loss of cations, constipation of itself is not debilitating, although mild abdominal discomfort and straining at stool are not salutary and tend to increase the severity of preexisting anorectal lesions. The acute onset of severe obstipation in an apparently normal person signifies that something has disturbed the neural, vascular, or muscular integrity of the gut or associated defecatory reflexes and muscles. Such disturbances may result from severe infections, particularly of the central nervous system, from acute mesenteric circulatory catastrophes, from renal colic, from cerebrovascular accidents, from mechanical obstruction of large or small intestine, from painful anal lesions, from certain drugs, or from fecal impaction. Of these, the last is the most embarrassing to overlook, since the puttylike mass filling the rectum makes the patient try to move his bowels and often results in frequent calls for a bedpan or visits to the toilet; such fruitless attempts at defecations may be called diarrhea, and the poor patient may receive antidiarrheal medications! Rapid but complete physical examination including a digital examination of the rectum and proctoscopy is called for in all cases of constipation of acute onset; if no other physical signs to explain the sudden constipation are elicited, a low-pressure barium enema should be given to establish the site of obstruction if present and appropriate measures taken.

A long history of intermittent bouts of constipation, accompanied by abdominal distress relieved by defecation and by passage of hard stools of small caliber, with or without much mucus, is characteristic of the *"irritable colon" syndrome,* one of the most common forms of anxiety met by the physician. The abuse of laxatives over many years is frequently added to the underlying emotional disturbance to aggravate the clinical picture. The symptoms are essentially exaggerations of normal physiologic activity of the colon and in mild degrees have probably been experienced by most healthy people as, for example, the constipation associated with travel. Extensive studies of sigmoid motility in patients with this syndrome have verified the clinical impression that disturbed motor function correlates closely with emotional conflicts. Proctoscopic examination of these patients demonstrates an unremarkable rectum and a rectosigmoid which is often spastic, the lumen smaller than normal, the veins prominent, and the mucus more abundant than usual. The stools are negative for blood, parasites, and pathogenic bacteria; the x-ray examination is usually not abnormal.

Another common form of constipation is also chronic and is not characterized by the triad of symptoms of the irritable colon syndrome. Whether as the result of childhood training or of a perverse understanding of the necessity for bowel movements occurring with chronometric precision, these patients have equated general health with "regularity." This leads to a dependence on laxatives or enemas to hasten the overdue evacuation, so that over the years they lose the sensitivity of the rectal defecatory reflexes. Consequently, they do not have a regular schedule for moving their bowels, which for most normal people is most easily accomplished after breakfast and, if needed, after the heaviest meal of the day; over the years they no longer demonstrate any rhythmicity in defecation, take laxatives whenever they feel "run down," and have stools which may be alternately voluminous and watery or small and hard. Lax abdominal muscles and a pelvic floor weakened by multiple deliveries may contribute to poor defecatory performance. On physical examination these patients often have a palpable colon filled with feces, and on rectal examination feces fill the ampulla, the patient being unaware of this. Such types of rectal insensitivity have been called *atonic constipation, dyschezia,* and *rectal constipation.*

In both the above types of constipation, it is obvious that a thorough analysis by the physician of dietary habits, defecatory habits, use of laxatives, mode of living, and emotional problems must be made before proper therapy can be instituted. At the same time it must be stressed that such patients are not immune to the development of neoplasms of the large bowel, and it is a most difficult task for the physician to decide how often complete studies should be carried out on patients with long-standing, apparently static, complaints. The simplest solution is to do repeated stool examinations for occult blood and digital and proctoscopic examinations, remembering also that in patients who have difficulty with evacuation, anal diseases—fissures, ulcers, and hemorrhoids—are more common than in the general population.

A lifelong history of obstinate constipation may be associated with the enormous dilatation of the large bowel seen in idiopathic or acquired megacolon. In the former condition, the rectosigmoid is contracted and obstructing, because of its lack of the ganglionic cells necessary to pass on the propulsive waves of the proximal colon; in the latter condition, severe contraction of the voluntary anal sphincter produces enormous dilatation of the rectal ampulla and colon. Radiologic studies are usually very helpful in differentiating these two conditions.

When constipation is of recent onset and progressive, the investigation should be thorough and extremely comprehensive. This is the optimal time to detect a neoplasm of the large bowel. General physical and psychiatric examination may reveal a systemic disorder: hypothyroidism, hyperparathyroidism, tuberculosis, urinary tract disease, congestive heart failure; a major psychosis, profound depression, parkinsonism, or recent cerebrovascular accident may be responsible for progressive constipation. A careful history of drug ingestion may reveal that the patient received ganglionic-blocking agents or opiates prior to onset of symptoms or large amounts of sedation. A marked change in dietary regimen, particularly in combination with sedative drugs, may produce a marked decrease in frequency of bowel movements.

If the digital and proctoscopic findings fail to explain the constipation, a barium enema and upper gastrointestinal x-rays are indicated. Tumors of the gastrointestinal tract comprise nearly half of all cancer, and patients with colonic cancers have a better prognosis for survival after surgical treatment than do those with gastric and esophageal lesions. A high index of suspicion for a neoplastic origin of changes in bowel habits, repeated tests for occult blood in the stools, and careful proctoscopy and x-ray studies will usually justify in salvaged lives the money and time spent.

PROCTALGIA. See Chap. 320.

REFERENCES

Davenport, H. W.: "Physiology of the Digestive Tract," 2d ed., Chicago, The Year Book Medical Publishers, Inc., 1966.

Mendeloff, A. I.: Chronic Diarrhea, Am. J. Dig. Dis., 3:801, 1958.

44   HEMATEMESIS AND MELENA

*Kurt J. Isselbacher and
Raymond S. Koff*

Hematemesis is defined as the vomiting of blood, and melena as the passage of black, tarry stools. These dramatic symptoms of gastrointestinal hemorrhage should not only bring the patient to prompt medical attention but, within certain limits, help define the anatomic site of bleeding. Only rarely will exsanguinating gastrointestinal hemorrhage occur without the appearance of altered or gross blood passed by mouth or rectum. The color of vomited blood will vary from red to black depending upon the duration of contact of the blood with gastric acid in the stomach. Thus if vomiting occurs shortly after the onset of bleeding, the vomitus is likely to be red; if there is delay in vomiting, the appearance will be dark-red, black, or of "coffee grounds" appearance. Since blood entering the gastrointestinal tract below the duodenum rarely reenters the stomach, hematemesis usually indicates that the bleeding is proximal to the jejunum.

Melena may occur independently of, or be associated with, hematemesis. Bleeding of sufficient volume to produce hematemesis usually results in melena. The altered color of the blood results from prolonged contact with gastric juice to produce hematin. In contrast to hematemesis, melena may result from hemorrhage into the jejunum or ileum provided that transit through the bowel is slow. At least 50 to 100 ml blood must rapidly enter the upper gastrointestinal tract to produce a single black, tarry stool. Following a single liter episode of hemorrhage, tarry stools will persist for 1 to 3 days. Subsequently the stools return to normal color, but tests for occult blood may be positive for 3 to 8 days.

The passage of red blood per rectum usually denotes lower intestinal bleeding, i.e., bleeding originating below the duodenum. However, if bleeding is massive and rapid enough, red blood may appear per rectum from an upper intestinal or gastric lesion.

Not all black or red stools are due to blood. Black stools may result from the ingestion of iron, charcoal, or bismuth. Red stools are occasionally seen after ingestion of beets or following intravenous sulfobromophthalein tests. The presence of gastrointestinal bleeding, even if detected only by positive tests for occult blood in the stool or clear aspirate of the gastric contents, indicates potentially serious disease and must be investigated.

The clinical manifestations of gastrointestinal bleeding are dependent upon the extent of hemorrhage, the rate of bleeding, and the presence of associated or coincidental diseases. Unless anemia is present prior to the onset of bleeding, loss of less than 500 ml blood is usually not associated with systemic symptoms. Rapid hemorrhage of greater volume will result in decreased venous return to the heart, decreased cardiac output, reflex vasoconstriction, and increased peripheral resistance. The patient may experience syncope, light-headedness, nausea, sweating, and thirst. He may appear anxious and restless. When blood loss approaches 40 percent of the blood volume, shock with tachycardia and a thready peripheral pulse are usually present. The skin is cold and clammy, and pallor is prominent. Initial hematocrits will not reflect the blood loss accurately until several hours later, when hemodilution has occurred. The platelet count rises, and leukocytosis is found 2 to 5 hr after the onset of bleeding. Occasionally the presence of blood in the intestinal tract is associated with mild fever (100 to 102°F), and the blood urea nitrogen becomes variably elevated 24 to 48 hr after bleeding because of the breakdown of blood proteins to urea by intestinal bacteria.

ETIOLOGY OF UPPER GASTROINTESTINAL BLEEDING

Swallowed blood resulting from epistaxis, hemoptysis, dental extractions, and tonsillectomy may be vomited or result in melena. A careful history and physical examination will exclude these sources.

The three most common causes of upper gastrointestinal hemorrhage are (1) esophageal or gastric varices, (2) peptic ulceration, and (3) erosive gastritis. These three entities encompass 90 to 95 percent of all cases of upper gastrointestinal bleeding in which a definite lesion can be found.

VARICEAL BLEEDING. Bleeding from esophageal or gastric varices is most frequently associated with portal hypertension due to cirrhosis of the liver. Although in the United States alcoholic cirrhosis is by far the most prevalent form of this disease, variceal hemorrhage may occur in other forms of cirrhosis associated with portal hypertension, especially postnecrotic cirrhosis. Portal vein thrombosis may also lead to variceal hemorrhage in the absence of cirrhosis. Bleeding from varices tends to be abrupt and often massive; however, minor bleeding may occur for days from esophageal varices before it is discovered. Upper gastrointestinal bleeding in a patient with cirrhosis suggests a variceal source, but because patients with cirrhosis have a higher incidence of peptic ulceration, bleeding from the latter must be excluded. Furthermore, in the alcoholic patient with cirrhosis who has continued to drink prior to the onset of bleeding, bleeding from gastritis is quite common.

PEPTIC ULCER. Peptic ulcer disease is probably the most common cause of upper gastrointestinal bleeding. The majority of these ulcers are situated in the duodenum. About 20 percent of patients with peptic ulcer will have at least one episode of significant gastrointestinal bleeding. When a patient with known peptic ulcer presents with gastrointestinal hemorrhage, the ulcer is the most probable site of bleeding.

GASTRITIS. Gastritis may be associated with recent heavy alcohol ingestion or with a history of ingestion of salicylates or other drugs. Similarly gastric erosions and ulcerations may occur in "stressful" situations and are not infrequently found in patients with intracranial disease, burns, or recent trauma. Erosive gastritis can rarely be diagnosed by radiologic techniques, and gastroscopy is necessary to confirm this diagnosis.

OTHER LESIONS OF THE UPPER GASTROINTESTINAL TRACT. Less common sources of upper gastrointestinal bleeding originating in the esophagus include esophagitis (with or without hiatus hernia), carcinoma, and peptic ulcer of the esophagus. Lacerations of the mucosa of the distal end of the esophagus associated with severe vomiting (the Mallory-Weiss syndrome) is suggested by a history of nonbloody vomiting followed by hematemesis. While sudden severe hemorrhage is seen in a small number of patients with carcinoma of the stomach, particularly in association with mucosal ulceration, chronic blood loss is a more frequent complication of gastric carcinoma.

Mesenteric venous or arterial occlusion by embolism or thrombosis may produce either occult or overt blood loss.

Lymphoma, polyps, and other tumors of the stomach and proximal small intestine are relatively uncommon lesions and are therefore unusual sources of hemorrhage. The Peutz-Jeghers syndrome of small intestinal polyposis and melanin pigmentation of the lips, mucosa, fingers, and toes may be associated with recurrent melena.

Saccular arteriosclerotic aortic aneurysms may rupture into the upper intestine and are almost invariably fatal. Most commonly rupture occurs into the third portion of the duodenum.

Primary blood dyscrasias including leukemia, thrombocytopenic states, and the hemophilias may result in significant gastrointestinal bleeding. Polycythemia vera, although associated with an increased incidence of peptic ulceration, may also result in gastrointestinal bleeding due to mesenteric or portal vein thrombosis. Periarteritis nodosa, Henoch-Schönlein purpura, and other vasculitides may lead to gastrointestinal blood loss.

Gastrointestinal bleeding, usually mild but occasionally persistent, may accompany amyloidosis, Osler-Rendu-Weber disease, pseudoxanthoma elasticum, Turner's syndrome, single or multiple intestinal hemangiomas, neurofibromatosis, Kaposi's sarcoma, and hemangiectatic hypertrophy. Although the occurrence of hematemesis and melena in uremia is unusual, mild occult intestinal bleeding is quite frequent.

ETIOLOGY OF LOWER GASTROINTESTINAL BLEEDING

ANAL LESIONS. The most common cause of small amounts of bright-red blood on the surface of the stool and on toilet tissue is bleeding from hemorrhoidal veins. Bleeding from internal or external hemorrhoids is frequently precipitated by straining or passage of hard stools. Anal fissures or fistulas likewise first may come to the attention of the patient as a result of rectal bleeding. The presence of an anal pathologic condition *does not preclude other causes and sources of bleeding, such as carcinoma, and these must be sought and excluded.*

RECTUM AND COLONIC DISEASE. Carcinoma of the rectum, rectal polyps, and ulcerative proctitis are the most common bleeding lesions of the rectum. Bleeding from carcinoma in any area of the colon may result in the appearance of gross blood, whether on the stool or mixed with the fecal contents. Bloody diarrhea is often the presenting feature of ulcerative colitis but is uncommon in granulomatous ileocolitis, although occult blood may be present in the stool. Bleeding may accompany bacterial and protozoan diarrhea, especially shigellosis and amebic colitis.

DIVERTICULITIS. Intestinal diverticula may occur in every part of the intestinal tract but are most commonly found in the sigmoid colon. Diverticulosis per se may rarely cause massive gastrointestinal hemorrhage. Bleeding, usually of minimal severity, may originate from these lesions but is more common when inflammation is pres-

ent, i.e., in diverticulitis. Meckel's diverticulum, a congenital anomaly occurring in about 2 percent of the population and located in the ileum usually 20 to 100 cm proximal to the ileocecal valve, is often associated with bleeding. Ectopic gastric mucosa may be present in about 15 percent of these diverticula and may ulcerate with profuse or recurrent rectal hemorrhage, particularly in children and young adults.

APPROACH TO THE PATIENT WITH GASTROINTESTINAL BLEEDING

The approach to the patient with gross bleeding from the gastrointestinal tract is dependent upon the site, extent, and rate of bleeding. In general the patient who presents with hematemesis is more likely to have bled greater amounts and is more likely to exsanguinate than the patient with melena. There is usually a sense of urgency in the immediate diagnosis and treatment of patients with upper gastrointestinal bleeding. When first seen, the patient may be in shock. Before a complete history and physical examination are undertaken, blood must be obtained for typing and cross matching, and an intravenous infusion of saline solution or other plasma expander must be started at once.

HISTORY. A history of epigastric pain relieved by food, milk, or antacids strongly suggests peptic ulcer disease. A history of jaundice and alcoholism suggests chronic liver disease. One must carefully inquire about a recent alcoholic binge or the ingestion of drugs such as aspirin, which may be associated with gastritis or precipitate bleeding from peptic ulcer. Attention must be directed to possible previous episodes of bleeding, vomiting, symptoms of gastrointestinal distress, diarrhea, cramps, weight loss, fever, bleeding from other sites such as the skin and mucous membranes, and a family history of intestinal disease or hemorrhagic diathesis.

PHYSICAL EXAMINATION. Physical examination is directed to excluding a nonintestinal source of blood (i.e., ruling out epistaxis, hemoptysis, pharyngeal lesions). Careful assessment of the skin may reveal the characteristic telangiectasia of Osler-Rendu-Weber disease, the diffuse melanin pigmentation of hemochromatosis, the localized pigmentation of Peutz-Jeghers syndrome, the soft tissue tumors and multiple sebaceous cysts of familial colonic polyposis, or the dermal neurofibromas of neurofibromatosis. The presence of peripheral stigmas of chronic liver disease with hepatosplenomegaly, ascites, and edema suggest the likelihood of portal hypertension and the possibility of bleeding from varices, gastritis, or peptic ulceration. One must look for the presence of abdominal tenderness or masses, determine the frequency and character of the bowel sounds, and look for evidence of malignancy such as a Virchow node or rectal shelf.

LABORATORY STUDIES. Initial studies include the hematocrit, hemoglobin, careful assessment of red cell morphologic features (the finding of hypochromic, microcytic red cells suggests that blood loss is chronic), and white cell count and differential. There should be a platelet count, or platelets should be estimated from the blood smear. Prothrombin time and coagulation studies may be in order to exclude primary or secondary clotting defects. While the initial studies are valuable and essential, it is important that there be *repeated evaluation* of the laboratory data as one follows the clinical course of the bleeding.

DIAGNOSTIC APPROACH

The diagnostic approach (see also Chap. 314 for a more detailed discussion) to the patient with gastrointestinal hemorrhage must necessarily be individualized. It must be emphasized that demonstration of a lesion of the intestinal tract in a patient with gastrointestinal bleeding should be accompanied by evidence that it is *the* bleeding lesion, since more than one potential bleeding lesion may be present. In recent years the number of experienced endoscopists has increased enormously, so that in many medical centers emergency endoscopy and upper gastrointestinal roentgenographic studies can be performed within hours of admission to the hospital. The patient who presents with melena or who has recently experienced hematemesis or is suspected of bleeding from the upper gastrointestinal tract initially should have a stomach tube passed to empty the stomach, to determine whether the bleeding is in the upper gastrointestinal tract and whether the bleeding is continuing.

The next step, provided that blood volume is maintained, will depend on the facilities available. In an increasing number of hospitals esophagoscopy and gastroscopy will be performed immediately thereafter, at the bedside if necessary, followed by emergency upper gastrointestinal roentgenograms. If the patient's condition does not permit these diagnostic measures and bleeding varices or peptic ulcer are strongly suspected, ice water lavage of the stomach may be attempted to slow bleeding, and, in the case of variceal bleeding, intravenous administration of vasopressin may permit hemostasis by reduction of portal venous pressure. Once bleeding is controlled, endoscopy and upper gastrointestinal x-rays are obtained.

If massive bleeding or hematemesis persists, it may be necessary to resort to esophageal tamponade with the Sengstaken-Blakemore tube or some variant of it. Although use of tamponade is extremely hazardous, even under the best of conditions, variceal hemorrhage may be controlled in the majority of patients and the patient's condition stabilized. The initial management of gastrointestinal bleeding may be controlled by the internist, but it is wise to call for the aid of the surgeon, early in the course, because surgical intervention may be necessary if bleeding cannot be controlled.

In the event that bleeding has stopped prior to admission or shortly thereafter and endoscopy and upper gastrointestinal series do not disclose the source of bleeding, one may resort to splenic pulp manometry and splenoportography, especially if varices are suspected. An elevated splenic pulp pressure (>25 to 30 mm Hg) correlates well with hemorrhage from varices. Although splenoportography is generally less useful than the combination of esophagoscopy and barium swallow in demonstrating varices, it provides exceedingly important information on the patency of the portal and splenic veins in the event that surgical decompression of the portal system is contemplated.

If endoscopic and radiologic studies are negative but slow bleeding from the upper intestinal tract persists, a radiopaque string or tape may be passed perorally to aid in localizing the site of bleeding. After the location of the string is checked by fluoroscopy, fluorescein or radioactive-labeled red cells may be injected intravenously; the string is then retrieved and examined for the location of occult blood, fluorescence, or radioactivity. Unfortunately, the string test is subject to a number of methodologic errors and has been of limited clinical value. Celiac angiography has also been used to localize bleeding from the small intestine, but its overall value remains to be determined.

The most important diagnostic procedure in the evaluation of rectal bleeding is digital rectal examination and proctosigmoidoscopy. Biopsy of lesions may be performed under direct vision through the sigmoidoscope, if necessary. Barium enema examination and air-contrast studies will aid in localizing lesions above the reach of the sigmoidoscope. Obviously bleeding must not be attributed to hemorrhoids or anal fissures unless other lesions are clearly excluded by adequate and repeated examinations. When appropriate, culture of stool specimens and examination of stools for ova and parasites complete the evaluation.

REFERENCES

Brick, I. B., and H. J. Jeghers: Gastrointestinal Hemorrhage, New Engl. J. Med., 253:458, 1955.

Conn, H. O., and J. A. Simpson: Excessive Mortality Associated with Balloon Tamponade of Bleeding Varices, J.A.M.A., 202:587, 1967.

Merigan, T. C., Jr., R. M. Hollister, P. F. Gryska, G. W. B. Starkey, and C. S. Davidson: Gastrointestinal Bleeding with Cirrhosis: A Study of 172 Episodes in 158 Patients, New Engl. J. Med., 263:579, 1960.

Peternel, W. W., A. E. Dagradi, A. I. Rogers, H. M. Nadal, E. B. Perin, and F. C. Jackson: Clinical Investigation of the Portacaval Shunt. III. The Diagnosis of Esophageal Varices, J.A.M.A., 202:1081, 1968.

45   JAUNDICE AND HEPATOMEGALY
Kurt J. Isselbacher

JAUNDICE

Jaundice, or *icterus*, refers to the yellow pigmentation of the skin or scleras by bilirubin. This in turn is a result of elevated levels of bilirubin in the bloodstream. Jaundice may be brought to the attention of the patient or the physician by a darkening of the urine or a yellow discoloration of the skin or sclera; the latter often is the site where clinical icterus may first be detected. Scleral pigmentation is attributed to richness of this tissue in elastin, which has a special affinity for bilirubin. Jaundice must be distinguished from other causes of yellow pigmentation such as carotenemia (see Chaps. 58 and 85), which is due to carotenoid pigments in the bloodstream and is associated with a yellowish discoloration of the skin but not the sclera. Atabrine treatment (see Chap. 241) may produce a yellow color of the skin and urine, but the scleras are usually only minimally discolored, and when pigment is present, it is only seen in the regions of the scleras exposed to light.

Normal serum bilirubin concentrations range from 0.5 to 1.0 mg per 100 ml, and normally most of this is unconjugated (see Fig. 45-1). The precise level at which jaundice becomes clinically evident varies, but usually it can be recognized when the total serum bilirubin exceeds 2 to 2.5 mg per 100 ml. Not infrequently in deep jaundice the skin may take on a greenish hue because of the conversion of bilirubin to biliverdin, an oxidation product of bilirubin. Oxidation occurs more readily with conjugated bilirubin, and hence a greenish hue is seen more frequently in conditions with pronounced conjugated hyperbilirubinemia.

Production and Metabolism of Bilirubin

NORMAL SOURCES OF BILIRUBIN (Fig. 45-2). The majority of the bilirubin is derived from the catabolism of hemoglobin present in senescent red cells. This normally accounts for about 80 to 85 percent of the daily bilirubin production. When a circulating red cell reaches the end of its normal life span of approximately 120 days, it is destroyed in the reticuloendothelial system. In the catabolism of hemoglobin, globin appears to be first dissociated from heme, after which the heme moiety is oxida-

Fig. 45-1. The chemical structures of conjugated (A) and unconjugated (B) bilirubin. Abbreviations: M = methyl, V = vinyl, P = propionic acid. The asterisk (*) refers to glucuronic acid.

tively cleaved and converted to biliverdin by a microsomal heme oxygenase. This enzyme system requires oxygen and a cofactor, reduced nicotinamide adenine dinucleotide phosphate (NADPH). Bilirubin is then formed from biliverdin by another enzyme, biliverdin reductase.

About 15 to 20 percent of the bilirubin is derived from sources other than senescent erythrocytes. One of these is the destruction of maturing erythroid cells in the bone marrow, or so called "ineffective erythropoiesis" (see Chap. 341). The other is from nonerythroid components, especially in the liver, and involves the turnover of heme and heme proteins (such as cytochrome, myoglobin, and heme-containing enzymes). These two sources of bilirubin are collectively referred to as the *"early labeled fraction,"* a term which is derived from experiments with labeled glycine and delta-aminolevulinic acid (ALA). Thus when labeled glycine is administered to a normal subject, approximately 15 percent of the label appears in stool stercobilinogen at about 120 days and reflects the bilirubin produced from the normal destruction of senescent red cells.

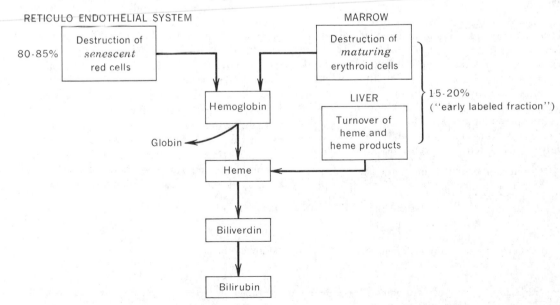

Fig. 45-2. The sources and precursors of plasma bilirubin.

TRANSPORT OF BILIRUBIN. Following liberation of bilirubin into the plasma virtually all the pigment is tightly *bound to albumin.* The maximum binding capacity is 2 moles of bilirubin per mole of albumin. Because in a normal adult this corresponds to plasma unconjugated bilirubin concentrations of 60 to 80 mg per ml, saturation of the binding capacity of the plasma almost never occurs. It is clinically relevant that certain organic anions, such as sulfonamides and salicylates, compete with bilirubin for common binding sites on albumin and may displace bilirubin from albumin, permitting it to enter tissues such as the central nervous system. Most of the evidence for albumin binding has been obtained from studies using unconjugated bilirubin. The conjugated pigment also appears to be bound primarily to albumin, although the binding forces may be different. Some conjugated bilirubin in the plasma is ultrafilterable.

Bilirubin is found in body fluids (cerebrospinal fluid, joint effusions, cysts, etc.) in proportion to the albumin content of the fluids and is absent from true secretions such as tears, saliva, and pancreatic juice. Scar tissue is rarely bilirubin-stained. The appearance of jaundice is also influenced by blood flow and edema. Paralyzed extremities and edematous areas tend to remain uncolored, and "unilateral" jaundice in patients with hemiplegia and edema may be seen if jaundice develops in such patients.

HEPATIC METABOLISM OF BILIRUBIN. The liver occupies a central role in the metabolism of the bile pigments. Three distinct phases are recognized: (1) *hepatic uptake,* (2) *conjugation,* and (3) *excretion* into bile. Of these three steps, excretion appears to be the rate-limiting step and the one most susceptible to impairment when the liver cell is damaged.

Uptake. Unconjugated bilirubin bound to albumin is presented to the liver cell, and upon entry the pigment and albumin became dissociated. Very little is known concerning the mechanism of the uptake phase, particularly whether it is an energy-dependent process. Hepatic uptake does, however, appear to be reversible.

Conjugation. Unconjugated bilirubin is water-insoluble and must be converted to a *water-soluble derivative* in order to be excreted by the liver cell into bile. This is accomplished by the process of conjugation whereby bilirubin is enzymatically converted to bilirubin glucuronide (actually diglucuronide). This reaction occurs in the microsomes or endoplasmic reticulum of the hepatocytes by action of the enzyme glucuronyl transferase. The action catalyzed by glucuronyl transferase is as follows:

Bilirubin + uridine diphosphate glucuronic acid →
  bilirubin diglucuronide + uridine diphosphate

As a result of this enzymatic reaction glucuronic acid is attached to the two carboxyl groups of bilirubin (Fig. 45-1). Glucuronyl transferase is also found in kidney and intestine, but the liver serves as the major site for conjugated bilirubin formation. The hepatic microsomal glucuronyl transferase system also is involved in the formation of glucuronides of other endogenous and exogenous substances (e.g., conjugates of steroids, antibiotics, and salicylates) (see Chap. 323).

The major product of conjugation is bilirubin diglucuronide, sometimes referred to as pigment II. Although some chromatographic evidence has suggested the existence of bilirubin monoglucuride, or pigment I, such a product appears to be a "complex" of unconjugated bilirubin and bilirubin diglucuronide and is perhaps an artifact produced in the course of isolating the pigments. While bilirubin sulfate has also been found in bile, the glucuronide conjugate is the major conjugated bile pigment excreted by the liver cells.

Excretion or Secretion into Bile. In order for bilirubin to be transferred from the liver cell into bile, *the pigment must be in the conjugated form.* Although the overall process is not well understood, the excretion of conjugated bilirubin into bile appears to be an energy-dependent process and the *rate-limiting* step in the hepatic metabolism of bilirubin. When this step is compromised, two consequences occur: (1) decreased excretion of bilirubin into bile and (2) "regurgitation," or reentry of conjugated bilirubin from the liver cells into the bloodstream.

INTESTINAL PHASE OF BILIRUBIN METABOLISM. After its appearance in the intestinal lumen, bilirubin glucuronide may be excreted in the stool or metabolized to urobilinogen and related products. Because of its polarity, conjugated bilirubin is not reabsorbed by the intestinal mucosa, a mechanism which may serve to rid the body of this pigment.

The formation of urobilinogen from conjugated bilirubin requires the action of bacteria and therefore occurs predominantly in the lower small intestine and colon. The bacteria, by stepwise enzymatic reductions, induce the formation of a series of colorless urobilinogens (Fig. 45-3) which react with Ehrlich's aldehyde reagent to produce red aldehyde complexes. Oxidation of the urobilinogens (i.e., *d*-urobilinogen, mesobilirubinogen, and stercobilinogen) leads to colored products, the urobilins. On mixing with Schlesinger's solution (zinc acetate in alcohol), zinc complexes are produced which have an intense green fluorescence. Because these compounds all have the same physiologic significance and are measured

Fig. 45-3. Chemical steps in the reduction of bilirubin to the urobilinogens and urobilins.

together in most quantitative analyses, they usually are referred to collectively as "urobilinogens" irrespective of their chemical structure or whether they are found in urine, feces, or bile.

In contrast to conjugated bilirubin, urobilinogen is readily reabsorbed from the small intestine into the portal blood and is thus subject to an enterohepatic circulation. Some urobilinogen is reexcreted by the liver into the bile, while the rest is excreted in the urine in an amount usually not exceeding 4 mg daily. When the hepatic excretory mechanism is impaired (e.g., in hepatocellular disease) or the production of bilirubin is greatly increased (e.g., in hemolytic anemia), the urinary urobilinogen may increase significantly.

The normal output of fecal urobilinogen ranges from 50 to 280 mg per day. Under conditions of decreased excretion of conjugated bilirubin into the intestine (e.g., liver disease, bile duct obstruction) or suppression of intestinal flora by antibiotics, fecal output will be diminished. In hemolytic anemia, both urinary and fecal urobilinogen excretion is greatly increased.

In a normal individual with a blood volume of 5 liters and a hemoglobin concentration of 15 gm per 100 ml, the total circulating hemoglobin is 750 Gm. Because approximately 1/120 of the red cells are destroyed daily, 6.3 Gm hemoglobin is released for catabolism. Assuming a quantitative conversion of heme to bilirubin and to urobilinogen, the expected daily output of urobilinogen would be approximately 250 mg plus the additional 15 to 30 mg which would be derived from the other sources described above (i.e., ineffective erythropoiesis, nonhemoglobin heme precursors). Often, however, the amount excreted is considerably less, and it appears likely that there are alternative pathways for hemoglobin degradation that may not involve the formation of bilirubin.

RENAL EXCRETION OF BILIRUBIN. Normally the urine is found to contain no bilirubin by the methods usually employed, although traces may be detectable by sensitive spectrophotometric procedures. In unconjugated hyperbilirubinemia, there is no bilirubinuria, whereas when conjugated hyperbilirubinemia occurs, bilirubin readily appears in the urine. The renal excretion of conjugated bilirubin may serve as a regulatory mechanism and probably accounts for the fact that in complete biliary tract obstruction the serum conjugated bilirubin level usually plateaus between 30 and 40 mg per 100 ml.

Although the renal mechanism for bilirubin excretion is not completely understood, most studies indicate that excretion of conjugated bilirubin occurs by glomerular filtration. The fraction of plasma conjugated bilirubin so filtered appears to be that small fraction which normally is both dialyzable and ultrafilterable. In the urine the dialyzable fraction seems to be associated with a non-albumin plasma constituent of low molecular weight, possibly a peptide. Bile salts enhance the dialyzability of conjugated bilirubin, and it has been suggested that in obstructive jaundice, the elevated plasma bile salts may be responsible for an increased renal excretion of conjugated bilirubin. Unconjugated bilirubin is neither dialyzable nor ultrafilterable, which probably accounts for its failure to be excreted in the urine.

Chemical Tests for Bile Pigments

The most widely employed chemical test for the bile pigments in serum is the van den Bergh reaction. In this reaction the bilirubin pigments are diazotized with sulfanilic acid, with initial conversion of the bilirubin from a tetrapyrrole to dipyrrole. The diazotized dipyrrole molecules are chromogenic and are measured colorimetrically. The van den Bergh reaction can be used to distinguish between unconjugated and conjugated bilirubin because of the different solubility properties of the pigments. When the reaction is carried out in an *aqueous* medium, the water-soluble conjugated bilirubin reacts to give the so-called *direct* van den Bergh reaction. When the reaction is carried out in *methanol*, both conjugated and unconjugated pigments react, giving a measure of the *total* bilirubin level. The total minus the direct-reacting bilirubin give the *indirect* value, which is a measure of the unconjugated bilirubin level.

In the direct van den Bergh reaction, the most accurate measurements are those carried out at 1 min. If the reaction is allowed to proceed longer, a small amount of the unconjugated pigment may begin to react in the aqueous medium. As a result, in a patient with unconjugated hyperbilirubinemia, if the direct reaction is carried out at 30 min, it may give falsely high values and conversely falsely low values for the indirect-reacting bilirubin. This serves to emphasize that the direct and indirect van den Bergh reactions represent *approximations* (not absolute measurements) of the conjugated and unconjugated pigments. A summary of the key differences in the properties and reactions of the bilirubin pigments is presented in Table 45-1.

Table 45-1. COMPARISON OF THE MAJOR DIFFERENCES BETWEEN CONJUGATED AND UNCONJUGATED BILIRUBIN

Properties and reactions	Bilirubin	
	Unconjugated	Conjugated (diglucuronide)
Water solubility...........	0	+
Affinity for lipids..........	+	0
Bound to serum albumin....	+++	+
Renal excretion...........	0	+
Van den Bergh reaction.....	Indirect (total minus direct)	Direct
Lipid membrane permeability	+	0

The measurement of bilirubin in the urine may be carried out by the Harrison spot test or with Ictotest[1] tablets. The foam test is also a simple and qualitatively valid procedure. When normal urine is vigorously shaken in a test tube, the foam is absolutely white. In a urine

[1] Trademark of Ames Company, Ames, Iowa.

containing bilirubin, the foam will be yellow. This difference may be subtle and may become evident only by comparing a normal urine and one containing bilirubin side by side. Urine urobilinogen may be estimated by the semiquantitative Watson-Schwartz test or the qualitative Diamond test. Fecal measurement must be quantitative to be of value.

Except for concentrated urine, the most common cause of a deep yellow-brown or dark urine is bilirubinuria. However, other mechanisms and diseases associated with a dark urine need to be considered. These include yellow urine due to drugs (e.g., azosulfapyridine); red urine due to porphyria, hemoglobinuria, myoglobinuria, or drugs (e.g., pyridium); and dark-brown or black urine due to homogentisic acid (in ochronosis) or melanin (with melanoma).

Classification of Jaundice

Once the presence of hyperbilirubinemia has been established, the underlying disorder should be approached by considering both (1) the *pathophysiology*

Table 45-2. CLASSIFICATION OF JAUNDICE BASED ON UNDERLYING DERANGEMENT IN BILIRUBIN METABOLISM

I. Predominantly *unconjugated* hyperbilirubinemia
  A. Overproduction
    1. Hemolysis (intra- and extravascular)
    2. Ineffective erythropoiesis
  B. Impaired hepatic uptake
    1. Gilbert's syndrome (constitutional hepatic dysfunction; familial nonhemolytic jaundice)
    2. Posthepatitis hyperbilirubinemia (probably the same as Gilbert's syndrome)
    3. Drugs
  C. Impaired glucuronide conjugation (decreased activity of glucuronyl transferase)
    1. Absence or deficiency (congenital) of transferase (Crigler-Najjar syndrome)
    2. "Immaturity" of transferase (neonatal jaundice)
    3. Deficiency or inhibition of transferase
      a. Inhibition by drugs (e.g., pregnanediol, chloramphenicol)
      b. Hepatocellular disease (e.g., hepatitis, cirrhosis)*
II. Predominantly *conjugated* hyperbilirubinemia
  A. Impaired hepatic excretion (functional or intrahepatic obstruction)
    1. Probable familial or hereditary disorders
      a. Dubin-Johnson, Rotor syndrome
      b. Recurrent (benign) intrahepatic cholestasis
      c. Cholestatic jaundice of pregnancy
    2. Acquired disorders
      a. Hepatitis and cirrhosis
      b. Drug-induced cholestasis
  B. Extrahepatic biliary obstruction (mechanical obstruction, e.g., stones, strictures, tumor of bile duct)

* In hepatitis and cirrhosis, there is usually interference in the three major steps of bilirubin metabolism—uptake, conjugation, excretion. However, excretion appears to be the rate-limiting step and is usually impaired to the greatest extent.

of bilirubin metabolism and (2) the underlying *disease* leading to this deranged metabolism. In many diseases there may be a derangement in *more than one* physiologic parameter of bilirubin metabolism. In any event, it is important first to determine whether the hyperbilirubinemia is predominantly of the *unconjugated* or *conjugated* type. A patient is considered to have predominantly unconjugated hyperbilirubinemia when less than *15 or 20 percent* of the total serum bilirubin is direct-reacting (with the 1-min van den Bergh reaction). A urine determination is important, because *bilirubinuria is found only in conjugated hyperbilirubinemia.*

In Table 45-2, jaundice is classified according to the fundamental derangements in bilirubin metabolism. These consist of (1) overproduction, (2) decreased hepatic uptake, (3) decreased hepatic conjugation, (4) decreased hepatic excretion (due to both intrahepatic and extrahepatic factors). Jaundice may also be described on the basis of the pathogenetic mechanism or disease process leading to deranged bilirubin function, and the terms *hemolytic jaundice, hepatocellular jaundice,* or *obstructive jaundice* are often used. In the past, *retention jaundice* has been used to refer to hemolytic jaundice and *regurgitation jaundice* for cases of hepatocellular or obstructive jaundice.

While these classifications and terms are helpful, in any one patient more than a single derangement or more than one "type" of jaundice may be present. For example, a patient with cirrhosis may have not only impaired liver cell function (and hence hepatocellular jaundice) but also hemolysis. Furthermore, obstructive jaundice may be due either to *mechanical* obstruction of the biliary radicles or to *functional* factors causing impaired hepatic excretion of bilirubin into bile.

In the present chapter a brief description of the major types of jaundice is given. A more detailed discussion of the individual disease entities is found in Chap. 325.

JAUNDICE WITH PREDOMINANTLY UNCONJUGATED BILIRUBIN IN THE SERUM. Overproduction of Bilirubin. When an increased amount of hemoglobin is released from red cells into either the bloodstream or tissues, the net result is an increased production of bilirubin. Hyperbilirubinemia will occur when the liver's capacity to remove the pigment from the circulation is exceeded. In most cases of hemolysis, the total serum bilirubin ranges from 3 to 5 mg per 100 ml. A slight increase in direct-reacting pigment may also be found, but this usually constitutes less than 15 percent of the total serum bilirubin. This finding is probably analogous to the slight elevations of direct-reacting bilirubin which occur when normal subjects are infused with unconjugated bilirubin. Both instances appear to be a reflection of the fact that the rate-limiting step in hepatic bilirubin metabolism is excretion and that when the liver's excretory capacity is exceeded, some reentry of conjugated bilirubin into the bloodstream occurs. For a detailed description of the causes of increased bilirubin production see Chap. 325.

Impaired Hepatic Uptake of Bilirubin. The entry of bilirubin into the liver cell entails a dissociation of the pigment from albumin, but the exact uptake mechanism has not been elucidated. In Gilbert's syndrome and some cases of drug-induced jaundice there may be a derangement in this phase of bilirubin metabolism (see Chap. 325).

Impaired Glucuronide Conjugation. Both acquired and genetic derangements in hepatic glucuronyl transferase occur. In the fetus and at birth, glucuronyl transferase activity is low and appears to account for the *neonatal jaundice* which normally is found between the second and the fifth day of life. There is also a rare congenital disorder associated with a deficiency of glucuronyl transferase, the Crigler-Najjar syndrome, in which marked unconjugated hyperbilirubinemia occurs.

Acquired defects in bilirubin glucuronyl transferase activity may be produced by drugs (i.e., enzyme inhibition) or intrinsic liver disease. However, in most diseases leading to liver cell damage, the excretory capacity of the liver is impaired to a greater extent than is the conjugating capacity. Therefore in most hepatocellular diseases, the hyperbilirubinemia is predominantly of the conjugated type (see Chap. 325).

JAUNDICE WITH PREDOMINANTLY CONJUGATED BILIRUBIN IN THE SERUM. Impaired Excretion of Bilirubin by the Liver. The impaired excretion of bilirubin into the biliary canaliculi, whether due to functional or mechanical factors, results in predominantly conjugated hyperbilirubinemia and bilirubinuria. The presence of *bilirubin in the urine is evidence of conjugated hyperbilirubinemia* and a most important point in the differential diagnosis of jaundice. Such findings are identical to those occurring in complete obstruction of the bile duct, emphasizing that *jaundice due to hepatocellular disease can seldom be differentiated from that due to extrahepatic obstruction solely on the basis of changes in bile pigment metabolism.* Indeed there are often instances when the two conditions are not distinguishable by any biochemical criteria and liver biopsy or laporotomy are needed for the definitive diagnosis.

When there is interference in the excretion of conjugated bilirubin into bile, by what mechanism does this pigment enter the systemic circulation? Several postulates have been proposed for this "reentry": (1) rupture of the bile canaliculi secondary to the necrosis of the hepatic cells that constitute their walls; (2) occlusion of the canaliculi by inspissated bile or their compression by swollen hepatic cells; (3) obstruction of the terminal intrahepatic bile ducts (i.e., cholangioles) by inflammatory cells; (4) altered hepatic cell permeability; and (5) that as a result of impaired excretion, conjugated bilirubin accumulates in the hepatocytes and secondarily diffuses into the plasma. Although some of these postulates are speculative, it is likely that several of these mechanisms occur. For example, occasionally in histologic sections escape of bile through rents in the walls of canaliculi in areas of necrosis is apparent. Also microscopic studies of the liver of rats injected with fluorescent dyes have shown reflux of bile from canaliculi into sinusoids. However, no anatomic damage needs to be invoked, because when unconjugated bilirubin is infused into normal subjects at high rates, conjugated hyperbilirubinemia occurs; this is explained most logically by passive diffusion.

Extrahepatic Biliary Obstruction. Complete obstruction of the extrahepatic bile ducts leads to jaundice with predominantly conjugated hyperbilirubinemia, bilirubinuria, and clay-colored stools. Failure of bile to reach the intestine results in virtual disappearance of urobilinogen from the stool and urine. The concentration of bilirubin rises progressively but then usually plateaus at a level of 30 to 40 mg per 100 ml. To some extent this plateau may be explained by a balance between renal excretion and diversion of bilirubin to other metabolites. In hepatocellular jaundice, such a plateau tends not to occur, and bilirubin levels in excess of 50 mg per 100 ml may be found.

Partial obstruction of the extrahepatic bile ducts can also give rise to jaundice but only if the intrabiliary pressure is increased, because the excretion of bilirubin does not diminish until the intraductile pressure approaches the maximal secretory pressure of approximately 250 mm bile. Jaundice may occur at much lower pressures if the obstruction is complicated by infection of the ducts or hepatocellular injury. Therefore, jaundice, bilirubinuria, and clay-colored stools are inconstant findings in partial biliary obstruction, and the amount of urobilinogen in urine and stool varies with the degree of occlusion.

The functional reserve of the liver is so great that *occlusion of the intrahepatic bile ducts* does not give rise to jaundice unless the drainage of bile from a large segment of the parenchyma is interrupted. Either of the two major hepatic ducts or a large number of secondary radicles may be occluded without production of jaundice. In experimental animals the ducts draining at least 75 percent of the parenchyma must be occluded before jaundice appears.

ADDITONAL POINTS OF TERMINOLOGY. In clinical practice, a patient may be described as having *obstructive,* or *cholestatic,* jaundice. By this is meant that clinically, and especially biochemically, there is little to suggest hepatocellular damage and that the main features point to interference with, or obstruction in, the flow of bile. Typically one would expect such a patient to show (1) predominantly conjugated hyperbilirubinemia, (2) minimal biochemical changes of parenchymal liver damage, and (3) a moderate to a marked increase in the serum alkaline phosphatase (usually greater than 15 Bodansky units). As emphasized in Chaps. 323 and 324, an *elevated alkaline phosphatase level* in a patient with jaundice or liver disease in the absence of other disorders such as bone disease is most suggestive of interference with bile secretion or an infiltrative process in the liver. However, often *laboratory tests alone may not permit differentiation of intrahepatic from extrahepatic cholestasis.*

Some clinicians reserve the term obstructive jaundice to those situations where anatomic obstruction can be demonstrated and use the term cholestatic jaundice for cases of parenchymal liver disease in which the obstructive phase is on a functional basis. Nevertheless, because these two entities frequently are indistinguishable by clinical and biochemical criteria, the terms obstructive jaundice and cholestatic jaundice are often used interchangeably.

Hepatocellular disorders in which jaundice associated with an obstructive, or cholestatic, phase occurs include (1) occasional cases of viral hepatitis, (2) drug reactions, especially those due to chlorpromazine and methyltestosterone, (3) some cases of alcoholic hepatitis or alcohol-induced fatty liver, (4) jaundice in the last trimester of pregnancy, (5) most cases of Dubin-Johnson or Rotor syndrome, (6) the disorder of so-called "benign recurrent intrahepatic cholestasis," and (7) certain types of postoperative jaundice. These and other conditions are discussed in Chaps. 325 and 326.

In summary, all forms of conjugated hyperbilirubinemia have by definition an impairment in the excretion of bilirubin into bile. In most cases of parenchymal liver disease, there is a broad derangement in the biochemical tests of liver function. However, when the major detectable alterations of liver function tests include (1) conjugated hyperbilirubinemia and (2) moderate to marked elevation of the serum alkaline phosphatase level, the terms obstructive or cholestatic jaundice may be appropriate. Additional procedures, including operation, are often needed to determine the cause of the cholestasis.

HEPATOMEGALY

In the supine position, the major part of the liver lies beneath the right rib cage. In some normal individuals the liver edge may be palpable 1 to 2 cm below the right costal margin, and a palpable liver edge by itself does not necessarily indicate hepatomegaly. In evaluating liver size by physical examination, two factors other than ability to palpate the liver edge need to be considered, namely, (1) the location of the upper border of liver dullness by percussion and (2) the body habitus.

Normally, the upper edge of liver dullness on the right side in the midclavicular line is at the level of the fifth rib, but in those of asthenic habitus it may be lower. The liver edge normally descends 1 to 3 cm with deep inspiration. In hypersthenic subjects, the liver may extend over to the left abdominal wall, with the lower edge high and not palpable; in hyposthenic subjects with a very acute costal angle the liver may lie in the right half of the abdomen, the edge being palpable by as much as 6 to 8 cm below the right costal margin lateral to the right rectus abdominis muscle. Thus, palpability does not necessarily imply hepatomegaly.

In determining liver enlargement by palpation, one should be certain that the liver is being palpated rather than other right upper quadrant masses such as gallbladder, colonic neoplasm, or fecal material in the colon. Liver enlargement is often confirmed by radiologic studies including hepatic scintiscans, celiac axis angiography, and splenic venography.

In many cases of generalized liver enlargement, the left lobe will be felt in the epigastrium between the xiphoid and umbilicus. The liver should be carefully palpated during deep inspiration to determine whether the edge is tender, regular or irregular, firm or soft, rounded and thickened or sharp. The edge is tender and often rounded with hepatic inflammation as in hepatitis or when the liver is acutely congested as in cardiac decompensation. Pulsation of the liver may be found with tricuspid valvular incompetence. A carcinomatous liver may be rocklike in hardness; the cirrhotic liver is very firm in consistency. The largest livers are often found with carcinoma (primary or metastatic), marked fatty infiltration, congestive cardiac decompensation, Hodgkin's disease, and amyloidosis. Rapid decrease in liver size may occur with improvement of congestive failure or mobilization of fat from the liver.

In a patient with hepatomegaly, auscultation is sometimes helpful. A friction rub may be audible (and palpable) in the right upper quadrant, usually due to a recent biopsy, tumor, or perihepatitis. In portal hypertension a venous hum may be audible between the umbilicus and the xiphoid. An arterial murmur or bruit over the liver may indicate tumor, usually hepatoma.

Table 45-3. CAUSES OF A PALPABLE LIVER AND HEPATOMEGALY

I. Palpable liver without hepatomegaly
   A. Right diaphragm displaced downward (e.g., emphysema, asthma)
   B. Subdiaphragmatic lesion (e.g., abcess)
   C. Aberrant lobe of liver (Riedel's lobe)
   D. Extremely thin or relaxed abdominal muscles
   E. Occasionally present in normal individuals
II. Hepatomegaly
   A. Vascular congestion (e.g., congestive heart failure, hepatic vein thrombosis)
   B. Bile duct obstruction (e.g., lesion in common duct leading to hepatomegaly and subsequently biliary cirrhosis)
   C. Infiltrative disorders
      1. Bone marrow and reticuloendothelial cells
         a. Extramedullary hematopoiesis
         b. Leukemia
         c. Lymphoma
      2. Fat
         a. Fatty liver (e.g., secondary to alcohol or toxins)
         b. Gaucher's disease and some other lipidoses
      3. Carbohydrate (especially glycogen; seen in some patients with diabetes, especially after insulin excess)
      4. Amyloid
      5. Iron (hemochromatosis and hemosiderosis)
      6. Granuloma (tuberculosis, sarcoid)
   D. Inflammatory disorders
      1. Hepatitis—due to drugs or infectious agents
      2. Cirrhosis—except in late stages when prolonged scarring may lead to a *small*, shrunken liver
   E. Tumor—primary or metastatic
   F. Cysts—polycystic disease, congenital hepatic fibrosis

Some of the causes of a palpable liver and hepatomegaly are given in Table 45-3.

REFERENCES

Castell, D. O., K. D. O'Brien, H. Muench, and T. C. Chalmers: Estimation of Liver Size by Percussion in Normal Individuals, Ann. Int. Med., 70:1183, 1969.

Gartner, L. M., and I. M. Arias: Formation, Transport and Excretion of Bilirubin, New Engl. J. Med., 280:1339, 1969.

Lester, R., and R. Schmid: Bilirubin Metabolism, New Engl. J. Med., 270:779, 1964.

Lester, R., and R. F. Troxler: Recent Advances in Bile Pigment Metabolism, Gastroenterology 56:143, 1969.

Sherlock, S.: Jaundice, Chap. 10, in "Diseases of the Liver," 4th ed. Philadelphia, F. A. Davis Company, 1968.

With, T. K.: "Bile Pigments: Chemical, Biological and Clinical Aspects," New York, Academic Press, Inc., 1968.

46 ABDOMINAL SWELLING AND ASCITES

*Kurt J. Isselbacher and
Robert M. Glickman*

Abdominal swelling or distension is a common problem in clinical medicine and may be the initial manifestation of a systemic disease or of otherwise unsuspected abdominal disease. *Subjective* abdominal enlargement, often described as a sensation of fullness or bloating, is usually transient and is often related to a functional gastrointestinal disorder when it is not accompanied by objective physical findings of increased abdominal girth or local swelling. *Obesity* and lumbar lordosis, which may be associated with prominence of the abdomen, may usually be distinguished from true increases in the volume of the peritoneal cavity by history and careful physical examination.

CLINICAL HISTORY. The development of abdominal swelling may be described by the patient as a progressive increase in belt or clothing size, the appearance of abdominal or inguinal hernias, or the development of a localized swelling. Often, considerable abdominal enlargement has gone unnoticed for weeks or months either because of coexistent obesity or because the ascites formation has been insidious, without pain or localizing symptoms. Progressive abdominal distension may be associated with a sensation of "pulling" or "stretching" of the flanks or groins and vague low back pain. Localized *pain* usually results from involvement of an abdominal organ (e.g., a passively congested liver, large spleen, or colonic tumor). Pain is uncommon in cirrhosis with ascites and when it is present, pancreatitis, hepatoma, or peritonitis should be considered. Tense ascites or abdominal tumors may produce increased intraabdominal pressure, resulting in *indigestion* and *heartburn* due to gastroesophageal reflux or *dyspnea*, *orthopnea*, and *tachypnea* from elevation of the diaphragm. A coexistent pleural effusion, more commonly on the right, presumably due to leakage of ascitic fluid through lymphatic channels in the diaphragm, may also contribute to respiratory embarrassment. The patient with diffuse abdominal swelling should be questioned about increased alcoholic intake, a prior episode of jaundice or hematuria, a change in bowel habits, or a past history of rheumatic heart disease. Such historic information may provide the needed clues to suspect an occult cirrhosis, a colonic tumor with peritoneal seeding, congestive heart failure, or nephrosis.

PHYSICAL EXAMINATION. *Inspection* of the abdomen is an important but often cursorily performed aspect of the abdominal examination. By noting the abdominal contour one may be able to distinguish localized from generalized swelling. The tensely distended abdomen with tightly stretched skin, bulging flanks, and everted umbilicus is characteristic of ascites. A prominent abdominal venous pattern with the direction of flow away from the umbilicus often is a reflection of portal hypertension; the presence of venous collaterals with flow from the lower abdomen toward the umbilicus suggests obstruction of the inferior vena cava; flow downward toward the umbilicus suggests superior vena cava obstruction. "Doming" of the abdomen with visible ridges from underlying bowel loops is usually due to intestinal obstruction or distension. An epigastric mass, with evident peristalsis proceeding from left to right, usually indicates underlying pyloric obstruction. A liver with metastatic deposits may be visible as a nodular right upper quadrant mass moving with respiration.

Auscultation may reveal the high pitched, rushing sounds of early intestinal obstruction or a succussion sound due to increased fluid and gas in a dilated hollow viscus. Careful auscultation over an enlarged liver occasionally reveals the harsh bruit of a vascular tumor, especially a hepatoma, or the leathery friction rub of a surface nodule. A venous hum at the umbilicus may signify portal hypertension and an increased collateral blood flow around the liver. A fluid wave and flank dullness which shifts with change in position of the patient are important signs that indicate the presence of peritoneal fluid. In the obese patient, small amounts of fluid may be difficult to demonstrate; on occasion the fluid may be detected by abdominal percussion with the patient on his hands and knees. Doubt about the presence of peritoneal fluid may be resolved by careful paracentesis with a small gauge (#19 or 20) needle. Careful percussion should serve to distinguish generalized abdominal enlargement from localized swelling due to an enlarged uterus, ovarian cyst, or distended bladder. Percussion can also outline an abnormally small or large liver. Loss of normal liver dullness may result from massive hepatic necrosis; it may also be a clue to free gas in the peritoneal cavity, as from perforation of a hollow viscus.

Palpation is often difficult with massive ascites, and ballottement of overlying fluid may be the only method of palpating the liver or spleen. A slightly enlarged spleen in association with ascites may be the only evidence of an occult cirrhosis. When there is evidence of portal hypertension, the finding of a soft liver suggests that obstruction to portal flow is extrahepatic; the presence of a firm liver suggests cirrhosis as the likely cause of the portal hypertension. A very hard or nodular liver is a clue that the liver is infiltrated with tumor, and when accompanied by ascites, it suggests that the latter is due to peritoneal seeding. A pulsatile liver and ascites may be found in tricuspid insufficiency.

An attempt should be made to determine whether a mass is solid or cystic, smooth or irregular, and whether it moves with respiration. The liver, spleen, and gallbladder should descend with respiration unless they are fixed by adhesions or extension of tumor beyond the organ. A fixed mass not descending with respiration may indicate that it is retroperitoneal. Tenderness, especially if localized, may indicate an inflammatory process such as an abscess; it may also be due to stretching of the visceral peritoneum or tumor necrosis. Rectal and pelvic examinations are mandatory; they may reveal otherwise undetected masses due to tumor or infection.

Radiographic and laboratory examinations are essential for confirming or extending the impressions gained on physical examination. Upright and recumbent films of the abdomen may demonstrate the dilated loops of bowel with fluid levels characteristic of intestinal obstruction or the diffuse abdominal haziness and loss of psoas margins suggestive of ascites. A plain film of the abdomen may reveal the distended colon of otherwise unsuspected ulcerative colitis and give valuable information as to the size of the liver and spleen. An irregular and elevated right diaphragm may be a clue to the presence of a liver abscess or hepatoma. Studies of the gastrointestinal tract with barium or other contrast media are usually necessary in the search for a primary tumor.

ASCITES

In most cases the clinical and laboratory evaluation of the patient with ascites is sufficient to reveal the cause of the fluid accumulation. Often the ascites is a component or complication of cirrhosis, congestive heart failure, nephrosis, or disseminated carcinomatosis. However, even when the cause of ascites seems obvious, it is often important to determine whether another separate or related disease process has supervened. For example, when the compensated cirrhotic with minimal ascites

Table 46-1. ASCITIC FLUID CHARACTERISTICS IN VARIOUS DISEASE STATES

Condition	Gross appearance	Specific gravity	Protein, Gm/100 ml	Cell count		Other tests
				Red blood cells, >10,000/mm^3	White blood cells/mm^3	
Cirrhosis	Straw colored or bile stained	<1.016(95%)*	<2.5(95%)*	1%	<250(90%)*; predominantly endothelial	
Neoplasm	Straw colored, hemorrhagic, mucinous, or chylous	Variable, >1.016(45%)	>2.5(75%)	20%	>1,000(50%); variable cell types	Cytology, cell block, peritoneal biopsy
Tuberculous peritonitis	Clear, turbid, hemorrhagic, chylous	Variable, >1.016(50%)	>2.5(50%)	7%	>1,000(70%); usually >70% lymphocytes	Peritoneal biopsy, stain and culture for acid fast bacilli
Pyogenic peritonitis	Turbid or purulent	If purulent, >1.016	If purulent, >2.5	Unusual	Predominantly polymorphonuclear leukocytes	+ gram stain, culture
Congestive heart failure	Straw colored	Variable, <1.016(60%)	Variable 1.5–5.3	10%	<1,000(90%); usually mesothelial, mononuclear	
Nephrosis	Straw colored or chylous	<1.016	<2.5(100%)	Unusual	<250; mesothelial, mononuclear	If chylous, ether extraction, Sudan staining
Pancreatitis, pseudocyst	Turbid, hemorrhagic, or chylous	Variable, often >1.016	Variable, often >2.5	Variable, may be bloodstained	Variable	Increased amylase in ascitic fluid and serum

* Since the conditions of fluid examination and patient selection were not identical in each series, the percentage figures (in the parentheses) should be taken as an indication of the order of magnitude rather than the precise incidence of any abnormal finding.

SOURCE: The data in this table are a composite of several large series (Refs. 1–5).

develops progressive ascites that is increasingly difficult to control with sodium restriction or diuretics, the obvious temptation is to attribute the worsening of the clinical picture to progressive liver disease. However, an occult hepatoma, portal vein thrombosis, or even tuberculosis may be responsible for the decompensation. The disappointingly low success of diagnosing tuberculous peritonitis or hepatoma in the patient with cirrhosis and ascites reflects the too-low index of suspicion for the development of such superimposed conditions. Similarly, the patient with congestive heart failure may develop ascites from a disseminated carcinoma with peritoneal seeding. The thorough evaluation of each patient with ascites, even in the presence of an "obvious" cause, will help avoid these errors.

Diagnostic paracentesis (50 to 100 ml) should be part of the routine evaluation of the patient with ascites. The fluid should be examined for its gross appearance, protein content, cell count, and differential, as well as gram and acid-fast stains and culture. Cytologic and cell-block examination may disclose an otherwise unsuspected carcinoma. Table 46-1 illustrates some of the features of ascitic fluid typically found in various disease states. In some disorders, such as cirrhosis, the fluid has the characteristics of a transudate (less than 2.5 Gm protein per 100 ml and a specific gravity less than 1.016); in others, such as peritonitis, the features are those of an exudate. Although there is variability of the ascitic fluid in any given disease state, some features are sufficiently characteristic to suggest certain diagnositic possibilities. For example, bloodstained fluid with more than 2.5 Gm protein per 100 ml is unusual in uncomplicated cirrhosis but consistent with tuberculous peritonitis or neoplasm. Cloudy fluid with a predominance of polymorphonuclear cells and positive gram stain is characteristic of bacterial peritonitis; if the cells are mostly lymphocytes, tuberculosis should be suspected. The complete examination of each fluid is most important for occasionally only one finding may be abnormal. For example, if the fluid is a typical transudate but contains more than 250 white blood cells per cu mm, the finding should be recognized as atypical for cirrhosis, nephrosis, or congestive heart failure and should warrant a search for tumor or infection.

Chylous ascites refers to a turbid, milky, or creamy peritoneal fluid due to the presence of thoracic or intestinal lymph. Such a fluid shows Sudan-staining fat globules microscopically, and an increased triglyceride content by chemical examination. A turbid fluid due to leukocytes or tumor cells may be confused with chylous fluid, and it is often helpful to carry out alkalinization and ether extraction of the specimen. Alkali will tend to dissolve cellular proteins and thereby reduce turbidity; ether extraction will lead to clearing if the turbidity of the fluid is due to lipid. Chylous ascites is most often the result of lymphatic obstruction from trauma, tumor, tuberculosis, filariasis (see Chap. 249), or congenital abnormalities. It may also be seen in the nephrotic syndrome.

The etiology of ascites may remain uncertain even after the usual diagnostic procedures have been carried out. Under those circumstances a high proportion of the cases will be due to (1) cirrhosis of the liver, (2) carcinomatosis with peritoneal involvement, (3) tuberculous peritonitis, or (4) hepatoma. In all of these conditions pronounced weight loss, wasting, anorexia, and fever may be found, and hepatomegaly, splenomegaly, and deranged liver function tests may be present. Procedures such as peritoneal biopsy, peritoneoscopy, liver biopsy, splenoportography, or laparotomy may be necessary to provide the diagnosis. Other less common causes of ascites include constrictive pericarditis, hepatic vein obstruction, myxedema and benign tumors of the ovary, particularly fibroma (Meigs's syndrome, with ascites and hydrothorax). The physiologic and metabolic factors involved in the production of ascites are described in Chap. 328.

REFERENCES

Berner, C. et al.: Diagnostic Probabilities in Patients with Conspicuous Ascites, Arch. Intern. Med., 113:687, 1964.

Burack, W. R., and R. M. Hollister: Tuberculous Peritonitis, Am. J. Med., 28:510, 1960.

Hyman, S., F. Villa, and F. Steigmann: Mimetic Aspects of Ascites, J.A.M.A., 183:651, 1963.

Levine, H.: Needle Biopsy of the Peritoneum in Exudative Ascites, Arch. Intern. Med., 120:542, 1967.

Paddock, F. K.: Diagnostic Significance of Serous Fluids in Disease, New Engl. J. Med., 223:1010, 1940.

Rovelstad, R. A. et al.: Helpful Laboratory Procedures in the Differential Diagnosis of Ascites, Proc. Mayo Clin., 34:565, 1959.

Sherlock, S.: Diseases of the Liver and Biliary System, 4th ed., Philadelphia, F. A. Davis Company, 1968.

Section 6
Alterations in Body Weight

47 LOSS OF WEIGHT
George W. Thorn

Weight loss as elicited by history or detected by physical examination constitutes a cardinal manifestation of disease or disordered bodily function, unless an otherwise normal individual has imposed on himself caloric restriction in an effort to reduce.

Under normal circumstances decreased food intake or total starvation initiates a constellation of metabolic changes designed to reduce energy expenditure and heat loss. Chief among these are reduced basal metabolic rate, lowered body temperature, restricted physical activity, and reduced peripheral blood flow (vasoconstriction). By these means the body attempts to maintain the function of vital organs such as the heart, brain, kidneys, liver, and lungs. These mechanisms are seriously impaired when complications such as fever, vomiting, diarrhea, and dehydration supervene.

Anorexia is a frequent accompaniment of chronic as well as acute disease processes. In the absence of specific abnormalities of gastrointestinal function, loss of appetite may be due to toxic products liberated by microorganisms, by breakdown products of tumor tissue, or by retention of metabolic end products as occurs in late-stage renal and hepatic disease. Hypoosmolarity of the body fluid compartment and increased cell water content may give rise to centrally mediated nausea and vomiting through its effect on specific hypothalamic centers. Thus, a patient with malignant hypertension may experience nausea as a consequence of hypertensive cerebrovascular changes in the absence of uremia or, later, as a result of retention of nitrogenous products with progressive renal failure.

In evaluating the implication of weight loss several considerations deserve special attention.

1. Is the patient's history concerning the magnitude and duration of weight loss reliable? Can it be documented by comparison with prior measurements or confirmed by physical examination?

2. Has there been a notable change in appetite or food intake?

3. Has there been evidence of disordered gastrointestinal function with a change in bowel habits?

4. Has there been evidence of polyuria, particularly nocturia?

The determination of the *magnitude of weight loss* is not always easy. Some patients follow changes in weight regularly on bathroom scales or weighing machines, or they have serial physical examinations. Other patients may be quite vague or uninformed regarding actual changes in weight. Questions regarding a change in waist measurement or collar, suit, dress, or shoe size may provide helpful clues. Physical examination should then confirm this, with its opportunity to detect adipose tissue loss and the presence or absence of edema or dehydration. Special consideration should be given to the valuation of overall weight loss in the presence of edema, as the actual tissue loss in such patients will, of course, greatly exceed the apparent decrease in total body weight.

Weight loss with anorexia and decreased food intake occurs in such a diversified range of acute and chronic diseases as not to be particularly helpful in differential diagnosis. The magnitude of weight loss may reflect either the *seriousness* or the *duration* of the underlying disorder. Thought should be given to the diagnosis of psychologic difficulties such as depression and anorexia nervosa, to generalized endocrine and metabolic disorders such as pituitary-adrenal insufficiency and hyperparathyroidism, and to hepatic and renal disease, as well as to chronic infection, neoplasm, and drug intoxication. Weight loss without a significant change in food consumption would suggest hypermetabolic states, such as thyrotoxicosis and anxiety or gastrointestinal hypermotility.

Of course, particular attention will be given in the history to any abnormality in gastrointestinal function as a cause of weight loss. Here again, one is concerned with *decreased food intake* such as might occur in partial intestinal obstruction; *decreased absorption,* which suggests pancreatic or hepatic disease, spruelike syndromes, regional enteritis, or severe food allergies; or *increased loss of food* and *fluids* through vomiting, diarrhea, or draining fistulas. Disorders of gastrointestinal function accompany systemic disorders so frequently that the physician must always maintain a high index of suspicion that what appears to be primarily a disorder of gastrointestinal function may actually reflect deep-seated infection, tumor, or renal, hepatic, cardiac, or pulmonary disease. On the other hand, *specific gastrointestinal disorders* may complicate systemic disease; thus, the patient with nausea, vomiting, and renal azotemia may have an associated peptic ulcer.

The presence of polyuria, and particularly nocturia, in association with anorexia and weight loss suggests diabetes mellitus, diabetes insipidus, chronic renal disease, and disorders giving rise to *hypercalcemia* or *hypokalemia*.

Physicians should encourage patients to weigh regularly and to maintain a lifelong record of changes in body weight, since alterations in weight so frequently mirror abnormalities in bodily function. Loss of weight may be the first indication of serious organic disease or psychologic disorder, the detection and significance of which may be measurably enhanced by carefully recorded changes in body weight.

48 GAIN IN WEIGHT
George W. Thorn

General Considerations

A gradual increase in weight may be secondary to either an accumulation of fluid (edema) or adipose tissue (obesity). However, weight gain in excess of 1 to 2 lb per day will almost invariably indicate excess fluid retention. Excess fluid accumulation or edema (see Chap. 34) should suggest underlying renal, cardiac, or hepatic insufficiency. Hypoalbuminemia usually suggests renal disease, but it may reflect nutritional deficiency or liver disease secondary to small-bowel pathology or inadequate protein intake. Occasionally, primary retention of water with hyponatremia will result from inappropriate antidiuretic hormone secretion. Excess salt intake, licorice, and drugs such as sex hormones, adrenal steroids, diphenylhydantoin, and reserpine may contribute to salt and water retention. The presence of edema and weight gain may mask a significant loss of body tissue. This is best exemplified by the cardiac or hypertensive patient who, following a brisk diuresis, becomes aware for the first time of the extent of body wasting.

Obese patients can retain rather large quantities of extracellular fluid without necessarily exhibiting edema. From a practical point of view, it should be assumed that a markedly obese patient has sequestered a significant volume of extracellular fluid. This can often be demonstrated by administering a diuretic agent; and, of course, this is the approach utilized by many "lose-weight-fast" schemes. Some appreciation of the salt- and water-retaining capacity of obese patients, or of patients with incipient edema, may be obtained by weighing the patient in the morning and again at night. It is not unusual for an obese individual, or a preedematous patient, to gain 4 to 8 lb during the day, particularly if he is up and about.

CYCLIC EDEMA

Idiopathic edema or "periodic swelling" constitutes a physicopsychologic syndrome which uniquely affects adult females. Physiologic mechanisms capable of modifying salt and water metabolism within the body include the antidiuretic hormone (ADH), aldosterone, "third factor," histamine, and the kinins. The intimate relationship between the secretory control of these humoral agents and the central nervous system is well established. Emotional and psychologic factors are readily capable of initiating the release of these agents and, hence, of inducing cyclical retention of fluid and electrolytes. Why the syndrome is limited to the female is still conjectural; however, cyclical retention of fluid and electrolytes occurs physiologically following menstruation and during pregnancy and lactation. Thus, a well-developed pathway is available in the female for psychologic disturbances to manifest themselves pathophysiologically. An understanding of the psychologic and emotional factors is basic to successful therapy. Judicious use of diuretic agents can correct the physiologic abnormalities in most instances; however, the basic symptomatology will not be relieved by diuresis alone. Of particular importance is the avoidance of excessive diuretic therapy with its predilection for inducing potassium and magnesium deficiency, which, in turn, may perpetuate the symptoms of weakness, fatigue, and irritability. The complex nature of this syndrome necessitates astute, thoughtful, and continued medical care.

OBESITY

Obesity occurs when the caloric intake exceeds the energy requirements of the body both for physical activity and for growth. As a result there is an accumulation of fat, which is stored in the adipose tissue. The excessive tissue may be distributed generally over the body, or it may be localized. The factors controlling the location of the fat are not all known, but pituitary, thyroid, and sex hormones play an important role. Obesity is a serious and common disease in those countries in which a combination of generous food supplies and sedentary occupations readily permit the assimilation of more food than is necessary. The excessive deposition of fat is associated with an increased incidence of degenerative diseases such as atherosclerosis, diabetes, and arthritis; indeed, the only common cause of death that does not strike earlier in the obese than in the lean population is suicide! The ill effects of obesity can be prevented and, to some extent, repaired by weight reduction. The treatment of obesity is one of the most serious problems in preventive medicine in the United States today.

Etiology

Under normal circumstances there is a very exact adjustment of food intake to body requirements. Unfortunately, in certain individuals this adjustment is deranged, and intake becomes excessive. The cause of the derangement is not understood, but several important factors are well known.

HYPOTHALAMIC RELATIONSHIPS. It has been known for years that lesions involving the hypothalamus may lead to obesity. Lesions in the ventromedial nucleus of the hypothalamus induce hyperphagia and obesity, whereas lesions in the lateral hypothalamic area lead to a cessation of eating. On the basis of these findings a dual mechanism has been postulated for the regulation of food intake: a "satiety" center in the ventromedial nucleus and a "feeding" center in the lateral hypothalamic area. Studies on gold thioglucose-treated mice have demonstrated fiber connections between these two centers.

Additional experimental studies relate to the theories of "glucostat," "lipostat," and "aminostat" control of food intake. It has been suggested that animals on a free feeding schedule begin to eat when a blood factor falls below a critical level and not because a "hunger" factor increases above a threshold level. Further support of a glucoreceptor is suggested by studies in which phlorhizin, a known inhibitor of glucose uptake in a wide variety of tissues, was tested for a similar effect on hypothalamic glucoreceptors in rats. The infusion of a minute quantity of phlorhizin into the lateral cerebral ventricle resulted in marked hyperphagia and gain in weight, whereas a similar quantity injected intraperitoneally had no demonstrable effect. These data suggest that cerebral glucoreceptors do indeed exist and are involved in the regulation of food intake.

Thus it appears that the basic cause of obesity is a derangement of the appetite-controlling mechanisms, permitting the assimilation of more food than is needed. It has been claimed that certain individuals are more efficient than others in their ability to digest, absorb, and utilize food and therefore that they become obese at lower caloric intakes than might be expected. Extensive balance studies on such patients have never substantiated this explanation; at equivalent levels of physical activity and basal metabolism, there seems to be little variation in the required caloric intake.

DECREASED BASAL METABOLIC RATE AND ACTIVITY. A decrease in basal metabolic rate and activity accompanies hypothyroidism and anterior pituitary deficiency. Some decrease in activity with an increased tendency for obesity occurs with primary gonadal failure—particularly in the female. Advancing age is characteristically attended by a progressive lowering of basal metabolic rate and, of course, in most instances with an appreciable reduction in physical activity. Disorders or diseases which limit ambulation, such as cardiac or pulmonary failure or bone and joint disease, will also predispose to weight gain unless caloric intake is appropriately readjusted.

HYPOTHYROIDISM. Hypothyroidism may be suspected in an individual who has developed intolerance to cold, whose skin has become dry and coarse, and whose reflexes are prolonged (see Chap. 89). Weight gain associated with a more severe degree of hypothyroidism or myxedema may be due to edema, ascites, and pleural effusion. Gordon and his colleagues believe that some obese patients have a specific block in the utilization of fatty acids by peripheral tissues that can be removed by administration of triiodothyronine.

ANTERIOR PITUITARY DEFICIENCY. Anterior pituitary deficiency of a mild degree such as that described by Sheehan (see Chap. 87) may be accompanied by weight gain. This syndrome is most frequently observed in women after childbirth. Hypopituitarism in males as well as in females may be caused by a chromophobe adenoma or cyst of the pituitary. In such instances, a clue to the disorder may present as a result of local pressure, i.e., headaches or visual disturbances. In all types of mild hypopituitarism, signs of target gland deficiency, i.e., thyroid, adrenal, or gonadal, should be looked for. Gonadal deficiency is characterized by impotence in men and oligomenorrhea or amenorrhea in women. The signs of secondary hypothyroidism do not differ appreciably from those of primary, except that thyroid enlargement is not expected. Secondary adrenal cortical insufficiency is *not* associated with hyperpigmentation and rarely presents as severe mineral (aldosterone) deficiency. Hypoglycemic manifestations are frequently observed.

A decrease in physical activity secondary to a change in occupation, to traumatic injury, to heart disease, or to other incapacitating illnesses will result in increased adiposity if normal caloric intake is maintained. This is of no pathologic significance other than the generally unfavorable effect of obesity on weight-bearing joints.

Increased Caloric Intake

Excessive food intake secondary to *organic* disease occurs most commonly in response to a hypoglycemic stimulus. When hypoglycemic symptoms occur under fasting conditions, hyperinsulinism and pancreatic tumor should be considered. When hypoglycemic manifestations occur 3 to 5 hr after a meal, the paradoxic hypoglycemic response of early diabetes mellitus may be suspected (see Chap. 96). In the latter case it is thought that the prolonged elaboration of insulin represents an inappropriate response to the initial postprandial hyperglycemia. Occasionally, traumatic lesions of the brain, localized encephalitis, and brain tumors appear to modify the satiety centers in the hypothalamus, with resulting stimulation of appetite over and above caloric needs.

FAMILIAL AND CULTURAL EATING HABITS. These are firmly implanted at an early age. In groups in which great emphasis is placed on food, there is a tendency to overeat. Sometimes the cultural pattern equates success with obesity (witness the common caricature of the obese banker) and encourages the ambitious person to achieve a comfortable corpulence. Moreover, when activity patterns change, eating habits may remain constant, so that the man who has previously been physically active may fail to reduce his caloric intake when he suddenly changes to a sedentary occupation. This tendency may be reinforced by the gradual decline of metabolic rate and of muscle activity, which ordinarily accompanies aging.

PSYCHOLOGICAL FACTORS. Certain individuals may have increased appetite for psychologic reasons. Under these circumstances food is used as a substitute for the satisfaction they should obtain from other emotional sources. In this respect, they are similar to alcoholics, who use alcohol as a substitute for such normal sources of satisfaction as their friends, their families, or success in their work.

Psychologists do raise the question, however, whether all individuals describe the changes as "hunger" and eat when the biologic machinery is activated. There is increasing evidence which suggests that major individual differences exist in the extent to which physiologic changes are associated with the desire to eat. Hilde Bruch, a psychoanalyst, has observed that her obese patients literally do not know when they are physiologically hungry. She has suggested that during childhood these individuals were not taught to distinguish between hunger and such states as fear, anger, and anxiety. If this is so, these individuals may be labeling any state of arousal as hunger. That the obese may not know when they are physiologically hungry has been substantiated by Stunkard (1961), who studied the relation of hunger sensation to gastric motility in obese and nonobese individuals. The results indicated that nonobese and obese do not differ in degree of gastric motility and that when the stomach was not contracting, the reports of both groups were similar. However, there was a significant difference between the two groups in the reported coincidence of hunger and gastric motility, i.e., nonobese, 21 percent; obese, 47 percent. Schachter, on the basis of these and many other experiments, suggests that the obese may be relatively insensitive to variations in the correlation of food deprivation but highly sensitive to environmental, food-related cues, and that this may provide one key to understanding the notorious long-run ineffectiveness of virtually all attempts to treat obesity. The use of the anorexigenic drugs such as amphetamine or of bulk-producing nonnutritive substances such as methylcellulose is based on the premise that such agents dampen the intensity of the physiologic symptoms of food deprivation. Probably they do, but these symptoms appear to have little to do with whether or not a fat person eats. Restricted, low-calorie diets should be effective just so long as the obese dieter is able to blind himself to food-relevant cues or so long as he exists in a world barren of such cues.

Therapeutic Considerations

CENTRAL DEPRESSION OF APPETITE. Unfortunately, there is no pharmacologic agent available at this time which acts primarily by depressing the "appetite center." This type of depression is seen regularly in disease states such as hepatitis and uremia and as a toxic manifestation of drugs such as digitalis.

SUBSTANCES WHICH DEPRESS APPETITE BY INDUCING A SENSE OF WELL-BEING. Amphetamine and its derivatives are the prototype of this group of substances. These agents are commonly referred to as "anorexigenic" or "anorectic." There is no evidence to show, however, that their action results from a depression of the appetite center. As a result of stimulation, or a "lift," the patient's drive toward overeating may be significantly modified and as far as he is concerned, the overall effect of the drug is "appetite-depressing." Obviously, drugs which create such a state of euphoria may lead to habituation in certain individuals.

Amphetamine and its derivatives have been shown to depress food intake in man as well as in experimental animals. Patients experience a sense of well-being after the ingestion of these drugs, and it is thought that the reduction in appetite is a consequence of distraction. At least in the hyperphagia which follows frontal lobotomy, no depression of appetite is induced by amphetamine or its congeners.

At present there is a large number of derivatives of amphetamine sulfate (Benzedrine) and closely related compounds available for clinical use, for example, dextroamphetamine sulfate (Dexedrine), levoamphetamine sulfate and phosphate, levoamphetamine alginate (Levonor), methamphetamine hydrochloride (Amphedroxyn, Desoxyephedrine, Desoxyn, Desyphed, Dexoval, Desoxyfed, Drinalfa, Efroxine, Methedrine, Norodin, Semoxydrine, Syndrox), phenylpropanolamine (Propadrine), phenmetrazine (Preludin), phenyl-*tert*-butylamine resin (Ionamin), and diethylpropion (Tenuate and Tepanil).

Although it is unfortunate that manufacturers avoid or disclaim the relationship of many of these substances with amphetamine, the fact is that the structural formulas differ very little (Fig. 48-1). The dextro form of amphetamine differs in its pharmacologic action from the levo form in that the cephalotropic effect is enhanced and the cardiovascular actions are less intense. However, this fact suggests that the dextro form might be expected to cause anxiety, restlessness or sleeplessness at the same dosage level. The action of methamphetamine differs little from dextroamphetamine except in its somewhat enhanced cardiovascular effects. Since phenylpropanolamine may be sold without prescription, it has become a common ingredient of many weight-reducing tablets. Although if given in adequate dosage phenylpropanolamine may reduce appetite, in the usual dosage found in most weight-reducing tablets (25 mg or less) it is no more effective than a placebo. Phenmetrazine, although subjected to intensive study and claimed to be quite different, is a typical congener of amphetamine with the effectiveness of dextroamphetamine. Phenyl-*tert*-butylamine resin is advertised as not being an amphetamine drug, although it clearly belongs to the amphetamine series, as a study of its structural formula indicates (Fig. 48-1).

The usual dosage of amphetamine sulfate (Benzedrine) or dextroamphetamine sulfate (Dexedrine) is 5 mg given 30 to 60 min before meals. It may be necessary in some patients to omit the evening dose because of increased nervousness or sleeplessness. Long-acting preparations which can be given in a single dose of 10 to 15 mg each morning are also useful. These substances may prove helpful for some patients during the early weeks of restricted food intake.

Although serious reactions are rarely encountered with amphetamine and its congeners, the physician

Ephedrine

Methamphetamine
(desoxyephedrine)

Amphetamine
(benzedrine)

Phenyl-tert butylamine
resin (Ionamin)

Fig. 48-1. Amphetamine and congeners.

must be alert to the sympathomimetic effect of these agents in causing a rise in blood pressure, increased cardiac rate and work, and the possible development of cardiac arrhythmias. Since tolerance to these drugs develops relatively rapidly, their usefulness is short-lived unless the dosage is increased. The possibility that continued use of amphetamine-like substances such as Menocil may induce pulmonary hypertension has been reported.

BULK PRODUCERS. Repeated attempts have been made to satiate the appetite by means of bulk of low caloric content. Leafy vegetables such as cabbage, spinach, and lettuce are helpful in many patients and constitute an important element in most low-calorie diets. Addition of calorie-free bulk to the diet does not automatically displace calorie-containing food unless specific restrictions are prescribed. Because of the significant reduction in fat content of the diet, patients may experience constipation; for this reason bulk producers such as dioctyl sodium sulfosuccinate (Colace), 50 to 200 mg daily, and agar may be required. However, as suggested earlier, neither appetite depressor nor bulk producer will be particularly effective in a weight-reduction program in an individual who does not normally equate increased gastric contractions with the sensation of hunger or a full intestinal tract with satiety.

METABOLIC STIMULANTS INCLUDING HORMONES. Repeated efforts have been made to discover a nontoxic agent which would maintain a normal metabolic level in the face of weight loss. Dinitrophenol has had the widest use. The consensus today is that its undesirable toxic side reactions make its use unjustified.

In most instances, substances of this type are being employed by physicians or patients in an attempt to induce *weight loss without caloric restriction*. To do this, it is obviously necessary to raise basal metabolic level *above normal*. There is no known substance which can be used safely to increase metabolic level above normal for prolonged periods of time without danger of toxicity.

In the mind of the lay public, "hormones" are the most important cause of obesity and are hopefully considered to be its cure. The well-informed physician recognizes to what a small extent disturbances in hormone secretion are primarily responsible for obesity and how futile most types of hormone therapy are as cures of obesity.

No pituitary preparation now available is useful in weight reduction. Male and female gonadal hormones and adrenal cortical hormones have no place in therapy unless specific deficiency of these hormones exists. Thyroid therapy has received wide application and merits special discussion.

Thyroid therapy is effective substitution therapy in patients with hypothyroidism. Unfortunately, however, the number of patients with hypothyroidism among the obese is relatively small. Thyroid therapy has a definite

Table 48-1. DESIRABLE WEIGHTS FOR MEN AND WOMEN, ACCORDING TO HEIGHT AND FRAME, AGES TWENTY-FIVE AND OVER, WEIGHT IN INDOOR CLOTHING

Height (in shoes)	Small frame	Medium frame	Large frame
	Men		
	lb.	lb.	lb.
5 ft. 2 in.	112–120	118–129	126–141
5 ft. 3 in.	115–123	121–133	129–144
5 ft. 4 in.	118–126	124–136	132–148
5 ft. 5 in.	121–129	127–139	135–152
5 ft. 6 in.	124–133	130–143	138–156
5 ft. 7 in.	128–137	134–147	142–161
5 ft. 8 in.	132–141	138–152	147–166
5 ft. 9 in.	136–145	142–156	151–170
5 ft. 10 in.	140–150	146–160	155–174
5 ft. 11 in.	144–154	150–165	159–179
6 ft.	148–158	154–170	164–184
6 ft. 1 in.	152–162	158–175	168–189
6 ft. 2 in.	156–167	162–180	173–194
6 ft. 3 in.	160–171	167–185	178–199
6 ft. 4 in.	164–175	172–190	182–204
	Women		
4 ft. 10 in.	92–98	96–107	104–119
4 ft. 11 in.	94–101	98–110	106–122
5 ft.	96–104	101–113	109–125
5 ft. 1 in.	99–107	104–116	112–128
5 ft. 2 in.	102–110	107–119	115–131
5 ft. 3 in.	105–113	110–122	118–134
5 ft. 4 in.	108–116	113–126	121–138
5 ft. 5 in.	111–119	116–130	125–142
5 ft. 6 in.	114–123	120–135	129–146
5 ft. 7 in.	118–127	124–139	133–150
5 ft. 8 in.	122–131	128–143	137–154
5 ft. 9 in.	126–135	132–147	141–158
5 ft. 10 in.	130–140	136–151	145–163
5 ft. 11 in.	134–144	140–155	149–168
6 ft.	138–148	144–159	153–173

and sustained effect on the metabolism of the hypothyroid case. Complete thyroid deficiency may require 0.2 Gm thyroid (USP) daily; 0.1 Gm thyroid (USP) daily should be adequate for milder cases. A given dose of thyroid will produce a predictable rise in basal metabolic rate in a patient with hypothyroidism, and a daily dose of thyroid will maintain the increase in basal metabolic rate indefinitely. It appears that certain patients with obesity can tolerate rather large doses of thyroid without undue symptoms but with sufficient increase in metabolic rate to assist appreciably in their weight-reduction program.

MAINTENANCE OF IDEAL WEIGHT

Patients should understand thoroughly when they undertake a reduction diet that, in all probability, some degree of dietary restriction or discretion will be necessary permanently after ideal weight (Table 48-1) has been attained. The degree of dietary restriction is best attained by establishing the custom of weighing in each morning and adjusting the day's intake of food to the changes in body weight. It may be necessary at this time for the physician to review the comparative caloric content of certain foods which may have been withheld during the diet regimen. It is usually desirable to discuss in detail the calories contained in alcoholic beverages.

Once ideal weight has been attained, a patient should be encouraged to visit his physician every 3 to 6 months for examination and advice. The continued interest of the physician is of paramount importance to the health and happiness of his patient.

REFERENCES

Arees, Edward A., and Jean Mayer: Anatomical Connections between Medial and Lateral Regions of the Hypothalamus Concerned with Food Intake, Science, 157:1574, 1967.

Davis, John, Robert Gallagher, and Robert Ladove: Food Intake Controlled by a Blood Factor, Science, 156:1247, 1967.

Glick, Zvi, and Jean Mayer: Hyperphagia Caused by Cerebral Ventricular Infusion of Phloridzin, Nature, 219:1374, 1968.

Gordon, E. S., E. M. Goldberg, J. J. Brandabur, J. B. Gee, and J. Rankin: Abnormal Energy Metabolism in Obesity, Trans. Assoc. Am. Physicians, 75:118, 1962.

Kekwick, A.: On Adiposity, Brit. Med. J., p. 407, Aug. 6, 1960.

Modell, Walter: Status and Prospect of Drugs for Overeating, J.A.M.A., 173:1131, 1960.

Rose, H. E., and Jean Mayer: Activity, Calorie Intake, Fat Storage, and the Energy Balance of Infants, Pediatrics, 41(1):18, 1968.

Rosenberg, B. A.: A Double-blind Study of Diethylpropion in Obesity, Am. J. Med. Sci., 242:201, 1961.

Schachter, Stanley: Obesity and Eating, Science, 161:751, 1968.

Section 7

Alterations in Genitourinary Function

49 DYSURIA, INCONTINENCE, AND ENURESIS

Bernard Lytton and Franklin H. Epstein

NORMAL MICTURITION

An appreciation of the anatomic and physiologic mechanisms involved in micturition is necessary for a rational approach to the difficult problems of urinary incontinence, enuresis, and other disorders of bladder function.

The bladder muscle, or detrusor, consists of interlacing bundles of muscle that arch around the internal vesicle orifice and continue down into the urethra, where they are interspersed with elastic fibers. The normal tone of these fibers constitutes the internal vesical sphincter. The bladder receives a dual nerve supply from the autonomic system. The sacral parasympathetic, via the pelvic nerves (second, third, and fourth sacral segments), provide the preganglionic fibers to ganglia of the pelvic plexus and bladder wall and these give off postganglionic fibers to the detrusor and posterior urethra. The sympathetic preganglionic fibers (last two dorsal and first two lumbar segments) pass via the lumbar splanchnic nerves to synapse in the paraaortic and pelvic plexuses. The postganglionic fibers supply mainly the blood vessels in the bladder wall and the muscles around the bladder neck. The sympathetic innervation has little influence on bladder function but is probably concerned with closure of the bladder neck at the time of ejaculation; removal of the first lumbar sympathetic ganglion bilaterally is usually followed by infertility due to retrograde ejaculation.

Afferent fibers subserving the sensations of distension and pain pass mainly via the pelvic nerves to the sacral segments of the spinal cord. Some of these fibers are said to pass via the sympathetic nerves, but it is probable that any residual sensation of bladder filling after section of the sacral nerves is due to stretching of the peritoneum overlying the bladder. The internal pudendal nerve supplies motor and sensory fibers from the second, third, and fourth sacral segments to the external sphincter muscle, urethra, and perineal muscles. The action of the detrusor and sphincter muscles is, therefore, both reflex and voluntary.

Micturition is normally a voluntary act. As the bladder fills, a fairly constant low pressure is maintained by the detrusor muscle as it accommodates itself to the increasing volume. When it reaches its capacity, 400 to 500 ml in the normal adult, the stretch receptors transmit impulses via the pelvic afferent nerves, the sacral reflex center, and the fasciculus gracilis to the brain. This initiates the desire to void. Impulses from the brain, which arise in the paracentral lobules, are transmitted via descending fibers just anterior to the corticospinal tracts to the micturition center in the sacral part of the cord and to the pelvic and pudendal nerves to initiate the act of micturition. An initial relaxation of the perineal muscles is followed by detrusor contraction. At this point there is usually tensing of the abdominal muscles and diaphragm, although the resultant rise in abdominal pressure alone cannot initiate voiding normally and is not essential for evacuation. The intravesical pressure rises rapidly to 18 to 43 cm water, the external sphincter relaxes, the bladder neck opens, and voiding occurs with a pressure of 50 to 150 cm. The opening of the bladder neck is the result of active detrusor contraction which widens the bladder neck and shortens the urethra, thus lowering the resistance of the bladder outlet. Closure of the bladder neck occurs with relaxation of the detrusor, which allows a return of the musculature to its normal position, assisted by recoil of the elastic fibers. It is apparent that any interference with detrusor activity or the anatomy of the bladder neck will interfere with the opening mechanism and lead to incomplete emptying or some loss of continence.

DYSURIA

Dysuria denotes difficulty or pain associated with voiding. It may result from a wide variety of pathologic conditions. Frequency, hesitancy, burning, urgency, and strangury (slow, painful emission of urine) are often referred to under the more general term dysuria.

Urgency occurs as a result of trigonal or posterior urethral irritation by inflammation, stones, or tumor. The urge may be so great and so sudden that a patient voids involuntarily.

Frequency of urination in bladder lesions occurs when there is a decreased capacity or when there is pain on distension. In acute inflammatory lesions, edema and loss of elasticity of the bladder wall cause pain or an urge to void when only a small quantity of urine is present in the bladder. Chronic inflammatory lesions such as tuberculosis produce a similar effect and may proceed to permanently diminished capacity from scarring. It can be an early presenting symptom of primary malignant disease of the bladder, due to induration of the bladder wall as a result of tumor invasion and reactionary inflammatory changes.

The majority of conditions producing these symptoms arise in the bladder and urethra. Diseases of other organs and systems may, by invading, compressing, or distorting the lower urinary tract, produce dysuria. Diseases of the nervous system, which involve the nerve supply of the bladder either centrally, as in tabes and multiple sclerosis, or peripherally, as in diabetic neuropathy, produce difficulty in voiding and sometimes pain when secondary infection occurs as a result of residual urine.

The evaluation of a patient with dysuria must include a complete history and physical examination, as well as a complete urologic examination, together with relevant radiologic or laboratory investigations suggested by abnormalities detected during the clinical examination.

Inflammatory lesions in the bladder, prostate, or urethra are the commonest causes of dysuria. These include acute bacterial infections, chronic prostatitis in men, and chronic posterior urethrotrigonitis in women. A great deal may be learned from examination of the external urinary meatus. About 20 percent of children with urinary complaints have a degree of *meatal stenosis*, which may interfere sufficiently with bladder function to result in recurrent infection. Meatal stenosis is often an important etiologic factor in the development and persistence of chronic prostatitis in men and chronic posterior urethritis and trigonitis in women. Unsuspected meatal stenosis of long standing may cause trabeculation of the bladder and other manifestations of obstructive uropathy. Meatotomy results in relief or considerable improvement.

A *urethral caruncle* may present with symptoms of severe discomfort on voiding. This tumor appears as a small cherry-red polyp which may or may not protrude from the posterior lip of the external meatus and which is generally exquisitely tender on palpation. The latter feature helps to distinguish it from the commoner condition of urethral prolapse. Simple excision is the treatment of choice.

Benign overgrowth of the prostate commonly causes frequency, hesitancy, straining, slowing of the stream, and dribbling in older men. Pain is uncommon unless the condition is complicated by infection or vesical calculi.

Frequency and urgency may follow *radiation injury* to the bladder. In the acute phase this may be amenable to treatment with bladder sedatives containing antispasmodics and with small doses of steroids to combat the inflammatory reaction. The persistence of symptoms or bleeding may necessitate surgical intervention. Malignant tumors of the bowel, diverticulitis, regional ileitis, or ulcerative colitis may involve the bladder and cause frequency. Fistula formation results in severe dysuria and pneumaturia.

Chronic interstitial cystitis, a nonspecific chronic inflammatory disease of the bladder wall manifested by small, shallow, stellate hemorrhagic ulcers (Hunner's ulcers), gives rise to a fairly characteristic pattern of dysuria. The patients, generally middle-aged women, complain of persistent frequency and often have severe suprapubic pain, relieved by voiding. There may be an associated terminal hematuria. The urine contains a few white cells and red cells but no bacteria. It may ultimately lead to fibrosis with permanent contraction of the bladder.

Frequency without discomfort on voiding may be associated with a normal bladder capacity and be due to the *polyuria* of diabetes, to conditions causing hypercalcemia or hypokalemia, to the *nocturia* of early congestive heart failure, or to loss of renal parenchyma resulting in the passage of a large volume of poorly concentrated urine. The absence of nocturia in a patient with frequency suggests that it may be of psychogenic origin or due to a polyp or irritative lesion in the posterior urethra that is relieved by recumbency. A patient who complains of recent onset of nocturia should be carefully questioned about diuretic medication.

It should always be remembered that frequency may be due to *paradoxic incontinence* (see below).

Expanding lesions in the pelvis that reduce bladder capacity by external compression are exemplified by pregnancy. Large ovarian cysts and uterine fibroids will have a similar effect. A retroverted gravid uterus or pelvic tumor which becomes impacted may result in stretching and elongation of the urethra and produce difficulty in voiding and finally complete retention.

INCONTINENCE

Paradoxic Incontinence

True incontinence must be distinguished from *paradoxic incontinence,* which accompanies bladder distension caused by mechanical or functional obstruction and is characterized by small, frequent, involuntary "overflow" voidings. In obstruction the increased power of the detrusor suffices to overcome the block, but as soon as a small quantity of urine is voided, the intravesical pressure drops and a large residual remains. Ultimately, the detrusor becomes paralyzed by overdistension, and complete retention ensues. With neurogenic bladders, small voidings occur, sometimes involuntarily, as the pressure of accumulating urine overcomes the resistance at the bladder outlet. With loss of a small amount of urine, pressure falls, and a large residual is left. Often both neurologic and obstructive elements contribute, as in elderly arteriosclerotic patients with prostatic enlargement or in cases of diabetic neuropathy with secondary bladder neck obstruction. The bladder in these patients is flaccid and painless, which may make it difficult to palpate, and the residual urine predisposes to infection. This response of the bladder muscle to obstruction might be compared to that seen in striated and heart muscle under an increased work load.

Congenital Incontinence

Congenital incontinence may be due to a congenital malformation, such as vesical extrophy, epispadias, ectopic ureteral openings in the female, patent urachus, and defects in the spinal cord which occur in association with spina bifida and meningomyelocele. The results of primary reconstructive surgery in cases of extrophy are cosmetically satisfactory, but sphincter control is rarely achieved. Furthermore, most of these children have persistent vesicoureteral reflux, which can lead to progressive renal damage. The majority therefore are still best treated by some form of urinary diversion with excision of the bladder. The results of urethral and bladder neck reconstruction in simple epispadias are better. The management of neurogenic bladder disturbance is principally directed toward the establishment of timed reflex voiding, diminution of residual urine, and control of infection. When there is progressive renal impairment, due to persistent infection and vesicoureteral reflux, urinary diversion is necessary.

Acquired Incontinence

This may occur as a result of disease or injury to the spinal cord, as in tabes, multiple sclerosis, and tumor, or following fractures of the spine. The disruption of the neural mechanism results in complete relaxation of the detrusor and bladder outlet or in ineffective contractions of the detrusor, so there may be overflow incontinence with a flaccid bladder or uncontrollable frequent voidings with a spastic bladder. Cerebral vascular accidents or senility can produce loss of voluntary control of bladder and bowel function.

Parturition can stretch and disrupt the structures of the pelvic floor and perineum to the point that urethral resistance, while sufficient to maintain continence at rest, gives way under stress of straining or coughing, and incontinence ensues. This is probably the result of loss of the urethrovesical angle and urethral shortening. This type of incontinence usually occurs in the erect posture.

Stress incontinence may be aggravated by urgency due to an associated urethrotrigonitis. Relief of the trigonitis will sometimes result in satisfactory control. Treatment is directed toward repair of the pelvic floor, restoration of urethral length, and correction of the urethrovesical angle.

Surgical or radiation injuries can produce vesicovaginal and ureterovaginal fistulas. Incontinence in ureterovaginal fistula occurs with normal voiding, but in vesicovaginal fistula there is generally no normal evacuation of the bladder. The treatment of these fistulas is always surgical. Temporary urinary diversion will enable spontaneous closure to occur in some instances. Excision and reconstruction of a damaged ureter is the treatment of choice, but implantation of the ureter into the bowel or substitution with an ileal segment may be necessary. Nephrectomy is the simplest procedure in the elderly or debilitated patient or when there are serious technical difficulties, provided there is adequate function in the other kidney.

Injury to the sphincter mechanism can occur with pelvic fractures or after prostatic or bladder neck surgery in elderly patients. Gradual improvement may occur for up to a year after injury. Postsurgical incontinence may be controlled with a penile clamp, but this has the disadvantage of producing edema and occasionally ulceration of the penis. A condom catheter may lead to maceration of the penile skin and is often difficult to apply. An indwelling catheter invariably leads to problems of chronic infection. A variety of surgical procedures have been devised to improve control, by using some mechanical means to increase urethral resistance, and are only partially successful. Urinary diversion may become necessary in certain cases.

ENURESIS

Enuresis is generally understood to mean the unintentional voiding of urine, usually at night, when it is synonymously referred to as bedwetting. The term should be restricted to those children in whom there is an absence of any gross urologic abnormality.

Micturition in infancy is governed by a simple spinal reflex. Maturation of the nervous system and development of control over the simple reflexes by the higher centers occurs during the second year of life. By the age of thirty months, most children have voluntary control over rectal and urinary sphincters. The child who persistently wets the bed after the age of three, or who, after a period of control, begins to wet the bed again presents a clinical problem. Enuresis then, may be a delay in the development or a loss of bladder control. It may be affected by physical and psychologic factors. There appears to be no constant single cause.

It is estimated that 15 percent of boys and 10 percent of girls at the age of five are enuretic, but by the age of nine only 5 percent of all children remain bedwetters. The majority of children with simple enuresis are dry by the time they reach puberty. It is more common among children with similarly affected siblings and in children of parents in the lower income groups. This latter finding could be due to the later institution of toilet training.

It is important to distinguish incontinence due to organic urologic disease from enuresis early in the management of these patients. Diabetes mellitus or insipidus may occasionally present with enuresis. Renal disease due to glomerulo- or pyelonephritis or sickle-cell disease producing papillary necrosis may cause bedwetting as a result of the increased volumes of urine passed by these patients. A careful evaluation at the outset should exclude chronic retention with dribbling incontinence due to either bladder neck obstruction or neurologic disease. Patients with organic disease of the bladder are usually incontinent during the day as well as at night, although enuretics may also exhibit this. Those with organic disease often have constant dribbling of urine. Occasionally, however, serious degrees of bladder neck obstruction present with nocturnal enuresis as the only symptom. A congenital decrease in bladder capacity may in part be responsible for enuresis, and is often familial. The enuresis generally ceases as the child gets older and spends less time asleep. Occasionally, a patient with petit mal epilepsy may present with wetting. Urinalysis will reveal any unsuspected infection. Enuresis occurring in retarded children or in those with serious psychiatric disturbances requires treatment directed to the management of their primary problem.

Contributory factors such as the child's general health, physical environment, and emotional state should be evaluated and the parents encouraged to adopt an understanding rather than a punitive attitude. Correction of minor urologic abnormalities such as meatal stenosis, balanitis, vulvovaginitis, posterior urethritis, and urethral valves will sometimes lead to relief, but this is perhaps attributable only to the dysuria following instrumentation or to the understanding interest shown by the physician. The administration of antiparasympathetic agents to reduce bladder activity, or amphetamines to lighten sleep, have been advocated, but the results are equivocal. Imipramine (Tofranil), a mood-elevating drug whose effect is reinforced by its anticholinergic and stimulant properties, has produced a favorable response in over half the children treated, but may require continuation of treatment for some time. The results of psychotherapy are unconvincing. Considerable success has been claimed for alarm systems which attempt to establish a conditioned reflex. The child is awakened when an electrical circuit is completed by wetting. This method seems to be worth a trial in older children who prove resistant to simpler therapy.

50 OLIGURIA, POLYURIA, AND NOCTURIA

Louis G. Welt

INTRODUCTION

The kidneys provide the main channel for the excretion of water and solutes, and the urine flow and composition is adjusted so as to maintain the internal environment of the body in a remarkably constant steady state. The volume and solute content of the urine in health may vary widely. It is largely dependent on the magnitude and characteristics of the fluid and food ingested and on the quantity of water lost from other routes such as perspiration and insensible water loss. There are many ways in which urine flow can be varied in both health and disease, and it appears essential to review briefly, and in a general fashion, the manner in which urine is formed so that the vicissitudes of life and the impact of disease on urine volume and osmolality may be better understood.

PHYSIOLOGIC CONSIDERATIONS

The final bladder urine represents the net effect of a host of reactions that begin with the formation of an almost protein-free ultrafiltrate of plasma in the glomeruli. The quantity of fluid filtered at the glomeruli per unit of time is the net effect of the difference in the chemical potential of the water of plasma and that of the ultrafiltrate as well as the surface area available for filtration. These factors apply to the filterable solutes as well. The volume of water excreted per unit of time is, then, the difference between the volume filtered and the volume reabsorbed. The quantity of solutes excreted per unit of time is the difference between that which is filtered and that which is reabsorbed or secreted by the renal tubules. Many things remain obscure about these mechanisms, but there is now a general concept around which a description may be presented and from which implications may be drawn with respect to the influence of a variety of circumstances and disease processes. We are indeed indebted to the brilliant micropuncture studies started by Richards and his group in Philadelphia, and continued more recently by Wirz, by Gottschalk and his colleagues, and now by many others.

The water filtered by the glomeruli is reabsorbed at several areas along the nephron by passive diffusion along osmotic gradients, which, in turn, are established by the active transport of solutes. The osmotic gradient is maximized in the medulla and papilla owing to the anatomic arrangement of the loops of Henle and their accompanying blood vessels, which permit the establishment of an ever-increasing osmolality as the papilla is approached. This latter mechanism is referred to as the *countercurrent multiplication system*.

The *initial* step in the reabsorption of water, and the step that represents the largest volume, occurs in the proximal convolution of the nephron. The active transport of solutes, which are primarily sodium, chloride, bicarbonate, and glucose, creates an osmotic gradient so that water follows immediately. In this fashion, approximately two-thirds to three-fourths of the filtered solutes and water are reabsorbed by the end of the proximal tubule. The characteristics of this fluid are altered considerably, not only in volume but in composition. However, it is still iso-osmotic with the parent filtrate.

Another phase in the reabsorption of water occurs in the more distal portions of the nephron, which include the loop of Henle, the distal convolution, and, lastly, the collecting ducts. Although the reabsorption at these levels is smaller in volume than that which occurs in the more proximal segment of the nephron, these latter mechanisms are responsible in one circumstance for the formation of a maximally concentrated urine, and in other circumstances for the formation of a dilute urine. There are, obviously, circumstances wherein the urine osmolality occupies positions intermediate between these polar extremes.

The formation of a *maximally concentrated* urine depends on the presence of antidiuretic hormone, which permits the distal convolution and collecting duct membranes to be completely permeable to water. The micropuncture data reveal that the fluid in the early part of the distal convolution is always hypotonic (whether or not there is maximal antidiuretic hormone activity) to plasma. Furthermore, water is lost between the end of the proximal convolution and the early distal convolution. This clearly implies that solutes have been transported in excess of water, and hence some part of the ascending limb is presumably impermeable to water in the presence or absence of the antidiuretic hormone.

In the presence of antidiuretic hormone activity, the fluid within the distal convolution becomes more concentrated. Where one distal convolution meets with another to form a collecting tubule, the fluid is invariably iso-osmotic (in the rodent) with the parent filtrate. As the fluid courses through the collecting duct (in the presence of antidiuretic hormone activity) and is exposed to a fluid with an ever-increasing osmolality, a passive movement of water causes the fluid within the collecting ducts to remain in osmotic equilibrium with the fluid in the interstitium; thus, it increases in concentration until it exits into the pelvis of the kidney and moves down into the bladder for excretion.

Allusion has been made to the mechanism whereby the fluid in the interstitium is rendered continuously more hyperosmotic from outer medulla to papillary tip. It is dependent upon the anatomic arrangement of the loops of Henle and their blood vessels and is achieved by the transport of sodium salts (in excess of water) from the ascending limb of the loop. This renders the fluid in the interstitium hyperosmotic to the fluid entering the descending limb of the loop of Henle. This difference in osmolality promotes a movement of water from the descending limb fluid; and, in addition, there is entry of solutes into this portion of the limb. The net result is an increase in the osmolality of the fluid in the descending limb. This same process is repeated over and over again, and the fluid in the limb and interstitium becomes more concentrated along its course. When the fluid reaches the ascending portion of the limb and solutes are transported out of the luminal fluid, this fluid and the interstitium become ever less concentrated and are, finally, made hypotonic by the time it reaches the early distal convolution.[1]

In this setting the fluid coursing through the collecting ducts is made more hyperosmotic. Since urea can presumably permeate the collecting ducts largely by passive diffusion, urea moves from the collecting system into the interstitium as water moves along the osmotic gradient. In this fashion, urea contributes significantly to the total solute concentration in the medullary and papillary interstitium and serves to counterbalance the concentration of urea within the collecting ducts.

In man, the maximal concentration of the final urine may be as high as 1,200 to 1,400 mOsm per kg water. This may be considerably higher in rodents, the experimental animals from which the data that permit this formulation have been obtained.

In contrast, in the "complete" absence of antidiuretic hormone, the fluid in the distal convolution is not only

---

[1] The antidiuretic hormone possibly serves to increase the rate of transport of solutes from the ascending limb in addition to its influence on the permeability of the distal tubular and collecting duct permeability.

hypotonic to plasma in the earliest portions but remains so and is excreted as bladder urine with the same or even lower osmolality. Data reveal that salt is transported from the distal convolutions and from the collecting ducts themselves. In the absence of antidiuretic hormone, this aids and abets formation of minimally concentrated urine.

In this fashion, one can visualize the manner in which a highly concentrated or a minimally concentrated urine can be formed. Varying amounts of antidiuretic hormone between none and maximal provide a graded response.

Furthermore, it must be pointed out that even in the two polar situations of maximal antidiuretic hormone activity, or none, the rate of excretion of solutes determines the volume and osmolality of urine. This is to state that a urine may have an osmolality approaching that of the plasma with no antidiuretic hormone activity in the face of a solute diuresis; in contrast, the urine volume may be large and the osmolality may approach that of plasma despite maximal antidiuretic hormone activity in the presence of a solute diuresis. The manner in which a solute diuresis influences the concentration and the volume of urine is not completely clear.

However, within the context of the discussion presented above, it is apparent that a good deal of the water removed from the initial volume of filtrate depends on the active transport of salt and other solutes from the luminal fluid. Even if a constant *percentage* of filtered salt were reabsorbed in the proximal tubule, an increased filtration *rate* would provide a larger volume of fluid to the descending limb of the loop of Henle. Furthermore, to the extent that limitations are placed on the transport of salt from the proximal tubule (owing to the presence in filtrate of a larger concentration of a poorly reabsorbable solute), less water will be reabsorbed. If less salt is transported out of the loop of Henle, or if the flow of fluid through the loop is hastened, the countercurrent multiplier system will operate less efficiently; hence, the maximal osmolality will not be achieved in the interstitium of the medulla and papilla. By the same token, if the reabsorption of solutes is diminished in the distal convolution (e.g., glucose is not reabsorbable at this site), less water will be reabsorbed and a greater volume will reach the collecting duct system. Hence, a large solute excretion will increase the volume and diminish the osmolality of the final urine despite maximal antidiuretic hormone activity.

In contrast, it will be recalled that the efficient transport of solutes prior to, in, and beyond the distal convoluted tubule, coupled with the relative impermeability to water of these latter structures in the absence of antidiuretic hormone, are responsible for the formation of minimally dilute urine. If reabsorption of solutes is less efficient, owing to the filtered load or to the presence of less readily reabsorbable solutes, it is clear that urine osmolality cannot reach minimally dilute levels. As the solute diuresis becomes more intense, urine osmolality will approach that of the plasma.

In summary, a small solute excretion in the absence of antidiuretic hormone would be anticipated to be accompanied by the most dilute urine, and in the presence of antidiuretic hormone, with the most maximally concentrated urine. Varying quantities of antidiuretic hormone will have obvious influences; and the character of the urine anticipated in the presence of maximal antidiuretic hormone activity or none will be modified by the quantity and character of the solute load destined for excretion.

PATHOLOGIC CONSIDERATIONS

Oliguria

DEHYDRATION. There are many causes for oliguria, and the commonest may well be simple dehydration. In the face of a diminished volume of body fluids (especially if the loss has been water in excess of salt to provide an osmotic as well as a volumetric stimulus for the secretion of antidiuretic hormone), one anticipates a diminished filtration rate and a reduced excretion of solutes owing to the influence of a plasma volume deficit on renal hemodynamics. The diminished rate of excretion of solutes accompanied by antidiuretic hormone activity should ensure a small volume of highly concentrated urine.

CONGESTIVE HEART FAILURE. Since the volume of the filtrate plays an important role in the rate of excretion of urine, any circumstance which causes a reduced glomerular filtration rate is likely to be associated with some diminution in the rate of flow of urine. The defective systolic emptying of the heart, which is a characteristic of congestive heart failure, is commonly associated with a reduced flow of blood to the kidney and with a reduced filtration rate. This becomes more and more intense as the failure becomes more profound. Furthermore, in congestive heart failure (see Chap. 34 for more details) the renal excretion of salt is diminished, and the combination is obviously likely to result in a small volume of urine. This may be a striking feature of heart failure.

CIRRHOSIS OF THE LIVER. Cirrhosis is frequently accompanied by diminished renal blood flow and filtration rate (despite a coexistent increase in cardiac output) and by a strikingly low urine flow. In cirrhosis of the liver, as in congestive heart failure, the renal tubular reabsorption of salt is presumably more efficient, and this contributes to a diminished urine volume.

ACUTE RENAL INSUFFICIENCY. A low urine volume is one of the cardinal manifestations of this condition. In acute glomerulonephritis (or disorders with the same basic pathology) this low volume is presumably almost entirely a consequence of the drastic reduction in filtration rate. In acute tubular necrosis there is almost certainly a reduced filtration rate, but other factors as well may contribute to the striking oliguria. It is quite possible that in this latter disorder, the necrotic epithelium represents a nonfunctioning and simply passive membrane. Under these circumstances the intraluminal fluid would be under the same influences with respect to the Starling forces as is the interstitial fluid of the kidney.

It could be anticipated, therefore, that the bulk of the diminished filtrate might be reabsorbed directly into the peritubular vessels, since the tubular walls no longer function as more than a passive diffusion barrier. In other instances the oliguria may be a consequence of nephron obstruction by casts. In many instances, the trivial formation of urine may be a consequence of a combination of these three mechanisms. In renal cortical necrosis, where all elements of the nephron are destroyed, total anuria is common. This may obtain because there is virtually no filtration whatsoever; what little does occur is likely to be subject to the influences suggested above in the context of acute tubular necrosis.

CHRONIC RENAL INSUFFICIENCY. The ability to form a maximally concentrated urine is disturbed early in chronic renal insufficiency. This is accredited to at least two factors. One suggestion is that with a reduced population of nephrons and an elevated concentration of urea the filtration rate and the filtered load of urea per nephron are increased, and in this circumstance there is an osmotic diuresis in those nephrons that contribute to the final urine. In the context of the discussion in the section on physiologic considerations, a framework was provided in an attempt to clarify the influence of the rate of excretion of solutes on the urine concentrating mechanism. Furthermore, if the destruction of renal mass occurs primarily in the medulla (as is so common in pyelonephritis) the nephrons with the longest loops of Henle are more likely to be destroyed. Since these longest loops of Henle set up the highest interstitial osmolality, it is apparent why urine concentrating defects are seen early. Hence, although chronic renal insufficiency may be associated with some polyuria, this is usually not striking. In the patient with end-stage kidney disease, striking reductions in urine flow are frequently observed. This is primarily a consequence of the magnitude of the destruction of renal mass.

OBSTRUCTION OF THE URINARY TRACT. Obstruction of the lower urinary tract, that is, from the bladder to the urethral meatus, is common and is due most frequently to stricture, to compression of the prostatic urethra by an enlarged gland, and, less commonly, to congenital malformations with valve formations that make emptying the bladder difficult. These patients may develop fairly striking acute reductions in urine flow, and this should always be a consideration when a patient is seen with oliguria.

Although it is less common to see oliguria as a consequence of obstruction of the upper urinary tract, it does occur. The reason for its rarity is that there are two kidneys and two ureters, and in order to achieve oliguria from obstruction above the bladder, both ureters must be compromised. However, this does occur in a variety of circumstances which include neoplastic infiltration of the ureters, and bilateral constriction consequent to a retroperitoneal sclerosing inflammatory process. On occasion constrictions may occur at the ureterovesical junctions bilaterally. Hence, although uncommon, bilateral obstruction of the upper urinary tracts may cause oliguria. Uni-

lateral ureteral calculus with ureteral spasm on the opposite side is also possible.

Polyuria

DIABETES INSIPIDUS. This condition results from inability to synthesize and secrete antidiuretic hormone and is the archetype of a disorder accompanied by the excretion of large volumes of dilute urine. In a compilation of several reports, intracranial tumors accounted for 40 percent of the variety of causes for diabetes insipidus, 33 percent were so-called *idiopathic,* and the remainder were scattered among a variety of disorders including trauma. Although not a rare disorder, diabetes insipidus is certainly uncommon. The primary condition from which it must be discriminated is primary polydipsia, which may be due to an intracranial organic lesion but perhaps more often accompanies a basic emotional disorder. These two disorders can be distinguished one from the other in a relatively simple fashion (see Chap. 88).

NEPHROGENIC DIABETES INSIPIDUS. Inability of the renal tubules to respond to antidiuretic hormone of endogenous or exogenous origin characterizes nephrogenic diabetes insipidus. It is a heritable disorder with full expression in males and partial expression in females, which manifests itself quite early in life; these patients are frequently referred to as "water babies." Their management is difficult since they do not respond to any of the available posterior pituitary preparations. However, they do respond to chlorothiazide drugs. The probable manner in which this agent influences the water turnover is by promoting a salt deficit. This, in turn, causes a smaller urine volume. This may be a consequence of a diminished filtration rate but is more likely to be associated with a larger fractional reabsorption of salt, and hence water, in the more proximal portions of the nephron. In this fashion less fluid is delivered to sites where it may escape into the bladder urine.

ACQUIRED RENAL LESIONS. There are acquired renal lesions associated with inability to concentrate the urine maximally.

Potassium depletion is commonly, if not invariably, associated with inability to concentrate the urine appropriately. The nature of the defect is not clear. Although it is at some risk that one translates data from rodents to human beings, information from rats and hamsters does exclude certain possibilities. Micropuncture data obtained by Gottschalk and his colleagues show that the osmolality of fluid in the distal convolution is the same in potassium-depleted rats as in control animals. Hence, there appears to be no lack of osmotic equilibration at this site. Furthermore, more recent data from the same laboratory utilizing normal and potassium-depleted hamsters reveal that there is no osmotic disequilibrium across the collecting duct epithelium. Other data indicate that the interstitial fluid deep in the papilla is not as hyperosmotic in potassium-depleted as in normal animals. The reasons for this are still unclear. Some published data on rats tend to deny the possibility that this is a consequence of a greater flow of fluid through the loop of Henle, since, if anything, the fractional reabsorption of water in the proximal convolution appears to be greater in a state of potassium depletion. Two obvious influences have not yet been evaluated, namely, the rate of medullary blood flow and the rate of active transport of salt in the ascending limb. An increase in medullary blood flow would tend to diminish the hypertonicity of the medullary and papillary interstitium; and a diminished rate of transport of salt across the ascending limb of the loops of Henle would diminish the efficiency of the countercurrent multiplier mechanism. The defect is reversible with potassium repletion.

Hypercalcemia has been known for some time to be accompanied by diminished ability to concentrate the urine maximally. In this instance as well, the precise mechanism is unknown. At this time the available data are somewhat similar to those discussed with respect to potassium depletion. There is no evidence of an osmotic disequilibrium across the collecting ducts and no evidence of an increased flow of fluid through the loop of Henle. The facets that have not been examined in the state of potassium depletion also raise questions about the hypercalcemic state.

Other examples of acquired renal lesions characterized by inability to concentrate the urine are seen frequently in patients with *chronic renal insufficiency,* as alluded to earlier. In addition, some rather striking examples of extreme polyuria have been seen in patients with multiple myeloma, amyloidosis, and, more commonly, after relief of an obstructive uropathy. Marked diuresis is commonly observed in the recovery phase of acute tubular necrosis from a variety of insults. This is frequently referred to as the "diuretic phase" of acute tubular necrosis and may be due in part to the delivery of accumulated fluid but very likely also due in part to renal tubular abnormalities with reference to the reabsorption of solutes and water.

SOLUTE DIURESIS. Large solute diureses, such as are noted in patients with uncontrolled diabetes mellitus and constant glycosuria, are almost always accompanied by large urine flows and complaint of polyuria. Solute diuresis may also occur in patients suffering a "reaction to injury" who are unable to utilize protein but are given large quantities of this foodstuff. In such instances protein is converted to a very large extent to urea and excreted. This increase in solute excretion promotes a large urine flow as described earlier.

Nocturia

The diurnal rhythm that applies to urine flow is such that a larger volume is excreted in the waking 12 hr than during the 12-hr period spent mostly asleep. The precise mechanisms underlying this particular rhythm are not clear, although the evidence suggests a correlation with filtration rate and solute excretion. This rhythm is lost in several circumstances, and in other instances it may appear to have been lost owing to mechanical problems.

The rhythm characterized by a relatively diminished volume of urine at night is frequently disturbed in patients with edema. This may very well be because edema accumulates more during the day owing to activity and the influence of gravity through posture. At night, when the patient is supine, some of the edema may be resorbed into the plasma volume, thereby promoting an alteration in renal hemodynamics that leads to increased excretion of urine.

Nocturia is common in patients with chronic renal insufficiency primarily because they excrete urine at a fairly constant rate, and hence the benefits to sleep of the normal diurnal rhythm are lost. The reasons for this may be similar to those relating to a concentrated urine. In this instance it may be due to a constant osmotic diuresis per nephron.

Partial obstruction of the bladder is often accompanied by nocturia simply because the stimulus to void is so frequently present.

For reasons that are certainly unclear, the patient with untreated adrenal cortical insufficiency loses the normal diurnal rhythm and hence may complain of nocturia.

Lastly, anything that causes dysuria is almost certain to promote nocturia. In this instance, as is the case with obstruction of the bladder, nocturia is characterized by frequent but *small* volumes in contrast to the other cases noted above.

APPROACH TO THE PATIENT

Carefully taken histories usually reveal evidence of disturbances characterized by excretion of small or large volumes of urine, or the presence or absence of nocturia. The associations with disease processes of this type of disturbance have been alluded to, and the questions suggested by these clues are, in a sense, implicit.

The point that bears some emphasis, perhaps, is that wide variations in urine flow exist in health as well as in disease, and a reasonable interpretation can be made only by careful evaluation of the characteristics of the symptom equated with other problems displayed by the patient. The specific evaluation of these disorders is discussed in other sections of this text.

REFERENCES

Gottschalk, C. W.: Osmotic Concentration and Dilution of the Urine, Am. J. Med., 36:670, 1964.

Kleeman, C. R., W. L. Hewitt, and L. B. Guzé: Pyelonephritis, Medicine, 39:3, 1960.

Pitts, R. F.: "Physiology of the Kidney and Body Fluids," Chicago, The Year Book Medical Publishers, Inc., 1963.

Strauss, M. B., and L. G. Welt, "Diseases of the Kidney," Boston, Little, Brown and Company, 1964.

51 HEMATURIA
Bernard Lytton and Franklin H. Epstein

Bleeding from the urinary tract, whether microscopic or gross, is a serious sign. It should be regarded with the same gravity as abnormal bleeding occurring from any other body tract. Hematuria is usually classified as initial, terminal, or total. Total hematuria indicates that the bleeding occurs throughout the urinary stream and suggests that the bleeding originates from either the kidney or the ureter. Initial bleeding is generally associated with lesions in the urethra distal to the bladder neck; terminal bleeding, with lesions in the bladder, usually in the area of the trigone. Severe hemorrhage from the bladder, however, will present as total hematuria. These distinctions as to the type of bleeding are, therefore, only rough indications as to the origin of the bleeding; too much reliance should not be placed on them. About 20 percent of patients who come to the physician with hematuria have it as the only symptom of their urinary tract disease; it is often difficult to persuade these patients to undergo a complete urologic investigation to establish the origin of the bleeding. Ureteral colic is often associated with renal bleeding and is due to the passage of clots.

The finding of an occasional red blood cell in a centrifuged specimen of urine is probably of no significance, since Addis showed that up to 500,000 red cells may normally be excreted in the urine in 12 hr. Vigorous exercise or even intense excitement may increase the numbers of red cells, epithelial cells, and casts in the urinary sediment of normal subjects. Microscopic hematuria may also be increased during certain febrile diseases without implying serious disease of the kidneys. The presence of red blood cell casts is pathologic and further indicates that the source of the bleeding is in the kidneys rather than the lower part of the urinary tract.

Certain dyes and pigments, such as phenolsulfonphthalein, azo dyes, and the indole alkaloids found in beet roots (betanin), may produce red discoloration of the urine which must be distinguished from bleeding. The appearance of the red dye from beet roots occurs only in certain individuals; it is thought to be related to the degree of absorption of the dye from the gastrointestinal tract. Pink or brown discoloration of the urine may occur as a result of hemo- or myoglobinuria. These may be precipitated by cold, exercise, or drug toxicity, especially in susceptible individuals such as those with sickle-cell trait (see Chap. 338).

Diseases of the renal parenchyma, such as glomerulonephritis, malignant hypertension, polycystic kidneys, renal infarction, periarteritis, or poisoning with a nephrotoxic agent, will in most instances be detected by a careful history, physical examination, and the usual laboratory tests. Hematuria may result from a *disorder of blood clotting*, produced by blood dyscrasias, scurvy, or anticoagulant drugs. The increased tendency to bleed in patients on long-term anticoagulant therapy may bring to light another, previously unsuspected, pathologic condition in the urinary tract. *Sickle-cell anemia* or sickle-cell trait may cause bleeding into the urine from disrupted capillaries and microinfarcts in the renal medulla. The aforementioned conditions account for only a small proportion of all patients with hematuria.

Tumors, urinary tract obstructions, calculi, and *infections* account for the bleeding in about 75 percent of patients with hematuria. Tumors alone account for some 20 percent of all cases. It is therefore mandatory in those patients in whom no other cause is found for the bleeding to visualize the upper part of the urinary tract by intravenous pyelography supplemented by retrograde pyelography as indicated and to visualize the bladder and urethra by instrumental examination. Retrograde pyelography may be supplemented by injections of air rather than opaque dye when one is trying to delineate suspected nonopaque calculi or small tumors in the renal collecting system. Doubtful lesions in the kidney may be further investigated by nephrotomography or aortography. The latter is probably best performed by the transfemoral route, which allows selective injections into individual renal vessels to be made if required. Renal tumors generally have greater opacification than the surrounding kidney tissue on tomography, and the aortogram shows the characteristic pooling of the dye in the venous sinusoids that occurs in these tumors and which is a result of the small arteriovenous communications which develop.

On cystoscopy, *acute* and *chronic cystitis*, interstitial cystitis, bladder tumors, and vesical calculi may be readily diagnosed. Bleeding from engorged veins in the prostatic urethra due to benign prostatic hypertrophy is a common source of hematuria. Like prostatitis in men and chronic nonspecific posterior urethritis in women, it should be accepted as the origin of the bleeding only if more serious conditions have been excluded.

Acute cystitis may produce gross hematuria, initially overshadowing all other symptoms. Chronic infections such as *tuberculosis* of the urinary tract or infection with *Schistosoma hematobium* may also have hematuria as their only presenting symptom. Schistosomiasis causes ulceration of the bladder mucosa at the site of deposition of the ova by the adult flukes which inhabit the venules of the bladder and pelvis. It is probably the commonest cause of hematuria in those areas in the Middle East and Africa where it is endemic.

Bleeding associated with the menses should suggest the possibility of *endometriosis* of the urinary tract, provided contamination from the vagina has been excluded.

Trauma to the kidney nearly always manifests itself as hematuria which is often painless and may persist for several days. The incidence of renal injury is increasing because of the increased number of serious automobile accidents. The majority of these cases may be treated conservatively with bed rest and careful observation. Follow-up intravenous pyelography should be carried out, as occasionally the renal injury may produce an anatomic deformity leading to either stone formation or hypertension. A blow on the lower part of the abdomen when the bladder is distended, particularly in children where the bladder is an abdominal organ, may produce a contusion of the bladder, giving rise to painless hematuria.

A group of about 6 to 8 percent of all cases seen have hematuria for which no obvious source can be detected. Further urologic and hematologic investigation 3 to 4 months after the first episode of bleeding will determine the cause in just under half of these. Patients in whom episodes of hematuria persist should have a renal biopsy at a time when they are bleeding. *A focal glomerulitis* has been found to be responsible for the bleeding in many of these cases. The condition appears to have a good prognosis as regards renal function. The severe bleeding which sometimes occurs may be controlled in some instances by the administration of steroids for 2 to 3 months. A small number of cases however, still remain undiagnosed and may have persistent hematuria over a period of many years for which no cause is found.

52 DISTURBANCES OF MENSTRUATION
George W. Thorn

Since normal menstrual cycles depend upon the integrated action of the endocrine and nervous systems, it is to be expected that abnormalities in the menstrual cycle may occur in association with a wide variety of systemic disorders as well as with specific pathologic changes in the reproductive organs. (See Chap. 98 for a discussion of disease of the ovaries and uterus.)

MENARCHE. In temperate climates the menstrual cycle usually begins between the ages of twelve to fifteen, whereas in tropical climates it may appear as early as nine or ten. During the first year or two, the menstrual cycles are likely to be irregular, since many are anovulatory.

Uterine bleeding in the newborn may be noted for 3 to 4 days following delivery and is thought to be due to the sudden decrease in circulating estrogen level which had previously induced endometrial growth in the fetus.

Vaginal bleeding in very young girls should suggest injury from a foreign body introduced into the vagina. Very rarely vaginal bleeding will occur in association with precocious development of breasts due to an ovarian or adrenal tumor.

The delayed onset of menses, beyond the age of sixteen years, suggests *abnormalities in the development of the reproductive system,* such as imperforate hymen, uterine hypoplasia, and ovarian agenesis; *endocrine dysfunction,* such as anterior pituitary or thyroid deficiency; or *psychologic disturbances,* which mediate their effect through neurohumoral pathways.

MENSES. Normally periods occur at intervals of 27 to 32 days, and flow lasts an average of 5 days. Approximately 60 to 250 ml blood is lost, with the greatest quantity lost during the first or second day. The volume of menstrual flow can be estimated by the fact that each well-soaked pad will contain approximately 30 to 50 ml blood.

MENOPAUSE. Naturally occurring menopause may be expected by age fifty. Menopause represents the period of change between the years of reproduction and the regression of ovarian function. A gradual reduction in the duration of the menstrual cycle is to be expected at this time. *Irregular bleeding* or *hypermenorrhea* is most often caused by anovulatory cycles, but *neoplasms* should always be suspected. Induced or artificial menopause follows extirpation or irradiation of the ovaries. *Premature menopause* may occur as early as thirty-five without definitive cause; occasionally a familial tendency for this will be noted. However, other causes of amenorrhea such as endocrine abnormalities and emotional factors must be excluded.

ABNORMAL UTERINE BLEEDING. During the reproductive cycle abnormal uterine bleeding should always suggest pregnancy and one of its complications, such as threatened abortion, ectopic pregnancy, or hydatid mole. Having excluded the complications of pregnancy by history, physical examination, and a rapid serologic test, one should consider uterine pathology such as polyps, leiomyomas, and carcinoma of the cervix or body of the uterus. For these a pelvic examination and diagnostic curettage will be required. Ovarian disease, pelvic inflammation, and hormonal abnormalities such as *hypothyroidism* also can induce abnormal uterine bleeding. Systemic disturbances, particularly those associated with anemia, leukemia, abnormalities in blood clotting, and circulatory disturbances such as hypertension should be excluded. The anemia that follows prolonged menstrual bleeding may predispose a patient to further excessive menstruation. In view of the widespread use of hormones, particularly estrogens, progesterone, and contraceptive pills, one should consider the *administration* or *withdrawal* of sex hormonal preparations as potential causes of abnormal uterine bleeding. Finally, disturbed emotional states or serious psychologic difficulties may predispose to abnormal uterine bleeding.

Hypermenorrhea, characterized by excessively long or too profuse menstrual bleeding, may result from delay in the repair of the endometrium and, of course, frequently accompanies anovulatory cyclic bleeding.

Polymenorrhea refers to regular menstrual cycles that occur more frequently than every 23 to 24 days. It is the least common of the menstrual irregularities and tends to occur very early or late in menstrual life. It is due to a shortening of the follicular or luteal phase of the menstrual cycle.

Intermenstrual bleeding refers to the occurrence of irregular bleeding between normally spaced periods. Spontaneous bleeding of this type is more likely to be endometrial in origin in contrast to bleeding of the cervix or vagina.

AMENORRHEA AND OLIGOMENORRHEA. Physiologic amenorrhea precedes the menarche, follows the menopause, and characterizes pregnancy and lactation. *Primary amenorrhea* indicates that menstruation has never occurred, whereas *secondary amenorrhea* refers to cessation of menstruation.

Uterine abnormalities such as agenesis or hypoplasia give rise to primary amenorrhea, whereas destruction of endometrium by irradiation or excessive curettage or removal of the uterus can induce secondary amenorrhea. *Vaginal abnormalities* include such conditions as imperforate hymen. The continued retention of blood may lead to hematometra, hematosalpinx, and eventually hematoperitoneum.

Ovarian agenesis or dysgenesis (Turner's syndrome) is a cause of primary amenorrhea, whereas polycystic disease of the ovary (Stein-Leventhal syndrome), masculinizing tumors of the ovary or adrenal, destruction of ovarian function by irradiation, and hormonal imbalance give rise in most instances to secondary amenorrhea or oligomenorrhea. Hypopituitarism with Simmond's cachexia, Sheehan's syndrome, or the Chiavi-Frommel syndrome will, of course, result in reduced ovarian function and predispose to oligomenorrhea or amenorrhea. With pituitary deficiency, one would expect associated evidence of reduced adrenal and thyroid function (Chap 87). Diabetes mellitus and hyperthyroidism may induce menstrual abnormalities characterized by oligomenorrhea or hypermenorrhea. Malnutrition, obesity, debilitating disease, intoxication, and severe anemia may be associated with oligomenorrhea or amenorrhea as well as with abnormal uterine bleeding. Fear, anxiety, and grief are frequent causes of temporary amenorrhea, and indeed psychologic factors acting on hypothalamic centers constitute one of the most frequent causes of secondary amenorrhea. Amenorrhea is almost an invariable accompaniment of anorexia nervosa.

DYSMENORRHEA. Some form of discomfort normally accompanies ovulatory menstruation in contrast to anovulation bleeding, which is almost never associated with pain. Dysmenorrhea may reflect itself as lower abdominal cramps, backache, headache, and occasionally nausea and vomiting. Of these symptoms, the commonest is abdominal cramps. Many women suffer some discomfort for a few hours on the first day of menstruation, but in the majority of cases this is not incapacitating. Obviously, the degree of pain and discomfort experienced by any individual will depend upon concurrent involvement of the pelvic organs in disease or anatomic abnormalities. The pain threshold of the patient and the effect of emotional and psychologic problems, particularly those related to ignorance or misconception about the significance of the menstrual cycle, are important factors in evaluating the pathogenesis of dysmenorrhea. In *primary spastic* or *intrinsic dysmenorrhea*, there is no evidence of pelvic pathology. It may gradually disappear later in reproductive life, and relief is usually afforded by the birth of a full-term fetus. *Characteristic of secondary dysmenorrhea is the onset of pain after several years of relatively painless periods.* Pain may begin several days before menstrual flow and radiate throughout the entire lower abdomen, into the lower back, and down the legs. It is more constant in nature and not as sharp or cramplike as that noted in the primary type. Secondary dysmenorrhea is usually associated with pelvic pathology such as endometriosis, retroversion of the uterus, pelvic neoplasm, or inflammatory disease such as salpingitis or parametritis. In rare instances intense pain at the time of menstruation may accompany the expulsion of a large mass of shaggy, uterine membrane, i.e., membranous dysmenorrhea. Such events are infrequent and isolated and do not occur with successive periods.

PREMENSTRUAL TENSION. This term is applied to a constellation of symptoms which increase in intensity for 5 to 10 days before menstruation. The most frequent complaints are a sense of abdominal bloating, breast tenderness, headache, irritability, mental depression, and an increase in weight which may be associated with edema of the legs. The abdominal distension and tight feeling may be present without any great increase in weight and ofttimes without gaseous distension of the intestines (Chap. 48). There is no doubt that the wide fluctuation in female sex hormone levels which occurs during the reproductive period, with their important effect on electrolyte and water metabolism as well as upon mood and drive, provide critical "triggering" mechanisms for pathophysiologic changes in peripheral tissues as well as in the central nervous system.

REFERENCES

Behrman, S. J., and J. R. G. Gosling: Fundamentals of Gynecology, chaps. 6–11, New York, Oxford University Press, 1959.

Rogers, J.: Menstrual Disorders, New Engl. J. Med., 270: 194, Jan. 23, 1964.

Thorn, G. W.: Approach to the Patient with Idiopathic Edema or Periodic Swelling, J.A.M.A., 206:333, 1968.

53 DISTURBANCES OF SEXUAL FUNCTION

George W. Thorn

GENERAL CONSIDERATIONS

In men disturbances in sexual function may result from alterations in one or all of three distinct entities.

1. Libido, or the sexual impulse
2. Potentia, or penile erection
3. Ejaculation of semen

In women aberrations of sexual function are more difficult to analyze. Lack or diminution of sexual drive or failure to attain orgasm (frigidity) is much more frequent than in men.

Alterations in Libido

LOSS OF LIBIDO. Loss of libido may occur as a result of either psychologic or somatic factors. It may be complete in the presence of serious organic disease or with advanced age. On the other hand, lost or diminished libido may occur only under particular circumstances or in relation to a particular person, indicating the predominance of psychologic factors. In instances such as these, it is not unusual for a patient to experience nocturnal penile erection and emission of semen. Although loss of libido may accompany serious endocrine disorders such as anterior pituitary deficiency, Addison's disease, or diabetic acidosis or ketosis, it is not likely to be a *primary com-*

plaint of the patient under these circumstances since the impairment in general health and activity is so overwhelming. Under these circumstances, it is more likely that the patient's spouse will have noted or called attention to the difficulty. For practical purposes it is important to bear in mind that the primary complaint of lost or decreased libido in male patients, in the absence of *severe* organic disease or *advanced* age, is almost certainly dependent *upon emotional or psychologic disturbances.*

FRIGIDITY. Inability on the part of women to consummate the sexual act is a distressing complaint of relatively frequent occurrence. The sexual drive of the normal woman is primarily conditioned by psychologic factors, with endocrine functions in a supporting role. The changes in sexual drive produced by alterations in hormonal level are of relatively little importance in contrast to the role of emotional and psychologic factors. Conditioning from birth or early childhood most often results in a woman's belief that she is frigid. Many experiences in childhood can, later in life, result in incapacity to consummate the sexual act. Such experiences develop a climate of fear, insecurity, and dread concerning the whole subject of sex. Because of these deep-seated emotional conflicts, most patients will require intensive psychotherapy. With an understanding of the real basis of the problem and in conjunction with medical and psychiatric assistance, a small dose of androgenic hormone such as methyl testosterone, 10 mg twice daily, may be given. This may increase sexual drive and more specifically increase the sensitivity of the clitoris. Its continued use, however, may result in menstrual irregularities as well as in hirsutism and acne.

EXCESSIVE LIBIDO. Excessive libido may occur in conjunction with serious neurologic disease such as encephalitis or brain tumor as well as with psychologic and emotional disturbances. *Nymphomania* refers to women who exhibit abnormal behavior that reflects greatly heightened libido.

Alterations in Potentia

IMPOTENCE. Impotence implies the presence of sexual desire in a patient who cannot attain or sustain penile erection. Impotence is rarely of endocrine origin. More frequently it accompanies a neurologic or emotional disorder. In neurologic disorders absence or impairment of parasympathetic nerve activity prevents the development of tumescence of the corpora cavernosa. Impotence is common among patients who suffer disease of the sacral cord segments and their afferent and efferent connections, e.g., cord tumor, tabes, and multiple sclerosis. Approximately one-fourth of male diabetics in the younger age group and about one-half in the fifth decade develop impotence as a consequence of diabetic polyneuritis. Loss of both sexual desire and erection may occur in hypopituitarism, hypothyroidism, and severe eunuchoidism as well as in association with many general debilitating diseases. Patients with trauma to the prostatic urethra and those subjected to perineal operations frequently

have reduced potentia. Malformation of the genitals such as extreme degrees of epispadias, pseudohermaphroditism, growths and edema of the penis, as well as large hernias, hydroceles, and elephantiasis may interfere with sexual function. In the majority of patients, however, impotence is of psychologic origin and fortunately temporary. Fears and phobias which arise about the sexual act, as well as feelings of guilt, may be responsible.

PRIAPISM. True priapism is a state of sustained erection of the penis not accompanied by sexual desire. It is most frequent in the third or fourth decades and is usually accompanied by pain. Two types are recognized: the sustained and the recurrent nocturnal type. Priapism may result from urethral inflammation, from new growth involving the corpora, or from systemic disease such as leukemia or sickle-cell anemia. Diseases of the spinal cord may be accompanied by penile erections, reflexly induced and sustained for long periods of time. The neural apparatus for the control of sexual function is organized through the lower spinal segments, and hence may function effectively even when completely removed from voluntary control by spinal cord lesions. Recurrent, nonsustained, painful priapism is of unknown etiology, although it is often associated with prostatitis. Since it frequently subsides spontaneously, the efficacy of therapy is difficult to document. The administration of amyl nitrite has been noted to cause relaxation during the early phase of priapism. It has also been suggested that an anticoagulant might be effective in minimizing the venous thrombosis which is likely to occur with prolonged priapism. For this, heparin is suggested intravenously in an initial dose of 100 mg, followed by subsequent doses of 50 mg every 6 hr.

Ejaculation

Another type of disturbance consists of *premature ejaculation* of semen, a common complaint in neurotic individuals, though by no means peculiar to them. After lumbar sympathectomy the semen may be ejected into the bladder because of paralysis of the periurethral muscle at the verumontanum.

Dyspareunia

Dyspareunia, or *pain on intercourse*, may be present for a short time at the onset of marriage or sexual intercourse. Pain that continues long after marriage or develops later in life suggests local disease or emotional disturbance. Vaginal and pelvic examination should be made to exclude pelvic inflammatory disease, endometriosis, or tumor. In the absence of demonstrable organic disease, psychologic or emotional factors must be considered. Fear of pregnancy, fear of cancer if contraceptives are used, and tension between husband and wife can prevent enjoyment of intercourse with consequent spasm of vaginal musculature. Explanation of these facts with reassurance by an understanding physician may be followed by appreciable improvement.

Sterility

In the male sterility may result from lack of or impairment of spermatogenesis due to testicular agenesis, hypogenesis, or cryptorchidism; to castration or exposure to roentgen rays or toxic substances; to injury or inflammation; or to endocrine or nutritional disorders. Obstruction of the seminal vesicles and epididymis and pronounced deformity of the penis interfere with the normal passage of the spermatozoa. Infection of the prostate or seminal vesicles may be injurious to the spermatozoa (Chap. 54).

In the female sterility may result from impaired oogenesis as a consequence of deficient ovarian tissue, e.g., ovarian agenesis or hypoplasia, polycystic disease of the ovary with thickened capsule; or as a consequence of the inability of the ovum to become impregnated due to disease of the fallopian tubes, such as infection and endometriosis; or to uterine, cervical, or vaginal abnormalities in structure and function. In addition, debilitating diseases, endocrine abnormalities, and nutritional deficiencies may impair ovulation as well as fertilization and implantation of the ovum.

Infertility

Infertility represents one of the most important and serious disturbances of sexual function. It is estimated that 10 percent of couples in the United States are involuntarily infertile. Of this number it is thought that approximately one-third of cases are due to infertility of the woman, one-third to infertility of the man, and one-third to *decreased fertility* of both partners. Absolute infertility is said to exist when there is complete aspermia or absent or rudimentary ovarian tissue. *Relative infertility* applies to men who have oligospermia, when conception has not taken place. In contrast to other disturbances of sexual function such as impotence, frigidity, and dyspareunia, which are so frequently dependent upon psychologic and emotional factors, sterility and infertility are due primarily to functional and organic disease of the urogenital tract. In most instances the problem of infertility or sterility will be presented by the woman.

The approach to the problem of infertility in both men and women as well as suggestions for corrective therapy are discussed in detail in Chap. 54.

The genesis of *sexual perversions* remains obscure. Endocrine, biochemical, and psychologic studies have failed thus far to clarify either their cause or their mechanism.

REFERENCES

Bell, W. R., and W. R. Pitney: Brief Recordings: Management of Priapism by Therapeutic Defibrination, New Eng. J. of Med., 280:649, 1969.
Calderone, M. S.: "Release from Sexual Tension," New York, Random House, 1960.
Grace, D. A., and C. C. Winter: Priapism: An Appraisal of Management of Twenty-three Patients, J. Urol., 99:301, 1968.
Hamm, F. C., and S. R. Weinberg: "Urology in Medical Practice," 2d ed., Philadelphia, J. B. Lippincott Company, 1962.
Schöffling, K., K. Federlin, H. Ditschuneit, and E. F. Pfeiffer: Disorders of Sexual Function in Male Diabetics, Diabetes, 12:519, 1963.

54 INFERTILITY
Melvin L. Taymor

DEFINITION. Infertility may be defined as the inability to conceive during the course of normal sexual activity. It is generally held that a marriage should not be considered infertile until a year of unprotected coitus has been allowed to pass. However, each couple's problems should be judged individually, and diagnosis and treatment instituted at an earlier or later date as indicated.

ETIOLOGY. The two fundamental concepts to be kept in mind are (1) the multiplicity of etiologic factors and (2) the equal responsibility of male and female partners. To delineate these possible factors working either singly or in concert, one need only review the pathways of conception in male and female and the disorders of these pathways that may ensue.

Deficiency of sperm production in quantity and quality accounts for the majority of the *male's* contribution to the problem of infertility. Sperm production may be adversely affected by congenital influences such as germinal aplasia or cryptorchidism, by hormonal deficiencies of the pituitary or thyroid glands, by infection such as mumps orchitis, and by environmental factors such as nutritional deficiencies, noxious chemicals and drugs, radiation, excess local heat, and altitude. Often the cause is not ascertainable by diagnostic methods available at present. Sperm transport is affected by congenital malformations, surgical trauma, and infections. Impotency, an important factor in many cases, is commonly on a psychologic basis, although local infection or general systemic disorders may play a contributory role.

Defects in the *female* are related to production of ova and interference with their union with spermatozoa. Vaginal causes are organic or functional. Very often these causes are a combination of organic and psychologic factors. The obstruction may be due to an unruptured hymen, or it may be functional due to hypertrophy and contraction of the levator ani muscles. Vaginitis itself is not a serious cause of infertility except in its role as a temporary deterrent to coitus. The cervix is one of the most important areas of obstruction to the passage of sperm. During the few days prior to ovulation the endocervical glands secrete a thin, watery mucus that is beneficial to sperm survival and migration. Infection or estrogen deficiency may decrease the quality of the mucus. Too often the offender is an overly zealous physician who cauterizes the cervix too deeply and destroys the endocervical glands. Uterine abnormalities are not a common cause of infertility. Infertility can be associated with an anomaly such as bicornate, or double, uterus. Uterine fibroids are more likely to result in repeated abortions rather than the failure to conceive. Tubal occlusion is usually secondary to gonorrheal salpingitis. Bacterial salpingitis, secondary to pelvic peritonitis, appendicitis, abortion, or instrumentation, is more likely to result in partial blockage of the fibrated end of the tube. Nongonorrheal infection is also more likely to result in what is called the peritoneal factor. In this condition adhesions may develop between the tube and ovary, or fixation of the ovary may occur. Under these circumstances the chances of union between the sperm and egg are significantly reduced. In addition to infection, the peritoneal factor can be due to endometriosis. Hormonal or endocrine factors are all-important; these may result in deficient corpus luteum function and absence of ovulation.

Immunologic factors may play a significant role in some cases of unexplained infertility.

Finally, emotional factors may play a vital role by interfering with ovulation or initiating tubal spasm or dyspareunia. However, the fact should be stressed that more often than not, the state of infertility with its accompanying diagnostic and therapeutic maneuvers is more likely to produce serious emotional reactions than are primary emotional factors likely to produce infertility.

TREATMENT. The treatment of any defects, minor or major, in both the husband or the wife should be carried out concomitantly so that the total fertility potential of the couple will be raised to an optimum level.

In the *male* with azoospermia, in whom spermatogenesis is normal as shown by testicular biopsy, and in whom a block has been demonstrated, epididymovasostomy can result in return of fertility in 10 to 20 percent of cases. When hormonal studies reveal a deficiency of pituitary gonadotropin, treatment with human chorionic gonadotropin (5,000 units APL intramuscularly twice weekly for 2 to 6 months) is indicated. However, sperm deficiencies not associated with specific pituitary defects will not respond to pituitary or pituitarylike extract. Azoospermia or severe oligospermia will not respond in any significant degree to the administration of hormones, vitamins, thyroid preparations, or diet unless a specific deficiency can be demonstrated. In the present state of knowledge, little can be offered in the vast majority of cases of azoospermia or severe oligospermia.

This degree of pessimism should not be carried over to the infertile male with moderate degree of oligospermia (10 to 30 million per ml) or to the male partner of an infertile couple with only a moderately lowered sperm count (30 to 60 million per ml), particularly if one considers the "couple as a unit" concept of infertility. A modest improvement in the sperm count or motility combined with attention to the factors in the female partner may raise the fertility of the couple above a critical level. Avoidance of excess alcohol and tobacco, sufficient sleep and exercise, an optimum diet, adjustment of local excesses of heat, administration of thyroid preparations in

minor degrees of hypofunction—all these singly or together may prove of definite benefit.

In the *female* specific attention should be directed to the cervical factor by correction of unfavorable coital habits, correction of retroversion of the uterus by a pessary, improvement in quality and quantity of preovulatory mucus by the daily administration of small dosages of estrogen (0.1 mg diethylstilbestrol daily for three or four cycles), by the use of plastic cervical cap, and by the correction of cervicitis by systemic and local antibotics or by cervical cauterization. Cauterization must be conservative lest more harm than good be produced by cervical stenosis or obliteration of mucus secreting glands. When cervical stenosis is found, dilatation under anesthesia is of definite value.

Attempts to overcome tubal occlusion by repeated insufflations, diathermy, and high dosage of estrogen occasionally meet with success. Plastic repair of tubes or cornual implantation is followed by success in only 10 to 20 percent of cases. Surgery for tube-ovarian blockade, due to ovaries fixed by endometriosis, peritubal or periovarian adhesions, but associated with essentially normal tubes, results in a higher percentage of success. Infrequent ovulation accompanied by gross irregularity will respond to thyroid preparations when specifically indicated and to the correction of a specific dietary or vitamin deficiency. Ovulation accompanied by an inadequate luteal phase should be treated with progesterone preparations (Medroxyprogesterone, 2.5 mg daily for 10 days) or injections of human chorionic gonadotropin (HCG, 1,000 units intramuscularly every other day for five doses). Treatment should begin on the fifth or sixth day after the mid-cycle rise in the basal body temperature. Absence of ovulation is rarely corrected by pituitary hormone preparations.

Additional approaches to the medical induction of ovulation, although still experimental and as yet commercially unavailable, show promise for future clinical application. The first is an extract of gonadotropins, high in FSH activity, prepared from the urine of postmenopausal females (HMG). The usual dosage is 150 to 200 FSH units administered intramuscularly daily for 5 to 12 days. When there is evidence of follicular activity, as indicated by increased levels of estrogen in the urine or increasing fern formation in cervical mucus, 8,000 IU of HCG is administered. Each patient responds differently. Overstimulation can result in enlarged cystic ovaries and multiple pregnancies, so each patient should be followed carefully. Polycystic ovaries are most susceptible to massive enlargement and possible rupture.

Clomiphene citrate, a chemical closely related to stilbestrol, also can stimulate ovulation. The mode of action is not completely clarified, but after a 3-to-5-day course of the medication, 100 mg daily, a burst of gonadotropins 3 to 10 days later often stimulates ovulation. It, too, should be used with caution in patients suspected of having polycystic ovaries.

Psychotherapy is of value in improving the coital habits of the couple, in reducing tubal spasm, and in correcting some deficiences of hormonal nature. Finally, the manner

Table 54-1. TESTS FOR INFERTILITY

I. In the male.
  A. Routine.
    1. Semen analysis. The semen is delivered into a clean glass container by withdrawal or masturbation. The following characteristics are considered normal:
      a. Volume—3 to 5 ml.
      b. Sperm count—above 60 million per ml is unquestionably normal, below 30 million per ml unquestionably indicates reduced fertility. The significance of counts between 30 million and 60 million depends upon the quality of motility and the degree of fertility in the female partner. A highly fertile female would be more susceptible to a count of borderline fertility.
      c. Motility—40 percent or more still actively motile 4 to 5 hr after collection.
      d. Morphology—at least 60 percent of the spermatozoa should be of normal size and shape.
    2. Examination of prostatic smear—excess leukocytes indicate that infection may play a contributory role.
  B. Special tests—for the male with reduced fertility as indicated by semen analysis.
    1. Evaluation of thyroid function by basal metabolic rate, protein-bound iodine, or radioactive iodine uptake.
    2. Testicular biopsy—in most cases this will result in a definitive diagnosis. In only a few cases, however, will it demonstrate a remediable defect.
    3. Urinary gonadotropins—these may be low in pituitary deficiency. Excretion is high in primary gonadal failure.
    4. Sex chromatin determination.
II. In the female.
  A. Routine.
    1. Postcoital test—examination of the cervical mucus for its preovulatory qualities of clarity, spinnbarkeit (ability of the mucus to form a thread 5 to 10 cm in length when stretched between slide and cover slip), ferning (ability of the mucus to form fernlike pattern when dried and examined under low power of microscope), and for the number of viable spermatozoa 8 to 12 hr after coitus.
      a. Good test—more than 20 active spermatozoa per high-power field.
      b. Fair test—5 to 20 spermatozoa per high-power field.
      c. Poor test—less than 5 spermatozoa per high-power field. A poor postcoital test in the presence of good preovulatory mucus suggests a semen deficiency, a deficiency of the coital method, or malposition of the cervix. A poor postcoital test combined with poor mucus in the preovulatory phase and a normal semen analysis indicates a hostile cervix either on an inflammatory or an endocrine basis.

Table 54-1. TESTS FOR INFERTILITY (*Continued*)

    2. The evaluation of tubal patency—initially by insufflation with carbon dioxide (Rubin test) and followed at a later date by hysterosalpingography in those cases which show failure of carbon dioxide to pass or who fail to conceive after an interval of time despite a normal Rubin test.
    3. Evaluation of ovulation and hormonal factors by:
      a. Measurement of basal body temperature, which characteristically shows a sustained rise after ovulation. Studies have shown that actual ovulation may occur as long as 2 days before or 2 days after the beginning of the temperature rise. The value of the temperature chart as an exact indicator of ovulation timing for purposes of timing coitus or insemination treatments can be overestimated.
      b. Endometrial biopsy with the demonstration of secretory changes in the endometrium is valid evidence that ovulation has occurred. The presence of endometrium out of phase with the time of biopsy is evidence of a progestational deficiency.
  B. Special tests should be carried out when indicated.
    1. Evaluation of thyroid function.
    2. Endocrine assays, such as urinary gonadotropin and 17 ketosteroid determination, in cases of anovulation or inadequate luteal function.
    3. Further studies of ovulation timing utilizing vaginal or urinary smears and studies of cervical mucus.
    4. Culdoscopy to detect early endometriosis, pelvic adhesions interfering with tube-ovarian function, or polycystic ovaries.

and attitude of the physician plays a role in the outcome by preventing undue feelings of guilt and depression from gaining the upper hand, and by instilling sufficient hope and fortitude to allow the couple to carry through with the tedious and sometimes painful diagnostic testing and therapeutic maneuvers.

REFERENCES

Gemzell, C. A.: Induction of Ovulation with Human Pituitary Gonadotropins, Fertility Sterility, 13:153, 1962.

Meeker, S. R.: "Human Sterility, Causation, Diagnosis and Treatment: A Practical Manual of Clinical Procedures," Baltimore, The Williams & Wilkins Company, 1933.

Stone, A., and M. E. Ward: Factors Responsible for Pregnancy in 500 Infertility Cases, Fertility Sterility, 7:1, 1956.

Taymor, M. L.: Gonadotropin Therapy, Possible Causes and Prevention of Ovarian Overstimulation, J.A.M.A., 203: 362, 1968.

——: Management of Infertility, Springfield, Ill. Charles C Thomas, Publisher, 1969.

Section 8
Alterations in the Integument

55 SKIN LESIONS
Faye D. Arundell and Eugene M. Farber

Examination of the skin should include a detailed history and thorough inspection of the entire surface encompassing the mucous membranes of the mouth and genital region, the hair, and the nails. The patient should be examined undressed, in order to carry out a thorough inspection of the hair, scalp, ears, eyes, mucosae of the nose, mouth, pharynx, teeth, all surfaces of the trunk and extremities, palms, soles, interdigital spaces, and nails. The examination should be performed in unobstructed daylight or artificial daylight illumination. Subtle color changes in the skin may be masked by inadequate artificial lighting. The routine use of a magnifying lens permits the perception of fine details and small lesions.

Orderly notation and description of the lesions are prerequisites to accurate diagnosis and judicious therapy (Chaps. 56 to 60, 400). Four fundamental changes in the skin can be detected by inspection and palpation. These abnormalities, which represent the basic pathologic reactions of skin, are changes in color, mass, fluid content, and texture. Color changes usually result from involvement of the vascular or pigmentary system. Changes in mass caused by cellular proliferation or infiltration result in palpable lesions that may project above the surface of the surrounding normal skin. Free fluid within the epidermis, or between the epidermis and dermis, creates *blisters;* increased free fluid within the dermis results in a solid *mass. Scales,* representing a change in texture of the outermost layers, are caused by defects in the formation or shedding of the horny layer. In any single lesion the changes may occur alone or in combination. The lesion which contains the fewest number of fundamental changes represents the *primary lesion.* The primary lesion should be identified, since its recognition makes it possible to diagnose an eruption. Evolutionary or secondary changes of the primary lesion, their arrangement or configuration, and their distribution on the body surface are additional diagnostic features. Many dermatoses are not accompanied by systemic changes, and their diagnosis is entirely dependent on the analysis of data obtained by observation and palpation of the skin.

PRINCIPAL PRIMARY LESIONS OF DISEASES AFFECTING THE SKIN. Macules.
Macules are small circumscribed changes in color of the skin unaccompanied by any change in mass or fluid content. If there is any palpable elevation or induration present in the colored lesion, it is not a macule. Circumscribed color changes in the skin larger than 1 cm in diameter are referred to as *patches.* Macular changes may be caused by deposition of extrinsic pigment as a consequence of trauma; increase or decrease of the intrinsic skin pigment, melanin, such as freckles and vitiligo; dilatation of cutaneous blood vessels, resulting in erythema; extravasation of erythrocytes to form petechiae or purpuric macules. Firm pressure with a glass slide over the dilated vessels of erythematous macules causes immediate blanching and readily differentiates them from purpuric macules. Erythematous macules are common in drug reactions and in exanthems such as roseola and rubella.

Papules. Papules are small (less than 0.5 cm in diameter) circumscribed increases in mass in the skin produced by tissue proliferation or infiltration. Papules are always palpable and may be accompanied by changes in color and texture. The color, shape, and configuration of papular lesions are characteristic in certain dermatoses. Papules which are violet in color, angular in shape, and have flat tops with adherent scales are the primary lesion of lichen planus. Erythematous papules arranged in rings and semicircles create the characteristic "nickels and dimes" lesions of secondary syphilis.

Papules may extend peripherally or coalesce to form large *plaques.* Erythematous plaques covered by layers of silvery scales are the hallmark of psoriasis (Chap. 400). Firm pebbled plaques occur in *lichen amyloidosis,* a type of amyloidosis confined to the skin.

Nodules. Deep circumscribed lesions that are firmer than the surrounding tissue are termed nodules when they are the result of tissue proliferation or inflammation. Red, hot, firm, tender nodules are present over the shins in erythema nodosum. *Tumors* are circumscribed indurated lesions which are arbitrarily defined as being larger than nodules.

Wheals (*hives, urticaria*) are a distinctive type of nodule caused by a localized collection of free fluid within the deeper layers of the skin. A hive has a central raised pale nodule surrounded by an erythematous patch, or flare. Wheals may enlarge to form alarmingly large swellings of an extremity or the face (*angioneurotic edema*). Hives, by definition, are transient itchy lesions which involute within hours, though new lesions continue to appear. The commonest causes of such acute urticarial reactions are food allergy, physical allergy, and drug reactions. Chronic urticaria is characterized by transient urticarial lesions that recur for periods longer than 6 weeks. Patients with chronic urticaria require a painstaking history regarding medications, chronic infections, food, environmental, physical, and psychologic factors. Individual urticarial lesions, which are not transient but persist for days or weeks, often form rings or bizarre figures. Persistent figurate urticarial lesions are the only primary lesions present in the chronic erythema group of diseases, such as *erythema annulare centrifugum*. Persistent urticarial lesions also occur as one of the primary lesions in association with blisters and patchy erythema in erythema multiforme (Chap. 400). The diseases characterized by persistent urticarial lesions require a thorough history and investigation for precipitating factors, such as drugs, infection, and neoplastic diseases. Urticarial lesions ordinarily respond to systemic antihistamine therapy. Life-threatening eruptions, such as severe bullous erythema multiforme, require systemic corticosteroid therapy. Under no circumstances should symptomatic therapy, whether antihistamines or corticosteroids, replace a search for and removal of the primary etiologic factor.

Vesicles and bullae. Vesicles are circumscribed small blisters containing free fluid. The free fluid may be located within the epidermis or between the epidermis and dermis. Inflammation of the skin due to chemical irritants, allergens, or physical agents often leads to cellular disintegration and accumulation of free fluid. Vesicles are the prime lesions of acute dermatitis. *Bullae* are vesicles larger than 0.5 cm in diameter. *Pustules* are vesicles containing purulent fluid. It is important for diagnosis to note the following features of the vesicles or bullae: (1) the contents (serous, sanguinous, or purulent fluid); (2) the roof (intact, tough, fragile, or umbilicated); (3) the tension (firm or flaccid); (4) the base (normal skin, erythema, or urticaria); and (5) the relationship of one vesicle to the others (grouped or isolated). These special features, combined with the distribution of the eruption, permit accurate clinical diagnosis of many vesicular diseases. *Herpes simplex* (Chap. 226) is characterized by a single lesion composed of clear or purulent, umbilicated, tough, tense, grouped vesicles on an erythematous base. Multiple lesions, each showing the features of herpes simplex, located in a linear pattern along a nerve root distribution are diagnostic of *herpes zoster* (Chap. 225). Isolated, tense, serous, or serosanguinous bullae on urticarial bases surrounded by concentric rings of normal skin and urticarial rings form the classic "target" or "iris" lesions of erythema multiforme. Isolated pustules surmounting purpuric macules at the tips of the digits represent septic emboli and are cutaneous signs of bacteremia.

SECONDARY LESIONS OF THE SKIN. The secondary lesions of the skin represent sequential or evolutionary changes in primary lesions.

Crusts. Crusts are the dried remains of exudates and may be composed of dried blood, serum, or pus. Crusts are usually situated on oozing erosions or ulcers that can be examined adequately only when the crusts are removed. Linear hemorrhagic crusts mark the sites of excoriations. Honey-colored, clear-yellow crusts are typical of *impetigo*. Impetigo is a superficial bacterial infection of the skin caused by staphylococci and/or beta hemolytic streptococci. Glomerulonephritis is a common accompaniment of impetigo when beta hemolytic streptococci are present in the cutaneous lesions.

Scales. Scales are visible and palpable fragments of the horny outer layer of skin, the stratum corneum. Special features of scales are helpful in diagnosis. Scales may be dry or greasy, lighter or darker than the normal skin, fine or platelike, loose or adherent. Scales may develop on primary lesions, macules, or papules, or on otherwise normal-appearing skin. The greasy yellow scales of seborrheic dermatitis, the silvery piled-up scales of psoriasis, and dark fishlike scales of ichthyosis are diagnostic features of three scaling dermatoses.

Erosions and Ulcers. Erosions are circumscribed superficially denuded areas of skin which usually heal without scarring. Ulcers occur when there is deeper destruction of the cutis and subcutaneous tissues. The etiologic factors concerned in the production of an ulcer may be single or multiple. Although repeated minor trauma is usually the primary cause of leg ulcers in elderly patients, the delayed healing and extension of the ulcer is a consequence of superimposed bacterial infection in individuals with peripheral vascular disease. Table 55-1 lists the conditions which are responsible for ulcers of the lower extremities, including physical agents, infections, vascular diseases, hematologic diseases, neurologic deficits, and neoplasia. The development of squamous cell carcinoma is a recognized risk in chronic ulcers from any cause. The presence of an ulcer demands a thorough investigation to elucidate the underlying causative factor. Biopsy of any ulcer which does not respond to specific therapy for the causative factor is mandatory in order to rule out superimposed neoplastic disease.

Lichenification. Thickening of the skin accompanied by an accentuation of the normal superficial skin markings is termed lichenification. The affected skin is studded with closely set papular elevations separated from each other by delicate furrows. Hyperpigmentation often is present in lichenified areas of skin. Since lichenification is produced by continued irritation of the skin, most commonly from scratching, it is found in many chronic pruritic dermatoses. In localized neurodermatitis (*lichen simplex chronicus*), lichenification and excoriations are the only skin changes to be found. The skin of the antecubital and popliteal fossae classically becomes lichenified in the juvenile and adult types of atopic dermatitis.

Scars. Scars are usually the result of severe dermal injury. In most cases, scars are preceded by ulcers, but dermal diseases, such as discoid lupus erythematosus, cause scars without previous ulceration. It is always dangerous to attempt to make a dermatologic diagnosis from scars alone. Hypertrophy, elevation, and pruritus are common in surgical or traumatic scars. *Keloids* are nodular, firm, generally linear masses of hyperplastic connective tissue which occur in the dermis and subcutaneous tissue after a traumatic injury or burn. The histologic changes in keloids and hypertrophic scars differ only in degree. In keloids the antecedent trauma is often trivial, and constitutional or hereditary factors play a predominant role.

Table 55-1. COMMON ULCERS OF THE
LOWER EXTREMITIES

I. Vascular disorders
   A. Large arteries
      1. Thromboangiitis obliterans
      2. Arteriosclerosis obliterans
      3. Acute arterial occlusion
   B. Small arteries and arterioles
      1. Livedo reticularis
      2. Chronic pernio
      3. Periarteritis nodosa
      4. Hypertensive ischemic leg ulcer
      5. Vasculitis—allergic, rheumatoid
   C. Veins
      1. Chronic venous insufficiency
   D. Arteries and veins
      1. Hemangioma
      2. Arteriovenous fistula
II. Blood dyscrasias
   A. Sickle-cell anemia
   B. Thalassemia
   C. Polycythemia vera
   D. Hereditary spherocytosis
III. Dysproteinemias
   A. Cryoglobulins
   B. Macroglobulins
IV. Infections
   A. Bacterial
      1. Tuberculosis
      2. Syphilis
      3. Chancroid
      4. Granuloma inguinale
      5. Amebiasis cutis
      6. Diphtheria cutis
      7. Pyodermas
      8. Leprosy
      9. Yaws
      10. Leishmaniasis
      11. "Tropical" ulcers
      12. Anthrax
      13. Tularemia
      14. Osteomyelitis
   B. Mycotic
      1. Blastomycosis
      2. Sporotrichosis
      3. Chromoblastomycosis
      4. Coccidioidomycosis
V. Neoplasms
   A. Squamous cell carcinoma
   B. Lymphoma
      1. Mycosis fungoides
      2. Hodgkin's disease
      3. Leukemia cutis
      4. Lymphosarcoma
   C. Melanoma
   D. Sarcoma
      1. Kaposi's sarcoma
      2. Dermatofibrosarcoma
VI. Neuropathic
   A. Trophic ulcers in diabetes, tabes dorsalis, polyneuritis
VII. Drug Reaction
   A. Iododerma
   B. Bromoderma

Table 55-1. COMMON ULCERS OF THE
LOWER EXTREMITIES (*Continued*)

VIII. Traumatic Factors
   A. Factitial
   B. Neurotic excoriations
   C. Insect bites
   D. Radiodermatitis
   E. Decubitus
   F. Physical injury
      1. Trench foot
      2. Immersion foot
      3. Frostbite
      4. Acute pernio
      5. Thermal burns
   G. Chemical burns
X. Miscellaneous
   A. Scleroderma
   B. Lupus erythematosus
   C. Pyoderma gangrenosum
   D. Relapsing febrile nodular nonsuppurative panniculitis

ARRANGEMENT OF LESIONS. Familiarity with the configuration or arrangement of multiple lesions is helpful in establishing a diagnosis of a dermatologic disease. Some dermatoses are characterized by the presence of discrete lesions; other dermatoses are characterized by special relationships or arrangements of multiple lesions in groups, annular or linear patterns, etc.

Grouping. Clusters or close aggregates of multiple vesicles are present in herpes simplex and herpes zoster. A symmetrical eruption of grouped, excoriated vesicles, papules, and scars clustered over the knees, elbows, sacrum, and scapulae occurs in *dermatitis herpetiformis* (Chap. 400).

Annularity. One of the most important configurations seen in the skin is the circle or arc of lesions surrounding normal skin. Annular, papular lesions occur in secondary syphilis, sarcoid, leprosy, discoid lupus erythematosus, and lichen planus. The characteristic lesion of granuloma annulare is a circle of papules or nodules on the extensor surfaces of joints. Evanescent annular erythematous macules occur over the joints in erythema rheumaticum, the cutaneous manifestation of rheumatic fever. Ringworm infections of the glabrous skin (tinea corporis) are characterized by papular, vesicular, scaling, annular lesions which clear centrally and extend peripherally. It is always possible to demonstrate the fungi in scrapings from the lesions of ringworm infections (see below).

Linearity. Linear arrangements of lesions occur in herpes zoster and warty linear epidermal nevi. Localized linear scleroderma may cause deformities by retarding the growth of underlying bones and muscles when it involves the face or extremities of children. Autoinoculation of warts along a scratch results in linear lesions. Similar linear lesions may occur in patients with psoriasis and lichen planus when their skin responds to nonspecific trauma by producing new lesions. Acute vesicular linear lesions aid in differentiating plant dermatitis (poison ivy or oak) from other types of contact dermatitis. Linear distribution of pink, scaling, oval lesions along the cleavage lines of the trunk result in the "Christmas tree" pattern of pityriasis rosea.

Chancriform Complex or Primary Inoculation Pattern. The special configuration of an initial inflammatory papule or ulcerative lesion at the site of inoculation, with the subsequent development of inflammatory nodules in a linear pattern along the lymphatic drainage or with regional adenopathy, is termed the chancriform complex. Primary cutaneous inoculation of bacteria as in syphilis, tuberculosis, and tularemia may follow this pattern (Chap. 155). Sporotrichosis is the commonest naturally occurring deep fungus infection that produces the primary inoculation pattern. Accidental cutaneous inoculation of blastomycosis and coccidiomycosis occurring in laboratory workers also causes a chancriform complex. The recognition of the primary inoculation pattern of reaction is important, since the specific organism can usually be detected in smears or cultures prepared from the primary lesion. Appropriate cultural procedures and biopsies confirm the diagnosis in tuberculosis and the deep mycoses.

DISTRIBUTION OF LESIONS. An important clinical feature of all eruptions is the distribution of lesions over the body. In some dermatoses the distribution is so characteristic of the eruption as to be diagnostic. The lesions may be localized or generalized. Generalized eruptions may be universal and involve the whole cutaneous surface or disseminated and composed of discrete lesions widely scattered over the skin. Disseminated eruptions may be symmetrical or asymmetrical. Areas of the body exposed to specific environmental factors or containing specialized epidermal appendages are the areas of involvement in certain eruptions.

Localized Distribution. In addition to the diseases occurring in linear or chancriform patterns, there are several dermatoses which primarily involve localized areas of the skin surface. Recurrent herpes simplex is characteristically a single lesion which repeatedly involves the same area, most commonly the lips or genitalia. The fixed drug eruption recurs as an acute urticarial or bullous lesion at the same "fixed" site with each exposure to the drug. The fixed site of acute reaction is marked by a hyperpigmented macule that persists between attacks. Certain compounds, such as phenolphthalein in proprietary laxatives, are notoriously associated with fixed drug reactions. Contact allergic dermatitis due to metals in solid objects characteristically causes a localized eruption at the sites of contact, e.g., ear lobes in earring dermatitis and discrete patches on the anterior and posterior thighs in garter dermatitis.

Universal Eruptions. Universal erythema with or without massive scaling is a reaction pattern of the skin. Investigation for the underlying precipitating factor in universal exfoliative erythrodermas is mandatory. Drug reactions, neoplastic diseases, especially the lymphomas, and aggravation of preceding dermatosis, such as psoriasis, may be the cause of universal erythroderma.

Disseminated Symmetrical Eruptions. In several dermatoses the distribution of lesions on one side of the body is an exact mirror image of the other side. Dermatoses due to intrinsic factors, such as drug eruptions, are commonly symmetrical eruptions. Psoriasis is a symmetrical eruption of erythematous silvery scaling plaques involving the elbows, knees, and scalp. Symmetrical, thickened, excoriated plaques of chronic dermatitis involve the antecubital and popliteal fossae in juvenile and adult patients with atopic dermatitis.

Special Areas of Involvement. Dermatoses related to environmental factors involve special areas. Distribution is limited to *exposed areas* in dermatitis where sunlight or air-borne pollens or chemicals play a causative role. Involvement of the face, neck, V-area of the chest, dorsum of the hands and arms, ending abruptly at the sleeve-level, occur in these eruptions. The anatomically shaded areas, the upper eyelids, retroauricular folds, and submental regions, are not involved in photosensitive eruptions, but are involved in air-borne dust dermatitis. *Sebaceous areas*, where sebaceous glands and hair follicles are abundant, are affected by acne, rosacea, and seborrheic dermatitis. In addition to the face, acne involves the neck, shoulders, and upper back and chest, but spares the scalp. Rosacea remains confined to the face, primarily to the flush areas. Seborrheic dermatitis involves the scalp, eyebrows, eyelid margins, sides of the nose, and external auditory canals. The *intertriginous areas, axillae*, inframammary, and anogenital regions, are also common sites of involvement in seborrheic dermatitis, psoriasis, erythrasma, and cutaneous moniliasis. The *pretibial region* is the characteristic site of four dermatoses: erythema nodosum, localized cutaneous myxedema, lichen amyloidosis, and necrobiosis lipoidica diabeticorum. These pretibial eruptions are usually bilateral. Involvement of *mucosal surfaces* is a common and diagnostically helpful feature in diseases which also involve the skin. A lacy white network on the buccal mucosa is pathognomonic of lichen planus. Vesicles and bullae rarely remain intact on mucosal surfaces. Erosions, the sequential lesions of bullae, occur on the tongue, gingiva, buccal, pharyngeal, nasal, and genital mucosa in erythema multiforme and pemphigus vulgaris.

DERMATOLOGIC LABORATORY PROCEDURES. In addition to the laboratory procedures used in general medicine, several special procedures are necessary in establishing or confirming the diagnosis of diseases of the skin.

Wood's Light. A special Wood's filter, which transmits ultraviolet light with wavelengths from 3100 to over 4000 Å, is used in conjunction with a hot quartz or fluorescent light source. Substances that are activated by the wavelengths transmitted through the Wood's filter will fluoresce. The demonstration of fluorescence of a specific color is an important test in porphyria cutanea tarda (Chap. 108), erythrasma, and tinea capitis (ringworm of the scalp hair). The urine in porphyria cutanea tarda fluoresces bright red with the light transmitted through a Wood's filter. Porphyrins produced by corynebacteria cause a distinctive coral-red fluorescence in the involved intertriginous areas in erythrasma (Chap. 400). The teeth are fluorescent in erythropoietic porphyria and in the dental abnormalities in infants caused by tetracyclines. The green-blue fluorescence of infected hairs is a useful screening procedure in epidemic scalp ring-worm.

Potassium Hydroxide (KOH) Preparations. The demonstration of hyphae in fungus infections and budding spores in moniliasis is an office procedure which rapidly establishes the diagnosis. The skin is cleansed with alcohol. Scrapings from scaling lesions, tops of vesicles, clippings from nails, or plucked hairs, are placed on a glass slide in a drop of 10% aqueous potassium hydroxide and covered with a cover slip. The KOH preparation is warmed gently over a match or alcohol lamp. Clearing occurs rapidly as the keratin structures dissolve. The fragile hyphae, spores, or budding yeasts are visible in the cleared preparation under "high dry" magnification. A positive KOH preparation is tantamount to a diagnosis. The investigation of all annular scaling or vesicular lesions, all thickened discolored nails, and hairs from

A

B

Fig. 55-1. A. Biopsy of cutaneous lesions requires the following equipment: a local anesthetic, biopsy punches, forceps, and scissors. Biopsy punches are available in graduated sizes from 2 to 6 mm in diameter. B. Skin sutures are ordinarily not necessary following punch biopsy. The tissue obtained by biopsy is placed in a formalin fixative.

patchy areas of hair loss, should include a KOH preparation. No dermatitis, nail dystrophy, or localized hair loss should be treated as a fungus infection unless positive KOH preparations have been obtained. The specific fungus or yeast responsible for the positive KOH preparation can be defined by culturing samples of the infected keratin (scales, hairs, nails) on Sabouraud's medium at room temperature. Since it takes approximately 3 weeks of growth to identify fungus cultures, the treatment of superficial fungus infections is ordinarily started on the basis of positive KOH preparations alone.

Cytologic Smears and Imprints. Diagnostic cytologic changes occur in pemphigus, herpes simplex, zoster, and varicella. The roof of the youngest vesicle or bulla is split with a scalpel and reflected. The inner surface of the reflected roof and the denuded floor of the vesicle are scraped gently with a scalpel. The white cellular material is transferred to a glass slide and rapidly air-dried. The slide is placed in Giemsa stain for 1 min, flushed with tap water, and examined microscopically. The giant multinucleated epidermal cells which are the diagnostic cytologic changes of herpes simplex, zoster, and varicella, are not present in vaccinia and variola. Loss of prickles (desmosomes), the basic cellular change in the epidermal cells in pemphigus, is referred to as *acantholysis*. The presence of many acantholytic cells, individual small rounded cells with large nuclei and basophilic peripheral condensations of cytoplasm, in smears from bullae is diagnostic of pemphigus. The definitive diagnosis of the type of pemphigus depends on clinical features and biopsies showing the level of the epidermis at which acantholysis first appears.

Cytologic imprints are prepared by firmly pressing the cut surface of an excised full-thickness piece of skin on a clean glass slide. Inflammatory and neoplastic cells in dermal infiltrates will adhere to the slide and may be stained with any hematologic stain. This procedure is particularly useful in defining the cellular type of lymphomatous lesions of the skin.

Biopsy. Since many cutaneous diseases have specific histologic changes, biopsies are useful in diagnosis. Biopsy is a mandatory procedure in the investigation of lesions suspected of being neoplastic. Tumors of sufficiently small size and suspected malignant melanomas regardless of size should be removed *in toto* by excision biopsy. With other tumors, a 4-mm punch biopsy yields sufficient tissue for histologic diagnosis. Multiple punch biopsies may be required to detect malignant changes in large ulcers. In order to establish the diagnosis in dermatoses, the youngest primary lesion, free from secondary or sequential changes, should be chosen for biopsy. Punch biopsies are particularly useful in the investigation of bullous eruptions; papular scaling eruptions, such as psoriasis and lichen planus; granulomatous diseases, such as tuberculosis, leprosy, and the deep mycoses; purpuric eruptions; and deposition diseases, such as xanthomas and amyloidosis. The characteristic histologic changes in cutaneous lesions aid in establishing the diagnosis in such systemic diseases as sarcoidosis, lupus erythematosus, scleroderma, and dermatomyositis.

Intradermal Tests. The detection of immediate urticarial reactions by scratch or intradermal tests of common pollens, foods, etc. is of limited usefulness in the study of skin diseases. The recognition of the delayed "tuberculin-type" of allergy (Chap. 68) is important dermatologically in the study of both systemic granulomatous and cutaneous granulomatous diseases. The most commonly used intradermal antigens are tuberculin, blastomycin, histoplasmin, and coccidioidin. Less commonly used antigens are mumps, trichophytin, trichenella, Frei antigen of lymphogranuloma venereum, lepromin, and Kveim. Negative reactions to mumps and trichophytin antigen are important in defining anergic states. Kveim antigen is a crude tissue homogenate prepared from lymph nodes or spleens involved with sarcoid. Patients with active sarcoidosis develop pure epithelioid tubercles which are detectable microscopically on skin biopsy of the site where the antigen had been injected intradermally 6 weeks previously.

Patch Tests. The patch test is a useful procedure in the diagnosis of contact allergic dermatitis. The diagnostic patch testing procedure is based on the principle that skin previously sensitized to an antigen will show an eczematous reaction at the site of subsequent applications of that specific antigen (Chap. 68). The suspected substance is applied to the skin and covered by an occlusive cellophane patch held in place by an adhesive plaster. The patch test is removed in 48 hr. A positive patch test, a reproduction of the disease in miniature, consists of erythema, papules, palpable edema, or vesicles. The intelligent use of patch testing depends on careful questioning to detect possible offenders. Known primary irritants such as strong acids, alkalis, soaps, and solvents must be used in only very dilute concentrations for patch testing. Patch tests should not be performed during acute episodes of dermatitis or while the patient is receiving systemic corticosteroid therapy.

PHYSICAL ALLERGY. The production of the disease in miniature by the application of the appropriate stimulus is a useful procedure in the investigation of physical allergies. Cold urticaria is confirmed by the development of an acute urticarial reaction at the site of contact of the skin with an ice cube. A hot bath or exercise induces a generalized eruption of small wheals surrounded by large erythematous flares in generalized cholinergic urticaria. Local heat hypersensitivity is confirmed by eliciting a wheal at the site of local heating of the skin. Photosensitivity testing is a specialized procedure requiring a hot quartz or carbon arc ultraviolet light source. Only small areas of skin should be exposed to light testing in order to avoid generalized or systemic reactions (Chap. 59).

56   ITCHING
Faye D. Arundell and Eugene M. Farber

Pruritus, or itching, is a unique cutaneous symptom that is best described as an unpleasant sensation which provokes the desire to scratch. It is specifically an epidermal sensation which depends on the presence of free unmyelinated nerve endings between the cells of the epidermis. Stimulation of these free nerve endings initiates impulses that travel the same nervous pathways as pain along the lateral spinothalamic tract to the thalamus. Itching evokes the purposive motor response of scratching. Pain, though an allied sensation, evokes reflex withdrawal.

Itching, unlike pain, occurs nowhere but in the skin. Removal of the epidermis abolishes the itching end organ but does not interfere with the perception of pain. Stimuli that will initiate itching are usually of milder degree than those which cause pain. Any mechanical, thermal, or chemical stimulus causing an appropriate degree of injury will induce itching if the epidermis is present. A number of chemicals, released or activated in various ways, appear to function as mediators of pruritus. Extremely low concentrations of proteases, kinins, and histamine cause itching.

Pruritus may be perceived, interpreted, and described by the patient as burning, prickling, stinging, or itching. There is a marked variation in individual itching thresholds. Atopic individuals in general are "itchy people" and have a low itch threshold. Pruritus causes a lowering of the threshold in the affected area, resulting in stimulation of itching by progressively milder stimuli. Scratching, the reflex response to itching, also decreases the itch threshold. A vicious cycle of itching, scratching, and itching may become established in cutaneous regions of lowered thresholds to itch. Vasodilatation lowers the itch threshold and may account for the circadian rhythm of itching, which is usually worse at night. Strong stimuli, such as pain and extremes of temperature, inhibit pruritus. Many severely itching patients learn to substitute pain for itch by pinching the skin adjacent to itching areas or by completely denuding the itchy region. Extremely cold applications give temporary relief which is promptly followed by aggravation of itching.

GENERALIZED PRURITUS

Generalized and persistent pruritus, which is not accompanied by demonstrable skin lesions other than excoriations, is associated with a variety of systemic diseases. Pruritus of sudden onset which is generalized and persistent demands a general medical investigation. The most commonly associated diseases are obstructive jaundice, lymphomas, internal cancers, severe renal insufficiency, and diabetes mellitus. Obstructive hepatic disease causing pruritus is detectable on physical examination, since the patients are invariably jaundiced. Pruritus may be out of proportion to the degree of jaundice, however; severe itching may occur with mild jaundice, and severe jaundice may be unaccompanied by pruritus. The severity of itching correlates better with the accumulation of bile salts than with increased bile pigments. (Chap. 45).

Lymphatic leukemia, Hodgkin's disease, lymphosarcoma, and mycosis fungoides are the lymphomas which cause generalized pruritus. Pruritus in the absence of any primary skin change may be the first manifestation of these diseases. Generalized exfoliative dermatitis, with an aggravation of the pruritus, may develop in the course of any of these lymphomas. The mechanism of the pruritus is unknown, but once specific tumors actually develop in the skin, they no longer itch. Other forms of internal neoplastic disease, such as carcinoma, may also be associated with generalized pruritus. Generalized pruritus in the absence of other systemic diseases always deserves complete study to detect hidden malignancies.

Persistent generalized itching occurs in advanced cases of uremia. Relief of renal failure gives prompt relief of the pruritus. Neither urea nor uric acid is responsible for pruritus, and the chemical mediator of uremic itching is unknown.

Generalized pruritus is usually out of proportion to the severity of diabetes mellitus. In a few diabetics pruritus cannot be explained on any other basis. Most commonly, however, diabetic itching is due to the excessive dryness of the skin rather than to the state of the diabetes. Xerotic skin, which has a decreased water-holding capacity, develops scaling, fine fissures or chapping, and a low itching threshold. Dry heat, cold winds, and frequent bathing aggravate the xerosis. Localized pruritus of the anogenital region of diabetics is usually caused by superficial *Candida albicans* infections.

ITCHY DERMATOLOGIC DISEASES

The cause of pruritus due to dermatologic diseases is evident on inspection of the skin. Since superficial damage causes itching, stimuli of sufficient degrees to cause pruritus usually leave a marker on the skin. Such stimuli may be extrinsic, as in infestations and infections, intrinsic as in immediate urticarial reactions, or a combination of these as in eczematous dermatitis.

INFESTATIONS AND INFECTIONS. Urticarial papules topped by puncta mark the sites of bites. The distribution of the bites depends on the living and feeding habits of the parasite. Flea bites are most common on the lower extremities because fleas are jumping rather than flying insects. The excoriated bites in pediculosis commonly become secondarily infected. The lice and their eggs are usually not found on the skin, since they only feed there, but are present on the hairs or clothing where they reside. A generalized eruption of excoriated papules is present in scabies, but the mite will be found only in burrows in the outer horny layer of the interdigital spaces, flexor surfaces of the wrists, axillary folds, buttocks, areola, and penis.

Pruritus is a common symptom in superficial fungus and yeast infections. Superficial candidiasis is extremely pruritic when it involves the intertriginous areas of the axillae, anogenital, and inframammary regions. The lesions of cutaneous moniliasis are sharply limited, macerated, red patches surrounded by loose epithelial fringes and satellite pustules. Tinea cruris and corporis (ringworm of the groin and body) cause itchy annular lesions with advancing raised scaling or vesicular borders. Potassium hydroxide–treated smears of the scales in moni-

liasis contain budding yeasts, and in tinea they reveal fragile hyphae.

URICARIA. The pathophysiology of the urticarial reaction is based on the liberation of histamine from mast cells around dermal blood vessels. The liberated histamine increases vascular permeability, and the accumulation of the transudate in the dermis causes visibly raised wheals, "hives." Sufficiently large accumulations compress the subepidermal vascular plexus resulting in a pale or blanched appearance of the wheal. A zone of reflex vasodilation creates an erythematous flare around the wheal. Wheals are transient; each lesion disappears within hours, though new lesions may continue to appear. All of these effects can be induced by injections of histamine intradermally. Amounts of histamine sufficient to cause wheals and flares also cause itching.

The stimuli which result in the release of histamine from mast cells are varied. In clinical medicine the important histamine-releasing stimuli are those which cause physical urticaria and allergic urticaria of the acute and chronic type. Physical stimuli, such as heat, cold, sunlight, and pressure, are causes of urticaria, and this can be confirmed by the reproduction of the lesion with appropriate applications of the stimulus to the skin. Certain drugs, such as morphine and codeine, cause histamine release and urticaria by their direct action on mast cells. Immediate types of allergic reactions are mediated by circulating antibodies which act indirectly through the activation of proteases and esterases to cause histamine release from mast cells. In general, the antigens responsible for these immediate allergic urticarial reactions reach the skin via the systemic circulation after they have been ingested or injected. Food and drug allergies are the commonest causes of acute urticaria. The detection of the underlying factors in chronic recurrent urticaria requires a thorough investigation of drug ingestion, physical factors, infections, parasites, ingested and inhaled allergens, and emotional factors.

ECZEMATOUS DERMATITIS. Itching is the predominant symptom of dermatitis. The hallmarks of acute dermatitis are erythema, vesicles, oozing, and crusting. Scaling and thickening of the skin develop as the dermatitis becomes subacute and chronic. Accentuation of the normal surface markings gives the skin a thick leathery appearance, which is referred to as *lichenification*. The basic histologic change in dermatitis is the accumulation of fluid between the cells of the epidermis. As the amount of fluid increases, disruption of the connections between epidermal cells occurs, and microscopic and macroscopic vesicles and bullae form. The reparative phases, subacute and chronic dermatitis, are marked by an accelerated rate of epidermal cell division and delayed cellular maturation. The number of cell layers in the epidermis increases, resulting in thickening. An imperfect keratin layer forms, and scaling results.

Several types of injury may initiate dermatitis. Physical injury, such as extremes of temperature, radiation, and mechanical trauma, may cause dermatitis. Chemicals, namely acids, alkalis, soaps, and detergents, damage the epidermis and cause dermatitis by their direct primary irritant action. These irritants are responsible for the common hand eczemas of housewives. Allergic mechanisms of the delayed type cause allergic contact dermatitis. Simple chemicals become complete antigens after conjugation with proteins in the skin. Once antibodies have been formed to the protein-chemical conjugate, the skin will react in an eczematous pattern on each subsequent contact between the skin and the chemical. The allergic eczematous reactions are of the delayed type, and 24 or more hours may elapse before detectable changes and itching appear. Contact allergic dermatitis is exemplified by poison ivy dermatitis. Simple chemicals, such as mercury, chrome, and nickel, are common contact antigens responsible for metal (jewelry, garters), leather, and cement dermatitis. More complicated chemicals, such as those in dyes, adhesives, and resins, are important antigens in occupational contact allergic dermatitis (See Chaps. 116 and 117). The most insidious type of contact dermatitis, that caused by antigenic constituents in topical medications, is commonly responsible for prolonging or aggravating dermatitis.

The same factors that initiate dermatitis will aggravate and prolong it. Mechanical damage caused by rubbing and scratching is an important factor. Primary irritation caused by excessive use of soap and water prolongs dermatitis. Excessive dehydration, brittleness, and chapping of the skin are aggravated by overbathing, which further decreases the skin's tolerance to primary irritants. Dryness of the skin aggravated by overbathing is an important factor in the winter, or senile, dermatitis which occurs on the extremities. Stasis in the venous system predisposes to dermatitis of the lower extremities and prolongs any dermatitis in these areas. Sweating tends to aggravate dermatitis, since sweating in the occluded sweat ducts in an area of dermatitis leads to rupture of the ducts and release of irritating sweat into the skin. Vigorous exercise and hot, humid atmospheres will aggravate dermatitis by superimposing *miliaria* ("prickly heat") on the involved areas.

Hereditary or constitutional factors predispose to a common clinical type of dermatitis. *Atopic dermatitis* is an eczematous dermatitis which occurs in individuals who have an inherited tendency to develop asthma and hay fever. The development of atopic dermatitis in these persons is a function of dry, sensitive, itchy skin and does not usually correlate with episodes of allergic rhinitis or asthma. In infants atopic dermatitis is characterized by vesicular crusted eczematous patches on the cheeks and extensor aspects of the extremities. The character and distribution of the eruption change with age. In atopic dermatitis of juveniles and adults the main areas of involvement are thickened, lichenified excoriated plaques of the antecubital and popliteal fossae, face, and neck. At all ages and in all stages atopic dermatitis is an exceedingly itchy eruption, and the patient must be protected from all of the factors which initiate or aggravate pruritus.

Persistent localized patches of chronic dermatitis are prone to develop in patients in whom the itch-scratch cycle has become firmly established. The lichenified

patches of *lichen simplex chronicus* are usually single or few in number. They are usually located in areas which the patient can conveniently reach for scratching purposes, namely, the ankles, calves, occiput, vulva, and perianal regions. Underlying factors responsible for initiating or prolonging the itch-scratch cycle should be investigated. Anal and vulvar pruritus may be initiated by seborrheic dermatitis, psoriasis, pinworm infections, moniliasis, reactions to oral antibiotics, diabetes mellitus, and contact dermatitis. Stasis factors, constricting clothing, and superimposed contact dermatitis from topical medications, prolong the itch-scratch cycle.

TREATMENT. Since itching is a symptom, the most effective approach is to detect and eliminate the cause. Removal of the offending parasite, drug, irritant, or antigen in dermatitis or urticaria and institution of appropriate treatment of the underlying systemic disease in cases of generalized pruritus are basic approaches. Ancillary and symptomatic care is directed toward the protection of the skin from all the factors which are known to aggravate and prolong dermatitis. Antihistamines and salicylates are useful oral medications for pruritus. It is inadvisable, however, to prescribe corticosteroids in the absence of a specific diagnosis.

Specific treatment in patients with generalized pruritus is dependent on treating the underlying systemic disease, such as obstructive jaundice, renal failure, diabetes, lymphomas, and malignancies. Such specific approaches offer the only chance for relief of pruritus in these disorders. Cholestyramine therapy, in oral doses of 10 g daily, is helpful in reducing the pruritus accompanying the jaundice of hepatic diseases which are not amenable to surgical relief of the obstruction (Chap. 45).

One application of a thin layer of 1 percent gamma benzene hydrochloride (Kwell) lotion or cream left on the entire skin surface for 24 hr is effective treatment for pediculosis and scabies. Tolnaftate (Tinactin) solution or undecylenic acid (Desenex) ointment applied twice daily to the affected areas is the treatment of choice in tinea pedis, cruris, and corporis. Griseofulvin, the systemic fungistatic agent, is reserved for the treatment of tinea capitis, resistant tinea corporis, and onychomycosis. The average dose of griseofulvin for adults is 1.0 Gm p.o. daily. Better absorption is obtained if the drug is taken at the end of a fatty meal or in the micronized form. Griseofulvin is fungistatic, not fungicidal, and is concentrated in keratin structures such as the hair, nails, and stratum corneum as they are formed. The antibiotic must be taken until the old infected keratin structures are shed and replaced by new keratin containing the drug. Griseofulvin is effective against dermatophytic fungi, but it is not effective against *C. albicans* and the organisms causing tinea versicolor, erythrasma, and the deep mycoses. Nystatin is an effective topical antimonilial agent. It is not absorbed from the gastrointestinal tract and must be applied locally as a lotion, cream, or powder.

Oral antihistamines are effective antipruritic agents and are the mainstay of the symptomatic treatment of urticaria. The specific treatment of the patient with urticaria depends on determining and eliminating the cause, whether it be a drug, food, physical factor, or infection. The most popular antihistamines are diphenhydramine (Benadryl) 50 mg t. i. d., dexachlorpheniramine (Polaramine), 2 mgm t. i. d., and cyproheptadine (Periactin), 4 mg q. i. d. Large doses, up to 600 mg Benadryl daily, are required to suppress severe urticarial drug reactions. Antihistamines may cause drug eruptions when they are administered parenterally. Since they are potent topical sensitizers, they should never be applied to the skin.

Eczematous reactions of the contact type respond to elimination of the offending antigen or irritant. The patient must permanently avoid contact with the antigen in order to remain free of the disease. Patch testing is a valuable investigative procedure in determining the offending antigens in the allergic type of contact dermatitis (Chap. 55).

The therapeutic program for all types of eczematous dermatitis includes symptomatic treatment of pruritus and discomfort and protection of the skin from all factors that aggravate or prolong dermatitis. Oral antihistamines relieve pruritus and prevent aggravation from scratching. Tepid tap water and open compresses relieve oozing, crusting, and vasodilation during the acute vesicular phases of dermatitis. Corticosteroid (0.5 percent hydrocortisone, 0.01 percent fluocinolone acetonide, or 0.025 percent triameinolone acetonide) lotions, creams, and ointments are potent antipruritics when they are applied as a thin layer q. i. d. to the affected areas in the subacute and chronic stages of dermatitis. Avoiding or limiting exposure to bathing and soap prevents aggravation of the dermatitis from excessive dehydration and primary irritation. The addition of bath oils to baths minimizes prolongation of chronic dermatitis. Bed rest and elevation of the legs relieve stasis factors in dermatitis of the lower legs. A uniform environmental temperature, loose clothing, and restriction of physical exercise prevents aggravation of dermatitis from overheating and sweating. The use of compounds which are known potent contact antigens, such as topical anesthetics, topical antihistamines, and certain topical antibiotics, should be minimized.

57   ALOPECIA AND HIRSUTISM
Faye D. Arundell and Eugene M. Farber

The cosmetic and psychologic significance of hair has increased as the biologic need for the protection from cold and trauma that hair provides has decreased. In Western societies, too much facial hair in women, too little scalp hair in men and women, and too much curl in the hair of Negroes are common endocrine and cosmetic concerns. The standards set by society outweigh those that are the physiologic norms determined by genetic and racial factors.

Genetic factors play an important role in determining the quantity, quality, and distribution of hair growth. The diameters of hairs from various body regions are the same in Caucasians and Japanese, but Orientals have scantier growth of beard, axillary, and pubic hair. The incidence of male baldness and female hirsutism is much lower in Japanese. This racial difference in hair growth may be attributable to a decreased sensitivity of the hair follicles to androgens, since there is no difference in the levels of plasma testosterone in Japanese and Caucasians. The ethnic differences in hair growth are striking in Caucasian women. The amount of facial hair and general hair growth which is normal for many women of Mediterranean stock would be grossly abnormal for most Nordics.

Hairs are cylindrical shafts composed of tightly fused hard keratin. The latter is a dead fibrous protein manufactured deep in the dermis. No trauma or treatment applied only to the dead hair can affect the vital proliferating hair follicle. Brushing, combing, shaving, cutting, bleaching, coloring, curling, or straightening may give psychologic and esthetic satisfaction to the individual, but none of these either stimulates or depresses hair growth. The epidermis cannot form new hair follicles after birth.

Hair follicles and sebaceous glands develop from the epidermis as a pilosebaceous unit in the third fetal month. Pilosebaceous units develop in all areas of the skin except the palms and soles. In some areas, such as the axillae and anogenital region, apocrine glands develop in association with the pilosebaceous unit.

The lower end of the hair follicle is expanded into the hair bulb, which lies deep in the dermis. An invagination in the base of the bulb contains a capillary loop in a connective tissue papilla. The papilla is an intrinsic part of the hair follicle that persists through all phases of the hair cycle. A viable dermal papilla is essential for growth of the hair. Melanocytes which furnish pigment for the growing hair are located over the dermal papilla in the bulb. The bulb contains the mitotically active cells of the hair matrix that form the hair. The rapid growth of the matrix pushes toward the surface the differentiating keratinizing cells which make up the hair.

The rate of cellular reproduction in the hair matrix is among the fastest in the body and is equaled only by that of the bone marrow. As many as 30 percent of the cells in the matrix may be in mitosis at any given time. Each scalp terminal hair follicle produces 0.35 mm hair per day. The total production of hair proteins by the approximately 100,000 scalp follicles per day is a phenomenal metabolic task. Metabolic activity of this degree is susceptible to many systemic stresses. Interference with the mitotic activity in the matrix is immediately reflected in disturbances in hair production. Radiation therapy, radiomimetic drugs, antimetabolites, and toxic chemicals, such as thallium, interfere with the cellular reproduction of the hair follicle. Transient interference with protein synthesis results in deformities of the hair shaft, while more prolonged interference causes complete inhibition of hair growth and loss of hair. Increased hair growth occurs with stimuli which increase the temperature or blood flow in the skin. Hair grows faster in summer, in constantly traumatized areas, in skin adjacent to healing bone fractures, and in sympathectomized skin.

Humans have three types of hair: lanugo, vellus, and terminal. *Lanugo* is the prenatal soft, silky, unmedullated, and usually unpigmented hair which normally is replaced by vellus and terminal hairs. In postnatal life, fine, pale, short vellus hairs cover the whole surface of the body except the palms and soles. *Vellus* hairs are almost imperceptible but they persist even in bald scalps, and they are the only hairs present on the glabrous skin. Tactile nerve endings are intimately associated with vellus hair follicles. Specialized tactile sensory end organs are present in the nonhairy areas of the palms, soles, and lips.

Terminal hairs are the coarse, dark, long hairs which develop only in certain areas, such as the scalp, beard, and axillae. The differences in terminal hairs of various regions depend on the growth rate, length of the hair cycle, and physiologic responsiveness. Terminal hairs can be classified into six regional types: (1) scalp, (2) eyebrow and eyelash, (3) beard, (4) axillary, (5) pubic, (6) body. The hairs which make up the secondary sexual characteristics, namely, the beard, axillary, pubic, and body hair, are controlled by androgens in both males and females. The other regional types of hair require no sexual hormone stimulus, although they may be modified by androgens. Androgenic stimulation in genetically predisposed men results in male-pattern baldness. Men who have been castrated before puberty never develop axillary, beard, or pubic hair, and never become bald. Replacement hormonal therapy in eunuchs results in the normal hair growth which comprises secondary sexual characteristics and may result in baldness in the genetically susceptible.

Human hair follicles do not produce hair indefinitely. Each hair follicle's active production of hair is independent of that in neighboring follicles. The activity of each individual follicle is cyclic (Fig. 57-1). A period of mitotic activity and production of hair is followed by a period of involution and rest. The hair in the resting follicle develops a bulbous nonpigmented root, or club, by which it remains attached in the follicle. The resting phase is termed the *telogen* phase and its hair, the club hair. When the follicle becomes active once more, that is, when the *anagen* phase begins, the old club hair is pushed out of the follicle by the newly developing hair beneath it. A certain number of club hairs are shed each day. Approximately 5 to 10 percent of scalp hairs are in the resting phase at any one time, and 20 to 100 club hairs are shed daily. Under normal physiologic circumstances the total population of hair remains constant, since no club hair is shed unless an actively growing hair expels it.

The final length of hair depends on the duration of the growth phase of the cycle in the follicle producing the hair. Follicles in different body regions have active and resting phases of varying lengths. The resting phase of scalp hair must last only a few months, since only 5 to 10 percent of scalp hairs are in the resting phase at any one time. The duration of the growth cycle of hairs on the rest of the body is shorter, probably only 2 to 6 months, and the resting phase of the cycle is of equal duration.

Stimuli which affect the duration of the active part of the hair cycle will obviously have a profound effect on the length of the hair produced and the relative proportions of active and club hairs. A change in the normal proportion of 90 to 95 percent growing hairs and 5 to 10 per-

Fig. 57-1. Stages in hair cycle. Progressive changes from a growing (anagen) hair to a resting club hair (telogen)—second from right. In the normal human scalp, some 10 percent of the hairs are in the resting phase. In various types of alopecia, this percentage rises sharply and may be easily determined by the number of hairs which are easily removed by gentle traction. (D. M. Pillsbury and W. B. Shelley)

cent resting hairs on the scalp indicates a change in the cycle of hair growth. If the growth period in many follicles is shortened simultaneously, an increased number of club hairs is formed, resulting in a sudden noticeable increase in the hairs shed daily in the succeeding months. Synchronized onset of the resting phase causes the physiologic alopecia seen in newborns and post-partum women. Severe febrile diseases, emotional shock, and debilitating diseases cause a similar synchronized resting phase and hair loss.

ALOPECIA

The psychologic trauma caused by too little hair may be greater than that caused by too much hair. Loss of hair may be the result of physiologic factors or it may be secondary to endocrinologic abnormalities, systemic diseases, cutaneous diseases, infections of the hairs and hair follicles, or physical or chemical trauma.

MALE-PATTERN BALDNESS. A gradual decrease of scalp hair accompanies aging in the human. Male-pattern baldness is inevitable in the presence of androgenic stimuli in men with a genetic predisposition to baldness. The age of onset and the amount of hair lost in men depends on genetic factors. When baldness begins in the late teens, the prognosis is for a significant baldness in the thirties. Some loss over the frontal regions, forming an M-shaped hairline occurs in most men. The loss may progress relentlessly to the parietal regions and vertex, but a marginal fringe of hair in the temporal and occipital regions persists. There is no topical or systemic therapy that will alter the inevitable course of male-pattern baldness. However, the hair follicles from the occipital area maintain their resistance to male-pattern baldness when transplanted into bald areas of the vertex. The success of hair transplants depends on the unique indifference or resistance of the occipital hair follicles. Female-pattern hair loss occurs in the frontal and parietal regions, but it rarely progresses to baldness. Genetic factors may be important in this type of hair loss, which usually begins in middle age. Any decrease of a woman's "crowning glory" may be a threat to her femininity resulting in concern and complaints out of proportion to the actual amount of hair lost.

NEONATAL HAIR LOSS. A marked shedding of scalp hair occurs in neonatal infants. Regrowth promptly begins, and within a few months the scalp is again covered with its normal complement of hairs.

POST-PARTUM HAIR LOSS. An increased proportion of club hairs and hair loss is a normal post-partum physiologic event. The prolonged growth phase resulting from hormonal stimulation during pregnancy ends after delivery, and a synchronized onset of the resting phase occurs in the scalp hair follicles. All women shed some hair in the post-partum period, but in some women the hair loss is pronounced. The prognosis for complete regrowth is good.

ENDOCRINE DISTURBANCES. The effect of individual hormones on the hair growth of various laboratory animals has been the subject of many investigations. In animals growth hormone appears to be responsible for the

increase in hair-shaft diameter, and luteotropin governs the change from infantile to adult pelage. Thyroxine in some species increases both the rate of hair growth and the proportion of hairs in the growing phase of the hair growth cycle. Adrenalectomy also increases the proportion of actively growing hairs, while oophorectomy accelerates the shedding of hairs.

In some types of human hair loss accompanying endocrinologic disturbances, the causes can be deduced from knowledge of the experimental effects of hormones in laboratory animals. However, there are many instances of hair loss associated with endocrine diseases which are unexplained in humans and for which no animal models exist. The hair loss and scanty hair growth in hypopituitarism are compatible with the failure of development or maintenance of adult hair growth in the presence of growth hormone deficiency. The hypopituitary dwarf may be completely hairless, and patients with acquired hypopituitary states and Sheehan's syndrome rapidly lose hair from the axillae, pubis, and at times, the scalp. The importance of the role of growth hormone in human hair growth is confirmed by the increased hair growth and coarse hair of acromegaly.

In congenital cretinism lanugo hair may be retained, and the scalp hair is sparse and dry. In adults, hypothyroidism causes a decrease in the secondary sexual or hormonal hair of the axillae, pubis, and beard, in addition to the characteristic loss of the lateral aspects of the eyebrows. These effects can be related to the retardation of the onset of the growing phase of the hair cycle which follows thyroidectomy in animals. The reason for the growth of long hair on the back, shoulders, arms, and legs of children with hypothyroidism is obscure, as is the hair loss of hyperthyroidism.

Abnormalities of the adrenal glands and ovaries usually are associated with changes in hair growth related to androgenic effects. In Addison's disease in women, the deficiency of adrenal androgens is responsible for the loss of sexual, or hormonal, hair of the axillae and pubis. Increased androgen production in women causes the loss of scalp hair in the pattern of male baldness and produces the increase of facial and body hair which accompanies adrenal hyperplasia and virilizing adrenal and ovarian tumors. The loss of scalp hair in a male pattern and the increased body and facial hair growth of Cushing's syndrome and exogenous ACTH administration probably are caused by increased production of adrenal androgens. The reason for the scalp hair loss and hirsutism of the face and body which occur with exogenous testosterone therapy is obvious, but the cause of the same pattern of abnormal hair growth associated with exogenous corticosteroid therapy is unexplained.

SYSTEMIC DISEASES. Prolonged febrile illnesses, systemic lupus erythematosus (LE), dermatomyositis, severe cachexia, and lymphomas are associated with hair loss. The transient hair loss after high fevers begins within 3 months of the acute illness and is followed by complete regrowth. This type of hair loss was seen more frequently in the preantibiotic era. The alopecia of systemic LE and dermatomyositis may be postfebrile and transient or permanent and associated with cutaneous involvement of the scalp by the disease. A patchy type of moth-eaten alopecia is an uncommon manifestation of secondary syphilis. Permanent hair loss on the extensor surfaces of the fingers is an early sign in systemic scleroderma. Occlusive peripheral vascular diseases are associated with loss of hair from the toes and feet.

PHYSICAL AND CHEMICAL AGENTS. Minor trauma may cause transient alopecia, but any physical damage which is severe enough to destroy the full thickness of the dermis also destroys hair follicles and results in permanent alopecia. The constant traction of certain hair styles causes a marginal alopecia of the frontal and temporal regions. Marginal alopecia occurs in girls and women who constantly wear their hair in braids or "ponytails." A change to a looser hair arrangement usually cures the alopecia. Third degree burns, whether from heat or chemical cauterants, results in permanent alopecia. Ionizing radiation in large doses (1,500r or more) causes permanent hair loss. Fractionated doses of x-rays in lower total doses (400r) result in temporary nonscarring alopecia. Radiomimetic drugs (such as nitrogen mustard), antimetabolites, thallium, heparin, coumarin, and excessive doses of vitamin A produce transient hair loss (Plate 1-2).

CUTANEOUS INFECTIONS. Superficial ringworm infections of the scalp cause patchy alopecia during the stage of active infection but rarely result in scarring and permanent alopecia. Deep pyogenic infections, namely boils and carbuncles, may cause permanent scarred alopecia, but folliculitis rarely does. Leprosy, cutaneous leishmaniasis, severe herpes zoster, and syphilitic gummas are associated with permanent hair loss in the affected area.

CUTANEOUS DISEASES. The permanent alopecia which occurs in lesions of discoid LE (Plate 1-5) localized scleroderma, and sarcoid is only apparent and important when the lesions involve the scalp and eyebrows. Scarring alopecia occurs in the rare dermatologic diseases *lichen planopilaris* and *pseudopelade*. Infants with congenital ectodermal defects characteristically have scanty scalp hair or areas of permanent alopecia. The scalp over nevi, tumors, and cysts may become bald.

TRICHOTILLOMANIA. Compulsive plucking of hairs from the scalp is a habit tic akin to nail-biting. Although the plucked areas may be large, they are never completely bald but contain a stubble of regrowing hairs of varying lengths as yet too short to be pulled.

ALOPECIA AREATA. Alopecia areata is characterized by the sudden development of single or multiple round bald patches of the scalp. The completely bald areas are slightly depressed, but no erythema or gross inflammatory changes are detectable. The patches may enlarge peripherally, and new areas may develop on the scalp, eyebrows, or beard region. Universal loss of all of the scalp and body hair sometimes occurs. The loss of the eyelashes, with the resultant loss of their sun-shading and dust-filtering actions is the only functional problem associated with alopecia areata. The general health is not affected, but the emotional stress caused by the cosmetic defect can be serious.

Although signs of inflammation in the areas of alopecia are grossly lacking, histologic examination reveals an infiltration of inflammatory cells in the papillae of the hair follicles. The cause of alopecia areata is unknown. A family history of the disease is not uncommon. Sudden emotional stress has been reported to precede some cases of alopecia areata, but it is certainly not a common finding. Nail changes, ranging from pitting to complete shedding, may occur. The severity of the nail changes roughly parallels the extent of the disease. The prognosis for spontaneous regrowth is good if the disease begins in adult life and involves only a few areas. If the disease begins in childhood or involves several areas or the whole body, the prognosis for regrowth is poor. Topical applications of corticosteroid creams covered by occlusive plastic dressings and intradermal injections of triamcinolone acetonide into the lesions may stimulate regrowth. Systemic corticosteroid therapy is not justified, since any results are usually transient. Massage, heat, ultraviolet light therapy, dessicated thyroid, and applications of irritants are of no value in the treatment of alopecia areata.

HIRSUTISM

The quantity and distribution of hair is dependent on genetic, racial, and hormonal factors, but the desirable amount of hair depends on cultural factors. The American culture views any hair on women other than on the scalp and pubis as cosmetically undesirable or unfeminine. Hair on the legs and axillae is removed as a matter of course by shaving or chemical depilatories. Hair on the face, breasts, and abdomen represents a threat to the American female's sexual identity for which cosmetic and medical help is commonly sought. Recognition of the psychologic problems created by hirsutism is an essential part of the management of these patients. Sympathetic explanations, reassurance, and cosmetic advice should be given by the physician to the woman whose hirsutism does not have a detectable and correctable endocrinologic basis.

The number of hair follicles in each anatomic region is the same in hirsute women, "normal" women, and men. The complaint of the woman who seeks medical help for hirsutism concerns the development of terminal hairs in regions where only lanugo hairs are usually present. The upper lip, chin, cheeks, chest, and abdomen, that is, the "hormonal" areas of hair growth, are those most commonly involved. Most hirsute women also have increased hair growth on the arms and anterior thighs and increased coarseness of hair. Androgens are known to increase the coarseness of hair and to stimulate the growth of terminal hairs in hormonal areas. A noticeable androgenic effect on hair can occur under three circumstances: (1) an increase in total androgen production, (2) an unusual sensitivity of the target organ (hair follicles) to normal amounts of androgen, (3) a relative preponderance of androgenic effects resulting from a decrease in estrogen. An increase in total androgens is present in virilizing syndromes of adrenal or ovarian origin. End organ insensitivity probably accounts for the decreased hair growth in the Japanese. Conversely, end organ hypersensitivity may account for the so-called "idiopathic" hirsutism of certain Caucasians, such as those of Mediterranean stock. Changes in androgen-estrogen balance may be responsible for the increased growth of facial hair and decrease in scalp hair in postmenopausal women. Hirsutism, once it is established, is relatively refractory to hormonal influences. A castrated man does not rapidly lose an established beard. The removal of a virilizing tumor in a woman stops the further progress of hirsutism but does not result immediately in a noticeable decrease in the established hirsutism.

A complete history and thorough physical examination are prerequisites to the correct diagnosis of the hirsute woman. A careful history of racial origins and family tendency to increased hair growth is important. Familial or genetic hirsutism occurs in 10 percent of Caucasian women. Some facial, abdominal, and chest hair is normal for many women of Mediterranean stock. A heavy growth of scalp hair, coarse hair, a low frontal hairline, and thick eyebrows are common in ethnic hirsutism. Familial hirsutism of this type begins at the menarche and continues to increase into the twenties.

Direct questioning is usually necessary in order to obtain evidence of excess androgen effect on other organs. A change in the voice, increased muscle mass and strength, decrease in breast size, increase in libido, and enlargement of the clitoris are indications of androgen excess. A detailed menstrual history is essential. Delayed onset of menarche, irregular or scanty periods, dysmenorrhea, infertility, or difficulty in conceiving or carrying to.

Table 57-1. CAUSES OF HIRSUTISM

I. Localized
   A. Congenital
      1. Hairy nevi
      2. Satyr's tail of spina bifida
      3. Congenital erythropoietic porphyria
   B. Acquired
      1. Occupational—sack carriers
      2. Porphyria cutanea tarda
II. Generalized
   A. Racial, idiopathic, familial
   B. Iatrogenic
      1. Testosterone
      2. ACTH
      3. Corticosteroids
   C. Adrenal Origin
      1. Congenital adrenal hyperplasia
      2. Delayed onset of congenital adrenal hyperplasia
      3. Borderline adrenal dysfunction
      4. Cushing's syndrome
      5. Virilizing adrenal tumors
   D. Ovarian
      1. Virilizing ovarian tumors
         a. Arrhenoblastoma
         b. Adrenal rest tumor
         c. Gynandroblastoma
         d. Hilus or Leydig cell tumor
      2. Polycystic ovary (Stein-Leventhal) syndrome

term may indicate excessive androgen production by the ovary or adrenals.

When an earlier photograph of the patient is available, it is often useful to compare it with the present appearance of the patient. A complete physical examination is in order in all women complaining of hirsutism whether or not ethnic factors are playing a role. The examination should be directed towards determining the degree of hirsutism and detecting signs of virilization or other adrenal or ovarian diseases (Table 57-1). It is not unusual for the hirsute woman to carefully remove excess hair from face before presenting herself for consultation. A cursory inspection of the face and trunk may result in overlooking obvious signs of virilism. The physical manifestations of androgen excess include a husky voice, male body habitus with broad shoulders and slim hips, coarse oily skin, acne, male-pattern baldness of the scalp, enlargement of the thyroid cartilage, hair growth on the chest, atrophy of breasts, male-pattern pubic hair growth, excess hair on the thighs, and enlargement of the clitoris. Palpable enlargement of the ovaries is a sign of polycystic ovaries (Stein-Leventhal syndrome, Chap. 98) or ovarian neoplasms. A plethoric complexion, acne, moon face, central obesity, etc. accompany the hirsutism of Cushing's syndrome (Chap. 92).

Any of these physical findings accompanying hirsutism of even mild degree or even in ethnically predisposed women demands further studies for laboratory evidence of androgen excess. Measurement of total urinary 17-ketosteroids, despite limitations, is a valuable screening test. The delineation of the underlying endocrinologic lesion may require extensive investigation of the physiologic relationships of the pituitary-adrenal-ovarian axis (Chap. 90) with alternate stimulation and suppression of these glands with ACTH, corticosteroids, and human chorionic gonadotrophin.

The problem of excess hair persists even after successful surgical or medical management of the endocrinologic lesion. Hirsutism secondary to the administration of ACTH, corticosteroids, or testosterone may persist for long periods after the medications have been discontinued. Since the expectation is for the hirsuitism present to remain unchanged, explanation and cosmetic advice must be supplied to the patient. Most women have an aversion to shaving the face, although they regularly shave their legs and axillae. Other means of removing or minimizing the excess hair should be discussed. Many excellent bleaches and depilatories, which can be used safely at intervals on the face and are more acceptable to the patient, are available. Electrolysis is the only method of permanently removing excess hairs. In the hands of expert technicians the results of electrolysis are excellent, although the procedure is time-consuming and expensive.

Localized Hirsutism. Localized hirsutism may be congenital or acquired. Congenital localized hirsutism is usually associated with pigmented nevi, which may disfigure large areas of the body. A localized patch of hairs, *Satyr's tail,* may occur in association with spina bifida.

Repeated prolonged trauma to an area may stimulate localized hair growth. This type of hirsutism occurs on the forearms of mentally defective patients who repeatedly bite the affected area, and on the shoulders of men whose occupation entails carrying heavy sacks or other burdens. The hirsutism which develops on exposed areas in porphyria cutanea tarda and erythropoietic porphyria may be related to prolonged trauma from exposure to ultraviolet light.

REFERENCES

Montagna, W. (Ed.): "Aging," New York, Pergamon Press, 1965.

Rogers, G. E.: Structural and Biochemical Features of the Hair Follicle, pp. 179–232 in "The Epidermis," W. Montagna, and W. C. Lobitz, Jr. (Eds.), New York, Pergamon Press, 1964.

Rook, A.: Endocrine Influences on Hair Growth, Brit. Med. J. (Lancet), 1:609, 1965.

Segro, E. J.: Androgens, Virilization and the Hirsute Female, Springfield, Ill., Charles C Thomas, Publisher, 1967.

58 PIGMENTATION
Faye D. Arundell and Eugene M. Farber

The color of normal skin depends primarily on its content of melanin, carotene, and blood. Pathologic changes in skin color result from the deposition of endogenous or exogenous pigmented compounds, such as bile pigments, hemosiderin, homogentisic acid, heavy metals, and tattoo pigments.

MELANIN

The biochemistry of melanin formation, the known mechanisms which influence its synthesis, and the various syndromes associated with decreased or increased amounts of melanin in the skin are discussed in detail in Chap. 109. A normal complement of melanin is the skin's prime protective mechanism against ultraviolet light radiation. Deficiency of melanin, either congenital or acquired, is associated with an increased incidence of photosensitivity and of skin cancer. Inability to form sufficient amounts of melanin in large areas of the skin prevents individuals with albinism and vitiligo from engaging in normal outdoor occupations and activities. The unpigmented patches of vitiligo in the deeply pigmented Africans and Asians are regarded as cosmetic defects and may be social stigmata as well. Excess melanin production associated with systemic diseases, such as Addison's disease and hemachromatosis, is more pronounced in areas of skin which are exposed to sunlight. Long-term treatment of chronic granulocytic leukemia with dimethanesulfonoxybutane (Myleran) causes diffuse hyperpigmentation in some patients.

Genetic factors are of great importance in controlling the function of the melanocytes. The number of melanocytes in the skin is the same in Caucasians and Negroes. Variations in skin color are due to genetically determined differences in the rate at which melanin granules are produced by the melanocytes and transferred to the surrounding epidermal cells. Reflectance spectrophotometry, which gives a quantitative description of skin color, is used in anthropologic studies of melanin pigmentation. The hue of normal skin, which varies from pale tan to black, is a combination of the amounts of melanin in the melanocytes, basal cells, Malpighian cells, and stratum corneum of the epidermis. A normal number of melanocytes is present in albino skin, but the melanocytes do not make pigment because of an inborn error of metabolism (Chap. 101).

Genetic factors also influence the response of melanocytes to a variety of stresses, including local trauma and hormonal, metabolic, and other systemic disturbances. With aging, a varying proportion of melanocytes in hair follicles lose their ability to form melanin. Premature graying of hair is often a familial characteristic. In normal skin an increase in pigmentation occurs after exposure to solar radiation. Individual variations in the amount of tanning developing after sun exposure are influenced by genetic factors. Dark-skinned individuals have very responsive melanocytes. They tan readily and well and have an increased tolerance to sunburn and an increased tendency to develop postinflammatory pigmentary changes in areas of trauma or dermatitis. The incidence of chloasma during oral contraceptive therapy and pregnancy is higher in dark-skinned women.

Unusual ashy, blue-black colors are produced by the presence of melanin outside the epidermis in the deeper layers of the skin. Because of the Tyndall light-scattering phenomenon, these melanin deposits create a gray to blue color in the overlying skin. Mongolian spots and blue nevi owe their unusual blue-black color to the presence of melanin-containing melanocytes in the dermis. Epidermal melanin granules which have been lost into the dermis secondary to epidermal damage may be held within dermal macrophages for prolonged periods of time. This phagocytized melanin gives the previously affected areas of skin a dark brown or ashy color.

PHENOTHIAZINE PIGMENTATION. A peculiar type of bluish-brown hyperpigmentation occurs in a small percentage of patients on long-term, high dosage chlorpromazine therapy. Most cases have occurred in female schizophrenics in mental institutions. The pigmentation occurs only after continuous large doses of 400 to 1,500 mg daily for 2 to 10 years. The pigmentation is blue-gray, violet, or brown and appears on the exposed areas of the face, neck, arms, and hands. Phenothiazines are photosensitizing drugs that bind to melanin in vitro. Drug-induced enhanced reaction to sunlight plays a significant role in the development of phenothiazine pigmentation. The pigment is present as brown granules, both free and within macrophages in the dermis. Melanin pigment is increased in the epidermis, and the dermal pigment is believed to be melanin or a complex of melanin and phenothiazine.

The cutaneous hyperpigmentation caused by phenothiazine drugs may be accompanied by fine stippling of the cornea and anterior capsule of the lens. The eye changes occur equally in males and females who have received large doses of chlorpromazine for prolonged periods of time. The stippling of the cornea and lens, which is visible on slit-lamp examination, and brown discoloration of light-exposed areas of the conjunctiva can occur without the skin pigmentation. Significant visual impairment rarely occurs in patients with phenothiazine eye changes. The skin and eye changes seem to be slowly reversible after the drug is withdrawn.

VARIOUS HEMOGLOBINS. The normal pink shade of skin is attributable to the amount and state of oxygenation of the blood in the skin. The red tint of oxyhemoglobin may be completely masked or almost indiscernible in dark brown or black skins. Cyanosis is due to the presence of reduced hemoglobin in the dermal blood vessels (Chap. 33). Abnormal hemoglobins produce diagnostic changes in the color of skin. Carboxyhemoglobin from carbon monoxide forms a cherry red color. Methemoglobin and sulfhemoglobin, which occur with the ingestion of sulfonamides, sulfones, acetanilid, or phenacetin, create various shades of blue that may mimic the cyanosis of cardiac or pulmonary disease. (Chap. 344).

CAROTENE. The normal yellow tint of skin is caused by carotene in the keratin layer of the epidermis and in the subcutaneous fat. Excessive carotene in the skin (Chap. 84) creates a striking yellow or orange color which is particularly noticeable in the heavily keratinized skin of the palms and soles. Sparing of the scleras is helpful in differentiating this condition from jaundice. The amount of carotene in the skin is increased in excessive dietary intake of yellow vegetables and fruits. Carotenemia is seen in infants, in adults on fad diets, male castrates, panhypopituitarism, myxedema, and diabetes.

JAUNDICE. The intensity of the yellow discoloration of the skin and scleras in jaundice is related to the concentration of bile pigments in the blood. The skin color in jaundice may vary from yellow to greenish-brown.

HEMOSIDERIN. Deposits of hemosiderin in the dermis cause relatively permanent pigmentation of the skin. The color changes created by hemosiderin range from copper to dark brown. Special stains for iron and melanin help to differentiate hemosiderin from melanin in skin biopsies (Chap. 109). Generalized hemosiderin deposits and increased melanin pigmentation occur in hemachromatosis. Localized hemosiderin deposits are common in the skin of the lower extremities in individuals with chronic vascular stasis and capillary fragility.

EXOGENOUS PIGMENTATION. The commonest type of exogenous pigmentation of the skin is the tattoo. The chief danger associated with tattooing is the accidental introduction of infections, such as tuberculosis, infectious hepatitis, and more rarely, syphilis and leprosy. The status symbol of the modern tattoo artist is the sterilizer, which is usually prominently displaced in the parlor. Lo-

cal dermatitis, photosensitivity, or granulomas may be caused by mercury or cadmium in the red areas of tattoos.

Diffuse metallic pigmentation from ingestion or local applications to mucosal surfaces of silver salts (argyria) and parenteral gold salts (chrysiasis) is rare today. The slate color of the pigmentation is usually accentuated in light-exposed areas. The metals can be seen in the dermis in microscopic sections of the affected skin.

A striking yellow pigmentation of the skin occurs with ingestion of quinacrine (Atabrine). During World War II, quinacrine was the most common prophylactic drug used in endemic malarial regions. The yellow pigmentation of the skin gradually disappeared within several months after the drug was discontinued. Absorption of dinitrophenol and tetryl by workers in the explosive industry also causes a marked yellow discoloration of the skin.

REFERENCES

Fox, H. M., and G. Vevers: "The Nature of Animal Colors," London, Sidgwick & Jackson, Ltd., 1960.

Greiner, A. C., and K. Berry: Skin Pigmentation and Corneal and Lens Opacities with Prolonged Chloroquine Therapy, Can. Med. Assoc. J., 90:663, 1964.

Montagna, W., and F. Hu: "The Pigmentary System," vol. 8, "Advances in Biology of Skin," New York, Pergamon Press, 1966.

59 SUNLIGHT AND PHOTOSENSITIVITY REACTIONS

Faye D. Arundell and Eugene M. Farber

Solar radiation is responsible for a number of diverse cutaneous disorders. In order for solar radiation to have an effect on the skin, it must fulfill the following criteria: (1) the radiation must reach the skin surface; (2) the radiation must penetrate the skin; (3) the radiation must be absorbed by some component of the skin; (4) the photon energy of the absorbed radiation must be great enough to initiate a photochemical reaction.

Wavelengths of sunlight shorter than 290 mμ do not reach the earth's surface. The solar radiation which reaches the earth's surface is composed of a continuous spectrum of wavelengths ranging from 290 to 1850 mμ. The shorter wavelengths of solar radiation, namely ultraviolet light (290 to 400 mμ), are responsible for cutaneous disorders. The longer visible and infrared wavelengths (400 to 1850 mμ) are rarely of clinical importance.

SUNBURN. The short "sunburn" wavelengths (290 to 320 mμ) penetrate the epidermis and upper corium. The long-wavelength ultraviolet and visible light penetrate deeply into the dermis and, perhaps, into the subcutaneous tissue. The absorption of long-wavelength ultraviolet light results in an immediate but transient pigmentation due to darkening of preformed melanin. The absorption of sufficient quantities of the sunburn wavelengths in the skin causes photochemical reactions which result in delayed erythema followed by persisting pigmentation. Sunburn erythema appears after a latent period of 6 to 8 hr, increases in intensity, and subsides in 72 to 96 hr. The normal sunburn inflammatory reaction varies from mild erythema to severe painful erythema and bullae. The intensity of the sunburn reaction is inversely proportional to the amount of protective melanin in the skin and directly proportional to the duration of exposure of the skin to solar radiation. Postinflammatory reparative processes are marked by thickening of the epidermis and stratum corneum. The delayed but persistent pigmentation caused by the sunburn spectrum of ultraviolet light is the result of new formation of melanin by melanocytes and upward migration of melanin in the epidermal cells. The new pigmentation begins in 2 days following sun exposure, reaches a maximum at 19 days and subsides over the next 9 months.

CHRONIC ACTINIC CHANGES. Prolonged excessive exposure to sunlight causes persistent leathery thickening of the skin. The collagen and elastin of the dermis degenerate, and the epidermis undergoes such changes as atrophy, hypertrophy, hyperkeratosis, and cellular atypism. These deleterious effects of excessive exposure to sunlight have been equated erroneously with aging. Comparison of the exposed skin of farmers, sailors, and sun worshippers with the protected skin of their trunks reveals that the striking changes are related to solar radiation and not to age. In time, premalignant actinic keratoses and carcinomas are induced in the actinically damaged exposed skin. There is a significant increase in the incidence of basal cell carcinomas and squamous cell carcinomas in individuals living in regions where the sun's radiation is intense. The incidence of skin cancers is greater in Texas than in Minnesota, greater in fair-skinned, freckled individuals than in those with dark complexions, and greater in farmers and ranchers than in office workers. Negroes almost never develop chronic actinic degeneration of the skin, actinic keratoses, or actinic skin cancers. Elderly Negroes look younger than their chronologic age, since their deeply pigmented skin does not undergo the same actinic changes which are commonly considered to be signs of aging in Caucasians.

It is obvious that the skin's main protections against solar radiation are hair and melanin. Actinic degeneration and carcinomas do not occur on the scalp which is shaded by hair but do occur in the exposed areas of the scalp of bald men. The tanning of the skin that results from increased melanin formation affords increased protection against solar radiation. Melanin gives protection by absorbing and scattering light. Greatly increased amounts of ultraviolet light are necessary to produce erythema (sunburn) in tanned skin.

PHOTOSENSITIVITY

Abnormal cutaneous reactions to ultraviolet light are referred to as photosensitivity reactions (Table 59-1).

Table 59-1. SKIN DISEASES RELATED TO SUNLIGHT

I. Phototoxic Eruptions
  A. Endogenous
    1. Congenital erythropoietic porphyria (Chap. 108)
    2. Porphyria cutanea tarda (Chap. 108)
    3. Erythropoietic protoporphyria (Chap. 108)
  B. Exogenous
    1. Drugs—furocoumarins, sulfanilamide, sulfonylurea, chlorpromazine, tetracycline
    2. Chemicals—coal tar, perfumes, chlorophylls, eosin and other dyes
II. Photoallergic Eruptions
  A. Endogenous
    1. Solar urticaria (some types)
  B. Exogenous
    1. Drugs—chlorothiazides, phenothiazines, griseofulvin, promethazine, sulfanilamide
    2. Chemicals—halogenated salicylanilides, bisphenol, para-aminobenzoic acid
III. Idiopathic
    1. Polymorphous light eruptions
    2. Solar urticaria (some cases)
IV. Intrinsic Abnormalities of the Skin
  A. Melanin Deficiency
    1. Albinism
    2. Vitiligo
  B. Idiopathic
    1. Xeroderma pigmentosum
    2. Epidermolysis bullosa
V. Dermatoses Precipitated or Aggravated by Light
    1. Herpes simplex
    2. Lupus erythematosus
    3. Dermatomyositis
    4. Pellagra (Chap. 80)
    5. Hartnup's disease (Chap. 101)
    6. "Photosensitive" psoriasis, lichen planus, seborrheic dermatitis, rosacea, pityriasis rubra pilaris, keratosis follicularis
VI. Excessive Sunlight Exposure
  A. Acute
    1. Sunburn
  B. Chronic
    1. Actinic degeneration of the dermis (farmer's and sailor's skin)
    2. Actinic keratoses
    3. Leukoplakia
    4. Squamous cell carcinoma
    5. Basal cell carcinoma

Photosensitivity is inevitable when the melanocytes of the epidermis are unable to form sufficient amounts of melanin, as in albinism and vitiligo. Photosensitivity in clinical practice most commonly is due to drugs and exogenous chemicals. In the photosensitive porphyrias the photosensitizing agent is an endogenous chemical (Chap. 108). Phototoxic disorders are those in which the basic mechanisms are nonimmunologic, such as porphyria, phototoxic drug eruptions, and phototoxic contact dermatitis. Photoallergic disorders are those photosensitivity reactions in which the basic mechanisms are clearly allergic, such as photoallergic drug reactions, contact photoallergic dermatitis, and some cases of solar urticaria. The pathogenetic mechanisms are unknown in other diseases which may be precipitated or aggravated by light, such as discoid and systemic lupus erythematosus, dermatomyositis, herpes simplex, and pellagra.

The four following groups of chemicals account for the majority of photosensitivity reactions seen in clinical practice:

1. *Sulfonamides,* including the sulfonylurea antidiabetic agents and the chlorothiazide diuretics, are common photoallergic agents.

2. *Phenothiazines,* such as chlorpromazine (Thorazine), promazine (Sparine), and promethazine (Phenergan), are phototoxic agents. Large doses of these drugs for prolonged periods of time may lead to severe hyperpigmentation.

3. *Tetracyclines,* especially demethylchlortetracycline, are phototoxic agents which may also induce shedding of the nails.

4. *Halogenated salicylanilides* and chemically related drugs, such as bisphenol (Bithionol), carbanilides, and hexachlorophene are common photoallergens. These chemicals are present in ever-increasing numbers of commercial antibacterial and deodorant soaps. The incidence of photoallergic dermatitis has shown a remarkable increase, especially in sunny climates, since the introduction of these new soaps in the 1960s.

PHOTOTOXICITY. The phototoxic reaction is similar to an exaggerated sunburn. The erythema begins earlier, and the local reaction is greater in intensity than in normal sunburn. The residual pigmentation is usually more intense and persistent. Phototoxicity can be likened to primary irritant reactions in the skin, since both types of reactions can be provoked in almost all adequately challenged individuals. An adequate challenge for phototoxicity includes two factors: (1) a sufficient amount of the chemical in or on the skin; (2) a concomitant exposure to a sufficient amount of light of the proper wavelength. Phototoxic drugs or chemicals presumably act by absorbing specific wavelengths of light, becoming activated, and passing the extra energy on to a component within the cell with resulting skin damage. The best-known phototoxic systemic drugs are the sulfonilamides, chlorpromazine, sulfonylurea, demethylchlortetracycline, and furocoumarins. Coal tar, perfumes, and furocoumarins are phototoxic agents which are applied topically to the skin. The phototoxicity of coal-tar preparations is used in the Goeckerman treatment for psoriasis, which employs topical applications of crude coal-tar ointment followed by exposure to ultraviolet light. The furocoumarin Tripsoralen (10 mg p.o. daily followed by measured sun exposure) is used to stimulate repigmentation in vitiligo.

PORPHYRIA. The photosensitivity which occurs in some types of porphyria is caused by endogenous phototoxic porphyrins. Severe photosensitivity and scarring occurs in infants and children with congenital erythropoietic porphyria (Chap. 108). In the chronic hepatic type, namely porphyria cutanea tarda, bullae occur on the hands and face following sun exposure and trauma. Urticarial and scarring vesicular lesions (hydroa vacciniforme) develop after sun exposure in erythropoietic protopor-

phyria. The photensitizing porphyrins are activated by long-wave ultraviolet light; hence, window glass gives these patients no protection.

PHOTOALLERGY. The photoallergic reactions have an immunologic basis which is most commonly a delayed "contact dermatitis" type. Only a small proportion of individuals exposed to the potential photoallergic agent become sensitized. The patient must be specifically sensitized by previous exposure to the chemical. After a latent period of several days, during which sensitization takes place, a delayed abnormal response occurs to specific wavelengths of light. The concentration of the photoallergen necessary to elicit the reaction in a sensitized person is usually much lower than that required for phototoxic reactions. The abnormal response may be urticarial, or papular and vesicular, i.e., a dermatitis. An adequate challenge for photoallergic reactions includes three factors: (1) a sufficient though small quantity of the antigen in or on the skin; (2) the presence of specific antibodies; (3) an exposure to a sufficient amount of the proper wavelengths of light.

Following repeated exposures to the allergen and light, the reaction time becomes shorter, and distant unexposed areas of skin may flare. Two groups of photoallergic patients are seen in clinical practice. The "transient light reactors" are photoallergic individuals in whom the eruption clears promptly when the sensitizing chemical is withdrawn. A small number of photoallergic patients become "persistent light reactors," and for unknown reasons the reaction to light persists for weeks or years after the chemical is withdrawn. Common photoallergic drugs which are administered parenterally include chlorthiazide, chlorpromazine, griseofulvin, and promethazine. Topically applied photoallergic drugs and chemicals include sulfanilamides, promethazine, para-aminobenzoic acid, and the antiseptic agents bisphenol, halogenated salicylanilides, and carbanilides. Photodecomposition products resulting from the action of ultraviolet light have been shown to be the actual sensitizers in the case of sulfanilamide and tribromosalicylanilide.

Clinical Manifestations of Phototoxicity and Photoallergy

The eruption is confined initially to the exposed areas of the face, neck, V-area of the chest, dorsal surfaces of the hands and arms, and the pretibial areas in women. Photoallergic reactions may become generalized, but the disease remains most pronounced in the exposed areas. Local regions which are anatomically shaded in the exposed areas (eyelids, submental regions, etc.) are spared. The primary lesions vary from exaggerated sunburn, bullae, and marked pigmentation in the phototoxic reactions to urticaria and eczematous dermatitis in photoallergic reactions.

Diagnostic tests for photodermatoses are based on the administration of known amounts of light of known wavelengths. There are three basic types of light tests which utilize a hot quartz or carbon arc light source.

1. *MED.* The minimal erythema dose (MED) is

determined by using measured time exposures from a given source of mixed short- and long-wave ultraviolet light. The MED is defined as the shortest exposure causing detectable erythema of the skin at 24 hr. The MED is shorter than normal in phototoxic and photoallergic reactions.

2. *Window-glass Test.* Window glass effectively blocks the short sunburn ultraviolet light wavelengths and provides a convenient method for irradiating the skin with only long wavelengths of ultraviolet light. Normal skin will not develop erythema after exposure to window-glass–filtered ultraviolet light. Prolonged exposures (10 times the MED) will elicit erythema in the phototoxic and photoallergic reactions which are related to long wave ultraviolet light.

3. *Photo Patch Test.* Patch testing with suspected photoallergens followed at 24 hr by exposure of the patch test sites to ultraviolet light is used in the investigation of contact photoallergic reactions. Reproduction of the disease in miniature by this procedure confirms the diagnosis.

The photosensitizer must be identified and eliminated from the patient's environment. These patients may react to light for some period of time after the drug has been withdrawn; therefore, confinement indoors, in darkened rooms and away from windows, may be necessary for several weeks in the more severe reactions. Topical corticosteroid creams give symptomatic relief during the acute stages. Protective clothing and sun-screening lotions or creams, such as red veterinary petrolatum and those containing benzophenones or titanium dioxide, should be used on all exposed skin of the photosensitive patient. The use of these sun-screening agents is necessary throughout the lifetime of patients with actinic degeneration of the skin and idiopathic photosensitive eruptions.

REFERENCES

Baer, R. L., and L. C. Harber: Light Sensitivity in Biologic Systems, Fed. Proc., 24: No. 1, Part III, 14, 15, 1965.

Epstein, S.: Masked Photo Patch Tests. J. Invest. Dermatol., 41:369, 1963.

Urbach, F.: Light Sensitivity, in Dermatologic Allergy: Immunology, Diagnosis, Management, L. H. Criep (Ed.), pp. 501–514, Philadelphia, W. B. Saunders Company, 1967.

60 SWEATING DISORDERS

Faye D. Arundell and Eugene M. Farber

Sweating is one of man's prime thermoregulatory mechanisms. In acclimatized individuals, cooling by evaporation of sweat accounts for 75 to 90 percent of the reduction of body heat. Sweating is a useful mechanism only if the sweat can evaporate and cause cooling of the body surface. The surface of the human body is covered with 3 million separate sweat units, namely, the eccrine sweat glands. The distribution of eccrine sweat glands over the whole body surface is found only in humans and simian primates. In other mammals, eccrine glands are present only in friction surface areas such as the footpads and prehensile tails. The number of sweat glands varies in different body regions of humans; the palms and soles have the greatest number per unit area. In addition to the number of glands, sweating ability depends on the size, output, and responsiveness of the individual glands.

The eccrine sweat gland is an epidermal appendage which develops independently of the pilosebaceous unit. The gland is a simple tubule with a coiled secretory portion located in the depths of the dermis. The duct extends as a straight tubule through the dermis and as a spiral coil through the epidermis to open in a pore on the surface. Two types of cells are present in the secretory portion of the gland: basophilic cells, which secrete mucin; and acidophilic cells, which secrete water and electrolytes.

When the ambient temperature exceeds 31 to 32°C, or 88 to 90°F, there is a sudden onset of visible sweating over the whole body surface. At lower temperatures, periodic insensible sweating occurs in alternate glands. This activity accounts for 10 to 30 percent of the body's total insensible water loss.

The innervation of sweat glands is by cholinergic postganglionic sympathetic fibers, and eccrine glands respond to all cholinergic drugs. Their response is enhanced by anticholinesterases and inhibited by cholinergic blocking agents such as atropine and methantheline bromide (Banthine). The central efferent pathway for sweating runs from the cortex via the hypothalamus, medulla, and lateral horn of the spinal cord to the sympathetic ganglia.

The main stimuli for sweating are psychic for the cortex and thermal for the hypothalamus. Emotion causes immediate, sudden sweating, primarily on the palms and soles but eventually all over the body. Hypothalamic thermoregulatory centers probably are stimulated by warmed blood arriving in the brain from the periphery of the body. Thermoregulatory sweating appears over the whole body surface, but the palms and soles are the last regions to show visible sweating. Axillary eccrine glands respond to both mental and thermal stimulation. In some individuals the axillary glands are as responsive as the palms and soles to mental stimuli. Gustatory sweating, accompanied by blushing, occurs over the lips and nose and may involve the whole face and head. The taste of spicy or acid food causes gustatory sweating in some normal individuals. Excessive gustatory sweating in certain regions (cheek and temple) may follow cervical sympathetic section and injury of the facial nerve (Chap. 355).

Intradermal injection of 0.1 ml of $1:10^5$ solution of acetyl-β-methylcholine (Mecholyl) or similar drugs causes sweating by a direct action on the glandular cells. A secondary, more widespread sweating occurring around the site of injection of these agents is the result of the nicotinic effect of these drugs which produce sympathetic axon-reflex sweating. Axonal reflex sweating is also caused by intradermal injections of nicotine and is abolished by infiltration anaesthesia. Intradermal injections of 0.1 ml Mecholyl ($1:10^3$ solution), nicotine sulfate ($1:10^5$ solution), and histamine diphosphate ($1:10^3$ solution) are useful methods for testing the integrity of the peripheral mixed nerves. Absence of the histamine flare indicates degeneration of peripheral sensory neurons. Absence of pilomotor (nicotine) and sweat (nicotine and Mecholyl) reflexes indicates degeneration of peripheral sympathetic neurons. All three axonal reflexes are absent in the lesions of tuberculoid leprosy (Chap. 175). Axonal reflex sweating may explain the local hyperhidrosis seen at the margin of inflammatory dermatoses. Sympathetic denervation is followed by failure of the eccrine glands in the affected area to respond to central thermal stimuli, emotional excitement, or axonal reflexes, but the glands are still able to respond to direct application of heat. This responsiveness to direct stimulation is not abolished by denervation, local anaesthetics, atropinization, or arrest of the circulation.

Eccrine sweat is a clear aqueous solution composed of 99 percent water and 1 percent solids. The normal value of 17 mEq per liter of chlorides in sweat accounts for 80 percent of the osmolality of sweat. The concentration of chlorides in sweat depends on many factors. In mucoviscidosis (cystic fibrosis) the eccrine gland functions at a lower level than normal (Chap. 334). In normal individuals, if the dietary intake of salt is high, the chloride content of the sweat is high. The salt content of sweat is decreased when the dietary intake of water or potassium is unusually high or when the salt intake is low.

The concentration of chlorides increases with time during a single episode of thermal sweating and during increased rates of sweating. With repeated episodes of profuse sweating, the glands begin to function at progressively lower temperatures, the sweat rate increases, and the salt content of the sweat decreases. This acclimatization process results from increased adrenal production of salt-retaining corticosteroids under the stimulus of thermal stress. The three important forms of heat exhaustion which occur in man are (1) heat stroke or hyperpyrexia due to central failure of thermoregulatory centers (Chap. 125); (2) salt-depletion heat exhaustion due to excess loss of salt and water in profuse sweating (Chap. 296); (3) sweat-retention syndrome due to plugging of sweat ducts and pores in hot humid environments.

The *apocrine gland* is a distinct type of epithelial gland which is unrelated anatomically or functionally to the eccrine sweat gland. Apocrine glands are present over the whole body surface in mammals, but they occur only in association with the pilosebaceous apparatus in the axillae, anogenital, and mammary regions of human beings. Specialized apocrine glands are present in the nose, eyelids (Meibomian glands), and external ear canals (where they secrete "ear wax"). The ducts of apocrine glands empty into the upper portion of hair follicles in the axillary, perianal, pubic, and mammary regions. These apocrine glands begin to function at puberty. Under emotional stress and other adrenergic stimuli they secrete a small amount of milky fluid which,

after decomposition by bacteria, creates distinctive regional odors. These odors can be controlled by regular bathing and topical antibacterial agents.

Chronic inflammation of axillary apocrine glands causes acute lesions resembling boils and the persistent draining sinus tracts of hidradenitis suppurativa (Chap. 139).

HYPERHIDROSIS

Thermal sweating performs an essential role in the regulation of body temperature. Emotional sweating, which is most apparent on the palms and soles, may have played an essential role in lubricating the friction surfaces of lower mammals; but in man, it is merely a source of embarassment.

GENERALIZED. The marked sweating during physical exertion, with defervescence, and in hot environments serves a useful function if it can evaporate and cause cooling. Alcohol, hot drinks, and aspirin accentuate any tendency to sweating.

Pain of any type and motion sickness also cause hyperhidrosis. A compensatory increase in the amount and rate of sweating occurs in patients who have undergone sympathectomy for hypertension.

LOCALIZED. Anxiety states are associated in many individuals with excessive outpouring of sweat from the palms, soles, and axillae. Hyperhidrosis of the hands may also occur in otherwise normal individuals. Direct stimulation of the sympathetic nerves causes local hyperhidrosis in inflammatory diseases, such as causalgia, nerve injuries, neuritis, and thrombophlebitis. The immersion foot syndrome is also associated with hyperhidrosis.

Normal amounts of sweating can be controlled with the commercially available antiperspirants containing astringent aluminum salts. Severe axillary hyperhidrosis may require local excision of the skin of the vaults of axillae. The use of systemic anticholinergic agents to control localized hyperhidrosis has been disappointing because uncomfortable side effects of these drugs occur at doses well below those required to stop sweating. Tranquilizers and explanatory reassurance may give some relief.

Diseases or injuries in the region of the parotid gland cause the localized hyperhidrosis which occurs in the auriculotemporal syndrome.

ANHIDROSIS

The confirmation of an inability to sweat depends upon sweat testing during mental or thermal stimulation. The starch-iodine test detects the arrival of sweat at the skin surface. A negative starch-iodine or filter paper test requires special testing procedures to determine whether sweat glands are present but occluded, present but not functioning, or absent. Poral occlusion is confirmed if the previously anhidrotic area sweats after Scotch-tape stripping of the stratum corneum. Sweating after intradermal injections of Mecholyl or nicotine confirms the integrity of the peripheral sympathetic nerves. Failure to sweat in the absence of poral occlusion and the presence of intact sympathetic nerves indicates deep duct occlusion or absence of eccrine glands. A full-thickness biopsy of the skin and subcutaneous fat may be needed to confirm the presence of sweat glands or deep plugging of the sweat duct.

GENERALIZED. Destruction of critical centers of the hypothalamus by tumors, vascular accidents, surgery, or trauma results in complete anhidrosis. Failure of the hypothalamic thermoregulatory centers causes heat stroke. Universal anhidrosis may accompany certain diseases of the peripheral nervous system (Chap. 354). Congenital absence of sweat glands occurs in the syndrome of anhidrotic ectodermal dysplasia. Generalized anhidrosis in which only the face is spared occurs in the *sweat-retention syndrome,* with deep poral occlusion in hot humid climates and in atabrine dermatitis when the sweat ducts are destroyed. Systemic diseases, such as myxedema, Simmonds' disease, and scurvy, may be accompanied by anhidrosis.

The individual with generalized anhidrosis, regardless of cause, is at a special risk during febrile illnesses, physical exertion, or high environmental temperatures. The loss of the evaporative cooling mechanism results in hyperpyrexia, exhaustion, and collapse. A controlled environment with cool temperatures and prevention of exertion and infections is a necessary lifelong pattern in all except the temporary "duct-occlusion" types of anhidrosis.

LOCALIZED. Interruption of the central or peripheral sympathetic nervous systems can result in localized anhidrosis. Syringomyelia, transverse myelitis, multiple sclerosis, tumors of the spinal cord, or interruption of peripheral nerves may cause the condition. Involvement of the peripheral nerves by leprosy, trauma, or other types of neuritis, and involvement of the peripheral sympathetic nerve by leprosy or degeneration secondary to diabetes or gout also cause local anhidrosis. Local anhidrosis due to sweat retention occurs in erythrodermia, psoriasis, atopic dermatitis, stasis dermatitis, and lichen planus. Sweat is still produced in these areas, but since it cannot reach the surface, miliaria and itching result.

REFERENCES

Herxheimer, A.: Excessive Sweating: A Review, Trans. St. Johns Hosp. Dermatol. Soc., 40:20, 1958.

Hurley, H. J., and W. B. Shelley: "The Human Apocrine Sweat Gland in Health and Disease," Springfield, Ill., Charles C Thomas, Publisher, 1960.

Montagna, W., et al. (Eds.): "Eccrine Sweat Gland and Eccrine Sweating," New York, Pergamon Press, 1962.

Shelley, W. B., P. N. Horvath, and D. M. Pillsbury: Anhidrosis: An Etiologic Interpretation, Medicine, 29:195, 1950.

Sulzberger, M. B., and F. Herrmann: "The Clinical Significance of Disturbances in the Delivery of Sweat," Springfield, Ill., Charles C Thomas, Publisher, 1954.

Section 9

Hematologic Alterations

61 PALLOR AND ANEMIA
M. M. Wintrobe and G. R. Lee

PALLOR

The color of the skin depends on many factors, which include the thickness of the epidermis, the quantity and type of pigment contained therein, and the number and degree of patency of the blood vessels, as well as the quantity and nature of the hemoglobin carried within them. Even the nature and fluid content of the subcutaneous tissue are significant factors. It is obvious, therefore, that pallor does not necessarily indicate that anemia is present.

A sallow complexion is present in certain individuals, as it was in their forebears before them, and may exist in the absence of any true anemia; the flush of excitement, on the other hand, or constant exposure to the sun and wind may produce an appearance which masks an underlying anemia. Physicians, at the turn of the present century, spoke of "rosy" chlorotics, as well as of green and pale ones. The number and pattern of distribution of the finer blood vessels vary in different individuals, and in the same person vasoconstriction may produce the appearance of pallor, whereas other factors, such as exercise, for example, may lead to the appearance of a "healthier" color. Certain disorders may affect the skin in such a way that a pallid appearance is produced, even though anemia is absent. These disorders include scleroderma, the various nephrotic states, and myxedema. The last two, however, may be accompanied by actual anemia.

ANEMIA

Definition and Detection

Anemia is most accurately defined as a reduction in the circulating red blood cell mass. However, since direct knowledge of the size of the red blood cell mass is not easily acquired, such a definition is of limited usefulness. It is more practical to define anemia in terms of concentrations per unit volume of blood. In these terms, anemia is a reduction below normal in the volume of packed red blood cells per 100 ml (VPRC), the blood hemoglobin concentration per 100 ml (Hb), and/or the red blood cell count per cubic millimeter (RBC). Under most clinical circumstances, these measurements accurately reflect changes in the red blood cell mass because the total blood volume tends to be kept within relatively narrow limits by a variety of physiologic mechanisms. It is rarely necessary to measure directly the blood volume, but in conditions in which blood volume deviates from normal, such as overhydration, dehydration, fluid retention, or significant blood loss, the usual measures of concentration may be misleading. An increase in the plasma volume may give a false impression of anemia. Of greater importance

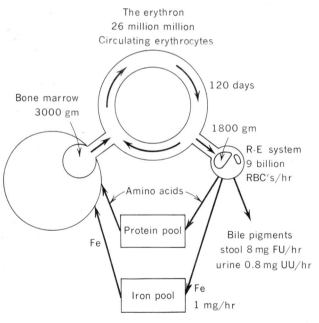

Fig. 61-1. The amount of blood in circulation represents the balance between production and destruction. In a 70-kg man the circulating red corpuscles carry approximately 770 Gm hemoglobin. Since the average life span of the red corpuscles normally is 120 days, the turnover rate per day is the total in the circulation divided by 120. In the average man this comes to approximately 2.16×10^{11} red corpuscles per day, or 9 billion per hour, and 6.4 Gm hemoglobin per day. From this are derived approximately 21 mg iron per day, 250 mg protoporphyrin, and 6.2 Gm globin. The iron and globin are reutilized. Of the protoporphyrin derived from the destroyed red corpuscles, somewhat less than 250 mg appears as fecal urobilinogen, since there are great variations in completeness of evacuation and also because of variations in the extent to which pigments giving this reaction are produced. Under normal conditions, through increased production and transformation of yellow marrow to red, the bone marrow is capable of approximately a seven- or eightfold increase in production capacity. Consequently, other things being equal, anemia will not develop as the result of increased blood destruction until the life span of the red corpuscles has been reduced to less than about 15 to 17 days.

is the fact that an extracellular fluid deficit may mask an underlying anemia.

The VPRC, as measured by the macro hematocrit method, is the simplest and most accurate of the three measures of red blood cell concentration in the blood and is therefore the one most suited for routine use. With relatively little extra effort, this method provides additional information which is extremely useful in the routine survey of a patient, such as the *erythrocyte sedimentation rate*, the *volume of packed white blood cells and platelets*, and the *icterus index*. The VPRC also may be determined by a micro method, and this and the measurement of blood hemoglobin concentration are satisfactory alternatives to the VPRC measured by the macro method when only a small volume of blood is available. Although the red blood cell count was the first available method for detecting anemia, it is rarely used for that purpose at present. When performed by the hemocytometer technique, the determination lacks accuracy; determination by more elaborate instruments, such as the Coulter counter, requires a relatively large initial investment and constant attention to accurate technique and machine maintenance. Consequently, the red blood cell count should be determined only for the purpose of calculating the corpuscular constants (p. 311).

The normal values for red corpuscles for persons at various ages are presented in the Appendix. These data are for persons living at sea level. At higher altitudes, higher values are found, roughly in proportion to the elevation above sea level. In general, the blood of normal persons tends to approach the mean for the sex. Provided the measurements are accurate, a deviation below the mean of more than 10 percent should be looked upon as representing anemia.

Pathologic Physiology

In normal subjects, erythrocytes are produced by the bone marrow and released to the circulation, where they survive approximately 120 days. They are then removed by the reticuloendothelial system, in which the hemoglobin is broken down to bile pigments, iron and globin. It is useful to think of the tissues involved in these processes as if they were one organ, the *erythron*, a concept which is illustrated diagrammatically in Fig. 61-1. It is apparent that the size of the circulating red blood cell mass is related to the rates of production and destruction. In a normal subject, the two rates are equal; therefore, the red blood cell mass remains constant in size, and the subject is said to be in equilibrium. When destruction exceeds production, the red blood cell mass decreases in size and anemia develops. When production exceeds destruction, the red blood cell mass increases.

ERYTHROCYTE PRODUCTION

Considerable evidence has accumulated which indicates that the rate of red blood cell production is under hormonal control. The major source of the hormone erythropoietin is the kidney, and its production appears to be stimulated by hypoxia. Erythropoietin acts to increase the number of immature red blood cell precursors in the bone marrow; the marrow becomes more cellular, fat is replaced by erythroid cells, and formerly inactive or "yellow" marrow becomes active or "red." Under maximum stimulation, the marrow is capable of increasing its production of red blood cells six- to eightfold.

Certain minerals, such as iron, copper, and cobalt, are essential to normal erythropoiesis, and anemia will develop in experimental animals when these are lacking. Certain of the B vitamins also have been shown experimentally to be essential to erythropoiesis, especially vitamin B_{12}, folic acid (pteroylglutamic acid), pyridoxine, ascorbic acid, pantothenic acid, and riboflavin. Nicotinic acid and vitamin E also may be concerned in erythropoiesis.

Since hemoglobin constitutes about 90 percent of the dry weight of the red blood cell, much of red blood cell production is concerned with hemoglobin synthesis. Hemoglobin, a compound of 64,458 mol wt, is made up of a colorless protein (globin) and a prosthetic group known as heme. The globin of adult hemoglobin (hemoglobin A) in man consists of two pairs of polypeptide chains, alpha chains and beta chains, which differ from one another in amino acid sequence. To each of the chains is attached one molecule of heme. Heme, which imparts the red color to the hemoglobin molecule, is a metal complex consisting of an iron atom in the center of a porphyrin structure (Fig. 61-2). The porphyrin has been designated protoporphyrin 9, type III. Like other porphyrin rings, it consists of four pyrrole nuclei connected to one another by methene (=C—) bridges. The iron, which has the capacity of binding oxygen reversibly, is linked to the nitrogen atom in each of the pyrrole groups and also to the imidazole nitrogen of one of the histidines in one of the polypeptide chains of globin.

The structure of heme is identical in all mammals, but the properties of hemoglobin with respect to electrophoretic mobility, solubility, and resistance to denaturation by alkali vary in different species, apparently because of differences in the amino acid composition of globin. In addition, in man a number of different types of hemoglobin, dependent on genetically determined differences in globin structure, have been discovered which in some instances govern the development of hematologic abnormalities and certain clinical manifestations (Chap. 339).

The source materials for the formation of porphyrin are the amino acid glycine and succinyl coenzyme A, which arises from the tricarboxylic acid cycle. In vitro as well as in vivo studies have clarified the steps in the synthetic process (Fig. 61-3). Acetate is transformed into α-ketoglutarate, and this, in the presence of coenzyme A, gives rise to succinyl CoA. This is one of the sites at which pantothenic acid functions in erythropoiesis, since this vitamin is a component of CoA. The vitamin pyridoxine is involved in the next step. The activated form of succinate condenses with a pyridoxal phosphate-glycine-enzyme complex to form delta-aminolevulinic acid

Fig. 61-2. Chemical structure of heme and its manner of union with globin to form hemoglobin. The carbon atoms derived from the alpha carbon of glycine are represented by ●, those supplied from the methyl carbon of acetate by ▼, and those derived from the carboxyl group of acetate by ✕. The unmarked carbons are those derived either from the methyl carbon atom of acetate or from the carboxyl atom.

(Δ-ALA) and carbon dioxide. Two molecules of Δ-ALA condense to form a monopyrrole, porphobilinogen. The subsequent steps leading to the formation of protoporphyrin are shown in the diagram. Ultimately protoporphyrin is converted to hemoglobin in the presence of iron, globin, and an enzyme, heme synthetase. The first and last steps in the heme biosynthetic chain occur in mitochondria; the other steps take place in the cytoplasm.

Globin is synthesized in the cell by a process common to the synthesis of all proteins. This requires messenger RNA, ribosomes, and "activated" amino acids (amino acids which are phosphorylated and attached to specific transfer-RNA molecules). Through a process known as translation, the ribosome travels along the strand of messenger RNA while simultaneously forming amino acids into a polypeptide chain. The specific amino acids selected depend on the sequence of purine and pyrimidine bases in the messenger-RNA molecule, the so-called "genetic code." Messenger RNA is synthesized in the nucleus by a process known as transcription, in the presence of a complementary strand of nuclear DNA (the "gene" or cistrone) and an enzyme, RNA polymerase.

RED BLOOD CELL DESTRUCTION

As noted previously, the normal red blood cell survives about 120 days. Since it contains no nucleus, all the enzymes necessary to maintain this life span must be in the cell when it enters the circulation. The principal factors essential to normal survival are (1) a source of energy, (2) the ability to maintain a stable fluid and electrolyte content, and (3) a system which protects the cell from endogenous and exogenous oxidants.

About 85 to 90 percent of the energy used by red blood cells is derived from the conversion of glucose to lactate by anaerobic glycolysis. The high-energy compound syn-

Fig. 61-3. Chemical steps in the biosynthesis of hemoglobin. The following abbreviations are used: *CoA*, Coenzyme A; *GTP*, guanosine triphosphate; *GDP*, guanosine diphosphate; *Pi*, inorganic phosphorus; *GSH*, glutathione; Δ-*ALA*, delta-aminolevulinic acid; Δ-*ALA-DH*, delta-aminolevulinate dehydrogenase; *PD*, porphobilinogen deaminase; *UI*, uroporphyrinogen isomerase; *UD*, uroporphyrinogen decarboxylase; *COx*, coproporphyrinogen oxidase; *HS*, heme synthetase; *Hgb*, hemoglobin. (*From M. M. Wintrobe, "Clinical Hematology," 6th ed., Philadelphia, Lea & Febiger, 1967.*)

thesized in this pathway is adenosinetriphosphate (ATP), two molecules of which are produced for each molecule of glucose broken down. The remaining 10 to 15 percent of erythrocyte energy is derived from the hexosemonophosphate shunt. Since no mitochondria are found in mature red blood cells, there is no tricarboxylic acid (Krebs) cycle, and energy from this pathway is not available.

The maintenance of the fluid and electrolyte content of the cell is primarily a function of its membrane. The total volume of the cell must be kept within relatively narrow limits despite an osmotic gradient, and a low sodium and high potassium concentration relative to plasma must be maintained in man. At least three different "pumps" capable of moving sodium out of the cell against an osmotic gradient exist in the erythrocyte membrane. Two of these utilize energy derived from ATP, require the enzyme adenosinetriphosphatase, and are inhibited by cardiac glycosides. They differ from each other in that one requires potassium in the external medium, and the other requires sodium. The third "pump" is inhibited by ethacrynic acid, but not by cardiac glycosides, and requires sodium in the external medium.

The principal components of the system which protect the red blood cell and its contents from oxidation are glutathione, reduced triphosphopyridine nucleotide (TPNH, NADPH), and the enzymes glucose 6-phosphate dehydrogenase, glutathione reductase, and glutathione peroxidase.

At the end of its life span, the red blood cell is removed by components of the reticuloendothelial system, principally the spleen. Within the reticuloendothelial cell, hemoglobin catabolism takes place. Iron and amino acids are extracted and subsequently are reutilized. The porphyrin ring is converted to bile pigments, which are excreted.

In the first step of hemoglobin catabolism, the iron atom is oxidized to the trivalent state, and methemoglobin is formed. Next, the linkage between the heme and the globin is severed, yielding **hematin.** Cleavage of the porphyrin ring is then accomplished by oxidation of the alpha methene bridge, a reaction which requires a ribosomal, mixed-function oxidase enzyme. Products of this reaction are iron, carbon monoxide, and **biliverdin,** a straight chain tetrapyrrole. Most of the liberated iron is transported as "plasma iron" via the transport protein, transferrin, a β_1-globulin, to the bone marrow, where it is used in the synthesis of new hemoglobin. Part of the iron may be retained within the reticuloendothelial cell as ferritin, a ferric iron-protein complex, or as hemosiderin, a ferric hydroxide polymer. The liberated globin is degraded and is returned to the body pool of amino acids. Biliverdin, as discussed earlier, is rapidly reduced to bilirubin, which is then transported from the site of hemoglobin breakdown to the liver via the blood plasma, where it is carried with albumin as a relatively stable protein-pigment complex. On reaching the liver, bilirubin is separated from albumin, conjugated with glucuronic acid, and excreted via the bile ducts in the form of protein-free di- and monoglucuronides.

Under pathologic conditions, free hemoglobin may escape into the circulation. This colors the plasma faint pink to deep red, depending on the concentration. The latter can be measured quantitatively by the benzidine reaction. Hemoglobinemia occurs in severe hemolytic states when there is intravascular hemolysis, as in erythroblastosis fetalis, blackwater fever, and *Clostridium welchii* (*C. perfringens*) sepsis (Chap. 172). Liberated hemoglobin is promptly bound by certain globulins with affinity for hemoglobin, the **haptoglobins,** and is carried to the reticuloendothelial system for breakdown there and conversion to bilirubin. The plasma haptoglobins can usually bind from 100 to 135 mg hemoglobin per 100 ml plasma. When this binding capacity is exceeded, other serum proteins which bind appreciable amounts of hemoglobin and its metabolites include (1) **hemopexin,** a heme-binding β_1-globulin, and (2) albumin which, by union with the ferric complex of protoporphyrin, hematin, forms **methemalbumin.** This compound reacts with benzidine and can be distinguished spectroscopically from other heme and pyrroll pigments. Demonstration of methemalbumin in plasma strongly suggests intravascular hemolysis. This compound may remain in the plasma for many hours or several days.

Hemoglobin liberated in the plasma escapes in the urine. The so-called "renal threshold" for hemoglobin is probably not a true renal barrier, but depends on the capacity of the binding proteins of the plasma and the reabsorptive capacity of the tubules. It is the free, unbound hemoglobin which appears in the urine. Hemoglobin usually appears in the urine if the plasma hemoglobin concentration exceeds the binding capacity of the various binding proteins of the plasma. Hemoglobinuria is then likely to continue until the plasma hemoglobin has fallen to 75 mg per 100 ml. The tubular epithelium of the kidney converts hemoglobin to hemosiderin, and hemosiderin is found regularly in the urine of patients with low concentrations of heme pigments in their plasma. The passage of hemoglobin by the kidney is accompanied and also followed by proteinuria, hemoglobin casts, and precipitates of hemoglobin. The color of urine ranges from pink to deep red with oxyhemoglobin, from purple to black from reduced hemoglobin.

Not all the bile pigment is derived from senescent erythrocytes. Studies of stercobilin excretion following the administration of ^{15}N-labeled glycine indicate that normally at least 10 percent (and in diseases such as pernicious anemia, thalassemia, and congenital porphyria, as much as 30 to 40 percent) is probably derived from heme or porphyrins produced in excess and not utilized in hemoglobin synthesis.

In the intestine, probably through the activity of the bacterial flora, bilirubin is converted to **urobilinogen.** Urobilinogen consists of three colorless chromogens, all of which are characterized by a strong Ehrlich aldehyde reaction, as well as by instability and ease of oxidation to three corresponding orange-yellow pigments which compose the urobilin group. The transition to urobilin can be hastened by mild oxidizing agents, such as iodine, and this is the basis of Schlesinger's qualitative test (alcoholic zinc acetate) for urobilin.

Although some investigators have maintained that the urobilinogens in urine come directly from bilirubin in the plasma, it is more generally held that they are derived from pigments absorbed from the colon into the portal circulation, most of which are returned to the liver and reexcreted in the bile, but a small proportion of which escape into the general circulation and are excreted by the kidney.

The amount of urobilinogen excreted in the urine in 24 hr (UU) by the normal adult is 0 to 3.5 mg, most frequently 0.5 to 1.5 mg. The normal range for fecal urobilinogen (FU), as calculated from a 4-day period of collection, is 40 to 280 mg per day, usually 100 to 200 mg. The expected values are related to the size of the circulating red blood cell mass; thus, lower values are found in young children. Mean values have been found to increase with age. An important qualification should be added. The oral administration of chlortetracycline (Aureomycin) causes a marked decrease in the concentration of fecal urobilinogen. This can be counteracted by the administration of aluminum hydroxide gel. The usefulness and limitations of urine and fecal urobilinogen determinations are discussed in a later chapter (Chap. 338).

Pathogenesis of Anemia

An *etiologic classification* of anemia is given in Table 61-1. The simplest mechanism by which anemia develops is blood loss. Anemia may also develop if red blood cell production is deficient or if red blood cell destruction is excessive. In anemias due to excessive destruction, a rather marked increase in rates of destruction must obtain before anemia occurs, since the normal bone marrow can compensate for a six- to eightfold increase by a like increase in production rates. In some anemias both decreased production and increased destruction play a role.

Anemia due to **blood loss** may be acute or chronic. When the blood loss is acute, the cause of the anemia is usually obvious, although sometimes a large hemorrhage may have occurred under conditions which do not reveal themselves readily. Hemorrhage in the gastrointestinal tract, e.g., from a peptic ulcer, may be dramatic in its symptoms and may be so severe as to cause shock; at other times it may be insidious in character and may occur without the development of pain or of symptoms pointing clearly to the gastrointestinal tract. Hemorrhage into one of the serous cavities may cause puzzling symptoms and signs: profound anemia may develop suddenly and icterus may even appear as the result of absorption of blood from a serous cavity.

Chronic loss of blood occurs most commonly from the pelvic organs in females and from the gastrointestinal tract in the male. A common cause of chronic posthemorrhagic anemia in certain parts of the world is infestation with the hookworm.

It is clear that in man anemia may occur as the result of iron **deficiency.** *Cobalt* deficiency has never been demonstrated in man, but a form of *copper* deficiency associated with hypoproteinemia and microcytic hypochromic anemia has been described in infants. Of the *B vitamins*, anemia due to deficiency has been demonstrated in man only in the case of folic acid and vitamin B_{12}. Deficiency of these substances is characterized by macrocytic anemia and megaloblastic bone marrow. Quite possibly the other B vitamins are available in such amounts, even under the extraordinary circumstances under which man sometimes finds himself, that anemia clearly attributable solely to lack of nicotinic acid, riboflavin, or pantothenic acid has not been demonstrated. Pyridoxine-deficiency anemia has only once been produced experimentally in the human infant, but anemia responding to the administration of pyridoxine has been reported in a number of patients, in whom it may have developed as the consequence of some metabolic defect. More frequently, deficiencies which result in anemia

in man are not due to lack of the substance in the diet but are "*conditioned*" by special circumstances. Thus lack of vitamin B_{12} in pernicious anemia results from an inability to absorb this vitamin because of lack of a gastric "intrinsic factor." Again, in sprue, vitamin B_{12} or folic acid deficiency may develop, presumably as the consequence of inadequate absorption. The same condition is occasionally encountered following extensive resection of the small bowel or in the case of a gastrocolic fistula. Excessive demands in pregnancy and greater needs for growth in childhood and adolescence may "condition" the development of various types of deficiency, and anemia will then ensue (see Table 337-1, p. 1598).

Severe deficiency of *protein* may lead to anemia in man and experimental animals. In the latter, anemia has been shown to be due to reduced production of erythropoietin.

The role of *ascorbic acid* in relation to anemia has not been established clearly; while anemia is seen in scurvy, it has not been shown that this is due directly to lack of vitamin C (see p. 410).

Anemia also results when the **bone marrow fails** for reasons other than the lack of specific nutrients. In these disorders, which are discussed in greater detail in Chap. 341, other bone marrow elements, the granulocytes and platelets, also tend to be reduced in number. Frequently, these "hypoplastic" anemias are due to toxins or drugs. In other instances, the cause of the marrow failure is not clear.

Hemolytic anemias (see Chap. 338) are anemias in which red blood cell destruction has increased to a degree that cannot be compensated for by the bone marrow. These anemias are characterized by certain unique features. Because of the excessive destruction of hemoglobin, there is an increased output of bile pigment. There may be mild to moderate jaundice, because of an increase in the unconjugated or "indirect" serum bilirubin fraction, and urine and fecal urobilinogen output are increased. There also is evidence of increased red blood cell production, the most reliable sign of which is an increase in the reticulocyte count.

Increased red blood cell destruction may result because the cell is *intrinsically defective* or because it is damaged by *extracorpuscular factors*. In a third category are the varieties of hemolytic anemia in which the *intrinsic erythrocytic defect* alone is not sufficient to lead to accelerated hemolysis, the latter occurring only *in the presence of an extraerythrocytic factor*. The various forms of hemolytic anemia are discussed in Chap. 338.

A number of disorders cannot be easily classified among the above three major groups. If red blood cell survival is measured, it is found to be moderately reduced, but not to a degree that would produce anemia. The capacity of the marrow to compensate for this increase in destruction is limited, however, and these two factors together lead to anemia. The extent to which the features of hemolytic anemia are found in these disorders depends on the degree of accelerated blood destruction.

The hemoglobinopathies are included in Table 338-1 among the hemolytic anemias attributable to intrinsic erythrocytic defects because they result from qualitative abnormalities of hemoglobin composition; **the thalassemia syndromes** are included because they are due to quantitative abnormalities of hemoglobin peptide synthesis (Chap. 339). The manifestations of these disorders are variable, however. In some, notably thalassemia major and sickle-cell anemia, there is a marked shortening of red blood cell survival, and it is in such cases that the usual features of hemolysis are present. In others, anemia appears to be due to a combination of reduced red blood cell production and a mild increase in destruction. Still others, including most of the heterozygous conditions, are not accompanied by anemia; in fact, some have been described in which polycythemia occurs as a result of abnormal hemoglobin oxygen binding. Consequently, the hemoglobinopathies and thalassemias may also be classified as disorders with both decreased production and increased destruction of red blood cells, as shown in Table 61-1.

Table 61-1. ETIOLOGIC CLASSIFICATION OF ANEMIA

I. Loss of blood
   A. Acute posthemorrhagic anemia
   B. Chronic posthemorrhagic anemia
II. Deficient red cell production
   A. Deficiency of factors concerned with erythropoiesis
     1. Iron deficiency
     2. Experimentally: copper and cobalt deficiencies
     3. Vitamin B_{12} or folic acid deficiency (pernicious anemia and related megaloblastic anemias)
     4. Experimentally: pyridoxine, riboflavin, pantothenic acid, vitamin E, and protein deficiencies
     5. Possible ascorbic acid deficiency
   B. Anemias of bone marrow failure
     1. Hypoplastic and aplastic anemia
     2. Refractory sideroblastic anemia
III. Excessive red blood cell destruction (hemolytic anemias) (see Chap. 338)
   A. Hemolysis principally attributed to intrinsic erythrocytic defects
   B. Hemolysis attributed to an intrinsic erythrocytic defect *plus* an extraerythrocytic factor
   C. Hemolysis principally attributed to extraerythrocytic factors
IV. Disorders with both decreased production and increased destruction of red blood cells
   A. Defective hemoglobin synthesis
     1. Thalassemias
     2. Hemoglobinopathies (sickle-cell anemia and related disorders)
   B. Anemias associated with chronic diseases (infection, cancer, rheumatoid arthritis)
   C. Anemia of renal disease
   D. Anemia of liver disease
   E. Anemia of myxedema and other endocrine disorders
   F. Anemias due to bone marrow invasion (myelophthisic anemias)

The **anemia accompanying chronic infection, cancer, and rheumatoid arthritis** (Chap. 340) is unique in that it is associated with a profound disturbance in iron metabolism. This is manifested by a low plasma iron concentration, reduced plasma iron-binding capacity, increased iron stores, and decreased marrow sideroblasts. The defect cannot be altered by iron administration, even if iron is given parenterally in large quantities. An increase in free erythrocyte protoporphyrin and in serum copper occurs at the same time. It is probable that the flow of iron to plasma from reticuloendothelial stores is restricted, but the way in which such a restriction is brought about is unknown. This metabolic defect is overcome and anemia is corrected when the underlying disease, e.g., infection, is treated appropriately.

In the **anemia of renal insufficiency** (Chap. 340), the decrease in red blood cell survival is, in part at least, the consequence of extracorpuscular factors. The nature of these factors has not been defined; there is no evidence of an autoimmune mechanism, nor is there a clear relation with any of the products which are retained in renal insufficiency. Since the kidney is concerned in erythropoietin production, attention has been directed to a possible defect in synthesis of this hormone as an explanation for the decrease in red blood cell production. Plasma erythropoietin levels have been found to be reduced in comparison with comparable degrees of anemia due to other causes. Furthermore, the radioiron marrow transit time, which becomes shortened as erythropoietin stimulates the marrow, is prolonged in renal disease. Unlike the anemia of other chronic disorders, the anemia of renal insufficiency is not characterized by hypoferremia as a constant feature.

Multiple factors are implicated in the pathogenesis of the **anemia of hepatic disease.** Blood loss from esophageal varices may lead to acute or chronic posthemorrhagic anemia. Nutritional folic acid deficiency not uncommonly accompanies cirrhosis in alcoholics. Alcohol itself has been shown to cause reversible depression of red blood cell production. In most cases, however, the cause of the anemia is not clearly defined. The red blood cells are normal or increased in size and tend to be thinner than normal, possibly because of the effect of bile salt retention on membrane lipids. Red blood cell survival is moderately shortened, and red blood cell production is decreased.

The pathogenesis of the anemia observed in **myxedema** is obscure. Defective absorption of vitamin B_{12}, uninfluenced by intrinsic factor, has been demonstrated in some cases. The anemia, which is usually only moderate in degree and is usually normocytic but may be macrocytic, disappears gradually as desiccated thyroid is given, but it seems unlikely that it is attributable directly to deficiency of the hormone. It has been suggested that it is brought about indirectly through the effect of the thyroid on the consumption of oxygen by the tissues. Moderate anemia is encountered in association with adrenocortical insufficiency and in hypopituitarism. The pathogenetic mechanisms are not understood, but in view of what is now known concerning the functions of the hormones secreted by the adrenal glands and the pituitary gland, it is at least plausible that the anemia is the consequence of some metabolic disturbance resulting from deficiency of these hormones.

The pathogenesis of the anemia in **leukemia, malignancy** with metastases to bone marrow (Chap. 340), **myelofibrosis** (Chap. 350), and other similar conditions is as yet obscure. Such anemia has been classified as myelophthisic. The term implies wasting away of the marrow, but it is usually used to refer to encroachment on or replacement of the bone marrow by leukemia or metastases. There is little or no evidence, however, that the erythropoietic tissue is crowded out in these myelophthisic anemias. Measurements of red blood cell production rates have at times yielded normal or increased values. It has been suggested that in some cases erythrophagocytosis contributes to the anemia. A number of studies have shown the "life span" of the red corpuscles to be reduced, and occasionally frank hemolytic anemia develops. It is possible that no single explanation for the anemia associated with these diseases will be found, but it is plausible, at least, that a metabolic fault related to the underlying disease is an important factor.

It should not be overlooked that in any given patient with a chronic ailment accompanied by anemia, more than one factor may play a role. Thus, in any longstanding illness there may be nutritional deficiency because of reduced intake, and sometimes also because of faulty absorption from the gastrointestinal tract. Blood loss may be an added factor. In addition, a metabolic disturbance, such as that which accompanies infection, may play a role as well. In some instances excessive blood destruction complicates the picture still further.

The Signs and Symptoms of Anemia

Anemia should never be thought of as a diagnosis in itself, but rather as a manifestation of an underlying disease process. Thus, the signs and symptoms found in the anemic patient are a mixture of those due to anemia and those due to the underlying disease. Only those symptoms common to all anemias will be discussed below; symptoms more specifically related to the underlying disease are dealt with in the chapters dealing with those entities.

Cardiorespiratory System. Hemoglobin is the vehicle and the cardiovascular system the means of delivery of oxygen to the tissues. When anemia is present, the oxygen-carrying capacity of the blood is reduced. If an equivalent amount of oxygen is to be delivered, blood flow must be increased by means of certain cardiovascular adjustments (Fig. 61-4). Many of the signs and symptoms of anemia reflect these changes in cardiovascular function.

An increased blood flow is accomplished by increases in cardiac stroke volume and heart rate. The patient may be aware of this increased cardiac activity and complain of palpitation. On examination, tachycardia and an increased pulse pressure may be found along with increased pulsations over the precordium and major arteries, and even a capillary pulsation in the fingertips may be detected. The circulation time may be shortened, and there may be a slight rise in right auricular pressure.

Still other signs of the "hyperkinetic syndrome" may be observed (Chap. 264).

The adequacy of the cardiovascular adjustments to anemia depends on the degree of the anemia, the rapidity with which it has developed, and the preexisting status of the cardiovascular system. Symptoms are usually present when the blood hemoglobin concentration is less than 7.5 Gm per 100 ml blood. If anemia has developed so rapidly that there has been little or no time for physiologic adjustment, symptoms are likely to be prominent and to appear comparatively early; on the other hand, if the anemia has been insidious in onset, the adjustment may be so good that the hemoglobin may be as low as 6 Gm per 100 ml, without sufficient functional embarrassment occurring for the patient to be seriously handicapped.

The cardiovascular changes necessarily encroach upon the cardiac reserve; consequently, exercise tolerance is decreased. There may be no symptoms at rest, but signs of oxygen want, such as easy fatigability and dyspnea, develop on exertion. When compensatory adjustments become imperfect or fail, either because of an extreme degree of anemia or because of a previously damaged heart, the clinical picture of cardiac failure ensues. There may be edema, congestion of the neck veins, hepatomegaly, and rales at the bases of the lungs.

Severe anemia may produce a systolic murmur, which is usually most marked at the pulmonic area, but may be heard elsewhere over the precordium, especially at the apex. Very rarely, diastolic murmurs are heard at the base. Over the vessels of the neck a curious humming sound, the *bruit de diable*, may be heard.

Neuromuscular System. Headache, vertigo, faintness, increased sensitivity to cold, tinnitus or roaring in the ears, black spots before the eyes, muscular weakness, and easy fatigability and irritability are common symptoms associated with anemia. Restlessness is an important symptom of rapidly developing anemia. Drowsiness develops in severe anemia. Headache due to anemia may be very severe. Delirium is seldom seen except in pernicious anemia and in the terminal stage of leukemia. Retinal hemorrhage is by no means infrequent.

Alimentary System. Loss of appetite is not unusual as an accompaniment of anemia. Nausea, flatulence, abdominal discomfort, constipation, diarrhea, vomiting, or abnormal appetite may also be found.

Genitourinary System. Menstrual disturbances (most often amenorrhea) in the female, and loss of libido in the male, are frequently encountered in severe anemia. In other instances, excessive menstrual bleeding accompanies anemia. Slight proteinuria and evidence of distinct renal function impairment may be seen in association with anemia.

Epithelial Tissues. The pallor which accompanies anemia has been discussed. The skin itself is an unreliable index of anemia; the mucous membranes (if not inflamed), the nail beds, and the palms of the hands are more dependable. The color of the conjunctiva may be very helpful, but one should not be misled by a coexistent conjunctivitis. The gums are not so useful as would be

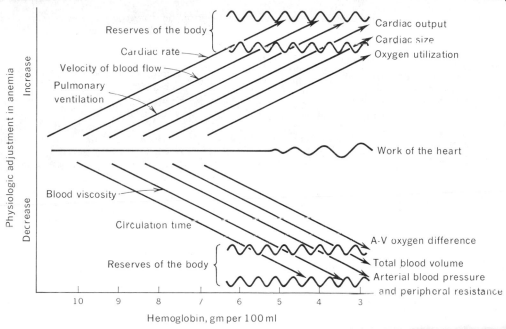

Fig. 61-4. Schematic diagram of physiologic adjustments to anemia. (*From M. M. Wintrobe, Blood,* 1:121, 1946.)

expected, for they may contain pigment or may be inflamed; furthermore, the pressure of the upper lip on the gums may produce some blanching if constriction of vessels results as the lip is retracted. Unless the hand has been held in an awkward position or has been exposed to cold or excessive heat, the nail beds and the palms of the hands will reveal anemia if much exists. In the palms the color of the creases is especially noteworthy, for they retain their red color even after the intervening skin of the palms has become definitely pale; when their color is lost, the hemoglobin may be judged as being below 7 Gm per 100 ml. In addition to pallor, loss of normal skin elasticity and tone, thinning of the hair, and purpura and ecchymoses may develop in the chronic forms of anemia.

The Approach to the Patient with Anemia

Anemia is not a diagnosis in itself, but a manifestation of disease. The challenge to the physician is to diagnose correctly and treat the underlying disease. Failure to appreciate this simple principle may lead to many serious errors in management of the condition. To cite a common example, a patient with anemia secondary to a bleeding cecal carcinoma may be treated with blood transfusions or iron-containing medications or even "hematinic" pills containing a mixture of nutrients and will apparently improve, but the carcinoma will progress to an inoperable stage.

Since literally hundreds of disorders may be associated with anemia, a rational approach to anemia requires that a classification of the causes of anemia be used which forms the basis of a systematic procedure leading to a diagnosis. Classifications of anemia have been based on etiology (as in Table 61-1), and such an approach may be effective in many cases. However, the necessary information is often difficult to obtain; accurate evaluation of rates of erythrocyte production and destruction often involves rather elaborate, time-consuming, and expensive procedures that needlessly delay proper management. An example is the determination of red blood cell life span. A more practical approach is based on a morphologic classification of anemia. The advantage is that the information necessary to make the classification is quickly obtained at little cost.

The first step in the morphologic classification of a given anemia is to categorize it as belonging in one of three major groups: (1) the macrocytic anemias, (2) the hypochromic and/or microcytic anemias, and (3) the normocytic, normochromic anemias. This is accomplished by the calculation of **corpuscular constants** (erythrocyte indexes) and the careful examination of the stained blood smear.

There are three corpuscular constants, *the mean corpuscular volume* (MCV), the *mean corpuscular hemoglobin concentration* (MCHC), and the *mean corpuscular hemoglobin* (MCH). They are calculated from ratios of the three measures of anemia. Thus,

$$\text{MCV } (\mu^3) = \frac{\text{VPRC}}{\text{RBC}}$$

$$\text{MCHC } (\%) = \frac{\text{Hb}}{\text{VPRC}}$$

$$\text{MCH } (\mu\mu g) = \frac{\text{Hb}}{\text{RBC}}$$

Table 61-2. MORPHOLOGIC CLASSIFICATION OF ANEMIAS

Class and severity	No. of red corpuscles	Mean corpuscular volume	Mean corpuscular hemoglobin	Mean corpuscular hemoglobin concentration	Summary
Macrocytic:					Red blood cells increased in volume; mean corpuscular hemoglobin proportionately increased; increase in size and hemoglobin content of red blood cells roughly inversely proportional to number of cells; mean corpuscular hemoglobin concentration remains normal throughout or may be slightly reduced.
Slight........................	−	+	+	0	
Moderate....................	− −	+ +	+ +	0 −	
Severe.......................	− − −	+ + +	+ + +	0 −	
Normocytic:					Reduction in the number of red blood cells without any, or at most only slight, increase in mean corpuscular volume and mean corpuscular hemoglobin; mean corpuscular hemoglobin concentration normal throughout.
Slight........................	−	0	0	0	
Moderate....................	− −	+0	+0	0	
Severe.......................	− − −	+0	+0	0	
Hypochromic and/or microcytic:					Reduction in hemoglobin characteristically more marked than reduction in number of cells.
Hypochromic................	−	0	−	−	
Microcytic..................	−	−	−	0	
Hypochromic, microcytic:					
Slight....................	0	−	− −	−	
Moderate................	−	− −	− − −	− −	
Severe...................	− −	− − −	− − − −	− − −	

+, increase; −, decrease; 0, no change from the normal; 0 −, no, or only slight, decrease; +0, slight or no increase. The amount of increase or decrease is indicated by the number of plus or minus signs, respectively.

Normal values for these constants are given in the Appendix. Their use in making a morphologic classification is outlined in Table 61-2.

Since the above determinations are subject to laboratory error, the morphologic impression should always be confirmed by examination of the blood smear. With experience, an accurate assessment of red blood cell size can be made by observing the average red blood cell diameter under the microscope. Hypochromia is seen as an increase in the area of central pallor. It is always wise to compare the observations made on the patient's blood with those made on a normal blood smear, since the magnification and illumination of microscopes vary. Uncommonly, distortions of red blood cell shape may lead to an erroneous impression from examination of the blood smear, especially when cells are unusually flat (leptocytosis), as they are in liver disease, in thalassemia, and after splenectomy. Such cells appear larger and more hypochromic than the corpuscular constants indicate.

The next step in the morphologic approach to anemia varies with the major morphologic category (Table 61-3). Macrocytic anemias are subdivided into two groups, **megaloblastic** and **nonmegaloblastic.** The megaloblastic anemias, of which pernicious anemia is the prototype,

result from defective synthesis of nucleic acids, usually because of a deficiency of vitamin B_{12} or folic acid. Certain morphologic features characterize the megaloblastic anemias. The earliest changes are seen in the blood smear and consist of the presence of *oval macrocytes* and *hypersegmented neutrophils.* In the bone marrow, characteristic alterations are seen in nucleated red blood cells; they are larger than normal, and the nuclear chromatin is finer and more particulate. These changes are discussed more fully in Chap. 330, along with a further subclassification of the megaloblastic anemias.

The *nonmegaloblastic* macrocytic anemias make up a heterogeneous group. Macrocytosis is found in patients with markedly increased rates of red blood cell production, because young erythrocytes are somewhat larger than mature erythrocytes; in addition, when demands upon the marrow are great, a "skipped generation" occurs—i.e., the nucleus is prematurely discharged and the red blood cell is released before maturation has progressed fully. Such cells are considerably larger than normal and, since hemoglobin synthesis has not been completed, may be somewhat hypochromic as well. Macrocytosis may also be observed in the anemia accompanying hypothyroidism, liver disease, or aplastic

Table 61-3. MORPHOLOGIC CLASSIFICATION OF ANEMIA

I. Macrocytic anemias (MCV, 94–160 cu μ; MCH, 32–50 $\mu\mu$g; MCHC, 32–36%)
   A. Those related to deficiency of vitamin B_{12} and folic acid (megaloblastic macrocytic anemias)
      1. Pernicious anemia
      2. Sprue and other conditions in which intestinal absorption is impaired
      3. Megaloblastic anemia of infancy
      4. Megaloblastic anemia of pregnancy
      5. Nutritional macrocytic anemias, refractory megaloblastic anemia, etc.
      6. Antimetabolites and increased demands for hematopoietic factors
   B. Where there is intense activity of the bone marrow and in other circumstances (nonmegaloblastic macrocytic anemias)
      1. Reticulocytosis (acute posthemorrhagic anemia, hemolytic anemias, and other conditions usually associated with normocytic anemia)
      2. Some cases of hypothyroidism, liver disease, aplastic anemia
II. Hypochromic, microcytic anemias (MCV, 50–82 cu μ; MCH, 12–27 $\mu\mu$g; MCHC, 24–32%)
   A. Iron deficiency due to
      1. Chronic blood loss
      2. Inadequate intake of iron together with
      3. Faulty absorption (achlorhydria, sprue, etc.) and
      4. Excessive demands for iron (growth, menstruation, pregnancies)
   B. Thalassemia and combinations with abnormal hemoglobinopathies
   C. Anemia of chronic disorders
   D. Sideroblastic (sideroachrestic, hypersideremic) anemias
III. Normocytic anemias (MCV, 82–92 cu μ; MCH, 28–32 $\mu\mu$g; MCHC, 32–36%)
   A. Acute blood loss
   B. Destruction of blood—acute and chronic hemolytic anemias
   C. Anemia of chronic disorders
   D. Anemia due to bone marrow failure
   E. Myelophthisic anemia
   F. Hydremia—not a true anemia

Note: MCV, mean corpuscular volume; MCH, mean corpuscular hemoglobin; MCHC, mean corpuscular hemoglobin concentration.

anemia, but the cause of the macrocytosis in these disorders is not understood.

The **hypochromic** and/or **microcytic anemias** are disorders in which hemoglobin synthesis is deficient. Normal hemoglobin synthesis requires iron, protoporphyrin, and globin, and an abnormality affecting the availability of any of the three may lead to a hypochromic and/or microcytic anemia. By far, the most common cause of this type of anemia is iron deficiency (see Chap. 336). Hypochromia and microcytosis are constant findings in thalassemia and may at times be seen in the hemoglobinopathies (see Chap. 339). The anemia of chronic disorders, such as infection, cancer, and rheumatoid arthritis, is usually normocytic and normochromic, but

at times is hypochromic and occasionally is both hypochromic and microcytic (see Chap. 340). The morphologic changes probably occur because of the disturbance in iron metabolism previously alluded to. Hypochromia and microcytosis are found also in sideroblastic anemias. These are comparatively rare and probably include a variety of entities, some acquired and some inherited. They have in common evidence of excessive iron stores, sometimes producing clinical manifestations of hemochromatosis.

Frequently, a final diagnosis in the hypochromic, microcytic group of anemias can be reached after a careful history and physical examination. Special attention should be given to the dietary history, to evidence of blood loss, and to the possibility of familial transmission. Evaluation of the status of iron metabolism will help to confirm the impression. The principal clinical tools used for evaluating iron metabolism are the serum iron level and iron-binding capacity and the quantitation of iron stores in marrow aspirates stained with the Prussian blue reaction and of iron in nucleated red blood cells (sideroblasts). Results of these procedures are indicated in Table 61-4.

Table 61-4. MEASURES OF IRON METABOLISM IN THE HYPOCHROMIC-MICROCYTIC ANEMIAS

Type of anemia	Serum iron	Serum iron-binding capacity	Marrow iron stores	Marrow sideroblasts
Iron-deficiency....	Decreased	Increased	Absent	Absent
Thalassemia.......	Normal or increased	Normal	Normal or increased	Normal or increased
Anemia of chronic disorders	Decreased	Decreased	Usually increased	Decreased
Sideroblastic anemias	Increased	Decreased	Markedly increased	Markedly increased

In evaluating the status of a patient with **normocytic, normochromic** anemia (Table 61-3, III), it is useful to try to draw some preliminary conclusions about the rates of erythrocyte production and destruction. It is rare that measurement of the red blood cell life span with ^{51}chromium is necessary; simpler methods usually provide the necessary information. The most useful, simple method for detecting increased red blood cell production is the reticulocyte count. Increased red blood cell destruction is detected by evaluating bile pigment metabolism by means of serum bilirubin and urinary and fecal urobilinogen determinations. The *anemia of acute blood loss* (Chap. 335) is associated with increased red blood cell production; consequently, the reticulocyte count is usually increased. The *hemolytic anemias* (Chap. 338) are characterized by evidence of both increased production and destruction. In the *anemia of chronic disorders* (Chap. 340), a moderate increase in erythrocyte destruction is accompanied by a modest decrease in production; the changes are subtle, so that the reticulocyte count and measures of hemoglobin catabolism remain within normal limits. The alterations in iron metabolism mentioned above may help to detect the condition. The *anemias due to bone marrow failure* are usually associated with a depressed reticulocyte count; there is no evidence of excessive hemoglobin catabolism, and leukopenia and thrombocytopenia also are present. The *myelophthisic anemias* are characterized by a bizarre blood smear: marked variations in erythrocyte size and shape, nucleated red blood cells, myeloid immaturity, and enlarged, bizarre platelets.

EXAMINATION OF THE BONE MARROW. In some of the above conditions, a final diagnosis is established by study of the bone marrow. This procedure is useful not only in the evaluation of the anemic patient, but also in disorders affecting other formed elements of the blood. There are two basic techniques by which marrow is obtained for study: *aspiration* from the sternum or iliac crest, and *biopsy* of the posterior iliac spine with the Westerman-Jensen needle. Thin smears are prepared from bone marrow aspirates, and such preparations, when stained with Wright's stain, are ideal for the study of fine morphologic details. These smears may also be stained with the Prussian blue reaction in order to assess the amount of iron in reticuloendothelial cells and sideroblasts. Fixed, thick sections of marrow obtained by biopsy are ideal for evaluating the cellularity of the marrow and for detecting fibrosis or granulomatous disorders.

When the patient's condition has been studied thoroughly in the manner indicated above, the number of instances in which examination of the bone marrow will be required is small. In Table 61-5 various types of reaction are listed which may be observed if differential counts on aspirated bone marrow are made. In such preparations, consideration should be given to the following:

Table 61-5. CONDITIONS IN WHICH VARIOUS TYPES OF REACTION MAY BE OBSERVED, AS DEMONSTRATED BY BONE MARROW ASPIRATION

M/E (myeloid/erythroid) ratio increased	*Nonmyeloid cells increased*
Myeloid forms of leukemia	Other forms of leukemia
The majority of infections	Multiple myeloma
Leukemoid reaction	Metastases from carcinoma, etc.
Decrease in nucleated red blood cells	Gaucher's disease, Niemann-Pick disease
	Aplastic anemia (usually relative increase only)
	Infectious mononucleosis

Normoblastic hyperplasia	*Megaloblastic hyperplasia*
Hemorrhagic anemias	Pernicious anemia
Iron-deficiency anemia	Sprue, idiopathic steatorrhea, resection of small intestine (certain cases)
Hemolytic anemias	
Thalassemia	
Cirrhosis of the liver	Tropical macrocytic anemia
Polycythemia vera	Nontropical nutritional macrocytic anemia
Plumbism	
Anemia of chronic renal disease	Macrocytic anemia with Diphyllobothrium infestation
Sideroblastic anemias	Megaloblastic anemia of infancy
	Megaloblastic anemia of pregnancy
	"Refractory megaloblastic" or "achrestic" anemia

1. The myeloid/erythroid (M/E) ratio. By this is meant the proportion of leukocytes of the myeloid series to nucleated red blood cells of all types. A decrease in the M/E ratio (i.e., a greater-than-normal proportion of nucleated red blood cells) may be the result of a decrease in the number of myeloid cells, or it may be the consequence of an increase in erythroid cells. In the latter event, one must differentiate between normoblastic and megaloblastic hyperplasia.

2. The presence of an increased number of cells other than those of the myeloid or erythroid series. These include lymphocytes, plasma cells, reticulum cells, and other forms (myeloma cells, carcinoma cells, Gaucher's cells, etc.).

3. Megakaryocytes. Since these form so small a proportion of the cells of the bone marrow, specific attention should be given them and a number of preparations of marrow should be examined. One should attempt to determine whether they appear to be increased or greatly decreased in number and whether their structure is normal.

4. The absence of marrow elements. In such cases, biopsy may be necessary.

In Table 61-6 are given normal values for the differential nucleated cell count of bone marrow obtained by puncture, and representative findings in a number of conditions are presented. These must be regarded only as examples of findings in typical cases; they do not give the range of variation in disease. The latter obviously depends on the stage of the disease and the presence or absence of modifying factors.

Although in all cases the material obtained by sternal puncture is of interest, bone marrow examination is an essential aid in diagnosis only in a limited number of conditions. These include aleukemic leukemia, multiple myeloma, Gaucher's and Niemann-Pick diseases, and unusual cases of macrocytic anemia. In the last-mentioned condition the demonstration of megaloblasts is very useful, since it suggests vitamin B_{12} or folic acid deficiency. In "aleukemic" leukemia, the bone marrow reveals numerous immature forms, thus dispelling the doubt raised by their absence or scarcity in the blood. In addition to these disorders, in disseminated tuberculosis and histoplasmosis, and in parasitic diseases such as kala-azar, the causative organisms may be discovered in the bone marrow when they cannot be found in any other way. Again, the cells of metastatic lesions may be demonstrated by sternal puncture.

In aplastic anemia it is the negative character of the aspirated marrow material which may be helpful. In cases suspected of being instances of "atypical leukemia," "agnogenic myeloid metaplasia," or "hypersplenism," sternal puncture followed by biopsy may support one of these diagnoses or, instead, may reveal myelosclerosis or myelofibrosis.

Management of Anemia

In the sense that by their administration a specific deficiency is corrected, vitamin B_{12}, folic acid, and iron

Table 61-6. REPRESENTATIVE DIFFERENTIAL COUNTS OF BONE MARROW OBTAINED BY PUNCTURE

Types of cells	Normal[1] average and range	Leukemia, acute[2,3]	Leukemia,[3] chronic myelocytic	Leukemia,[3] chronic lymphocytic	Multiple myeloma[4]	Pernicious anemia	Hemolytic anemias	Iron-deficiency anemia	I.T.P.[7]
Myeloblasts.......	2.0 (0.3–5.0)	*50–95*[5]	4.0	. . .	0.5	0.8	0.8	0.5	
Promyelocytes.....	5.0 (1.0–8.0)	. . . . . .	*10.0*	0.8	1.8	2.7	3.0	2.0	1.5
Myelocytes									
Neutrophilic.....	12.0 (5.0–19.0)	. . . . . .	*26.0*	1.5	1.8	7.7	8.0	9.0	8.0
Eosinophilic.....	1.5 (0.5–3.0)	. . . . . .	2.0	0.7	. . .	0.8	2.0	0.8	
Basophilic.......	0.3 (0.0–0.5)	. . . . . .	0.4	0.2	. . .	0.3			
Metamyelocytes....	22.0 (13.0–32.0)	. . . . . .	22.0	8.0	3.3	14.5	18.0	15.0	15.3
Polymorphonuclear neutrophils......	20.0 (7.0–30.0)	. . . . . .	29.0	8.5	62.0	14.5	9.0	28.0	31.0
Polymorphonuclear eosinophils......	2.0 (0.5–4.0)	. . . . . .	0.8	1.0	3.5	0.5	0.6	0.2	0.5
Polymorphonuclear basophils........	0.2 (0.0–0.7)		0.4	3.0	1.2	0.2	. . .	. . .	0.2
Lymphocytes......	10.0 (3.0–17.0)		1.4	*60.0*	13.0	9.5	10.0	1.0	2.5
Plasma cells.......	0.4 (0.0–2.0)	. . . . . .	. . .	. . .	*4.3*[4]	0.2	0.4	0.7	0.8
Monocytes........	2.0 (0.5–5.0)	. . . . . .	0.2	. . .	0.2	0.3			
Reticulum cells....	0.2 (0.1–2.0)	. . . . . .	1.2	1.5	1.0	2.0	2.6	0.8	
Mitotic figures.....	0	. . . . . .	0.2	0.3	. . .	2.7	1.0		
Abnormal cells.....	0								
Megakaryocytes....	0.4 (0.03–3.0)		. . .	. . .	. . .	. . .	. . .	. . .	0.2[6]
Megaloblasts......	0	. . . . . .	. . .	. . .	. . .	*40.0*			
Pronormoblasts....	4.0 (1.0–8.0)	. . . . . .	. . .	0.2	. . .	. . .	5.0	. . .	4.0
Normoblasts.......	18.0 (7.0–32.0)	. . . . . .	2.4	14.3	9.0	3.0	*43.0*	*40.0*	36.0
M/E ratio........	4:1 (3–5:1)	. . . . . .	40:1	1.5:1	8:1	1:1.5	*1:1*	1.4:1	1.5:1

[1] Adapted from M. M. Wintrobe "Clinical Hematology," 6th ed., Philadelphia, Lea & Febiger, 1967.

[2] The immature forms are listed in the table as myeloblasts merely as a matter of convenience. In acute lymphoblastic leukemia the cells are lymphoblasts, not myeloblasts. Often it is difficult to distinguish the various immature abnormal cells seen in acute leukemia. The essential point is the great preponderance of very young forms.

[3] The bone marrow picture in *aleukemic leukemia* is similar to that of leukemia of the various types, whether or not changes can be demonstrated in the blood.

[4] The characteristic cells in multiple myeloma differ somewhat from typical plasma cells in that the nuclear chromatin is relatively fine and the wheel-spoke arrangement of the chromatin is not present; the cytoplasm is basophilic and bright blue, not blue-green as in the plasma cell. A perinuclear clear zone is unusual.

[5] The most significant changes are shown in *italics*.

[6] Although the number of megakaryocytes may not appear to be increased, in typical idiopathic thrombocytopenic purpura the majority (64 percent in the case cited) have no platelets about them and most of the remainder (32 percent) have very few.

[7] Idiopathic thrombocytopenic purpura.

may be considered to be specific agents for the treatment of certain types of anemia. In macrocytic anemias characterized by megaloblastic bone marrow, of which pernicious anemia is the commonest example, the administration of **vitamin B$_{12}$** corrects the deficiency and the anemia is relieved. In certain rare instances of macrocytic megaloblastic anemia, **folic acid** rather than vitamin B$_{12}$ relieves the anemia. Examples are the megaloblastic anemia of infancy, "refractory megaloblastic" or "achrestic" anemia, many cases of "pernicious anemia of pregnancy," and some cases of sprue. These agents are valueless in anemias other than those in which the bone marrow is megaloblastic.

Likewise **iron** therapy is effective in iron-deficiency anemia and is useless in all other types of anemia. Such therapy is almost always effective by mouth, and only in the rare instances of severe gastrointestinal intolerance and in cases of chronic ulcerative colitis with iron deficiency is it justifiable to give iron parenterally. Under such circumstances, iron-dextran or iron-sorbitol may be given intramuscularly with reasonable safety.

Whether or not desiccated thyroid and ascorbic acid should be classed as specific therapeutic agents, as they are in Table 61-7, is debatable. It is clear that the anemia accompanying hypothyroidism is relieved only by the administration of thyroid, but whether this is the direct consequence of the relief of a deficiency is less certain. The relationship of ascorbic acid therapy to the anemia of scurvy is even less apparent.

Anemias which are neither due to deficiency of iron

Table 61-7. THERAPEUTIC AGENTS FOR ANEMIA

I. Specific: Vitamin B₁₂, folic acid, iron
   Desiccated thyroid (?), ascorbic acid (?)
II. Nonspecific: Blood transfusions
   Irradiation and chemotherapy (in leukemia, etc.)
   ACTH, adrenocorticosteroids, androgens
   Splenectomy

nor caused by lack of vitamin B₁₂ or folic acid are most difficult to manage. Iron or liver therapy, vitamins, or combinations of these, given orally or parenterally, are useless and wasteful of the patient's funds and the physician's time. These anemias cannot, in the present state of our knowledge, be relieved without the elimination of the underlying cause. Thus, the anemia of chronic renal disease is difficult to treat because the renal disease itself is usually so unremittent in character. Likewise, the anemia of chronic infection persists as long as the underlying infection continues. Aplastic anemia in which the bone marrow has been damaged in general carries a very poor prognosis. In some instances the destruction of hematopoietic tissue may not be complete, and in such cases the maintenance of life by transfusion may ultimately be followed by some, or even occasionally by complete, regeneration of bone marrow. The anemia of leukemia is relieved if the leukemic process can be checked by irradiation or chemotherapy. The same is true of the anemia of Hodgkin's disease and other disorders of the lymphoid tissue. In all these conditions the administration of iron, vitamin B₁₂, and folic acid or liver is valueless, and the giving of transfusions is but a temporary measure of limited value.

The use of blood transfusions in the treatment of anemia and other hematopoietic disorders is discussed in a separate chapter (Chap. 342).

Adrenocorticosteroids and corticotropin may be very useful in the management of acquired hemolytic anemias, and indirectly, when they affect the leukemic process, they serve to relieve anemia temporarily in acute lymphoblastic leukemia. The corticosteroids and **androgens** also have some value in other instances of anemia, e.g., certain instances of aplastic anemia.

Splenectomy produces permanent relief of the anemia of hereditary spherocytosis and may be valuable in some cases of acquired hemolytic anemia. This is especially true in the more chronic cases and when leukopenia and thrombocytopenia also are present. This operation is also valuable in certain cases characterized by "hypersplenism" (Chap. 350). However, splenectomy should not be undertaken without a thorough diagnostic study and full knowledge of the risks involved—the operative mortality rate, the possibility of postoperative atelectasis or other complications, such as postoperative thrombosis (in association with the marked thrombocytosis which may develop after operation). Finally, one must consider the likelihood of failure to achieve the result desired by this operation.

Details of the management of anemia will be discussed in later chapters in connection with the various types of anemia. In dealing with cases of anemia, the value of a diet containing food factors especially useful in blood regeneration, such as animal protein, the B vitamins, and iron, should not be overlooked. Such a diet offers much more than can be gained from vitamin capsules. The diet should also include all other nutritional essentials, such as ascorbic acid. In addition, the physician should ensure a reasonable balance between rest and activity, and attention should be given to the need for reassurance and the necessity of providing the patient with some understanding of his illness. Palliative measures may also be required for various complaints as they arise.

It should be apparent from what has been said already that adequate management of anemia is impossible without a thorough study of the patient and discovery of the nature and cause of the anemia.

REFERENCES

Gordon, A. S., G. W. Cooper, and E. D. Zanzani: The Kidney and Erythropoiesis, Seminars Hematol., 4:337, 1967.

Lester, R., and R. Schmidt: Bilirubin Metabolism, New Engl. J. Med., 270:779, 1964.

Mauzerall, D.: Normal Porphyrin Metabolism, J. Pediat., 64:5, 1964.

Wintrobe, M. M.: "Clinical Hematology," 6th ed., Philadelphia, Lea & Febiger, 1967.

62 BLEEDING
T. C. Bithell and M. M. Wintrobe

Except for that which occurs during menstruation, spontaneous bleeding is abnormal, and blood loss from even large injuries is usually insignificant. This is a consequence of the efficiency with which vascular integrity is normally maintained and the rapidity with which it is restored following injury. In general, both of these phenomena reflect the function of the hemostatic apparatus. Rapid and voluminous bleeding may develop spontaneously or following trivial trauma, when any of the components involved in hemostasis is lacking.

It must be recognized, however, that the adequacy of the hemostatic apparatus is relative. A ruptured esophageal varix will usually result in serious hemorrhage, while the erosion of blood vessels by a gastric tumor will produce less dramatic but continued bleeding, despite the presence of a normal hemostatic mechanism. Thus, bleeding may result from either a failure of the hemostatic apparatus or from localized pathologic processes which produce vascular erosion or malformation. In either case, this symptom is one of the most serious and significant of the cardinal manifestations of disease.

Localized pathologic processes are by far the most common causes of bleeding; such disorders will be discussed here from a general standpoint only. Although less common, bleeding which results from disorders of hemostasis will be covered in more detail.

Fig. 62-1. A simplified diagram of the hemostatic process. Subscript *a* denotes the activated forms of the respective factors; PL denotes phospholipid; solid arrows denote transformation; interrupted arrows denote action.

THE PHYSIOLOGY OF HEMOSTASIS

Hemostasis is the process which stops the flow of blood from injured vessels. Completely efficient hemostasis requires normal blood vessels and extravascular tissue, numerically and functionally normal platelets, and a normal coagulation mechanism. A simplified diagram of the hemostatic process is seen in Fig. 62-1, which for descriptive purposes is divided into vascular, platelet, and coagulation "phases."

THE VASCULAR PHASE. The most immediate consequence of injury to small vessels is a reduction of blood flow as a result of vasoconstriction and extravasation of blood. Vasoconstriction tends to markedly reduce blood flow through an injured area. The escape of blood into normal tissue is limited by the extravascular supporting tissue, and the increased tissue pressure which results tends to collapse venules and capillaries which may then rapidly cohere and even become obliterated. These virtually instantaneous phenomena are quickly supplemented by the events of both the platelet and coagulation phases, which are initiated by the process of contact activation, and by various substances released from injured tissues, the most important being tissue *thromboplastins*, and *adenosine diphosphate* (ADP).

THE PLATELET PHASE. Within seconds after injury, the platelets begin to adhere to the surface of the injured vessel (adhesion) and to one another (aggregation). These processes are greatly facilitated by the retarded blood flow which results from the events of the vascular phase, and rapidly produce a small platelet "plug" or thrombus. The processes of *platelet adhesion and aggregation* are complex and poorly understood, and numerous substances appear to be involved. These include a poorly defined plasma factor (the anti-VW factor) which is lacking in von Willebrand's disease (Chap. 346) and ADP derived from injured tissues, including erythrocytes, and the platelets themselves.

Like the vessels, the platelets play both a mechanical and a biochemical role in hemostasis. This involves the release of various substances which are involved in the coagulation phase. In this regard, the platelet has been likened to a sponge, since despite its small size, it contains a remarkable variety of hemostatically important ingredients. These include, in addition to ADP and ATP, various coagulation factors and the substance which is uniquely responsible for the phenomenon of clot retraction. Most important are various *phospholipids* (generically termed *platelet factor* 3) which become active in coagulation before the platelet membrane is visibly altered. It is probable that such phospholipids become activated *in situ*, the platelet membrane serving as a catalytic surface; some may also be released into the plasma in the form of lipid micelles.

In small injuries, the formation of a platelet thrombus alone may suffice to arrest bleeding, and in larger injuries, it may provide "temporary" hemostasis. However, it is generally agreed that "permanent" hemostasis depends on the formation of a firm, impermeable fibrin thrombus as a result of the process of blood coagulation.

THE COAGULATION PHASE. Blood coagulation is the process by which fluid blood is converted into a coagulum or a clot. This process involves the interaction of various poorly defined trace plasma proteins, the "coagulation factors." The *nomenclature* of the coagulation factors has now been standardized by designating each with a Roman numeral (Table 62-1). Factor III originally referred to tissue thromboplastin, factor IV to calcium, and factor VI to the activated form of factor V. These terms are seldom used. The descriptive terms *fibrinogen* and *prothrombin* are generally preferred to the Roman numerals.

The mechanism by which the coagulation factors interact is still uncertain. Evidence suggests that they are proenzymes which are normally inert, but which are transformed into proteolytic enzymes when activated, each sequentially activating the proenzyme next in line (*the* "cascade," or "waterfall," hypothesis). *Calcium* is essential for most steps in the coagulation process, but remarkably little is known concerning its mechanism of action.

Table 62-1. SYNONYMS FOR VARIOUS COAGULATION FACTORS

International nomenclature	Common synonyms
Factor I	Fibrinogen
Factor II	Prothrombin
Factor V	Proaccelerin, labile factor, accelerator globulin (AcG), thrombogen
Factor VII	Proconvertin, stable factor, serum prothrombin conversion accelerator (SPCA), autoprothrombin I
Factor VIII	Antihemophilic factor (AHF), antihemophilic globulin (AHG), thromboplastinogen, platelet cofactor I, plasma thromboplastic factor A, *facteur antihémophilique* A
Factor IX	Christmas factor, plasma thromboplastin component (PTC), platelet cofactor II, autoprothrombin II, plasma thromboplastic factor B, *facteur antihémophilique* B
Factor X	Stuart factor, Prower factor
Factor XI	PTA (plasma thromboplastin antecedent), antihemophilic factor C
Factor XII	Hageman factor
Factor XIII	Fibrin stabilizing factor, Laki-Lorand factor, fibrinase

Several of the coagulation factors are utilized or consumed during in vitro coagulation (factors V, VIII, XIII, fibrinogen, and prothrombin), whereas the remainder are found in the serum.

The coagulation phase begins with the phenomenon of *contact activation*. Indirect evidence suggests that this involves a molecular rearrangement of factor XII, which as a result acquires enzymatic properties and converts factor XI into its enzymatic form. In the test tube, contact activation occurs when shed blood is exposed to electronegative surfaces, such as glass. In vivo, a similar effect may be produced by skin, collagen, and other "foreign" extravascular surfaces.

The activated form of factor XI (factor XI*a*) initiates the next two steps involving factors IX and VIII, which lead to the conversion of factor X into its enzymatic form. Activated factor X forms a particulate complex (prothrombinase) with factor V and phospholipid from the platelets, which then initiates the conversion of prothrombin into thrombin.

Prothrombinase can be produced by the aforementioned sequence of reactions beginning with contact activation and involving factors XII, XI, IX, and VIII. This is termed the *intrinsic pathway*. The production of prothrombinase by means of this pathway is relatively slow but requires neither tissue thromboplastin nor factor VII. A functionally identical prothrombinase can be produced in a matter of seconds by tissue thromboplastins. This involves a sequence of reactions termed the *extrinsic pathway* which, in addition to factors X and V, requires only factor VII. Consequently this pathway bypasses the steps initiated by contact activation involving factors XII, XI, IX, and VIII. Thus, blood coagulation is initiated by only two processes, i.e., contact activation and tissue thromboplastin; it proceeds initially via two separate pathways, i.e., the tissue-activated extrinsic pathway and the contact-activated intrinsic pathway; later steps leading to the formation of fibrin proceed via a *common pathway*, requiring factors X, V, phospholipid, prothrombin, and fibrinogen.

The final step in the coagulation phase, the *thrombin-fibrinogen reaction*, involves the transformation of fibrinogen into fibrin, which is the physical basis of all blood clots. This occurs in three separate steps; viz., the enzymatic proteolysis of fibrinogen by thrombin which removes four peptides (fibrinopeptides), the formation of a visible but unstable fibrin polymer (soluble fibrin), and finally the formation of a stable fibrin polymer (insoluble fibrin) as the result of the action of factor XIII (fibrin-stabilizing factor). Structurally, fibrin resembles the proteins of muscle and skin and provides an extremely strong and stable framework for the "permanent" hemostatic plug.

CLOT RETRACTION. This is the result of the mechanical shrinkage of fibrin strands within a clot. The platelets supply both the energy (ATP) and the contractile apparatus required for this process (thrombasthenin, a protein which functions like actomyosin of muscle). Despite the teleologic view that clot retraction may constitute a "physiologic" ligature which pulls the edge of a wound together, the hemostatic significance of the process remains uncertain.

PHYSIOLOGIC INHIBITORS OF COAGULATION AND FIBRINOLYSIS. Mechanisms which maintain the normal fluidity of the blood, restrict the processes of hemostasis to the site of injury, and remove the resulting "debris" when its function has been served, are homeostatically as important as the processes which lead to hemostasis. The *physiologic inhibitors of coagulation* are poorly understood substances which neutralize the various enzymes produced during blood coagulation and thus prevent the propagation of a thrombus beyond the wound site. They include the antithrombins, the antithromboplastins, inhibitors of prothrombinase, and numerous others. Activated coagulation factors may also be removed from the circulation by cellular mechanisms in the liver and reticuloendothelial system.

Fibrinolysis is usually considered to be the major physiologic means of disposing of fibrin after its hemostatic function has been fulfilled. This process is thus of great importance in wound-healing, and in the recanalization of thrombosed vessels. Fibrinolysis (Fig. 62-2) is accomplished by the leukocytes and by a proteolytic enzyme (plasmin) which, like the coagulation factors, is formed from an inert precursor in the plasma (plasminogen). Various substances activate plasminogen in vitro, including tissue extracts, certain bacterial enzymes, factor XIIa, and thrombin. The mechanism of plasminogen activation in vivo is poorly understood, but fibrinolysis can be initiated by a variety of stimuli, including stress, hypoglycemia, anoxia, and even vigorous exercise. Plasminogen is avidly bound to fibrin (Fig. 62-2, step 1), and when activated (step 2), is present in both a bound form and free in the plasma. The antiplasmins in the plasma rapidly destroy free plasmin but are relatively ineffective against bound plasmin, which is thus free to carry out its physiologic function, fibrinolysis (physiologic proteolysis) (step 3). If plasmin is activated in amounts which exceed the capacity of the antiplasmins, however, other proteins in the plasma, including fibrinogen and most of the coagulation factors, may be destroyed. This abnormal process (pathologic proteolysis) (step 4) may lead to a serious coagulation disorder (Chap. 346).

The process of hemostasis is considerably more complicated than the stepwise reactions illustrated in Fig. 62-1 would suggest, and many of the complexities are of

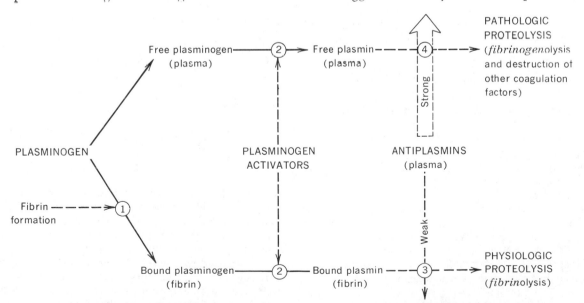

Fig. 62-2. A simplified diagram of the fibrinolytic enzyme system. Plasminogen is synonymous with profibrinolysin; plasmin with fibrinolysin. Solid arrows denote transformation; interrupted arrows denote action.

fundamental homeostatic importance. For example, although the production of thrombin is a relatively slow process at first, when once formed in even trace amounts, this enzyme alters platelets to further their aggregation and also activates factors V and VIII. As a result of such "autocatalytic" feedback mechanisms, the hemostatic process proceeds at an ever-accelerating rate, and once initiated, fibrin formation is virtually instantaneous. This is of great importance in arresting blood loss from a major injury. In this, and in many other respects, the hemostatic apparatus functions in a remarkably interdependent manner. As a result, hemostatic function compatible with life is maintained even when an essential component is completely lacking. The physiologic inhibitors of coagulation and the fibrinolytic enzyme system are also closely integrated with the hemostatic process. For example, fibrin, which provides the basis for the permanent thrombus, also restricts the extent of the thrombus by absorbing large amounts of thrombin. Fibrinolysis may be activated by factor XIIa as a result of the process of contact activation or by thrombin. Thus, the mechanism which activates the process of coagulation also initiates fibrinolysis, and the products of coagulation are themselves potent inhibitors of the process. These relationships are of fundamental importance when homeostasis is threatened by intravascular coagulation.

THE CLINICAL EVALUATION OF BLEEDING

In the evaluation of bleeding, particular attention should be directed to (1) the signs and symptoms of blood loss; (2) the location or source of the bleeding; (3) the appearance and amount of the blood; and (4) certain bleeding manifestations which suggest the presence of a disorder of hemostasis.

The *signs and symptoms* of blood loss per se depend on the amount and the rapidity of the bleeding. Acute and severe blood loss occurring within a matter of a few minutes usually results in syncope, whereas the loss of a comparable amount over a period of hours results in the picture of peripheral circulatory collapse (Chap. 36). In hemorrhage into the serous cavities; e.g., fractures of the pelvis or ribs, rupture of the spleen, ectopic gestation, and hemophilia, large amounts of blood may accumulate in the pleura, peritoneum, or retroperitoneal space, and shock may develop rapidly without external evidence of bleeding. Slow continuous blood loss results in the insidious development of the symptoms of iron deficiency anemia (Chap. 336).

The most common *locations* and *sources of bleeding*, together with the most common causes of each, are summarized in Table 62-2. Bleeding into the skin and from the bodily orifices is usually obvious to the patient. An exception is blood loss in the stools, which may be unnoticed but is a common source of significant blood loss.

Hemorrhage into the confined spaces of the central nervous system rapidly produces definite symptoms and neurologic signs. Intracerebral hemorrhage is a common

Table 62-2. THE CAUSES OF COMMON BLEEDING MANIFESTATIONS

Location or source of bleeding	Most common causes
Gastrointestinal tract (Chap. 44)	Peptic ulcers (Chap. 314), tumors (Chap. 315), gastritis, hiatal hernia, esophageal varices (Chap. 328), colitis, hemorrhoids
Respiratory tract (Chap. 38)	Tumors (Chap. 292), pulmonary emboli (Chap. 285), tuberculosis, mitral stenosis (Chap. 270), bronchiectasis (Chap. 291), other infections
Urinary tract (Chap. 51)	Stones (Chap. 307), glomerulonephritis, infections (Chap. 303), cystitis, tumors (Chap. 310), prostatic hypertrophy
Central nervous sytems (Chap. 26)	Trauma, hypertension, vascular malformations
Vagina (Chap. 52)	Endocrine disorders, tumors, obstetrical complications
Nose and paranasal sinuses	Trauma, hypertension, tumors, polyps, inflammation, perforation of nasal septum, hereditary hemorrhagic telangiectasia (Chap. 347)
Ears	Trauma, basal skull fracture
Serous cavities	Trauma, rupture of spleen, ectopic gestation
Nipples	Fissure, breast tumor
Intraocular (Chap. 401)	Hypertension, nephritis, diabetes, trauma, leukemia
Skin (petechiae and ecchymoses)	Thrombocytopenia or other disorders of blood vessels or platelets (Chap. 345)
Dissecting intramuscular and soft-tissue hematomas	Hemophilia or other coagulation disorders (Chap. 346)
Synovial joints	Hemophilia or other coagulation disorders (Chap. 346)

terminating event in hypertension, and spontaneous bleeding into the subarachnoid space from a congenital aneurysm of the circle of Willis may occur in young persons. Subdural hemorrhage must always be kept in mind in patients who have suffered even trivial head trauma.

The *appearance and the amount of blood* should be carefully noted. The appearance of blood originating from the lungs and bronchi varies with the degree of aeration and the presence or absence of mucus, pus, etc. It is usually bright red and frothy in appearance; e.g., hemoptysis in tuberculosis, but if it originates in areas of consolidation or congestion, it appears dark; e.g., the "rusty" sputum of pneumococcal pneumonia. In most infectious processes, the blood is mixed with pus or mucus and is seldom large in amount. An exception is tuberculosis, where hemoptysis from arteriobronchial fistulas may be alarming. Mitral stenosis may lead to massive pulmonary bleeding when bronchial varicosities rupture (bronchial "apoplexy").

Due to the conversion of red hemoglobin into brown acid hematin by the gastric acid, the appearance of blood from the gastrointestinal tract depends on its site of origin. That originating from the upper gastrointestinal tract, e.g., peptic ulcer, gastritis, resembles coffee grounds if vomited, and if sufficient to discolor the stools, produces a black tarry appearance (melena). In the presence of achlorhydria or when hematemesis is massive, however, the blood may appear red. Blood which originates in the intestinal tract below the ligament of Treitz imparts a bloody red or brown color to the stools (hematochezia) rather than a tarry appearance. In ulcerative colitis, intussusception, volvulus, and mesenteric thrombosis, a bloody mucoid discharge is usually seen. It must be remembered that blood from the nose, sinuses, or lungs may appear in the stools if swallowed, or may be swallowed and then vomited.

Gastrointestinal bleeding from peptic ulcers, Meckel's diverticula, and esophageal varices may be massive, while that which occurs from most polyps, tumors, and infectious processes is seldom so. Esophageal hiatal hernias and hookworm infestation usually produce slow and continued bleeding which is insufficient to change the color of the stools (occult bleeding).

In epistaxis from nasal polyps, various inflammatory processes which produce engorgement of Kiesselbach's plexus, and hypertension, the blood is bright red, and bleeding may be rapid. In epistaxis associated with perforation of the cartilagenous nasal septum, e.g., syphilis, small amounts of blood mixed with mucus are usually seen. Profuse epistaxis is frequently the initial and often the sole symptom in patients with hereditary hemorrhagic telangiectasia.

Small amounts of blood often impart a smoky color to the urine, e.g., glomerulonephritis, whereas in prostatic hypertrophy, renal stones, etc., the urine may appear grossly bloody, and when bleeding is rapid, clots may be passed per urethra. With the exception of renal tuberculosis, infections of the urinary tract, e.g., pyelonephritis, are rarely associated with gross bleeding but commonly produce hematuria which is discovered in the examination of the urine sediment (microscopic hematuria).

Abnormal vaginal bleeding is exceedingly common, and may be manifest as an abnormally heavy menstrual period (hypermenorrhea, menorrhagia), e.g., anovulatory cycle bleeding, or may occur between menses (metrorrhagia), e.g., adenocarcinoma of the uterus. Blood originating from the uterus is usually dark and fluid, but may appear bright red and be mixed with clots if bleeding is rapid, e.g., abruptio placentae. Bleeding from disorders of the cervix, e.g., carcinoma or polyps, is usually intermittent and small in amount.

Clinical Manifestations of Disordered Hemostasis

Although any of the varieties of bleeding summarized in Table 62-2 may be encountered, certain *bleeding manifestations* are more or less *characteristic of the disorders of hemostasis*. For example, bleeding into the synovial joints (hemarthrosis) in the absence of obvious trauma and spontaneous bleeding into the skin are rarely encountered in patients with normal hemostatic function. Moreover, such signs and symptoms fall into two relatively distinct patterns, i.e., those which are most common in disorders of vessels and platelets, and those which are more frequently seen in disorders of coagulation (Table 62-3). *Hemarthrosis* and its sequelae, for

Table 62-3. THE CLINICAL DISTINCTION BETWEEN DISORDERS OF VESSELS AND PLATELETS AND DISORDERS OF BLOOD COAGULATION

Findings	Disorders of coagulation (Chap. 346)	Disorders of platelets and vessels ("purpuric" disorders) (Chap. 345)
Hemarthroses..	Characteristic	Rare
Petechiae......	Rare	Characteristic
Positive family history......	Common	Rare
Sex..........	95% of hereditary forms occur only in males	Relatively more common in females
Traumatic bleeding.....	Onset often delayed; rapid and voluminous	Onset immediate; slow and persistent oozing

example, are almost diagnostic of a severe hereditary coagulation disorder, e.g., hemophilia, and are exceedingly rare in vascular and platelet disorders. Recurrent crops of *petechiae*, on the other hand, are strongly suggestive of an abnormality of the vessels or platelets, e.g., thrombocytopenia, and are rare in the coagulation disorders. Ecchymoses may occur in any disorder of hemostasis, but if they are the result of abnormal blood coagulation, they are large, characteristically dissect deeper structures, and may spread to involve an entire limb.

Profuse and often life-threatening hemorrhage following trivial trauma or surgical procedures is a hallmark of the coagulation disorders, and the onset of bleeding is often delayed for several hours. This phenomenon of *delayed bleeding* is rare in disorders of vessels or platelets, where slow but persistent oozing begins immediately following trauma.

The *sex* of the patient, the *age* when abnormal bleeding was first noted, and the *family history* are of particular importance in evaluating the disorders of hemostasis, since most disorders of vessels and platelets are acquired, whereas most serious coagulation disorders are hereditary, and among these, over 90 percent occur only in males. The absence of a family history of bleeding, however, does not exclude the presence of a hereditary coagulation disorder.

The history remains the best single "screening" test for the presence of a hemorrhagic disorder, and the corollary to this statement is no less true. A history of surgery, major injury, or even multiple tooth extractions without abnormal bleeding is good evidence against the presence of a hereditary coagulation disorder.

THE LABORATORY EVALUATION OF BLEEDING

Laboratory Findings in Acute Bleeding

The acute loss of blood stimulates the hematopoietic system (Chap. 335), resulting in leukocytosis with an increase in immature neutrophils and an elevation of the platelet count (thrombocytosis) and the reticulocyte count (reticulocytosis). Other evidence of accelerated red cell production may be seen in the blood smear (polychromasia and stippling of the erythrocytes), and even nucleated red cells of the normoblastic type may occasionally be found following acute hemorrhage. The erythrocyte sedimentation rate and the indirect reacting serum bilirubin may be increased as a result of bleeding into the tissues. The laboratory findings in anemia are described elsewhere (Chaps. 61, 335, 336). The various procedures which are valuable in the differential diagnosis of the causes of bleeding, other than those concerned with disorders of hemostasis, are considered in the appropriate chapters, as indicated in Table 62-2.

Laboratory Diagnosis of Disorders of Hemostasis

There is no single test which is suitable for the laboratory evaluation of the hemostatic process, but numerous methods of varying complexity and utility are now available for testing the vascular, platelet, and coagulation phases of hemostasis.

TESTS OF THE VASCULAR AND PLATELET PHASES. *The enumeration of the platelets* is considerably more difficult than is the case with erythrocytes or leukocytes. This difficulty is due to the tendency of platelets to aggregate in vitro and the difficulty of visualizing these small highly refractile structures. Among the numerous techniques which have been used, the so-called indirect methods and those hemocytometer methods which employ an ordinary microscope (Rees-Ecker) are very inaccurate and are seldom used. The only satisfactory methods presently available require a phase-contrast microscope (Brecher-Cronkite method) or automated counting equipment, e.g., the Coulter counter. In view of the many variables involved and the relatively large error of even the best methods, the platelet count should always be verified by the examination of a well-prepared peripheral blood smear.

Clot retraction is a specific function of intact platelets. It is usually deficient in thrombocytopenia and in a rare disorder of platelet function (Glazmann's disease) (Chap. 345). The determination of the presence or absence of clot retraction is seldom necessary in the diagnosis of thrombocytopenia, however, since the platelets can now be enumerated with reasonable accuracy. Qualitative estimates of the extent of clot retraction can be made by incubating one of the samples obtained for the clotting time, where retraction is normally apparent within 2 hr.

Hemostasis in a small superficial wound, such as that produced in measuring *the bleeding time*, depends on the rate at which a stable platelet thrombus is formed and thus measures the efficiency of the vascular and platelet phases. Unfortunately, the bleeding time leaves much to be desired in terms of reproducibility, since no two skin areas are exactly the same and it is impossible to produce a truly standard wound. Despite these intrinsic limitations, the bleeding time is valuable when carefully performed. It is prolonged in the majority of patients with von Willebrand's disease and disorders of platelet function. Although usually prolonged in thrombocytopenia, the bleeding time is seldom of diagnostic importance. Contrary to theory, this test is only inconstantly abnormal in the various disorders attributed to dysfunction of the vessels. The bleeding time is occasionally prolonged in severe coagulation disorders.

In the *tourniquet test*, a "standard" increase in venous and capillary pressure is produced for a short time. Normally, the vessels are unaffected by this procedure, but in the presence of vascular abnormalities or insufficient or abnormal platelets, small capillary hemorrhages (petechiae) may develop. Their number and size is an extremely crude index of the efficiency of the vascular and platelet phases. However, many normal subjects will develop some petechiae and many patients with bleeding due to vascular or platelet disorders will not. The tourniquet test correlates poorly with the platelet count, and although it is usually positive in severe thrombocytopenia, petechiae are usually apparent on physical examination of such patients in any case. The bleeding time, tourniquet test, and platelet count are usually normal in disorders of coagulation.

TESTS OF THE COAGULATION PHASE. Great care must be used in the collection of blood samples for coagulation studies, and foaming and contamination of the specimen with tissue juice, in particular, must be avoided. Because of the innumerable technical variations which are employed in even the simplest tests, only the "normal" range for the particular laboratory and technique utilized is meaningful.

In Fig. 62-1, it can be seen that in addition to the coagulation factors normally present in the plasma, the production of fibrin via the intrinsic pathway requires contact activation, phospholipids from platelets, and calcium. The *partial thromboplastin time* (*PTT*) is a simple test of this pathway, where contact activation is provided by a glass tube and phospholipid is added in the form of a crude cephalin fraction (platelet substitute, e.g., Thrombofax–Ortho). In the activated PTT, contact activation is further standardized by the addition of various particulate silicates, e.g., Kaolin, Celite. When such a mixture is recalcified, fibrin forms at a normal rate only if the factors involved in the intrinsic pathway (i.e., factors XII, XI, IX, and VIII) as well as those required in the common pathway (i.e., factors X, V, prothrombin, and fibrinogen) are present in normal amounts (Fig. 62-3). Cephalin provides an excess of phospholipid, and the PTT is thus unaffected by the platelets. Since it bypasses the tissue-activated extrinsic pathway, this test is also unaffected by factor VII. The PTT will be prolonged if the level of any of the required factors is below 15 to 20 percent of normal. Since, in severely affected patients coagulation factor levels are as low as 1 or 0 percent, the PTT detects many mildly affected patients. The test is also prolonged by heparin and by inhibitors of any of the essential factors.

The production of fibrin via the extrinsic pathway (Fig. 62-1) requires only tissue thromboplastin and calcium, in addition to the coagulation factors normally present in the plasma. This pathway is measured by the *plasma prothrombin time*, in which plasma is recalcified in the presence of an excess of tissue thromboplastin. Fibrin forms at a normal rate in such a mixture only if the factors involved in the extrinsic pathway (i.e., factor VII) and the common pathway (i.e., factors X, V, prothrombin, and fibrinogen) are present in normal amounts (Fig. 62-3). This test bypasses the intrinsic pathway and the factors concerned there, i.e., factors XII, XI, IX, and VIII. Since tissue thromboplastin contains phospholipids, the prothrombin time is also insensitive to platelets. Of the five coagulation factors measured in the prothrombin time, three (i.e., factors VII, X, and prothrombin) are depressed by coumarin-like drugs (Chap. 346). As a result, the prothrombin time is the most widely used test for controlling anticoagulant therapy with such drugs. The prothrombin time is relatively more sensitive to deficiencies of factors VII and X than to deficiencies of fibrinogen and prothrombin and is prolonged by inhibitors of any of the essential factors or of tissue thromboplastins and by heparin. The expression of the prothrombin time as a "percentage" of normal is not recommended, since the dilution curves used to arrive at this figure often are misleading.

The *clotting time of whole blood* is the most frequently used and most commonly misinterpreted coagulation test. In theory, it would seem that the rate of fibrin formation in whole blood would provide a measurement of the same coagulation factors as the PTT, as well as the platelets, since the coagulation of blood collected without contaminating tissue thromboplastins is initiated by contact with glass, bypasses the extrinsic pathway, and depends on the contained platelets as a source of phospholipid. In fact, the coagulation time measures only the time required to form the first traces of thrombin which suffice to produce a visible clot. Even the small amounts of phospholipid which are available in severe thrombocytopenia are sufficient to produce these requisite traces of thrombin, and consequently, the clotting time is unaffected by the platelet count. For the same reason, the

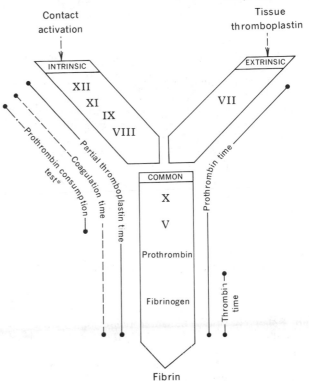

Fig. 62-3. The interpretation of screening tests of blood coagulation.
*Platelet phospholipid is also required for normal prothrombin consumption.

clotting time is significantly prolonged only in severe deficiencies of the factors involved in the intrinsic and common pathways (Fig. 62-3) and is usually normal when these factors are present in amounts which exceed 1 percent of normal plasma levels. The clotting time is unaffected by the level of factor VII and remains the most widely used test to control heparin therapy.

Although the clotting time may be normal when only small amounts of prothrombinase are produced, a large amount of unconverted prothrombin will remain; i.e., it will not have been normally utilized or consumed. The qualitative or quantitative measurement of residual prothrombin in serum after a standard interval is thus an indirect measurement of the amount of prothrombinase formed and is the essence of the *prothrombin consumption test*. This test measures only those factors in the intrinsic pathway required to form prothrombinase, i.e., factors XII, XI, IX, VIII, X, and V (Fig. 62-3). Although more sensitive than the clotting time in that it is abnormal when any of the essential factors are below 2 to 3 percent of normal, the prothrombin consumption test is less sensitive than the PTT and, like the clotting time, fails to detect mildly affected patients. Prothrombin conversion is incomplete and the prothrombin consumption test is abnormal in the presence of thrombocytopenia and qualitative abnormalities of the platelets.

In the *plasma thrombin time*, preformed thrombin is added to plasma, and the time required to form a clot thus indicates the rate at which the first visible fibrin polymers (soluble fibrin) are formed. The thrombin time is prolonged when the fibrinogen level is low and when the fibrinogen is functionally defective, but is unaffected by the levels of any of the other coagulation factors. It is prolonged by heparin, and by abnormal amounts of antithrombins.

The Fi test is a simple test for hypofibrinogenemia which utilizes latex particles coated with specific antibody to human fibrinogen. When this reagent (Hyland) is mixed with normal blood, visible fibrinogen-latex aggregates are formed which are lacking when the fibrinogen concentration is low. Primarily because it can be quickly performed, this is a valuable test in the diagnosis of the hypofibrinogenemias (Chap. 346).

The *rate of whole blood clot lysis* is a gross measurement of the fibrinolytic enzyme, plasmin. This test requires only the incubation and observation of one of the samples obtained for the clotting time. If fibrinolysis is rapid, the whole blood clot lysis time may be helpful, but otherwise the time required for lysis, which is normally in excess of 72 hr, is usually too long to be of diagnostic help. Relatively simple but more definitive tests, such as the euglobulin lysis time, are available for the study of abnormal fibrinolysis.

All the aforementioned tests of blood coagulation are usually normal in disorders of the vessels or the platelets.

INITIAL LABORATORY STUDY OF THE DISORDERS OF HEMOSTASIS

The definitive diagnosis of the disorders of hemostasis often requires a specially equipped laboratory and relatively elaborate methods. However, the most essential information can usually be obtained from the four simple tests summarized in Table 62-4. The platelet count and the bleeding time together provide the most reliable and reproducible test of the vascular and platelet phases. The PTT measures all of the coagulation factors involved in the intrinsic and common pathways and is generally accepted as the best single screening test for disorders of blood coagulation. This test, and its various modifications, when accurately performed, will be abnormal in over 90 percent of patients with abnormalities of blood coagulation. When supplemented with the plasma prothrombin time, which assesses the extrinsic as well as the common pathway, the abnormality can usually be localized to one of the three pathways and the factors involved therein. In view of their availability, simplicity, and low cost, these four tests are admirably suited to serve as primary screening tests. They should be the first laboratory tests obtained, since they direct further laboratory study, and when interpreted in the light of a careful history, a thorough physical examination, and the laws of probability, they provide a valuable "presumptive" diagnosis, i.e., whether the bleeding is due to a coagulation disorder, to thrombocytopenia, or to a disorder of the vessels or a qualitative disorder of the platelets. Further details concerning the clinical picture, differential diagnosis and treatment of the various hemorrhagic disorders will be found in subsequent sections concerned with the disorders of blood coagulation (Chap. 346) and disorders of vessels and platelets (Chap. 345).

REFERENCES

Biggs, Rosemary, and R. G. MacFarlane: "Human Blood Coagulation," 3d ed., Philadelphia, F. A. Davis Company, 1962.

Cartwright, G. E.: "Diagnostic Laboratory Hematology," 4th ed., New York, Grune & Stratton, Inc., 1968.

Ratnoff, O. D.: "Bleeding Syndromes. A Clinical Manual," Springfield, Ill., Charles C Thomas, 1960.

Williams, W. J.: Biochemical Aspects of Blood Coagulation and Hemostasis, Med. Clinics N. Am., 50:1257, 1966.

Wintrobe, M. M.: "Clinical Hematology," 6th ed., Philadelphia, Lea & Febiger, 1967.

Table 62-4. THE INITIAL LABORATORY EVALUATION OF HEMOSTATIC FUNCTION

Vascular and Platelet Phases		Coagulation Phase		"Presumptive" diagnosis
Platelet count	Bleeding time	Partial thromboplastin time	Prothrombin time	
Reduced	Prolonged	Normal	Normal	Thrombocytopenia (Chap. 345)
Normal or increased	Normal or prolonged	Normal	Normal	Vascular or qualitative platelet disorder (Chap. 345)
Normal	Usually normal	Usually prolonged	Normal or prolonged	Coagulation disorder (Chap. 346)

63 ENLARGEMENT OF LYMPH NODES AND SPLEEN

M. M. Wintrobe and D. R. Boggs

There are some 500 to 600 *lymph nodes* in the body, varying from less than 1 mm to 1 to 2 cm in size. These structures afford mechanical filtration for the lymph stream, removing cellular debris, foreign particles, and bacteria which may have gained access to the lymph from the various structures drained by the lymph channels. In the normal individual very few lymph nodes are palpable, even on careful physical examination. However, the access of disease-producing bacteria and certain viruses sets up an inflammatory reaction in the nodes, and various types of malignant cells can proliferate there. It has been aptly stated that in the exercise of their function the lymph nodes may sacrifice their own integrity for the welfare of the organism as a whole. One may wonder whether they do not mistakenly also nourish neoplastic tissue at their own expense.

These structures are also the site of formation of lymphocytes and of antibodies. Furthermore, in certain diseases, lymph nodes may be the site of formation of erythrocytes, neutrophils, and platelets. This is known as myeloid metaplasia and is a reflection of embryonal hematopoietic potentialities. This reaction also is accompanied by lymph node enlargement.

On physical examination the cervical, supraclavicular, axillary, and inguinal nodes are those most often found to be enlarged. Other lymph nodes which may be found to be enlarged on palpation are the epitrochlear, brachial, and very rarely, the popliteal. Enlargement of mediastinal nodes is detected by chest roentgenography. *Lymphangiography* is a technique in which a radiopaque dye is injected into lymphatic channels in the feet. The dye drains into abdominal and even mediastinal lymph node chains, thereby permitting enlarged nodes to be visualized. Roentgenography is the most reliable nonsurgical technique for demonstrating nonpalpable enlargement of abdominal nodes.

CAUSES OF LYMPH NODE ENLARGEMENT

Enlargement of the lymph nodes may be purely local, or it may be widespread. Such enlargement may be accompanied by all the signs of acute inflammation, such as heat, reddening of overlying skin, and tenderness. The nodes may remain discrete or they may fuse with one another as the result of perilymphangitis. Necrosis may even ensue and may be followed by rupture of the nodes and the formation of a sinus. Rapidly enlarging nodes are likely to be tender, but tenderness usually reflects a response to antigen or actual infection within the node. Inflammation of the skin overlying the tender nodes is usually indicative of an infected node. On the other hand, very great enlargement of the lymph nodes may take place in the absence of any signs of inflammation.

Enlarged lymph nodes may be discrete or matted together; they may be extremely hard or only moderately so or they may even be soft or feel cystic. Nontender nodes which feel hard and matted together usually contain metastatic carcinoma or a very aggressive intrinsic neoplasm such as reticulum cell sarcoma. Noninflamed, enlarged lymph nodes usually do not produce serious symptoms unless their enlargement obstructs some vital passageway. Thus, mediastinal lymphadenopathy may be very great and yet produce no symptoms unless the vena cava or bronchi are obstructed.

The chief causes of lymph node enlargement are listed in Table 63-1.

Infection may cause lymph node enlargement as a result of antibody response, granulomatous hyperplasia in response to infection within the node, or because of suppurative infection of the node. Localized infections ordinarily induce lymph node enlargement which is

Table 63-1. CHIEF CAUSES OF LYMPH NODE ENLARGEMENT

I. Antigenic challenge
  A. Infection
    1. Regional lymph node enlargement in the area draining a localized infection
    2. Generalized lymph node enlargement with systemic infection
  B. Allergic reactions such as serum sickness
  C. Diseases associated with "autoimmunity" such as systemic lupus erythematosus
II. Suppurative infections of lymph nodes [e.g., streptococcus, staphylococcus, *Pasteurella tularensis*, *Treponema pallidum*, virus of lymphogranuloma venereum, *Pasteurella pestis* (plague)]
III. Granuloma formation
  A. Due to infections such as tuberculosis, syphilis, and histoplasmosis.
  B. Diseases of unknown etiology such as sarcoid
IV. Primary lymph node diseases: Hodgkin's disease, lymphosarcoma, reticulum cell sarcoma, etc.
V. Leukemia
VI. Metastases from malignant disease in breast, stomach, etc.
VII. Congenital abnormalities (lymphangiomas)

limited to the regional nodes draining the infected area. If infection is systemic, whether due to steady "seeding" of the bloodstream with bacteria, as in bacterial endocarditis, or due to a systemic virus infection such as infectious mononucleosis, measles, or chicken pox, generalized lymph node enlargement may be present. This, however, is not of the same degree in all parts of the body. In infectious mononucleosis, for example, generalized lymph node enlargement is characteristic, but cervical glandular enlargement is often more striking than that found elsewhere in the body.

Of the *chronic infections*, tuberculosis and syphilis are the commonest causes of lymphadenopathy. In tuberculosis the cervical, mediastinal, or mesenteric glands are most often involved. The enlargement usually is slowly progressive and is easily confused with that caused by Hodgkin's disease. However, tuberculous glands frequently are tender and firm and adhere to one another. Sometimes breakdown of the overlying skin occurs, leading to the production of a stubborn draining sinus. Rarely the lymph node enlargement is acute and rapidly developing, and in such cases the glands may remain discrete and freely movable. In relation to syphilis, mention may be made of the firm, painless swelling in the regional lymph nodes draining the primary lesion; the generalized, firm, shotty, nontender nodes which accompany the secondary stage; and the glandular swelling of various degrees which may accompany the late stages or the congenital form. Other chronic infections in which glandular swelling may be prominent include fungous infections and filariasis.

Serum sickness should not be overlooked as a cause of lymphadenopathy, particularly since it is usually accompanied by fever.

Hodgkin's disease, lymphosarcoma, reticulum cell sarcoma, and giant follicular lymphoma are frequently classed under the single heading of primary lymph node diseases or "*lymphomas*" because, clinically, they are very similar. In these conditions the lymph node enlargement is characteristically localized at first; only as the disease progresses does wider dissemination occur. The node enlargement usually is discrete and firm and ranges greatly in degree. When the adenopathy becomes widespread, nodes may be discovered in locations where the presence of lymphoid tissue may not have been suspected. Such cases of lymph node enlargement are distinguished from those due to leukemia chiefly by the changes in the blood characteristically seen in the latter condition, but also by the asymmetry of the swellings which is often seen in the lymphomas. In leukemia, lymph node enlargement usually is generalized and symmetric, although especially in acute leukemia, adenopathy may be much more prominent in the neck than elsewhere. Tenderness of lymph nodes suggests infection rather than one of the lymphomas, leukemia, or metastatic involvement. However, some degree of tenderness, as well as pain, may be encountered when the glands have enlarged rapidly, especially in Hodgkin's disease. In the last condition, the presence of connective and fibrous tissue in the nodes may cause them to be harder than usual; occasionally they may have the consistency of cartilage.

In *sarcoidosis* the pre- and postauricular lymph nodes, the submaxillary, submental, epitrochlear, and paratracheal glands, are more often affected than in Hodgkin's disease. A history of involvement of the eyes and of the parotid glands (uveoparotid fever) suggests sarcoid, and punched-out areas in the small bones of the hands and feet may be demonstrable by roentgenography (see Chap. 254).

Treatment of convulsive disorders with various *hydantoin or hydantoinlike drugs* may produce a clinical and pathologic syndrome which closely mimics the lymphomas. Lymph node hyperplasia also is encountered in Addison's disease, hyperthyroidism, and hypopituitarism.

Lymph node enlargement due to *metastatic* carcinoma, as a rule, is distinctly localized, and the glandular swelling ordinarily is very hard. Such enlargement may involve nodes which are easily discovered, such as those of the axilla in cases of carcinoma of the breast. Or, the lymphadenopathy may be more often heard about than seen, such as Virchow's sentinel node above the clavicle in cases of carcinoma of the stomach or other abdominal organs. When the adenopathy is present in some region of the body inaccessible to physical examination, it is discoverable only by roentgenography or through the indirect effects of pressure produced by enlargement of the nodes.

Of congenital abnormalities which may lead to lymphoid enlargement, simple or capillary lymphangiomas, cavernous lymphangiomas, and the cystic form (cystic hygroma) may be mentioned.

DIFFERENTIAL DIAGNOSIS OF LYMPH NODE ENLARGEMENT

It should be evident from this discussion that the discovery of the cause of lymph node enlargement requires a thorough examination of the patient.

The location of the glandular enlargement may suggest the site of origin of the disease and may sometimes give some clue to its nature. Acute cervical adenitis should direct attention to the mouth and pharynx, mastoid adenitis to scalp infections, axillary adenitis to the upper extremity and the breast, epitrochlear enlargement to involvement of the ulnar side of the hand or forearm, and inguinal swelling to the lower extremities and genitalia. The examination of the patient must be painstaking, for sometimes secondary glandular enlargement may be much more prominent than the primary cause. Thus, for example, cervical metastases from a nasopharyngeal tumor usually overshadow the primary growth, which is characteristically small and easily overlooked unless a careful nasopharyngoscopic examination is made. The study of the patient should include careful palpation of the sternum for tenderness and of the abdomen for splenic enlargement, as well as examination of the chest for evidence of mediastinal tumor. Rectal and pelvic examination must not be overlooked.

Important laboratory procedures include the serologic test for syphilis; examination of the blood for agglutination reactions; and blood culture and culture of the throat, sputum, and other possible sources which might reveal infection; as well as examination of the blood and sometimes of the bone marrow for morphologic evidences of disease. Skin tests, such as tuberculin, histoplasmin, and coccidioidin, may also need to be performed.

If a disease known to be associated with lymph node enlargement is uncovered by the above studies, it is reasonable to assume that the enlarged nodes are due to this cause. However, if a definitive diagnosis is not made or if doubt exists, a *lymph node biopsy* should be performed. In addition to microscopic examination of the node, culture for bacteria and fungi may be helpful. As a general rule, if more than one area of lymph node enlargement is present, the cervical and supraclavicular areas are better sites for a lymph node biopsy than are the axillary and inguinal areas. Pathologic interpretation of an inguinal node biopsy often proves difficult, presumably because of the frequency with which this area is called upon to respond to the challenge of chronically traumatized feet and legs of man. The surgeon may have difficulty finding axillary nodes unless they are quite enlarged.

In patients with pulmonary lesions of unknown etiology or with a known but apparently localized carcinoma of the lung, scalenus fat pad biopsy may be required (Chap. 292).

THE SPLEEN

A palpable spleen is always a somewhat alarming finding to the physician because of the association of splenomegaly with leukemia and lymphoma. If the spleen is palpable, it is presumed to be enlarged. However, a palpable spleen does not necessarily always imply the presence of disease. Thus, McIntyre and Ebaugh, as a part of a routine physical examination, were able to palpate the spleen in 3 percent of entering college freshmen. Three years later, 30 percent of these students still had a palpable spleen and had no discernible disease.

Structure and Function of the Spleen

The pulp of the spleen is composed of (1) anastomosing strands of lymphoid tissue (white pulp), (2) a reticular network and branching multipolar cells which are placed about blood sinuses and intermingle with the strands of lymphoid tissue (red pulp), and (3) lymphocytes, granulocytes, and erythrocytes. The spleen is a very vascular organ and is capable of changing substantially in size, depending on its content of blood. It is also contractile; its capsule contains a small amount of elastic tissue. The circulation of the spleen is unique. In the lymphatic sheath, capillaries branch at right angles from arterioles. These capillaries rarely contain blood cells but rather appear to "skim" plasma from the arteriole. They serve as afferent lymphatics terminating within the lymphatic sheath. The sinusoidal structure of the red pulp consists of wide sinuses through which blood flow is rapid. These alternate with much narrower sinuses, termed *cords*, in which only a small amount of blood is normally present. The large sinuses and the cords are separated by a basement membrane containing regularly spaced perforations which provide direct communication between the two types of sinuses.

Arterioles terminate in the marginal zone of concentric flattened cells which loosely separates the white and red pulp. Erythrocytes course through the spleen by filtering through these flattened cells and then enter and rapidly traverse the large sinuses. A lesser number of red cells circulate slowly through the smaller sinuses (cords). These cells enter the cords from a few arterioles which terminate in the cords or from the marginal zone or the large sinuses through perforations of the basement membrane. Normally, only a small proportion of the blood, perhaps 20 ml, is present outside the main channel of blood flow.

The spleen, as a lymphoid organ, participates in the cellular events leading to antibody formation. However, splenectomy leads to no detectable defect in antibody production in adults or adolescents. It has been claimed that children who have been splenectomized are more than normally susceptible to infection.

If the spleen is removed, certain characteristic changes in blood cells are observed. Immediately following splenectomy, normoblasts, target cells, and erythrocytes with Howell-Jolly bodies, diffuse basophilia, basophilic stippling, and siderotic granules appear in the blood. Howell-Jolly bodies and target cells are usually demonstrable indefinitely in such patients, but other erythrocyte abnormalities tend to disappear. Neutrophilia and thrombocytosis are present immediately after splenectomy but disappear in a few weeks in most patients. Changes in the blood following splenectomy have been cited as evidence that the spleen exerts an inhibitory action on the bone marrow. Definitive experimental evidence for any humoral influence by the spleen on the bone marrow has not been forthcoming. Insofar as the red cell changes

are concerned, there is experimental evidence to support the view that the spleen normally removes the forms which are not usually seen in the blood. The primary site of destruction of senescent erythrocytes is the spleen.

Approximately one-third of the blood platelets are within the splenic circulation, a much higher figure than that for erythrocytes. There is evidence to suggest that the youngest and presumably most viable platelets are preferentially sequestered by the spleen. When the spleen is enlarged, the proportion of the total body pool of platelets which is in the spleen may increase, resulting in thrombocytopenia. Thrombocytopenia due to accelerated rates of platelet destruction by the spleen occurs when platelets are coated with antibody. There is no evidence that the normal spleen sequesters a significant number of neutrophils, and the mechanism of neutropenia which may develop in association with splenomegaly has not been determined.

During embryonic life the spleen plays an important part in blood formation, and the potentialities of this organ for blood formation persist even in adult life. In certain circumstances, foci of extramedullary blood formation can be found in the spleen; thus, when the functional activity of the bone marrow is impaired, the hematopoietic potentiality of the spleen may become an important asset.

ENLARGEMENT OF THE SPLEEN. This may occur under a great variety of circumstances. The chief ones are listed in Table 63-2.

Of greatest frequency is the enlargement of the spleen which occurs in association with infections. The *"acute splenic tumor"* accompanying various systemic infections such as typhoid fever and septicemia are examples. Like lymph node enlargement, splenic enlargement is frequently encountered in various contagious diseases and is often seen in infectious mononucleosis. Likewise, various subacute infections, notably bacterial endocarditis, are characteristically accompanied by enlargement of the spleen. *Abscess* of the spleen is rare and is usually secondary to pyemia arising from some other site. Frequently multiple and unrecognized, it is unusual for a splenic abscess to achieve prominence and produce local symptoms such as pain, elevation of the left leaf of the diaphragm, or rupture into the peritoneal cavity.

Malaria is, perhaps, the commonest cause of splenic enlargement when the world population is considered. Infection with other parasites which leads to splenic enlargement includes leishmaniasis, trypanosomiasis, and schistosomiasis. In kala-azar the spleen may be huge.

Primary tuberculous splenomegaly is extremely rare, but slight enlargement of the spleen accompanying a widespread tuberculous infection is by no means unusual. Splenomegaly may occur in connection with syphilis, especially congenital syphilis. Enlargement of this organ may also accompany the late stages of syphilis in association with gummas or amyloidosis. Rheumatoid arthritis, brucellosis, and sarcoidosis are other chronic diseases which may be accompanied by splenic enlargement. Splenic enlargement has been observed in about 25 percent of cases of disseminated lupus erythematosus.

Table 63-2. CHIEF CAUSES OF SPLENOMEGALY

I. Inflammatory splenomegaly
   A. "Acute splenic tumor": many acute and subacute infections
      1. Bacterial (typhoid, septicemias, subacute bacterial endocarditis, abscess, etc.)
      2. Viral and miscellaneous (contagious diseases, infectious mononucleosis)
   B. Chronic infections (tuberculosis, syphilis, brucellosis, histoplasmosis, malaria, schistosomiasis, leishmaniasis, trypanosomiasis, etc.)
   C. Miscellaneous diseases (lupus erythematosus, rheumatoid arthritis, sarcoidosis, histiocytosis X, etc.)
II. Congestive splenomegaly (Banti's syndrome)
   A. Cirrhosis of liver
   B. Thrombosis or stenosis, portal or splenic veins
III. Hyperplastic splenomegaly
   A. Hemolytic anemias, congenital and acquired
   B. Thalassemia and certain hemoglobinopathies
   C. Myelofibrosis, myelophthisic anemias
   D. Polycythemia vera
   E. Miscellaneous chronic anemias (pernicious anemia, chronic iron deficiency, "pyridoxine-responsive anemia," etc.)
   F. Thrombocytopenic purpura
   G. Obscure disorders ("big spleen syndrome," "primary splenic neutropenia," and "panhematopenia")
IV. Infiltrative splenomegaly
   A. Gaucher's disease, Niemann-Pick disease
   B. Amyloidosis, hemosiderosis
V. Neoplasms and cysts
   A. True cysts (dermoid, echinococcus, etc.)
   B. False cysts (hemorrhagic, serous, inflammatory, degenerative)
   C. Benign tumors (lymphangioma, hemangioma, etc.)
   D. Leukemia, lymphomas
   E. Malignant tumors (direct invasion or metastatic)

The vascularity of the spleen and its location in the portal bed make this organ liable to swelling as the result of increased venous pressure in that region. Such types of enlargement of the spleen can be classed under the general heading of "congestive splenomegaly" and include the syndromes known as *Banti's disease* and *splenic anemia,* as well as the splenic enlargement which accompanies cirrhosis of the liver and thrombosis of the splenic or portal vein (Chap. 350) and that which may be associated with cardiac failure.

The functions of the spleen in relation to the hematopoietic system result in enlargement of this organ when there is increased blood destruction (acute and chronic hemolytic anemias) or in the presence of chronic anemia of various types such as pernicious anemia, chronic hypochromic anemia, myelophthisic anemia, thalassemia, hemoglobin-C disease, and other hemoglobinopathies. Again, the spleen is enlarged, as a rule, in leukemia. In polycythemia vera splenomegaly is often encountered, and this finding helps to distinguish the primary disorder from secondary forms of polycythemia, where splenic enlargement is rare. The lymphatic hyperplasia which is associated with hyperthyroidism may be accompanied by splenomegaly. The spleen is also enlarged in myelofibrosis, primary splenic neutropenia, and primary splenic panhematopenia (Chap. 350).

Certain rare diseases such as Gaucher's disease and Niemann-Pick disease are characterized by splenic enlargement. In these conditions the swelling of the organ is probably due to the excessive storage of normal and abnormal metabolic products in the cells of the spleen (see Chap. 350).

Like other organs, the spleen may be enlarged as the consequence of the presence of neoplasms of various types. Hodgkin's disease, lymphosarcoma, reticulum cell sarcoma, and giant follicular lymphoma, however, are far commoner causes of splenomegaly than other types of new growth. Carcinoma is the most frequent type of metastatic tumor, but even this is extremely rare. Direct extension from carcinoma of the stomach and hematogenous spread from the stomach, lung, pancreas, and breast and from malignant melanoma may occur. Other tumors that may involve the spleen include lymphangioma, hemangioma and endothelial sarcoma (lymphangiosarcoma), fibrosarcoma, leiomyosarcoma, and myoma. A subcapsular cavernous hemangioma may rupture into the peritoneal cavity and produce acute hemorrhagic shock.

Cysts of the spleen may be of parasitic origin or nonparasitic. Of the latter, those containing serous or hemorrhagic fluid and due to trauma are commonest. They can sometimes be identified roentgenographically because of calcification of the wall. Echinococcus cysts occur more rarely in the spleen than in the liver. "True" cysts are formed from embryonal defects or rests and include dermoids and mesenchymal inclusion cysts.

DIFFERENTIAL DIAGNOSIS OF SPLENOMEGALY

A thorough physical examination, together with the history and the examination of the blood, will serve to differentiate many of the causes of splenomegaly which have been outlined. Sometimes additional procedures may be required, such as blood culture, sternal puncture, a roentgenogram of the chest, serologic tests including thoses for syphilis, liver function tests, and spleen or lymph node biopsy. Since certain of the causes of splenomegaly do not induce diagnostic pathologic changes in the spleen, a splenic aspiration or splenic biopsy will not necessarily yield a diagnosis. In most instances the cause of splenomegaly is not determined by studying the spleen itself but by detecting diseases which are known to be associated with splenomegaly.

The absence of fever is more helpful in differential diagnosis here than is its presence, since most of the conditions which have been mentioned may be accompanied by fever. However, at times, as in malaria and in undulant fever, the characteristic temperature curve is very helpful in making the diagnosis. In the septicemias the splenic enlargement is, as a rule, obviously only a minor feature of the whole clinical picture. The exanthemas are recognized by the respective characteristic changes in the skin. In their absence the skin should be inspected carefully for evidence of the pete- chiae which may accompany acute leukemia, thrombo- cytopenic purpura, or other hematopoietic disorders; the red petechiae occurring in crops together with the larger, slightly nodular and tender Osler nodes so characteristic of subacute bacterial endocarditis; or the spider telangiectases which accompany long-standing liver diseases. The plum-red "cyanosis" of polycythemia vera can hardly be overlooked.

Moderate lymph node enlargement accompanying sple- nomegaly is seen in many infectious diseases as well as in leukemia, but an asymmetric enlargement should arouse suspicion of Hodgkin's disease or lymphosarcoma. Great enlargement of the lymph nodes is seen in the last- named conditions as well as in chronic leukemia, espe- cially in the lymphocytic form. The discovery of icterus suggests hemolytic anemia as a cause or, if there is little or no anemia and the splenic enlargement is only slight, infectious hepatitis. The splenomegaly associated with the Banti syndrome (congestive splenomegaly) and with cir rhosis of the liver is usually substantial in degree, and jaundice is not the rule under these circumstances. Ma- laria must be kept in mind among the causes of hemo- lytic anemia.

Lesions in the mucous membranes accompanying sple- nic enlargement are seen in measles (Koplik's spots), secondary syphilis (mucous patches), infectious mono- nucleosis (infection of the throat, tonsillar enlargement, sometimes signs of Vincent's angina), and acute leukemia (swollen, thickened gums which may be bleeding or pur- plish in color). In the leukemias, sternal tenderness may be quite pronounced.

The discovery of very great enlargement of the spleen tends to rule out the acute splenic tumor of various sys- temic infections, although sometimes the spleen may ex- tend 4 to 6 cm below the costal margin in septicemia and in subacute bacterial endocarditis. Huge spleens are en- countered in the chronic leukemias, in the Banti syn- drome, in kala-azar, in schistosomiasis, in Gaucher's dis- ease, in Hodgkin's disease and lymphosarcoma, in myelo- fibrosis, and in many instances of chronic hemolytic ane- mia.

Examination of the blood may indicate at once the nature of the disorder, as in malaria, the frank leukemias, or infectious mononucleosis. The discovery of icterus will lead to a reticulocyte count, examination of the stools and urine for the products of blood destruction, an eryth- rocyte fragility test, and other studies (see Chap. 338) to rule out the various hemolytic anemias. The discovery of leukopenia should lead to the consideration of malaria, "aleukemic" leukemia, the Banti syndrome, typhoid fever, histoplasmosis, and leishmaniasis, but it must be kept in mind that the white cell count may sometimes be low also in infectious mononucleosis and in some cases of chronic hemolytic anemia. The demonstration of throm- bocytopenia, as well as prolonged bleeding time, poor clot retraction, and positive tourniquet test, is an important finding, for it suggests acute leukemia. In that condition immature leukocytes will be found in the blood. In the "aleukemic" form, immature cells are absent from the

blood or very scarce, but they are readily demonstrated by sternal puncture. In idiopathic thrombocytopenic pur- pura, the spleen is barely palpable in about 33 percent of cases, but it is never very large. Thrombocytopenia only very rarely accompanies infectious mononucleosis and, while present in other conditions such as pernicious anemia, chronic hypochromic anemia, chronic hemolytic anemias, myelophthisic anemia, the Banti syndrome, Hodgkin's disease, and the related lymph node disorders, it is rarely severe in these diseases.

Sternal puncture may be very helpful if "aleukemic" leukemia, leishmaniasis, or Gaucher's disease is being con- sidered seriously, for the characteristic cells or causative organisms may be demonstrated in this way. Sternal puncture does not often reveal malaria when the parasites have eluded careful study of the blood, but sometimes positive blood cultures for bacteria are obtained by this means when the usual method has failed. Splenic punc- ture is helpful when parasites, storage cells, signs of mye- loid metaplasia, or granulomas are found, but this pro- cedure should not be undertaken when hemorrhagic man- ifestations are present or in the absence of evidence of distinct splenic enlargement.

Various disorders of the spleen are discussed in a later chapter (Chap. 350).

REFERENCES

Jandl, J. H., and R. H. Aster: Increased Splenic Pooling and the Pathogenesis of Hypersplenism, Am. J. Med. Sci. 253:383–398, 1967.

McIntyre, O. R., and F. G. Ebaugh, Jr.: Palpable Spleens in College Freshmen, Ann. Intern. Med. 66:301–306, 1967.

Saltzstein, S. L., and L. V. Ackerman: Lymphadenopathy In- duced by Anticonvulsant Drugs, Cancer, 12:164, 1959.

Wintrobe, M. M.: "Clinical Hematology," 6th ed., Philadel- phia, Lea & Febiger, 1967.

64 ALTERATIONS IN LEUKOCYTES
Dane R. Boggs and M. M. Wintrobe

Unlike the red corpuscles, the leukocytes do not carry out their chief functions in the circulating blood. For them the circulation is mainly a transport system through which they pass from the sites where they are formed to the locations where they are needed. The time that the leukocytes spend in the blood does not reflect their life span, and exact life spans for different types of leukocytes are not known. Their fate, like that of soldiers, probably depends as much on external factors as on the ultimate wearing out of internal metabolic activities.

Little is known about the factors which normally main- tain the leukocyte count and the proportion of different types of leukocytes within a rather narrow range of values, nor is much known about the factors which cause these to change. However, it has been possible

Table 64-1. NORMAL VALUES FOR CONCENTRATION*
OF BLOOD LEUKOCYTES

Cell type	Mean (cells per cu mm)	95% Confidence limits (cells per cu mm)
Neutrophil........	3,650	1,830–7,250
Lymphocyte......	2,500	1,500–4,000
Monocyte........	430	200–950
Eosinophil........	150	0–700
Basophil..........	30	0–150

* Total leukocyte counts from venous blood samples were done in a "Coulter counter," and 200 leukocytes were differentiated on Wright's stained blood smears made on cover glass.

to infer a great deal about the functions of the leukocytes by observing the alterations which are associated with various physiologic states and with different disease entities. In many respects the leukocyte and differential counts serve as mirrors which reflect changes taking place in the body, and thereby, these determinations have proved to be of immense value in differential diagnosis.

The only known function of the leukocytic systems is to defend the body from foreign material by means of phagocytosis and antibody formation. These are interrelated functions; phagocytosis is enhanced by the presence of antibody specific for the substance being phagocytized, and phagocytosis of antigen may be an initiating step in antibody production. Neutrophils, monocytes, eosinophils and basophils are phagocytes, while lymphocytes and plasma cells are concerned with antibody production. Each of these six types of leukocytes probably plays a distinct and unique role in body defense mechanisms, although the role of basophils and eosinophils is unclear.

The concentration in blood of each specific type of

leukocyte is a much more meaningful value than is total white cell count (total leukocyte concentration). The mean and 95 percent confidence limits of various blood leukocytes as found in 291 prisoners from the Utah State Prison are given in Table 64-1. The number of eosinophils and basophils in the blood is so small that the normal range encompasses zero. Thus, eosinopenia and basopenia cannot be determined from results of routine blood examination.

In this chapter current concepts of the physiology of each of the leukocytic systems will be reviewed, and the diagnostic and clinical significance of changes in the concentration of the various blood leukocytes will be considered.

THE PHAGOCYTIC SYSTEM

Neutrophils

NEUTROPHIL PHYSIOLOGY

During the first half of the last century a number of investigators noted that leukocytes within the confines of blood vessels often are marginated along venule and capillary walls. Modern techniques have made it possible to show that in man approximately one-half of the intravascular neutrophils are marginated and one-half circulate freely (Fig. 64-1B). Blood neutrophil concentration, as determined in venous samples, measures the circulating but not the marginal pool.

Neutrophils enter the blood from a storage reservoir in the bone marrow and leave the blood in random fashion after an average intravascular sojourn of 10 hr (Fig. 64-1A). They do not return to the blood after leaving it. There are many more neutrophils and neutrophil precursors in the bone marrow than are present in the blood. Bone marrow neutrophils consist of two pools of cells, the mitotic production pool and the postmitotic maturation and storage pool (Fig. 64-2). Morphologic subdivisions within these pools necessarily are somewhat arbitrary. The production pool can be considered as consisting of three compartments of increasing maturity: myeloblasts, promyelocytes, and myelocytes. The postmitotic maturation and storage pool consists of metamyelocytes, "bands" or "juveniles," and segmented neutrophils. Under ordinary circumstances, metamyelocytes are not released to the blood. Bands and segmented neutrophils are readily released to the blood, although segmented neutrophils are released in preference to bands. These cells constitute the storage compartment of bone marrow neutrophils.

From this marrow reserve of neutrophils the rate of cell entry to the blood can be accelerated upon demand before an increase in the rate of cell production occurs. In normal individuals there are enough postmitotic neutrophils to replace those in the blood for approximately 10 days at normal rates of marrow release. Approximately 60 percent of the postmitotic neutrophil pool of normal marrow consists of bands and segmented neutrophils. Thus the effective storage reservoir is approximately 15 times as large as the blood pool (Fig. 64-2).

The fate of neutrophils leaving the blood has not been

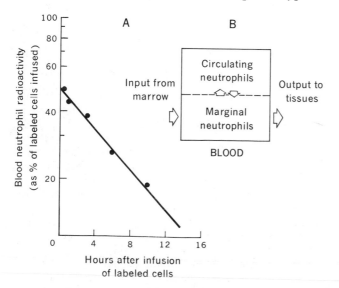

Fig. 64-1. Disappearance of ^{32}DFP-labeled neutrophils in a normal subject (*A*) and a model of blood neutrophil kinetics (*B*).

Fig. 64-2. Diagrammatic model of neutrophil kinetics. Neutrophils share with platelets and erythrocytes a common precursor (pluripotential stem cell). The marrow mitotic pool is the site of production. The postmitotic pool consists of cells which continue to mature (metamyelocytes and bands) and a marrow reserve of mature neutrophils. From this, cells enter the blood for a brief sojourn on their way to tissues and body cavities. Only the circulating pool is measured in the traditional leukocyte count of the blood. Data for the size of the system and the transit times through various compartments are based upon studies of neutrophils labeled with radio-active diisopropyl fluorophosphate in normal volunteers from the Utah State Prison. Cell ratios, indicated by the numbers posted on each compartment, are based upon 500 cell differential counts of neutrophils and neutrophil precursors in smears of marrow aspirates from 12 such volunteers.

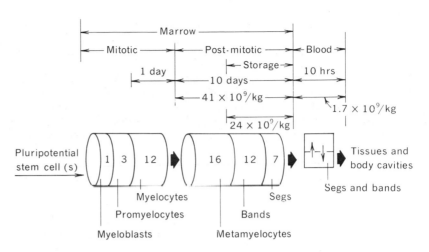

entirely clarified. In a normal subject, neutrophils appear in bronchial secretions, in urine, and in the lumen of the gut. Whether these sites of egress account for the majority of neutrophils leaving the blood each day or represent but a small proportion of these cells is not known. Following initiation of tissue injury, neutrophils marginate along the walls of the capillaries and venules adjacent to the injured area and by diapedesis traverse the intervening tissue. They enter the area of beginning exudate formation within 1 or 2 hr following the inflammatory stimulus. Diapedesis takes place between endothelial cells of the blood vessel. Neutrophils are delayed for some time at the basement membrane and then move in a seemingly directed fashion through the intervening tissue to enter the exudate. Turnover of neutrophils through an established exudate is almost as rapid as the turnover of neutrophils through the blood.

Neutropenia and neutrophilia may develop by a variety of kinetic mechanisms. Transient changes in blood neutrophil concentration may develop without any change in the rate at which cells enter or leave the blood; rapid shifts of cells between marginal and circulating pools can take place. Since this mechanism does not induce a change in the total number of neutrophils in the confines of the vascular system, it may be designated as producing "pseudoneutrophilia," or "pseudoneutropenia." Strenuous exercise or the administration of epinephrine and perhaps a variety of other stimuli leads to transient demargination of neutrophils with a brief but sometimes striking episode of neutrophilia.

Persistent neutrophilia is usually accompanied by an accelerated rate of entry of new cells from the bone marrow and is of necessity accompanied by increased production. Conversely, in most instances of persistent neutropenia, the storage pool of the bone marrow is exhausted, and usually, production is found to be decreased.

However, changes in egress of neutrophils from the blood can also be the primary cause of changes in blood neutrophil concentration. Administration of pharmacologic doses of hydrocortisone induces neutrophilia, at least in part by reducing the rate of cell loss from the blood. Certain instances of neutropenia, such as those

induced by overwhelming infection, by injection of endotoxin, or by administration of antineutrophil antibody, reflect a very marked acceleration in the rate of cell loss from the blood. This acceleration is so great that input from the marrow and increased production cannot keep pace, and neutropenia develops primarily because of accelerated cell loss.

NEUTROPHILIA

An increase in blood neutrophil concentration accompanies most *bacterial infections*. With the exception of a few diseases, such as tuberculosis, brucellosis, and typhoid fever, neutrophilia develops during the inception and persists through the acute phases of bacterial infection. Neutrophilia may be present in some fungal infections, such as actinomycosis; a few viral infections, such as rabies and herpes zoster; and a variety of parasitic and rickettsial infestations. The highest neutrophil levels, often exceeding 30,000 per cu mm, commonly are observed in pneumococcal pneumonia or with localized abscesses. Neutrophilia may not persist as infections become chronic. In some chronic infections, such as bacterial endocarditis and pyelonephritis, neutrophil concentration may be normal.

The presence or absence of neutrophilia is a useful diagnostic sign, and serial determination of neutrophil concentration provides prognostic information during the course of infection. The proportion of blood neutrophils which are not segmented (band/segmented ratio) is of equal or even greater diagnostic and prognostic significance. In the early stages of infection the rate of release of neutrophils from the marrow storage pool to the blood is accelerated in response to demand for phagocytes at the infected site. As the storage pool is reduced, a greater proportion of bands is released, and the band/segmented ratio in the blood increases, leading to a moderate "shift to the left." As the infection is controlled, or as it stabilizes, the demand for neutrophils is reduced or marrow production accelerates to meet continued increased demands. In these circumstances neutrophilia may persist for some time, but as the marrow storage pool is reconstituted, the band/segmented ratio returns toward normal.

On the other hand, if the infection is spreading, the demand for neutrophils may steadily increase and may exceed the ability of the marrow to increase production, so that the storage pool either remains small or may actually become exhausted. In such a patient the shift to the left becomes increasingly more pronounced. Thus the characteristic pattern of early infection is neutrophilia with a modest shift to the left; of healing or well-controlled infection, neutrophilia with little or no cell immaturity; and of severe continuing infection, neutrophilia or even neutropenia with an increasing proportion of bands in the blood.

The magnitude of neutrophilia varies with its cause, being greater as a rule in localized in contrast to systemic infections and in highly virulent infections in otherwise healthy patients as compared with debilitated individuals.

The *transient episodes of neutrophilia* induced by injecting *epinephrine* or by *strenuous exercise* are due to demargination of intravascular neutrophils and are not attended by any change in the band/segmented neutrophil ratio. It is likely that the brief episodes of neutrophilia which are observed in such conditions as *paroxysmal tachycardia, convulsive seizures,* and *delirium tremens* are the result of demargination.

Neutrophilia accompanying many other noninfectious processes probably is produced by accelerating the rate of release of marrow neutrophils, since a modest increase in band/segmented ratio is observed as the neutrophilia develops. This is seen following *acute hemorrhage* and in *acute hemolytic anemia.* The neutrophilia which develops in many diseases can be attributed to the influence of a combination of factors. In some, such as acute *gout, myocardial infarction* or *pulmonary embolism* and *infarction, burns,* and *spider* and *snake bites,* the stimulus for neutrophilia is tissue damage, inflammation, and sterile exudate formation. From what is known about the effects of pharmacologic doses of *hydrocortisone,* described above, it is likely that increased hydrocortisone blood levels, whether resulting from increased production due to stress or decreased degradation, as in hepatic failure, may be, at least in part, responsible for the neutrophilia. Patients with *Cushing's disease* often have mild neutrophilia.

Neutrophilia also is seen in *diabetic acidosis, uremia, eclampsia,* in *Hodgkin's disease,* and sometimes in association with rapidly growing malignant neoplasms. The excessive production of neutrophils, eosinophils, basophils, and platelets, as well as of erythrocytes, so characteristic of *polycythemia vera* may be due to an abnormally functioning pluripotent stem cell compartment.

Unexplained or extreme *neutrophilia* or significant numbers of myelocytes and metamyelocytes and other immature cells in the blood suggests leukemia. The diagnosis of leukemia and its differentiation from "leukemoid reactions" is considered in Chap. 348.

NEUTROPENIA

Neutropenia may be present when the white count (total leukocyte concentration) is decreased, normal, or increased. It should be obvious that the percentage of neutrophils in differential leukocyte counts is relatively meaningless unless it is multiplied by the total leukocyte count to obtain neutrophil concentration.

CLINICAL MANIFESTATIONS. Of itself, neutropenia causes no symptoms unless infection supervenes. However, patients with neutropenia of any cause may suffer from frequent and severe bacterial infections. When neutropenia is related to some disease, the clinical manifestations will be those of the underlying disorder.

The decrease in resistance to infection which attends neutropenia was dramatically exemplified by the syndrome of *agranulocytosis* or *agranulocytic angina,* first recognized in 1922. This disorder is characterized by severe sore throat, marked prostration, and extreme reduction or even complete disappearance of the neutrophils from the blood. Although there may be a prodromal period marked by malaise or moderate fever, the onset is usually acute and fulminating. When first described, agranulocytosis often ended in sepsis and death. It was later recognized that the appearance of this syndrome corresponded with the introduction of certain coal-tar derivatives as therapeutic agents, in particular the antipyretic, aminopyrine (Pyramidon). The course of events was shown to consist of (1) neutropenia; (2) loss of resistance to infection, development of sore throat; and (3) overwhelming sepsis and death. Recognition of the etiologic basis of the syndrome, prohibition of further use of the offending drug, and prompt antibiotic therapy have greatly altered the prognosis.

The symptoms and physical signs directly attributable to neutropenia of any cause are those produced by the infections which attend neutropenia. Infection usually begins in the skin, especially the perineal and axillary areas, the throat, or the lungs, but may be first noted in virtually any area of the body. Initial infections usually are due to common bacteria such as pneumococci, staphylococci, streptococci, and coliform organisms. In patients with recurrent infections, or in patients who receive repetitive courses of antibiotics, more unusual organisms and those resistant to antibiotics, such as *Pseudomonas,* are observed, and infection with fungi, such as *Candida,* becomes more common. With very severe neutropenia infections spread rapidly and bacteremia is common. Patients with a small but significant number of neutrophils in the blood often suffer from chronic, indolent infections which can be contained with proper local and systemic measures but often defy complete cure.

The relationship between the severity of neutropenia and the frequency of infection is far from exact. However, as a general statement, patients with idiopathic neutropenia rarely develop life-threatening infections unless the neutrophil concentration is less than 1,000 per cu mm. In patients with a count of less than 500, this complication is usually observed.

Absolute numbers of monocytes and eosinophils may be increased, and hypergammaglobulinemia is present in some patients with neutropenia. These changes may be due to a physiologic response of other protective systems in compensation for the decreased resistance to infection secondary to the neutropenia or may merely represent the reaction to repeated or chronic infections. Blood lymphocyte concentration is quite variable and may be decreased, normal, or increased.

ETIOLOGY. Neutropenia may exist as an isolated hematologic abnormality or may be associated with anemia and/or thrombocytopenia. All of the causes of aplastic anemia (Chap. 341) are also causes of neutropenia. The major causes of neutropenia can be categorized as (1) drug induced, (2) secondary to known diseases (or syndromes), (3) familial, (4) antibody induced, and (5) idiopathic. Examples of each are given in Table 64-2.

Table 64-2. CAUSES OF NEUTROPENIA

I. Drugs and physical agents (see Table 64-3)
II. Diseases
   A. Infections
      1. Bacterial, e.g., overwhelming infections of any type; also certain other, not necessarily overwhelming infections, e.g., typhoid, paratyphoid, brucella
      2. Viral and rickettsial, e.g., influenza, measles, rubella, hepatitis, Colorado tick fever, psittacosis
   B. Nutritional deficiency, e.g., starvation, selective deficiency of folic acid or vitamin B_{12}
   C. Hematopoietic diseases, e.g., acute leukemia, chronic lymphocytic leukemia, lymphosarcoma, aplastic anemia, paroxysmal nocturnal hemoglobinuria, thymic alymphoplasia, deficient immunoglobulin production
   D. Diseases producing splenomegaly, e.g., congestive splenomegaly, Gaucher's disease, Felty's syndrome
   E. Other diseases, e.g., lupus erythematosus, pancreatic exocrine deficiency
III. Familial chronic neutropenia
IV. Antibody induced neutropenia, e.g., autoantibodies and transplacental antibodies
V. Idiopathic neutropenic syndromes, e.g., cyclic neutropenia, hypoplastic neutropenia, hyperplastic neutropenia

Neutropenia induced by *drugs or by physical agents*, such as x-ray, is probably the most common form of neutropenia (Table 64-3). Drugs which induce neutropenia can be divided into two broad classes, those in which neutropenia can be expected if enough of the drug is given and those in which neutropenia is an unpredictable, "hypersensitivity" reaction. Neutropenia is a common side effect of antitumor therapy, since the alkylating agents, antimetabolites, stathmokinetic agents (those which poison the mitotic spindle, thereby leading to cell death in metaphase), and x-ray (Chap. 348 and 351) all produce neutropenia if given in sufficient dosage. This effect appears to be due to a decrease in neutrophil production, and recovery will usually follow discontinuation of the drug. Certain chemicals, such as benzene, can be added to the above list of agents which produce dose-related neutropenia.

In addition to those listed in Table 64-3, many other drugs have been suspected as a cause of neutropenia. Neutropenia with certain of the above drugs has been accompanied by virtual absence of neutrophil precursors from the bone marrow, while with others mitotic neutrophil precursors have been abundant in marrow aspirates.

Thus it appears that different pathogenetic mechanisms, increased destruction and decreased production, are involved in hypersensitivity reactions.

Certain drugs, notably aminopyrine, appear to destroy mature neutrophils by an immunologic mechanism in sensitized patients. Patients who have recovered from aminopyrine-induced neutropenia become neutropenic again within a few hours following administration of a very small challenging dose of the drug. Blood, withdrawn from such patients 3 hr after a test dose of the drug, induces transient neutropenia when transfused into normal subjects.

Table 64-3. DRUGS AND PHYSICAL AGENTS
PRODUCING NEUTROPENIA

Group I—regularly produce neutropenia if given in sufficient amounts
  Physical agents:
    Radiation with roentgen rays, gamma rays, beta rays, and neutrons.
  Antitumor drugs:
    Alkylating agents (nitrogen mustard, busulfan, chlorambucil, cyclophosphamide, etc.), antimetabolites (methotrexate, 6-mercaptopurine, etc.), stathmokinetics (vinblastine, etc.), antibiotics (daunomycin, etc.).
  Benzene
  Colchicine
Group II—produce leukopenia in "sensitive" persons only
  Analgesics (aminopyrine, dipyrone, phenylbutazone, etc.)
  Phenothiazines (chlorpromazine, promazine, mepazine, etc.)
  Antithyroid drugs (thiouracil, methimazole, etc.)
  Anticonvulsants (trimethadione, phethenylate, etc.)
  Sulfonamides and derivatives [carbutamide, sulfisoxazole (Gantrisin) etc.]
  Antihistamines (Pyribenzamine, etc.)
  Antimicrobial agents (organic arsenicals, chloramphenicol)
  Tranquilizers (meprobamate, etc.)
  Miscellaneous (dinitrophenol, gold salts, etc.)

Neutropenia associated with sensitivity to such drugs as the phenothiazines apparently is due to interference with neutrophil production in the bone marrow rather than to destruction of mature neutrophils. In such cases few or no neutrophil precursors are demonstrable in the bone marrow. The phenothiazine, chlorpromazine, inhibits in vitro nucleic acid synthesis of suspensions of marrow cells.

Many classes of disease are associated with neutropenia (Table 64-2). Mild neutropenia is common in a variety of *viral and protozoal infections* and in infections such as typhoid fever and brucellosis. Neutropenia may also be observed in response to acute, severe, bacterial infections in which neutrophilia is the rule. In the last circumstance neutropenia should be viewed as a very poor prognostic sign for recovery from the infection. In experimental studies of induced pneumococcal pneumonia in dogs, neutropenia developed only in those animals in which the infection was so overwhelming that the marrow reserve of neutrophils was exhausted. If an infected patient runs out of phagocytes, a poor prognosis can be expected. Such patients are not only neutropenic, but very few of their remaining neutrophils are fully mature.

Neutropenia often accompanies *diseases of the hematopoietic system* (Table 64-2). Neutropenia was reported to be the first hematologic change in rare instances of copper deficiency in infants, and mild neutropenia occasionally accompanies severe iron-deficiency anemia. Neutropenia may accompany deficient immunoglobulin production (Chap. 69).

A number of children with pancreatic exocrine insufficiency which is not due to cystic fibrosis also have neutropenia. Since neutropenia is not common in cystic fibrosis, the relationship of the pancreatic dysfunction to the neutropenia is unclear.

Removal of the spleen leads to transient neutrophilia, and in certain diseases the presence of neutropenia seems to be correlated with an *enlarged spleen*. Patients with cirrhosis of the liver often have neutrophilia, but when the spleen is congested and enlarged as a result of increased portal pressure in cirrhosis, neutropenia is more common. Congestive splenomegaly of any cause and splenomegaly due to such diseases as Gaucher's disease may be associated with neutropenia. Neutropenia is rarely observed in rheumatoid arthritis unless the spleen is enlarged (Felty's syndrome). In other diseases, such as systemic lupus erythematosus, the presence of neutropenia correlates poorly with the presence of splenomegaly. The role of the spleen in neutrophil kinetics remains to be clarified, but it is likely that in certain of the above circumstances the spleen traps and destroys an abnormally large number of neutrophils.

Familial neutropenia probably exists in at least two forms: severe neutropenia inherited as an autosomal recessive trait, and a milder form inherited as an autosomal dominant.

Antineutrophil antibodies developing in the absence of such drugs as aminopyrine (autoimmune antineutrophil antibodies) may be responsible for many instances of idiopathic neutropenia, but there is no fully satisfactory in vitro test for detecting their presence. The observation that children born of neutropenic mothers may suffer from transient neutropenia suggests the presence of such antibodies.

Transient neonatal neutropenia also has been observed in children born of multiparous mothers without neutropenia. This suggests that maternal sensitization to fetal neutrophil antigens may occur, resulting in a situation somewhat analagous to erythroblastosis fetalis.

Idiopathic forms of neutropenia are separable into various syndromes, but none of these syndromes is common, and none is very well understood. Neutropenia occurring in regular cycles and sometimes persisting for years has been reported in a number of patients. In some instances the neutropenia has recurred at roughly 3-week intervals. In others the intervals were longer or more irregular. Such cycling of blood levels suggests a disturbance in the regulatory mechanism for neutrophil production. Other examples of chronic idiopathic neutropenia include those with few or no neutrophil precursors (*hypoplastic*) and those with abundant neutrophil precursors in the bone marrow (*hyperplastic neutropenia*).

KINETIC MECHANISM OF NEUTROPENIA. The changes in neutrophil kinetics which can lead to neutropenia are indicated in Fig. 64-3. Blood and/or bone marrow neutrophils can be labeled with radioactive diisopropyl fluorophosphate, and from such in vivo studies the rate of neutrophil production, destruction, blood and marrow transit times, and the sizes of the circulating and marginal pools can be determined. Short-term cultures of bone marrow can be used to study rates of maturation or of proliferation as judged by incorporation of tritiated thymidine into DNA of neutrophil precursors. Neutrophil migration from the blood into induced inflammatory exudates on the skin can be measured. Administration of epinephrine results in demargination of blood neutrophils, and the resultant increase in neutrophil concentration in venous blood samples provides a rough estimate of the size of the marginal pool. Administration of endotoxin, etiocholanolone, or hydrocortisone "flushes" neutrophils from the marrow storage pool into the blood. If the expected increase in blood neutrophil concentration following administration of these drugs does not take place, it is assumed that the patient's storage pool is exhausted.

Either increased cell loss with compensatory increase in production or decreased production can result in exhaustion of the marrow storage pool. In either case, most

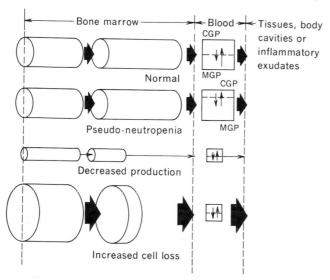

Fig. 64-3. Changes in neutrophil kinetics resulting in neutropenia. The bone marrow is represented as two connected tubes which contain the mitotic and postmitotic compartments, as described in Fig. 64-2. The diameters of the tubes reflect the sizes of the pools, and their length represents their morphologic integrity. The normal neutrophil system is shown at the top of the figure, and three types of change in the system which may lead to neutropenia are illustrated diagrammatically below. In pseudoneutropenia there is a change in the ratio of the circulating (CGP)/marginal (MGP) pools, but the bone marrow is normal. Both when there is decreased production or increased cell loss, the storage compartment of the postmitotic pool is drained, leaving only young metamyelocytes. However, the mitotic pools differ greatly in size in these two neutropenic states.

of the neutrophils in the blood will be "bands." If the bone marrow is examined in these patients, the ratio of mitotic to postmitotic neutrophil precursors is found to be increased. Assuming that the patient is not anemic, the myeloid/erythroid ratio of the bone marrow should distinguish between an increase or a decrease in the size of the marrow mitotic pool of neutrophils. With neutropenia due to increased cell loss, abundant mitotic neutrophil precursors and metamyelocytes should be observed in the bone marrow, producing a pattern which has been termed *maturation arrest*. This is a misnomer because such a pattern probably signifies the reverse of maturation arrest; except in leukemia, it reflects a marrow in which the storage pool is exhausted and from which bands are released to the blood as soon as they are formed.

Careful examination of the blood smear is very useful in interpreting kinetic changes in patients with neutropenia. If the storage pool is exhausted, band form neutrophils are released to the blood as soon as they are formed, and very few will have had time to mature into segmented neutrophils. In this circumstance there will be an increase in the band/segmented cell ratio in the blood. In contrast, if pseudoneutropenia resulting from increased margination of neutrophils along vessel walls is present, the band/segmented cell ratio in blood should be normal.

THERAPY. There is no known method of therapy which will safely and reproducibly accelerate the rate of neutrophil production in a neutropenic patient. Administration of such agents as bacterial endotoxin leads to an accelerated rate of neutrophil production in experimental animals and probably in normal man. However, this acceleration of production appears to be a physiologic response to the acute neutrophil depletion induced by endotoxin. Neutropenic patients would be expected to be under maximal or near maximal stimulation of neutrophil production through normal physiologic mechanisms. Through the years a number of agents have been reported as efficacious in the therapy of neutropenia, but to date none can be considered to be of proven benefit.

If the patient is receiving any drugs or has been exposed to any other agents which might possibly be injurious, further exposure to these drugs and agents should be avoided. Drug-induced neutropenia usually responds to discontinuance of the offending agent, although a few patients die of infection before recovery can occur, and a few others develop chronic neutropenia for reasons which are not clear.

Neutropenia secondary to known diseases such as those listed in Table 64-2 improves or is corrected if general improvement in the disease is brought about.

In a limited proportion of cases of neutropenia, improvement has followed splenectomy, particularly in cases with splenomegaly; for example, in patients with congestive splenomegaly secondary to obstruction in the portal circulation. However, the advisability of the operation must be weighed in the light of the many other problems and complications which may develop. At present there is no means of predicting which patients will respond favorably to splenectomy. Experience with splenectomy in patients who have few neutrophil precursors observable in the bone marrow and who do not have palpable spleens has generally been unfavorable. Only a few of the reported splenectomized cases of idiopathic neutropenia have benefited from the procedure.

Pharmacologic doses of corticosteroids induce neutrophilia in normal human subjects but do so in part by reducing the rate of cell egress from the blood, and such therapy has little or no effect on the rate of neutrophil production. Administration of 40 mg prednisone per day to normal human subjects reduces the number of neutrophils migrating into induced inflammatory exudates to about 10 percent of normal despite doubling of the number of neutrophils in the blood. Even in some patients with neutropenia blood neutrophils may increase with corticosteroid therapy. However, if the mechanism of increase in these patients is the same as it is in normal subjects, the neutrophil increase in the blood is at the expense of neutrophil outflow to the tissues. In that event, steroid therapy would have to be looked upon as dangerous in neutropenic patients.

ALTERATIONS IN NEUTROPHIL MORPHOLOGY AND FUNCTION

MORPHOLOGIC ABNORMALITIES. Microscopically identifiable abnormalities of neutrophils characterize or are associated with a variety of inherited conditions. Most patients, such as those with hereditary hyposegmentation (Pelger-Huët anomaly), hereditary hypersegmentation, or increased, fat-containing azurophilic granulation (Alder's anomaly), do not suffer from frequent infections. It is reasonable to assume that these anomalies do not interfere significantly with neutrophil function. On the other hand, patients who inherit the *Chediak-Higashi syndrome* usually die in childhood of fulminant infection. This anomaly, characterized by the presence of enormous granules (giant lysosomes) in neutrophils and in other leukocytes, is inherited as an autosomal recessive and is associated with partial albinism, hepatosplenomegaly, and development of lymphoid neoplasms. The anomalous leukocytes phagocytize bacteria in an apparently normal fashion. However, the giant lysosomes seem to be functionally defective in killing bacteria, thus reducing the resistance of these patients to infection. Also in the *May-Hegglin anomaly* (cytoplasmic crescent- or spindle-shaped inclusions, dominantly inherited) leukocyte dysfunction at inflammatory sites has been described.

CHRONIC GRANULOMATOUS DISEASE OF CHILDHOOD. Neutrophils of normal morphologic appearance but with decreased ability to kill phagocytized bacteria appear to be responsible for this syndrome. Recurrent infections with bacteria of low virulence develop shortly after birth, and death due to sepsis occurs before adulthood. Chronic lymphadenitis and infected eczematoid dermatitis are usually found in these children. The name of the disease is derived from the granulomas observed in lymph nodes, lungs, liver, spleen, and other viscera. Most patients with the syndrome have been males, and inheritance appears to be sex linked. However, two girls with normal families have been described, and thus, there may be more than one form of disease responsible for this syndrome. Neutrophils from these patients phagocytize bacteria normally, but certain types of bacteria survive for an abnormally long time after being phagocytized. The exact defect in lysosome-phagocytic vacuole interaction in the neutrophils has not been determined.

The environment of the neutrophil may limit its bactericidal capacities. Phagocytosis of bacteria by neutrophils in vitro is inhibited by high concentrations of glucose in the suspending medium. The inhibitory concentrations are within the range of glucose observed in patients with *diabetic acidosis*. The propensity of such patients for developing bacterial infection possibly is explained by inhibition of phagocytosis.

Monocytes

The origin of the monocyte and its relationship to tissue macrophages have been the subject of long-standing controversy. However, recent studies suggest that most exudate macrophages are derived from blood monocytes and that blood monocytes are in turn derived from the bone marrow. Monocyte precursors have not been identified morphologically. Cogent arguments can be raised suggesting their origin from lymphoid or granulocytic systems.

Monocytes migrate into inflammatory exudates at a slower rate and/or in a later phase of inflammation than do neutrophils. Monocyte maturation continues in the inflamed tissue, and the monocyte enlarges, synthesizes enzymes, and assumes the morphologic and chemical characteristics of a macrophage. Macrophages are avid phagocytes and probably play a scavenging role, clearing the exudate of dead neutrophils and other debris in addition to engulfing and killing bacteria.

Macrophages may play some role in the initiation of antibody production under certain circumstances, although there is little to suggest that the monocyte itself is capable of antibody production (Chap. 68). Soluble and particulate antigens are pinocytized and phagocytized by macrophages. Small lymphocytes accumulate around the antigen-bearing macrophage and some form of transfer of antigen or antigen-related material occurs.

Monocytosis is often observed in chronic inflammatory disorders due to infection (tuberculosis, subacute bacterial endocarditis, brucellosis) or other causes, during recovery from infection, in many protozoan (e.g., malaria, trypanosomiasis) and some rickettsial infections (Rocky Mountain spotted fever), in some patients with Hodgkin's disease, and in patients with neutropenia.

Eosinophils

Knowledge concerning the physiology and function of eosinophils is fragmentary. The site of eosinophil production is the bone marrow. If the eosinophilic cells of rodents are the same types of cells as the eosinophils of man, the kinetics of eosinophils probably are similar to those of neutrophils. Eosinophils migrate into induced

inflammatory exudates in man, and eosinophil/neutrophil ratios in the exudate approximate those in the blood.

A modest degree of *eosinophilia* (from 600 to 2,000 eosinophils per cu mm) is common in overtly allergic conditions such as seasonal hay fever and asthma, in some skin diseases such as pemphigus, in a variety of parasitic infestations, and in such diseases as periarteritis nodosa. It is also seen in Hodgkin's disease and in Addison's disease. Hereditary eosinophilia, unassociated with overt disease, has been described.

Marked eosinophilia, up to and even exceeding 50,000 eosinophils per cu mm, has been observed in an occasional patient with carcinoma, during acute phases of tissue invasion with parasites such as *Trichina,* and in idiopathic states described as Loeffler's syndrome, tropical eosinophilia, pulmonary infiltration with eosinophilia, and eosinophilic leukemia (Chap. 348).

Eosinophilia usually is present in chronic myelocytic leukemia, myelofibrosis, and polycythemia vera. In these diseases the degree of eosinophilia often parallels the degree of neutrophilia, although in an occasional patient the eosinophilia may be so striking as to overshadow other leukocytic changes. The presence of eosinophilia is useful in distinguishing chronic myelocytic leukemia from leukemoid reactions and polycythemia vera from secondary polycythemia.

During acute bacterial infections eosinophils usually disappear from the blood. Hydrocortisone is known to produce transient eosinopenia.

Basophils

This least common member of the family of normal blood leukocytes is even less well understood than the eosinophil. Whether it is closely related or entirely distinct from tissue mast cells is unclear. However, these two cells are both rich in histamine and may play a role in the allergic response.

Elevated blood basophil concentration is commonly observed in chronic myelocytic leukemia, myelofibrosis, and polycythemia vera. Basophilia is a useful diagnostic sign in distinguishing chronic myelocytic leukemia and polycythemia vera from leukemoid reactions and secondary forms of polycythemia, respectively. A modest increase in basophils may be observed in myxedema, ulcerative colitis, and other chronic inflammatory diseases.

IMMUNOCYTES

Lymphocytes and plasma cells are concerned with the production of antibody rather than with phagocytosis. The exact relationship of plasma cells to lymphocytes is unsettled, but it seems probable that the plasma cell develops directly from the lymphoid system as a specialized cell concerned with the production of circulating antibody.

LYMPHOCYTE KINETICS

Most of the small lymphocytes of the blood, thoracic duct, and lymph nodes constitute a relatively long-lived population, while lymphocytes in the thymus, in the germinal centers of lymph nodes, and in the bone marrow are relatively short-lived. How long the long-lived population may survive without dividing is indicated by studies in patients who have been irradiated. Chromosome defects of a type which induce cell death upon division can be detected for a number of years following therapeutic irradiation. From such studies an estimate of an average intermitotic time of more than a year has been derived.

Lymphocytes do not remain in the blood for this long a period of time but seem to migrate from blood to lymphoid tissue and back to the blood. Vascular exit is through specialized cells in the postcapillary venules of lymph nodes. In the node, recirculating lymphocytes constitute the majority of cells in the cuff surrounding the germinal centers, and from this cuff they migrate into lymph channels and reenter the blood through the thoracic duct or the right lymphatic duct. The number of lymphocytes entering the blood from the thoracic duct is sufficient to replace the total number in the blood several times each day. Such a recirculatory pattern for cells is indicative of very complex cellular kinetics. Any shift or change in the recirculatory pattern at any point in the circuit can induce a profound change in the concentration of lymphocytes in the blood. However, a change in the rate of lymphocyte production may or may not be reflected by a change in blood lymphocyte concentration, and certainly no conclusions can be drawn concerning lymphocyte production from blood levels. The independence of blood lymphocyte levels in relation to events occurring elsewhere in the lymphocyte system is most dramatically illustrated by the pattern of lymphocyte changes which often accompanies hydrocortisone therapy of chronic lymphocytic leukemia. Therapeutic doses of hydrocortisone and its derivatives usually lead to a reduction of the total number of lymphocytes within the body, but for the first few weeks of therapy blood lymphocyte concentration increases.

Injected antigen is delivered to lymph nodes via lymphatics, when it becomes attached to reticular surfaces in the cortex of the node or may be phagocytized by macrophages in the medulla. A new antigen or the product of antigen cellular interaction stimulates conversion of small "uncommitted" lymphocytes to large cells synthesizing DNA. These large blastlike cells may be capable of antibody production or they or their progeny may mature into plasma cells or lymphocytes specialized for antibody production. Immunoglobulins are synthesized by plasma cells as well as by cells which are morphologically similar to the large lymphocyte. Certain studies suggest that most 7s immunoglobin is produced by plasma cells while most 19s immunoglobin is produced by large lymphocytes.

From such cellular proliferation in response to an antigenic challenge, a small lymphocyte eventually emerges. This small lymphocyte is not concerned directly with producing antibody, but carries the capacity ("immunologic memory") to produce a specific antibody. Small lymphocytes of this "committed" compartment may remain dormant for years unless once again exposed to the antigen for which they carry antibody-specific "memory." Faced with a second antigenic challenge, these cells hypertrophy and again develop into or produce antibody-producing cells.

The role of the thymus in the development of the immunocyte system and details concerning the formation of antibody are found in Chap. 68.

The size of the immunocyte system depends, at least in part, upon the degree of antigen exposure. Germ-free animals have fewer lymphocytes than conventional animals but rapidly develop a lymphoid system of normal size when removed from the germ-free environment.

LYMPHOCYTOSIS

The diagnostic significance of lymphocytosis depends in part upon whether the increase is due to normal- or abnormal-appearing lymphocytes. Lymphocytosis due to an increase in normal-appearing small lymphocytes may accompany recovery from acute infections and may be present during *chronic infections*, especially in *tuberculosis* and *syphilis*. In *pertussis* and in a rare syndrome of children and young adults termed **infectious lymphocytosis** very striking increases in the concentration of small lymphocytes may occur. Persistent, unexplained lymphocytosis with normal-appearing small lymphocytes in older patients usually proves to be due to *chronic lymphocytic leukemia* (Chap. 348).

Infectious mononucleosis (Chap. 255) is usually accompanied by lymphocytosis as well as by the appearance of abnormal-appearing lymphocytes in the blood. Known viral diseases, such as *measles*, may be accompanied by lymphocyte changes somewhat similar to those seen in infectious mononucleosis. *Acute lymphoblastic leukemia* (Chap. 348) is characterized by very immature lymphoblasts in the blood, and these cells are easily distinguished from those of infectious mononucleosis by their fine, granular chromatin and prominent nucleoli.

LYMPHOPENIA

Lymphopenia occurs as a relatively nonspecific response to various forms of *stress*, such as *trauma, acute infection,* or *hemorrhage*. Such lymphopenia usually disappears within a few days. Chronic lymphopenia should raise the suspicion of *Hodgkin's disease*.

Plasma Cells

These are but rarely observed in the blood of normal subjects but may appear in small numbers during severe *antigenic challenges*, as in certain *infections* or in *serum sickness*. Large numbers of plasma cells appear in the blood of a few patients with *multiple myeloma* (plasma cell leukemia Chap. 348). Plasma cells constitute less than 1 percent of the nucleated cells of normal bone marrow, but they are not distributed uniformly throughout the marrow, so that the range of normal is quite wide (up to 5 percent in counts of 500 cells from marrow aspirates of normal nonalcoholic inmates of the Utah State Prison). An increased percentage of plasma cells on smears of marrow aspirates should raise the suspicion of multiple myeloma or some other protein-secreting tumor, but may also be observed in such conditions as *liver disease*, during antigenic challenge and in *aplastic anemia*. *Absence of plasma cells* on smears of marrow aspirates usually is indicative of one of the diseases associated with inadequate production of serum antibody, such as *sex-linked hypogammaglobulinemia* or *chronic lymphocytic leukemia*.

REFERENCES

Boggs, D. R.: The Kinetics of Neutrophilic Leukocytes in Health and in Disease, Seminars in Hematology, 4:359, 1967.

Kauder, E., and A. M. Mauer: Neutropenias of Childhood, J. Pediat., 69:147, 1966.

Wintrobe, M. M.: "Clinical Hematology," 6th ed., Philadelphia, Lea & Febiger, 1967.

65 THE ERYTHROCYTE SEDIMENTATION RATE

M. M. Wintrobe

Measurement of the erythrocyte sedimentation rate (ESR) differs from many other types of laboratory examination because it serves only to indicate a deviation from normal without providing a clue to its cause. Nevertheless, this limitation does not detract from its utility. The procedure has the merit of simplicity and can be classed with the measurement of temperature and pulse rate as an index of disease. The ESR is especially useful as a disease indicator because it may be elevated in the absence of fever.

The blood is a suspension of red corpuscles in plasma. The ESR is a measure of the rate of settling of the red corpuscles, as determined by placing blood, to which an anticoagulant has been added, into a vertical tube and noting the distance the upper level of the column of red corpuscles has fall in a specific period of time, usually an hour. The test is most easily carried out in the "macro" hematocrit (Wintrobe), using blood collected for counts and determination of volume of packed red cells. It is only necessary to allow the tube to stand in a vertical position and to read the level to which the red corpuscles have fallen in an hour. Following this the specimen, after appropriate centrifugation, can be used for measurement of packed red cell volume and for inspection of the plasma (icterus, turbidity) and layers of white cells and platelets. The Westergren method has the advantage of a wider bore and is less likely to give an occasional misleading result, but it entails a special step in the laboratory, rather than being only the first step in a simple screening procedure.

Various technical factors affect the ESR, but if a standard procedure is employed, few will be of great importance. The tube must be placed in a vertical position or the rate of sedimentation will be accelerated. The degree of anemia or polycythemia affects the result, but *correction for this is not entirely satisfactory and is not recommended*. In the presence of severe anemia, the ESR is of limited value.

Normal values for ESR are given in the Appendix. The difference between those for men and for women is largely due to the sex difference in numbers of red corpuscles.

Alterations in ESR depend mainly on the concentration of macromolecules in the plasma, particularly plasma proteins of high molecular weight, such as the α_2 and γ, macroglobulins, and especially fibrinogen. The ESR is more rapid when these macromolecules are present in amounts greater than normal. Under these circumstances, and probably because of changes in the surface charge of the red corpuscles, aggregation of the red corpuscles is increased, and corpuscular aggregates of large volume and relatively small surface area are formed, which causes the ESR to be accelerated.

The only physiologic state in which the ESR is significantly increased is *pregnancy*. The rate gradually increases, beginning about the tenth to twelfth week, and is greater than is attributable to the gradual decrease in volume of packed red cells. It does not return to normal until the third or fourth week post partum. This increase is perhaps a reflection of the tissue changes which take place during delivery and the post-partum period.

The ESR is increased in all acute general infections, but in localized acute inflammatory conditions, variations depend on the nature and severity of the process. Usually the ESR is increased in localized acute suppurations even when the temperature and pulse are normal. In chronic localized inflammation the ESR varies with the extent and nature of the inflammatory process. Uncomplicated new growths are not necessarily associated with rapid sedimentation, even when malignant. When the tumor is very vascular or is undergoing necrosis, the rate may be increased.

The ESR is useful (1) in calling attention to the presence of more or less occult disease; (2) if very rapid, it may be an important clue to collagen vascular disease, notably polymyositis, in a patient with nonspecific complaints, such as headache, muscle aches and pains, and only slight fever; (3) occasionally in differential diagnosis (e.g., pelvic inflammatory disease versus uncomplicated ovarian cyst, psychosomatic versus organic disease), and most important, (4) as a guide to the progress of a disease already recognized (e.g., pulmonary tuberculosis, rheumatic carditis, Hodgkin's disease) when fever or other signs are normal or equivocal. On the other hand, the ESR may be normal when otherwise it might be expected to be accelerated, in patients with multiple myeloma complicated by the presence of cryoglobulin, when there is hypofibrinogenemia, and in circumstances in which rouleau formation does not take place (sickle-cell anemia, hereditary spherocytosis).

Section 10

Other Laboratory Manifestations of Disease

INTRODUCTION

George W. Thorn

There is an increasing interest in the identification of occult disease and in the prevention of ill health, but the acute shortage of physicians compels the recruitment of assistance from "paramedical" personnel and the full exploitation of the potential contributions of improved technology. The basis of good medical practice is, and undoubtedly always will be, a careful history and physical examination. These, in turn, will dictate the specific or appropriate laboratory tests. The automation of quantitative biochemical determinations and the "read-out" potential of computerized data will permit broad scale screening of large segments of our population, and it is important that these technical advances be fully utilized. Physicians, however, will continue to provide the expert consultation needed to plan and evaluate such programs.

In the practice of medicine, it is common for a specific disease process to present initially with nonspecific symptoms, for example, the weakness and increased fatigability of a patient with hypercalcemia secondary to hyperparathyroidism. The classical approach to diagnosis and treatment does not always suggest the appropriate laboratory tests, and the underlying disorder may remain undetected for a long period. It is in this setting that a selected group of biochemical tests may provide an early clue to the correct diagnosis or the presence of an unsuspected "carrier state." This clinical approach is not to be confused with indiscriminate laboratory testing, but accepts the fact that a group of determinations which are known to be frequent harbingers of disease can now be carried out on a single specimen of blood at low cost to the patient. It is also probable that the ready availability of multiple biochemical determinations at relatively low cost will increase the number of individuals who will utilize more regularly scheduled appointments for periodic examinations.

The succeeding chapters describe biochemical analyses and other tests which in the present state of knowledge and technology are feasible for use by physicians in private practice or for public health screening programs.

66 BIOCHEMICAL DETERMINATIONS
George W. Thorn

Serum Electrolytes and Metabolites

With present-day instrumentation, it is possible to determine on a single specimen of blood the concentration of sodium, potassium, calcium, magnesium, chloride, inorganic phosphate, and carbon dioxide–combining power. The possibility of comparing values for several electrolytes on a single specimen is especially useful. For example, an elevated serum sodium value with elevated serum chloride suggests dehydration if serum potassium is normal or elevated; however, if serum sodium is elevated and serum chloride and potassium are low, alkalosis and primary hyperaldosteronism should be considered. Low serum sodium and potassium suggest excessive hydration, serious tissue hypoxia, or excessive diuretic therapy (Thiazide). This last possibility is further strengthened by the finding of elevated serum uric acid and blood glucose levels. If serum calcium level is moderately elevated and serum inorganic phosphorus is low, then primary hyperparathyroidism is almost a certainty— whereas elevated serum calcium with normal or elevated serum phosphate suggests disorders such as breast cancer, multiple myeloma, and sarcoid as possible causes for the hypercalcemia. Tetany and convulsive seizures require determination of blood sugar, serum calcium, and magnesium levels as possible causes.

When screening for diabetes mellitus, blood sugar values should be checked postprandially (2 hr). For detecting disorders associated with hypoglycemia, blood sugar determinations made in the fasting state are more informative. Elevated uric acid with a normal blood-urea-nitrogen suggests gout or other diseases associated with high urate production, e.g., polycythemia, lymphoma, or the effect of x-rays or chemotherapy. Elevated uric acid with elevated blood-urea-nitrogen indicates primary renal disease or severe dehydration.

The level of total serum protein is another very useful determination. An increase in total serum protein with elevated blood-urea-nitrogen and hematocrit suggests dehydration. In the absence of dehydration, elevated total serum protein almost always reflects hyperglobulinemia, whereas lowered total serum protein values usually indicate hypoalbuminemia.

An elevation of serum cholesterol or serum lipids can identify an individual with increased susceptibility to coronary vascular disease, particularly if these abnormalities are associated with an elevated blood glucose.

The most useful and practical screening battery includes the measurement of blood-urea-nitrogen, glucose, serum sodium, potassium, calcium, magnesium, chloride, inorganic phosphate, uric acid, CO_2-combining power, cholesterol and other serum lipids, and total plasma proteins. The time at which blood is taken should be carefully recorded, and stasis should be avoided in obtaining venous samples.

Blood Enzyme Levels

Release of enzymes into the circulation follows injury of any type. In mild or early organic disease, an elevated blood enzyme level may be the sole indicator of underlying pathology. The extent to which the blood enzyme level will reflect the pathologic process depends upon the nature and degree of tissue injury and the capacity of cells to produce enzymes; hence, a diffuse but mild disease may be associated with a significant elevation in blood enzyme level, whereas extensive destruction of cells may be associated with little or no rise. For example, a large increase in plasma alkaline phosphatase level may be observed in the presence of relatively mild intrahepatic cholestasis (Thorazine, methyltestosterone), whereas acute yellow atrophy with widespread total destruction of hepatic parenchymal cells may be accompanied by relatively low levels of alkaline phosphatase, lactic dehydrogenase, and serum glutamic oxalacetic transaminase.

The ability to measure isoenzymes, which are most specific for a particular tissue, will increase appreciably the diagnostic value of blood enzyme levels, particularly since it is possible to observe an increase in the level of a particular isoenzyme without necessarily observing a significant rise in total blood enzyme level.

The capacity to carry out multiple biochemical determinations on a single blood specimen not only is of great value in confirming a clinical impression or detecting an unsuspected disorder or carrier state, but it is also probable that a computer analysis of the different values obtained simultaneously may suggest further possible diagnoses under circumstances in which the magnitude of the deviation of a single biochemical determination is not great enough to be considered abnormal.

67 OTHER SCREENING TESTS
George W. Thorn

Although the following procedures are well recognized as essential components of the complete examination of a patient, their tabulation and a few comments may be found useful. These examinations will provide (1) additional diagnostic potentiality, (2) an initial screen which may suggest more elaborate or definitive examinations, and (3) a point of reference against which changes in the future may be compared and interpreted.

URINALYSIS. Routine examination will include tests for glucose and protein and an examination of the sediment. If the specific gravity is greater than 1.020 and no substances which will elevate it artifactually, such as glucose, large amounts of protein, or organic dyes (an intravenous pyelogram, for example), are present, renal function can be assumed to be normal. On the other hand, a low urine specific gravity is of no clinical significance because in most instances it reflects only greater than average fluid intake. It should be checked with some specific renal func-

tion tests such as blood-urea-nitrogen or serum creatinine.

BLOOD EXAMINATION. By collecting 5 ml blood in an anticoagulant which will not alter the size or hemoglobin content of the red corpuscles or injure the leukocytes or platelets (e.g., Sequestrene), together with a few blood smears made directly from the collecting needle, one can determine (1) sedimentation rate, (2) volume of packed red cells, (3) icterus index, (4) volumes of packed white cells and platelets, (5) leukocyte count, (6) platelet count, and (7) differential leukocyte count. The usefulness of these as screening procedures has been discussed in Chap. 61.

STOOL ANALYSIS. Determination of the presence or absence of occult blood is a very important primary screen. In certain parts of the world screening of the stool for parasites is essential.

ELECTROCARDIOGRAM AND CHEST ROENTGENOGRAM. These should be made at the time of the initial examination. In addition to their diagnostic value, they will prove invaluable as a basis for comparison with potential changes in the future.

TIMED VITAL CAPACITY. Timed vital capacity is an essential measurement for the early determination of impaired pulmonary function and for monitoring patients with pulmonary and cardiovascular disease.

TUBERCULIN TEST. The tuberculin test is a valuable determination, particularly in the young or those whose occupation includes a high exposure rate. A negative tuberculin test in a very ill patient requires that other skin tests be carried out to exclude the possibility of anergy.

OCULAR PRESSURE. Since glaucoma is a frequent cause of blindness, measurement of ocular pressure should be carried out routinely on all adult patients.

PAPANICOLAOU EXAMINATION. This should be carried out regularly on the cervical smear of every adult female patient. A similar examination should be made of the sputum, gastric washings, and urine of patients with symptoms suggesting specific organ disease.

SIGMOIDOSCOPY. Although in the asymptomatic patient this procedure will yield a relatively low incidence of serious pathology, it does offer a unique opportunity to detect curable neoplasm in the rectosigmoid region.

It is important from the public health viewpoint as well as that of the individual physician to note that almost all of the procedures included in this and the preceding chapter do not require a physician's participation. A well-trained technician can analyze the urine, stool, and blood specimens as well as the Papanicolaou smears. Ultimately, electrocardiograms and chest roentgenograms will be screened by computer techniques and only those showing significant abnormalities will be referred for professional review and evaluation. Technicians can be trained to administer and evaluate tuberculin tests and vital capacity measurements, as well as to measure ocular pressure. Only sigmoidoscopy, among those procedures outlined above, requires high-level professional skill. Thus, technical advances in instrumentation, coupled with the supervised training of an increased number of paramedical personnel, should permit the physician to devote more time to his individual patient's needs, both physical and emotional.

Nationally, these same developments could facilitate the regular screening of large segments of our population and, hence, increase the possibility of identifying "carrier states" or incipient disease with its exciting remedial possibilities.

Part Four

Disorders Due to Hypersensitivity and Altered Immune Response

68 INTRODUCTION TO CLINICAL IMMUNOLOGY

K. Frank Austen

The immunologic response not only constitutes the principal means of man's defense against pathogenic microorganisms, but also is capable of mediating adverse clinical reactions. Whether an immune response is defined clinically as immunity or hypersensitivity is determined by its effect on the host; the distinction does not necessarily imply different mechanisms of elicitation. The components of the immune system may be considered in terms of the sequential manner in which they contribute to the immune response. The principal features include immunogens, capable of initiating the immune response; cellular processing of immunogenic material; products of the immune response; control mechanisms of the response; and consequences, both beneficial and detrimental, of the immune response. Consideration of the immunologic response in terms of these arbitrary divisions affords a basis for a clinical approach to the diagnosis and management of immune deficiency states and hypersensitivity syndromes.

INITIATION OF THE IMMUNE RESPONSE

A substance must ordinarily be recognized as foreign in order to elicit an immune response. The ability of a substance to evoke such a response is termed *immunogenicity;* the capacity to react specifically with the antibodies induced is termed *antigenicity.* The distinction is useful because many simple substances of less than 1,000 mol wt are not immunogenic unless coupled convalently or by large numbers of ionic bonds to macromolecules but can react with antibodies of appropriate specificity; such simple substances are termed *haptens.*

Deliberate initiation of the immune response is accomplished most reliably by injection of the immunogen. Feeding is not usually effective because being proteins, most immunogens are digested in the gastrointestinal tract. The oral route may, however, be utilized under certain circumstances, such as with attenuated poliomyelitis virus. Natural immunization to environmental substances may occur by such diverse routes as inhalation of plant or tree pollens, ingestion of certain foods or drugs, and skin contact with drugs or natural chemicals such as the catechols of poison ivy plants.

CELLULAR PROCESSING OF IMMUNOGENTIC MATERIALS

After injection, the immunogen is most conspicuous in the macrophages of the reticuloendothelial system, and a variety of observations involving particulate immunogens indicate that ingestion by the macrophage may be an essential step in the immune response. It appears that the macrophage complexes fragments of the immunogen to a unique ribonucleic acid moiety, and that the complexed immunogen is considerably more immunogenic than in the free form. The macrophage ribonucleic acid associated with the immunogenic fragments is distinguished by several criteria, including: (1) low molecular weight, insufficient to contain the base sequence information of messenger RNA; (2) an appreciable representation in the DNA template, as assessed by hybridization techniques, contrasting with the small representation observed with ribosomal RNA; and (3) physicochemical characteristics which do not appear to change as a result of exposing the macrophage to various immunogens, implying a nonspecific carrier function.

Following an immunogenic stimulus the regional lymph nodes (or spleen) become hyperplastic and increase severalfold in weight, and the specific antibody levels in the efferent lymph exceed those in the afferent lymph entering the regional node. Net antibody synthesis by isolated lymph node tissue also has been demonstrated in vitro. The evidence that the plasma cell is particularly active in antibody synthesis includes (1) the prominence of plasma cells as lymphoid tissue becomes hyperplastic in response to an immunogenic stimulus; (2) the approximate relationship between the antibody extractable from such tissue with the plasma cell content; (3) the demonstration by immunofluorescent staining procedures of gamma-globulin in the cytoplasm of plasma cells; and (4) the clinical observations of increased numbers of plasma cells in circumstances of gamma-globulin overproduction and the virtual absence of such cells in heritable disorders of antibody production.

The steps between "activation" of the immunogen by the macrophage and production of specific antibody by the plasma cell are not completely understood but seem to involve the small lymphocyte. In the resting lymph node, plasma cells are rare and about three-fourths of the cells are small lymphocytes while the remainder are large lymphocytes. The population of small lymphocytes is believed to be heterogeneous and is presumed to be capable of several different functions. From their paucity of ribosomes and mitochondria and relatively long generation time of months, certain small lymphocytes seem to be "resting." Directly or, more likely, following processing by the macrophage, the immunogen appears to stimulate these small lymphocytes to differentiate into rapidly dividing, large, ribosome-rich cells termed *immunoblasts*. The immunoblasts are then presumed to differentiate either into plasma cells or back into small lymphocytes which persist as "memory" cells, primed to respond to subsequent encounters with the same or related immunogens. Although the plasma cell is the most active in synthesizing and secreting antibody, both small and large lymphocytes have on occasion been shown to produce antibody.

PRODUCTS OF THE IMMUNE RESPONSE

STRUCTURE OF GAMMA-GLOBULINS. The gamma-globulins are a group of serum proteins with a distinct electrophoretic mobility and the capacity to behave as antibodies. On the basis of different physicochemical and immunochemical properties, these proteins, termed immunoglobulins, have been divided into a number of major classes. The fundamental molecular unit of all classes of immunoglobulins as determined by the employment of reducing and denaturing agents consists of two heavy (H) and two light (L) polypeptide chains linked by interchain disulfide bonds and non-covalent bonds. Disulfide bonds (two or more in man) join the two H chains, and each H chain is linked to its respective L chain by single disulfide bonds. The non-covalent bonds between the polypeptide chains are predominantly hydrophobic bonds. When the enzyme papain is employed, human IgG is split into three fragments; two, termed Fab, are identical and contain the antigen combining sites, and the third, Fc, can be crystallized and is responsible for the unique biologic activities of a class. The Fab fragment consists of an L chain and the N-terminal half of the H chain, termed the Fd fragment, joined by their interchain disulfide bond; the Fc fragment consists of the C terminal portions of the two H chains held by their interchain disulfide bonds. The molecular basis of the specificity of bivalent antibody for antigen resides in the Fab fragments. The combining site is probably constructed predominantly from the Fd fragment of the H chain, while the L chain contributes indirectly by interacting with and stabilizing the neighboring Fd fragment. Differing antibody specificities depend on differing primary amino acid sequences in the region of the combining site; these differences exist in both the H and L chains, which vary in the combining site region but are constant in the C terminal ends of the chains.

For the L chain the constant portion is approximately one-half the chain, whereas in the H chain the invariable portion includes the Fc piece and about one-half of the Fd fragment. It is the antigenic differences in the invariable portion of the H chain which permit division of the human immunoglobulins into five major classes (IgG, IgA, IgM, IgD, and IgE). The constant portion of the L chain allows recognition of two types (kappa and lambda), which occur in combination with all five H chains (gamma, alpha, mu, delta, and epsilon). The molecular formulas for the preponderant immunoglobulin class, IgG, would thus be gamma$_2$ lambda$_2$ ($\gamma_2 \lambda_2$) and gamma$_2$ kappa$_2$ ($\gamma_2 \kappa_2$). IgG is further subdivided into four subclasses, IgG 1 to 4, on the basis of minor intraclass antigenic differences. In addition to the designation of class and subclass by structural differences, there are genetic differences within a class, termed allotypy, expressed by additional discrete structural differences. Genetic control of structural differences in three of the gamma chain subclasses, 1 to 3, has been related to the Gm loci, while allotypic differences in the kappa chain reside in the Inv locus.

PRIMARY IMMUNE RESPONSE. The immune response to the first introduction of an immunogen is termed primary. In a primary response, possibly because of the differential sensitivity of the methodology employed, the IgM antibodies are recognized somewhat earlier than those of the IgG class. The IgM antibodies are observed within the first week of immunization and decline thereafter as the titer of IgG antibodies increases. This relationship and the finding that formation of IgM antibodies requires appreciable levels of immunogen have been interpreted to indicate that IgG antibodies inhibit synthesis of antibodies of the IgM class. Antibodies of the IgA class may be observed following prolonged and rather intensive immunization. The view that IgM antibodies represent a primitive product of the immune response is supported by the predominant synthesis of this antibody class in the newborn and by phylogenic observations. In addition to sequential changes in immunoglobulin class, heterogeneity of the primary response occurs within the IgG class, expressed as an increasing affinity for the antigen. This may be explicable in terms of continued formation of new antibodies capable of interacting with increasing numbers of diverse antigenic determinants on the macromolecular immunogen.

SECONDARY IMMUNE RESPONSE. When the antibody levels have diminished following initial immunogenic exposure, a subsequent encounter will evoke an enhanced response, termed secondary or anamnestic. The anamnestic response requires a lower threshold dose of immunogen for elicitation and is characterized by a shortened lag phase for appearance of detectable product and a higher and more persistent antibody response. Although the quantity of antibody produced per unit time is usually much greater in the secondary response, the doubling time appears to be about the same as in the primary, which is consistent with the participation of more cells rather than an augmentation in the rate of synthesis per cell. The antibodies formed after the secondary stimulus have a much higher affinity for the corresponding antigenic determinant than those appearing after a comparable time during the primary response. The high-affinity antibodies characteristic of the secondary response are of the IgG class.

DETERMINATION OF ANTIBODY SYNTHESIS. Studies by immunofluorescent techniques have demonstrated that individual lymph node cells produce only a single class of heavy and light chains at any one time. Preliminary evidence suggests that L chains are made on small polyribosomes and H chains on large ones; and it is held that half the immunoglobulin molecules, consisting of single L and H chains, are assembled through attachment of free L chains to the polyribosomal-bound H chains, and that the product then is released for assembly into a bivalent immunoglobulin molecule. Although it has been demonstrated that antibody specificity is determined by amino acid sequence, there is no real insight into the molecular basis by which a flexibility sufficient to recognize the vast array of potential immunogens is maintained. Theories of antibody production ranging from instructive, in which the immunogen helps shape the corresponding antibody, to selective, in which the immunogen selectively stimulates a cell or portion of the gene already capable of producing the desired product, continue to be assessed; this theory seems most consistent with the data at hand.

The consequences of the immune response grouped as cellular immunity are of great biologic importance but cannot be presented in physicochemical terms. Accordingly, these cellular phenomena, along with the humoral responses, will be examined in the sections dealing with control mechanisms and the biologic consequences of the immune response.

CONTROL MECHANISMS OF THE IMMUNE RESPONSE

Wide variations usually are observed in the amounts of specific antibody formed in different individuals of the same species in response to a similar immunogenic stimulus. A heritable basis for different responses to certain synthetic immunogens has been well documented in highly inbred strains of guinea pigs and mice. In man there is evidence that the capacity to make antibodies of the IgE class in response to inhaled pollens is associated with an increased incidence of a similar immunoglobulin response to drugs and other environmental antigens.

ROLE OF THE THYMUS. The development of the capacity to respond to an immunogen is dependent on a functioning thymus gland as well as on other lymphoepithelial structures arising embryologically as outpouchings of the gut wall and eventually consisting of lymphocyte populations in close proximity to epithelial cells of endodermal origin. Experimental studies have revealed that neonatal thymectomy interferes with the development of the lymphoid system, profoundly impairs the immunologic capabilities termed "cellular immunity" (such as rejection of foreign-tissue grafts and delayed hypersensitivity), and also under certain circumstances diminishes humoral responses. The manner in which the thymus mediates the development of these aspects of immunologic competence is not entirely clear but may include (1) an environment in which "stem" cells, possibly of bone marrow origin, differentiate to become immunologically competent before being distributed peripherally to populate node tissue; (2) elaboration of a humoral factor regulating the maturation of peripheral lymphocytes; and (3) the exertion of "censorship," whereby potentially self-reacting clones are eliminated. The consequences of thymectomy are less dramatic in the adult animal, but there is evidence that the thymus continues to provide a mechanism whereby immunologically uncommitted cells acquire the capacity to respond to specific immunogens.

In birds there is an anatomic separation of the central control of the capacity to develop cellular and humoral immunity, the former is regulated by the thymus and the latter by the bursa of Fabricius. In mammals the precise equivalent of the bursa has not been established, but it is assumed to be some portion of the gut-associated lymphoid tissue. The evidence in man for some division of central control resides in the existence of patients with hereditary lesions expressed predominantly as defects in cellular immunity, humoral immunity, or both.

TOLERANCE. The capacity of an individual's immune response to distinguish between his own and foreign macromolecules was termed "horror autotoxicus" by Ehrlich and "self-tolerance" by Burnet. An operational definition of tolerance sufficient to include a variety of terms developed from special experimental circumstances is "a state of specific immunologic nonreactivity to an immunogenic stimulus which would be followed by a recognizable response in a normal animal." Though moderate doses of an immunogen can initiate the immune response, an excessive dose is followed by a state of tolerance or specific nonreactivity to any subsequent dose of the immunogen, although unrelated immunogens, in appropriate dose, are fully active. Tolerance is more easily established in the neonate than in the adult, is maintained by persistence of the immunogen, and can be manifested by impairment of either humoral or cellular immunity. Tolerance to an immunogen has been shown experimentally to be associated with the functional absence of the specifically responding cells or clone. It is held that the excess immunogen destroys the relevant clones as they arise, possibly by bypassing the "activation" step in the macrophage and presenting to the small lymphocyte as free immunogen or as an immune complex in the region of great antigen excess.

AUTOIMMUNITY. The appearance of antibodies in man directed against self represents an autoimmune response. These autoantibodies may reflect a normal response to tissue antigens, which are separated anatomically from the immune system during fetal development and appear later as a consequence of tissue breakdown. Autoantibodies also may arise following abrogation of tolerance in a normal immune system by an exogenous antigen cross-reacting with self or because an abnormal immune system has lost the capacity to distinguish self. Autoantibodies do not necessarily indicate an autoimmune disease. This term must be restricted to situations in which the autoimmune response, humoral or cellular, is responsible for tissue injury.

CONSEQUENCES OF THE IMMUNE RESPONSE: HOST RESISTANCE

The consequences of the immune response are termed *immunity* when beneficial to the host and *hypersensitivity* or *allergy* when detrimental. This is a clinical judgment and does not imply that the basic pathways leading to immunity or hypersensitivity are different.

The constituents of host defense in normal man are both nonimmunologic and immunologic, while those developing as a result of deliberate immunization or overt infection are exclusively immunologic. The nonimmunologic lines of defense include the extrinsic barriers to pathogen penetration, both mechanical and enzymatic, and the intrinsic cellular elements—circulating polymorphonuclear leukocytes and monocytes and fixed mononuclear phagocytic cells. Although these cellular elements are effective in the absence of an immune response, they clearly operate much more effectively in its presence. The so-called *natural antibodies* are present in normal persons who have not been subjected to deliberate immunization or overt infection; these natural antibodies would appear to result from the host's subclinical exposure to the specific pathogen or some cross-reacting pathogen. This makes it possible to consider the role of the immune response in host defense without further reference to a subclinical or overt encounter with the immunogen.

SERUM COMPLEMENT. The humoral immune response participating in host resistance appears to involve a supporting system, known as serum complement; hence it is relevant to examine this system before evaluating the role of the various immunoglobulin classes in host defense. The complement system (C') consists of distinct serum proteins, numbered 1 through 9, which interact in a well-defined sequence as cytotoxins for target cells and yield a series of by-products representing the essential ingredients of an inflammatory response. When an immune aggregate, or a target cell sensitized by interaction with specific antibody against some cell-surface antigen, interacts with normal serum, the first component of complement (C'1) binds to the complex and is converted from an inactive precursor form to an active enzyme. Complex-bound C'1 then acts on its natural substrates, the fourth and second components of complement, yielding a new cell-bound enzymatic activity consisting of C'4 and the fragment C'2a; the 4,2a unit is termed C'3 convertase. The action of C'3 convertase on C'3 results in the binding of the major portion of the molecule, C'3b, to the complex, leaving the lesser fragment, C'3a or anaphylatoxin, in the fluid phase. The complex, having achieved the 1,4,2a,3b state, can attach to a specific receptor on primate red blood cells or polymorphonuclear leukocytes, a phenomenon known as *immune adherence*, which enhances phagocytosis. The subsequent interaction of the fifth, sixth, and seventh complement components with the complex yields a chemotactic factor for polymorphonuclear leukocytes. The sequential action of the eighth and ninth components to complete the reaction leads to osmotic lysis of the target cell with disruption of the cell membrane by electron microscopy. The system has biologic meaning because it is lethal for some target cells and results in the elaboration of various by-products capable of mediating an inflammatory response. These include *anaphylatoxin,* which produces a local increase in vascular permeability, bringing more antibody and complement to the site of the lesion; the *chemotactic factor,* which attracts polymorphonuclear leukocytes; and a *complex carrying C'3a,* which promotes immune adherence and enhanced phagocytosis. The complement reaction may be beneficial or detrimental to the host, depending entirely on the location of the antigens against which the antibody mediating the reaction is directed.

ANTIBODY. IgG comprises 70 to 80 percent of the serum antibodies of man and is almost exclusively responsible for the antibodies to viruses, toxins, and gram-positive pyogenic bacteria. It is transported across the placenta, while other maternal immunoglobulins mostly are excluded from the fetal circulation. The interaction of IgG with antigen to activate the complement system leads to the development of anaphylatoxin, a release of chemotactic factor, and the capacity of the complex to undergo immune adherence and enhanced phagocytosis; it may be of great importance in controlling man's pyogenic environment.

Between 5 and 10 percent of the total serum antibody is IgM. Antibodies of this class commonly are directed against lipopolysaccharide antigens typified by the somatic O antigens (endotoxins) of gram-negative bacteria. The sensitization of a site on a target cell for subsequent lysis by the nine components of complement can be accomplished either by a single IgM molecule or an IgG doublet. The doublet reduces the efficiency of IgG in mediating cytotoxic reactions, and there is ample evidence that the bactericidal activity of human serum against gram-negative bacteria is mainly dependent on the diverse pool of natural IgM antibodies.

Antibodies of the IgA class comprise about 10 to 20 percent of serum immunoglobulins and are the predominant immunoglobulin in parotid saliva, tears, colostrum, nasal and bronchial secretions, bile, succus entericus, and urine. Secretory IgA has activity against viruses and bacteria, and a specific immune response to experimental virus infection has been demonstrated in the saliva, nasal secretions, and tears of human volunteers. While serum IgA has a sedimentation coefficient of 7S, secretory IgA is principally 11S protein because of an additional structural unit, the T (transport) piece. The T piece probably is responsible for the movement of the molecule into secretions; and it is presumed that such molecules in the external secretions of the respiratory, gastrointestinal, and genitourinary tract contribute to host resistance. The functions in host resistance of the trace immunoglobulins IgD and IgE are unknown.

SPECIFIC CELLULAR IMMUNITY. Specific cellular immunity to intracellular pathogens has been demonstrated experimentally in several models, the most direct of which has involved *Listeria monocytogenes* infection in the mouse. Mice infected with a sublethal dose of this organism developed resistance to a dose 100 times the LD_{50}. Resistance was not associated with the appearance of antibody because agglutination titers were negligible and protection could not be conferred by passive transfer serum; resistance was, however, correlated in time with the development of delayed-type skin hypersensitivity to listeria culture filtrate. Furthermore, monolayer cultures of normal mouse peritoneal macrophages are destroyed readily by innoculation with listeria, while cultures obtained from resistant animals, previously infected with a sublethal challenge, are capable of eliminating the organism. These peritoneal macrophages are demonstrating specific cellular immunity because their activity is not diminished by repeated washing nor enhanced by the addition of normal or immune serum to the culture. Furthermore, these macrophages are capable of destroying intracellular pathogens, other than those used to initiate the immune response such as *Brucella abortus* or *Salmonella typhimurium,* indicating that cellular immunity may be expressed in nonspecific fashion. On the other hand, the induction of cellular immunity is specific because recall can be initiated only by an organism which has previously been used to initiate a primary response. *Induction* of cellular immunity is immunologically specific, while the *expression* by the "activated" macrophage is nonspecific. The association of cellular immunity with the cutaneous reaction of delayed hypersensitivity suggests that the specificity resides in the sensitized lymphocyte, which then "activates" the macrophage to exhibit a nonspecific increased resistance to intracellular pathogens. This is somewhat analogous to humoral immunity, wherein specificity resides with the antibody produced by the plasma cell while the execution involves the nonspecific complement system.

The experimental data considered above imply that a deficiency of IgG would predispose to pyogenic infection, an absence of IgM to infection with gram-negative enteric flora, and a defect in cellular immunity to infection with intracellular pathogens. These generalizations are supported by clinical observations in patients illustrating such heritable or acquired defects (Chap. 69).

CONSEQUENCES OF THE
IMMUNE RESPONSE: HYPERSENSITIVITY

The adverse or allergic manifestations of the immune response traditionally have been divided on the basis of their time course following antigen challenge into *immediate, subacute,* and *delayed* hypersensitivity. Clear differences exist in the mechanisms whereby these three broad categories of clinical responses arise; and even differences within a category, such as immediate hypersensitivity, are being appreciated.

IMMEDIATE HYPERSENSITIVITY. Immediate hypersensitivity consists of all the allergic responses that begin within minutes of antigen-antibody interaction and may be divided into *cytotoxic* and *anaphylactic* on the basis of the mediation of the clinical response. In a cytotoxic reaction, such as an acute hemolytic transfusion reaction in man, the critical damage is to the primary target cell

selected because the responsible complement-fixing antibody is directed against some cell-surface antigen. In an anaphylactic reaction, the interaction of antigen with antibody results in the formation and/or release of chemical mediators which act at secondary sites, namely, smooth muscle and vascular tissue.

ANAPHYLAXIS. The chemical mediators of anaphylactic tissue injury known to be specifically formed and/or released from mammalian tissue by antigen-antibody interaction include amines, such as histamine and serotonin, small peptides such as the nonapeptide, bradykinin, and an acidic lipid known as slow-reacting substance of anaphylaxis (SRS-A). Each mediator is capable of causing contraction in a particular group of smooth muscles and of increasing vascular permeability. While the amines, histamine and serotonin, are released from tissue stores, in which they exist in their biologically active form, bradykinin and SRS-A must be formed as well as released as a result of antigen-antibody interaction. SRS-A is the only member of the group without an established chemical structure, but it can be recognized because of a unique combination of chemical and pharmacologic characteristics. This lipid is elaborated in large amounts when lung tissue from individuals with allergic or extrinsic asthma is exposed in vitro to pollen antigen; SRS-A also profoundly constricts the isolated human bronchiole in the presence of specific pharmacologic antagonists of histamine and serotonin.

The anaphylactic reaction may be divided further into cytotropic and aggregate to indicate whether the critical interaction of antigen with antibody leading to release of chemical mediators occurs on a primary target cell, such as a mast cell, or in the fluid phase. The sensitization of human polymorphonuclear leukocytes with antibody of the IgE class for the subsequent antigen-induced release of histamine is an example of a cytotropic reaction. An example of aggregate-induced immediate hypersensitivity is the immune reaction in the fluid phase leading to histamine release via formation of anaphylatoxin. Such a pathway requires IgG and IgM antibodies, which in turn are necessary to activate complement. Not only can the same chemical mediator be released by distinctly different antibody-mediated pathways, but experimental work in the rat has revealed that different chemical mediators of immediate hypersensitivity are released by interaction of the same specific antigen with different homologous immunoglobulins residing on different target cells.

Because an animal or man can respond to an immunogen by making antibodies of several immunoglobulin classes, the clinical picture termed systemic anaphylaxis, which follows a subsequent challenge with specific antigen by a route or dose sufficient to bring about an immediate reaction, represents a composite response to the interaction of antigen with several different immunoglobulins. It is not surprising, therefore, that man exhibits at least three distinct reaction patterns within the anaphylactic syndrome, perhaps reflecting genetic differences in the immune response or variation in the pattern of exposure to the immunogen. Patients may experience respiratory distress due to edema of the hypopharynx and larynx or as a result of intractable bronchospasm. Hypotension then occurs secondary to the hypoxia. Alternatively, a primary vascular collapse without antecedent respiratory difficulty may ensue. It is possible to speculate on the basis of minimal experimental data in man that the pattern of laryngeal edema is mediated by histamine, the intractable bronchospasm by SRS-A, and primary vascular collapse by bradykinin. However, the critical point is that the anaphylactic syndrome has a variable presentation, probably determined by the relative amounts of the different antibodies involved.

ARTHUS REACTION. Subacute hypersensitivity reactions, depending on the deposition of immune complexes, activation of the complement system, and infiltration of polymorphonuclear leukocytes, are termed *Arthus lesions* when produced in the skin and *serum sickness* when they occur systemically. In contrast to the immediate clinical wheal of cutaneous anaphylaxis mediated by the release of chemical mediators, the Arthus lesion is a hemorrhagic reaction which develops over 4 to 10 hr and is associated with a marked polymorphonuclear leukocyte infiltrate of venules with surrounding edema and hemorrhage with or without secondary thrombosis. The reaction is not elicited by precipitating antibodies which do not activate complement and is absent in inborn or acquired complement deficiencies or in acquired leukopenia. The mechanism of the Arthus lesion appears to be as follows: (1) antigen-antibody aggregates are deposited in vessel walls; (2) the complement system is activated, and the chemotactic principle is elaborated; (3) polymorphonuclear leukocytes enter, resulting in (4) enhanced phagocytosis of the aggregates, which, in turn, (5) leads to release of lysosomal enzymes with secondary focal necrosis of the vessel wall.

SERUM SICKNESS. Serum sickness (Chap. 74) may be considered a disseminated form of the Arthus lesion, although the polymorphonuclear leukocytic infiltrate is less striking in the arteritis or glomerulitis of serum sickness than in the classical Arthus lesion. When man or an experimental animal receives a foreign or heterologous protein, the disappearance curve is characterized by three phases: (1) distribution throughout the extracellular compartment; (2) metabolic degradation; and (3) immune elimination due to an immune response with the appearance of specific antibody. The manifestations of serum sickness appear just prior to the onset of the immune elimination phase and are attributed to circulating antigen-antibody complexes formed in the region of antigen excess; these complexes apparently escape the usual clearance mechanisms effective against complexes formed at equivalence or in the zone of antibody excess and are trapped at vascular sites. For example, in experimental glomerular lesion the complexes appearing in association with the complement components are deposited on the epithelial side of the basement membrane. Similarly, immunofluorescent and electronmicrographic techniques have shown deposition of complexes and development of glomerulitis in acute poststreptococcal nephritis and systemic lupus erythematosus in man. However, this is not the only recognized immunologic mechanism of renal disease in man; in Goodpasture's syndrome and certain other instances of nephritis an anti-basement membrane antibody is deposited on the endothelial side of the basement membrane and may produce direct cytotoxic injury.

DELAYED HYPERSENSITIVITY. These reactions are exemplified in the skin by the tuberculin skin test or contact sensitivity and are implicated in the classical allograft rejection reaction of the unmodified recipient. The cutaneous response of erythema and induration is evident within 12 hr and reaches a peak in 24 to 48 hr. Granulocytes about small blood vessels are abundant in 12 hr, but by 24 hr a massive accumulation of mononuclear cells predominates. The delayed hypersensitivity response differs from the cutaneous anaphylactic or Arthus lesion because it is not transferred by serum but requires the transfer of viable lymphocytes in experimental animal models. The lymphocyte plays an essential role because (1) transfer of the delayed reaction can be achieved with thoracic duct cells, (2) the reaction can be suppressed in animals or man treated with an antiserum against the lymphocyte, and (3) the capacity to show contact sensitivity or allograft rejection in heritable or acquired lymphocyte deficiency states is absent. In man, the delayed reaction has been transferred with an extract of peripheral blood cells termed *transfer factor,* which has a molecular weight of less than 10,000. Elicitation of the delayed skin reaction requires a larger portion of the antigen than does interaction with humoral antibody; this phenomenon, referred to as hapten-carrier specificity, means that the specificity for eliciting a delayed response exceeds that of the reaction requiring humoral antibodies. Although this specificity seems to reside in the sensitized lymphocyte, it is only part of the reaction mechanism. Special studies of a skin test site have revealed that the vast majority of the accumulated mononuclear cells are nonsensitive. Studies on the inhibition of macrophage migration in the presence of sensitized lymphocytes and specific antigen have demonstrated an excellent correlation with all aspects of delayed hypersensitivity in vivo and have shown also that the antigen stimulates the lymphocyte to produce a soluble, nondialyzable protein which activates the macrophage. Therefore, the clinical absence of delayed hypersensitivity in acquired diseases such as Hodgkin's disease, sarcoidosis, or measles, may be due not only to defects of the afferent or efferent arcs of the immune response but also to defects in the effector cells.

CONCLUDING COMMENTS

In understanding both heritable and acquired defects in host resistance, it is important to appreciate not only the elements of the immune response contributing specificity, such as the immunoglobulins and the sensitized lymphocyte, but also the role of the nonspecific elements, such as the complement sequence, the polymorphonuclear leukocyte, and the macrophage. These nonspecific elements provide the killing mechanism after a specific immunoglobulin or sensitized lymphocyte has interacted with cell-surface antigens of the pathogen. Defects may occur at any point in the sequential steps in the afferent and efferent arcs of the immune response as well as in the nonspecific humoral and cellular systems which are activated in the final expression of the response. Similarly, in considering hypersensitivity to an exogenous immunogen or an autoantibody, immunochemical and immunopathologic definition of the lesion will assist materially in understanding its mechanism and in arriving at a rational course of therapy, which then may be directed at any point in the afferent and efferent arcs of the immune response or at the nonspecific participants involved in its expression.

REFERENCES

Austen, K. F., and E. L. Becker: "Biochemistry of the Acute Allergic Reactions," Oxford, Blackwell Scientific Publications, Ltd., 1968.

Davis, B. D., R. Dulbecco, H. N. Eisen, H. S. Ginsberg, and W. B. Wood, Jr.: "Microbiology," (see sec. II, Immunology), New York, Hoeber Medical Division, Harper & Row, Publishers, Incorporated, 1967.

David, J. R.: Delayed Hypersensitivity (sec. A, VI), in "Textbook of Immunopathology," P. A. Miescher and H. J. Muller-Eberhard (Eds.), New York, Grune & Stratton, Inc., in press.

Gottlieb, A. A.: The Antigen-RNA Complex of Macrophages, in "Nucleic Acids in Immunology," W. Braun and O. Plescia (Eds.), Berlin, Springer-Verlag, 1968.

Haber, E.: Recovery of Antigenic Specificity after Denaturation and Complete Reduction of Disulfides in a Papain Fragment of Antibody, Proc. Nat. Acad. Sci., 52:1099, 1964.

Janeway, C. A., F. S. Rosen, E. Merler, and C. A. Alper: "The Gamma Globulins," Boston, Little, Brown and Company, 1967.

Mackaness, G. B., and R. V. Blanden: Cellular Immunity, Progr. Allergy, 11:89, 1967.

Muller-Eberhard, H. J.: Chemistry and Reaction Mechanisms of Complement, Advan. Immunol., 8:1, 1968.

Wolstenholme, G. E. W., and R. Porter: "Ciba Foundation Symposium on the Thymus," Boston, Little, Brown and Company, 1966.

69   IMMUNOLOGIC DEFICIENCY DISEASES

(Hypogammaglobulinemia and Related Disorders)

James C. Allen

The greatest benefit of the immune response in man is enhanced resistance to infection. This resistance is impaired in immunologic deficiency states, and repeated or severe infections in patients with immunologic deficiencies bring them to medical attention. The immunologic

defenses in man and animals are divided into two categories: (1) those defense mechanisms mediated by immunoglobulins (antibodies), and (2) those mediated by cells of the lymphocytic series (Chap. 68). Lymphocyte-mediated defense mechanisms are frequently called cellular immunity and are evaluated clinically by delayed hypersensitivity reactions. Immunoglobulins are produced primarily by plasma cells which derive from lymphoid germinal centers and Peyer's patches of the gastrointestinal tract, while the lymphocytes which are of significance in cellular immunity arise from the thymus. Congenital deficiencies in immunoglobulin production usually are associated with poorly developed germinal centers in lymphatic tissue and marked reduction in the usual numbers of plasma cells, while congenital deficiencies in cellular immunity are generally accompanied by lymphopenia and improper development of the thymus. Although the exact significance of each type of immunity in mediating resistance to infection is imperfectly understood, antibodies are of major importance when microbial agents or their products are localized primarily in the bloodstream or extracellular tissues, while cellular immunity may be of greater importance when the microbial agents exist primarily within cells. Exceptions to this generalization probably exist.

Several attempts have been made to categorize the immunologic deficiency diseases, but an entirely satisfactory and logical classification is not available. This apparent confusion exists because the etiology of various deficiency syndromes is not known and the basic defects are not fully defined. In this presentation an attempt is made to organize these disorders according to their immunologic defect: impaired antibody production or impaired cellular immunity.

IMPAIRED ANTIBODY PRODUCTION

The majority of immunoglobulins present at birth are the gamma-G-globulins transferred across the placenta from the maternal circulation. As the neonate catabolizes these proteins, the serum concentration falls to a low of 300 to 500 mg per 100 ml within 4 to 12 weeks. Normally, endogenous production of immunoglobulins gradually increases, the serum level of these proteins rises, and adult levels are attained by the second year. Occasionally, the increases of immunoglobulin synthesis are delayed, and the concentration will fall as low as 75 to 100 mg per 100 ml. In these infants, repeated infection may occur until autogenous production of immunoglobulin reaches satisfactory levels. This syndrome, termed *physiologic hypogammaglobulinemia*, resolves spontaneously.

A sex-linked recessive disease, *familial hypogammaglobulinemia (Bruton's)*, is characterized by immunoglobulin levels of 50 mg per 100 ml or less. Repeated infections occur usually within the first 2 years of life. *Acquired hypogammaglobulinemia* may occur in either sex and may begin at any age. Generally, immunoglobulin concentrations are somewhat higher than those found in the congenital type, and are between 50 and 150 mg per 100 ml. Impaired antibody production and increased susceptibility to infections may be *secondary* to the replacement of lymphoid tissue by neoplastic or granulomatous disease, as in *chronic lymphocytic leukemia,* or in association with other reticuloendothelial malignancies such as *reticulum cell sarcoma, multiple myeloma,* or *Waldenström's macroglobulinemia.* In addition, *idiopathic* cases of hypogammaglobulinemia occur in which a specific underlying disease cannot be demonstrated; heredity may play a role in these patients. An entity encompassing increased susceptibility to infection associated with hypogammaglobulinemia, thymoma, and absence of eosinophils has been described.

PATHOLOGY. The outstanding pathologic finding in primary and idiopathic forms of hypogammaglobulinemia is the paucity of plasma cells in the bone marrow, lymph nodes, and other tissues. Lymph nodes from patients with congenital hypogammaglobulinemia show ill-defined germinal centers and a thin cortex. Peyer's patches in the gastrointestinal tract are diminished or absent, but the thymus is relatively normal histologically and shows only involution compatible with the patient's age and previous state of health. Pathologic changes associated with the secondary type of hypogammaglobulinemia are those of the underlying disease.

MANIFESTATIONS. The symptoms are a direct consequence of the inability to synthesize protective antibodies in the face of antigenic challenges. There is marked increase in susceptibility to infections, with recurrent and often life-endangering episodes of pneumonia, otitis media, meningitis, sinusitis, septic arthritis, and various infections of the skin. The causative organisms usually are the common pyogenic bacteria, pneumococci, staphylococci, meningococci, and streptococci, but infectious hepatitis, generalized vaccinia, and pneumocystis carinii pneumonia also occur. Approximately one-third of children with congenital sex-linked hypogammaglobulinemia have developed disorders similar to collagen diseases. Recurrent arthritis which is indistinguishable clinically from rheumatoid arthritis is most common, but dermatomyositis, scleroderma, and polyarteritis-like diseases have been reported. Patients with acquired hypogammaglobulinemia also may have recurrent enterocolitis, with marked malabsorption. "Hypersplenism" with leukopenia, thrombocytopenia, and anemia has been described, especially in the idiopathic acquired type of hypogammaglobulinemia. Some studies have shown abnormalities of the immunoglobulins and an increased incidence of collagen vascular disease in relatives of patients with congenital hypogammaglobulinemia.

LABORATORY FINDINGS. The outstanding laboratory finding in these patients is a significant reduction in the concentration of all immunoglobulins which may be demonstrated qualitatively by immunoelectrophoresis or quantitatively by appropriate immunochemical studies. The total immunoglobulin concentration is usually less than 100 mg per 100 ml. Isoagglutinins are lacking or present in low titer, and the expected antibody response to immunization with bacterial antigens is absent. For example, the Dick test is positive, and the Schick test remains positive after immunization with diphtheria toxoid. The demonstration of limited antibody activity does not exclude the diagnosis; small amounts of antibodies to selected antigens are often detectable in serums from these patients. Rarely there is a selective inability to form specific antibodies even though concentration of "normal" immunoglobulins is within the expected range or is only slightly reduced, as in *multiple myeloma* and *Waldenström's macroglobulinemia.* In these instances, specific antibody titers are often low irrespective of the amount of monoclonal immunoglobulin or concentration of the nonmonoclonal immunoglobulins in the patient's serum, and resistance to infection may be impaired. The peripheral blood counts are normal and reflect only intercurrent infections; specifically, chronic lymphopenia is not demonstrable.

IMPAIRED CELLULAR IMMUNITY

Impaired cellular immunity of the familial form classically is associated with imperfect development of the thymus. Two types of *thymic alymphoplasia* without immunoglobulin deficiency have been recognized; they may represent variants of the same disorder. That described by *Nezelof* is associated with normal concentrations of serum immunoglobulins and normal antibody response; in the *dysgammaglobulinemic* form there is an increased concentration of γ_M-globulins with a decrease in the γ_G- and γ_A-globulins. Careful evaluation of antibody production in this disorder is not yet available, but the evidence suggests that no gross deficit exists.

The third and fourth pharyngeal pouches are the embryonic origin of the parathyroid glands and thymus. Failure of these pouches to develop results in congenital absence of the parathyroids and the thymus, leading respectively to hypoparathyroidism and immunologic deficiency. This constellation of defects has been termed the *DiGeorge syndrome.* Cellular immunity is markedly impaired even though lymphopenia may or may not exist. Deliberate immunizations show decreased formation of antibodies, but immunoglobulin levels are normal.

PATHOLOGY. The thymic alymphoplasias are characterized by improper development of the thymus, which is quite small weighing 1 Gm or less at autopsy and is located atypically, often in the area of the thyroid, as a result of improper developmental descent. Histologically, the gland is organized poorly; Hassall's corpuscles and cortical-medullary differentiation are lacking. The primary cell type is epithelial, and the thymus, as well as the spleen, lymph nodes, tonsils, and gastrointestinal lymphoid tissue, has a markedly reduced content of lymphocytes.

MANIFESTATIONS. Increased susceptibility to infections is the hallmark of impairment in cellular immunity. Compared with deficient antibody formation, however, susceptibility to mycotic and viral infections, especially candidiasis, herpes simplex, and cytomegalovirus disease, is more marked. On physical examination, detectable lymphatic tissue (tonsils, peripheral lymph nodes) is diminished markedly, and no thymic shadow is demonstrable radiographically.

LABORATORY FINDINGS. Serum immunoglobulins are grossly normal, although the dysgammaglobulinemic form of thymic alymphoplasia is associated with increased γ_M-globulins and decreased γ_A- and γ_G-globulins in the serum. Antigenic challenge produces a humoral antibody response in these patients. Deficient cellular immunity and deficient delayed hypersensitivity are most easily demonstrated by skin testing with antigens which effectively show this type of immunity, e.g., mumps, trichophyton, histoplasmin, tuberculin (especially PPD—purified protein derivative), Candida, and streptokinase-streptodornase. These patients lack reactivity to the chemical and show delayed or absent rejection of homologous skin grafts. *Lymphopenia* is always present but varies markedly in magnitude, possibly because of differences in expression of the genetic defect. Lymphocyte counts often are less than 2,000 per cu mm; levels as low as 500 per cu mm have been reported.

COMBINED DEFICIENCY OF ANTIBODY PRODUCTION AND CELLULAR IMMUNITY

A combined defect in antibody production and cellular immunity is more common than either alone. Among the most severe of these disorders is *reticular dysgenesis,* a rare disease in which death from infections supervenes shortly after birth. Profound, though poorly studied, immunologic deficits in this disease probably result from failure of a primordial stem cell important to the development of immunologic competence. It is associated with profound leukopenia, lymphopenia, and thymic aplasia.

Two types of thymic alymphoplasia with hypogammaglobulinemia have been described, the autosomal Swiss type and the sex-linked disease, which are both inherited as recessive traits. Aside from the different modes of inheritance, the two diseases are similar and are characterized by hypogammaglobulinemia, impaired antibody response, vestigial thymus glands, and impaired delayed hypersensitivity reactions. Pathologically, sparse plasma cells and diminished lymphatic tissue are characteristic.

Ataxia telangiectasia is a congenital disorder with progressive cerebellar ataxia, cutaneous and conjunctival telangiectasia, and recurrent pulmonary and paranasal sinus infections. It is associated with normal levels of γ_G-γ_M-globulins but very low γ_A-globulins and impaired antibody production. An occasional patient is found to have a greatly elevated concentration of γ_A-globulin. Significant impairment of cellular immunity is also characteristic of this disorder.

The *Wiskott-Aldrich* syndrome is a poorly understood variant of the immunologic deficiency diseases which is characterized by abnormalities of antibody production and cellular immunity. The classical clinical picture is one of eczematoid dermatitis, thrombocytopenia with bleeding diathesis, and increased susceptibility to infections with bacteria, viruses, and fungi. The disease is inherited as a sex-linked recessive trait. The concentra-

tion of γ_M-globulins in the serum is reduced and that of γ_A-globulins may be increased, although there is a selective impairment of antibody response to polysaccharide antigens. Germinal centers and plasma cells are present in normal amount. Lymphopenia is characteristic, but histologically the thymus is within normal limits. Progressive loss of small lymphocytes from lymphatic tissue in males with this disease suggests that it may represent secondary or acquired dysfunction of the immunologic system. A number of patients have developed reticuloendothelial malignancies.

Depression of both antibody production and delayed hypersensitivity reactions may occur in association with the clinical use of *cytotoxic drugs,* either in therapy for malignancy or when these drugs are used as immunosuppressive agents during organ transplantation. In many instances, the occurrence of life-threatening infections is the major limiting factor to the use of these drugs.

DIAGNOSIS OF DISEASES ASSOCIATED WITH THE IMMUNOLOGIC DEFICIENCY STATE

The diagnostic hallmark of this group of diseases is increased susceptibility to infections. When infections occur in association with hypogammaglobulinemia, impaired antibody response, diminished hypersensitivity reactions, lymphopenia, or deficient lymphatic tissue, one of this group of disorders may be involved. It is often difficult to decide with certainty which of the specific syndromes is present, but the age and sex of the patient, the family history, the age at onset, the type of immunologic deficit, the pathologic findings in lymph nodes and bone marrow, and associated findings such as eczema, ataxia with telangiectasia, hypoparathyroidism, or dysgammaglobulinemia are helpful.

TREATMENT

Treatment of these disorders has had limited success. Infections are almost uniformly the presenting problems, and successful management involves accurate microbiologic diagnosis, specific chemotherapeutic or antibiotic treatment, drainage of pus, and general supportive measures. In addition, recognition of the underlying immunologic deficiency state is important. When hypogammaglobulinemia is involved, immediate and chronic replacement therapy with concentrated human γ-globulin is indicated. Fortunately, the half-life of isologous γ-globulin in these patients is generally normal or slightly prolonged. Empirically, resistance to infections in most patients is adequate when the concentration of γ-globulin is about 150 mg per 100 ml. A practical approach is to estimate the amount of γ-globulin which will increase the serum concentration by 100 mg per 100 ml. On the basis of a life of 30 days, monthly administration of 200 mg γ-globulin per kilogram of body weight will maintain this level. Whether therapy is successful should be judged by ensuing resistance to infections, not by the concentration of circulating γ-globulin. Rarely, recurrent infections with the same organism require the use of specific immune γ-globulin. In secondary acquired hypogammaglobulinemia, treatment also is governed by the underlying disease.

Immunologic deficiency states associated with impaired cellular immunity are not amenable to prolonged treatment. Transfer of immunologically competent cells in the form of spleen tissue, bone marrow, or neonatal thymus from normal individuals will restore cellular immunity. Except for one report, however, the use of such transplantation therapy has been followed by a graft-versus-host reaction in which the donor cells reject and destroy the host's tissues.

ABNORMALITIES OF IMMUNE SYSTEMS WITHOUT INCREASED SUSCEPTIBILITY TO INFECTION

That resistance to infection involves many factors is witnessed by the occurrence of immunologic abnormalities without a concomitant increased susceptibility to infections. For example, congenital absence of the $γ_A$-*globulins* has been reported in a number of clinically normal individuals. Significant immunoglobulins may be lost in the urine in patients with the *nephrotic syndrome* who usually are not unduly susceptible to infections but who may have an increased incidence of pneumococcal disease.

Intestinal lymphangiectasia is a disease of unknown cause which is characterized by dilated intestinal lymphatics and a protein-losing enteropathy with hypoproteinemia and edema. Serum immunoglobulin concentrations are reduced, but antibody response to immunization is impaired only modestly. Significant lymphopenia (levels to 800 per cu mm is characteristic, and there is profound depression of delayed hypersensitivity reactions, with prolonged homograft survival. Increased susceptibility to infection, however, is not characteristic of this disease. In the nephrotic syndrome and in intestinal lymphangiectasia, the basic mechanisms of antibody formation and cellular immunity are intact. In nephrosis, the detectable defect in immunity is due to loss of immunoglobulins in the urine, while in intestinal lymphangiectasia, both immunoglobulins and lymphocytes are lost in the stool. In both instances, however, there is no significantly increased susceptibility to infections.

Sarcoidosis and *Hodgkin's disease* are classically associated with cutaneous anergy to delayed hypersensitivity reactions. In sarcoidosis, increased susceptibility to infections is unusual, while the occurrence of infection in Hodgkin's disease is dependent on activity of the disease, the type of treatment, and the patient's general condition. Certainly, profound anergy occurs in the course of Hodgkin's disease without clinically apparent increased susceptibility to infection. That passive transfer of delayed hypersensitivity is possible in Hodgkin's disease but not in sarcoidosis suggests different mechanisms for the anergy seen in these instances.

Transient cutaneous anergy may occur during the course of a variety of *acute febrile disorders*, particularly those of viral origin, and in association with *uremia*. Transient anergy to tuberculin may also be demonstrated in association with *miliary or serosal tuberculosis*. In none of these instances has diminution in delayed hypersensitivity reactions paralleled increased susceptibility to infections.

REFERENCES

Cooper, M. D., H. P. Chase, J. T. Lowman, W. Krivit, and R. A. Good: An Immunologic Deficiency Disease Involving the Afferent Limb of Immunity. Wiskott-Aldrich Syndrome: Clinical Studies, Am. J. Med., 4:499, 1968.

Gitlin, D., C. A. Janeway, L. Apt, and J. M. Craig: Agammaglobulinemia, in "Cellular and Humoral Aspects of the Hypersensitive States," H. S. Lawrence (Ed.), New York, Hoeber Medical Division, Harper & Row, Pub., Inc., 1959.

Good, R. A., W. D. Kelly, J. Rotstein, and R. L. Varco: Immunologic Deficiency Diseases, Progr. Allergy, 6:187, 1962.

Hitzig, W., and H. Willi: Hereditary Lymphoplasmocytic Dysgenesis ("Alymphocytosis with Agammaglobulinemia"), Schweiz. Med. Wochschr., 91:1625, 1961.

Hoger, J. R., M. D. Cooper, E. C. Gabrielsen, and R. A. Good: Lymphopenic Forms of Congenital Immunologic Deficiency Diseases, Medicine, 47:201, 1968.

Peterson, R. D. A., W. D. Kelly, and R. A. Good: Ataxia-telangiectasia: Its Association with a Defective Thymus, Immunologic-deficiency Disease, and Malignancy, Lancet, 1:1189, 1964.

Rosen, F. S., S. V. Kevy, E. Merler, C. A. Janeway, and D. Gitlin: Recurrent Bacterial Infections and Dysgammaglobulinemia: Deficiency of 7S Gamma Globulin in the Presence of Elevated 19S Gamma Globulins: Report of 2 Cases, Pediatrics, 28:182, 1961.

Seligmann, M., H. H. Fudenberg, and R. A. Good: A Proposed Classification of Primary Immunologic Deficiencies, Am. J. Med., 45:817, 1968.

Strober, W., R. D. Wochner, P. P. Carbone, and T. A. Waldmann: Intestinal Lymphangiectasia: A Protein-losing Enteropathy with Hypogammaglobulinemia, Lymphocytopenia and Impaired Homograft Rejection, J. Clin. Invest., 46:1643, 1967.

70 IMMUNOGLOBULINS AND SOME OF THEIR DISORDERS

Edward C. Franklin

INTRODUCTION AND CLASSIFICATION

Antibodies with different specificities are known to be dissimilar in their primary structure. Hence, it is not surprising that antibody activity is associated with a heterogeneous group of proteins which are collectively known as the immunoglobulins. Though the bulk of antibody activity resides in the slowly migrating γ-globulin fraction, small amounts of protein related to the immunoglobulins have been identified by serologic tech-

Table 70-1. SOME PROPERTIES OF IMMUNOGLOBULIN

Property	Immunoglobulin class-γ				
	G	A	M	D	E
Molecular weight	145,000	$\pm$160,000	900,000	$\pm$160,000	200,000
Sedimentation coefficient (Svedberg's)	7	7(9, 11, 13, 15)	19	7	8
Electrophoretic mobility	γ	γ-β	γ-β	γ-β	γ-β
Approx. concentration (mg/100 ml)	1,200	200	100	3	0.03
Carbohydrate (%)	2.5	10	10	?	10
Valence	2	2(?)	5(?)	?	?
"Paraprotein"	G myeloma	A myeloma	Macroglobulin	D myeloma	E myeloma

niques in the β- and the α_2-globulins. In addition to antibodies, the immunoglobulins include a group of structurally related proteins ("paraproteins"), which include myeloma proteins and macroglobulins and are found in several proliferative disorders of plasma cells and lymphocytes. Although these proteins generally appear to be devoid of antibody activity, their structural similarities to classical antibodies have led to their use as models of antibodies. The discovery of antibody activity in some of these paraproteins has raised the possibility that all of them may be antibodies to some as yet undefined antigens.

In spite of the enormous variability among different antibodies, the immunoglobulins show certain properties which permit their grouping into at least five major classes and a limited number of subclasses. Table 70-1 summarizes the relative concentrations and the major physical, chemical, and antigenic features of the five currently recognized classes of immunoglobulins. Though their ultracentrifugal and electrophoretic properties have been of great value in classification, it is their antigenic properties which have been especially useful in clinical practice. In particular, certain unique antigenic determinants which distinguish each class from the others have resulted in the development of class-specific antiserums which are widely used to quantitate and characterize the immunoglobulin fractions in various body fluids by immunoelectrophoretic and immunodiffusion techniques.

Antibodies have been identified in the γ_G-, γ_A-, and γ_M-globulin fractions; the γ_D-fraction has not been shown to possess antibody activity, but its structure suggests that it, too, may contain antibodies. The discovery that reaginic antibodies exist in the hitherto undescribed γ_E-globulin fraction suggests that additional classes of immunoglobulins may be found.

Table 70-1 also lists the paraproteins corresponding to each of the major immunoglobulin classes. When large series of patients with paraproteinemia are studied, the frequency of each paraprotein is closely related to the relative concentration of the corresponding fraction in normal serum. For example, G myeloma proteins occur more frequently than A myeloma proteins, which, in turn, are seen more often than macroglobulins, while D and E myeloma proteins occur only rarely.

The five well-characterized classes of immunoglobulins show striking differences in their distribution in the body and in some of their biologic properties. For example, the γ_G fraction is the only one to cross the placental barrier and thereby provides passive immunity to the newborn infant. During intrauterine life and early infancy, both γ_M and γ_G antibodies are formed by the fetus, while synthesis of γ_A-globulins does not commence until later.

Following an antigenic stimulus later in life, γ_M antibodies generally appear rapidly—the primary response—and production continues only as long as the antigen persists; γ_G antibodies are formed somewhat later, persist for a longer period, and are largely responsible for "immunologic memory," i.e., the ability of the individual to respond more strongly and rapidly to subsequent encounters with the same antigens. However, a clear-cut separation between the properties of these two classes of antibodies is not feasible.

Though all immunoglobulins are widely distributed in the intravascular and, in some instances, the extravascular compartments, the γ_A-globulins are unique in being the major, if not the sole, immunoglobulin fraction in external secretions, such as bronchial and intestinal mucus, saliva, colostrum, and lacrimal fluid, where they provide a first line of defense against bacterial and viral antigens. The γ_A-globulins in these secretions differ from those in the blood in being larger and in containing an extra structural unit with a molecular weight of about 50,000. This unit, known as a "transport piece" or "secretory piece," is synthesized in the epithelial cells of the exocrine glands, and appears to play an important role in the secretion of antibodies into these fluids or possibly in protecting them from proteolysis. The transport piece differs in structure from any of the immunoglobulin subunits, and appears to be under separate genetic control, because it is present in patients with agammaglobulinemia who cannot produce significant amounts of γ-globulins.

STRUCTURAL UNITS OF THE IMMUNOGLOBULINS

The immunoglobulins, like many other complex proteins, are made of multiple polypeptide chains, each of

Fig. 70-1. Schematic diagram of γ_G-globulin. Heavy chains H consist of an Fc fragment, which is the same in all molecules of given subclass, and an Fd fragment, part of which is constant and part of which varies in composition in different myeloma proteins. Similarly, light chains L have a constant and a variable half. A light chain and an Fd fragment make up the Fab fragment. S—S = disulfide bond. N and C are N and C terminal ends. Gm and Inv are genetic factors associated with H and L chains respectively.

which is under separate genetic control. Consequently, similarities in the classes of immunoglobulins may be attributed to the existence of certain structural units found in all of them, while differences among the classes are considered due to structural units unique to each class. In general, each of the immunoglobulins consists of a basic subunit composed of four polypeptide chains held together by disulfide (covalent) and non-covalent bonds (Fig. 70-1). Two of these polypeptide chains have molecular weights of 22,000 and are called light chains. There are two major types, known as κ and λ, which are common to all classes of immunoglobulins. The other two polypeptide chains have molecular weights between 55,000 and 70,000, and are, therefore, called heavy chains. Because the heavy chains are different in each class of immunoglobulin, they are identified by the Greek letter corresponding to the class (γ, α, μ, δ, ε, for the γ_G, γ_A, γ_M, γ_D, and γ_E fractions, respectively). The γ_M, or macroglobulin, fraction has a molecular weight of about 850,000, compared with 160,000 to 200,000 for the others. It is composed of five such subunits, each of which is probably made of two heavy and two light chains. The disulfide bonds, joining these subunits, can be cleaved readily by sulfhydryl reagents, often with a concomitant loss of antibody activity. This inactivation of antibodies by gentle reduction has been used clinically to identify antibodies in this fraction, but the method appears not to be infallible.

The antigen-binding sites include only a small region of the total molecule and appear to involve both the heavy and light polypeptide chains. They reside in the amino terminal half of the molecule (the Fab fragments) (Fig. 70-1), while many of the other properties generally associated with antibodies reside in the Fc fragment, which constitutes the carboxy terminal end of the heavy

chain. Each γ_G molecule, as well as probably all the other 7S immunoglobulins, has two antigen-binding sites. It is not known whether 5 or 10 combining sites exist in the intact γ_M-macroglobulin, although it appears likely that 10 sites are potentially available to react with antigens. The elucidation of the amino acid sequence of a number of Bence Jones (light-chain) proteins and parts of several myeloma proteins has demonstrated clearly that both the heavy and light chains contain regions which differ in composition for different proteins. These "variable" regions are located in the amino terminal half of the molecule and, consequently, appear to contribute to the specific conformation required by the antigen-binding sites. Studies of the relatively homogeneous "paraproteins" have extended the knowledge regarding the synthesis and genetic control of the normal immunoglobulins. It has been demonstrated that each class and subclass of heavy and light chains appears to have certain unique structural features in the region of the molecule known as the "constant" region. This region is similar for all molecules belonging to a particular immunoglobulin class and occupies the carboxy terminal half. The synthesis of each of the immunoglobulin chains appears to be under the control of a specific genetic locus. Because of difficulties in the assay system used to define them, not all these loci have been identified. Nevertheless, at least five loci are now known to be involved in the synthesis of the immunoglobulin chains. The constant region of the κ chains is under the control of the Inv locus; the Oz locus may play a similar role for the λ chains. A series of closely linked loci, collectively known as the Gm loci, determine the structure of the different subclasses of γ heavy chains and are known as the γ_1, γ_2, and γ_3 loci. Analogous genetic factors for γ_4, α, μ, δ, and ε chains undoubtedly exist but remain to be identified. Multiple alleles exist at each of these loci. In the case of the Inv factors, where studies have progressed furthest, differences between the constant regions of κ chains that are Inv (a+) or Inv (b+) consist of a single amino acid residue. It seems likely also that in other instances the differences between chains under the control of alleles at each of these loci will be limited to only a few amino acid residues. Though all classes of light and heavy chains exist in any one individual, studies of the more homogeneous paraproteins suggest that individual molecules are always symmetric and contain two identical heavy and two identical light chains. Consistent with this finding is the observation that each plasma cell can synthesize only one type of heavy chain and one type of light chain at any one time. Studies with mouse plasma cell tumors in vitro have shown that the synthesis of heavy and light chains occurs on separate polyribosomes, and that, in general, synthesis of light and heavy chains

is approximately equal. The small excess of light chains may be stored in the cell and may play a role in the orderly release of completed antibody molecules.

DISORDERS OF IMMUNOGLOBULINS

Several diseases are associated with quantitative alterations in the immunoglobulins. A diffuse increase in all immunoglobulins (Fig. 70-2B) is the most frequent abnormality and generally reflects an increase in γ-globulin synthesis. This is a common nonspecific manifestation of many chronic diseases such as infections, liver disease, "connective tissue" diseases, and sarcoidosis. This type of diffuse hypergammaglobulinemia is entirely nonspecific and of little aid in diagnosis. Occasionally, one or another class of immunoglobulin may be increased out of proportion to the others. A decrease in one or more of the immunoglobulins (hypogammaglobulinemia) is usually

Fig. 70-2. Paper electrophoretic patterns of A. normal serum; B. serum with diffuse hypergammaglobulinemia; C. serum with G myeloma protein ("paraproteinemia"); D. urine with light-chain (Bence Jones) protein.

the result of a decrease in synthesis and is only rarely due to excessive catabolism or loss via the urine or gastrointestinal tract (Chap. 69). This abnormality is most pronounced in the many types of congenital or acquired agammaglobulinemia or hypogammaglobulinemia. Another type of disorder involves the production of antibodies which react with an antigen present in the host and which have been called "autoantibodies." It seems likely that in many instances, autoantibodies are induced initially by foreign antigens and cross-react with tissue or serum constituents of the host. "Autoantibodies" may be directed against nucleoproteins, autologous or isologous γ-globulin (rheumatoid factors), or against red blood cells, white blood cells, platelets, thyroid antigens, and intrinsic factor. Though "autoantibodies" may be demonstrable in many diseases, their role in the pathogenesis of most of them remains unclear.

A third group of disorders is characterized by the production of immunoglobulin components which appear as homogeneous "spikes" in the electrophoretic pattern of serum or urine (Fig. 70-2C and D). It is not known whether these proteins are abnormal or whether they simply represent a quantitative increase in a normal subfraction. These diseases include a number of neoplastic processes involving plasma cells and lymphocytes, including multiple myeloma, macroglobulinemia, and "heavy-chain" disease. The abnormal proteins range in electrophoretic mobility from the slow γ-globulin to the fast α$_2$-globulin fraction. Precise identification is not possible from the appearance or mobility of the spike on paper electrophoresis and requires immunoelectrophoretic and, in some instances, ultracentrifugal analyses. In about 5 percent of patients with plasma cell dyscrasias, there is no detectable serum or urine abnormality or only a decrease in the γ-globulin level.

The abnormal proteins produced in the so-called dysproteinemias may be viewed best in the light of the normal immunoglobulins and their structural units (Table 70-2). For each normal immunoglobulin there is a

Table 70-2. DISORDERS OF γ-GLOBULIN SYNTHESIS

Heavy and light-chain synthesis	Resultant immunoglobulin disorder
Balanced	Serum paraprotein (myeloma or macroglobulin)
Light only	Urine "L chain" (Bence Jones protein)
Excess light	Serum paraprotein and urine "L chain" (Bence Jones protein)
Heavy-chain or fragment only	"Heavy-chain" fragment in serum and urine
Excess heavy-chain or fragment*	Serum "paraprotein" plus "heavy-chain" fragment in serum and urine

* Not yet observed.

corresponding class of paraprotein. However, the precise nature of the proteins elaborated is determined by the relative rates of synthesis of the constituent polypeptide chains. For example, in a patient with multiple myeloma or macroglobulinemia, a myeloma protein or macroglobulin is found in the blood if the synthesis of light and heavy chains remains balanced. In certain instances, asynchronous production of heavy and light chains occurs. If only light chains are produced, a homogeneous protein spike, often with the thermal properties of Bence Jones protein, appears in the urine, and no abnormal protein is found in the serum. Bences Jones proteins are defined by their insolubility when heated to 56°C and their resolubilization at 100°C. Since they represent the light polypeptide chains and since many of them fail to demonstrate the characteristic thermal properties, it seems preferable to refer to them as light-chain proteins and to rely on electrophoretic and immunologic methods for their identification. These cases cannot be classified as belonging in any of the major classes of paraproteinemia. If light chains exceed the quantity of heavy chains, both a serum "paraprotein" spike, related to one of the major classes of immunoglobulins, and a light-chain spike are found in the urine. Occasionally, because of the existence of larger polymers or because of decreased catabolism, light chains accumulate in the serum and also can present a spike.

In patients with "heavy-chain disease," a fragment of the heavy chain resembling the Fc fragment is produced and can be identified in both serum and urine (see also Chap. 349). Most of these patients have produced a fragment of the γ chain. However, at least one patient with α heavy-chain disease has been described, and it seems likely that similar disorders of μ, δ, and ε chains will be found. The coexistence of a myeloma protein in the serum and a heavy-chain disease protein in serum and/or urine in patients with asynchronous production of the two types of chain seems conceivable but has not been described.

As judged by a variety of chemical and serologic techniques, these "paraproteins" have significantly greater homogeneity than the normal immunoglobulin fractions. When examined in pure form, they possess only one class of light chain and one subclass of heavy chain, and invariably carry only the genetic markers controlled by one allele at the pertinent locus, even when they occur in an individual who is heterozygous for these factors. In most instances, the proteins produced in these disorders are devoid of antibody activity. However, cold agglutinin and rheumatoid factor activity have been found associated with some macroglobulins, and a few myeloma proteins have shown other antibody activities.

As emphasized in Chap. 349, dealing with the clinical features of the paraproteinemias, the manifestations of macroglobulinemia and multiple myeloma rarely are related to the abnormal proteins, but reflect the existence of a malignant disease. However, in some patients large amounts of the abnormal proteins, the existence of proteins with unusual solubility or antibody properties, and occasionally the marked depression of normal γ-globulins may be responsible directly for certain clinical features, as described below.

Hyperviscosity Syndrome

The presence in serum in high concentrations of a protein, most often a macroglobulin, may cause a marked rise in viscosity, which in turn may interfere with efficient circulation to the brain, digits, kidneys, or eyes. The fundi may show a characteristic appearance, with very dilated venules and many hemorrhages. The hyperviscosity syndrome often results in the sudden onset of confusion, which frequently progresses to severe organic central-nervous-system disturbances. Progressive signs of cardiac and peripheral vascular insufficiency result from the impaired circulation in the small capillaries. The diagnosis may be confirmed by demonstration of increased serum viscosity with an Ostwald viscosimeter. Treatment must be instituted immediately, with repeated plasmaphereses until the viscosity is diminished and symptoms subside. Subsequently, viscosity may be maintained within normal limits by regular plasmaphereses; therapy must be continued indefinitely. Plasmapheresis is particularly successful in patients with macroglobulinemia because these high molecular weight proteins are confined largely to the intravascular space.

Cryoglobulins

Somewhat similar clinical findings may result from the presence of cryoglobulins, which are proteins that precipitate in the cold and redissolve on warming. While cryoglobulins are often detected accidentally in asymptomatic patients, they may on occasion cause peripheral vascular insufficiency and even gangrene after exposure to low temperatures. Cryoglobulins are most often associated with multiple myeloma and macroglobulinemia, but they may occur in systemic lupus erythematosus or other "connective tissue" diseases or even in the absence of any overt illness. About one-third of cryoglobulins are G myeloma proteins, one-third are macroglobulins, and about one-third are mixtures of γ_G- and γ_M-globulins. These mixtures are most often found in patients with one of the "connective tissue" diseases and are associated with purpura and progressive, often fulminant, renal lesions reminiscent of those seen in nephritis caused by antigen-antibody complexes. The precise mechanism for cryoprecipitation is not known, and in general, there is little correlation between symptoms and the amount of cryoglobulins or the temperature at which precipitation occurs. There is evidence that many cryoglobulins may, in fact, be antibodies to γ-globulins.

Cold Agglutinins

Another disorder directly related to an unusual group of abnormal macroglobulins is the hemolytic anemia induced by cold agglutinins (Chap. 338). Though antibodies which cause hemolysis after exposure to the cold may be seen transiently in certain infections, such as infectious mononucleosis or atypical pneumonia, they rarely cause severe hemolysis in any disease other than macroglobulinemia or lymphosarcoma. The cold ag-

glutinins causing hemolysis are generally directed against the I antigen of the red blood cell and usually possess only κ light chains. Unlike antibodies which interact with red blood cells at body temperature, cold agglutinins usually appear free in the circulation because they frequently can be eluted spontaneously from the red blood cells after reacting with certain components of complement.

Bence Jones Proteins

Another abnormality directly related to abnormal proteins is the renal disease seen in patients with Bence Jones proteinuria. The filtration of large amounts of these proteins through the glomeruli exposes the tubules to an enormous reabsorptive load, which may cause degeneration of tubular cells, deposition of proteinaceous inclusions in the cells, and the formation of tubular casts. This is often referred to as "myeloma kidney," and may result in renal failure with uremia or in the appearance of the nephrotic syndrome. Severe dehydration preceding certain diagnostic procedures such as intravenous pyelograms may be sufficient to precipitate acute renal failure in these patients.

Miscellaneous

On rare occasions paraproteins may interact with other substances, such as calcium and some of the clotting factors, or may coat blood platelets and intefere with the normal mechanisms of blood coagulation and hemostasis. There is some evidence that these disorders may be associated with amyloidosis, but it is unlikely that γ-globulins are an integral part of amyloid. Amyloid appears to be a fibrillar protein with several unique properties (Chap. 114).

Hypogammaglobulinemias

The recurrent infections often seen in patients with hypogammaglobulinemias (Chap. 69), are not directly caused by the presence of abnormal proteins but are probably attributable to the decrease in the immune response which is followed by diminished production of immunoglobulins.

SIGNIFICANCE OF PARAPROTEINEMIAS

In rare instances, the paraproteins contribute directly to the pathogenesis of some symptoms. More often they merely provide important clues in the diagnostic classification of these disorders. Evidence in support of the minor role generally played by the paraproteins in the production of clinical symptoms is provided by the ever-increasing number of elderly persons who are found to have a "paraprotein" during a routine study for an unrelated disease, who have no other symptoms, and who cannot be diagnosed as having multiple myeloma or related diseases.

REFERENCES

Cohen, S., and C. Milstein: Structural and Biological Properties of Immunoglobulins, Advan. Immunol., 7:1, 1967.

Fahey, J. L.: Serum Protein Disorders Causing Symptoms in Malignant Neoplastic Diseases, J. Chronic Dis., 16:703, 1963.

——, R. Scoggins, J. P. Utz, and C. Szwed: Infection, Antibody Response and γ-Globulin Components in Multiple Myeloma and Macroglobulinemia, Am. J. Med., 35:698, 1963.

Meltzer, M., and E. C. Franklin: Cryoglobulinemia—A Study of 29 Patients. I. IgG and IgM Cryoglobulins and Factors Affecting Cryoprecipitability, Am. J. Med., 40:828, 1966.

——, ——, K. Elias, R. T. McCluskey, and N. Cooper: Cryoglobulinemia—A Clinical and Laboratory Study. II. Cryoglobulins with Rheumatoid Factor Activity, Am. J. Med., 40:837, 1966.

Osserman, K., and K. Takatsuki: Plasma Cell Myeloma—γ-Globulin Synthesis and Structure—A Review of Biochemical and Clinical Data with the Description of a Newly Recognized and Related Syndrome Hγ₂ Chain (Franklin's) Disease, Medicine, 42:357, 1963.

Solomon, A., and J. L. Fahey: Bence Jones Proteinemia, Am. J. Med., 37:206, 1964.

71 TRANSPLANTATION

John P. Merrill

Transplantation of the human kidney is now a justified procedure for the treatment of advanced chronic renal failure. An analysis of more than 2,000 cases performed as of July, 1968, shows a 2-year survival rate of 80 percent for transplants between siblings done since January, 1966. For a similar period, 2-year survival rates for parent-to-child transplants are 60 percent and those for cadaver kidneys, 40 percent. The data show a striking improvement in results since the first successful kidney transplant in 1954, and further improvement can be expected. The results compare favorably with such accepted procedures as open heart surgery for acquired valvular heart disease. Human liver, pancreas, bone marrow, heart, and endocrine glands also have been transplanted but with less success. Even for these tissues, however, the problem does not appear insurmountable.

IMMUNOLOGIC CONSIDERATIONS

Necessary to the understanding of transplantation immunity are the following terms: *autograft*—the transplantation of tissue from one part of an individual to another part of that same individual; *isograft*—the transplantation of tissues between two individuals of the same inbred strains. Because in these cases the antigens of the donor and recipient are identical, no *histocompatibility* difference exists and no immune response to the graft occurs. A case in point in man is transplantation between identical twins. In an *allograft*, i.e., a graft of tissues between two individuals of the same species, histocompatibility differences may be strong or weak, depending on the individual and the species. A *xenograft* is a graft between individuals of two different species. The term "heterograft" is still used synonomously with xenograft.

Most of the knowledge of the biology of human tissue transplantation stems from experimental work in animals. Though species differences do exist, a justifiable analogy to data from animal experiments may be made and can be summarized by the following generalizations. The rejection of an allograft in man is due to an immune response in the recipient against an antigen present on the tissues of the donor and absent in the host. In man, it is probable that the three major antigenic mosaics of the human histocompatibility system (HU-1) are strong antigens. These antigens not only are detectable by serologic techniques but also may, by virtue of their presence or absence in the donor and recipient pair, modify the course of transplants and the amount of immunosuppressive therapy necessary. In experimental animals, by long and careful inbreeding it is possible to control histocompatibility, and the immune response between animals of different histocompatibility can be delineated by carefully controlled experiments involving grafting in a large number of lower mammals. For obvious reasons this is not true for man. However, it is possible in man to transplant skin, to inject peripheral leukocytes and platelets, to study the reactions of peripheral leukocytes from various individuals to a single anti-human leukocyte serum, and to correlate this information with the results in kidney transplantation.

HOST VERSUS GRAFT REACTION. If a piece of skin is transplanted from A to B, ingrowth of capillaries from the host into the graft occurs and the graft becomes vascularized in a normal fashion for 3 or 4 days. During this time it is probable that antigens of the graft reach the host by way of both the lymphatics and the bloodstream. The graft antigens appear to consist of lipoprotein complexes. The recipient becomes sensitized to the antigens released by the graft in the following fashion: Fig. 71-1 (1) Antigen from the graft reaches the regional lymph nodes by the afferent lymphatic vessels and reacts with a macrophage. Here the antigen acquires an RNA component, which is then transfered to an unsensitized or "uncommitted" lymphocyte. This small lymphocyte enlarges into a large pyroninophilic cell (lymphoblast), which divides repeatedly, giving rise to many sensitized lymphocytes, i.e., lymphocytes containing antibody directed against the graft. These cells then reach the vasculature of the graft, causing damage to its vascular endothelium, and eventually pass through the wall of the vessels where they infiltrate the interstitium of the graft. (2) It is possible that this process also takes place outside the lymph nodes, including the kidneys and other directly vascularized grafts, where lymphocytes or macrophages come in direct contact with antigens of the graft. Once these sensitized cells reach lymphatic tissue anywhere in the body, they may stimulate the process described above. It is probable also that cell-free or soluble antibody in the form of gamma-globulin (IgG)

Fig. 71-1. (1) Unsensitized lymphocyte (2) Lymphocyte sensitized by passage through kidney (3) Antigen released from kidney (4) Macrophage (5) Processed antigens (6) Lymphocyte (7) Lymphoblast (8) Sensitized lymphocyte (9) Antibody globulin (10) PMN leukocyte (11) Macrophage (12) Complement (13) MIF factor.

There are two current concepts of the mode of sensitization of a recipient to a transplanted kidney. In the first, antigens of the kidney (3) may be engulfed by the macrophage system (4) of the recipient and the processed antigen (5) induces transformation of some of the lymph node lymphocytes (6) into lymphoblasts. Alternatively, circulating lymphocytes (1) may become sensitized directly as they pass through the kidney (2). Either way, the result is production of lymphocytes (8) particularly sensitized to the graft. When these cells arrive at the vasculature of the graft along with antibody globulin (9), which is also produced by the lymph nodes, they attach to antigenic binding sites on the wall of the vessel. Complement is bound at the antibody sites and the complement (12) sequence is initiated. As a result of this initiation, the polymorphonuclear (PMN) chemotactic factor is released and PMN's (10) are attracted to the graft where the release of lysosomal enzymes from the leukocytes may result in damage to the vascular wall. Similarly the interaction of sensitized lymphocytes and antigens at the graft site releases macrophage migration inhibitory factor (MIF) (13) which causes the accumulation of cells (11) at the graft site. Some mononuclear cells migrate through the vessel wall and are seen as perivascular accumulations. Intravascular accumulation results in slowing of flow, stasis, and graft ischemia. Not shown here are platelet deposition and small thrombi, which may accompany this reaction.

may react directly with the vascular endothelium of the graft. When this occurs, the cellular reaction is secondary. An example in man is the accelerated rejection that occurs when an individual (*B*) who has been sensitized by a previous skin graft from *A* receives a second skin graft; if the second graft is placed a certain length of time following the initial transplant, it may be rejected in an "accelerated fashion." Under these circumstances the second graft never becomes vascularized. Small-vessel thrombosis occurs with rapidity. No lymphocytes are seen at the site of the rejected graft, and the polymorphonuclear leukocytes that appear seem to be due to a response to necrosis rather than to an immune reaction. Alternatively, it is possible that sensitized lymphocytes

reach the vascular endothelium but are destroyed upon contact with it, liberating proteolytic enzymes which cause further endothelial destruction and injury. Finally, both mechanisms may be operative in previously sensitized individuals. Soluble antigens from the graft encounter a sensitized lymphocyte at the vessel wall. The antigen combines with the cell-bound antibody, and a protein factor is released which interferes with the migration of monocytes by making them adhere to the vessel wall and injure its endothelial lining. The monocytes activated by this migration-inhibitory factor (MIF) are transformed into macrophages which force themselves through the endothelium of the vessel wall, releasing lysosomal hydrolases which attack both the vessel wall and the parenchymal elements. Many similarities between the rejection of transplanted tissue and the so-called delayed hypersensitivity reaction have been noted, and graft rejection is thought to be a manifestation of delayed hypersensitivity.

IMMUNOSUPPRESSIVE TREATMENT

When histocompatibility differences exist between donor and recipient, it is necessary to modify or suppress the immune response in order to enable the recipient to "tolerate" a graft. Immunosuppressive therapy in general suppresses all immune responses, including those to bacteria, fungi, and even malignant tumors. Agents used in man to suppress the immune response are the following:

TOTAL-BODY IRRADIATION. Lethal doses of x-irradiation in animals destroy the lymphopoietic system and the ability to reject a tissue graft. However, because irradiation also destroys the bone marrow, it is necessary to transplant bone marrow in order to enable the animal to survive. Attempts to utilize this technique in man generally have been unsuccessful, but one patient at least has done well.

DRUGS. *Azathioprine* (Imuran), an analogue of 6-mercaptopurine, is the keystone of immunosuppressive therapy in man. This agent inhibits synthesis of deoxyribonucleic acid (DNA) or ribonucleic acid (RNA) or both. Because cell division and proliferation result as part of the immune response to antigenic stimulation, suppression may be mediated by the inhibition of mitosis of immunologically competent lymphoid cells interfering with synthesis of DNA. Alternatively, inhibition may occur by blocking the synthesis of ribonucleic acids (possibly messenger RNA) which is thought to play an important role in the processing of antigens prior to lymphoid stimulation. Therapy with azathioprine is generally instituted 2 to 10 days prior to transplantation of the kidney and is continued as long as the allograft functions. Because the drug is excreted by glomerular filtration, the dose must be varied according to the functional status of the kidney. Bone marrow depression may occur as a result of excess dosage of azathioprine, as may jaundice, anemia, and alopecia. *Actinomycin C* formerly was employed in the treatment of rejection crises but because of its toxicity is used infrequently.

The *corticosteroids*, usually in the form of prednisone, are important adjuncts to immunosuppressive therapy. Of all the agents employed, the effect of prednisone is easiest to assess, and in large doses it is unquestionably the most effective agent for the reversal of rejection. In general, 150 to 200 mg prednisone is given immediately prior to or at the time of transplantation, and the dosage is reduced to maintenance levels, over a period of 2 weeks. The well-known side effects of the corticosteroids, particularly impairment of wound healing and predisposition to infection, make it desirable to taper the dose as rapidly as possible in the immediate postoperative period. Prednisone should be used in large doses (200 to 500 mg) immediately upon detection of beginning rejection. When the drug is effective, the results are

usually apparent within 24 to 48 hr, and the dose then may be reduced again. Although most patients whose renal function is stable after 6 months or a year do not require large doses of prednisone, maintenance doses of 20 mg per day are the rule.

THORACIC DUCT FISTULA. Lymphocyte depletion by cannulation and drainage of the thoracic duct appears to lessen the number of rejection crises in the early posttransplant period in man.

EXTRACORPOREAL IRRADIATION. Irradiation of blood as it passes through an extracorporeal source connected to the patient by the arteriovenous cannula usually utilized for dialysis with the artificial kidney, has resulted in lymphocyte depletion and is an adjunct to other forms of immunosuppressive therapy but not a substitute for them. It is particularly useful in maintaining immunosuppression when toxicity of other agents requires their temporary discontinuance.

ANTILYMPHOCYTE SERUM. When serums from animals made immune to host lymphocytes are injected into the recipient, they destroy lymphoid cells and suppress the immune response to tissue grafts. Antilymphocyte serum is unquestionably effective in prolonging grafts in experimental animals, but its efficacy in human beings is somewhat less clear. In practice, peripheral human lymphocytes or lymphocytes from cadaver spleens or thoracic duct fistulas are injected into horses to produce antilymphocyte serums, from which the specific globulin is then separated. The globulin is injected intramuscularly into patients 5 days to a week prior to transplantation, and injections are continued for 2 to 3 weeks thereafter. Pain and swelling occur at the site of injection, and occasional anaphylaxis has been reported. No deaths attributable to the use of horse serum have occurred. When an effective preparation of antilymphocyte globulin is used, delayed-type hypersensitivity skin tests disappear in the recipient. There is suggestive but not conclusive evidence that the mortality rate of patients treated in this fashion is decreased and that when antilymphocyte serum is used, smaller doses of azathioprine and steroids will prevent rejection. Although antilymphocyte serum should be used with extreme caution in man, it seems probable that further exploration of this preparation may yield an effective agent which can be used with relatively little hazard of serum sickness or nephrotoxic nephritis.

Other techniques of immunosuppression, including thymectomy, splenectomy, and local irradiation of the kidney, have not influenced the course of human kidney transplants favorably.

COMPLICATIONS OF RENAL TRANSPLANTATION

The complications of human renal transplantation often result from the use of *immunosuppressive therapy*. Wound infection with gram-negative organisms is common, as is breakdown of wounds, particularly the ureteral anastomosis. Pulmonary infections with a variety of unusual organisms, including *Candida* (Chap. 190), *Aspergillus* (Chap. 193), *Nocardia* (Chap. 192), *Pneumocystis*

(Chap. 245), and cytomegalovirus (Chap. 232), also occur. Their relationship to a general defect in immunologic integrity is clear. The complications of *corticosteroid* therapy are well known and include gastrointestinal bleeding, hemorrhagic pancreatitis, and impairment of wound healing. Leukopenia, anemia, and jaundice occur as a result of azathioprine administration.

Even identical twins who do not require immunosuppressive therapy develop complications. In 18 sets of identical twins, whose original disease was glomerulonephritis, 11 developed a similar histologic lesion in the transplanted kidney. The glomerular lesion is not, however, limited to the isograft, nor is it necessarily a question of "catching" the disease in the transplant because of continuing antiglomerular activity. A number of patients with true allografts treated with immunosuppressive therapy have developed typical glomerular lesions over a period of years. One patient who received a successful allograft from his mother developed a classical nephrotic syndrome with glomerulonephritis 2½ years after transplantation. Because the reason for transplantation initially was the accidental removal of a single normal ectopic kidney, the development of glomerulonephritis in the transplant cannot be attributed to "continuing activity."

Another long-term complication of renal allografting has been the development of *nephrosclerosis* with proliferation of the vascular intima of renal vessels, intimal fibrosis, and marked decrease in the lumen of the vessels. The result is renal ischemia, hypertension, widespread tubular atrophy, interstitial fibrosis, and glomerular atrophy with eventual renal failure. Both the long-term vascular lesions and the glomerular lesions are probably the result of subclinical episodes of rejection with damage to capillary and vascular endothelium and resultant healing with fibrosis and sclerosis.

Sensitization of the human recipient to subsequent skin grafts from any donor may occur following the intradermal injection of donor leukocytes, and uremic recipients, particularly when maintained for long periods on hemodialysis, require repeated transfusions and thus have repeated exposure to formed elements in the blood which are capable of sensitizing the recipient to subsequent tissue grafts. Rapid rejection of a first kidney allograft has been documented in a number of patients who presumably have been sensitized by platelets or leukocytes in transfusions administered prior to operation. Antibodies to human leukocytes have been demonstrated in the serum of these patients and are associated in a significant number of instances with a rapid rejection of the renal transplant.

Tumor cells have been transplanted inadvertently with kidneys taken from cadaver donors dying from bronchogenic carcinoma and other malignancies. The immunosuppressive therapy which allows the kidney to be tolerated in the recipients also apparently permits survival and propagation of the malignant tumor. With cessation of immunosuppressive therapy both the renal allograft and the tumor are destroyed.

TISSUE TYPING

In the experimental animal the duration of allograft survival depends on the "strength" of the difference in histocompatibility between the donor and the recipient. A number of techniques for "typing" tissue have been developed. Of these, the most important are (1) serotyping of leukocytes and (2) use of mixed lymphocyte cultures. In serotyping, serums obtained from patients who have been immunized inadvertently to human leukocytes (either multiparous women or patients who have received repeated transfusions) are evaluated with respect to their ability to agglutinate leukocytes and to elicit a cytotoxic effect. In the performance of both tests, donor and recipient cells are tested against a single antiserum; as many different antiserums as feasible are used. If agglutination or cytotoxicity is detected for both sets of cells, antigenic configurations are said to be similar; the same holds true if neither is affected. If one set of cells is affected and the other is not, a difference is assumed to be present. Serial dilutions of serum may sharpen differences in agglutination or cytotoxicity. By cross absorption of antiserums it is theoretically possible to obtain monospecific antiserums capable of recognizing a single leukocyte antigen. Five of these antigen groups have been characterized and predict important histocompatibility antigens in man. In general, there has been a good correlation between close histocompatibility and transplant survival. Predictably, the correlation has been better between siblings and parent-child combinations than with cadaver kidneys, probably because not all antigens recognized by these techniques are related to true histocompatibility. The *mixed lymphocyte culture technique* involves culturing peripheral blood lymphocytes from donor and recipient. When these cells are stimulated, they are transformed into large basophilic blastlike cells, presumably an indication of antibody synthesis which can be quantitated either by a number of morphologic changes or by the uptake of tritiated thymidine or iodouridine. Stimulation to form antibody will be greater when histocompatibility difference between donor and recipient is marked. Inhibition of the immunologic potential of cells at a certain point in their inactivation by mitromycin interferes with the ability of cells to react, but these cells still can be stimulated, making it possible to predict how strongly a potential recipient may be stimulated by donor cells. These techniques in selecting donor recipient pairs are promising and may lead to a rational decrease in the dose of toxic immunosuppressive therapy which must be utilized to prevent rejection.

SELECTION OF RECIPIENTS FOR KIDNEY TRANSPLANTATION

Table 71-1 lists practical considerations in the selection of a recipient for a human renal allograft. Such a procedure should be undertaken only when conservative treatment has failed, when there are no reversible ele-

TRANSPLANTATION

Table 71-1. CONTRAINDICATIONS TO HUMAN KIDNEY TRANSPLANTATION

1. Absolute contraindications:
   a. Reversible renal involvement
   b. Ability of conservative measures to maintain useful life
   c. Major extrarenal complications (cerebrovascular or coronary disease; neoplasia)
   d. Active infection
   e. Active glomerulonephritis
   f. Previous sensitization to human tissue
2. Relative contraindications:
   a. Age
   b. Presence of vesical or urethral abnormalities
   c. Iliofemoral occlusive disease
   d. Diabetes mellitus
   e. Inactive lupus erythematosus
   f. Psychiatric problems

ments in the patient's renal failure, and when he is too sick to be maintained comfortably with the usual methods of treatment. However, the considerable success with kidneys transplanted from blood relatives, reports of success with second or third kidney transplants, and the ability to maintain patients who have had transplant failures on hemodialysis justify consideration of kidney transplantation before the patient is critically ill and possibly even before it is obvious that hemodialysis is the only other course. The recipient should be free of life-threatening extrarenal complications such as cancer, severe coronary artery disease, and cerebrovascular disease. Provided that diffuse vascular involvement is not present, diabetes itself is not a contraindication. Although age may be a limiting factor, the "physiologic" age rather than the chronologic age contraindicates transplantation. A cadaver transplant into an eighty-two-year-old patient is on record, and adult renal allografts have been transplanted into recipients as young as three. Although abnormalities of the bladder and urethra present additional hazards, successful renal allografts have been placed in individuals with these abnormalities by prior construction of an artificial bladder (i.e., ileal conduit) into which the donor ureter is placed. The demonstration of "preformed antibodies" in the potential recipient prior to transplantation is a contraindication when it can be shown that these antibodies react specifically to donor cells.

DONOR SELECTION

Donor sources are cadavers or volunteer blood-related living donors. Living volunteer donors should be found completely normal on physical examination and should be of the same major ABO blood group, because there is good evidence that crossing major blood group barriers prejudices survival of the allograft. It is, however, possible to transplant a kidney of a type O donor into an A or B recipient. Selective renal arteriography should be performed on volunteer donors to rule out the presence of multiple or abnormal renal arteries, because the sur-

gical procedure is inordinately difficult and the ischemic time of the normal kidney prohibitively long when vascular abnormalities exist. Cadaver donors should be free of malignant neoplastic disease because of possible transmission of cancer to the recipient. Tissue typing of donor and prospective recipient and direct crossmatching are mandatory.

CLINICAL COURSE OF THE RECIPIENT

Usually, but not invariably, bilateral nephrectomies are performed prior to transplantation, and the recipient is maintained on intermittent hemodialysis. Removal of the patient's own diseased kidneys obviates a source of infection in the postoperative period and facilitates the diagnosis of rejection of the allograft, because variations in renal function and urine sediment are then related only to changes in the allograft.

Psychologic complications following transplantation are common. Depression and anxiety may reflect both the difficult and stressful postoperative course and the anxiety and uncertainty of the physician.

THE REJECTION CRISIS. Early diagnosis of rejection is imperative because prompt institution of vigorous therapy may reverse renal function and prevent irreversible damage due to fibrosis. Clinical evidence of rejection is characterized by fever, swelling, and tenderness over the allograft, and by oliguria. In patients whose renal function is good initially, oliguria may be accompanied by decreased urinary sodium concentration and increased urine osmolarity. These changes may not be present in more chronic stages of rejection or when renal function is impaired at the onset of rejection. A transplanted cadaver kidney more often than not undergoes a period of anuria which may last as long as 3 months without prejudicing the eventual function of the graft. In this instance, the reversible lesion is presumably due to ischemia, and the diagnosis of rejection becomes more difficult. Renal arteriography and radioactive Hippuran renograms may be useful in ascertaining changes in the renal vasculature and in renal blood flow even in the absence of urine flow. When renal function has been good initially, a rise in the blood urea nitrogen level and a decrease in the creatinine clearance may herald the onset of rejection. The creatinine clearance is perhaps more reliable, because fever and the administration of prednisone may influence the concentration of blood urea nitrogen without necessarily reflecting a decrease in urea clearance. Increase in the 24-hr excretion of urinary lysozyme has been helpful. Increase in proteinuria may reflect rejection, but when it occurs later in the course of the postoperative period, predominant glomerular disease may be present. Hypertension is also a concomitant of rejection. When hypertension responds to prednisone, it is likely that rejection has been responsible for the elevation of blood pressure, because other forms of hypertension usually do not improve with corticosteroid therapy. The measurement of the intrarenal distribution of blood by the xenon washout technique has been valuable in assessing rejection both in man and in experimental animals. It is possible at operation to leave in the renal artery a small polyvinyl catheter through which these studies may be done repeatedly.

TRANSPLANTATION OF OTHER VISCERAL ORGANS

Organs other than the kidney which have a potential for clinical transplantation are the liver and heart. Two possible indications for *liver transplantation* are chronic hepatic failure and malignancy which is localized to the liver. Two techniques for liver transplantation have been utilized in man: (1) *Orthotopic*—the recipient's own liver is removed and the transplant is substituted for it in the anatomic position. (2) *Auxiliary*—the recipient's liver is left in place and the allograft is placed in the right paravertebral gutter. The donor's vena cava then is interposed in the recipient terminal inferior vena cava, and the hepatic artery is anastomosed to the right common iliac artery. Finally, the end of the allograft portal vein is anastomosed to the recipient's superior mesenteric vein.

Immunosuppressive regimens are similar to those in kidney transplantation. There is some suggestion that the use of antilymphocyte globulin is more effective in liver allografting. Obviously, the donor source must be a cadaver. Complications of liver transplantation have been strikingly different from those encountered with renal allografts. In many instances an initial hemorrhagic diathesis with fibrinolysis ocurs. This is followed by a phase of hypercoagulability in the successfully transplanted recipient, which in one instance resulted in fatal pulmonary emboli. Infections also seem to present a greater problem than with renal allografts. These complications are not insurmountable, and although no patient with a liver transplant has survived for more than 1 year, the prospects for the future are promising.

Transplantation of the heart has been accomplished successfully in man in a number of instances. Early results suggest that it is comparable to transplantation of the kidney and that results certainly will improve. Indications for cardiac transplantation are myocardial insufficiency, usually due to severe coronary artery disease and myocardial fibrosis, and failure to respond to the most rigorous medical measures. The donor must be a cadaver and is usually an individual whose death has resulted from trauma or suicide. The question of the ethics and morals raised by the removal of a heart capable of sustaining life in another individual has been discussed by many medical and lay authors. It seems eminently reasonable that if "death" of the brain has occurred, as evidenced by lack of electrical activity in the electroencephalogram over a period of 24 to 36 hr, dilated pupils, failure of spontaneous respiration, and lack of peripheral reflexes, the ability to maintain respiration or cardiac output by artificial methods is academic. Nevertheless, the decision as to when to discontinue these efforts should be made independently by the physician caring for the prospective donor in consultation with one or two colleagues. The question of whether or not the heart is to be used for transplantation should not affect this decision. Once the decision has been made, the donor can be maintained until the recipient is prepared for operation.

Human *spleen* and *pancreas* have been transplanted with limited success. If it could be shown that normal spleen can produce a useful amount of antihemophilic globulin, transplantation of that organ to some patients with hemophilia would provide a distinct advantage over standard substitution therapy. Transplantation of lymphoid tissue (including spleen) for total agammaglobulinemia has resulted in temporary improvement, but eventually the transplanted lymphoid tissue rejects the host (graft versus host reaction). Temporary success in transplanting pancreas in diabetics also has been reported, but substitution therapy seems more feasible.

Various other *endocrines*, including parathyroid, adrenal, and thyroid, have all been transplanted, with only temporary success. A large percentage of *corneal grafts* survive as allografts in man, primarily because the cornea is not vascularized, which excludes immunologically competent cells. Grafts of bone and blood vessels do not survive as living allografts but act as a "scaffolding" over which host tissue may grow.

Transplantation of allogenic marrow in man is of particular interest because when allogenic marrow is transplanted successfully following irradiation, the marrow recipient "tolerates" skin grafts from animals isologous with the marrow donor.

The obvious application of marrow transplantation to patients with leukemia and aplastic anemia has resulted in a number of attempts at human marrow transplantation. When identical twin donors have been used, the results have been uniformly promising. For example, marrow transplants were carried out in four patients with leukemia following lethal total-body irradiation. In every instance the transplant was successful and the patient died later of recurrent leukemia. Also using identical twin donors, successful marrow transplants have been performed in at least four patients with acute bone marrow failure and in one patient following accidental lethal whole-body irradiation. In these cases the transplants were successful and appear to have been lifesaving. A complication of marrow transplantation is a reaction of the grafted cells against the host whose immunosuppressive potential has been ablated by irradiation or nitrogen mustard. This reaction is characterized by fever, anorexia, diarrhea, dermatitis, and alopecia and is similar to that demonstrated in animals who have been treated in this fashion. Encouraging results in preventing the "graft versus host reaction" by the early administration of Amethopterin and cyclophosphamide have been reported.

ORGAN PRESERVATION

If it were possible to remove cadaver organs and to store them for a period of days or longer under conditions permitting their successful replantation, one of the difficult problems in organ procurement would be solved. Bone marrow is the only organ that can be stored easily for prolonged periods. The hope of kidney, heart, or liver banks in which suitably typed organs could be stored for subsequent transplantation to a suitable recipient is still a long way from reality. The most effective technique for preservation is hyperbaric, hypothermic perfusion, but organs treated in this fashion must be transplanted within 24 to 36 hr.

XENOGRAFTS

Kidneys, lungs, and hearts have been transplanted to human beings from various primates, including chimpanzees and baboons. Although one chimpanzee kidney graft functioned well for more than 7 months, clinical efforts in this area have been abandoned. It seems quite possible, however, that continuing efforts to find other species whose tissues may be more compatible to man's (e.g., the pig) may result eventually in a source of organs which might eliminate many of the present problems. In fact, it might be possible to breed pigs for histocompatibility with man in the same fashion that mice were bred to produce purebred lines with predictable tissue antigenicity.

REFERENCES

Amos, B.: Immunologic Factors in Organ Transplantation, Am. J. Med., 44:767, 1968.

Merrill, J. P.: Human Tissue Transplantation, in F. J. Dixon and H. G. Kunkel (Eds.), Advan. Immunol., 7:276, 1968.

Rapaport, F. T., and J. Dausset: "Human Transplantation," New York, Grune & Stratton, Inc., 1968.

Russell, P. S.: Kidney Transplantation, Am. J. Med., 44:776, 1968.

Starzl, T. E.: "Experience in Renal Transplantation," Philadelphia, W. B. Saunders Company, 1964.

72 ASTHMA, HAY FEVER, AND OTHER MANIFESTATIONS OF ALLERGY

Philip S. Norman

ASTHMA

DEFINITION. Asthma is characterized by paroxysms of expiratory dyspnea and wheezing, overinflation of the lungs, cough, and rhonchi. The onset of paroxysms may be sudden or insidious; their duration may be brief or they may last weeks. Symptoms are due to generalized bronchial airway obstruction, which occurs as a result of contraction of bronchial smooth muscle, hypertrophy of the bronchial wall, edema of the bronchial mucosa, and accumulation of secretions in the bronchial lumens.

MANIFESTATIONS AND PATHOPHYSIOLOGY. In asthma, it is probable that bronchospasm, mucosal edema, and bronchial secretions are the principal mechanisms producing airway obstruction, which is localized primarily in the small bronchioles. Normally, the bronchial lumens enlarge upon inspiration and narrow upon expiration. Dyspnea, therefore, is most pronounced, and wheezing and rhonchi are audible, during expiration. The expiratory phase of respiration is prolonged, and inspiration characteristically is not as difficult as expiration. Expiratory dyspnea requires the use of accessory muscles to deflate the lung, increasing the intrathoracic pressure. During inspiration, on the other hand, the negative intrathoracic pressure is accompanied by retraction of the intercostal, suprasternal, and supraclavicular spaces. The expiratory airway obstruction leads to hyperinflation or reversible emphysema of the lungs.

Asthma characteristically occurs in attacks of variable duration; between attacks pulmonary function is normal or nearly normal and patients are relatively free of symptoms. Such spasmodic asthma is more frequent at night, and attacks usually last several minutes to several hours. Occasionally spasms last several days, and some asthmatic patients maintain an almost continuous state of airway obstruction nearly every day.

The precise mechanism of dyspnea in asthma is not known, but it probably results from a combination of conscious recognition of obstruction to breathing, hyperinflation, changes in intrapleural pressure, and increased work. Wheezing, dyspnea, and cough are worse with effort, are exaggerated by anxiety, and tend to be most severe at night. During a paroxysm, the patient is usually most comfortable while sitting with the trunk forward and the arms elevated to rest at shoulder level. Elevation of the diaphragm while the patient is recumbent reduces the respiratory reserve. The sitting posture reduces intra-abdominal pressure and allows the viscera to move downward and forward.

The physical properties of the bronchial secretions undoubtedly influence the manifestations of asthma, but very little is known of the changes that may occur in sputum viscosity, elasticity, and stickiness. The ease with which sputum can be evacuated from the bronchi, however, obviously is an important factor in the severity of airway obstruction. Cough frequently becomes more severe during recovery from an asthmatic attack, when sputum seems more liquid and is raised in larger quantities. Syncope may occur when prolonged periods of increased intrathoracic pressure associated with paroxysms of coughing interfere with venous return to the heart. The sputum usually is white and mucoid and contains no blood or pus. Microscopic examination often shows eosinophils and Charcot-Leyden crystals. In addition, as an asthmatic attack subsides, mucous casts of the bronchi or bronchioles may be seen in the sputum (Curschmann's spirals). Purulent sputum indicates bronchial or pulmonary infection.

There is no fever unless asthma is caused by or associated with infection. After a prolonged attack the patient may complain of soreness in the chest or abdomen as well as tiredness, but otherwise there are no systemic manifestations of the disease.

During a mild attack the sensation of obstruction to breathing may lead the patient to overcompensate by hyperpnea and there will be a reduction in blood CO_2 tension. If airway obstruction becomes more severe, there may be a fall in oxygen tension with cyanosis and a rise in CO_2 tension due to ventilatory failure. Such rises in P_{CO_2} are often uncompensated and are accompanied by a low plasma bicarbonate concentration. There is also an altered ventilation/perfusion ratio in asthma which arises from regional defects in ventilation due to bronchial plugging. These ventilation defects may reflexly cause transient regional reduction in blood flow, which can be detected during asthmatic attacks by pulmonary scanning techniques.

When an asthmatic episode is prolonged for many hours or days and is resistant to therapy, it is defined as *status asthmaticus*. The chest is greatly distended, the patient works desperately to move air through the obstructed airways, using the accessory muscles of respiration, and breath sounds and wheezes may become very faint because movement of air is poor. Cough is virtually impossible, and the patient is often volume-depleted and extremely fatigued. If status does not resolve, the chest becomes almost silent and severe respiratory acidosis ensues. Death from respiratory arrest is possible, and vigorous emergency treatment is necessary.

Asthmatic episodes may be complicated by *atelectasis* due to mucoid plugging of bronchi with subsequent extraction of gases from the unventilated portion of the lung. *Pneumonia* may supervene in poorly ventilated or atelectatic portions of lung. *Spontaneous pneumothorax* and *mediastinal emphysema* are rare complications of an asthmatic attack. Ordinarily, asthma does not affect cardiac function unless the attack is protracted or is accompanied by irreversible emphysema. Under these circumstances, cor pulmonale may develop.

ETIOLOGY. Asthma begins before age ten in about one-half of cases and before age thirty in another third, but it may begin *de novo* even in old age. Before age ten, asthma is twice as frequent in boys, but by age thirty the incidence is equal in men and women. Asthma is present in members of the immediate family of about one-third of patients.

In most asthmatics four main factors are thought to interact to a variable degree in producing attacks: (1) allergy to external inhaled allergens; (2) respiratory infections; (3) psychophysiologic reactions to life stress; and (4) air pollution. Although asthma is regarded as an allergic disease, hypersensitivity is found to be the predominant cause in only about one-third of cases and a contributing factor in perhaps another third.

Hay fever and urticaria sometimes precede development of asthma, or occur simultaneously, suggesting that asthma is attributable to inhaled or ingested antigens in an individual with reaginic or atopic allergy. This type of asthma is observed most commonly in young persons and usually is seasonal. The same inhaled pollens, molds, dusts, danders, etc., described further on in this chapter under Allergic Rhinitis (Hay Fever) are implicated in allergic asthma. The relationship to seasonal exposure, positive skin tests, and family history of allergy are the same as in hay fever. Nonseasonal asthma may also be due to allergy to dust, feathers, animal danders, foods, or drugs.

A syndrome of chronic sinusitis, nasal polyps, poorly remitting asthma, and unusual sensitivity to aspirin has been observed in some adults. These individuals have onset of symptoms as adults and may have rapidly developing life-threatening paroxysms of bronchospasm after a single aspirin tablet.

Respiratory infections appear to be the predominant etiologic factor in about 40 percent of cases and are most common in the very young, the elderly, and those with the most serious disease. Initially these infections may appear to be no more than a common cold, but they may set off a train of asthmatic symptoms lasting days or weeks. There has been no systematic attempt to isolate and identify the specific bacteria or viruses which initiate these infections; presumably the same organisms implicated in respiratory infections in normal individuals are involved.

Allergic bronchopulmonary aspergillosis is a specific infection occurring in asthmatic patients in whom endobronchial growth of *Aspergillus fumigatus* is accompanied by prolonged asthma, expectoration of small brown "plugs" of mycelia, transient pulmonary infiltrates, and eosinophils in the sputum and blood. The diagnosis may be suspected from the character of the pulmonary infiltrates and the appearance of the sputum and is established by demonstration of mycelia on microscopic examination of the sputum and positive cultures for *A. fumigatus*. These infections have been recognized repeatedly in Great Britain but appear to be rare in the United States. They respond to the usual measures for asthma but may recur.

In about a third of patients, emotional strain and specific stressful life situations appear to be important factors in initiating asthmatic episodes. It would be presumptuous to identify a specific kind of psychologic stress as generating asthma or to describe an "asthmatic personality." Nevertheless, many asthmatic episodes occur when there are no detectable external factors except psychologic stress.

"Tokyo-Yokohama asthma" or *"New Orleans asthma"* refers to a greatly increased rate of asthmatic attacks which have appeared at times of heavy air pollution in highly industrialized urban areas in individuals not otherwise troubled with asthma. The relationship to industrial air pollution is suggestive but not proved. Nevertheless, several surveys in large cities have indicated that emergency room visits by patients with known asthma are much more frequent on days of increased air pollution. The specific pollutants acting as irritants in these situations are unknown.

The etiologic factors which have been incriminated in asthmatic episodes may be acting in individuals with an underlying physiologic defect which predisposes them to bronchospasm. For example, asthmatic patients will react with a greater degree of bronchospasm for a longer period to drugs such as acetylcholine, mecholyl, histamine, serotonin, or cholinesterase inhibitors than normal, and are also unusually sensitive to nonspecific irritants such as dusts, cooking odors, and gaseous air pollutants. They will respond to vigorous exercise with bronchospasm and react more vigorously to the above-mentioned stimuli after treatment with β-adrenergic blocking agents such as propranolol. Therefore, these drugs are contraindicated in asthmatic patients. If there is an acquired or innate physiologic defect in some or all asthmatic patients, its nature is unknown.

DIAGNOSIS. Certain specific causes of local or generalized airway obstruction must be considered when a patient comes initially to the physician with asthma. Generally, wheezing and rhonchi are heard throughout the chest; localized wheezing indicates endobronchial disease, such as foreign body aspiration, neoplasm, or stenosis. The symptoms of airway obstruction in localized endobronchial disease are at times spasmodic and may mimic asthma closely. "Cardiac asthma" or wheezing occurring during cardiac failure or pulmonary edema usually can be differentiated from paroxysmal asthma by the presence of moist rales, blood-tinged sputum, and other signs of heart failure (Chap. 264). Asthma occasionally is a presenting manifestation of polyarteritis nodosa (Chap. 391). Reactions to drugs, particularly aspirin, are an occasional cause of severe asthma. Loeffler's allergic pneumonitis, caused by parasitic infestation of the lungs, is often accompanied by asthma.

Poisoning with cholinergic drugs or insecticides may induce bronchoconstriction and expiratory dyspnea that can be specifically relieved with atropine (Chap. 116). Carcinoid tumors which elaborate serotonin may be associated with asthma (Chap. 105). Sometimes, cerebral trauma may result in asthmatic symptoms.

Chemical pneumonias such as silo filler's disease (Chap. 289) may be accompanied by difficult breathing resembling asthma. On the other hand, allergic interstitial pneumonitis, which is a hypersensitivity reaction to inhaled organic dusts, usually is not accompanied by bronchospasm.

LABORATORY FINDINGS. Skin tests used for the diagnosis of allergic asthma are no different from those used for the diagnosis of hay fever (see below). There are no specific laboratory tests that define the allergic etiology, but finding an increased number of eosinophils in sputum and blood occasionally will suggest an allergic cause of asthma. Measurements of pulmonary function will demonstrate increased airway resistance and hyperinflation which are almost completely reversible between attacks. Frequent measurements of arterial P_{O_2} and P_{CO_2} may be crucial in assessing the severity of status asthmaticus and the response to therapy.

THERAPY. Specific Treatment. As is the case in hay fever, elimination of the offending antigen from the patient's environment is the most successful means of preventing and treating allergic asthma. Mechanical obstruction of the tracheobronchial tree should be corrected, and infection of the sinuses should be treated.

Specific desensitization or hyposensitization of the patient with asthma due to inhaled antigens is performed as in hay fever but may be less effective, and improvement usually does not persist when desensitization is discontinued.

The frequent occurrence of bronchial infection in adults with nonseasonal or chronic asthma necessitates special consideration. The pneumococcus and *Hemophilus influenzae* are the microorganisms most often isolated from the bronchi and sputum of patients with asthma and chronic bronchitis, and exacerbations of cough and dyspnea may be associated with an increase in the number of these bacteria. These patients may be treated with tetracycline, 0.5 to 1.0 Gm per day, or ampicillin, 1.0 Gm per day, continuously during the winter months or at the earliest sign that symptoms are increasing. This approach may lead to a significant decrease in the severity and frequency of exacerbations.

Nonspecific Treatment. Treatment of acute asthma is most effective when begun soon after onset of the paroxysm. Mild attacks may be readily relieved by inhalation of 50 to 150 μg of nebulized isoproterenol. A variety of commercial products which furnish a measured dose of isoproterenol with inert freon as a propellant are available. The smallest amount consistent with relief should be employed, and administration should not be repeated more often than every 3 hr. With a rapidly developing severe paroxysm, 0.3 to 1.0 ml of 1:1,000 epinephrine should be injected subcutaneously; this dose may be repeated as needed but no more often than every 30 min. Both isoproterenol and epinephrine may become ineffective after repeated use in a prolonged asthmatic attack. There are reports that a single inhalation of isoproterenol may have caused paradoxic bronchospasm (following an initial transient decrease in airway resistance) in a few patients who had used the drug excessively for unremitting asthma over several days. Some asthmatic deaths may be associated with overuse of isoproterenol, as its effectiveness in relieving bronchospasm becomes progressively less.

Early in attacks, a sedative such as amobarbital, 50 or 100 mg, may be desirable to allay agitation and relieve anxiety. As the attack becomes more severe and prolonged, sedatives become less desirable because the patient needs every faculty for the work of breathing. Respiratory arrest has been reported in severely asthmatic patients shortly after injections of sedative or tranquilizing drugs. Drugs which depress respiration such as morphine have been the apparent cause of sudden death and should never be used during asthmatic episodes.

Aminophylline is an active bronchodilator and may be used with, or in preference to, epinephrine. It may be given intravenously or rectally; a dose of 0.5 Gm is usually required for adequate bronchodilatation. It is ordinarily not possible to give this dose orally without gastric irritation. Intravenous aminophylline must be given slowly, and it is desirable to dilute 0.5 Gm in 50 ml of 5 percent glucose and to administer it in a drip over a 20-min period. Hydration to prevent inspissation of mucus is important, and it is often convenient to follow intravenous medication with a liter or more of 5 percent glucose.

When epinephrine and aminophylline are poorly effective in relieving bronchospasm or there is prompt recurrence, administration of corticosteroids is necessary. Daily doses will range between 15 and 80 mg prednisone, and a favorable response cannot be expected for several hours. Considerable foresight is required to select those patients who will require steroids for adequate control, because the physical signs of asthma are often misleading. Early determination of arterial P_{O_2} and P_{CO_2} often will help to recognize those patients who are on the verge of ventilatory failure and who will require prompt and vigorous therapy. Increasing carbon dioxide tension despite treatment is a grave prognostic sign and may mean that tracheostomy and mechanical ventilation will be necessary to prevent death.

When steroids are required, 100 to 300 mg hydrocortisone may be given intravenously, although this route probably is no more effective than the oral route. Once initiated, steroids should be continued to maintain improvement, and then tapered as rapidly as is consistent with continued control of asthma.

Continuous administration of adrenal steroids to patients with chronic asthma or asthmatic bronchitis has been effective and safe in preventing paroxysms. The dose required is usually less than 20 mg prednisone or its equivalent per day. This regimen has been continued for several years in many patients without serious side effects or complications. In fact, patients with severe asthma accompanying infections often have fewer episodes of infection while receiving adrenal steroids continuously.

Prophylactic management of asthmatic patients involves the use of drugs to abort paroxysms. Oral ephedrine, 25 to 50 mg, and phenobarbital, 30 to 60 mg, may be given three or four times a day when the patient is most likely to develop asthma. Recommended doses of oral theophylline or aminophylline preparations contain too little drug to be effective, and effective doses usually cause gastric irritation. Smoking is undesirable in asthmatics, as are obesity, excessive exertion, fatigue, and dietary indiscretion.

ALLERGIC RHINITIS (Hay Fever)

DEFINITION. Allergic rhinitis is characterized by sneezing, rhinorrhea, swelling of the nasal mucosa, itching of the eyes, and lacrimation. Hay fever is the common term for allergic rhinitis due to seasonal spread of pollens in the air, but the disease is not necessarily seasonal and may result from exposure to antigens other than pollen. *Vasomotor rhinitis* designates those diseases without allergic or infectious etiology which resemble hay fever.

ETIOLOGY. Plants that spread large amounts of airborne pollen are common sources of antigens responsible for hay fever, but those pollinated by insects, including most flowering plants such as roses and goldenrod, are not. Ragweed pollen is the principal offender

in the United States. It is prevalent in the central, eastern, and southeastern part of the country, but virtually absent west of the Rocky Mountains. Ordinarily ragweed pollinates between early August and late October, the most likely season for hay fever.

In the northern half of the United States, grasses pollinate from May to July, while in the South grass may pollinate throughout the year. Although the time of year when trees pollinate may vary, they ordinarily do so in early spring, and earlier in the South than in the North. Some widespread airborne pollens are nonallergenic; pine pollen, for instance, almost never causes hay fever. Certain widespread molds, found most frequently on decaying vegetation, which also propagate by means of airborne spores, appear in definite seasons. *Hormodendrum* has a peak incidence in July and *Alternaria* in October; both may cause seasonal allergic rhinitis.

Most pollen particles are about 25 to 40 μ in diameter and settle promptly from the air. The settling properties of pollen are used for crude estimations of the "pollen count" in the air by collecting and enumerating particles on a greased glass slide. There is an approximate but regular correlation between the pollen count and the frequency and severity of hay fever in the exposed population. Pollen particles from plants, grasses, or trees of varying types can be differentiated by microscopic examination, permitting precise definition of the airborne pollens responsible for hay fever.

Pollen particles are relatively large and, when inhaled, will impinge on and be deposited within the nose. Very few particles would be expected to reach the terminal bronchioles. House dust, fungus spores, animal danders, feathers, broken insect parts, facial powders, vegetable dusts, insecticides, and food particles disseminated during cooking also have been incriminated as causes of hay fever; the etiologic relationship between ingested food and respiratory allergy has been difficult to document.

PATHOGENESIS. When pollens and mold spores land on the nasal mucosa, their carbohydrate coat is digested by the lysozyme of respiratory mucus, which releases the protein contents. Careful analysis reveals that the grains of ragweed and grass pollens contain several specific proteins, referred to as *allergens*, which account for the sensitizing potential of the pollen. The allergens are of relatively low molecular weight (10,000 to 40,000) and consist of 1 percent or less of the extractable solids of the pollen. The biologic potency of these allergens is such that intradermal injection of 1 $\mu\mu$ will cause a wheal and erythema reaction when injected intradermally in a sensitive patient. Other pollen, mold, and dander allergens are less well characterized but appear to have similar properties. Presumably, it is the unusual ability of allergic individuals to become sensitized following release of these allergens in the respiratory tract that leads to allergic disease.

The sensitivity in hay fever is not confined to the mucous membranes but is general and is exemplified by the ability of the entire skin to react. Furthermore, the granulocytic leukocytes in vitro will respond to the addition of pollen extract by secreting histamine into the surrounding medium. This process requires living metabolizing cells and is independent of the presence of complement. These reactions are conferred by the fixation to cells of "reaginic" antibodies, a special type of antibodies which are usually of the IgE class, which have a particular affinity for cells, and which are usually detected by the Prausnitz-Küstner test (see below). Allergen-induced release of histamine from mucosal tissue mast cells sensitized by reaginic antibody probably accounts for the major manifestations of respiratory allergies. The ability to synthesize reagins is not confined to allergic individuals; nearly everyone will develop wheal and erythema skin reactivity to repeated intradermal injections of antigens such as ascaris extract and bovine ribonuclease. Allergic individuals, however, are likely to develop such reactions to antigens instilled into the nose, while normal individuals rarely do. The nature of the defect responsible for this phenomenon is unknown, but it is probably hereditary, because there is a strong tendency for allergic disease to run in families. The mode of inheritance has not been determined, but when both parents have "atopic" disease, the allergy in the offspring is apt to be unusually severe. In all, from 5 to 15 percent of individuals are atopic—i.e., they are capable of developing allergy to inhaled antigens.

The nasal mucosa of patients with hay fever or allergic rhinitis also appears to be more susceptible to the effects of irritants than is the nasal mucosa of normal persons. Furthermore, studies in volunteers indicate that persons with allergic rhinitis are more susceptible to infection by respiratory viruses than are normal persons. This enhanced reactivity of the nasal mucosa to a variety of stimuli also may explain the effects of emotional disturbances in exaggerating and possibly initiating symptoms of rhinitis in the allergic individual.

MANIFESTATIONS. Pruritus about the eyes, nose, throat, and mouth, nasal discharge, sneezing, and lacrimation are the characteristic features of hay fever or allergic rhinitis. Particularly troublesome to the patient is mucosal swelling with occlusion of the airway, making breathing difficult and often causing insomnia. Symptoms vary in severity from day to day.

Occlusion of the nasal passages by swelling of the turbinates and mucous membranes may result in obstruction of the sinus ostiums or the eustachian tube, and infection of the sinuses and middle ear is a relatively common complication of perennial allergic rhinitis but is uncommon in seasonal hay fever. In addition, infection of the sinuses or nose in patients with allergic rhinitis results in formation of nasal polyps. These polyps further obstruct the nasal passages, increase symptoms, and exaggerate infection.

Many persons with hay fever or allergic rhinitis subsequently develop asthma. Retrobulbar neuritis, laryngeal edema with hoarseness, angioedema, urticaria, and other allergic illnesses occasionally accompany allergic rhinitis.

DIAGNOSIS. Symptoms of allergic rhinitis or hay fever occur in situations where allergy cannot be incriminated. For example, sneezing, watery nasal discharge, and lacrimation may develop upon exposure to an atmosphere heavily contaminated with smoke, dust, or other irritants. Similarly, these symptoms often herald the onset of a viral upper respiratory tract infection. The symptoms of hay fever are attributable to nonsuppurative inflammation of the nasal mucosa, and any situation resulting in inflammation of the nose can produce an illness which is indistinguishable from allergic rhinitis. Ingestion of alcoholic beverages and emotional stimuli may also produce hyperemia of the nasal mucous membranes, exaggerating the symptoms of allergic rhinitis. Polycythemia vera may occasionally be recognized initially because of nasal and conjunctival hyperemia, resulting in symptoms resembling those of hay fever. Certain drugs, particularly rauwolfia derivatives, may have similar effects.

The pale and edematous appearance of the nasal mucosa helps to distinguish allergic rhinitis or hay fever. The conjunctivas and the skin about the eyes, nose, and occasionally the mouth are reddened. In addition, nasal polyps are characteristic of allergic nasal disease, although infection in the nose or sinuses may also be present. Microscopic examination of nasal secretions shows many eosinophils.

Of great importance in the diagnosis of hay fever is its seasonal occurrence, which coincides with pollination of weeds, grasses, or trees. Allergic rhinitis due to local contamination of the patient's environment is diagnosed by carefully correlating the patient's symptoms with exposure to potential allergens at home, at work, and at play. The continuous character of perennial allergic rhinitis makes an allergic etiology less readily recognizable. Examination of nasal secretions for eosinophils, however, is often helpful. Blood eosinophilia also is found occasionally in patients with allergic rhinitis.

Skin Tests. Approximately 25 percent of the normal population will develop wheal and erythema skin reactions following intracutaneous inoculation of common airborne antigens. Not all persons with positive skin reactions, however, have allergic rhinitis. The allergic patient commonly has positive skin reactions to many antigens when from the history only one or two are incriminated as the cause of symptoms. Skin tests with allergenic antigens, therefore, are of more value in detecting an allergic propensity than in detecting the specific antigen responsible for the patient's symptoms. Only careful correlation of the skin reactivity with the environmental circumstances will delineate the responsible antigen.

Tests are performed with crude aqueous extracts of pollen, dust, foods, animal dander, insects, and other substances. These extracts are commercially available, but their potency varies considerably. No method of standardization is very reliable, because the extracts are crude and the measurement of specific antigen has not been possible.

Skin tests are done by applying a drop of antigen to a skin scratch or by intradermal inoculation of 0.01 to 0.02 ml. In the beginning, very dilute extract should be used. The concentration may be increased gradually until there is certainty that the patient has a negative reaction. Ordinarily, it is unwise to test a patient repeatedly on the same day or to test with many extracts at one time. Positive reactions appear within 15 to 20 min and are characterized by wheal and erythema formation and local pruritus. If large doses of extract are given, symptoms of hay fever or even a generalized reaction may be produced. Extracts of foods are available for skin testing, but their use should be limited because it is preferable to diagnose allergy to foods by history and by elimination diets. Identification of bacteria in the respiratory tract which are potentially responsible for infection is more valuable than skin testing with bacterial extracts.

When it is undesirable to perform skin tests in young children or in persons with generalized skin disease, passive transfer of the patient's serum to normal recipients may be performed (Prausnitz-Küstner, or P-K test). Ordinarily, 0.05 to 0.1 ml of the patient's serum is injected intradermally into the recipient, and 24 hr later normal skin and sites injected with serum are tested with the antigenic extracts.

Epinephrine and ephedrine greatly reduce the wheal and erythema response to intradermally injected antigen, as do large doses of antihistamines; these drugs should not be administered before skin testing. Adrenocortical steroids have little effect on these reactions.

THERAPY. Specific Treatment. Elimination of the offending antigen from the patient's environment is the most effective means of controlling allergic disease. This is not always easy, even when the antigen is known. If it is determined that dander from dogs or cats is responsible, for example, then animals should be avoided. When feathers are found to be responsible for allergic symptoms, a feather pillow should be replaced by one of foam rubber. Air filtration is often useful in controlling symptoms due to airborne pollens, but occasionally it may be necessary to advise the patient to live in a pollen-free area during the hay fever season. Mechanical obstruction of the nasal airway, which may aggravate the symptoms of rhinitis, should be corrected, and infection should be treated with an antibacterial drug capable of eradicating the specific microorganism. Alleviation of emotional disturbances by the use of drugs, correction of the environment, or psychiatric guidance occasionally will alleviate the symptoms of allergy.

Desensitization, hyposensitization, or immunization with the antigens recognized as specifically responsible for allergic respiratory disease may be effective. Controlled studies of desensitization in patients with hay fever due to ragweed pollen have shown that approximately 80 percent of patients are partially relieved of their symptoms, while only 25 percent of patients given a placebo improved. Improvement appears to be related to two factors: the development of normal circulating IgG antibodies ("blocking" antibodies) which can combine with the antigen and block its ability to trigger cellular histamine release, and an actual reduction (sometimes complete abolition) of the cellular sensitivity which confers the allergic reaction. The reasons for the reduction in cellular sensitivity are not clear, because the patient continues to have circulating reaginic antibody, although in reduced titer.

Treatment by desensitization may be perennial, coseasonal, or preseasonal. Continued therapy throughout the year probably is preferable to intermittent treatment, but the dose of antigen in some patients must be reduced considerably during the season of the year when symptoms are expected to occur. The beneficial effects of desensitization persist for some months after treatment is discontinued, but the allergic symptoms tend to recur eventually.

Bacterial vaccines have been employed in desensitizing patients with allergic rhinitis. Because of the lack of evidence for bacterial hypersensitivity as a cause of allergic respiratory disease and the lack of data that such treatment is effective, it cannot be recommended.

Nonspecific Treatment. Many patients can be relieved of their complaints with symptomatic therapy. The severity, recurrence, and refractoriness to symptomatic treatment will determine whether or not specific desensitization should be attempted. Antihistamines, such as tripellenamine, 50 mg; diphenhydramine, 50 mg; chlorpheniramine, 4 mg; and many others, often are effective in controlling hay fever. Their repeated use frequently is associated with gradually decreasing effectiveness, but when one drug fails, another may be effective. In addition they may produce drowsiness and reduce physical and mental dexterity.

Oral adrenocortical steroids are extraordinarily effective in relieving the symptoms of most patients with allergic respiratory disease and were it not for their side effects, could be generally recommended as the drugs of choice in hay fever. Nevertheless, they can be used to manage acute symptoms, and in some patients small daily doses will suppress symptoms completely during an entire season. Hydrocortisone, 25 to 100 mg, prednisone 5 to 20 mg, and methylprednisolone, 4 to 12 mg each day, are all usually quite effective. Adrenal steroids can cause a remarkable disappearance of nasal polyps when used in patients with perennial rhinitis. The benefit derived from adrenal steroids always must be balanced against the potential side effects of these potent drugs.

Small doses of the water-soluble steroid dexamethasone sprayed into the nose three or four times a day effectively suppress the symptoms of all but the severest hay fever without danger of systemic side effects. The effect of the steroid is local and cannot be duplicated by the same dose given orally. As further experience accumulates, intranasal dexamethasone may become accepted as the treatment of choice in allergic rhinitis. Shrinkage of polyps also can be achieved by this treatment.

A variety of agents are available for shrinking the nasal mucous membrane to relieve obstruction of the nasal airways. Aqueous phenylephrine (0.25 or 0.5 percent) is an effective nasal decongestant that is useful in patients who are very uncomfortable from hay fever or allergic rhinitis until other remedies can correct the underlying disease. Repeated use of the drug, however, may cause reactive hyperemia of the nasal mucosa, further exaggerating the symptoms of rhinitis. Orally administered ephedrine, 25 mg, or pseudoephedrine, 60 mg, may also be used to shrink nasal mucous membranes, but they have limited effectiveness. Atropine-like drugs may help to dry up excessive nasal secretions, if there is no concomitant asthma.

ALLERGIC SKIN DISEASE

There are many dermatologic manifestations of allergy, including contact dermatitis, urticaria, angioedema, erythematous rashes, and eczema. These are roughly divisible into those related to "delayed" and "immediate" hypersensitivity. Urticaria and angioedema usually are manifestations of immediate hypersensitivity, while contact dermatitis and many instances of eczematous dermatitis are attributable to delayed hypersensitivity. At times an antigen may induce and elicit both immediate and delayed hypersensitivity reactions, resulting in both urticaria and eczema.

Urticaria, angioedema, contact dermatitis, and erythematous rashes are the principal forms of allergy in which the skin is the major target organ. Many other rashes are attributed to systemic allergic disease, including erythema nodosum, erythema multiforme, exfoliation, bullae, purpura, "fixed" drug eruptions, and photosensitivity. Certain supposed immunologic diseases such as systemic lupus erythematosus, dermatomyositis, rheumatic fever, and scleroderma also are characterized by "allergic" skin lesions.

CONTACT DERMATITIS. See Chap. 400.

URTICARIA. Urticaria (hives) is characterized by white or red evanescent wheals, papules, or macules that are surrounded by erythema and are pruritic. They may be generalized, but they commonly appear in areas of skin covered by clothing. Urticaria also may involve mucous membranes such as the stomach and mouth and frequently is accompanied by eosinophilia. It often occurs in serum sickness (Chap. 74) or in combination with hay fever and allergic asthma. Emotional tension, increased heat, and physical exercise may exaggerate urticaria. Urticaria can be induced by histamine and acetylcholine, and good evidence indicates that liberation of histamine during an allergic reaction is responsible for hives. Urticaria may occur from ingestion, inhalation, injection, or contact with the offending antigen. Foods and drugs frequently are responsible, but hives also have been related to a great variety of inhalants and contactants, such as pollen, dander, dust, feathers, and wool. As in other allergic diseases, the responsible antigen may be detected by careful history, skin test, or elimination diets.

If a specific cause of urticaria is found, it should be corrected or the antigen eliminated from the environment. Acute symptoms usually respond to antihistamines, but adrenal steroids may be needed. Epinephrine, 0.2 to 0.5 ml of 1:1,000 aqueous solution intramuscularly, provides prompt but transient relief. Chronic, idiopathic urticaria is often refractory to treatment, and many of these patients require psychiatric assistance. Prolonged use of adrenal steroids in chronic urticaria is inadvisable.

When first seen, subacute lupus erythematosus occasionally resembles recurrent urticaria.

Angioedema is characterized by edema of the eyelids, lips, external genitalia, and the mucous membranes of the mouth, tongue, or gastrointestinal tract. The swelling may be localized to one area or may be diffuse, and commonly is acompanied by urticaria elsewhere. When the respiratory tract is involved, the patient may have laryngeal edema with hoarseness, stridor, and cyanosis, and rarely death may ensue. Generally, angioedema is attributed to food allergy; shellfish very commonly are incriminated. In addition, the reaction may occur from the many antigens responsible for urticaria. The treatment of angioedema is the same as for urticaria. If respiratory tract obstruction occurs, tracheostomy may prove lifesaving.

A rare form of angioedema is inherited as an autosomal dominant trait and begins in childhood. Nonpruritic angioedematous swellings in the skin characteristically are acompanied by angioedema of the gut, which may result in abdominal pain and lead to unnecessary laparotomy. The diagnosis is made by demonstrating a specific deficiency of a serum protein that inhibits the first component of complement and the proteolytic enzyme kallikrein. There is no specific treatment.

REFERENCES

ALLERGIC RHINITIS

Lowell, F. C., and W. Franklin: A "Double-blind" Study of Treatment with Aqueous Allergenic Extracts in Cases of Allergic Rhinitis, J. Allergy, 34:165, 1963.

Norman, P. S.: Treatment of Allergic Rhinitis, Johns Hopkins Med. J., 121:49, 1967.

Samter, M., and H. L. Alexander: "Immunological Diseases," Boston, Little, Brown and Company, 1965.

ALLERGIC SKIN DISEASE

Waughan, W. T., and J. H. Black: "Practice of Allergy," St. Louis, The C. V. Mosby Company, 1954.

ASTHMA

Bates, D. V., and R. U. Christie: "Respiratory Function in Disease," Philadelphia, W. B. Saunders Company, 1965.

Gay, L. N.: The Pathology of Asthma, Clinics, 5:347, 1946.

Williams, D. A., E. Lewis-Fanning, L. Rees, J. Jacobs, and A. Thomas: Assessment of the Relative Importance of the Allergic, Infective and Psychologic Factors in Asthma, Acta Allergol, 12:376, 1958.

73 REACTIONS TO DRUGS
Leighton E. Cluff

The incidence of adverse reactions to drugs has paralleled the growing use of pharmaceuticals, and with continued introduction of new drugs, this problem has become even more serious.

DEFINITION. Classification of drug reactions is not easy, but undesired responses to therapeutic agents have certain specific features that facilitate categorization. Nearly any drug can elicit pharmacologic effects other than those for which it is usually administered, and when these appear, they are referred to as *side effects*. Some patients show unusual susceptibility to the pharmacologic actions of a drug and are said to have an *idiosyncrasy*. Reactions not explained by the pharmacologic properties of a drug, and therefore indicative of altered reactivity of the patient, are termed *allergic*. Pharmacologic effects, as a rule, are intensified by increasing dosage or cumulative action (*toxic effects*), and readministration is not associated with increased reactivity of the patient. For example, nausea, hyperpnea, and tinnitus in a person given aspirin are side effects, and reduction in dosage will usually alleviate the situation. The occasional patient who displays these symptoms after taking a small amount of aspirin has an idiosyncrasy to the drug. However, if ingestion of aspirin is followed by bronchial asthma or urticaria, reactions not explainable by the pharmacologic action of the drug, the patient is allergic to it. This type of reaction is likely to be associated with symptoms commonly ascribed to hypersensitivity (rash, asthma, pruritus, arthritis, fever, leukopenia, etc.), frequently recurs promptly on readministration of the drug, and is not closely dependent on dosage or cumulative action.

The clinical importance of differentiating side effects, idiosyncrasy, and allergy relates to the hazard of readministration of a drug or to its probable safety in lower dosage.

ETIOLOGY. Allergy to drugs is attributed to immunologic mechanisms and may be manifested by immediate or delayed hypersensitivity. Most pharmacologic agents, however, are incapable of initiating an immunologic response by themselves, and the actual antigen is a conjugate of the drug or its derivatives with autologous proteins. Under such circumstances, the drug acts as a *hapten*, is nonantigenic by itself, but confers antigenic specificity to the protein, which is able to combine with the antibody or react with cells of the sensitized person. Many drugs are bound by body proteins, and there is experimental evidence that the ability of chemical compounds to elicit allergic contact dermatitis can be correlated with their affinity for sulfhydryl-containing proteins of skin. Practically all drugs bind to serum protein, particularly albumin, after absorption, but there is little to suggest that these protein-drug conjugates are important in drug allergy. Other tissue proteins also may bind drugs, but those specifically responsible for rendering a chemical antigenic are not known. The firmness of the combination of a drug or chemical to protein is a determinant of the antigenicity of the complex. Furthermore, the administered drug may be less important in inducing an immunologic response than its degradation products. For example, penicillenic acid and penicilloic acid, degradation products of penicillin, are believed to be responsible for most instances of penicillin allergy. Identification of penicilloyl derivatives in penicillin allergy was predicated upon the knowledge that they could conjugate firmly to proteins.

Serum antibody has been demonstrated in some persons with drug allergy involving cellular elements of blood, as in agranulocytosis, hemolytic anemia, and thrombocytopenia. In other types of drug hypersensitivity, however, precipitation, hemagglutination, or complement fixation tests with a patient's serum may be negative, and direct intradermal or passive transfer tests of the Prausnitz-Küstner type are often unrevealing. In addition, demonstration of agglutination by serum of erythrocytes sensitized with a drug such as penicillin may fail to differentiate the allergic from the nonallergic individual. These results however, are more indicative of the inadequacy of present methods of testing than an argument against an immunologic basis for hypersensitivity to drugs. Demonstration of penicilloyl derivatives associated with penicillin hypersensitivity has provided an important diagnostic test for penicillin allergy. A significant proportion of persons who have penicillin allergy will have a positive wheal and flare skin test to penicilloyl conjugated to a polylysine carrier. Moreover, a positive skin test to minor determinants (which is usually elicited by penicillin G) reflects individuals with the greatest propensity to develop serious systemic anaphylaxis. Though these skin tests indicate that some progress has been made in detecting drug reactions, particularly those to penicillin, the lack of effective testing methods is a great handicap to clinical investigation of these reactions.

Most types of allergic reactions to drugs are nonfamilial; however, anaphylaxis may occur more commonly in persons with other allergic disease, such as hay fever, asthma, or urticaria. Certain diseases seem to predispose to the development of drug allergy. For example, patients with inflammatory or necrotizing gastrointestinal lesions appear to be particularly susceptible to orally administered drugs. Furthermore, the patient acquiring a reaction to one drug often develops allergic reactions to other drugs, but manifestations may differ.

The likelihood of a patient developing an adverse reaction to a drug is directly related to the number of different medications administered. Approximately 5 percent of hospitalized individuals receiving fewer than six different drugs will experience a drug-induced illness. Over 40 percent of hospitalized patients receiving more than 16 different drugs will have an adverse reaction. In part this is attributed to an additive effect, but pharmacologic interactions or incompatibilities also account for the increased rate of adverse reactions when many drugs are given.

Five percent of patients admitted to a hospital have a drug-induced illness; they are three times more likely to acquire another drug-induced illness during hospitalization than patients admitted without an adverse drug reaction. Similarly, a prior history of untoward drug effects is associated with predisposition to subsequent drug-induced illness. In part, this predisposition may be due to genetic differences between patients, exemplified by the susceptibility of individuals with glucose-6 phosphate dehydrogenase deficiency to hemolytic anemia following administration of primaquine and nitrofurans.

Renal and liver dysfunction obviously influences drug metabolism and excretion, and may affect the frequency of adverse reactions to certain drugs. The dosage of many drugs, particularly antibiotics, should be adjusted in the presence of renal and hepatic disease.

Sedatives and tranquilizers most often are incriminated as causes of adverse drug reactions in hospitalized patients. The antibiotics, digitalis, and diuretics are next in importance. Penicillin is the drug most frequently incriminated as a cause of drug allergy, particularly anaphylaxis.

EPIDEMIOLOGY. The incidence of adverse reactions to drugs is not known accurately because there have been few efforts to relate the number of adverse reactions observed to the patients at risk who are taking the drug. From the information available, it appears that most adverse reactions to drugs are not serious and that reactions vary in frequency among drugs. Women are more likely to show adverse reactions to drugs than men. With a few exceptions, exemplified by adverse drug reactions related to genetically abnormal erythrocytes, race and age in adults do not affect the incidence of reaction to drugs. Most reactions develop within 7 to 10 days of drug administration. There appears to be an increased likelihood of adverse drug reaction when multiple drugs are taken by the same patient.

MANIFESTATIONS. Adverse effects of drugs attributed to their pharmacologic action are drug-specific. Allergic reactions, however, are often the same irrespective of the incriminated drug. Some presumed allergic reactions, however, are more common with certain drugs than with others.

The commonest manifestations of allergy to drugs are no different from hypersensitivity reactions of other types and include rashes, asthma, and the symptoms of serum sickness. These are easily recognized clinically as allergic in origin. Other features of drug allergy are less easily characterized. The tabulation in Table 73-1 of common drugs and reactions they may elicit includes some effects that may not be allergic at all.

Skin. Morbilliform, urticarial, and maculopapular rashes are probably the most common skin reactions, but many others are observed, including vesicular, bullous, exfoliative, eczematous, and purpuric eruptions. Pruritus is frequent. Although the type of skin lesion usually will not help identify the causative drug, certain skin reactions are relatively specific. Erythema multiforme or nodosum is seen in allergy to Dilantin, bromides, iodides, trimethadione, and sulfonamides. "Fixed" drug eruptions are most frequently due to aminopyrine, phenolphthalein, or atabrine. Photosensitization during drug therapy occurs characteristically with chlorpromazine, phenothiazine, sulfonamides, and tetracycline derivatives.

Fever. Fever may be an isolated manifestation of drug allergy, and most pharmaceuticals in common use can produce a febrile reaction, including most antibiotics and chemotherapeutic agents. However, the tetracycline derivatives are uncommon causes of drug fever, and digitalis has rarely, if ever, been incriminated as the cause of a pyrogenic reaction. Elevation of temperature may appear abruptly after treatment begins, or it may develop in a stepwise fashion during or after the second week of drug administration. Drug fever is often associated with chills and constitutional symptoms and may be accompanied by leukocytosis. Discontinuing therapy usually results in defervescence within a short period, although several days may be required for return of temperature to normal.

Blood. Changes in the formed elements of the blood are common during drug allergy and may have no specificity. Some drugs have been found to have limited or no effects on the blood, while others produce specific abnormalities. For example, penicillin has not been incriminated as a cause of serious hematologic abnormalities. In therapeutic doses, acetanilid is probably not a cause of anemia, agranulocytosis, thrombocytopenia, or aplastic anemia; in high dosage, however, it may produce leukocytosis, methemoglobinemia, and acute hemolysis. *Methemoglobinemia* also occurs with antipyrine, nitrites, sulfonamides, primaquine, and pamaquine, but this reaction is probably not allergic in origin. Barbiturates, salicylates, and para-aminosalicylic acid rarely, if ever, produce agranulocytosis. *Eosinophilia* may accompany allergic reactions of many types, but it occurs with such frequency as an isolated finding during therapy with streptomycin or nirvanol that it has no significance. *Lymphocytosis* is common in patients receiving Dilantin and nirvanol, and polymorphonuclear leukocytosis may be found in individuals taking Dilantin or atropine. Studies of the erythrocyte abnormality responsible for the *acute hemolytic anemia* induced by primaquine, sulfonamides, and nitrofurans in certain individuals indicate that what was thought to be drug allergy is actually a genetically determined enzyme deficiency. Jaundice due to pharmaceutical agents is discussed elsewhere (Chap. 327).

Nervous System. A variety of neurologic manifestations may appear during drug therapy, but in the majority of instances there is little evidence to incriminate allergy as a cause. The commonest reaction is delirium, seen particularly with digitalis, atropine, thiocyanates, and sedatives. Other drugs that produce adverse effects on the nervous system (ranging from paresthesias and peripheral neuritis to deafness) are streptomycin, hydralazine, chlorpromazine, Diamox, isoniazid, polymyxin, neomycin, and kanamycin.

Others. Nausea, vomiting, and diarrhea are exceedingly common drug reactions. In addition, *abdominal pain* in the absence of other symptoms may be produced by quinidine, chlorpromazine, and primaquine. *Albuminuria* and *cylindruria* occur particularly with heavy metals, bacitracin, polymyxin, and colimycin. Dilantin, chloral hydrate, sulfonamides, trimethadione, Phenurone, colchicin, thiocyanate, and amphotericin B occasionally produce renal dysfunction, probably because of their direct toxic action. Amphotericin B may produce tubular necrosis and renal calcification, but this is only occasionally associated with significant evidence of renal insufficiency and nitrogen retention. Hypersensitivity to sulfonamides has resulted in acute hemorrhagic nephritis.

Histologic lesions indistinguishable from those of *polyarteritis nodosa* have been found in the tissues of patients who have experienced allergic reactions to iodides, Dilantin, sulfonamides, and penicillin. Manifestations of

Table 73-1. ADVERSE REACTIONS TO DRUGS

Drug	Gastro-intestinal				Cutaneous							Hematologic (Marrow failure)							Metabolic			Neurologic				Ear and eye		Allergic			Cardi-orenal				
	Nausea-vomiting	Diarrhea	GI bleeding	Jaundice	Dermatitis	Acneiform eruption	Erythema multiforme	Urticaria	Purpura	Fixed eruption	Photosensitization	Red blood cells	White blood cells	Platelets	Hemolysis	Leukocytosis	Eosinophilia	Hypoprothrombinemia	Hypokalemia	Hyperuricemia	Hyperglycemia	Delirium	Convulsions	Peripheral neuropathy	Extrapyramidal syndrome	C_8 nerve damage	Ocular damage	Anaphylaxis	Fever	"Serum sickness"	Arrhythmia	Hypotension	Renal disorder	Collagen-vascular syndromes	Fetal and neonatal effects
Acetazolamide					+						+	+	+	+					+										+				+		
Acetophenetidin					+			+	+	+		+	+	+	+	+													+				+		
Alkylating agents	+	+	+	+	+			+			+	+	+	+						+									+				+		+
Aminopyrine					+			+		+			+		+														+		+				
Aminosalicylic acid	+	+	+	+	+								+	+	+	+	+	+										+	+	+	+				
Amphotericin B	+	+										+												+					+				+		
Anabolic steroids	+			+		+																													+
Antihistamines	+				+			+				+	+	+														+	+	+	+				
Antimetabolites	+	+	+	+					+			+	+	+						+									+						+
Barbiturates					+		+	+	+	+		+										+							+	+					
Belladonna alkaloids					+											+						+							+						
Benzothiadiazines	+			+	+						+		+	+					+	+	+												+		+
Bromides	+					+	+	+														+							+				+		
Chloral hydrate	+				+			+	+																								+		
Chloramphenicol	+		+	+	+			+				+	+	+															+						+
Chlordiazepoxide				+												+	+					+							+		+				
Chloroquine	+	+			+						+				+												+								
Chlorpropamide	+			+				+				+	+	+															+						
Cocaine (derivatives)	+				+																	+	+					+	+						
Codeine	+				+			+																											
Colchicine	+	+										+	+	+										+					+				+	+	
Colistin and polymyxin								+																+					+				+		
Corticosteroids			+			+										+			+		+	+					+								+
Coumarin derivatives	+	+	+		+			+										+																	+
Diethylstilbestrol	+				+											+																			
Digitalis	+	+			+		+	+								+	+					+	+												
Dimercaprol (BAL)	+				+			+							+	+													+		+				
Ergot alkaloids	+																							+											
Erythromycin	+	+		+	+																								+						
Ethynyl estradiol	+			+	+						+																								
Gold		+		+	+		+	+	+	+		+	+	+								+	+										+	+	
Griseofulvin	+	+			+			+														+		+									+		
Guanethidine		+			+																										+	+	+		
Heparin			+												+														+	+		+			
Hydantoin derivatives				+	+	+		+				+	+	+	+	+	+							+					+	+				+	+
Hydralazine	+	+	+		+		+					+	+											+					+	+		+		+	
Imipramine and amitriptyline				+	+								+												+		+				+	+			
Insulin					+			+																				+							
Iodides	+	+			+	+	+	+	+	+		+	+	+			+											+	+	+				+	+
Isoniazid	+			+	+			+					+				+					+	+	+					+						
Kanamycin and neomycin	+																+									+							+		
Meperidine	+							+																								+			+
Meprobamate					+							+	+	+														+							

Table 73-1. ADVERSE REACTIONS TO DRUGS (Continued)

Drug	Nausea-vomiting	Diarrhea	GI bleeding	Jaundice	Dermatitis	Acneiform eruption	Erythema multiforme	Urticaria	Purpura	Fixed eruption	Photosensitization	Red blood cells	White blood cells	Platelets	Hemolysis	Leukocytosis	Eosinophilia	Hypoprothrombinemia	Hypokalemia	Hyperuricemia	Hyperglycemia	Delirium	Convulsions	Peripheral neuropathy	Extrapyramidal syndrome	C8 nerve damage	Ocular damage	Anaphylaxis	Fever	"Serum sickness"	Arrhythmia	Hypotension	Renal disorder	Collagen-vascular syndromes	Fetal and neonatal effects
Mercurials	+				+		+	+		+		+							+										+	+	+				+
Methyldopa		+		+	+							+																	+				+	+	
Methimazole				+	+			+				+					+												+						
Methylphenidate	+					+																	+								+	+			
Methyltestosterone				+	+																														+
Morphine	+				+			+													+														+
M.A.O. inhibitors				+	+								+									+		+							+				
Nitrofurantoin	+			+				+								+	+							+					+	+					
Novobiocin	+	+		+	+																								+						+
Penicillins					+		+	+	+							+						+	+					+	+	+				+	
Phenformin	+	+																																	
Phenindiones	+	+	+	+	+								+				+	+											+	+					
Phenolphthalein		+			+		+	+		+									+										+	+					
Phenothiazines	+			+	+			+	+		+	+				+	+					+	+		+			+	+		+	+			+
Phenylbutazone		+	+	+	+			+				+	+	+															+	+			+	+	
Primaquine	+	+		+								+	+	+	+							+					+								
Probenecid	+			+	+											+													+	+					
Procaine amide	+	+			+			+		+		+										+						+	+	+	+	+		+	
Progesterone	+																																		+
Propoxyphene	+				+																														
Propylthiouracil				+	+			+					+				+	+											+	+				+	+
Quinidine/quinine	+	+			+			+	+	+		+	+	+			+					+					+		+	+	+	+	+		
Rauwolfia	+	+	+		+																				+							+			+
Salicylates	+		+		+		+	+	+							+	+				+	+					+	+	+	+	+	+			
Spironolactones					+																	+									+	+			
Streptomycin	+	+			+			+				+	+				+					+				+		+	+	+			+		
Sulfonamides				+	+		+	+	+	+	+	+	+	+	+		+					+		+				+	+				+	+	+
Sympathetic amines					+			+									+				+	+	+					+							
Tetracyclines	+	+		+	+			+		+																			+				+		+
Tolbutamide	+	+	+					+	+		+	+	+	+																			+		
Trimethadione		+		+	+		+					+	+	+																			+	+	
Vancomycin					+																					+			+				+	+	
Xanthine derivatives	+		+		+					+													+						+	+		+	+		

systemic lupus erythematosus have appeared during therapy with gold, hydralazine, and a few other drugs. The manifestations of lupus associated with drug reactions usually have been reversible following discontinuation of the drug (Chap. 392).

Anaphylaxis may follow the parenteral administration of a variety of drugs, but the agent incriminated most often is penicillin. The risk of any particular patient's developing anaphylaxis to penicillin is very small, but because a large number of patients (20 to 30 percent in general hospitals) receive the drug, this reaction may be observed relatively frequently. Radiopaque iodinated dyes, particularly those used for intravenous pyelography, and Bromsulphalein are two other common diagnostic agents which have been incriminated in anaphylaxis.

TREATMENT AND PROPHYLAXIS. Allergic reactions to drugs usually subside promptly when the agent is discontinued. For reasons that are not understood, however, the reaction occasionally persists for prolonged periods despite withdrawal of the drug. Recurrent urticaria for many months after a penicillin reaction is a common example.

The management of serum sickness is described in Chap. 74. In the event of persistent or severe manifestations of drug allergy, the use of adrenocortical steroids is indicated. Adrenal steriods, antihistamines, and epinephrine are usually ineffective in alleviating reactions due to idiosyncrasy or side effects of a drug. Reactions of this type are best managed by withdrawing the offending drug and administering other drugs with appropriate pharmacologic actions, e.g., sedatives for excitability, stimulants for depression, etc.

Although it is usually not possible to predict the occurrence of drug allergy in a patient, the fact that hypersensitivity to drugs may be commoner in individuals with other allergic reactions makes it reasonable to inquire about this before beginning treatment with any agent. A specific history of hypersensitivity to a given drug contraindicates its readministration unless the clinical situation is serious. When confronted with such a situation, the procedure of choice is to look for an alternative agent which is just as efficacious. For example, vancomycin may be used as effectively as a penicillin in staphylococcal endocarditis. In a number of instances when it has been judged necessary to prescribe a drug to which a patient is known to be allergic, the concomitant administration of adrenal steroids has completely suppressed the manifestations of hypersensitivity. The third alternative, namely "desensitizing the patient" by administering progressively increasing dosages of a drug such as penicillin, should be used only as a last resort. Though desensitization is often successful, there are occasional examples of an individual who was believed to have been "desensitized" and who experienced a fatal anaphylactic reaction upon receiving a large systemic dose of the drug in question.

Although it is said that sensitivity to a drug will subside if its administration is continued, this is not a regular occurrence and should not be accepted as a basis for further therapy with the incriminated agent.

The U.S. Food and Drug Administration and the Council on Drugs of the American Medical Association are accumulating information on adverse drug reactions. They solicit the cooperation of all physicians in reporting reactions to them.

REFERENCES

Alexander, H. L.: "Reactions to Drug Therapy," Philadelphia, W. B. Saunders Company, 1956.

Carr, E. A., Jr.: Drug Allergy, Pharmacol. Rev., 6:365, 1954.

Cluff, L. E., and J. E. Johnson: Drug Fever, Progr. Allergy, 8:149, 1964.

Eisen, H. N.: Hypersensitivity to Simple Chemicals, in "Cellular and Humoral Aspects of Hypersensitivity," New York, Hoeber Medical Division, Harper & Row, Publishers, Incorporated, 1959.

Landsteiner, K.: "The Specificity of Serological Reactions," Cambridge, Mass., Harvard University Press, 1945.

Seidl, Larry G., G. F. Thornton, J. W. Smith, and L. E. Cluff: Studies on the Epidemiology of Adverse Drug Reactions: III. Reactions in Patients on a General Medical Service, Bull. Johns Hopkins Hosp., 119:299, 1966.

Smith, J. W., L. G. Seidl, and L. E. Cluff: Studies on the Epidemiology of Adverse Drug Reactions: V. Clinical Factors Influencing Susceptibility, Ann. Intern. Med., 65:629, 1966.

74 SERUM SICKNESS AND RELATED DISORDERS

Leighton E. Cluff

DEFINITION. Serum sickness is a systemic illness which occurs in individuals allergic to foreign serum or serum protein. An identical illness may also develop from allergic reactions to drugs. The reaction is characterized by fever, skin eruptions, lymphadenopathy, and arthralgia.

ETIOLOGY AND PATHOGENESIS. Serum sickness was first recognized when the use of immune horse serum for prophylaxis and therapy of diphtheria became widespread. With advances in chemotherapy, foreign serum is employed less and less frequently, and its use is now limited for the most part to diphtheria, tetanus, gas gangrene, botulism, envenenation by reptiles, and rabies. The increasing availability of human immune globulin for treatment and active immunization in many diseases has decreased significantly the importance of allergic reactions to foreign serum. For reasons not entirely clear, transfusion of blood is occasionally followed by serum sickness. Though whole foreign serum is more likely to elicit a reaction, purified fractions are also capable of producing illness. The incidence and severity of serum sickness increase with dosage of the antigen.

Serum sickness is an immunologic reaction dependent on antigen and serum antibody. Following an initial injection of foreign serum, serum fraction, or some drugs, antibody will develop within 7 to 10 days. The reaction leading to illness occurs while the antibody is appearing in the serum and antigen is present in excess of available antibody. Circulating antigen-antibody complexes may be found in the blood. As the reaction develops, serum complement declines. An individual previously exposed to an antigen and possessing specific serum antibody may develop an immediate reaction with anaphylactic shock upon subsequent exposure to the antigen. The previously exposed person who possesses no specific serum antibody may have an accelerated reaction after a second exposure to the antigen, because the booster or anamnestic response results in rapid reappearance of antibody. Depending on the degree of prior sensitization and the level of serum antibody, a severe reaction may occur within minutes or hours.

Apparent relapses or recurrences of serum sickness are not unusual. Serum is not a single antigenic substance, and such a course results from a series of reactions to different antigenic components of the injected material.

The mode of injury to tissue, the release of histamine, serotonin, acetylcholine, etc., by antigen-antibody union are discussed in Chap. 68. The elicitation of illness by nonprotein drugs involves immunologic mechanisms also. These are discussed in Chap. 73.

PATHOLOGY. Serum sickness is rarely fatal. However, examination of tissues of patients dying of other causes during or shortly after an episode of serum sickness often shows lesions indistinguishable from those of periarteritis nodosa. Similar lesions are readily produced in rabbits by injection of foreign protein. The finding of vasculitis in allergic reactions is one of the several factors that have led to the idea that hypersensitivity may be important in the causation of periarteritis nodosa, rheumatic fever, systemic lupus erythematosus, and other diseases characterized by vascular damage.

MANIFESTATIONS. After an incubation period of 4 to 10 days (it may be much shorter in sensitized persons or as long as 21 days in others), there is the onset of *pruritus,* followed shortly by *rash.* The rash may take the form of erythematous, morbilliform, or petechial eruption, but by far the commonest pattern is urticaria. Often, the skin lesions appear at the local site of injection of the serum several hours before the rash becomes generalized. *Lymphadenopathy,* most prominent in the area draining the injection site, is usual, as is *edema* of the face, lips, eyelids, or, rarely, the glottis. Most patients with serum sickness have fever which is often accompanied by arthralgia and at times by arthritis, with effusion into one of the large joints. The joint manifestations may be, in fact, the overshadowing feature of serum sickness. Other symptoms include headache, nausea, vomiting, abdominal pain, diarrhea, cardiac arrhythmias, and pericarditis.

The most disabling complications of serum sickness are neurologic disorders, which occur in a minority of cases. Unilateral mononeuritis which involves the shoulder girdle or arm and is characterized by weakness and sensory deficit, may appear. Isolated facial palsy occurs, and occasionally, there may be extensive polyneuritis or meningoencephalitis.

LABORATORY FINDINGS. There is usually a mild peripheral neutrophilic leukocytosis, and the bone marrow shows an increase in number of plasma cells. Eosinophilia is not a feature of classical serum sickness, but it occasionally accompanies the drug-induced syndrome. The urine may contain protein, casts, and erythrocytes. Electrocardiograms sometimes show transient conduction defects. Slight pleocytosis in the cerebrospinal fluid is frequent even in the absence of demonstrable neurologic dysfunction.

COURSE. Serum sickness is a benign, self-limited disease which subsides within 1 to 3 weeks. In patients with neuropathy, residual weakness may require several weeks to abate, but complete restoration of function is the rule. Rare deaths from edema of the glottis are recorded, but a fatal outcome is more often a result of the intercurrent disease.

TREATMENT. Urticaria usually responds to small doses of epinephrine and can be controlled with ephedrine and antihistaminics. Joint pains are usually relieved promptly by aspirin or other salicylates.

For severely ill and uncomfortable patients, adrenal steroids offer prompt relief, and the great efficacy of these compounds has led to their increasing use for symptomatic treatment. They need to be given for only 4 to 7 days in most patients.

Tracheostomy or tracheal intubation is needed at times for sudden respiratory obstruction by edema, and equipment for these procedures should be at hand during the early stages of the disease. Adrenal steroids relieve incipient respiratory obstruction promptly.

In patients who have developed serum sickness as a result of administration of tetanus or diphtheria horse antiserum, active immunization with toxoid should be initiated before the patient is released from medical care. Once a foreign serum has produced serum sickness it should never be given again.

ANAPHYLAXIS. Occasional patients given an injection of serum, of skin-test antigen, or a drug will become profoundly ill and may collapse and die within minutes. Asthmatic wheezing, cyanosis, and severe pruritus involving the hands often occur at the onset of illness. This reaction is the human counterpart of anaphylactic shock in lower animals. Because it rarely occurs in individuals who give no history of hypersensitivity and because fatalities have followed the injection of tiny amounts of serum for the purpose of determining a patient's state of sensitization, prevention is very difficult. Perhaps the most important step in reducing the incidence of anaphylaxis is to follow the dictum that no serum product or drug should be given to any patient without clear indications. Although most severe reactions occur after parenteral administration of the antigen or drug, fatalities have been reported after oral ingestion.

Treatment consists of the intravenous or intracardiac administration of epinephrine and vigorous support of respiration and circulation. Adrenal steroids may be given parenterally but are of little or no value in treating this acute situation. When the injection site permits, a tourniquet may be applied to slow absorption of the antigen.

ARTHUS REACTION. When experimental animals are sensitized to foreign serum or other proteins, reinjection of antigen into the skin often elicits transient erythema and edema, similar to a "positive" skin test in man. If animals are highly sensitive or if the dose of antigen is large, the skin lesion may progress to hemorrhage and necrosis, with eventual ulceration and scarring. This irreversible tissue damage after local application of antigen in a sensitive animal is the classic Arthus phenomenon. Rarely, a similar type of hemorrhagic necrosis occurs at sites of injection of serum or drugs in man. These Arthus-like reactions are unusual, however, and are far outnumbered by inflammatory reactions at injection sites attributable to the intrinsic irritating properties of a drug, to hemorrhage in patients with hemophilia, thrombocytopenia, or drug-induced coagulation defects, or to secondary bacterial infection. Until these disorders have been ruled out, an Arthus reaction should not be invoked as the cause of tissue damage in man.

SHWARTZMAN REACTION. Appropriately timed intradermal injections of bacterial endotoxins or endotoxins in combination with various other substances can elicit in rabbit skin a hemorrhagic necrosis that resembles the Arthus reaction. The mechanism of the reaction is not clear, but it may have a pathogenesis similar to that of immunologic reactions. Numerous attempts have been made to demonstrate the importance of this reaction in the pathogenesis of human disease, including peptic ulcer, acute pancreatitis, and focal reactions in tuberculosis, but it remains, for the most part, a dramatic laboratory phenomenon. The confluent purpura and the adrenocortical hemorrhage of meningococcemia may be the human counterpart of a Schwartzman reaction (Chap. 142).

REFERENCES

Austen, K. F.: Systemic Anaphylaxis in Man, J.A.M.A., 192: 116, 1963.

Dixon, F. J., J. J. Vazquez, W. O. Weigle, and C. G. Cochrane: Pathogenesis of Serum Sickness, A.M.A. Arch. Pathol., 65:18, 1958.

Kojis, F. G.: Serum Sickness and Anaphylaxis, Am. J. Dis. Child., 64:93, 313, 1942.

Longcope, W. T.: Serum Sickness and Analogous Reactions from Certain Drugs, Particularly the Sulfonamides, Medicine, 22:251, 1943.

v. Pirquet, C., and B. Schick: "Serum Sickness," Baltimore, The Williams & Wilkins Company, 1951.

Part Five

Nutritional, Hormonal, and Metabolic Disorders

Section 1

Basic Considerations

INTRODUCTION

Nutrition, the science of food, is concerned with types and amounts of foodstuffs with respect to their basic components (minerals, amino acids, lipids, carbohydrates, or vitamins) and the ways they are carried through the processes of digestion, absorption, transport utilization, and excretion. It is a widely held view among the laity that all health is somehow attributable to poor food habits, and patients will expect physicians to be attentive to this possibility and to give knowledgeable advice.

The term *nutrition*, however, does not confine one necessarily to a consideration of dietary or exogenous materials. Even though the diet may contain all of the 40-odd essential nutrients, a variety of causes may precipitate conditioned deficiency states which will prevent the fulfillment of all the nutritional requirements of the cells and tissues of the body. In nations in which technology, education, social security, medical services, food, clothing, housing, and many other socioeconomic factors are highly developed and food of all types is abundant, disorders of nutrition generally are due to factors which interfere with assimilation or absorption of nutrients, produce excess loss, or cause excess elimination of an adequate intake. Psychic factors, such as those which play an important role in anorexia nervosa or food fads, also are important considerations.

In less favored societies ("developing nations") reduced intake of calories and essential nutrients is likely to be the most important cause of nutritional deficiency—the result of poverty, insufficient education, and cultural and religious practices. In such countries the classical nutritional diseases are seen.

Nutritional lack finds expression in various ways, and the physician must recognize and understand its effects. He must bear in mind that malnutrition will often complicate an illness and may aggravate it. On the other hand, good nutrition can facilitate the management of disease, and thus, food habits and diet therapy become inextricably a part of diagnosis and therapeutics.

In medical centers the availability of dieticians, specialized dietary services, and a large variety of laboratory facilities has eased the application of nutrition science for physicians early in their careers. A hidden danger is that such readily available assistance leaves them relatively unprepared for their possible subsequent isolation from such facilities. This section reviews the essential elements of nutrition and metabolism and discusses the application of the principles of nutrition science to diagnosis and management. The classical deficiency states are described, but the emphasis is upon the more relevant matter of relating nutritional disturbances to the prevention and management of other illnesses.

75 INTERMEDIARY METABOLISM OF PROTEIN, FAT, AND CARBOHYDRATE

George F. Cahill, Jr. and Frederic L. Hoch

Life may be defined as a system of matter having heritability and mutability; as such, it requires continued or intermittent capture of both energy and matter. The processes maintaining life in the cell may be divided accordingly: the transformation of captured energy into forms useful to and usable by cells, and the transformation of matter (molecules) to make more available their energy content or to use the matter to replace the machinery of the cell or to synthesize new machinery for growth or reproduction. Disturbances in transformation of energy or molecules may become manifest as disease processes, though our knowledge of the precise metabolic events in most cases is as yet fragmentary.

These functions of the cell are carried out in specialized subcellular compartments: maintenance and renewal of cell structure is governed by information contained in nuclear deoxyribonucleic acid (DNA); energy transformations are performed mainly by mitochondria; and synthetic and degradative processes are accomplished in microsomes and in the surrounding soluble fluid or cytoplasm.

ENZYMES

The functioning unit of the cell which catalyzes all the molecular changes is a protein molecule, an *enzyme*. A biochemist's view has been summarized: "Except for those rare phenomena in biology which are purely physical, the 'aliveness' of cells is basically the summation of enzymatic catalysis and its regulation" (Anfinsen). Enzyme function is localized to a small portion of the usually large polypeptide sequence, the active site E. This site binds the substrate molecule S transiently during the act of catalysis to form the enzyme-substrate complex ES, which then dissociates to liberate free enzyme and product P. The process of catalysis by the enzyme can be formulated as a set of rates maintaining a chemical equilibrium:

$$E + S \underset{k_{-1}}{\overset{k_1}{\rightleftharpoons}} ES \overset{k_2}{\to} P + E \qquad (1)$$

The velocities are expressed by the constants k_1, k_{-1}, and k_2 and are properties of the enzyme molecule arising from its three-dimensional structure and from the arrangement of its active sites. The overall chemical equilibrium $S \rightleftharpoons P$, which in the absence of the catalytic enzyme might be reached only after a prolonged period of time, is accelerated by the enzyme, which, by forming complexes as in Eq. (1), imparts much higher velocities to some of the individual steps of the reaction. An interrelationship between these velocity constants can be expressed through a constant that depends on the features of the enzyme and the conditions of the reaction:

$$K_m = \frac{k_{-1} + k_2}{k_1} \qquad (2)$$

K_m is the Michaelis constant. When k_2 is small compared with k_{-1}, K_m is also the measure of the affinity of the active site for the substrate, the dissociation constant of the enzyme-substrate complex; K_m can also be thought of as the concentration of substrate that half-saturates the active enzyme sites. These concepts are of increasing importance in understanding normal and disease mechanisms, since controls can be exerted on enzymes which catalyze "rate-limiting" steps in a sequence of reactions

Adenosine-3′, 5′-Monophosphate
(Cyclic-3′, 5′-AMP)

Fig. 75-1. The structure of cyclic-3′,5′-adenosinemonophosphate (cyclic-3′,5′-AMP or cyclic adenylate). It is produced in the cell from adenosinetriphosphate (see Fig. 75-2).

or on enzymes at points in the pathways of intermediary metabolism (or of energy transfer) which are "switching stations," where more than one path is possible. The mechanism of control at these points may be a chemical reaction between the controlling agents and the effector molecule, and is governed by the properties of the enzyme and agent and their interactions, much the same way as the reactions shown in Eq. (1).

CONTROL MECHANISMS

The state of simple chemical equilibrium is probably seldom attained in reactions in the living cell. Since the product is usually being removed by another process, the reaction, although potentially bidirectional, usually carries substrate in only one direction. In certain cases, the nature of the reaction catalyzed by the enzyme is so heavily favored in one direction, because of loss of free energy in the reaction (exergonic), that the enzyme catalyzes a reaction which is essentially unidirectional. Wherever this occurs, there appears to be an important site of overall metabolic control, as by a hormone or some other regulatory process, which by changing the activity or quantity of the enzyme is able to alter profoundly the rate of the reaction and therefore the flow of substrate over this and subsequent reactions.

Knowledge of enzymes has so far been of medical value in two areas: the empiric use of enzyme activity measurements as diagnostic aids and the recognition that certain genetically transmitted diseases or disease traits are the result of a single discrete biochemical lesion, due to a defect either in the synthesis or in the action of an enzyme. The usefulness of diagnostic enzymology is being increased by observations that *isozymes*, enzymes catalyzing the same reaction but possessing different structural or functional (e.g., K_m) properties, can be identified in body fluids as originating in a specific organ or tissue. The catalytic nature of enzymes (some enzymes handle the alteration of more than 5 million substrate molecules per min per molecule of enzyme) makes them key control points for the regulation of metabolic flux by hormones, vitamins, trace metals, pharmacologic agents and toxins, and specific metabolites which can bind to an enzyme and either alter the three-dimensional conformation of the enzyme (allosteric transitions) or compete with the substrate and cause inhibition.

Other control mechanisms include (1) changes in the state of polymerization of enzyme molecule structure, e.g., the transformation of inactive phosphorylase dimers into the active tetramer under the indirect influence of a unique molecule, cyclic-3′,5′-adenosinemonophosphate (Fig. 75-1); (2) the availability of oxidized or reduced coenzymes; (3) actions on membrane permeability. There is also evidence that hormones act on membranes that enclose and partition the interiors of cells to control the transport of substrates or cofactors from one compartment to another. With the discovery that the membrane of the mitochondrion, for instance, contains oriented enzymes, this distinction may lose some of its sharpness. Nevertheless, the phenomena of diffusion, active membrane transport, and pinocytosis (an action engulfing external particles or molecules, in which part of the membrane forms a shell around the object of transport) have been shown to be affected by hormone action. (4) The amount of an enzyme present in the cell also controls the catalytic action exerted. Enzymes are made via the usual routes of synthesis of proteins, but there are more specific influences on enzyme synthesis than those governing the general production of proteins. In primitive unicellular organisms, where the supply of substrates can be controlled, production of an enzyme can be induced *de novo* by supplying a new substrate. The role of enzyme induction in mammals is not so clear, although some examples of adaptation of tissues to metabolize certain compounds more rapidly have been reported. When an enzyme contains a special organic or inorganic prosthetic group that is not synthesized via the ordinary metabolic routes, interference with the supply of the prosthetic group may decrease the amount of active enzyme synthesized; conditioned or dietary deficiencies of vitamins and inorganic elements may also cause such defects.

Energy Transformation

The energy that allows living protoplasm in heterotrophic cells to maintain its structure and growth and therefore its function against the demands of the less-organized environment is derived from the potential energy inherent in the chemical bonds of large, moderately complex organic molecules—biologic fuels. This energy is transformed by various catalytic mechanisms partly into heat, which in homotherms maintains a constant body temperature higher than that of the environment, facilitating enzyme catalyses. In autotrophic cells, energy for useful work is derived not from organic molecules, but from sunlight, which is used to fix carbon dioxide from the air and to synthesize carbohydrate; this is the ultimate source of the substrates needed by heterotrophic cells to survive.

High-energy Bonds

The carrier molecule for the free energy derived from foodstuffs (or from sunlight) is adenosinetriphosphate (ATP) (Fig. 75-2). In the cells, the terminal phosphate groups are transferred to "activate" other molecules; the free energy of the ATP molecule is conserved in part in this transfer so that the activated acceptor molecule can thereafter participate in energy-requiring processes such as muscle contraction or syntheses. The high-energy bond of ATP is the pyrophosphate linkage of its terminal phosphate groups ($\sim$P), and the free energy content of each $\sim$P is about 8 kcal per mole. This may be thought of as the energy evolved when the phosphate ester linkage is simply hydrolyzed in solution. Ordinary "energy-poor" phosphate ester linkages have a free energy content of approximately 2 kcal per mole. The high energy is apparently imparted to the bond by the other resonant chemical bonds immediately adjacent to the phosphate group: it is as if they supplied negative charges like the

Adenosine-5'-Triphosphate (ATP)

Fig. 75-2. The structure of adenosinetriphosphate. Energy is stored in the two terminal high-energy phosphate bonds (denoted in the text as $\sim$P) and is released or transferred to support reactions requiring energy (endergonic).

negative poles of a magnet, kept together only by the phosphate bond; when hydrolysis or transfer occurs, this highly "stressed" bond releases or transfers its potential energy content.

High-energy bonds are not found solely in ATP, although it is probably the principal source of these bonds in the cell. In mammalian muscle, the main storage form of high energy is in the phosphoamide bond of creatine phosphate (in lower animals, in arginine phosphate). Other forms are the phosphoenols like phosphoenolpyruvate and acetyl phosphate; pyrophosphate and polypyrophosphate; thioesters like acetyl coenzyme A; and sulfonium compounds like S-adenosylmethionine, which activate methyl groups for the synthesis of choline, creatine, N-methylnicotinamide (for coenzyme I or DPN$^+$),[1] and norepinephrine.

There are two major pathways by which high-energy bonds in ATP are generated. (1) *Intra*molecular H transfer (hydrogen atom transfer), which is performed by single or complex soluble enzymes in the cytoplasm or in the free fluid inside mitochondria. (2) *Inter*molecular H transfer, which is performed by solid-state, insoluble complexes of oriented enzymes in mitochondrial membranes. Mitochondria transduce energy in heterotrophic cells, transforming substrate energy to ATP bonds through the use of over 90 percent of the O_2 consumed by the cell.

In mitochondria, the enzymes, starting with that one specific for the substrate being utilized, transfer H atoms or electrons stepwise to each other (diphosphopyridine nucleotide, flavins, cytochromes) in the membrane portion, and at the same time esterify inorganic phosphate to make an (as yet hypothetic) high-energy intermediate compound, $X \sim P$ (Fig. 75-3). In the presence of adenosinediphosphate (ADP) the high-energy phosphate is transferred from the intermediate compound on the mito-

[1] Diphosphopyridine nucleotide (DPN$^+$) and reduced diphosphopyridine nucleotide (DPNH) have been renamed nicotinamide adenine dinucleotide (NAD$^+$ and NADH), and the respective triphosphopyridine nucleotide compounds TPN$^+$ and TPNH have been renamed nicotinamide adenine dinucleotide phosphate (NADP$^+$ and NADPH).

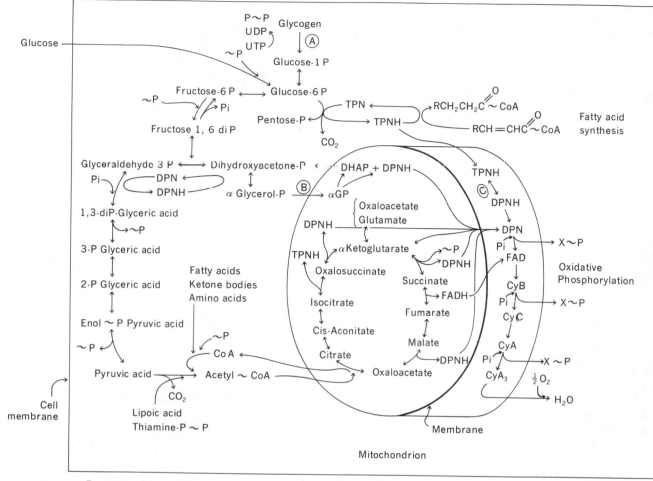

Fig. 75-3. A general scheme of energy and molecular transformations in compartments of the cell. Glucose is transported across the cell membrane, phosphorylated through use of a high-energy phosphate bond ($\sim P$), and then transformed either to store its energy content (upward, glycogenesis) or to release its energy content (downward) via (1) breakdown of glycogen by phosphorylase (*A*); (2) oxidation through the glycolytic cycle to form acetyl CoA; (3) hydrogen transfer (*B*) to enter the mitochondrial apparatus; (4) oxidation through the pentose pathway. Energy is transformed into useful form via the consumption of O_2 in mitochondrial membranes, with concomitant esterification of inorganic phosphate (P_i) to form a (hypothetic) high-energy phosphate intermediate compound ($X \sim P$), which can be used to synthesize ATP (see Fig. 75-2); this mitochondrial process is oxidative phosphorylation. The mitochondrial matrix contains enzymes catalyzing the Krebs (tricarboxylic acid) cycle, transforming the energy released from acetyl CoA produced from glucose, amino acids, ketone bodies, or fatty acids. Further details are discussed in the text.

chondrion to make ATP; three ATP molecules are produced for each atom of oxygen used in oxidizing most substrates. This process is *oxidative phosphorylation*. The mitochondrial apparatus, besides transforming energy, also contains its own control mechanism for respiration. When the high-energy intermediate remains *in situ*, i.e., when no ADP is present to accept the high-energy bond from $X \sim P$, oxidation proceeds at a relatively slow rate; when acceptor ADP is added, the oxidative rate increases up to tenfold or more as substrate is consumed. The demand for useful energy thus controls the generation of useful energy, a mechanism of *respiratory control*. Living cells, surprisingly perhaps, respire at the lower rate and so are in a state of controlled respiration. The oxygen consumption of man, measured as the BMR, is predominantly due to this basal mitochondrial oxygen utilization. The coupling between oxidation and phosphorylation in the normal cell may be compared to the clutch of a car, which engages and harnesses the consumption of fuel and oxygen to rotating the wheels; the phosphate-acceptor function of ADP is like releasing a set brake and advancing the throttle.

The transformation of energy by oxidative phosphorylation in mitochondria can be inhibited by chemical agents in vitro and in vivo. Dinitrophenol and salicylates act this way, reducing phosphorylation but allowing oxidation to continue. Indeed, when this "uncoupling" of phosphorylation occurs, the rate of oxidation increases severalfold, as if the clutch of the car had been disengaged while the throttle was still advanced, allowing the motor to run faster and overheat without doing useful work. This accounts for the toxic actions of dinitrophenol and salicylates, which raise the BMR and eventually the body temperature; toxic amounts of thyroid hormone induce a similar change.

INTERMEDIARY METABOLISM

Mitochondrial Oxidation

Mitochondria can oxidize a number of substrates as fuel for generation of high-energy bonds, through the presence of enzymes specific for the substrate; the H atoms so obtained all traverse the common mitochondrial membrane pathway of electron transport and H transport to produce useful energy. The following metabolic fuels or molecules derived from them can be oxidized by mitochondria to serve as the important sources of energy (Fig. 75-3): (1) glucose, (2) amino acids, (3) ketone bodies, and (4) fatty acids. As detailed below, the proportion and amount utilized of each of these is under physiologic and biochemical control. Products of the metabolism of glucose and amino acids (after transamination) enter the Krebs cycle in the soluble matrix of the mitochondrion mainly as acetyl CoA, an activated thioester of acetate and coenzyme A, which contains the vitamin pantothenic acid. The esterification proceeds from energy derived from ATP. Fatty acids and ketone bodies are also oxidized by mitochondria as CoA esters. Studies suggest that the fatty acid molecules enter mitochondria combined with carnitine, a known growth factor. There is a complex mitochondrial fatty acid oxidation cycle, whereby fatty acids are activated using CoA and ATP. Dehydrogenation is accomplished by flavoproteins which contain the vitamin riboflavin and the metals Cu or Fe. The unsaturated fatty acid is then hydrated, dehydrogenated (using DPN^+, containing the vitamin nicotinamide); and split by a molecule of CoA, liberating acetyl CoA to enter the Krebs cycle and generate ATP). From this process there remains a fatty acid two carbons shorter than the original, which in turn re-enters the fatty acid cycle to repeat the above sequence. In the cycle, the reducing equivalents obtained from the two dehydrogenation steps may also enter the electron-transport chain to generate high-energy bonds.

Glucose Metabolism

Mitochondrial generation of ATP is not the only source of utilizable energy in the cell, though it accounts for more than 90 percent. Anaerobic glycolysis in the cytoplasm also produces via intramolecular H-atom transfers two ATP molecules per molecule of glucose oxidized, as indicated in Fig. 75-3. The efficiency of energy transformation, the amount of useful energy obtained per unit of fuel burned, is much lower in glycolysis than in mitochondrial oxidative phosphorylation; in other words, glycolysis is a relatively inefficient means of supplying large amounts of energy.

In the utilization of glucose by a cell, it is first phosphorylated to glucose 6-phosphate by the enzyme hexokinase. Adenosinetriphosphate is utilized in the process, yielding ADP and glucose 6-phosphate. Thus a high-energy phosphate bond is transferred to form a low-energy bond with loss of heat, which makes the reaction essentially unidirectional and therefore a potential site of metabolic control. Glucose 6-phosphate occupies a strategic position with reference to several biochemical pathways (see further on).

GLYCOLYSIS. This sequence of reactions is the most important route of glucose 6-phosphate metabolism. The first step is the conversion of glucose 6-phosphate to fructose 6-phosphate by phosphoglucose isomerase. Then another high-energy phosphate is added from ATP by phosphofructokinase to form fructose 1,6-diphosphate. This is another exergonic or unidirectional step, and it has been suggested that this step controls the entire glycolytic pathway. Phosphofructokinase action is opposed by another enzyme, fructose 1,6-diphosphatase, which converts fructose 1,6-diphosphate back to fructose 6-phosphate. This latter enzyme, as expected, is located in tissues which *produce glucose, and therefore is found* in liver; there its activity is increased by any one of a numerous group of metabolic stimuli which accelerate gluconeogenesis, e.g., glucocorticoids. Conversely, fructose 1,6-diphosphatase is essentially lacking in tissues such as muscle, adipose tissue, or brain, where the only route of glucose metabolism is via glycolysis to pyruvate and lactate and then via acetate and the Krebs cycle to CO_2, in the presence of oxygen.

After formation of fructose 1,6-diphosphate, the hexose unit is split into two interconvertible 3-carbon phosphorylated sugars. One of these, glyceraldehyde 3-phosphate, is dehydrogenated and phosphorylated to form DPNH (NADH)[1] and 1,3-diphosphoglyceric acid, which through a series of reactions yields pyruvate and two high-energy phosphate bonds. Thus the overall reaction is:

$$\text{Glucose} + 2 \sim P + 2\,\text{Pi} + 2\,\text{DPN}^+ \rightarrow 2\,\text{pyruvate} \\ + 4 \sim P + 2\,\text{DPNH} + 2\,\text{H}^+$$

If oxygen is lacking and the DPNH cannot be oxidized to DPN^+, its hydrogen atom can be disposed of in the conversion of pyruvate to lactate, and thereby DPN^+ is replenished for further glycolysis. Thus the overall reaction is:

$$\text{Glucose} + 2 \sim P \rightarrow 2\,\text{lactate} + 4 \sim P$$
or
$$\text{Glucose} \rightarrow 2\,\text{lactate} + 2 \sim P \qquad (3)$$

This sequence, termed *anaerobic glycolysis* since it can occur in the absence of oxygen, can provide a small but, in an emergency, significant and necessary amount of energy. *Anaerobic glycolysis is limited, however, by the accumulation of lactic acid which eventually lowers the pH to a degree not compatible with cellular function.*

GLYCOGENESIS. Glucose 6-phosphate can alternatively be converted to glycogen by first being altered to glucose 1-phosphate by phosphoglucomutase. The glucose 1-phosphate is condensed with uridine triphosphate (UTP) to form uridine diphosphoglucose (UDGP) and pyrophosphate, which in turn is hydrolyzed to free inorganic phosphate. Thus two high-energy phosphate bonds are utilized, an exergonic reaction. As expected, the activity of this system is a site of metabolic control, being increased in muscle by insulin, and possibly also in liver. The UDP-glucose is then condensed with one of the many outer chains of an already existing glycogen molecule to form one more glucose unit attached by a 1,4 link. The glycogen chain can be modified by the "branching" enzyme to form another chain. In the opposite direction, glycogen is broken down to glucose 1-phosphate by another enzyme, phosphorylase (Fig. 75-3,A). This also is an exergonic process and essentially unidirectional. Phosphorylase activity is increased by different hormones in different tissues, e.g., epinephrine and glucagon in liver, epinephrine in muscle, norepinephrine and epinephrine in adipose tissue, and probably others. The precise activations of phosphorylase are different in various tissues, i.e., in muscle a condensation of two proteins takes place, in liver a phosphate is joined to the inactive enzyme. In all tissues, cyclic-3',5'-adenosinemonophosphate (Fig. 75-1) appears to be the intermediate effector molecule between the stimulator and the activation of phosphorylase. The end result is glycogenolysis and presentation of extra fuel for glycolysis in whatever tissue is activated. These reactions are discussed in further detail in Chap. 111.

DIRECT OXIDATIVE PATHWAY. In several tissues (adipose, liver, adrenal, mammary) reduced TPN^+ (TPNH or NADPH) is required to provide the hydrogen and electrons for synthesis of lipid. Thus a certain proportion of glucose 6-phosphate and TPN^+ is oxidized by glucose 6-phosphate dehydrogenase to TPNH and 6-phosphogluconic acid, and the last in turn to a compound which loses carbon-1 as CO_2 and produces another TPNH and a pentose phosphate, ribulose 5-phosphate. Through a complicated series of reactions, the pentose phosphates return to the main glycolytic sequence as fructose 6-phosphate or triose phosphate.

GLUCOSE 6-PHOSPHATASE. This enzyme comprises yet another pathway of glucose 6-phosphate metabolism and is located only in those tissues capable of producing glucose: liver and kidney, and also placenta. In the liver, it is the final common pathway for glucose production, and opposes the activity of the glucose-phosphorylating system. The activity of glucose 6-phosphatase in liver is increased in states associated with increased glucose production (diabetes, excess adrenal glucocorticoids) and is decreased in those associated with increased insulin or carbohydrate intake. Again there are two "unidirectional" enzymes at an important site of metabolic control, the production or uptake of glucose by liver. The role of the enzyme in kidney is apparently different and may be related to the process of reabsorption of metabolic intermediates which are converted to glucose 6-phosphate and then released into the bloodstream. It is clearly not related to the renal tubular reabsorption of glucose, since this process does not involve phosphorylation or dephosphorylation.

GLUCURONIC ACID PATHWAY. An alternative route of glucose 6-phosphate metabolism is the oxidation of carbon-6 of glucose, the glucose having been condensed with UTP to form uridinediphosphate glucose, similar to its route to glycogen. The glucuronic acid thus formed may become a moiety in many of the complex carbohydrates which serve as structural units (glycoproteins) or may be used to conjugate and detoxify endogenous and exogenous compounds prior to their elimination from the body. As part of this pathway, carbon-6 of UDPG can be cleaved to form CO_2 and a 5-carbon sugar which, through a series of reactions, enters the glycolytic pathway. One of the intermediates in this sequence, l-xylulose, may accumulate and be excreted in the urine in the benign disease, essential pentosuria, which is due to lack of the enzyme which catalyzes the subsequent step in the sequence (Chap. 95).

Acetate and Pyruvate Metabolism

Just as glucose 6-phosphate occupies a position at the crossroads of many metabolic reactions, so do acetate and its closely related products. Pyruvate, the terminus of the previously mentioned pathways, to be further metabolized, must be decarboxylated in the presence of DPN^+ and coenzyme A (thiamine or vitamin B_1 and lipoic acid are essential cofactors) to form CO_2 and acetyl CoA (see Chap. 81). Free acetate itself is of only minor importance in nonruminants as a metabolic fuel. It is the acetyl CoA, therefore, which can enter the subsequent metabolic routes.

In the process of fatty acid synthesis, the acetyl CoA accepts CO_2 to form malonyl CoA and through a series of reactions involving condensations and reductions [TPNH derived from glucose oxidation via the direct oxidative pathway or via transhydrogenation from DPNH (Fig. 75-3C) is the reducing agent] a 16-carbon, saturated, long-chain fatty acid, palmitic acid, is formed; this can then be extended or unsaturated by other enzyme systems. This sequence takes place primarily in adipose tissue but also in liver and to a lesser extent in other tissues. Another route open to acetyl CoA is the formation of ketone bodies, a reaction which occurs exclusively in liver. There is some question as to whether ketones are formed by direct condensation of two acetyl CoA's or via an intermediate comprised of three acetyl CoA's, namely, β-hydroxy-β-methylglutaryl CoA. A third route for acetyl CoA metabolism, via β-hydroxy-β-methylglutaryl CoA, is in the formation of the steroid nucleus and the various compounds derived from it by further metabolic changes, such as cholesterol, steroid hormones, and bile salts. The fourth and perhaps most important route is the condensation of acetyl CoA with oxaloacetate to form citrate, the first step in the sequence of intramitochondrial reactions involving the Krebs or citric or tricarboxylic acid cycle, as previously described.

Another pathway of pyruvate metabolism is the direct

condensation with CO_2 to form oxaloacetate. This sequence is unique in liver and is catalyzed by an enzyme, pyruvic carboxylase. In fasting, or in diabetes mellitus in which fat breakdown to acetyl CoA occurs at a rapid rate, the high level of acetyl CoA accelerates this reaction. Normally oxaloacetate would accept the acetyl CoA to form citrate for oxidation via the citric acid cycle, but this reaction is apparently blocked under fasting conditions or diabetes, and under these conditions the oxaloacetate is phosphorylated and decarboxylated to form phosphoenolpyruvate by another enzyme unique to liver, phosphoenolpyruvate carboxykinase. By this sequence, pyruvate is converted to phosphoenolpyruvate and then to glucose, a reaction which cannot proceed directly in this direction because of the energy differential.

Hydrogen Shuttles

H atoms (reducing equivalents) can be shunted between different metabolic or structural compartments or pathways which eventually generate ATP. Thus, H atoms can be transferred from the low-efficiency glycolytic-cytoplasmic pathway to the high-efficiency mitochondrial apparatus, increasing the generation of ATP. Any metabolite that is reduced in the cytoplasm to a product which is a substrate for an intramitochondrial oxidation can act as an H carrier. One such system is the α-glycerophosphate-dihydroxyacetone shuttle:

$$\alpha\text{-Glycerophosphate} + DPN^+ \rightleftharpoons$$
$$\text{dihydroxyacetone phosphate} + DPNH + H^+ \quad (4)$$

A soluble cytoplasmic α-glycerophosphate dehydrogenase uses DPN^+ to oxidize α-glycerophosphate (αGP) to dihydroxyacetone phosphate (DHAP) (both produced by the glycolytic cycle) and DPNH. DPNH cannot apparently enter mitochondria to act as a carrier of H equivalents from the cytoplasm, but α-glycerophosphate can (Fig. 75-3B). Then a distinctly different α-glycerophosphate dehydrogenase within mitochondria oxidizes αGP to DHAP, producing intramitochondrial DPNH, which in turn generates mitochondrial ATP. The DHAP then diffuses into cytoplasm to reenter the shuttle cycle. In rats, thyroid hormone rapidly produces a marked increase in the activity of only the mitochondrial dehydrogenase, making possible increased H-shuttle activity, which in turn increases metabolic ATP generation. A similar H shuttle exists between the fatty acid synthetic cycle and mitochondria, consisting of two β-hydroxybutyric acid dehydrogenases, DPN^+, β-hydroxybutyric acid, and acetoacetate.

A different sort of H shuttle can transfer H atoms between the two coenzymes for dehydrogenation, DPN^+ and TPN^+ (Fig. 75-3C). This is of importance in that H atoms carried into the mitochondrial electron-transport system by DPNH generate ATP; H atoms carried into extramitochondrial oxidizing systems by TPNH generate no high-energy phosphate bonds but are available for the reductive steps of fatty acid and other syntheses.

These transhydrogenations between DPN^+ and TPN^+ are thus a switching point where reducing equivalents generate useful energy, are used in syntheses directly, or are dispelled as heat. A specific transhydrogenase enzyme is found in mitochondrial membranes, and there are probably many additional *de facto* transhydrogenases. Any enzyme that has a coenzyme specificity broad enough so that it can react with both DPN^+ and TPN^+, e.g., glutamic dehydrogenase in mitochondria or steroid dehydrogenase in microsomes, can act as a molecular H shuttle.

Uses of ATP

A detailed listing of specific reactions into which ATP enters may be found in standard biochemical texts. A selected few are of illustrative interest. Studies indicate that the mitochondrion, a self-sufficient apparatus in many ways, transforms energy, and also has a capacity to maintain high internal electrolyte concentrations when it is functioning in its energy-producing role. Mitochondria can accumulate K^+, Ca^{++}, Mg^{++}, Mn^{++}, and phosphate ions while oxidizing and phosphorylating, but not when phosphorylation is uncoupled. The purpose of the accumulation is as yet obscure, for Ca^{++} ions, for instance, are themselves uncoupling agents. However, demonstrations that parathyroid hormone is capable of affecting phosphate and Ca^{++} exchanges in mitochondria in vitro are of obvious importance in understanding the mechanism of action of the hormone. The contribution of the osmotic work done by mitochondria toward that of the whole cell is not yet clear.

A major role of ATP in the body is to serve as the ultimate energy source for muscle contraction. The detail of the molecular events concerned with this physical process is still a matter for investigation, but ATP is necessary for the relaxation phenomenon, whereby the contracted actomyosin fibrils resume their more elongated form, primed for the next contraction. Indeed, so definite is the association between the use of ATP and muscle contraction that the actomyosin molecule is called an "ATPase." The dependence of muscle contraction on ATP is reflected in the demands of the myocardium, for instance, for a continued supply of utilizable energy derived from oxidation. The myocardium is supplied with large intricate mitochondria, and interference with the supply of oxygen by a decrease in blood flow produces *noncontracting* myocardial areas with differences in electric potential (see Chap. 260). Such changes probably increase cellular permeability so that enzymes (e.g., lactic dehydrogenase and the transaminases from cytoplasm, and intramitochondrial enzymes such as malic dehydrogenase) leak into the circulation to provide biochemical diagnostic criteria of impaired myocardial function. Biochemical lesions of the myocardium that interfere with the generation of ATP occur in anemia, thyrotoxicosis, and beriberi, and result in a myocardial contractile defect which is not susceptible to the beneficial action of digitalis, ordinarily so effective when the contractile mechanism itself operates at a disadvantage but has an adequate energy supply. Defects in energy transformation in *skeletal* muscle appear to be present in at least two diseases, as demonstrated by functional and structural changes in muscle mitochondria in patients with thyrotoxicosis, and in a reported case of hypermetabolism in a euthyroid woman.

Another significant use of ATP is the generation of heat to maintain body temperature. In the synthesis of ATP by oxidative phosphorylation, for example, only 60 percent of the energy liberated from oxidation of its substrates is transformed by the mitochondrion to phosphate bond energy. An appreciable portion of the liberated energy is evolved as heat, which assists in maintaining body temperature. When the external environment increases the need for heat production, the body responds with an increased rate of oxygen consumption. Fat depots may function actively in controlling body temperature, not only as an insulator but possibly by increased heat production. The free fatty acids liberated under hormonal control from adipose tissue are reesterified and reincorporated through a burst of O_2 consumption and ATP utilization, and heat is generated concomitantly. The major toxic symptom of agents that uncouple oxidative phosphorylation is hyperthermia, seen with salicylates and dinitrophenol, and in thyroid crisis.

The syntheses of the polymeric compounds that store energy in the body require ATP, e.g., the condensation of glucose 1-phosphate to form glycogen, of acetyl CoA to form fatty acids, of soluble RNA–amino acid complexes to form polypeptides and proteins, and of nucleosides to form nucleotides.

ENERGY TRANSFORMATION

To survive, a species must possess mechanisms whereby it can deposit and store fuel during periods of availability, and be able to mobilize this fuel at times of increased need, in addition to storing and mobilizing fuel for the necessary chemical reactions required to maintain the integrity of its structure.

The human body contains numerous organic compounds with energy potential: lipids, carbohydrates, proteins, and nucleic acids. The lipids are by far the most quantitatively important form of storage of fuel, in addition to providing other functions such as insulation of the body as a whole or as essential components in the structure of cell walls, myelin, and other membranes. Carbohydrates serve as a lesser form of fuel storage except for the nervous system. Protein serves as the structural basis for all enzymes, as well as for contracting elements such as muscle or supporting structures such as collagen, and as a fuel, as a precursor for carbohydrate in the process of gluconeogenesis. Nucleic acids form fundamental components in the hereditary and synthetic mechanisms and, fortunately, are not available as fuels. The body can be divided into four main metabolic compartments, adipose tissue, nervous tissue, muscle, and liver.

Adipose Tissue

Adipose tissue is composed of between 60 and 90 percent triglyceride and thus contains 6 to 8 kcal per Gm tissue. A normal 70-kg male may have 10 kg adipose tissue and thereby a potential fuel reserve of approximately 75,000 kcal, which theoretically could support life for well over 2 months. In obesity, 100 kg of adipose tissue may be present—an entire year's supply!

Adipose tissue metabolism (Fig. 75-4) is controlled by many factors, which may be grouped into two general classes, anabolic and catabolic. A rise in blood glucose level following ingestion of carbohydrate stimulates insulin production; insulin directly increases glucose uptake into adipose tissue, where, in the process of lipogenesis, it is metabolized via acetate into fatty acids, which are then esterified with glycerol to form triglycerides. Thus the individual has converted a less efficient fuel on a weight basis (carbohydrate) to a more efficient form of energy storage (lipid). Some of the ingested glucose may be converted to glycogen in liver, muscle, and adipose tissue. These carbohydrate stores serve two ancillary purposes: (1) as a temporary storage site during ingestion of large amounts of carbohydrate until the lipogenetic process can store the energy as fat; (2) as an emergency store of quickly available glucose for anaerobic glycolysis during periods of stress. The increased economy of storage of energy as lipid far surpasses that as carbohydrate, since triglyceride is deposited in an extraaqueous phase, whereas glycogen is stored with water and electrolytes; 1 Gm glycogen-containing tissue yields only 1 to 1½ kcal and it is therefore one-fourth to one-sixth as efficient for storage of energy as an equivalent unit of lipid-containing tissue.

Insulin appears to exert other effects on adipose tissue. Following a fatty meal, triglycerides enter the bloodstream as particulate aggregates—chylomicrons—via the thoracic duct. They may then enter the liver and be chemically remodified and released into the circulation or they may be directly incorporated into adipose tissue where they are hydrolyzed into free fatty acids and reesterified into triglyceride. These many rearrangements of the originally ingested fat may be the animal's mechanism to ensure that the fat which it stores in its adipose tissue contains the correct number and types of fatty acids. Insulin in the fed individual apparently plays an important role in the uptake of circulating triglycerides into adipose tissue, in addition to its role in promoting lipogenesis from glucose.

Fuel stored as adipose tissue triglyceride is released in only one form, free fatty acids. Adipose tissue free fatty acid concentration is in equilibrium with the fatty acid bound to albumin in the circulation; thus, a rise in adipose tissue free fatty acids induces a release of these into the circulation. The level of free acids in adipose tissue is controlled by several factors. Insulin decreases this level by providing increased glucose uptake, which supplies increased glycerol acceptor for esterification of fatty acids in the cell. Insulin also inhibits the breakdown of triglyceride into free fatty acid.

ADIPOSE TISSUE

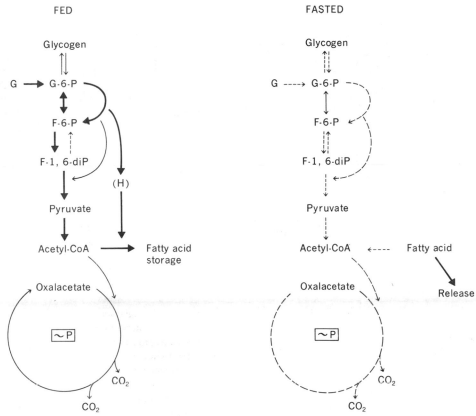

Fig. 75-4. Comparison of flow of substrate across metabolic pathways in adipose tissue in the fed and fasted state. In the former, glucose (G) is metabolized to acetyl CoA, which is then resynthesized to fat and stored. During fasting, glucose metabolism is limited and fatty acids are released for fuel for the remainder of the body.

Conversely, lack of insulin, as in fasting, increases adipose tissue free fatty acid by a reversal of these processes and thereby augments fatty acid release. Among other substances which increase fatty acid production by adipose tissue are norepinephrine, epinephrine, and growth, thyroid, and adrenal hormones. The action of epinephrine on free fatty acid mobilization depends on the thyroid status, being increased in hyperthyroidism and decreased or absent in hypothyroidism.

Nervous Tissue

Nervous tissues require glucose as fuel at all times (Fig. 75-5). This glucose utilization is independent of insulin, or of glucose concentration (as long as it is adequate), or of the state of nervous activity. Only in severe metabolic derangements producing coma is there a significant decrease in the use of glucose (except for a gradual slight decrease with age).

During prolonged starvation, however, and probably in individuals who have been on a very high fat (ketogenic) diet, the brain may decrease its glucose utilization without loss of function because of its capacity to

adapt to utilization of acetoacetate and β-hydroxybutyrate.

In nervous tissue glucose is totally glycolyzed and then oxidized to CO_2 by the tricarboxylic acid cycle. Thus glucose and oxygen must always be available; if their supply is interrupted, brain function ceases immediately.

Muscle

Muscle tissue is versatile in that it can utilize several different fuels to support activity (Fig. 75-5). Glucose is readily removed by muscle from the circulating fluids under the stimulus of insulin, although increased muscular activity or anoxia can also increase glucose uptake. The glucose in muscle is readily glycolyzed to lactic acid and, if there is adequate oxygen, to CO_2 and water. The glucose may also be stored to be used as emergency fuel for glycolysis when oxygen is unavailable or relatively inadequate.

Muscle mitochondria also readily utilize fat as fuel. The fat can come from several sources, from circulating particulate fat (triglyceride) derived from the diet or

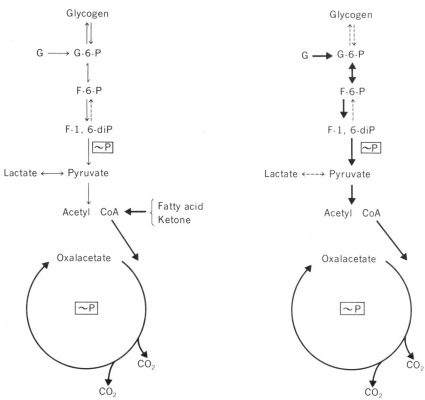

Fig. 75-5. Muscle tissue utilizes predominantly fatty acid or ketone as a source of fuel, but it is also able to derive limited amounts of energy ($\sim$P) from the conversion of glucose to lactate (anaerobic glycolysis). Nervous tissue is able to utilize only glucose as its metabolic fuel, and requires a constant supply of oxygen for total combustion of the glucose to CO_2 in order to derive energy for adequate function.

secondarily from the liver, from free fatty acids circulating in the blood, having been released from adipose tissue, or from a third source, fat stored directly in the muscle itself. Whatever the origin, the fatty acid is oxidized completely to CO_2 and water, and it is fat which serves as the major contributor of energy to muscle metabolism.

A third type of fuel for muscle is derived from the liver as a product of the incomplete combustion of fatty acids, namely, acetoacetic and β-hydroxybutyric acids, which, with acetone, form the *ketone bodies*. These two acids are also completely metabolized to CO_2 and water in muscle and in certain circumstances can provide a major share of muscle fuel.

By mechanisms not yet clarified, muscle selectively metabolizes ketone bodies, then fatty acids, and, as a last resort, glucose. If ketones are unavailable and free fatty acid concentration is low, as after carbohydrate or insulin administration, muscle will then readily metabolize glucose. Conversely, if ketone or fatty acid concentrations are high, glucose metabolism is minimized, even in the presence of insulin and the glucose which is taken into the tissue is converted to and stored as glycogen.

One major role of muscle is to serve as a storehouse

for amino acids. It is now accepted that a primary site of insulin action is to stimulate the incorporation of circulating amino acids into muscle protein. This action is biochemically distinct from the effect on glucose. If insulin is lacking, this process is decreased or even reversed, and amino acids are mobilized. Adrenocortical hormones oppose the insulin effect. In fasting, amino acids are mobilized from muscle, and during feeding, when insulin increases, amino acids are incorporated into muscle protein. Removal of both insulin and adrenal hormones achieves a new balance, but one without flexibility in either direction.

Liver

Of the four groups of tissues playing a major role in body fuel economy, liver (Fig. 75-6) serves as the director of traffic and, as such, is more complicated than adipose, nervous, and muscle tissues. During fasting, it must provide glucose for those tissues requiring glucose for survival (mainly the brain), and during times of carbohydrate ingestion, it stops producing glucose and, instead, removes glucose and stores it as glycogen, transiently if the glycogen reserve is already adequate, or more permanently if the glycogen reserve has been previously depleted by prolonged fasting or other stress.

Unlike peripheral cells, the liver cell is freely permeable to glucose, and the concentration of glucose in the blood is approximated by the concentration in the liver cell, being slightly greater if glucose is being produced by the liver and slightly less if glucose is being removed. The net flow of glucose inside the liver cell into and out of the metabolically activated pool of glucose, glucose 6-phosphate, is a function of two enzymes unique to liver, glucokinase and glucose 6-phosphatase. The activity of the former of these is increased by insulin or carbohydrate feeding, and that of the latter by fasting, insulin insufficiency, or adrenal steroids. Thus the activities of these two opposing systems direct the net flow of glucose into and out of the liver, and are a control over the concentration of glucose in the circulating fluids.

Liver is also unique in possessing other enzymes which are located at metabolic control sites in the sequence of reactions between amino acids and glucose and which increase in activity during times of increased gluconeogenesis, as associated with fasting, diabetes, or adrenal steroid administration, and are decreased by carbohydrate feeding or insulin administration.

During fasting, liver must provide glucose for fuel for those tissues requiring glucose, primarily brain, but also spinal cord, peripheral nerve, leukocytes, erythrocytes, renal medulla, and probably others. This it does by synthesizing new glucose (gluconeogenesis) from glycogenic amino acids released into the circulation from muscle, and, to a lesser extent, from lactate or pyruvate returning to the liver from peripheral tissues, as well as from glycerol arising from lipolysis in adipose tissue. Normally liver contains only 70 to 80 Gm glycogen, less than one-half a day's supply of carbohydrate, should gluconeogenesis not be stimulated to provide the glucose needed by the organism. The liver in a fasting normal man produces approximately 180 Gm glucose daily, of which approximately 144 Gm is oxidized to CO_2 and water and 36 Gm is returned as lactate and pyruvate. To accomplish this, about 75 Gm muscle protein is metabolized to amino acids, which are removed by the liver as precursors for the bulk of the glucose which has to be synthesized. Although net conversion of fat into carbohydrate has not been shown in mammalian tissues, 128 Gm glucose (glycerol from adipose tissue mobilization of triglyceride provides about 16 Gm) cannot be synthesized from 75 Gm protein; many explanations for this process have been offered, such as utilization of fat or ketones or utilization of a small amount of the stored glycogen for a brief period of time.

The liver in the normal fed individual uses as its source of fuel mainly amino acid. During fasting, the amino acid which is presented to the liver is diverted, for

Fig. 75-6. As described in the text, the liver in the fed animal stores glucose as glycogen and derives its own energy from amino acid metabolism. During fasting, its energy ($\sim$P) is derived from the conversion of fatty acids to ketone, and amino acids are diverted into glucose synthesis.

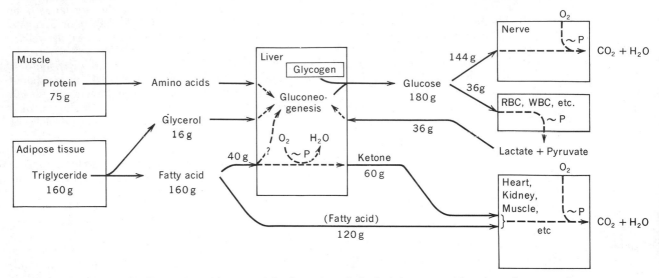

ORIGIN OF FUEL   FUEL CONSUMPTION

Fig. 75-7. Quantitative estimation of the flow of metabolic fuels by a normal fasted man for a period of 24 hr, utilizing 1800 kcal.

FED MAN

FUEL INTAKE   FUEL DISPOSITION

Fig. 75-8. Quantitative estimation of the flow of metabolic fuel of a man eating a theoretic meal containing 200 Gm carbohydrate (100 Gm as glucose, 20 Gm galactose, and 80 Gm fructose), 75 Gm protein, and 75 Gm fat and disposing of the meal in peripheral depots in 4 hr.

economical reasons, into glucose synthesis, and the liver now uses for its own energy needs the partial oxidation of fatty acids to ketone bodies, from which one-third of the total potential energy of the fatty acid is derived. Thus the process of gluconeogenesis, amino acid metabolism (and therefore urea production), and the production of ketone bodies are intimately related.

When the animal is fed, liver metabolism is grossly altered through a number of complicated mechanisms. Gluconeogenesis ceases, those amino acids which enter the liver are metabolized, providing the needed energy for the liver's own metabolic processes, and ketone production ceases. The level of free fatty acids in the circulation falls, since their release from adipose tissue is inhibited. The liver, however, continues to remove about one-fourth of the total turnover of free fatty acids, but now, since its own energy is adequately provided by amino acid oxidation via its citric acid cycle, esterifies these free fatty acids and returns them to the periphery instead of converting them to ketone bodies. In other words, during fasting, amino acid carbon is diverted into gluconeogenesis, the liver citric acid cycle is inoperative, and the liver's energy is derived from ketogenesis. During feeding, the citric acid cycle predominates, amino acids are deaminated, and their products are oxidized via the cycle, and ketone production essentially ceases.

Total Organism

Figures 75-7 and 75-8 summarize the two metabolic phases of fasting and feeding in a normal man at rest. The basal metabolic expenditure, that amount of fuel as determined by the oxygen consumed to burn it, is a function of body surface, age, and sex and is remarkably constant in a single person and, more important, between persons of similar age, size, and sex. The basal metabolic rate (BMR) is expressed as a percentage variation of the mean oxygen consumption obtained from a normal population of similar sex and surface area, or substituting for surface area, height and weight, from which surface area is derived. The appetite mechanism in a normal individual appears to be exquisitely set so as to maintain the body at constant weight and to be able to compensate for the increased fuel consumption during muscular work. Thus the weight normally varies little from year to year. For example, if an additional 100 kcal, i.e., one slice of bread, were to be stored daily as adipose tissue, at the end of the year there would have been over a 10-lb weight gain. The sensitivity of the appetite mechanism and, obviously, of the capacity to expend the calories beyond those required to maintain basal metabolism, and the equality between these two processes in the normal individual are overtly disturbed

SEVERE DIABETES

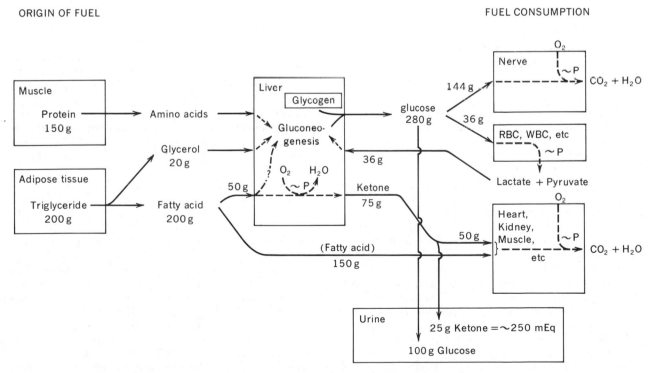

Fig. 75-9. Quantitative estimation of the flow of metabolic fuel for a period of 24 hr in a subject with diabetes mellitus; the subject was losing 25 Gm ketone and 100 Gm glucose in the urine. This glucose is in addition to that amount lost in the urine if the subject were eating and spilling the ingested carbohydrate. Thus a net negative carbohydrate balance of this degree is the causative factor which necessitates increased gluconeogenesis and the resultant ketosis. Net energy loss is 2400 kcal.

in states of abnormal energy storage such as anorexia nervosa, or its antithesis, obesity (discussed further in Chaps. 42 and 48).

Diabetes Mellitus

The metabolic changes of the normal fasted man may be extrapolated into those of the subject with diabetes, who loses glucose in the urine because of hyperglycemia (Fig. 75-9). Thus, muscle protein is mobilized at a faster rate to supply precursors for the accelerated gluconeogenesis. Fatty acids are released more rapidly from adipose tissue, and concomitantly ketones are produced more rapidly by the liver, and these also are spilled in the urine; being relatively strong acids, their loss is associated with sodium and potassium loss, thereby producing a metabolic acidosis. The entire sequence progresses (as described in Chap. 94) until reversed by the administration of insulin.

REFERENCES

Anfinsen, C.: "The Molecular Basis of Evolution," New York, John Wiley & Sons, Inc., 1959.

Lehninger, A. L.: "The Mitochondrion," New York, W. A. Benjamin, Inc., 1964.

Stanbury, J. B., J. B. Wyngaarden, and D. C. Fredrickson: "The Metabolic Basis of Inherited Disease," 2d ed., McGraw-Hill Book Company, New York, 1966.

76 ESSENTIAL NUTRIENTS: REQUIREMENTS
George V. Mann

Only 40 of the thousands of substances involved in human metabolism are essential—meaning that these materials must be supplied in the diet. All the remaining compounds can be derived through the metabolic processes of the body. The requirement for the essential nutrients is highly specific. It varies among species and among human individuals, and it is influenced by differing physiologic circumstances, such as growth and periods of high activity or relative physiologic quiescence. These variations make definitions of nutritional requirements only approximations.

The nutritional requirements of man have been identified during the past 70 years by use of an experimental technique employing "purified diets." Experimental animals or human beings were fed chemically defined diets; when growth failure or other signs of debility appeared, food concentrates or synthetic materials were tested for the essential nutrient responsible. It has been possible by this method to produce in animals disorders which mimic human disease and to isolate the essential organic factors (vitamins). The vitamins were first named alphabetically and were then, when they were identified, given chemical names. Systematic studies with purified diets

were begun about 1900 by F. G. Hopkins and E. V. McCollum and were extended by H. C. Sherman, H. Steenbock, the Mellanbys, C. Elvejhem, and many others. This immensely useful work has been reviewed by McCollum, a pioneer in the field who died in 1967.

The major nutrients, fat, protein, and carbohydrate, were first defined, and then certain of the bulkier minerals which are indispensable for growth and health were identified. The vitamins, the essential amino acids, and the essential trace elements were recognized later. Estimates of daily requirements have been summarized and published since 1943 by the Food and Nutrition Board of the National Research Council of the United States. These recommendations are intended to serve as standards of reference rather than final judgments. They are sometimes misinterpreted because of failure to note that the *Recommended Dietary Allowance* (RDA) includes a generous margin of safety above the current estimates of minimal daily requirements. It does not follow that all persons taking less than the RDA are malnourished. The RDA attempts to set a goal which will ensure good nutrition in healthy individuals under current living conditions in the United States.

Other official agencies have published similar recommendations for nutrient intake which are more applicable to their particular needs or national situations. The differences among these recommendations do not imply that various racial and ethnic groups have different nutritional requirements. While there are differences of requirement due to variations in body size, physical activity, and environmental conditions, all human beings of whatever race or cultural group have similar, average nutritional requirements.

The tabulations in the RDA represent an average of the best available information concerning requirements. For most nutrients the procedure has been to add to the observed mean twice the standard deviation of the distribution of minimal requirement for the subject measured. Depending upon how representative the subjects were and how reliable the measurements, the RDA should be applicable for at least 95 percent of a similar population. The recommendations do tend to obscure individual differences in requirement, and they also tend to be generous.

Another widely used reference table has been published, with periodic revisions, since 1941 by the U.S. Food and Drug Administration. This is called the *Minimum Daily Requirement* (MDR). It was intended for use in the regulation of food products in commerce. The tabulations of the MDR are important for physicians and patients because they are often used in advertising and on the labels of food products, and since they are lower than the RDA, they sometimes tend to inflate the nutritional value of a product. Patients more often have been informed about the MDR than the RDA.

The 40 essential elements and compounds necessary in the human diet are listed in Table 76-2. The essentiality of a nutrient is determined by species, by individual constitution, and by the metabolic circumstances.

Ascorbic acid is necessary for primates and a few ro-

Table 76-1. RECOMMENDED DAILY DIETARY ALLOWANCES, FOOD AND NUTRITION BOARD,
NATIONAL ACADEMY OF SCIENCES, NATIONAL RESEARCH COUNCIL

	Age,[1] years	Weight kg	Height cm	Kcal[2]	Protein, Gm	Fat soluble vitamins			Water soluble vitamins							Minerals				
						A[5] IU	D, IU	E, IU	Ascorbic acid, mg	Folic acid, mg	Nicotinic acid,[3] mg.Eq.	Riboflavin, mg	Thiamine, mg	Vitamin B6, mg	Vitamin B12, μgm	Ca, Gm	P, Gm	I2, μg	Fe, mg	Mg, mg
Infants[4].......	0–1	4–9	55–72	kg × 120	kg × 2	1500	400	5	35	0.05	6	0.4	0.3	0.3	1.5	0.6	0.5	40	10	100
Children......	1–10	12–28	81–131	1100–2200	25–40	2500	400	10	40	0.2	10	1.0	0.7	1.0	4	0.8	0.8	80	10	200
Adolescent																				
Male.......	10–18	35–59	140–170	2500–3000	45–60	5000	400	20	50	0.4	18	1.4	1.2	1.8	5	1.4	1.4	135	18	350
Female.....	10–18	35–54	142–160	2250–2300	50–55	5000	400	20	50	0.4	15	1.4	0.9	1.8	5	1.3	1.3	115	18	350
Adult[6]																				
Male.......	18 up	67–70	175 up	2800	60 up	5000	....	30	60	0.4	17	1.7	1.0	2.0	5	0.8	0.8	130	10	350
Female.....	18 up	58 up	163 up	2000	55 up	5000	....	25	55	0.4	12	1.7	0.8	2.0	5	0.8	0.8	100	18	300
Pregnant......	......	......	......	+200	65	6000	400	30	60	0.8	15	1.8	1.0	2.5	8	+0.4	+0.4	125	18	450
Lactating.....	......	......	......	+1000	75	8000	400	30	60	0.5	20	2.0	1.2	2.5	6	+0.5	+0.5	150	18	450

[1] The age ranges are more abridged here than in the original table.

[2] Calorie adjustment must be made for size and expenditure.

[3] Nicotinic acid equivalents include preformed nicotinic acid and tryptophane, 60 mg.Eq. to 1 mg nicotinic acid.

[4] Allowances for calcium, thiamine, riboflavin, and nicotinic acid are proportional to calorie requirement.

[5] Assuming one-fifth from preformed vitamin A and four-fifth from beta-carotene.

[6] These allowances will include a range of individual requirements for individuals living in the United States under usual environmental conditions. They can be achieved with a variety of common foods which will also supply other nutrients for which human requirements are uncertain.

SOURCE: This table is adapted from the more detailed table of the "Recommended Dietary Allowances" of the National Research Council, Food and Nutrition Board, 7th ed. Publication 1694 Price $1, NAS Printing and Publications Office, 2101 Constitution Ave. N.W., Washington, D.C. 20418.

dents and birds because they lack the enzyme necessary for one step in the formation of ascorbic acid from glucose. The essential amino acids illustrate the relativity of the term *essential*. Arginine and histidine are essential for growing children but not for human adults. Glycine and L-cystine are essential for chickens during periods of feather growth but not at other times.

DIET MIXTURES. The energy for growth, metabolism, and physical activity is supplied by the major foodstuffs, fat, carbohydrate, and protein. In the United States ap-

Table 76-2. ESSENTIAL NUTRIENTS FOR
HUMAN BEINGS

Elements	Major	Ca, P, Na, Cl, K, Mg
	Minor	Fe, I, Mn, Mb, Co, Zn, Cu
	Uncertain	Se, Cr, Fl
Vitamins	Water soluble	Thiamine, riboflavin, pyridoxine, niacin, folacin, pantothenic acid, cobalamine, biotin, ascorbic acid
	Fat soluble	Vitamin A-carotene, D, E, K essential fatty acids (linoleic, arachidonic)
Nitrogenous	Essential amino acids	Lysine, threonine, leucine, isoleucine, methionine, tryptophane, valine, phenylalanine (for children, arginine and histidine)
	Nonessential nitrogen	

Notes—Carbon and oxygen are essential. Choline is not considered a vitamin. When optimal amounts of cobalamine, serine, and methionine are available, choline is synthesized from them.

proximately 15 percent of the calories of this fuel mixture is derived from protein, 40 percent from fat, and 45 percent from carbohydrate. These proportions are strongly influenced by cultural and socioeconomic conditions. The proportion of fat and protein in the diet mixture has tended to increase since 1900 in the United States as the proportion of carbohydrates, especially the complex polysaccharides from foods such as potatoes and cereal flours, has decreased.

The human organism has an astonishing versatility in adapting to different food mixtures. Thus, the hunters and pastoralists of the world exist in good nutritional health on meat or milk diets which contain less than 50 Gm carbohydrate daily, whereas agriculturists and vegetarians maintain good health on diets with only 30 to 40 Gm protein and 25 Gm or less fat daily. It is important to recognize that dietary adequacy can be obtained with widely different fuel mixtures (Fig. 76-1).

CALORIES. The recommended dietary allowances include energy allotments according to age, size, sex, and activity. These recommendations are more useful for economic planners than for physicians because of the wide variation of individual calorie requirement. It has been useful to define a reference man who is twenty-two years old and weighs 70 kg and a reference woman age twenty-two and weighing 58 kg. Resting metabolism is related to size as body weight in $kg^{0.72}$. This energy requirement declines with age at the rate of about 2 percent per decade after age twenty. Energy costs are also increased by deviations from ambient temperature below 14°C and above 30°C.

Pregnancy requires the accumulation of about 55,000 Cal, an average of 200 Cal per day. The production of 850 ml milk per day requires about 1000 Cal. The re-

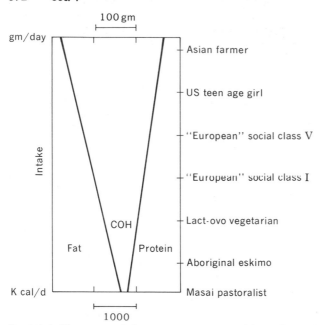

Fig. 76-1. The range of dietary mixtures compatible with good nutrition encountered in various groups of individuals. Social classes I to V are those designated by the Registrar General of the United Kingdom in accordance with socioeconomic status. Class I refers to professional persons, and Class V to unskilled laborers.

maining energy cost for adult persons is attributable to physical activity, and this is almost always the critical determinant of the amount of adipose tissue. The preoccupation with appetite as the cause and with restriction of food in the treatment of obesity to the neglect of expenditure rates has been a major error of nutritional science (See Chap. 48). The cost of maximal physical activity for man can be increased by exertion to twenty times the resting level of 65 Cal per hr. Cultural attitudes and technical developments have largely abolished such high and protracted levels of energy expenditure in the Western world, and the consequences are increasing obesity and health problems of many kinds.

The energy cost of fever is discussed in Chap. 16.

CARBOHYDRATE. With the exception of ascorbic acid there are no particular carbohydrates known to be essential in the human diet. Despite statements to the contrary, there are no persuasive reasons to believe that refined carbohydrates in the diet are damaging or predispose to disease. There is evidence that the ability of some individuals to metabolize lactose is progressively impaired with age, probably through a loss of intestinal lactase. The increasing evidence of intolerance to milk in older persons is explained on this basis. The amount of carbohydrate in the diet has a distinct but transitory influence on the plasma level of triglycerides.

FAT. The dietary fat furnishes 9 Cal per Gm, while protein and carbohydrate supply only 4 Cal per Gm. Fats add palatability to food. The fat content of the diet in the United States has steadily increased over the last 50 years, more in the content of polyunsaturated vegetable

fatty acids than in saturated animal fat. It has not been established that the kind of dietary fat is a factor in the development of disease, although it is widely assumed, on the basis of circumstantial evidence, that saturated animal fat contributes to hypercholesteremia and atherosclerosis (see Chap. 275).

Two unsaturated fatty acids, linoleic and arachidonic, have been shown to be essential nutrients for experimental animals and for children, but essential fatty acid deficiency is unknown in human adults. Diets low in fat have an additional significance because dietary fat is the vehicle for absorption of other fat-soluble nutrients, especially vitamin A and carotenes. Fatty acids with 8 to 12 carbons are absorbed directly into the portal system. Mixtures of triglyceride made with these "medium chain" fatty acids are useful because they are better absorbed than the long-chain fatty acids more prevalent in natural foodstuffs. They are useful in the management of intestinal malabsorption (Chap. 316).

PROTEIN. Protein is a dietary essential because of its component amino acids. Food proteins contain various combinations of the 20 natural amino acids, of which 10 have been shown to be essential for human beings. Arginine and histidine are essential only for growing children.

The amino acids recovered from the hydrolysis of dietary protein are either used for the synthesis of body protein or they are catabolized for energy. The energy requirements of the body take priority so that catabolism can supersede anabolism, thus accounting for the interdependence of amino acid requirement and energy supply. As described in Chap. 79, there is a spectrum of protein-calorie malnutrition ranging from protein deficiency with sufficient calories to a dietary energy deficiency which is not relieved even by high quality protein in the diet.

Genetic determinants govern the formation of proteins. The body protein can only be formed or replaced with the amino acid mixture appropriate for the protein being synthesized, and all the constituent amino acids must be present simultaneously. Lacking one or more of the amino acids, the body cannot make proteins, since it cannot make incomplete ones, and it has a limited ability to conserve an incomplete mixture until the missing amino acids can be obtained. The 10 to 12 nonessential amino acids are part of this mixture and differ in the capability of the body to synthesize them from simpler available substrates. The actual essential chemical substances are not the amino acids themselves but the alpha-keto acids which are readily aminated to furnish amino acids. This fact is important in the search for a nutritionally adequate dietary mixture which will minimize the urinary nitrogen in patients with uremia. Thus, in addition to the nutritional requirement for each of the essential amino acids there is a need for nitrogen which can be used for aminating the nonessential alpha-keto acids as they are synthesized.

Deficiencies of essential amino acids in human beings result in no specific signs or symptoms. The requirements for the essential amino acids have been established by measurement of nitrogen balance. Balance is a statement of the net economy of a substance, positive during retention, negative during loss. The major nitrogen loss from the body is in the urine, and this amount is highly dependent upon protein intake. Urea nitrogen tends to predominate in the urine with high protein diets and become negligible on protein-free diets. The fecal nitrogen is relatively constant, averaging about 1 Gm per day in adults. With sweat and desquamation a small loss of nitrogen occurs through the skin.

The *nutritional quality of a dietary protein* can be determined in several ways. The most useful experimental method has been the measurement of *biological value*, which is the percent nitrogen absorbed from a given protein which is retained in the body. For identifying the essential amino acids and measuring the minimum daily requirement of each in man, determination of the minimal protein level necessary to maintain nitrogen balance has been more useful. The measurements must be precise, the observational periods long, and the environmental conditions carefully controlled. These technical requirements make the method tedious and costly, and it has not been applied to large numbers of subjects. A third method for evaluating nitrogen requirement is to sum up nitrogen losses through the urine, the feces, and the skin while the test subject is fed a protein-free diet. When allowances are made for growth, the requirement is the sum of all these channels. Because the nitrogen content of protein is about 16 percent, the sum of the excreted nitrogen × 6.25 (100/16) equals the daily protein requirement in grams.

If minimal total body nitrogen loss in adults and children is 3.2 mg per basal Cal energy exchange, then the daily maintenance requirement is 20 mg (3.2 × 6.25) of protein per basal Cal. Assuming the basal energy requirement for the reference man is 1750 Cal, then (1750 × 20)/1000 gives a minimal requirement of 35 Gm of an ideal protein daily. However, because the coefficient of variation among individuals for protein required per basal Cal is about 15 percent, twice this, or 30 percent of 35 Gm, is added, giving a daily requirement of the ideal protein of 45 Gm. This is the generous margin of the estimate. On the average, dietary proteins are only about 70 percent utilized because of limitations of absorption and retention. Consequently 45 × 100/70 equals 65 Gm daily as the requirement for ordinary protein. This amounts to 0.93 Gm protein per kg of body weight for the reference man and is the basis for the commonly used estimate of requirement (1 Gm protein per kg body weight per day). Growing children and pregnant or lactating women are given additional allowances for growth and secretion of protein.

The quality of dietary protein is critically important. Proteins which are low in one or more of the essential amino acids must be taken in large amounts in order to furnish the amino acid mixture necessary for synthesis of body protein. This relationship has additional nutritional significance. Two or more proteins, each deficient in different essential amino acids, can complement one another when eaten together. Between them they may furnish a high-grade protein. This is one reason for advising people to eat a variety of foods to ensure a sound diet. It is also the basis for the search for indigenous food proteins in areas of the world where protein malnutrition is prevalent in order to find a combination of native proteins which will yield an adequate mixture of high biological value. This usually is a more economical and feasible solution than importing a complete protein or introducing entirely new foods.

Generally, the available amino acid pattern of plant proteins is less like that of human tissues than proteins from animal sources. Whole egg protein has a high biologic value and is often used as a reference standard. However, since animal proteins require that time, labor, plant proteins, and other foodstuffs be used to feed livestock for their production, a long-term goal has been to find ways in agriculture, food technology, and cookery to make mixtures of complementary plant proteins which will be as nutritious as the animal proteins which approximate the composition of human proteins.

It is possible in animals to produce imbalances of amino acid intake which lead to growth failure, but this has not been shown to be important in man. There is no known dietary requirement for any whole protein or polypeptide. There is probably some upper limit of dietary nitrogen intake, although this must be very high. Some pastoralists are well nourished on a diet of milk and meat which entails a daily protein intake of 300 Gm and an equal amount of fat.

ESSENTIAL ELEMENTS. In addition to the elements which are furnished as components of the major foodstuffs (O, H, N, S, C), there are 16 others which are known or suspected to be essential. These are shown in Table 76-2.

CALCIUM AND PHOSPHORUS. Calcium and phosphorus are particularly important during growth. They are especially abundant in bone and are also essential ionic components of soft tissues. There is accumulating evidence that the mass of bone mineral accumulated in young adult life is steadily depleted thereafter and that the appearance of subsequent disorders involving demineralization may be a function of this starting mass.

Calcium is not absorbed efficiently from the intestine. Vitamin D is required for this process. Circumstances which produce malabsorption as well as dietary phytates, oxalates, and excessive phosphate may compromise absorption of calcium. The obligatory loss of calcium in the urine of an adult is about 175 mg per day, while the fecal loss of endogenous calcium is 125 mg daily. An additional 10 to 20 mg is lost each day through the skin, making the total loss about 300 mg daily. Only about 40 percent of the dietary calcium is absorbed, so that an allowance of 800 mg per day in the food is necessary to replace this loss. Nevertheless, it has been shown that many individuals can, by adaptive processes, come into balance on as little as 300 mg daily intake. It is not established that a long-continued intake which is low or marginal in calcium is a cause of osteoporosis (Chap. 381). During growth, pregnancy, and lactation, additional allowances of 100 to 600 mg daily are recommended.

SODIUM AND CHLORIDE. While sodium and chloride are essential ions, they often are consumed in great excess. The best estimate of the usual adult intake in the United States is between 6,000 and 18,000 mg sodium chloride daily. This is in contrast to an estimated sodium chloride requirement of 800 to 1,000 mg daily. That this excess intake contributes to ill health is not clear. The intake of sodium chloride in the United States has tended to decline as other methods for preserving food have been developed. A drive for eating salt occurs in animals which subsist on a vegetarian diet low in sodium and high in potassium. Carnivores have no craving for salt because they obtain sufficient sodium from the meat they eat. The ratio of K to Na intake of herbivores is 20, as compared with 5 for most carnivores and 1.0 for human beings in the Western world.

Only severe and prolonged heat exposure requires supplementary salt, since dietary intake usually is high, and because of the efficient adaptation reaction mediated by aldosterone secretion (Chap. 92) which diminishes the sodium in sweat and urine after heat exposure. Disorders of sodium homeostasis occur where the adaptation is overwhelmed or, as in mucoviscidosis (Chap. 334), when full adaptation cannot be achieved. The availability of potent saluretic drugs has diminished but not abolished the need for salt-restricted diets (see Chap. 264). Sodium depletion is generally the consequence of a restricted intake and urinary wastage caused by either a saluretic agent or renal disease (see Chap. 300).

POTASSIUM. The principal intracellular cation is potassium. Appreciation of the clinical significance of potassium was delayed because the plasma concentration of potassium is not a sensitive index of changes in intracellular concentration. Disorders attributable to hyper- or hypokalemia are described in Chaps. 92, 264, and 300.

There are no recommended dietary allowances for sodium, potassium, or chloride because they are widely distributed in food, and disorders are more commonly the result of excessive losses or retention than of dietary deficiency.

IRON. Iron is an indispensable element which is often taken in marginal or low amounts in human diets. Iron deficiency will be discussed in Chap. 336. Iron toxicity can occur (Chap. 107), especially when iron intake is high in the face of a low protein diet. Since only 10 percent of dietary iron is absorbed and absorption varies with the source of iron, the RDA ranges from 12 to 18 mg per day for men, pregnant women, and growing children. The three physiologic conditions which require particular attention to iron intake are infancy and adolescence, when growth is rapid; menstruation, which causes a loss of an average of 15 mg of iron during each cycle; and pregnancy, when maternal iron-bearing tissues are enlarging and the fetus is accumulating iron as well.

MAGNESIUM. Magnesium is a cofactor for many body enzymes. Adult tissues contain about 20 to 25 Gm magnesium, about half of which is in bone. The RDA is 350 mg per day for men and 300 mg per day for women. This is readily obtained in ordinary diets. The average American diet contains about 120 mg of magnesium per 1000 Cal.

Experiments with a small group of human subjects fed a diet deficient in magnesium but adequate in other respects produced a nonspecific spectrum of neurologic, muscular, and gastrointestinal manifestations which seemed related to a marked decrease in serum calcium and potassium levels. It appeared in these studies that magnesium is well conserved by both the kidney and the bowel when the supply is limited, but it is poorly stored so that a regular intake is necessary to avoid deficiency. The manifestations of magnesium depletion are described in Chap. 85.

HALOGENS. The daily requirement of *iodine* is 50 to 70 μg. It is an essential part of the thyroid hormones. Its metabolism is discussed in Chap. 89. An efficient way to assure this intake, especially in areas with soil depleted of iodine, is by the use of iodized salt. In the United States such salt is offered optionally with 100 ppm of iodide. Since 1920, this practice has dramatically reduced the prevalence of goiter. Some nations by mandate require iodinization of salt.

While *fluoride* is not known to be essential, its administration during the formative years of life at a rate of about 1 ppm in drinking water will approximately halve the rate of dental caries. An excess of fluoride, above 3 to 5 ppm in water, leads to cosmetic disfigurement of teeth, and larger excesses cause osteopetrosis and ossification of ligaments. It has been proposed that a fluoride intake of 1 to 5 ppm may diminish the prevalence of osteoporosis in adult life. The fluoride ion is thought to change the crystalline structure of apatite in bone by replacing an hydroxyl ion. This action in bone may resemble its effect on teeth.

COPPER. Copper is known to be essential in man, but deficiency is thought to be very rare. An adult man's tissues contain 75 to 150 mg copper. The concentration is highest in the liver at birth. Most of the serum copper is bound to the protein ceruloplasmin. Copper intoxication is well known in Wilson's disease (Chap. 110). A daily intake of 2 mg copper maintains balance and is easily obtained even in relatively poor diets. Deficiency is usually associated with an iron deficiency or with major malabsorptive disorders.

TRACE ELEMENTS. The trace or microelements include chromium, cobalt, manganese, molybdenum, selenium, and zinc.

Chromium may influence carbohydrate metabolism, since chromium-deficient rats show abnormal glucose tolerance. *Cobalt* appears to function in man only as a component of vitamin B_{12}. *Manganese* is a component of several enzyme systems and is also found in bone, but deficiency of this element in man has not been recognized. *Molybdenum* is essential for experimental animals, but a deficiency in man is unknown. *Selenium* has been shown to have functions like those of vitamin E, and clear-cut deficiency has been produced in animals. Selenium intoxication is also well known in animals raised in areas with a high selenium content in the soil and vegetation.

Zinc deficiency has been demonstrated in animals, but

the existence of definite human deficiency is still uncertain. In patients with cirrhosis, low levels of plasma zinc and high urinary levels have been reported, but the relation of these changes to the disease is not established.

The vitamins are discussed in the chapters which follow.

REFERENCES

DuBois, E. F.: "Basal Metabolism in Health and Disease,"

pp. 410–442, chap. 18, Philadelphia, Lea & Febiger, 1936.

Holt, P. R.: Medium Chain Triglycerides. A Useful Adjunct in Nutritional Therapy, Gastroenterology, 53:961, 1967.

McCollum, E. V.: "A History of Nutrition," Boston, Houghton Mifflin Company, 1964.

Shils, M. E.: Experimental Human Magnesium Depletion, Medicine, 48:61, 1969.

Underwood, E. J.: "Trace Elements in Human and Animal Nutrition," 2nd ed., New York, Academic Press Inc., 1962.

Section 2
Nutritional Deficiency States

77 NUTRITIONAL DEFICIENCY STATES

George V. Mann

Malnutrition in Western developed countries has two aspects, overnutrition and undernutrition. Sporadic instances of scurvy and rickets in United States children usually result from some combination of misinformation or ignorance and are not indicative of widespread deficiency. Lamentations about the nutrition of teenagers are often heard, but these are more often based on the misapplication of generous dietary allowances rather than on the documentation of physical or chemical signs of nutritional deficiency.

THE PATHOGENESIS OF NUTRITIONAL DISEASE. Human beings cannot select an adequate diet from a variety of foods by instinctive reliance upon taste or the other senses, but require nutrition education. Moreover, poor food habits are very difficult to change. Margaret Mead has observed that one can change religion more easily than food habits.

Dietary deficiencies result from two kinds of changes. Thus the food supply may change as with the introduction of maize into Europe, which led to pellagra, or the change to polished rice in the Orient, which led to endemic beriberi. Another cause of dietary deficiency is a shift from a wide to a narrow assortment of food choices. When a varied diet gives way to alcohol, when meat is replaced by crackers and tea, when fresh vegetables are replaced by a few canned foods, or when civilization and northerly migration bring smoke and clothing which prevent the exposure of the skin to sun, then nutritional deficiencies may occur.

Seven principles should be kept in mind in relation to the causes and management of nutritional disease.

1. Animals, including man, adapt to the available food. This adaptation occurs for many nutrients, but that for protein is better understood. When the protein supply is low, the organism becomes more efficient in nitrogen utilization and it can come into nitrogen balance on as little as 20 to 30 Gm protein per day.

2. Culture determines food behavior. A child learns the way his culture has dealt with food and he follows this through life. The most important teacher of nutrition is the mother. Elementary schools offer an important opportunity to correct or modify food habits.

3. Food deprivation alters behavior. This is a conspicuous effect, especially during periods of calorie deprivation. Starvation causes profound deterioration of personality, whether caused by cancer, famine, or the faddist treatment of obesity.

4. Foods complement one another in their nutrient content. Two proteins, each incomplete in content of essential amino acids, may when taken together, serve as a complete protein. The incidence of nutritional deficiency increases when the diet has been restricted in variety.

5. Nutrient deficiencies are generally multiple because a diet of natural foods rarely will be low in only one essential nutrient. This is important in therapy for treatment with a single nutrient will often aggravate coexistent deficiencies of other nutrients.

6. The nutrient requirements of human beings are known. While this may seem an overconfident statement, it is a reasonable assumption. There is no foundation for the faddists' argument which advocates bizarre foods for managing ill health because it is contended that "unknown essential nutrients" are supplied by these crude or unprocessed foods.

7. Frank deficiency disease appearing in a few individuals usually is indicative of subclinical or occult disease in others of the same family or social group.

The patterns of nutritional disease can be seen in two quite different social circumstances (Figs. 77-1 and

77-2). In the technically developed countries and among affluent classes, and even in underdeveloped areas, the pattern is one of "malnutrition amid plenty." Despite abundance of food, misguided or misinformed choices and consumption of highly refined and processed foods can result in dietary imbalance and nutritional deficiency. In the underdeveloped areas of the world and among the poor and underprivileged classes of all countries, the problems of too little food and too little choice are compounded by lack of judgment in the selection of food or its optimal preparation. The stress of parasitic infestation and infection often aggravates the already marginal intakes of energy and nutrients in these groups. There is no doubt that nutritional deficiency may be precipitated by other diseases, but it is not well established that malnutrition predisposes to other diseases. The morbidity and mortality from infectious disease is higher in malnourished populations than in the well nourished, but it has been difficult to show that malnutrition increases the incidence of infections.

FACTORS LEADING TO THE DEVELOPMENT OF DEFICIENCY STATES. These are six in number.

1. A low dietary intake of essential nutrients. This may be a result of poverty, ignorance, social isolation, or food faddism or the result of other behavioral abnormalities.

2. Low intakes may be caused by a disorder of the oral or pharyngeal cavities which impairs food intake.

3. Deficiency states may be the consequence of malabsorption. They will often be seen as a complication of sprue or of other malabsorption syndromes (Chap. 316).

4. Deficiency states may result from poor utilization of a nutrient of which intake is adequate. For example, the utilization of carotene, the provitamin A, is poor in the presence of hypothyroidism, and carotene is poorly absorbed if the diet is exceptionally low in fat. Vitamin K is poorly absorbed in the absence of bile in the intestinal tract, and the synthesis of prothrombin is often impaired in the presence of advanced liver disease.

5. Nutrient wastage may account for malnutrition, as

Fig. 77-1. The pattern of malnutrition in underdeveloped cultures.

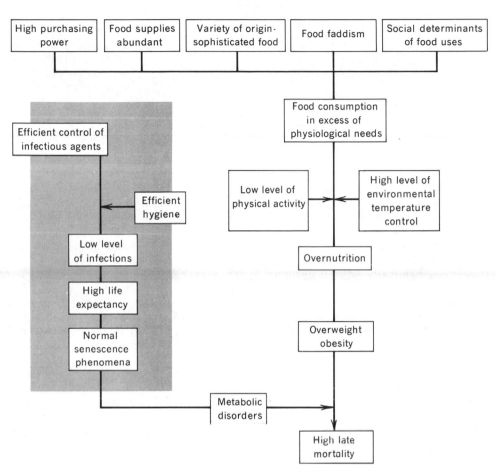

Fig. 77-2. The pattern of malnutrition in technically advanced cultures.

in the aminoacidurias or phosphaturias associated with renal tubular disease.

6. The utilization of a nutrient may be impaired even though intake is adequate, as when goitrogens impair iodine utilization. Substances with antivitamin activity are well known in experimental nutrition. Certain drugs impair the utilization of pyridoxine (Chap. 336).

REFERENCES

Behar, M., F. Viteri, R. Bressani, G. Arroyave, R. L. Squibb, and N. S. Scrimshaw: Principles of Treatment and Prevention of Severe Protein Malnutrition in Children (Kwashiorkor), Ann. N.Y. Acad. Sci., 69:854, 1959.

Mitchell, H. H.: Nutritional Adaptation, chap. 6 in "Nutrition," vol. 2, "Vitamins, Nutrient Requirements and Food Selection," G. H. Beaton, and E. W. McHenry (Eds.), New York, Academic Press Inc., 1964.

Scrimshaw, N. S., C. E. Taylor, and J. E. Gordon: Interactions of Nutrition and Infection, World Health Organ. Monogr., 1965.

78 EVALUATION OF NUTRITIONAL STATUS
George V. Mann

The diagnosis of malnutrition depends on the diet history, the recognition of distinctive physical signs, the demonstration of biochemical abnormalities, and the response to therapeutic trials.

DIET HISTORY. Of the several ways of measuring dietary intake, only the dietary history is likely to be applicable for physicians. In dietary surveys measurements of food intake often are made in the home by a household food inventory method. Dietitians may use the patient's 3- or 7-day food diary, and economists rely on evidence from commodity balance sheets and food available for consumption.

Obtaining a dietary history is simplest when food choice and variety have been limited. The inquiry must determine food habits over a period of weeks and months rather than a few days because the long-term intake is

Table 78-1. A SYNOPSIS OF U.S. BASIC FOOD GROUPS AND THEIR NUTRIENT CONTRIBUTION

Food group	Essential nutrient contribution											
	Calories	Protein	Ca	P	Fe	Vitamin A and carotene	Vitamin D	Vitamin C	Nicotinic acid Thiamine Riboflavin Pyridoxine	Folic acid	B_{12}	Vitamin E
Dairy..........	−	+	+	+	−	−	+	−	+	−	+	−
Meat...........	+	+	+	+	+	−	−	−	+	−	+	+
Cereal and bread	+	−	−	+	−	−	−	−	+	+	−	+
Vegetables......	+	+	+	−	+	+	−	−	+	+	−	−
Fruit..........	−	−	−	−	+	+	−	+	−	−	−	−

important. The dietary history of children and of many adults must be obtained from the parent or spouse who actually purchases, prepares, and serves the food. Leading questions should be avoided because many patients know what they *should* eat and will tell the questioner this rather than what they actually *do* eat. The interviewer should have some familiarity with the cultural environment of the patient in order to obtain an adequate history. The possibility of many deficiency states can be eliminated at once by establishing certain food practices of the patient. Thus citrus fruits or meat taken once or twice a week or consumption of enriched bread or cereal daily eliminate the possibility of a deficiency of vitamin C, protein, or thiamine.

The diet history is best obtained by first determining the meal pattern (number and timing of meals and the kinds of food eaten in a typical day) and then asking about individual items of the five major food groups in Table 78-1. This type of cross-check will bring to light inconsistencies that should be explored. The physician's needs are met by ruling out possibilities rather than by aiming for quantification of intake of nutrients.

PHYSICAL SIGNS. The diagnostic specificity of the physical signs of nutritional disease, such as cheilosis, perleche, nasolabial seborrhea, follicular hyperkeratosis, conjunctival injection, dry hair, swollen gums, and even bowed extremities or bossed skulls, as evidence of past or present nutritional disease has been exaggerated.

The posture and muscle tone and the patient's attitude may be helpful in the appraisal of malnutrition, but these signs are not specific. The amount of subcutaneous fat can be useful in appraising calorie deficiency and can be quantitated with standard calipers. By using the principles of isotopic dilution, it is possible to calculate the size of the body compartments, and body composition can be measured, but such measurements are not practical for physicians. Body fat can also be derived from measurements of body density, but inspection and palpation of subcutaneous fat will serve almost as well.

There are a few changes in mucous membranes and the skin and hair which are useful because they are fairly specific for nutritional deficiency. *Bitot's spot* (Chap. 84) generally indicates deficiency of vitamin A. Other vascular and membranous changes in the conjunctival sac are apt to be misleading. The *perifollicular hemorrhages* and the unique *"corkscrew" hair* associated with adult scurvy are fairly specific, but phrynoderma, or *follicular hyperkeratosis* without hemorrhage, which has been associated with vitamin A deficiency, is not a specific sign. *Nasolabial seborrhea* and *scrotal dermatitis* are suggestive but not diagnostic of pyridoxine deficiency or ariboflavinosis. The pigmentary changes and dermatitis associated with kwashiorkor and pellagra are typical and almost diagnostic. *Papillary atrophy and reddening of the tongue* should suggest nutritional deficiency, although these may be seen in any of several individual deficiency states, including those of iron, nicotinic acid, vitamin B_{12}, and folic acid. The *gum changes* in scurvy often are typical because of the great hypertrophy of the interdental papillae and their fragility to mechanical injury. These changes do not appear in edentulous persons. Enlargement of the salivary glands is seen in malnutrition, but it is not a specific sign.

Neuropathy is a feature of many deficiency states, including those of thiamine, pyridoxine, cobalamine, and nicotinic acid. Thiamine deficiency is associated with peripheral weakness, wasting, and paresthesia, as well as Wernicke's ophthalmoplegia and psychosis. Pyridoxine deficiency often leads to convulsions in infants and in experimental animals to lesions of sensory neurons. Deficiency of cobalamine may cause subacute degeneration of the spinal cord. Psychosis is a common complication of pellagra (Chap. 363).

The *radiologic signs* of rickets, osteomalacia, and juvenile scurvy often are decisive in the acute stages of the disorder. The intestinal mucosal pattern formerly described as a *deficiency pattern* is misnamed. Although the changes are often seen in sprue as a result of atrophy of the villi and changes in the mucous secretions, they do not reflect any specific vitamin deficiency.

There are no typical electrocardiographic signs of vitamin deficiency, but the changes in the ECG during hyper- and hypokalemia are typical. These are described in Chap. 265.

BIOCHEMICAL TESTS. The many biochemical tests for assessing nutritional status are summarized in Table 78-2.

Table 78-2. BIOCHEMICAL AIDS IN DIAGNOSING NUTRITIONAL DEFICIENCY

Nutrient	Test	Level suggesting nutritional disorder	Normal range
Protein	Plasma total protein	< 6.0 Gm%	6.5–8.0 Gm%
	Serum albumin	< 3.5 Gm%	4.0–5.2 Gm%
	Plasma Essential amino acid/ Total amino acid	< 0.3	0.3–0.5
Vitamin A and carotene	Plasma vitamin A	< 20 µg%	50–100 µg%
	Plasma carotenoids	< 30 µg%	100–200 µg%
	Response to 200,000 IU Vitamin A	Plasma level increases × 2	< × 1
Vitamin D	Serum Ca	< 3.5 mEq/L	4.5–6 mEq/L
	Serum P	< 0.8 mEq/L	1.0–1.5 mEq/L
	Serum alkaline phosphatase	> 15 units—adults	5–13 K-A units
		> 20 units—children	10–20 K-A units
Vitamin C	Whole blood	< 0.20 mg%	0.4–1.0 mg%
	Buffy coat	< 10 mg%	25–40 mg%
Thiamine	Blood lactate	> 15 mg%	9–15 mg%
	Plasma pyruvate	> 2.0 mg%	0.8–2.0 mg%
	Transketolase (TK) RBC	< 850 µg hexose/ml/hr.	900–1500 µg hexose/ml
	Thiamine pyrophosphate effect on TK	> 15%	< 15%
	Urinary thiamine	< 50 µg/Gm creatinine	100–500 mg/Gm creatinine
Riboflavin	Plasma flavin adenine dinucleotide	< 1.5 µg	2–3 µg%
	Urinary riboflavin	< 50 µg/gm creatinine	100–500 µg/Gm creatinine
Pyridoxine	Urinary xanthurenic acid after 10 Gm dl-tryptophane	> 50 mgm/24 hr	trace
Vitamin B$_{12}$	Plasma B$_{12}$ level (Euglena gracilis in serum)	< 100 µµg/ml	200–900 µµg/ml
	Schilling test	< 8% ^{60}Co B$_{12}$	> 8% nucleide following 1 mg B$_{12}$ IM
Pantothenic acid	Serum	< 50 mµ Gm/ml	100 mµ Gm/ml
Folic acid	Serum level (L. casei)	< 5 mµg/ml	5–20 mµg/ml serum
	Formimino glutamic acid (Figlu) after 20 Gm l-histidine HCl p.o.	> 75 mg/12 hr in urine	0–55 mg/12 hr
Iron	Serum iron	< 60 µg/100 ml	60–190 µg%
	Serum iron-binding capacity	> 400 µg	250–400 µg%
Magnesium	Serum	< 1.5 mEq/L	1.5–3.0 mEq/L
Copper	Serum	< 85 µg%	114 µg%
Zinc	Plasma	< 80 µg%	120 µg%
Vitamin K	Plasma Prothrombin Time	> 20 sec	10–15 sec
Tocopherol	Plasma	< 0.4 mg%	0.5–2.0 mg%
Sodium	Serum	< 132 mEq/L	132–142 mEq/L
Potassium	Serum	< 3.5 mEq/L	3.5–5.0 mEq/L

Sampling for these tests must be done promptly, before the hospital diet or dietary suggestions alter the findings and confuse the diagnosis.

A practical strategy in nutritional diagnosis is to use the dietary history to establish the possibility of nutritional deficiency, to use the results of physical examination and appropriate laboratory tests to establish a tentative diagnosis, and to employ the therapeutic trial to confirm it.

THERAPEUTIC TRIALS. The urgency of circumstances, coupled with unavailability or delays in obtaining biochemical tests, sometimes forces the immediate application of a therapeutic trial as a diagnostic measure. In following this course, three precautions should be observed: (1) If therapy includes multiple nutrients, the patient's recovery may not be attributable to a single cause, and if such information is lacking, the disorder may recur because of failure to correct the cause. (2) The ease with which the deficiency is treated and with which recovery occurs may prevent adequate explanation or nutrition education and invite recurrences. (3) There are certain definite hazards associated with nutrient therapy because both vitamins A and D are toxic in excessive dosages. Vitamin A given in amounts over 25,000 units per day will in time produce anorexia, irritability, decalcification of bone, headache, and loss of hair. For vitamin D the margin between requirement and toxicity is lower. Doses of over 2,000 international units (IU) per day are potentially dangerous and may cause hypercalcemia. The vitamin D intake should not exceed 400

IU per day. Another hazard in vitamin therapy is the danger of administering folacin to a person with vitamin B_{12} deficiency. This will lead to relief of anemia, but neurologic lesions of vitamin B_{12} deficiency will persist and may progress to irreversible stages before B_{12} deficiency is recognized (Chap. 337).

Vitamin Supplements. Multivitamin preparations are readily available without prescription and are aggressively promoted. They often are used wastefully. A physician may be tempted to prescribe them because they are thought to be harmless or because he looks upon this as a simple way to protect patients against the small chance of developing a deficiency state. This practice is undesirable on three counts: it is wasteful; the use of unnecessary medication is to be deplored; and such use of vitamins lulls many patients and a few doctors into neglecting needed diagnostic studies.

With the exception of occasional pregnant or lactating women, well people do not need supplemental vitamins in their diets.

The Council on Nutrition of the American Medical Association has published suggestions for composition of therapeutic vitamin mixtures. Multiple vitamin mixtures should contain only those nutrients known to be essential for man. Supplements should not include such natural mixtures as liver, yeast, or wheat germ. The available multivitamin preparations fall into three general categories according to the amount of nutrients supplied. The first class should supply about one-half of the RDA and is indicated as a supplement in the prophylaxis of nutritional deficiencies for persons with minor disturbances of dietary intake or with unusually large temporary requirements. The second class should contain about 1½ times the recommended dietary allowance and is intended as a therapeutic supplement for proven or suspected deficiency states. The third type of multivitamin supplement should contain from three to five times the RDA and is recommended for use in disorders of absorption, retention, or excessive vitamin losses. This type should not be used as a dietary supplement for protracted periods. The levels of individual nutrients in the mixtures should be proportionate multiples of the recommended dietary allowances.

There is no justification for the widespread marketing of multivitamins to families for their purported value in preventing colds or infections. This effect cannot be documented. The tendency among food merchants to increase the vitamin content of breakfast cereals to therapeutic levels is an insidious marketing device that cannot be justified.

Cereal Enrichment. During World War II a program of enrichment of certain basic cereal foods was begun in the United States, and it has since been continued. Because one-half or more of the food energy supply of the majority of human beings comes from carbohydrate, the National Research Council recommended the enrichment of white flour and bread. It is estimated that about 90 percent of all white breads presently sold in the United States are enriched. The significant addition of nutrients to the composition of those products is indicated in Table

Table 78-3. NUTRIENT LEVELS IN FLOUR, UNITED STATES (in mg/lb)

	Thiamine	Riboflavin	Nicotinic acid	Iron
Whole wheat flour..	2.49	0.54	19.7	15.0
White flour........	0.28	0.21	4.1	3.6
Enriched white flour	2.00	1.20	16.0	13.0

78-3. Five southern states also require that corn meal and grits be enriched. South Carolina requires that rice be enriched.

The most dramatic demonstration of enrichment as a means of preventing nutritional disease is the Philippine experiment with enriched rice. The project demonstrated in Bataan that enrichment of rice with thiamine and riboflavin was feasible, economically desirable, acceptable, and a highly efficient way of preventing sickness and death from beriberi.

In addition to these required enrichments, a number of other common foods in the United States are permitted to contain nutrient additives. An early additive was milk powder to bread, which significantly increased its protein and vitamin content. With the development and patenting of the process for obtaining vitamin D_2 by irradiating ergosterol, whole milk was allowed to be enriched to a level of 400 IU per quart, and represents an important source of vitamin D for children.

REFERENCES

Pearson, W. N.: "Assessment of Nutritional Status: Biochemical Methods," chap. 7 in "Nutrition, A Comprehensive Treatise," vol. 3, G. H. Beaton, and E. W. McHenry (Eds.), New York, Academic Press Inc., 1967.

Quiogue, E. S.: The Rice Enrichment Project in Bataan, Philippines, Am. J. Public Health, 42:1086, 1952.

White, P. L.: Vitamin Preparations as Dietary Supplements and as Therapeutic Agents, J.A.M.A., 169:41, 1959.

Young, C. M., and M. F. Trulson: Methodology for Dietary Studies in Epidemiological Surveys. II. Strengths and Weaknesses of Existing Methods, Am. J. Public Health, 50:803, 1960.

79 STARVATION AND PROTEIN MALNUTRITION

George V. Mann

STARVATION. Starvation emphasizes the importance of the principle of adaptation in nutrition. As people starve, their physiologic processes change in ways to conserve energy. Their surfaces become smaller and cooler, their pulses slower, and their spontaneous activity lessens. Secondary sexual characteristics disappear and personality is altered as all interests become preoccupied with food.

The changes consequent to starvation are the same whether in sick patients or in starving populations. They have been recorded systematically in two scientific studies, Benedict's experiment in 1919 and that of Keys in 1950.

The compositional changes in simple starvation are largest for body fat because fat comprises the main energy reserve. The stores of energy available to a well-nourished man of average composition are summarized in Table 79-1. It is significant that such a man, with the usual

Table 79-1. ENERGY STORES IN A "STANDARD" MAN

Component	Cal/g, kcal	Total weight, Gm	Caloric equivalent	Available as energy
Protein.......	4	11,000	44,000	8,000
Fat..........	9	9,000	81,000	72,000
Carbohydrate.	4	500	2,000	800
Water........	...	45,000		
Mineral......	...	4,500		
Total......	...	...	...	81,000*

* 81,000/1,200 = 67 days

adaptation to starvation, might reduce his daily resting metabolism from 1750 to 1200 Cal or less. With these stores he would be predicted to survive about 67 days, when he would have exhausted his fuel supply. In fact, this is about the survival time of adult men during famines. Women, starting with more body fat, have typically survived longer than men. Chassat's Rule is that recovery from starvation is doubtful after half the normal weight has been lost.

Starvation often is associated with fluid retention, the *hunger edema* which still is unexplained. It is probably due in part to the hypoproteinemia consequent to the profound negative nitrogen balance, this leading to alterations in the osmotic concentrations of the body, especially in the renal interstitial tissues, which in turn result in impaired excretion of water and salt. The edema may also reflect some alteration in the functions of adrenal corticoid hormones with starvation.

Contrary to previous belief, rehabilitation can be achieved with an abundance of almost any balanced diet. Starvation and episodes of malnutrition, especially in the young, have been shown to impair physical and intellectual growth in experimental animals. Whether periods of malnutrition may produce permanent intellectual damage, analogous to the arrests and opacities seen in bone by x-ray after these nutritional disorders, is presently unknown. If this were true, it might contribute to the backwardness of human beings in the so-called "underdeveloped areas" at home and abroad.

Clinical Changes. The changes occurring with starvation are most clearly seen in anorexia nervosa where the usual sociologic and physical disturbances of famine are not present. Anorexia nervosa is discussed in Chap. 42. The increased pigmentation of a starving person is prob-

Fig. 79-1. An example of marasmus. (*Photograph courtesy of Nevin S. Scrimshaw*)

ably due to closer juxtaposition of melanocytes in the skin. The prevalence of infection in famine probably is due to the usual deterioration of housing facilities and public health barriers to infection rather than to a decline of individual resistance.

The current fad of using total starvation in the treatment of obesity requires the reminder that these starving patients do not develop deficiencies of the micronutrients and do not require supplementary vitamins.

MARASMUS AND KWASHIORKOR. *Marasmus* is the term applied to a child with exhaustion of protein and energy stores (Fig. 79-1). It is the end stage of both protein and calorie insufficiency. *Kwashiorkor* is primarily a protein deficiency. It was first identified, described, and recorded by Dr. Cicely Williams in Ghana in 1931. The name is that used by the Ga people, to whom the disorder was well known. Kwashiorkor is protein deficiency occurring in the presence of sufficient energy intake. The child is edematous, although its muscles are wasted. It is apathetic and often anorexic, and may present a characteristic dermatosis (Fig. 79-2). The hair often is depigmented, assuming a reddish hue with thinning and straightening of the kinky texture normal in Negro children. There are profound deficiencies of intestinal enzymes. The liver is fatty and enlarged, and persistent

Fig. 79-2. A child with kwashiorkor. (*Photograph supplied by Nevin S. Scrimshaw*)

diarrhea is typical. The disorder often is precipitated by an infection in a child weaned from breast milk to a pablum of cassava meal in water which, although supplying energy, is disastrously low in protein. Initially this disorder was confused with adult pellagra. Since World War II, it has been clearly established as a major cause of death and disability in children throughout the world.

The term *protein-calorie malnutrition* has been widely used to designate collectively the spectrum ranging from pure protein deficiency to total energy deficiency. The hungry, emaciated, marasmic child can usually be distinguished from the sullen, anorexic, edematous child with a dramatic dermatosis. There are, however, all shades of intermingling of these classical extremes of marasmus and kwashiorkor. The relationship of calorie and protein de-

ficiency to this terminal state is shown graphically in Fig. 79-3. Marasmus and kwashiorkor are not always separable as the diagram suggests. These children waste away without the typical physical signs of any particular nutrient deficiency, although vitamin A deficiency is a common complication and many other stores of nutrients are depleted. Kwashiorkor represents one end of this spectrum, marasmus the other.

There is no efficient biochemical indicator of protein-calorie malnutrition. The serum albumin will generally be reduced. Levels of 3.50 to 2.75 Gm per 100 ml indicate a probable protein deficiency, and levels below 2.75 Gm per 100 ml are highly probable indicators. In time the plasma total protein becomes reduced although the tendency to hyperglobulinemia in persons who live in underdeveloped areas tends to obscure this sign. The ratio of essential to nonessential amino acids in plasma will decline, but this has not been a dependable sign.

Extracellular fluids tend to increase until frank edema develops. The diagnosis largely depends upon the dietary history and the clinical appearance. The skin and hair changes in children with kwashiorkor are often dramatic, while in adults such skin changes are rarely seen, although apathy, wasting, and great weakness are found. Even though some intestinal enzymes may be depleted, the disorder responds to hydration and refeeding with an abundance of protein of high biologic value. Because of the frequency with which infection is seen as the immediate precipitating cause, broad-spectrum antibiotics are used immediately, along with therapeutic levels of vitamins. Even with optimum treatment the death rate in children remains high. Malnourished children tend to have repeated bouts of malnutrition unless the mother can be made to understand the relationship between the poor diet and the illness.

Trauma. The metabolic response to trauma is characteristic and predictable (Chap. 92). Even in well-nourished persons the stress of injury, infection, or surgery will induce a sequence of catabolism that entails loss of body fat, nitrogen, potassium, magnesium, sulfur, and calcium and retention of water and sodium. The reactions appear to be mediated hormonally. It is not established that any amount of forced feeding will abolish this sequence. The metabolic wasting that occurs with a combination of starvation and infection has been termed *sep-*

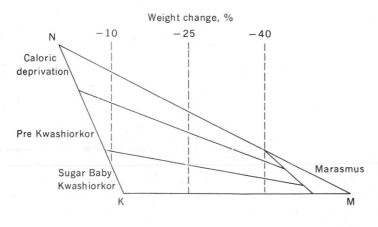

Fig. 79-3. The relationship of marasmus (*M*) and kwashiorkor (*K*). The energy depletion is indicated along the abscissa, the extent of protein depletion, along the ordinate. The classical example of kwashiorkor, the sugar baby fed a pablum of starch, will show but little weight loss because his energy stores are preserved. The child with marasmus is greatly underweight and protein depleted. Infection may move a child rapidly toward *K* and *M*. (*Adapted from Scrimshaw and Behar*)

tic starvation. Intracellular water diminishes, but the total body water increases. The wasting may reach a rate of 1.5 kg tissue daily. As minimal trauma as a venesection of 500 ml produces similar but lesser changes. The wasting disorder called *cardiac cachexia* is seen in patients with chronic heart failure (Chap. 264).

Ethanol. The role of ethanol in causing or contributing to nutritional disease is exceedingly important. Ethanol yields about 7 Cal per Gm and is often an important source of calories in the diet. There is a tendency for light drinkers to become obese because they seem not to compensate for this increased caloric intake. Heavy drinkers tend to decrease their intake of foods as their intake of alcohol increases and to lose weight. It has been widely supposed that the malnutrition associated with alcoholism is a consequence of replacement of food by alcohol, but this is not true. The pathologic effects of ethanol are discussed in Chaps. 118 and 328. Ethanol is toxic to many tissues.

REFERENCES

Brock, J. F.: Dietary Protein Deficiency, Ann. Intern. Med., 65:877, 1966.

Keys, A., et al.: "The Biology of Human Starvation," vol. 1, chap. 1, the University of Minnesota Press, 1950.

Lieber, C. S.: Metabolic Derangement Induced by Alcohol, Ann. Rev. Med., 18:35, 1967.

Moore, F. D., et al.: "The Body Cell Mass and its Supporting Environment Body Composition in Health and Disease," Philadelphia, W. B. Saunders Company, 1963.

Scrimshaw, N. S., and M. Behar: Malnutrition in Underdeveloped Countries, New Engl. J. Med., 272:137, 1965.

Terris, M.: Epidemiology of Cirrhosis of the Liver: National Mortality Data, Amer. J. Public Health, 57:2076, 1967.

80 PELLAGRA
Richard H. Follis, Jr. and George V. Mann

HISTORY. During the eighteenth century, a new disease began to appear with increasing frequency in northern Spain and Italy. First called *mal de la rosa* by Casal (from the erythematous skin lesions), the malady soon came to be known as *pelle agro* (skin, rough), from which the present-day name, *pellagra*, is derived. Casal described the prominent features: "a horrible crust" involving the skin, particularly of the hands and neck; "painful burning of the mouth"; "perpetual shaking of the body"; and "mania." He noted the prominence of maize in the diet of the people whom he had studied. During the nineteenth century, the principal focus of the disease was northern Italy, where in some areas as many as 5 percent of the population in a given area might be affected. A number of explanations were advanced for the cause: that maize acquired toxic properties as a result of infestation with molds or fungi; that a material present

Fig. 80-1. Pellagra in a young girl. (*Photograph courtesy of Dr. J. G. Prinsloo and the American Journal of Clinical Nutrition*)

in the grain was transformed into a poisonous substance in the intestinal tract of man; that maize contained some chemical that sensitized the skin to the photodynamic action of sunlight; that some specific microorganism was present; or that a diet predominantly of maize was a poor source of nourishment.

Pellagra began to appear in epidemic proportions in the southern United States in the early 1900s. Joseph Goldberger, of the U.S. Public Health Service, soon showed in classic studies that diet alone could cure, prevent, or cause the disease. He demonstrated the importance of protein in the diet and for a time he favored the idea that lack of specific amino acids was the cause. His interest then shifted to the curative effects of yeast and to the identification of an antipellagra vitamin. In 1937, Elvehjem and his coworkers showed that nicotinic acid would cure black tongue, a pellagra-like disease, in dogs. Shortly thereafter nicotinic acid proved effective in the therapy of clinical pellagra. When it was found that the essential amino acid, tryptophan, is a precursor of nicotinic acid, it became clear that pellagra results from a deficiency of dietary tryptophan and/or nicotinic acid; deficiency of other nutrients, such as riboflavin, thiamine, folic acid, and vitamin B_{12}, may complicate the disease. The persistent relationship of dietary maize to the development of pellagra is not explained. Pellagra is rare in populations consuming other grains with even lower content of nicotinic acid and tryptophan than maize. It has not been possible to demonstrate the significance of substances binding nicotinic acid in maize, which may interfere with its utilization.

PREVALENCE. After 1940, the prevalence of endemic pellagra diminished greatly in the United States. The disease is still important in Yugoslavia, Rumania, Egypt, India, South Africa, and Yucatan. Cases of sporadic pellagra are rarely observed in the United States; when encountered, they often accompany chronic disease states, particularly those affecting the gastrointestinal tract. In addition, pellagra occurs in individuals who consume large quantities of alcohol and whose diets are restricted with respect to a number of essential nutrients.

CLINICAL FINDINGS. Before pellagra becomes clinically manifest and the patient seeks the help of a physician, certain prodromal symptoms may be present. These include loss of appetite leading to weight loss, indigestion, diarrhea or constipation, generalized weakness, lassitude, burning sensations, headache, and insomnia. These symptoms are usually followed after varying periods of time by the manifestations of full-blown pellagra, which affect the skin, alimentary tract, nervous system, and to a lesser extent, the blood. Pellagra is a seasonal disease with acute exacerbations in the spring, when a combination of the winter's impairment of diet and a new exposure to sun and heavier work seem to precipitate the acute episodes.

The *skin lesions* may begin as an erythema that looks very much like sunburn. Burning or itching may be intense. The initial changes may be followed by the formation of vesicles or by peeling. The erythematous skin may assume a dirty-brown color and then becomes rough and scaly. This stage, which may not necessarily be preceded by erythema, may remain for prolonged periods. Characteristically, the skin lesions are symmetric and tend to be localized over exposed areas: backs of hands in adults and backs of feet in children, on the face, neck, elbows, and knees. In addition, the scrotum, vulva, and perianal region may be involved. Unilateral dermatitis is usually associated with local pressure, trauma, heat, or sunlight. The evolution of the lesions may differ; erythema of the hands may appear while hyperkeratosis of the legs is already present. Seborrhea about the nose with comedo formation may be conspicuous in some patients.

Sore mouth is a common complaint. Changes in the tongue are conspicuous, and glossitis is thought by some to be a more sensitive gauge of the disease than skin lesions. The tip and margins of the tongue become hyperemic, a change that may spread to involve the entire surface so that the structure acquires a beef-red appearance. Small ulcers sometimes appear. Inflammatory lesions may be found in the mucous membrane of the mouth. Secondary infection is common, particularly with fusospirochetal organisms. In advanced stages of the disease, the tongue may be pale with complete atrophy of the papillae. Angular lesions, i.e., gray macerated or ulcerated areas at the corners of the mouth, are frequently present. Pain on swallowing is common. Anorexia, accompanied by epigastric discomfort, is a frequent complaint. *Diarrhea* has always been a prominent part of the pellagra syndrome. Stools are small, frequent, and watery, quite different from those in sprue. The liver ordinarily is not enlarged.

Neurologic signs rarely appear at the beginning of the disease but are common when skin or alimentary manifestations are prominent. Subjectively, the patient may complain of vertigo, weakness, headache, paresthesia, anesthesia, and general aches. Severe pain of the hands and feet may be present. Objectively, tendon reflexes are abnormal, usually diminished. Coarse tremors of the tongue, head, or extremities may be noted on examination. Muscular spasms are sometimes prominent. Mental disturbances have always been a feature of endemic pellagra; they include general "nervousness," confusion, depression, insomnia, apathy, and delirium. The picture is a varied one.

The above clinical manifestations account for the old description of pellagra as the disease of the four D's: "dementia, diarrhea, dermatitis, and death."

LABORATORY FINDINGS. Chemical examinations of the blood are of little help in pellagra. Occasionally hypoproteinemia, with low serum albumin values, is found. Gastric analysis reveals achlorhydria in about one-half the cases. On examination, the stools may show the presence of hookworm ova or other parasites in areas where infestations are prevalent. The content of N-methyl nicotinamide in the urine is helpful in assessing tryptophan-nicotinic acid nutriture in population groups, but this determination is of little help in the individual case. The urinary excretion of riboflavin may be decreased in pellagra.

Anemia is present in approximately one-half the cases of pellagra, but in only about one-quarter is it of any consequence. The anemia is not particularly specific.

PATHOLOGY. The earliest skin lesions show dilatation of the superficial blood vessels and proliferation of their endothelial cells. The superficial connective tissue elements of the corium assume a spongy appearance. The epidermis, which may already show hyperkeratosis, separates from the corium with the formation of a vesicle. There may be increased pigmentation of the superficial hyperkeratotic layer with decrease in pigment cells in the basal region. Chronic lesions merely show hyperkeratosis. The epithelium of the tongue is atrophic, with loss of papillae; a subacute inflammatory reaction may be present. The esophagus is commonly the site of acute inflammation with loss of epithelium. Alterations in the remainder of the intestinal tract are not particularly noteworthy, save in the colon. Here small ulcers may be present with abscess formation in the submucosa. Cystic dilatations of the mucous glands are prominent. The liver may contain excessive fat, which is usually periportal in distribution. The lining of the vagina frequently is acutely inflaméd with superficial ulceration. The neurologic changes are variable and consist of atrophy of cerebral neurones, degeneration of peripheral nerves, nerve roots, and tracts in the spinal cord. Bone marrow, if abnormal, may show a megaloblastic response or erythroblastic hyperplasia.

Pathogenesis. When man subsists on a diet of which the main staple is maize and in which there is little other protein, pellagra is likely to ensue. Maize is nutritionally inferior to other foods in a number of ways, particularly when modern milling procedures are employed. Its protein is low in quantity and, more important, in quality because it is low in two essential amino acids. Maize protein contains only a trace of tryptophan and low levels of lysine. Although maize contains appreciable quantities of nicotinic acid when assayed chemically, much of this vitamin is unavailable, since it cannot be assimilated from maize in the intestinal tract. Nicotinic acid is found in high concentrations in liver, yeast, red muscle meats, fish, and wheat germ. Vegetables and cereals contain much less. Coffee is a significant source of nicotinic acid.

In India, in contrast to many other countries, the use of millet and sorghum (jowar) in the diet, rather than maize, has been associated with the development of pellagra.

Meat protein, dairy products, and eggs are generally limited or entirely lacking in the pellagrin's diet. Furthermore, diets that have been associated with pellagra have been deficient not only in protein, but also in available nicotinic acid, riboflavin, thiamine, and vitamin B_{12}.

The multiple nutrient deficiency aspects of pellagra have been recognized for some time, and they cause one to ask: What is the definition of pellagra? Some workers would be restrictive and define the disease as pure tryptophan–nicotinic acid deficiency. The argument is that since the cardinal symptoms respond to nicotinic acid, pellagra should be regarded as a deficiency of this vitamin. Since, however, some of the classic symptoms and signs are alleviated not by nicotinic acid therapy but by other nutrients, it may be preferable to define pellagra as a multiple deficiency syndrome produced principally by deficiencies of tryptophan–nicotinic acid, riboflavin, and thiamine, and occasionally by folic acid, vitamin B_{12}, and possibly pyridoxine.

It is generally agreed that exposure of the skin to ultraviolet radiation may precipitate the appearance of dermal lesions or may increase the severity of those already present. In addition, the exposure of pellagrous subjects to sunlight may lead to effects in areas other than the skin; for instance, glossitis may be induced, nausea and vomiting may occur, or diarrhea may appear. The effect of sunlight helps to explain the seasonal variations in the prevalence of pellagra in the north temperate zones.

Individuals of different age groups are not equally affected by the disease. The greatest prevalence is in females, aged twenty to forty-five, i.e., the childbearing, lactating group. The next most common prevalence is usually found in children aged nine to fifteen years, but this statement must be qualified since these data come from Goldberger's studies in the southern United States at a time when child labor was extensive.

Sporadic cases of pellagra, not associated with a maize diet, are important, for today they comprise in the United States the commonest group of pellagrins. "Secondary" or "conditioned" pellagra may develop in persons who have some other disease. Disturbances of the gastrointestinal tract are the most common cause, e.g., gastric ulcer or carcinoma and various disturbances of the large and small intestine, particularly those which lead to diarrhea. The second most important group are the chronic alcoholics, although it is more usual for the chronic alcoholic to develop symptoms of thiamine deficiency. Polyneuritis, as well as the skin and other signs characteristic of pellagra, may be observed in the same individual.

DIAGNOSIS. Signs in endemic pellagra often are diagnostic. The dietary history is especially important. The diagnosis of incipient pellagra or the recognition of cases without skin manifestations ("pellagra sine pellagra") is more difficult. Here it may be necessary to evaluate the response to therapy with nicotinic acid and other nutrients. The estimation of N^1-methylnicotinamide concentration in the urine may be of help. The possibility of overt or subclinical pellagra should be considered in every person with a compatible diet history who suffers from gastrointestinal disease, particularly those conditions which lead to the malabsorption syndrome (Chap. 316). So, too, with any chronic alcoholic, the question of adequate nutrition with respect to nicotinic acid and other vitamins must always be considered.

Three forms of disorder with pellagra-like skin lesions, though uncommon, are worthy of mention. The first is an hereditary affliction called *Hartnup's disease* (Chap. 96). This syndrome consists of a pellagra-like skin rash following exposure to sunlight, intermittent cerebellar ataxia, renal aminoaciduria, and the excretion of large amounts of indole-3-acetic acid and indican in the urine. Increased quantities of protoporphyrin are found in the stool. Other manifestations of pellagra, such as glossitis, stomatitis, or gastrointestinal symptoms, are not present. The skin lesions respond to nicotinic acid therapy, suggesting that the metabolic disorder results from diversion of tryptophane from its normal route of degradation to pyrrole metabolites.

A second form of pellagra-like disease has been reported in patients receiving isoniazid, the *tuberculostatic* drug which is also a vitamin B_6 antagonist. In such patients peripheral neuritis and pellagra-like skin lesions appear and may not regress even when the drug is discontinued. Treatment with nicotinic acid often is efficacious in curing the skin lesions. Pyridoxine or B-complex preparations will usually relieve the neurologic manifestations.

The third disturbance in which pellagra-like skin lesions have been observed is associated with malignant carcinoid tumors (*malignant argentaffinomas*). These tumors produce such large amounts of 5-hydroxytryptamine (serotonin) from tryptophan that a conditioned form of tryptophan deficiency results. In addition to skin lesions, the patients may exhibit other characteristics of pellagra: mental confusion, diarrhea, and glossitis.

TREATMENT. Severely ill pellagrins, particularly those with diarrhea and dementia, should be treated as emergencies. Water and electrolyte deficits must be corrected immediately. Intravenous administration of nicotinic acid or nicotinamide in doses of 100 mg two or three times a day is recommended. These amounts can be added to physiologic salt solution containing 5% glucose. Nicotinamide is free from the unpleasant vasomotor effects of nicotinic acid. Other nutrients, particularly riboflavin, also are necessary. A practical, economical form of therapy is the administration of ½ to 1 oz debittered brewer's yeast in tomato juice three times a day. A high (3000 to 4000) calorie, high protein diet is desirable. Frequent feedings are advocated at first. Stomatitis, diarrhea or constipation, and oozing or ulcerated lesions of the skin will necessitate symptomatic medication.

PROGNOSIS. Until the advent of yeast and vitamin therapy, the prognosis of pellagra was grave, but now the prognosis is excellent. The glossitis begins to decrease in 24 hr; the papillae of the tongue will begin to regenerate by the end of the first week. Lesions of the lips begin to heal in 2 to 3 days. Gastrointestinal symptoms improve in 24 to 48 hr, and diarrhea will usually have ceased by the end of the first week. Demented patients usually become rational after 3 or 4 days, unless, of course, damage to the brain is irreversible. Polyneuritis, if present, may take some time to improve.

REFERENCES

Bean, W. B., T. D. Spies, and M. A. Blankenhorn: Secondary Pellagra, Medicine, 23:1, 1944.

FAO Nutritional Stuidies, "Maize and Maize Diets," no. 9, Rome, 1953.

Gillman, J., and T. Gillman: "Perspectives in Human Malnutrition: A Contribution to the Biology of Disease from a Clinical and Pathological Study of Chronic Malnutrition and Pellagra in the African," New York, Grune and Stratton, Inc., 1951.

Goldsmith, G. A., H. P. Sarett, V. D. Register, and J. Gibbens: Studies of Niacin Requirement in Man: I. Experimental Pellagra in Subjects on Corn Diets Low in Niacin and Tryptophan, J. Clin. Invest., 31:533, 1952.

Sydenstricker, V. P.: The History of Pellagra, Its Recognition As a Disorder of Nutrition and Its Conquest, Am. J. Clin. Nutrition, 6:409, 1958.

Terris, M. (Ed.): "Goldberger on Pellagra," Baton Rouge, La., Louisiana State University Press, 1964.

81 BERIBERI
Richard H. Follis, Jr. and George V. Mann

HISTORY. During the seventeenth, eighteenth, and nineteenth centuries, as a result of the increasing contacts of

European physicians with the Far East, a disease peculiar to that area became known to Western physicians. The principal characteristics of this disease, oriental beriberi, as described by a nineteenth-century physician, were "a feeling of numbness, sense of weight and weakness" in the legs, "edema of the feet," "unsteady and tottering walk" with "almost total palsy," "rigidity and various affections of the nerves," "oppression and weight in the precordium," and, occasionally, "sudden death." The disease was endemic throughout South China, Southeast Asia, the Philippines, the East Indies, and parts of India.

Studies soon revealed the close relationship of rice in the diet to the disease. Beriberi was eradicated from the Japanese Navy by Takaki, who added meat, vegetables, and condensed milk to the rice diet of the common sailor. In Batavia (now Djakarta), Eijkman observed a beriberi-like disease in fowl fed polished rice; the birds could be cured with unpolished grain. In Malaya, differences were noted in the prevalence of beriberi among persons who consumed parboiled rice and those who were accustomed to eat highly polished grain. By 1912, the therapeutic effectiveness of rice polishings had been demonstrated, particularly in patients with acute cardiac manifestations of beriberi. This led E. B. Vedder, a U.S. Army physician, to recommend to R. R. Williams, a chemist then working in Manila, that the protective substance be isolated. As a result, 20 years later Williams and his coworkers announced the chemical structure and synthesis of the active principle, thiamine. The metabolic role of thiamine was demonstrated at once.

PREVALENCE. Today the prevalence of clinical beriberi in the Far East is much reduced. One may encounter occasional cases of the disease, particularly in infants and pregnant or lactating women. Thiamine deficiency in the United States is most often seen in alcoholics. The presence of thiamine in enriched flour and white bread has no doubt diminished the prevalence of this disorder. The dramatically successful rice enrichment program in the Philippines has been discussed (Chap. 78). The desirability of enriching wines, beers, and whiskeys with thiamine has been considered but thought to be an undesirable endorsement.

CLINICAL FINDINGS. Three main types of beriberi have been recognized in the Orient: a chronic form in which neurologic involvement is prominent, an acute form with heart failure, and a less acute state in which edema is the most characteristic manifestation. The onset of the chronic neurologic form is insidious. Over the course of days or weeks, the patient comes to be easily fatigued and experiences heavy feelings in the legs, together with stiffness and aching in the muscles. In time the muscles become weaker, acutely painful, and then atrophic. The extensors of the foot usually are first affected, then the muscles of the calf and thigh. Pain followed by atrophy soon occurs in the muscles of the arms; the muscles of the trunk may be affected later. Associated with these signs and symptoms are foot drop and wrist drop, together with loss of reflexes at the ankle and knee. Paresthesias and anesthesias may be demonstrated, particularly over the lower extremities. Circumoral anesthesia may be present. Aphonia is sometimes a symptom. Walking becomes difficult, and the patient can only shuffle about with a cane or is forced to hold on to objects about him to keep from falling. Evidences of neurologic involvement may fluctuate. In time, however, the patient becomes completely bedridden. Involvement of the cerebrum is absent.

All the while, weight loss will have been progressing, and anorexia usually is persistent. Diarrhea may be more or less continuous. Evidences of cardiac involvement may accompany these neurologic disturbances or may appear suddenly in the absence of any evidence of involvement of the nervous system. The cardiac manifestations consist of palpitation, precordial pain, and dyspnea which may come on in paroxysms without warning. The heart is found to be enlarged and tachycardia is present. Prominent venous pulsations are noted in the neck. Edema usually is present. The blood pressure is not elevated, but the pulse pressure is increased and venous pressure is elevated. Death may result suddenly, with or without exertion.

Beriberi in infants has been and continues to be a health problem in the Far East. In babies the clinical classifications are the aphonic, in which the child loses his voice; the cardiologic, a sudden episode of cyanosis and cardiac arrest leading to death; and the pseudomeningitic with the manifestations of meningitis. These babies are typically born of mothers with low dietary intakes of thiamine and consequently low levels in their milk. The baby seems to flourish until quite suddenly it is stricken, usually at three to six months of age. The disorder is prevented by giving the mother thiamine and treated by the administration of thiamine to the infant. This will often bring a dramatic cure in a matter of hours.

In the mid-1930s, observers in large urban clinics in the Occident began to recognize instances of cardiac and neurologic disease occurring predominantly in alcoholics. In some areas the prevalence of these forms of *Occidental beriberi*, as these entities came to be called, was high. The clinical aspects of this form of heart disease are described in Chap. 264.

The symptoms and signs relative to neurologic involvement in alcoholics have the characteristics of a progressive polyneuritis with sensory and motor defects (Chaps. 118 and 363). Almost invariably there is a history of excessive consumption of alcohol and poor dietary intake. In addition, such patients frequently exhibit manifestations of delirium tremens, Korsakoff's syndrome, or Wernicke's disease. To such examples of neurologic involvement in poorly nourished, chronic alcoholics have been added other syndromes in recent years, such as amblyopia, central pontine myelinolysis, and corticocerebellar degeneration. None of these changes, including Wernicke's disease, has been described in beriberi occurring in Oriental peoples.

Thiamine is involved in a number of key reactions in glycolysis. Consequently, disturbances of lactate metabolism and of pentose phosphate shunt reactions would be expected to reflect alterations of these functions. However, the significance of elevated plasma levels of lactate and pyruvate in the diagnosis of thiamine deficiency is limited by the sensitivity of these to other factors, particularly physical exercise or the hypoxia associated with congestive failure. More useful is the measurement of the transketolase content of red blood cells. This enzyme functions in the pentose phosphate shunt and requires thiamine as a cofactor. Thus it is sensitive to deficiency states. The test is combined with an assessment of the effect of thiamine pyrophosphate added to the in vitro system, the so-called "TPP Effect." This amounts to an in vitro therapeutic trial. It is proving to be a most useful diagnostic procedure.

PATHOLOGY. From the above account of the clinical manifestations of beriberi, anatomic alterations might be expected in the nervous tissues and heart. Post-mortem examinations performed on patients dying with neurologic manifestations of beriberi at the turn of the century in the Orient revealed myelin degeneration of the peripheral nerves, with loss of axoplasm. Lesions in the brain and spinal cord have not been reported from the Orient. Among the sporadic cases designated as neurologic beriberi encountered in the Occident, usually among alcoholics, lesions of peripheral nerves have also been described. More prominent, however, are changes in the brain. Alterations characteristic of Wernicke's disease— bilateral hemorrhagic necrotic foci in the mammillary bodies, the hypothalamic nuclei, and midline structures —are found. Damage to the optic nerve and lesions in the spinal cord have been reported.

The heart is usually described as enlarged, but this increase in size is usually due to dilatation, although hypertrophy of the right ventricle has sometimes been noted. The myocardial fibers do not exhibit necrosis, although swelling and vacuolization may be prominent. No cellular infiltration is present.

PATHOGENESIS. Rice is the principal foodstuff of one-half or more of the inhabitants of the world. The introduction of power milling machinery at the end of the nineteenth century led to a great increase in beriberi in the Far East. When rice is highly milled, most of its vitamin content, such as thiamine, riboflavin, nicotinic acid, pantothenic acid, and pyridoxine, is removed. Lipids and minerals, such as calcium, iron, and iodine, which are present in the outer portions of the grain, are lost as well. Rice is milled to preserve its storage quality and, as with highly milled flour in the Western world, the refined product has come to be preferred by consumers. The protein content of rice is low, though its quality is good.

Although the rice eater's diet is deficient in a number of nutrients, the principal manifestations of beriberi— the derangements in cardiac and neurologic function— appear to be related to thiamine deficiency. The therapeutic response of the patient with cardiac beriberi, whether infant or adult, to thiamine is good evidence for this relationship. The development of anatomic lesions in the heart of experimental animals deprived of thiamine is further proof for the relation of this vitamin to the integrity of the myocardium. Thiamine is involved in several enzymatic transformations involving pyruvate, alpha-ketoglutarate and in the transketolase reaction mentioned above. The explanation for the edema probably is two-fold; heart failure and protein malnutrition.

The precise relationship of thiamine to maintenance of the integrity of the peripheral nervous system is uncertain. The predilection of the nervous system for injury in thiamine deficiency suggests that the vitamin is especially crucial for those tissues which depend upon carbohydrate metabolism exclusively for their energy sources. The clinical response to thiamine usually is not rapid, though this can be explained on the basis that damage has been severe enough to have caused structural loss. Hence, regeneration is necessary if function is to be restored. Lesions of the peripheral nerves have been difficult to produce in experimental animals. In contrast, the manifestations of Wernicke's disease may clear up in a few hours after thiamine administration, and lesions similar to those observed in Wernicke's disease have been demonstrated in the brains of thiamine-deficient animals. The enigma of the absence of Wernicke's disease in the Orient (except among Western prisoners of war) remains.

DIAGNOSIS. In the Orient, the symptoms are characteristic enough. Certain simple tests are helpful: pain when the calf muscles are squeezed, anesthesia to pinprick over the anterior surface of the tibia, loss of patellar reflex, and inability to rise from the squatting position. The presence of pitting edema and manifestations of cardiac involvement help with the diagnosis when they are present.

The diagnosis of the occasional case in the Occident is more difficult. Here the dietary history, particularly if alcoholism has been present, is important. Evidence of neurologic involvement usually is the most prominent symptom.

TREATMENT. When there is cardiac involvement in infants or adults, beriberi becomes a medical emergency. The immediate administration of thiamine is important. Intravenous administration of 10 to 20 mg thiamine, two or three times a day, is recommended. Doses of thiamine, 3 to 5 mg orally two or three times a day, should be adequate for the ordinary patient. A balanced diet is important in prevention.

PROGNOSIS. The response of infants and adults with cardiac beriberi in the Orient is one of the most dramatic in medicine. Cardiac symptoms improve rapidly. Diuresis begins within the first 12 hr. In the Occident such dramatic responses are not seen as often. When neurologic involvement is present, response to therapy is much more gradual. However, as mentioned above, the ophthalmoplegia, ataxia, and nystagmus of Wernicke's disease respond to thiamine, as do mental symptoms such as apathy and drowsiness. Amentia responds less rapidly.

REFERENCES

Brin, M.: Erythrocyte Transketolase in Early Thiamine Deficiency, Ann. N.Y. Acad. Sci., 98:528, 1962.

Kinney, T. D., and R. H. Follis, Jr. (Eds.): Nutritional Disease: Beriberi, Fed. Proc., 17: Supp. 2, 3, 1958.

Vedder, E. B., "Beriberi," New York, William Wood & Company, 1913.

Victor M., and R. D. Adams: On the Etiology of the Alcoholic Neurological Diseases, Am. J. Clin. Nutrition, 9:379, 1961.

Williams, R. R.: "Toward the Conquest of Beriberi," Cambridge, Mass., Harvard University Press, 1961.

82 SCURVY
Richard H. Follis, Jr. and George V. Mann

HISTORY. Although accounts of a disease which might be construed as scurvy are found in ancient writings, the first clear-cut descriptions appear in records of the Crusades. When the long sea voyages of discovery began toward the end of the fifteenth century, scurvy became commonplace and soon ranked first among causes of disability and mortality in sailors. Scurvy on land appeared among military and civilian population groups as a result of the many European wars which led to troop movements and civilian displacement.

In 1747 James Lind, a British naval surgeon, in a model experiment, studied the effects of several types of treatment, including one composed of "two oranges and one lemon given every day" on sailors with typical signs of scurvy: "putrid gums, the spots and lassitude, with weakness of their knees." The curative efficacy of these citrus fruits was clear.

Infantile scurvy began to receive attention after 1883, when Barlow described the syndrome as it is recognized today: the swollen, tense, exquisitely painful, flexed lower extremities; crepitus at the ends of the shafts of the bones; swollen, bleeding gums; and subcutaneous hemorrhages. With increasing use of breast milk substitutes, scurvy became common in the urban areas of Europe and the United States at the turn of the century.

A disease of the growing bones of guinea pigs, quite like that seen in children, was produced by dietary means in 1907. Investigators then had a way to assay antiscorbutic materials, and 25 years later, C. G. King and his associates isolated from lemon juice a biologically active, crystalline material. This compound was later synthesized and shown to be ascorbic acid.

PREVALENCE. In previous times scurvy in adults tended to occur in epidemic-like outbreaks. Scurvy now is seen in isolated individuals, usually lonely men whose diet is grossly unbalanced and devoid of sources of ascorbic acid (*bachelor scurvy*). Each year in urban clinics in the United States and Europe such examples of adult scurvy are encountered. Occasional cases of scurvy continue to appear in pediatric clinics, usually a result of maternal error or ignorance.

CLINICAL FINDINGS. There are three principal manifestations of scurvy in the adult: swollen gums with loss of teeth, skin lesions, and pain and weakness in the lower extremities. The clinical course of the disease is understood as a result of studies on volunteers in whom ascorbic acid deficiency was deliberately produced. The first change, which was observed after approximately 140 days, was prominence of the hair follicles, usually those over the back and thighs. This prominence is due to plugging of the lumens with an excessive amount of keratin, which leads to an impediment to hair growth so that the hair becomes coiled upon itself within the follicle. The epithelium surrounding each follicle becomes hyperemic, and blood cells extravasate into the tissues. These disappear leaving deposits of pigment, so that the perifollicular area becomes discolored. Large confluent ecchymoses appear over the seat in a saddle pattern. Petechiae tend to appear on the dorsal surfaces with application of a tourniquet. Lesions in the mouth appear after approximately 200 days of deprivation. Reddening and swelling of the interdental papillae occur first, soon followed by hemorrhage. The time of appearance and degree of severity of the gum changes are related to the state of oral hygiene. Pain and weakness in the extremities have been prominent in experimental studies. Old scars become tender and livid, and new injuries heal slowly.

The clinical picture in children is very different from that observed in adults. The peak incidence is 8 months; few cases are seen after the first year. The most prominent sign on physical examination is tenderness of the lower extremities, which are also usually somewhat swollen. The legs are characteristically partially flexed and guarded. Involvement of the upper extremities is less common. The extremities are obviously painful; the child screams when approached. The costochondral junctions may be enlarged. Crepitus of the epiphyseal areas of the ankles and wrists may be felt. The gums are swollen and hemorrhagic when teeth are present, but show little change before teeth erupt. Subcutaneous hemorrhages may be observed; these tend to be in the form of ecchymoses, not the pinpoint hemorrhages seen about the follicles in the adult. Follicular lesions are uncommon in children. Hemorrhages occur elsewhere: suborbital with proptosis, epistaxis, hematuria, or signs of subdural bleeding.

LABORATORY FINDINGS. The concentration of ascorbic acid may be determined in samples of plasma or in the buffy coat layer. Zero levels may be present in the plasma of adults for months before tissue stores are depleted. The plasma level mirrors the recent intake of ascorbic acid. Even if minimal or zero concentrations of ascorbic acid are present in plasma, the clinical syndrome will likely not be present. When adults subsist on an intake of 10 mg ascorbic acid per day, the concentrations of the vitamin in the buffy coat average about 2 mg per 100 ml. In such instances no clinical evidence of scurvy is present. On a vitamin C-deficient diet, the ascorbic acid concentration in the buffy coat falls to 1 mg or less after 4 to 6 months. At these values clinical scurvy may become manifest.

Saturation or load tests may be of some help in evaluating ascorbic acid nutriture. When adequate amounts of the vitamin are being ingested, the urinary output will be about 25 to 75 mg per 100 ml. Urinary output will be virtually zero when the body stores are depleted. If 200 mg ascorbic acid is administered each day and urinary excretion of the vitamin is small during the first 3 or 4 days, this indicates that the stores are reduced.

PATHOLOGY. In adults studied at autopsy, the most conspicuous finding is the presence of generalized hemorrhage. The perifollicular lesions and ecchymoses noted clinically are conspicuous. In addition, extravasations of blood are found in the pericardial or pleural cavities, walls of the intestinal tract, bladder, and renal pelves. In young adults separation of the epiphyses or costochondral junctions may be present, as well as subperiosteal hemorrhage.

In children the most characteristic changes at autopsy are in the skeleton. The periosteum has separated or may be easily stripped from the shaft of a bone; the costal or epiphyseal cartilages have separated from the shaft of the rib or a long bone. Microscopic examination at the cartilage-shaft junction shows a dense "lattice" of spicules of calcified cartilaginous matrix, many of which have fractured. Little bone has formed on this lattice, which furthermore, has not been destroyed. In less advanced cases, fractures occur only at the edges or corners of the bone. Hemorrhage may be observed in the marrow or beneath the periosteum. As a result of decreased osteoid formation, the cortex and trabeculae of the shaft are reduced in thickness. Aside from hemorrhages elsewhere—subdural, subpleural, and subcutaneous—little else is found that is specific for scurvy. Rickets frequently coexists in such children.

PATHOGENESIS. Scurvy represents the reaction of particular hosts, such as man, other primates, and the guinea pig, to a lack of ascorbic acid in the diet. Most mammalian species can synthesize the vitamin. Ascorbic acid is found in high concentrations in citrus and other fruits, leafy vegetables, tubers, most grasses, and sprouting plants. The vitamin content of human milk varies, since the mother is dependent on dietary sources. Milk from a well-nourished woman contains 5 to 7 mg per 100 ml. Fresh cow's milk contains 1.0 to 2.6 mg per 100 ml; however, storage and sterilizing reduces this to virtually zero in dairy milk. Scurvy is virtually unheard of in breast-fed infants unless the mother is deficient. On the other hand, the use of sterilized infant formulas prepared from cow's milk or proprietary foods may be expected to produce scurvy in infants if the diet is not supplemented with a source of ascorbic acid.

Scurvy is, broadly speaking, a genetic disease in that the tissues of these species appear to have lost their ability to synthesize ascorbic acid. The chemical steps in the formation of the vitamin are well known:

a. D-glucuronate + TPNH + H$^+$ → L-gulonate + TPN$^+$

b. L-gulonate + DPN$^+$ → L-gulonolactone + DPN$^+$ + H$^+$

c. L-gulonolactone → L-ascorbate + H$_2$O

Liver and kidney tissues of all mammalian species so far studied can carry out reactions *a* and *b*. Only liver cells can form L-ascorbate via reaction *c*, but the hepatic tissues of man, other primates, and guinea pigs cannot carry this out.

The basic structural disturbance in scurvy is the failure of various types of connective tissue cells to form their respective collagenous matrices. Fibroblasts are unable to elaborate collagen; osteoblasts and odontoblasts do not synthesize osteoid and dentine. The lack of formation of these matrices explains the failure of wounds to heal, the changes in the growing bone of infants and children, and the alterations in the teeth of experimental animals. What is the underlying biochemical lesion? Collagen is characterized chemically by large amounts of glycine, proline, and hydroxyproline. The presence of the latter, a hydroxy-amino acid, and of hydroxylysine make collagen unique, since these amino acids are not found in other proteins. Hydroxyproline is not synthesized in the absence of ascorbic acid. This is most important when it is recalled that exogenous hydroxyproline is normally not incorporated into collagen. All the hydroxyproline in the basic

Fig. 82-1. The film shows four characteristic changes of scurvy. A large subperiosteal hemorrhage is being calcified. The epiphyseal margin shows a translucent line medially, the "corner sign" of Park. The epiphyseal plates are dense, and the bone shaft shows a ground-glass appearance with lack of trabecular detail. (*Photograph courtesy, Dr. Henry Burko, Vanderbilt University*)

collagen molecule is derived from the hydroxylation of proline in vivo. The point in collagen synthesis at which hydroxylation of proline takes place is not clear at this time. In ascorbic acid–deficient organisms, the connective tissue cells can proliferate. However, their microscopic appearance implies their functional impotency. Their cytoplasm is scanty, and virtually no stainable RNA is present. What this means in terms of altered synthetic mechanisms is obscure at this time.

The role of ascorbic acid in the integrity of blood vessels is not clear. The characteristic perifollicular hemorrhages indicate a defect in the vascular wall. Under the biomicroscope, capillary dilatation may be observed. Since the integrity of collagen is affected as a result of ascorbic acid deficiency, it is possible that the blood vessels may lose the support provided by these fibers and, hence, become more liable to the effects of minor trauma.

Certain other metabolic defects may be observed as a result of ascorbic acid deficiency, though these are not usually considered part of the scurvy syndrome. One of the most interesting aspects of ascorbic acid function is its nonspecific relation to metabolism of the aromatic amino acids, phenylalanine and tyrosine. Premature infants deficient in ascorbic acid excrete relatively large amounts of parahydroxyphenyllactic acid and parahydroxyphenylpyruvic acid in the urine when excess phenylalanine and tyrosine are administered. The defect appears to be an inability to metabolize the tyrosine. Ascorbic acid is implicated in the secretion of the aqueous humor. The vitamin also plays a role in the metabolism of folic acid, i.e., in the transformation of this material to folacin (citrovorum factor). Occasionally, scurvy is associated with a macrocytic anemia which responds to citrovorum factor.

DIAGNOSIS. The clinical features of full-blown scurvy in adults or infants are characteristic. A most important point to emphasize is the feeding history in infants. If an infant four to six months or older has been bottle-fed with boiled milk or milk substitutes from birth or shortly after and has received no supplemental ascorbic acid, the possibility of scurvy should be considered. The feeding history of adults is likewise important because the disease often is observed in individuals subsisting on diets obviously low in ascorbic acid content. The history relative to vitamin C intake is easy to obtain.

X-ray examination in the adult is not of particular help in diagnosing scurvy, except that one may see alterations in the lamina dura of the jaws. In infants, x-ray examination of the skeleton may be helpful. At the junction between the epiphyseal cartilage and shaft of the long bones, there may be a zone of increased density, which represents the area of excess spicules of calcified cartilaginous matrix, some of which may have fractured (Fig. 82-1). There may also be defects, i.e., areas of rarefaction, at the "corners" of the bones, and these result from fractures at the periphery of the junction between cartilage and shaft. The formation of spurs or projections of the periosteum about the margins of the cartilage also are characteristic. In addition, the bone film will show a "ground glass" appearance, which reflects the decrease in density due to diminished width of the cortices and size of the medullary trabeculae.

TREATMENT. In infants the administration of fresh orange juice in single or multiple doses per day is advised. This may be sweetened with sugar. If orange juice is refused, twice the amount of tomato juice is the next choice. Synthetic ascorbic acid may be employed orally, 100 to 300 mg per day. There is little need for parenteral therapy. In view of the changes that have taken place in the skeleton, children in whom the disease is in the stage of healing should be handled as little and as gently as possible. It is not necessary to manipulate any bony deformities, nor should splints or casts be applied.

Treatment in adults involves administration of orange juice or ascorbic acid in divided doses up to 500 mg per day. A diet rich in vitamin C should be initiated and continued in both children and adults.

PROGNOSIS. Under therapy gum lesions, if present in infants and in adults, begin to regress in 2 to 3 days. Periosteal shadows, resulting from new bone formation, begin to appear in the long bones of infants after approximately a week. Hemorrhages in the skin usually disappear in 2 to 3 weeks.

REFERENCES

Barlow, T.: On Cases Described as "Acute Rickets" Which Are Probably a Combination of Scurvy and Rickets, the Scurvy Being an Essential and the Rickets a Variable Element, Med. Chir. Trans., 66:159, 1883.

Gould, B. S.: Collagen Formation and Fibrogenesis with Special Reference to the Role of Ascorbic Acid, Int. Rev. Cytol., 15:301, 1963.

Hess, A. F.: "Scurvy, Past and Present," Philadelphia, J. B. Lippincott Company, 1920.

Medical Research Council: Vitamin C Requirements of Human Adults, Spec. Rep. Ser., no. 280, London, 1953.

Park, E. A., H. G. Guild, D. Jackson, and M. Bond: The Recognition of Scurvy with Special Reference to the Early X-ray Changes, Arch. Dis. Child., 10:265, 1935.

83 VITAMIN D DEFICIENCY AND HYPERVITAMINOSIS D

George Nichols, Jr.

VITAMIN D DEFICIENCY

INTRODUCTION. Deficiency of vitamin D, whether the result of dietary inadequacy, lack of exposure to sunlight, failure of absorption, or defective metabolism and utilization, results in either rickets or osteomalacia—conditions which differ from each other only because of the presence or absence of active bone growth. Thus rickets begins in childhood, although its manifestations may persist throughout life, while osteomalacia begins after skeletal growth has been completed.

HISTORY. These diseases have been known since an-

tiquity, with references to soft, waxy bones being found in Plato's writings. The prevalence of these diseases seems to have increased when people began living in cities, presumably because of dietary lack or inadequate exposure to ultraviolet light rather than poverty; even Charles I of England and his second daughter were severely afflicted with rickets. The first complete description of the disease is usually attributed to Glisson, in whose book, published in 1650, the well-known physical signs, "swellings and knotty excrescences about some of the joynts," "tumors in the tops of the ribs where they are conjoyned with gristles in the breast," "breasts of a hen or capon," and "crooked bones" are described. However, an equally careful description was published 5 years earlier by Whistler, then a medical student at Leiden.

The true nature and origins of these diseases were not understood until Mellanby produced, by dietary means, a ricketslike condition in dogs which could be prevented by an antirachitic vitamin found in certain fats and oils. Between 1918 and 1927 the pathogenesis of rickets was virtually completely elucidated: The disease was induced and studied histologically in experimental animals; the importance of the concentrations of calcium and phosphorus relative to one another was demonstrated; the antirachitic vitamin was proved to be a specific compound, vitamin D, which by 1927 had been chemically identified; the role of ultraviolet radiation in activating a provitamin in foods and in the skin was demonstrated; deranged concentrations of calcium and phosphorus in the serum of rachitic children were described and found to return to normal after therapy with vitamin D; healing processes in the bones were followed roentgenographically and histologically; and calcification of rachitic cartilage *in vitro* was produced by suitable concentrations of calcium and phosphorus in the incubation medium.

PREVALENCE. Vitamin D enrichment of animal and human food has effectively prevented rickets so that the disease in its florid forms has become a rarity in technically advanced countries. Rickets was found only in 1 in 2,800 North American pediatric admissions in 1962. However, rickets has persisted in North Africa and other underdeveloped areas, and the disease is still seen in urban areas in the United Kingdom, where migratory populations from the West Indies and Pakistan, especially, have come from a sunny to a clouded climate and have not taken advantage of the preventive measures.

While the most common type of rickets continues to be that due to vitamin D deficiency, abnormalities of calcium and phosphorus metabolism are beginning to be recognized more and more frequently as causes of so-called "endogenous," or "conditioned," rickets.

Osteomalacia is now uncommon in both developed and developing countries. In the past, however, famine accompanying war gave rise to many cases of osteomalacia, particularly in women. In North China, osteomalacia has been common as a result of low calcium intake, insufficient sunlight, and many pregnancies. A similar situation has been described in Moslem women in *purdah*. Virtually all instances of osteomalacia encountered in the

Western World now are due to some conditioning factor related to abnormal vitamin D or calcium and phosphorus metabolism, such as poor absorption, excessive intestinal loss, disordered metabolic turnover, or increased renal excretion.

CLINICAL FINDINGS. Uncomplicated Rickets. The cardinal signs of *uncomplicated rickets* are muscular hypotonia and skeletal deformities. The pattern of the skeletal deformities is influenced largely by the age at which the disease becomes manifest. If it begins when the infant is recumbent, the effects of pressure due to gravity tend to produce flattening of the skull, thorax, and pelvic girdle. If the child has been able to sit up, kyphosis or deformity of the forearms and anterior bowing of the lower legs are found if the extremities have been crossed or if the feet hang over the edge of a chair. When the child can walk, further vertebral and pelvic deformity may ensue, as well as curvatures of the lower extremities such as bow legs, knock-knees, and even fractures.

Among the first physical signs of rickets to appear in the infant are softened areas in the skull, *craniotabes*. The bone may be readily depressed because of lack of rigidity, resulting from decreased deposition of inorganic materials. Craniotabes is not a specific sign of rickets, however, and may be observed in other diseases such as osteogenesis imperfecta and hydrocephalus. There may also be thickening and/or bossing of the cranial bones, particularly the parietal or frontal structures. Costochondral swellings, or beadings (*rachitic rosary*),

Fig. 83-1. The x-ray changes of the long bones in juvenile rickets. The shaft of the tibia is deformed; the metaphysis is widened, irregular, cupped, and translucent. (*Photo courtesy, Dr. Henry Burko, Vanderbilt University.*)

are among the cardinal signs of rickets, but similar changes may be observed in scurvy. With the development of the rachitic rosary, the lateral configuration of the thorax becomes flattened, and the sternum is pushed forward to form the so-called *"pigeon breast."* The ribs are deformed by inward stress at the points of attachment of the diaphragm and form *"Harrison's grooves."* These deformities reduce the volume of the thorax sometimes to such a degree that ventilation may be seriously impaired. Kyphosis of the lower thoracic and upper lumbar spine is found if the child has begun to sit up but disappears if the infant is suspended. Bilateral swellings of the ankles, and particularly the wrists, are characteristic. The shafts of the long bones may be thickened. Greenstick fractures may occur. Curvatures, either outward (bowlegs, *genu varum*) or inward (knock-knees, *genu valgum*) are prominent, and bending of the lower leg may lead to anterior curvature. Twisting of the metaphysis may result in *coxa vara.*

Primary dentition is delayed, and the order of tooth eruption may be abnormal. The enamel of the permanent teeth may show pits or grooves. In severe cases enamel may be virtually absent.

Hypocalcemic tetany can occur in rickets, usually appearing near the onset of the disease and sometimes in the healing stage. The lowered serum calcium concentration may on occasion be sufficient to lead to laryngeal spasm, convulsions, and death.

Both growth and weight gain generally are normal in uncomplicated rickets. There is, however, an extreme form of this disorder known as *dystrophic rickets,* or *osteomalacic rickets,* which apparently also is due to vitamin D deficiency. Here the muscular hypotonia and bony deformities are extreme, growth and weight gain cease, and multiple fractures as well as severe anemia and hepatosplenomegaly can occur. Whether other nutritional deficiencies besides vitamin D are involved in this condition is not clear, but like the more common form of rickets, dystrophic rickets responds dramatically (if more slowly) to treatment with vitamin D.

Osteomalacia. The clinical aspects of *osteomalacia* in adults are not as dramatic as those seen in the growing child. Weakness and/or vague aches and pains in various parts of the skeleton, back, pelvis, ribs, and extremities usually are the earliest signs. When skeletal pain is present, it tends to be generalized and persistent in contrast to the episodic "lumbago" of osteoporosis. As the disease progresses, weakness becomes sufficiently severe to confine the patient to bed, and spontaneous fractures or collapse of vertebras can occur. Tetany may be encountered, and, if the disease has been present for a long time, curvatures of the extremities may be present. Bone pain on pressure may also be present. As noted, osteomalacia due solely to dietary deficiency is rare, so that the presence of conditions such as intestinal malabsorption or certain renal or other abnormalities which create an increased demand for vitamin D should be suspected, and vice-versa.

LABORATORY FINDINGS. The serum calcium concentration in rickets generally is normal or at the lower limit of normal, while serum phosphorus values are reduced from the normal childhood level of 5 to 6 mg to 2 to 4 mg per 100 ml. In some individuals, serum calcium and not phosphorus may be reduced. In premature babies both calcium and phosphorus concentration may be lower than normal. Adults with vitamin D–deficient osteomalacia show similar changes, with serum calcium values being normal, while serum phosphorus concentration usually is somewhat reduced below the normal level of 3 to 4 mg per 100 ml. Serum alkaline phosphatase activity generally is elevated in both disorders, although normal values are occasionally encountered in mild cases. Other abnormalities include mild metabolic acidosis, amino aciduria, glycosuria, and increased excretion of hydroxyproline in the urine. Reductions in plasma and urinary citrate values together with increased fecal excretion of calcium and phosphate may be observed.

RADIOLOGY. The radiologic signs of rickets reflect the inadequate mineralization and overproduction of osteoid which are the hallmarks of the skeletal pathology in this disease. Thus, in the growing child, the metaphyses of the long bones are wide, their upper surfaces tend to be cupped, and the span of the growth cartilage is markedly widened. The epiphyses are small and irregular and the trabeculae are indistinct. Thinning of the cortex, bowing, fractures (especially of the greenstick type), and other deformities are present (Fig. 83-1).

In osteomalacia, the epiphyseal changes are not seen because the disease develops after they have closed. Therefore, thinning of the cortex of the long bones; deformities, including marked bowing, especially of the weight-bearing bones of the lower extremities; fractures, and pseudofractures are the distinguishing features. "Pseudofractures," or *Looser's zones*, are characteristic bands of decalcification which are perpendicular or oblique to the surface of the bone. They are considered pathognomonic of osteomalacia but are seen in rickets as well. While usually straight, they may zigzag. On either side of the band, a denser shadow of callus often helps make the band more obvious. Looser's zones tend to be symmetrical, and their distribution is fairly constant: the neck of the humerus and femur, the pubic rami, the ribs, and especially the axillary borders of the scapulae. In addition, subperiosteral erosions, similar to those found in hyperparathyroidism, have been reported to occur in as many as 50 percent of cases.

Although the reversal of radiologic changes with treatment is relatively slow in osteomalacia, reversal begins quite promptly in rickets, the first change being the appearance of a dense band of calcification midway between the epiphysis and metaphysis. This becomes quite distinct between the eighth and thirteenth day following the onset of vitamin D therapy. Mineralization begins in this area and ultimately spreads to involve the entire uncalcified metaphyseal area. After several months, complete healing may be found; alternatively, the cortical bone in the concavity of bowed bones may remain thickened, resulting in some narrowing of the normal marrow cavity. Islands of cartilage which fail to calcify adequately occasionally are trapped in the diaphysis and

appear as translucent defects in otherwise healthy tissue.

The radiologic changes found in rickets and osteomalacia generally are quite easy to distinguish from other conditions, although in the absence of pseudofractures, osteomalacia may not be easily differentiated from osteoporosis by radiologic criteria alone. Biopsy will show a striking excess of osteoid in osteomalacia which is not found in osteoporosis, thus establishing the diagnosis in doubtful cases.

PATHOLOGY. The distinguishing features of the skeletal changes in both rickets and osteomalacia are defective mineralization and a relative overabundance of new uncalcified bone matrix or osteoid. The relative undermineralization of the skeleton is manifested *chemically* by a reduction in the mineral ash content of the dried bone solids from more than 60 to less than 50 percent. In addition to excess osteoid there is a greater than normal number of osteoblasts. Widened osteoid seams are noted in the cortical bone in areas which have been remodeled recently. The trabeculae have prominent borders of osteoid. In some patients, evidence of excessive destruction of the bone formed before the disease began or of newly produced osteoid may be observed; the number of osteoclasts may be increased as well as osteoblasts. In addition, in the growth cartilage defective calcification along the columns of hypertrophic cells is found.

In rickets, the degree of involvement of the different parts of the skeleton is related to the rate of growth of the different bones. Because the anterior ends of middle ribs grow fastest, the disease is most marked there. For the same reason, the epiphyses about the knee, shoulder, and wrist show more change than the opposite ends of these bones. Since osteomalacia is rickets in adults in whom epiphyseal growth has ceased, the conspicuous change is found only in the bone biopsy, where the osteoid seams noted above are seen.

As healing of rickets occurs, inorganic material appears in the matrix about the most recently matured hypertrophic cartilage cells (Muller's line). Calcification of the oldest osteoid seems to occur first in membranous bones. Healing of osteomalacia is indicated by disappearance of the osteoid borders and ultimately of the osteoid seams in the dense cortical bone.

In cases of classic vitamin D–deficiency rickets, little that is specific besides bone lesions is to be found at autopsy. A fairly constant finding in cases of long-standing rickets and osteomalacia is enlargement and increased cellularity of the parathyroid glands. However, when rickets or osteomalacia is secondary to malabsorption or renal disease, pathologic changes in the gastrointestinal tract, including obstruction of the bile or pancreatic ducts may be present. The kidney may show abnormalities in the structure of the nephron; such as the shortening of the renal tubules which has been reported in cases of phosphate diabetes with aminoaciduria. In addition, chronic renal disease in the form of chronic glomerulonephritis, interstitial, or pyelonephritis may be present.

PATHOGENESIS. Rickets may be defined as a disease of the developing skeleton characterized by defective mineralization of the organic matrices of the cartilage and bone. Because osteomalacia is rickets in adults in whom cartilagenous growth has ceased, it may be defined as the skeletal disease in adults which is characterized by defective mineralization of the bone matrix.

Several lines of evidence indicate that both rickets and osteomalacia are due to lack of vitamin D specifically and not just to a decreased calcium-phosphorus ion concentration product in the body fluids as was once thought. In brief, experimental rickets characterized by increased osteoid and decreased mineralization can be produced in animals by vitamin D–deficiency alone and occurs regardless of the levels of calcium and phosphate which are fed. Indeed, calcium deficiency alone inhibits bone growth (and has been cited as a cause of osteoporosis), but the osteoid which is laid down is normally calcified and excessively wide osteoid seams are never seen. It is important to note that *phosphate deficiency* (with or without lowered serum phosphate concentrations) and ingestion of a number of foreign ions, notably strontium, beryllium, and fluoride, can produce bone disease with many of the outward features of rickets and osteomalacia. These differ in several important respects, however, from the condition produced by vitamin D deficiency; parathyroid enlargement is absent, serum calcium concentrations are almost invariably normal, and vitamin D is not curative.

Vitamin D is a sterol derivative formed in nature by the irradiation of ergosterol or 7-dehydrocholesterol, with ultraviolet light of a wave length between 250 and 312 mμ. This opens the B ring to produce either ergocalciferol (vitamin D$_2$) when ergosterol from plant sources is irradiated, or cholicalciferol (vitamin D$_3$) when 7-dehydrocholesterol, the precursor found in normal human skin, is exposed. The sterol derivative, AT-10 has vitamin D activity but offers no advantage over vitamin D$_2$ and is more expensive.

The international unit of vitamin D activity is defined as the amount that is equal in potency to 1 mg of the international standard of the irradiated ergosterol. This is equivalent to 0.025 μg of pure crystalline calciferol (40,000 units = 1 mg of calciferol). Thus two related substances with vitamin D activity are available to the organism: Vitamin D$_2$ is less effective biologically in birds and at least some of the New World primates, but the two forms appear to be equally effective in human beings.

Vitamin D occurs only in very small amounts in common foods such as cereals, vegetables, and fruit. Liver, butterfat, and egg yolk contain small amounts (8 to 20 units per 100 grams). Human and cow's milk also are poor sources, but most marine fish contain appreciable amounts and liver oils are particularly high in vitamin D content. Cod-liver oil contains 8,500 units; halibut, 60,000; and the oil from the liver of the blue-fin tuna, some 4,000,000 units per 100 ml. In many countries, including the United States, dietary sources, usually milk, margarine, or butter are fortified with additional vitamin D. The required level in this country is 400 international units per quart of milk.

The high fat solubility of vitamin D and its insolubility in water explain the failure of dietary sources to provide adequate amounts of the vitamin under a variety of pathological conditions; an example is steatorrhea due to intestinal malabsorption, blockade of the bile ducts, or pancreatic disease. Occasionally rickets or osteomalacia occurs in individuals ingesting excessive amounts of mineral oil. Similarly, the need for exposure to sunlight explains the geographical prevalence of these disorders in northern countries and the particular susceptibility of Negroes to these diseases, because the pigment in their skins tends to absorb much of the ultraviolet radiation before it can reach the Malpighian layer where the vitamin D precursor is found.

The absorption of dietary vitamin D from the gastrointestinal tract has been studied with isotopically labeled materials. Vitamin D is absorbed with the chylomicrons and very low density lipoproteins into the lymph. Thus the presence of fat and bile salts in the gastrointestinal tract is of great importance to normal absorption of vitamin D. The vitamin is transported via the circulation to the liver, where it is converted to the metabolically active form, 25-hydroxycholecalciferol. From there it is distributed to its target organs, gut, skeletal tissue, and kidney. The highest concentrations per cell are found in the intestine and skeleton.

The presence of vitamin D is apparently of critical importance to the absorption of calcium by the intestinal mucosa. This action seems to be particularly important in the upper part of the small intestine, the major site of active transport. The exact biochemical mechanism involved in this action has yet to be identified. However, DeLuca and Avioli, while searching for an explanation of the delay in the onset of vitamin D action following its administration, were able to demonstrate metabolic conversion of the vitamin to a biologically active form during this interval. Other work in which binding of the metabolically active derivative of vitamin D (25-hydroxycolicalciferol) to the nuclear membrane in the cells of target tissues (bone and gut) and the induction of RNA synthesis in these tissues under its influence, suggest that the primary action of the metabolic derivative is upon the synthesis of messenger RNA and thereby, perhaps, the synthesis of a specific calcium-binding protein.

For many years, it was thought that the sole action of vitamin D was on the intestine, but it is now clear that it acts on the skeleton as well, in two ways. First, without vitamin D normal calcification of the osteoid laid down during remodeling does not occur in vitro or in vivo, regardless of the calcium and phosphate concentration. Some vitamin D also seems to be required for the calcium-mobilizing action of parathyroid hormone on the skeleton. In addition, *large* doses of vitamin D appear to mimic the action of parathyroid hormone because they cause mobilization of mineral from the skeleton, resulting in increases in serum calcium concentration and urinary calcium excretion, both to abnormally high levels.

Less information is available concerning the action of vitamin D on the kidney. Both increases and decreases in tubular absorption of calcium have been reported, although the most recent and well-controlled studies suggest that calcium reabsorption in the proximal tubule is probably increased as a result of the action of the vitamin. On the other hand, it is clear that phosphate excretion may be increased by vitamin D just as it is by parathyroid hormone.

Vitamin D–deficient Rickets and Osteomalacia. With these facts in mind, the mechanism of the development of rickets and osteomalacia secondary to a deficient supply of vitamin D can be understood. Calcium absorption from the gut is decreased, and its excretion in the feces is increased by taking with it larger amounts of phosphate. Decreased mineralization of the growing cartilage of bone occurs partly because the availability of calcium is inadequate, but more importantly, because the mechanism for calcium deposition in the plate is somehow blocked. Failure of adequate intestinal absorption of calcium together with deficient resorption of bone tends to lower the serum calcium, and this in turn stimulates the parathyroid gland to excessive secretion. While the parathyroid hyperactivity maintains the serum calcium at normal concentration, it is also accompanied by decreased concentration of serum phosphate because of increased urinary excretion of that ion. This secondary hyperparathyroidism is probably responsible for the interesting effects of feeding phosphate to rachitic children. Ingestion of 100 mg per kg of this ion is without effect in normal children but often sharply lowers the calcium concentration in the serum of rachitic children, sometimes to tetanic levels. Indeed an acute illness which causes tissue lysis with release of tissue phosphate into the circulation may produce hypocalcemic tetany in rachitic children. The mechanism for the developement of osteomalacia is presumably identical to that described for rickets.

"Conditioned" or Secondary Rickets and Osteomalacia. Because diets in the United States are quite adequate in vitamin D, the presence of rickets or osteomalacia should call attention to the possibility that the disease is secondary to some other disorder. If calcium intake is relatively low and there is an inadequate supply of sunlight, multiple pregnancies may lead to vitamin D and calcium deficiency and the early appearance of osteomalacia, presumably related to losses of vitamin D, calcium, and phosphorus with lactation. Other factors such as the pH of the intestinal contents, the presence of certain insoluble compounds, such as phytic acid from cereals, which bind calcium, or the presence of excessive nonmetabolized or absorbed lipids in the diet (for example, mineral oil) may restrict the absorption of vitamin D and/or calcium and produce rickets or osteomalacia.

Either glomerular or tubular *renal disease* may be accompanied by clinical rickets in children and by evidence of osteomalacia in adults. Hypocalcemia and hyperphosphatemia are commonly found. While hyperphosphatemia can be partially reduced by feeding the patient compounds which bind phosphate in the gastrointestinal tract, thus controlling absorption of phosphate, the hypocalcemia of renal disease is notoriously resistant to the usual therapeutic doses of vitamin D (*vitamin D resistance*). In patients with chronic renal disease the plasma concentration of the metabolically active derivative of vitamin D is decreased because of accelerated destruction or loss and increased turnover. Furthermore, serum calcium concentrations are not restored to normal by secondarily increased parathyroid function because of a lack of the amounts of metabolically active derivative of vitamin D required for the normal functioning of the skeletal cellular mechanisms responsible for maintaining serum ionized calcium concentrations at their normal level (Chap. 379).

At the renal tubular level, disturbances of renal hydrogen ion excretion (renal tubular acidosis) may lead to excessive losses of calcium through the kidneys with secondary nephrocalcinosis and hypocalcemia, in addition to metabolic acidosis. Although the mechanism of this syndrome is not clear at the present time, it is generally thought to result from the excretion of acid metabolites in association with sodium, potassium, calcium, and other "fixed" cations.

Phosphate Deficiency. Although a lack of dietary phosphorus probably is sufficiently rare as to have no clinical significance in normal man, failure to absorb adequate phosphate from the gastrointestinal tract, with or without excessive urinary losses, may lead to a condition which strongly resembles rickets or osteomalacia with respect to its biochemical alterations and the microscopic appearance of the skeletal tissues, though the mechanisms which underlie its appearance are still unclear. Like renal tubular acidosis, this condition appears most commonly to result from defects in renal tubular function. These may involve phosphate reabsorption only (*phosphate diabetes*) or be multiple, involving in addition to phosphate, glucose and amino acids (*Fanconi's syndrome*). The most striking features of these conditions are the abnormal amounts of phosphate and the other materials in the urine and the resistance of the conditions to the therapeutic effects of usually curative doses of vitamin D.

Hypophosphatasia. This condition is another, probably genetically determined disorder which leads to defective mineralization of skeletal tissues. It is easily identified by the low levels of alkaline phosphatase activity which are found in the plasma together with the excessive excretion of phosphoethanolamine in the urine.

A list of the various conditions which may underlie or appear in conjunction with rickets and osteomalacia with or without associated secondary hyperparathyroidism is given in Table 83-1.

DIAGNOSIS. The diagnosis of both rickets and osteomalacia must be made on clinical grounds because a suitably sensitive, convenient assay for vitamin D activity in the circulating fluids still is not available. However, the diagnosis is generally not difficult and can be made on the basis of history, the presence of characteristic clinical and radiologic features, and the concentration of serum calcium, phosphorus, and alkaline phosphatase activity. The presence of widened osteoid seams on histologic examination of samples of bone obtained at biopsy provides important confirmatory evidence. Finally, a prompt therapeutic response to orally or paren-

Table 83-1. THE PATHOGENESIS OF RICKETS
AND OSTEOMALACIA

I. Vitamin D deficiency
  A. Defective endogenous formation in skin
  B. Exogenous dietary deficiency
  C. Decreased absorption
    1. Malabsorption syndromes
    2. Absence of bile or pancreatic juice
II. Phosphorus deficiency
  A. Dietary deficiency
  B. Formation of insoluble complexes
  C. Malabsorption syndromes
  D. Phosphate diabetes (vitamin D–resistant rickets)
  E. Fanconi syndrome
    1. With glycosuria
    2. With glycosuria and aminoaciduria
    3. With cystinosis
    4. With glycinuria
    5. Associated with heavy-metal toxicity
    6. Associated with Wilson's disease
    7. Associated with multiple myeloma
    8. Associated with neurofibromatosis
    9. Lowe's syndrome
III. Miscellaneous
  A. Hypophosphatasia
IV. Contributing causes
  A. Calcium deficiency
    1. Dietary deficiency
    2. Poor absorption (vitamin D deficiency)
    3. Insoluble complex formation
    4. Increased pH of intestinal contents
    5. Steatorrhea and malabsorption syndromes
    6. Idiopathic hypercalcuria
    7. Chronic renal disease
    8. Renal tubular acidosis
    9. Pregnancy and lactation
    10. Excessive sweating

terally administered vitamin D can serve to confirm the diagnosis, especially in vitamin D–deficiency rickets.

TREATMENT. Simple rickets requires less than 5 mg vitamin D by mouth given in doses of 0.05 to 0.1 mg (2,000 to 4,000 units) each day for 6 to 12 weeks. Even smaller doses may be quite adequate; larger doses may be detrimental (see below) and are required only in specific instances where a therapeutic response is not obtained due to relative resistance to vitamin D. However, if rickets is complicated by tetany, large doses of vitamin D as well as intravenous infusion of calcium chloride or calcium gluconate may be required in the early stages of treatment.

The addition of calcium to the therapeutic regimen usually is desirable, partly to provide the calcium needed for mineralization of previously uncalcified osteoid, partly to avoid the complication of hypocalcemia, which occurs not infrequently in the early days of treatment. Because the normal human diet contains excessive amounts of phosphate, the particular calcium salt employed probably is of relatively little significance; many prefer to use calcium phosphate salts ($CaHPO_4$) with the thought that both calcium and phosphate will be provided in this way in adequate amounts.

Prevention of rickets can be achieved by feeding as little as 400 units vitamin D daily to infants until the age of two years and by also giving this amount until full growth is achieved if sunshine is absent during the winter months. The absolute amount required varies considerably from individual to individual and with the circumstances of living, especially the amount of exposure to ultraviolet radiation and sunshine. Premature infants probably have no store of vitamin D at birth and require larger amounts (2,000 to 3,000 units daily for the first 2 or 3 months of life), and darkskinned people, who are relatively insensitive to ultraviolet radiation and hence have lower rates of endogenous vitamin D production, also may require larger amounts.

In cases of Vitamin D resistance, the use of 25-hydroxycholecalciferol may be effective.

HYPERVITAMINOSIS D

INTRODUCTION. Vitamin D, like vitamin A, can cause toxic manifestations if administered in excessive amounts. The dangers of excessive dosage came to light soon after the crystalline form of the vitamin became available and began to be used, often in huge doses, in the unsuccessful treatment of such varied conditions as rheumatoid arthritis, psoriasis, and tuberculosis of the skin. Recognition of the syndrome of hypervitaminosis D in the late 1940s led to a marked reduction in the number of cases. Now, the condition is relatively rare, occurring only through inadvertent excessive intake, as in the "idiopathic" hypercalcemia of infants which proved to be secondary to excessive fortification of cow's milk with vitamin D. Vitamin D intoxication also has occurred in the course of treatment of vitamin D–resistant rickets, renal osteodystrophy, and hypoparathyroidism.

The exact amount of the vitamin needed to cause intoxication varies from patient to patient as well as with age, renal function, and calcium intake, but as little as 50,000 units per day has been reported to be toxic in some patients.

CLINICAL FEATURES. The signs and symptoms of vitamin D intoxication are largely those of hypercalcemia and include weakness, lethargy, anorexia, nausea and vomiting, weight loss, polyuria and polydipsia, irritability, mental depression, and calcific keratitis (band keratitis). Albuminuria and casts are often present, and the signs and symptoms of renal stones or uremia, secondary to nephrocalcinosis, may ultimately appear. Diarrhea with cramping abdominal pain and acute pancreatitis also can occur. Hypertension, secondary to renal damage, is a frequent late complication.

LABORATORY FINDINGS. Elevations of serum calcium, which may be marked, and phosphorus concentrations, with depression of serum alkaline phosphatase activity, are found. In addition, alkalosis with decreased serum potassium concentration is frequent. Increased urine calcium excretion is present in the early phases of the disease, but calcium excretion may fall to normal or low levels as renal failure secondary to nephrocalcinosis develops. Despite increased calcium absorption from the gut, the total body balance of calcium is negative.

RADIOLOGY. In advanced cases of vitamin D intoxication, especially in children, increased density of the metaphysis of the long bones may occur in association with decreased density in the shafts. Lines, not unlike those seen in lead poisoning, have been reported in the metaphyseal region and correspond to the time of peak vitamin D ingestion.

Much more striking when it is present is soft-tissue metastatic calcification. Although the diffuse calcium deposits in the kidney usually are not easy to see, calcification in the media of the larger vessels, deposits of calcium adjacent to joints, and renal stones may be very prominent.

PATHOLOGY. Significant pathologic changes are found in kidneys, arteries, and bones. In the kidneys, deposits of calcium are found first in the tubular basement membranes, especially near the corticomedullary junction, and gradually extend to involve the tubular cells and even the membrane of Bowman's capsule. Hyaline and calcium-containing casts also are found in the tubules. Inflammatory changes and fibrosis develop in later stages.

Surprisingly, the bony trabeculae show increased osteoid borders reminiscent of rickets. However, other features of bone histology are generally normal in man, although changes strongly resembling those of hyperparathyroidism have been induced in animals with vitamin D.

In addition to these changes, deposits of calcium may be found in the skin, heart, pancreas, stomach, lung, thyroid, and other tissues.

PATHOGENESIS. The precise roles played in the development of this syndrome by the various vitamin D–sensitive mechanisms are not yet clear. While increased calcium absorption from the gut doubtless plays some role, excess mobilization of calcium and phosphorus from skeletal stores accounts for most of the elevation of serum calcium.

TREATMENT. The treatment of this disorder clearly is to stop excessive intake of vitamin D. This usually is sufficient to reverse the process. However, dehydration and electrolyte imbalance secondary to disturbed renal function may demand attention. Details concerning treatment of the acute hypercalcemic syndrome will be found in Chap. 90.

PROGNOSIS. Generally, the prognosis is favorable if the condition is recognized early and vitamin D is withdrawn. The serum calcium falls to normal over a period of days. Gradually the skeleton becomes normal, metastatic calcification disappears, and normal renal function returns. However, in young children or in adults in whom the process has advanced to renal fibrosis and hypertension, the prognosis may be grave.

REFERENCES

Avioli, L., Birge, S., Lee, S. W., and Slatopolsky, E.: The Metabolic Fate of Vitamin D_3-^{3}H in Chronic Renal Failure, *J. Clin. Invest.*, 47:10, 1968.

Blunt, J. W., De Luca, H. F., and Schnoes, H. K.: 25-Hydroxycholecalciferol. A Biologically Active Metabolite of Vitamin D_3, Biochemistry, 7:10, 1968.

Fourman, P., and Royer, P.: "Calcium Metabolism and the Bone," Philadelphia, F. A. Davis Company, 1968.

Loomis, W. F.: Skin-pigment Regulation of Vitamin D Biosynthesis in Man, *Science*, 157:3788, 1967.

Wasserman, R. H.: "Transport Proteins from Animals, Proceedings of the Symposium on Membrane Proteins, New York Heart Association, New York, Nov., 1968.

84 VITAMIN A DEFICIENCY, XEROPHTHALMIA, NIGHT BLINDNESS AND HYPERVITAMINOSIS A

Richard H. Follis, Jr. and
George V. Mann

HISTORY. Inability to see in subdued light, called *night blindness*, and dryness, haziness, and spontaneous necrosis of the cornea are abnormalities which have been recognized for many years. Over a century ago, Bitot called attention to the simultaneous occurrence of night blindness and lesions of the conjunctiva. By the turn of the century, Mori had suggested that ocular lesions in Japanese children might be related to a lack of fat in the diet. Soon a fat-soluble material (later to be called vitamin A) was shown to enhance the growth of rats and prevent the development of ocular lesions that histologically resembled those which had been observed in man. During the second decade of this century, investigators in Denmark clearly established the relationship of vitamin A to xerophthalmia in children. In 1930 carotene was demonstrated to be provitamin A. Vitamin A was chemically identified in 1931 and synthesized in 1936.

PREVALENCE. Today the areas of greatest prevalence of endemic vitamin A deficiency are found in Indonesia, particularly Java and parts of Sumatra; India; the Near East; and North Africa. Isolated instances of conditioned vitamin A deficiency have been described in Europe and the United States.

Vitamin A deficiency is the first cause of blindness in the world, and yet this occurs mostly in tropical areas where the carotenes which would prevent it are plentiful. The real need is for nutrition education.

CLINICAL FINDINGS. The term *xerophthalmia* is used here in an inclusive sense to refer to certain anatomic abnormalities of the eye resulting from vitamin A deficiency. The lesions usually exhibit a definite sequence of stages in development. The initial change, which is called xerosis (*xerosis epithelialis conjunctivae*), consists of dryness and opacity of the bulbar conjunctiva. Secretion of tears is decreased. At the lateral margin of the cornea, a triangular-shaped accumulation of sticky secretion may appear. This is the Bitot spot, which resembles a plaque or pseudomembrane filled with bubbles (Fig. 84-1). As the photograph indicates, the lesion has the appearance of a fleck of meringue. This material is difficult to scrape off. Fine pigmentation may also be present throughout the conjunctiva. These alterations are either accompanied or soon followed by haziness and dryness of the cornea (*xerosis corneae*). The tarsal glands along the eyelid frequently are enlarged. Photophobia may be marked. The most serious consequence is the appearance of small epithelial erosions on the cornea. These soon become infected and enlarged. If this ulceration continues, destruction of the cornea (*keratomalacia*) occurs, a process that may be extremely rapid. Thus a child with conjunctivitis and photophobia may open his eyes one morning to reveal the lens extruded, the bulb collapsed, and vision irrevocably lost (Fig. 84-2). Short of this, the cornea may heal but with a scar that greatly limits vision.

As already noted, visual acuity in subdued light is reduced as a result of vitamin A deficiency. This disturbance is called night blindness. Two other terms, *nyctalopia* and *hemeralopia*, have been used to refer to this condition. Nyctalopia means an inability to see in subdued light. Hemeralopia refers to a decrease in vision that follows exposure to bright light. Defective ability to see in subdued light may be established by certain tests; however, these are difficult to perform under routine conditions and are particularly unsuited for children. An instrument, the electroretinogram, has been developed for objective testing in research.

The nonocular manifestations of vitamin A deficiency are not conspicuous and are usually obscured by signs of general malnutrition or the presence of some conditioning disturbance, such as obstruction of the pancreatic or biliary ducts, which may lead to poor absorption of the vitamin. Tracheitis, bronchitis, and pneumonia are the commonest clinical manifestations.

LABORATORY FINDINGS. Vitamin A nutriture may be assessed by determining the carotene and/or vitamin A content of blood serum. Values are expressed in International Units (IU) or micrograms per 100 ml. One IU is equivalent to 0.3 µg vitamin A or 0.6 µg β-carotene. Vitamin A concentration is decisive; carotene values may be misleading, since other pigments may be present.

Fig. 84-1. Bitot's spots showing the characteristic meringue texture. (*Photograph courtesy of Professor D. S. McLaren and the American Journal of Clinical Nutrition*)

Serum values for carotene and vitamin A are usually considered to be normal if over 40 and 20 µg per 100 ml, respectively. When values for carotene and vitamin A fall below 20 and 10 µg per 100 ml, respectively, the deficient state is probably present. Valuable information on vitamin A nutriture among population groups has been obtained from analyses of liver tissue. For instance, among well-nourished groups in Great Britain, values averaging 450 IU per Gm have been obtained. In contrast, data derived from Chinese subjects indicate much lower levels, averaging 79 IU per Gm.

PATHOLOGY. The tissues chiefly affected are epithelial in nature, principally those which ordinarily are not keratinized. These include the lining epithelium of the upper and lower respiratory passages, genitourinary tract, eye and paraocular glands, salivary glands, accessory glands of the tongue and buccal cavity, and pancreas. The fundamental change is metaplasia of the normal nonkeratinized lining cells into a keratinizing type of epithelium. The cornea becomes dry, wrinkled, and hazy due to intrinsic changes as well as to lack of tears as a result of obstruction of the ducts. The ciliated epithelium of the respiratory tract is replaced by a keratinizing lining so that the important mechanical effects of the cilia are lost. The basal cells in all areas retain, however, their potentiality for reverting to normal if their supply of vitamin A is restored.

At autopsy other changes may be found that are responsible for conditioned vitamin A deficiency. For instance, obstruction to the biliary tract or pancreatic duct may interfere with fat absorption. Liver disease may have interfered with storage.

PATHOGENESIS. At least two forms of vitamin A alcohol are known (A_1 and A_2), together with acid and aldehyde derivatives. The vitamins A are intimately related to provitamins, the carotenes, and certain other pigmented compounds. A part of ingested carotene is absorbed by the cells of the intestinal mucosa and transformed into vitamin A. Bile is important in this process. Vitamin A is usually present in ester form in foods; it is hydrolyzed in the intestinal tract and absorbed as the alcohol (*retinol*). Within the cells of the intestinal mucosa, vitamin A is esterified, usually with palmitic acid, and transported via the thoracic duct as the ester to the liver, where it is stored. As needed, vitamin A ester is hydrolyzed to the alcohol and transported, attached to plasma protein, to the tissues. Vitamin A aldehyde (*retinal* or *retinene*) is found in the retina and is important in the visual process. The interrelations between alcohol, acid, and ester forms of vitamin A have been greatly clarified. It is possible that vitamin A acid (*retinoic acid*) may be the "active form." The alcohol (retinol) is converted to aldehyde (retinal or retinene). The latter may be converted to the acid by an enzyme in the liver. The reverse reaction, i.e., acid to alcohol or aldehyde, does not appear possible. The acid is more effective for growth in experimental animals than is the aldehyde. The acid is not active in the visual process.

The greatest concentration of vitamin A in man is found in the liver. Concentrations are also appreciable in kidneys, adrenals, lungs, and the retina. Fat depots contain a small amount of the vitamin.

Vitamin A deficiency may result from an insufficiency of this vitamin or its precursors in the diet or because of some process which interferes with absorption from the intestinal tract, transport, or storage in the liver. Obstruction of the biliary tract or pancreatic ducts in children or adults may lead to diminished absorption of vitamin A. Diarrhea and the various types of malabsorption syndromes are accompanied by vitamin A malnutrition. Of particular importance is the interrelation of vitamin A and protein nutrition, since vitamin A alcohol appears to be transported by plasma albumin. Transport to and mobilization from the liver may be impaired as a result of protein malnutrition.

The intricate reactions whereby vitamin A enters into the visual process may be briefly summarized. Vitamin A aldehyde (retinal or retinene) is found in the retina bound to a protein called *opsin*. Together these form the compound *rhodopsin*, the red pigment of the retinal rods. Under the influence of light, *rhodopsin* breaks down into its two components, thereby initiating a nerve impulse. The mechanism of this reaction was worked out by the Nobel Prize-winning studies of George Wald and his associates.

How vitamin A maintains the integrity of epithelial structures remains a mystery. Vitamin A appears to be implicated in the metabolism of intracellular structures, the lysosomes, in mucopolysaccharide metabolism, and in steroid hormone formation. While the integrity of specialized epithelial structures does require vitamin A, it has not been shown that high intakes of vitamin A will prevent infections. The old remark that carrots are good for vision applies only to persons with vitamin A deficiency and nyctalopia.

DIAGNOSIS. McLaren observed that the eye changes and biochemical findings in vitamin A deficiency often are poorly correlated. The diagnosis and treatment must not wait for all the confirmatory information. A dietary history suggesting a low carotene intake, and especially if the diet is also low in fat and thus one which causes poor absorption of carotene, should be suggestive. Protein deficiency appears to aggravate vitamin A deficiency by impairing transport of the vitamin in vivo. Sprue and diarrheal states will also predispose to vitamin A deficiency.

Measurements of plasma carotene may be misleading because of the presence of other carotenes which are poor provitamins. Vitamin A levels below 20 μg per 100 ml signalize the need for immediate therapy. Distinctive eye changes demand therapy even without laboratory confirmation.

THERAPY. Oral administration of 500,000 IU vitamin A daily as the palmitate or acetate for 3 or more days is recommended. In addition, it may be well to administer similar-sized doses intramuscularly. The diets of children with vitamin A deficiency are usually also lacking in other nutrients and hence should be improved, particularly with respect to protein.

PROGNOSIS. The outcome as far as sight is concerned

Fig. 84-2. The destruction of the eye by colliquative necrosis of the cornea. The lens is about to drop out. (*Photograph courtesy of Professor D. S. McLaren*)

will depend on the degree of involvement of the ocular structures before therapy is instituted. If only clouding of the cornea has occurred, prognosis is excellent. However, if perforation and infection of the anterior chamber have taken place, restoration of sight is virtually unknown.

Hypervitaminosis A

The ingestion of large amounts of vitamin A, in doses ranging from 75,000 to 500,000 IU daily to infants or adults, results in a variety of signs and symptoms that sometimes may be extremely confusing, particularly if a history of ingestion has not been elicited. Ignorance is usually the reason for taking excessive amounts of vitamin A.

In infants, the effects of acute toxicity are drowsiness, vomiting, and bulging of the fontanels as a result of increased intracranial pressure. More chronic evidences of toxicity include failure to gain weight, alopecia, coarseness of hair texture, hepatomegaly, and evidences of bone pain. X-ray examination of the skeleton reveals characteristic areas of periosteal new bone formation, particularly prominent in the shafts of the long bones.

In adults, headache, blurred vision or diplopia, nausea, and vomiting all may be present. Bone pain and osseous changes similar to those occurring in children may be observed. In addition, calcification of ligaments and tendons may be seen on x-ray examination. Peeling of the skin, neuritis, fissures and sores at the corners of the mouth, coarsening of the skin, alopecia, and localized areas of hyperpigmentation of the epidermis are common. As might be expected, the level of vitamin A in the serum is elevated; values as high as 2,000 μg per 100 ml have been reported. Fortunately, the prognosis is good when vitamin A ingestion halts.

Mention should be made of *carotenemia*, because it may be confused with jaundice. When large amounts of carotene-containing foods are ingested, the blood plasma may contain a high enough concentration of pigment to impart a yellowish color to the skin (especially the palms of the hands and the nasolabial folds) but not the conjunctivas.

REFERENCES

Dowling, J. E. and G. Wald: Vitamin A Deficiency and Night Blindness, Proc. Nat. Acad. Sci., 44:648, 1958.

McLaren, D. S.: "Malnutrition and the Eye," New York, Academic Press, Inc., 1963.

Medical Research Council: Vitamin A Requirements of Human Adults, Special Report Series no. 264, 1949.

Moore, T.: "Vitamin A," New York, Elsevier Publishing Company, 1957.

Oomen, H. A. P. C.: An Outline of Xerophthalmia, Int. Rev. Trop. Med., 1:131, 1961.

85 OTHER DEFICIENCY STATES
George V. Mann

There are a number of nutritional deficiencies other than those discussed already which often appear as complications of other diseases or of therapy. These will be considered in the present chapter.

SODIUM DEPLETION. Although the usual intake of sodium chloride is five to ten times the daily requirement, there are a few disorders in which excessive losses of sodium produce depletion of body stores. The excessive losses in Addison's disease result from failure of the hormone-conditioned retrieval of sodium in the kidney (Chap. 92).

Diarrhea, especially when coupled with fever and salt loss from excessive sweating, may produce salt depletion. This is most often seen in children and may be aggravated by excessive replacement of fluids without adequate attention to serum sodium levels. Thus hyponatremia may reflect either depletion of sodium or excessive dilution of the serum.

Some stages of chronic nephritis are associated with excessive urinary loss of sodium. This may be complicated by low sodium diets and the use of diuretic agents. Diagnosis and management are discussed in Chap. 301.

The normal organism has a remarkable ability to adapt to sodium deprivation so that either low-salt diets, as used in the treatment of hypertension, saluretic agents or heat exposure lead to a hormonal response which conserves sodium. This reaction cannot be efficient in the presence of congenitally absent or diseased sweat glands, as in mucoviscidosis or in renal or adrenal disease. The signs of hyponatremia are weakness, apathy, confusion, nausea, muscle cramps, and azotemia. The diagnosis depends upon the presence of clinical manifestations of dehydration and appropriate biochemical measurements.

POTASSIUM DEPLETION. The potassium of the body is predominantly intracellular so that serum measurements are poor criteria for the level of body stores. Hypokalemia may be associated with nausea, weakness, and confusional states in addition to paralytic ileus and cardiac irregularities, such as flattening of T waves and prolongation of the Q-S intervals in the ECG. A common cause of hypokalemia is the use of diuretic agents which cause the kidney to lose potassium as well as sodium. Potassium losses also can be great from the gastrointestinal tract and during metabolic acidosis, during starvation, or in any wasting disorder. Excessive adrenal steroids induce potassium loss. Potassium deficiency leads to necrosis of muscle fibers and vacuolization of renal epithelium. In familial periodic paralysis the potassium disturbance is associated with a shift of the ion among body compartments rather than loss in the urine.

Potassium is rich in plant foods. The requirement for potassium is influenced by the sodium intake because the sodium/potassium ratio appears to be critical. Repletion of potassium losses involves two possible hazards. Excessive parenteral potassium may cause cardiac irregularities and standstill if the plasma level is raised too rapidly. Oral preparations of potassium, especially enteric coated pills, have been a cause of intestinal ulceration, bleeding, and stenosis. The proper management of potassium deficiency is prevention by ensuring an adequate intake of potassium-rich foods, especially when potassium-wasting drugs are given. Readily available foods such as bananas, orange juice, tomato juice, or meat broth are good sources of potassium for this purpose. Repletion of stores may require parenteral administration but this should be carried out very cautiously in the presence of oliguria or anuria and serum levels should be checked at frequent intervals (see Chaps. 296 and 297).

MAGNESIUM DEPLETION. Magnesium deficiency in man is well known as a complication of alcoholism and of intestinal malabsorption. It occurs occasionally as a complication of diabetes mellitus, of kwashiorkor in children, and of disturbances in parathyroid and adrenal function. Magnesium is predominantly an intracellular cation. The serum contains only 2 mEq per liter, but there is a total of 25 Gm in the body of which about half is in the skeleton (Chap. 76). Like deficiencies of sodium and potassium, magnesium depletion may occur from deficient intake, poor absorption, and increased renal excretion. A syndrome characterized by vertigo, weakness, distension, positive Chvostek sign, and convulsive seizures with or without tetany has been ascribed to a decrease in serum concentration of magnesium (Chap. 21). The deficiency signs respond quickly to magnesium therapy but not to calcium. The typical symptoms of Tetany may even be aggravated by calcium in such cases.

RIBOFLAVIN DEFICIENCY. It is something of a paradox that riboflavin deficiency has not produced more profound or characteristic signs because flavoproteins play a central role in many metabolic processes. In young experimental animals, riboflavin deficiency causes cessation of growth and extensive skin changes. In adult animals fatty changes in the liver and sudden death may occur. Dietary deficiency has been produced in a number of human trials and has been shown to cause only mild angular lesions of the lips (cheilosis) and a scrotal, seborrheic dermatitis. Riboflavin deficiency also has been produced by feeding human subjects the riboflavin antagonist galactoflavin. This procedure caused an anemia, a change not seen in dietary riboflavin deficiency. The level of flavine-adenine-dinucleotides in the plasma in riboflavin deficiency is a good index of deficiency, but this measurement is not widely available. Diagnosis depends upon the dietary history, the suggestive skin signs and a therapeutic trial.

PYRIDOXINE DEFICIENCY. Vitamin B_6 denotes a group of three compounds, pyridoxine, pyridoxal, and pyridoxamine. The first is found in plant foods and the last two are found in animal products. All are unstable to heat and light, but they are so widely distributed that simple dietary deficiency is very unusual in man. In experimental animals a deficiency of vitamin B_6 causes cachexia and scaling of the skin, as well as a profound, microcytic hypochromic anemia. Convulsive seizures may be seen, and sensory neurone degeneration develops. In babies fed diets deficient in vitamin B_6 convulsive seizures occurred. The diagnosis of deficiency can be substantiated by the disappearance from the urine of the metabolite 4-pyridoxic acid or by measuring the amount of xanthurenic acid in the urine before and after administering l-tryptophan. In pyridoxine deficiency, the conversion of this amino acid to nicotinic acid is impaired, and xanthurenic acid excretion is increased.

A number of drugs interfere with vitamin B_6 utilization. Isoniazid and hydralazine form inactive derivatives and increase the pyridoxine requirements. Polyneuritis may appear as a complication of therapy with these agents and can be relieved by supplying large amounts of the coenzyme.

Certain microcytic anemias have been found to be partially responsive to pyridoxine therapy (Chap. 336). Convulsive seizures have been described in infants receiving normal diets which could be relieved by administration of pyridoxine. Such observations have lead to the concept of *pyridoxine dependency* arising from a genetically determined requirement for unusually large amounts of pyridoxine. Such dependency may represent an example of a metabolic "in-born error" caused by a deficiency of the coenzyme pyridoxine, which contrasts with the metabolic error caused by deficiency of the protein apoenzyme in phenylketonuria. The latter can only be managed by dietary reduction of the enzyme substrate phenylalanine in order to minimize accumulation of an injurious metabolite (Chap. 102).

PANTOTHENIC ACID DEFICIENCY. This deficiency is well known in experimental animals and has been produced in mild form in human beings by feeding a pantothenate antagonist. The vitamin is widely available in foods. A natural deficiency has not been described in man, but pantothenic acid deficiency may contribute to multiple deficiency states observed with grossly defective diets or with severe malabsorption. A daily intake of 5 to 10 mg is considered adequate. The American diet supplies an average of 10 to 15 mg daily.

BIOTIN DEFICIENCY. This deficiency occurs only when the diet contains large amounts of a protein called *avidin* which binds biotin and prevents absorption from the intestine. Avidin occurs especially in raw egg white. It is inactivated by heating. An experimental deficiency of biotin in human beings causes a dermatitis, malaise, anxiety, hyperesthesia, and nonspecific ECG changes. The vitamin is widespread in animal food products. Deficiency in man must be very rare.

VITAMIN E DEFICIENCY. There is a widespread misconception that vitamin E facilitates reproductive function. While it is true that a deficiency of alphatocopherol in rats and certain other species has led to resorption of fetuses, it does not follow that vitamin E will augment lagging reproductive activity in man. A number of isomeric tocopherols, which are abundant in vegetable oil, have vitamin E activity. Deficiency of these materials typically causes muscular degeneration and creatinuria in several species. Because storage capacity for the vitamin is large, experimental deficiency develops slowly and requires 400 to 600 days in Rhesus monkeys. In these animals the red blood cells became fragile and an anemia developed. Anemia responding to tocopherol has also been reported in malnourished infants. It appears that the requirement for vitamin E is determined in part by the amount of polyunsaturated fatty acid in the diet. Diets rich in polyunsaturated fat may increase the requirement for alphatocopherol, but the two substances generally occur in the same food sources, so that in practice, these diets should not require supplementation with vitamin E.

FOLIC ACID DEFICIENCY. *Folic acid* or *folacin* refers to a group of substances widely distributed in both vegetable and animal foods. It exists in several forms, either free or conjugated, with one or more molecules of glutamic acid. The vitamin acts with vitamin B_{12} in the transfer of single carbon units which are essential for hematopoiesis and mucosal proliferation. The pathogenesis and clinical manifestations of folic acid deficiency are discussed in Chap. 337. Megaloblastic anemia due to folate deficiency has been more commonly recognized than previously as biochemical techniques for assays of blood folate (Chap. 78) have improved. In the United Kingdom the ratio of anemia caused by folate deficiency to pernicious anemia is about 1:1.25. The deficiency tends to be commoner in the aged, in pregnancy, and in persons with malabsorptive disorders. Lacking biochemical confirmation, the diagnosis is confirmed by a therapeutic trial by following the reticulocyte response after treatment with folate (Chap. 337). Occasionally a response to folic acid will be seen in the anemia of scurvy, and sometimes folate deficiency will respond incompletely to vitamin B_{12} therapy. These must represent multiple deficiency states.

An average United States diet supplies 150 to 200 μg of folic acid daily. While the minimal requirement may be only 50 μg per day, some of the dietary supply is lost in food preparation, and the efficiency of absorption is variable. The recommended dietary allowance (RDA) is 400 μg per day, and this should be doubled in pregnancy.

The sale of vitamin preparations containing more than

100 μg folic acid in the daily dose is now prohibited by federal regulations which are aimed at preventing inadvertent treatment of pernicious anemia while the neurologic manifestations progress. This amount of folate will supply the daily requirement for a normal adult.

VITAMIN K DEFICIENCY. The family of substances with vitamin K activity occurs in plants (phylloquinones) and in bacteria. They are essential for blood clotting because they are needed for the production of prothrombin and several other clotting factors (Chap. 62). Vitamin K deficiency may occur in the newborn before the intestinal flora and the diet begin to supply the vitamin (Chap. 346). This is prevented by prepartum treatment of the mother with the vitamin, thus assuring the infant a normal clotting mechanism during birth trauma. The natural vitamin derived from plants is called vitamin K_1 (phylloquinone) and that derived from bacteria, K_2 (farnoquinone). A commonly used therapeutic agent is menadione, or vitamin K_3, which is the synthetic compound 2-methyl 1,4 napthoquinine. The dosage given premature infants should be no more than 1 to 2 mg per day or kernicterus may develop. Because vitamin K_1 does not show this toxicity for premature infants, the present regulations prohibit the inclusion of menadione in over-the-counter vitamin supplements available to expectant mothers. Water-miscible forms of vitamin K are available for parenteral use especially to reverse the hypoprothrombinemia and bleeding caused by excessive therapy with anticoagulants.

Because the supply of vitamin K is derived from the intestinal flora as well as the diet, treatment with antimicrobials by depressing intestinal flora may diminish the vitamin supply and lead to hypoprothrombinemia. This is particularly likely to occur when there is concomitant administration of anticoagulants. Vitamin K deficiency rarely occurs from simple lack in the diet. No recommended dietary allowance has been established.

REFERENCES

Folic Acid and Pregnancy, Nutr. Rev., 25:325, 1967; 26:5, 1968.
Fomon, S. J., et al.: Vitamin K Compounds and the Water Soluble Analogues, Pediatrics, 28:501, 1961.
Horwitt, M. K.: Nutritional Requirements of Man with Special Reference to Riboflavin, Am. J. Clin. Nutr., 18:458, 1966.
Mason, K. E., et al.: Symposium—Hematological Aspects of Vitamin E, Am. J. Clin. Nutr., 21:1, 1968.
Raskin, N. H., and R. A. Fishman: Pyridoxine Deficiency Due to Hydralazine, New Engl. J. Med., 273:1182, 1965.
Wacker, W. E. C.: Magnesium Metabolism, J. Am. Diet. Ass., 44:362, 1964.

Section 3

Hormonal Disorders

86 GENERAL CONSIDERATIONS AND MAJOR SYNDROMES

George W. Thorn

INTRODUCTION

Isolation, purification, identification, and synthesis of new hormones continue at a rapid rate, and it is reasonable to assume that within the near future those few remaining unidentified principles will also succumb to the technical advances of chemistry and biophysics. Noteworthy among recorded achievements are the determination of the structure and amino acid sequence of adrenocorticotropin, melanocyte-stimulating hormone, and insulin; the synthesis of posterior pituitary hormone and a host of adrenal and gonadal steroid hormones; and the isolation of several new thyroid substances as well as the isolation, identification, and synthesis of glucagon and calcitonin.

Coupled with these chemical advances is a rapidly expanding body of knowledge concerning the regulation of hormonal secretion and the precise locus of hormonal action. Although this latter field has barely been opened, the effect of insulin on permeability to certain sugars, the mechanism whereby estrogens provide energy for the growth of their target organs, and the physical modification of mitochondrial particles by thyroxin illustrate the type of information rapidly becoming available.

It is now generally agreed that hormones do not initiate new events in the complicated biochemistry of metabolic processes, but rather produce their effects by regulating enzymatic and other chemical reactions already present. In view of the relatively large number of hormones, their diverse chemical structures, and their multiple sites of action, it can be assumed that scarcely a single important metabolic event can escape the effect of their primary or secondary action. From this one may conclude that a true understanding of any disease process or physiologic disorder must encompass an appreciation of the possible etiologic role of hormones and the factors regulating their synthesis, release, and degradation. In this regard, one can point to such widely diverse actions as the effect of catechol amines (adrenal medulla) on brain metabolism and psychologic behavior; the effect of adrenal steroids on the inflammatory reaction associated with infection, trauma, surgery, or burns; the effect of insulin on adipose tissue metabolism; and the importance of growth hormone on the fabrication of body proteins.

MECHANISMS OF ENDOCRINOPATHIES

Characteristically, endocrine abnormalities arise as a consequence of increased or decreased hormone secretion. In the majority of patients, the clinical manifestations derive from an excess of or deficiency of the *normally* secreted hormone. However, in certain syndromes, such as some cases of adrenal virilism, the endocrinopathy may result from secretion of an abnormal hormone. In addition, hormonal disorders may result from aberrations in the metabolism or degradation of hormones. For example, a deficiency of plasma proteins may decrease the quantity of hormone-carrying protein in the blood and hence modify significantly the balance between "free" and "bound" thyroid hormone; liver disease may alter the conjugation or degradation of steroid hormones, giving rise to abnormal blood and tissue hormone levels. In such types of abnormalities, however, serious endocrine disorders will result only if the "servo-regulating" mechanism, or feedback response, fails to stimulate the appropriate reaction in the trophic gland. Endocrine abnormalities may also develop when local tissues are unable to respond to a normal hormonal level. For example, localized myxedema over the tibia may occur in the presence of thyrotoxicosis or euthyroidism; in cases of pseudohypoparathyroidism, the abnormalities observed in hypoparathyroidism occur despite the presence of normal parathyroid glands. In some endocrinopathies, heightened tissue susceptibility to hormone action is the determining factor in the genesis of the syndrome, for example, hirsutism in young women with a minimal abnormality in androgenic steroid secretion, or extreme degrees of hyperpigmentation observed in patients with early adrenal insufficiency and increased melanin pigmentation on a racial basis.

Hormonal secretions in general show wide fluctuations throughout the 24-hr period, periods of high activity often alternating with those of reduced secretion; for example, in the early morning the level of adrenal cortical secretory activity is high. Evidence is accumulating that endocrinopathy may result from a loss of cyclic diurnal pattern due to a more or less constant hormonal elaboration throughout the day and night, resulting in only a slight increase, if any, in total secretion. Two important considerations have been derived from these observations: (1) Interpretation of single determinations of hormone content—of blood, tissues, or urine—reflecting instantaneous or relatively short collection periods may be unreliable; for final evaluation, repeated determinations, longer collection periods, or isotopic "turnover" studies may be required. (2) Clinical application of the cyclic method of hormone administration has been quite successful in minimizing undesirable hormone side effects while maintaining control of the underlying disease process.

DIAGNOSTIC APPROACH TO ENDOCRINE ABNORMALITIES

The suspicion that an endocrine abnormality may play a role in a patient's illness will often derive initially from the gross physical appearance of the patient, as in myxedema, hyperthyroidism, pituitary dwarfism or gigantism, acromegaly, hypogonadism, carotenemia (diabetes mellitus or hypothyroidism), Addison's disease, Cushing's syndrome, and the adrenogenital syndrome. Although a careful history and physical examination will in most instances provide presumptive evidence of an underlying endocrine disorder, the definitive diagnosis will almost invariably depend upon the values obtained from laboratory examinations. Here, accuracy in diagnosis depends upon the specificity of the laboratory test, its precision and its reproducibility, the care and understanding with which specimens are collected, and the reliability of the laboratory that carries out the procedures. In the past, endocrine abnormalities were established for the most part on the basis of nonspecific laboratory examinations such as the basal metabolic rate; roentgenograms; glucose tolerance test; and blood sugar, calcium, sodium, and potassium determinations. Today, tests of endocrine dysfunction are employing more and more frequently measurement of the specific hormones under consideration, for example, protein-bound iodine level, blood and urinary steroid values, urinary gonadotropins, and blood ACTH or insulin levels. It is essential for the practicing physician to realize, however, that a single determination of a specific hormone (in blood, urine, or tissue) does not necessarily establish or exclude an endocrine abnormality. The addition of hormonal "turnover" or "secretory" measurements by means of isotopic techniques represents a great step forward. The use of stressful situations or specific substances such as ACTH (adrenocorticotropin) for the adrenal, thyroid-stimulating hormone (TSH) for the thyroid, and glucose for the detection of early diabetes permits one to test the functional reserve of these endocrine systems and thereby facilitates the diagnosis of potential endocrine deficiency at a time when prophylactic measures may prove effective. In the succeeding chapters, particular attention will be devoted to indicating the usefulness and limitations of diagnostic methods and the degree of specificity attached to the procedure. Because of its great practical importance, the source of common errors related to these determinations will also be emphasized.

ENDOCRINE SYNDROMES

Although secretions of the endocrine glands govern widespread metabolic activities throughout the body, from the viewpoint of the internist, major endocrine disorders present over and over again as a limited number of syndromes. These will be reviewed briefly in relation to the cardinal manifestations of disease.

WEAKNESS AND INCREASED FATIGABILITY (see also Chap. 19). These are without doubt the most frequent presenting symptoms of adult patients seeking assistance from the internist or general practitioner. Although in the majority of instances these complaints derive primarily from emotional or psychologic disturbances, underlying organic disease must always be considered. When endocrine abnormalities are suspected, one should inquire first whether the symptoms have been accompanied by *weight loss*—if so, adrenal cortical insufficiency, hyperthyroidism, and diabetes mellitus should be considered. Adrenal cortical insufficiency, if present, should be accompanied by some increase in pigmentation, hypotension, gastrointestinal disturbances, and perhaps salt craving. Hyperthyroidism would be suggested by goiter, eye changes, tremor, intolerance for heat, etc., and diabetes mellitus by polyuria and polydipsia.

Without weight loss, but with symptoms of weakness and fatigability, one would consider hypothyroidism, hypopituitarism, hyperparathyroidism, and hyperaldosteronism. The first of these is characteristically associated with delayed reflexes, intolerance to cold, dry skin, and carotenemia. Hypopituitarism is suggested by oligomenorrhea or amenorrhea in the female, impotence in the male, decreased tolerance to cold, hypoglycemic episodes, and hypotension. Hyperparathyroidism is suggested by the association of bone pain, renal calculi, and polyuria. Hyperaldosteronism might be accompanied by significant hypertension, demonstrable muscular weakness, polyuria, and electrocardiographic changes that suggest potassium depletion.

MENSTRUAL IRREGULARITIES (see also Chap 98). In addition to pregnancy and local disease of the uterus, menstrual irregularities are associated with four major endocrine disturbances: (1) *primary ovarian failure*, prior to natural menopause and characterized by hot flashes, gain in weight, increased emotional instability, and elevated urinary values of follicle-stimulating hormone; (2) *secondary ovarian failure*, associated with reduced or absent urinary gonadotropins and evidence of other target gland deficiencies, i.e., thyroid and adrenal; (3) *hypothyroidism*, in which menorrhagia as well as oligomenorrhea frequently occur; (4) *adrenogenital syndrome*, in which oligomenorrhea or amenorrhea is seen in combination with increased muscular development, hirsutism, and other signs of masculinization.

HIRSUTISM (see also Chap 57). Increased body hair in females and decreased scalp hair in both sexes is a frequent disorder for which patients seek medical attention. Unfortunately, to date, most female patients with increased hair do not have a demonstrable excess of adrenal or ovarian androgens. Increased androgenic secretion should be considered when *hirsutism* is associated with menstrual irregularities and amenorrhea, or with other evidence of virilism, i.e., increased muscular development and increased size of clitoris.

Although loss of scalp hair and baldness is almost never due to a specific endocrinopathy, a receding hair line in female patients associated with *increased* body hair should always suggest excessive androgenic hormone secretion of adrenal or gonadal origin. Thinning of the hair is frequent in patients with Cushing's syndrome, hypothyroidism, or hypopituitarism. It is rare, however, to observe disturbances in hair growth as a manifestation of serious endocrine abnormality in the absence of rather well-defined signs and symptoms of adrenal, pituitary, or gonadal dysfunction.

IMPOTENCE AND DECREASED LIBIDO (see also Chap. 53). Although these cardinal manifestations of functional disorder are a frequent basis for medical consultation, they are rarely due primarily to endocrinopathies. In addition to primary disease of the generative organs, however, *anterior pituitary deficiency*, especially associated with chromophobe adenomas, should be considered. Evidence of local tumor (changes in vision, headache, etc.) and associated target gland deficiencies (adrenal, thyroid, and gonadal) should be sought. Patients with diabetes mellitus will often exhibit both impotence and decreased libido, but in most instances this occurs after the disease has been present for some time.

OBESITY (see also Chap. 48). Obesity suggests the possibility of an underlying endocrine disturbance, which in practice rarely is causative. However, two serious disorders must be considered in patients with marked, generalized obesity. The first is diabetes mellitus, and this should be investigated with a postprandial glucose determination and a glucose tolerance test, if fasting blood glucose levels are within the normal range and if sugar is not present in the urine. The second serious disorder is insulinoma. Hunger, increased appetite, and weight gain are characteristic of patients with insulinoma as well as those with "reactive" hypoglycemia. The former experience greatest hunger and symptomatology after prolonged fast, the latter shortly after eating, particularly a meal of high carbohydrate content. In both instances appetite and food intake are stimulated by absolute or relative hypoglycemia, and the vicious cycle is continued.

Hypothyroidism and mild hypopituitarism may be associated with moderate obesity. The final diagnosis of the former will require laboratory tests of thyroid function; the latter requires tests for the adequacy of target gland function.

Gross obesity in Cushing's syndrome is rare—what is more common is loss of adipose tissue in the extremities with an increase in abdominal fat pad, striae, and "buffalo hump."

There is no doubt that castration or ovarian failure predispose to obesity. This is not only well-established in man but of practical significance to poultry and cattle raisers. However, in young women there often occurs a reversal of this cycle; namely, rapid weight gain secondary to excess food intake, stress, and anxieties, which may be *followed* by oligomenorrhea or amenorrhea. Whether the weight gain itself is of primary importance in the genesis of the ovarian dysfunction, or whether weight gain and altered gonadal function are both secondary to changes in the hypothalamic centers is not known. However, it is well established that with improvement in emotional status and with weight loss, normal ovulation and menstruation will often ensue. In contrast, primary ovarian failure from organic disease is usually attended by hot flushes and other evidence of vasomotor instability as well as by elevated urinary gonadotropin levels.

HYPERTENSION (see also Chaps. 92, 93, and 276). Hypertension is another frequent disorder encountered in medical practice that should suggest an underlying endocrine abnormality. The hypertensive patient with minimal abnormalities in urinary constituents but with polyuria and nocturia suggests hypokalemia (hyperaldosteronism) or hypercalcemia (hyperparathyroidism). Clinically the hypokalemic patient with *hyperaldosteronism* rarely presents with the malignant form of hypertension and characteristically exhibits neuromuscular weakness. The electrocardiogram will often reveal changes consistent with potassium depletion, whereas serum sodium concentration is usually *elevated*. The problem is to exclude hypokalemia induced by diuretic administration, especially the thiazides, and the ensuing secondary hyperaldosteronism.

The patient with hypertension, polyuria, and hypercalcemia associated with *hyperparathyroidism* will frequently give a history of urinary calculi or bone pain. He may also present the stigmas of psychoneurosis as a consequence of sustained hypercalcemia. Band keratopathy is rare except with long-continued elevated serum calcium level. A palpable tumor in the neck, unfortunately, is usually a thyroid nodule.

Two characteristic findings in patients with hypertension secondary to *pheochromocytoma* are the cyclic nature of hypertension in the classic syndrome and the absence of obesity. Unfortunately, most tumors secrete predominantly norepinephrine; hence, the textbook picture of tachycardia, nervousness, sweating, and glucosuria is infrequent. Catechol amine excretion may be within normal values between episodes.

Hypertension and moderate obesity, particularly of the truncal type, suggest the possibility of underlying *Cushing's syndrome*. This possibility is greatly increased if diabetes mellitus, easy bruisability, and pink abdominal striae are present. Every hypersensive patient with diabetes mellitus should be screened for adrenal overactivity. The simplest test is a direct eosinophil count. With a count of more than 100 per cu mm, Cushing's syndrome can be reasonably excluded; with a value under 50, definitive tests should be carried out.

Hypertension as an early manifestation of diabetes mellitus is uncommon. However, since hypertensive-vascular disease is such a frequent complication of diabetes mellitus, hypertensive patients—especially those who are obese—should have postprandial blood glucose determinations evaluated and glucose tolerance tested.

Hypertension as a manifestation of *adrenogenital syndrome* should be considered in young subjects with associated evidence of virilism.

ABNORMALITIES IN GROWTH (see also Chaps. 87 and 89). Abnormalities in growth, particularly in children, are associated with *hypothyrodism* and *cretinism*. The latter must be detected within the first few weeks after birth if serious damage to the central nervous system is to be prevented. All babies with *persistent* umbilical hernia should be screened for possible *hypothyroidism*. Untreated diabetes mellitus will result in retarded growth as will excess cortisol and androgen secretion. Long-standing renal disease will impair skeletal growth and mimic an endocrinopathy because of the frequent coexistence of secondary hyperparathyroidism.

Closely related to abnormalities in growth among adolescent boys is the problem of undescended testes. A conservative approach is urged, and the reader is referred to Chap. 97 for details as to the management of this important problem.

Other cardinal signs that should call attention to possible endocrine abnormalities include the following:

1. Changes in the skin (see also Chaps. 58–60). Dryness in hypothyroidism and Addison's disease; thin, atrophic skin with "wrinkles" in pituitary and gonadal failure; easy bruisability in Cushing's syndrome; moist, fine, warm skin in hyperthyroidism; coarse, reduplicated skin in acromegaly; hyperpigmentation in Addison's disease.

2. Arthropathies are not infrequent in acromegaly, gigantism, myxedema, and primary gonadal failure.

3. Tetany and convulsive seizures (see Chap. 28) may indicate hypoglycemia (insulinoma, reactive hypoglycemia, Addison's disease, hypopituitarism), hypocalcemia (hypoparathyroidism), or hypokalemia (hyperaldosteronism, Cushing's syndrome).

4. The presence of edema (see Chap. 34) should suggest hypothyroidism or myxedema as well as secondary hyperaldosteronism and Cushing's syndrome.

5. Psychologic abnormalities (see Chap. 18) are frequently observed in Addison's disease and Cushing's syndrome as well as in hypopituitarism, hypothyroidism, hyperthyroidism, hyperparathyroidism, and acromegaly.

IATROGENIC ENDOCRINOPATHIES

With the general use of the corticosteroids, thyroid, and the sex hormones as nonspecific therapeutic agents, new and difficult problems present themselves to the internist and endocrinologist. One may be faced on the one hand with iatrogenic Cushing's syndrome, hyperthyroidism, or virilism—or severe adrenal insufficiency or hypothyroidism if hormone therapy is discontinued rapidly or completely. Special problems relating to these phenomena will, because of their seriousness, be discussed at length in relation to each of the specific hormones so implicated. The use of hormones as nonspecific therapeutic agents, while offering great promise in many serious and often fatal diseases, is fraught with difficulties and requires, in addition to a thorough knowledge of the endocrine preparations a comprehension of their physiologic and pharmacologic effects, the exercise of sound judgment on the part of the physician, and complete cooperation on the part of the patient. Without these the end result accompanying endocrine pharmacotherapeutics may be more disabling than the untreated cause of the primary disease.

87 DISEASES OF THE ANTERIOR LOBE OF THE PITUITARY GLAND

Don H. Nelson and George W. Thorn

The pituitary gland lies at the base of the brain in a bony cavity, the sella turcica, within the sphenoid bone. The normal gland measures $10 \times 13 \times 6$ mm and weighs approximately 0.6 Gm. Anatomically it is divided into the anterior lobe, which constitutes three-quarters of the weight of the gland, a rudimentary intermediate lobe, and a posterior or neural lobe. The classic histology of the anterior lobe divides the cells into three types, depending on the presence and staining characteristics of the intracellular granules. These are the chromophobes, which are agranular, the eosinophils and the basophils, in the proportions of approximately 52, 37, and 11 percent, respectively. More detailed studies suggest that some of the agranular cells may contain fine acidophilic and basophilic granules; hence the term "amphophils."

The anterior lobe secretes a variety of peptide hormones, of which six are clearly defined. Growth hormone (HGH) has a generalized somatic effect on growth; adrenocorticotropin (ACTH) stimulates the secretory activity of the adrenal cortex; thyroid-stimulating hormone (thyrotropin, TSH) stimulates the formation and release of thyroid hormones; follicle-stimulating hormone (FSH) stimulates growth of the graafian follicle and estrogen secretion in the female and spermatogenesis in the male; luteinizing hormone (LH) initiates ovulation and luteinization of the mature follicle in the female; in the male, this hormone is the testicular interstitial cell-stimulating hormone (ICSH), responsible for male hormone secretion. Prolactin or lactogenic hormone (LtH) is responsible for secretion of milk by the properly developed mammary gland. Although production of the melanocyte-stimulating hormone (MSH) is classically ascribed to the intermediate lobe, this hormone may also be a secretion of the anterior lobe.

According to classic concepts, the chromophobe cells are considered to be nonsecretory, the eosinophilic cells responsible for secretion of GH, LH, and LtH, and the basophilic cells producing ACTH, TSH, and FSH. Such a simple classification, however, does not now seem probable; some pituitary tumors associated with Cushing's syndrome have been found to be composed of chromophobe as well as eosinophilic cells, although the largest number are small basophilic tumors. Similarly, eosinophilic tumors are most often associated with increased growth hormone production, but tumors of other cell types may occasionally be responsible.

PITUITARY TUMORS

Pituitary tumors account for approximately 10 percent of all intracranial tumors. By far the commonest pituitary tumor is the *Chromophobe adenoma*, which is usually nonsecretory in nature. Active pituitary tumors usually secrete only one pituitary hormone in excess.

Tumors secreting GH, ACTH, MSH, TSH, and LtH have all been described, although the last three types of tumor are very rare. FSH- or LH-secreting tumors are notable by their absence.

In addition to producing the *signs and symptoms* of hormone excess, discussed in later sections on the specific hormones, these tumors may compress and destroy normal pituitary tissue within the sella turcica and produce hormonal deficiency states, or they may extend out of the sella turcica to compress the optic nerves, hypothalamus, and other nervous structures in the vicinity. Pressure on the optic chiasma most often involves the decussating nerve fibers supplying the nasal retinal fields and leads to loss of the temporal fields of vision and classical bitemporal hemianopsia. Further extension of the tumor may involve one or both optic nerves and result in loss of visual acuity and even in complete blindness. These tumors may also compress the hypothalamus and result in disturbances in sleep, temperature control, appetite, and autonomic nervous functions. Curiously, these tumors are not known to damage the supraopticohypophyseal tract to a degree to cause diabetes insipidus. Involvement of the third, fourth, and sixth cranial nerves is rare but may occur. Headache is a frequent complaint in patients with this condition and has no well-defined pattern.

Clinical evaluation of these patients should include roentgenograms of the skull and visual fields, ophthalmoscopic examination, spinal fluid examination (particularly for increased protein content), and pneumoencephalography, especially in patients with severe optic nerve compression, increased intracranial pressure, or signs of hypothalamic and brain involvement. Carotid angiography may also be useful in delineating any extension of a tumor out of the sella.

Therapy of pituitary tumors generally involves a choice between pituitary irradiation or surgery. Postponement of specific treatment is justifiable in occasional patients with small, localized chromophobe adenomas, in which case specific hormonal replacement therapy should be initiated and the patient carefully observed for signs of tumor growth and extension. Surgical resection of tumor tissue is indicated when there is rapid deterioration of vision, ventricular obstruction, or significant brain compression. Although surgery provides the greatest opportunity for arrest of tumor growth, there is a calculated morbidity and mortality, particularly with the large tumors extending outside the sella turcica.

Radiotherapy in tissue doses of 3,500 to 4,500 r is often associated with regression of the tumor and relief of local signs and symptoms. In these doses, normal pituitary tissue and surrounding nervous structures are unharmed. Some tumors recur and may require further x-ray therapy, or surgery. Further experience with such experimental techniques as cryohypophysectomy, high-voltage and proton-beam irradiation, and radioactive implantations offers hope for better methods of treating these tumors.

Hemorrhage into a tumor, so-called "pituitary apoplexy," may result in an acute catastrophe accompanied by severe headache, blindness, hypotension or shock, fever, and signs of meningeal irritation or brain involvement. Emergency treatment is required, which may include surgical aspiration of the sella turcica, use of adrenal-steroids, and other supportive measures. Pituitary apoplexy may occur spontaneously and is occasionally observed following irradiation.

The craniopharyngioma, which is usually suprasellar in position, is the most common type of tumor involving the pituitary gland in childhood and thus the most common cause of prepuberal hypopituitarism. The tumor represents a secretory vestige of Rathke's pouch cut off from its origin in the roof of the pharynx and carried cephalad by the migrating pituitary anlage. The viscous, cholesterol-containing fluid of such suprasellar cysts is prone to calcification, which provides a useful diagnostic sign on x-ray examination. Although these tumors are more frequent in the younger age group, occasionally they are slow-growing and may not be clinically apparent until adult life. These patients often mature normally and come to the physician with an adult form of hypopituitarism. These tumors usually require surgical intervention. *Other tumors* which may involve the pituitary or the suprasellar area include meningiomas, epidermoid or dermoid tumors, primary or metastatic carcinomas, and granulomatous disorders such as sarcoidosis, gummas, tuberculomas, and Hand-Schüller-Christian disease.

GROWTH HORMONE

Growth hormone, unlike the other anterior pituitary hormones, does not have a specific "target organ" but has a generalized effect on all tissues and organs. This hormone has a molecular weight of 22,000, although there is some indication that an "active core" may be considerably smaller. Though once thought to be solely concerned with growth in the early years of life, growth hormone has been found to exert significant physiologic functions throughout life. It has been shown to facilitate amino acid transport and incorporation into protein, to mobilize free fatty acids from peripheral fat stores, and to reduce lipid synthesis. Growth hormone also causes renal retention and body storage of calcium, phosphorus, sodium, potassium, and nitrogen as part of its generalized anabolic action. It has an anti-insulin or diabetogenic action and, in large doses, can produce glucosuria, impaired glucose tolerance, and insulin resistance. Growth hormone is responsible for the elevated level of serum inorganic phosphorus and alkaline phosphatase observed in growing children.

Growth hormone is species-specific, and only primate growth hormone has been found to have significant physiologic effects in man and to be capable of stimulating growth in pituitary dwarfs.

Concentration of plasma growth hormone can now be determined with immunologic techniques, and elevated levels have been found in most patients with acromegaly. Significantly, growth hormone levels have been shown to increase following exercise, prolonged fast, and during hypoglycemia, which suggests a dynamic physiologic role for this hormone throughout life, in addition to its growth-promoting effects in childhood.

Other substances which may produce an increase in plasma growth hormone are arginine, vasopressin, pyrogens, and estrogens. The latter, due to their widespread use in contraceptive preparations, may give falsely high growth hormone values in patients suspected of having acromegaly.

Growth Hormone Secreting Tumors

Marie, in 1886, first described the classical clinical manifestations of acromegaly. One year later, Minkowski reported a case with a pituitary tumor, and Benda subsequently showed that such tumors were eosinophilic in nature. In 1895, Brissaud and Meige suggested an association between gigantism and acromegaly, and Hutchinson subsequently reported the pathologic findings in three cases of gigantism associated with pituitary tumors. Acromegaly and gigantism are now recognized as identical disturbances of growth hormone secretion, differing only in the age of onset of the disorder.

GIGANTISM

Prior to puberty, excess growth hormone secretion results in a generalized overgrowth of the skeleton and soft tissues. Early in the course of the disorder, these patients are usually physically strong and alert. Later in the disease, however, pituitary insufficiency may develop, with its associated weakness and easy fatigability. Hypogonadism of the pituitary type develops during the course of the disease.

The underlying lesion is generally an *eosinophilic or mixed cell adenoma of the anterior lobe* which is usually visible radiologically. The condition, although rare, presents no difficulty in diagnosis and needs only to be differentiated clinically from the tall stature of primary gonadal failure. Persons with the latter condition exhibit the characteristic eunuchoid habitus and associated gonadal failure and, unlike the patient with gigantism, have increased titers of urinary follicle stimulating hormone characteristic of primary hypogonadism. Treatment of pituitary gigantism is similar to that for acromegaly.

ACROMEGALY

In adults, the same type of pituitary tumor producing excess growth hormone results in the clinical picture of acromegaly. The disease is usually first manifested by changes in facial features and overgrowth of the head, hands, and feet which may necessitate an increase in hat, glove, or shoe size (Fig. 87-1). In other instances, headache or visual disturbances from local effects of the expanding pituitary tumor may be the first indications of the disorder.

The fully developed syndrome is easily recognized, but in the earlier stages, comparison of serial photographs over a span of years may be extremely helpful in documenting a gradual and progressive change in features.

The hands and feet are broad and greatly enlarged, the ends of the digits are square, and prognathism may be so marked as to interfere with mastication (Fig. 87-2). Arthritic manifestations are not unusual, and widespread osteoarthritic-like changes in the bones and joints are often demonstrable. Patients with acromegaly are particularly subject to psychologic disturbances and almost always exhibit considerable emotional instability.

Among the associated endocrine disturbances, enlargement of the thyroid and an increased basal metabolic rate are frequently found. Hyperthyroidism, however, occurs in only a small percentage of cases. Although frank diabetes mellitus is present in only 10 to 15 percent of these patients, glucose tolerance is impaired in the majority of patients during the active phase of the disease. Diabetes mellitus, when present, is typically mild but may be relatively resistant to insulin therapy. Libido may be increased at the onset but is lost subsequently, and gonadal atrophy may occur late in the disease. The course of the disease is usually one of benign chronicity, but fatal termination may occur as a result of cardiac failure, diabetic acidosis, local complications of the tumor, or unrecognized hypopituitarism.

Fig. 87-2. Characteristic tufting or "arrowhead" appearance of the terminal phalanx in acromegaly (right). Normal phalanx for comparison (left). Note also the thickness of the acromegalic finger.

Diagnosis

Diagnosis is made by the typical changes in body configuration, possible demonstration of a pituitary tumor by x-ray or visual field defects, and most importantly, by an elevated basal plasma growth hormone level which does not decrease during a standard glucose tolerance test. Because the skeletal changes are permanent, it is important in the treated as well as the untreated case to determine whether there is continual hypersecretion of growth hormone, or whether a deficiency of growth hormone and perhaps of other hormones has resulted from pituitary destruction from pressure, hemorrhage, or earlier x-ray therapy. Activity of the process is implied by continued skeletal and soft-tissue growth, by the presence of diabetes mellitus or a significantly impaired glucose tolerance test, by elevated levels of serum inorganic phosphorus and alkaline phosphatase, and by increased excretion of hydroxyproline in the urine. The basal plasma growth hormone determination is usually necessary for final determination of activity. Patients with active acromegaly may show a hyperactive increase in urinary 17-ketosteroid excretion following intravenous ACTH while 17-hydroxysteroid excretion is normal.

There is one familial condition without evidence of increased growth hormone, the Touraine-Solenti-Golé syndrome, in which afflicted individuals present acromegalic features. Particularly suggestive of acromegaly

Fig. 87-1. A forty-four-year-old woman with arrested acromegaly. Onset of the disease occurred when patient was twenty-four years of age, when enlargement of the sella turcica was demonstrated. Following x-ray therapy of the pituitary no further progression of the disease has been observed.

in this condition are the skin changes; thus its common designation, pachydermoperiostitis (idiopathic hypertrophic osteoarthropathy). Although the fingers are often clubbed, the periosteal thickening of the bones is not what one would expect to see in acromegaly. The amount of growth hormone is of course not increased.

TREATMENT. Eosinophilic adenomas may respond to irradiation, but in general this form of therapy is not presently considered to be so effective as an ablative procedure of the pituitary gland. The presence of hypopituitarism must be suspected and the appropriate substitution therapy instituted (adrenal, thyroid, and gonadal hormones), particularly if surgery is contemplated. Because of the permanent disfigurement which acromegaly produces, the progress of the disease must be watched closely, particularly in women, and earlier surgical intervention should be considered in an attempt to minimize the cosmetic complications. Although successful therapy will not reverse the bony changes, the decrease in hypertrophy of the skin and subcutaneous tissues may produce an important improvement in appearance.

ADRENOCORTICOTROPIN (ACTH)

This hormone is a polypeptide composed of 39 amino acids with a molecular weight of approximately 4,500. The primary structure has been elucidated, and small quantities have been synthesized (Fig. 87-3).

The principal physiologic effect of this hormone is to stimulate the secretion of hydrocortisone from the adrenal cortex. Under the stimulus of ACTH, the adrenal gland also secretes corticosterone, aldosterone, estrogens, and certain so-called "adrenal androgens." In the case of aldosterone, ACTH is not the chief controlling factor regulating its secretion. As part of its adrenal stimulating effect, ACTH promotes an increase in adrenal blood flow and hypertrophy of the gland. Certain extra-adrenal actions of ACTH of obscure physiologic significance include a lipid-mobilizing effect and a hypoglycemic action. ACTH has intrinsic melanocyte-stimulating activity because of similarities between its N-terminal amino acid sequence and the structure of MSH (Fig. 87-3).

Secretion of ACTH is regulated by the concentration of hydrocortisone in plasma and by various parts of the brain, particularly the anterior median eminence of the hypothalamus. Nerve cells in this area are thought to produce one or more peptide neurohormones, termed corticotropin-releasing factors (CRF), which are released into the pituitary portal circulation and stimulate the secretion of ACTH by the anterior pituitary cells. Higher centers of the brain may act to stimulate or inhibit ACTH secretion.

Central-nervous-system activity maintains a diurnal rhythm of ACTH secretion, which results in highest levels in early morning and lowest levels at night. There is a considerable increase in plasma ACTH concentration in adrenal insufficiency because of loss of the normal reciprocal relationship between plasma hydrocortisone concentration and ACTH secretion. Substantial increases in ACTH secretion occur during stress irrespective of the plasma steroid level. Prolonged administration of corticosteroids depresses the secretion of ACTH and results in adrenal atrophy indistinguishable from that observed in spontaneous hypopituitarism.

CUSHING'S DISEASE

(Also see Chap. 92.) In 1932, Cushing described the clinical disorder of pituitary basophilism associated with adrenocortical hyperplasia. This concept led to consid-

Fig. 87-3. Amino acid sequences of corticotropin and melanocyte-stimulating hormones. (Modified from I. Harris.)

erable controversy and a voluminous literature on the presence and significance of basophilic adenomas in patients with adrenocortical hyperfunction.

Relatively few patients with adrenocortical hyperfunction first come to the physician with definite enlargement of the pituitary gland; however, the incidence of pituitary tumor is significantly increased in those patients subjected to total adrenalectomy. Since bilateral total adrenalectomy has only been widely practiced for little more than a decade, it is possible that more patients will develop clinically evident pituitary tumors in due time. Curiously, most of the postadrenalectomy pituitary tumors have proved to be chromophobe adenomas. Eosinophilic and mixed-type tumors have also been found in Cushing's disease, but the largest number are associated with small basophilic tumors or hyalinization of the basophils.

Biologic tests for the measurement of ACTH in plasma, and more recently immunoassay techniques, may be of value in establishing the cause of adrenocortical hyperfunction. The finding of an elevated plasma ACTH level suggests a pituitary origin, but such an elevation may also be found in patients who have nonendocrine carcinomas that also secrete ACTH-like substances. In a series that we have undertaken, an elevated plasma ACTH level was found more often in those patients with a nonendocrine tumor, e.g., in the lung or pancreas, than in patients with Cushing's syndrome and adrenal hyperplasia. In an adrenalectomized patient with Cushing's disease, an abnormal elevation in ACTH, exceeding the level observed in Addison's disease or in patients adrenalectomized for other diseases, is highly suggestive of an ACTH-secreting pituitary tumor. These patients often show intense pigmentation of the skin which may be due to the MSH-like activity of ACTH referred to above or to actual secretion of MSH by the tumor.

Increased Plasma ACTH in Addison's Disease and Congenital Adrenal Hyperplasia

Elevated plasma ACTH levels are apparent within 24 hr of steroid withdrawal in patients with Addison's disease and fall to normal several hours after a physiologic dose of steroid. This excess production of ACTH is not pathologic and has not been associated with pituitary tumors. It may be, at least in part, responsible for the hyperpigmentation which occurs in this disease.

Patients with congenital adrenal hyperplasia also have elevated plasma ACTH level, because of a similar mechanism, deficient secretion of hydrocortisone. As far as is known, the pituitary gland is normal in this disease. The excess secretion of ACTH is also easily suppressed by physiologic doses of corticosteroids (see Chap. 92).

Increased ACTH Secretion in Tumors of Nonendocrine Origin

A number of patients with Cushing's syndrome secondary to the release of ACTH-like substances from non-

endocrine neoplasms has been reported. Carcinoma of the lung is the most frequent type of tumor associated with this syndrome. Of particular interest has been the association of Cushing's syndrome with benign bronchial adenomas as well as malignant tumors. In a few cases the substance produced by the tumor has been shown to be, in all probability, ACTH. It is possible that neoplastic tumors could also secrete an ACTH-releasing factor which would in turn stimulate the secretion or release of ACTH. The latter could be detected biologically by its effectiveness in the presence of an intact pituitary-adrenal system and its ineffectiveness in the absence of the anterior pituitary gland. To date, there is no evidence that these nonendocrine neoplasms secrete adrenal steroids; hence, removal of both adrenals should result in a cure of the Cushing's syndrome in circumstances which prevent the complete removal of the primary neoplasm.

THYROTROPIN (TSH)

(See Chap. 89). Thyrotropin is a glycoprotein of approximately 26,000 molecular weight. It stimulates the uptake of iodide by the thyroid gland and the synthesis and release of thyroid hormones. Continued stimulation results in hypertrophy of the gland and an increase in the vasculature. Thyrotropin deficiency results in glandular atrophy and depressed thyroid function. The administration of thyroid hormone depresses the secretion of thyrotropin and produces similar changes in thyroid function. There is good evidence that the ventral medial nuclei and paraventricular nuclei of the hypothalamus are involved in the control of TSH secretion, and that destruction of these areas depresses thyroid hormone synthesis.

The role of the anterior pituitary in the causation of primary hyperthyroidism is not clear. Although elevated levels of TSH in the blood of patients with hyperthyroidism have been reported, the results have not been consistently reproducible. A long-acting thyroid stimulator (LATS) has been demonstrated in the plasma of a high proportion of patients with hyperthyroidism.

The anterior pituitary gland may also secrete an exophthalmos-producing substance which may be responsible for the ocular manifestations of exophthalmic goiter.

The occurrence of hyperthyroidism following hypophysectomy or pituitary stalk section suggests that TSH may not be essential for the development of hyperthyroidism. It does appear, however, that certain pituitary tumors may secrete excess TSH and result in thyroid hyperplasia and hypersecretion. Since TSH secretion may be increased by stimuli arising in the hypothalamus, it is thought that a mechanism acting through higher central nervous system centers may be related to the not-infrequent development of thyrotoxicosis following major emotional or psychic trauma. It is also probable that increased TSH secretion is involved in the hyperthyroidism associated with acromegaly.

GONADOTROPINS

(See Chap. 98). The gonadotropins, FSH and LH, are large protein hormones of approximately 30,000 molecular weight. These hormones regulate the development, reproductive functions, and hormonal secretions of the ovary and testicle. Prolactin (LtH) is also classed as a gonadotropin; however, its primary action is on the mammary gland and though it may be luteotrophic (i.e., sustaining the function of the corpus luteum) in lower animal species, this action has not been shown to be of physiologic significance in man.

The secretion of gonadotropins is influenced by the rate of sex hormone production and by certain areas of the hypothalamus. Castration increases and estrogens decrease the secretion of FSH, probably by modifying the hypothalamic centers which control FSH secretion by the anterior pituitary. The secretion of LH is also increased by castration but is less sensitive to inhibition by estrogens. Progesterone depresses LH secretion in some species. Testosterone is a poor inhibitor of FSH secretion but does block the secretion of LH.

Secretion of LH has been clearly shown to be regulated by the posterior hypothalamus. This area is also important in prolactin secretion, probably by producing a hormone that inhibits the production and release of LtH by the anterior pituitary. Lesions in this area block LH secretion and result in enhanced secretion of prolactin and pathologic lactation.

Gonadotropins are not found in the urine until puberty. Thereafter, they are present in significant quantities throughout life, with peaks of excretion appearing at the time of ovulation and greatly increased levels occurring after the menopause or following castration. Although relatively crude, the bioassay for urinary gonadotropins (FSH assay) is the most widely used direct assay of a pituitary hormone in general use. The assay is not specific for FSH, since even small quantities of LH appear to be necessary for the biologic action of FSH. Low urinary FSH levels are occasionally found in normal individuals, and several determinations are necessary for accurate clinical evaluation. Increasing availability of radioimmunassay of these and other pituitary hormones makes diagnosis of gonadotropin abnormalities much more reliable.

Chorionic gonadotropin (HCG) is derived from the placenta and appears in the urine in large quantities during pregnancy. Preparations from human pregnancy urine are available for clinical use. This hormone has predominantly an LH action and is used clinically to stimulate Leydig cell function and ovulation (Chap. 98).

Sexual Precocity

No definite pituitary disorders are associated with increased secretion of LH or FSH. There are cases of isosexual precocity, often familial, in which premature but normal sexual development occurs, probably on the basis of early maturation of central nervous system centers regulating gonadotropin formation and release. Lesions of the hypothalamus or pineal gland also may result in premature secretion of gonadotropic hormones and precocious puberty (Chap. 100).

Galactorrhea

Abnormal lactation is sometimes observed in patients with acromegaly or chromophobe adenomas and also may occur after pituitary stalk section. A condition associated with persistent post-partum lactation and amenorrhea is referred to as the Chiari-Frommel syndrome. The galactorrhea in these disorders is most likely the result of excess prolactin secretion. If a pituitary tumor is found, it should be treated. In the absence of evidence of a tumor, galactorrhea may be suppressed by estrogen administration.

PANHYPOPITUITARISM

PREPUBERAL. Prepuberal panhypopituitarism, which was first described in 1871 by Lorrain, is a rare condition usually associated with suprasellar cyst or craniopharyngioma. The disease is characterized by dwarfism and subnormal sexual development but normal mentality. The impairment of growth is symmetric and the body proportions are normal. As in other cases of hypopituitarism, the skin often has a pale yellowish appearance and increased wrinkling. Sexual maturation is delayed, and in rare cases there may be obesity from hypothalamic involvement. Diabetes insipidus is not an infrequent accompaniment.

If the tumor is of sufficient size to affect the optic chiasma, there may be bitemporal hemianopsia or complete blindness. X-ray studies reveal delayed fusion of the epiphyses, supresellar calcification, and, often, destruction of the sella turcica. The condition must be distinguished from genetic dwarfism and from hypothyroidism. Children with a familial type of dwarfism have isolated deficiency of growth hormone secretion but normal production of other pituitary hormones and development of epiphyses consistent with chronologic age. Hypothyroid children have subnormal mentality, infantile body proportions, dwarfism, and the characteristic epiphyseal dysgenesis.

Treatment with cortisone, thyroid, and sex hormones, described in more detail in the next section, should be instituted, with dosage adjusted for body size and age. Although limited by the availability of material, human or monkey growth hormone in doses of 1 to 3 mg weekly has had considerable success in producing growth in these patients. Because of the psychologic and sociologic importance of reaching normal stature, every attempt should be made to obtain such therapy for these patients if the epiphyses have not closed. Growth hormone from nonprimate sources has had no effect on growth in human beings.

POSTPUBERAL PANHYPOPITUITARISM. The common causes for panhypopituitarism in the adult include chromophobe adenoma, post-partum pituitary necrosis, craniopharyngiomas, and the end stages of acromegaly. Less common lesions include gliomas, basilar meningitis, head injuries associated with hemorrhage into the pituitary or the suprasellar region, and granulomatous disorders such as sarcoidosis and Hand-Schüller-Christian disease.

Post-partum pituitary necrosis (Sheehan's syndrome) is due to extensive thrombosis of the pituitary circulation during delivery, usually associated with uterine hemorrhage but occasionally developing after a bout of hypotension without blood loss. Characteristically, these patients fail to lactate in the puerperium and do not have a recurrence of menstrual function. The association of these signs should always suggest this diagnosis. There follows the insidious onset of a host of vague symptoms, including asthenia, lethargy, loss of libido, loss of axillary and pubic hair, and cold intolerance (Fig. 87-4). Some patients appear quite healthy and often are classified as psychoneurotic until the true diagnosis is revealed. Others gradually lapse into a far-advanced state of anterior pituitary insufficiency involving gonadal, thyroid, and adrenal function in approximately that order of development. Physical signs consist of bradycardia, hypotension, loss of axillary, pubic, and scalp hair, premature wrinkling and pallor of the skin, which is fine and atrophic, and a general loss of secondary sex characteristics, with atrophy of the breasts and genitalia.

Irrespective of the cause of panhypopituitarism, the secondary effects on the endocrine glands are similar. There is marked atrophy of the thyroid, adrenals, and gonads. Interference with growth occurs if the lesion appears prior to epiphyseal closure. The pituitary gland has a large reserve, and substantial amounts of pituitary tissue must be damaged before significant hormone deficiency develops. Not all patients develop hypofunction of all three target glands; isolated gonadal failure is relatively common, or gonadal failure may be associated with either thyroid or adrenal insufficiency. Isolated growth hormone deficiency, TSH or ACTH deficiency may also be seen although the latter is quite rare.

LABORATORY FINDINGS. Laboratory findings reflect decreased function of the target endocrine glands. Thus, the serum protein-bound iodine and thyroidal radioiodine uptake are low, and there is a decrease in the basal metabolic rate. The level of serum cholesterol, unlike that in primary myxedema, is rarely elevated, despite lowered thyroid function. Levels of urinary 17-ketosteroids, 17-hydroxycorticosteroids, and 17-ketogenic steroids are depressed, and urinary gonadotropins are subnormal or absent. Blood levels of ACTH and growth hormone are depressed. A normochromic anemia is often present, and there may be leukopenia and relative lymphocytosis in the presence of adrenal insufficiency. Fasting hypoglycemia is rarely found but may occasionally be severe enough to produce coma. The serum sodium concentration is usually normal, but hyponatremia may occur during periods of stress. The serum potassium level and BUN are usually normal, in contrast to increases seen in the patient with Addisonian crisis.

DIAGNOSIS. The diagnosis of hypopituitarism is generally not difficult to establish once it is suspected, but because of the insidious onset and the variable signs and symptoms, the disorder may escape detection for many years. These patients often come to the physician with acute medical emergencies associated with infection or trauma and fail to respond normally to the usual therapeutic measures. In such instances, clinical evidence of gonadal, thyroid, or adrenal insufficiency should be sought; if present, it will quickly suggest the diagnosis.

Patients with pituitary myxedema must be differentiated from those with primary thyroidal failure. Patients with the pituitary form often do not appear to be so myxedematous as those with primary hypothyroidism. An enlarged thyroid gland is indicative of primary hypothyroidism, since the thyroid is atrophic in hypopituitarism. In the absence of clear evidence of a primary thyroid disorder such as might result from radioiodine therapy, thyroidectomy, or thyroiditis, pituitary insufficiency should be ruled out in every patient with hypothyroidism. The response to TSH is helpful in differentiating primary from pituitary hypothyroidism. In contrast to the lack of response to TSH in the patient with primary hypothyroidism, a marked increase in the protein-bound iodine and the radio-iodine uptake will be produced in the patient with the pituitary type of hypothyroidism by the administration of 10 units of TSH intramuscularly daily for 2 days. Some patients with pituitary myxedema may not respond to TSH, probably because of advanced thyroidal atrophy.

The patient with adrenal failure secondary to pituitary disease will usually show an increase in the 24-hr urinary excretion of 17-ketosteroids, 17-hydroxycorticosteroids, and 17-ketogenic steroids with administration of ACTH. These patients often do not respond to a single day's infusion of ACTH, but administration of 40 units intravenously over an 8-hr period on three or four successive days characteristically will reveal a step-wise increase in steroid excretion by the third or fourth day of administration. Hypopituitary patients secrete near-normal quantities of aldosterone and thus are usually in sodium balance. Hyponatremia, when it does occur, however, may be due to sodium depletion as well as to extracellu-

Fig. 87-4. Photographs of a forty-year-old woman when first seen for hypopituitarism (Simmond's disease) and after 6 months' therapy.

lar dilution. The hyponatremia seen secondary to hypopituitarism is easily corrected by the intravenous administration of cortisol in contrast to hyponatremia secondary to the inappropriate secretion of antidiuretic hormone.

Measurement of urinary steroids following the administration of 2-methyl-1,2 bis-(3-pyridyl)-1-propane [SU 4885 (Metopirone)] provides a particularly useful index of the ability of the pituitary gland to increase ACTH secretion. This compound inhibits the 11-hydroxylation of the steroid molecule in the adrenal gland and leads to decreased secretion of 17-hydroxycorticosterone (hydrocortisone) and increased secretion of 17-hydroxy-11-deoxycorticosterone (substance S). The hydrocortisone deficiency results in increased ACTH secretion from the anterior pituitary gland, a marked increase in the adrenal secretion of substance S, and a resultant increase in the urinary excretion of 17-hydroxycorticosteroids and 17-ketogenic steroids. Patients with normal pituitary-adrenal function will show an increase in these urinary steroids with this drug, but patients with either primary or secondary adrenal insufficiency will fail to demonstrate such an increase in urinary 17-hydroxycorticosteroids (Fig. 87-5). This test is of particular value in assessing pituitary ACTH reserve in patients who have normal or only slightly depressed basal urinary steroid levels. It is a hazardous test in patients with obvious deficiency in adrenal steroid secretion and can induce adrenal crisis in patients with primary adrenal insufficiency or those with adrenal atrophy secondary to deficient ACTH production. For this reason the test is best performed on hospitalized patients. If adrenal insufficiency occurs, it can be relieved quickly by IV cortisol.

Hypogonadism secondary to pituitary disease is characterized by decreased or absent urinary gonadotropins, in contrast to the increased titers found in primary gonadal failure. The prolonged amenorrhea observed in many patients with chronic illness and especially in those with anorexia nervosa is often confused with that due to panhypopituitarism. Urinary gonadotropin concentration may be low in these patients, but adrenal and thyroid function is usually normal. Thus, detailed study of each target gland will often be necessary to establish or rule out pituitary insufficiency in patients with obscure hypogonadism, hypothyroidism, or hypoadrenalism.

Other physiologic tests which have been employed in the past in establishing a diagnosis of hypopituitarism, such as the insulin tolerance test and the water test are less specific and may be life-threatening if not carried out under close supervision.

Patients with pituitary-adrenal insufficiency excrete administered water at a depressed rate, similar to the rate of excretion in patients with primary adrenal failure; however, this test may be falsely positive in the presence of renal, hepatic, or cardiac disease. These patients may develop water intoxication during the test and should be carefully observed for this complication and treated with I.V. cortisol if required.

TREATMENT. The use of pituitary hormones would be true replacement therapy for panhypopituitarism. However TSH and ACTH must be given daily by intramus-

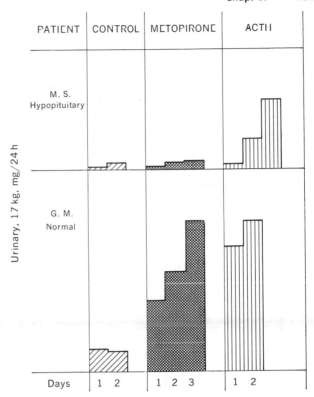

Fig. 87-5 Response of urinary 17-ketogenic steroids in a hypopituitary patient (M.S.) and a normal subject (G.M.) to Metopirone (750 mg every 6 hr for 48 hr) and ACTH (40 units intravenously over 8 hr on two or three successive days). Note the lack of response to Metopirone and delayed response to ACTH in the hypopituitary patient.

cular injection, and pituitary gonadotropins cannot be used successfully for any prolonged period because of the tendency to antibody formation. In practice, excellent results are obtained by oral replacement therapy with the target gland hormones. Thyroxin should be given at first in a dose of 0.05 mg a day, with the amount gradually increased over a period of several weeks to a total daily dose of 0.2 to 0.3 mg. Cortisone acetate should be initiated at a level of 5 to 10 mg per day and increased to 15 to 30 mg as needed. Since the administration of thyroid hormone alone in a patient with associated pituitary-adrenal insufficiency may precipitate a serious adrenal crisis, it is important to initiate cortisone therapy prior to or at least simultaneously with thyroxin therapy in these patients. Salt-retaining hormone therapy is generally not needed, but if required, can be achieved with the oral administration of 0.05 to 0.1 mg fluorohydrocortisone daily.

A long-acting testosterone preparation should be given intramuscularly in doses of 100 to 200 mg every 2 to 4 weeks to male patients; proportionately smaller doses are often beneficial in female patients. In the female patient, estrogens may be given daily by mouth or at intervals of 2 to 4 weeks by injection. If desired, cyclic therapy with estrogens and progesterone may be given to induce artificial menstrual function.

It should be emphasized that hormonal therapy is intended only to provide normal replacement of physiologic levels for proper body function. Although the harmful effects of large-dose corticosteroid administration may not be observed with this schedule, psychic disturbances of various kinds are occasionally noted in patients suddenly exposed to full replacement therapy after a long period of adrenal or thyroid hormone deficiency. Another problem often noted is that of excessive appetite in some patients receiving even small doses of cortisone. In this instance, it may be necessary to institute a restrictive diet or to decrease cortisone dosage to bare minimum levels.

OTHER SYNDROMES OF POSSIBLE PITUITARY ORIGIN

Froehlich's syndrome and the Laurence-Moon-Biedl syndrome are two disorders associated with failure of gonadal development in which disturbances in anterior pituitary gonadotropin secretion are postulated. However, no consistent lesions have been observed in the anterior pituitary; and it is thought that the primary disturbance is in the hypothalamus.

Froehlich's syndrome is associated with adiposity and sexual infantilism. In addition to truncal obesity, there are underdevelopment of the gonads and an absence of the secondary sex characteristics. The condition may be associated with mental retardation, visual disturbances, diabetes insipidus, and impaired skeletal growth. It is important to differentiate between cases of Froehlich's habitus (obesity and apparently delayed genital development) and true Froehlich's syndrome. The former condition is often observed in normal prepuberal boys who may have normal sex organs hidden in the adipose tissue. With the onset of puberty, these boys develop normally and often lose their adiposity and assume normal adolescent body proportions. Froehlich's syndrome may be associated with tumors or other disorders of the hypothalamic-pituitary area. The obesity may be caused by damage to hypothalamic centers regulating appetite.

The Laurence-Moon-Biedl syndrome is a hereditary disease characterized by adiposity, genital atrophy, mental retardation, skull deformities, retinitis pigmentosa, and associated congenital malformations such as polydactyly and syndactyly. Fewer than 100 cases have been reported, and there is no evidence of pituitary lesions in these patients. The adiposity and genital atrophy are assumed to be caused by hypothalamic-pituitary dysfunction.

INTERMEDIATE LOBE OF THE PITUITARY GLAND

The intermediate lobe of the pituitary gland is the probable site of production of melanocyte-stimulating hormone (MSH). Two types of MSH have been identified. Alpha-MSH is a polypeptide composed of the same 13 amino acids found in the N-terminal position of ACTH (Fig. 87-3). Human β-MSH contains 22 amino acids and is closely related structurally to α-MSH as well as to ACTH. Because of the common N-terminal sequence, ACTH preparations have intrinsic melanocyte-stimulating effects; however, pure MSH does not stimulate adrenal cortical secretion. It is of interest that cortisone administration may suppress MSH as well as ACTH secretion from the pituitary gland.

There have been descriptions of MSH-secreting tumors of the pituitary gland. These rare tumors are associated with a generalized increase in pigmentation similar to that observed in patients with pituitary tumors following adrenalectomy for Cushing's syndrome. The hyperpigmentation observed in patients with Addison's disease may be due to increased production of MSH as well as ACTH. Increased MSH secretion may also be responsible for the hyperpigmentation observed in some cases of hyperthyroidism, biliary cirrhosis, sprue, and other chronic diseases. Conversely, it is probable that the decreased pigmentation often apparent in patients with panhypopituitarism is due to decreased production of MSH.

REFERENCES

Antoniades, H. N.: "Hormones in Human Plasma," Boston, Little, Brown and Company. 1960.

Brasel, J. A., J. C. Wright, L. Wilkins, and R. M. Blizzard: An Evaluation of Seventy-five Patients with Hypopituitarism Beginning in Childhood, Am. J. Med., 38: 484, 1965.

Harris, G. W., and B. T. Donovan: "The Pituitary Gland," London, Butterworths, 1966.

Lerner, A. B.: Hormonal Control of Pigmentation, Ann. Rev. Med., 11:187, 1960.

Liddle, G. W., D. Island, and C. K. Meader: Normal and Abnormal Regulation of Corticotropin Secretion in Man, Recent Progr. Hormone Res., 13:125, 1962.

Nelson, D. H., J. W. Meakin, and G. W. Thorn: ACTH-producing Pituitary Tumors Following Adrenalectomy for Cushing's Syndrome, Ann. Intern. Med., 52:560, 1960.

Odell, W. D., G. T. Ross, and P. L. Rayford: Radioimmunassay for Human Luteinizing Hormone, Metabolism, 15: 287, 1966.

Poppen, J. L.: Changing Concepts in the Treatment of Pituitary Adenomas, Bull. N.Y. Acad. Med., 39:21, 1963.

Purnell, D. C., R. V. Randall, and E. H. Rynearson: Postpartum Pituitary Insufficiency (Sheehan's Syndrome): Review of Eighteen Cases, Proc. Staff Meetings Mayo Clin., 39:321, 1964.

Rabkin, M. T., and A. G. Frantz: Hypopituitarism: A Study of Growth Hormone and Other Endocrine Functions, Ann. Intern. Med., 64:1197, 1966.

Rimoin, D. L., T. J. Merimee, and V. A. McKusick: Growth Hormone Deficiency in Man: An Isolated, Recessively Inherited Defect, Science, 152:1635, 1966.

Roth, J., S. M. Glick, P. Cuatrecasas, and C. S. Hollander: Acromegaly and Other Disorders of Growth Hormone Secretion, Ann. Intern. Med., 66:760, 1967.

Utiger, R. D.: Radioimmunassay of Human Plasma Thyrotropin, J. Clin. Invest., 44:1277, 1965.

88 DISEASES OF THE NEUROHYPOPHYSIS

Joseph F. Dingman and
George W. Thorn

Oliver and Schaefer in 1894 demonstrated a pressor effect of pituitary extracts, and in 1897 Howell showed that the pressor principle resided in the posterior lobe. The oxytocic action of posterior pituitary extracts was described by Dale in 1909 and the antidiuretic action by von den Velden in 1913. Fisher, Ingram, and Ranson in 1938 demonstrated a functional relationship between certain hypothalamic nuclei and the posterior pituitary. The studies of Scharrer and Scharrer since 1928 concerning the secretory activity of nerve cells (neurosecretion), the demonstration by Bargmann in 1949 of secretory granules in the neurones of the supraoptic and paraventricular nuclei of the hypothalamus, and the successful synthesis of oxytocin and vasopressin by du Vigneaud and coworkers represent important advances in current understanding of the endocrine functions of the neurohypophysis.

General Considerations

The principal effects of posterior pituitary extracts are to enhance the reabsorption of water by the renal tubules (antidiuretic effect); stimulate uterine contraction (oxytocic effect); promote the secretion of milk from the lactating breast (milk-ejecting effect); and, only in anesthetized mammals, produce a rise in blood pressure (vasopressor effect). The neurohypophyseal hormones are vasopressin (antidiuretic hormone, ADH) and oxytocin. The former is predominantly responsible for pressor and antidiuretic actions, whereas the latter is most potent in uterine stimulation and milk ejection. The neuroendocrine unit responsible for production and secretion of these hormones has been designated the neurohypophysis (Fig. 88-1) which includes the neurones of the supraoptic and paraventricular nuclei of the anterior hypothalamus, the axones that form the supraopticohypophyseal tract, and the posterior lobe of the pituitary body, the pars nervosa, in which the axone endings terminate.

Classic concepts of the endocrine function of the neurohypophysis ascribed the role of hormone production to parenchymatous secretory cells in the posterior lobe; however, an impressive body of evidence has been accumulated to show that vasopressin is actually secreted by the neurones of the supraoptic nuclei and oxytocin by the paraventricular nuclei. Gomori's chrome hematoxylin stain for the beta cells of the pancreatic islets demonstrated the presence of secretory granules within the cytoplasm of these neurones. These granules migrate along the axones and accumulate in the perivascular axone endplates in the posterior pituitary. The bulk of neurohypophyseal hormone is contained in the posterior lobe and only a small fraction of total activity is found in the tuber cinereum, stalk, and hypothalamic nuclei. The posterior pituitary then serves mainly as a reservoir of hormone readily available for rapid release into the systemic circulation.

Removal of the posterior lobe will lead to hormonal deficiency only if most of the axones of the hypothalamohypophyseal tract are severed and retrograde degeneration of the hypothalamic neurones occurs. With severance of the stalk close to the posterior pituitary body, short axones terminating at a higher level may escape injury and the remaining viable neurosecretory cells apparently

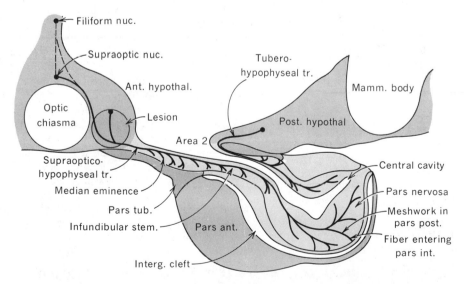

Fig. 88-1. Diagram of a midsagittal section through the hypothalamus and hypophysis. The broken lines indicate proposed filiform-supraoptic connections and the tractus paraventricularis. The gray circle indicates the position of a typical lesion designed to produce diabetes insipidus. (*Fisher, Ingram, and Ranson: "Diabetes Insipidus and the Neuro-Hormonal Control of Water Balance," Fig. 2, Ann Arbor, Mich., J. W. Edwards, Publisher. Incorporated, 1938.*)

can maintain secretion and release of hormones, probably into the vessels of the stalk and the hypothalamus.

The physiologic significance of the peculiar anatomic location of this neurosecretory organ, in which hypothalamic neurones extend their processes over relatively great distances into the posterior pituitary, is obscure. Such an arrangement may have been necessary, teleologically, in order to provide a ready route for hormone release into the systemic circulation through the highly vascularized posterior pituitary. In addition, posterior lobe extracts contain one or more hypothalamic neurohormones, which regulate the release of ACTH from the anterior pituitary (corticotropin-releasing factor, CRF), and oxytocin may play a role in regulating the secretion of prolactin (lactogenic hormone). Thus, the neurohypophysis may provide an important link between the central nervous system and the secretion of anterior pituitary tropic hormones which so profoundly influence the body economy.

In view of this evidence, consideration of the posterior pituitary as an endocrine gland warrants revision, and reference should be made to the neurohypophysis when discussing this endocrine system. However, the terms posterior pituitary gland and posterior lobe hormone are still in common usage at the present time.

Fig. 88-2. Oxytocin. (*B. Berde: "Recent Progress in Oxytocin Research," Fig. 1, Springfield, Ill., Charles C Thomas, Publisher, 1959.*)

Nature of Neurohypophyseal Hormones

Extracts of the neurohypophysis are assayed biologically with reference to oxytocic, vasopressor, and antidiuretic activities. One international USP or BP unit is defined as the activity of 0.5 mg of an international standard bovine posterior pituitary powder. In crude extracts of the posterior lobe the biologic activity appears to reside in a homogeneous protein or polypeptide fraction having a molecular weight of the order of 30,000 and an isoelectric point of pH 4.8. Such fractions show approximately equal vasopressor and oxytocic activities in terms of the reference powder, of the order of 16.6 IU per milligram. It has not been conclusively established whether this protein represents the natural secretion of the neurohypophysis or whether vasopressin and oxytocin loosely bound to the protein by electrostatic forces are released in a free form into the circulation.

Using modern technics of ion exchange chromatography and countercurrent distribution, highly purified preparations of *vasopressin* (600 IU per milligram) and oxytocin (500 IU per milligram) have been obtained from posterior lobe extracts. Both vasopressin and oxytocin contain eight amino acids and 3 moles of ammonia. The peptide structure of each hormone has been determined, and both hormones have been successfully synthesized by de Vigneaud and his coworkers, representing a milestone in peptide chemistry and hormone research. Both hormones are composed of five amino acids arranged in the form of a ring closed by the disulfide linkage of cystine, with a side chain of three amino acids. Oxytocin contains cystine, tyrosine, isoleucine, glutamine, and asparagine in the ring, with proline, leucine, and glycinamide in the side chain (Fig. 88-2). Vasopressin differs from oxytocin by only two amino acids. Phenylalanine replaces isoleucine in the ring, and leucine in the side chain is replaced by arginine (human, beef vasopressin, Fig. 88-3) or lysine (hog vasopressin). The molecular weight of oxytocin is 1,007 and of arginine vasopressin, 1,084. Both are ampholytes, oxytocin having an isolectric point of pH 7.7, and arginine vasopressin being considerably more basic, with an IP of pH 10.9.

Oxytocin has been shown to possess slight but definite pressor and antidiuretic effects, whereas vasopressin contains not only equal pressor and antidiuretic activities but also significant intrinsic oxytocic and milk-ejecting properties. Partially purified posterior pituitary preparations available commercially include Pitocin (oxytocin) and Pitressin (vasopressin), each fraction being slightly contaminated by the other in pharmaceutical preparations. Synthetic oxytocin (Syntocinon) is now available, and synthetic lysine vasopressin should soon become available for clinical use.

Physiology of Neurohypophyseal Secretion

Secretion of vasopressin is regulated by the total solute concentration or osmolality of plasma (osmoregulation),

Fig. 88-3. Vasopressin. (B. Berde: "Recent Progress in Oxytocin Research," Fig. 2, Springfield, Ill., Charles C Thomas, Publisher, 1959.)

the intravascular or extracellular fluid volume (volume regulation), and by central nervous system activity (neural regulation). Secretion of oxytocin has been demonstrated during labor and milk release, consistent with the known uterotonic and milk-ejecting actions of the hormone. (Other factors regulating oxytocin secretion will be discussed below).

The osmoregulatory mechanism controlling vasopressin release is exquisitely sensitive to slight changes in plasma osmolality. Dilution of the plasma solutes by administration of water inhibits the secretion of vasopressin, and rapid excretion of water by the kidneys ensues; secretion is restored when plasma osmolality returns to normal. An increase in plasma osmolality resulting from a deficit of water or a relative increase in the ratio of extracellular to intracellular solutes stimulates the secretion of vasopressin and maximum conservation of water by the kidneys. This mechanism is probably the first line of defense in day-to-day preservation of water balance and is mediated principally by changes in the concentration of sodium in the extracellular fluid.

A poorly understood auxiliary mechanism regulating vasopressin secretion, which may be more important than plasma osmolality, especially in pathologic conditions, is the influence of the volume of the body fluids on neurohypophyseal function. Various procedures which reduce effective blood volume such as quiet standing, venous congestion, and hemorrhage are known to stimulate vasopressin secretion. The acute release of vasopressin with graded hemorrhage in the dog can be effectively blocked by severance of the vagi and maintenance of carotid sinus perfusion pressure. Thus, it appears that a contrac-

tion of blood volume activates afferent neural pathways to the neurohypophysis which arise in the carotid and aortic baroreceptors and the stretch receptors in the wall of the left atrium.

Of the two vascular modalities, osmolality and volume, the former apparently operates effectively in most normal situations by retaining or releasing body water to suit the needs of the body. However, in pathologic conditions characterized by a decrease in intravascular or extracellular fluid volume or in cardiac output, volume regulation supersedes osmoregulation. In this situation, vasopressin secretion may persist despite the simultaneous occurrence of hypotonicity. A primary decrease in osmolality, such as that seen in the hyponatremia of Addison's disease, salt-losing nephritis, or long-standing congestive heart failure, would severely deplete body water if osmolality were the only factor governing vasopressin secretion. A regulator of secretion sensitive to the volume of the body water or the fullness of the vascular compartment or both would protect against desiccation and vascular collapse in these situations, the body giving up an optimal osmotic state for the vital requirements of the tissues for water. This antidiuretic mechanism, although protective in nature, may lead to serious complications, particularly in disorders already characterized by fluid retention and edema, since persistent water retention in salt-restricted subjects may lead to severe hyponatremia, water intoxication, and further compromise of circulation and renal function (Chap. 296).

Since neurohypophyseal hormones represent secretions of the central nervous system, studies of the central neural control of the neurohypophysis have assumed great importance in neuroendocrine physiology. There is little doubt that the central nervous system has a dominant role in regulating vasopressin secretion. Secretion of vasopressin has been produced in man and monkeys by electrical stimulation of the hypothalamus and components of the "limbic system" including the hippocampus, the amygdala, the septal nuclei, and the mesencephalic reticular formation. Electrical stimulation of various areas of the cerebral cortex, however, has been shown not to evoke vasopressin release. These findings suggest that neural reflexes to the neurohypophysis may be transmitted primarily via the more primitive areas of the brain rather than through neocortical pathways.

Studies of neurohypophyseal physiology have been significantly advanced by the development of specific assay methods for arginine vasopressin and oxytocin in plasma using cation exchange resin columns to isolate the polypeptide hormone fraction and glass paper chromatography to separate vasopressin and oxytocin from each other. The concentrations of these hormones in normal human plasma after overnight dehydration range from 2.5 to 10 microunits per ml for vasopressin and 300 to 1,000 microunits per ml for oxytocin. Forced hydration inhibits vasopressin secretion, but oxytocin levels increase two- to threefold over fasting levels. Nicotine and hypertonic saline stimulate vasopressin secretion, but oxytocin secretion is acutely inhibited in most subjects. Specific increases in oxytocin secretion accompanied by an abrupt cessation of vasopressin secretion have been observed both during active labor as well as during breast feeding.

The release of vasopressin with increased plasma osmolality and contracting blood volume and its inhibition with plasma dilution are consistent with this hormone's physiologic role in water metabolism. The release of oxytocin during labor and breast feeding is also representative of specific physiologic responses. However, the inhibition of oxytocin secretion during vasopressin release and the converse response during active oxytocin secretion suggest a reciprocal relation in neurohypophyseal hormone secretion which may have important but still undefined implications in health and disease. Of obscure physiologic significance are the findings of measurable oxytocin levels in mildly dehydrated subjects of both sexes and the increase in oxytocin secretion observed with hypotonic expansion of the body fluid volume.

Normal to elevated plasma oxytocin levels have been found in most patients with spontaneous diabetes insipidus, and oxytocin deficiency has been observed only in patients subjected to hypophysectomy or pituitary stalk section. These findings corroborate the experimental evidence for separate sites of secretion of vasopressin and oxytocin by the supraoptic and paraventricular nuclei respectively. Lesions of the median eminence or anterior hypothalamus which interrupt the supraoptico-hypophyseal tract apparently spare certain paraventricular axons which enter the stalk from more lateral and caudal areas of the hypothalamus. Severance of the pituitary stalk would be expected to interrupt all nerve tracts to the posterior pituitary and thus lead to combined vasopressin and oxytocin deficiency.

Numerous centrally acting substances stimulate the neurohypophysis. These include emotional stresses such as fright, noise, and pain; fainting, which may also act through volume regulators; coitus, suckling, and changes in environmental temperature; and numerous drugs such as nicotine, acetylcholine, and many hypnotics and sedatives. Alcohol inhibits ADH secretion. Of the various hormones and endogenous substances, small doses of epinephrine inhibit and large doses stimulate the release of vasopressin, at least in animals. Ferritin, the iron-containing hepatic vasodepressor substance, and bradykinin have been shown to be antidiuretic by virtue of stimulating the neurohypophysis, and the hydrocortisone-like adrenal steroids have been shown to inhibit vasopressin secretion (see below).

Thus it is readily apparent that the neurohypophyseal hormones are secreted under diverse and seemingly inexplicable situations. With the availability of specific assay methods for these hormones in human plasma, their importance in the body economy and in the pathogenesis and the complications of disease should soon be more clearly defined.

Physiologic Actions of Neurohypophyseal Hormones

VASOPRESSIN (ADH). The pressor and antidiuretic activities of vasopressin are properties of a single molecule. The antidiuretic action is of profound importance in regulating water balance. The current hypothesis as to the mechanism of action of vasopressin on water reabsorption by the kidney, based on experiments with various biologic membranes, such as frog skin and toad bladder, is that it renders the cells of the distal portions of the nephron permeable to water, permitting passive diffusion of tubular water along an osmotic gradient across the cell and into the peritubular vessels. The antidiuretic action of vasopressin is best demonstrated during water diuresis; *this effect represents the true physiologic role of the hormone on water metabolism, which is to prevent the bulk of the filtered water entering the distal tubular segment from escaping into the urine.* The effect of vasopressin during hypertonic urine flow is extremely variable and limited by the maximum rate of water reabsorption which the concentrating mechanism of the collecting tubules can achieve.

An interesting aspect of the studies of the action of vasopressin on biologic membranes has been the demonstration that this hormone has a pronounced effect on transport of sodium as well as water across cell boundaries. The effect of vasopressin on sodium excretion by the kidney is, however, extremely variable and depends upon experimental conditions. It is probable that vasopressin does not have a direct effect on sodium excretion and that any observed change in sodium balance is secondary to the modifying influence of this hormone on the total volume and distribution of body water.

Vasopressin has been shown to exert a pressor effect in persons with postural hypotension, and large intravenous doses may also produce transient increases in blood pressure even in normal man. The significance of this observation in relationship to blood pressure regulation in normal persons is unknown. Generally, posterior lobe preparations used therapeutically in man have no consistent effect on blood pressure, probably because of compensatory adjustments elsewhere in the circulation.

Lysine vasopressin has also proved to be of value as a means of assessing adrenocorticotropin secretion by the anterior pituitary. Although other corticotropin-releasing factors (CRF) differing from vasopressin have been extracted from the hypothalamus and posterior lobe, vasopressin itself has been shown to be a potent CRF. In clinical investigation, large intramuscular doses of 5 to 10 units are required to produce measurable increments in plasma steroid levels; however, intravenous doses as low as 50 to 80 microunits have been shown to produce significant increments in ACTH secretion in the rat. Since these vasopressin levels fall well within the physiologic range of stressed animals, it is possible that vasopressin may serve a physiologic role as an ACTH releasing neurohormone in addition to its direct peripheral actions.

OXYTOCIN. Recent studies with purified and synthetic oxytocin have significantly advanced understanding of the role of this hormone in uterine function and milk secretion. Oxytocin has been shown to be the hormonal substance of posterior lobe extracts responsible for release of milk from the lactating breast, as little as 0.5 units, or 1 μg, synthetic hormone producing a copious flow of milk within 30 sec of intravenous injection. Synthetic oxytocin has also been used successfully to initiate labor, and as previously mentioned, there is some evidence that oxytocin stimulates or sustains the secretion of prolactin by the anterior pituitary. Oxytocin, therefore, appears to play a very important and fundamental role in reproduction. Vasopressin also possesses oxytocic and milk-ejecting properties but is much less potent than oxytocin in this regard.

Other effects of oxytocin that warrant consideration include its marked but evanescent vasodepressor action demonstrable both in human beings and experimental animals and its effect on water excretion and renal function. In appropriate experimental situations, oxytocin has been shown to antagonize the antidiuretic action of vasopressin and to increase renal plasma flow and sodium excretion. The latter effect is currently attributable to an action of the hormone on the brain, which is abolished by hypophysectomy or the induction of diabetes insipidus. The demonstration that some of the actions of oxytocin are directly opposed to those of vasopressin implies a physiologic system for regulation of the volume and composition of the body fluids as well as the arterial pressure under the control of the central nervous system and the hypothalamus, which, although obscure at this time, may prove to be of clinical significance in the future.

Adrenocortical-neurohypophyseal Relationships

Patients with primary and secondary adrenocortical insufficiency characteristically show increased body water, hyponatremia and an inability to excrete a water load. These patients have been shown to have in the fasting state abnormally elevated plasma vasopressin levels which remain above the normal range despite forced hydration and further dilution of the plasma solutes. Curiously, plasma oxytocin is immeasurable both in the fasting and overhydrated state. Administration of hydrocortisonelike steroids to dehydrated patients is accompanied by a fall in plasma vasopressin and an increase in oxytocin levels into the range of fasting normal subjects. Water administration in the steroid-treated patient is accompanied by a normal osmoreceptor response to hemodilution with a fall in plasma vasopressin to zero and an increase in oxytocin levels to those observed in hydrated normal subjects. The inhibition of vasopressin secretion is accompanied by a normal water diuresis. Thus, it is apparent that the abnormal water metabolism of adrenocortical insufficiency is related to increased and sustained vasopressin secretion despite hypotonicity of the body fluids. Glucocorticoids restore normal water metabolism in this disease by a direct inhibitory action on vasopressin secretion and restoration of a normal osmoreceptor response to induced expansion of the body water. The observed changes in oxytocin secretion in untreated and steroid-treated patients suggest that the adrenal cortex influences oxytocin release either directly or indirectly through its effect on vasopressin secretion.

Hydrocortisone induces a transient water diuresis within the first few hours of administration even in subjects with normal adrenocortical function, an effect which is probably due to an acute decrease in vasopressin secretion. The resulting loss of body water would lead to relative hypertonicity of the body fluids and reactivation of vasopressin release via osmoregulatory pathways, even though blockade of neural pathways for ADH secretion may persist. The physiologic significance of this effect of hydrocortisone on the secretion of a hormone of prime importance in regulating water metabolism has not been delineated, but it may represent a hormonal mechanism for independently regulating the body content of sodium and water, which may be of fundamental importance in clinical disorders of sodium and water metabolism.

The adrenal steroids have not been shown to modify the antidiuretic effect of vasopressin in man. Thus, it has been shown that the diuretic effect of adrenal steroids is mediated not through a direct effect on the renal tubular reabsorption of water but by an indirect pathway involving inhibition of vasopressin secretion and a decrease in antidiuretic hormone action on the kidney.

In patients with partial neurohypophyseal insufficiency, a more complete state of diabetes insipidus can be induced with hydrocortisone administration, and a greater loss of solute-free water from the kidney occurs. Patients with a complete absence of vasopressin secretion do not have a true water diuresis with adrenal hormone administration. Since these hormones, at times, increase solute excretion by the kidney, there may be a concomitant increase in water excretion because of an inability of the kidney, in the absence of vasopressin, to increase solute concentration of the urine.

Adrenal steroids affect water metabolism in several other ways. Prolonged steroid therapy may occasionally result in extensive potassium depletion and the development of kaliopenic nephropathy associated with isosthenuria and a two- to threefold increase in urine flow. Very rarely, adrenal steroids may produce a striking polydipsic syndrome with urine volumes as high as 15 to 20 liters per 24 hr. Steroid effects on thirst-regulating centers in the anterior hypothalamus or other parts of the brain may be implicated in this disorder.

The adrenal steroids thus appear to influence water metabolism in man (1) by inhibiting the central neural control of vasopressin secretion and decreasing vasopressin action on the kidney; (2) by increasing solute excretion and the obligatory excretion of water in patients with vasopressin deficiency; (3) by producing the sensation of thirst, possibly by an effect on hypothalamic and other central nervous system thirst centers; (4) by producing potassium deficiency and kaliopenic nephropathy.

Vasopressin Deficiency— Diabetes Insipidus

Diabetes insipidus is a chronic symptom complex characterized by the passage of large quantities of pale, dilute urine, with secondary polydipsia. It results from a defect in the chain of events by which vasopressin is released from the neurohypophysis and acts on the cells of the renal tubules. The classic anatomic and physiologic studies of Fisher, Ingram, and Ranson, revealed that the disease may be caused by interference with the functional integrity of the neurohormonal unit comprising the supraoptic and paraventricular nuclei of the hypothalamus, the supraoptico hypophyseal tract, and the posterior lobe of the hypophysis. The full-blown disease occurs only when the tract is interrupted close enough to the hypothalamus to cause degeneration of at least 85 percent of the supraoptic and paraventricular neurones. There is also a relatively rare disorder, nephrogenic diabetes insipidus, which is mostly familial. This disorder may be due to a hereditary refractoriness of the renal tubules to vasopressin, and it is presumed that there is no neurohypophyseal disease in this group.

The incidence of classic diabetes insipidus following hypophysectomy may be significantly diminished if damage to the supraoptic neurones is minimized by careful severance of the pituitary stalk as close to the pituitary gland as possible. The polyuria of hypophysectomized human beings has been shown to vary with the magnitude of vasopressin deficiency. Patients who lack this secretion demonstrate persistent polyuria despite withdrawal of adrenocortical replacement therapy. These observations illustrate the important role of vasopressin in determining the rate of water excretion and corroborate the concept that the diuretic effect of adrenal steroids is mediated indirectly through an effect on vasopressin secretion. The adrenal steroids may increase urine volume in such patients, however, by increasing solute excretion.

The thyrotropic and growth hormones of the anterior pituitary are necessary to maintain polyuria, probably by influencing the nutritional state and solute turnover as well as by sustaining renal function. A peripheral antagonism of vasopressin by thyroid hormone has been demonstrated, but this effect may not be a direct one.

INCIDENCE. Diabetes insipidus is a rare disease, with a slightly greater incidence in youth and in males. In 1924 Rowntree reported 10 and 16 cases, respectively, in two series of 100,000 admissions to the Mayo Clinic. With the advent of hypophysectomy in recent years for the treatment of far-advanced breast carcinoma and other serious disorders, the disease is becoming much more prevalent in the general hospital population.

ETIOLOGY. As shown by Fink's pathologic studies in 107 cases, the great majority of instances of this disease are due to anatomic lesions involving the hypothalamic-hypophyseal system and, hence, presumably interfering with vasopressin production. In clinical practice, it will often be impossible to elicit any other evidence of such a lesion; while the label *idiopathic* may be justifiable for such cases antemortem, the finding of an anatomic lesion at autopsy generally may be predicted.

PATHOLOGY. The primary pathologic processes associated most frequently with the syndrome have been tumors of the diencephalopituitary region, basilar meningitis, sarcoidosis, and the histiocytic disorders. Transitory and occasionally permanent polyuria may follow severe head injuries. Pathologic changes consist of those due to the primary disorder, such as tumor, brain injury, and inflammation, and secondary changes in the urogenital tract, such as dilatation and hypertrophy of the bladder with megaloureter.

CLINICAL PICTURE. The chief symptoms of diabetes insipidus are polyuria and polydipsia. The loss of large amounts of pale, dilute urine, occasionally as much as 15 to 29 liters per day, results in dehydration and, consequently, in such related symptoms and signs as dry skin, constipation, and an intense, almost insatiable thirst. Water deprivation to the limit of tolerance does not prevent polyuria, nor does it lead to a significant increase in urine concentration. Thus, in this disease, polydipsia is secondary to polyuria, in contrast to patients with psychogenic polydipsia, who pass large quantities of urine as an aftermath of a large fluid intake. In patients with diabetes insipidus, no consistent physical or chemical changes are noted other than those of dehydration. However, there may be symptoms referable to the localized disease process causing the syndrome.

The role of trauma in the production of diabetes insipidus deserves special comment, since the polyuria that sometimes follows head injury is not infrequently transient, as contrasted with the chronicity of most other forms of the disease. A similar syndrome may develop subsequent to cerebrovascular accidents or intracranial surgery, and in association with other forms of cerebral disease. When the full-blown syndrome develops under these conditions, serious dehydration may occur before the diagnosis is suspected, particularly in the incontinent patient or in the patient with clouded sensorium who is unable to request or partake of an adequate volume of fluids. The dehydration, which is due principally to water loss, may be accentuated by the administration of isotonic saline or solutions containing large amounts of protein. Such large solute loads will aggravate the renal loss of water in these patients because of an inability of the kidney to increase the solute concentration of the urine in the absence of vasopressin.

DIAGNOSIS. The symptoms plus the large urine volume, with specific gravity below 1.010 and urinary osmolality less than that of plasma, unassociated with a history or other findings of diabetes mellitus or of chronic renal disease, will quickly suggest diabetes insipidus. Since this diagnosis commits the patient to sustained replacement therapy for an indefinite period, it is not to be made lightly, and the clinical impression should be supported by careful studies made under hospital conditions. All cases of diabetes insipidus, moreover, should be studied carefully for active intracranial lesions, which should be presumed to be present until proved otherwise. Thus, examination should include, in addition to the differential tests of water excretion outlined below, a study of the spinal fluid, roentgenograms of the skull and chest (metastatic disease), electroencephalogram, serologic test (syphilis), the serum protein level, sternal marrow aspiration (multiple myeloma), and visual fields.

DIFFERENTIAL DIAGNOSIS. The syndrome must be differentiated from psychogenic polydipsia, chronic nephritis, and diabetes mellitus as well as from the polydipsia and polyuria so characteristically associated with the hypochloremic alkalotic syndrome and the hypercalcemia of hyperparathyroidism and vitamin D intoxication. Chronic nephritis may be excluded by the absence of protein or formed elements in the urine, a normal blood urea nitrogen level, and normal kidney function tests. Often the most difficult differential diagnosis is that between diabetes insipidus and psychogenic polydipsia. Other procedures helpful in making a differential diagnosis are the following:

1. Dehydration for 8 to 12 hr should be performed cautiously during the day, with close observation of the patient for signs of vasomotor collapse, which can occur with sudden severe dehydration. An inability to increase the specific gravity and osmolality of the urine to hypertonic levels is characteristic of diabetes insipidus and serves to differentiate this syndrome from psychogenic polydipsia but not from chronic nephritis. Great care must be taken in suspected psychogenic cases to be certain that the patient does not have access to water or other fluids.

2. Alleviation of symptoms will follow repeated small doses of aqueous vasopressin, i.e., 5.0 units intramuscularly every 3 to 4 hr. This differentiates diabetes insipidus from chronic nephritis but not from psychogenic polydipsia. The possibility of vasopressin-resistant diabetes insipidus must always be kept in mind, since 5 to 15 percent of cases of diabetes insipidus fall into this category.

3. Secretory function should be tested. Since the secretion of vasopressin can be initiated by either neurogenic or osmotic stimuli, both the hypothalamic neurones and the osmoregulators must be stimulated in turn for the integrity of this neurohormonal unit to be properly evaluated. In addition, the adequacy of renal tubular responsiveness to vasopressin must also be measured to understand fully the nature of the polyuria. The functional integrity of the neurohypophyseal-renal system may be evaluated within a few hours by serial intravenous injections of nicotine, hypertonic saline solution, and vasopressin under constant water-loading conditions. Acute changes in urinary osmolality and free water clearance (C_{H_2O}) during water diuresis reflect the action of vasopressin on the renal tubular reabsorption of water and may be regarded as a useful index of the secretory capacity of the neurohypophysis.[1]

Technique for Studying Neurohypophyseal Function. The patient is hydrated with 20 ml water per kg body weight over 30 to 60 min. Preliminary dehydration is unnecessary and may be dangerous. Urine is collected at 15- to 30-min intervals by spontaneous voiding if at all possible or else through an indwelling catheter. In the latter case, it is worthwhile to administer 0.5 Gm tetracycline by mouth several hours before catheterization to prevent urinary tract infection. A constant state of hydration is maintained by oral or intravenous administration of a volume of fluid equal to that excreted during the preceding collection period. When a sustained high rate of urine flow is reached (over 5 ml per min), 1.0 mg nicotine in solution is injected intravenously over a period of 0.5 to 2 min. The dose of nicotine is gradually increased by 0.5 to 1.0 mg at intervals of 30 min until a clear-cut antidiuretic response ensues or symptoms of nicotine intoxication (i.e., vertigo, nausea, vomiting) preclude further administration. As an alternative, the subject can smoke one to three cigarettes rapidly and with deep inhalation.

The normal antidiuretic response to nicotine, which occurs within 15 to 30 min after injection, is a decrease in urine flow and free water clearance, accompanied by an increase in urinary creatinine, chloride, and total solute concentrations (Fig. 88-4). Patients with diabetes in-

---

[1] The urine volume, V, is equal to the algebraic sum of the osmolal clearance, C_{osm}, and the free water clearance, C_{H_2O}.

$$V = C_{osm} + C_{H_2O}$$
$$C_{osm} = V \frac{\text{total solute conc. urine}}{\text{total solute conc. plasma}}$$

C_{osm} represents the volume of water required to contain the urinary solutes in a solution isosmotic with plasma. C_{H_2O} represents the net excess or deficit of water beyond the osmolal clearance; it will be positive during a water diuresis and negative when urine is concentrated by the abstraction of solute-free water, as in antidiuresis. C_{H_2O} usually parallels urine flow during water diuresis studies, since osmolal clearance remains relatively constant. This index is particularly useful in determining the changes in water excretion occurring during the solute diuresis usually observed with hypertonic saline administration. Not infrequently, a large increase in C_{osm} may mask a concomitant decrease in C_{H_2O}. In this instance, urinary flow may fall only slightly or may actually increase, even though an increase in water reabsorption may be under way under the influence of released vasopressin.

Fig. 88-4. See text and footnote. Patient, J. H., a nonsmoker, was given twice the usual dose of nicotine.

sipidus usually do not show a fall in water excretion with normal doses of nicotine; however, some may have a minimal antidiuretic response with much larger amounts (5 to 6 mg nicotine base), which may be due to residual neurohypophyseal activity or transient hemodynamic effects on the kidney. When urine flow returns to control levels, 15 to 25 milliunits aqueous vasopressin is injected intravenously. The response to vasopressin differentiates renal disease from true diabetes insipidus.

The administration of water is discontinued with the vasopressin injection to decrease the volume of retained water in preparation for the intravenous administration of hypertonic saline solution, since excessive hydration may abolish the osmotic response by diluting the hypertonic saline as it enters the circulation. When the antidiuresis to vasopressin is completed, 3 percent saline (10 ml per kilogram) is infused rapidly over 30 to 45 min. In normal persons a marked antidiuretic response will occur during the infusion or within the following 60 min. In patients with diabetes insipidus, this antidiuresis does

not occur and a rise in free water clearance is frequently observed due to the associated solute diuresis (Fig. 88-4). Patients with psychogenic polydipsia demonstrate normal antidiuresis to the hypertonic saline infusion, but, curiously, many do not respond normally to nicotine, suggesting some derangement in hypothalamic function and neural regulation of vasopressin release in this disorder.

The response to nicotine, to hypertonic saline solution, and to vasopressin may be used to differentiate the locus of the functional disturbance responsible for the polyuria, i.e., hypothalamus, osmoregulators, and renal tubules. Patients with vasopressin-deficient diabetes insipidus classically do not respond to hypertonic saline. However, certain patients with diabetes insipidus apparently have secreting neurohypophyseal tissue that responds to normal doses of nicotine but not to hypertonic saline solution. Post-mortem studies on one such patient with metastatic breast carcinoma demonstrated an abundance of secretory granules within the neurones of the intact supraoptic nuclei, but the posterior pituitary and stalk were devoid of neurosecretion and completely destroyed by tumor. This phenomenon suggests that isolated posterior pituitary damage may lead to a selective failure of the osmoregulatory control of vasopressin secretion and a clinical syndrome of vasopressin-deficient diabetes insipidus despite the presence of functioning neurohypophyseal tissue.

TREATMENT. Treatment of diabetes insipidus may be divided into two phases: (1) correction of the underlying intracranial difficulty, if present; (2) replacement therapy with vasopressin, which usually must be continued throughout life.

Pitressin is a partially purified vasopressin fraction obtained from animal posterior lobes supplied as an aqueous solution in 0.5- and 1-ml ampuls with a strength of 20 IU pressor activity per milliliter. The quantity of Pitressin required to ameliorate polyuria is very small (0.1 to 0.2 ml), but the evanescent action of the aqueous preparation necessitates repeated injections at 3- to 4-hr intervals, making this form of treatment impractical for prolonged periods. Synthetic lysine vasopressin solution for parenteral use is comparable in action to aqueous Pitressin.

Nasal insufflations of dried posterior pituitary powder (supplied in 5- and 30-Gm bottles) every 3 to 6 hr accomplish the same purpose and are more easily administered, but most patients develop a chronic rhinopharyngitis and even gastritis from swallowed powder. Systemic allergic reactions are rare but have been observed.

A synthetic *lysine vasopressin* solution containing 50 pressor units per milliliter in 5-ml plastic spray vials is available for intranasal use as a spray or as drops. Its activity is as rapid and as prolonged as posterior lobe powder, but this preparation has the decided advantage of eliminating the local or systemic allergic reactions to the foreign protein in posterior pituitary preparations of animal origin. This material currently is the treatment of choice for ambulatory patients.

Pitressin tannate in oil is supplied in 1-ml ampuls with a strength of 5 IU per milliliter. This preparation provides relatively prolonged hormonal action; a single injection is usually effective for 24 to 72 hr. A test dose of 0.3 to 0.5 ml (1.5 to 2.5 IU) should be given initially to determine the effectiveness of treatment and to guard against the serious, but fortunately rare, occurrence of excess fluid retention and water intoxication in particularly sensitive individuals. For practical purposes chronic treatment with 1.0-ml doses of hormone should be tried and the frequency of injection gauged by the recurrence of polyuria. Most patients will retain 1 to 2 kg water following an injection, and the dissipation of effective hormone levels will be attended with a sudden polyuria and loss of body weight before onset of polydipsia. In general, injections should be timed to coincide with the onset of polyuria in order to prevent marked fluctuations in body water content and fluid compartmental shifts. Abnormal fluid retention may be mitigated by instructing the patient to guard against excessive fluid ingestion after treatment. The hormone is preferably given in the evening to ensure a restful night. *It is very important to instruct the patient to warm the vial and to shake it thoroughly, since the active material has a tendency to precipitate out in the vial.* This is the commonest cause of so-called "vasopressin resistance."

Occasionally, patients with vasopressin-sensitive diabetes insipidus may develop resistance to the action of the hormone, in some cases accompanied by allergy either to the hormone or to the oily menstruum. Allergy to the latter may be easily corrected by use of a different medium, and hormone allergy may be overcome by desensitization. Vasopressin resistance is also observed in patients with hypokalemia and hypercalcemia or hypercalciuria, either of which blocks the full action of ADH on the renal tubules. Serum and urinary calcium and potassium measurements should be made in all patients with vasopressin-resistant polyuria and appropriate investigations and treatment carried out.

Both *chlorothiazide* and *hydrochlorothiazide* have been shown to increase free water reabsorption in diabetes insipidus. These drugs, however, will decrease urine flow by no more than about 30 to 50 percent, and most patients usually will continue to require vasopressin therapy as well to prevent abnormally large urine volumes. The thiazide derivatives may have their greatest usefulness in lessening polyuria in the rare form of vasopressin-resistant diabetes insipidus. The average daily dose of chlorothiazide is 0.5 to 1.0 Gm and of hydrochlorothiazide, 0.05 to 0.1 Gm given in divided doses. Since the thiazides may produce potassium depletion, which can impair the concentrating ability of the kidney, it is worthwhile to administer 1.0 to 2.0 Gm KCl syrup by mouth with each dose of thiazide drug. Simultaneous administration of spironolactone (Aldactone^R) with the thiazide may prevent hypokalemia by blocking the aldosterone-mediated NaK exchange in the distal renal tubule.

Chlorpropamide in doses of 250 to 500 mg per day is also effective antidiuretic therapy in some patients. The value of this drug is that the volume depletion and hypokalemia from thiazides can be avoided. The possible development of hypoglycemia from chlorpropamide should be investigated and corrected by decreasing the dose or discontinuing therapy if necessary. The mechanism of action of this drug on renal water reabsorption has not been clarified.

The prognosis of diabetes insipidus is determined by the outcome of the primary disease process. With regular treatment, patients with isolated neurohypophyseal atrophy can lead normal lives.

Excess of Antidiuretic Hormone

Abnormally elevated levels of antidiuretic substances in blood and urine have been reported in a variety of disease states associated with edema or defects in water diuresis, including cardiac failure, cirrhosis with ascites, nephrosis, and Addison's disease. While the hypothesis that excessive antidiuretic activity may be responsible for the water retention observed in edematous patients is quite attractive, proof has not been clearly established.

It is generally agreed that patients with these disorders do not show excessive sensitivity to or delayed inactivation of administered vasopressin. Some studies with nicotine stimulation of endogenous vasopressin secretion in patients with edema have yielded normal results, but some patients whose disease is associated with severe hyponatremia have shown enhanced neurohypophyseal response to nicotine and other stimuli. Many of the studies that minimize a role of vasopressin in edema formation are based upon data observed in patients in equilibrium with their fluid retention who can excrete water loads, albeit at a somewhat depressed rate. It is obvious that vasopressin release mechanisms should be evaluated during the active phase of edema formation, but studies have been hampered by the fact that such patients frequently cannot excrete administered water, which automatically vitiates the only reliable biologic end point of vasopressin action, i.e., antidiuresis. Further advances in this field will depend upon the application of precise and reliable methods for measuring vasopressin levels in the plasma.

The level of vasopressin in the body fluids need not necessarily be increased to account for water retention, since even physiologic amounts effectively halt a water diuresis. The abnormality in water metabolism may be primarily related to a *persistence* of vasopressin secretion despite the presence of excess body water or hypotonicity, both of which normally should induce water diuresis. It appears that the distribution rather than the total quantity of body water may determine the secretory activity of the neurohypophysis, and more extensive studies of the precedence of volume versus osmolal regulation of vasopressin secretion should shed more light on the nature of fluid retention in these disorders.

Inappropriate ADH Syndrome

The above discussion is particularly pertinent in understanding the nature of the antidiuretic factors responsible for the *inappropriate ADH syndrome,* described in patients with oat cell carcinoma of the lung, acute intermittent porphyria, various central nervous system disorders, etc. Antidiuretic assays of whole plasma and urine purport to show increased ADH levels in several patients. The situation is made more complex by the finding of antidiuretic activity in extracts of primary and metastatic tumor tissues. These antidiuretic substances have not been confirmed as ADH, however; the bioassay methods employed are not specific for vasopressin and may be interfered with by vasoactive peptides other than ADH in the biologic extracts or by a nonspecific release of ADH by the assay animal following injection of noxious substances or heterologous tissue extracts. The fact that the characteristic syndrome is also observed in nontumorous conditions suggests that abnormalities in neurohypophyseal secretion of vasopressin may well prove to be the common denominator in these diverse clinical disorders. Proof of vasopressin synthesis by these nonendocrine tumors must await results of tissue culture of tumor cells or specific radioimmunologic or ultramicrochemical measurements of arginine vasopressin in the tumors.

The interrelationships between neurohypophyseal secretion and the adrenal secretion of aldosterone are not well defined. Patients with aldosterone-secreting tumors do not usually develop edema, and normal subjects treated with aldosterone have been shown to escape readily from sodium and water retention. Furthermore, patients with diabetes insipidus will retain sodium with aldosterone therapy but will not retain isosmotic quantities of water unless they receive vasopressin simultaneously.

Aldosterone secretion may be inhibited by expansion of body fluids despite the presence of hyponatremia. In this respect, the regulation of aldosterone secretion resembles that for vasopressin secretion, the influence of fluid volume having precedence over osmolal concentration. It is probable that there is an intimate physiologic interrelation between aldosterone, which governs sodium metabolism, and vasopressin, which regulates water metabolism. Both vasopressin and aldosterone are probably necessary for the isosmotic retention of fluid, and persistent secretion of both hormones could be responsible for the development of edema in patients with fundamental derangements in circulation.

REFERENCES

Ahmed, A. B. J., B. C. George, C. Gonzalez-Auvert, and J. F. Dingman: Increased Plasma Arginine Vasopressin in Clinical Adrenocortical Insufficiency and Its Inhibition by Glucosteroids, J. Clin. Invest., 46:111, 1967.

Bartter, F. C., and W. B. Schwartz: The Syndrome of Inappropriate Secretion of Antidiuretic Hormone, Am. J. Med., 42:790, 1967.

Dingman, J. F., and J. Hauger-Klevene: Treatment of Diabetes Insipidus: Synthetic Lysine Vasopressin Nasal Solution, J. Clin. Endocrinol. Metab., 24:550, 1964.

du Vigneaud, V.: Trail of Sulfur Research: From Insulin to Oxytocin, Science, 123:967, 1956.

Symposium on Antidiuretic Hormones, Am. J. Med., 42:651, 1967.

Verney, E. B.: Absorption and Excretion of Water: Antidiuretic Hormone, Lancet, II:739, 1946.

89 DISEASES OF THE THYROID
Herbert A. Selenkow and Sidney H. Ingbar

Diseases of the thyroid gland are manifested by increases in gland size (goiter, neoplasm), alterations in hormonal secretion, or both. Changes in gland size and weight (normally 15 to 35 Gm) are associated with toxic or nontoxic goiter, adenomas, thyroiditis, or malignancies. Symptoms may arise from local compression in the neck and superior mediastinum, from disturbances in hormonogenesis resulting in hypothyroidism or hyperthyroidism, or from malignancy. Alterations in thyroid hormone secretion produce a wide variety of anatomic, physiologic, and metabolic effects, characteristic of which are increased oxygen consumption (hypermetabolism) from excessive secretion and decreased oxygen consumption (hypometabolism) from thyroid insufficiency.

In 1891, Murray, an English physician, administered thyroid substances to a myxedematous patient, who subsequently improved remarkably. The material employed was a glycerin extract obtained from sheep thyroids. Magnus-Levy, in 1895, observed that administration of thyroid extract to patients with hypothyroidism was followed by an increase in basal metabolic rate. In 1896, Baumann obtained an acid hydrolyzate of thyroid tissue in powder form that contained 10 percent iodine, thus establishing the high iodine content of this hormone. Oswald, 8 years later, prepared iodothyroglobulin, which indicated that thyroid hormone was a protein substance. *Thyroxin* was first isolated by Kendall in 1915 and subsequently synthesized by Harington and Barger in 1927. The potent homologue of thyroxin, 3,5,3'-triiodothyronine, was isolated chromatographically from plasma and thyroid tissue and identified simultaneously in 1952 by Gross and Pitt-Rivers and by Roche, Lissitsky, and Michel.

ANATOMY AND EMBRYOLOGY

The human thyroid originates embryologically from an invagination of the pharyngeal epithelium with some cellular contributions from the lateral pharyngeal pouches. Progressive descent of the midline thyroid anlage gives rise to the thyroglossal duct, which extends from the foramen cecum at the base of the tongue to the isthmus of the thyroid. Remnants of tissue may persist along the course of this tract as "lingual thyroid," as thyroglossal cysts and nodules, or as a structure contiguous with the thyroid isthmus, called the *pyramidal lobe.* The cephalad portion of the pyramidal lobe in adults is usually a vestigial structure consisting of a thin fibrous cord. The remnant close to the thyroid isthmus may contain significant amounts of thyroid tissue that can be identified by careful palpation as the pyramidal lobe. This lobe usually extends from the thyroid cartilage to the thyroid isthmus and is more commonly located to the left than to the right of the midline. Hypertrophy of this lobe is found in disorders of diffuse thyroid enlargement such as hyperthyroidism, diffuse hyperplasia of adolescence or pregnancy, and in lymphoid thyroiditis. Ectopic thyroid tissue may occur rarely in the trachea or esophagus.

The human fetal thyroid becomes detectably functional around 14 to 16 weeks and during the latter part of gestation develops the capacity to synthesize and secrete thyroid hormones. The extent to which fetal requirements for thyroid hormones are met by secretion from the maternal or fetal thyroid is not clear. The thyroid gland enlarges progressively during fetal development and neonatal life and reaches the adult size of about 20 to 25 Gm. The precise weight of the "normal" adult thyroid gland varies considerably with geographic, genetic, and environmental factors.

BIOCHEMICAL PHYSIOLOGY

The hormonal activity of the thyroid gland is controlled mainly by the thyrotropic or thyroid-stimulating hormone (TSH) of the anterior pituitary gland (see Chap. 87). Release of TSH from the pituitary is regulated, at least in part, by hypothalamic centers and generally depends upon the quantity of thyroid hormones available to the tissues. A reduction in the availability of thyroid hormones stimulates TSH output, which, in turn, tends to increase the secretion and size of the thyroid gland. Conversely, in normal persons, an excess of available thyroid hormones tends to depress secretion of TSH and so, in turn, to reduce thyroid activity and size. Certain chemical compounds, as well as congenital or acquired enzymatic defects within the thyroid, reduce hormonal secretion leading to increased TSH secretion and goiter formation (goitrogenesis). Conversely, thyroid hormones inhibit secretion of TSH and thus act as antigoitrogenic agents.

Pathways of iodine metabolism are schematically represented in Fig. 89-1. Approximately 100 to 200 μg dietary iodide is absorbed daily via the gastrointestinal tract, and a similar amount is excreted in the urine. Circulating inorganic iodide is usually present in serum in minute amounts of the order of 0.5 μg per 100 ml. This ionic iodide is available to the thyroid, kidneys, and exocrine glands. That portion not concentrated by the thyroid is rapidly cleared by the kidneys. Iodide extracted by the exocrine glands is recirculated via intestinal resorption. The intrathyroidal processes leading to synthesis and secretion of thyroid hormones may be divided into four sequential stages (Fig. 89-2). Iodine in the plasma is available to the thyroid gland for hormonal synthesis only as inorganic iodide. This is derived from two major sources, the peripheral degradation and deiodination of hormonal as well as nonhormonal iodinated compounds and, more importantly, the diet. In most areas of the world the dietary intake of iodine is sufficiently low so that the concentration of iodide in plasma is well below 1 μg per 100 ml. The first step in hormonal biosynthesis is active transport of iodide from plasma at a rate exceeding efflux from the gland, with the result that a concentration gradient for iodide is maintained. Thyroid/serum gradients may vary from 10 to 500, or more, under varying physiologic conditions. The activity of the iodide transport or trapping mechanism is increased directly by TSH or indirectly via low thyroidal iodine stores. Next, through a reaction apparently mediated by an intrathyroidal peroxidase, iodide is oxidized to a higher valence form, possibly iodine or hypoiodite. This highly reactive form of iodine exists only momentarily, as it combines rapidly with tyrosyl groups in thyroid proteins (organification) to form monoiodotyrosine (MIT) and diiodotyrosine (DIT). These iodotyrosines then undergo oxidative condensation (coupling), possibly again through the mediation of a thyroidal peroxidase, to yield a variety of iodothyronines, including thyroxin (T4) and 3,5,3'-triiodothyronine (T3). The latter compound (hereafter referred to as triiodothyronine) and thyroxin are the major hormonally active products secreted by the thyroid gland. These, as well as the other iodinated amino acids, are formed within the thyroglobulin molecule and stored as such in the thyroid follicle. Under physiologic condi-

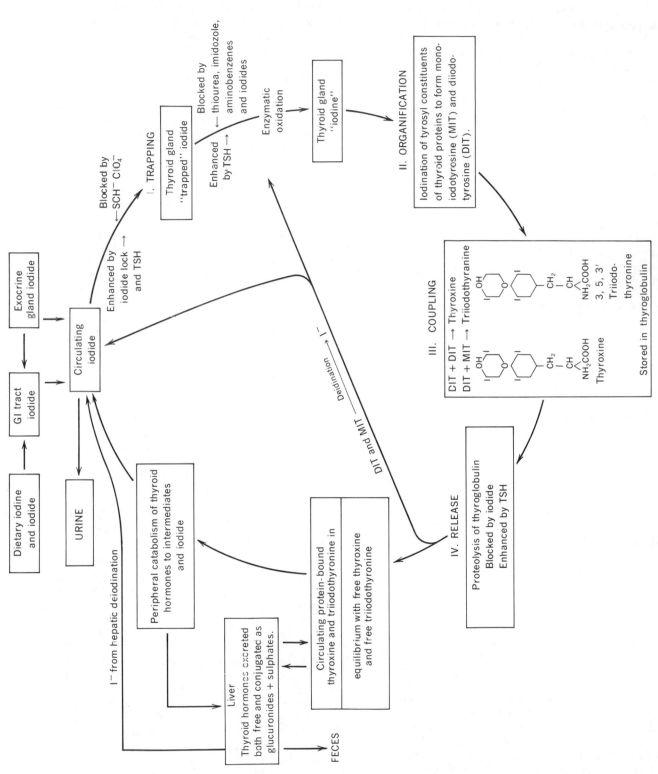

Fig. 89-1. Simplified schematic representation of pathways of iodine metabolism.

I. TRAPPING

II. ORGANIFICATION

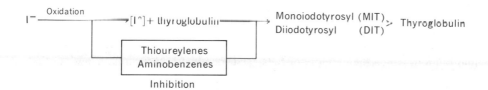

III. COUPLING

$$2 \text{ DIT} \longrightarrow \text{Thyroxinyl} \quad (T4)$$
$$1 \text{ MIT} + 1 \text{ DIT} \longrightarrow \text{Triiodothyroninyl (T3)} \Big\} > \text{Thyroglobulin}$$

IV. RELEASE

Fig. 89-2. Sequential stages of intrathyroidal synthesis and secretion of thyroid hormones.

tions, thyroglobulin does not enter the circulation. Secretion of hormonally active materials requires hydrolysis of thyroglobulin (release), which is effected by thyroidal proteases and peptidases. The thyroid hormones released by proteolysis of thyroglobulin are free to enter the bloodstream, whereas MIT and DIT are prevented from entering the circulation by action of an iodotyrosine deiodinase, which removes their iodide. This iodide is in part reutilized for synthesis of hormone and in part lost from the thyroid gland into the circulation.

The foregoing reactions are subject to inhibition by a variety of chemical compounds. Such agents are generally termed *goitrogens,* since, by virtue of their ability to inhibit hormonal synthesis, they induce goiter formation. Certain inorganic anions, notably perchlorate and thiocyanate, inhibit the iodide transport mechanism and thus either prevent thyroid cells from concentrating iodide or cause release at thyroidal iodide into the circulation. The goiter and hypothyroidism that follow chronic depletion of intrathyroidal iodide, such as these agents induce, can be prevented or relieved by doses of iodide sufficiently large to enable adequate quantities to enter the gland by simple diffusion. The commonly employed antithyroid agents, such as the derivatives of thiourea and mercaptoimidazole, exert more complex actions upon pathways of hormonal biosynthesis. These agents, as well as certain aniline derivatives, inhibit the initial oxidation (organic binding) of iodide, decrease the proportion of DIT relative to MIT, and block coupling of iodotyrosines to form the hormonally active iodothyronines. The latter reaction is the most sensitive to inhibition by these agents. It is therefore possible for the synthesis of hormonally active iodothyronines to be decreased greatly, although the total incorporation of iodine by the thyroid is inhibited but little. Excessive concentrations of intrathyroidal iodide, such as follow acute administration of large quantities of iodide, also inhibit these oxidative reactions. Normally, this effect is transient; however, in a few peculiarly sensitive individuals, the antithyroid effect of iodide may persist and lead to development of goiter and myxedema. Pharmacologic quantities of iodide can also inhibit proteolysis of thyroglobulin. This effect is most readily demonstrable in hyperfunctioning thyroids and is responsible for the rapid ameliorative action of iodides in thyrotoxicosis.

In the bloodstream, T4 and T3 are almost entirely bound to plasma proteins. Electrophoretic analyses indicate that T4 is bound primarily to an interalpha-globulin termed *thyroxin-binding globulin,* or TBG, to a prealbumin, *thyroxin-binding prealbumin,* or TBPA, and to albumin in decreasing order of intensity. The interaction between T4 and its binding proteins conforms to a reversible binding equilibrium in which the majority of the hormone is bound and a very small proportion (normally less than 0.1 percent) is free. Since only the free or unbound hormone is available to tissues, the metabolic state of the patient will correlate more closely with the concentration of free hormone than with the total concentration of hormone. Furthermore, homeostatic regulation of thyroid function will be directed toward maintenance of a normal concentration of free rather than total hormone. Disturbances of the thyroid hormone–plasma protein interaction are of two general types (see Table 89-2). In the first, the thyroid-pituitary axis is intrinsically normal, and the homeostatic control of thyroid secretion is intact. Under these circumstances, disordered binding interactions result from primary alterations in the concentration or avidity of the thyroxin-binding proteins. For example, an increase in binding activity will lower the concentration of free hormones and thus diminish the quantity of hormones available to tissues. Total hormonal concentration in serum will then increase until the *concentration* of free hormones is restored to normal, but at this time, the proportion of hormones which is free will be decreased. The increase in total hormonal concentration counterbalances the decrease in the proportion which is free, with the result that the concentration of free hormones is normal and the metabolic state of the patient is unchanged. Converse changes occur when the binding of T4 by plasma proteins declines. The binding activity of TBG is increased in serum of normal pregnancy, during administration of estrogens, in patients with estrogen-secreting tumors, and in some patients with acute idiopathic porphyria. Binding activity of TBG is decreased in serum of patients given androgenic steroids, some anabolic drugs, or large doses of glucocorticoids; in nephrosis (where substantial quantities of TBG are lost in the urine); and in patients receiving hydantoins that are competitive inhibitors of T4-binding by TBG. Rarely,

the binding activity of TBG may be either increased or virtually absent for unknown reasons. Such idiopathic disorders of hormonal binding appear to be familial. The thyroxin-binding activity of TBPA is not known to be enhanced in any disease but is increased by anabolic steroids. It is decreased in patients with a wide variety of systemic diseases and by competitive inhibitors such as salicylates, dinitrophenol, or their congeners.

The second type of disturbance of thyroid hormone binding interaction results from primary alterations in the concentration of thyroid hormones in the blood such as occur in hypothyroidism or thyrotoxicosis. Here, homeostatic control of thyroid hormone secretion is disrupted and pathologic factors regulate hormonal secretion independent of the thyroid-pituitary axis. Under these circumstances, the activity of the thyroxin-binding proteins is changed little, if at all, and the concentration of free hormones will vary directly with the total concentration. Since such changes in circulating hormone usually result from intrinsic thyroidal disease, homeostatic mechanisms cannot restore the concentration of free hormones to normal. Primary changes in thyroidal function are therefore associated with persistent changes in the concentration of both total and free hormone, and therefore, with alterations in the anabolic status of the patient. In these disorders, the relative change on the *concentration* of free hormones is greater than the change in total hormones, with the result that the proportion of free hormones varies *pari passu* with the total hormonal concentration.

Because the free thyroid hormones in blood represent only a very small proportion of the total, even in abnormal states, the concentration of protein-bound hormone will closely reflect the total concentration of thyroid hormones in the blood. This is generally measured as the protein-bound iodine (PBI) or the serum thyroxin (serum T4). Direct measurement of the proportion of free thyroid hormones can be accomplished by dialysis techniques. The mathematical product of this value and the serum PBI or T4 will indicate the concentration of free T4. Dialysis methods for determining free T4 are technically difficult; however, a reflection of the proportion of free hormones can be obtained from one of the several in vitro triiodothyronine "uptake" methods such as the Resin sponge ^{131}I-triiodothyronine uptake test (Resin-T3, Triosorb). In a manner analogous to calculation of the absolute concentration of free T4, the product of the Resin-T3 and the PBI (or serum T4) yields the *free thyroxin index.* This value is proportional to the free T4 concentration and, like the free T4, by dialysis varies with the metabolic state of the patient.

Triiodothyronine is not bound by TBPA and is bound by TBG only weakly. As a consequence, the unbound proportion of T3 is normally eight to ten times greater than T4. T3 is, therefore, removed from the blood much more rapidly than T4, which accounts for its failure to contribute materially to the total hormonal iodine concentration in the blood and possibly for its more rapid onset and offset of action. Its binding characteristics, however, do not account fully for the fact that it has a three-to fourfold greater metabolic potency than thyroxin when administered orally.

In the normal individual, the metabolic state reflects a summation of the action of T4, which contributes substantially to PBI, and of T3, which does not. Therefore, when exogenous hormones are employed to treat hypothyroidism or to suppress endogenous thyroid function, a normal metabolic state will be associated with a slightly elevated PBI if T4 is used and with a subnormal PBI if T3 is employed. Under physiologic circumstances, normal levels of free thyroxin in serum are maintained via an intact thyroid-pituitary axis through a negative feedback (servo) relationship with TSH. However, under pathologic circumstances, such as in the thyrotoxicosis of Graves' disease or autonomous thyroid tumors, pituitary thyrotropin is inhibited fully by the elevated serum levels of free T4 and the excessive thyroidal hormone secretion results from stimulatory factors which are not suppressed by even high levels of free T4. In Graves' disease, the persistently excessive thyroid secretion appears to be mediated via a circulating immunoglobulin with prolonged TSH-like properties known as LATS (long-acting thyroid stimulator). Thyrotoxicosis also results from excessive secretion of autonomous thyroid tumors (as in single or multiple hyperfunctioning nodules) and, rarely, from multiple metastases of thyroid cancer. Thyroidal independence of pituitary thyrotropic activity in patients with thyrotoxicosis forms the basis for the thyroid suppression test. A separate serum factor has been postulated to be etiologically responsible for the ophthalmopathy associated with Graves' disease, but to date this has not been identified or characterized with certainty.

DIAGNOSTIC LABORATORY TESTS

Availability of a variety of useful laboratory tests makes possible accurate evaluation of thyroid hormone economy under diverse clinical circumstances (Table 89-1). For simplicity, such tests may be divided into two major categories: the first, *thyroid indices,* includes those which measure some aspect of thyroid hormone metabolism involving iodine, such as hormonal synthesis, secretion, or plasma concentration. The second category, *metabolic indices,* includes those tests which measure some metabolic action of thyroid hormones on cellular metabolism. Unfortunately, the latter are to a large extent influenced by a variety of nonthyroidal factors and therefore tend to be less specific.

The *basal metabolic rate* (BMR) measures oxygen consumption in the basal state and is expressed as a percentage of values found in normal individuals of the same age, sex, and body surface area. Nonthyroidal disorders that alter oxygen consumption must be excluded if this test is to be of diagnostic value. Febrile illnesses, leukemia, neoplasms, hypertension, congestive heart failure, aortic stenosis, diabetes, pheochromocytoma, chronic pulmonary insufficiency, polycythemia, or perforated eardrums may be associated with an increased BMR. The BMR is most helpful in following changes in oxygen con-

sumption in the same individual during therapy. Similarly, the serum cholesterol, creatine tolerance tests, photomotogram, and electrocardiogram are of ancillary but limited diagnostic value because of their nonspecificity.

The *serum protein–bound iodine* (PBI) usually reflects the concentration of circulating thyroid hormones and represents an excellent diagnostic laboratory test for estimating thyroid function in the absence of interfering substances. Under abnormal circumstances, the PBI may include iodinated materials of either endogenous or exogenous origin. These may be either iodinated proteins, as in lymphoid thyroiditis, or iodinated organic compounds, such as radiopaque contrast drugs, which bind to plasma proteins (usually albumin). The iodinated proteins can be separated physically from the thyroid hormones by a butanol extraction procedure (BEI). On the other hand, most organic iodinated compounds are also extracted by butanol and therefore measured by the BEI. Thyroid hormones can be distinguished from iodinated proteins and most organic iodinated compounds by column chromatographic techniques, particularly when the latter are not present in high concentration.

Serum Thyroxin (serum T4) can be assayed directly by a method which depends upon the ability of thyroxin (T4) extracted from serum to displace radioactive T4 from a protein mixture containing TBG (binding displacement analysis). This test requires no chemical determination of iodine and is therefore not influenced by iodinated contaminants or heavy metals such as mercury. Furthermore, the high specificity of TBG for T4 renders this test independent of endogenous iodinated substances other than T4. In view of this remarkable specificity, the serum T4 test is more widely applicable for most clinical situations than the PBI or BEI. The designation serum T4 will be used hereinafter for the measurement obtained by this method.

Serum "free" thyroxin (free T4) is an important constituent of the metabolically active T4 pool. The small fraction of the total serum T4 which circulates free can be measured directly by dialysis techniques using radioactive T4 added to serum samples. The product of free T4 *fraction* and the total serum T4 gives the *concentration* of free T4. According to current concepts, the free T4 concentration relates directly to the patient's metabolic status and to regulation of thyroid gland secretion via pituitary thyrotropin in most circumstances.

The *Resin-Triiodothyronine uptake* (Resin-T3) is used commonly as a diagnostic test of thyroid function. This in vitro test depends upon competitive binding for radioactive T3 between serum TBG and a resin. If the thyroid hormone binding sites on TBG are saturated with endogenous T3 and T4 or are not available for binding, the radioactive T3 added to the system will be bound preferentially by the resin and Resin-T3 "uptake" will be high, as in thyrotoxicosis or congenital TBG deficiency. The converse occurs when the TBG binding sites are undersaturated or available in excessive amounts as in myxedema or pregnancy. The Resin-T3 uptake is directly proportional to the fraction of free T4 in serum and inversely

Table 89-1. COMPARATIVE VALUES COMMONLY OBTAINED FOR TESTS OF
THYROID FUNCTION IN VARIOUS CLINICAL SITUATIONS

Diagnostic and Clinical Status	24-hr ^{131}I uptake, %	Serum PBI,* μg/100 ml	Serum T4† μg/100 ml	BMR, % normal standard	Resin T3‡ uptake, % normal control
Euthyroidism:					
Normal values.........................	15–50	4–8	4–11	−15–+15	85–115
Pregnancy............................	Normal/high	High	High	+20–+25	Low
Iodide deficiency......................	High	Normal/low	Normal/low	Normal/low	Normal/low
Iodide therapy, 3.0 mg/day.............	Low	High	Normal	Normal	Normal
Thyroid, USP, >120 mg/day............	Low	Normal/high	Normal/high	Normal/high	Normal/high
L-thyroxin, >0.4 mg/day..............	Low	Normal/high	Normal/high	Normal/high	Normal/high
L-triiodothyronine, >0.1 mg/day........	Low	Low	Low	Normal/high	Normal/high
Congestive heart failure................	Variable	Normal/low	Normal/low	Variable	Normal/high
Hyperthyroidism:					
Untreated............................	50–100	7–20	11–20	High	115–160
Pregnancy............................	High	High	High	High	Normal/high
Iodide therapy, >2.0 mg/day...........	Low	>20	5–15	High/normal	High/normal
Thyroid, USP, >120 mg/day§..........	>20	High	High	High	High
L-Thyroxin, 0.4 mg/day§..............	>20	High	High	High	High
L-Triiodothyronine, 0.1 mg/day§.........	>20	High	High	High	High
Antithyroid drug therapy (euthyroid).....	Variable	Normal	Normal	Normal	Normal
Thyroiditis (acute):.....................	Low	Normal/high	Normal/high	Normal/high	Normal/high
Myxedema (primary):					
Untreated............................	0–15	0–4	0–4	−20–−50	Low‡
Thyroid USP, 120 mg/day (euthyroid)	Low	Normal¶	Normal¶	Normal	Normal
L-Thyroxin, 0.4 mg/day-euthyroid........	Low	Normal/high	Normal/high	Normal	Normal/high
L-Triiodothyronine, 0.1 mg/day (euthyroid)	Low	Low	Low	Normal	Normal

* The presence in serum of trace quantities of mercurial salts will render values for the PBI and BEI factitiously low by the usual methods. Normal values for the serum butanol–extractable iodine (BEI) and the serum T4 by column are 3.2 to 6.5 μg%.

† Serum T4 designates values obtained by the binding displacement method of Murphy and Pattee (J. Clin. Endoc. 26: 247, 1966).

‡ The Resin-T3 values listed here are for the resin sponge method (Triosorb, Abbott) expressed as a percent of a standard control serum. This test is also expressed as an absolute percent uptake with normal values ranging from 25 to 35 percent (See JAMA 202: 135, 1967). The Resin-T3 test is not generally diagnostic of hypothyroidism because of excessive overlap of values in the low normal range with those in hypothyroidism.

§ Suppression test (see text).

¶ The PBI and serum T4 values may be lower than normal in patients receiving some lots of desiccated thyroid, USP, or thyroglobulin (Proloid).

proportional to the available TBG binding sites. It is more readily performed than the direct measurement of the fraction of free T4 by dialysis and serves as a useful indirect measure thereof. Unfortunately, this test depends upon the integrity of the thyroxin-binding proteins and is thus influenced by factors which modify the quantity or binding affinity of these proteins. Common among these are wasting diseases, hepatitis, acidosis, pulmonary insufficiency, renal diseases, and supraventricular tachycardias. A "free T4 index" can be derived from the mathematical product of the concentration of serum T4 (or PBI) and the Resin-T3 uptake (see Table 89-2) in a manner analogous to calculating the actual concentration of free T4 in serum.

The *thyroidal* (^{131}I) *uptake* indicates the *proportion* of ingested iodide accumulated by the thyroid gland. A normal value suggests a physiologic rate of hormone synthesis if it is assumed that the total quantity of iodide being metabolized is normal and that the iodide, once accumulated by the thyroid, is incorporated into active hormonal products. When body iodide stores are expanded, the ^{131}I uptake will almost invariably decrease, although the patient remains metabolically normal. The converse will occur in iodide deficiency.

The *thyroid suppression test* has come into wide clinical usage. This test reflects the integrity of the pituitary-thyroid mechanisms that maintain homeostasis, as described in an earlier section. It is based on the fact that when normal homeostatic mechanisms are disrupted, exogenous thyroid hormone will not suppress the patient's thyroid function. Abnormal tests are therefore found in patients with thyrotoxicosis resulting from hormonal overproduction, whatever its cause. In addition, abnormal tests reflect the physiologic disturbance which, in Graves'

Table 89-2. CLASSIFICATION OF THE VARIETIES OF
DISORDERED THYROID HORMONE-PLASMA
PROTEIN INTERACTIONS

Clinical condition	Total T4 (serum T4 or PBI)	Proportion free T4 (Resin-T3)	Concentration free T4 (free T4 index)
1. Primary Abnormality in Thyroid Binding Proteins			
a. Increased Binding	↑	↓	N
b. Decreased Binding	↓	↑	N
2. Primary Disorder of Thyroid Function			
a. Myxedema	↓	↓	↓
b. Thyrotoxicosis	↑	↑	↑

disease, may exist in the absence of thyrotoxicosis. Examples occur in some patients whose hyperthyroidism has been treated and in some exhibiting solely the ophthalmic manifestations of Graves' disease (hyperophthalmic Graves' disease).

The test is usually performed using a standard dose of liothyronine (sodium L-triiodothyronine). After an initial radioactive iodine uptake (usually at 24 hr), the patient is given a course of liothyronine, 100 μg daily. On the seventh day of liothyronine administration, the radioactive iodine uptake is repeated. If, after appropriate correction for residual radioactivity, the 24-hr radioactive iodine uptake is less than 20 percent, thyrotropin suppression is presumed. Values above 20 percent in 24 hr indicate a disturbance of homeostatic control such as in Graves' disease or autonomous thyroid tumors. Since technical factors vary, the test should be standardized for each laboratory. Desiccated thyroid or sodium L-thyroxin in calorigenically equivalent doses can also be used. It is generally inadvisable to undertake this test in patients over the age of fifty or in those with potential or actual cardiac or vascular disease, since the excessive metabolic activity induced by thyroid hormone stimulation may induce atrial fibrillation, cardiac failure, or vascular accidents. The thyroid suppression test is particularly helpful in the differential diagnosis of various forms of goiter in young adults. It is also useful in evaluating whether the homeostatic disturbance persists in thyrotoxic patients who have been treated.

The *thyrotropin stimulation test* (TSH test) is useful to distinguish primary thyroidal failure, either complete or partial (decreased thyroid reserve) from thyroid hypofunction caused by inadequate TSH stimulation. The latter may result from either intrinsic pituitary disease or from pituitary suppression by exogenous hormone. An increase in radioactive iodine uptake of 10 to 15 percent or more or a rise in serum PBI of more than 1.5 to 2.0 μg per 100 ml indicates that the thyroid gland can re-

spond to exogenous TSH stimulation. The usual dosage of thyrotropin, USP (Thytropar, Armour) is 5 or 10 units given as a single intramuscular injection to determine primary thyroid insufficiency or diminished thyroid reserve. In pituitary failure, this dosage may be insufficient due to thyroidal refractoriness, and doses of 15 to 30 units can be given over a 24 to 48 hr period, 5 to 10 units each 12 to 24 hr. The second uptake test or PBI is obtained 24 hr after the last dose of TSH. Absence of a measurable response to TSH may be caused by several factors but is most commonly the result of primary thyroid failure.

Immunoreactive thyrotropin (TSH) can be measured in serum directly by radioimmunoassay. Although this assay has been of assistance in confirming pathophysiologic concepts of thyroid-pituitary interaction, it is not available generally for clinical testing.

Values for the 24-hr thyroidal radioactive iodine uptake, serum PBI, and serum T4 as well as the in vitro resin-triiodothyronine uptake test are listed in Table 89-1 for common clinical situations. Despite the specificity of these tests, numerous factors may alter their absolute value and yield a result inconsistent either with other results or with the clinical condition of the patient. Modification of test results by extraneous factors most commonly follows administration of iodine, in either organic or inorganic form. Here, high values for tests measuring serum iodine levels and low thyroidal uptakes of ^{131}I are seen. Under such circumstances, the tests of serum T4 and hormonal binding (RBC-T3 and Resin-T3 are useful, since they are not influenced by nonhormonal iodinated compounds. The presence of mercury in serum will produce factitiously low values for PBI and BEI but will not alter the serum T4 or binding tests. On the other hand, systemic disorders and drugs that alter protein binding also affect the values for the RBC-T3 and Resin-T3 tests. Liver disease, cachexia, pulmonary insufficiency, acidosis, androgens, anticoagulants, and anticonvulsants produce increases in the RBC-T3 or Resin-T3 uptake test. Contrariwise, estrogens and pregnancy reduce these uptake tests. Under these circumstances, the values reported differ from the patient's clinical status. When there is some apparent contradiction in the values for different tests, the explanation can usually be found by a careful history of drug ingestion and by a physiologic interpretation of the observed facts.

SIMPLE (NONTOXIC) GOITER

There is considerable confusion concerning the descriptive terms *endemic* and *sporadic goiter*. Endemic implies an etiologic factor or factors common to a particular geographic region. The term has been defined as the presence of generalized or localized thyroid enlargement in over 10 percent of the population. The connotation of sporadic is that goiter arises in nonendemic areas as a result of a stimulus that does not affect the population generally. Since these terms fail to define or distinguish the causes of such goiters and since thyroid enlargement of diverse etiology may exist in both endemic and nonendemic regions, it seems prudent to employ a general term such as *simple* or *nontoxic goiter*. This all-inclusive category can be further subdivided into specific etiologic groups as defined by objective procedures. Simple or nontoxic goiter may be defined as any enlargement of the thyroid gland that does not result from an inflammatory or neoplastic process and does not lead to thyrotoxicosis or myxedema.

HISTORY. Goitrous enlargement of the thyroid gland has been recognized since antiquity by many cultures in diverse parts of the world. Its existence has been documented in historic accounts dating back to the fifteenth century B.C. and has been incorporated into the art, literature, and folklore of many cultures. By the nineteenth century, goiter became recognized medically as a common entity in many geographic areas, particularly in mountainous regions such as the Pyrenees, Alps, Carpathians, Himalayas, Sierras, and Andes. Cretinism was described in many goitrous regions of the world and, in the Americas, was noted in pre-Columbian art forms.

Iodine was discovered in the residue of burned seaweed by Courtois in 1812 and identified as a new element by Gay-Lussac. It has been used empirically for therapy of goiter since ancient times. In 1896, iodine was found to be a normal constituent of the thyroid gland by Baumann, but it was not until 1915 that Kendall isolated L-thyroxin. The chemical structure of this hormone was determined and proved by chemical synthesis in 1927 by Harington and Barger. A second hormonal constituent of the thyroid gland, L-triiodothyronine, was isolated and identified in 1952 by Roche, Lissitsky, and Michel in France and by Gross and Pitt-Rivers in England. Coindet in 1820 first described in scientific fashion the results of iodide therapy before the Swiss Society of Natural Sciences. However, because of complications of overdosage and the poor comprehension of thyroid disease prevalent at that time, iodine therapy failed acceptance by most physicians for the next century. The important relationship of iodine deficiency to goiter was renewed through the devoted labors of Marine who in 1905 began a systematic investigation of this association. His research reached a peak of excellence in 1917 when Marine and Kimball initiated the now classic controlled study of elementary school children in Akron, Ohio and concluded several years later that iodide deficiency was a major cause of goiter and that such goiters could be prevented by supplementation of dietary iodine. Despite this remarkable discovery, most nations have yet to pass adequate legislation to guarantee this important dietary mineral to all people. It was estimated by the World Health Organization in 1960 that approximately 200 million people were goitrous. The incidence varies with the prevalence of dietary iodine and has tended to decrease with the introduction of iodine as a public health measure. It is, however, still a major public health problem even in highly industrialized countries, despite a concerted, albeit inadequate, effort to reduce the high incidence of goiter by dietary measures.

ETIOLOGY. Although the causes of simple goiter are manifold, their clinical manifestations reflect the operation of a common pathophysiologic mechanism. Simple goiter results when one or more factors impair the capacity of the thyroid, in the basal state, to secrete sufficient quantities of physiologically active hormones to meet the needs of peripheral tissues. Under these conditions, secretion of TSH is enhanced, and this stimulates both glandular growth and the activity of all intrathyroidal reactions involved in synthesis and secretion of thyroid hormone. Such compensatory increases in functioning thyroidal mass and stimulation of cellular activity are sufficient to overcome mild or moderate impairments of hormonal synthesis, and the patient remains metabolically normal although goitrous. When, however, impairment of hormonal synthesis is severe, compensatory responses are inadequate and the patient is both goitrous and more or less severely hypothyroid. Thus, the entity of simple goiter cannot be separated clearly, in the pathogenetic sense, from goitrous hypothyroidism. Specific causes of simple goiter are included in Table 89-3 and may exist with or without hypothyroidism.

PATHOLOGY. The histopathology of the thyroid in simple goiter will vary with the severity of the etiologic factor and the stage of the disorder at which the examination is made. In its initial stages, the gland will reveal a uniform hypertrophy, hyperplasia, and hypervascularity. As the disorder persists or undergoes repeated exacerbations and remissions, uniformity of thyroidal architecture is usually lost. Occasionally, the greater part of the gland may display a reasonably uniform degree of involution or hyperinvolution with colloid accumulation. More often such areas are interspersed with patchy areas of focal hyperplasia. Fibrosis may demarcate a variable number of nodules, which may be hyperplastic or involuted; these may resemble, but do not really represent, true neoplasms (adenomas). Areas of hemorrhage and calcification may be present.

CLINICAL PICTURE. In simple goiter, the clinical manifestations arise solely from enlargement of the thyroid, since the metabolic state of the patient is normal. In goitrous hypothyroidism, symptoms caused by thyromegaly are similarly present but are accompanied by signs and symptoms of hormonal insufficiency. Mechanical sequelae include compression and displacement of the trachea or esophagus, occasionally with obstructive symptoms if the goiter becomes sufficiently large. Superior mediastinal obstruction may occur with large intrathoracic goiters. Signs of compression can be induced in the case of large cervical goiters when the patient's arms are raised above the head (Pemberton's sign); suffusion of the face, giddiness, or syncope may result from this maneuver. Compression of the recurrent laryngeal nerve leading to hoarseness is rare in simple goiter and suggests neoplasm. Sudden hemorrhage into a nodule may lead to an acute, painful swelling in the neck and may produce or enhance compressive symptoms. Hyperthyroidism not uncommonly supervenes in long-standing multinodular goiter (toxic multinodular goiter). It is not known whether this represents the superimposition of Graves' disease upon a chronic nontoxic goiter or a separate disease entity.

In geographic regions where iodine deficiency is severe,

acquired goitrous enlargement may also be associated with varying degrees of hypothyroidism. Cretinism, both goitrous and nongoitrous, occurs with increased frequency in the children of goitrous parents, and contributes a significant sector of the socially dependent population in many countries where goiter is common. The association of deaf-mutism, goiter, and varying degrees of mental retardation has been termed *Pendred's syndrome*.

DIAGNOSIS. The *diagnosis* of simple goiter can often be suspected on clinical grounds. However, other goitrous conditions such as forms of chronic thyroiditis, drug or iodide goiter, or primary thyroid neoplasms, cannot always be excluded by the consistency, size, or symmetry of the enlargement. A careful history is important to determine the prevalence of thyroidal pain and tenderness, drug ingestion, rapid changes in size, or hoarseness. High titers of circulating thyroglobulin antibodies suggest but do not necessarily indicate lymphoid thyroiditis (Hashimoto's struma). At times, needle biopsy of the thyroid is indicated to confirm or exclude the diagnosis of thyroiditis, but it should not be used if thyroid cancer is suspected. Laboratory tests of thyroid function in the inhabitants of countries where goiter is highly endemic (greater than 10 percent of the population) may vary considerably. An elevated thyroidal uptake of radioactive iodine often accompanies low levels of inorganic serum and urinary iodide. Serum T4 (and PBI) levels are usually in the low normal range or may be moderately reduced if hypothyroidism coexists.

TREATMENT. The object of treatment is to remove the stimulus of thyroidal hyperplasia, either by relieving external encumbrances to hormone formation or by providing sufficient quantities of exogenous hormone to inhibit TSH and thereby put the thyroid gland almost completely at rest. In disorders characterized by decreased thyroidal iodide stores, such as iodine deficiency or impairment of the thyroidal iodide–concentrating mechanism, small doses of iodide may prove effective. Occasionally, a known extrinsic goitrogen can be withdrawn. Most commonly, however, no specific etiologic factor can be detected, and *suppressive thyroid therapy* is required. For this purpose, desiccated thyroid in dosage usually ranging from 120 to 180 mg is the agent of choice. Purified hormones such as the sodium salts of thyroxin or triiodothyronine are equally effective metabolically but may render it difficult to assess overdosage through measurement of the PBI. Suppression of endogenous thyroid function is most readily assessed by serial measurements of the 24-hr thyroidal uptake of ^{131}I. Partial suppression is indicated when ^{131}I uptake is reduced below control values and complete suppression when the 24-hr uptake falls below 10 percent. In multinodular, nontoxic goiter, lack of complete suppression usually indicates the presence of autonomously functioning foci, demonstrable by scanning techniques. Radioactive iodine uptake studies can be obtained at appropriate intervals and the dose of exogenous hormone gradually adjusted as needed to achieve maximum suppression. Occasionally, physiologic replacement doses of

exogenous hormones will induce mild but usually transient symptoms of thyrotoxicity. In such patients, more prolonged intervals between dosage changes will usually permit achievement of full thyroid suppression without inducing symptoms of toxicity.

Reported results of therapy vary widely. There is general agreement that the early diffuse, hyperplastic goiter responds well, with regression or disappearance in 3 to 6 months. In the authors' experience, the later, nodular stage responds less favorably, and significant reduction in gland size is achieved in approximately half the cases. Internodular tissue regresses more often than do nodules themselves. The latter may therefore become more prominent during treatment. After maximum regression of the goiter, suppressive medication may be maintained for prolonged periods, reduced to minimal levels, or at times withdrawn. In an unpredictable manner, goiter will in some cases remain relieved while in others it will recur. In the latter instances, suppressive therapy should be reinstituted and should be continued indefinitely. When treatment is initiated in patients of childbearing age, it should probably be continued through the menopause.

Surgical therapy of simple goiter is physiologically unsound, but it may occasionally be necessary to relieve obstructive symptoms, especially those which persist after a conscientious trial of medical therapy. Surgical exploration of nodular goiter may be indicated in some individuals when evidence suggests carcinoma. However, the suggestion that subtotal resection of multinodular, nontoxic goiter affords effective prophylaxis against the development of thyroidal carcinoma is unsound. If for some reason subtotal thyroidectomy has been performed, use of physiologic replacement doses of desiccated thyroid, 120 to 180 mg daily, is recommended to inhibit regenerative hyperplasia and further goitrogenesis.

HYPOTHYROIDISM

HISTORY. The concept that sporadic cretinism is caused by absence of the thyroid gland was first expressed by Dr. C. H. Fagge at Guy's Hospital in 1871. In 1874, Gull described adult myxedema, stating that it resembled cretinism but occurred in adult life. The term *myxedema*, or *mucous edema*, has been credited to Ord (1878). During the subsequent 4 to 5 years, the Reverdin brothers, of Geneva, and Kocher, of Berne, observed that following thyroidectomy for goiter there appeared what they termed *postoperative myxedema* or *cachexia strumipriva*. The striking effects of thyroid replacement therapy in myxedematous patients were described in 1891 by Murray, who was the first to administer a glycerin extract of animal thyroid. The next year, Mackenzie and Fox noted independently that animal thyroid was equally effective by mouth, and for over 75 years this natural hormone has been used extensively. Standardization of desiccated thyroid was introduced into the U.S. Pharmacopoeia in 1915 and persists to the current edition. Synthetic L-thyroxin was reintroduced into therapy around 1953 after a commercially feasible synthesis was devised by Hems and his associates. Use of L-triiodothyronine (liothyronine) followed shortly thereafter.

INCIDENCE. Cretinism is rare. The incidence of myxedema (juvenile and adult) is estimated to be 1 in every 1,500 hospital admissions. Adult myxedema occurs about five times as frequently in women as in men and most frequently between the ages of thirty and sixty years.

ETIOLOGY. Hypothyroidism may be either primary (thyroid gland failure) or secondary (anterior pituitary failure) (Table 89-3). Primary hypothyroidism dating

Table 89-3. CLASSIFICATION OF HYPOTHYROIDISM

I. Primary (sporadic and endemic)
   A. Nongoitrous
      1. Idiopathic
      2. Postablative (surgery, radiation)
      3. Postinflammatory
   B. Goitrous
      1. Congenital and hereditary defects
         a. Trapping
         b. Organification
         c. Coupling
         d. Dehalogenation
         e. Release
         f. Maternal-induced (iodide, antithyroid compounds)
      2. Acquired
         a. Iodides (excess or lack)
         b. Drugs (thiocyanates, PASA, butazolidine, cobalt)
         c. Natural goitrogens (food, milk)
         d. Thyroiditis (Hashimoto's)
II. Secondary
   A. Pituitary failure
   B. Transport abnormalities
   C. Utilization defects (hypothetic)

from birth results in a clinical picture characteristic of cretinism. Two varieties of cretinism can be distinguished, athyreotic and goitrous. In areas of endemic goiter, cretinism is common and is usually, but not invariably, goitrous. The sporadic cretinism of nonendemic areas is usually athyreotic but may be goitrous. In the latter patients, hereditary disorders of thyroid hormone biogenesis can usually be identified. Deaf-mutism is a common accompaniment of cretinism and, when associated with goiter, has been termed *Pendred's syndrome.*

The occurrence of primary thyroid deficiency later in life gives rise to the syndromes of juvenile and adult myxedema. Under these circumstances, inadequate production of thyroid hormones results from destruction of the thyroid gland by disease, atrophy, or ablative procedures (thyroidectomy, radioactive iodine therapy, or external radiation). Secondary hypothyroidism results from a deficiency of pituitary TSH and may occur at any age as a consequence of anterior pituitary failure (Chap. 87).

A classification of the more important pathophysiologic etiologies of hypothyroidism is presented in Table 89-3.

The most frequent cause of spontaneous hypothyroidism is idiopathic atrophy of the thyroid gland. In children, this may result from developmental abnormalities. In adults, such atrophy may represent the final stage of an autoimmune response to thyroglobulin or other thyroid antigens and may therefore be related to one form of chronic thyroiditis, struma lymphomatosa (Hashimoto's struma). Circulating thyroid antibodies may be detected in a majority of patients with spontaneous hypothyroidism (see under Thyroiditis). Postthyroidectomy and postradiation hypothyroidism occur more frequently than the spontaneous varieties, and radioactive iodine therapy of hyperthyroidism is currently the most common cause of hypothyroidism. Occasionally, in patients who have undergone thyroid ablative procedures or have experienced chronic thyroid inflammation, thyroid function is not completely abolished but is insufficient to meet peripheral hormonal needs. Such patients, who may have mild symptoms of hypothyroidism, can be distinguished by their failure to respond to TSH and have been described as having decreased thyroid reserve.

CLINICAL PICTURE. The general appearance of children with hypothyroidism varies considerably, depending on the age at which the deficiency begins and the promptness of replacement therapy. Signs and symptoms of cretinism may be clinically evident at birth, or more commonly, within the first several neonatal months, depending upon the completeness of thyroid failure. These children are dwarfed, stocky, and somewhat overweight, with a broad flat nose, eyes set apart because of failure of nasoorbital development, coarse features with thick lips, protruding tongue, pale mottled skin, poor muscular tone and intestinal activity, spadelike stubby hands with x-ray evidence of retarded bone age and epiphyseal dysgenesis, delayed eruption of teeth, and malocclusion resulting from macroglossia. *In infancy, the characteristic facies, the hoarse cry, the large tongue, the "potbelly" and the presence of an umbilical hernia should call attention to the diagnosis of severe degrees of thyroid deficiency. Diagnosis and treatment at the earliest possible date in infancy are important,* since the extent of mental retardation may be related to the age at which treatment is instituted. Good results are obtained only when the diagnosis is established early and adequate therapy is instituted at once. If therapy is delayed, most of the clinical features of cretinism may still be reversed but some degree of mental retardation usually persists.

The adult and older child with myxedema have a typical facies, characterized by a dull, uninterested expression and puffy eyelids, often with alopecia of the outer third of the eyebrows. The skin of the face exhibits creamy pallor, and occasionally there is palmar yellowing. The changes in coloring result from anemia combined with carotenemia. The skin elsewhere on the body is dry and rough. The subcutaneous tissue is indurated and doughy because of interstitial fluid of high protein content. The hair is brittle and dry. There is swelling of the tongue and larynx and a halting, slurred, hoarse speech with slowing of physical and, seemingly, of mental activity. Anemia, constipation, and increased sensitivity to cold are present as well as increased capillary fragility, as evidenced by susceptibility to bruising. Women with myxedema during the active ovarian cycle usually note prolonged or excessive menstrual bleeding. Some patients with hypothroidism complain of constant rhinorrhea, coryza, or deafness. There may also be arthralgia, symptoms indistinguishable from those of peripheral neuropathy, signs and symptoms of cerebellar disturbance, muscular weakness, or myotonia.

The cardiac silhouette is usually larger than normal, partially because of dilation but mostly from pericardial effusion, which is commonly present. Rarely, the cardiac silhouette may be small; if so, pituitary myxedema should be considered. Thyroid tissue is rarely palpable except in presence of chronic thyroiditis, endemic goiter, goitrogen ingestion, or goitrous cretinism. Skeletal growth is usually normal in the adult patient with myxedema, but in children or adolescents both growth and skeletal maturation are usually retarded significantly. The relaxation time of the deep tendon reflexes is characteristically slowed in patients with myxedema. Severe ileus with a picture of megacolon is also seen. Rarely, psychoses (myxedema madness) may dominate the clinical picture in patients with myxedema. Untreated patients with profound degrees of myxedema may exhibit hypothermic coma (myxedema coma), a serious and usually fatal complication. Some features of myxedema coma are related to respiratory depression and consequent CO_2 narcosis. Occasional hyponatremia, not responsive to glucocorticoids, is present and may represent a form of refractive dilutional hyponatremia. Hydrothorax, ascites, and pericardial effusions of high protein content are not uncommon.

DIAGNOSIS. Laboratory examinations in primary thyroid atrophy usually reveal a low basal metabolic rate, elevated serum cholesterol level, low plasma protein-bound iodine or serum T4, low resin T3 uptake of labeled triiodothyronine, and decreased radioiodine uptake in the thyroid. Extraneous factors that may modify the plasma PBI level or the radioiodine uptake of the gland are enumerated in Table 89-2. In some varieties of goitrous hypothyroidism, the thyroid uptake of radioactive iodine may be increased. In those in whom ^{131}I remains unbound, it may be discharged from the gland after administration of potassium thiocyanate or perchlorate.

It is noteworthy that the spinal fluid protein concentration may be elevated in patients with profound myxedema. There may be a significant normocytic or slightly macrocytic anemia as well as gastric achlorhydria. When losses of iron are excessive, such as may occur with menorrhagia, a picture of hypochromic anemia may predominate. The electrocardiograph may reveal a marked decrease in voltage with flattened or inverted T waves. Serum enzyme levels are often increased in myxedema, the lactic dehydrogenase (LDH) usually being elevated to a greater extent than the creative phosphokinase (CPK) or glutamic oxaloacetic transaminase (SGOT). These findings may be confusing when myocardial infarction is

suspected as a complication in myxedema, particularly since this elevation results principally from the cardiac isoenzymes of LDH. Serum uric acid may also be elevated in myxedema.

The signs and symptoms of mild or moderate hypothyroidism are less striking. The symptoms are similar to those in frank myxedema but are less severe. Such symptoms are, however, readily confused with those of many other organic or psychogenic disturbances. Even the BMR may be low for reasons other than the presence of thyroid disease. It is important, therefore, to establish the diagnosis of true, mild hypothyroidism on the basis of objective criteria. Such criteria may be met either by the finding of subnormal values for serum T4, PBI, Resin T3 uptake, and the thyroidal ^{131}I uptake or, in the presence of marginal values for these tests, by their failure to increase after TSH.

Hypothyroidism secondary to anterior pituitary deficiency may present a picture indistinguishable from that of primary myxedema. However, the accumulation of subcutaneous fluid (myxedema fluid) is usually not so pronounced in patients with pituitary myxedema as in those with primary myxedema. Careful investigation will usually reveal associated gonadal and adrenocortical deficiency out of proportion to that seen in primary myxedema. In general, the serum cholesterol level is within, or close to, normal limits in patients with hypothyroidism secondary to anterior pituitary failure, whereas it is usually elevated in primary myxedema. Patients with primary myxedema respond readily and satisfactorily to thyroid replacement therapy. In contrast, administration of this hormone to patients with pituitary myxedema is usually less effective and may precipitate adrenal crisis. The administration of TSH to patients with pituitary hypothyroidism is usually followed in 24 hr by a rise in the thyroidal uptake of radioactive iodine and in serum protein–bound iodine or serum T4.

DIFFERENTIAL DIAGNOSIS. Little difficulty will be experienced in diagnosing classic cretinism or juvenile and adult myxedema. Occasionally, a mongoloid infant may be confused with a cretin. However, the characteristic mongoloid eyes, hyperextensibility of the finger joints, and normal skin and hair texture distinguish the mongoloid imbecile from the hypothyroid cretin. Chronic nephritis and especially nephrosis may simulate myxedema. This is particularly true of the chronic uremic patient with retarded mental acuity and characteristic facial expression. In nephrosis, the basal metabolic rate is usually below normal as is the level of the serum PBI, or serum T4. Since the nephrotic patient may also exhibit anemia, hypercholesterolemia, and anasarca (simulating myxedema fluid), the differential diagnosis may be confusing. However, the uptake of radioactive iodine is usually normal in nephrotic patients, the low level of serum PBI or serum T4 being caused by a decrease in throxin- binding proteins in the blood, resulting from proteinuria. The hyperactive deep tendon reflexes of the uremic patient, as contrasted with the slowed relaxation phase of the reflexes in patients with myxedema, may aid in distinguishing the two conditions. Not infrequently hypothyroid patients exhibit anemia and clinically resemble patients with pernicious anemia. Though usually separate, myxedema and pernicious anemia may coexist; recent evidence suggests that they may share related immunologic abnormalities.

Patients with secondary hypothyroidism, because of attendant adrenocortical failure, must be distinguished carefully from patients with primary myxedema. Urinary 17-ketosteroid and 17-hydroxycorticoid excretion may be reduced in both conditions, and the response to the 2-day ACTH test may occasionally be misleading in differentiating these conditions (see Chap. 87). The finding of elevated levels of urinary FSH, a normal water-loading test, and a good response to metyrapone (SU-4885) helps distinguish primary myxedema from anterior pituitary failure. In addition, the rise in serum immunocreative growth hormone (HGH) in response to insulin-induced hypoglycemia or arginine infusion is characteristically absent in panhypopituitarism, but present in primary myxedema. Although the patient with Addison's disease is frequently hypometabolic, absence of excessive pigmentation, a normal water-loading response, and low values for PBI, serum T4, and radioactive iodine uptake help distinguish myxedema from Addison's disease.

Table 89-4. APPROXIMATE EQUIVALENT DOSES OF VARIOUS THYROID PREPARATIONS

Preparation	Average daily oral maintenance dose, mg*	Serum PBI†
Thyroid, USP.........	120–180	Normal
L-Thyroxin (T4).......	0.3–0.4	Slightly elevated
L-Triiodothyronine (T3)...............	0.075–0.125	Depressed
L-T4+L-T3........... (Liotrix)	L-T4:0.20–L-T4:0.180 L-T3:0.030–L-T3:0.045	Normal

* Infants and children require proportionally larger doses of thyroid preparations than adults.

† Serum levels of PBI vary according to preparation used and may not be a direct measure of thyroid hormone effect (see text).

TREATMENT. Desiccated thyroid (thyroid, USP) is the most commonly used preparation and is usually administered in 30-, 60-, 120-, or 180-mg tablets. Its major disadvantage is inadequate standardization of hormonal content. Sodium L-thyroxin is available as 0.05-, 0.1-, 0.2- and 0.3-mg tablets (Synthroid, Flint), and sodium L-triiodothyronine is marketed in 0.005-, 0.025-, and 0.050-mg tablets (Cytomel). A new combination containing synthetic sodium L-thyroxine and sodium L-triiodothyronine in a ratio of 4:1 by weight (Euthroid) has been introduced to obviate some of the problems inherent in the standardization of thyroid, USP. Serum T4, PBI, and resin T3 uptake tests in patients receiving this synthetic

thyroid combination are usually representative of their metabolic status. The average daily maintenance dosages of these preparations are listed in Table 89-4. Some commercially available lots of UTP thyroid, as well as some lots of a thyroglobulin preparation (Proloid) give levels of PBI lower than anticipated by the patient's metabolic status. This is presumably a result of increased ratio of triiodothyronine to thyroxin in these preparations.

In all instances, except perhaps in myxedema coma, it is desirable to institute therapy with relatively small doses of a thyroid substance, since sudden changes in metabolic level may induce undesirable psychologic or cardiovascular disturbances, especially in elderly patients. The occurrence of angina pectoris or congestive heart failure during therapy for myxedema is an indication to proceed with caution, since rapid changes in metabolic rate may precipitate as well as increase the severity of these conditions. In adults, one may begin with a dose of 15 mg USP thyroid or less per day, gradually increasing the dosage at weekly or biweekly intervals. In patients over forty or fifty years of age, thyroid therapy should be given cautiously with longer intervals between increments in dosage. The usual daily dose of desiccated thyroid necessary to maintain an athyreotic patient in euthyroidism is 90 to 180 mg. In the presence of any evidence of cardiovascular disease, the total dosage should not exceed 30 to 60 mg daily until the patient has been followed for several weeks at this level. The maximum effect from a given dosage level will not be obtained for at least 7 to 10 days, and thyroid hormone action will persist for several weeks after the last dose. It is not necessary to give desiccated thyroid more than once daily. Because of its relatively more rapid onset and shorter duration of action, triiodothyronine may be given in divided doses.

In many patients, generalized muscular aching follows initiation of therapy regardless of the dosage of thyroid hormone, and occasionally coryza is noted. It is essential in patients with cretinism or juvenile myxedema to maintain therapy at close to toxic levels in order to ensure the desired growth response. The requirement for optimum bone growth appears to be higher than that usually needed for satisfactory maintenance of the overall clinical status. Children need somewhat more thyroid in proportion to their size than do adults. Dosage usually must be adjusted according to clinical evaluation of the effects obtained, at the same time avoiding symptoms of overdosage such as tachycardia, irritability, continuous weight loss, diarrhea, or sweating. In panhypopituitarism, thyroid hormone therapy should *not* be instituted until after adrenocortical replacement therapy has been initiated. The initial dose of desiccated thyroid should be small and increased gradually by 15-mg increments at 3-week intervals.

It should be noted that patients with untreated myxedema, like patients with Addison's disease, are extremely sensitive to the pharmacologic actions of many drugs such as narcotics, barbiturates, and tranquilizers as well as to most stressful situations such as operations. Patients with myxedema coma should be treated with parenteral triiodothyronine, adrenocortical steriods, artificial respiration (if CO_2 narcosis exists), and correction of any electrolyte disturbances.

HYPERTHYROIDISM

The terms *hyperthyroidism* and *thyrotoxicosis* usually denote the complex of physiologic and biochemical disturbances that result when the tissues are exposed to excessive quantities of thyroid hormones. This occurs most commonly in association with diffuse hyperplasia of the thyroid gland often accompanied by specific ophthalmic abnormalities and is usually designated *Graves' disease.* It is also termed *Parry's* or *Basedow's disease.* It should be recognized, however, that hyperthyroidism may result from overproduction of thyroid hormone by a hyperfunctioning adenoma, multinodular goiter (Plummer's disease), or ectopic thyroid tissue. The peripheral features of hyperthyroidism also result when thyroid medication is taken in excess (thyrotoxicosis factitia). The following discussion will deal mainly with Graves' disease. In addition, features of other disorders that may produce hyperthyroidism will be discussed.

HISTORY. In 1786, Dr. Caleb Parry described a disease characterized by thyroid enlargement, dilatation of the heart, palpitation, exophthalmos, and nervous as well as menstrual symptoms. Graves and Basedow, between the years 1835 and 1843, published treatises independently on the syndrome that now bears their names. That hyperthyroidism was the fundamental disorder in Graves' disease was formulated by Möbius in Germany in 1887. The use of iodine in the treatment of thyrotoxicosis was popularized by Plummer. Recent advances in the medical therapy of hyperthyroidism include the introduction in 1942 of antithyroid substances such as derivatives of thiourea and imidazole. Radioactive iodine, introduced in 1942, now occupies a prominent position as a therapeutic agent in the treatment of thyrotoxicosis.

INCIDENCE. Graves' disease is a relatively common disorder which may occur at any age but occurs especially in the third and fourth decades. The disease is much more frequent in women than in men. In nongoitrous areas the ratio of predominance in females may be as high as 8:1. In endemic goitrous areas the ratio is lower. Hyperthyroidism is comparatively rare in children. When it occurs, there is usually a diffuse goiter free of nodules.

ETIOLOGY. Basic to Graves' disease is a derangement of those homeostatic mechanisms that normally adjust thyroid hormone secretion to meet the physiologic needs of the peripheral tissues. In the past, it was suggested that this homeostatic disruption resulted from either overproduction of TSH by the pituitary or development of autonomous hyperfunction within the thyroid itself. The weight of evidence now indicates, however, that neither is the case. Rather, thyroidal hyperfunction in Graves' disease appears to result from the action of an hormonotropic serum globulin called the "long-acting thyroid stimulator" (LATS). Under appropriate bioassay conditions, LATS is demonstrable in the serum of approximately 90 percent of thyrotoxic patients with Graves'

disease. Its designation as LATS derives from the fact that in the test system its action is more prolonged than that of TSH. The initial action of LATS on thyroidal iodine metabolism is to stimulate hormonal release, but it is also capable of increasing ^{131}I uptake and inducing thyroidal hyperplasia. Like thyrotropin, it stimulates several aspects of thyroid intermediate metabolism. It has not been possible, by means of available fractionation techniques, to separate LATS from other 7S gamma-globulins of plasma. Furthermore, the action of LATS on the thyroid is inhibited by antibodies to normal human 7S gamma-globulin, but not antibodies to TSH. Although the nature of the putative antigen is unknown, these findings suggest that LATS is itself an antibody to some cytologic component of the thyroid. If so, Graves' disease should be included among those disorders associated with, if not necessarily caused by, autoimmune phenomena. Titers of LATS in the patient's serum do not correlate completely with the presence or absence of thyrotoxicosis or with its degree of severity. Indeed, some authorities believe that titers of LATS correlate best with the presence and severity of ophthalmopathy or pretibial myxedema. Hence, it is likely that factors other than LATS also serve to condition the state of thyroid function in Graves' disease.

PATHOLOGY. In Graves' disease the thyroid gland is diffusely enlarged bilaterally, soft, and vascular. The essential pathology is that of parenchymatous hypertrophy and hyperplasia, characterized by increased height of the epithelium and redundancy of the follicular wall, giving the picture of papillary infoldings and cytologic evidence of increased activity. Such hyperplasia is usually accompanied by lymphocytic infiltration. In hyperthyroidism associated with nodular goiters (Plummer's disease), the major part of the thyroid tissue shows colloid involutional changes with hyperplastic paranodular areas that exhibit the functional changes responsible for the hyperthyroidism. This type of gland is thought to represent the end stage of an involuted nodular goiter and is erroneously termed *toxic adenoma.* True thyroid tumors (adenomas) that produce hyperfunction occur only rarely; in these, the paranodular tissue is inactive. Following iodine medication, there is colloid storage, which sometimes causes enlargement and increased firmness of the gland. Graves' disease is associated with generalized lymphoid hyperplasia and infiltration. Thyrotoxicosis may lead to degeneration of skeletal muscle fibers, enlargement of the heart, fatty infiltration or diffuse fibrosis of the liver, decalcification of the skeleton, and loss of body tissue (including fat deposits, osteoid, and muscle).

CLINICAL PICTURE. Common manifestations of Graves' disease include exophthalmos, goiter, fine tremor (especially of the extended fingers and tongue), increased nervousness as well as emotional instability, excessive sweating and heat intolerance, palpitations, and hyperkinesis. Loss of weight and of strength usually exist, often despite increased appetite. Hyperdefecation and occasionally anorexia, nausea, and vomiting may occur. Dyspnea, paroxysmal arrhythmias, and in individuals over the age of forty, cardiac failure occur not infrequently.

Oligomenorrhea and amenorrhea are commoner than menorrhagia. In general, nervous symptoms dominate the clinical picture in younger individuals, whereas cardiovascular and neuromusuclar symptoms predominate in older subjects.

The skin is warm and moist with a velvety texture, and palmar erythema is often found. The hair is fine and silky. Occasionally, increased loss of hair from the temporal aspects of the scalp may be noted. Excessive melanin pigmentation is not uncommon. Ocular signs include a characteristic stare with widened palpebral fissures, blinking, lid lag, failure of convergence, and failure to wrinkle the brow on upward gaze. These signs are thought to result from sympathetic overstimulation and usually subside when the thyrotoxicosis is corrected. The *infiltrative ophthalmopathy* characteristic of Graves' disease will be discussed in a later section.

The diffuse toxic goiter may be asymmetric and lobular. A bruit heard best directly over the gland is not found invariably. When heard, it usually signifies that the patient is thyrotoxic, but may also rarely be present in association with other disorders in which the thyroid is markedly hyperplastic. Venous hums and carotid souffles should be distinguished from true thyroid bruits. A hyperplastic pyramidal lobe of the thyroid may often be palpable if carefully sought.

Cardiovascular findings include a wide pulse pressure, sinus tachycardia, atrial arrhythmias (especially atrial fibrillation), systolic murmurs, increased intensity of the apical first sound, cardiac enlargement, and at times, overt heart failure. A to-and-fro, high-pitched sound may be audible in the pulmonic area and may simulate a pericardial friction rub (Means-Lerman scratch).

DIAGNOSIS. When severe, Graves' disease (as well as other thyrotoxic disorders) is so striking that the diagnosis presents little difficulty. Goiter, eye signs, loss of weight despite good appetite, tachycardia, sweating, psychic instability, tremor, increased basal metabolic rate, high serum PBI and T4 increased resin uptake of radioactive triiodothyronine, and a rapid, increased thyroidal uptake of radioiodine all serve to establish the diagnosis (Table 89-2).

In a few patients the clinical picture may be one of apathy rather than of hyperactivity, and the basal metabolic rate elevation may be relatively slight. In such instances the clinical detection of underlying thyrotoxicosis is difficult, but the thyroidal uptake or radioactive iodine and the serum PBI levels are usually diagnostic. A barium swallow may be helpful in demonstrating displacement of the esophagus or trachea by substernal enlargement of the thyroid. All patients with unexplained cardiac failure or irregularities in rhythm, especially atrial fibrillation, should be surveyed carefully for underlying thyrotoxicosis. In patients with preexisting cardiac disease, even mild thyrotoxicosis may induce severe disability. The circulation time may be rapid or normal in the presence of an elevated venous pressure, and the response to digitalis is usually poor.

Although eye signs are important, it should be recognized that infiltrative ophthalmopathy may occur antecedent to or in the absence of thyrotoxicosis. Prominent eyes and wide palpebral fissures without infiltrative ophthalmopathy occur normally in some individuals. Proptosis and occasionally mild degrees of conjunctival hyperemia are seen in advanced uremia, Cushing's syndrome, cirrhosis of the liver, and malignant hypertension; in such instances, thyroid function is normal and the ophthalmopathy is not of thyroidal origin.

DIFFERENTIAL DIAGNOSIS. Signs and symptoms in a number of nonthyroidal disorders may simulate certain aspects of the thyrotoxic syndrome. *Anxiety* is a prominent feature of hyperthyroidism, and there is thus some overlap in the symptomatology of this disorder with pure anxiety states of emotional origin. Such symptoms as tachycardia, tremulousness, irritability, weakness, and fatigue are common to the anxiety of both disorders. In anxiety of emotional origin, however, the peripheral manifestations of excessive thyroid hormones are absent; thus, the skin of the extremities is usually cold and clammy rather than warm and moist. *Weight loss,* when present in emotional anxiety, is characteristically accompanied by anorexia, whereas in hyperthyroidism it is generally but not invariably accompanied by excessive appetite. Hyperthyroidism can occasionally be confused with such disorders as metastatic carcinoma, cirrhosis of the liver, hyperparathyroidism, sprue, and neuromyopathies such as *myasthenia gravis* and *periodic paralysis.* These conditions may be mimicked by hyperthyroidism or, rarely, may coexist with it. Sympathetic activity of thyrotoxicosis may result in an overlap of signs and symptoms with those of *pheochromocytoma,* including heat intolerance, excessive perspiration, tachycardia with palpitations, and a hypermetabolic state, which may often be severe. In all the above disorders, as well as other conditions considered in the differential diagnosis of hyperthyroidism, careful evaluation of one or more of the specific laboratory procedures previously described will usually distinguish hyperthyroidism from the others.

Hyperthyroidism is a disorder of so many diverse clinical manifestations that it may masquerade as one of many seemingly unrelated disorders. Signs and symptoms directing the physician's attention to gastrointestinal, cardiovascular, or neuromuscular diseases are not infrequent, particularly in older individuals. This differential diagnosis is extremely important in patients with heart disease in whom thyrotoxicosis must be considered in the etiology of atrial fibrillation and congestive heart failure. Subacute bacterial endocarditis, myocarditis, pericarditis, acute rheumatic fever, and coronary heart disease may be mimicked by uncomplicated hyperthyroidism.

TREATMENT. Graves' disease is a disorder often characterized by cyclic phases of exacerbation and remission. Occasionally, patients with forms of the disease may recover spontaneously. This characteristic of Graves' disease has important implications in the choice of and response to therapy.

There are two major approaches to the treatment of hyperthyroidism; both are directed to limiting the quantity of thyroid hormones the gland can produce. The first major therapeutic category, the use of antithyroid agents, interposes a chemical blockade to hormone synthesis, the effect of which is operative only as long as the drug is administered or until a spontaneous remission occurs. Thus, the agents can control successfully a single phase of active thyrotoxicity but probably will not prevent exacerbation at some subsequent period. The second major approach is ablation of thyroid tissue, thereby limiting hormone production. This may be achieved either surgically or by means of radioactive iodine. Since these procedures induce permanent anatomic alterations of the thyroid, they can control the individual active phase and are more likely to prevent recurrence of thyrotoxicity during a later exacerbation. On the other hand, the permanency of the effects of surgery or radiation makes these modes of therapy capable of leading to hypothyroidism, either shortly after treatment or with the passage of years.

Each major mode of therapy has advantages and disadvantages, indications and contraindications. The latter are more often relative than absolute. In general, a trial of long-term antithyroid therapy is desirable in children, adolescents, young adults, and pregnant women, but it may also be employed in older patients. Indications for ablative procedures include relapse or recurrence following drug therapy, a large goiter, drug toxicity, and failure of the patient to follow a medical regimen or to return for periodic examinations. Subtotal thyroidectomy is usually elected for patients under the age of forty in whom ablative therapy is required. With older patients, radioactive iodine is clearly the ablative procedure of choice, as it is for patients who have had previous thyroid surgery or those in whom serious systematic disease contraindicates elective surgery.

In those patients selected for *long-term antithyroid therapy*, satisfactory control can almost always be achieved if a sufficient dosage of the drug is administered. Most patients can be managed successfully by propylthiouracil, 100 mg every 8 hr. Methimazole is at least as effective as propylthiouracil when administered in one-tenth the dosage. Once euthyroidism is achieved, the initial daily dosage may be reduced to the smallest doses that control the thyrotoxicosis fully. In many clinics, however, the initial dose is continued and is supplemented with 120 to 180 mg USP thyroid or its equivalent in synthetic thyroid preparations. By this latter regimen, hypothyroidism resulting from overdosage of antithyroid drugs can be prevented. This is especially important in pregnant patients. Furthermore, the undesirable consequences of hypothyroidism, such as enhancement of oculopathy and enlargement of the goiter, may thereby be forestalled. The precise duration of therapy is difficult to predict in the individual patient and may be a function of the spontaneous course of the disease itself. If this is the case, the longer the course of therapy, the more likely it is that the patient will remain well when the drug is discontinued. In general, however, an 18- to 24-month course is usually employed. A normal suppressive response to exogenous thyroid hormone when the antithyroid compound is discontinued indicates that the patient is likely to remain well for some time. Following a regimen of this type, approximately 50 percent of patients will remain well for a prolonged period or indefinitely.

The *treatment of hyperthyroidism during pregnancy* is a subject of disagreement. Most physicians agree that antithyroid therapy is preferable to subtotal thyroidectomy, and this is particularly true during the first and third trimesters. The major disadvantage of antithyroid therapy is the possibility of inducing goiter and hypothyroidism in the fetus, since antithyroid agents readily traverse the placenta. Maintenance of a metabolic state in the mother consistent with the pregnant state greatly decreases the likelihood that fetal hypothyroidism will ensue. Antithyroid therapy should therefore be adjusted to permit maintenance of a serum protein–bound iodine of between 7 and 11 μg per 100 ml throughout pregnancy with a resin-T3 level below 85 percent and a basal metabolic rate of +25 to +30 percent during the last half or trimester. This can be achieved by careful regulation of dosage, but some authorities regularly supplement the antithyroid regimen with replacement doses of thyroid hormone. The latter program is highly successful, provided that a false sense of assurance does not lead to administration of excessive doses of antithyroid agent or neglect of frequent observation of the patient.

Leukopenia is the principal undesirable side effect of antithyroid drugs. Mild transient leukopenia may occur in approximately 10 percent of patients treated and is not necessarily an indication for discontinuing therapy. When the absolute number of polymorphonuclear leukocytes reaches 1,500 or less, antithyroid medication should be discontinued. Allergic rashes and drug sensitivity develop in a small percentage of patients. These may disappear with antihistamine therapy at the same or reduced dosage of antithyroid agent, but it is probably preferable, when sensitivity reactions occur, to change to another drug. On rare occasions (in less than 0.2 percent), agranulocytosis may occur. This may be sudden in onset.

Iodides inhibit the release of thyroid hormones from the thyrotoxic gland, and their ameliorative effects occur more rapidly than those of antithyroid compounds. However, response to iodides is often incomplete and transient. Furthermore, by expanding the thyroidal stores of hormones, iodides may prolong greatly the latency of response to subsequently instituted antithyroid therapy. Therefore, in the medical therapy of hyperthyroidism, iodides are mainly useful as an adjunct to other therapeutic measures in those cases in which rapid control of thyrotoxicosis is mandatory. Only rarely will contraindication to other forms of therapy dictate the use of iodides alone.

Radioactive iodine (^{131}I) affords a relatively simple, effective and economical means of treating thyrotoxicosis. Its major advantage is that it can produce the ablative effects of surgery without the immediate operative and postoperative complications. The principal disadvantage of ^{131}I therapy, in the dosage which has usually been employed, is its tendency to produce hypothyroidism with a frequency that increases progressively with time. As many as 30 to 70 percent of patients may develop this complication by 10 years after treatment. Although hypothyroidism is readily treated, once diagnosed, the insidious onset of the disorder may obscure the diagnosis until serious complications of hypothyroidism have developed. Hence, some recommend that all patients be treated with large doses of ^{131}I to ensure relief of thyrotoxicosis and then be placed on permanent physiologic replacement doses of thyroid hormone.

To date, studies have provided no evidence of a significant carcinogenic or leukemogenic effect of radioiodine in those doses commonly used in treating hyperthyroidism. Nevertheless, many physicians prefer to reserve radioiodine therapy for patients over forty years of age, thinking that it is currently not justifiable to administer an agent of undetermined radiation potentialities to younger persons, particularly those of childbearing potential. Patients with recurrent thyrotoxicosis following surgery, those who refuse surgery, or those who have complicating illnesses contraindicating surgery are excellent candidates for radioiodine therapy. The usual therapeutic dose for diffusely enlarged thyroid glands ranges between 120 to 140 μc per estimated Gm thyroid tissue (approximately 4 to 8 mc total dose). Nodular goiters may require somewhat larger doses, usually 8 to 12 mc. Repeated doses are sometimes required, and these may be given at intervals of 3 to 6 months until euthyroidism is achieved.

The foregoing doses are those which have been used commonly and are intended to produce relief of thyrotoxicosis within a few months of treatment. Smaller doses (approximately half as much ^{131}I) may not induce delayed hypothyroidism as frequently, but are also less likely to relieve thyrotoxicosis within a relatively short period. Antithyroid agents can be employed, however, to maintain metabolic control while the effect of the ^{131}I is taking hold.

Radiation thyroiditis from radioiodine may contraindicate its use in patients with large substernal goiters likely to induce respiratory embarrassment upon swelling. Patients exhibiting severe hyperthyroidism, heart failure, or progressive ophthalmopathy may first be rendered euthyroid by the use of methimazole or prophylthiouracil; by discontinuing antithyroid treatment for 2 or 3 days, or longer, and then administering radioactive iodine, a good therapeutic response may be obtained and the potential complication of radiation thyroiditis avoided.

Before radioactive iodine was introduced, subtotal thyroidectomy was the classic form of ablative therapy and it is still widely employed in younger patients in whom antithyroid therapy is unsuccessful. Although precise preoperative programs differ, several general principles should be emphasized. Patients should first be rendered fully euthyroid by means of antithyroid agents. Only then should iodides (5 to 10 drops Lugol's solution three times a day for approximately 2 weeks) be administered concomitantly to effect an involutional response in the gland. Antithyroid drugs should not be discontinued merely because treatment with iodides is instituted.

Hazards of *subtotal thyroidectomy* include immediate operative complications such as anesthetic accidents, hemorrhage sometimes leading to respiratory obstruction, and hypoparathyroidism. As time progresses, wound infection, cord paralysis, and hypothyroidism may occur. In experienced hands, surgery is an effective and relatively safe mode of therapy. Postoperative recurrences are quite uncommon. However, carefully conducted follow-up studies reveal that hypothyroidism follows surgery more frequently than previously suspected, although not as commonly as following ^{131}I.

Thyrotoxic Crisis

The clinical picture of thyrotoxic crisis or storm is that of a fulminating increase in all the signs and symptoms of thyrotoxicosis. In the past, this disturbance was most often observed postoperatively in patients poorly prepared for surgery. However, with the preoperative use of antithyroid drugs and iodide and with appropriate measures directed to control of metabolic factors, weight, and nutritional status, postoperative thyrotoxic crisis should not occur. At present, so-called "medical storm" is more common and occurs in untreated or inadequately treated patients. It is precipitated by surgical emergency or complicating medical illness, usually sepsis. The syndrome is characterized by extreme irritability, delirium or coma, hyperpyrexia to 106°F or more, tachycardia, restlessness, hypotension, vomiting, and diarrhea. Rarely, the clinical picture may be more subtle, with apathy, severe prostration, and coma with only slight elevation of temperature. Such postoperative complications as sepsis, septicemia, hemorrhage, and transfusion or drug reactions may mimic thyrotoxic crisis. It is thought that in certain patients thyrotoxic crisis is associated with or precipitated by adrenocortical insufficiency. The possibility of this complication gains support from evidence indicating increased adrenocortical hormone requirements in thyrotoxicosis and from evidence indicating reduced adrenocortical reserves in this disorder.

TREATMENT. Treatment of thyroid crisis should include the intravenous administration of large quantities of hypertonic glucose, hydrocortisone, and iodide; the intramuscular administration of B-complex vitamins, particularly thiamine, and where indicated, reserpine, guanethidine, or propranalol. Large doses of antithyroid drugs should be continued or instituted. The patient should be placed in a cooled, humidified oxygen tent and the hyperpyrexia treated as indicated. Full digitalization should be employed only in the presence of cardiac failure. If shock exists, intravenous pressor agents may be employed with extreme caution since patients with hyperthyroidism are particularly sensitive to pressor amines.

Ophthalmopathy

The clinical signs associated with the ophthalmopathy of Graves' disease may be divided into two components: the spastic and the mechanical. The former includes the stare, lid lag, and lid retraction that accompany thyrotoxicosis and account for the "frightened" facies and classic eye signs previously described. These findings need not be associated with actual proptosis and usually return to normal after appropriate correction of thyrotoxicosis. The mechanical component includes proptosis of varying degrees with ophthalmoplegia and congestive oculopathy characterized by chemosis, conjunctivitis, marked periorbital swelling, and the resultant complications of corneal ulceration, optic neuritis, and optic atrophy. These changes are associated with and may result from an increase in retrobulbar volume and pressure produced by accumulation of fat, water, and inflammatory cells in the retroorbital connective tissue and ocular musculature. When exophthalmos progresses rapidly and becomes the major concern in Graves' disease, it is usually referred to as *progressive* and, if severe, *malignant* exophthalmos. The term *exophthalmic ophthalmoplegia* refers to the ocular muscle weakness that so commonly accompanies this disorder and results in strabismus with varying degrees of diplopia. Exophthalmos may be unilateral early in the course of the disorder but usually progresses to symmetric involvement. It must be differentiated from retrobulbar tumors of various types as well as from a rare granulomatous disorder, *pseudotumor oculi*. Exophthalmos can be familial, is more common in some ethnic groups, and is seen in other endocrine disorders such as Cushing's syndrome and acromegaly, as well as in uremia, malignant hypertension, severe aortic stenosis, and superior mediastinal obstruction. Where doubt as to the cause of exophthalmos exists, an abnormal thyroid suppression test affords strong presumptive evidence that the oculopathy takes its origin in Graves' disease.

It is probable that the ophthalmopathy of Graves' disease results from some factor or factors of the anterior pituitary gland or the hypothalamus, although the genesis of this disorder is not known definitely. The exophthalmos may stabilize or decrease after treatment of hyperthyroidism but usually follows a course independent of the metabolic response to therapy. Rapid progression of exophthalmos with marked chemosis and edema is generally a grave prognostic sign and should serve as a warning that progressive eye changes may be anticipated. In treating this type of exophthalmos it is important to bring the thyrotoxicosis under control gradually and to prevent the development of hypothyroidism. Subtotal thyroidectomy or radioactive iodine therapy early in the course of this disease may enhance the progression of exophthalmos. Although there appears to be little difference in the incidence of progressive eye changes following the various forms of therapy of hyperthyroidism, antithyroid drug therapy seems to be the least provocative of severe or malignant exophthalmos. The long-continued administration of thyroid to forestall hypothyroidism may favor the regression of exophthalmic changes.

In mild forms of the disorder, considerable benefit may be derived from simple measures, such as elevating the head of the bed at night, administration of mercurial or thiazide diuretics or spironolactone to reduce edema, and provision of tinted glasses for protection from wind and foreign bodies. A 1% solution of methylcellulose or plastic shields may help to prevent corneal drying in patients unable to appose the lids during sleep. In more severe cases, as evidenced by progressive exophthalmos, increasing chemosis, ophthalmoplegia, or loss of vision, large doses of prednisone (120 to 140 mg daily) may be administered. Following improvement, the dosage is reduced to the lowest effective level. Prolonged administration is usually not feasible because of undesirable glucocorticoid side effects. In cases that appear to progress despite these measures, orbital decompression, if performed sufficiently early, will at times halt progression of the disease and preserve vision.

Localized or Pretibial Myxedema

Localized myxedema, a circumscribed deposition of mucinous material in the deeper layers of the skin over the lower portion of the legs or dorsa of the feet, occurs in patients with past or present Graves' disease and is not a manifestation of hypothyroidism. The affected area of skin may be pruritic with increased pigmentation, hirsutism, and a *peau d'orange* appearance that is sharply delineated from the normal skin. The clinical course resembles that of exophthalmos, with which it is associated frequently. It may also be associated with clubbing of the fingers. About half the cases occur during the active stage of thyrotoxicosis, and in the remainder the lesions develop after treatment. The activity of the disorder is usually self-limited. No form of therapy is entirely satisfactory, although the local injection of hyaluronidase or hydrocortisone has been beneficial transiently in some cases.

Thyrotoxic Heart Disease

The cardiac manifestations of hyperthyroidism have been described. Many elderly patients may exhibit obvious cardiac disease but without the usual clinical appearance of hyperthyroidism. These thyrocardiac patients have been called *apathetic* or *masked*. Occasionally they represent difficult diagnostic problems, but if one maintains a constant awareness of thyrotoxicosis in patients with heart disease, the correct diagnosis is almost always suspected. In these patients hyperthyroidism is usually associated with a toxic multinodular goiter. Although the basal metabolic rate may not be grossly abnormal, the PBI (in the absence of antecedent mercurial therapy) or the serum T4 and the radioactive iodine uptake of the thyroid are usually diagnostic.

In patients with cardiac decompensation and thyrotoxicosis, the cardiac output is frequently above normal, with a rapid or normal circulation time in spite of an elevated venous pressure. This condition is one of several examples of so-called "high-output failure." Even though elevated, the cardiac output is unable to satisfy the high metabolic requirements of the body, and thus heart failure occurs. It is probably wise to obtain such thyroid studies as the PBI or serum T4 and the radioactive iodine uptake in all patients with atrial fibrillation or congestive heart failure of undetermined etiology, since the finding of thyrotoxicosis affords a remediable form of cardiac disease.

Evidence suggests that the production of hypothyroidism and, consequently, hypometabolism is beneficial in appropriately selected *euthyroid* patients with congestive heart failure from any cause or in those with angina pectoris or intractable supraventricular tachycardia. Hypothyroidism may be produced readily by the administration of radioactive iodine.

Thyrotoxic Myopathy

Weakness, impairment of muscular function, and wasting of varying severity often accompany thyrotoxicosis and may suggest the presence of a primary muscular disorder. In certain patients, severe myopathy may be the dominant feature of thyrotoxicosis. Creatinuria is present under these circumstances, as it is in nonthyrotoxic myopathies. Myasthenia gravis and periodic paralysis occur more commonly with, or may be exacerbated by, thyrotoxicosis. A moderately beneficial response to prostigmine and related drugs may occur in thyrotoxicosis and does not of itself indicate the presence of myasthenia gravis (see Chap. 377).

Thyrotoxic Bone Disease

Skeletal demineralization is a not uncommon manifestation of thyrotoxicosis and is associated with hypercalcuria and hyperphosphaturia even when loss of bone salts is not demonstrable radiologically. Serum calcium, phosphorus, and alkaline phosphatase levels are usually normal. In some patients, however, serum calcium and alkaline phosphatase may be elevated. The latter findings may be purely a manifestation of uncomplicated thyrotoxicosis rather than associated hyperparathyroidism, but at times the two diseases coexist. Clinically, significant degrees of skeletal demineralization are rarely seen except in elderly patients in whom thyrotoxicosis may accentuate the effects of preexisting osteoporosis (see Chap. 380).

THYROID NEOPLASMS

Adenomas

True adenomas, as contrasted with localized adenomatous areas, are encapsulated and usually compress contiguous thyroid tissue. Such adenomas are generally present in the thyroid gland but may also occur ectopically. They vary greatly in size and histologic characteristics. Adenomas are often classified into three major types: papillary, follicular, and Hürthle cell. The follicular adenomas can be subdivided according to the size of the follicle into colloid or macrofollicular, fetal or microfollicular, and embryonal varieties. There is considerable variation in physiologic differentiation as judged by their ability to concentrate radioiodine. Generally, the more highly differentiated adenomas (follicular) are most likely to mimic the function of normal thyroid tissue. Function-

ing adenomas are usually independent of TSH stimulation and may produce sufficient thyroid hormone to suppress completely the activity of the remainder of the thyroid gland. Ultimately, production of hormone by the adenoma may be sufficient to produce thyrotoxicosis (toxic adenoma). Such lesions can be distinguished by isotopic scanning procedures, which reveal localization of

Table 89-5. CLASSIFICATION OF THYROID TUMORS

I. Tumors of low malignancy
    A. Adenomas with blood vessel invasion
    B. "Histologic carcinoma" (small tumors found incidentally at operation; without symptoms, recurrence, or metastases)
    C. Papillary adenocarcinoma (occurs in young age group; lymphangioinvasive)
II. Tumors of moderate malignancy
    A. Nonpapillary, solid, or alveolar, adenocarcinoma (occurs in older age group; hemangioinvasive; histologically the metastases may appear benign—"benign metastasizing struma")
    B. Hürthle cell adenocarcinoma (occurs in middle age group; usually locally invasive, occasional skeletal or pulmonary metastases)
    C. Medullary carcinoma with amyloid stroma (usually occurs after the age of 50, usually metastasizes via both lymphatics and bloodstream, may be familial and associated with other endocrine and mesodermal disorders)
III. Tumors of high malignancy (rare)
    A. Small-cell carcinoma (simplex)
    B. Giant-cell carcinoma
    C. Epidermoid carcinoma
    D. Fibrosarcoma
    E. Lymphoma

radioiodine solely in the area of the adenoma ("hot nodule"). In such instances, function in the suppressed portion of the thyroid can be restored by exogenous TSH, and this can be demonstrated by isotopic scanning. Following excision of a "hot" nodule, endogenous TSH usually restores function in the previously suppressed tissue. This uncommon disorder should not be confused with Graves' disease. When the toxic adenoma is ablated by surgery or radioiodine, the remainder of the thyroid tissue almost always resumes entirely normal function. The incidence of adenomas varies considerably and is usually increased in areas of endemic goiter. The etiology of true encapsulated adenomas is unknown and doubtless differs from that of adenomatous goiter. As in other organs, the role of benign adenomas as forerunners of carcinoma is uncertain.

Ectopic thyroid tissue, both encapsulated and nonencapsulated, can occur along the thyroglossal tract from the base of the tongue to the diaphragm. Lingual goiters, thyroglossal duct cysts, pyramidal lobe adenomas, and both esophageal and tracheal rests have been described. Ectopic thyroid tissue in the ovary (struma ovarii) may produce thyroid hormone and has been alleged to cause thyrotoxicosis. Isotopic scanning techniques can be helpful in diagnosing ectopic thyroid tissue if it is sufficiently differentiated to concentrate radioiodine.

Carcinoma

Cancers of the thyroid gland are pathologically pleomorphic and seldom of a pure type. Definitive pathologic classification is difficult, and the degree of malignancy as determined histologically is not necessarily consistent with the clinical course of the disease. A modification of Warren's classification is given in Table 89-5.

From a clinical point of view, primary thyroid carcinomas are of four major types: (1) A small number are highly anaplastic and histologically undifferentiated. These are often quite malignant and for the most part not amenable to surgical or radiation therapy. (2) A similarly uncommon type is the follicular carcinoma, whose structure so closely mimics that of normal thyroid tissue that it has been termed *benign metastasizing thyroid carcinoma.* This variety has a predilection for metastases to bone and is often first discovered radiologically or when a metastatic lesion is biopsied. (3) Medullary or solid carcinoma with amyloid stroma is the most distinctive type of malignant thyroid neoplasm. It occurs after the age of fifty and metastasizes via both lymphatic and blood vessel invasion. The disease is sometimes familial and may be associated with pheochromocytoma, intestinal polyps, or fibromata. An unusual association with Cushing's syndrome and a syndrome similar to that produced by carcinoid tumors has been reported. Convincing evidence that amyloid tumors may secrete thyrocalcitonin, sometimes in huge quantities, has been presented and some patients develop severe hypocalcemia. (4) The largest number of thyroid cancers present with varying degrees of differentiation. The most common of these is papillary adenocarcinoma, which is generally of low virulence, metastasizes to regional lymph nodes, and is the most amenable to therapy.

DIAGNOSIS AND MANAGEMENT. The diagnosis and management of malignancies of the thyroid gland present several problems, each of which must be taken in proper perspective. In the past, statistical analyses of the incidence of thyroid cancer in surgical specimens led to a concept upon which was based the rationale for surgical removal of thyroid nodules in the prophylaxis or therapy of thyroid cancer. This concept proposes that goiters be removed surgically to prevent cancer and is predicated upon the finding of a high incidence of cancer in surgical specimens of goiters containing either a single nodule or multiple nodules. Recent reappraisal of this concept has shown that, although the incidence of thyroid cancer in surgical specimens appears to be increasing, the actual incidence of thyroid cancer in the general population is quite low, somewhere in the range of 2.5 cases per 100,000 population per year. This is in contrast to the high incidence of nodular goiter in the population. The death rate from thyroid cancer is quite low, probably less than 0.6 per 100,000 population per year. The low death rate from this disease has suggested that the high

incidence of carcinoma in surgical specimens results from effective selection of high-risk patients and that the pathologic criteria of thyroid malignancy may not truly reflect the natural history of this lesion.

Signs and symptoms most suggestive of more virulent varieties of thyroid cancer are rapid and progressive growth (not to be confused with overnight enlargement of a nodule, which is usually the result of hemorrhage or infarction), hoarseness caused by recurrent laryngeal nerve paralysis, presence of lymph node enlargement in the neck or supraclavicular area, or fixation of the thyroid gland to contiguous structures. Papillary and follicular adenocarcinoma of the thyroid are often clinically indolent. Thyroid nodules or lymph nodes harboring these varieties of thyroid cancer may not show clinical evidence of growth over periods of years. Follicular carcinoma of the thyroid is frequently diagnosed for the first time by the finding of skeletal or pulmonary metastases on routine x-ray. Hyperthyroidism or hypothyroidism is rarely associated with thyroid cancer. Needle biopsy of the thyroid is considered by some physicians to be contraindicated in the diagnosis of thyroid malignancy because of the tendency of these neoplasms to "seed" in the incised area.

The relative degree of functional differentiation can be determined by use of the scintigram obtained after administration of radioactive iodine. The degree of ^{131}I uptake in the nodule can thus be determined and compared to that present in the normal tissue. In this manner, thyroid nodules may be divided arbitrarily into "hot" or "cold," depending upon whether or not they take up more or less ^{131}I than the normal portions of the gland. Generally speaking, the "cold" nodules have a greater likelihood of being malignant. However, it must be remembered that many benign nodules and cysts are likewise "cold" and that this test should not be used as the sole determinant of malignancy or operability. There appears to be an etiologic relationship between radiation therapy directed to the head and neck regions of children and young adults and the later development of thyroid cancer.

Conservative treatment of most thyroid malignancies is a growing trend in the approach to this problem. Such conservatism stems from several factors. First, thyroid cancer of a high degree of malignancy usually progresses so rapidly that it is frequently beyond any form of treatment at the time diagnosis is established. Second, nodular goiter is common, while carcinoma of the thyroid is rare; hence, indiscriminate operation on all nodular goiters in the hope of uncovering the occasional malignancy may result in a greater morbidity and mortality than would be produced by the carcinoma if left untreated. However, as indicated above, a presumptive diagnosis of carcinoma in the thyroid can usually be made with a reasonable degree of accuracy on the basis of the criteria previously mentioned. Therefore, it should be possible to select a group of high-risk patients in whom surgery may be indicated. When such a high-risk patient is young, most authorities agree that surgery should be performed. There is less agreement as to the benefits of surgery when similar lesions are detected in older patients. When, at surgery, a carcinoma is found, excision with a generous portion of surrounding normal tissue is recommended. Removal of lymph nodes in which cancer is obviously present is justified. In addition, selected nodes from areas of drainage should be removed to provide information concerning the extent and localization of distant metastases. Radical neck dissections do not appear to be justified at this time.

Although ablation of thyroid carcinoma with large therapeutic doses of radioactive iodine is theoretically possible and has been used occasionally, instances are rare in which the primary or metastatic lesions concentrate sufficient radioiodine to make this possible. External radiation may be helpful especially when metastases are localized to a single accessible area.

The use of suppressive doses of exogenous thyroid hormone to inhibit tumor growth is being evaluated further. Because of the virtual absence of serious side effects from such medication (120 to 240 mg USP thyroid daily), all patients with thyroid cancer, regardless of whether or not surgery has been undertaken, should be treated with thyroid suppression.

THYROIDITIS

Thyroiditis is a comparatively rare disease. It may be specific (suppurative or nonsuppurative), nonspecific (acute or subacute), or chronic (Hashimoto's or Riedel's struma).

Specific Thyroiditis

This condition may be caused by almost any known pathogenic organism, pyogenic or nonpyogenic, and is relatively rare compared to the nonspecific varieties. It may occur after infection of the mouth, pharynx, upper respiratory tract, or cervical lymph nodes. Very rarely tuberculosis, actinomycosis, syphilis, or infection with pyogenic organisms may result in single or multiple abscesses. Classically, redness, swelling, and tenderness of the skin over the thyroid occur together with fever and other systemic signs of infection. Treatment consists, for the most part, of specific antibiotic or chemotherapeutic agents along with surgical drainage where indicated.

Nonspecific Thyroiditis

This variety of thyroiditis is of unknown etiology, is probably not an autoimmune disorder, and may be viral in origin. It is usually self-limited, with repetitive episodes of progressively less severity. It is seen predominantly in middle-aged women and rarely progresses to hypothyroidism. The most common form of acute or subacute thyroiditis is associated histologically with giant-cell formation (de Quervain's thyroiditis). The onset of symptoms may be dramatic and often seems to follow an upper respiratory tract infection. There is usually progressive swelling and tenderness in the thyroid gland, with radiation of pain to the ears or jaw, associated with systemic manifestations of fever, nervousness, myalgia, and headache. Laboratory investigation often shows an elevated sedimentation rate, a normal or low leukocyte count, and a slightly increased PBI and BMR. The thyroidal ^{131}I uptake is characteristically depressed but may at times be normal. Each lobe of the thyroid can be affected separately, but the entire gland is involved as the disease progresses. A needle biopsy is helpful if the diagnosis is not clear and may be necessary to differentiate thyroiditis from hemorrhage or from a suppurative process.

Therapy should be conservative, since complete spontaneous recovery is the general rule. Hypothyroidism only rarely results from this inflammatory process. Rest, fluids, and aspirin often suffice. When symptoms are severe, a short course of steroid therapy (50 mg cortisone or its equivalent every 6 hr) usually will relieve them, but they often return upon withdrawal of the steroid. X-ray therapy in doses of 300 to 400 r has been reported to be efficacious in this disorder.

Chronic Thyroiditis

Two varieties of chronic thyroiditis of undetermined etiology may be diagnosed histologically: *Hashimoto's struma* (struma lymphomatosa, lymphadenoid goiter) and *Riedel's struma*. Struma lymphomatosa, by far the more common of the two, occurs predominantly in middle-aged women. It is characterized by a firm, rubbery, lobular swelling of the thyroid, simulating multinodular goiter. The serum of patients with this disorder may contain increased amounts of gamma-globulin, and the thymol turbidity and cephalin flocculation tests may be abnormal.

In the early stages of this disorder, the patients are metabolically normal, and thyroid function studies are either normal or may reveal a slightly elevated ^{131}I uptake. Occasionally there are abnormal, noncalorigenic, iodinated proteins in the blood. As a result, the PBI may be inordinately high compared to the metabolic state of the patient and to the serum T4 concentration. Such dissociation between the PBI and the serum T4, although occasionally seen in other nontoxic goiters, most commonly occurs in Hashimoto's disease. Ultimately, hypothyroidism results from replacement of the functional thyroid structures by lymphoid or fibrous tissue. At this time, the serum protein–bound iodine and the 24-hr radioactive iodine uptake are usually low, and there is often no response in these indices to TSH administration.

Of particular interest in this disorder is the detection of circulating autoantibodies to thyroglobulin as well as to cellular antigens. A variety of antibodies has been described, certain of which may be measured by gel diffusion or fluorescent antibody techniques or by the tanned erythrocyte hemagglutination assay. It has been postulated that Hashimoto's struma is an example of an autoimmune disease in which the damaging effects of the antigen-antibody combination in the thyroid gland lead to destruction of functional thyroid tissue. Proof of this is lacking, however. Detection of circulating antibodies to thyroglobulin is not specifically diagnostic of Hashimoto's struma, however, since they may be found in other thyroidal disorders.

Diagnosis of Hashimoto's struma is suspected on clinical grounds when nodular goiter is present with hypothyroidism. Definitive diagnosis depends upon histologic confirmation, which may be obtained by needle biopsy, and by the presence of high titers of thyroglobulin antibody. Treatment consists of replacement doses of 120 to 180 mg USP thyroid daily to correct or avoid hypothyroidism and, in some patients, to reduce the size of the goiter. When Hashimoto's disease is first diagnosed following subtotal thyroidectomy, it is particularly important to institute thyroid substitution therapy to avoid the unusually common postoperative consequences of hypothyroidism.

Riedel's struma produces a firm, ligneous swelling of the thyroid, which may involve surrounding neck structures. This disorder is exceptionally rare and must be differentiated from thyroid neoplasia.

REFERENCES

Forester, C. F.: Coma in Myxedema: Report of a Case and Review of the World Literature, A.M.A. Arch. Intern. Med., 111:734, 1963.

Hazard, J. B.: Thyroiditis: A Review, Am. J. Clin. Pathol., 25:289, 399, 1955.

Ingbar, S. H., and N. Freinkel: Hypothyroidism, Disease-a-Month, September, 1958.

——: Physiological Considerations in Treatment of Diffuse Toxic Goiter, A.M.A. Arch. Intern. Med., 107:932, 1961.

—— and K. A. Woeber: The Thyroid Gland, chap. 4 in "Textbook of Endocrinology," R. H. Williams (Ed.), Philadelphia, W. B. Saunders Company, 1968.

Lindsay, S.: "Carcinoma of the Thyroid Gland," Springfield, Ill., Charles C Thomas, Publisher, 1960.

McGill, D. A., and S. P. Asper, Jr.: Endocrine Exophthalmos. A Review and a Report on Autoantibody Studies, New Engl. J. Med., 267:133, 188, 1962.

Means, J. H., L. J. DeGroot, and J. B. Stanbury (Eds.): "The Thyroid and Its Diseases," 3d ed., New York, McGraw-Hill Book Company, 1963.

Pitt-Rivers, R. (Ed.): "Advances in Thyroid Research," London, Pergamon Press, 1961.

—— and W. R. Trotter (Eds.): "The Thyroid Gland," vols. 1 and 2, London, Butterworth & Co., Publishers, Ltd., 1964.

Selenkow, H. A., and C. S. Hollander: Physiologic, Pharmacologic and Therapeutic Considerations in Surgery for Hyperthyroidism, Anesthesiology, 24:425, 1963.

Veith, F. J., J. R. Brooks, W. P. Grigsby, and H. A. Selenkow: The Nodular Thyroid Gland and Cancer: A Practical Approach to the Problem, New Engl. J. Med., 270:431, 1964.

Werner, S. C. (Ed.): "The Thyroid," New York, Harper & Row Publishers, Inc., 1962.

90 DISEASES OF THE PARATHYROID GLANDS

Daniel S. Bernstein and George W. Thorn

The parathyroid glands were first recognized as separate structures and described by Sandstrom in 1880. Shortly thereafter Gley (1881) and others performed extirpation experiments demonstrating that tetany ceased with the intravenous injection of calcium. Further proof of the endocrine nature of these glands followed from the preparation of parathyroid extracts by Collip in Canada, and by Hanson and Berman in the United States, and from the demonstration that these extracts could induce elevation of plasma calcium level.

ANATOMY

The parathyroid glands originate from the posterior halves of the third and fourth pairs of pharyngeal pouches. Therefore, like the thyroid, the parathyroids are entodermal in origin. In man the parathyroids are reddish- or yellowish-brown and are flattened, ovate, or pyriform bodies located on the posterior surfaces of the lateral lobes of the thyroid. There are normally 4 glands. The number may vary from 2 to 10, and their location is extremely variable. They have been found within the thyroid gland, in the mediastinum, and in scattered regions of the neck. The average size of a human parathyroid gland is $5 \times 3 \times 3$ mm, and the combined weight of 4 glands averages about 120 mg.

In the adult, the parathyroid gland contains chief cells and oxyphil cells. The chief cells are more numerous and are the source of the parathyroid hormone. These cells are 6 to 8 μ in diameter and contain glycogen. The oxyphil cells appear in the human gland at about the tenth year of life. They contain no glycogen, and their nuclei are somewhat pyknotic. They may represent a more mature or inactive chief cell. Another cell, the large water-clear cell (*wasserhelle* cell) derived from the chief cell, is the commonest cell type observed in hypertrophy and hyperplasia of the parathyroids.

EFFECTS OF PARATHYROID HORMONE

The function of parathyroid hormone is to maintain a normal level of plasma calcium. In the normal human being, the hormone performs this action so well that the plasma calcium varies only slightly from time to time even though the entry and egress of calcium to and from the body may vary widely. This regulation is mediated by an effect on the skeleton, the largest reservoir of calcium in the body. The significance of the phosphaturic effect of parathyroid hormone is unknown, although it may be a factor in stabilizing the plasma calcium.

Bone

Parathyroid hormone causes dissolution of the relatively stable fraction of bone mineral as well as the bone matrix, releasing calcium, phosphate, magnesium, and hydroxyproline to the extracellular fluid. The precise mechanism is unknown, but it has been shown that the major portion of bone mineral and matrix resorption is normally a function of the osteocyte (and, to a smaller extent, of the osteoclast), which under abnormal situations such as hyperparathyroidism, becomes the predominant cell causing bone resorption. Thus, the mobilization of bone mineral is a product of bone cellular metabolism, perhaps because of changes in bone mineral solubility produced by metabolic organic end products or by release of lysosomal enzymes stored intracellularly and released at appropriate times secondary to hormonal influences or other substances which labilize lysosomal membranes.

There is little doubt now that the action of parathyroid hormone on bone is a direct one. Bone tissue culture implants can be seen actively to resorb bone after minute amounts of parathyroid hormone are added. Parathyroid glands transplanted directly to bone cause local resorption around the area of transplantation. Histologically, the end product of parathyroid hormonal activity is a cystic space in the bone filled with fibrous tissue, i.e., osteitis fibrosa cystica. Any theory explaining the action of parathyroid hormone on bone must account for this pathologic picture.

Urinary Inorganic Phosphate

Since the advent of a more purified parathyroid preparation, arguments over the major site of the phosphaturic action of the hormone have been, for the most part, resolved. It is apparent that the hormone inhibits the well-documented process of renal tubular reabsorption of phosphate. There is, however, a small group who maintain that the hormone causes an increase in tubular secretion of phosphate, although the evidence for this process of tubular secretion of phosphate is scanty. The site in the kidney for tubular phosphate absorption is the proximal tubule, and the hormone exerts its effect on this function with little, if any, action on glomerular filtration rate.

Urinary Calcium

Renal handling of calcium is a complex process complicated by an interrelationship with sodium excretion. Calcium is probably actively resorbed from the distal tubule, although there may be some passive diffusion of calcium in the proximal tubule. In human beings with hypocalcemia, it appears that the TR Ca^{++} (TR = tubular reabsorption, Ca = calcium) is decreased. When parathyroid hormone is given, the TR Ca^{++} increases somewhat, although the evidence for this has not been sufficiently documented as yet. It would fit the scheme that parathyroid hormone tends to maintain the plasma Ca^{++} level within narrow limits. Excessive calcium loads presented to the kidney cause increased excretion of sodium, and vice versa, although mechanisms are not well understood. One may conclude that the majority of

investigators now feel that parathyroid hormone effects an increase in the renal tubular reabsorption of calcium, although additional evidence is needed to substantiate this hypothesis.

Gastrointestinal Absorption and Secretion

The effect of parathyroid hormone on the intestinal transport of calcium is probably to increase the amount of calcium absorbed against the mucosal-serosal gradient. The experimental evidence for this effect is disputed, and, even if substantiated, probably is of such small magnitude as to be relatively insignificant in affecting the overall calcium balance.

Lactation

It has been postulated that parathyroid hormone controls the amount of calcium in breast milk in animals, although there are no data regarding this point in human beings. Experimentally, parathyroidectomy in a lactating animal increases the calcium content of breast milk, and parenterally administered parathyroid extract given to such animals will restore the calcium content by reducing the amount of calcium secreted by the tubular epithelium of the breast. Therefore, parathyroid hormone may act to conserve blood calcium not only by its action on bone, kidney, and gut, but also on another portal of egress of calcium, the breast.

Lens

It has long been recognized that the incidence of cataracts is high in untreated hypoparathyroidism. Some experimental evidence suggests that the lens calcium is increased in hypoparathyroidism at a time when extracellular fluid calcium is reduced. Incubation of the lens in vitro with parathyroid hormone can reduce the lens calcium.

In summary, parathyroid hormone has an effect on any organ system involved in the handling of calcium. This action, at any specific site, is designed to maintain a constant level of plasma calcium. The exact manner by which the parathyroid hormone exerts its effects on single organ systems remains an enigma, however, and a fertile field of future research.

CHEMISTRY OF PARATHYROID HORMONE

In recent years major progress has been made in purifying parathyroid hormone. The purest preparation has been made by phenol extraction of bovine parathyroid glands and subsequent purification by gel filtration. Various estimates of the molecular weight range from 8,400 to 9,400. All the common amino acids, with the exception of cystine, 17 in number, are represented. Methionine accounts for the sulfur content of the polypeptide. The absence of cystine and the isolation of a single N-terminal amino acid, alanine, support the conclusion that the hormone is a single-chain polypeptide. Parathyroid extracts can be reversibly inactivated by oxidation (as by hydrogen peroxide) and the biologic activity restored or increased above preinactivation values by reducing agents (mercaptoethanol; cysteine). Other agents, such as heparin, oil, and gelatin, appear to stabilize the activity of the hormone. The active, purified hormone contains both calcium-mobilizing and renal-tubular-phosphate–blocking properties. Parathyroid extract is available commercially. Parathyroid extract, USP, is standardized by biologic assay so that 1 ml contains 100 to 120 USP units. The USP unit is defined as $1/100$ of the amount required to raise the plasma calcium level of a normal male dog weighing 10 to 12 kg by 1.0 mg per 100 ml within 16 to 18 hr after a single subcutaneous injection.

REGULATION OF PARATHYROID ACTIVITY

The parathyroid glands do not appear to be under direct control of a tropic hormone elaborated by the anterior pituitary, nor is there evidence of nervous control of their secretory activity. However, a number of observations point to an indirect relationship to other endocrine organs. Parathyroid hyperplasia has been reported in cases of acromegaly, Cushing's syndrome, Addison's disease, and pancreatic islet cell adenomas. Experimentally, hypophysectomy in animals causes some involution of the parathyroids, whereas growth hormone, adrenocorticotropin, crude anterior pituitary extracts, and adrenal steroids cause hyperplasia. It is possible that these changes are secondary to the alteration in serum mineral levels mediated by the pituitary, thyroid, adrenal, gonadal, and islet cell hormones. A number of cases of multiple tumors involving the anterior pituitary, pancreatic islet tissue, and the parathyroids have been reported. Since tumors of these glands are quite rare, their association can scarcely be explained as a matter of chance. Also the familial occurrence of multiple tumors of this type has been noted. Although unexplained, the association of these tumors is of clinical importance.

The parathyroid glands alter their production of hormone in response to change in the **plasma level of ionized calcium.** It is generally agreed that hormone production is stimulated by hypocalcemia and decreased by hypercalcemia. Hyperplasia of the parathyroids is found in those conditions in which there is a tendency toward a low plasma calcium level, namely, rickets (or osteomalacia), calcium deprivation, and renal insufficiency with acidosis. There is conflicting evidence concerning an increase in parathyroid hormone production in patients with hyperphosphatemia in the absence of hypocalcemia.

With the application of newer methods of radioimmunoassay techniques, it has been shown that there is probably not a normal circadian rhythm to parathyroid synthesis or release. As measured by radioimmunoassay, parathyroid hormone levels in man respond proportionally to changes in plasma calcium concentration as produced by EDTA (ethylenediaminetetraacetic acid). Extraordinarily high plasma levels of parathyroid hormone occur in hypocalcemia associated with chronic renal disease. Concentrations of parathyroid hormone in cases of parathyroid adenoma show considerable variation, with an appreciable proportion of such patients showing a normal plasma parathyroid hormone concentration. However, such a finding in the presence of hypercalcemia, which ordinarily would decrease plasma immunoreactive parathyroid hormone levels, suggests an autonomously functioning nonsuppressible gland. In patients with azotemic renal disease and hypocalcemia the values are uniformly higher than in primary hyperparathyroidism. These findings only point out the difficulty in deciding whether a patient with severe renal impairment and a high normal plasma calcium level in the presence of elevated serum phosphate has a primary parathyroid adenoma and secondary renal disease or primary renal disease and secondary or autonomous parathyroid hyperplasia ("tertiary hyperparathyroidism"). Since the consequences of "tertiary hyperparathyroidism" are extensive osteitis fibrosa cystica and metastatic soft-tissue calcification, subtotal (seven-eighths) parathyroidectomy may be justified, especially if future renal homotransplantation is contemplated. Although measurements of plasma parathyroid hormone have added a new tool aiding in the diagnosis of hyperparathyroidism, it may be seen from the above discussion that changes in the plasma calcium, phosphate, and alkaline phosphatase levels are still reliable and important indicators of parathyroid function.

HYPOPARATHYROIDISM
History

One of the causes of tetany is total or extensive parathyroidectomy. Tetany received its name from Corvisart in 1852. MacCallum and Voegtlin in 1908 showed that the mechanism of this type of tetany was dependent upon hypocalcemia. The Swiss surgeons Reverdin and Kocher in 1882 described postoperative tetany after a complete thyroidectomy for goiter without realizing that the condition was due to parathyroid deficiency.

Etiology and Pathology

Primary parathyroid deficiency is extremely rare, usually occurring in patients under the age of sixteen, but often persisting throughout adult life. In most instances, clinical evidence of parathyroid deficiency is secondary to thyroidectomy. During the past decade increased knowledge and experience in surgical techniques have decreased the incidence of permanent parathyroid deficiency secondary to thyroidectomy. Transient deficiency is not unusual and is attributed to trauma, edema, hemorrhage, and temporary interference with the blood supply to the remaining parathyroid glands. There have been no documented cases of hypoparathyroidism secondary to the administration of radioactive iodine in the treatment of thyrotoxicosis.

Pathologic Physiology

There is a pronounced disturbance of calcium and phosphate metabolism as reflected by plasma calcium levels as low as 2.5 mEq per liter (5 mg per 100 ml) and plasma inorganic phosphate levels as high as 3 to 4 mM per liter (9.3 to 12.4 mg per 100 ml). The decrease in calcium facilitates the transmission of impulses across the myoneural junction, which is responsible for much of the clinical picture.

Clinical Picture

The most striking symptom is an increased neuromuscular excitability resulting from a decrease in the plasma ionized calcium. The presenting complaint in most (70 percent) of these patients is tetany or tetanic equivalents. Tetany is manifested by carpopedal spasm in which the stiff, hollowed hand with rigid fingers is flexed at the metacarpal-phalangeal, wrist, and elbow joints and the legs and feet are extended. The tetanic equivalents include tonic and clonic convulsions, laryngeal stridor (spasm) which may be fatal, paresthesias, numbness, muscle cramps, dysphagia, dysarthria, muscular palsies, and cardiac irregularities. Spasm may involve the smooth muscle of the eye, gastrointestinal tract, bladder, and blood vessels. About 40 percent of these patients are seen because of epileptic seizures. The electroencephalographic findings in these patients suggest that occasionally underlying factors unrelated to plasma calcium levels play an important part in lowering the threshold for convulsive seizures. Mental changes are frequent and include anxiety, depression, increased irritability, and psychoses. Acute symptoms may be precipitated by infection, undue fatigue, menstruation, and emotional upsets and by an increase in the phosphate content of the diet. In some cases, the symptoms may be quite mild, varied, and even vague. Patients have manifested fatigue, muscular weakness, palpitations, numbness and tingling of the extremities, and other signs of latent tetany for as long as 30 years before a diagnosis of chronic hypoparathyroidism was established.

On examination, increased neuromuscular excitability may be demonstrated by contraction of the facial muscles in response to a light tap over the facial nerve in front of the ear (Chvostek's sign). This test is almost always positive in untreated hypoparathyroidism; however, it does occur occasionally in normal individuals. Dorsal flexion and abduction of the foot may be elicited by tapping the lateral surface of the fibula just below its head (peroneal sign). If the circulation to the arm is occluded by inflation of a blood pressure cuff above the level of systolic pressure, the hand may assume the typical position seen in carpopedal spasm within 3 min (Trousseau's sign). This sign is sometimes negative in marked hypoparathyroidism. Extensive tropic changes of the ectoderm may be seen. The hair is likely to be sparse, prematurely gray, and is occasionally absent in the axillary and pubic regions. Generalized or patchy erythema may be found. The skin is rough, dry, and scaling, and

there may be papules, vesicles, or bullae. A number of skin diseases have been described in association with hypoparathyroidism, including moniliasis of the skin, nails, tongue, and mouth. However, no etiologic relationship has been established. The nails are deformed and brittle, showing transverse ridging. In children one finds evidence of faulty dentition, including pitting and ridging of the enamel. Cataracts are frequently present, their extent being related to the duration and severity of the hypocalcemia. Early lens changes, not apparent on ophthalmoscopic examination, can usually be found with the aid of a slit lamp. Papilledema has been observed. The electrocardiogram usually shows a prolongation of the Q-T interval. The density of the bone may appear normal or increased. Abnormalities of dentition, such as deformed or absent roots, may be helpful in determining the age of onset of the disease. The pronounced disturbance of calcium and phosphate metabolism is reflected by lowered plasma calcium and elevated plasma inorganic phosphate levels. The alkaline phosphatase is normal or low. Hypocalcuria may be present, as shown by a negative Sulkowitch test (see p. 470). The spinal fluid may be under increased pressure without other abnormalities. When this occurs in the presence of papilledema, the diagnosis of a brain tumor may be made incorrectly. In primary hypoparathyroidism, bilateral symmetric calcification of the basal ganglions is commonly seen on the skull film. Other areas, such as the cerebellum and choroid plexus, are occasionally calcified.

Differential Diagnosis

The principal causes of tetany are hypocalcemia and alkalosis. Of the nonparathyroid causes of hypocalcemia, rickets, osteomalacia, steatorrhea, and renal insufficiency are the most common. Recently, there has been described a new syndrome of "decreased tissue calcium with tetany." This condition is manifested by severe tetany with normal plasma levels of calcium, magnesium, potassium, and carbon dioxide content. It has been demonstrated by radioactive calcium studies that the tissue calcium pool is lower than normal and that treatment with vitamin D will tend to bring the level of calcium in this pool toward normal. Extreme caution must be employed since the difference between the therapeutic and toxic dose of vitamin D is narrow.

In rickets, osteomalacia, and steatorrhea, a low value for plasma calcium is almost invariably associated with a normal or low value for plasma phosphate. In late-stage renal insufficiency with hypocalcemic tetany, the elevation in plasma phosphate level is disproportionately higher than that which occurs with a given level of hypocalcemia in parathyroid tetany. Nitrogen retention, as evidenced by an elevated blood urea nitrogen or nonprotein nitrogen, is early always present and differentiates the two conditions. A lowered plasma magnesium can also produce tetany. Magnesium salts have been used to eliminate hypocalcemic tetany. Furthermore, the level of plasma potassium plays an important part in the clinical manifestation of hypocalcemic tetany. The relationship of these three ions in the serum as regards tetany can be formulated as follows: calcium $\times$ magnesium/potassium. This is especially important in the treatment of renal failure, in which all three of these ions are drastically altered.

In addition to general renal insufficiency, two specific tubular lesions are to be considered. The first is a failure of reabsorption of certain amino acids (Fanconi syndrome, Chap. 103) in which there is increased excretion of phosphate and low-phosphate rickets, and the second is a rare selective failure of calcium reabsorption accompanied by metabolic acidosis and often by renal calcinosis.

Alkalosis causes tetany with no demonstrable change in the concentration of calcium in the plasma. It may be due to hyperventilation, to prolonged vomiting of acid gastric contents, or to excessive alkali ingestion. With hyperventilation, the carbon dioxide *content* of the plasma is reduced; whereas with vomiting, and alkali ingestion, the carbon dioxide–combining power of the plasma may be increased greatly (see Chap. 297) Alkalotic tetany occurs most frequently in association with acute infection, particularly in children.

Treatment

The object of treatment is to increase and maintain the plasma calcium at an approximately normal level.

MANAGEMENT OF ACUTE HYPOPARATHYROIDISM. Immediate correction of hypocalcemia may be accomplished by intravenous injections of calcium gluconate (10 ml of a 10 percent solution) or calcium chloride (10 ml of a 5 percent solution or an intravenous drip of 500 ml of 0.2 percent solution over a 1-hr period) (see Table 90-1). The effect is transitory, lasting only a few hours, and additional calcium may have to be administered. Caution should be exercised with patients on digitalis, since rapid infusion of calcium may cause cardiac arrest. Parathyroid extract injection may be instituted along with the infusion of calcium and will give more prolonged action (12 to 24 hr). Parathyroid extract is available in injectable form containing 80 to 120 USP units per milliliter. From 100 to 200 units should be administered intravenously. Administration should proceed slowly initially since anaphylactoid reaction may occur and necessitate discontinuance. From 25 to 50 units of parathyroid extract may be given every 6 to 12 hr during the acute phase of hypoparathyroidism.

Dihydrotachysterol should be administered in doses of 1 to 3 ml (1.25 to 3.75 mg) one to three times daily by mouth until calcium appears in the urine, as indicated by the Sulkowitch test. The dose is then adjusted to maintain a normal serum calcium level. Treatment may be continued with this preparation or with a cheaper but just as adequate preparation of calciferol (vitamin D_2). Supplementary calcium preparations should be given orally as soon as possible. Calcium chloride is most effective, since it forms an acid solution which favors calcium absorption and also contains a higher percentage of available calcium. It may be administered in doses of 10 ml of a 30 percent solution, well diluted, three times a day after meals (see Table 90-1). A licorice syrup medium will conceal the taste of calcium chloride solution.

MANAGEMENT OF CHRONIC HYPOPARATHYROIDISM. The objective of therapy in chronic hypoparathyroidism is to reduce the plasma phosphate and raise the plasma calcium levels. This is best accomplished by a combination of dietary and drug therapy. The diet should include as much calcium as can be tolerated, but there is nothing to be gained by reducing the amounts of phosphate in the diet unless it is eaten in excess. From 4 to 8 Gm of the various calcium salts shown in Table 90-1 should be given.

Parathyroid hormone is rarely used except in critical situations since it must be given daily and may be associated with local reactions. There is no evidence that antibodies will develop to chronically administered parathyroid hormone. It is almost always advantageous to administer vitamin D_2 (calciferol) in ranges of 50,000 to 150,000 units daily, in order to enhance plasma calcium levels. Dihydrotachysterol, a synthetic derivative of ergosterol, may also be used, but while its action is sim-

Table 90-1. CALCIUM-REGULATING COMPOUNDS

Type	Route of administration	Dosage	Effect on plasma calcium
Calcium gluconate (USP).....	Intravenous Intramuscular Oral	5 to 20 ml of 10% aqueous solution (IV) 10 ml of 5% solution (1 to 2 times daily IM) 10 to 25 Gm daily	Immediate but of only short duration
Calcium chloride (USP).......	Intravenous Oral	55 ml of 0.2% over 1 hr (IV) or 10 ml of 5% aqueous solution slowly (IV) 10 ml of 30% aqueous (2 to 3 times daily)	Immediate but of only short duration
Calcium lactate.............	Oral	10 to 15 Gm daily (as a clear solution)	Immediate but of only short duration
Dihydrotachysterol (AT 10)...	Oral	3 to 4 ml (1.25 mg per ml) daily initially; 1 ml (3 to 5 times weekly) as maintenance	Delayed, with a maximum in 48–96 hr. Prolonged effect
Calciferol (vitamin D_2).......	Oral	50,000 to 200,000 units daily (1.25 to 5 mg)	Delayed. Prolonged effect
Parathyroid................	Subcutaneous or intramuscular	100 to 200 units in severe tetany and then 25 to 50 units every 6 to 12 hr. Not recommended maintenance	Moderately rapid, with maximum in 8 to 18 hr

ilar to that of vitamin D_2 in all respects, it is much more expensive and rarely must be resorted to in favor of vitamin D_2. When vitamin D_2 or AT 10 (dihydrotachysterol) is used in therapy, the plasma calcium should be determined at frequent intervals, because persistent hypercalcemia and hypercalcuria may lead to deleterious effects. Since vitamin D_2 or AT 10 will cause an increase in the urine calcium before affecting a rise in blood calcium levels, it is important to check the urine level of calcium often as well as the plasma calcium, either by total 24-hr calcium excretion or by the Sulkowitch test. The Sulkowitch solution has the following composition:

Oxalic acid	2.5 Gm
Ammonium oxalate	2.5 Gm
Glacial acetic acid	5.0 ml
Distilled water q.s. ad	150.0 ml

The test is performed by adding 5 ml of the reagent to 5 ml urine in a test tube and noting the speed of appearance and the density of the precipitate. The result is graded 0, 1, 2, 3, or 4+. Routine use of the test for a short time enables one to become familiar with a normal response. The calcium intake (e.g., quantity of milk) as well as marked concentration or dilution of the urine should be taken into account. A negative test after a week on a diet free of milk and cheese suggests hypocalcemia —less than 3.5 mEq per liter (7.0 mg per 100 ml)—and a 3 to 4+ test suggests hypercalcemia—more than 5.2 mEq per liter (10.4 mg per 100 ml). Although this test can be run by the patient, it is important to check plasma levels from time to time. A 2+ Sulkowitch reaction is the most desirable.

An adjunctive mode of therapy is the use of probenecid (Benemid) by mouth in doses ranging from 0.5 to 1.5 Gm (daily). This agent is most useful in treating the tetany seen directly after inadvertent surgical removal of the parathyroids but is of little help in the chronic treatment of hypoparathyroidism. Rarely can Benemid be used alone. It acts on the kidney, blocking the reabsorption of phosphate by the renal tubule in a similar manner to the way it blocks the tubular reabsorption of uric acid. If epilepsy is evident, Dilantin or other antiepileptic drugs should be employed.

PSEUDOHYPOPARATHYROIDISM

The first description of this rare condition was given by Albright and his coworkers in 1942. This disease presents the same clinical and chemical features as hypoparathyroidism, except that these patients have round faces and short, thick figures. Subcutaneous centers of ossification are seen. There is a characteristic shortening of some of the metacarpal and metatarsal bones as a result of early epiphyseal closure, so that a dimple rather than a knuckle shows upon clenching of the fist. Most of the patients show some degree of mental deficiency. Not all these characteristics are necessarily present; any one

or a combination of them may be found. The apparent parathyroid deficiency in these patients appears to be due to a lack of end organ response. This is supported by the failure to respond to parathyroid extract, the finding of normal or hyperplastic glands where biopsy specimens have been obtained, and the failure to demonstrate antibodies to parathyroid hormone in the serum of patients in whom studies were done. The failure of these patients to respond to parathyroid extract need not be complete, and there are patients who have almost normal response to injected hormone. The finding of a 100-fold increase in thyrocalcitonin in the thyroid of one such pseudohypoparathyroid patient may provide an important clue in the pathogenesis of this disease.

It was suggested that the abnormalities seen in pseudopseudohypoparathyroidism and which are also found in pseudohypoparathyroidism are probably due to separate genetic factors, which may penetrate independently. Subsequent reports support this concept. Albright and his group have reported a case of a young woman with a rounded face, thickset figure, characteristic smile, shortened fingers and toes, and subcutaneous calcium deposits. However, the plasma calcium and phosphate levels were normal, and the Chvostek and Trousseau signs were absent.

Diagnosis

Because of the frequent history of convulsions, the condition may be incorrectly labeled epilepsy. The symptoms, chemical findings, and physical signs are those of hypoparathyroidism. The relative resistance to parathyroid extract as measured by failure to produce a phosphate diuresis (Ellsworth-Howard test) serves to distinguish it from hypoparathyroidism.

THE ELLSWORTH–HOWARD TEST. The test is performed as follows: The patient, in the fasting state, is given 2 ml (200 units) of parathyroid extract intravenously, and the urinary phosphate content is determined hourly for 3 hr prior to, and for 3 to 5 hr following, the injection. Occasional anaphylactoid reactions to the extract make slow and careful administration necessary. Parathyroid extracts are assayed by their effect on the plasma calcium level, and recent preparations have not been so effective in producing an increased phosphate excretion as those previously available. It is best to compare the response of the patient to that of a normal control given the same amount of hormone. The degree of phosphate diuresis induced by parathyroid hormone is dependent upon both the level of endogenous parathyroid secretion and the responsiveness of the phosphorus-reabsorbing mechanism of the renal tubules. Following the injection of a standard amount of parathyroid extract, there is a five- to sixfold increase in urine phosphate in normal persons, a tenfold or greater increase in patients with hypoparathyroidism, and at the most a twofold increase in patients with pseudohypoparathyroidism (parathyroid hormone resistance). Patients with hyperparathyroidism show a variable response to the extract.

Treatment

The therapy is the same as that outlined under chronic hypoparathyroidism.

PRIMARY HYPERPARATHYROIDISM

History

Generalized osteitis fibrosa cystica, a generalized disease of bones, was described in 1891 by von Recklinghausen. Askanazy associated this condition with a parathyroid tumor in 1904, and in 1925 Mandl removed a parathyroid adenoma from a patient suffering from this disease and noted a remarkable improvement. The occurrence of hyperparathyroidism without bone disease was pointed out by Albright in 1934. The clinical and metabolic studies subsequently carried out by Albright, Bauer, Aub, and Cope are classic.

Incidence

The exact incidence of the disease is unknown, but thanks to the work of Albright and his colleagues there has been a deliberate search for the disease, with a consequent increase in the frequency of diagnosis. The disease occurs most often in middle life, and about 70 percent of the patients reported are women. It has been shown that hyperparathyroidism can exist without evident disease of bone and that skeletal involvement represents a relatively late development. Involvement of the urinary tract is much more common than bone disease in the United States, presumably because of the high calcium intake, and in several series of cases more than 5 percent of all kidney stones have been associated with hyperfunction of these glands. Many cases of hyperparathyroidism in the United States are "masked" by insignificant or atypical alterations in plasma calcium and phosphate levels resulting from a high phosphate intake.

Etiology

Hypersecretion of the parathyroid glands may be caused by adenoma, hyperplasia, or carcinoma. The most common cause of primary hyperparathyroidism is an adenoma (90 percent of cases), hyperplasia is rather infrequent, and carcinoma is rare.

Pathology

Adenomas are usually limited to one gland. Norris collected from the literature 322 cases of parathyroid adenoma, with only 20 cases (6.2 percent) having multiple tumors. The pathologic overactivity of these tumors is not closely associated with their size. The adenomas are encapsulated, soft, orange-brown masses embedded in fat. They are occasionally lobular. The appearance, grossly, differs from that of the hyperplastic gland, which is irregular in shape and a darker, mahogany brown in color. The adenoma usually involves the entire gland but may involve only part of it. Adenomas are found in all the locations of the normal parathyroid glands. In one large series, 75 percent were found in the mediastinum. All cell types may be present, forming cords, glands, and solid masses. Cyst formation is common.

In primary diffuse hypertrophy and hyperplasia all the glands are involved but not necessarily to the same extent. The glands show a uniformity of structure, with a predominance of very large *wasserhelle* cells and a tendency to gland formation. There is a good correlation of size to the degree of overactivity.

Carcinoma of the parathyroid gland is extremely rare, accounting for 1 percent of functioning parathyroid tumors. They are generally larger than adenomas and in most cases have been clinically palpable. All these tumors have been associated with severe hyperparathyroidism with bone disease. They are generally slow-growing, tending to recur locally when excised, and are very resistant to x-ray therapy. Metastases to the regional lymph nodes, lungs, and liver may occur. Evidence indicates that carcinoma may develop from an adenoma.

The skeletal lesions observed in conjunction with long-standing hyperparathyroidism are discussed in Chap. 380, Osteoporosis. Degenerative changes occur in the renal tubular epithelium, heart muscle, and gastric mucosa and are often followed by calcification. About 80 percent of the cases show some evidence of renal damage such as nephrolithiasis, pyelonephritis, and calcium deposits in and around the tubules.

Mineral Levels

Characteristically, the plasma calcium is elevated and may attain values as high as 10 mEq per liter (20 mg per 100 ml). The plasma inorganic phosphate level is reduced below 1 mm per liter (3.1 mg per 100 ml) unless renal damage has resulted in secondary phosphate retention. In the presence of a high phosphate intake, many patients with hyperparathyroidism have plasma phosphate levels which fall within normal limits, with minimal elevation in plasma calcium levels. The excretion of calcium and phosphate in the urine is increased. With extensive bone involvement, the alkaline phosphatase may reach levels as high as 20 to 30 Bodansky units.

Clinical Picture

The earliest symptoms rarely lead to a diagnosis. They may be recognized in retrospect as an accompaniment of hypercalcemia. The symptoms include muscular weakness, anorexia, nausea, and constipation. Polyuria and polydipsia accompany the excessive calcium, phosphate, sodium, and potassium excretion as well as the renal lesions, which cause a loss of the ability of the kidney to concentrate urine even before structural changes have occurred. Often the first indication of hyperparathyroidism is renal colic or a spontaneous fracture. Deafness, paresthesias, and bone pain have been observed, and weight loss may be marked. On examination one may find hypotonia, muscular weakness, calcific keratitis (band keratitis), skeletal deformities, fractures, and tumor masses, especially in the jaw (epulis). When bone disease is present, x-ray studies may show a generalized decrease in bone density, cysts, tumors, fractures, and deformities, which are most marked in the hands, long bones, vertebras, pelvis, skull, and jaw. Bone marrow depression is common, with anemia, leukopenia, and occasionally thrombocytopenia. Peptic ulcer occurs in many patients with this disorder.

Diagnosis

Classic cases of chemical hyperparathyroidism with von Recklinghausen's disease (osteitis fibrosa generalisata or osteitis fibrosa cystica) are diagnosed easily from the clinical picture and the chemical findings of hypercalcemia, hypophosphatemia, hypercalcuria, and an increased plasma alkaline phosphatase (Table 90-2). It is important to carry out simultaneous calcium and total protein determinations, as marked hypoproteinemia (with accompanying decrease in calcium proteinate) may mask an increase in diffusible ionized calcium, the fraction of importance in this disease. It is also important to obtain plasma calcium levels on several occasions, particularly if the first determination is not elevated. The ion activity of calcium can be accurately and rapidly measured by the use of a special calcium ion activity electrode. Usually the calcium ion activity is about 48 to 50 percent of the total calcium, with 49 percent bound to protein and 2 to 3 percent bound to complexes such as citrate and phosphate. Bone lesions may be absent or minimal when calcium and protein intake have been high or when the disease is relatively mild or of short duration. In such cases the plasma alkaline phosphatase level may not be elevated. The diagnosis of hyperparathyroidism should be carefully ruled out in all patients with renal stones. Lithiasis often occurs in mild cases in which no other symptoms are present and plasma mineral levels show minimal changes.

Although hypercalcuria occurs in the absence of hyperparathyroidism, particularly in patients with nephrolithiasis, it is helpful in establishing the diagnosis from other causes. If after 7 to 14 days on a diet of 200 mg calcium the patient excretes more than 200 mg calcium in the urine in 24 hr, hypercalcuria is present. In the presence of avitaminosis D or renal insufficiency, hypercalcuria may not be found in hyperparathyroidism. An approximation of the urinary calcium concentration may be made with the Sulkowitch test.

The early diagnosis of hyperparathyroidism in the absence of renal and skeletal lesions may be extremely difficult, and several procedures have been devised to facilitate diagnosis.

INTRAVENOUS CALCIUM TEST. When a calcium load is administered intravenously, the normal individual responds with a rise in the plasma phosphate level and a fall in the urinary phosphate excretion. This is due to the fact that calcium will "shut off" the parathyroids if the plasma level is high enough. Theoretically, patients with hyperparathyroidism should not show the decrease in urinary excretion of phosphate, but the results are often inconclusive. Patients with hypoparathyroidism show a

Table 90-2. SUMMARY OF CHEMICAL FEATURES OF DISEASES WITH DISTURBED PLASMA CALCIUM AND PHOSPHATE

Disease	Serum			Urine		Feces*	
	Calcium	Phosphate	Alkaline phosphatase	Calcium	Phosphate	Calcium	Phosphate
Hyperparathyroidism	Increased	Decreased	Normal or increased	Increased	Increased	Normal	Normal
Paget's disease	Normal	Normal	Increased	Normal	Normal	Normal	Normal
Hypoparathyroidism	Decreased	Increased	Normal	Decreased	Decreased	Normal	Normal
Renal insufficiency	Decreased	Increased	Normal or increased	Decreased	Decreased	Normal	Increased
Osteomalacia	Decreased or normal	Decreased	Increased	Decreased	Decreased	Normal or increased	Decreased
Senile osteoporosis	Normal	Normal	Normal	Normal	Normal	Normal	Normal
Multiple myeloma	Normal to increased	Normal	Normal	Normal to increased	Normal to decreased	Normal	Normal
Milk-alkali syndrome	Increased	Normal to increased	Normal	Normal to decreased	Normal to decreased		
Vitamin D intoxication	Increased	Increased	Normal	Increased	Decreased	Decreased	Decreased
Metastatic carcinoma	Normal to increased	Normal	Normal to increased	Increased	Normal		
Sarcoidosis	Increased	Normal to increased	Normal to increased	Increased	Decreased	Decreased	Decreased
Hyperventilation (alkalosis)	Normal	Normal	Normal	Normal	Normal		

* On low-calcium diet.

marked phosphate diuresis, and this test is probably most useful in diagnosing true hypoparathyroidism.

TUBULAR REABSORPTION OF PHOSPHATE. Parathyroid hormone decreases the tubular reabsorption of phosphate in the renal tubules, and it has been found that patients with hyperparathyroidism have a tubular reabsorption of phosphate which is distinctly lower than normal. This can be best demonstrated by giving these patients an oral phosphate load (1 mM phosphate per kg body weight, made up of buffered mono- and dibasic sodium phosphate at pH 7.4), following which the tubular maximal transport of phosphate can be calculated (expressed as tubular reabsorption of phosphate in micromoles per 100 ml glomerular filtration rate per minute). Normal values range from 110 to 150. It can be shown that when there is a normal inulin clearance, this type of determination is valid and is further evidence for the tubular blocking action for phosphate by parathyroid hormone.

CORTISONE TEST. The action of cortisone on the normal subject is to decrease the absorption of calcium from the

MULTIPLE MYELOMA. This condition may show sharp demarcation of bone lesions by x ray, with increased plasma and urine calcium, possible stones, a variable phosphate level, increased globulin, Bence-Jones protein (50 percent), and plasma cells in the bone marrow. Even though massive bone disease may be seen by x-ray, the alkaline phosphatase usually remains within normal limits.

METASTATIC MALIGNANCIES. These may present a variable roentgenogram, depending on whether the origin of the primary tumor is the breast, prostate, kidney, bronchus, or thyroid. Plasma calcium and alkaline phosphatase may be increased. An increase in the prostatic fraction of the total acid phosphatase is presumptive evidence for carcinoma of the prostate. The acid phosphatase level may be elevated in other types of metastatic cancer to bone.

RENAL OSTEITIS FIBROSA. In this condition there exists a history of onset of renal difficulties prior to skeletal changes. However, this differentiation is often extraordinarily difficult to ascertain. It should be stated that

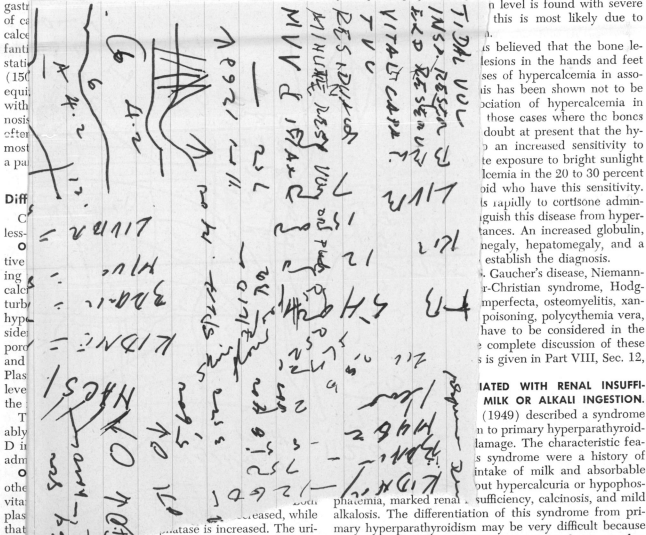

n level is found with severe
this is most likely due to

is believed that the bone le-
lesions in the hands and feet
ses of hypercalcemia in asso-
his has been shown not to be
ociation of hypercalcemia in
those cases where the bones
doubt at present that the hy-
an increased sensitivity to
te exposure to bright sunlight
lcemia in the 20 to 30 percent
oid who have this sensitivity.
ds rapidly to cortisone admin-
guish this disease from hyper-
tances. An increased globulin,
negaly, hepatomegaly, and a
establish the diagnosis.

Gaucher's disease, Niemann-
-Christian syndrome, Hodg-
mperfecta, osteomyelitis, xan-
poisoning, polycythemia vera,
have to be considered in the
complete discussion of these
is given in Part VIII, Sec. 12,

IATED WITH RENAL INSUFFI-
MILK OR ALKALI INGESTION.
(1949) described a syndrome
to primary hyperparathyroid-
amage. The characteristic fea-
syndrome were a history of
intake of milk and absorbable
out hypercalcuria or hypophos-
phatemia, marked renal insufficiency, calcinosis, and mild alkalosis. The differentiation of this syndrome from primary hyperparathyroidism may be very difficult because of the high incidence of ulcer symptoms in hyperparathyroidism. Treatment consists of a low-milk, low-alkali diet

and a high fluid intake. The azotemia and hypercalcemia may diminish and the chemical imbalance may be restored to normal, but residual renal damage may persist.

VITAMIN D INTOXICATION. Excessive vitamin D administration induces a clinical and pathologic picture similar to that of hyperparathyroidism. The symptoms of intoxication are those secondary to hypercalcemia and hypercalcuria already described. Recovery depends on prompt diagnosis and on the severity of the toxicity. Cortisone is the treatment of choice, as well as complete elimination of all sources of vitamin D, in moderate to severe cases of poisoning. The dosage of cortisone should range from 75 to 150 mg per day and should be maintained at this level until a normal plasma calcium is attained. The severe manifestations of the hypercalcemia will recede in a week to 10 days under such treatment, but other minor side effects, such as lassitude, weakness, and loss of appetite, may linger weeks or months before disappearing.

HYPERCALCEMIA IN CARCINOMA WITHOUT METASTASES. Recently there have been numerous instances in which a picture resembling hyperparathyroidism was abolished by removing a cancer locally. These cases were not associated with any demonstrable bony metastases. The cause of the hypercalcemia is not evident, although it has been presumed that these tumors have secreted a substance with plasma calcium–raising properties. The cortisone test is often a useful tool in differentiating this cause of hypercalcemia from hyperparathyroidism.

IMMOBILIZATION. Any patient with diffuse skeletal disease or chronic disease, if immobilized, may develop hypercalcemia and hypercalcuria, unless appropriate measures to prevent its occurrence are taken. No patient with Paget's disease should be put to bed for any long interval, since such a patient is especially likely to develop hypercalcuria.

IDIOPATHIC HYPERCALCEMIA OF INFANCY WITH FAILURE TO THRIVE. This is a new syndrome first described in Great Britain by Lightwood and his associates. These infants often have mental retardation, elfin facies, elevated cholesterol levels in the plasma, and hypercalcemia with all its secondary effects on the kidney and elsewhere. They will respond to cortisone or a diet devoid of vitamin D and calcium. It has been postulated that these children have an abnormal sensitivity to vitamin D similar to that found in sarcoidosis.

IDIOPATHIC HYPERCALCURIA. A large group of patients in whom renal calculi occur characteristically have hypercalcuria, low plasma phosphate, and normal plasma calcium. They may or may not have a lowered tubular reabsorptive rate for phosphate. Bone lesions and elevation of the alkaline phosphatase level are absent. Though the etiology of this syndrome is not clear at the present time, it is possible that these patients have a variant of hyperparathyroidism, and their condition should be followed carefully. Should they develop hypercalcemia at any time in their clinical course, neck exploration for an adenoma should be considered seriously.

OTHER CAUSES OF HYPERCALCEMIA. Thyrotoxicosis has been described in association with hypercalcemia, although this is a rare phenomenon.

Treatment

Once the diagnosis of primary hyperparathyroidism is established, fluids should be forced, intake of calcium restricted, and surgical consultation obtained with a view toward neck exploration. Difficulty in locating the offending gland or glands because of inconstant anatomic positions, and because the noninvolved glands show compensatory atrophy, may necessitate not only extensive but also repeated surgical exploration. Careful x-ray studies of the neck, including the esophagus and the mediastinum, may be helpful in locating the tumor before exploration, but they are often misleading. Removal of an adenoma or removal of all except a portion of one gland in case of hypertrophy and hyperplasia may be expected to cure the condition. When plasma alkaline phosphatase level is markedly elevated, large quantities of calcium may be required postoperatively to prevent recurrent tetany, since the bone will avidly remove calcium from the plasma in order to recalcify the bone lesions. The treatment of postoperative tetany is similar to that described in the treatment of hypoparathyroidism except that more vigorous treatment may have to be continued for some time to control the acute manifestations. A diet high in calcium and phosphate should be given postoperatively, but there is no need for increased doses of vitamin D over the normal intake unless there is a problem of chronic tetany. Under normal circumstances great improvement may be noted in the skeletal lesions as well as the renal function.

ACUTE HYPERCALCEMIC SYNDROME

Hypercalcemia caused by acute parathyroid intoxication or nonendocrine tumor constitutes an acute medical emergency. Acute parathyroid intoxication, with marked elevation of the plasma calcium level, occurs occasionally as a complication of hyperparathyroidism. It is characterized by weakness, lethargy, intractable nausea and vomiting, coma, and sudden death. The oral, rectal, or intravenous administration of phosphate is probably the most effective medical therapy for the treatment of hypercalcemia. A solution containing NaH_2PO_4 and Na_2HPO_4 (Fleet's Phospho-Soda), each 5 ml containing 3.3 Gm sodium phosphate, may be given orally. The usual dose is 10 to 20 ml (diluted with water or juice) daily, and the maintenance dose depends on the level of plasma calcium. The hypocalcemic effect of phosphate is apparent usually in 12 to 24 hr. If the patient is anorectic or comatose, a Fleet's Phospho-Soda enema may be used, since phosphate is readily absorbed through the sigmoid colon. One to three enemas daily may be used until the patient is able to swallow liquids. Intravenously, one may administer 500 ml of 0.1 M phosphate (0.08 mole Na_2HPO_4 plus 0.02 mole KH_2PO_4 per liter) over a 4- to 8-hr period, followed, if necessary, by an additional 500 ml INPHOS (Davies, Rose-Hoyt), a commercial preparation, available for intravenous use. One should be extremely cautious when using intravenous phosphate in azotemic patients, since profound hypocalcemia with tetany and convulsions has been reported. Great care should be taken as well to prevent infiltration of the phosphate infusion, since this will lead to subcutaneous calcification at the site of infiltration. It should be pointed out that early operation is indicated, because phosphate administration is not indicated as permanent treatment for hypercalcemia.

SECONDARY HYPERPARATHYROIDISM
History

Enlargement of the parathyroid glands secondary to another disease process in the body was first noted in 1905 by MacCallum in a case of nephritis. One year later, Erdheim noted similar findings in rickets, and since that time the syndrome of secondary hyperfunction of the parathyroids has been recognized.

Incidence

As a complication of advanced renal disease, hyperfunction of the parathyroids is relatively common. In 1933 Pappenheimer and Wilens reported that in a series of 21 cases of nephritis the mean parathyroid weight was 50 percent greater than in a control group.

Etiology

The most common cause of this condition is chronic, long-standing renal disease, as in glomerulonephritis and pyelonephritis. The term *renal rickets* does not apply to cases of secondary hyperparathyroidism and should be reserved for those cases seen most often in children in whom true rickets is secondary to prolonged and chronic renal disease and the supervening acidosis. Both secondary hyperparathyroidism and rickets have been described in the same patient as a complication of chronic renal disease. Reports of secondary hyperparathyroidism have been noted in a variety of diseases, such as osteogenesis imperfecta, Paget's disease, multiple myeloma, carcinoma with bone metastases and pituitary basophilism.

Pathology

The parathyroid glands are enlarged diffusely and are hyperplastic. No single adenomas are visible. The cells are normal in size and easily differentiated from those seen in primary hyperparathyroidism. The former are principally chief cells with some increase in oxyphil cells, as opposed to the huge, water-clear cells of primary hyperparathyroidism due to hypertrophy and hyperplasia. The bone lesions are entirely similar to those seen in primary hyperparathyroidism, namely, generalized decalcification and bone cysts, with or without outright fracture.

Pathologic Physiology

It is unclear at the present time what the precise mechanisms for the development of parathyroid hyperplasia are in renal disease. It was believed that long-standing phosphate retention was the *sine qua non* for the development of the syndrome. The metabolic acidosis which invariably accompanies chronic renal disease leads to a negative calcium balance, since bone mineral constitutes in effect an important homeostatic mechanism for the neutralization of fixed acid, and an effective, although costly, device for the defense against progressive acidosis in patients whose kidneys have lost their capacity to regulate the acid balance of the body. Whether or not acidosis affects the skeleton by modifying the physiologic actions of vitamin D, parathyroid hormone, or thyrocalcitonin has not, as yet, been determined. Correction of the acidosis by alkali administration, vitamin D, or renal homotransplantation has led to variable degrees of bone repair.

Clinical Picture

The symptoms are usually those of the primary disease process before any evidence of hyperparathyroidism is noted. Classic glomerulonephritis or pyelonephritis, uremia, and evidence of renal insufficiency dominate the clinical picture. In children, dwarfism and pathologic fractures may be the presenting complaints.

Diagnosis

The chemical findings of normal or low-normal plasma calcium with hyperphosphatemia and high alkaline phosphatase, with the classic skeletal roentgenograms of bone cysts and generalized demineralization, lead to the diagnosis of parathyroid hyperfunction with renal disease. The history of early renal disease is often the only differential diagnostic point, since the primary cases are often complicated late in the disease by renal failure secondary to long-standing hyperparathyroidism. An elevated plasma calcium level in the presence of uremia indicates autonomous parathyroid hyperfunction due either to a primary adenoma or to "tertiary" parathyroid hyperplasia.

Treatment

Of greatest importance is a correct diagnosis. Once this is established, all therapy is directed at the primary disease, and an attempt is made to correct the acidosis by the administration of alkaline salts, such as bicarbonate or citrate. Attempts to elevate the plasma calcium level by large amounts of vitamin D (calciferol, in doses of 50,000 to 150,000 units per day, or the equivalent in vitamin D_3 or dihydrotachysterol) are often indicated when the plasma calcium is reduced in order to suppress excessive parathyroid hormone secretion. However, this type of therapy is extremely dangerous and must be carefully regulated, since the difference between therapeutic and toxic doses of vitamin D is quite narrow. Certain patients with chronic renal disease and severe secondary hyperparathyroidism have had subtotal parathyroidectomy followed by vitamin D therapy. Though the bone disease is strikingly cured by such means, the basic renal disorder is unaltered and the patients have ultimately died of uremia.

NONFUNCTIONING TUMORS OF THE PARATHYROID GLANDS

Nonfunctioning carcinoma of the parathyroids has been reported, but these cases have not been generally accepted, because of the difficulty in establishing the origin of the tumor. Other nonfunctioning tumors include oxyphil adenomas which may be burned-out primary adenomas), metastatic carcinoma, and cysts. Microscopic cysts are common in hyperplastic and adenomatous glands, whereas gross cysts are quite rare. Symptoms, when present, are due to pressure on local structures, including the recurrent laryngeal nerve. Most tumors have been found in the lower glands.

REFERENCES

Baker, W. H.: Abnormalities in Calcium Metabolism in Malignancy: Effects of Hormone Therapy, Am. J. Med., 21:714, 1956.

Bernstein, D. S., and C. D. Guri: Hyperparathyroidism and Hypoparathyroidism: Preoperative and Postoperative Care, Anesthesiology, 24:448, 1963.

Bogdonoff, M. D., A. H. Woods, J. E. White, and F. L. Engel: Hyperparathyroidism, Am. J. Med., 21:583, 1956.

Bourne, G. H.: "The Biochemistry and Physiology of Bone," New York, Academic Press, Inc., 1956.

Bronsky, D., D. S. Kushner, A. Dubin, and I. Snapper: Idiopathic Hypoparathyroidism and Pseudohypoparathyroidism, Medicine, 37:317, 1958.

Chambers, E. L., G. S. Gordan, L. Goldman, and E. C. Reifenstein, Jr.: Tests for Hyperparathyroidism: Tubular Reabsorption of Phosphate, Phosphate Deprivation, and Calcium Infusion, J. Clin. Endocrinol. & Metab., 16:1507, 1956.

Goldsmith, R. S., and S. H. Ingbar: Inorganic Phosphate Treatment of Hypercalcemia of Diverse Etiologies, New Eng. J. Med., 274:1, 1966.

Heaney, R. P., and G. O. Whedon: Radiocalcium Studies of Bone Formation Rate in Human Metabolic Bone Disease, J. Clin. Endocrinol. & Metab., 18:1246, 1958.

Munson, P. L., P. F. Hirsch, and A. H. Tashjian: Parathyroid Gland, Ann. Rev. Physiol., 25:325, 1963.

Rasmussen, H.: Purification of Parathyroid Polypeptides, J. Biol. Chem., 235:3442, 1960.

Underdahl, L., L. B. Woolner, and B. M. Black: Multiple Endocrine Adenomas: Eight Cases Involving Parathyroids, Pituitary, and Pancreatic Islets, J. Clin. Endocrinol. & Metab., 13:20, 1953.

91 CALCITONIN

Daniel S. Bernstein and
Menelaos A. Aliapoulios

Historical Development

That precise regulation of plasma calcium is mediated by parathyroid hormone acting on bone, intestine, and kidneys has been recognized over the past 40 years. In 1961, this classic concept was challenged as a result of the demonstration of a second substance involved in calcium homeostasis by Copp and his coworkers, who showed that perfusion of the thyroparathyroid glands with a hypercalcemic solution produced a rapid fall in plasma calcium level. In 1963, Hirsch and colleagues demonstrated a fall in plasma calcium and phosphate in rats given a crude extract of hog thyroid. They appropriately named this new hormone *thyrocalcitonin*. The presence of the new hormone originating in the thyroid gland was established in other species as well as in man.

Anatomy and Physiology

Initially it was thought that thyrocalcitonin originated in the epithelial cells of the thyroid gland. It is now known that thyrocalcitonin is derived from the ultimobranchial bodies which fuse with the thyroid in mammals. These bodies, whose function hitherto was obscure, remain as separate structures in birds, fish, reptiles, and amphibians. They develop from the ventral part of the pharyngeal entoderm immediately behind the last pair of gill pouches. Their cells have a particular microscopic appearance, which is now recognized to be similar to that of the thyroid "C" cells. These "C" cells were identified long ago as differing from the thyroid follicular cells and now have been shown to be the site of production of thyrocalcitonin. Stimulation of the thyroid by TSH produces no increase of thyrocalcitonin, and propylthiouracil administration induces no decrease in the secretion of this substance. The term *thyrocalcitonin* can now be discarded because this hormone is derived from ultimobranchial tissue which is not necessarily confined to the thyroid.

Chemical Structure

The chemical structure of calcitonin (porcine) was determined independently by three groups of investigators. Following this, the total synthesis of the hormone was accomplished. Calcitonin is a 32-chain polypeptide with a disulfide bridge and a molecular weight of approximately 3,600. The amino acid composition is unique in the absence of isoleucine and in the high content of glycine, proline, and serine. Calcitonin is highly potent, and its biologic activity is demonstrable in microgram quantities.

Physiologic Action

It has been established that calcitonin, when injected into various test animals as well as humans, induces a rapid fall in plasma calcium, with ionized calcium and phosphate levels rarely lasting longer than 3 to 4 hr. It has been shown that the fall in plasma calcium and phosphate levels following injection of calcitonin is not dependent upon the presence of the parathyroid gland. Calcitonin has no significant effect on calcium transport across the duodenum, and nephrectomy does not alter its hypocalcemic effect. Investigators, using varied experimental models, have shown that calcitonin has a direct inhibiting effect on bone resorption which is proportional to the concentration of calcitonin employed. With decreased bone resorption, there is an associated decrease in the excretion of urinary hydroxyproline. In long-term use, calcitonin has been shown to increase trabecular bone formation in parathyroidectomized rats. The extent to which calcitonin can inhibit bone resorption is probably dependent upon the existing rate of bone resorption, a greater response being evoked in the presence of increased bone resorption. Calcitonin also produces a decrease in the urinary excretion of calcium, magnesium, and hydroxyproline, whereas the effect on renal phosphate excretion has not been clearly elucidated.

Clinical Significance

Human thyroid tissue has been shown to contain significant amounts of calcitonin. The presence of calcitonin in the plasma of two normal persons at rest has been detected by rat bioassay and by radioimmunoassay. This implies that the hormone has a physiologic role other than combating periodic hypercalcemia. Furthermore, the concentration of calcitonin is increased in response to an infusion of calcium. In two cases of pseudohypoparathyroidism, calcitonin concentration 100 times greater than normal was found and deserves attention as a possible factor responsible for the alteration in calcium metabolism observed in this syndrome. In cases of thyroid goiter, adenoma, and hyperplasia, calcitonin is absent or found in decreased amounts. In hyperparathyroidism, there is decreased calcitonin in the thyroid gland.

Several patients have been described with medullary carcinoma of the thyroid and an excess of hypocalcemic activity in the blood or tumor. A variety of laboratory techniques as well as radioimmunoassay of serum in one instance confirmed that the active substance was calcitonin. Only one patient was noted to have hypocalcemia and hypophosphatemia, and none was reported to have dense bones on x-ray examination. It now appears certain that medullary carcinoma results from malignant proliferation of thyroid "C" cells. No other syndrome in man has been formally proved to result from abnormal production of calcitonin, but studies in cows with hypocalcemia and hypophosphatemia at parturition showed that excess release of calcitonin might be responsible for this condition.

The practical importance and the possible clinical application of this new hormone are speculative at present. There may be pathogenetic significance in the elevated levels of calcitonin found in pseudohypoparathyroidism and in medullary carcinoma of the thyroid. The direct effect of calcitonin in decreasing bone resorption could be of benefit to patients with osteoporosis, hypercalcemia of diverse etiology, bone fractures, Paget's disease, and other demineralizing bone disorders accompanied by excessive bone resorption. Calcitonin administration has produced a temporary fall in plasma calcium level in a patient with hypercalcemia due to metastatic carcinoma.

In a patient with hypercalcemia associated with a malignant parathyroid tumor, calcitonin administration for periods of approximately 2 to 3 weeks on two occasions resulted in a decrease in serum calcium level and a reduction in urinary calcium excretion.

REFERENCES

Aliapoulios, M. A., D. S. Bernstein, and M. C. Balodimos: Thyrocalcitonin: Its Role in Calcium Homeostasis, Arch. Intern. Med., 123:88, 1969.
——, and P. L. Munson: Thyrocalcitonin, Surg. Forum, 16:55, 1965.
Dambacher, M. A., J. Guncaga, T. Lauffenburger, and H. G. Haas: Human Calcitonin, Germ. Med. Mth., 14:356, 1969.
Foster, G. V.: Calcitonin (Thyrocalcitonin), New Engl. J. Med., 279:349, 1968.
Galante, L., T. V. Gudmundsson, E. W. Matthews, E. D. Williams, A. Tse, N. J. Y. Woodhouse, and I. MacIntyre: Thymic and Parathyroid Origin of Calcitonin in Man, Lancet, p. 537, September 7, 1968.
Hirsch, P. F., and P. L. Munson: Thyrocalcitonin, Physiol. Rev., 49:548, 1969.
Pechet, M. M.: Symposium on Thyrocalcitonin, Am. J. Med., 43:645, 1967.

92 DISEASES OF THE ADRENAL CORTEX

David P. Lauler, Gordon H. Williams, and George W. Thorn

INTRODUCTION

Thomas Addison's description in 1849 of a clinical syndrome resulting from destruction of the adrenal glands first attracted attention to these organs. Seven years later Brown-Séquard demonstrated that removal of both adrenals from experimental animals caused death soon after operation, whereas control animals subjected to a sham operation survived. Subsequent investigations established that the life-maintaining hormone was elaborated by cells in the cortex, since destruction of all medullary tissue was not accompanied by the classic signs and symptoms of adrenal insufficiency noted after complete removal of the glands.

Between 1927 and 1930, Hartman and his associates, Rogoff and Stewart, and Pfiffner and Swingle all independently described methods for preparing potent adrenocortical extracts. During the following decade, crystalline steroid substances were isolated from these extracts by Kendall, by Grollman, and by Reichstein. In 1937, Steiger and Reichstein synthesized the first natural corticosteroid, 11-deoxycorticosterone, a year before it was identified in adrenal extracts. From 1940 to 1950, the synthesis of several 11-oxygenated compounds was achieved, including cortisone and hydrocortisone. The contributions of Sarett and his collaborators, Reichstein et al., and Kendall and his coworkers were outstanding in this regard. In 1954 aldosterone, the principal salt-retaining hormone of the adrenal, was identified by Simpson and Tait in collaboration with the Swiss group under Reichstein.

Since 1954, a number of remarkable advances have occurred. ACTH has been isolated, its amino acid sequence determined, and the complete molecule synthesized. A number of substances which interfere with the action of adrenal steroids have also been synthesized. For example, amphenone and 2-methyl-1,2-bis-(3-pyridyl)-1-propanone (metyrapone) interfere with the synthesis of hydrocortisone. Spironolactone and 2,4,7-tri-amino-6-phenylpteridine (triamterene) block the physiologic effects of aldosterone. Among the most significant advancements have been the refinements in the ease and accuracy with which steroids and their metabolic products may be measured, e.g., by double isotope derivative, competitive protein-binding radioassay, and radioimmunoassay techniques.

BIOCHEMISTRY AND PHYSIOLOGY

Steroid Nomenclature

The adrenal steroids contain as their basic structure a cyclopentanoperhydrophenanthrane nucleus consisting of three 6-carbon hexane rings and a single 5-carbon pentane ring (D). The carbon atoms are numbered in a predetermined sequence beginning with ring A (Fig. 92-1). The Greek letter Δ indicates a double bond, as does the suffix -ene. The position of a substituent below or above the plane of the steroid molecule is indicated by the letters α and β respectively. The α-substituent is drawn with a broken line (--OH), and the β-substituent is drawn with a solid line (—OH). The C_{19} steroids are those which have substituent methyl groups at positions C-18 and C-19. C_{19} steroids that also have a ketone group at C-17 are termed *17-ketosteroids*. These C_{19} steroids have predominant androgenic activity. The C_{21} steroids are those which have a 2-carbon side chain (C-20 and C-21) attached at position 17 of the D ring and, in addition, have substituent methyl groups at C-18 and C-19. C_{21} steroids that also possess a hydroxyl group at position 17 are termed *17-hydroxycorticosteroids* or *17-hydroxycorticoids*. The C_{21} steroids may have either predominant glucocorticoid or mineralocorticoid properties. *Glucocorticoid* signifies a C_{21} steroid with predominant action on intermediary metabolism, and *mineralocorticoid* indicates a C_{21} steroid with predominant action on the metabolism of the body minerals, sodium and potassium.

Biosynthesis of Adrenal Steroids

Cholesterol, derived from the diet and from endogenous synthesis via acetate, is the principal starting compound in steroidogenesis. The three major adrenal biosynthetic pathways lead to the production of glucocorticoids (cortisol), mineralocorticoids (aldosterone), and adrenal androgens (dehydroepiandrosterone) (Fig. 92-2).

GLUCOCORTICOID PATHWAY. $\Delta 5$-Pregnenolone is formed after cleavage of the side chain of cholesterol. $\Delta 5$-Pregnenolone is converted to progesterone by the action of the enzymes 3β-hydroxydehydrogenase and $\Delta 5, \Delta 4$-isomerase. These enzymes transform the 3β-hydroxy group of $\Delta 5$-pregnenolone to a C-3-ketonic group and transform the double bond between C-5:C-6 of $\Delta 5$-pregnenolone to position C-4:C-5 of progesterone. A series of hydroxylations mediated by specific hydroxylating enzymes then occurs in sequential fashion at C-17, then at C-21, and finally at C-11. With the introduction of a hydroxyl group at position C-17 of progesterone by the enzyme C-17 hydroxylase, 17α-hydroxyprogesterone is formed, which in turn has a hydroxyl group introduced at C-21 by the enzyme C-21 hydroxylase, producing 11-deoxycortisol (Compound S), the major precursor of cortisol. Finally, a third hydroxyl group is introduced at the C-11 position of 11-deoxycortisol by the enzyme C-11 hydroxylase, to produce cortisol (Compound F, hydrocortisone), the major glucocorticoid. The chemical name for cortisol is 11β,17α,21-trihydroxy-4-pregnene-3,20-dione.

MINERALOCORTICOID PATHWAY. Progesterone, after transformation from $\Delta 5$-pregnenolone, is hydroxylated at the C-21 position to form 11-deoxycorticosterone. This C-21 hydroxylase, rather than being identical to the enzyme used to form 11-deoxycortisol, may be an isoenzyme of it; 11-deoxycorticosterone is then hydroxylated at the 11 position to form corticosterone, compound B. A hydroxyl group is then introduced at the 18 position to form 18-hydroxycorticosterone, the immediate precursor of aldosterone. With conversion of the hydroxyl group at C-18 to an aldehyde group, the major mineralocorticoid, *aldosterone,* is formed. The 18-aldehyde group exists free

Basic steroid nucleus

C-19 Steroid

C-21 Steroid

17-Ketosteroid

17-Hydroxycorticosteroid

Fig. 92-1. Basic steroid structure and nomenclature.

Fig. 92-2. Biosynthetic pathways for adrenal steroid production. Major pathways to mineralocorticoids, glucocorticoids, and androgens. Circled letters and numbers denote specific enzymes: *DE* = debranching enzyme; *3β* = 3β-ol-dehydrogenase with Δ4–Δ5 isomerase; 11 = C-11 hydroxylase; 17 = C-17 hydroxylase; 21 = C-21 hydroxylase.

or in the hemiacetal form. The chemical designation for aldosterone is $11_\beta,21$-dihydroxy-18-aldo-4-pregnene-3,20-dione.

ANDROGEN PATHWAY. By the enzymatic action of 17_α-hydroxylase, $\Delta5$-pregnenolone is converted to 17_α-hydroxypregnenolone, which on cleavage of its C-20:C-21 side chain forms the 17-ketosteroid dehydroepiandrosterone. The $\Delta5,$-3 hydroxyl grouping of this compound is transformed to a $\Delta4,$-3 oxo- grouping by the enzymes 3_β-hydroxydehydrogenase and $\Delta5,\Delta4$ isomerase to produce the 17-ketosteroid androstenedione. Androstenedione can undergo direct transformation to testosterone as a result of hydrogenation at position C-17, and androstenedione also is converted to 11_β-hydroxyandrostenedione by hydroxylation at position C-11. Note that the adrenal androgens require a preliminary hydroxylation at C-17 prior to their formation and, also, that 17-ketosteroids with an oxygen group at position C-11 are of adrenal origin.

It is unlikely that the adrenal gland can convert testosterone or androstenedione to estradiol and estrone, as had been previously thought. These conversions probably take place from adrenal precursors in the liver.

Steroid Transport

In the analysis of the metabolic actions of steroids, an important feature is the mechanism of transport from origin to site of action. Many hormones, including some of the steroid hormones, e.g., testosterone and cortisol, appear to circulate to a considerable extent bound to plasma proteins. Aldosterone, however, seems to have a relatively poor binding affinity for any serum protein. Cortisol, after release into the systemic circulation, occurs in the plasma in three forms: free cortisol, protein-bound cortisol, and cortisol metabolites. *Free cortisol* refers to that quantity which is physiologically active but not protein bound and, therefore, represents a form of cortisol acting directly on tissue sites. Normally, less than 5 percent of circulating cortisol is free. *Protein-bound cortisol* is that portion of cortisol which is reversibly bound to circulating plasma proteins. There are two distinct cortisol-binding systems of plasma. One is a high-affinity, low-capacity globulin termed transcortin or cortisol-binding-globulin (CBG), and the other is a low-affinity, high-capacity protein, albumin. Cortisol-binding globulin in normal man can bind approximately 20 to 25 μg cortisol per 100 ml plasma. As the amounts of cortisol released by the adrenal gland exceed this level, the excess becomes bound in part to albumin. The CBG level may be increased by administration of natural or synthetic estrogens. This endogenous rise in CBG is accompanied by a parallel rise in protein-bound cortisol, with the result that the level of plasma 17-hydroxycorticosteroids is elevated. However, free cortisol levels remain normal, and thus signs of cortisol excess do not appear. This effect of estrogen on steroid binding is most evident in pregnancy.

Cortisol metabolites such as tetrahydrocortisol also circulate in the plasma. These metabolites are biologically inactive and bind only weakly to circulating plasma proteins.

It is evident that the protein binding of steroids exerts a major influence on the equilibrium concentration of cortisol across membrane barriers. For example, by this mechanism, urine loss of steroids is minimized, since only the unbound cortisol and its metabolites are filtrable at the glomerulus. Furthermore, cortisol binding to proteins serves as a reserve buffer mechanism capable of binding excess cortisol when the plasma free cortisol is high, and conversely, capable of releasing bound cortisol when the free cortisol level is low.

Considerable evidence has accumulated for a testosterone-binding globulin with as strong an affinity for testosterone as cortisol-binding globulin has for cortisol. It is unclear whether these two globulins are entirely separate proteins or represent different sites on the same protein moiety. Testosterone-binding globulin is likewise markedly increased by estrogens and pregnancy.

Aldosterone appears to be bound to proteins to a much smaller extent than either testosterone or cortisol. It has been shown that an ultrafiltrate of plasma probably contains as much as 50 percent of the circulating aldosterone. Aldosterone, like other steroids, is bound to albumin. There is also some evidence that a separate protein, other than albumin- or cortisol-binding globulin, may participate in partially binding aldosterone. The limited binding of aldosterone by plasma protein may be significant in the metabolism of this hormone.

Steroid Metabolism and Excretion

GLUCOCORTICOIDS. The principal glucocorticoids secreted by the normal adrenal gland are cortisol and corticosterone. The daily adrenal secretion of cortisol ranges between 15 and 30 mg, with a pronounced diurnal cycle, and that of corticosterone between 2 and 4 mg. Cortisol is distributed in a volume of body fluids approximating the total extracellular fluid space. The total plasma concentration of cortisol in the morning hours is approximately 15 μg per 100 ml, with more than 90 percent of this cortisol appearing in the protein-bound fraction. The plasma concentration of cortisol is determined by the rate of secretion, the rate of inactivation, and the rate of excretion of free cortisol. The biologic half-life of cortisol is between 60 and 120 min. Cortisol is inactivated by means of six major biotransformations: (1) 11-dehydrogenation; (2) reduction at C-20; (3) reduction of ring A; (4) cleavage of the C-20:C-21 side chain; (5) 6_β-hydroxylation; and (6) conjugation. The 11-dehydrogenase system converts cortisol to the inactive cortisone. This reversible system is one of the major factors in regulating the level of circulating cortisol under normal circumstances. The enzyme is strongly influenced by the level of circulating thyroid hormone, with hyperthyroidism markedly accelerating the oxidative reaction. The second mechanism of inactivation, C-20 hydroxylation, is brought into play by the addition of two hydrogen atoms at C-20. Further reduction elsewhere in the molecule is possible, and the products are the cortols and the cortolones. The third mechanism is the reduction of ring A. The initial saturation of the C-4:C-5 double bond in ring A by the introduction of two hydrogen ions produces *dihydrocortisol* (Fig. 92-3). Next the C-3 ketonic group of dihydrocortisol is reduced by further addition of two hy-drogen atoms to form *tetrahydrocortisol* (THF). Furthermore, cortisone may go through a similar reduction process to produce tetrahydrocortisone (THE). From 5 to 10 percent of the secreted cortisol is metabolized in the liver by cleavage of the C-20:C-21 side chain to form

Fig. 92-3. Metabolism of cortisol to tetrahydrocortisol, tetrahydrocortisone, cortol, and cortolone. Conjugation occurs with glucuronic acid at C-3 position. Note interconversion of cortisol and cortisone.

the corresponding 11-oxyketosterol. Finally, in normal man, 6_β-hydroxylation of cortisol represents a relatively minor metabolic transformation. However, under certain circumstances, in infancy and toxemia of pregnancy and with certain drugs, the formation of this product becomes important. The first four transformations produce compounds which are not water-soluble. These compounds are conjugated in the liver with glucuronic acid at position C-3 to produce water-soluble products. Sulfation appears to be a relatively minor process, except perhaps in infancy. The 6_β-hydroxycortisol is sufficiently water-soluble that it can clear the kidney without conjugation. The average amounts of metabolites excreted per 24 hr. are as follows: free cortisol, 0.05 mg; glucuronides of cortols and cortolones, 3 mg; 17-ketosteroids derived from cortisol and cortisone, 1.5 mg.

MINERALOCORTICOIDS. In normal subjects on a normal salt intake, the average daily secretion of aldosterone ranges between 50 and 250 μg, and the plasma concentration ranges between 5 and 15 mμg per 100 ml. Since aldosterone is only weakly bound to proteins, its volume of distribution is larger than that of cortisol and approximates 35 liters. Under normal circumstances, greater than 75 percent of circulating aldosterone is inactivated during a single passage through the liver. However, under certain conditions, such as congestive failure, this percentage is markedly reduced.

Under steady-state conditions, aldosterone exists as the 11-18-hemiacetal form rather than the 18-aldehyde form. Most transformations of this compound are reductive in nature. There has been no substantial evidence of oxidative reactions involving aldosterone, in contrast to cortisol metabolism. Of the numerous reductive metabolites that may be formed, 50 percent of aldosterone is transformed into the tetrahydro derivative produced by ring A reduction. This reaction appears to occur only in the liver, and because this metabolite is water-insoluble, it is conjugated with glucuronic acid before it is excreted in the urine. From 7 to 15 percent of aldosterone appears in the urine as a glucuronide conjugate, from which free aldosterone is released on standing at pH 1. This *acid-labile conjugate* appears to be formed both in the liver and in the kidney. The relative proportions appear to be related to relative blood flow to the two organs and the state of the general circulation. The acid-labile conjugate is also referred to as the *3-oxo conjugate,* because the 3-oxo grouping is not irreversibly reduced, as it is in tetrahydroaldosterone. Ninety percent of the acid-labile conjugate is excreted within 6 hr, whereas comparable tetrahydroaldosterone excretion requires 24 to 36 hr. For average salt intake, the 24-hr urine excretion of the acid-labile conjugate ranges from 1 to 10 μg, that of the tetrahydro derivative from 25 to 35 μg, and that of the nonconjugated, nonreduced free aldosterone from 0.2 to 0.6 μg. Aldosterone excretion, like cortisol excretion, exhibits diurnal variations, with daytime excretion predominating.

ADRENAL ANDROGENS. The major androgenic compound secreted by the adrenal gland is dehydroepiandrosterone (DHEA) and its C-3 sulfuric acid ester.

From 15 to 30 mg of these compounds is secreted daily. Much smaller amounts of Δ4-androstenedione and 11_β-hydroxyandrostenedione and testosterone are secreted. The major fraction of dehydroepiandrosterone is found in the urine as the sulfate. However, only a small portion of the secreted compound reaches this stage without other metabolic alterations. The first step, which is irreversible, is the conversion to Δ4-androstenedione (Fig. 92-4). This compound is then interconvertible with testosterone and shares with testosterone a common group of metabolites, consisting of androsterone, epiandrosterone, and etiocholanolone. The second major route of transformation is the formation of the 16_α-hydroxyl derivative of either dehydroepiandrosterone or its sulfate. In pregnancy, this compound performs a vital role as a precursor in the placental production of estriol.

Fig. 92-4. Metabolism of adrenal androgens. Δ4-androstenedione and testosterone contribute to the same metabolites.

Two-thirds of the urine 17-ketosteroids in the male are derived from adrenal metabolites, and the remaining one-third comes from testicular androgens. In the female, almost all urine 17-ketosteroids are derived from the adrenal gland. It is improbable that estrogens are synthesized by the adrenal gland. There has been no substantial proof of aromatic enzymes being present in adrenal tissue. The increased estrogens in ovariectomized patients and in feminizing adrenal tumors are probably secondary to the action of liver enzymes on androgenic precursors secreted by the adrenal glands.

ACTH Physiology

The adrenocorticotropin hormone (ACTH) (see Chap. 87) is an unbranched long-chain polypeptide containing 39 amino acids. It is stored in and released from the anterior pituitary gland, where histologically it appears to be localized to basophil cells. Only 50 units, or roughly 0.25 mg, of the active peptide are stored in the anterior pituitary. Much of the potential for producing the corticotropic actions of ACTH is present in smaller polypeptide fragments. It appears that the significant structure necessary for high adrenocorticotropin activity is the unusual sequence of basic amino acid lys-lys-arg-arg occurring in the 15 to 18 position. The biologic half-life of ACTH is less than 10 min. The release of ACTH from the anterior pituitary gland is governed by a "corticotropin-releasing center" in the median eminence of the hypothalamus, which upon stimulation releases a chemical mediator (corticotropin-releasing factor, CRF) that travels via the pituitary-stalk portal bloodstream to the anterior pituitary gland, where it effects the release of stored ACTH (Fig. 92-5). CRF is thought to be a short-chain polypeptide whose release is facilitated by a large number of nervous stimuli, including those arising from higher centers. The principal regulator of CRF release is the plasma free cortisol level, which by a negative feedback mechanism causes increased release of CRF when plasma cortisol level is low and a decreased release of CRF when plasma cortisol concentration is elevated. This servomechanism establishes the primacy of blood cortisol concentration and serves to buffer deviations in blood cortisol levels from a supposed optimal level. It also appears that cortisol feeds back directly on the pituitary gland and higher brain centers, and perhaps even on the adrenal cortex as well.

Besides its major action in stimulating the biogenesis and release of steroid hormones by the adrenal gland, ACTH can stimulate melanocytes of amphibians and can increase adipokinetic activity in a number of species. Both these extraadrenal actions have been verified with synthetic ACTH molecules.

The action of ACTH on the adrenal gland itself is rapid; within minutes of its release, there is an increased concentration of steroids in the adrenal venous blood. It produces a number of biochemical changes: (1) an increase in adrenal weight; (2) a decrease in amount of adrenal lipids, cholesterol, and ascorbic acid; (3) an increase in protein synthesis and oxidative phosphorylation; and (4) an accelerated rate of glycolysis. The molecular basis of ACTH action has not been elucidated. Some investigators suggest that ACTH accelerates the production of Δ5,pregnenolone from cholesterol in a rate-limiting manner; others have suggested that ACTH acts by

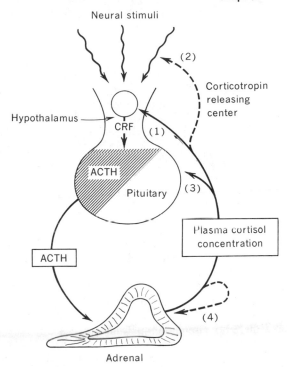

Fig. 92-5. Hypothalamic-pituitary-adrenal axis. *CRF* = corticotropin-releasing factor. (1) Dominant feedback control on the hypothalamus; (2) possible feedback of plasma cortisol on higher nerve centers; (3) feedback on the pituitary gland; and (4) possible direct feedback on the adrenal gland itself.

increasing the formation and availability of adenosine-3',5'-monophosphate in the adrenal gland, which would lead to an increase in the synthesis of reduced coenzymes needed for steroid biosynthesis. Evidence has been obtained which suggests that activation of protein biosynthesis is an important if not an essential part of the action of ACTH and possibly of other tropic hormones. ACTH apparently increases protein biosynthesis either by stimulation of messenger ribonucleic acid or by enzyme activation.

Renin-Angiotensin Physiology
(See Chap. 276)

Renin is a proteolytic enzyme with an approximate molecular weight of 35,000 to 40,000. It has been semi-purified. It is produced and stored in the granules of the juxtaglomerular cells surrounding the afferent arterioles of the cortical glomeruli. The juxtaglomerular apparatus consist of both the juxtaglomerular cells and the cells of the macula densa. The latter area also contains some renin. Renin acts on the basic substrate angiotensinogen (a circulating alpha$_2$-globulin) made in the liver, to form the decapeptide angiotensin-I. Various inhibitors of intrarenal renin formation are believed to exist (Fig. 92-6). Angiotensin-I is then enzymatically converted by converting enzyme to the octapeptide angiotensin-II by the splitting off of the two C-terminal amino acids. Angiotensin-II is the most potent pressor compound (on a milli-

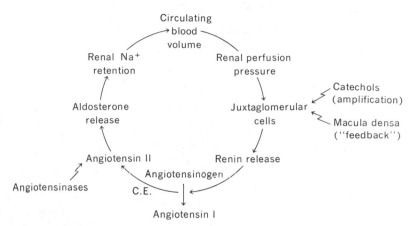

Fig. 92-6. Renin-angiotensin-aldosterone volume regulation in normal man.

gram-for-milligram basis) made in the body, and it exerts this pressor action by a direct effect on arteriolar smooth muscle. In addition, angiotensin-II is the most potent direct stimulus to the production of aldosterone by the zona glomerulosa of the adrenal cortex. Various peptidases, collectively termed "angiotensinases," in organ tissue, vessel walls, and circulating plasma are responsible for the ultimate biochemical degradation of circulating angiotensin-II. Angiotensin-II may also play a role in modifying the renal tubular transport of sodium. Such a direct tubular effect, independent of its effect on renal hemodynamics, remains controversial.

Renin release is controlled both by extrarenal and intrarenal mechanisms. The extrarenal mechanism is capable of overiding the intrarenal mechanism, although in many situations they act synergistically in series. The common denominator for the release of renin by the *extrarenal* mechanism is that of volume depletion. Volume depletion may be induced (by hemorrhage, ganglionic blockade, diuretic administration, salt restriction) or may exist on a chronic basis, as in certain disorders associated with edema.

The juxtaglomerular cells, which are specialized myoepithelial cells cuffing the afferent arterioles, act as miniature pressure *transducers,* sensing renal perfusion pressure and corresponding changes in afferent arteriolar perfusion pressures. The changes in pressure are perceived as distortions in the existing stretch on the arteriolar walls. For example, under conditions of a reduction in circulating blood volume, there will be a corresponding reduction in renal perfusion pressure and, therefore, in afferent arteriolar pressure. This will be perceived by the juxtaglomerular cells as a decreased stretch exerted on the afferent arteriolar walls. The juxtaglomerular cells will then release increasing quantities of renin within the kidney circulation, leading to the formation of angiotensin-II. Angiotensin-II leaves the kidney both by a renal lymphatic and a renal venous outflow. It directly stimulates the adrenal cortex to release increasing quantities of aldosterone. (At higher levels, angiotensin may have a direct pressor effect.) Increasing plasma levels of aldosterone lead to increasing renal sodium retention and thus result in expansion of extracellular fluid volume, which, as it is completed, dampens the initiating signal for renin

release. Within this context, the renin-angiotensin-aldosterone system is subserving volume control by appropriate modifications of renal tubular sodium transport. Circulating catecholamines, and perhaps the renal sympathetic nerves, are capable of amplifying the response of the juxtaglomerular cells to changes in perfusion pressure. The renal nerves per se are not a prerequisite for such an amplification, however, since the denervated kidney can successfully adapt to salt restriction.

An *intrarenal* control mechanism for renin release has been postulated. Such a theory centers on the macula densa cells. These are a group of special-staining distal convoluted tubular epithelial cells found in direct apposition to the juxtaglomerular cells. It has been suggested that they may function as chemoreceptors, monitoring the sodium load presented to the distal tubule, and that such formation, while it is being monitored, is directly fed back to the juxtaglomerular cells where appropriate modifications in renin release may take place. Such an intrarenal renin-release mechanism is said to be capable of operating independently of changes in renal perfusion pressure. Under conditions of increased delivery of filtered sodium to the macula densa, such feedback may occur to the juxtaglomerular apparatus, resulting in a release of increasing quantities of angiotensin, which could then be capable of decreasing glomerular filtration rate, thereby reducing the filtered load of sodium (hypothesis of Thurau). The evidence for the hypothesis is conflicting.

The pressor response to infused or circulating angiotensin is conditioned by at least two factors: (1) it is inversely related to the circulating levels of angiotensin; (2) it is modified by the concentration of plasma sodium. Pressor response is dampened by a decrease in plasma sodium concentration.

Glucocorticoid Physiology

The division of adrenal steroids into glucocorticoids and mineralocorticoids is somewhat arbitrary in that most glucocorticoids have some mineralocorticoid-like properties, and vice versa. The descriptive term *glucocorticoid* is applied to those adrenal steroids having a predominant action on intermediary metabolism. The principal glucocorticoid is cortisol (hydrocortisone). The actions of the glucocorticoids on intermediary metabolism include the regulation of protein, carbohydrate, lipid, and nucleic acid metabolism. Their actions appear mainly to be catabolic in effect, with an increased protein breakdown and nitrogen excretion. Glucocorticoids also increase hepatic glycogen content by increasing hepatic glucose synthesis. This is brought about by increasing the quantity of intermediary metabolites, especially those derived from glycogenic amino acids. Hepatic trapping and deamination of amino acids derived from peripheral supporting structures, such as bone, skin, muscle, and connective tissue, appears to be essential to the process. The increased mobilization of protein results in increased plasma amino acid levels and increased urinary nitrogen excretion. Glucocorticoids are capable of directly increasing the level of specific hepatic enzymes, such as tryptophan pyrrolase and tyrosine-α-ketoglutarate transaminase. The elevated levels of these hepatic enzymes can influence the balance of serum amino acids, which in turn can be responsible for diminished protein metabolism and subsequent cytolysis of lymphoid tissues and muscle. Cortisol enhances the release of free fatty acids from adipose tissue during fasting or adrenergic stimulation. The action of cortisol on structural protein and adipose tissue varies considerably in different parts of the body. For example, depletion of protein matrix of the vertebral column may be striking, whereas long-bone structure may be affected only minimally; peripheral adipose tissue may diminish, whereas abdominal and interscapular fat may accumulate. Cortisol has a major effect on body water in both its distribution and its excretion. It subserves the extracellular fluid volume by a retarding action on the inward migration of water into cells. It affects renal water excretion in a dual manner, by increasing the rate of glomerular filtration and by a direct action on the renal tubule, both of which summate to increase solute-free water clearance. Glucocorticoids, in general, will increase renal tubular sodium reabsorption and cause an increased urine potassium excretion. Cortisol is also necessary for normal vascular reactivity, ensuring the response of vascular smooth muscle to circulating vasoconstrictor factors. The glucocorticoids have significant anti-inflammatory effects, producing lysis of lymphoid tissues and diminishing circulating eosinophils. Some of these actions may be due to the ability of the glucocorticoids to stabilize lysosomal membranes. In this way, cortisol can suppress the release of acid hydrolases which are stored within the lysosomes. The integrity of personality is enhanced by cortisol, and emotional disorders are common with either excesses or deficits of cortisol. Lastly, cortisol is the major determinant of pituitary ACTH release by its direct effect on the hypothalamic corticotropin-releasing center.

Mineralocorticoid Physiology

Three major mineralocorticoids are produced by the human adrenal cortex: 11-deoxycorticosterone (DOC), corticosterone, and aldosterone. DOC and corticosterone are the immediate precursors in the biosynthetic pathway for aldosterone, and the production of DOC and corticosterone is governed by ACTH levels. Production rates for these hormones on a normal sodium intake are DOC, 50 to 250 μg per day; corticosterone, 900 to 4,500 μg per day; and aldosterone, 50 to 250 μg per day. The effects of these various mineralocorticoids on sodium and potassium metabolism are indistinguishable, but the potency of aldosterone is much greater than that of the other compounds. For this reason, aldosterone is considered the principal mineralocorticoid.

Aldosterone has two important physiologic functions: (1) it is the prime regulator of extracellular fluid volume, and (2) it is a major determinant of potassium metabolism. It regulates volume through a direct effect on the renal tubular transport of sodium. Aldosterone acts predominantly at the site of the distal convoluted tubule, where it accelerates the exchange of tubular sodium ions for secreted potassium and/or hydrogen ions. Aldosterone increases the efficiency of this distal tubular sodium-potassium exchange site. The reabsorbed sodium ions are then transported out of the tubular epithelial cells into the interstitial fluid volume of the kidney and from there into the renal capillary circulation. Since sodium ions are the prime determinant of extracellular fluid volume, aldosterone, through its regulation of renal sodium transport, may be said to be the prime regulator of extracellular fluid volume. Water will passively follow the aldosterone-mediated transported sodium. In effect, through the agency of aldosterone, extracellular fluid can be expanded by a mechanism analogous to an endogenous infusion of normal saline solution.

Aldosterone, under conditions of extracellular fluid volume depletion, also markedly influences the iso-osmotic reabsorption of proximal tubular sodium. Contrariwise, expansion of extracellular fluid volume, with the associated suppression of aldosterone release, will be characterized by a decrease in the percentage of the filtered sodium load reabsorbed by the proximal tubules. A definitive action of aldosterone on the transport of sodium in the ascending limb of Henle has not been clearly documented.

Aldosterone also acts directly on the epithelium of the salivary ducts and sweat glands and on the mucosal cells of the gastrointestinal tract to cause direct reabsorption of sodium in exchange for potassium ions. A direct cellular action, as on muscle cells, of aldosterone has been difficult to prove. It has been reported that in the absence of aldosterone, sodium tends to leave the extracellular fluid base by migrating into cells, onto tendon and bone surfaces, and increasing sodium wasting by the kidneys will occur. The d-isomer of aldosterone is the biologically active form.

There are three well-identified control mechanisms for aldosterone release, and in all probability several as yet undiscovered control systems also exist. The recognized control systems are renin-angiotensin system, potassium, and ACTH. The renin-angiotensin system is the major system for control of extracellular fluid volume, via regulation of aldosterone secretion. In effect, the renin-angiotensin system attempts to maintain circulating blood volume constant by causing increasing aldosterone-induced sodium retention during periods registered as volume deficiencies, and by decreasing aldosterone-dependent sodium retention under conditions in which volume is registered as being ample. In clinical medicine, volume deficits are much more common than volume excesses. Such deficits are repaired by stimulation of the renin-angiotensin-aldosterone system and its consequent effect on the renal retention of sodium and water. Volume regulation in the absence of the renin-angiotensin system (renoprival man) is extremely difficult and is characterized by marked oscillations of blood pressure. Such information documents that the renin-angiotensin system is the major control system for aldosterone-mediated volume regulation.

Potassium ions can regulate aldosterone secretion independently of the renin-angiotensin system. If a solution of potassium ions is injected into the adrenal artery, immediate increase in adrenal venous aldosterone levels can be documented. It appears that potassium has a direct stimulatory effect on adrenocortical production of aldosterone, presumably via a transmembrane effect. Adrenocortical cells act as if they monitor the flux of potassium across their membranes, and under conditions of increased flux to the cell, there is an increase in aldosterone production and release; contrariwise, under conditions of decreased potassium influx, there is a decrease in aldosterone release. This potassium-mediated control system for aldosterone release operates in parallel with the renin-angiotensin system and can be of comparable potency. When the renin-angiotensin system may be impaired, as in acute and chronic renal failure, this potassium-aldosterone control system assumes even greater importance.

Potassium stimulation of aldosterone release may be a protective mechanism against potassium intoxication. When the human organism receives an acute load of potassium, aldosterone release will be stimulated, and the released aldosterone, by accelerating the potassium-sodium distal tubular exchange, will result in increased urinary loss of potassium, thus minimizing the increase in plasma potassium concentration. Under conditions of potassium depletion and hypokalemia, there is a marked diminution in aldosterone production and release. Adrenal responsiveness to potassium stimulation can be potentiated by activation of the renin-angiotensin system through sodium restriction.

ACTH plays a permissive role in aldosterone release. Hypophysectomized patients, or patients with pituitary insufficiency, have a suboptimal aldosterone response to sodium restriction. In normal persons, with ACTH administration, there is an acute rise in aldosterone secretion to levels three to four times above the base line. However, with the continued administration of ACTH, aldosterone production rates return to control levels, providing suggestive evidence that ACTH is not an important control mechanism in day-to-day physiologic conditions. Such a control mechanism would assume importance, however, under conditions of acute stress, burns, hemorrhage, etc. More recently, it has been suggested that there may exist pituitary factors other than ACTH which are necessary

for a maximal adrenal aldosterone response. When normal individuals are given a long-term course of aldosterone (or a comparable mineralocorticoid, such as parenteral DOC), an initial period of sodium retention is followed by a natriuresis, and sodium balance is reestablished. As a result, clinical edema formation does not develop. Thus, with continuous administration of the potent sodium-retaining hormone aldosterone, patients reachieve sodium homeostasis and do not continue to exhibit sodium retention. This phenomenon is referred to as the "escape phenomenon," signifying an "escape" by the renal tubules from the sodium-retaining action of chronically administered aldosterone. The mechanism responsible for the escape phenomenon has remained elusive. It does appear to be dependent on normal renal hemodynamics, and it has been suggested that an as-yet-unidentified natriuretic principle may be involved. Such an "escape" phenomenon is also exhibited by patients with essential hypertension (primary aldosteronism) but is characteristically absent in patients with edema disorders.

Androgen Physiology

The principal adrenal androgens in terms of quantitative secretion are dehydroepiandrosterone (DHEA), androstenedione, and 11-hydroxyandrostenedione. Of these, androstenedione is the major androgen, five times more active than DHEA. Testosterone, which is interconvertible with androstenedione peripherally and which has been isolated from the adrenal gland, exhibits an additional fivefold increase in androgenic potency when compared to androstenedione, pointing up that DHEA, androstenedione, and 11-hydroxyandrostenedione are biologically weak androgens. The release of adrenal androgens is stimulated by ACTH and not by gonadotropins. With ACTH stimulation urine 17-ketosteroids increase but to a much lesser extent than do urine 17-hydroxycorticoids. Part of this increment in 17-ketosteroid excretion is due to the metabolism of the increasing 17-hydroxycorticoids by the mechanism of C-20:C-21 side chain cleavage, producing 11-oxy-17-ketosteroids. Adrenal androgens are suppressed by exogenous glucocorticoid administration, as judged by decrements in urine 17-ketosteroid excretion. Additional specific control mechanisms for adrenal androgen release may exist independently of the ACTH system.

The major effects of these androgenic hormones are on protein metabolism and on secondary sexual characteristics. Androgens increase the synthesis of protein from amino acids, and this anabolic action leads to increased muscle mass and strength. Linear growth is accelerated by androgens prior to epiphyseal closure, which is hastened by androgen excess. The secondary sexual characteristics are affected through inhibition of the female characteristics (defeminization) and accentuation of the male characteristics (masculinization). These are seen clinically as hirsutism and virilization in the female with amenorrhea, atrophy of breasts and uterus, enlargement of the clitoris, deepening of the voice, acne, increased muscle mass, increased heterosexual drive, and receding hairline. In the male there are increased body and sexual hair and enlargement of the sexual organs.

The bioassay of androgens has been largely replaced by more specific analytic techniques, such as double isotope derivative analysis using S-35 thiosemicarbazide, electron capture gas-liquid chromatography, and competitive protein-binding radioassay. The first two techniques require a great deal of biochemical and electronic sophistication in order to achieve reliable results. However, the competitive protein-binding method requires fewer technical skills and, therefore, may become the more practical way of determining adrenal androgen levels.

LABORATORY EVALUATION OF ADRENOCORTICAL FUNCTION
Blood Levels

ACTH. Before 1964, blood ACTH levels were determined by bioassay preparations. However, since then it has been possible in a number of laboratories to determine ACTH by radioimmunoassay. Problems of specificity and sensitivity have limited the general application of this technique. Plasma ACTH levels show a diurnal cycle, with lower blood levels detected in late afternoon and early evening. In normal man, the morning ACTH concentration is between 0 and 10 mμg per ml.

ANGIOTENSIN–RENIN. Chemical measurements of plasma angiotensin levels have been attempted, but because of problems of extraction and precise chemical identity, such methods have been largely abandoned. Radioimmune assays for angiotensin are being developed by the production of antibodies to the octapeptide angiotensin-II by linkage to a larger molecule, such as albumin or poly-1-lysine. By such methods, values for normal subjects on a low salt diet have been found to be supine, 40 $\mu\mu$g per ml; upright, 60 $\mu\mu$g per ml.

Measurements of the enzyme renin are made by several laboratories utilizing a purified renin substrate. The majority of clinical determinations of the renin-angiotensin system, however, involve measurements of peripheral "plasma renin activity" (PRA) in which the renin activity is gauged by the generation of angiotensin during a standardized incubation period. This method depends on the presence of sufficient angiotensinogen in the patient's plasma as substrate. The generated angiotensin then is measured in a standardized rat pressor bioassay. Plasma renin activity levels will depend on dietary intake of the patient and whether or not the patient is ambulatory. Values for resting supine patients on a normal salt intake range between 100 to 300 (angiotensin produced, mμg/ml/4 hr).

CORTISOL. Blood levels of cortisol can be measured in a number of ways; the most sensitive of these is the double isotope derivative technique. However, the level of plasma cortisol determined by competitive protein-binding radioassay also appears to be reliable. A less-sensitive and specific method is measuring Porter-Silber

chromogens in the blood by a fluorimetric technique. The morning plasma levels of 17-hydroxycorticoids range between 10 and 20 μg per 100 ml. These blood levels exhibit a marked diurnal pattern, with highest values between 6 and 8 A.M. and the lowest value at 10 P.M. to 12 midnight.

ALDOSTERONE. Because of the minute quantities of plasma aldosterone present, it has been difficult to determine it directly. Only a few laboratories, utilizing double isotope dilution techniques, can measure peripheral plasma levels. On normal salt intake, the values range from 5 to 15 mμg per 100 ml.

ANDROGENS. Testosterone in plasma has been measured by isotopic and competitive protein-binding means; the range for nonhirsute females is 30 to 100 and for males 400 to 1,000 mμg per 100 ml.

Urine Levels

The principal determinations are of urine 17-hydroxycorticoids, 17-ketosteroids, 17-ketogenic steroids, free cortisol, and aldosterone. The urine 17-hydroxycorticoids are determined as Porter-Silber chromogens, i.e., these steroids react with the reagent phenylhydrazine to produce a characteristic color. This reaction is specific for steroids with a "dihydroxy acetone" C-17 side chain, i.e., with hydroxyl groups on C-17 and C-21 and a ketone group on C-20 (Fig. 92-7). Therefore, this determination will include cortisol, cortisone, tetrahydrocortisol, tetrahydrocortisone, and 11-dexoycortisol but not cortols, cortolones, and pregnanetriol. Normal values for 24 hr range from 1 to 10 mg per day, with daytime (7 A.M. to 7 P.M.) excretion exceeding night values (7 P.M. to 7 A.M.). It is of extreme importance that the completeness of any and all urine steroid collections be checked by urine creatinine determinations.

The urine 17-ketosteroids are those containing a ketone group at C-17; two-thirds of these originate from the adrenal gland and the remainder from the testes. Their measurement depends on the Zimmerman reaction, whereby color is produced when 17-ketosteroids are condensed with m-dinitrobenzene. This reaction is specific for steroids with a ketone substituent with an adjacent unsubstituted carbon atom. The major urine 17-ketosteroids are dehydroepiandrosterone, epiandrosterone, androsterone, etiocholanolone, 11-oxoetiocholanolone, 11-hydroxyetiocholanolone, and 11-hydroxyandrosterone (Fig. 92-8). Normal values for males range between 7 and 25 mg per day and for females between 5 and 15 mg per day. The diurnal pattern for 17-ketosteroid excretion is definite but less accentuated than that for 17-hydroxysteroids. Urine 17-ketosteroid values are highest in young adults and decline with age.

The total urine 17-ketosteroids may be subdivided into those having either an oxygen or hydroxyl substituent at position C-11 (11-oxy-17-ketosteroids) and those having no such groups (11-deoxy-17-ketosteroids). The 11-oxy-17-ketosteroids include 11-oxoetiocholanolone, 11-hydroxyetiocholanolone, and 11-hydroxyandrosterone. These

11-oxy-17-ketosteroids are uniquely derived from the adrenal gland, since other tissues do not possess the enzymes for active C-11 hydroxylation, whereas the 11-deoxy-17-ketosteroids may arise from adrenal, testicular, and ovarian tissue.

Ketogenic steroids is a descriptive term for those C-21 hydroxycorticoids potentially capable of transformation into 17-ketosteroids in vitro. After the excreted 17-ketosteroids are reduced to noninterfering compounds, the side chains of C-21 hydroxycorticosteroids are oxidized to 17-ketonic groups, which then can be measured by the Zimmermann reaction as 17-ketosteroids. The Norymberski technique for ketogenic steroid analysis is specific for compounds containing the following groups:

17-HYDROXY-CORTICOIDS (Porter-Silber chromogens)

17-KETO-STEROIDS (Zimmerman reaction)

17-KETOGENIC-STEROIDS (Norymberski technique)

Fig. 92-7. Key reactive groups (enclosed by dashed circle) in urine steroid determinations.

17,21-dihydroxy-20-keto; 17,20,21-trihydroxy-; and 17,20-dihydroxy-21-deoxy-. It may be seen that the first of these groupings represents those compounds capable of reacting as *Porter-Silber chromogens;* the second, or trihydroxy, grouping would include the cortols and the cortolones; and the third, or 21-deoxy, grouping would include pregnanetriol. Thus, urine 17-ketogenic steroid determination includes all steroids determined as 17-hydroxysteroids by the Porter-Silber method and, in addition, includes the cortols, cortolones, and pregnanetriol. The normal range for urine **17-ketogenic steroids** is 5 to 20 mg per day.

11-DEOXY-17-KETOSTEROIDS

Dehydroepiandrosterone

Androsterone

Etiocholanolone

Epiandrosterone

11-OXY-17-KETOSTEROIDS

11-Oxo-etiocholanolone

11-Hydroxy-etiocholanolone

11-Oxo-androsterone

11-Hydroxy-androsterone

Fig. 92-8. Principal urine 17-ketosteroids, 11-oxy-17-ketosteroids derived from the adrenal glands.

The determination of either urine free cortisol or aldosterone excretion is more difficult, usually requiring double isotope derivative techniques. Urinary free cortisol may also be determined by partition chromatography or competitive protein-binding radioassay. Normal subjects excrete less than 100 μg per day.

Aldosterone excretion rate is tested by determining the excretion of a major metabolite, usually the acid-labile conjugate. A carefully timed urine collection is a prerequisite for all excretory determinations. Normal values for the 24-hr aldosterone excretion rate range between 2 and 10 μg.

Steroid Secretion Rates

The basic assumption in the interpretation of urine steroid values is that excreted adrenal steroid metabolites (17-hydroxycorticoids, 17-ketogenic steroids) accurately reflect adrenal secretory rates of that steroid (cortisol). Measurement of the actual adrenal secretory rate of a given steroid would, of course, be preferable, and such methods are finding increasing clinical application. The adrenal secretory rate is calculated by the dilution that an administered radioactive steroid undergoes as a consequence of the admixture of endogenously secreted nonradioactive steroid hormone with the exogenous radioactive steroid. In practice, a major metabolite of the steroid is isolated and purified by chromatography; from a determination of its specific activity (counts per minute per microgram of steroid) and knowledge of the specific activity of the administered steroid one may calculate by the dilution principle the actual amount of the steroid secreted by the adrenal gland during the period of urine collection (usually 24 hr). Such secretory rate determinations have been standardized for cortisol and aldosterone. The average daily cortisol secretory rate determined by such methods is 8 to 30 mg per day, and the average aldosterone secretory rate 50 to 250 μg per day on a normal sodium intake.

The determination of secretion rates of the adrenal androgens is complicated by two facts: most androgens are derived from two different sources (adrenals and gonads), and they are readily interconvertible after secretion. Because of this, classic secretory techniques are probably not applicable. Instead, androgen production rates are usually determined by the use of metabolic clearance rates and plasma concentrations of the particular steroid. Because these methods are more cumbersome, less information has been obtained about androgen metabolism.

Stimulation Tests

Stimulation tests are useful in documenting the existence of a hormonal deficiency state. A standardized and specific stimulus for the production and release of a given hormone is applied, and the quantity of the released hormone is then measured.

GLUCOCORTICOID STIMULATION TESTS. Within minutes after initiating an infusion of ACTH, increased cortisol levels are noted in adrenal venous blood. This responsiveness of the adrenal gland to ACTH is utilized as an index of the "functional reserve" of the gland to produce cortisol. Under maximal ACTH stimulation the cortisol secretion increases tenfold to 300 mg per day. Such maximal stimulation is obtainable only with prolonged ACTH infusions. For clinical purposes, the functional adrenal reserve for cortisol production is standardized with a shorter infusion time (8 hr). The standard intravenous ACTH test is performed by administering 40 units of aqueous ACTH in 500 ml normal saline solution intravenously over an exact 8-hr interval (from 8 A.M. to 4 P.M.) on two successive days and collecting the complete 24-hr urine output for analysis of creatinine, 17-hydroxycorticoids (or 17-ketogenic steroids), and 17-ketosteroids. The patient may be ambulatory during this period. With such a method of testing, an average increment of 15 mg (range, 5 to 25) has been noted in urine 17-hydroxysteroids on the first day of testing and an average increment of 25 mg (range, 15 to 35) on the second infusion day, by one commonly used method. Much smaller rises in urine 17-ketosteroid excretion are noted, with average increments of 4 to 8 mg per day on the first and second day of testing, respectively. In the performance of the test the duration of the infusion must be strictly adhered to. Screening tests utilizing the intramuscular injection of ACTH (40 to 80 units twice daily) have been employed and offer the occasional advantage of ease of performance, but they have a more serious disadvantage in that the responses often vary because of irregular absorption of the ACTH from the injection site.

Occasionally it is necessary to prolong the ACTH infusion in order to separate primary from secondary adrenal insufficiency. This can be accomplished by using an 8-hr infusion on four or five consecutive days or by a continuous 48-hr infusion. The 48-hr infusion is given as 80 units of ACTH in 1,000 ml 5 percent dextrose in water or dextrose in normal saline every 24 hr for two consecutive days. Fluid retention due to the contamination of most commercial preparations of ACTH with ADH is a problem in some patients.

MINERALOCORTICOID STIMULATION TESTS. Standardized aldosterone stimulation tests have been devised utilizing a protocol of programmed volume depletion. Volume depletion may be engendered by sodium restriction, diuretic administration, or venesection. The simplest stimulation test involves the modality of sodium restriction. The patient is placed on a constant diet containing 200 mEq sodium and 100 mEq potassium, with defined physical activity. After a 5-day equilibration period on this diet, dietary sodium intake is abruptly lowered to 10 mEq per day and held constant. The diet-physical activity program is left unchanged. After 3 to 5 days of such sodium deprivation, aldosterone secretion rates (or excretion rates) should exhibit a two- to threefold increase.

Stimulation tests may also be carried out by the administration of a potent diuretic, such as ethacrynic acid or furosemide, with measurements of aldosterone secretion being made on the day preceding, the day of, and the day after diuretic administration. The diuretic is administered throughout a 24-hr period in doses sufficient to cause an increase in urine output (over control) of

1,500 ml and/or a weight loss of 3 lb in 24 hr. The test may be carried out while the patient has a high or low sodium intake. Again, a two-to threefold rise in aldosterone production should be observed. The difficulty with this testing procedure is that the diuretic will induce variable losses of potassium, which will tend to dampen the hypersecretion of aldosterone that otherwise would have occurred for a corresponding degree of volume depletion.

Hemorrhage, either functional or induced, may also be used as an aldosterone-stimulating test. As measurements of plasma aldosterone become available, this may become the preferred method of stimulating the aldosterone system via the renin-angiotensin mechanism. Functional hemorrhage may be tested by making measurements of plasma aldosterone before and after 4 to 5 hr of ambulation. There is a minimum of three- to sixfold rise in plasma aldosterone levels under such conditions, which is presumably a response to transthoracic volume depletion which occurs with assumption of the upright position. Aldosterone secretion or excretion rates can be made on the day before and the day of acute venesection, with withdrawal of 400 to 600 ml of venous blood over a period of 30 to 40 min. The normal response is a two-fold rise in aldosterone secretion/excretion.

Because of adverse effects on the coronary circulation, angiotensin infusions have not found favor as a means of performing tests of adrenal aldosterone responsiveness.

Suppression Tests

Suppression tests are used to document hypersecretion of adrenocortical hormones and are based on the demonstration of a decrease in the target hormone following standardized suppression of its tropic hormone. Thus, suppression testing for cortisol hypersecretion would involve suppression of ACTH release, with the documentation of an appropriately normal decrease in cortisol production, while suppression testing of aldosterone would involve demonstration of a decrease in aldosterone secondary to suppression of the renin-angiotensin system.

GLUCOCORTICOID SUPPRESSION TESTS. The hypothalamic-pituitary ACTH release mechanism is sensitive to the circulating blood level of glucocorticoids. When such blood levels are increased in the normal individual, the corticotropin-releasing center decreases its production of the corticotropin-releasing factor (CRF), and consequently less ACTH is released from the anterior pituitary; secondarily, less steroid will be produced by the adrenal gland. The integrity of this feedback mechanism can be tested clinically by giving a potent glucocorticoid and judging suppression of the corticotropin-releasing center by analysis of urine steroid excretory values. A potent glucocorticoid such as dexamethasone is utilized in order that the administered compound may be given in such small amounts that it will not contribute significantly to the steroids to be analyzed.

One or more of three standard tests are usually employed. The simplest is the overnight dexamethasone suppression test. This involves the measurement of plasma corticoid levels at 8 A.M. and/or the urine 17-hydroxycorticoid and creatinine excretion between 7 A.M. and 12 noon following the oral administration of 1 mg dexamethasone the previous midnight. The 8 A.M. value for plasma corticoids in normal subjects should be less than 10 μg per 100 ml, and the ratio of urine Porter-Silber chromogens per milligram of creatinine in the 5-hr urine specimen should be less than 0.004.

The usual method of testing adrenal suppressibility is to administer 0.5 mg dexamethasone every 6 hr for two successive days while collecting urine over a 24-hr period for determination of creatinine, 17-hydroxysteroids, and 17-ketosteroids. In patients with a normal hypothalamic-pituitary ACTH release mechanism, a fall in the urine 17-hydroxycorticoids to less than 3 mg a day on the second day of dexamethasone administration is seen.

An intravenous dexamethasone suppression test is used less often. One milligram of dexamethasone is administered intravenously per hour for a total of 3 hr, and blood is collected for plasma glucocorticoid determinations. A 50 percent fall in plasma cortisol at the end of 3 hr of infusion is normally expected. Normal response to any of the suppression tests implies that the ACTH control of the adrenal glands is physiologically normal. However, an isolated abnormal result, particularly when the overnight suppression test is being used, does not in itself imply pituitary and/or adrenal disease.

MINERALOCORTICOID SUPPRESSION TESTS. Mineralocorticoid suppression testing procedures have been devised using saline infusions, oral salt loading, or DOCA administration as the means for expansion of the extracellular fluid volume. With expansion of extracellular fluid volume, there will be a decrease in renal renin release, a decrease in circulating plasma renin activity, and a decrease in aldosterone secretion and/or excretion. This would be the appropriate "normal" response. Varied tests differ in the rate at which extracellular fluid volume is expanded. The "normal saline suppression test" involves the intravenous administration of 2 liters of normal saline solution over a 4-hr period from 9 A.M. until 1 P.M. on two consecutive days. Aldosterone secretion or excretion rate is measured the day before and on the second day of saline loading. The patient previously has been permitted to come into equilibration on a 10 mEq sodium/100 mEq potassium constant diet. Normal response of suppression of aldosterone secretion by this maneuver is to a value of less than 200 μg per day. The "oral salt-loading suppression test" is conveniently carried out by abruptly increasing the patient's sodium intake from a constant level of 10 mEq per day to 200 mEq per day for a period of 3 to 5 days, with measurements of aldosterone secretion on the fourth or fifth day, at which time a 24-hr secretion rate should be less than 200 μg per day. Potassium intake is held constant throughout the test, since potassium will cause aldosterone secretion to vary independently of the renin-angiotensin system. The "DOCA suppression test" is carried out by placing the patient on a normal (100 mEq) or high (200 mEq) sodium intake. After the patient is in sodium balance, deoxycorticosterone acetate is administered intramuscularly

(10 mg every 12 hr) for a period of 3 to 5 days. Normal subjects on a sodium intake of 100 mEq daily demonstrate a 70 percent decrease in aldosterone excretion rate, when compared with control levels, which means that the aldosterone excretory value should be less than 5 μg per day.

Test of Pituitary Responsiveness

A number of stimuli, such as insulin hypoglycemia, arginine vasopressin, and pyrogen, will cause release of ACTH from the pituitary by an action on higher nerve centers, the hypothalamus, or the pituitary gland itself. By measuring plasma ACTH, or urine or blood glucocorticoids, the status of pituitary ACTH can be evaluated.

Metyrapone [SU4835 (Metopirone)] is a drug that selectively inhibits the enzyme action of 11-beta-hydroxylase in the adrenal gland. As a result, the conversion of 11-deoxycortisol (Compound S) to cortisol is interfered with and increased amounts of 11-deoxycortisol accumulate while blood levels of cortisol decrease (Fig. 92-2). Since 11-deoxycortisol is a weak suppressor of the hypothalamic-pituitary axis, the anterior pituitary responds to the declining cortisol blood levels by releasing larger quantities of ACTH in an attempt to stimulate the adrenal gland to release additional cortisol, which attempt, however, is thwarted by the metyrapone-induced enzymatic blockade. The metabolites of 11-deoxycortisol are excreted in increasing amounts in the urine, where they are measured as 17-hydroxycorticoids. *Note that the adrenal glands must be capable of being stimulated by ACTH, since assessment of the response depends on adrenal steroid production.*

The metyrapone response has been standardized for clinical evaluation of the reserve capacity of the anterior pituitary gland to release ACTH. Every 4 hr over a 48-hr period 750 mg metyrapone is administered orally, and daily urine collections for 17-hydroxycorticosteroids are obtained the day before testing, the 2 days of testing, and the day after the last dose of metyrapone. The peak response of increased urine 17-hydroxysteroid excretion may be seen on the day after completion of metyrapone administration, and normal individuals will respond with at least a doubling of their basal 17-hydroxysteroid excretion.

Tests for Renin Responsiveness

Attempts have been made to standardize measurement of renin responsiveness by the acute induction of volume depletion and/or hypotension. Acute hypotension, induced either by diazoxide or by hydralazine, has been tried, but the results have been variable. Standardization has been improved by controlled volume depletion, induced by diuretics or by the assumption of the upright position. Diuretic-induced volume depletion is limited by patient-to-patient variability to the same dose of diuretic.

The most widely accepted test, suggested by Conn, is based on postural augmentation of plasma renin activity. This test involves determination of plasma renin activity in the supine patient before and immediately following 4 hr of ambulation. The normal response is a two- to threefold rise in plasma renin activity. In normal persons, a diurnal rhythm for plasma renin activity is characterized by peak values occurring between 10 A.M. and 12 noon, with decreases in activity in the afternoon.

HYPERFUNCTION OF THE ADRENAL CORTEX

Distinct clinical syndromes are produced when excess amounts of the principal adrenocortical hormones are secreted. Thus, excess production of the principal glucocorticoid cortisol is associated with Cushing's syndrome; excess production of the principal mineralocorticoid aldosterone with clinical and chemical signs of aldosteronism; excess production of adrenal androgens with adrenal virilism. As would be expected, these syndromes do not always occur in the "pure" form but may have overlapping features.

Cushing's Syndrome

From an analysis of the clinical and pathologic findings in a series of 12 patients, Harvey Cushing, in 1932, established a syndrome characterized by truncal obesity, hypertension, fatigability and weakness, amenorrhea, hirsutism, purplish abdominal striae, edema, glucosuria, and osteoporosis. As knowledge of this syndrome increased and as clinical tests of adrenocortical function became standardized and readily available, the diagnosis of Cushing's syndrome has been broadened into the following classification:

CAUSES OF CUSHING'S SYNDROME

I. *Adrenal hyperplasia,* 70 percent of cases
   A. Secondary to hypothalamic dysfunction
   B. Secondary to ACTH-producing tumors
      1. Pituitary tumors
      2. Nonendocrine tumors (bronchogenic carcinoma)
II. *Adrenal adenoma,* 15 percent of cases
III. *Adrenal carcinoma,* 10 percent of cases
IV. *Exogenous,* iatrogenic
   A. Prolonged use of glucocorticoids
   B. Prolonged use of ACTH

It is apparent that, regardless of etiology, all cases of Cushing's syndrome are due to increased production of cortisol by the adrenal gland. The majority of cases are due to *bilateral adrenal hyperplasia,* in which the adrenal gland weight usually exceeds the normal combined total weight of 10 Gm. Harvey Cushing originally postulated that the adrenal hyperplasia in these patients was attributable to the presence of pituitary basophilic adenomas. However, many cases are found without basophilic adenomas. Some are due to ACTH-producing chromophobe adenomas, but these cases represent a small fraction of the total. In the remaining cases attention has focused also on the elaboration of increased amounts of ACTH in the absence of pituitary tumors, possibly as a result of hypothalamic dysfunction, whereby the cortico-tropin-releasing center is reset to respond to a higher level of circulating cortisol. Proof of such a theory may now be possible with the availability of sensitive methods for determining plasma ACTH. Such cases of Cushing's syndrome due to adrenal hyperplasia, presumably due to excessive ACTH stimulation, always affect both adrenal glands.

In some 15 percent of cases of Cushing's syndrome, unilateral *adrenal adenomas* are found. On occasion they may occur bilaterally. These adenomas may or may not function in autonomous manner; i.e., they may or may not be independent of ACTH stimulation and control. In addition, approximately 10 percent of cases of Cushing's syndrome are associated with *adrenal carcinomas*, most often unilateral and most often functioning autonomously. In those cases of Cushing's syndrome due to unilateral adrenal adenomas or carcinomas functioning independently of ACTH, atrophy of the contralateral gland is often found, attributable to suppression of ACTH release by the high levels of cortisol secreted by the tumors. A small number of patients with Cushing's syndrome are found to have *adrenal rest tumors*, i.e., aberrant adrenocortical tissue occurring outside the adrenal gland. These embryologic remnants may be in the perirenal area, ovaries, or testes and exhibit histologic features of hyperplastic or adenomatous changes.

Nonendocrine tumors secreting polypeptide fractions that have an ACTH-like action are also occasionally responsible for Cushing's syndrome secondary to bilateral adrenal hyperplasia. The major association of a nonendocrine tumor has been with primitive "oat-cell" carcinomas of the lung. Hypokalemic alkalosis is often prominent in such cases, whereas many of the distinctive physical findings usually associated with Cushing's syndrome may be absent.

INCIDENCE. As steroid analyses have become more available, increasing numbers of patients with Cushing's syndrome are being detected among persons undergoing evaluation for such diverse entities as diabetes mellitus, hypertension, obesity, and osteoporosis. Many of these patients exhibit mild degrees of adrenal hyperfunction. The incidence of Cushing's syndrome in the female is three times that in the male. The most frequent age of onset is the third or fourth decade.

CLINICAL SIGNS AND SYMPTOMS. The frequency of clinical findings is listed in Table 92-1. Knowledge of

Table 92-1. INCIDENCE OF SIGNS AND SYMPTOMS IN 35 CASES OF CUSHING'S SYNDROME, PERCENT

Typical habitus	97	Amenorrhea	77
Increased body weight	94	Cutaneous striae	67
Fatigability and weakness	87	Personality changes	66
		Ecchymoses	65
Hypertension (above 150/90)	82	Edema	62
		Polyuria, polydipsia	23
Hirsutism	80	Hypertrophy of clitoris	19

the physiologic effects of glucocorticoids shows that many of the signs and symptoms logically follow. As a result of mobilization of peripheral supportive tissue, there are muscle weakness and fatigability, osteoporosis, and cutaneous striae. The latter involve a weakening and rupture of collagenous fibers in the dermis, so that the heavily vascularized subcutaneous tissues are exposed. Likewise, because of the loss of perivascular supporting tissue, there is easy bruisability, and ecchymoses often appear at sites of mild trauma. The osteoporosis may be so severe that collapse of vertebral bodies and pathologic fractures of other bones are frequently encountered. As a result of increased hepatic gluconeogenesis from these mobilized precursors, there may be frank diabetes with polydipsia and polyuria. More frequently, with the presence of an adequate reserve of insulin, there is deposition of this excess glucose in fat depots. This is observed most notably in the upper part of the face, the classic "moon" facies; in the interscapular area, the "buffalo" hump; and in the mesenteric bed, where it produces the classic "truncal" obesity (Fig. 92-9). Rarely, there may be episternal fatty tumors and mediastinal widening secondary to fat accumulation. The reason for this peculiar distribution of lipid is not known. The face also appears plethoric, even in the absence of any increase in red blood cell concentration. Hypertension is most always present, and frequently there are profound emotional changes, ranging from irritability or emotional lability to severe depression, confusion, or even frank psychosis. Acne and hirsutism are frequent in female patients, hirsutism often appearing as a fine "downy" coat over the face, forehead, and upper part of the trunk. Likewise in women patients, oligomenorrhea or amenorrhea is a frequent disturbance.

LABORATORY FINDINGS. With rare exceptions, plasma and urinary 17-hydroxycorticoid levels are elevated. Cir-

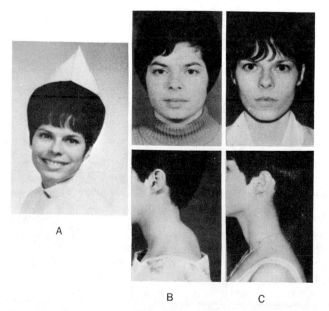

Fig. 92-9. A twenty-year-old female with Cushing's syndrome due to a right adrenal cortical adenoma: *A*, 2 years prior to surgery, age eighteen; *B*, 1 month prior to surgery, age twenty; and *C*, 1 year after surgery, age twenty-one.

culing eosinophils are below 100 cells per cu mm in 90 percent of cases, and patients characteristically show a mild neutrophilic leukocytosis. In spite of markedly plethoric facies, the hematocrit is usually within the normal range, but occasionally erythemia with higher hematocrits is encountered, particularly when the syndrome is associated with excessive production of 17-ketosteroids. Serum sodium concentration is usually normal; however, with marked excess secretion of cortisol, there may be hypokalemia, hypochloremia, and metabolic alkalosis. More than three-fourths of patients exhibit intermittent glucosuria, and nearly all have a decreased rate of disappearance of infused glucose from the circulation. Some patients may have frank diabetes, necessitating insulin therapy. X-ray studies usually reveal generalized osteoporosis, most marked in the spine and pelvis, but also frequently found in the skull, with disappearance of the lamina dura, and fractures are often seen in the ribs and vertebras. Intravenous pyelography and laminograms with or without retroperitoneal insufflation may demonstrate

adrenal enlargement, particularly when an adenoma or carcinoma is the pathologic cause of the disease. More sophisticated x-ray techniques, such as selective adrenal arteriography or venography, may make the localization and diagnosis more specific. However, in many cases, these sophisticated procedures are probably not necessary, particularly since they are not without risk. The increased friability of the adrenal veins in Cushing's syndrome makes venography particularly hazardous.

DIAGNOSIS. The diagnosis of Cushing's syndrome depends on the direct or indirect demonstration of increased cortisol production in the absence of stress. Once this is established, further testing is carried out to determine whether or not the excess cortisol is being produced in an autonomous manner, since such knowledge will permit a more specific etiologic diagnosis.

For initial screening purposes, 24-hr urine 17-hydroxy- and 17-ketosteroid determinations are carried out, since values in excess of 10 mg per day for urine 17-hydroxysteroids (Porter-Silber) justifies further evaluation (Ta-

Table 92-2. LABORATORY EVALUATION AND TESTING OF ADRENOCORTICAL FUNCTION IN NORMAL SUBJECTS AND IN PATIENTS WITH CUSHING'S SYNDROME*

Normal values	Plasma ACTH	Plasma cortisol	Cortisol secretory rate	Urine values		Control base line	Days of ACTH stimulation		Days of dexamethasone suppression, mg q 6h			
									0.5		2.0	
							1	2	1	2	1	2
	N	N	N	17-OH	:	1–10	18–40	25–50	1–6	0–3	0–3	0–3
	N	N	N	17-KS	:	5–25	15–30	20–40	6–18	5–15	4–12	4–8
Cushing's syndrome:												
Hyperplasia.................	N–I	I	I	17-OH	:	15	50	90	12	10	8	5
				17-KS	:	20	50	90	18	15	12	10
Adenoma:												
Complete autonomy........	D	I	I	17-OH	:	30	30	30	30	30	30	30
				17-KS	:	12	14	18	12	10	8	6
Incomplete autonomy..............	N–D	I	I	17-OH	:	15	50	90	15	15	12	10
				17-KS	:	12	14	16	12	10	10	10
Carcinoma:												
Adrenal.................	D	I	I	17-OH	:	50	50	50	50	50	50	50
				17-KS	:	60	60	60	60	60	60	60
Extraadrenal (ACTH-producing tumor)	I	I	I	17-OH	:	30	65	80	30	30	30	30
				17-KS	:	25	55	70	25	25	25	25
Exogenous steroids (iatrogenic)	D	D	D	17-OH	:	1	1	2	1	1	1	1
				17-KS	:	4	5	6	5	4	4	4

* Clinical status charted vertically and *representative* values for steroid tests charted horizontally. 17-OH, 17-KS refer to 24-hr urine 17-hydroxycorticosteroid and 17-ketosteroid excretion. 17-KS base-line excretion higher in males than in females. All laboratory values given in milligrams per day. Urine ketogenic steroid values will be approximately twofold greater than those listed for urine 17-OH (except in adrenogenital syndrome). See text for normal blood steroid values. Note that only in the iatrogenic form of Cushing's syndrome are both the plasma ACTH and plasma cortisol levels decreased. ACTH stimulation causes brisk rise in *both* 17-OH and 17-KS in hyperplasia; disproportionate rise in 17-OH in adenoma; and no change in steroid excretion in adrenal carcinoma. Dexamethasone suppression is usually incomplete at the 2-mg daily dosage level in hyperplasia but complete with 8-mg dosage; incomplete at both 2- and 8-mg daily dosage in both adenomas and carcinomas with complete autonomy; incomplete in Cushing's syndrome secondary to extraadrenal ACTH-producing tumors. Abbreviations: N = normal; I = increased; D = decreased.

ble 92-2). An ancillary screening procedure is to determine the diurnal excretion pattern for urine 17-hydroxysteroids by collecting urine between 7 A.M. and 7 P.M. and 7 P.M. to 7 A.M. The patient with Cushing's syndrome will generally excrete an equivalent or greater amount of the 17-hydroxysteroids in the night collection, in contrast to most normal subjects. Creatinine determinations are of critical importance to demonstrate the accuracy and adequacy of the collection procedure. An adult female excretes approximately 1,000 mg creatinine daily, with about 50 to 60 percent found in the daytime collection; an adult male excretes approximately 1,800 mg daily. Day-to-day variation in creatinine excretion by a patient should not exceed 20 percent. If it is demonstrated that the diurnal cycle for steroid excretion is "reversed," i.e., night urine 17-hydroxysteroids are almost equal to or greater than daytime excretion, one then knows that excessive cortisol is being released continuously "around the clock." These urine steroid determinations, which reflect the metabolites of cortisol, are indirect but adequate proof of excessive cortisol production. A direct method is available utilizing radioisotopic cortisol to determine the actual cortisol secretory rate, which in cases of Cushing's syndrome is in excess of 30 mg per day. Another method of direct confirmation of excess cortisol is the determination of the free cortisol in the urine, which reflects the active free cortisol in the blood. Normal persons excrete less than 100 μg daily of free cortisol, whereas patients with Cushing's syndrome may excrete up to ten times this amount. The sensitivity of this urine free cortisol test resides in the fact that only free cortisol of the plasma is freely filtrable at the glomerulus, and thus increments in the plasma level of this biologically active form are magnified in terms of urine excretory values.

Owing to a marked diurnal variability plasma 17-hydroxycorticoid determinations are not meaningful when performed in isolated fashion, but demonstration that the expected normal fall in late afternoon blood levels does not occur is increasingly used as a diagnostic measure. Normally, the plasma level declines by half or more; if such a decrease is not noted, one assumes that continuous hypersecretion of cortisol is occurring.

An additional screening procedure involves the use of the rapid dexamethasone suppression test.

Specific diagnosis of the type of lesion causing Cushing's syndrome can usually be made by the combined use of ACTH-stimulation and dexamethasone-suppression tests. Adrenal hyperplasia, whether caused by hypothalamic dysfunction or by an ACTH-producing tumor, is characterized by hyperreactivity to exogenous ACTH. The continuous stimulation of the hyperplastic glands by endogenous ACTH appears to "prime" the adrenals to this hyperactive response to exogenous ACTH testing. This hyperactive response is evidenced in the parallel rise of both urine 17-hydroxy- and urine 17-ketosteroids. Whereas adrenal cortisol production is suppressed in normal subjects given dexamethasone 0.5 mg every 6 hr for 48 hr, no suppression occurs in patients with bilateral adrenal hyperplasia given this dosage. Suppression of

cortisol production in normal subjects is judged by a decrease in urine 17-hydroxysteroids to less than 3 mg per day, demonstrating that the hypothalamic-pituitary axis is appropriately responsive to increases in blood glucocorticoid levels, with a resultant decline in ACTH release. Lack of suppression in patients with adrenal hyperplasia given 2 mg daily of dexamethasone suggests that their hypothalamic-pituitary axis is "reset" to a higher blood level of glucocorticoids. On higher doses of dexamethasone (2 mg every 6 hr) suppression of urine 17-hydroxysteroid levels to values less than half the base-line levels can be demonstrated, consistent with the view that the hypothalamic-pituitary axis in these patients is reset upward and is responsive only to higher blood levels of glucocorticoids, at which point an appropriate decline in ACTH release does occur. The finding of a normal plasma ACTH level in these patients is an abnormal sign, since with the elevated blood cortisol levels one would expect a decreased blood ACTH level. On metyrapone testing, patients with adrenal hyperplasia due to hypothalmic dysfunction will again demonstrate a hyperactive response. In patients with adrenal hyperplasia secondary to an *ACTH-producing tumor*, such as an oat-cell bronchogenic carcinoma, no suppression will occur after dexamethasone administration and an abnormally depressed metyrapone test results, since the ACTH production by the tumor functions in an autonomous manner.

In patients with Cushing's syndrome secondary to an *adrenal adenoma*, hyperreactivity to exogenous ACTH testing may or may not occur, depending on whether the adenoma is functioning in an autonomous manner; if it is, it will be found ACTH-insensitive and thus fail to demonstrate a brisk rise in urine 17-hydroxycorticoids on ACTH stimulation. The diagnosis of adrenal adenoma is suggested by the disproportionate elevation in base-line urine 17-hydroxycorticoids with only a modest rise in 17-ketosteroids. Those adenomas which function autonomously fail to suppress after administration of dexamethasone at either the 2- or 8-mg daily dosage schedule, whereas the ACTH-sensitive adenomas most often fail to suppress with the lower, 2-mg daily dosage but may demonstrate suppression at the higher, 8-mg daily dosage. The variability of dexamethasone suppression testing is greater at the higher dose levels, and the distinction between adenomas and carcinomas is as a result less decisive. Another entity in the differential diagnosis is multinodular ("adenomatous") adrenal hyperplasia, which is an uncommon condition characteristically having features of both hyperplasia and of adenomas. Response to ACTH stimulation is abnormally brisk, but patients with multinodular adrenal hyperplasia most often do not show suppression after dexamethasone. Bilateral enlargement of the adrenals may be noted in such patients on the roentgenogram, and some patients excrete high levels of 3β-hydroxy-Δ5-steroids. Such patients usually do not show suppression with the standard doses of dexamethasone. However, with large doses, such as 4 to 8 mg every 6 hr, suppression often occurs.

Metyrapone testing is useful in differentiating adrenal tumors (adenoma or carcinoma) from adrenal hyperplasia, since the adrenal tumors by their autonomy suppress the ACTH-releasing capacity of the pituitary, with the result that on metyrapone challenge testing the pituitary fails to release ACTH in an appropriate manner and the usual rise in urine 17-hydroxycorticoids fails to occur. This finding of impaired response to metyrapone challenge separates adrenal tumors from adrenal hyperplasia, in which normal or hyperactive responses occur.

The diagnosis of *adrenal carcinoma* as a cause of Cushing's syndrome is suggested by markedly elevated baseline values of *both* urine 17-hydroxycorticoids and urine 17-ketosteroids. Adrenal carcinoma is usually resistant to both ACTH stimulation and dexamethasone suppression because of the autonomy of the tumor tissue itself and because of extreme atrophy of the normal remaining adrenal tissue. Virilization is often present. Functioning adrenal carcinomas that produce Cushing's syndrome are most often associated with elevated urine excretory values for the metabolites of the intermediates of steroid biosynthesis (such as tetrahydro-11-deoxycortisol) in addition to the cortisol metabolites, suggesting inefficient conversion of the intermediates to the final product. This is in contrast to Cushing's syndrome associated with adrenocortical hyperplasia, where the elevation of urine steroids is largely accounted for by cortisol metabolites.

Cushing's syndrome is being reported with increasing frequency in association with *nonendocrine tumors* producing an ACTH-like material in an autonomous manner, with the resultant development of adrenal hyperplasia. Approximately half these cases have been associated with the primitive small-cell type of bronchogenic carcinoma, and the remainder have been reported chiefly with tumors of thymus, pancreas, ovary, or thyroid. The onset of Cushing's syndrome is distinctively sudden in these patients, and this partly accounts for their failure to exhibit all the classic physical findings of the syndrome. Extracts of some of these nonendocrine tumors have produced a compound that is biologically, physiochemically, and immunologically similar to pituitary ACTH. Since such tumors often produce large amounts of this ACTH-like material, base-line urine steroid values are usually markedly elevated, and increased skin pigmentation is almost always present. These changes may be due to a MSH- or CRF-like material produced by the tumor. Hypokalemic alkalosis is much more common in these patients than in patients with Cushing's syndrome due to other causes. Edema and hypertension are also seen with greater frequency in these patients. On being tested, these patients will demonstrate a hyperactive response to ACTH stimulation but no suppression with dexamethasone and no increment in urine 17-hydroxycorticoid excretion after metyrapone administration. Plasma ACTH levels are most often markedly elevated in these patients, a helpful diagnostic finding, since plasma ACTH levels in other categories of Cushing's syndrome are at most modestly elevated.

Hyperpigmentation in patients with Cushing's syndrome always points to an extraadrenal tumor, either in an extracranial location, as discussed in the previous paragraph, or within the cranium. In the first 100 cases reported of Cushing's syndrome associated with pituitary tumors the majority had associated basophilic adenomas; chromophobe adenomas were in a distinct minority. Since this original series, chromophobe adenomas and carcinomas are being reported in much greater frequency than are basophilic adenomas. Basophilic adenomas do not cause enlargement of the sella turcica, whereas chromophobe tumors are the commonest cause of ballooning of the sella. The chief complaint of patients with chromophobe tumors is decreasing visual acuity, often with blurred vision and always with headaches. The chromophobe adenomas are asymmetric in growth, and as they progress upward, pressure on the optic nerve tracts results in visual field defects in most patients, with earliest losses occurring in the superior temporal quadrants; later a full bitemporal hemianopsia results. Headaches would appear to be caused by traction on surrounding dural structures or on the diaphragma sella. This association of pituitary tumors with Cushing's syndrome has generated interest as to whether all cases of adrenal hyperplasia may be caused by extraadrenal tumors and has led further to the speculation that chronic hypothalamic dysfunction may lead to the development of anterior pituitary tumors. A limitation to such interpretation has been the finding that approximately one-tenth of patients undergoing bilateral adrenalectomy for Cushing's syndrome have developed enlarged sella turcica and pituitary tumors, clinically evident only *after* the surgery, strongly suggesting that the loss of adrenal tissue, and consequent loss of the usual negative cortisol feedback on ACTH release, may be instrumental in the genesis of such tumors. Since intrasellar tumors may be present at an early stage in many patients *without* sellar enlargement, a decisive opinion as to their role in the genesis of Cushing's syndrome, or in the sequelae of its surgical therapy, must be withheld for further investigation. Clinically, all patients suspected of having Cushing's syndrome must be carefully examined for visual field defects and enlargement of the sella turcica; if defects are found, further diagnostic procedures may be warranted, such as sellar tomography, pneumoencephalography, and angiography.

DIFFERENTIAL DIAGNOSIS. Patients with exogenous obesity, hypertension, and diabetes mellitus, occurring singly or in combination, present major problems in diagnosis. Extreme *obesity* is uncommon in Cushing's syndrome; furthermore, with exogenous obesity, the adiposity is generalized, not truncal. On adrenocortical testing, abnormalities, if noted in patients with exogenous obesity, are never extensive but only modest. Basal urine steroid excretion levels in obese patients are either normal or slightly elevated, a finding similar to their cortisol secretory values. Some patients demonstrate an increased percentage of conversion of secreted cortisol into excreted metabolites. Blood cortisol levels are normal, and, of greater importance, a normal diurnal pattern in blood and urine levels is seen. On ACTH stimulation some of the patients will demonstrate a brisk response; however, in most cases this response is suppressed easily with dexamethasone. It would appear that exogenous obesity may *cause* alterations in the secretion and metabolism of steroids, pointing up the secondary nature of altered steroid testing patterns sometimes encountered. These patients are best treated by a concerted weight reduction program with periodic retesting of adrenal function.

Patients with *hepatic disease,* notably cirrhosis, often with obesity, may exhibit some of the manifestations of Cushing's syndrome. The reason for this resides in their impaired ability to inactivate circulated steroids, owing to decreased hepatic blood flow, with the result that blood levels may increase but secretory rates generally are found in the normal range. The defect is in inactivation of steroids, not in excessive secretion, so that therapy is initiated only for the underlying hepatic disease.

Iatrogenic Cushing's syndrome, induced by the administration of either glucocorticoids or ACTH, is indistinguishable by physical findings from the endogenous forms of adrenocortical hyperfunction. On occasion one may wish to rule out an underlying endogenous form of Cushing's syndrome that may be clinically magnified by exogenous therapy. This is accomplished by changing the patient's therapy to 1.0 mg dexamethasone daily while collecting base-line and diurnal split urine output for corticosteroid analysis. Patients with a pure exogenous form of Cushing's syndrome due to prolonged suppression of their hypothalamic-pituitary axis by administered steroid will demonstrate low base-line steroid excretion, predominantly in the daytime, a finding in distinct contrast to that in patients with endogenous Cushing's syndrome. Patients receiving long-term ACTH therapy, in addition to the features of Cushing's syndrome, may also have melanodermia. The production of iatrogenic Cushing's syndrome is related both to the total steroid dose and to the duration of therapy. Also, patients on afternoon and evening doses of steroid develop Cushing's syndrome more readily and on smaller daily steroid doses than do patients on a steroid program limited to morning doses only. In addition, there appears to be a marked interpatient difference in the enzymatic disposition of administered steroid. Several cases have been reported in which a spontaneous remission of Cushing's syndrome occurred; some have been characterized by intermittent abnormalities in adrenal testing. It is difficult to know whether such abnormalities are functional in nature or true pathophysiologic processes.

THERAPY. When an adenoma or carcinoma is suspected, adrenal exploration is performed, with excision of the tumor. Since cortisol production by the tumor generally causes atrophy of the contralateral gland, if an atrophied gland is noted on the initial side of exploration, the tumor must be on the opposite side. Because of this probable atrophy of the contralateral adrenal, the patient is prepared and treated pre- and postoperatively for total adrenalectomy even when a unilateral lesion is suspected, the routine being similar to that for an Addisonian patient undergoing elective surgery (Table 92-3).

The possibility of chemically inhibiting adrenocortical hyperfunction due to carcinoma is under active investigation. The principal antitumor drug under evaluation is *o,p'*-DDD [2,2-bis-(2-chlorophenyl,4-chlorophenyl)-1,1-dichloroethane], an isomer of the insecticide DDT. *o,p'*-DDD originally was demonstrated to induce adrenal atrophy of the "cytotoxic type" in experimental animals. This drug suppresses cortisol production and decreases plasma and urine steroid levels. It also suppresses peripheral enzyme systems responsible for steroid transformations. Daily dosage of *o,p'*-DDD has ranged from 2 to 12 Gm. Its cytotoxic action appears specific for adrenal glandular tissue, but histologic hepatic abnormalities have

Table 92-3. STEROID THERAPY SCHEDULE FOR PATIENTS WITH CUSHING'S SYNDROME UNDERGOING ADRENALECTOMY*

	Steroid							
	Cortisone acetate (intramuscularly)		Cortisone acetate (orally)				Fluorohydrocortisone (orally)	Hydrocortisone infusion
	7 A.M.	7 P.M.	8 A.M.	12 M.	4 P.M.	8 P.M.	8 A.M.	Continuous
Day before operation.........	...	100						
Day of operation............	100	50	...	...	...	...	...	300
Postoperative day 1..........	50	50	...	...	...	...	...	200
" 2..........	50	50	...	...	...	...	...	150
" 3..........	50	50	...	...	...	...	...	100
" 4..........	50	25	25	25	25	25	...	
" 5..........	50	...	25	25	25	25	0.1	
" 6..........	...	...	50	25	25	25	0.2	
" 7..........	...	...	25	25	25	25	0.2	
" 8..........	...	...	25	12.5	25	12.5	0.2	
" 9–14.......	...	...	25	12.5	25	...	0.1	
" 15–21......	...	...	25	12.5	12.5	...	0.1	
" 22–........	...	...	25	...	12.5	...	0.1	

* Both intravenous and intramuscular routes are utilized to minimize hazards of infusion infiltration. All steroid doses are in milligrams.

been reported. Almost all patients experience side effects of anorexia, diarrhea, or vomiting, and patients on long-term therapy must be observed closely for signs of adrenal insufficiency. For this reason patients may be placed on long-term glucocorticoid replacement therapy. In some patients dramatic regression of both tumor and metastases may occur, but long-term survival remains discouragingly limited. Predictability of expected response is poor. Investigation of this drug, however, has expanded the search for a more perfect chemical inhibitor of hyperactive adrenal tissue. For example, aminoglutethamide appears to inhibit steroid synthesis at a step between the conversion of cholesterol to pregnanelone. Because of this, it has been used in the treatment of Cushing's syndrome. However, it also may induce hypothyroidism and has moderate to severe side effects, severely limiting its usefulness. Another compound is DL-2-(p-aminophenyl)-2-phenylethylamine. At present, there has been little clinical experience with this compound, but it seems to exert its effect by blocking 11_β-hydroxylation thereby offering promise as an effective inhibitor of adrenal biosynthesis.

In patients with a severe form of Cushing's syndrome due to adrenal hyperplasia, with features of hypertension, overt diabetes, psychosis, and osteoporosis with pathologic fractures and in the absence of an enlarged sella turcica, a complete total bilateral adrenalectomy is preferred. Since, as mentioned earlier, one-tenth of these patients develop pituitary tumors after surgery, pituitary irradiation is also indicated in any patient who develops increased pigmentation or in whom the sella turcica size increases postoperatively. In patients past the reproductive years, pituitary irradiation may be carried out prophylactically in conjunction with complete adrenalectomy. It cannot be stressed too strongly that the status of all patients with bilateral adrenalectomy must be followed diligently with periodic reexaminations for evidence of increasing sellar size or pigmentary changes.

If patients with adrenal hyperplasia are noted to have signs of pituitary tumor (melanodermia, increased sellar size, visual field defects), specific therapy directed at the pituitary gland must be undertaken. In general, the type of therapy is either surgery or some form of radiation. Complications of surgical therapy include cerebrospinal fluid rhinorrhea, optic nerve and posterior pituitary injury, as well as removal of all tropic hormones. The morbidity and mortality rates are greater than with radiotherapy, and therefore surgery is often reserved for those cases not amenable to treatment with radiation. There are three major methods of directing radiotherapy at the pituitary gland. (1) The classical approach is the use of conventional external radiation at a dose of 3,000 to 5,000 r delivered over several weeks. The total dosage is limited by possible damage to surrounding neural structures and by the loss of additional pituitary tropic function. Treatment has been successful in fewer than one-third of the patients with Cushing's syndrome who were treated solely by this method. (2) The second method is internal pituitary irradiation by the stereotactic implantation of ^{90}yttrium pellets in the pituitary via the transnasosphenoid route. Possible limitation of this form of

therapy may be found once long-term evaluation on the effects of the radiation on perisellar structures (such as the internal carotid artery) has been made. (3) The most recent development has been the use of the alpha particle or proton beam as a source of external radiation. By this method as much as 12,000 r can be directed at the pituitary gland without evident damage to surrounding structures. This is because the beam can be focused more sharply than the more commonly used gamma radiation and because multiple portals of entry can be used. Even with this therapy there is a significant incidence of ocular motor palsies. This form of therapy holds great promise because of its ease of application, insignificant mortality rate, and low morbidity rate. However, final evaluation awaits long-term follow-up studies on treated subjects.

In patients with milder forms of adrenal hyperplasia without serious steroid-induced complications, several methods of approach are available, such as unilateral adrenalectomy with or without pituitary irradiation, or external or internal pituitary irradiation. Unilateral adrenalectomy without pituitary irradiation must be reserved for those patients with the mildest forms of adrenal hyperplasia.

If Cushing's syndrome redevelops after bilateral adrenalectomy, excessive stimulation of a remnant of adrenocortical tissue must be occurring. In very rare instances an embryologic extraadrenal remnant may be stimulated to produce excess cortisol. Surgical exploration has not been rewarding because of the difficulty in identifying small adrenocortical remnants. What is needed is an isotopic detection method whereby radioactive incorporation into the aberrant tissue can be monitored, and thus identification secured, at the operative field.

Aldosteronism

Aldosteronism is a syndrome associated with hypersecretion of the major adrenal mineralocorticoid aldosterone. *Primary* aldosteronism signifies that the stimulus for the excessive aldosterone production resides within the adrenal gland, whereas in *secondary* aldosteronism the stimulus is of extraadrenal origin.

PRIMARY ALDOSTERONISM

The constellation of signs and symptoms of excessive inappropriate aldosterone production was first summarized by Conn in 1956. The disease results from an aldosterone-producing adrenal adenoma (Conn's syndrome) or, in some cases, an adrenal carcinoma; cases have occurred with adrenal hyperplasia, and in rare instances the disease has occurred in the absence of pathologic changes in the adrenal gland as judged by light microscopy.

The majority of cases (75 percent) involve a unilateral adrenal adenoma, usually small and occurring with equal frequency on either side. It is twice as common in women as in men, presenting between the ages of thirty and fifty.

INCIDENCE. Primary aldosteronism is an uncommon disease. An estimated 400 cases have been reported worldwide in the first 10 years after its description. The incidence in unselected hypertensive patients is less than 0.5 percent. Because of special diagnostic procedures involved, diagnosis has been largely restricted to symptomatic patients. With greater availability of these procedures an increased incidence may be seen.

SIGNS AND SYMPTOMS. The continual hypersecretion of aldosterone increases the renal distal tubular exchange of intratubular sodium for secreted potassium and hydrogen ions, with progressive depletion of body potassium and development of hypokalemia. Almost all patients have diastolic hypertension, usually not of marked severity, and complain of headaches. The hypertension is related in some unknown manner to the increased sodium reabsorption. *Potassium depletion* is responsible for the major complaints of muscle weakness and fatigue and is related to the effect of intra- and extracellular potassium ion depletion on muscle membrane. The muscle weakness is most striking in the legs and may progress to transient paralysis. Muscles innervated by cranial nerves are usually spared. Most patients have nocturnal polyuria due to a vasopressin-insensitive, potassium-depletion-induced nephropathy. The polyuria results from impairment of concentrating ability and is often associated with polydipsia. These patients may have electrocardiographic and roentgenographic signs of left ventricular enlargement secondary to their hypertension, and hypertensive retinopathy is often seen but papilledema is absent. Electrocardiographic signs of potassium depletion such as prominent U waves are often present. In the absence of associated congestive heart failure, mental disease, or preexisting abnormalities (such as thrombophlebitis), edema is characteristically absent in these patients.

In cases of long duration, potassium-depletion nephropathy becomes manifest, with azotemia, often with superimposed bacilluria, and in some instances with congestive heart failure and edema.

LABORATORY FINDINGS. Laboratory findings are dependent on both the duration and the severity of the potassium depletion. On examination of the urine, negative to trace amounts of protein are found, sometimes with superimposed pyuria and bacilluria, presumably because of the predilection of potassium-depleted kidneys for infection. Urine specific gravity is low (less than 1.015), and an overnight concentration test with simultaneous vasopressin administration reveals impaired ability to concentrate the urine. Urine pH is often neutral to alkaline, because of excessive secretion of ammonium and bicarbonate ions; potassium depletion may lower the maximal tubular transfer rate for bicarbonate. Urine 17-hydroxycorticosteroid and 17-ketosteroid excretion levels are always within the normal range in patients with aldosteronomas but may occasionally be elevated in those rare instances of primary aldosteronism due to adrenal carcinoma. Mild azotemia is an inconstant finding.

Serial blood sampling usually reveals *hypokalemia* and *hypernatremia*. Serial blood sampling is stressed. The hypokalemia may be severe (less than 3.0 mEq potassium per liter) and reflects significant body potassium depletion, usually in excess of 300 mEq. *Hypernatremia* is due

to both sodium retention and a concomitant water loss from polyuria. The serum bicarbonate level may be elevated as a result of hydrogen ion loss into the urine and migration into potassium-depleted cells, with alkalosis then developing. The alkalosis is perpetuated with potassium deficiency, since such deficiency increases the capacity of the proximal convoluted tubule to reabsorb filtered bicarbonate. This alkalosis predisposes to signs and symptoms of tetany. If hypokalemia is severe, serum magnesium levels will be reduced. In the absence of azotemia, serum uric acid concentration is normal.

Salivary sodium potassium ratios are reduced in the majority of cases, as is thermal sweat sodium concentration.

Total body sodium content is increased but not to the degree seen in edematous states. Total exchangeable sodium is moderately elevated, and total exchangeable body potassium is usually, but not invariably, reduced. The volume of extracellular fluid is expanded in most cases, with expansion of plasma volume in many. The expanded extracellular fluid volume is thought to be responsible for the reversed diurnal excretory pattern for salt and water that many of these patients exhibit, with predominant salt and water excretion occurring during the night. Polyuria contributes to the nocturia.

DIAGNOSIS OF PRIMARY ALDOSTERONISM. The major criteria which permit the clinician to derive an unequivocal diagnosis of primary aldosteronism are (1) diastolic hypertension without edema; (2) hypersecretion of aldosterone which fails to be suppressed appropriately during volume expansion (salt loading); (3) hyposecretion of renin (as judged by low plasma renin activity levels) which fails to increase appropriately during volume depletion (upright posture); (4) hypokalemia and/or inappropriate urine potassium loss.

Diastolic hypertension is a prerequisite for the diagnosis of primary aldosteronism, even though transient periods of relative normotension may be observed during long-term evaluation. Diastolic hypertension exhibited by patients with primary aldosteronism does not differ from the labile variety of essential hypertension. Blood pressure readings characteristically become reduced after hospitalization, but moderate to severe rises may occur in hospital and are often related to emotional situations. Accelerated (sustained) diastolic hypertension is uncommon but has been reported.

Patients with primary aldosteronism characteristically *do not have edema,* since they are exhibiting a perpetuated "escape" phenomenon. Since they are in a chronic state of escape from the sodium-retaining aspects of mineralocorticoids, they characteristically excrete an administered salt load with a greater rapidity than do normotensive subjects, a characteristic which is shared by patients having essential hypertension. Only a limited sodium retention occurs when patients with primary aldosteronism are given sodium-retaining hormones parenterally. Rarely in patients with associated potassium-depletion nephropathy and azotemia, pretibial edema may be present.

Since hypersecretion of aldosterone may occur either in primary or in secondary aldosteronism, documentation of this parameter alone is not sufficient to arrive at a diagnosis of primary aldosteronism. It must be further documented that this hypersecretion of aldosterone *fails to be suppressed* normally during volume expansion of a sufficient degree to suppress the renin-angiotensin system. It is to be noted that the autonomy exhibited by aldosterone tumors in these patients refers only to their resistance to suppression of hypersecretion during volume expansion; such tumors can and do respond either in normal or supernormal fashion to the stimuli of potassium loading or ACTH infusion. Patients with primary aldosteronism do not respond to volume expansion since their renin-angiotensin system is already suppressed. Appropriate suppression testing may be carried out by saline loading, oral salt loading, or DOCA administration (see Mineralocorticoid Suppression Tests, earlier in this chapter). The autonomy of these tumors to volume expansion is not necessarily complete; many patients with primary aldosteronism will demonstrate some decrease of hypersecretion of aldosterone during volume expansion maneuvers, but such decreases are significantly less than the expected normal response.

The finding of a *low plasma renin activity level* which fails to respond appropriately to volume depletion, in conjunction with documentation of hypersecretion of aldosterone, constitutes the unique biochemical finding for a diagnosis of primary aldosteronism (see Fig. 92-10). Since some patients with essential hypertension, for reasons not known, have low plasma renin levels, it is essential to demonstrate that these low levels in patients with suspected primary aldosteronism fail to respond appropriately to volume depletion (see pp. 485 to 486). (This finding is comparable to the situation of long-term pituitary ACTH suppression resulting from hypersecretion of cortisol.)

A major criterion for the diagnosis of primary aldosteronism is the demonstration of *hypokalemia* associated with an inappropriately high urine potassium excretion. Judgments as to the significance of a given degree of hypokalemia for a given rate of urine potassium excretion must take into account the patient's potassium and sodium intake. Patients with hypokalemia secondary to diuretics, laxatives, etc., will generally have a 24-hr urine potassium excretion of less than 40 mEq per day, and often the value is markedly less than this. Most patients with primary aldosteronism, on the other hand, with a potassium intake of 100 mEq per day always have a 24-hr urine potassium excretion of greater than 40 mEq per day. Since potassium excretion can be modified by manipulations in sodium intake, this latter factor must be taken into consideration. During periods of high sodium intake, delivery of sodium ions to the distal tubular sodium-potassium exchange site will be increased, resulting in a rise in potassium excretion over control values. Contrariwise, potassium excretion can be minimized for any degree of hypokalemia by restriction of sodium intake, which limits the amount of sodium reaching the

Primary aldosteronism

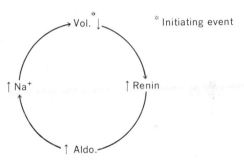

Secondary aldosteronism

* Initiating event

Fig. 92-10. Responses of the renin-aldosterone volume control loop in primary versus secondary aldosteronism.

distal tubular exchange site. Patients with primary aldosteronism will always exhibit inappropriate urine potassium losses during either saline or oral salt loading procedures.

Precise localization of aldosterone-producing adenomas may be determined preoperatively in many cases by the technique of percutaneous transfemoral bilateral adrenal vein catheterization with simultaneous adrenal arteriography and venography. Such a technique permits radiologic localization, and, in addition, the adrenal vein sampling may demonstrate a two- to threefold increase in plasma aldosterone concentration on the involved side compared with the uninvolved side.

DIFFERENTIAL DIAGNOSIS. All patients with *accelerated hypertension* and hypokalemia must be evaluated for unilateral renal disease. If such a diagnosis is confirmed, an additional diagnosis of primary aldosteronism is unlikely, although in rare instances both have been recorded to occur simultaneously. A useful maneuver in distinguishing between secondary aldosteronism due to accelerated hypertension and primary aldosteronism is to monitor serum potassium levels and aldosterone secretion (or excretory rates) prior to and following therapeutic correction of the hypertension. In patients with accelerated hypertension and secondary aldosteronism, the aldosteronism will subside with successful antihypertensive therapy, i.e., aldosterone parameters will return to normal and the hypokalemia and/or alkalosis will disappear. In distinct contrast, patients with primary aldosteronism in

Table 92-4. CHARACTERISTICS OF VARIOUS HYPERMINERALOCORTICOID STATES

Disorder	Blood pressure	Edema	Serum Na$^+$	Serum K$^+$	Plasma renin activity	Aldosterone
Primary aldosteronism	↑	0	↑,N	↓	↓↓	↑
Secondary aldosteronism:						
Accelerated hypertension	↑↑	0	↓,N	↓	↑↑	↑↑
Edema disorders	N,↓	+	↓,N	N,↓	↑	↑
DOC tumor	↑	0	↑,N	↓	↓↓	↓,N
Licorice ingestion	↑	0	↑,N	↓	↓	↓,N
Cushing's syndrome	↑	0,+	N,↑	↓,N	N,↓	N,↓
Bartter's syndrome	N,↓	0	N,↓	↓	↑↑↑	↑↑

whom successful blood pressure reduction is undertaken will continue to exhibit hypokalemic alkalosis with hypersecretion of aldosterone. An additional maneuver is sometimes useful. This is based on the observation of Melby that the majority of patients with primary aldosteronism become normotensive when treated with the aldosterone antagonist, spironolactone (Aldactone A), when given in a dose of 50 mg every 6 to 8 hr daily over a period of 2 to 5 weeks, whereas a minority of patients with essential hypertension become normotensive. Such therapy in patients with accelerated hypertension and secondary aldosteronism often will correct the electrolyte abnormalities, but hypertension will persist. It is of interest that patients with primary aldosteronism have been successfully managed medically for as long as 6 years through the chronic use of spironolactone therapy.

Primary aldosteronism must also be distinguished from other *hypermineralocorticoid states.* In a few instances, hypertensive patients with hypokalemic alkalosis have been found to have DOC-secreting adenomas. Such patients will have reduced plasma renin activity levels, but **aldosterone measurements will be either normal or reduced,** suggesting the diagnosis of mineralocorticoid excess due to a hormone other than aldosterone (see Table 92-4).

Licorice ingestion produces a syndrome mimicking primary aldosteronism. Licorice contains a sodium-retaining principle, glycyrrhizinic acid, which causes sodium retention, expansion of the extracellular fluid volume, hypertension, depressed plasma renin levels, and suppressed aldosterone levels. The diagnosis is excluded by a careful history.

Hypokalemic alkalosis is a prominent feature of *Bartter's syndrome* (juxtaglomerular hyperplasia). Patients with this disorder are easily distinguished by the finding of normotension and moderate to marked increases in plasma renin levels.

Base-line measurements of plasma renin activity and aldosterone secretion/excretion rate are not sufficient for a diagnosis of primary aldosteronism, since a small segment of the hypertensive population has been documented to have low-level plasma renin activity for undetermined reasons. Such patients may demonstrate an appropriate response in terms of plasma renin levels to volume depletion but display a subnormal rise in aldosterone secretion. Data are not available as to the response of this group of patients to the maneuver of volume expansion. It should also be pointed out that autonomous hypersecretion of aldosterone *without* demonstration of a low plasma renin level is not of sufficient accuracy to permit the diagnosis of primary aldosteronism, since it may occur in either secondary or "tertiary" aldosteronism.

SECONDARY ALDOSTERONISM

Secondary aldosteronism refers to an appropriately increased production of aldosterone by the adrenal gland in response to stimuli originating outside the gland. The adrenal production rates of aldosterone are often higher in patients with secondary aldosteronism than in those with primary aldosteronism. Most patients with secondary aldosteronism exhibit this syndrome either as an associated feature of the accelerated phase of hypertension (regardless of the primary disease) or on the basis of an underlying edema disorder.

The majority of patients in the *accelerated phase* of hypertensive disease exhibit a secondary aldosteronism characterized by hypokalemic alkalosis, absence of edema, moderate to severe increases in plasma renin levels, and moderate to marked increases in aldosterone secretion/ excretion rates. It has been postulated that the profound renal vasoconstriction which may be present in such patients is responsible for the excessive release of renin and hence initiates the state of secondary aldosteronism. Such a suggestion is supported by the observation that therapeutic correction of the hypertension results in the disappearance of the hyperaldosteronism.

Secondary aldosteronism is present in most *edema* disorders. Edema may be said to be the cardinal finding on physical examination for the presence of secondary aldosteronism. Hypersecretion of aldosterone in such clinical states correlates best with the phases of rapid accumulation of edema fluid. During phases of stable body weight, aldosterone measurements are often reported to be within the normal range. Patients with secondary aldosteronism due to edema disorders differ qualitatively from normal subjects and from patients with primary aldosteronism, in that they fail to exhibit a normal "escape" pattern in response to the chronic administration of DOC. These patients are exquisitely sensitive to the sodium-retaining properties of the mineralocorticoids and will exhibit a profound decrease in urine sodium excretion, often to barely detectable levels. They retain excess salt and water, but this retained fluid is ineffective in terms of reexpanding what is registered by the renin-angiotensin system as a deficient circulating blood volume. Instead, the excess salt and water that are retained accumulate in increasing quantities as edema fluid. Diuretic therapy often exaggerates the features of secondary aldosteronism via the mechanism of acute volume depletion; when this happens hypokalemia and on occasion alkalosis become prominent features.

Increased aldosterone secretion rates have been amply documented in patients who form edema as a result of either cirrhosis or the nephrotic syndrome. In congestive heart failure, however, elevated aldosterone secretion is a variable finding. The stimulus for aldosterone release in these clinical conditions appears to be *arterial hypovolemia*. Arterial blood volume may be depleted in cirrhosis as a result of decreased hepatic protein synthesis and protein loss into ascitic fluid; likewise, urine protein losses in the nephrotic syndrome may lead to arterial hypovolemia. Despite venous congestion, arterial hypovolemia may occur in congestive heart failure as a result of a failing cardiac output. The finding of normal aldosterone secretory rates in some patients with congestive heart failure requires explanation. It has been shown that approximately 95 percent of the circulating blood aldosterone is removed from the plasma and metabolized or extracted by the liver during a single passage. The rate of removal of aldosterone from plasma is termed its *metabolic clearance rate*, and since aldosterone is almost exclusively "cleared" by the liver, hepatic blood flow will approximate the aldosterone clearance rate. Since the blood level of circulating aldosterone is presumed to be the critical factor in its biologic activity, it is to be appreciated that the blood level will be determined by both the aldosterone secretion rate and the rate of hepatic inactivation. Thus, in clinical states characterized by reduced hepatic blood flow, such as congestive heart failure, an increased blood circulating aldosterone level can occur and result in sodium retention, even though the secretion rate of the hormone is within the normal range. Some of the patients currently being reported as having primary aldosteronism due to bilateral adrenocortical hyperplasia may in the future be classified as having secondary aldosteronism. Such a possibility would have to await the demonstration of an extraadrenal stimulus to aldosterone production other than ACTH and angiotensin. It is postulated that if such patients were to have secondary aldosteronism, they would have hypersecretion of aldosterone because of this unidentified stimulus. The excess aldosterone would then suppress plasma renin activity to a low level, thus mimicking primary aldosteronism.

"TERTIARY" ALDOSTERONISM

An increasing number of patients are being reported who do not fulfill precise criteria for either primary or secondary aldosteronism. This is analogous to the clinical evolution of our concepts of parathyroid disease, and one may predict that some of these patients will in time be classified as having "tertiary" aldosteronism. Such a diagnosis implies that in the initial phase of their disease, hyperaldosteronism occurs as an appropriate response to an extraadrenal stimulus but that at a later stage, hypersecretion of aldosterone becomes independent of the initiating stimulus. For example, a patient has been observed who had profound hypovolemia due to abnormal capillary permeability; after a decade of diuretic therapy he was found to have an aldosteronoma.

Adrenal Virilism

The adrenal virilizing syndromes result from excessive productions of adrenal androgens, such as dehydroepiandrosterone and Δ4-androstenedione which are converted to testosterone, the elevated testosterone levels account for most of the virilization. As in other states of adrenocortical hyperfunction, the syndrome may result from hyperplasia, adenoma, or carcinoma. It also may arise in a congenital form, termed *adrenogenital hyperplasia*, due to enzymatic deficits. The adrenal virilizing syndromes may be associated with secretions of greater or smaller amounts of other adrenal hormones and may, therefore, present as a "pure" syndrome of virilization or a "mixed" syndrome associated with excessive production of glucocorticoid and some of the characteristics of Cushing's syndrome. In *congenital* adrenal hyperplasia the virilizing syndrome may be associated with either excessive or decreased secretion of mineralocorticoid or decreased production of glucocorticoid.

The enzymatic composition of the adrenal as determined by heredity (and perhaps other factors as well) determines the relative rate of synthesis of hormones with glucocorticoid activity and of hormones with androgenic activity.

Since in man hydrocortisone is the principal adrenal steroid regulating ACTH elaboration, and since ACTH stimulates both hydrocortisone and adrenal androgen production, it stands to reason that an enzymatic interference with hydrocortisone synthesis may result in the enhanced secretion of adrenal androgens. In severe congenital virilizing hyperplasia, the adrenal output of hydrocortisone may be so compromised as to cause clinical evidence of glucocorticoid deficiency despite anatomic adrenal hyperplasia. Conversely, a high hydrocortisone output as the result of primary adrenal pathology (adenoma) may inhibit ACTH secretion and thus result in a low adrenal androgen output.

INCIDENCE. Congenital bilateral adrenocortical hyperplasia is by far the most common adrenal disorder of infancy and childhood. It has also been described later in life, predominantly in women. Its appearance in postpuberal men would obviously not be as clinically apparent; nevertheless, it has been reported. In its various forms, adrenogenital hyperplasia is thought to be related to a defective autosomal recessive gene. The most common form of significant "noncongenital" adrenal virilization is that seen with bilateral adrenocortical hyperplasia and is most frequently associated with various degrees of excessive production of glucocorticoid hormone and the clinical signs and symptoms of Cushing's syndrome.

CLINICAL SIGNS AND SYMPTOMS. In the adult female, regardless of etiology, the clinical signs and symptoms are those anticipated from excessive androgen production. These include hirsutism, acne, increased sebum production, temporal baldness, deepening of voice, increased muscle mass and strength, decreased breast size, atrophy of the uterus, amenorrhea, enlargement of the clitoris, increased heterosexual drive, and development of a male habitus. The clinical distinction between excessive hair growth (hirsutism) and virilization is useful. Virilization signifies that multiple signs of androgen excess are present in addition to hirsutism, and one of the more easily recognized of these signs is hypertrophy of the clitoris. Hirsutism in the absence of other signs of virilization is uncommon in these patients. The virilizing syndromes are difficult to document in the adult male, for obvious reasons.

The congenital form of adrenal hyperplasia is secondary to a defect in steroid enzymatic activity. To date, defects have been described in the C-21, C-18, C-17, and C-11 hydroxylase enzymes, as well as in the 3β-ol-dehydrogenase enzyme. Most of these defects produce virilization. However, the C-17 hydroxylase defect may actually produce sexual immaturity. These enzymatic deficits may occur singularly or in combination. Adrenal virilization at birth is almost always due to congenital adrenal hyperplasia; however, the disease may not become apparent until many years later, and sometimes only in adult life. In the most common form of congenital adrenal hyperplasia, that due to impairment of *C-21 hydroxylation*, there will be reduced conversion of 17-hydroxyprogesterone to 11-deoxycortisol and thus reduced formation of cortisol from 11-deoxycortisol (Fig. 92-2). In addition to cortisol deficiency, there may or may not be an associated reduction in aldosterone secretion as a result of impaired C-21 hydroxylation of progesterone to 11-deoxycorticosterone, a precursor of aldosterone. Thus, with congenital adrenal hyperplasia secondary to C-21 hydroxylase deficiency, adrenal insufficiency will be present with or without an associated salt-losing tendency due to aldosterone deficiency. It is probable that the C-21 hydroxylase enzymes, rather than being identical, are isoenzymes.

Therefore, the difference between the salt-losing variety and the non-salt-losing variety resides in whether the genetic abnormality involves one or both of these isoenzymes. As a result of the C-21 hydroxylase deficit, precursor products accumulate and are shunted into alternate pathways of metabolism, chiefly the androgen pathway, accounting for the production of excessive androgens. The accumulation of progesterone may also exaggerate any salt-losing tendency, since progesterone has an antialdosterone effect on renal tubular salt conservation. Since a cortisol deficiency exists, the adrenal glands become hyperplastic because of excessive ACTH stimulation.

With a *C-11 hydroxylase* deficiency a "hypertensive" variant of congenital adrenal hyperplasia develops with cortisol deficiency, since there is impaired conversion of 11-deoxycortisol to cortisol. Hypertension occurs because of the impaired conversion of 11-deoxycorticosterone to corticosterone, resulting in the accumulation of 11-deoxycorticosterone, a potent mineralocorticoid. Increased shunting again occurs into the androgen pathway.

Recently, two new enzymatic defects have been reported. One is a pure C-17 hydroxylase deficiency. The other is a combined C-17 hydroxylase and C-18 hydroxylase deficiency. In those patients with a C-17 hydroxylase deficiency alone, there is increased production of progesterone and its metabolite pregnanediol, with decreased production of cortisol and shunting into the mineralocorticoid pathway. This leads to the characteristic clinical picture of excess aldosterone secretion with low plasma renin activity. The effects of an increased aldosterone secretion are also noted, in that hypertension and hypokalemia are frequent. Because C-17 hydroxylation is also necessary for androgen formation, virilization has not been described with this defect. C-17 hydroxylation is also important in gonadal biosynthesis, and defects in gonadal biosynthetic pathways have been described. With the combination of C-17 and C-18 hydroxylase deficiency, a similar clinical picture is seen except that there is a decrease in aldosterone synthesis. Most, if not all, of these patients with combined deficiencies have gonadal enzymatic abnormalities and an exaggerated salt-losing tendency because of the accumulation of progesterone behind the block (Table 92-5).

Table 92-5. URINE EXCRETORY PRODUCTS IN CONGENITAL ADRENAL HYPERPLASIA

	17-KS	17-OH	THS	Pregnanetriol	Pregnanediol	THDOC	THB	Aldosterone
C-21 hydroxylase deficiency:								
Salt-losing	I	N–D	N–D	I	I	D	D	D
Non-salt-losing	I	N–D	N–D	I	N–I	N–I	N–I	N–I
C-11 hydroxylase deficiency	I	I	I	I	N–I	I	D	D
C-17 hydroxylase deficiency	N–D	N–D	N–D	N–D	I	I	I	I
C-17 and C-18 hydroxylase deficiency	N–D	N–D	N–D	N–D	I	I	I	D
3β-ol-Dehydrogenase deficiency	I	N–D	N–D	N–D	N–D	N–D	N–D	N–D

Note: THS, tetrahydro 11-deoxycortisol; THDOC, tetrahydro 11-deoxycorticosterone; THB, tetrahydrocorticosterone; I, increased; N, normal; D, decreased.

With 3_β-ol-dehydrogenase deficiency, there is impaired conversion of pregnenolone to progesterone, with the result that pathways to both cortisol and aldosterone are "blocked," with shunting then occurring into the adrenal androgen pathway via 17_α-hydroxypregnenolone to dehydroepiandrosterone.

Clinically adrenal virilism due to congenital adrenal hyperplasia manifests itself as *pseudohermaphroditism* of females and *premature virilization* of males. The age of onset of virilization is most probably prenatal, after the fifth month of embryonic development. At birth there may be macrogenitosomia in the male infant and enlargement of the clitoris, partial or complete fusion of the labia, and sometimes a urogenital sinus in the female. If the labial fusion is nearly complete, the female infant will have external genitalia resembling a penis with hypospadias, changes consistent with female pseudohermaphroditism. Chromosomal sex can be determined by skin biopsy or examination of oral mucosal smears. Those infants with a salt-losing tendency often crave salt, and episodes of acute adrenal insufficiency are common. This salt-losing variant of congenital adrenal hyperplasia is often associated with vomiting, diarrhea, and hypotension. Hypertension is, of course, a key feature of the hypertensive variant of congenital adrenal hyperplasia, and its severity may dominate the clinical picture. In the *postnatal period* from infancy through adolescence, congenital adrenal hyperplasia will be associated with virilization in the female and isosexual precocity in the male. The excessive androgens produced will result in accelerated growth before fusion of epiphyses occurs, with skeletal growth exceeding the chronologic age. With epiphyseal closure, which is hastened by excessive androgens, growth stops but truncal development continues, giving the characteristic appearance of a child of short stature with a well-developed trunk. Incomplete variants of congenital adrenal hyperplasia sometimes occur in adult life, with virilization occurring in the female. It is not apparent why the adrenogenital syndrome should be dormant until adult life. One possibility may be that only a partial deficiency of an enzyme system such as C-11 hydroxylase was inherited and that the production of androgens in adult life may further inhibit the action of this enzyme, with consequent overproduction of adrenal androgens.

DIAGNOSIS. The diagnosis of adrenal virilism due to congenital adrenal hyperplasia should be considered in all infants exhibiting "failure to thrive," particularly those having episodes of acute adrenal insufficiency or having sustained hypertension. The diagnosis is further suggested by the finding of hypertrophy of the clitoris, fused labia, or urogenital sinus in the female and isosexual precocity in the male infant. In infants and children with a *C-21 hydroxylation block*, increased urine 17-ketosteroid excretion is typically associated with an increase in the excretion of pregnanetriol, which is a metabolite of 17_α-hydroxyprogesterone. These children will show low urine 17-hydroxycorticoid excretion levels and elevated levels of plasma ACTH. Ketogenic steroid excretion will be elevated, since the depressed 17-hydroxycorticoid excretion is more than offset by increments in pregnanetriol excretion, which metabolite is included in the analysis. On testing with ACTH, the altered metabolic pathways

Table 92-6. LABORATORY EVALUATIONS AND TESTING OF ADRENOCORTICAL FUNCTION **IN THEORETICAL CASES** OF ADRENAL VIRILIZING SYNDROMES*

Syndromes	Plasma ACTH	Plasma cortisol	Cortisol secretory rate	Urine values	Control base line	Days of ACTH stimulation		Days of dexamethasone suppression, mg q 6h			
								0.5		2.0	
						1	2	1	2	1	2
Benign androgenic hyperplasia.............	N†	N	N	17-OH :	7	20	35	4	2	1	1
				17-KS :	17	35	50	10	5	4	3
Virilizing carcinoma.........	N–D‡	N–I	N–I§	17-OH :	12	24	35	10	5	4	4
				17-KS :	150	150	150	150	150	150	150
Virilizing adenoma...........	N	N	N	17-OH :	8	17	30	6	4	3	3
				17-KS :	150	160	170	150	140	130	120
Congenital adrenal hyperplasia.............	I	D	D	17-OH :	3	12	20	3	4	5	5
				17-KS :	40	60	90	25	20	15	10

* Clinical status charted vertically and representative values for steroid tests charted horizontally. 17-OH, 17-KS refer to 24-hr urine 17-hydroxycorticosteroid and 17-ketosteroid excretion. All laboratory values given in **milligrams per day**. Base-line urine 17-KS are either at upper limits of normal or slightly elevated in benign androgenic hyperplasia, whereas they are markedly elevated with virilizing carcinoma or adenoma. With ACTH stimulation, in benign androgenic hyperplasia, there is disproportionate rise in 17-KS; in virilizing tumors, there is no increment in 17-KS; in congenital adrenal hyperplasia, there is a rise in 17-KS (unless base-line 17-KS are very high). With dexamethasone suppression, in benign androgenic hyperplasia, there is complete suppression; in virilizing tumors, no suppression; in congenital adrenal hyperplasia, complete suppression.

† N, normal.

‡ D, decreased.

§ I, increased.

are exaggerated, with sharp rises occurring in 17-keto-steroid excretion and little or no rise in 17-hydroxycorti-coid excretion (Table 92-6).

The diagnosis of a *salt-losing form* of congenital adrenal hyperplasia due to defects in both C-21 hydroxylase enzymes is suggested by episodes of acute adrenal insufficiency with hyponatremia, hyperkalemia, dehydration, and vomiting. These infants and children often "crave" salt and exhibit laboratory signs of concomitant deficits in both cortisol and aldosterone secretion.

With the *hypertensive form* of congenital adrenal hyperplasia due to impaired C-11 hydroxylation, the precursor 11-deoxycortisol will accumulate. As a result, both urine 17-keto- and 17-hydroxycorticoid excretion may be elevated, since 11-deoxycortisol would be included in the analysis of Porter-Silber chromogens. The diagnosis is secured by demonstrating increased amounts of tetrahydro-11-deoxycortisol in the urine with decreased amounts of tetrahydro metabolites of cortisol.

The finding of very high levels of urine dehydro-epiandrosterone with low levels of pregnanetriol and of cortisol metabolites is characteristic of patients with congenital adrenal hyperplasia due to 3β-ol-dehydrogenase deficiency. These patients also exhibit marked salt wasting.

The C-17 hydroxylase deficiency results in low levels of all cortisol precursors up to progesterone and its metabolite, pregnanediol, which are increased. Also, there is increased excretion of aldosterone and corticosterone. Patients with the combined C-17 and C-18 hydroxylase deficiencies have a similar excretion pattern except that corticosterone excretion is elevated while aldosterone secretion is decreased (see Table 92-5).

The adrenal virilizing syndrome in adults is most often due to noncongenital causes, namely, adrenal hyperplasia or tumor. *Benign androgenic adrenal hyperplasia* refers to those patients with hirsutism with normal or slightly elevated urine 17-ketosteroids and normal 17-hydroxycorticosteroids (Table 92-7). With ACTH stimulation there is a brisk rise in the urine 17-ketosteroids when compared to the 17-hydroxysteroids. Base-line 17 keto-steroids are easily suppressed on 2 mg daily of dexamethasone. An estimated one-third of patients with the polycystic ovarian syndrome and one-third of females with idiopathic hirsutism have findings consistent with benign androgenic adrenal hyperplasia. In adrenocortical hyperfunction of Cushing's syndrome, both urine 17-ketosteroid

Table 92-7. CAUSES OF HIRSUTISM IN FEMALES

1. Idiopathic
2. Familial
3. Ovarian
   a. Polycystic ovaries
   b. Tumor: arrhenoblastoma, hilus cell, adrenal rest
4. Adrenal
   a. Benign androgenic hyperplasia
   b. Congenital adrenal hyperplasia
   c. Virilizing carcinoma
   d. Virilizing adenoma
   e. Noncongenital adrenal hyperplasia (Cushing's)

and 17-hydroxysteroid base-line values will be elevated, the latter separating Cushing's syndrome from benign androgenic hyperplasia.

Adrenal adenomas and *carcinomas* may also cause a pure or mixed virilizing syndrome. Since adrenal androgens are weak androgens compared with gonadal androgens, adrenal virilization is characterized by large increments in urine 17-ketosteroids, often with less impressive clinical signs of virilism. Virilizing adrenal cortical adenomas are rare. They produce very high levels of urine 17-ketosteroids, often greater than 200 mg per day, and are associated with no rise or only a slight rise in urine 17-hydroxysteroids. They may or may not be sensitive to ACTH stimulation and likewise may or may not be sensitive to dexamethasone suppression. *Virilizing adrenal carcinomas* are the most common adrenal tumor causing virilization. They are also associated with very high urine 17-ketosteroid excretion and may have normal 17-hydroxycorticoid excretion or a moderate rise in 17-hydroxysteroid excretion. They characteristically show no increase in steroid excretion upon stimulation with ACTH and also characteristically fail to be suppressed with dexamethasone administration. These tumors are often associated with marked virilization of sudden onset. The very high ketosteroid excretion of both virilizing adenomas and carcinomas is made up in large part of the weak androgen dehydroepiandrosterone, which has approximately 5 percent of the androgenicity of testosterone. The clinical differentiation between virilizing adrenal adenoma and carcinoma is tenuous and cannot be made with certainty preoperatively.

DIFFERENTIAL DIAGNOSIS. The chief consideration in the differential diagnosis of adrenal virilization is virilization due to ovarian causes (Table 92-6). The low to slightly elevated urine 17-ketosteroid values associated with "idiopathic" hirsutism are in sharp contrast to the very high values with adrenal virilization. The hirsutism associated with polycystic ovaries is associated with other signs of virilization in 10 to 15 percent of patients. The association of amenorrhea with bilaterally large ovaries suggests polycystic ovaries, although some polycystic ovaries are of normal size. Urine 17-ketosteroid excretion in polycystic ovarian syndrome is either normal or slightly increased and characteristically fails to exhibit normal suppression with dexamethasone administration. In some of these patients a modest rise in urine 17-ketosteroids is shown on ACTH administration and purified FSH preparations cause a rise in the 11-deoxy-17-ketosteroid fraction with no or little change in the urine 11-oxy-17-ketosteroids. Hirsutism in these patients is thought to be due to defective ovarian aromatization whereby the androgen precursors, Δ4-androstenedione and testosterone, are not completely aromatized to the estrogens, estrone and estradiol, with the result that the blood level of the androgens will increase.

The most common *ovarian tumor* causing virilization is the arrhenoblastoma, but other ovarian tumors such as adrenal rest tumor, granulosa cell tumor, hilar cell tumors, and Brenner tumors have been associated with virilization. These masculinizing ovarian tumors may secrete testosterone as the major androgen, and the secretion of a few milligrams of testosterone, in view of its high androgenicity, can cause overt hirsutism. As a result, urine 17-ketosteroids are within the normal range in half these patients, and moderate elevations occur in the remainder. Urine base-line 17-ketosteroid excretion in excess of 40 mg per day is rare, with the exception of adrenal rest tumors. Urine 17-hydroxycorticoid excretion is normal. These ovarian tumors characteristically fail to be suppressed with dexamethasone; with the exception of adrenal rest tumors, they are largely independent of ACTH stimulation. Adrenal virilization due to *adrenal tumor* is characterized by high urine 17-ketosteroid excretion representing metabolites of weak adrenal androgens (such as dehydroepiandrosterone), whereas virilization due to ovarian tumors is characterized by normal or moderate elevation of urine 17-ketosteroids, since the ovaries are secreting the extremely potent androgen, testosterone. The principal difference between biosynthesis of androgens by the ovaries and by the adrenals is that tropic control is exerted principally by gonadotropins in the former and by ACTH in the latter case.

Direct inspection of the ovaries by culdoscopy is a valuable means of differentiating between ovarian and adrenal causes of hirsutism. Polycystic ovaries have a characteristic "oyster" appearance, and varying degrees of bilateral enlargement may be seen. Unilateral ovarian enlargement suggests ovarian tumor. If on culdoscopic examination "normal" ovaries are found, this, of course, strengthens the probability of an adrenal etiology for virilization. Suprarenal and ovarian tomography, with or without contrast studies, is helpful in delineating this problem.

With the finding of isosexual precocity in young boys, in addition to congenital adrenal hyperplasia, one must consider the possibility of hyperplasia of adrenal rest tissue occurring in the epididymis or testes. These *testicular adrenal rests* secrete high quantities of ketosteroids and operate under ACTH control. The aberrant adrenal rest tissue usually causes bilateral testicular enlargement, in contrast to the unilateral testicular enlargement with contralateral atrophy usually seen with true interstitial cell tumors. Further differentiation from interstitial testicular cell tumors is afforded by the insensitivity of the latter to ACTH stimulation.

TREATMENT. Treatment of adrenal virilism is dictated by the type of lesion suspected. The patients with *congenital adrenal hyperplasia* have the fundamental defect of cortisol deficiency with resultant excessive ACTH stimulation producing hyperplasia of the adrenal glands and causing additional "shunting" into the adrenal androgen pathway. Therapy in these patients consists of daily glucocorticoid (dexamethasone, prednisone, cortisone, etc.) administration to suppress pituitary ACTH secretion. In children, this not only suppresses urinary ketosteroid excretion but also ends virilization and the associated problems of hyperandrogenicity. The dosage schedule is governed by repetitive analysis of the urine 17-ketosteroids and by skeletal growth and maturation. Those children born with abnormalities of external genitalia may require

surgical correction of labial fusion, urogenital sinus, etc. Response of these children to steroid therapy is gratifying in that normal growth and development occur and the menarche and onset of spermatogenesis occur at the appropriate age. Many females with this disorder have married and borne children. Steroid therapy is indicated throughout the life span of these patients.

Some infants and children with the associated defect of salt wasting require vigorous correction of salt deficits in conjunction with small doses of a potent mineral corticoid such as 9_α-fluorohydrocortisone.

In patients with adrenal virilization due to adrenal tumors, prompt surgical intervention with complete excision of the tumor is, of course, indicated. One cannot postpone surgical intervention in patients suspected of having virilizing adrenal adenomas, since such adenomas are practically indistinguishable from adrenal carcinomas, both clinically and biochemically. Preoperative localization of adrenal tumors is attempted with renal tomography or selective adrenal angiography. Since "pure" virilizing adrenal tumors do *not* cause contralateral adrenal atrophy, thorough inspection and exploration of both suprarenal areas is mandatory. If metastases have occurred, one may consider the use of antitumor drugs such as *o,p'*-DDD with or without local irradiation. *o,p'*-DDD in some patients has been associated with striking regression in peripheral metastases paralleled by a decrease in urine 17-ketosteroid and 17-hydroxycorticoid excretion; however, long-term survival is rare. In some patients given a trial of *o,p'*-DDD, regression of metastases is not seen but a fall in urine 17-hydroxycorticoids occurs. The explanation resides in the fact that *o,p'*-DDD can alter the extraadrenal metabolism of cortisol so as to decrease the metabolism and excretion of the usual metabolite, tetrahydrocortisol, causing the decrease in Porter-Silber chromogens; yet at the same time, there is increased conversion to and excretion of 6_β-hydroxycortisol, a steroid not included routinely as a Porter-Silber chromogen because of its poor solubility in the preliminary extracting solvent (dichloromethane).

Adrenal Feminization

Adrenal feminization is an exceedingly rare entity and, when present, is almost always due to adrenal tumor. These adrenal tumors will cause feminization in the male, with development of gynecomastia (often with breast tenderness), change in body habitus, testicular atrophy, feminizing hair changes, and loss of libido. They may occur in "pure" form, i.e., with normal levels of urine 17-ketosteroids, or in "mixed" form, with feminization despite high 17-ketosteroid excretion. They are always associated in the male with increased excretion of estrogen metabolites, such as estrone and estradiol. These adrenal tumors secrete increased amounts of androstenedione, which undergoes conversion, either in the adrenal or peripherally in the liver, into the estrogens, estrone and estradiol. Some patients have had elevated urine values for pregnanetriol, suggesting that 11_β-hydroxylation may be impaired.

The majority of adrenal tumors causing feminization are carcinomas. They are most common in the age group twenty-five to forty-five. These tumors are almost always unilateral and occur with equal frequency on either side. In rare instances they have occurred in an extraadrenal locus such as the testis. The feminizing adrenal carcinomas are large tumors (weighing several hundred grams) and often are easily palpable on physical examination, whereas feminizing adrenal adenomas are characteristically small tumors. Metastases occur most often to the liver and lungs. Feminizing adrenal tumors do not cause contralateral adrenal atrophy, which makes bilateral exploration mandatory if the initial adrenal explored is normal. Almost all cases of feminizing adrenal carcinoma are evident on suprarenal tomography studies. Patients with feminizing adrenal tumors usually have normal to moderately elevated 17-ketosteroid excretion levels. If the urine 17-ketosteroid excretion is greater than 100 mg per day, the diagnosis of a feminizing adrenal carcinoma is almost certain. Urine 17-hydroxycorticoid excretion is usually within the normal range or slightly elevated. Associated Cushing's syndrome is rare. ACTH stimulation causes little change in 17-ketosteroid excretion. The chemical determination of urine estrogen titers always demonstrates an elevated value. The elevated urine estrogen excretion level is principally due to increased estriol and also to increments in estradiol and estrone. Since the estrogens produced by adrenal feminizing tumors are conversion products from androgen precursors, the amount of estrogens elaborated will depend both on the amount of androgen precursors formed and on the efficiency of the androgen-to-estrogen conversion process.

Radiotherapy has not been helpful in treatment. Despite operative intervention, most patients with adrenal feminizing carcinoma die within 3 years of diagnosis. With successful operative removal of feminizing tumors, the urine estrogen titer falls; a failure of the titer to fall or a recurrence of elevated urine titers indicates functioning tumor tissue.

The diagnosis of adrenal feminization in the male is strongly suggested by the onset of gynecomastia associated with a flank mass. The additional finding of increased urine estrogen titers confirms the diagnosis. Gynecomastia may also be seen with *testicular tumors* (chorioepithelioma, Sertoli cell, seminoma, interstitial cell tumor) because of increased production by the tumors of chorionic gonadotropin, with an associated elaboration of estrogens by the testes. Adrenal feminization in the female is more difficult to detect, but it has been reported.

HYPOFUNCTION OF ADRENAL CORTEX

Adrenocortical hypofunction includes all conditions in which the secretion of adrenal steroid hormones falls below the requirements of the body. Various types of adrenal insufficiency are encountered and may be divided into two general categories: (1) those associated with primary inability of the adrenal to elaborate sufficient

quantities of hormone and (2) those associated with a secondary failure due to a primary failure in the elaboration of ACTH (Table 92-8).

Table 92-8. CLASSIFICATION OF CAUSES OF ADRENAL INSUFFICIENCY

I. Primary adrenal insufficiency
  A. Anatomic destruction of gland (chronic and acute)
    1. Infection
    2. Invasion: metastatic, fungal, etc.
    3. Hemorrhage
    4. "Idiopathic" atrophy, autoimmune
    5. Surgical removal
  B. Metabolic failure in hormone production
    1. Virilizing hyperplasia, congenital (certain types)
    2. Enzyme inhibitors
      a. Specific: metyrapone
      b. Nonspecific: amphenone
    3. Cytotoxic agents: o,p'-DDD, aminoglutethamide
II. Secondary adrenal insufficiency
  A. Hypopituitarism due to pituitary disease
  B. Suppression of hypothalamic-pituitary axis
    1. Exogenous steroid
    2. Endogenous steroid from tumors after tumor removal
    3. Pharmacologic agents

Chronic Adrenocortical Deficiency

This disorder is also called Addison's disease or chronic glucocorticoid deficiency. Addison's classic description in 1855, namely, "general languor and debility, remarkable feebleness of the heart's action, irritability of the stomach, and a peculiar change of the color of the skin," summarizes the dominant clinical features of the disease. Advanced cases usually cause little difficulty in diagnosis, but recognition of the disease in its earlier phases may present a real challenge. The disease, when unrecognized and untreated, carries an almost uniformly poor and frequently fatal prognosis. Early diagnosis is important, since present-day therapy may provide complete correction of the metabolic derangement.

INCIDENCE. Primary adrenocortical insufficiency is relatively rare. It may occur at any age in life and affects both sexes with equal frequency. Because of increasing therapeutic use of exogenous steroids, secondary adrenal insufficiency is seen with increasing frequency.

CLINICAL SIGNS AND SYMPTOMS. Adrenocortical insufficiency is most frequently characterized by an insidious onset with slowly progressive fatigability, weakness, anorexia, nausea and vomiting, weight loss, cutaneous and mucosal pigmentation, hypotension, and occasionally hypoglycemia. These signs and symptoms compose the classic syndrome of Addison's disease; however, the spectrum may vary, depending on the duration and degree of adrenal hypofunction, from a complaint of mild chronic fatigue to the fulminating shock associated with acute massive destruction of the glands in the type of syndrome described by Waterhouse and Friderichsen. Table 92-9 lists the incidence of symptoms and signs noted in cases of Addison's disease.

Table 92-9. INCIDENCE OF SYMPTOMS AND SIGNS IN
125 CASES OF ADDISON'S DISEASE, PERCENT

Weakness	99	Hypotension (below	
Pigmentation of skin	98	110/70)	87
Pigmentation of mucous		Abdominal pain	34
membranes	82	Salt craving	22
Weight loss	97	Diarrhea	20
Anorexia, nausea, and		Constipation	19
vomiting	90	Syncope	16
		Vitiligo	9

Asthenia is the cardinal symptom of Addison's disease. Early it may be sporadic, usually most evident at times of stress; as adrenal function becomes more impaired, the weakness progresses until the patient is continuously fatigued, necessitating bed rest. Even the voice may fail, so that speech finally becomes listless and indistinct.

Pigmentation is the most striking sign of the disease. It commonly appears as a diffuse brown, tan, or bronze darkening of both exposed and unexposed points such as elbows or creases of the hand and in areas normally pigmented such as the areolas about the nipples. In many patients, bluish-black patches appear on the mucous membranes. Some patients develop dark freckles, and occasionally irregular areas of vitiligo may appear paradoxically. As an early sign, patients may notice an unusually persistent tanning following exposure to the sun.

Arterial hypotension is also extremely frequent, and in severe cases blood pressures may be in the range of 80/50 or less. Postural accentuation is common, and syncope may occur.

Abnormalities of gastrointestinal function are not only extremely frequent but often are the presenting complaint. Symptoms may vary from mild anorexia with weight loss to fulminating nausea, vomiting, diarrhea, and various types of ill-defined abdominal pain, which at times may be so severe as to be confused with an acute condition of the abdomen requiring surgery. Rarely a Landry's type of ascending paralysis with flaccid quadriplegia and mixed sensory defects accompanied by ascending muscular weakness has been noted in conjunction with a high serum potassium level. In these instances, the electrocardiogram may reflect the hyperkalemia. In addition, patients with adrenal insufficiency frequently have marked personality changes, usually in the form of excessive irritability and restlessness. Enhancement of the sensory modalities of taste, olfaction, and hearing is often present and is reversible with therapy.

LABORATORY FINDINGS. In the milder forms, sometimes called *partial* or *incomplete* Addison's disease, there may be no demonstrable abnormalities in any of the parameters measured in the routine laboratory, and even plasma and urinary steroid determinations may indicate values relatively low yet within normal range. However, definitive studies of adrenal stimulation with ACTH show abnormalities even in this stage of the disease. In the more advanced stages, levels of serum sodium, chloride, and bicarbonate are reduced while serum potassium is elevated. The hyponatremia is due to extravascular loss of sodium both into the urine (due to aldosterone defi-

ciency) and from the vascular compartment into tendon, cartilage, and bone. This extravascular sodium loss depletes extracellular fluid volume and accentuates hypotension. Elevated plasma levels of vasopressin and angiotensin have been reported, and these may be contributing factors to hyponatremia through impairment of free-water clearance. The hyperkalemia is due to a combination of factors including aldosterone deficiency, impaired glomerular filtration rate, and acidosis. These patients may show marked reduction in heart size, and in about one-quarter of the patients suprarenal calcification is seen but is unfortunately not pathognomonic. The electrocardiogram may show nonspecific changes and the electroencephalogram a striking reduction and slowing of the predominant activity. The basal metabolic rate may be low, but other thyroid indexes are usually normal. There may be a normocytic anemia, a relative lymphocytosis, and usually a moderate eosinophilia.

DIAGNOSIS. The diagnosis of adrenal insufficiency requires demonstration either directly or indirectly of decreased cortisol production by the adrenal in the basal state (*complete* adrenal insufficiency) or the unmasking of decreased cortisol production only in the stimulated state (*incomplete* adrenal insufficiency) (Table 92-10).

In all cases of *complete* adrenal insufficiency the cortisol secretory rate is markedly decreased, and this may be ascertained indirectly by the finding of low to absent 24-hr urine 17-hydroxycorticoids and urine 17-ketosteroids. Because of the contribution of the male gonads to urine 17-ketosteroids, basal excretory values in complete adrenal insufficiency will be higher for males than females. With incomplete adrenal insufficiency, urine steroid excretion values overlap into the normal range; because of this, a diagnosis of adrenal insufficiency cannot be made solely on the values of basal urine steroid determinations. Plasma cortisol values are from zero to the lower range of normal. Aldosterone secretion is very low judged by isotopic secretory rate determinations, as are aldosterone excretory values. In patients with primary adrenal insufficiency, plasma ACTH levels are elevated because of loss of the usual cortisol-hypothalamic feedback relationship, whereas in secondary adrenal insufficiency plasma ACTH values are low, a finding consistent with the absence of increased pigmentation in patients having the latter condition.

The specific and definitive diagnosis of adrenal insufficiency can be made only with the ACTH stimulation test to assay the adrenal reserve capacity for steroid production. In addition, ACTH testing is helpful in establishing whether adrenal insufficiency is primary or secondary. In patients undergoing ACTH testing as a diagnostic method for adrenal insufficiency, saline solution should be utilized as the diluent for the ACTH to be infused, since on occasion patients may experience an acute febrile episode when glucose is used. An additional advantage of using saline diluent is that a clinical estimate of adrenal responsiveness may be made by the presence or absence of weight gain during the infusion period, weight gain commonly occurring when adrenocortical function is intact. The potential dangers of ACTH testing in patients

Table 92-10. LABORATORY EVALUATION AND TESTING OF ADRENOCORTICAL FUNCTION IN ADRENAL INSUFFICIENCY*

	Plasma ACTH	Plasma cortisol	Cortisol secretory rate	Urine values	Control base line	Days of ACTH stimulation			
						1	2	3	4
Primary:									
Complete..................	I†	D‡	D	17-OH :	0–2	0–2	0–2	0–2	0–2
				17-KS :	3–6	3–6	3–6	3–6	3–6
Incomplete................	I	D	D	17-OH :	1–4	5–10	6–12	5–10	5–10
				17-KS :	5–7	7–10	8–12	7–10	7–10
Secondary:									
Complete..................	D	D	D	17-OH :	0–2	2–6	5–10	7–14	10–20
				17-KS :	0–6	4–8	5–8	6–10	8–15
Incomplete................	D	D	D	17-OH :	1–4	5–10	7–14	10–20	20–30
				17-KS :	5–7	5–8	6–10	8–15	15–20

* Clinical status charted vertically, and representative values for steroid tests charted horizontally. 17-OH, 17-KS refer to 24-hr urine 17-hydroxycorticosteroid and 17-ketosteroid excretion. All laboratory values given in milligrams per day. Note that plasma ACTH values are increased in primary forms and decreased in secondary forms. Note also that differentiation between primary and secondary forms on ACTH stimulation testing becomes greatest on day 3 and day 4 of stimulation.

† I, increased.

‡ D, decreased.

with limited adrenal reserves may be minimized by the prior **administation of 1 mg of a potent steroid such as dexamethasone.** The excretory products of 1 mg of this compound will not add appreciably to the amount of 17-hydroxycorticoids measured in the urine and therefore will not interfere with the test. For testing purposes, 40 units of ACTH is infused in the standard manner for 4 to 5 successive days, with daily urine collections tested for creatinine, 17-hydroxycorticoid, and 17-ketosteroid levels. Alternatively, a continuous 48-hr ACTH infusion may be used by giving 40 units of ACTH in 500 ml of 5 percent dextrose in normal saline solution every 12 hr for four consecutive 12-hr periods. In patients with complete primary adrenal insufficiency, ACTH stimulation by either method will cause a rise in steroid excretion of less than 2 mg per day.

In *incomplete* adrenal insufficiency, ACTH testing carried out by either method will result in subnormal increments in urinary 17-hydroxycorticoids. A variant of this response is sometimes seen in which small increments in steroid excretion occur on the first 3 days of the 5-day infusion test, while on the last 2 days, there is an actual decline in the level of steroids. Alternately, the last 12 hr of the continuous 48-hr infusion will show a decline in 17-hydroxycorticoid excretion. These results suggest that the limited adrenal tissue has been maximally stimulated and has insufficient steroid reserve capacity. In patients with adrenal insufficiency secondary to *anterior pituitary hypofunction,* a "staircase" response in steroid excretion is seen on successive days of ACTH stimulation, signifying that the adrenal can respond to exogenous ACTH and that the deficit must reside in the failure to produce and/or release endogenous ACTH.

Patients receiving long-term steroid therapy, despite physical findings of Cushing's syndrome, develop adrenal insufficiency both because of prolonged suppression of the hypothalamic corticotropin-releasing center and because of actual adrenal atrophy. Adrenal atrophy results from the loss of endogenous ACTH stimulation, which stimulus is prerequisite for maintaining normal adrenal size. Thus, these patients acquire two deficits, a loss of adrenal responsiveness to ACTH and a failure of pituitary ACTH release. These patients are characterized by low blood cortisol and ACTH levels, low base-line steroid excretion, and abnormal ACTH and metyrapone test results. On testing these patients with ACTH, one looks for the "staircase" response, with successive daily increments in steroid excretion; however, *prolonged ACTH testing* may be needed to elicit such a response. The urine steroid pattern, when adrenal reactivation does occur, often reveals increments in 17-hydroxycorticoids without parallel increments in 17-ketosteroids. Practically all patients with steroid-induced adrenal insufficiency will eventually respond to ACTH testing, but individual response time is most variable, ranging from days to months. Once such patients are shown to have reacquired adrenal sensitivity to exogenous ACTH, their ability to release endogenous pituitary ACTH must be determined. The standard metyrapone test is utilized for this purpose. For a valid metyrapone test, it must be previously documented that the patient's adrenal glands are sensitive to ACTH, since the metyrapone test response depends on adrenal responsiveness to released ACTH. For this reason the test is *contraindicated* in patients with suspected or proved adrenal insufficiency. In patients with steroid-induced adrenal insufficiency, abnormal (low) metyrapone tests usually continue for several months after the adrenal glands have regained responsiveness to ACTH. In interpreting the metyrapone test it is useful to consider it as an endogenous ACTH stimulation test and compare the peak urine 17-hydroxycorticoid excretion with the maximal values previously obtained with exogenous ACTH stimulation.

Plasma ACTH levels help distinguish between primary

and secondary adrenal insufficiency, since they are elevated in the former and decreased to absent in the latter.

Indirect tests of adrenocortical function include (1) a delay in water excretion following an acute water load; (2) defective renal conservation of sodium when a low sodium, high potassium diet is imposed; (3) a tendency toward hypoglycemia during fasting and hypoglycemic unresponsiveness following the intravenous administration of insulin. Since ACTH is available for direct evaluation of adrenocortical function, these procedures are *rarely* indicated; furthermore, in a patient with adrenocortical insufficiency, water intoxication, sodium deprivation, or hypoglycemia may all be life-threatening situations.

DIFFERENTIAL DIAGNOSIS. Since weakness and fatigue are such common complaints, clinical diagnosis of early adrenocortical insufficiency is frequently difficult (Table 92-9). However, mild gastrointestinal distress with weight loss, anorexia, and a suggestion of increased pigmentation make mandatory ACTH stimulation testing to rule out adrenal insufficiency, particularly before steroid treatment is begun. Weight loss is useful in evaluating the significance of weakness and malaise. Racial pigmentation in Negroes, Orientals, Indians, Spanish Americans, and Latins and hyperpigmentation in other diseases represent a major problem. These diseases include hemochromatosis, acanthosis nigricans, porphyria, thyrotoxicosis, polyostotic fibrous dysplasia, chronic metal poisoning (bismuth, lead, arsenic, silver), chronic malnutrition (starvation, anorexia nervosa, sprue syndrome, pellagra), progressive malignancy, chronic anemia, salt-losing nephritis with hypotension, renal tubular acidosis, scleroderma, excess nicotinic acid, and hepatic cirrhosis. In most cases, differentiation from Addison's disease is not difficult, but when doubt exists, ACTH administration ordinarily provides clear-cut differentiation.

ETIOLOGY AND PATHOGENESIS. Addison's disease results from progressive adrenocortical destruction, which must involve more than 75 percent of the glands before clinical signs of adrenal insufficiency appear. The adrenal is a frequent site for chronic infectious diseases of the granulomatous variety, predominately tuberculosis but also including fungal infections such as histoplasmosis, coccidioidomycosis, and cryptococcosis. In previous years, tuberculosis was found at postmortem examination in 70 to 90 percent of cases; however, the most frequent finding at present is *idiopathic* atrophy, and it has been suggested that an autoimmune mechanism may be responsible for this process. Rarely, other lesions are encountered, such as bilateral tumor metastases, amyloidosis, or sarcoidosis.

The possibility that some patients may have primary adrenal insufficiency on an *autoimmune basis* has been strengthened by the finding that one-half of patients with Addison's disease have circulating adrenal antibodies, tested by the indirect Coons method. These antibodies appear species-specific but lack organ specificity. Certain of these patients also have additional circulating antibodies to thyroid or parathyroid tissue, a finding of inter-

est because of the increased incidence of hypothyroidism and hypoparathyroidism in Addison's disease.

ADDISON'S DISEASE ASSOCIATED WITH OTHER ENDOCRINE DYSFUNCTIONS. In 1926, Schmidt described two patients with nontuberculous Addison's disease and chronic lymphocytic thyroiditis. Subsequent reports have documented association of thyroid insufficiency and Addison's disease, and the possibility of a common autoimmune process has been raised as the etiologic factor responsible for *Schmidt's syndrome.* More than 20 patients have been described with concomitant parathyroid and adrenal insufficiency. In most of these patients, autoantibodies have been discovered, raising the possibility that these two diseases may be related to a common event. Diabetes mellitus has now been reported as being associated with Addison's disease in more than 100 cases. Again, what role genetic predisposition and/or autoimmunity may play in the occurrence of these two diseases in the same individual is unknown. Rarely, the combination of Addison's disease, myxedema, and diabetes mellitus has been described. Between 3 and 4 percent of patients with Addison's disease have coexistent hyperthyroidism. The presence of both disorders in the same individual poses a difficult diagnostic problem, since many of the clinical manifestations are similar. Furthermore, the hyperthyroid state may change a subclinical insufficiency to complete adrenal insufficiency, because of the effect, mentioned above, of thyroid hormone on cortisol metabolism.

Further study of patients with combined endocrine dysfunction may prove valuable in revealing the cause of spontaneous adrenal destruction.

TREATMENT. All patients with Addison's disease should receive specific hormone replacement therapy. Like diabetics, these patients require careful and persistent education in regard to their disease. Since the adrenal gland elaborates three general classes of hormone, of which two, glucocorticoids and mineralocorticoids, are of primary clinical importance, replacement therapy should correct both deficiencies. Cortisone (or hydrocortisone) is the mainstay of treatment; however, its mineralocorticoid effect, when it is given in sufficient dosage to replace the endogenous hydrocortisone deficiency, is inadequate for complete electrolyte balance; therefore, the patient usually requires other supplementary hormone. Cortisone dosage varies from 12.5 to 50 mg daily, with the majority of patients taking 25 to 37.5 mg in divided doses. Because of its direct local effect on gastric mucosa, patients are advised to take their cortisone with meals or, if this is impractical, with milk or an antacid preparation. In addition, the larger proportion of the dose (25 mg) is taken in the morning and the remainder (12.5 mg) in the late afternoon, to simulate somewhat the normal diurnal adrenal rhythm. Some patients may exhibit insomnia, irritability, mental excitement, and even frank psychosis soon after initiation of therapy; in these the dosage should obviously be reduced. Other indications for maintaining the patient on smaller amounts are hypertension, diabetes, or active tuberculosis.

Since, as mentioned earlier, this amount of cortisone or

hydrocortisone fails to replace the mineralocorticoid component of the adrenal gland, supplementary hormone is usually needed. The simplest means is daily oral administration of 0.1 to 0.2 mg of 9α-fluorohydrocortisone. If parenteral administration is indicated, 2.0 to 5.0 mg deoxycorticosterone acetate in oil may be given every day intramuscularly. An alternative method of therapy is an injection of 25 to 50 mg deoxycorticosterone trimethylacetate in oil intramuscularly every 3 to 4 weeks, but as with the previous use of subcutaneous implantation of pellets of deoxycorticosterone which lasted for 8 to 10 months, most patients prefer the simplicity of daily oral administration of the 9α-fluorohydrocortisone.

Complications of cortisone therapy, with the exception of peptic disease, particularly ulcer or gastritis, are *extremely rare* in the dosage used in the treatment of Addison's disease. However, overtreatment with deoxycorticosterone preparations or 9α-fluorohydrocortisone is more frequent and may present as edema, hypertension, cardiac enlargement, or even congestive failure due to sodium retention. Overtreatment may also present as weakness, progressing to total paralysis, due to hypokalemia. In the management of patients with Addison's disease, regular measurements of body weight, serum potassium, heart size, and blood pressure, and serial electrocardiograms are useful.

All patients with adrenal insufficiency, including bilaterally adrenalectomized patients, should carry medical identification, should be educated and instructed in the parenteral self-administration of steroids, and should be registered with a national medical alerting system.

SPECIAL THERAPEUTIC PROBLEMS. During periods of intercurrent illness, the dose of cortisone or hydrocortisone should be increased to levels of 75 to 150 mg per day. When oral administration is not possible, parenteral routes should be employed. Likewise, before surgery or dental extractions, excess steroid should be administered. For a representative program of steroid therapy for an Addisonian patient or an adrenalectomized patient undergoing a major operation, see Table 92-11. The patients should all be advised of these facts and should carry an identification card bearing detailed instructions for the administration of steroid in case of acute illness or injury. Patients should also be advised to increase the dose of 9α-fluorohydrocortisone and add excess salt to their otherwise normal diet during periods of excessive exercise with sweating, during extremely hot weather, or during periods of gastrointestinal upsets. In spite of animal studies demonstrating an increased susceptibility to tubercular spread associated with excess steroid administration, patients with Addison's disease and tuberculosis may be maintained safely on 12.5 to 25 mg cortisone daily.

COURSE AND PROGNOSIS. Untreated Addison's disease characteristically runs a chronic and relentless course. In some patients, its advance is relatively slow, but in all patients the condition may rapidly deteriorate into adrenal crisis. With treatment, the prognosis of the disease is extremely favorable. In fact, some of the degenerative vascular problems such as hypertension or congestive failure are more easily handled in an Addisonian patient than in one with intact adrenal glands.

Acute Adrenocortical Insufficiency

Acute adrenocortical insufficiency may result from several processes. One of these, usually termed *adrenal crisis,* is a rapid and overwhelming intensification of chronic adrenal insufficiency. Another process involves an acute hemorrhagic destruction of both adrenal glands, usually associated with an overwhelming septicemia. Adrenal hemorrhage due to excessive anticoagulants is being seen with increasing frequency. A third, and probably the most

Table 92-11. STEROID THERAPY SCHEDULE FOR ADDISONIAN PATIENT UNDERGOING A MAJOR OPERATION*

	Cortisone acetate (intramuscularly)		Cortisone acetate (orally)				Fluorohydrocortisone (orally)	Hydrocortisone infusion
	7 A.M.	7 P.M.	8 A.M.	12 M.	4 P.M.	8 P.M.	8 A.M.	Continuous
Routine daily medication.....	...	...	25	...	12.5	...	0.1	
Day before operation........	...	50	25	...	12.5	...	0.1	
Day of operation............	100	50	...	...	...	...	...	200
Postoperative day 1..........	50	50	...	...	...	...	...	100–150
" 2..........	50	50	...	...	...	...	...	50–100
" 3..........	50	50	25	...	...	25	...	
" 4..........	50	...	25	25	25	...	0.1	
" 5..........	...	...	25	25	25	25	0.1	
" 6..........	...	...	25	25	25	...	0.2	
" 7..........	...	...	25	12.5	25	...	0.2	
" 8..........	...	...	25	12.5	25	...	0.2	
" 9–13.......	...	...	25	12.5	12.5	...	0.1	
" 14.........	...	...	25	12.5	...	...	0.1	

* All steroid doses are given in milligrams.

frequent, cause of acute insufficiency results from the rapid withdrawal of steroids from patients with adrenal atrophy secondary to chronic steroid administration.

Adrenal Crisis

The long-term survival of patients with Addison's disease largely depends upon prevention and treatment of adrenal crisis. Consequently, the occurrence of infection, trauma (including surgery), gastrointestinal upsets, or other forms of stress requires an immediate increase in hormone. In previously untreated patients, preexisting symptoms are intensified. Nausea, vomiting, and abdominal pain may become intractable. Fever is frequently severe but may be absent. Lethargy deepens into somnolence, and the blood pressure and pulse fail as hypovolemic vascular shock ensues. In contrast, patients previously maintained on hormone therapy may not exhibit severe dehydration or hypotension until preterminally, at which time there is an extremely rapid decline.

Treatment is primarily directed toward the rapid elevation of circulating adrenocortical hormone, in addition to the replacement of the sodium and water deficit. Hence, an intravenous infusion of 1,000 ml 5 percent glucose in normal saline solution containing 100 to 200 mg of any of several soluble hydrocortisone preparations is begun rapidly, with the first 250 ml infused in the first ½ to 1 hr and the remainder over the ensuing 4 to 8 hr. If the condition is extreme, immediate intravenous infusion of 100 mg hydrocortisone in the first few minutes is suggested, followed by a rapid infusion as described above. Epinephrine, 0.2 mg intravenously, may also be indicated. In any case, it is also advisable to administer 100 mg cortisone acetate intramuscularly in case the infusion becomes infiltrated or inadvertently stopped. If the crisis was preceded by prolonged nausea, vomiting, and dehydration, several liters of saline replacement is indicated. With large doses of steroid, as, for example, 200 mg cortisone or hydrocortisone, the patient receives a maximal mineralocorticoid effect, and supplementary deoxycorticosterone is superfluous. After the initial infusion, depending on the patient's condition, a second similar infusion may be given; if there has been marked improvement, the patient may be offered oral fluids and be given 50 mg cortisone acetate intramuscularly every 12 hr until gastrointestinal absorption is guaranteed, at which time the steroid can be given orally. Steroid dosage is then tapered over the next few days to maintenance levels, with reinstitution of supplementary mineralocorticoid if needed.

Adrenal Hemorrhage

Adrenal hemorrhage (adrenal apoplexy) is usually associated with overwhelming septicemia (Waterhouse-Friderichsen syndrome); however, it may also occur in the absence of sepsis. Occasionally, massive bilateral adrenal hemorrhage results from birth trauma. The infant may either be stillborn or die soon after birth of shock and hyperpyrexia. Adrenal hemorrhage also occurs in patients with advanced hypertension and arteriosclerosis, during pregnancy, following idiopathic adrenal vein thrombosis, during convulsions in epilepsy or during electroconvulsive therapy, with excessive anticoagulant therapy, and after trauma or surgery. Pain in the flank and epigastrium is frequent, and if the hemorrhagic process ruptures into the abdomen, signs of peritoneal inflammation are present.

The adrenal hemorrhage associated with septicemia is most frequent with meningococcemia but is also seen with overwhelming infections due to pneumococcus, staphylococcus, or *Hemophilus influenzae*. The onset is often explosive, with a shaking chill, violent headache, vertigo, vomiting, and prostration. A petechial rash appears on the skin and mucous membranes and progresses rapidly to a confluent, extensive purpura. Large areas of skin may become grossly hemorrhagic. Body temperature may be subnormal but is usually markedly elevated. Circulatory collapse rapidly ensues, and death may occur within 6 to 48 hr. Specific diagnosis requires immediate identification of the organism. Frequently, the septicemia is so massive that organisms may be seen in peripheral blood smears or petechial scrapings. Time is not sufficient for determination of adrenal function; however, a plasma sample for later determination of 17-hydroxysteroid level may be of academic interest.

Treatment must be immediate and intensive. Control of the infection by vigorous administration of parenteral, preferably intravenous, antibiotics is indicated in addition to the steroid schedule delineated for adrenal crisis. Intravenous norepinephrine (4 to 8 mg per liter) may also be required to maintain vascular tone. Since shock may also be associated with massive septicemia without adrenal hemorrhage, one is never completely certain whether adrenal insufficiency is contributing to the patient's decompensation; however, the authors think that because of the increasing frequency of survival of patients treated with steroid, some degree of adrenal insufficiency, whether relative or absolute, is present and that steroid treatment is therefore indicated in all patients in whom fulminating septicemia is associated with shock.

Adrenal Insufficiency Due to Metabolic Failure in Hormone Production

This group of patients includes those with congenital adrenal hyperplasia and those receiving one of several pharmacologic agents which are capable of inhibiting hormone synthesis in the gland. These include Amphenone, which appears to inhibit synthesis of all hormones early in the sequence of reactions from cholesterol and concomitantly results in hypertrophy of the gland; and various derivatives of diphenyl dichloroethane, of which the o,p-dichloro-derivative is the most active [o,p'-DDD (Perthane)] and causes atrophy and even necrosis of adrenocortical tissue. Three other compounds specifically block an enzymatic step in the formation of cortisol: 2-methyl-1,2-bis-(3-pyridyl)-1-propanone (metyrapone, SU-4885) and p-aminophenyl-2-phenylethylamine selectively inhibit 11-hydroxylation of the steroid nucleus, and aminoglutethamide appears to block the conversion of cholesterol to pregnanelone. Furthermore, thyroid hormone, increases the conversion of cortisol to the biologically inactive cortisone and thereby can produce a state of relative adrenal insufficiency.

Hypoaldosteronism

Patients with *isolated* aldosterone deficiency are rare. Such a deficiency accompanied by normal cortisol production has been reported as a congenital biosynthetic defect; postoperatively following removal of aldosteronoma; during protracted heparin or heparinoid administration; in pretectal disease of the nervous system; in severe postural hypotension; and in association with complete heart block.

In severe cases urine sodium wastage is present on a normal salt intake, whereas in milder forms excessive urine sodium losses occur only during salt restriction. The patients always develop hyponatremia and hyperkalemia, the latter often to a severe degree.

A biosynthetic defect has been noted in some patients who are unable to transform the angular C-18 methyl group of corticosterone to the C-18 aldehyde grouping of aldosterone. This C-18 transformation requires first the formation of 18-hydroxycorticosterone from corticosterone, and then, secondly, dehydrogenation of the C-18 hydroxyl group to form the characteristic C-18 aldehyde group of aldosterone. These patients will manifest low to absent aldosterone secretion and excretion in association with elevated secretion and excretion values for corticosterone and 18-hydroxycorticosterone.

The feature common to all patients with hypoaldosteronism has been their inability to *increase* aldosterone secretion appropriately during severe salt restriction. An additional feature has been the reversal of the signs of salt wasting, hyponatremia and hyperkalemia, with the administration of potent mineralocorticoids. For practical purposes the oral administration of 9_α-fluorohydrocortisone in a dose of 0.1 to 0.3 mg daily restores electrolyte balance.

NONSPECIFIC USE OF ACTH AND ADRENAL STEROIDS IN CLINICAL PRACTICE

The widespread application of ACTH and adrenal steroid therapy in many branches of medicine and surgery emphasizes the need for a thorough understanding of the metabolic effects of these agents if clinical use is to be most effective and if undesirable side reactions are to be minimized. Before instituting adrenal hormone therapy, a physician should weigh carefully the gains that can reasonably be expected versus the potentially undesirable metabolic actions of the particular hormone. Accurate appraisal will require familiarity with the reports of others in similar instances, a critical evaluation of the statistical significance of such reports, as well as a clear understanding of the chemical, physiologic, and psychologic changes

Table 92-12. ADRENAL PREPARATIONS

Commonly used name	Other names	Estimated potencies*	
		Glucocorticoid	Mineralocorticoid
Hydrocortisone......................	Cortisol, hydrocortone Compound F, 17-hydroxycorticosterone PREGN-4-ene-11_β,17_α,21-triol-3,20-dione	1	1
Cortisone...........................	Cortone, compound E 11-Dehydro-17-hydroxycorticosterone PREGN-4-ene-17_α,21-diol-3,11,20-trione	0.8	0.8
DOC...............................	Percorten, cortexone, 11-deoxycorticosterone PREGN-4-ene-21-ol-3,20-dione	0	15
Aldosterone........................	Electrocortin PREGN-4-ene-11^β, 21-diol-18-al-3,20-dione	0.3	400
Prednisolone.......................	Meticortelone, Δ1-hydrocortisone PREGN-1,4-diene-11_β,17_α,21-triol-3,20-dione	4	0.25
Prednisone.........................	Meticorten,Δ1-cortisone PREGN-1,4-diene-17_α,21-diol-3,11,20-trione	4	0.25
Methyl prednisolone.................	Medrol, 6-methyl-Δ1-hydrocortisone	5	±
Triamcinolone......................	Aristocort, Kenacort 16_α-Hydroxy-9_α-fluoro-$Δ^1$-hydrocortisone	5	±
Dexamethasone......................	Decadron, Hexadrol 16_α-Methyl-9_α-fluoro-$Δ^1$-hydrocortisone	30–40	±
Fluorohydrocortisone................	Florinef, Fluoro-F 9_α-Fluorohydrocortisone	10	300

* Relative milligram comparisons to cortisol, setting the glucocorticoid and mineralocorticoid properties of cortisol as 1. Sodium retention insignificant in usual doses employed of methyl prednisolone, triamcinolone, and dexamethasone.

Table 92-13. CONSIDERATIONS PRIOR TO THE USE OF CORTICOSTEROIDS AS PHARMACOLOGIC AGENTS

1. How serious is the underlying disorder?
2. How long will therapy be required?
3. What is the anticipated effective dose range?
   a. To ameliorate symptoms?
   b. To suppress effectively the signs and symptoms of the disorder?
4. Is the patient predisposed to any of the known hazards of steroid therapy by virtue of having:
   a. Hypertension or cardiovascular disease?
   b. Peptic ulcer, gastritis, or esophagitis?
   c. Osteoporosis?
   d. Diabetes mellitus?
   e. Tuberculosis or other infections?
   f. Psychologic difficulties?
5. Which adrenal preparation is preferable?
   a. Choice of steroid preparation?
   b. ACTH versus steroids?
   c. Steroids by mouth versus steroids by injection?
6. Alternate day therapy.
7. Supplementary adjuvants employed to minimize metabolic disabilities.
8. A schedule for withdrawing corticosteroids.
9. Summary.

that hormone preparations of this type are known to induce (Table 92-12).

Perhaps an approach to the problem presented by a particular patient may be facilitated by reviewing the specific considerations outlined in Table 92-13.

How Serious Is the Underlying Disorder?

The use of any nonspecific or "symptomatic" pharmacologic agent must be weighed against the seriousness of the underlying disorder. Each pharmacologic agent has a "price tag," which must be evaluated carefully before a therapeutic program is begun. With the antibiotic agents this price tag may consist of the possibility of inducing drug-sensitivity reactions or the development of antibiotic-resistant strains of pathogenic organisms; with the agents employed for hypertensive cardiovascular disease the price tag may consist of disturbing side effects referable to the autonomic nervous system. With the corticosteroids, effective therapy may be purchased at the risk of inducing undesirable side reactions such as peptic ulceration, osteoporosis, or psychologic abnormalities. Clearly, in a patient whose life is threatened by unexplained shock or in whom other measures have failed to modify the course of disseminated lupus erythematosus, the physician need not hesitate to employ massive steroid therapy. On the other hand, one should exercise restraint in administering suppressive steroid therapy to a patient with early rheumatoid arthritis who as yet has not received the possible benefits of physiotherapy and a well-organized program of general medical care.

How Long Will Therapy Be Required?

The problems which arise in connection with evaluating the seriousness of the underlying disorder naturally involve the expected or anticipated duration of therapy. Thus the use of intravenous hydrocortisone for 24 to 48 hr in the treatment of severe status asthmaticus or acute serum sickness or a drug reaction does not present the same problem as the treatment of chronic, lifelong asthma or psoriasis. In general, contraindications to steroids for severe, short-lived disorders will be few, whereas in suppressive therapy for chronic, persistent disorders one must envisage the serious problem presented by Cushing's syndrome, which results from prolonged ingestion of exogenous glucocorticoid.

What Is the Anticipated Effective Dose Range?

Hormone therapy may be employed in a relatively low dosage schedule calculated to achieve clinical improvement but not necessarily complete suppression of all signs and symptoms of the disorder. In the former case, 50 to 75 mg cortisone or hydrocortisone (or the equivalent amount of one of its derivatives) may be adequate to attain worthwhile clinical improvement, whereas 150 to 300 mg cortisone or hydrocortisone may be needed to suppress all evidences of activity of the disease. At the 50- to 75-mg dosage of cortisone or hydrocortisone, it might be feasible to embark on long-term therapy with minimal risk of serious complications resembling Cushing's syndrome, whereas at the 150-mg dosage level, relief of one disease may be attained only at the risk of inducing another (Cushing's syndrome). In general, doses of hydrocortisone or cortisone of 75 mg or less may be tolerated by most patients for prolonged periods of time with a minimum of underlying metabolic disabilities, whereas doses of cortisone or hydrocortisone of 100 mg or more will usually be associated with progressive metabolic aberrations. Dosage of cortisone or hydrocortisone in the range of 25 to 50 mg daily can, in all probability, be tolerated by most patients for life.

Is the Patient Predisposed to Any of the Known Hazards of Steroid Therapy by Virtue of Having Any of the Following Conditions?

HYPERTENSION OR CARDIOVASCULAR DISEASE. In general, the sodium-retaining propensity of most adrenal steroid preparations requires that caution be used when they are given to patients with preexisting hypertension or cardiovascular or renal disease. The availability of preparations in which sodium-retaining activity is minimal (triamcinolone and dexamethasone), restriction of dietary sodium intake, and the use of resins, diuretic agents, and particularly supplementary potassium salts will permit the safe use of steroid therapy where important indications exist. Of course, in congestive failure or pericardial effusion associated with acute rheumatic activity or in patients with nephrotic edema, steroid hormone preparations may act as effective diuretic agents.

For all patients in whom prolonged steroid therapy is contemplated cardiovascular-renal status should be carefully evaluated, with a chest film for *heart size* and an electrocardiogram included.

PEPTIC ULCER, GASTRIC HYPERSECRETION, OR ESOPHAGITIS. Patients with a history of gastric hypersecretion or peptic ulcer are likely to experience aggravation of their symptoms while receiving adrenal hormone therapy. It is not known for certain whether aggravation of peptic ulceration and complicating gastrointestinal hemorrhage reflect the increased gastric secretory activity so frequently associated with adrenal hormone therapy or whether the nitrogen-depleting effect of these hormones accelerates the process of ulceration and perforation. Antacid therapy and an ulcer diet are useful precautions in susceptible patients. *The development of anemia in a patient on ACTH or cortisone therapy should immediately suggest gastrointestinal bleeding,* and patients should be cautioned to note black or tarry stools. A clear-cut history of peptic ulcer is a contraindication to ACTH and cortisone therapy unless extreme precautions are taken.

OSTEOPOROSIS. All patients on prolonged cortisone-like steroid therapy are likely to develop some degree of osteoporosis. Obviously a considerable change in bone structure must occur before it is radiologically demonstrable. For this reason patients should have standard films of the spine and pelvis in order to establish the status of the bony framework before therapy and for comparative purposes later. Postmenopausal women and men and women of advanced age will be predisposed to the earlier development of serious changes of this type. The skin also participates in the depletion of body protein, becoming thin and atrophic and easily bruisable. It is possible that ACTH may cause less osteoporosis for a given level of steroid therapy because of a concomitant increase in adrenal androgen secretion. This possible advantage of ACTH over crystalline steroids is offset by the difficulty with which an exact pharmacologic dosage of endogenous steroid is maintained with the tropic hormone. Since corticosteroids, in general, exert an anti-vitamin-D-like action, all patients on adrenal steroids should receive a generous supplement of vitamin D, i.e., 1,500 IU daily. Supplementary calcium therapy in the form of calcium lactate, 1 Gm three times daily, and estrogen and androgen therapy should be considered in those patients known to be susceptible to the catabolic action of adrenal steroids. Sodium fluoride therapy (3 mg daily) may also be beneficial. Of course, any degree of osteoporosis a priori would constitute evidence against the desirability of prolonged high-dosage adrenal hormone therapy.

DIABETES MELLITUS. Prolonged ACTH or cortisone-like steroid therapy may unmask latent diabetes mellitus and aggravate preexisting disease. For this reason a careful history is important to exclude familial incidence of diabetes, as well as an examination of the blood and urine for excess glucose levels. It is more valuable to carry out these examinations following a test load of carbohydrate. A convenient method consists in measuring blood and urinary glucose 2 to 3 hr after the ingestion of a breakfast containing approximately 100 Gm carbohydrate (see Chap. 94). Obviously the presence of frank diabetes mellitus or the demonstration of impaired glucose tolerance will affect the physician's decision to institute adrenal hormone therapy. However, if such therapy appears necessary or desirable in the presence of latent diabetes, the judicious use of supplementary insulin should be seriously considered. The insulin requirement of known diabetics will usually need to be increased with ACTH or cortisone-like therapy except in those rare instances in which the diabetic patient is suffering from some degree of insulin-protein reaction in which the anti-inflammatory or antiallergic effect of cortisone enhances the metabolic effectiveness of the insulin sufficiently to balance off the diabetogenic action of the former.

TUBERCULOSIS OR OTHER INFECTIONS. Before prolonged steroid therapy is seriously considered, it is imperative to exclude tuberculosis and other infections. Continued steroid therapy, without a specific antibiotic agent, can lead to serious spread of infection. A chest film is essential before prolonged steroid therapy is begun, and the desirability of cultures from the nose and throat and of the urine and feces, if symptoms point to any disturbances, is evident.

PSYCHOLOGIC DIFFICULTIES. From time to time steroid therapy may be complicated by severe psychologic disturbances, and, of course, less-severe abnormalities are relatively frequent. In general, serious psychologic disturbances are more closely related to the patient's personality structure than to the actual dose of hormone, although, as might be anticipated, larger doses of hormone will be associated with more frequent serious reactions. At present there is no reliable method of determining beforehand a patient's psychologic reaction to steroid therapy. Patients with known psychologic difficulties undoubtedly experience more frequent and more severe disturbances. Further difficulty arises because previous tolerance of steroids does not necessarily ensure immunity from subsequent courses of therapy, and untoward psychologic reactions on one occasion do not invariably mean that the patient will respond unfavorably to a second course of treatment. This is one area in which the physician must follow his patient carefully during the early period of steroid therapy and one in which he must take a responsible member of the patients' family into his confidence.

Consideration of the foregoing conditions will produce important data on which the physician's ultimate decision for or against hormone therapy will rest.

Which Adrenal Preparation Is Preferable?

CHOICE OF STEROID PREPARATION. Four considerations need to be taken into account in deciding which steroid preparation to use. The first of these is the biologic half-life of the particular compound. The rationale behind every-other-day therapy is to decrease the metabolic effects of the steroids for a significant amount of time over the 2-day period, yet at the same time to produce pharmacologic suppression of sufficient duration to maintain the disease in remission. Too long a half-life would defeat the first purpose, and too short a half-life would defeat the second. In general, the more potent the steroid, the longer its biologic half-life tends to be. The second consideration is whether the mineralocorticoid effects of the steroid are important. The newer synthetic steroids have much less mineralocorticoid effect relative to their glucocorticoid effect than cortisol or cortisone (Table 92-12). This may be an important consideration in certain disease states. Thirdly, cortisone and prednisone, in contrast to the other glucocorticoids, have to be converted into their biologically active equivalents before any anti-inflammatory effects can occur. Finally, the cost of the medication needs to be considered seriously, particularly if chronic administration is to be undertaken. Per tablet, prednisone is the least expensive of all adrenal steroids. However, the physician should be aware that there are probably a number of steroid preparations whose formulation is inferior, so that they result in less than the optimum therapeutic effect.

ACTH VERSUS STEROIDS? In most cases, the only decision of major consequence is whether to use ACTH rather than one of the adrenal steroid preparations. In general, adrenal steroid therapy is effective by mouth and can be regulated more accurately than ACTH therapy. The latter will fluctuate considerably in the amount of steroid produced from day to day, depending on the rate and extent of absorption of ACTH and on the state of the adrenal cortex. ACTH therapy does stimulate the secretion of adrenal androgens as well as hydroxysteroids. The former may have advantages in certain diseases, such as dermatomyositis, in which the adrenal androgens may prove helpful in maintaining the muscle mass while the inflammatory reaction is being suppressed by the 17-hydroxycorticosteroids. Combined androgen and corticoid therapy may, of course, attain the same objective. Sodium retention with ACTH has often been more marked than with cortisone or, particularly, with prednisone therapy.

There is little support for the belief that ACTH stimulates the production of naturally useful steroids qualitatively different from those available commercially. The use of ACTH, of course, presupposes a normally responsive adrenal cortex, an assumption that cannot always be verified in serious or prolonged disorders. Both ACTH and steroid administration induce pituitary inhibition. In addition, steroid therapy also induces adrenal suppression. For practical purposes ACTH is used to initiate a therapeutic response and to activate the adrenal cortex before steroid therapy is discontinued. It has, of course, a very important use in the diagnostic approach to disorders of adrenal function.

STEROIDS BY MOUTH VERSUS STEROIDS BY INJECTION. In acute emergencies such as brain tumor, allergic reactions, and shock, steroids will be administered intravenously in large doses, i.e., 300 to 500 mg hydrocortisone or 10 to 20 mg dexamethasone in 24 hr. For patients on long-term steroid therapy who develop gastrointestinal bleeding or symptoms of peptic ulcer, it may prove helpful in addition to the usual medical measures, to administer the daily steroid requirement *intramuscu-*

larly. This reduces the concentration of steroid reaching the gastrointestinal tract, without impairing the systemic effect.

"Alternate-Day" Therapy

It has been shown that twice the daily maintenance dose, given every other day, may minimize pituitary and adrenal atrophy as well as reduce the degree of Cushingoid changes. Such a schedule is well worth considering for any patient destined to receive corticosteroids for prolonged periods.

Supplementary Adjuvants Employed to Minimize Metabolic Disabilities

Since the continued use of ACTH or adrenal steroids induces a hypokalemic, hypochloremic metabolic alkalosis, supplementary potassium therapy should be given daily to patients receiving these hormone preparations. Potassium may be given as an elixir of potassium chloride, 2 to 3 tsp three times daily with meals (4 mEq potassium per tsp). Potassium chloride has a great theoretical and practical advantage over "mixed" potassium salts, particularly those containing potassium bicarbonate or citrate. Renal insufficiency is the primary complication in which supplementary potassium medication must be monitored carefully.

Antacid therapy and an ulcer-type diet *should be instituted* for all patients on steroid or ACTH therapy who give evidence of past or present increased gastric acidity, peptic ulceration, or upper gastrointestinal bleeding.

In patients who will require long-term ACTH or steroid therapy, the attending physician should make repeated efforts to ascertain whether the major manifestations of the underlying disorder cannot be held in satisfactory abeyance with a reduced hormone dosage. The ultimate development of Cushing's syndrome and its serious complications may prove more disastrous 3 to 5 years hence than the disease for which steroids were initially prescribed. Therefore *any* reduction in hormone dosage, however small, may be important in postponing the day of reckoning.

It is often possible to effect a considerable reduction in steroid maintenance dosage, if very small decrements are made, such as 5 percent per month. *Percentage* reduction should always be employed, as a reduction of 5 mg prednisone per day from a level of 100 mg to 95 mg is quite different from a reduction from 30 to 25 mg. It is also important for both patient and physician to appreciate that steroid therapy in general creates some degree of "euphoria" and hence a tendency to addiction. Thus a reduction in steroid dosage will initially be accompanied by a decrease in "energy" or sense of well-being. This may reduce the patient's threshold for tolerating the symptoms of his underlying disease without necessarily representing a true exacerbation. With a very small percentage decrease in dosage and with reassurance by the physician and understanding on the part of the patient, it is remarkable what can be accomplished in reducing the steroid level over a prolonged period. Patients are extremely grateful for any help that they can be given in this direction, when the long-range threat of steroid-induced complications is carefully explained.

When carrying out a slow, gradual reduction in steroid dosage, it must be realized that a sudden exacerbation of the underlying process may occur in conjunction with an acute infection or unusual stress. Under these circumstances the steroid dosage must be increased immediately, but it can usually be reduced promptly to the former dosage level once the precipitating factor is alleviated.

A Proposed Schedule for Attempting Withdrawal of ACTH or Corticosteroids Following Their Long–term Use as Pharmacologic Agents

Corticosteroid therapy induces both pituitary and adrenal suppression, whereas ACTH therapy affects only the former. For practical purposes it should be assumed that the majority of patients on prolonged steroid therapy will ultimately regain sufficient pituitary-adrenal activity to meet everyday needs. Regardless of how far in the past prolonged steroid therapy was given, in case of emergencies such as surgery, injuries, and severe infections, *supplementary cortisol or cortisone should always be employed*. It will also be apparent that regardless of the stepwise manner in which complete withdrawal of steroids is accomplished, there must always be a period of relative hypoadrenalism before endogenous ACTH-adrenal activity is restored. This is a point that must be seriously considered in patients with systemic lupus or widespread skin diseases, in which temporary hypoadrenalism may precipitate a serious or life-threatening exacerbation and hence is contraindicated. In such patients, Addisonian maintenance therapy for the long term may be indicated. For those patients, however, in whom it would appear advantageous to withdraw steroid therapy, the following schedule is suggested. *Steroid medication should not be withdrawn* until a patient's daily requirement is less than 50 mg hydrocortisone, 10 mg prednisone, or 1 to 1.5 mg dexamethasone.

The patient's steroid is changed to dexamethasone in a dosage equivalent to that of the steroid being employed, i.e., 1 mg dexamethasone for each 25 to 30 mg hydrocortisone; 1 mg dexamethasone for each 5 to 8 mg prednisone.

After 3 to 5 days on dexamethasone alone, base-line 24-hr urinary hydroxysteroid levels are determined (dexamethasone at this dosage level does not add appreciably to urinary steroid values).

While dexamethasone therapy is continued, ACTH is added in relatively large doses, i.e., 40 units intravenously over 8 hr daily for 3 to 5 successive days, or 80 units given in a continuous 24-hr infusion for 2 days or 80 units intramuscularly twice daily until urinary hydroxysteroids have attained a value at least three times the normal base line.

With evidence of adequate adrenocortical response, the maintenance dose of dexamethasone should be appropriately reduced and discontinued.

During this entire period the patient remains vulnerable to undue stress and must be protected on such occasions by administration of ACTH or an appropriate dose of glucocorticoid.

When a patient being maintained on dexamethasone and receiving ACTH in the larger dose as outlined above, fails to display a brisk adrenal response, he must be returned to a maintenance dose of steroid. ACTH can then be given intramuscularly two to three times weekly in a dose of 80 units in addition to the maintenance dose of steroid, and at a later date (4 to 6 weeks) the original schedule may be tried again. Failure to observe a satisfactory adrenal response on the second occasion implies, for practical purposes, permanent primary adrenocortical insufficiency, and the patient should be treated as for Addison's disease.

Summary

Several general facts should be considered in the management of patients receiving prolonged steroid therapy.

1. There is real danger of inducing acute adrenal failure if steroid therapy is suddenly withdrawn. Furthermore, adrenal reserve may be inadequate for a *prolonged* period after steroid therapy ends. Under these circumstances, patients must be warned about the additional risk of acute stress reactions such as injuries, operations, and infections. Both the patient and his doctor should be aware of this problem, and supplementary corticoid therapy should be readily available at all times.

2. Patients being maintained on a constant dose of steroid over a prolonged period should be protected by an increase in hormone therapy during a period of surgery or endocrine stress. It may be necessary to increase the basic dose of glucocorticoid by the equivalent of 100 mg cortisone per day.

3. When steroids such as prednisone, which usually do not invoke appreciable sodium retention or edema, are being used, one must be on the alert for more subtle evidence of overdosage during a prolonged therapeutic program. Special attention should be given to disturbance in the gastrointestinal tract, as indicated by the appearance of digestive symptoms or occult blood in the stool. Signs suggestive of bone pain due to the development of underlying osteoporosis should be carefully watched for.

4. All patients receiving prolonged steroid therapy should have periodic checks, which should include body weight, blood pressure, urine sugar, and appraisal of the cardiovascular, digestive, and skeletal systems. The possibility of the development of posterior subcapsular cataracts must be considered.

Adrenal hormone therapy constitutes a potent pharmacologic agent in the armamentarium of every practicing physician. As with all potent medicaments, a physician's responsibility must include an adequate knowledge of the pharmacologic actions of these agents as well as of the indications and contraindications for their use.

REACTION TO INJURY AND STRESS

A febrile response, leukocytic changes, and alterations in the erythrocyte sedimentation rate are well recognized indexes of injury and the body's reaction to it. It is now recognized, however, that the reaction to injury involves a series of integrated responses which affect the whole organism. Changes in the circulation are accompanied by important psychologic and neuromuscular alterations. These are mediated via a group of chemical and metabolic reactions initiated by neurohormonal mediators and chemical substances—the latter derived from injured tissue. These reactions involve the pituitary and adrenal gland secretions, as well as the liver, kidney, and hematopoietic tissues. Alterations in protein, carbohydrate, and fat metabolism occur, as well as significant changes in electrolyte concentration and distribution. In addition, immunologic changes accompany the general reaction to stress and represent important defense mechanisms for the organism (see Chap. 68).

Selye has applied the descriptive title of "the alarm reaction" to the series of events which may be initiated by such varied stresses as emotional disturbances, infection, hemorrhage, trauma, or undue exposure to heat and cold. Injury such as occurs with full-thickness burns gives rise to the most intense pattern of reaction.

In the original hypothesis, it was assumed that the increased liberation of adrenal hormones, both medullary and cortical, was largely responsible for initiating the widespread metabolic changes characteristic of this syndrome. Indeed, by the use of highly purified ACTH preparations or synthetic adrenal steroids, it has been possible to reproduce many of the changes characteristic of this general response. Thus, increased excretion of nitrogen, potassium, and phosphorus, retention of sodium chloride and water, reduction in circulating eosinophils and lymphocytes, increase in polymorphonuclear leukocytes, elevation of blood sugar level with decreased glucose tolerance, changes in important plasma constituents such as cholesterol and globulin, and alterations in gastrointestinal secretions, as well as fundamental changes in psychologic behavior and neuromuscular function, have all been observed in patients and in normal persons given large quantities of ACTH or cortisol. Although widespread effects of this type can be induced by stimulating the intact adrenal gland of man with purified ACTH preparations or by the administration of the appropriate adrenal steroids, there is evidence that mechanisms other than those related to activation of the pituitary-adrenal axis are capable of inducing similar metabolic and chemical changes. In fact, only in severe stress or tissue injury is a measurable increase in blood or urine adrenal steroid level demonstrable. Thus, it appears more correct to interpret the total response of the organism to stress as representing the effects of pituitary–adrenal cortical stimulation acting in combination with a variety of other metabolic and immunologic alterations.

REFERENCES

Addison, T.: "On the Constitutional and Local Effects of Disease of the Suprarenal Capsules," London, S. Highley, 1855.

Afifi, A. K., R. A. Bergman, and J. C. Harvey: Steroid Myopathy. Clinical, Histologic, and Cytologic Observations, Johns Hopkins Med. J., 123:158, 1968.

Beisel, W. R., V. C. DiRaimonde, and P. H. Forsham: Cortisol Transport and Disappearance, Ann. Intern. Med., 60:641, 1964.

Berson, S. A., and R. S. Yalow: Radioimmunoassay of ACTH in Plasma, J. Clin. Invest., 47:2725, 1968.

Biglieri, E. G., M. A. Herron, and N. Brust: 17-Hydroxylation Deficiency in Man, J. Clin. Invest., 45:1946, 1966.

Blizzard, R. M., R. W. Chandler, M. A. Kyle, and W. Hung: Adrenal Antibodies in Addison's Disease, Lancet, II:901, 1962.

Conn, J. W., and L. H. Louis: Primary Aldosteronism, A New Clinical Entity, Ann. Intern. Med., 44:1, 1956.

Cushing, H.: The Basophil Adenomas of the Pituitary Body and Their Clinical Manifestations (Pituitary Basophilism), Bull. Johns Hopkins Hosp., 50:137, 1932.

Dexter, R. N., L. M. Fishman, R. L. Ney, and G. W. Liddle: Inhibition of Adrenocortical Steroid Synthesis by Amino Glutethamide: Studies of Mechanisms of Action, J. Clin. Endocrinol. & Metab., 27:473, 1967.

Graber, A., R. L. Ney, W. E. Nicholson, D. P. Island, and G. W. Liddle: Natural History of Pituitary Adrenal Recovery Following Long-term Suppression with Corticosteroids, Trans. Assoc. Am. Physicians, 77:296, 1964.

Hellman, L., H. L. Bradlow, B. Zumoff, and T. F. Gallagher: The Influence of Thyroid Hormone on Hydrocortisone Production and Metabolism, J. Clin. Endocrinol. & Metab., 21:1231, 1961.

Herrera, M. G., G. F. Cahill, Jr., and G. W. Thorn: Cushing's Syndrome: Diagnosis and Treatment, Am. J. Surg., 107:144, 1964.

Hutter, A. M., Jr., and D. E. Kayhoe: Adrenocortical Carcinoma: Clinical Features in 138 Patients, Am. J. Med., 41:572, 1966.

Lauler, D. P.: Preoperative Diagnosis of Primary Aldosteronism, Am. J. Med., 41:855, 1966.

Luetscher, J.: Primary Aldosteronism: Observations in Six Cases and Review of Diagnostic Procedures, Medicine, 43:137, 1964.

Maeda, R., M. Okamoto, L. C. Wegienka, and P. H. Forsham: A Clinically Useful Method for Plasma Testosterone Determination, Steroids, 13:83, 1969.

Murphy, B. E.: Some Studies of the Protein Binding of Steroids and Their Application to the Routine Micro and Ultramicro Measurements of Various Steroids in Body Fluids by Competitive Protein Binding Radioassay, J. Clin. Endocrinol. & Metab., 27:973, 1967.

Paris, J.: On the Diagnosis of Addison's Disease and Cushing's Syndrome by Laboratory Methods, Mayo Clinic Proc., 39:26, 1964.

Ross, E. J.: Aldosterone and Its Antagonists, Clin. Pharm. & Therap., 6:65, 1965.

Thorn, G. W.: Clinical Considerations in the Use of Corticosteroids, New England. J. Med., 274:775, 1966.

93 PHEOCHROMOCYTOMA

Roger B. Hickler and George W. Thorn

The first pheochromocytoma was described by Frankel in 1886, with the term subsequently given by Pick to describe tumors which are selectively colored by chromium salts. The syndrome of paroxysmal hypertension due to this tumor was first clearly described by Labbe, Tinel, and Coumier in 1922. In 1926 Roux and in 1927 Mayo performed the first successful surgical removals of the tumor. In 1936 Beer, King and Prinzmetal determined that the characteristic paroxysmal rise in blood pressure was associated with the release of hormone from the tumor into the blood. *Persistent* hypertension was first attributed to the tumor in the same year by Kremer.

INCIDENCE. It is estimated that over 1,000 cases of pheochromocytoma have been identified, the incidence rising with improved diagnostic techniques. Anatomic statistics from the Mayo Clinic showed 15 of these tumors in 15,984 autopsies, an overall incidence of 0.1 percent. Smithwick estimated the incidence in a hypertensive population explored for sympathectomy to be 0.5 percent.

ANATOMY. Embryologically two cell types differentiate from a common stem cell, the sympathogonia of the primitive neuroectoderm, to form the adrenal medulla: the chromaffinoblast and the neuroblast, which mature into the chromaffin cell and sympathetic ganglion cell, respectively. These medullary cells are richly supplied with preganglionic fibers from the splanchnic nerves.

The chromaffin cell is so named because of its capacity to show brown intracytoplasmic granules on treatment with chromium salts, a result of oxidation and polymerization of the catecholamine stored in the granules. Chromaffin cells are found in widely dispersed sites at birth: the adrenal medulla, the paraganglia (along the retropleural and retroperitoneal sympathetic chains), the organs of Zuckerkandl (paired structures lying anterior to the bifurcation of the abdominal aorta), chemoreceptor areas ("glomic tissue" at the carotid bifurcation, along the aortic arch, and at the jugular bulb), and the human dermis. Many of the extraadrenal sites undergo progressive involution until puberty, but remnants account for the extraadrenal occurrences of pheochromocytomas, reported in all of the areas cited with the exception of the skin.

PATHOLOGY. Over 50 percent of pheochromocytomas occur in the region of the adrenals, sometimes bilaterally, and over 90 percent lie between the diaphragm and pelvic floor. As indicated by metastases, 6 percent are malignant and 7 percent occur simultaneously in more than one focus. Metastases may be functional and have occurred in liver, lungs, and central skeleton, as well as paraaortic lymph glands. The tumor weight may vary from a gram to several thousand grams (averaging about 100 Gm) and correlates poorly with the severity of the symptomatology. The tumors are round, frequently lobulated, and highly vascular. They may show hemorrhagic and necrotic areas with cystic degeneration, particularly large tumors. On section they appear brown or gray. Histologically they resemble the adrenal medulla; the nuclei are often multiple, cytoplasmic vacuolization is common, and dark staining with chromium salts is characteristic. Benign tumors may invade the capsule and are difficult if not impossible to distinguish from malignant forms on purely histologic grounds.

PHYSIOLOGY. The chromaffin cells of the adrenal medulla synthesize, store, and secrete epinephrine and norepinephrine. The biosynthesis of these hormones proceeds as follows: conversion of phenylalanine to tyrosine; oxidation of tyrosine to dopa (3,4-dihydroxyphenylalanine); decarboxylation of dopa to dopamine (3,4-dihydroxyphenylethylamine); and oxidation of dopamine to norepinephrine; epinephrine is formed by methylation of norepinephrine (Fig. 93-1). Epinephrine is the major hormone of the adrenal medulla, constituting 80 percent of its stored content of catecholamine; the major source of norepinephrine is the postganglionic sympathetic neurone, where it acts as the neurotransmitter.

The catecholamines are stored in cytoplasmic granules in the medullary chromaffin cells, which also contain a high content of adenosine triphosphate (ATP). It has been suggested that hydrolysis of adenosine triphosphate in the granules by an adenosine triphosphatase disrupts the granules and permits release of the hormone, which is normally released by cholinergic preganglionic sympathetic nerve impulses. A number of agents can directly stimulate chromaffin cells or the adrenergic neurones to release catecholamines, including acetylcholine, nicotine, histamine, 5-hydroxytryptamine, tyramine, and reserpine. A number of physiologic stimuli cause an increase in the release of both epinephrine and norepinephrine such as severe muscular work, asphyxia and hypoxia, and hemorrhagic hypotension. Insulin hypoglycemia causes a selective release of epinephrine alone, favoring the concept of separate cells for the synthesis and separate control of the release of adrenomedullary epinephrine and norepinephrine.

The physiologic effects of the adrenomedullary hormones may be characterized as preparing the organism to meet an emergency situation. Both epinephrine and norepinephrine have a direct inotropic and chronotropic effect on the heart. However, the purely vasoconstrictor effect of norepinephrine results in diastolic and systolic hypertension, producing reflex slowing of the heart, so that cardiac output is generally unchanged or reduced. The net peripheral vasodilator effect of physiologic doses of epinephrine (due primarily to vasodilatation of resistance vessels of skeletal muscle) permits a rise in cardiac output, with widening of pulse pressure through a rise in systolic pressure; diastolic pressure may fall slightly. Cutaneous and renal vasoconstriction is common

Fig. 93-1. The degradation of epinephrine and norepinephrine by catechol-O-methyl transferase (CMT) and monamine oxidase (MAO). All the above compounds appear in the urine in the free form or conjugated to glucuronide or sulfate. The heavier arrows indicate the major pathways. 3-Methoxy-4-hydroxy-mandelic acid is also designated as vanil mandelic acid (VMA).

to both hormones. Both increase the rate and depth of respiration and stimulate the release into plasma of non esterified fatty acids from neutral fat depots. Other metabolic effects characteristic of epinephrine and, to a lesser extent, of norepinephrine, include increased formation of active phosphorylase in liver and skeletal muscle, resulting in accelerated hepatic glycogenolysis and release of lactic acid from muscle. These effects lead to hyperglycemia, increased oxygen consumption, and a high respiratory quotient.

CATECHOLAMINE METABOLISM. Figure 93-1 shows the major paths of metabolism of norepinephrine derived from sympathetic nerve endings, and of norepinephrine and epinephrine derived from the adrenal medulla. Most of the norepinephrine which is synthesized is converted *in situ* to metabolically inactive dihydroxymandelic acid by the action of intraneuronal monamine oxidase (MAO) before it can exert any biologic effect. This is discharged into the circulation and may be further metabolized by the enzyme catechol O-methyl transferase (COMT), present in high concentration in liver and kidney, to 3-methoxy, 4-hydroxy mandelic acid (vanil mandelic acid or VMA). Of the catecholamine which is released "intact," a small fraction interacts with receptor sites. The rest is either recovered and again bound in the storage granules, or carried in the circulation and rapidly converted by catechol O-methyl transferase to inactive

methoxy derivatives: norepinephrine to normetanephrine and epinephrine to metanephrine (collectively referred to as *metanephrines*). A portion of the metanephrines so formed may, in turn, be oxidized by monamine oxidase, present in most tissues, to vanil mandelic acid. Bilateral adrenalectomy results in only a minor depression of urinary catecholamines, since 80 percent is normally norepinephrine, largely derived from sympathetic nerve endings. The high activity of these two enzyme systems (MAO and COMT) is indicated by the fact that, by weight, the daily urinary content of the metanephrines (after hydrolyzing the major conjugated fraction free of its glucuronide or sulfate) is approximately seven times, and of VMA approximately thirty times that of the total catecholamines. Half of the catecholamine is in the "free" form and half as glucuronide or sulfate conjugates.

Crout and Sjoerdsma have defined the abnormal turnover and metabolism of catecholamines in patients with pheochromocytoma. Individual tumors vary widely in rates of production and turnover of catecholamines. Small tumors tend to release in active form (and rapidly replace) a comparatively high proportion of their relatively small total content of stored catecholamines. This relates to a low rate of oxidation by the tumor of stored catecholamines to inactive metabolites, as judged by a comparatively low urinary VMA catecholamine ratio. By contrast, large tumors tend to metabolize a considerable portion of their relatively large catecholamine stores prior to release, thus generating a high urinary VMA/catecholamine ratio. The latter probably escape detection until they grow to a size large enough to permit a significant level of release of free catecholamines despite their high rate of inactivation by the tumor. Reports of "asymptomatic" pheochromocytomas, found incidentally at laparotomy or autopsy, may be explained by these phenomena.

CLINICAL MANIFESTATIONS. In a review of 507 cases of pheochromocytoma, Hermann and Mornex report that 26 percent of cases presented with paroxysmal hypertension and 60 percent with permanent hypertension; of the latter, nearly half had crises superimposed on their sustained hypertension. The remaining 14 percent had atypical features or absent clinical signs. Thus, *the characteristic hypertensive crisis is found in only about one-half of all cases.* Thomas, Rook, and Kvale reviewed the symptoms in 100 patients with the paroxysmal hypertensive form of the disease. The triad of headache, excessive perspiration, and palpitations was found in about three-quarters of instances. Commonly associated manifestations were pallor, nausea, tremor, weakness, nervousness, and epigastric pain. Less common complaints were chest pain, dyspnea, flushing, numbness, visual blurring, tightness of the throat, and dizziness. Bradycardia is found in approximately 20 percent of cases. Paroxysms are frequently spontaneous but may be precipitated by physical exertion, abdominal palpation, and emotional upset. They may occur several times a day or at rare intervals, and may last for only a minute or for as long as a week. Blood pressure levels frequently exceed 250/150 mm during an attack in association with the paroxysmal release of catecholamine, as shown in Fig. 93-2. Shock and renal failure may attend or follow a paroxysmal attack. During a paroxysm death may occur from pulmonary edema, ventricular fibrillation, or cerebral hemorrhage.

Cases of *persistently* secreting tumors may be difficult to distinguish from cases of essential hypertension, but hyperglycemia and hypermetabolism (elevated BMR) are found in approximately 50 percent of patients with these tumors. Progressive weight loss and the demonstration of postural hypotension are further suggestive clinical evidence of sustained catecholamine secretion by a tumor. Frank retinopathy (grade 3 to 4 funduscopic changes) is found in more than half of these patients, an appreciably higher incidence than is found in the purely paroxysmal variety. This underscores the gravity of this form of hypertension and the importance of early clinical detection.

Special Features. Several unique aspects of the disease deserve emphasis. The tumor may first appear in early childhood or old age, but the average age of onset is during the fourth decade. In childhood pheochromocytoma the hypertension is almost always of the sustained variety, and the tumor tends to be bilateral and show a higher incidence of malignancy than in the adult. Distinct genetic factors are implicated in some instances by the prevalence of the tumor in certain families, sometimes in association with other congenital disorders of the neuroectoderm such as neurofibromatosis and central nervous system hemangioblastoma. A number of reports deal with the familial coincidence of pheochromocytoma and thyroid cancer, which is usually the medullary or solid type with amyloid production. This complex also has been coupled with parathyroid tumors as in the form of "multiple endocrine neoplasia" (Chap. 87).

Chromaffin-positive norepinephrine-secreting tumors of the glomic tissue of the carotid body and jugular bulb have been reported. These may represent further examples of the relationship between dysplasia of the neuroectoderm and the paroxysmal syndrome. There is an isolated case report of unilateral adrenal medullary hyperplasia in which removal of the hyperplastic gland resulted in complete amelioration of the signs and symptoms of excessive catecholamine secretion.

True polycythemia has been reported in association with the tumor, with return of the red cell mass to normal after successful surgery. Pheochromocytoma of the bladder wall produces a unique syndrome of paroxysmal symptoms, particularly throbbing headache, on micturition. While the majority of pheochromocytomas produce more norepinephrine than epinephrine (in contradistinction to the normal adrenal medulla), a few have been reported which are predominantly epinephrine secretors. These tend to be of the paroxysmal type and to produce hypotension and shock during a paroxysm, perhaps due to the vasodilating effect of the beta-adrenergic stimulation on the peripheral vasculature. The frequency of a diabetic tendency increases as the proportion of the epinephrine to the total catecholamine content of the tumor increases, perhaps because of the greater glycogenolytic activity of epinephrine. However, impaired carbohydrate tolerance has been found in pure norepinephrine secretors, and recent evidence indicates that the associated excessive alpha-adrenergic stimulation will inhibit insulin release to account for the impairment.

Over 50 percent of patients dying with a pheochromocytoma have an active myocarditis at autopsy. In the

M.A., ♀, 49 YRS.
Pheochromocytoma

Fig. 93-2. The plasma epinephrine and norepinephrine levels before, during, and after a spontaneous paroxysm. The change in levels illustrates the intermittent secretory activity shown by some tumors and underlines the importance of obtaining samples for diagnostic purposes at the height of a spontaneous or induced attack.

majority of these instances there was prior clinical evidence of left ventricular failure. In all probability this is a direct, "toxic" effect of the high levels of catecholamines on the myocardium.

Finally, a hypertensive response to smoking, to anesthesia, or to therapy with ganglionic blocking agents and guanethidine should raise the strong suspicion of a pheochromocytoma.

DIAGNOSIS. The clinical picture of essential hypertension with marked vasomotor lability strongly suggests pheochromocytoma, but pheochromocytoma with sustained hypertension in the absence of paroxysms may be indistinguishable from essential hypertension. Thus, routine laboratory screening of all patients with significant hypertension is desirable for this potentially curable form of hypertension.

Urinary Assay for Catecholamines and Their Methoxy Derivatives. Modern chemical methods for the determination of 24-hr urinary catecholamines and their methoxy derivatives have largely replaced the older pharmacologic tests in routine screening because of their safety and greater accuracy. Current chemical methods for determining urinary free catecholamines involve modifications of the trihydroxyindole (THI) method of Lund. The urinary-free catecholamines are adsorbed on an alumina or resin column, eluted with acid, oxidized to form "chromes," which, in turn, are tautomerized in alkali to form strongly fluorescent trihydroxyindoles. Free epinephrine and norepinephrine may be measured separately from fluorometric readings at different wave lengths. After acid hydrolysis to free the conjugated fractions, metanephrine (MN) and normetanephrine (NMN) may be isolated on resin and converted to trihydroxyindoles for fluorometric assay or oxidized to vanillin and read photometrically. VMA is measured by isolation and oxidation to vanillin, which may be read photometrically directly or after color development with added indole.

With these techniques Sjoerdsma and associates determined, simultaneously, the 24-hr urinary free catecholamines, metanephrines, and vanilmandelic acid on 64 patients with proven pheochromocytoma. The results are shown in Fig. 93-3 and indicate that the values obtained for all three assays were above the upper limit of normal in all but a few instances, giving an overall diagnostic reliability in the range of 90 percent. The upper limits of normal are (1) free catecholamines (epinephrine plus norepinephrine), 100 μg; (2) metanephrine plus normetanephrine, 1.3 mg; (3) VMA, 6.5 mg. Therapy with alpha-methyl dopa will produce false elevations in the free catecholamines and, potentially, in the metanephrines. Dietary sources of p-hydroxy-mandelic acid such as bananas produce false positives in the VMA determination. In general, *it is important to discontinue sympathomimetic agents and monamine oxidase inhibitors when performing these assays.* The relative diagnostic merits of the three different indices is debated, and it is probable that any one of them, carefully done, will serve equally well.

Pharmacologic Tests for Pheochromocytoma. In the absence of facilities for these chemical determinations, re-

liance may be placed on the various intravenous pharmacologic tests. Along with the phentolamine (Regitine[R]) test, which produces a precipitous fall in blood pressure in pheochromocytomas, there are now in use three "provocative" tests: the older histamine and the newer tyramine and glucagon tests. Unfortunately, deaths have occurred after both phentolamine and histamine in pheochromocytomas, and the pharmacologic approach probably fails to detect as many as 25 percent of cases. The matter is further complicated by the prevalence of false positives with these agents. The intravenous tyramine test has the advantage over histamine and glucagon of causing a milder rise in blood pressure in the presence of a pheochromocytoma, but, by the same token, the end point of a positive reaction is less succinct. It is strongly contraindicated in any patient receiving amine oxidase inhibitor therapy, where the administration of tyramine may precipitate a hypertensive crisis. Histamine and probably glucagon should not be used if the control pressure is 170/110 mm or above, and phentolamine should be ready for immediate administration in the advent of a precipitous rise in blood pressure when these tests are performed. With pressures in the range of 170/110 mm or above, the tyramine and phentolamine tests are the ones of choice.

In a small percentage of patients, particularly during a normotensive period in those with intermittently secreting tumors, 24-hr urinary assay for catecholamines (or derivatives thereof) may not be clearly elevated into a diagnostic range. If suspicion is still strong on clinical grounds, the tumor may be provoked to secrete with 0.01 to 0.025 mg histamine base, given intravenously. This should be followed by the rapid injection of 5 mg phentolamine intravenously, should an alarming rise in blood pressure ensue. Blood may be drawn during the control period and at intervals of 2 min in the immediate posthistamine period for plasma assay for catecholamines, or a timed urine specimen (after prior emptying of the bladder) may be collected for a period of 6 hr for analysis for catecholamines or methoxy derivatives which may be expressed as amount excreted per milligram of creatinine.

The upper limit of normal for plasma epinephrine and norepinephrine varies with the method employed (trihydroxyindole or ethylenediamine condensation) and must be established in a given laboratory to determine a diagnostic rise following histamine administration. The upper limit of normal for urinary catecholamines (epinephrine plus norepinephrine) is 0.05 μg per mg creatinine; for metanephrine plus normetanephrine, it is 2.1 μg per mg creatinine; for VMA, it is 9.5 μg per mg creatinine. Levels above these following histamine administration are diagnostic. If a spontaneous attack should occur while a patient is under observation, blood and urinary determinations should be made immediately (Fig. 93-2). The plasma ethylenediamine condensation method for plasma catecholamines is invalid in the presence of uremia.

Localization of Tumor. While rarely palpable, a tumor mass may be detected on a plain film of the abdomen. Traditional and more specialized techniques for tumor localization have been tomography of the suprarenal areas

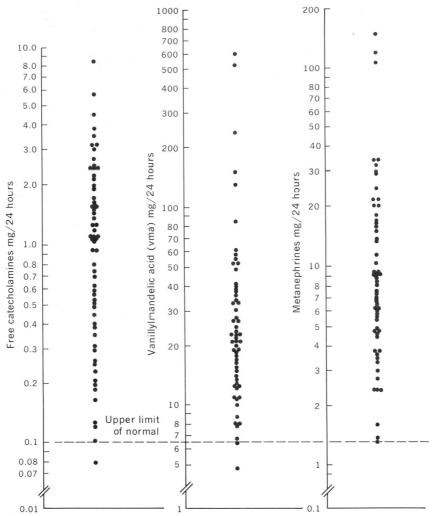

Fig. 93-3. Urinary excretion of catecholamines and metabolites in 64 patients with proved pheochromocytoma. (*By permission of The Annals of Internal Medicine 65: 1966, Fig. 2, p. 1306. Sjoerdsma, A., Engelman, K., Waldmann, T. A., Cooperman, L. H., and Hammond, W. G., Combined Clinical Staff Conference at the National Institutes of Health. Pheochromocytoma: Current Concepts of Diagnosis and Treatment.*)

during an intravenous pyelogram, and abdominal filming following the contrast afforded by presacral carbon dioxide insufflation. More recently, the advent of selective renal and adrenal angiography has afforded superb information in this regard; in some hands, these newer radiologic procedures are proving to be the ones of choice. The hazards attending these contrast techniques (including the potential for direct tumor stimulation) are apparent, and phentolamine should be ready for immediate administration during their performance. The analysis of catecholamines in plasma obtained by catheter at different levels in the venous system under fluoroscopic control has also been useful. Thoracic tumors, while rare, may be seen on a plain chest film.

Crout and Sjoerdsma report that the separate determination of urinary epinephrine and norepinephrine is of predictive value in tumor localization. If there is a significant elevation of epinephrine as well as norepinephrine

(42 percent of all cases), the tumor may be expected to lie in or adjacent to one of the adrenal glands or, rarely, in the organs of Zuckerkandl. If the urine contains elevated norepinephrine alone (58 percent of all cases), the tumor, of course, may still be found in one of the adrenal areas. Less than 10 percent of tumors are extra-abdominal, and these will generally show only an elevation of urinary norepinephrine and probably reflect a deficiency of N-methylating enzyme, present in the normal adrenal medulla and necessary for the conversion of norepinephrine into epinephrine.

DIFFERENTIAL DIAGNOSIS. Incorrect diagnoses in the presence of a pheochromocytoma have included diabetes mellitus, thyrotoxicosis, anxiety neurosis, "vascular" headache, epilepsy, and hypertensive crises due to lead poisoning and porphyria.

Patients with "nonchromaffin" sympathetic tumors, i.e., ganglioneuromas and, particularly, neuroblastomas have shown elevated levels of norepinephrine in the urine as well as increased excretion of its precursors (dopa and dopamine) and of its methoxy metabolites (metanephrines and VMA). Since some of these patients have associated hypertension, these tumors are to be distinguished from true "chromaffinomas." Another condition in which hypertension may be associated with markedly elevated urinary catecholamine excretion in the absence of a pheochromocytoma is Guillain-Barre syndrome, which perhaps results from a pathologic alteration in the sympathetic nervous system.

TREATMENT. In patients in whom surgical resection of the tumor cannot be performed, as with functioning metastases, the regular oral administration of the alpha-adrenergic blocking agent phenoxybenzamine (Dibenzyline[R]) has been reported to have controlled most of the disturbing signs and symptoms for a period of many months. This approach has also been recommended routinely for a period of several weeks in order to get patients into an optimum condition in preparation for surgery, as in the presence of malignant hypertension with congestive heart failure. The use of beta-adrenergic blockers, such as propranolol, may also be useful in protecting against beta-adrenergic mediated cardiac arrhythmias from high circulating levels of catecholamines. The use of inhibitors of catecholamine synthesis is another approach to the pharmacologic treatment and preoperative control of patients with pheochromocytoma; preliminary reports of the use of alpha-methyl-para-tyrosine in this regard are very encouraging.

Surgical removal of the tumor is the treatment of choice for this potentially lethal disease. Since over 90 percent of all such tumors are located in the abdomen, a careful abdominal exploration through a generous transverse upper abdominal incision may be undertaken, even without the certain exclusion of a rare extraabdominal site. To avoid extremes of hypertension during induction of anesthesia and surgical manipulation, an intravenous drip of phentolamine should be ready at all times. To avoid extremes of hypotension on clamping the blood supply of the tumor and following its removal, an intravenous drip of norepinephrine or other pressor amine should also be prepared in advance. *Administration of whole blood or plasma on removal of the tumor may be of paramount importance in preventing postoperative shock*, since the sudden relief of the prolonged vasoconstriction attending the disease produces a state of disparity between the vascular capacity and effective blood volume.

REFERENCES

Crout, J. R., and A. Sjoerdsma: Turnover and Metabolism of Catecholamines in Patients with Pheochromocytoma, J. Clin. Invest., 43:94, 1964.

Hermann, H., and R. Mornex: Human Tumours Secreting Catecholamines: Clinical and Physiopathological Study of the Pheochromocytomas, Oxford, Pergamon Press, 1964.

Mitchell, P. L., and E. Meilman: The Mechanism of Hypertension in the Guillain-Barre Syndrome, Am. J. Med., 42:986, 1967.

Page, L. B., and R. B. Copeland: Pheochromocytoma, Disease-a-Month, January, 1968.

Sjoerdsma, A., K. Engelman, T. A. Waldmann, L. H. Cooperman, and W. G. Hammond: Combined Clinical Staff Conference at the National Institutes of Health. Pheochromocytoma: Current Concepts of Diagnosis and Treatment, Ann. Intern. Med., 65:1302, 1966.

Sheps, S. G., and F. T. Maher: Histamine and Glucagon Tests in Diagnosis of Pheochromocytoma, J.A.M.A., 205:895, 1968.

Steiner, A. L., A. D. Goodman, and S. R. Powers: Study of a Kindred with Pheochromocytoma, Medullary Thyroid Carcinoma, Hyperparathyroidism and Cushing's Disease: Multiple Endocrine Neoplasia, Type 2, Medicine, 47:371, 1968.

Thomas, J. E., E. D. Rooke, and W. F. Kvale: The Neurologist's Experience with Pheochromocytoma: A Review of 100 Cases, J.A.M.A., 197:754, 1966.

Wurtman, R. J.: Catecholamines, New England Journal of Medicine Medical Progress Series, Boston, Little, Brown and Company, 1966.

94 DIABETES MELLITUS

Jurgen Steinke and George W. Thorn

Knowledge of diabetes is important because of its high prevalence, it has been estimated that there are 200 million diabetics in the world, and because the treated diabetic individual has the potential for a nearly normal life-span. Diabetes has metabolic and vascular components, which are both probably interrelated. The metabolic syndrome is characterized by an inappropriate elevation of blood glucose, associated with alterations in lipid and protein metabolism for which a relative or absolute lack of insulin is responsible. The vascular syndrome consists of accelerated nonspecific atherosclerosis and a more specific microangiopathy particularly affecting the eye and kidney.

HISTORY

Diabetes has been recognized from antiquity. Chinese medical writings mentioned a syndrome of polyphagia, polydipsia, and polyuria. Aretaeus (*ca.* A.D. 70) described the disease and gave it its name, meaning in Greek "to run through."

The study of the chemistry of diabetic urine was initiated by Paracelsus in the sixteenth century; however, he mistook the residue of the boiled urine for salt instead of sugar. Some 100 years later, Thomas Willis described the sweetness of the diabetic urine, "as if imbued with honey or sugar," which Dobson proved to be sugar. This led to a rational dietary approach, introduced by Rollo 29 years later. Morton (1686) noted the hereditary character of diabetes. In 1859, Claude Bernard demonstrated the increased glucose content of diabetic blood and recognized hyperglycemia as the cardinal sign of the disease. In 1869, Langerhans, still a medical student, described the islet cell formation in the pancreas, which now bears his name. Kussmaul characterized the air hunger and labored breathing of the patient in diabetic coma in 1874. The careful work by clinicians such as Bouchardat, Naunyn, von Noorden, Allen, and Joslin led to a significant therapeutic success with diet. Von Mering and Minkowski carried out their studies in 1889, demonstrating that dogs could be made diabetic by pancreatectomy. However, it took more than 30 years before Banting and Best were able to prepare an extract from dog pancreas capable of reducing an elevated blood glucose level. In 1939, the first long-acting insulin was introduced by Hagedorn. The chemical structure of ox insulin was established by Sanger in 1953; Nicol and Smith described the chemical structure of human insulin in 1960. The basic unit contains two polypeptide chains united by disulfide bridges. In 1964, Katsoyannis in the United States and Zahn in Germany completed the synthesis of both the A and B chains of insulin and were able to combine both chains into biologically active material. In 1967 Steiner described a large "proinsulin" molecule which is converted by enzymatic cleavage into the smaller biologically active insulin.

The accidental discovery of the hypoglycemic action of carbutamide by Franke and Fuchs in Germany, in 1955, and the earlier experimental work of Loubatieres in France initiated the use of oral hypoglycemic agents.

PREVALENCE

Diabetes mellitus is a disease of worldwide distribution. If it is more frequent in some countries than in others, it will have to be established when diagnostic criteria are agreed upon and uniformly controlled detection drives are executed. In the United States there are approximately 4 million persons with diabetes, close to 2 percent of the total population. Diabetes is more frequent in older people. The United States Public Health Service estimates that there are 2 diabetics for every 1,000 people up to age twenty-four, 10 between the ages of twenty-five and forty-four, 33 in the age group forty-five to fifty-four, 56 between ages fifty-five and sixty-four, and 69 per 1,000 between sixty-five and seventy-four years of age. Unless a cure or some preventive measure is found for diabetes, this number will continue to increase for the following reasons: (1) the population grows and becomes older; (2) the life expectancy of the treated diabetic is close to normal, or is at least two-thirds that of the general population at a given age; (3) since more diabetics live long enough to have children, an increasing number of children will inherit the diabetic gene; and (4) obesity, which appears to precipitate diabetes among those predisposed to it, is also on the rise, thus allowing more potential diabetics to emerge.

The undiagnosed adult diabetic presents a major challenge to the practicing physician. Not infrequently diabetic symptoms are minimal, and the patient does not seek medical advice. In the United States, approximately 50 percent of the 4 million diabetics are unidentified. Because early treatment prolongs life, these undiagnosed diabetics must be found. As it is not feasible to test the entire population, it is advisable to concentrate on those individuals with predisposition for the disease. They are (1) relatives of known diabetics, among whom diabetes is 2½ times more frequent than in the general population; (2) obese persons, since 85 percent of diabetic patients are, or were at one time, overweight; (3) persons in the older age groups, as four out of five diabetics are over forty-five; and (4) mothers delivered of large babies, since the birth of a large infant may be an indication of maternal prediabetes.

Apart from these high-risk groups, routine testing for diabetes should be performed whenever a new patient visits a physician's office or is admitted to a hospital. Furthermore, it would be desirable to include testing for diabetes in preemployment examinations and to retest employees at yearly intervals.

INHERITANCE

It is well-established that diabetes mellitus is inherited; the *mode* of inheritance is still under discussion.

The acceptance of heredity for diabetes is based on the greater frequency of diabetes among blood relatives of known diabetics. The pattern of inheritance is characterized by (1) a more frequent occurrence in the mates of identical than of nonidentical twins; (2) the equilateral transmission of the trait by either affected parent; and (3) the susceptibility of both sexes. However, genetic study is complicated by the fact that susceptibility to diabetes is inherited, but the disease itself may not become apparent clinically for years. Genetic studies are based on occurrence of clinical diabetes (phenotype), not on presence of the genetic predisposition (genotype), for the latter cannot be detected at the present time. It is possible that the diabetic trait may be dominant and the manifest diabetic disease recessive. There is further confusion because diabetes is a syndrome; for example, chronic pancreatitis may be associated with hyperglycemia indistinguishable from that observed in genetic diabetes. This could lead to false designation of an individual as affected with genetic diabetes. Diabetes has a variable age of onset (youth onset and maturity onset), each with a characteristic clinical pattern. This has led, on the one hand, to the hypothesis of multifactorial inheritance and to the hypothesis that the mode of inheritance in juvenile diabetes is homozygous, whereas the hereditary factor in maturity onset diabetes is heterozygous. On the other hand, Steinberg has reviewed all available genetic data and expressed the belief that diabetic inheritance is consistent with homozygosity for a recessive gene at a single locus, with variable penetrance.

CLASSIFICATION

It is helpful to classify the diabetic patient not only according to the type of his diabetes but also according to his present stage of carbohydrate decompensation.

The latter implies that progression or regression from one stage to the next occurs and may be very rapid, may proceed slowly, or may never take place. The following *stages* of diabetes are almost universally accepted: (1) Overt or clinical diabetes: this is frank diabetes either of the ketosis-prone (juvenile) or ketosis-resistant (adult) type. Fasting and random blood glucoses are definitely elevated, symptoms related to hyperglycemia and glycosuria can usually be elicited. (2) Chemical or asymptomatic diabetes: the fasting blood glucose level is usually normal, but the postprandial level is frequently elevated. An oral or intravenous glucose tolerance test performed in the absence of stress is clearly abnormal. There are no diabetic symptoms. If observed in children, this stage is usually of short duration, as they progress rapidly to overt diabetes; in adults it may be present for years, and some patients never progress beyond it. Despite this, diabetic angiopathy may be present. (3) Latent or stress diabetes: present in a person who at the *present* time has a normal glucose tolerance but who is known to have been a diabetic at some *previous* time, i.e., during pregnancy (gestational diabetes), during infection, when obese, or when under stress, such as cerebrovascular accident, myocardial infarction, extensive burns, or endocrinopathies. Patients with such temporary carbohydrate intolerance should be watched closely, particularly when there is a family history of diabetes. (4) Prediabetes: this is a conceptual term, a retrospective diagnosis, applied to the period of time preceding any glucose intolerance. By definition it cannot be diagnosed with certainty in the current state of our knowledge except in the nondiabetic identical twin of a diabetic patient and possibly in the offspring of two diabetic parents.

As to the *types* of diabetes, the following etiologic classification can be applied:

1. *Genetic (hereditary, idiopathic, primary, essential) diabetes,* subdivided according to the age of onset into juvenile and adult diabetes.

2. *Pancreatic diabetes,* where the carbohydrate intolerance can be attributed directly to destruction of the pancreatic islets by chronic inflammation, carcinoma, hemochromatosis, or surgical removal.

3. *Endocrine diabetes,* when the diabetes is associated with endocrinopathies such as hyperpituitarism (acromegaly, basophilism), hyperthyroidism, hyperadrenalism (Cushing's syndrome, primary aldosteronism), pheochromocytoma, and pancreatic islet cell tumor of the A-cell type. Under this category can also be included the gestational diabetes and the various forms of stress diabetes listed above.

4. *Iatrogenic diabetes,* when precipitated by administration of corticosteroids, certain diuretics of the benzothiadiazine type and possibly also by estrogen-progesterone combinations.

PATHOLOGY

Pancreas

With the use of special stains with the light microscope and with the availability of the electron microscope, it now appears very likely that almost all diabetic patients exhibit a correlation between severity of their diabetes, on the one hand, and reduced total mass of beta cells and degree of beta cell degranulation, on the other. These two factors correlate with the amount of extractable pancreatic insulin. Generally speaking, after several years of established clinical diabetes, the patients with youth-onset diabetes shows essentially no extractable pancreatic insulin, whereas the pancreas of the adult-onset diabetic still contains some insulin, approximately half that found in control pancreases. Patients with maturity-onset diabetes studied at autopsy reveal a significant incidence of hyalinization of pancreatic islets. It has been suggested that this material is related to amyloid (Lacy).

Of special interest is the finding that some juvenile diabetics who come to autopsy shortly after clinical onset of diabetes show large islets of Langerhans. This would support the concept that the *initial* lesions is not necessarily decreased insulin production by the pancreas.

There is also the admittedly rare patient with recent onset of diabetes whose pancreatic islets indicate lymphocytic infiltration (insulitis), a lesion again found only in young diabetics. This raises the possibility of an infection or autoimmune mechanism.

Blood Vessels

Atherosclerosis in the diabetic patient is not different from that commonly observed, but it is equally present in both sexes and occurs earlier in life. Coronary artery disease is a frequent cause of death, and cerebrovascular accidents are significantly more common. In addition, these patients usually have small-vessel disease, or microangiopathy, of which the initial lesion is a thickened basement membrane.

Retina

Microaneurysms, small hemorrhages, and exudates are frequently seen in patients with long-standing diabetes. Frequently, there is also a striking dilatation of venules. Hemorrhage into the vitreous may be the cause of sudden loss of vision. Proliferative retinopathy is found frequently in juvenile diabetes of long duration. There is formation of new blood vessels around the optic disc. If, in response to hemorrhage into the vitreous, scar tissue forms, it may upon retracting produce retinal detachment. In proliferative retinopathy, a secondary hemorrhagic glaucoma is often the final step leading to total blindness. At the present time, in the United States, diabetic retinopathy is the third most frequent cause of blindness, after cataracts and glaucoma.

A better understanding of the mechanism of early vascular changes has been made possible by the introduction of the in vitro trypsin digestion of the flattened retina. Cogan and Kuwabara describe two types of vascular cells, the endothelial and the mural cell. In diabetics, there is a specific loss of mural cells, resulting in loss of tone with formation of microaneurysms and some diffuse distension with consequent ischemia of adjacent areas. This theory is supported by in vivo findings employing fluorescein, injected intravenously in the general circulation, followed by serial photographs of the fundus. In diabetics, there is not only delayed emptying but also leakage of the dye from blood vessels in areas where exudates and hemorrhages are occurring.

Kidney

Specimens for histologic study can be obtained by open or percutaneous biopsy or, of course, at autopsy. The specific diabetic lesion is the nodular glomerulosclerosis described by Kimmelstiel and Wilson. The lesions consist of PAS-positive material, believed to accumulate first in the mesangial region. With time, nodules form. In addition, the basement membrane of the glomerular loops becomes diffusely or focally thickened, and furthermore, the effects of arterial and arteriolar sclerosis become manifest. Pyelonephritis, a frequent complication, is a local manifestation of the generalized increased susceptibility to infection. The combination of these lesions constitutes diabetic nephropathy and manifests itself clinically with proteinuria, edema, and hypertension.

Link Between Metabolic and Vascular Changes

Some of the pathologic changes observed in diabetic patients are obviously secondary to hyperglycemia, such as deposition of glycogen in the renal epithelium, especially in the proximal convoluted tubule and the loop of Henle, where it is directly correlated to the glucose concentration in the urine. Hyperglycemia also results in deposition of glycogen in non-insulin-dependent organs, such as skin, heart muscle, iris, and ciliary bodies of the eye. The liver of the diabetic patient, except in the terminal stages, contains normal amounts of glycogen; however, the distribution may be abnormal within the nuclei of the hepatic parenchymal cells. Occasionally the liver is enlarged and infiltrated with fat, mainly in untreated or poorly treated diabetics.

The relationship between derangement of intermediary metabolism and microangiopathy has not been clarified and is the subject of controversy. Except for the patient with mild diabetes, perfect control is almost impossible to achieve in the immediate postprandial state, and therefore, most patients present varying shades of insufficient control.

Biochemically it is possible that excessive synthesis of mucopolysaccharides from glucose, via an insulin-dependent pathway, leads to derangement of the basement membrane, with secondary infiltration by materials from the bloodstream. It has been questioned whether such a derangement is necessarily the consequence of an abnormal glucose metabolism or if both the level of blood glucose and the state of the basement membrane could be influenced by a third factor. On the other hand, it is now well documented that all the complications of genetic diabetes can occur in secondary forms of diabetes in man

and furthermore that they can be reproduced in animals with experimental diabetes (Bloodworth).

Pathophysiology

In all likelihood the diabetic syndrome develops as a consequence of an imbalance between insulin production and release, on the one hand, and hormonal or tissue factors modifying the insulin requirement, on the other.

Insulin is absolutely lacking in those forms of secondary diabetes where destruction or removal of the pancreas has taken place. Similarly overt growth-onset diabetes is characterized by insulin deficiency. There is essentially no extractable pancreatic insulin, no response to oral hypoglycemic agents of the sulfonylurea type, a marked tendency to ketoacidosis, and therefore dependence on exogenous insulin for survival. It is assumed that diabetes in the child begins when the pancreatic production of insulin declines. However, this is not always irreversible, as at least one-third of all juvenile diabetics will develop a phase of remission, usually within 3 months after the acute onset of the disease. If present, the remission may last from several days to several months; it rarely exceeds 1 year. Often during such a remission no insulin treatment is necessary, and a glucose tolerance test may be normal. Nevertheless, after this remission the juvenile diabetic progresses rapidly to a state of total insulin deficiency.

The patient with adult-onset diabetes develops his disease considerably more slowly. At the early stage no symptoms may be present, and diagnosis is suspected by discovery of elevated blood glucose levels 1 or 2 hr postprandially. Measurement of serum insulin may indicate close to normal fasting levels; however, the insulin response to administered glucose is abnormal in that it occurs late. This is responsible for the elevated blood glucose 1 to 2 hr postprandially. As insulin release increases with the rising blood glucose, the blood glucose declines; with excess insulin, the blood glucose may fall precipitously, provoking the symptoms of reactive hypoglycemia between the *third and fifth hour* postprandially. As the disease progresses further, the insulin release becomes less pronounced, the episodes of reactive hypoglycemia tend to disappear; finally the amount of circulating insulin is insufficient to return the blood glucose to normal levels between meals. In maturity-onset diabetes the pancreatic insulin reserve is decreased, but rarely totally absent. Thus the occurrence of diabetic ketoacidosis is uncommon.

Although in many patients the contrast between growth-onset and maturity-onset is initially at least quite sharp, there are crossovers between these two types and the above comments must be considered only as generalizations.

Regardless of the type of diabetes, by definition, the cardinal sign is hyperglycemia, frequently associated with glycosuria. The hyperglycemia has two components: hepatic overproduction and peripheral underutilization. The source of the glucose released from the liver is dietary carbohydrate, liver glycogen, and gluconcogenesis from protein. Underutilization of glucose in the peripheral tissue takes place mainly in adipose tissue and muscle, both of which are insulin-sensitive, and is attributed to a lack of circulating insulin. Impaired glucose uptake by muscle leads to loss of muscle glycogen and release of amino acids for gluconeogenesis. Impaired glucose uptake by adipose tissue causes impaired triglyceride synthesis. In addition, with lack of insulin, there is release of free fatty acids from adipose tissue into the bloodstream. In the liver, the fatty acids are metabolized to ketone bodies. Although they can be utilized by certain tissues, they are formed in excess in the diabetic person. They accumulate in the blood and lead to ketonuria. As they are strong acids, it is necessary for the kidney to excrete a fixed base with them, leading to both sodium and potassium loss. Therefore, the diabetic organism loses glucose, water, ketone bodies, and base. This will result in dehydration, ketoacidosis, and weight loss, and in extreme cases, may proceed to diabetic coma and death.

The exact mechanism by which insulin acts remains unknown. However, it is well established that tissues vary widely in sensitivity and responsiveness to insulin. For example, in muscle and adipose tissue, insulin probably acts on cell membrane permeability and so facilitates the entry of glucose into the cell. On the other hand, liver cells exhibit no demonstrable permeability barrier to glucose. The insulin effect on liver appears to be on the phosphorylating mechanism. It has recently been suggested that the liver contains two enzymes for phosphorylation of glucose: hexokinase and glucokinase. Hexokinase is insulin-*independent*, and glucokinase is insulin-*dependent*. In addition, insulin affects glycogen synthesis. The effect of insulin on fatty acids has been mentioned above. It is noteworthy that this antilipolytic action requires a lower level of insulin than that for glucose uptake. Therefore an absolute deficiency of circulating insulin as in juvenile diabetes will lead to hyperglycemia and marked lipolysis with resultant ketosis, whereas only a decrease of circulating insulin such as in adult-onset diabetes will lead to hyperglycemia without ketosis.

In diabetes the primary inherited defect responsible for the failing insulin production remains unknown. The recent discovery of proinsulin may be a step forward. Proinsulin is a larger molecule than insulin (molecular weight 9000, versus 6000) because of some 30 additional amino acids, but it exhibits considerably less biological activity. Controversy exists whether proinsulin is an inactive storage form or a precursor of insulin. It is transformed into insulin by cleavage of the intermediate chain.

It is conceivable that in some diabetic patients there is a failure to activate proinsulin. As large quantities of proinsulin would be required to meet the body's insulin demand, this failure could eventually lead to pancreatic exhaustion and thus to frank diabetes.

PRECIPITATION OF DIABETES BY EXTRAPANCREATIC FACTORS

Obesity is frequently associated with diabetes, though it should not be inferred that all obese individuals are potential diabetics. Biopsy studies have shown that adult onset obesity is associated with hypertrophy of adipose cells and that the larger the cell, the less responsive to insulin it becomes. As less glucose can be disposed of, the resulting hyperglycemia will lead to hyperinsulinemia. In patients genetically predetermined, this may lead to pancreatic exhaustion or at least to a relative insulin deficiency.

Pregnancy also exerts a definite diabetogenic action in women so predisposed. Initially, diabetes may become apparent only during pregnancy and disappear following delivery; rarely it remains; frequently, years or decades later, permanent diabetes develops. There is evidence that hormonal factors, such as placental lactogen and marked destruction of endogenous insulin by the placenta, may play a role in precipitating diabetes. It is speculated that the higher frequency of diabetes in adult females may be due to pregnancies and obesity.

Recently, the diabetogenic action of certain *diuretics* of the benzothiadiazine type has been noted. There is evidence that these drugs mediate such mechanism by inhibiting pancreatic insulin release. This effect is reversible, contrary to the damage produced by the administration of alloxan. Growth hormone is diabetogenic by decreasing peripheral glucose utilization and by increasing release of free fatty acids. Excess epinephrine causes increased hepatic glycogenolysis and, in addition, inhibits pancreatic insulin release. The steroids act by increasing hepatic gluconeogenesis and decreasing glucose uptake by adipose tissue. Thyroxin increases hunger and food intake and generally heightens the level of metabolic activity. Infection of any sort will impair glucose tolerance and may unmask the tendency to diabetes. The diabetogenic mechanism of infection is probably nonspecific and consists of elevated levels of corticosteroids, fever that increases the general metabolic load, and possibly catecholamine release, all of which decrease the effectiveness of circulating insulin. In rare instances inflammation of the pancreatic islets takes place.

DIAGNOSIS

The diagnosis of diabetes mellitus is frequently suggested by a history of polydipsia, polyuria, and polyphagia, associated with weight loss. A clinical suspicion of diabetes is confirmed by finding glucose in the urine *and* by detecting an abnormally elevated blood glucose. If hyperglycemia is associated with glycosuria *and* with ketonuria, the diagnosis of diabetes mellitus is certain.

In the patient without any obvious symptoms suggestive of diabetes, the following procedures are recommended as screening tests for diabetes. By far, the simplest tests is to obtain a urine specimen 1 to 2 hr after a heavy carbohydrate meal. However, in older persons with an elevated renal threshold, the blood glucose may be elevated without being associated with glycosuria; furthermore, the finding of urinary sugar alone is not diagnostic of diabetes. Therefore, determination of blood glucose not only is preferable as a screening procedure but is mandatory to establish the diagnosis of diabetes. Unfortunately much confusion exists as to what represents an abnormal blood glucose value. Whereas there is general agreement that a 1-hr postprandial blood glucose of 200 mg per 100 ml or higher indicates diabetes, there is considerable discussion if abnormality starts above a value of 160, 170, or 180 mg per 100 ml. It has become apparent that clinical information and follow-up studies as well as the methodology of the blood glucose determination have to be taken into account. In general terms it can be stated that upper limits of normalcy increase with age and during pregnancy. As to methodology, the physician needs to know (1) if capillary or venous blood was used (the capillary blood glucose will be higher); (2) if the blood glucose was determined on whole blood or plasma (plasma or serum will render higher values than whole blood; on the other hand, severe anemia will give falsely elevated values with whole blood); (3) which particular technique for measuring blood glucose was employed. A rather less specific method such as Folin-Wu will give the highest values as it measures in addition to glucose also fructose, lactate, pyruvate, etc. The glucose oxidase method will reflect the "true" glucose content and therefore yield the lowest value. The autoanalyzer employs the ferricyanide method which is slightly higher than the glucose oxidase technique. It is apparent that the possible variations are many, therefore the best advice is to be familiar with the methods and normal range in a given hospital. When blood glucose values are reported to outlying institutions or life insurance companies, the type of blood and the technique employed should be noted.

Fasting and Postprandial Blood Glucose

The normal range for fasting blood glucose as measured by the autoanalyzer is between 70 and 110 mg per 100 ml whole blood. An elevated fasting blood sugar is highly suggestive of diabetes; on the other hand, diabetes can never be ruled out by presence of a normal fasting blood sugar. Therefore, it is advisable to obtain a blood sugar determination 1 or 2 hr after a meal which has

Table 94-1. 100-GM CARBOHYDRATE BREAKFAST

Food	Quantity	Carbohydrate, Gm
Orange juice............	8 oz	24
Cooked cereal..........	4 oz	
or		16
Dry cereal.............	1 oz	
Bread.................	2 slices	32
Egg..................	1	
Butter...............	2 pats	
Milk.................	6 oz	9
Cream...............	3 oz	4
Sugar...............	3 tsp	15
Coffee or tea..........	ad lib.	
		100

contained approximately 100 Gm carbohydrate, as indicated in Table 94-1, or a regular breakfast to which 50 Gm glucose have been added. A 1-hr value of 170 mg per 100 ml or higher is highly suspicious of diabetes, as is a 2-hr value above 120 mg per 100 ml. If the level is borderline, or especially if one wishes definitely to rule out diabetes, then a formal 3-hr glucose tolerance test is indicated.

Oral Glucose Tolerance Test

Following a fasting blood glucose determination, 100 Gm glucose (available commercially in solution) is given and the blood glucose measured at ½ hr, 1 hr, 2 hr, and 3 hr; the urine is examined for the presence of sugar. The following are considered upper normal values obtained with venous blood as measured by the autoanalyzer method: Fasting, 110 mg per 100 ml; ½ hr (or peak value), 170 mg; 1 hr, 170 mg; 2 hr, 120 mg; and 3 hr, 110 mg per 100 ml. There should be no glucose in the urine at any time. The result of the glucose tolerance test in an apparently healthy subject is influenced by at least three factors: diet, physical activity, and age. It is mandatory that the patient be on a preparatory diet containing 250 to 300 Gm carbohydrate for 3 days before testing; otherwise a decreased carbohydrate tolerance can be observed, known as *starvation diabetes*. Physical inactivity also decreases carbohydrate tolerance, and therefore prolonged bed rest may give false-positive results. Finally, age exerts an effect on glucose tolerance. Although standards are not available for individuals of different decades, especially over the age of fifty, Fajans suggests that between the ages of fifty and fifty-nine the 2-hr level can be considered normal up to 130; between the ages of sixty and sixty-nine, up to 140; between the ages of seventy and seventy-nine, up to 150; and above age eighty, above 160 mg per 100 ml. Additional factors known to affect glucose tolerance are fever, infection, endocrinopathies, liver disease, myocardial infarction, cerebrovascular accident, and certain medications such as diuretics of the benzothiodiazine type.

Intravenous Glucose Tolerance Test

As intestinal absorption of glucose may interfere with a glucose tolerance test, it is occasionally desirable to perform an intravenous glucose tolerance test. This is especially indicated if there is a history of gastrointestinal surgery. Accelerated intestinal absorption of glucose, as in the "dumping syndrome" may result in a diabetic-type oral glucose tolerance curve; however, the intravenous glucose tolerance may be well within normal limits.

The dose of glucose is 0.5 Gm per kg body weight as a 25 percent solution. It is administered intravenously within 2 to 4 min, and blood is collected every 10 min for 1 hr. Under these conditions, the rate of blood glucose decreases in an exponential manner, and the glucose disappearance can be calculated. Disappearance rate = $70/t\frac{1}{2}$, where $t\frac{1}{2}$ = number of minutes it takes for the blood glucose to fall 50 percent. In normal individuals it usually exceeds 1.5 percent of the administered dose per minute, and values below 1 percent are clearly diabetic.

If glucose tolerance tests are performed routinely in a large hospital population, many patients afflicted with chronic diseases like rheumatoid arthritis, cancer, or amyotrophic lateral sclerosis may exhibit impaired glucose tolerance curve without any clinical evidence of diabetes. Because many of these patients with "chemical diabetes" will not progress to a state of overt clinical diabetes, one has to be careful not to overdiagnose diabetes.

Cortisone Glucose Tolerance Tests

Fajans and Conn have proposed performing the oral glucose tolerance test after priming with cortisone in an attempt to establish the diagnosis of chemical diabetes at a time when the conventional oral glucose tolerance test is still within normal limits. The technique consists of administering 50 mg cortisone acetate 8 and 2 hr before the glucose tolerance test. The cortisone glucose tolerance test may detect carbohydrate intolerance earlier than the standard oral glucose tolerance test.

DIFFERENTIAL DIAGNOSIS OF GLYCOSURIA (See Chap. 95)

The presence of glucose in the urine should be considered to indicate diabetes until an alternate diagnosis can be definitely established. Glycosuria may indicate a low renal threshold, which is present in pregnancy, in patients with chronic renal disease, and in patients with idiopathic renal glycosuria. In the latter, glucose is present in most urine specimens, including a second voided specimen after an overnight fast, but the glucose tolerance test is normal. The transient glycosuria that occurs occasionally in apparently healthy persons under conditions of stress or infection or following ingestion of a high carbohydrate meal is usually associated with an abnormal glucose tolerance test and, therefore, indicates chemical diabetes.

CLINICAL PICTURE

Growth-onset Type

The growth-onset type of diabetes if characterized by a rapid onset with symptoms, such as polydipsia, polyuria, polyphagia, loss of weight and strength, marked irritability, and in children frequently, recurrence of bedwetting. The diabetes is apt to be of the unstable or brittle type, being quite sensitive to the administration of exogenous insulin and easily influenced by physical activity. The patient is prone to ketoacidosis. For adequate treatment, diet and insulin therapy are mandatory. Since the introduction of insulin therapy, diabetic ketoacidosis has been markedly reduced as a major cause of death; the primary causes of death in diabetic patients are now cardiovascular and renal. Diagnosis of diabetes in the growth-onset-type patient is usually not difficult. However, occasional children and adolescents have asymptomatic diabetes demonstrable only by glucose tolerance test. In these patients the disease appears to progress very slowly.

Maturity-onset Type

The maturity-onset diabetic patient has a less stormy beginning, frequently symptoms are minimum or absent. The chief complaint may be moderate weight loss or occasionally, weight gain. There may be some nocturia. A female patient might consult her gynecologist because of vulvar pruritis. Frequently, however, the patient seeks medical attention because of vascular complications. As a consequence of blurred or decreased vision, the patient may see an ophthalmologist first, who may diagnose diabetic retinopathy. Fatigue and anemia may be caused by fairly advanced diabetic nephropathy. Diabetic neuropathy may present as paresthesias, loss of sensation, impotence, nocturnal diarrhea, postural hypotension, or neurogenic bladder. Not infrequently, the patient presents with an ulcer or gangrene of his toes or heel and on examination has a pulseless or painless foot. Thus the patient with maturity-onset diabetes usually does not present with the dramatic, acute metabolic syndrome observed in the juvenile patient but rather with a chronic vascular syndrome. It is therefore important to suspect diabetes as an underlying disease under a wide variety of circumstances.

TREATMENT

The aims of managing diabetes are (1) correction of the underlying metabolic abnormalities by diet, oral hypoglycemic agents, or insulin; (2) attainment and maintenance of ideal body weight; and (3) prevention, or at least delay, of complications commonly associated with the disease.

Successful therapy will depend upon the thoroughness with which the physician understands the particular problems in each individual case, upon how well the patient has been instructed, and upon how conscientious the patient is about following instructions.

On initiating treatment of a patient with diabetes, it is essential to be certain that there is no active focus of infection, as it will aggravate the diabetic state. Infection of the urinary tract should be looked for particularly, and a chest x-ray is imperative. It is also advisable to obtain careful baseline evaluations of the state of the cardiovascular, nervous, and renal systems and of the eye grounds to serve as subsequent points of reference.

Diet

Dietary treatment of diabetes still constitutes the basis for management. The principal considerations in designing diabetic diets are (1) the basic nutritional requirements of a patient with diabetes are the same as those of a nondiabetic patient; (2) the diet should be varied and palatable.

THE BASIC CALORIC REQUIREMENT. This is dictated by the desirable, or ideal, weight, the age, and the occupation of the patient. If he is obese, the diet will be restricted in calories; if the patient is undernourished, the diet initially will exceed the basic caloric requirement. The desired weight is calculated from the height, taking frame size into consideration. For an approximate calculation of the basic caloric requirement, the ideal weight is multiplied by 10. Example: A patient's ideal weight is 180 lb, his total caloric requirement will be 1800 Cal. Additional calories should be allowed according to the patient's occupation and activities. Calories may be reduced for patients over fifty years of age who are less active.

PARTITION OF CALORIES. The average American diet consists of carbohydrate, 40 to 45 percent; protein, 15 to 20 percent; and fat, 35 to 40 percent. The diabetic diet can approximate this distribution. The caloric value of carbohydrate and protein is approximately 4 Cal per Gm and of fat, 9 Cal per Gm.

CARBOHYDRATE. To prevent acetonuria, a minimum of 1 Gm per lb body weight is necessary, or in the example of the patient weighing 180 lb, 180 Gm. This minimum requirement should be increased if indicated by occupation or during the growth period in children. It is obvious that regulation of diabetes will be simpler with a greater number of feedings involving smaller quantities of carbohydrate than with three large meals. In particular, diabetic patients receiving insulin or oral hypoglycemic agents should receive a midafternoon and bedtime snack in order to minimize fluctuation of the blood glucose.

PROTEIN. A *minimum* of 0.5 Gm per lb body weight is indicated. This is increased during pregnancy and during childhood and decreased only in the presence of azotemia.

FAT. It can be metabolized without the direct influence of insulin. However, dietary fat, particularly of animal origin, together with other factors such as decreased physical activity, seems to play an important role in the pathogenesis of atherosclerosis; therefore, fat intake should be kept to a minimum. The amount prescribed is calculated by subtracting calories allowed for carbohydrate and protein from the total caloric requirement.

Example: Total Calories based on an ideal weight of 180 lb are 1800. Assigned for carbohydrate $180 \times 4 = 720$, for protein $90 \times 4 = 360$ Cal, there remain $(1800 - 720 - 360) = 720$ Cal. These are given as fat, or $720/9 = 80$ Gm fat. The final diet then consists of carbohydrate 180 Gm, protein 90 Gm, and fat 80 Gm. It is probably advisable to reduce the total amount of cholesterol and to supply some of the fat as unsaturated fatty acids.

The American Diabetes Association and the American Dietetic Association have published a booklet on meal planning with exchange lists. In it all the available foods are divided into six types. Foods cannot be switched between the lists but can be interchanged within each list. Food is subdivided into (1) milk exchanges; (2) (*a*) essentially unlimited vegetables, (*b*) somewhat limited vegetables; (3) fruits; (4) bread exchanges which in-clude apart from bread also cereal, rice, spaghetti, potato, etc.; (5) meat exchanges which include meat, cold cuts, egg, fish, cheese; and (6) fat exchanges. In Tables 94-2 and 3 these exchange lists are presented in more detail. Food can be weighed or measured with a standard 8-oz measuring cup, teaspoon, and a tablespoon.

Oral Hypoglycemic Agents

These have a definite place in the treatment of maturity-onset diabetes, provided it is of the nonketotic type and that dietary treatment alone is unsuccessful in achieving adequate control. Patients falling into this category constitute approximately two-thirds of all maturity-onset diabetics. It should be emphasized that none of the oral hypoglycemic agents is insulin, nor can they replace it in conditions such as diabetic ketoacidosis. The agents presently in use are of two types: the sulfonylureas and the biguanides.

SULFONYLUREAS. The sulfonylureas available by prescription are tolbutamide (Orinase), acetohexamide (Dymelor), chlorpropamide (Diabinase), and tolazamide (Tolinase). Although there is some evidence that they directly decrease hepatic glucose output, they act primarily by enhancing the secretion of endogenous insulin. Thus, to be effective, at least residual function of the beta

Table 94-2. FOOD EXCHANGES

LIST 1. MILK[1]
Calories 170, Carbohydrate 12 Gm, protein 8 Gm, fat 10 Gm per serving.

Food	Approximate measure 1 exchange	Weight, Gm
Milk, plain.............	1 cup (8 oz)	240
Milk, evaporated........	½ cup	120
Milk, powder, skim[2]......	⅓ cup (5⅓ tbsp level)	48
Milk, powder, whole......	½ cup (8 tbsp level)	35
Buttermilk[2].............	1 cup	240
Milk, skim[2].............	1 cup	240

LIST 2. VEGETABLES
One or more fat exchanges from the diet allowance may be used to season the vegetables.
Carbohydrate 7 Gm, protein 2 Gm, fat negligible
One exchange equals ½ cup.

Beets	Peas, green	Squash, winter
Carrots	Pumpkin	Turnip
Onions	Rutabagas	

[1] Modified from Meal Planning with Exchange Lists. Obtainable from the American Diabetes Association, Inc., New York, N.Y.

[2] Add 10 Gm fat (2 fat exchanges). Most commercial buttermilk is skimmed. Check local supplies.

All other vegetables, except those listed under Bread Exchanges, contain negligible carbohydrate, protein, and fat. They may be used as desired.

Table 94-2. FOOD EXCHANGES (Continued)

LIST 3. FRUITS

Fresh, cooked, canned, or frozen *unsweetened*. Carbohydrate 10 Gm per exchange; protein and fat negligible.

Fruit	Approximate measure 1 exchange	Weight, Gm
Apple, 1 small	2″ diameter	80
Applesauce	½ cup	100
Apricots, dry	4 halves	20
Apricots, fresh	2 medium	100
Banana	½ small	50
Berries (blackberries, raspberries, and strawberries)	1 cup	150
Blueberries	⅔ cup	100
Cantaloupe	½ (6″ diameter)	200
Cherries	10 large or 15 small	75
Dates	2	15
Figs, dried	1 small	15
Figs, fresh	2 large	50
Grapefruit	½ small	125
Grapefruit	½ cup	100
Grapes	12	75
Grape juice	½ cup	60
Honeydew melon	⅛ (7″ diameter)	150
Mango	½ small	70
Nectarines	1 medium	100
Orange	1 small	100
Orange juice	½ cup	100
Papaya	⅓ medium	100
Peach	1 medium	100
Pear	1 small	100
Pineapple	½ cup, cubed	80
Pineapple juice	⅓ cup	80
Plums	2 medium	100
Prunes, dried	2 medium	25
Raisins	2 tbsp level	15
Tangerine	1 large	100
Watermelon	1 cup diced 1 slice 3″ × 1½″	175

LIST 4. BREAD EXCHANGES

Carbohydrate 15 Gm, protein 2 Gm, fat negligible.

Food	Approximate measure 1 exchange	Weight, Gm
Bread, baker's	1 slice	25
Biscuit, roll	2″ diameter	35
Muffin	2″ diameter	35
Cornbread	1½″ cube	35
Cereals, cooked	½ cup, cooked	100
Cereals, dry (flakes, puffed, and shredded varieties)	¾ cup, scant	20
Rice, macaroni, noodles, spaghetti	½ cup, cooked	100
Crackers:		
Graham	2 (2½ × 2¾″)	20
Oyster	20 (½ cup)	20
Saltines	5 (2″ square)	20
Soda	3 (2½ × 2½″)	20
Round, thin varieties	6–8 (½″ diameter)	20
Vegetables:		
Beans, peas, dried (cooked) Includes limas, navy, kidney beans, black-eyed peas, cowpeas, split peas, etc.	½ cup, scant	100
Corn	⅓ cup or ½ ear	80
Parsnips	½ cup	125
Potatoes:		
White, baked	2″ diameter	100
White, boiled, mashed	½ cup	100
Sweet or yam	¼ cup	50
Ice cream, vanilla[3]	⅛ qt	70
Sponge cake, no icing	1½″ cube	25

[3] Omit 2 fat exchanges.

cells is necessary. They are indicated in the maturity-onset diabetic patient in whom diet alone has failed, acetonuria has not been demonstrated, and there is no history of diabetic ketoacidosis. Such a patient can be started on sulfonylureas without the prior use of insulin, or he can be transferred from insulin to sulfonylureas. The chance of therapeutic success with these agents is better when clinical diabetes has been present for a relatively short period of time, if the patient is over the age of forty, and if he or she is overweight. A large initial loading dose is now not considered necessary for the sulfonylureas. In general, side effects are rare; and except for chlorpropamide in high doses, these agents have a good record, especially with respect to hepatic function. Alcohol intolerance has been observed under treatment with sulfonylureas. Occasionally, in elderly undernourished patients, severe hypoglycemia may follow their ad-ministration. Apart from this, prolonged hypoglycemia is frequently observed when a sulfonylurea is administered to a patient with uremia, as renal excretion of the drug will be delayed. This is the case particularly with chlorpropamide and acetohexamide, as the former is not metabolized to any significant extent and the latter is transformed by the liver to hydroxyhexamide, which also exhibits a potent hypoglycemia property. In both instances, elevated blood levels of the respective drug will lead to severe and protracted hypoglycemia. If this occurs, prolonged and intensive treatment with intravenous glucose (i.e., 200 Gm within 24 hr) and close medical supervision for at least 48 to 72 hr is mandatory.

Between 20 to 30 percent of diabetic patients initially considered to be good candidates for treatment with sulfonylurea will fail to respond after several months or years. This secondary failure can often be attributed to

Table 94-2. FOOD EXCHANGES (*Continued*)

LIST 5. MEAT EXCHANGES
Carbohydrate negligible, protein 7 Gm, fat 5 Gm per serving.
All items expressed in cooked weight.

Food	Approximate measure 1 exchange	Weight, Gm
Meat: Beef, fowl, lamb, veal (medium fat), liver, pork, ham (lean).......	1 oz	30
Cold cuts: Salami, minced ham, bologna, cervelat, liver sausage, luncheon loaf..................	1 slice 4½″ diam. × ⅛″	45
Frankfurters (8 to 9 per lb)	1	50
Fish:		
Cod, haddock, halibut, herring, etc...........	1 oz	30
Salmon, tuna, crab-meat, lobster........	¼ cup	30
Shrimp, clams, oysters (medium)..........	5	45
Sardines..............	3 medium	30
Cheese:		
Cheddar type.........	1 oz	30
Cottage..............	3 tbsp level	45
Peanut butter[4].........	2 tbsp scant	30
Egg....................	1	50

[4] Limit to one serving per day unless adjustment is made to balance carbohydrate content.

LIST 6. FAT EXCHANGES
Carbohydrate and protein negligible, fat 5 Gm per serving. Fat exchanges utilized in cooking should be accounted for.

Food	Approximate measure 1 exchange	Weight, Gm
Avocado...............	⅛ (4″ diam.)	24
Butter or margarine......	1 tsp level	5
Bacon, crisp............	1 slice	10
Cream, light, sweet, or sour—20%...........	2 tbsp level	30
Cream, heavy—40%......	1 tbsp level	15
Cream cheese...........	1 tbsp level	15
French dressing.........	1 tbsp level	15
Mayonnaise.............	1 tsp level	5
Nuts...................	6 small	10
Oil or cooking fat........	1 tsp level	5
Olives.................	5 small	50

poor adherence to a prescribed diet, the presence of infection, or the gradual progression of the diabetes to a more insulin-deficient state. Sometimes, a secondary failure is due to destruction of the pancreatic islets by carcinoma or hemochromatosis.

Table 94-3. EXAMPLE OF AN 1800 CALORIE DIABETIC DIET ORDER
(CARBOHYDRATE 181 GM, PROTEIN 90 GM, FAT 80 GM)

Exchange	Breakfast	Lunch	Snack	Supper	Snack
Milk.............	½	1	—	—	½
Bread............	2	2	1	2	1
Meat............	1	2	1	3	1
Fat.............	1	1	—	2	—
Fruit............	1	1	—	1	—
Vegetable........	—	1	—	1	—
Partition in Gm:					
Carbohydrate......	46	52	15	47	21
Protein...........	15	26	9	27	13
Fat..............	15	25	5	25	10

TOLBUTAMIDE. This is the most widely used oral hypoglycemic agent. Each tablet contains 500 mg. The biologic half-life is approximately 6 hr. It is administered before breakfast *and* before supper, the total daily dose ranging from 1 to 3 Gm. The excretory product in the urine may give a false positive test for albumin, since it is precipitated by acidifying the urine.

ACETOHEXAMIDE. Tablets are available in strengths of 250 and 500 mg. Its half-life is longer and, therefore, a *single* dose may be effective. Recently, a moderate uricosuric property has been attributed to acetohexamide, which would make it a useful drug in subjects with coexisting diabetes and gout.

CHLORPROPAMIDE. Tablets are available containing 100 or 250 mg. The biologic half-life is approximately 36 hr, and daily administration may result in a cumulative effect. The recommended daily dose is 100 to 250 mg before breakfast; it should not exceed 500 mg. Because of its long action, a bedtime snack containing carbohydrate, protein, and fat, e.g., milk with crackers, is advisable. As it has a slightly greater toxic effect on the liver than has tolbutamide or acetohexamide, and since its long half-life may occasionally result in hypoglycemia

Table 94-4. ORAL HYPOGLYCEMIC AGENTS

Generic name	Available form	Average dose	Duration of action
Tolbutamide	500 mg	500–1,000 mg b.i.d.	6–12 hr
Acetohexamide	250 mg 500 mg	250–1,000 mg A.M.	12–24 hr
Tolazamide	100 mg 250 mg	100–500 mg A.M.	16–24 hr
Chlorpropamide	100 mg 250 mg	100–500 mg A.M.	24–36 hr
Phenformin	25 mg tablet 50 mg capsule	25 mg b.i.d. 50 mg b.i.d.	4–6 hr 8–12 hr

in the early morning, it is advisable to keep the daily dose as low as possible.

TOLAZAMIDE. This is available in 100 and 250 mg tablets with a half-life of approximately 12 hr. It is administered in a single or divided dose, not exceeding 500 mg per day.

Biguanides

PHENFORMIN. Of the biguanides, *phenformin*, a phenethyl biguanide (DBI), is commercially available as a 25-mg tablet with a biologic half-life of 3 to 4 hr and as a 50-mg time-disintegration capsule of longer half-life. The mechanism of action differs fundamentally from that of the sulfonylureas in that it can correct hyperglycemia in the pancreatectomized animal and the hypoglycemic effect cannot be produced in nondiabetic-fed subjects. The mechanism of action is still poorly understood, but it appears that phenformin influences the anaerobic pathway of glucose and inhibits hepatic gluconeogenesis. As phenformin makes a diabetic patient occasionally more sensitive to exogenous insulin, it has been suggested that phenformin inhibits an insulin antagonist. The use of phenformin as the only antidiabetic agent is limited because the effective dose is frequently associated with gastrointestinal side effects such as anorexia, nausea, vomiting, and diarrhea. Furthermore, phenformin may contribute to excess lactic acid; it should not be used in those circumstances in which marked tissue hypoxia might be expected to occur, i.e., myocardial infarction, hypotension, low arterial blood oxygen saturation, etc. Fatalities have been reported in which severe lactic acidosis apparently facilitated by the administration of phenformin constituted an important contributory effect. The indications for its use are (1) the very rare diabetic patient of maturity onset who is allergic to the sulfonylureas (the daily recommended dose of phenformin ranges from 50 to 200 mg, to be given either as tablets t.i.d. or as capsules b.i.d.); (2) in combination with sulfonylurea in the elderly patient who fails to respond to a maximum dose of a sulfonylurea; (3) in the brittle diabetic on insulin with frequent hypoglycemic reactions, in whom the addition of phenformin might result in reduction of the insulin requirement and thus facilitate control. Unfortunately, the use of phenformin in this type of patient is often disappointing; (4) in the obese overeating non-insulin-dependent diabetic in whom the sulfonylureas have failed.

The adult-onset diabetic patient can often be controlled by diet alone, and he should be given an adequate trial for several weeks, unless dictated otherwise by clinical circumstances such as acute infection. The multitude of oral agents available, each with somewhat different dosages and durations of actions, make it difficult to master them all; therefore, it is recommended to become familiar with a short-acting drug such as tolbutamide and a longer acting, more powerful agent such as chlorpropamide. A summary of all the available agents is given in Table 94-4. In general, the safety record of the sulfonylureas has been good, however potentiation of their actions by other drugs such as Gantrisin, Butazolidin, and Dicumarol have been reported; therefore, the physician should be aware of such possibilities.

Insulin

The use of insulin is clearly indicated in the youth-onset diabetic and in those patients with maturity-onset diabetes in whom diet and oral hypoglycemic agents have proved inadequate to maintain satisfactory levels of blood glucose in both the fasting and the postprandial state. Furthermore, the use of insulin is mandatory in diabetic ketoacidosis.

TYPES OF INSULIN. In the United States the animal sources for insulin are beef and pork. As human insulin has a structure similar to that of pork, the use of pure pork insulin rather than a beef-pork mixture may be preferred. Apart from the species difference, seven types of insulin are commercially available. They can be divided into insulins of fast, intermediate, and long action. Their properties are summarized in Table 94-5.

Each of the insulins is available in two different strengths, namely, 40 or 80 units per milliliter. The choice between the two is governed according to the amount of insulin required by the patient. If only a small amount is necessary, for example, 16 units, the use of U 40 will allow a more accurate dosage; if a larger amount is required, U 80 has the advantage of a smaller volume.

CHOICE OF INSULIN. (1) Crystalline insulin is best for emergencies, such as the treatment of diabetic ketoacidosis or the achievement of fast control in the patient with

Table 94-5. INSULIN ACTION CURVES

Action	Insulin	Modifier	Duration of action, hr	Maximum effect, hrs postinjection
Fast......................	Crystalline zinc (regular)	None	6	2–3
Intermediate...............	Semi-Lente	Zinc	12	3–6
	Globin	Globin	18	6–8
	NPH	Protamine	24	8–10
	Lente	Zinc	24	8–10
Long.....................	Ultralente	Zinc	36	12–20
	Protamine zinc	Protamine	36	12–20

marked hyperglycemia; it is also employed for daily use in combination with an intermediate insulin to bring on earlier action. (2) Intermediate insulins in a single dose injected before breakfast will control the majority of diabetics. The dosage will be gauged by the prelunch, midafternoon, and fasting blood sugar values. The midafternoon blood glucose corresponds to the peak of insulin action and will dictate the maximum morning dose. It is advisable that all patients receiving an intermediate insulin be given a midafternoon snack. If the midafternoon blood glucose level is between 80 and 120 mg per 100 ml, and the prelunch value is still unduly elevated, the addition of a small amount of crystalline insulin at breakfast time is indicated. It can be mixed with NPH or lente in the same syringe. Almost all maturity-onset diabetics can be adequately controlled by intermediate insulins alone or in combination with crystalline insulin administered before breakfast.

The patient with youth-onset diabetes often develops nocturnal hyperglycemia and, consequently, will exhibit a high fasting blood glucose associated with glycosuria. Further increase in the morning dose of intermediate insulin will often lead to hypoglycemia in the midafternoon. To reduce the fasting blood glucose to normal levels, a long-acting insulin can be tried, but often a second small dose of the intermediate insulin before supper or at bedtime is preferable. The latter regime is eminently satisfactory in the 24-hr control of the juvenile diabetic, and usually patients do not complain about the second injection because they feel so much better. Very rarely, sugar is spilled at bedtime but none before supper. Then the addition of a small amount of crystalline insulin to the evening dose of NPH is indicated, and both are given before supper. As a general rule, it can be stated that whenever insulin is given in the evening in addition to the morning dose, the latter should be reduced. (3) The use of long-acting insulin with the hope of establishing control with a single morning injection, in general, has been disappointing.

INITIATION OF INSULIN THERAPY. If the patient has massive glycosuria and elevated blood glucose, insulin therapy is begun immediately with crystalline insulin. The following schedule is recommended: 20 units for a 4+, 15 units for a 3+, and 10 units for a 2+ urine test. Once the acute syndrome is under reasonable control, or if the metabolic derangement is less dramatic, a longer acting insulin can be started. It is best to start with 10 or 20 units of NPH or lente and increase this by 5 units per day, as indicated by urine tests and blood glucose levels. Most diabetic patients will require between 30 and 50 units of insulin daily.

COMPLICATIONS OF INSULIN THERAPY. Insulin Reactions. These are commonly caused by excess insulin dosage, delayed food intake, or unusual physical activity. Very rarely, an increased sensitivity to insulin is due to early adrenal or pituitary hypofunction and, even more exceptionally, to development of a functioning islet cell tumor. Occasional insulin reactions are almost unavoidable, especially in the juvenile insulin-sensitive diabetic, but they are harmless if recognized and treated early. To reduce them to a minimum, it is essential that the patient knows how to test his urine for glucose and, provided he does not have an elevated renal threshold for glucose, how to reduce his insulin dose when his urine tests indicate absence of glucose for several days. The patient also has to be instructed to eat his meals on time and, when unusual physical activity is anticipated, either to reduce his morning insulin dose or to ingest extra calories to compensate for the blood-sugar-lowering effect of exercise.

The signs and symptoms of an insulin reaction vary with the type of insulin used. *Crystalline insulin produces a characteristic reaction* of rapid onset consisting of hunger, a peculiar abdominal sensation, sweating, palpitation, tremor, tachycardia, weakness, irritability, and pallor. Patients usually recognize these symptoms early, and they are relieved within minutes by ingestion of carbohydrate: sugar, orange juice, candy, etc. To prevent any awkward situation, every diabetic patient on insulin should carry several lumps of sugar with him at all times. As a patient in insulin reaction may act as though he were intoxicated, *it is further recommended that all diabetics carry a card identifying them as such.* This is especially important in patients with a long history of diabetes. Due to neuropathy, sympathetic nervous system signs may gradually be lost, and thus the patient lacks indications of impending reaction and may exhibit only impairment of cerebral functions. *The intermediate and long-acting insulins produce a more gradual decline in blood glucose* with consequently less release of epinephrine; symptoms are produced by deficient glucose metabolism of the higher nervous centers. They consist of headache, blurred or double vision, fine tremor, uncontrollable yawning, hypothermia, mental confusion, incoordination, and eventually, unconsciousness. In elderly persons an insulin reaction may mimic a cerebrovascular accident. Treatment is administration of glucose by mouth or by vein. In severe and prolonged insulin reactions it is advisable to administer a glucocorticoid to produce maximum stimulation of gluconeogenesis. Relatives of diabetic patients prone to severe insulin reactions, and especially parents of diabetic children, should be instructed in the use of glucagon. It can be injected subcutaneously, just as insulin, and will lead to a transient rise in blood glucose that is long enough to wake the patient up and enable him to receive some carbohydrate by mouth.

Recurrent hypoglycemic attacks, with their attendant anxiety, headache, loss of concentration power, etc., constitute a nuisance to the diabetic patient, but only *severe and prolonged* attacks of hypoglycemia will lead to intellectual deterioration as a result of irreversible damage to cortical neurones.

An insulin reaction initiates a counterregulatory mechanism characterized by release of epinephrine, adrenal corticosteroids, and growth hormone. This will result in a rebound hyperglycemia, for "hypoglycemia begets hyperglycemia." Knowledge of this physiologic defense mechanism will prevent the physician from administering extra insulin to combat this hyperglycemia. If the insulin reaction is due to excess insulin, the patient will benefit from a reduced insulin dosage.

Reactions at the Site of Insulin Injection

Such reactions are not uncommon at the beginning of treatment. They are characterized by redness, swelling, pain, and nodule formation. As they usually disappear within a few days or weeks, the patient can be reassured, and no treatment is indicated. If the local reaction persists, it can be improved by changing to an insulin of the lente type, which does not contain protamine. Skin infections at the site of injection are extremely rare.

Insulin Lipodystrophy

This reaction is characterized by either hypertrophy or atrophy of the subcutaneous adipose tissue at the site of insulin injection. This is frequent and affects children and females more than males. If the patient is bothered by the esthetic aspect of this complication, injection of insulin into other sites is recommended until the lesion improves; then the atrophic area may again be used in the hope of inducing lipogenesis.

Insulin Resistance

Almost all diabetic patients treated with insulin for several months will develop circulating antibodies to insulin. However, only a few (approximately 1 in 1,000 insulin-treated diabetics) will develop insulin resistance. By definition it is present if the daily insulin requirement in the absence of ketoacidosis exceeds 200 units. Patients with insulin resistance may require several thousand units daily. When insulin resistance is associated with hemochromatosis, severe infections, Cushing's syndrome, acromegaly, or hyperthyroidism, it is secondary. Frequently, no obvious cause can be detected. Examination of serum will demonstrate the presence of large quantities of antibodies to insulin and an increased insulin-binding capacity. In such patients a trial with pure pork insulin is always justified, and very often a sizable reduction in insulin requirement can be achieved. If such a simple measure fails, the use of steroids is indicated, for their anti-insulin effect is outweighed by their antiallergic effect. Rarely the sulfonylureas are helpful. The natural course of idiopathic insulin resistance is characterized by spontaneous remission within several weeks or months. Frequently, the resistance breaks abruptly and the patient exhibits episodes of severe hypoglycemia as the antibody-bound insulin is released and becomes suddenly available.

COMPLICATIONS OF DIABETES

Diabetic Ketoacidosis and Coma

Lack of insulin is the cause of diabetic ketoacidosis. The patient may be (1) an undiagnosed diabetic, (2) a known diabetic who fails to increase his insulin dose despite poor urine tests, or (3) a known diabetic who suffers from nausea and vomiting and, as he does not eat, reasons that he does not need his daily insulin. Omission of insulin probably constitutes the single largest cause of diabetic acidosis.

DIAGNOSIS. Among clinical signs and symptoms, vomiting is present in approximately two-thirds of patients with acidosis. Abdominal pain and tenderness may be related to nausea and vomiting or sodium depletion and may be so severe as to mimic an abdominal emergency ("pseudoappendicitis" of diabetic acidosis). Air hunger and heavy labored breathing as described by Kussmaul are expressions of the acidosis and correlate with the reduction in serum CO_2. There is dehydration as evidenced by soft eyeballs, dry skin, poor urinary output, and hypotension. Laboratory findings include the following: the urine usually contains massive amounts of glucose and acetone; frequently there is also transient albuminuria. The diagnosis of diabetic ketoacidosis is made, however, by finding hyperglycemia, ketonemia, and reduction of serum CO_2 content. The acidosis is metabolic and is caused by accumulation of ketone bodies associated with loss of sodium and potassium. The azotemia is due partly to dehydration and partly to tissue protein breakdown. Serum lipids are generally increased. The rise in hematocrit indicates dehydration; usually there is leukocytosis.

DIFFERENTIAL DIAGNOSIS. On clinical grounds alone it is sometimes difficult to distinguish between diabetic acidosis and an insulin reaction. If any doubt exists, blood should be drawn for laboratory tests and 50 ml of 50 percent glucose injected intravenously. If the coma is due to insulin reaction, the patient will wake up immediately; if he is in diabetic coma, no harm has been done. Among diagnoses to be considered are salicylate poisoning; lactic acidosis; hyperglycemic, hyperosmolaric, nonketotic coma; or far-advanced renal failure—all conditions which can occur in a diabetic patient.

TREATMENT. This will vary greatly from patient to patient; however, the general principles are as follows: (1) through a large needle blood is withdrawn for laboratory tests (blood glucose, BUN, Na, K, Cl, CO_2 Hct, plasma acetone), and the vein is kept open with an infusion of normal saline. The rationale for this rests on the observation that patients in diabetic coma may decompensate very rapidly, and precious time will be lost in finding a vein and performing a venous cutdown. (2) Crystalline insulin is administered both subcutaneously and intravenously. The average dosage of insulin required for patients in diabetic coma is 200 units, 100 units intravenously and 100 units subcutaneously. The dosage, of course, will vary from patient to patient and may have to be larger for an obese diabetic and less in a frail, elderly diabetic. If the patient has been in diabetic coma previously and required 300 units to respond, chances are he may require a similar dose again. Severe acidosis necessitates reevaluation of blood glucose, serum CO_2, and serum acetone levels every 2 hr; if less severe, every 4 hr will suffice. If the blood glucose level remains above 500 mg per 100 ml and serum acetone is positive at 1:4 dilution, another 100 units of insulin should be given. If the patient does not respond at all or if he deteriorates, successive doses are increased rapidly and given at hourly intervals. An occasional patient may require 5,000 or 10,000 units within the first 24 hr of treatment. If, on the other hand, at the fourth hour the level of blood glucose has decreased but remains above 400 mg per 100 ml, administration of another 50 units of insulin is indicated. (3) All patients in diabetic acidosis are severely dehydrated and depleted of sodium and potassium. They will require a large amount of fluid, usually a total of 4 to 8 liters during the first 24 hr. Many electrolyte formulas have been proposed for adequate replacement, and though their value is not doubted, it is important to start fluid therapy *immediately*, which is best done with the universally available normal (0.9 percent) saline solution. Once treatment is under way and the laboratory has reported values for blood glucose, serum CO_2, and electrolytes, finer adjustments can be made. The addition of bicarbonate is certainly indicated if the acidosis is severe (CO_2-combining capacity less than 10). It may also counteract the inhibitory effect a lowered pH has on insulin activity and therefore restore the patient's sensitivity to insulin. Once the blood glucose approaches 200 mg per 100 ml, the intravenous fluid should be changed to 5% glucose in saline in order to avoid hypoglycemia. Usually there is also a deficiency of potassium, and this should be replaced, starting at the second or third hour, at a rate not exceeding 20 mEq per hour; rarely more than 80 mEq is needed during the initial 24 hr of treatment. The need for and administration of potassium can be monitored with an electrocardiograph. Signs of hypokalemia are flattening or inversion of T waves and prolongation of the Q-T intervals. (4) There are useful accessory procedures in treatment of diabetic acidosis. If the patient is unconscious, gastric lavage should be performed to prevent aspiration pneumonia. If the patient is in obvious circulatory collapse, blood, plasma, or a plasma volume expander should be given. Finally, the precipitating cause for the development of diabetic acidosis has to be established for each patient before specific treatment can be initiated. (5) The acute phase of diabetic acidosis is considered ended once the patient is completely responsive, the blood glucose is below 200 mg per 100 ml, the undiluted serum shows no evidence for acetone, serum CO_2 is normal, and the urine shows minimal glycosuria and not more than 1+ acetone. Now is the time to start the patient on intermediate insulin in a small dose to prevent a relapse into ketosis and also, if needed, to give crystalline insulin in amounts dictated by urine sugar levels. A soft diet should be started. It is essential to begin with frequent small feedings. Intravenous fluid administration may be discontinued as soon as the patient is able to retain liquids by mouth. The overall mortality of patients with diabetic acidosis is approximately 5 percent. A very rare but serious complication of diabetic ketoacidosis is facial mucormycosis, see Chap. 191.

Hyperglycemic Nonketotic Coma

This entity is characterized by extreme elevation of blood glucose (values of 1,000 mg per 100 ml or higher are not rare; "syrupy" blood), and absence of ketonemia or acetonuria. The marked hyperglycemia and the associated hypernatremia secondary to water loss lead to an increase in extracellular fluid osmolarity with consequent intracellular dehydration, the effect of which on the central nervous system accounts for the neurologic symptoms and coma. Serum osmolarity can be estimated by multiplying the Na concentration times 2 and adding 5.5 for each 100 mg of glucose (molecular weight of glucose is 180, therefore $100/18 = 5.5$). Normal values range between 290 and 310 mOsm per liter. A patient with values of Na of 160 mEq per liter and of blood glucose of 1,000 mg per 100 ml exhibits an approximate serum osmolarity of $320 + 55 = 375$ mOsm per liter. The highest level recorded is 458 mOsm per liter.

It is observed usually in the middle-aged or older person, frequently associated with corticosteroid therapy or peritoneal dialysis and may be the first indication of diabetes. Awareness of this syndrome is important, as a comatose patient seen for the first time may be misdiagnosed, as he will show massive glycosuria but no acetone, and therefore it is reasoned that the cause for his coma is not diabetic ketoacidosis and no antidiabetic treatment is initiated. Thus valuable time may be lost. Treatment consists of intravenous fluid, preferably hypotonic saline and insulin. Some patients are markedly sensitive to insulin, and 25 to 50 units may suffice, whereas others may require 200 or more units. According to the literature the mortality of this diabetic complication approximates 50 percent; however, in our personal experience with eight patients only one patient died. After recovery not all patients will require insulin. Some can be carried with oral agents or diet alone.

Diabetic Retinopathy

This can be detected in varying degrees in more than 90 percent of diabetic patients after 20 years of clinical diabetes.

The earliest recognizable lesions on fundoscopy are dilatation of veins and "microaneurysms" which actually consist of small punctate hemorrhages. Unless they occur within the macula, the vision will not be impaired. Other relatively early lesions are waxy exudates. This stage of the retinopathy can remain stationary for many years. It is the long-term juvenile diabetic who may progress to a more malignant stage, that of neovascularization and proliferative retinopathy. The new blood vessels usually emanate from the disk and grow toward the vitreous. If a preretinal hemorrhage occurs, organization takes place with formation of fibrous and collagenous tissue. Shrinkage of the scar tissue will produce retinal detachment (Fig. 94-1 and color plate). Advanced diabetic retinopathy is frequently associated with retinal lesions caused by atherosclerosis, arterial hypertension, and renal insufficiency.

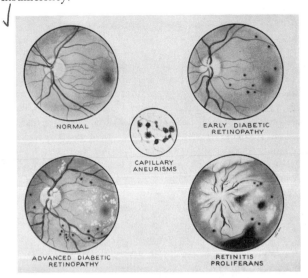

Fig. 94-1. Note the early dilatation of the venules and the punctate hemorrhages *in early diabetic retinopathy* actually representing capillary aneurysms surrounded by hemorrhages, as shown in a microscopic preparation of the retina (*center*). In *advanced diabetic retinopathy*, note in addition the typical hard, waxy exudates. In *retinitis proliferans* is seen the spread of connective tissue, revealed as a white material emanating from the optic disk, together with endovascularization in the form of small irregular vessels. Note the detachment of the retina at the top of the figure, and the larger hemorrhages.

The appearance of retinopathy is fundamentally related to duration of diabetes; one of the reasons for strict chemical control of the metabolic component of diabetes is the possibility of delaying its onset and if possible, making it less severe. If incapacitating retinopathy is present, pituitary ablation should be considered, either by stalk section, total hypophysectomy, or irradiation. Poor vision in one eye and rapidly progressing retinopathy in the other eye constitute the major indication. However, the patient needs to be carefully selected as to emotional stability, long-term willingness to cooperate, and relative freedom from coronary artery disease or nephropathy. As hypoglycemia presents a major hazard after pituitary intervention, the patient should preferably not be living alone. After ablation of the pituitary, preliminary results indicate that two-thirds of patients have stabilized or improved their vision. The factor responsible for improvement has not been identified. Whereas pituitary manipulation represents a last effort to salvage vision, and is associated with the iatrogenic induction of thyroid, adrenal, and gonadal deficiency, newer forms of treatment are directed towards the affected eyes themselves. They are photocoagulation, introduced by Meyer-Schwickerath, and laser beam treatment of the retina. Preliminary results indicate that these procedures may be applied to *early* retinal lesions, and the results obtained are encouraging.

Diabetic Nephropathy
(See Chap. 311 for discussion.)

Diabetic Neuropathy

This is a common, distressing, and therapeutically unsatisfactory complication of diabetes at any stage. Although it most frequently involves peripheral nerves, it may involve any portion of the nervous system and, thus, has an almost unlimited range of manifestations (Table 94-6). The peripheral neuropathy is characterized by a

Table 94-6. DIABETIC NEUROPATHIES

Peripheral:
    Sensory: loss of vibratory sense, paresthesias, pain, loss of pain
    Neuromuscular: weakness, paralysis, absent tendon reflexes, diabetic amytrophy (thighs), extraocular muscle palsies
Autonomic:
    Eye: pupillary changes
    Gastrointestinal: delayed gastric emptying, gallbladder dysfunction, nocturnal diarrhea
    Genitourinary: sexual impotence, atonic urinary bladder, retrograde ejaculation
    Vascular: orthostatic hypotension
    Bones and joints: neuropathic joint (Charcot)
    Skin: neurogenic ulcer, absent sweating, dependent edema

nonsegmental distribution. An interesting differential diagnosis is presented by the patient with severe headache and ocular palsy. If an intracranial aneurysm can be ruled out by angiogram, diabetic neuropathy may be the underlying cause. The neuropathy may be primarily metabolic, which is potentially reversible, or primarily vascular, which is less amenable to treatment.

Treatment of diabetic neuropathy consists of careful control of the diabetes; however, it is not specific, and weeks or months may pass before improvement takes place. If the neuropathy is associated with hyperlipemia, a trial with Clofibrate, 2 Gm daily, is justified.

Gangrene of the Feet

This is a serious and frequent complication of diabetes, especially in the older age group. It may be due to vascular lesions ("pulseless" foot) or to neuropathy ("painless" foot), usually with a superimposed infection or injury. Gangrene may also be associated with small vessel disease in which pedal pulses are not decreased. Arterial insufficiency is diagnosed by a history of claudication and by finding, on examination, weak or absent pedal pulses, blanching of the foot when raised above a 45° angle, and delayed venous filling when the foot is dependent. An arteriogram is indicated. Amputation is the treatment; hence, prevention, or at least delay of onset, of gangrene is of paramount importance. Simple rules for prevention include (1) washing the feet with warm but never *hot* water each evening; (2) applying lanolin two or three times weekly if the skin is dry; (3) inserting lamb's wool between overlapping toes; (4) avoiding injuries to feet (the patient should never go barefoot); (5) not cutting toenails if vision is poor; (6) treating of corns and calluses by a qualified podiatrist or surgeon.

SURGERY AND DIABETES MELLITUS

Diabetic patients may be affected by any surgical disease, but there are certain conditions, such as gangrene of the foot and cholelithiasis, to which they are more prone than the average person. There is also a strong association between cancer of the pancreas and diabetes. In addition, surgical problems may be unrelated to diabetes, such as repair of a hernia. As diabetes is a relatively common condition, from time to time every surgeon and anesthesist will be confronted with a diabetic patient.

The present surgical mortality in diabetics is approximately that of the general population. The surgical risk is increased in diabetics in the presence of poor regulation, obesity, arteriosclerosis, and cardiovascular-renal disease. However, even for the uncomplicated diabetic patient, operation and anesthesia constitute an additional metabolic stress, which will accentuate the predisposition to hyperglycemia and ketosis. Nevertheless, diabetes constitutes no contraindication to surgery; and if the case is an emergency, only a few hours are generally needed to evaluate and prepare such a patient for operation.

On admission for elective or emergency surgery, the patient with diabetes presents in either of two ways: either he is a known diabetic under treatment with varying degree of metabolic control, or the diagnosis of diabetes is suggested by routine preoperative testing. If the scheduled surgery is elective in nature and the diabetes requires further regulation, surgery should be postponed until glycosuria is minimal, acetonuria absent, and preprandial blood glucose close to normal. If, on the other hand, surgery is urgent and there is marked hyperglycemia and ketosis, vigorous treatment is started immediately with intravenous fluid and insulin. The majority of diabetic patients will not present in this dramatic way; most of them are under reasonable metabolic control. Their management during surgery will vary according to the severity of their condition. As a general principle, one should aim to prevent acetonuria and excessive protein breakdown by providing an adequate carbohydrate intake. This is done on the day of surgery by replacing the oral feedings with intravenous 5% or 10% glucose in water or saline, the volume being dictated by the cardiac state and fear of overhydration. Usually, 1,000 to 1,500 ml of 5% glucose in saline is sufficient. By history and laboratory evaluation three types of diabetes are encountered: (1) mild diabetes, treated with diet alone; only close surveillance with frequent urine testing and daily blood glucose is required. (2) Patients on oral agents, such as tolbutamide, acetohexamide, tolazamide, chlorpropamide; or phenformin. As oral intake is usually impossible on the day of surgery, these patients are best changed to a small amount of intermediate-acting (lente or NPH) insulin, for example, 10 to 20 units. Once oral feedings are resumed in the postoperative period, insulin is discontinued and the respective tablets restarted at the former dose. (3) Patients previously on insulin and well controlled receive on the day of surgery two-thirds of their usual *total* dose, preferably divided into a preoperative and postoperative dose, and omitting crystalline insulin. Example: Preoperative insulin dose = 10 units crystalline insulin, 35 units NPH, total dose 45 units. Therefore, on the day of surgery, one-third, or 15 units, of NPH is given preoperatively, and 15 units of NPH is given postoperatively. It is customary in some centers not to give any preoperative insulin, presumably due to fear of hypoglycemia, and only to administer crystalline insulin according to urine test in the postoperative period. In our experience, hypoglycemia occurs rarely if the preoperative insulin is only NPH or lente, provided the total dose is reduced by one-third and, furthermore, if glucose is administered intravenously throughout the operative period. The benefits of this regimen are that the patient does not escape into severe hyperglycemia or ketosis with resultant electrolyte imbalance during surgery or the immediate postoperative period.

PREGNANCY AND DIABETES MELLITUS

The problem of management during pregnancy has assumed increasing importance, as young diabetic patients now survive longer and are thus capable of procreation. Infertility in female diabetic patients, common before insulin therapy, is rarely seen with good control of the diabetes. The problems engendered by pregnancy in diabetics concern maternal survival, fetal salvage, and prevention of diabetes in the offspring.

Today pregnancy carries but slightly added risk to the well-managed diabetic mother; the maternal survival is 99.7 percent (White). In contrast, fetal mortality is still high. Stillbirths among diabetics are six times as common as among nondiabetics. Fetal salvage will depend on the duration of the mother's disease and presence or absence of vascular lesions such as nephropathy.

Diagnosis

In patients not previously known as diabetic, pregnancy may induce a temporary state of diabetes. The diagnosis may offer some difficulty, since with the lowered renal threshold of pregnancy, glycosuria is not uncommon even among nondiabetic pregnant women. If urinary glucose is found during pregnancy and there is, in addition, a history of frequent miscarriages, of babies with a birth weight exceeding 9 lb, or a family history of diabetes, diabetes should be suspected. The diagnosis can be firmly established only by the presence of abnormal blood glucose levels, whether fasting or postprandial. If they are borderline, performance of a glucose tolerance test is definitely indicated.

Treatment

The best results are obtained by close cooperation between the patient, the internist, and the obstetrician. The treatment of pregnant diabetic patients entails the same general health measures as those recommended for nondiabetic pregnant women. It is desirable to maintain a high intake of protein (i.e., at least 2 Gm per kg body weight per day) with a total caloric intake of 30 Cal per kg body weight and an adequate intake of calcium and iron. To prevent edema and minimize hydramnios, a low-salt diet is indicated, and the liberal use of diuretics is advisable. In most women, diabetes is regulated throughout pregnancy with insulin. Because of the lowered renal threshold for glucose one should not attempt to keep the urine sugar-free. It is admittedly often difficult to avoid excessive weight gain, but at least 200 Gm carbohydrate must be utilized to prevent ketosis.

Care of a diabetic patient through the first trimester may be difficult because of nausea and vomiting. If antiemetic drugs fail to control nausea and vomiting and frequent small feedings are not well tolerated, intravenous glucose must be administered. In the last trimester the insulin requirement usually increases concurrently with a rise in adrenal cortical activity, the presence of hormonal anti-insulin factors of placental origin, and placental destruction of insulin. It is of utmost importance to detect preeclamptic toxemia and hydramnios, since treatment will reduce fetal mortality. Timing of delivery is also important. The more advanced the diabetic state of the mother, the earlier the delivery should be attempted. Patients with only chemical diabetes can be delivered at term, patients with vascular complications should be delivered at the thirty-sixth week. The child may be delivered vaginally or by section. Early delivery has the advantage of removing the infant before it becomes too large and before placental circulation is impaired. The latter may be either the cause or the effect of the tendency to toxemia. A sudden decrease of insulin requirement to prepregnancy level usually follows delivery; therefore, it is advisable to omit the insulin dose on the day of delivery and to administer glucose intravenously.

CARE OF THE NEWBORN

Special attention has to be paid to the predisposition of newborn infants of diabetic mothers to develop the respiratory distress syndrome (hyaline membrane disease) and hypoglycemia.

The incidence of diabetes later in life in a child delivered of a diabetic mother is 22 percent and thus not essentially different from that of the general population with either a diabetic mother or a diabetic father.

REFERENCES

Bressler, R.: Investigative Issues in Diabetes Mellitus, Arch. Int. Med., 123:219, 1969.

Butterfield, W. J. H., and W. Van Westering: Tolbutamide after Ten Years, Excerpta Med., 1967.

Clarke, B. F., and Duncan, L. J. P.: Comparison of Chlorpropamide and Metformin Treatment of Weight and Blood Glucose Response of Uncontrolled Obese Diabetics, Lancet, I:123, 1968.

Duncan, L. J. P.: Diabetes Mellitus, Edinburgh, University Press, 1966.

Goldberg, M. F., and S. L. Fine: Symposium on the Treatment of Diabetic Retinopathy, Public Health Service Publication No. 1890, 1969.

Grodsky, G. M., and P. H. Forsham: Insulin and the Pancreas, Ann. Rev. Physiol., 28:347, 1966.

Halmos, P. B., J. K. Nelson, and R. C. Lowry: Hyperosmolar Non-ketoacidotic Coma in Diabetes, Lancet, I:675, 1966.

Hirsch, J., and P. W. Han: Cellularity of Adipose Tissue: Effects of Growth, Starvation, and Obesity, J. Lipid. Res., 10:77, 1969.

Lacy, P. E.: The Pancreatic Beta Cell, Structure and Function, New Engl. J. Med., 276:187, 1967.

Special Report: Classification of Genetic Diabetes Mellitus, Diabetes, 16:540, 1967.

Steiner, D. F., D. Cunningham, L. Spigelman, and B. Aten: Insulin Biosynthesis, Evidence for a Precursor, Science, 157:697, 1967.

U.S. Department of Health, Education, and Welfare: "Diabetes Source Book," No. 1168, May, 1964.

Warren, S., P. M. LeCompte, and M. A. Legg, "The Pathology of Diabetes Mellitus," 5th ed., Philadelphia, Lea & Febiger, 1966.

White, P. (ed.): "Diabetes," Med. Clinics N. Am., 49:4, 1965.

95 NONDIABETIC MELITURIA
Alexander Marble

DEFINITION. Nondiabetic melituria includes a variety of conditions in which, apart from diabetes mellitus, sugar appears in the urine in amounts large enough to yield positive tests by methods in common clinical use. It is, therefore, not a precisely defined entity. Certain of the conditions appear to be inborn errors of metabolism, and most, though not all, are asymptomatic anomalies with no apparent influence on longevity.

CLASSIFICATION. The nondiabetic meliturias may be classified by whether or not the sugar found in the urine is glucose, as shown in Table 95-1.

GLUCOSURIC MELITURIA

PHYSIOLOGY. Normally, the concentration of glucose in the glomerular filtrate is the same as that in the plasma water. Glucose is reabsorbed in the proximal convoluted tubules, chiefly in their proximal portions. Since the passage of glucose through the tubular mucosa takes place against an ever-increasing gradient, the reabsorption involves an active transport process requiring energy. As the concentration of glucose in the plasma increases, the amount of glucose absorbed by the tubules reaches a

Table 95-1. TYPES OF NONDIABETIC MELITURIA

I. Glucosuric melituria
   A. Renal glucosuria
      1. Hereditary
         a. "True" renal glucosuria with glucosuria invariably
            present even during fasting
         b. Associated with other renal tubular defects, as in
            the Fanconi syndrome
      2. Nonhereditary
         a. Pregnancy
         b. Nephropathy, with damage to proximal tubules
   B. Transient glucosuria in diverse conditions in which there
      is temporary hyperglycemia considered not to be due to
      diabetes
II. Nonglucosuric melituria
   A. Pentosuria
   B. Fructosuria
      1. Essential fructosuria
      2. Hereditary fructose intolerance
   C. Lactosuria
   D. Galactosuria
   E. Mannoheptulosuria
   F. Other conditions

transfer maximum (Tm_G), which in the normal adult is about 300 to 350 mg per minute. When the arterial blood glucose exceeds a certain level (usually about 150 to 180 mg per 100 ml) and the amount of glucose presented to the tubules for reabsorption is greater than the Tm_G, glucose appears in the urine. However, this concentration of blood glucose, often called the *renal threshold,* is not rigidly fixed and is not the sole factor concerned. Changes in the glomerular filtration rate alter the total quantity of glucose reaching the proximal tubules per unit of time and variations in the activity of tubules of individual nephrons influence the composite effect.

RENAL GLUCOSURIA. "True" renal glucosuria with glucose in the urine constantly and persistently even during the fasting state (with blood glucose levels below 100 mg per 100 ml) is a rare condition. Among approximately 50,000 patients with melituria, this type and degree of renal glucosuria was recognized in only 85 cases. However, if the designation of renal glucosuria is made more loosely so as to include situations in which the renal threshold is lower than average but not below 100 mg per 100 ml, the number of cases may be large. Whether or not there is any basic difference in the situations responsible for these varying degrees of lowering of the renal threshold, and whether or not one is justified in considering "true" renal glucosuria an entity, cannot be answered with the information available. Indeed, the cause and nature of the tubular abnormality in renal glucosuria remain obscure. Renal biopsy studies, admittedly few in number and limited in scope, have failed to demonstrate any specific anatomic or enzymatic defect.

Renal glucosuria is a condition set apart from diabetes mellitus. Glucosuria is invariably present, and the blood glucose is unquestionably normal both on random sampling and during an oral glucose tolerance test. Measures

designed to evaluate carbohydrate utilization yield normal results, and ketosis develops during starvation rather than after dietary excesses. Symptoms characteristic of diabetes are lacking, and without treatment the condition is not progressive.

Renal glucosuria has been thought to be inherited as a dominant trait. However, the results of certain family surveys suggest that it is transmitted as a single autosomal gene which, in its homozygous expression, is manifested by persistent, gross glucosuria and in its heterozygous expression by slight or no glucosuria. Although, as stated above, it appears to be unrelated to diabetes mellitus, diabetes seems to occur in the families of persons with renal glucosuria with a frequency greater than expected. There is no evidence that diabetes develops later among persons with "true" renal glucosuria to a greater extent than would be expected in the general population. Care must be taken at the time of original study to exclude those persons in whom glucose tolerance tests yielded borderline results. It is important that persons thought to have renal glucosuria be observed closely, particularly for the first few years in order to establish with reasonable certainty the diagnosis of a benign condition.

Decreased capacity of the renal tubules to reabsorb glucose may be part of a more extensive disturbance of tubular function, as in the *Fanconi syndrome,* which is characterized also by defective reabsorption of amino acids, phosphate, and bicarbonate (see Chap. 103 and 104).

Temporary renal glucosuria occurs frequently in *pregnancy,* particularly during the latter half. The mechanism is poorly understood. The chief responsibility of the physician is to make sure that the condition is benign glucosuria and not diabetes mellitus, which may well have its onset or be recognized first during pregnancy. "Screening" tests should be made by determining the level of blood glucose at 1 hr after 50 Gm glucose, after a meal liberal in carbohydrate, or after the intravenous administration of glucose (see Chap. 94).

Glucosuria of varying degree and duration may also occur in nephropathies in which there is tubular damage and impaired absorption of glucose. These include certain nephritides and particularly nephrosis resulting from the administration of chemical agents such as heavy metals and (in animals) phlorhizin.

Patients with diabetes mellitus may also have a renal threshold lower than normal. When insulin is used in treatment, the dosage must be chosen carefully with special attention to the blood glucose. Parallel studies of blood and urine glucose will furnish a practical guide as to what degree of glucosuria must be allowed to prevent episodes of hypoglycemia.

TRANSIENT GLUCOSURIA IN DIVERSE CONDITIONS. Glucose may appear in the urine transiently and intermittently in a wide variety of conditions, including disorders of the pituitary (acromegaly, pituitary basophilism), adrenals (Cushing's syndrome, pheochromocytoma), and thyroid (hyperthyroidism); stimulation of intracranial nerve centers as with brain tumors, cerebral hemorrhage, and injuries of the skull; infections, toxemias, anesthesia, and asphyxia; administration of carbohydrate following starvation ("hunger glucosuria"); following subtotal gastrectomy; acute myocardial infarction; and malignant disease. In most of these conditions hyperglycemia is present temporarily and affords a satisfactory explanation for the glucosuria. However, recent studies and experience suggest that often diabetes mellitus is actually present in early or latent form and has been brought to the level of clinical recognition by the stressful situation. Accordingly, patients with temporary hyperglycemia and glucosuria require careful observation and periodic examinations for years so that if overt diabetes should develop, it may be recognized early. Such individuals should be encouraged to keep the body weight throughout life at a level appropriate for age, height, and body build.

NONGLUCOSURIC MELITURIA

In patients with persistent normoglycemic melituria it is important to ascertain the type of sugar excreted. In most instances the reducing substance will be found to be glucose, but in a number of cases sufficiently large to make special study definitely worthwhile, the sugar is not glucose but pentose, fructose, or some other sugar less commonly encountered. These sugars bear no relation to diabetes mellitus, and their recognition has practical importance as regards eligibility for employment, life insurance, etc., since for the most part these conditions are benign. A systematic study includes the following procedures:

1. Benedict's test, or a modification (Clinitest). This is positive for all sugars found in the urine. The ketoses, particularly fructose, the pentoses, and mannoheptulose, reduce Benedict's solution after a few hours at room temperature (i.e., without heating) and within 10 min at 50 to 60°C.

2. Glucose oxidase test (specific for glucose). Paper strips (Tes-tape and Clinistix) are available for quick testing.

3. Bial (orcinol hydrochloride) reaction. It is positive for pentose.

4. Seliwaroff (resorcinol hydrochloride) reaction. It is positive for fructose.

5. Paper chromatography to confirm the identity of the sugar.

6. Formation of characteristic osazone crystals with phenylhydrazine or (in the case of fructose) methylphenylhydrazine. This may be carried a step further by determination of the melting point of the crystals (glucosazone, 205°C; pentosazone, 157 to 160°C).

7. Fermentation with baker's yeast. Glucose and fructose are always, galactose usually, lactose occasionally, and pentose and mannoheptulose never fermented.

PENTOSURIA. Essential pentosuria is a benign condition inherited as an autosomal recessive trait. Its rarity is indicated by the fact that among 50,000 patients with melituria, only 11 cases of essential pentosuria were recognized. It is characterized by the constant presence in the urine of pentose 1-xylulose in small amounts varying from 1 to 4 Gm daily. With Benedict's method one usually obtains a constant green test. Most reported cases have been in Jews, although some have been in Lebanese families. Although pentosuria was thought formerly to occur predominately in males, recent studies suggest that the sex distribution may be more nearly equal. Most of the families of pentosurics in the New York City area studied by Lasker came originally from geographic foci of relatively limited extent, largely Poland and Germany. The condition is harmless, asymptomatic, and unrelated to diabetes. It requires no treatment

The enzymatic defect concerned in pentosuria appears to be related to the metabolism of glucuronic acid. Normally, uronic acids are converted to a pentose (1-xylulose), then to a sugar alcohol (xylitol), and finally through a series of steps to hexose. In individuals with pentosuria the enzyme responsible for the conversion of 1-xylulose to xylitol apparently is deficient. As a result, 1-xylulose accumulates and is excreted in the urine.

FRUCTOSURIA. Essential Fructosuria. Like pentosuria, this is a benign, asymptomatic anomaly of metabolism, probably inherited as an autosomal recessive trait. All reported cases have been in Jews. Fructosuria appears in males and females with about equal frequency. Fructosuria is rarer than pentosuria. Among 50,000 persons seen with melituria, only 4 cases of fructosuria, 2 in males and 2 in females, were recognized. Two of the patients were brother and sister.

Following the ingestion of fructose by persons with essential fructosuria, the concentration of that sugar in the blood reaches higher levels and remains high longer than in the normal individual. As a consequence, some 10 to 20 percent of the amount administered is excreted in the urine. Furthermore, the rise of the respiratory quotient is less than normal and the blood lactic and pyruvic acid concentrations remain unchanged. Available evidence strongly suggests that the faulty metabolism is due to a primary deficiency of hepatic fructokinase, an enzyme that catalyzes the conversion of fructose to fructose 1-phosphate.

Hereditary Fructose Intolerance. Hereditary fructose intolerance is an uncommon error of metabolism characterized by symptomatic hypoglycemia and vomiting after the ingestion of fructose. In this condition, thought to be inherited as an autosomal recessive trait, the primary defect is a deficiency of fructose 1-phosphate aldolase in the liver. The accumulation of fructose 1-phosphate supposedly inhibits fructose phosphorylation by fructokinase and this results in fructosemia and fructosuria. The mechanism for the secondary hypoglycemia is not clear. Indirect evidence favors inhibition of glucose production or release by the liver by fructose 1-phosphate, although the details of this action have not been clarified.

Treatment consists of elimination of fructose-containing foods from the diet. The outlook is excellent if the condition is recognized early in infancy and appropriate steps taken. If fructose is not avoided, long-term effects may include liver damage, renal impairment, and finally, cachexia and death.

LACTOSURIA. Lactose appears in the urine toward the end of pregnancy and during lactation. It may be considered as a physiologic event and need cause no concern. However, particularly during pregnancy, the finding of sugar in the urine should prompt the determination of the blood glucose at 1 hr after 50 Gm glucose or a meal liberal in carbohydrate in order to detect diabetes if present. Lactose gives a positive test with Benedict's solution. It is best identified by paper chromatography.

GALACTOSURIA. (See Chap. 112).

MANNOHEPTULOSURIA. Mannoheptulose appears in the urine of certain persons in small amounts after the eating of avocado. It is of no importance clinically.

OTHER MELITURIAS. Maltosuria has been reported rarely but has not been shown to be of clinical significance. Sucrose is promptly excreted in the urine following its administration intravenously, since under these conditions there is no provision in the body for hydrolyzing it to simpler sugars. Alimentary sucrosuria of slight degree may occur in normal individuals following a loading dose of cane sugar. Endogenous sucrosuria, difficult to explain, has been noted rarely and then only in association with disease of the pancreas. In reported cases the specific gravity of the urine reached values as high as 1.070. One must be on guard for cases of deception in which patients add cane sugar to urine brought for examination, not realizing that sucrose will not reduce Benedict's solution. An unusually high specific gravity of the urine leads one to think of the possibility of sucrose in the urine.

REFERENCES

Freeman, J. A., and K. E. Roberts: A Fine Structural Study of Renal Glycosuria, Exper. Mol. Pathol., 2:83, 1963.

Froesch, E. R., H. P. Wolf, H. Baitsch, A. Prader, and A. Labhart: Hereditary Fructose Intolerance. An Inborn Defect of Hepatic Fructose 1-phosphate Splitting Aldolase, Am. J. Med., 34:151, 1963.

Khachadurian, A. K., and L. A. Khachadurian: The Inheritance of Renal Glycosuria, Am. J. Human Gen., 16:189, 1964.

Marble, A.: Nondiabetic Melituria, pp. 717–738 in E. P. Joslin, H. F. Root, P. White, and A. Marble: "The Treatment of Diabetes Mellitus," 10th ed., Philadelphia, Lea & Febiger, 1959.

Stanbury, J. B., J. B. Wyngaarden, and D. S. Fredrickson: "The Metabolic Basis of Inherited Disease," 2d ed., New York, McGraw-Hill Book Company, 1966; see chapts. on Pentosuria by H. H. Hiatt, p. 109; Fructosuria by E. R. Froesch, p. 124; and Renal Glycosuria by S. M. Krane, p. 1221.

96 HYPERINSULINISM, HYPOGLYCEMIA, AND GLUCAGON SECRETION

Stefan S. Fajans and
George W. Thorn

INTRODUCTION

The maintenance of a constant blood glucose level is an essential part of homeostasis. The blood glucose level at any given time reflects the balance of two groups of physiologic processes: (1) those which add glucose to the blood, namely, (*a*) mobilization of glucose from glycogen stores, (*b*) formation of carbohydrate from nonglucose sources (gluconeogenesis), and (*c*) absorption of ingested carbohydrate; and (2) those which remove glucose from the blood, namely, utilization of glucose by liver, adipose tissue, muscle, brain, and other tissues.

CLASSIFICATION. Hypoglycemia may be produced by a variety of factors. In some the mechanism is poorly understood. Hence, a complete classification based on pathologic physiology is difficult. Nevertheless, the common causes of spontaneous hypoglycemia can be grouped as listed in Table 96-1. From the clinical view, patients with

Table 96-1. ETIOLOGIC CLASSIFICATION
OF SPONTANEOUS HYPOGLYCEMIA

I. Organic hypoglycemia*
  A. Pancreatic islet cell tumor, functioning
  B. Nonpancreatic tumors associated with hypoglycemia
  C. Anterior pituitary hypofunction
  D. Adrenocortical hypofunction
  E. Acquired extensive liver disease
II. Hypoglycemia due to specific hepatic enzyme defect
  A. Glycogen storage diseases*
  B. Hereditary fructose intolerance
  C. Galactosemia
  D. Familial fructose and galactose intolerance
III. Functional hypoglycemia
  A. Reactive functional
  B. Reactive secondary to mild diabetes
  C. Alimentary hyperinsulinism
  D. Transient postnatal hypoglycemia in infant of diabetic mother*
  E. Transient hypoglycemia in the newborn of low birth weight*
  F. "Idiopathic hypoglycemia" of infancy and childhood*
  G. Alcohol and poor nutrition*
IV. Exogenous hypoglycemia*
  A. Iatrogenic ⎱ insulin or sulfonylurea compounds
  B. Factitious ⎰

*Fasting hypoglycemia.

hypoglycemia can be divided into two groups, according to the usual relationship of hypoglycemia to the fasting or postprandial state. Regardless of etiology, the conditions listed in Table 96-1 interfere with the homeostatic mechanism, which regulates the blood glucose level. Such interference may take place at different levels, even if the underlying cause of hypoglycemia is a single one. For example, in patients with functioning islet cell tumors, hypoglycemia is the result not only of increased glucose uptake in insulin-sensitive tissues and decreased hepatic glucose output but also of decreased inflow to the liver of substrates needed for gluconeogenesis. For example, the mobilization of amino acids from muscle is reduced.

CLINICAL PICTURE. The clinical symptoms and signs of hypoglycemia are the same regardless of the underlying cause. The symptoms which occur in any given patient vary with the degree and the rate of decline of blood glucose levels and with the variable and individual susceptibility of the underlying state of the central and autonomic nervous systems. Symptoms associated with a rapid decline in blood glucose levels are due in part to activation of the autonomic nervous system and the ensuing release of epinephrine. These symptoms are sweating, shakiness, trembling, tachycardia, anxiety, nervousness, weakness, fatigue, hunger, nausea, and vomiting. Other symptoms of hypoglycemia result from decreased uptake of glucose and decreased utilization of oxygen by the brain and usually occur when the decline in blood glucose levels is slow and/or when hypoglycemia is severe or prolonged. These symptoms are headache, visual disturbances, lethargy, yawning, faintness, restlessness, and difficulty with speech and thinking. Other manifestations may be agitation, mental confusion, somnolence, stupor, prolonged sleep, loss of consciousness, coma, and hypothermia. Twitching, convulsions, "epilepsy," and bizarre neurologic signs, motor as well as sensory in nature, may occur. Prominent signs observed in patients with alcohol-induced hypoglycemia are hypothermia, conjugate deviation of eyes, extensor rigidity of extremities, positive Babinski signs, and trismus. Repeated hypoglycemic episodes may lead to loss of intellectual ability and personality changes characterized by outbursts of temper or queer, bizarre, and psychotic behavior. Extensive and permanent mental or neurologic damage may result from frequent and prolonged episodes of hypoglycemia.

FUNCTIONING ISLET CELL TUMORS
Pathology

Approximately 90 percent of functioning islet cell tumors are benign adenomas; approximately 10 percent are definitely malignant with identified metastases. Hyperplasia of the islet cells has not been proved to occur in adults. Functioning islet cell tumors may be diagnosed at any age, with a majority of cases occurring between thirty and sixty years. Benign islet cell adenomas vary in size from 0.14 to 15 cm in diameter, but the majority are between 0.5 and 3.0 cm. They are usually encapsulated, firmer than the normal pancreas, highly vascular, purplish and occasionally whitish in color, and they present an irregular surface. They are found to be equally distributed throughout the head, body, and tail of the pancreas. Benign adenomas of islet cell tissue rarely occur outside the pancreas. Multiple adenomas are found in approximately 5 to 10 percent of cases. Multiple adenomas of islet cells may be associated with adenomas of the pituitary, parathyroids, and other endocrine glands and with peptic ulceration. In recent years it has been emphasized that this association frequently has a familial basis. A family history of diabetes has been found also in 25 to 30 percent of patients with functioning islet cell tumors.

Clinical Picture

Symptoms of hypoglycemia due to islet cell adenoma may develop insidiously, with periodic hypoglycemic attacks becoming more frequent and more severe. Fasting and exercise precipitate attacks. Attacks usually occur in the early morning hours, during the longest daily fasting period, or they may occur in late afternoon, especially if the noon meal is missed. Symptoms may also occur 2 to 5 hr after meals. Symptoms and signs secondary to decreased cerebral oxygen utilization usually predominate over symptoms secondary to hyperepinephrinemia. The pattern of symptoms is usually repetitive in the same patient, but it may differ from patient to patient. Many patients learn to avert symptoms by taking frequent feedings, including a feeding at 2:00 or 3:00 A.M. Obesity may thereby result. Chronic hypoglycemia may not only produce profound personality changes but may result also in damage to anterior horn cells of the spinal cord, with progressive muscular atrophy.

Diagnosis

A typical symptomatic attack with demonstrated hypoglycemia and relief of symptoms and signs by administration of glucose constitute the diagnostic criteria outlined by Whipple. This *triad of Whipple* is not specific for patients with functioning tumors of the pancreas, as it may occur in patients with other types of hypoglycemia. The level of the overnight fasting blood glucose is usually below normal. More prolonged fasting is the most helpful diagnostic procedure and will cause a fall in blood sugar below 30 to 35 mg per 100 ml (true blood glucose method). In the majority of cases, a typical attack with associated hypoglycemia can be induced within the first 24 hr of fasting. If hypoglycemia and typical symptoms are not induced, fasting should be prolonged for up to 72 hr, at which time the patient should be exercised vigorously. In patients with insulinomas, or other types of fasting hypoglycemia, exercise produces a further fall in blood sugar levels, but it produces a rise in blood glucose in patients with functional hypoglycemia.

Assays of serum insulin (Chap. 94) performed in conjunction with fasting blood glucose levels may be valuable in diagnosing insulinoma. Elevated fasting levels of serum insulin in peripheral blood are found in only two-thirds of patients with functioning islet cell tumors. Thus, diagnosis of insulinoma is strengthened by an elevated fasting insulin level, but a "normal" level does not rule out this diagnosis. When fasting insulin levels are measured daily for several days in the same patient, an elevated level can frequently be found in at least one specimen. A serum insulin level in the "normal range" associated with a fasting blood sugar level in the hypoglycemic range is also significant. In addition, when the overnight fast is prolonged for 4 hr or more in patients with fasting blood sugar levels in the borderline range, the blood glucose level may fall into the hypoglycemic range, while the level of serum insulin remains constant or rises, indicating an abnormal glucose-insulin homeostatic relationship. This is good evidence for the presence of an autonomous insulin-producing tumor. An elevated fasting level of plasma insulin after an overnight fast is not specific for insulinoma as it is also seen in obese patients and has been reported in patients with galacto-semia and familial fructose and galactose intolerance.

The intravenous tolbutamide test is valuable in the differential diagnosis of spontaneous hypoglycemia. After blood for a fasting blood glucose determination is obtained, 1 Gm sodium tolbutamide dissolved in 20 ml distilled water is injected intravenously over 2 min. Subsequently blood levels of glucose are determined every 15 min for the first hour and every 30 min during the second and third hours of the test. If plasma levels of insulin can be obtained during the test (see below), blood samples for insulin assay should be obtained every 5 min during the first 15 min after administration of tolbutamide. The greatest usefulness of the test is in obtaining evidence against a diagnosis of insulinoma in patients suspected of having functional hypoglycemia but whose history is unusual or in whom fasting blood glucose levels are in the lower range of normal. In such patients a normal 3-hr intravenous tolbutamide test (return of blood glucose to 70 percent or more of fasting blood sugar level) may obviate hospitalization and determination of blood glucose during prolonged fasting. In patients suspected of harboring insulinoma the test can be used for confirmation, but it should be carefully performed with the patient in the hospital. Tolbutamide-induced hypoglycemia persisted for 3 hr in 50 of 55 patients subsequently proved to have insulinomas. In these 55 patients fasting blood sugar levels were 50 mg per 100 ml or above. The lower the fasting blood sugar, the more frequently will the test have to be terminated early because of severe neurologic symptoms. False positive responses can occur in association with severe liver disease, alcoholic hypoglycemia, idiopathic hypoglycemia of infancy, severe undernutrition, and azotemia. They also may occur in some patients with nonpancreatic tumors and associated hypoglycemia, particularly in those patients in whom blood sugar levels decrease rapidly on fasting. In contrast, no false positive responses have occurred in patients with functional hypoglycemia, diabetes mellitus with reactive hypoglycemia, or patients without spontaneous hypoglycemia. Obviously the test is of little help if the fasting blood glucose level is very low.

Assays of blood insulin in conjunction with the intravenous tolbutamide test increase the value of the test. The finding of excessive increases in plasma insulin levels (above 190 μ U per ml) within the first 15 min after intravenous administration of tolbutamide and/or prolonged elevation of plasma insulin thereafter (1) increases the specificity of this test in patients with insulinoma; (2) increases the usefulness of the test in patients with low fasting blood sugar levels, since it allows termination of the test when necessary; and (3) may differentiate insulinoma patients from patients with false positive blood glucose responses. Approximately 80 percent of patients with islet cell tumors exhibit an abnormal insulin response to intravenously administered tolbutamide. However, an increase in levels of insulin in the high normal range after intravenous tolbutamide does not rule out the existence of an insulinoma.

Sensitivity to leucine may be useful diagnostically. In adult patients a large decrease in blood glucose (over 25 mg per 100 ml) and a large increase in plasma insulin (over 30 μU per ml) after administration of leucine strongly suggest diagnosis of an insulinoma. Approximately 70 percent of patients with functioning islet cell tumors exhibit an exaggerated response to leucine. In childhood, sensitivity to leucine does not differentiate between idiopathic hypoglycemia and insulinoma. Severe leucine-induced hyperinsulinemia and hypoglycemia will also be obtained in factitious hypoglycemia due to surreptitious administration of sulfonylureas, since profound sensitivity to leucine-hypoglycemia can be produced in normal subjects by pretreatment with such compounds. A negative response to leucine does not rule out the existence of an insulinoma.

An exaggerated increase in serum levels of insulin over 160μU per ml after the intravenous administration of 1 mg of glucagon is observed in 50 to 75 percent of patients with proven islet cell tumors. When this occurs, the hyperglycemic effect of glucagon may be subnormal and followed by a profound fall in blood glucose.

In patients with suspected islet cell tumors all three provocative tests should be employed, since an abnormal response may be obtained with one but not another of these tests. Obese patients have an exaggerated rise in plasma insulin with any of these stimuli to insulin secretion, but the hyperinsulinemia is not accompanied by abnormal secondary hypoglycemia.

The oral glucose tolerance test (Chap. 94) may give a relatively flat curve with rapid return of the blood glucose into the hypoglycemic range due to excessive insulin release from the tumor in response to a rising concentration of blood glucose. Occasionally a high plateau curve may be found due to factors counterregulatory to chronic hypoglycemia and normal or subnormal release of insulin from the tumor in response to a rising blood glucose level. The intravenous glucose tolerance test with calculation of an index of glucose utilization is also of limited usefulness, as variable results are obtained in patients with functioning islet cell tumors.

TREATMENT. When the diagnosis of functioning islet cell tumor is made, relief of hypoglycemia by early surgery is indicated to prevent any further damage to the central nervous system and to prevent obesity, which makes surgical management more difficult. Identification of the tumor at the time of surgery may present a problem, particularly in the case of a relatively small tumor not located on the anterior surface of the pancreas. Selective pancreatic arteriography has made it possible to localize some of these tumors preoperatively. It was successful in locating a tumor radiographically in 5 of 11 patients with proven islet cell tumors. Of these five tumors three were located in the head of the pancreas and could not be palpated by the surgeon at the time of laporatomy.

Glucocorticoids have been used as an adjunct in the preoperative preparation of patients with insulinomas or in patients with persistent hypoglycemia following unsuccessful surgery. Cortisone, 100 to 200 mg per day, may be required preoperatively, but of course, continued administration at this level will lead to increased obesity and signs of Cushing's syndrome.

The benzothiadiazine compound, diazoxide, particularly when used in conjunction with one of the diuretic thiazides, such as trichlormethiazide, has been useful to elevate blood levels of glucose into the normoglycemic or hyperglycemic range prior to operation. Diazoxide causes increases in blood glucose by decreasing the secretion of insulin. In addition, diazoxide and the diuretic thiazides elevate blood glucose by one or more extrapancreatic mechanisms. Effective dosage ranges between 150 and 450 mg for Diazoxide and 2 and 3 mg for trichlormethiazide. The drugs should be discontinued 2 days before surgery.

The surgical approach to insulinomas may be complicated by difficulty in identifying the tumor, by difficulty encountered in "shelling out" completely all tumor tissue, and by the fact that multiple tumors are not at all uncommon. In the absence of a definite insulinoma, resection of first the tail and then the body of the pancreas is justified, as a significant proportion of tumors are located in these areas. After excision of the adenoma or subtotal pancreatectomy to find the adenoma, the patient is usually cured except in cases of multiple tumors or unlocated tumors in the head of the pancreas. Difficulty in shelling out the complete tumor is undoubtedly a significant factor in tumor recurrence. In approximately 20 percent of cases diagnosed histologically as carcinoma, follow-up observations have failed to reveal a recurrence of symptoms or tumor for several years.

Patients with nonresectable metastatic islet cell tumors present a management problem, as their hypoglycemia may be so severe as to respond only poorly to oral and even intravenous glucose administration. Since diazoxide is a potent and consistent inhibitor of pancreatic insulin release, it has proved to be an effective agent for the alleviation of symptomatic and biochemical hypoglycemia in many of these patients. To counteract the sodium-retaining effect of diazoxide administered in a dose of 600 to 1000 mg per day, a naturetic thiazide, such as trichlormethiazide, should be used in a dose of 2 to 3 mg per day.

In patients with metastatic islet cell carcinoma who do not respond to the hyperglycemic effect of diazoxide, the use of streptozotocin may be indicated. Streptozotocin, an antibiotic and an experimental antitumor agent, is a highly effective cytotoxic agent for pancreatic beta cells. Although not devoid of renal and hepatic toxicity, it has considerably greater specificity for normal or abnormal beta cells than is true for alloxan. Two patients with metastatic islet cell cacinoma who were teated with streptozotocin have had complete relief from hypoglycemia and regression of tumor mass.

The use of glucocorticoids and injections of glucagon may also be valuable.

NONPANCREATIC TUMORS ASSOCIATED WITH HYPOGLYCEMIA

Severe hypoglycemia has been reported in more than 100 patients harboring nonpancreatic tumors of meso-thelial, epithelial, or endothelial origin. Most of these tumors are mesothelial in type and are classified as fibromas, sarcomas, or fibrosarcomas. They are usually situated in the thorax, the retroperitoneal space, or the pelvis. They may be attached to the diaphragm or found within the liver. Other cases of nonpancreatic tumors associated with severe hypoglycemia include 28 patients with primary hepatic carcinoma, 14 patients with carcinoma of the adrenal cortex, 5 patients with gastrointestinal carcinomas, 2 patients with pseudomyxoma peritonei, 2 patients with bronchogenic carcinoma, and 1 with a bronchial carcinoid tumor. The common clinical characteristics of these tumors, particularly of the fibrosarcomas, are their slow growth and their massive size (up to 9 kg). Hypoglycemia disappears after resection or occasionally after irradiation of the tumor. Many theories have been advanced to explain the mechanism by which these tumors cause hypoglycemia, but none of these is applicable to all patients. A block in hepatic glucose output, excessive glucose consumption by tumor tissue with a high rate of anaerobic glycolysis, and inhibition of lipolysis have been reported in some of these patients. In the majority of patients immunoreactive insulin and insulinlike activity in serum or extract or tumor tissue have been normal or subnormal. High levels of serum insulin have been reported in one patient with severe hypoglycemia due to a large fibrosarcoma and in another patient with a bronchial carcinoid tumor with metastases. Only rarely have tumor extracts contained immunologically recognizable insulin. Twelve reports indicate that extracts of tumors from some of these patients contain an insulinlike substance stimulatory in either isolated rat diaphragm or epididymal fat pad systems. It is possible that some of these tumors synthesize a polypeptide closely related to insulin, but which in the majority of instances is not recognized immunologically as insulin.

OTHER CAUSES FOR FASTING HYPOGLYCEMIA

Although it is infrequent, fasting hypoglycemia may occur in patients with hypofunction of the anterior pituitary (Chap. 87) or hypofunction of the adrenal cortex (Chap. 92). Usually, other stigmas of these disorders enable one to make a diagnosis. In infants and children hypoglycemia due to isolated growth hormone deficiency has been reported.

Alcohol ingestion superimposed upon an inadequate dietary intake can precipitate acute hypoglycemia. Blood glucose levels as low as 10 or 20 mg per 100 ml have been observed. Inhibition of gluconeogenesis is primarily responsible for hypoglycemia in conjunction with depletion of liver glycogen stores.

Occasionally, diffuse hepatic disease (Chap. 323) may be associated with hypoglycemia. Very seldom, fasting hypoglycemia can be traced to a glycogen-storage disease (Chap. 111) or to galactosemia (Chap. 112).

In children the most common type of fasting hypoglycemia is that classified as *idiopathic hypoglycemia of infancy and childhood*. This entity is probably heterogeneous. Fasting hypoglycemia may begin in early postnatal life or in the first 2 years of life. The hypoglycemia may be mild and intermittent or more persistent and severe. Usually by seven to nine years of age these children "outgrow" the occurrence of hypoglycemia. Differentiation from functioning islet cell tumor is most difficult, although the occurrence of insulinoma is rare in this age group.

POSTPRANDIAL HYPOGLYCEMIA
Reaction Functional Hypoglycemia

Reactive functional hypoglycemia occurs almost uniformly in patients with emotional problems. It has been thought to be due to excessive secretion of insulin in response to a normal rise of blood glucose following meals. This is not a consistent finding. The diagnosis is suspected by a history of hypoglycemic symptoms occurring 2 to 4 hr after ingestion of a meal rich in carbohydrates, and it is confirmed by an oral glucose tolerance test extended for 4 or 5 hr, blood samples being obtained at half-hour intervals. It is not unusual in such patients to find blood glucose levels of 30 or 40 mg per 100 ml between the second and fourth hour of the test.

However, the usual symptoms produced by reactive hypoglycemia are transitory and often subside spontaneously in 15 to 30 min. Weakness, hunger, inward trembling, sweating, and tachycardia are the most common symptoms in these patients. Loss of consciousness or convulsions do not occur, and the severity of symptoms is not progressive. In patients with functional hypoglycemia attacks are more frequent when emotional stress and anxiety are greater. A 72-hr fast is well tolerated, and the concentration of blood glucose rarely drops below 45 mg per 100 ml. The intravenous tolbutamide test is normal. A family history for diabetes mellitus is usually absent.

In some patients with advanced cerebrovascular disease, reactive functional hypoglycemia may be the trigger which initiates a cerebral ischemic episode and its subsequent potential chain of events. Similarly, in patients with a hypersensitive carotid sinus or with postural hypotension, the same procedures that do not induce the vascular response at other times may do so during an episode of reactive hypoglycemia. Likewise, there are a number of patients with ectopic tachycardias of various types in which an episode of reactive hypoglycemia is either the sole "trigger" initiating the attacks, which is quite rare, or one of several "triggers," which is quite common. Episodes of reactive hypoglycemia may precipitate attacks of angina as well as bouts of acute pulmonary edema in predisposed cardiac patients. For this small but important group of patients serious cerebral and cardiovascular complications may be minimized by *recognizing* the possible role that reactive functional hypoglycemia may play as an initiating factor.

TREATMENT. The distressing symptoms experienced by patients with functional hypoglycemia may be prevented by a diet low in carbohydrate and high in protein, with adequate fat to maintain caloric requirements. The diet is divided into three to six feedings, with protein and carbohydrate proportions divided equally among the meals. In patients with a history suggestive of reactive hypoglycemia but in whom the diagnosis cannot be substantiated by a glucose tolerance test, diet therapy may be tried. An important approach is to improve the psychologic and emotional status of the patient with functional hypoglycemia. In this regard the use of sedatives such as Phenobarbital, 30 mg at 10:00 A.M., 3:00 P.M.; and bedtime, as well as tranquillizers such as Librium, 10 mg two to three times daily, may prove useful. The prognosis is good, as usually it is a self-limiting disease within a few months or years.

Reactive Hypoglycemia Secondary to Mild Diabetes

This condition has to be distinguished from reactive functional hypoglycemia, for both the underlying mechanism and the prognosis are different. Whereas in patients with reactive functional hypoglycemia the pancreatic insulin release is thought to be excessive but well-timed in response to the rising postprandial blood glucose, in patients with mild diabetes the insulin release is delayed. It is not until the blood glucose rises to frank diabetic levels that insulin is secreted in excess. Measurements of serum insulin during glucose tolerance tests in such patients have demonstrated that relatively large amounts of insulin are released, albeit late; the blood glucose then decreases from diabetic to normal levels and further to hypoglycemic levels. This type of hypoglycemic response is most likely to occur between the third and the fifth hours. It is apparent that these patients have only mild diabetes, as endogenous insulin is available and their fasting blood glucose is within normal limits. Their carbohydrate intolerance can only be detected by a postprandial blood glucose determination or an oral glucose tolerance test. Frequently there is a family history of diabetes mellitus.

Treatment consists of a diabetic diet with frequent feedings. Weight reduction in the obese patient may normalize glucose tolerance, with disappearance of reactive hypoglycemia. Contrary to the relatively benign prognosis of reactive functional hypoglycemia, the disorder is not self-limiting and such patients may eventually progress to a more advanced state of insulin deficiency and the clinical syndrome of diabetes mellitus (Chap. 94).

Alimentary Hypoglycemia

In patients with gastroenterostomy or subtotal gastrectomy, hypoglycemia is due to excessive insulin release in response to excessive postprandial hyperglycemia (alimentary hyperinsulinism). The diagnosis is made by history of abdominal surgery, an *abnormal oral glucose tolerance test* with elevation of the peak blood glucose level, but a *normal intravenous glucose tolerance test.*

Other Causes of Postprandial Hypoglycemia

Leucine sensitivity in the adult is extremely rare. Approximately 70 percent of patients with functioning islet cell tumors and 30 percent of patients with idiopathic hypoglycemia of infancy and childhood may be sensitive to leucine. Recently, hypoglycemia following the ingestion of fructose has also been described, due to an inborn error of metabolism in which there is a deficiency of the enzyme hepatic fructose 1-phosphate aldolase. It is very infrequent.

EXOGENOUS HYPOGLYCEMIA

The possibility of factitious hyperinsulinism as a result of surreptitious administration of insulin or sulfonylureas should always be considered, particularly in nurses, other medical personnel, and relatives of diabetic patients. If self-administration of insulin is suspected, presence of *insulin antibody in serum* from such patients may point to the proper diagnosis, provided there is no history of previous insulin administration.

In the case of ingestion of tolbutamide (Orinase) in large amounts, acidification of the urine will disclose a white precipitate which is a crystallization of the carboxylated excretion product of tolbutamide.

REGULATION OF GLUCAGON SECRETION AND EFFECTS OF GLUCAGON
Source and Characteristics

Glucagon is a polypeptide hormone secreted by the alpha cells of the islets of Langerhans. The hormone is made up of 29 amino acids in a straight chain and has a molecular weight of 3485. With a sensitive radioimmunoassay employing an antiserum specific for glucagon, its concentration can be assayed in pancreatic tissue and in blood. From different portions of the gastrointestinal mucosa (stomach, but particularly small intestine) extracts have been prepared which have immunological characteristics similar to but not identical with pancreatic glucagon. This immunoreactive material, called "gut glucagon," "entero-glucagon," or "glucagon-like immunoreactive material," has been found to be separable into two fractions, one of molecular weight of approximately 7000 and the other with a molecular weight of 3500. The former differs from glucagon in biologic activity (see following). The plasma concentrations of pancreatic glucagon in peripheral blood is approximately 100 pg per ml in the basal state.

Factors Influencing Secretion of Glucagon

Unger and associates have demonstrated that insulin-induced hypoglycemia is followed by increases in the concentration of glucagon in pancreatic and peripheral blood. Starvation is another stimulus to increased secretion of glucagon. On the other hand, hyperglycemia due to orally or intravenously administered glucose causes suppression of glucagon secretion. The ingestion of protein meals or the intravenous or oral administration of certain amino acids (arginine) are other potent stimuli to the secretion of pancreatic glucagon. Administration of pancreozymin, a gastrointestinal hormone released after protein ingestion, has also been found to increase plasma levels of glucagon and to augment the effect of amino acids on glucagon secretion.

The oral but not the intravenous administration of glucose is followed by a significant increase in immunoreactive glucagon in peripheral blood which is due to release of "gut-glucagon."

Metabolic Effects of Glucagon

Glucagon exhibits a marked effect on carbohydrate, protein, and lipid metabolism in vivo and in vitro. Glucagon stimulates hepatic glycogenolysis by increasing cyclic 3′, 5′ adenosine monophosphate (AMP) which leads to increased phosphorylase activity. Increased glycogenolysis and inhibition by glucagon of hepatic glycogen synthetase (also via cyclic AMP) cause hyperglycemia. Glucagon stimulates gluconeogenesis by promoting the hepatic uptake of amino acids,. It inhibits the incorporation of amino acids into liver protein and increases excretion of nitrogen. Glucagon, by activating the adenyl cyclase systems, also promotes lipolysis in liver and adipose tissues. The resulting increased hepatic concentration and oxidation of free fatty acids stimulate hepatic gluconeogenesis and ketogenesis.

In addition to these effects of glucagon on hepatic and adipose tissues, glucagon has a direct effect on stimulating increased release of insulin from the pancreatic beta cells independent of the increases in blood glucose. Glucagon's effect on pancreatic beta cells may also be mediated by activation of the adenyl cyclase system. "Gut glucagon" of molecular weight 7000 also increases the secretion of insulin but does not have the hepatic effects of pancreatic glucagon.

Other extrahepatic effects of glucagon are a positive inotropic effect upon cardiac muscle, a stimulation of adrenal medullary secretion, and a slight lowering of serum levels of calcium and phosphate.

Physiologic Role of Glucagon

The extreme sensitivity of hepatic and adipose tissues to glucagon and the fact that increased secretion of glucagon is stimulated by fasting and hypoglycemia suggest that glucagon is released in order to provide for increased distribution of energy substrates during periods of glucose need. Glycogenolysis and gluconeogenesis will lead to increased levels of blood glucose, and increased lipolysis will furnish free fatty acids for energy and will stimulate gluconeogenesis. In contrast to the effects of fasting and hypoglycemia, rapid increases in blood glucose inhibit the secretion of glucagon. In birds the removal of the pancreas, rich in alpha cells and glucagon, is followed by the development of severe hypoglycemia. This hypoglycemia can be alleviated by the injection of glucagon. Amino acid–induced glucagon release after protein feeding may be an important factor in preventing hypoglycemia which might otherwise occur during amino acid–induced insulin release.

Whether or not pancreatic glucagon plays a physiologic

role in mediating increased release of insulin is still to be demonstrated. It is possible, although not established, that release of "gut glucagon" after ingestion of carbohydrate is one of the mediators of insulin secretion when glucose is ingested.

Abnormalities of Glucagon Secretion

McGavran and his associates have reported a patient with a malignant tumor of the alpha cells of the pancreas who also had diabetes. There was an increase in concentration of glucagon in tumor tissue and plasma. Removal of part of the tumor resulted in decreased concentration of plasma levels of glucagon and in amelioration of the hyperglycemia. At the present time there is no evidence that abnormalities of glucagon secretion play a role in diabetes of genetic origin. Some patients with familial multiple endocrine adenomatosis have been described to have elevated levels of plasma glucagon in addition to evidence of hyperinsulinism, hyperparathyroidism, and other hormonal hypersecretion. A syndrome caused by decreased secretion of glucagon has not been described as yet. However, it can be anticipated that a hypoglycemic state due to glucagon deficiency will eventually be documented. Some infants and children with so-called "idiopathic hypoglycemia" may be found to be deficient of glucagon. Decreased plasma levels of glucagon and decreased glucagon reserve have been reported in some patients with severe chronic pancreatitis and associated diabetes. The plasma glucagon response to intravenously administered arginine should prove to be a valuable test for pancreatic glucagon reserve.

Clinical Usefulness of Glucagon Administration

In the presence of normal glycogen stores glucagon produces a hyperglycemic effect when given subcutaneously, intramuscularly, or intravenously. The acute administration of glucagon has been used clinically most frequently in the treatment of severe insulin-induced hypoglycemia of labile diabetics when oral or intravenous administration of glucose is not possible. More prolonged administration of a repository form of glucagon (zinc glucagon) has been of some help in the treatment of some patients with inoperable pancreatic islet cell tumors. Recently, large amounts of glucagon have been administered to selected patients with severe heart failure and cardiogenic shock. A beneficial effect has been obtained in some patients due to the positive inotropic effect exerted by glucagon.

Glucagon Tests

Several types of glucagon tests have been employed. One test takes advantage of the glycogenolytic properties of glucagon as a means for assessing adequacy of hepatic glycogen stores and the competency of enzymes in producing glycogenolysis. One milligram of glucagon is in-

jected intravenously over 4 min and blood specimens are obtained at 0, 20, 30, 45, 60, 90, and 120 min. In healthy subjects the blood sugar level rises from 30 to 90 mg per 100 ml 20 to 30 min after injection of glucagon. In patients with cirrhosis or glycogen storage disease there is a subnormal or no rise in blood sugar.

Another glucagon test takes advantage of the insulin-releasing property of glucagon. In patients with functioning pancreatic islet cell tumors, injection of 1 mg glucagon may be followed by excessive increases in plasma insulin. Blood samples are obtained at −15 min and 0 time, and again 3, 5, 10, 15, 30, 45, 60, 90, 120, 150, and 180 min after injection of glucagon. Excessive increases in plasma insulin (over 160 microunits per ml) may occur during the first few minutes after injection of glucagon in 50 percent or more of patients with insulin secreting tumors. This may be associated with a subnormal rise in blood glucose but may be followed by excessive secondary decreases in blood glucose. The test may have to be interrupted if severe hypoglycemic symptoms develop. Such patients should be treated with intravenous glucose.

Intravenous administration of 0.5 to 1.0 mg of glucagon has also been used as a provocative test in patients suspected of harboring pheochromocytoma. In patients with pheochromocytoma glucagon evokes release of excessive quantities of pressor amines, resulting in a hypertensive paroxysm.

REFERENCES

Black, J.: Diazoxide and the Treatment of Hypoglycemia, Ann. N. Y. Acad. Sci., 150:194, 1968.

Conn, J. W., and H. S. Seltzer: Spontaneous Hypoglycemia, Am. J. Med., 19:460, 1955.

Dormandy, T. L., and R. J. Porter: Familial Fructose and Galactose Intolerance, Lancet, 1:1189, 1961.

Fajans, S. S., J. C. Floyd, Jr., R. F. Knopf, J. Rull, E. M. Guntsche, and J. W. Conn: Benzothiadiazine Suppression of Insulin Release from Normal and Abnormal Islet Tissue in Man, J. Clin. Invest., 45:481, 1966.

Field, J. B., H. Keen, P. Johnson, and B. Herring: Insulin-like Activity of Nonpancreatic Tumors Associated with Hypoglycemia, J. Clin. Endocrinol. & Metab., 23:1229, 1963.

Floyd, J. C., Jr., S. S. Fajans, R. F. Knopf, and J. W. Conn: Plasma Insulin in Organic Hyperinsulinism: Comparative Effects of Tolbutamide, Leucine and Glucose, J. Clin. Endocrinol. & Metab., 24:747, 1964.

Freinkel, N., D. L. Singer, R. A. Arky, S. J. Bleicher, J. B. Anderson, and C. K. Silbert: Alcohol Hypoglycemia: I. Carbohydrate Metabolism of Patients with Clinical Alcohol Hypoglycemia and the Experimental Reproduction of the Syndrome with Pure Ethanol, J. Clin. Invest., 42:1112, 1963.

Froesch, E. R., H. P. Wolf, H. Baitsch, A. Prader, and A. Labhart: Hereditary Fructose Intolerance: An Inborn Defect of Hepatic Fructose-1-Phosphate Splitting Aldolase, Am. J. Med., 34:151, 1963.

Graber, A. L., D. Porte, Jr., and R. H. Williams: Clinical Use of Diazoxide and Mechanism for Its Hyperglycemic Effects, Diabetes, 15:143, 1966.

Lawrence, A. M.: Glucagon Provocative Test for Pheochromocytoma, Ann. Int. Med., 66:1091, 1967.

McGavran, M. H., R. H. Unger, L. Recant, H. C. Polk, C. H. Kilo, and M. E. Levin: Glucagonoma: The Identification of A Glucagon-Secreting-Alpha-Cell Carcinoma of the Pancreas, New Eng. J. Med., 274:1408, 1966.

Murray-Lyon, I. M., A. L. Eddleston, R. Williams, M. Brown, B. M. Hogbin, A. Bennett, J. C. Edwards, and K. W. Taylor: Treatment of Multiple-Hormone-Producing Malignant Islet-Cell Tumour with Streptozotocin, Lancet, 2:895, 1968.

Ohneda, A., E. Aguilar-Parada, A. M. Eisentraut, and R. H. Unger: Characterization of Response of Circulating Glucagon to Intraduodenal and Intravenous Administration of Amino Acid, J. Clin. Invest., 47:2305, 1968.

Ohneda, A., E. Aguilar-Parada, A. M. Eisentraut, and R. H. Unger: Control of Pancreatic Glucagon Secretion by Glucose, Diabetes, 18:1, 1969.

Pek, S., S. S. Fajans, J. C. Floyd, Jr., R. F. Knopf, and J. W. Conn: Effects upon Plasma Glucagon of Infused and Ingested Amino Acids and of Protein Meals in Man, Diabetes, 18:328, 1969.

Samols, E., and V. Marks: Insulin Assay in Insulinomas, Brit. Med. J., 1:507, 1963.

Samols, E., G. Marri, and V. Marks: Promotion of Insulin Secretion by Glucagon, Lancet, 2:415, 1965.

Shames, J. M., N. R. Dhurandhar, and W. G. Blackard: Insulin-Secreting Bronchial Carcinoid Tumor with Widespread Metastases, Am. J. Med., 44:632, 1968.

Unger, R. H., A. M. Eisentraut, and L. L. Madison: The Effects of Total Starvation Upon the Levels of Circulating Glucagon and Insulin in Man, J. Clin. Invest., 42:1031, 1963.

Unger, R. H., A. Ohneda, I. Valverde, A. M. Eisentraut, and J. Exton: Characterization of Response of Circulating Glucagon-Like Immunoreactivity to Intraduodenal and Intravenous Administration of Glucose, J. Clin. Invest., 47:48, 1968.

97 DISEASES OF THE TESTES

John F. Crigler, Jr., Eugenia Rosemberg, and George W. Thorn

History

Androgen deficiency resulting from loss of testicular tissue was undoubtedly recognized by prehistoric man, as was the associated sterility; indeed, testicular tissue was recommended for impotence over 30 centuries ago. This dual function of the testes, as both the site of spermatogenesis and the primary site of male hormone production, was clearly defined in the middle of the nineteenth century when Berthold returned to the capon the characteristics, both physical and behavioral, of the cockerel by testicular grafts, and when his contemporaries, the anatomists von Kolliker, Leydig, Sertoli, and Schweigger-Seidel, defined the morphology of the gland. They recognized the spermatogonia, spermatids, the Sertoli (or sustentacular) cells, and cells located interstitially between the tubules (the Leydig or interstitial cells).

The tropic role played by the anterior pituitary gland in the development and maintenance of testicular function was demonstrated by Smith and Engle in 1927, and several years later Butenandt isolated androsterone from male urine. By 1935, testosterone had been synthesized from cholesterol and isolated in crystalline form from bull testes. In addition, it was conclusively shown to be the most significant natural androgenic material.

Embryologists had debated for many years the relative importance of sex chromosomal pattern, hormones or "determiners" secreted by the embryonic gonads, and maternal hormones on sex differentiation. In 1917, Lillie described the role of sex hormones in the development of freemartins. Wiesner proposed in 1935 that there is an autonomous tendency which results in female development unless opposed by male hormone. However, it was not until the late 1940s and early 1950s that Alfred Jost (1947) and other experimental embryologists clearly demonstrated that secretions of the fetal testes are necessary for development of male genital ducts and external genitals and that female development occurs in the absence of gonads. About the same time, Barr and Bertram (1949) described sex chromatin masses at the periphery of the nucleus in resting ganglion cells of female cats, a distinguishing characteristic of the female sex subsequently shown to be present in the peripheral cells of most mammalian species. The application of this simple cytologic means of assessing the number of X chromosomes and, more recently, of more sophisticated cytogenetic techniques, to the study of patients with sexual abnormalities has added to our advances in the fields of embryology and cytogenetics, which have been of great importance in elucidating the pathophysiology of testicular disorders.

Development

EMBRYOGENIC. In the fourth to sixth weeks of fetal development, the primitive genital ridge differentiates into cortical and medullary components capable of becoming either a testis or an ovary. If the primordial germ cells which migrate from the dorsal endoderm of the yolk sac to the urogenital ridge have a Y chromosome, the primary sex cords of the medulla undergo proliferation to form seminiferous tubules, which subsequently link up with convoluted tubules of mesonephric origin (rete testis and epididymis) and channel into the Wolffian duct. Ingrowths of coelomic epithelium carry germ cells to the seminiferous tubules. The cortex of the primitive gonad becomes isolated by the tunica albuginea and involutes. Interstitial cells of Leydig are abundant by the age of eight weeks and secrete fetal masculinizing hormones necessary for development of Wolffian duct structures (vas deferens, seminal vesicles), involution of the Müllerian system (appendix testis), and enlargement of the genital tubercle and fusion of the urethral and labioscrotal folds to form male external genitalia. If the primordial germ cells have two X chromosomes, the medullary component of the primitive gonad involutes and the cortical component proliferates and persists as the future ovary. In the absence of masculinizing factors of the interstitial cells of the fetal testis, development presumably evoked by the presence of a Y chromosome, normal female development of genital ducts and external genitalia takes place, with the formation of the fallopian tubes, uterus and upper vagina from the Müllerian ducts, regression of the Wolffian system, and persistence of the small genital tubercle and unfused urethral and labioscrotal folds.

POSTNATAL. Shorty after birth the testes measure 1.5 to 2.0 cm in length and 0.7 to 1.0 cm in width and weigh approximately 0.5 Gm each. The interstitial cells, active during uterine life as a result of chorionic gonadotropin, undergo differentiation and remain quiescent or semiquiescent until puberty. Studies using sufficiently sensitive techniques, however, demonstrate measurable levels of both gonadotropic and sex steroid hormones at all ages. It is recognized, also, that hypogonadal children show an earlier rise of gonadotropins than normal children, indicating a restraining influence of the prepuberal gonad upon the gonadotropic activity of the pituitary. At birth, 10 percent of male infants have incompletely descended testes, but after the first year, this figure drops to 2 to 3 percent. Late prepuberal descent further decreases the number, so that only 0.3 to 0.4 percent of males have either unilateral or bilateral undescended testes, postpuberally, unilateral undescended testes being four to five times more frequent.

During adolescence, each testis increases in size, as a result chiefly of changes in the seminiferous tubules under the stimulation of pituitary follicle–stimulating hormone (FSH) and androgens produced locally by developing interstitial cells. The fully developed testis measures 3.5 to 5.5 cm in length and 2.1 to 3.2 cm in width, and weighs 15 to 20 Gm each. Interstitial cell–stimulating hormone (ICSH) induces interstitial cell differentiation, with the production of male sex hormones, genital enlargement, and the development of secondary sexual characteristics. Normal function, including demonstrated fertility, has been noted when testes were less than half the mean size.

ABERRATIONS IN EMBRYONIC DEVELOPMENT. It is currently postulated that sex-determining genes on the X and Y chromosomes are responsible, through their effects on cellular function of the primitive cortex or medulla, for gonadal differentiation of these tissues into either a testis or an ovary. Embryologic studies have indicated that normally functioning fetal testes are required for male differentiation of genital ducts and external genitalia. The fetal testis appears to produce, at least, two types of substances: (1) a "duct-organizing substance," which stimulates development of the Wolffian system and involution of the Müllerian duct; and (2) an androgen, which may play a role in Wolffian duct development but is required for masculinization of the external genitalia. The correlation between chromosomal patterns, gonadal differentiation, and subsequent genital development in human beings has been quite consistent. Some cases, however, remain unexplained by the above stated concepts, although they do not disprove the hypothesis, since current techniques do not detect all chromosomal anomalies (mosaicism, interchange of sex-determining factors between X and Y chromosomes, etc.) or measure directly fetal gonadal function.

If gonadal tissue does not develop (gonadal dysgenesis, genotypic XO, X isochromosome X, X deleted X, etc.) or interstitial cells are nonfunctioning before differentiation of genital ducts in a genotypic male (XY), **both internal and external genitalia are entirely female.** Partial failure in testicular development or in the elaboration of fetal masculinizing hormones (genotypic XY or mosaics having a cell line with a Y chromosome) results in ambiguous internal and external genital development, the type of abnormality reflecting the age of onset and degree of fetal gonadal dysfunction. Patients with abnormal fetal testes, therefore, may have genital development ranging from almost complete feminization through incomplete fusion of the urethral and labioscrotal folds with some enlargement of the genital tubercle and various degrees of development of the Müllerian ducts to mild degrees of hypospadias. In addition, if testicular tissue exists unilaterally (true hermaphrodite, mixed gonadal dysgenesis), male development of genital ducts occurs on the side of the testes and Müllerian duct structures develop on the side with the ovary or missing gonad. These findings are consistent with observations in other animal species which demonstrate a local effect by diffusion of fetal masculinizing hormones (Chap. 4).

Some genotypic males (XY) who have histologically normal-appearing testes before puberty show total **feminization of external genitalia although internal genitals are masculinized** (syndrome of testicular feminization). This abnormality is inherited as either a sex-limited recessive or a sex-limited autosomal dominant mutant gene, as half of the genotypic males are affected. The lack of masculinization of external genitals (but not of internal genitalia), the absence of sexual hair (present in approximately one-third of the patients), and the occurrence of feminization at adolescence with normal plasma and urine testosterone concentrations indicate an abnormality in the response of tissues to androgens. Decreased reduction of testosterone to 17β-hydroxyandrostane urinary metabolites and activity of the Δ^4-5α-reductase of skin, which catalyzes the transformation of testosterone to 17β-hydroxy-5α-androstan-3-one (dihydrotestosterone), a metabolite with biological activity comparable to testosterone, has been demonstrated in these patients. Intramuscular administration of dihydrotestosterone to a patient with testicular feminization, however, failed to produce the changes in urinary nitrogen, phosphorus, and citric acid excretion observed in a control individual. Nevertheless, these new biochemical observations are consistent with the hypothesis that the basic defect is an inability of end-organ tissues to metabolize testosterone in a normal manner. Feminization of the external genitals of these patients may be so complete that the abnormality is only discovered later in life when primary amenorrhea, the absence of sexual hair, or the appearance of inguinal masses make the diagnosis apparent. Surgical exploration of these patients reveals the presence of vas deferens, epididymis, and testes, the latter showing variation in histologic findings with age and the completeness of the defect. After adolescence, tubular adenomas and hyperplasia of Leydig cells (often adenomatous) are common.

Finally, **masculinization** of **external genital development of a genotypic female** fetus (XX) may be induced by excess fetal adrenal androgens (patients with congenital adrenal hyperplasia) or by excess androgens produced or taken (usually synthetic progestational steroid hormones) by the mother during pregnancy. Defects induced by these extragonadal androgens are limited to the external genitalia (hypertrophy of the genital tubercle with various degrees of fusion of the urogenital and labioscrotal folds), so that if the condition is recognized, an appropriate sex assignment can be made and the genital abnormality surgically corrected.

Physiology

The role of fetal testicular function on genital development has been described above. The precise interrelationships of hypothalamic-pituitary and testicular functions (Fig. 97-1) at adolescence and in adult life are not completely defined. The hormone elaborated by the anterior pituitary gland that appears to induce development and then functional maintenance of the testicular interstitial (Leydig) cells has been appropriately labeled interstitial cell–stimulating hormone (ICSH) and reportedly is identical to luteinizing hormone (LH) in the female. Pituitary FSH stimulates development of the seminiferous tubules. At the moment, the role of ICSH and testosterone in seminiferous tubular development and spermatogenesis is not well defined. It is generally accepted that the Leydig cell is the principal site of synthesis of steroid hormones (testosterone, estrogens, and others). The probable role of ICSH and the Leydig cell in hormonal production in human beings is illustrated by observations on so-called "fertile eunuchs," patients who show spermatogenesis but lack masculine secondary changes and in whom testicular biopsies show an absence of Leydig cells.

FSH and *ICSH* have been measured by specific bioassays and radioimmunoassays in the urine and serum of prepuberal children. It has been suggested that sexual maturity is accompanied by a marked increase in the excretion of LH, with a relatively smaller increase in FSH. Though these changes in gonadotropins at adolescence have been demonstrated, the factors, probably neural, initiating pubery are still unknown. Nevertheless, production of androgenic hormones by the testes at puberty effects the numerous somatic changes noted in the adolescent male. These include enlargement and increased pigmentation of the external genitalia, hypertrophy of the larynx with lowering of the voice, a generalized increase of amount of hair to hirsutism with growth of a beard and a typical masculine pelvic escutcheon and forehead hair line, enlargement of the prostate and seminal vesicles,

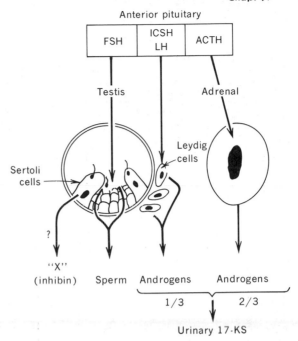

Fig. 97-1. Scheme showing anterior pituitary–testis relationship.

and an overall increase in muscular development. Metabolic balance studies demonstrate retention of electrolytes, nitrogen, and phosphorus; and radiologic examination shows acceleration of osseous development with subsequent epiphyseal fusion.

The testes of the normal, young male secrete between 4 and 8 mg testosterone daily and, approximately 40 μg of estradiol, another 20 to 25 μg of estradiol being formed from testosterone and androstenedione in other tissues. Approximately half the testosterone appears in the urine as measurable 17-ketosteroids, primarily androsterone and etiocholanolone (Fig. 97-2). The total 17-ketosteroid daily excretion for males, which includes the steroid derivatives from the testes and adrenal cortex, is 8 to 18 mg, of which approximately 4 mg is derived from the testes and the remainder from the adrenals. Plasma testosterone concentrations in young adult males vary from 0.4 to 1.0 μg per 100 ml (mean 0.7 μg per 100 ml), whereas normal females of similar age have plasma concentrations between 0.02 and 0.07 μg per 100 ml. Recent studies of testosterone production rates in normal men aged sixty-six to eighty-six years suggest that with advancing years, there may be a significant fall in testosterone secretion. It is well known that urinary 17-ketosteroid excretion diminishes with increasing age. It seems unlikely, however, that a sudden cessation in gonadal function analogous to the process in the female ever occurs in the male.

TESTICULAR DISORDERS

The principal abnormalities of testicular function, listed according to their effect on both interstitial and seminiferous tubular activity, are summarized in Table 97-1.

Fig. 97-2. Synthesis and metabolism of androgens. The broken line between cholesterol and pregneno-lone signifies a series of reactions, all of which, including the conversion to 17α-hydroxyprogesterone to Δ4-androstenedione (Δ) and to testosterone (T), occur in the testis. More recently there is evidence that dehydroisoandrosterone (D), principally secreted by the adrenal, is also normally synthesized by gonadal tissue. In addition, it is now well recognized that D, Δ, and T are peripherally interconvertible, as shown by the arrows. Further metabolism of these compounds to the principal urinary metabolites (italicized in the diagram) occurs mainly in liver, where they are also conjugated to excretion as glu-curonides or sulfates.

Hypogonadism

The clinical term *hypogonadism* as most often used refers to failure in interstitial cell function which results in decreased or absent production of male sex hormones. Seminiferous tubular failure, however, often is associated and, indeed, may occur without significant changes in testicular hormonal production (Sertoli-cell-only syndrome and postpuberal abnormalities). Both testicular functions may be decreased either primarily by a developmental or destructive lesion of the testes or secondarily by failure in production of pituitary gonadotropins.

PREPUBERAL HYPOGONADISM. The clinical picture of hypogonadism is directly related to the time of development of androgen deficiency. Prepuberal deficiency results

in varying degrees of failure to develop the expected secondary sexual characteristics associated with maturity. Total lack of androgen production by the testes is associated with persistent infantile structure, a high voice, partial or total lack of facial, axillary, and pubic hair, infantile genitalia, and a barely palpable prostate. Because of lack of osseous maturation, epiphyseal closure is delayed, resulting eventually in a tall "eunuchoid" habitus with long arms and legs and a span 2 in. greater than height. Gynecomastia, wide hips, and girdle obesity may also be present. The skin is pale and delicate and may show early wrinkling. Acne and seborrhea are absent.

Prepuberal hypogonadism remains inapparent (unless there are gross anomalies of the testes, which may signal

Table 97-1. ABNORMALITIES OF TESTICULAR FUNCTION

I. Hypogonadism (decreased androgen production and/or spermatogenesis).
 A. Primary (increased urinary gonadotropins).
  1. Developmental abnormalities.
   a. Klinefelter's syndrome (seminiferous tubule dysgenesis). Classic form—eunuchoidism, gynecomastia, mental retardation, and small firm testes. Buccal smear—chromatin-positive. Leukocyte karyotype usually XXY or XXYY but may have other poly X and Y chromosomal constitution and mosaicism with combination of many cell lines.
   b. Reifenstein's syndrome (male pseudohermaphroditism). Hereditary testicular disorder with hypospadias, varying degrees of gynecomastia and eunuchoidism, and postpuberal seminiferous tubular atrophy. No chromosomal abnormality.
   c. Male Turner's syndrome. Somatic anomalies of phenotypic female Turner's syndrome. Leukocyte karyotype usually XY, although occasionally show abnormal chromosomes or mosaicism. Variable testicular histology and function.
   d. Sertoli-cell-only syndrome (germinal aplasia). Normal development. Infertility. No chromosomal abnormality. Etiology unknown.
   e. Anorchia. Cryptorchid with no somatic anomalies. No chromosomal abnormality. Etiology unknown.
  2. Postpuberal abnormalities.
   a. Seminiferous tubule failure.
    1. Orchitis (mumps, tuberculosis, leprosy, gonorrheal infection, brucellosis, syphilis, etc.), hyperpyrexia, irradiation, trauma, neoplasm, or surgical castration.
    2. Congenital disorders—myotonia dystrophica, cystic fibrosis, Laurence Moon-Biedl syndrome.
    3. Idiopathic.
   b. Leydig cell failure (male climacteric).
 B. Secondary (decreased urinary gonadotropins).
  1. Isolated gonadotropin deficiency. Often associated with congenital anomalies including anosmia or hyposmia, harelip, cleft palate, etc. May be inherited as a sex-linked recessive or sex-limited autosomal dominant.
  2. Isolated ICSH deficiency (fertile eunuch).
  3. Multiple pituitary deficiencies (panhypopituitarism).
   a. Idiopathic prepuberal.
   b. Secondary to neurohypophyseal lesions—neoplasm (chromophobe, astrocytoma, hamartoma, teratoma), cyst (craniopharyngioma) or granulomatous process (sarcoid, etc.).
   c. Congenital disorders—Laurence-Moon-Biedl syndrome.
II. Hypergonadism (excess androgen production).
 A. Primary (functioning interstitial cell tumor).
 B. Secondary (measurable urinary gonadotropins).
  1. Familial.
  2. Tumor in region of third ventricle (pinealoma, astrocytoma, hamartoma, teratoma, and craniopharyngioma).

pathologic changes at an earlier age) until the expected time of puberty. A total absence of any of the usual changes of adolescence at approximately age fourteen or fifteen suggests that interstitial cell function may be abnormal. However, as in other developmental states, there is a wide range of normal variation, so that puberal changes may not be noticeable in some normal boys until the sixteenth or seventeenth year, when genital and secondary sexual changes may begin to be apparent. This delay in adolescent development causes much concern to patient, family, and physician, and not infrequently some form of hormonal therapy is given, followed by somatic changes that undoubtedly would have occurred without treatment.

POSTPUBERAL HYPOGONADISM. Postpuberal hypogonadal changes decrease or are minimized when the hypogonadal state develops late in adult life; thus castration of elderly men may cause none of the alterations seen in younger individuals. In young males, there are usually diminished beard growth and thinning axillary and other body hair. The skin becomes smoother, the prostate atrophies to the point of being barely palpable, and sexual desire and performance wane. The genitalia lose pigmentation and may decrease somewhat in size. The voice does not change, but gynecomastia may appear. In older men none of these changes may be noted; beard and body hair growth usually persist, and there may be no noticeable change in libido or sexual function.

PRIMARY HYPOGONADISM. The causes of primary hypogonadism in males are listed in Table 97-1. The testicular abnormality may be present at birth as either a genetic or an embryologic defect, or it may occur at any time later in life as a result of either testicular infections (such as mumps, tuberculosis, brucellosis, leprosy, syphillis) or following trauma, irradiation, neoplasm, or castration, either surgical or accidental. Beginning in early adolescence, even before the appearance of the obvious physical characteristics of hypogonadism, the patient may have increased serum concentrations of pituitary gonadotropin hormones (measured by radioimmunoassay) and may excrete excessive quantities in the urine. The immature mouse uterine weight assay, which measures both ICSH and FSH, is used most frequently for determination of total urinary gonadotropin content. In addition, because of lack of testosterone synthesis, plasma testosterone concentrations as well as urinary 17-ketosteroid excretion of adult patients are significantly decreased. It should be stated here with emphasis, however, that the patient's own tissues clinically observed frequently provide the most significant assay of androgen production. The following syndrome is an example of primary hypogonadism.

KLINEFELTER'S SYNDROME (Seminiferous Tubule Dysgenesis). Klinefelter, Reifenstein, and Albright described in 1942 a clinical syndrome of hypogonadism that includes gynecomastia, eunuchoidism, elevated level of urinary gonadotropins, and decreased testicular size associated with hyalinization of the tubules. Barr demonstrated that many of these patients were *chromatin-positive*, exhibiting nuclei similar to those seen in females (see Chap. 4). Culture of marrow cells and leukocytes in vitro in the presence of colchicine has permitted direct

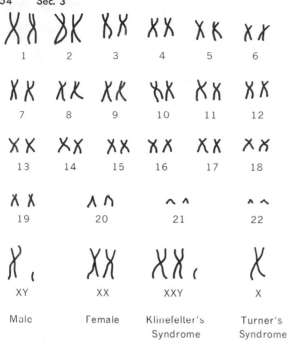

Fig. 97-3. Schematic drawing of 22 pairs of autosomes and sex chromosomes, including two aberrant forms of sex chromosomes as seen in patients with Klinefelter's or Turner's syndrome.

chromosomal counting and classification (see Fig. 97-3); and indeed, many patients with the triad described by Klinefelter et al. have been shown to possess an extra sex chromosome, resulting in a karyotypic classification of 22 autosomes plus 2 X chromosomes and 1 Y chromosome (See Chap. 4). Thus, they have 47 instead of 46 chromosomes, and it is therefore not surprising that many of these patients also have various degrees of mental deficiency. A clue to the diagnosis of this disorder often lies in the behavior and personality of the Klinefelter patient. Talkativeness with little substance to the content is an outstanding behavioral trait. Klinefelter's syndrome in some patients who lack the classical chemical findings of gynecomastia, eunuchoidism, and small testes may be discovered only when they appear in an infertility clinic. In addition, Klinefelter's syndrome is not infrequently discovered when the patient seeks medical care for chronic pulmonary disease, obesity, diabetes mellitus, varicose veins, and thrombophlebitis, disorders which appear to be more prevalent in these individuals; thus, the spectrum of Klinefelter's syndrome is broad, including obviously feminized males on one end and, on the other end, normally virilized men with only abnormal microscopic testicular anatomy but often with the associated diseases listed above.

SECONDARY HYPOGONADISM. Secondary hypogonadism results from failure of pituitary elaboration of the necessary tropic hormones, specifically ICSH and FSH (Table 97-1, I-B). Isolated deficiencies of gonadotropic hormones without demonstrable loss of other pituitary hormones have been described in males in association with anosmia or hyposmia by Kallman. The condition is inherited either as a sex-linked recessive defect or as a sex-

limited autosomal dominant one. Very rarely, an isolated ICSH deficiency occurs. In most cases, however, there is an associated loss of other pituitary tropic hormones, resulting in growth failure before adolescence and in decreased thyroid, adrenal, and gonadal function at all ages. When there is a progressive loss of hypothalamic-pituitary function because of a neoplasm (chromophobe, astrocytoma, hamartoma, teratoma), cyst (craniopharyngioma), or granulomatous process (sarcoid), a decrease of gonadotropins is often the first deficiency observed, and the patient, therefore, may appear in the clinic with isolated hypogonadism. Prepuberal hypopituitarism is usually recognized because of the dwarfism that results from growth hormone deficiency. Occasionally, however, testes of preadolescent boys with other evidences of pituitary dysfunction are significantly small. Froehlich in 1901 described such an obese hypogonadal boy with signs of a tumor in the hypothalamic area. Since then, Froelich's name has been inappropriately applied to the condition of a large group of overweight boys with slightly retarded maturation but with normal linear growth and no demonstrated hypothalamic lesion; in such cases the delay in maturation is without any real clinical significance. Patients with the Laurence-Moon-Biedl syndrome have been described with both primary (germinal aplasia) and secondary (hypogonadotropic) hypogonadism.

The absence of serum and urinary gonadotropins after the age of adolescence in patients with diminished gonadal function is diagnostic of secondary hypogonadism. Studies of growth, thyroid, adrenal, and antidiuretic hormones may reveal clinically unsuspected deficiencies. Skull roentgenogram may also show intracranial calcification, enlargement of the sella turcica, or erosion of the clinoid processes, and visual field examination may demonstrate early involvement of the optic nerves.

TREATMENT OF HYPOGONADISM. Patients with primary hypogonadism (increased urinary gonadotropins) require testosterone replacement therapy. Preparations commonly used are listed in Table 97-2. The usual method of ther-

Table 97-2. HORMONAL THERAPY FOR HYPOGONADISM

Preparations	Route and Dosage
Methyltestosterone (linguets)	Sublingual 5–10 mg, 4 times daily.
Testosterone propionate	Intramuscular 25–50 mg, 3 times weekly.
Testosterone enanthate Testosterone cyclopentyl- propionate Testosterone phenylacetate	Intramuscular 100–200 mg every 1–2 weeks for maximum effect, 200 mg every 3–5 weeks for maintenance.
Human chorionic gonadotropin	Intramuscular 1,000–4,000 IU 3 times weekly for 6 to 9 months. Repeated courses as required.

apy is to start with relatively small doses of the long-acting depot preparations of testosterone, giving either 50 mg every 2 weeks or 150 mg every 3 to 4 weeks. The dosage subsequently (after epiphyseal fusion in adolescent boys) is increased to 200 mg every 2 weeks to obtain full androgen effect, including deepening of the voice and increased facial hair. Final adult maintenance requirements are usually satisfied by 200 mg of the depot preparations every 3 to 5 weeks. Excessive acne formation, edema from retention of sodium, and undesirable personality changes all indicate overtreatment, and the dosage should be diminished appropriately.

In patients with secondary hypogonadism, a trial on human chorionic gonadotropin (HCG) may be indicated. Usually 6 to 9 months of 1,000 to 4,000 IU of HCG are given as a single course. If regression to a hypogonadal state occurs when HCG is discontinued, either a second course of HCG may be given or testosterone therapy as outlined above may be begun. In the past, long-term therapy with HCG has not proved practical. A gonadotropin preparation rich in FSH has been obtained from human menopausal urine. Experience with this preparation in gonadotropin-deficient postpuberal males indicates that it can restore spermatogenesis to normal. The prepuberal testes seem to require stimulation with HCG before spermatogenesis can be induced by administration of the human menopausal gonadotropin preparation.

Hypergonadism

The production of excessive quantities of androgenic hormones in the adult male results in little, if any, morphologic or functional change. However, in the child, the somatic changes associated with puberty may be induced at an early age and therefore become clinically apparent (precocious puberty). The causes of hypergonadism and isosexual precocity in the male are listed in Table 97-1. Hypergonadism may be due to excessive androgen production from a functioning testicular tumor, the Leydig, or interstitial, cell carcinoma. Children with these tumors show all the changes associated with puberty, such as increased hair growth and phallic enlargement, and usually have a palpable testicular tumor. However, the presence of the tumor may be difficult to determine if the testes are undescended, or if the tumor is extremely active in producing hormone but is very small. Plasma testosterone concentrations are increased. Urinary 17-ketosteroids, however, may be normal or only slightly increased, because of the marked potency of testosterone. Urinary pituitary gonadotropins are usually absent. Hypergonadism may also result from an early onset of puberty due to altered hypothalamic-pituitary function. The sequence of development is similar to that observed in adolescence, with enlargement of genitalia, appearance of pubic and axillary hair, deepening of the voice, and appearance of acne and seborrhea occurring in that order and beginning at two to three years of age or earlier. The testes are large for the patient's chronologic age but are in accord with the size expected for the degree of maturity exhibited by the remainder of his somatic development. Gonadotropins may be present in the urine but are not invariably measurable by routine assay procedures. In the early stages, the level of 17-ketosteroids may not be significantly elevated for the patient's chronologic age (in contrast to virilism produced by adrenal abnormalities), but

subsequently it rises to a degree appropriate for his developmental age. Isosexual precocity of this type in males, although uncommon, is often familial, in contrast to the more frequently occurring true precocity in females, from whom a family history of early puberty is seldom obtained. When true precosity occurs in males without a family history, it is almost always associated with space-occupying lesions in the region of the third ventricle (pinealoma, astrocytoma, hamartoma, and rarely a craniopharyngioma). The continued production of androgens excessive for their age in these patients results in accelerated growth during childhood, followed by early closure of the epiphyses, ending in an adult who frequently is smaller than his contemporaries.

Isosexual precocity in the male may also result from excessive quantities of adrenal androgens. The pattern of accelerated growth and development is similar to that produced by testicular hormones. The testes remain, however, infantile and atrophic; and gonadotropins are invariably absent. The diagnosis is made on the basis of markedly elevated level of urinary 17-ketosteroids. For further discussion, see Chap. 92.

NEOPLASMS OF THE TESTES

Neoplasms of the testes are relatively uncommon. It is generally believed that they occur more often in the cryptorchid testis (1 in 2,000) than in the normal testis (1 in 100,000). They may be classified as follows, in their relative order of frequency:

1. Seminoma (germinoma)
2. Teratocarcinoma
3. Embryonal carcinoma
   a. Chorioepithelioma
4. Teratoma
5. Interstitial cell tumor
6. Fibroma, lipoma, adrenoma, myxoma
7. Unclassified varieties

In addition, lymphoma, plasmacytoma, leukemia, and carcinoma of other tissues occasionally produce secondary tumors in the testes. The incidence of teratocarcinoma is roughly constant throughout life, whereas the incidence of seminoma tends to rise with age. One-year survival is rare for patients with embryonal carcinomas and chorioepitheliomas, not uncommon for those with teratocarcinomas and teratomas, and the rule for those with seminomas.

Endocrine changes (such as gynecomastia and increased secretion of gonadotropins, giving a positive Aschheim-Zondek test result) are occasionally seen with chorioepitheliomas, as well as with embryonal carcinomas and teratocarcinomas. The endocrine effects of interstitial cell tumors have been discussed.

Diagnosis

The diagnosis is made by palpating a mass, usually firm, smooth, and painless. Neoplasms must be distinguished from the changes induced by tuberculosis or gonorrheal epididymitis, from syphilis (usually accompanied by a positive serologic test and a response to specific therapy), and from the various fluid-containing cysts (hydrocele, spermatocele), which may be transilluminated. The diagnosis may be aided also by increased urinary excretion of 17-ketosteroids, estrogens, or gonadotropins; the latter give a positive Aschheim-Zondek test. Rarely, tumor cells may be identified in the semen.

Treatment

Surgical removal is always indicated in any tumor of the testes and will usually effect a cure in the benign varieties. If the tumor is malignant, a radical operation, followed by irradiation, should be employed. X-ray therapy has been shown to effect a cure in the majority of cases of seminoma. Results of therapy may be followed by repeated determinations of the 17-ketosteroids or estrogens or by the Aschheim-Zondek test, if it was originally positive. Certain testicular tumors, particularly the chorioepitheliomas, have been shown to be exquisitely sensitive to certain antimetabolic agents such as 4-amino-N^{10}-methylpteroylgutamic acid (Methotrexate).

DISEASES OF THE PROSTATE

Benign Prostatic Hypertrophy

This pathophysiologic disorder, which affects a high proportion of elderly men, is a significant cause of dysuria and incontinence (see Chap. 49) and urinary tract obstruction (see Chap. 302). It has been also considered a potentially precancerous lesion. Hormonally, the prostate is significant as a clinical indicator of androgen secretion, since appreciable reduction in prostatic size accompanies either primary or secondary hypogonadism as well as those disorders of liver function characterized by excessive estrogen activity.

Carcinoma of the Prostate

Adenocarcinoma of the prostate is one of the most common tumors of men. It is rare before the age of forty; the incidence rises rapidly with advancing age, with the condition occurring microscopically in 10 to 15 percent of men in the fifth decade and in as many as 40 percent of those in the eighth decade. However, only one-fourth of these cases may become clinically apparent before death. Three-fourths of these tumors arise in the posterior lobe. The majority are easily palpable; hence, frequent routine rectal examinations are indicated to demonstrate early, operable tumors. Although the whole gland need not be enlarged, the presence of stony, hard, indurated nodules or masses strongly suggests an adenocarcinoma. Frequently, there may be an elevation in the "prostatic" fraction of serum acid phosphatase while the tumor is still located within the prostatic capsule, and elevation of this enzyme may serve to differentiate a benign hypertropic nodule from a malignancy. Once the tumor has spread locally from the gland, particularly after it has

metastasized, total serum acid and alkaline phosphatase levels may be greatly elevated.

Therapy consists of radical prostatectomy; irradiation by x-ray, radium, or radioactive isotopes (colloidal gold); and estrogen hormonal treatment (especially when metastatic disease develops). Androgens are decreased by orchidectomy and by adrenalectomy or adrenocortical suppression following dexamethasone administration (1 to 2 mg given orally in divided doses); estrogen levels are increased by administering diethylstilbestrol, 10 to 15 mg daily, or the equivalent dosage of other estrogenic products.

REFERENCES

Albert, A.: Bioassay and Radioimmunoassay of Human Gonadotropins, J. Clin. Endocrinol. & Metab., 28:1683, 1968.

Albert, A., L. O. Underdahl, L. F. Greene, and N. Lorenz: Male Hypogonadism: I, II, III, IV, V, VI, VII, Proc. Staff Meet. Mayo Clinic, 28:409, 557, 698, 1953; 29:131, 317, 368, 1954; 30:31, 1955.

Dorfman, R. I., and R. A. Shipley: "Androgens–Biochemistry, Physiology and Clinical Significance," New York, John Wiley & Sons, Inc., 1956.

Federman, D. D.: "Abnormal Sexual Development. A Genetic and Endocrine Approach to Differential Diagnosis," Philadelphia, W. B. Saunders Company, 1967.

Howard, R. P., R. C. Sniffen, F. A. Simmons, and F. Albright: Testicular Deficiency: A Clinical and Pathological Study, J. Clin. Endocrinol., 10:121, 1950.

Klinefelter, H., E. Reifenstein, Jr., and F. Albright: Klinefelter Syndrome Characterized by Gynecomastia, Aspermatogenesis without A-Leydigism, and Increased Excretion of Follicle-stimulating Hormone, J. Clin. Endocrinol., 2:615, 1942.

McCullagh, E. P., J. C. Beck, and C. A. Schaffenburg: A Syndrome of Eunuchoidism with Spermatogenesis; Normal Urinary FSH and Low or Normal ICSH ("Fertile Eunuchs"), J. Clin. Endocrinol. & Metab., 13:489, 1953.

Patton, J. F., D. N. Seitzman, and R. A. Zone: Diagnosis and Treatment of Testicular Tumors, Am. J. Surg., 99:525, 1960.

Paulsen, C. A.: The Testes, p. 405 in "Textbook of Endocrinology," R. H. Williams (Ed.), Philadelphia, W. B. Saunders Company, 1968.

Strickland, A. L., and F. S. French: Absence of Response to Dihydrotestosterone in the Syndrome of Testicular Feminization, J. Clin. Endocrinol., 29:1284, 1969.

98 DISEASES OF THE OVARY
Janet W. McArthur

HISTORY

The ovulatory function of the ovaries was first described by a Dutch physician, Reinier de Graaf, in 1673. He recognized small fluid blisters, now known as *graafian follicles,* which had succeeded in reaching the surface of the ovaries before ovulation. The hormonal function of the ovaries was first demonstrated in 1896, by the German biologist, Knauer, who showed that ovarian grafts in the dog would prevent the uterine atrophy that follows castration. It was next observed, by Marshall and Jolly, that the ovarian secretion which produced estrus differed from that which was formed by the corpus luteum. The presence of estrogens in the follicles was proved by R. T. Frank, and their occurrence in urine was established by Allen and Doisy, who demonstrated the effectiveness of potent urinary extracts in producing estrus in the vaginal mucosa of rodents. This relatively simple biologic assay method became of incomparable help in the isolation and synthesis of estrogenic compounds. In 1929, Butenandt and Doisy and associates isolated estrone in a crystalline form from the urine of pregnant women. In 1930, estriol was identified by Browne in human placentas, and in 1936, MacCorquodale obtained estradiol, the most potent natural estrogen, from ovarian follicular fluid. The progestational activity of the corpus luteum hormone was first demonstrated by Corner and Allen in 1929. Five years later progesterone was isolated and identified simultaneously and independently by Butenandt, Allen, Slotta, and Hartmann.

INTRODUCTION

The ovary is a specialized organ of reproduction which serves (1) as an exocrine gland which liberates gametes for fertilization, and (2) as a complex of endocrine glands which secretes hormones responsible for (a) the growth and cyclic function of the reproductive tract, and (b) a variety of metabolic effects in nongenital tissues. During mature reproductive life a new endocrine gland, the follicle, is activated each month. After ovulation the follicle undergoes transformation into a second gland of internal secretion, the corpus luteum. To the extent that the formation of the corpus luteum requires the prior existence of a follicle, the two structures are interdependent. Nevertheless, differences of fundamental significance obtain between their secretory products. Both structures are embedded in an interstitium, or stroma, which constitutes a third endocrine gland.

A major difference between the ovary and the testis is that the former is endowed with a finite stock of germ cells, whereas the latter proliferates gametes continuously. The number of ova reaches a maximum 5 months before birth. Thereafter the number declines, mainly as the result of atresia, until by the end of the fifth decade the original complement of germ cells is exhausted. An inexorable, though less-rapid, decline in follicular hormone secretion begins in the fifth decade. In addition, the secretion of luteal hormones becomes more and more erratic as the incidence of anovulatory cycles increases. By old age, only the ovarian stroma retains any semblance of functioning tissue.

DEVELOPMENT

The formation of the gonads begins at a very early stage, when the embryo has attained a crown-rump length of 5 mm (twenty-one to twenty-eight days of age). The genetic sex of the conceptus is identifiable even earlier, at the age of fifteen days, by the presence of nuclear sex chromatin in the female. During the seventh week, the ovarian destiny of the "indifferent gonad" can be inferred histologically by the absence of the epithelial cords which characterize the developing testis.

Four major phases in the development of the ovary are recognized: (1) migration of primordial germ cells from their site of origin in the endoderm of the primitive gut to bilateral thickenings (the "germinal ridges") of the coelomic epithelium ventral to the developing mesonephros, (2) proliferation of the germinal and nongerminal cells in the genital ridges, (3) division of the gonads into a peripheral cortex and a central medulla, and (4) sex differentiation, consisting of proliferation of the cortex and involution of the medulla in the female, and the reverse process in the male. A complex sex-determining mechanism, the details of which are obscure, is responsible for the conversion of the "indifferent gonad" into an ovary or testis. The cortical germ cells (oogonia) increase rapidly in number as a result of mitotic division, whereupon they enter the meiotic prophase, to become, by definition, oocytes. Each is soon invested by a single layer of smaller supporting cells to form the primordial follicles. In this resting phase the oocytes remain throughout childhood and adult life until either preovulatory maturation or pseudomaturation with atresia occurs. The oocytes appear to exert an inductive influence upon the surrounding granulosa cells, since follicles fail to develop in ovaries which lack oocytes, and oocyte atresia is followed by granulosal degeneration.

COMPARTMENTS

The complexity of the tasks devolving upon the ovary is reflected in the heterogeneity of its structure. Throughout active reproductive life, morphologic and biochemical events are occurring simultaneously in the follicular, luteal, and interstitial compartments. Anatomic specialization in the ovary is paralleled by a degree of biochemical specialization. Thus, although in vitro studies reveal that upon incubation with acetate, each of the compartments is capable of synthesizing all the major categories of gonadal steroids, in vivo there is a preferential formation of estrogen by the follicle, of progestogens by the corpus luteum, and of androgens by the stroma.

Follicle

Follicular growth comprises two phases. During the first, the oocyte enlarges rapidly to virtually adult dimensions while the investing cortical cells (the membrana granulosa), which convert the germ cell into a primordial follicle, grow very slowly. During the second phase, further growth of the oocyte is minimal but the follicle enlarges rapidly and develops an antrum, which fills with fluid secreted by the granulosa cells. The antrum first appears when the follicle attains a diameter two or three times that of the contained oocyte. Once a follicle has acquired an antrum it becomes, by definition, a graafian follicle.

Maturation falls short of completion in all but that minute proportion of graafian follicles destined to ovulate. Periodically, in response to gonadotropin stimulation (see below), the elected follicle exhibits an intense preovulatory growth spurt, accompanied by increasing antral distension, the loosening of the cumulus oophorus (those granulosa cells which hold the egg in suspension), and the hypertrophy and hyperemia of the theca interna. As the follicle enlarges, its wall thins and presently ruptures, releasing the ovum into the peritoneal cavity. A complex of satellite follicles enlarges concomitantly, but to a lesser extent; and after ovulation they undergo rapid atresia.

Growth of the follicle is paralleled by biochemical processes resulting in the secretion of estrogen and, during the immediately preovulatory phase, of small amounts of progesterone. At the peak of follicular activity, the secretion rate of estradiol varies from 0.2 to 0.5 mg per 24 hr. The prime locus of estrogen synthesis has not been directly identified but is believed to be the theca interna.

Corpus Luteum

Following ovulation the ruptured follicle is converted into a corpus luteum, which likewise has a limited anatomic and biochemical life span. This is divisible into stages of proliferation and hyperemia, vascularization, maturity, and retrogression. The secretion of estrogen is continued and is supplemented by the secretion of progesterone. Biosynthetic activity increases steadily and becomes maximal on days 21 to 22 of the menstrual cycle, when implantation of the fertilized ovum occurs. Estimates of the progesterone secretion rate, though discrepant, agree qualitatively in that they reveal a phenomenal increase in the biosynthetic capacity of the transformed follicle, to the vicinity of 20 to 40 mg progesterone per day.

How the follicular-to-luteal change in the pattern of hormone synthesis is effected is the subject of much speculation. One view is embodied in the so-called "two-cell" theory. This postulates that the cells of the theca interna are endowed with the full enzyme complement required for the synthesis of estradiol-17β, whereas the cells of the granulosa possess little or no 17-desmolase activity and only weak 17-hydroxylase activity. During the follicular phase, the well-vascularized theca internal cells synthesize estrogens, which have ready access either to the follicular fluid or the systemic circulation, whereas the granulosa cells, lacking a blood supply, are presumably deprived of the nutrients required for hormone synthesis. After ovulation, the granulosa cells become richly vascularized, undergo enlargement, and form the corpus luteum. However, in consequence of their enzymic endowment, they are ill equipped to synthesize estrogen in quantity and secrete mainly progesterone.

In the event that conception occurs, the trophoblast of the implanted ovum secretes a complex of proteins known collectively as "human chorionic gonadotropin" (HCG) into the maternal circulation. By a luteotropic action, HCG then prolongs the life of the corpus luteum until the placenta gains secretory competency. If conception fails to occur, the corpus luteum undergoes rapid regression and over the course of 7 to 10 months is replaced by a hyaline remnant, the corpus albicans.

Interstitium

The interstitium, or stroma, acts as a supporting matrix for the follicles, corpora lutea, and corpora albicantia, and, in addition, it secretes steroids. Qualitative and quantitative changes in its structure occur in association with various reproductive processes. During pregnancy there is increasing luteinization of the stroma, and during the postmenopausal years stromal proliferation and luteinization are frequent. In extreme old age, the stroma tends to lose its stimulated appearance. The higher grades of stromal luteinization are sometimes associated with clinical indications of androgen hypersecretion.

The hilus may come eventually to be regarded as a fourth ovarian compartment, but at present it is generally treated as a specialized portion of the interstitium. It contains elements resembling testicular Leydig cells, which occur in nests, the size of which varies at different ages. Hyperplasia of these cells may occur during pregnancy, and the larger hilus cell complexes are more frequent in elderly women.

Androstenedione and dehydroepiandrosterone can be extracted from normal ovarian stroma, the highest concentrations being found in the hilus.

PHYSIOLOGIC CONTROL OF THE OVARY

The **follicles of the ovary** can develop to the antrum stage in the absence of pituitary function. However, maturation of the follicles and the sequential changes which characterize the normal menstrual cycle are contingent upon the release of the gonadotropins from the anterior lobe of the pituitary. The pituitary, in turn, is subject to the control of the hypothalamus. When stimulated by pituitary follicle–stimulating hormone (FSH) the follicles acquire an investment of multiple layers of granulosa cells, and they secrete estrogen in response to the joint action of FSH and luteinizing hormone (LH). Preovulatory growth of the follicle, ovulation, and transformation of the spent follicle into a corpus luteum are effected by LH, possibly in conjunction with FSH. Once formed, the human **corpus luteum** requires no additional gonadotropin support in order to secrete estrogen and progesterone. The in vitro synthesis of steroids by the stroma is increased by LH and human chorionic gonadotropin, (HCG), which, in the female as in the male, appear to be interstitial cell–stimulating hormones.

The central nervous system controls the synthesis and release of FSH and LH by the pituitary via two mechanisms. The first is a system which is localized in the ventromedial arcuate nuclear region of the hypothalamus. By discharging tonic quantities of the so-called FSH- and LH-releasing factors into the hypophyseal-portal circulation, this system assures the basal secretion of gonadotropin in quantities sufficient to maintain estrogen production. However, the ovulatory surge of gonadotropin cannot be independently initiated at this level. The second system comprises sex steroid–sensitive (and perhaps gonadotropin-sensitive) neural elements which are located mainly in the preoptic region of the anterior hypothalamus, the thalamohypothalamic border region, and the limbic system. Afferent pathways from the external environment also converge upon this region of the hypothalamus, which integrates all the relevant information. Under proper hormonal and environmental conditions, the preoptic region activates the more terminal infundibular region and evokes an ovulatory discharge of gonadotropins from the pituitary (Fig. 98-1).

HORMONES OF THE OVARY

The ovary secretes a water-soluble nonsteroid hormone or hormone complex known as relaxin and three types of steroid hormones: estrogens, progestogens, and androgens.

Nonsteroid (Relaxin)

Relaxin has not been isolated as a chemical entity, but its activity is associated with a water-soluble polypeptide structure. In conjunction with estrogens and progestogens, it facilitates parturition in certain mammals by loosening the symphysis pubis and sacroiliac joints. Relaxin has also been reported to soften the cervix, increase the uterine content of glycogen, nitrogen, and water, decrease the tone and motility of the uterus, increase uterine responsiveness to oxytocin, and promote lobuloalveolar growth of the mammary gland. In human pregnancy, blood relaxin values reach a maximum during the thirty-sixth week and remain high until delivery, whereupon a precipitous fall occurs. The cellular source in the ovary is unknown, and since the hormone can apparently be formed in other organs of the reproductive tract, its specificity as an ovarian secretion is in doubt.

Steroids

The ovarian steroids are synthesized from acetate via cholesterol and pregnenolone by essentially the same pathways as exist in other steroid-producing organs, the testis, adrenal cortex, and placenta.

ESTROGENS. The term *estrogen* refers strictly to substances capable of inducing estrus, or sexual receptivity, in female mammals. However, it has been extended to include compounds which produce certain uterine changes and to the steroid metabolites of true estrogens, whether or not these possess biologic activity. In the nonpregnant female, the ovary is the principal site of estrogen formation; during pregnancy, placental estrogen formation gradually increases until, by the third trimester, it may exceed ovarian production by a thousand fold.

Estradiol-17$_\beta$ is believed to be the primary secretory product of the human ovary, and to be interconvertible

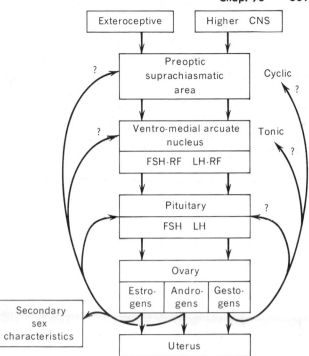

Fig. 98-1. The central nervous system–pituitary–ovarian–uterine chain. (*Adapted from R. Hertz, W. D. Odell, and G. T. Ross, Ann. Int. Med., 65:800, 1966.*)

with estrone by dehydrogenases which are present in the ovary and in many other tissues. Estrone and estradiol are, in turn, irreversibly converted to estriol, an estrogen of human urine that is quantitatively important, especially during pregnancy. Additional estrogenic metabolites of low biologic activity have been isolated in great number from human tissues and from the urine of pregnant and nonpregnant women.

The natural estrogens are all 18- or 19-carbon steroids which are characterized by the aromatic nature of ring A, the oxygen substituent at C-17, and the phenolic hydoxyl group at C-3. Many nonsteroidal estrogens have been synthesized for clinical use; they produce biologic effects resembling those of the natural estrogens. Representative examples from both the natural and synthetic categories are depicted in Fig. 98-2.

The liver is the principal site of the interconversion of estradiol and estrone, and is largely responsible for the inactivation of estrogen in the body. Protein-bound estrogen is abstracted from the plasma and excreted into the bile, from which it returns to the liver via the enterohepatic circulation. Degradation of estrogen is accomplished by (1) conversion to relatively inactive estrogenic compounds, (2) conjugation with glucuronic and sulfuric acids for excretion in the urine as water-soluble complexes, and (3) oxidation to unknown nonestrogenic substances.

PROGESTERONES. The term *progestogen* refers to substances which serve to prepare the uterus for the reception and development of the fertilized ovum. It has been extended to include compounds capable of duplicating, in

NATURAL

Estradiol-17β   Estrone   Estriol

SYNTHETIC

Diethylstilbestrol   17α-Ethinyl estradiol   3-Methoxy-17α-ethinyl estradiol (mestranol)

Fig. 98-2. The structural formulas of some important estrogens, natural and synthetic.

whole or in part, the effects produced by the corpus luteum secretions.

Progesterone is synthesized by all the steroid-producing glands. When secreted by the corpus luteum and placenta it exerts powerful physiologic effects in its own right; in addition, it is thought to serve as the key intermediate from which the androgens, estrogens, and corticosteroids are ultimately derived.

The ovarian progestogens consist of progesterone, the most important and abundant compound, and at least two other steroids: 20_α- and 20_β-dihydroprogesterone. Both of these partially reduced compounds have been detected in human follicular fluid and in the corpus luteum and placenta, the 20_α isomer in higher concentration than the

Acetate
↓
Cholesterol
↓
Pregnenolone → Progesterone
↓   ↓
17-Hydroxypregnenolone → 17-Hydroxyprogesterone
↓   ↓
Dehydroepiandrosterone → Androstenedione
              ↓
              Testosterone
      ↓   ↓
    Estrone ⇌ Estradiol

Fig. 98-3. Biosynthetic pathways for the synthesis of ovarian estrogens in the human female. (*Adapted from O. W. Smith and K. J. Ryan, Am. J. Obstet. & Gynecol., 84:141, 1962.*)

20_β. The basic molecule consists of 21 carbon atoms, two of which are contained in the side chain at C-17. These compounds are secreted by the follicle just prior to ovulation and are produced in much larger amounts by the corpus luteum. The quantity of progesterone which can be isolated from the corpus luteum is small compared with the amounts of progesterone secreted during the luteal phase of the cycle, indicating that progesterone is secreted almost as rapidly as it is produced.

A number of progestational steroids which mimic various facets of natural progesterone action have been synthesized. Many exhibit androgenic or estrogenic as well as progestational properties and, in these qualitative differences from the natural hormone, differ materially from the synthetic estrogen compounds. The short half-life of progesterone and the large doses consequently required to elicit biologic effects have prompted efforts to alter the progesterone molecule so as to increase its potency. Two groups of progestogens far surpassing the natural hormone in oral activity have been synthesized: (1) derivatives of testosterone (ethisterone) and of 19-nortestosterone (e.g., norethynodrel and norethindrone), the latter exhibiting the marked enhancement of oral potency which results from the removal of the angle-methyl group (C_{19}) attached to C_{10}, and (2) compounds derived from 17-hydroxyprogesterone [e.g., medroxyprogesterone (Provera), chlormadinone]. Esterification of 17_α-hydroxyprogesterone by caproic or other long-chain fatty acids yields long-acting preparations useful for parenteral administration.

The structural formulas of some representative synthetic progestational steroids are shown in Fig. 98-4, together with allied natural compounds.

The liver is largely responsible for the inactivation of progesterone, which it first reduces to pregnanediol and then conjugates with glucuronic acid for excretion in the urine. These processes are aided by an enterohepatic circulation which differs from that of the estrogens in that approximately 30 percent of progesterone or its metabolites are lost in the feces, whereas the estrogens are almost completely absorbed from the intestine. Some 10 to 15 percent of exogenously administered progesterone can be accounted for by urinary pregnanediol, and a small additional percentage by several isomers and closely related pregnane derivatives. The major degradation products of progesterone are unknown.

ANDROGENS. That the ovary possesses the biochemical potential for androgen production has long been evident from physiologic and clinical observations. In vitro incubations reveal, moreover, that testosterone is a product of the stroma and of no other ovarian compartment. However, in vivo studies are bringing to light an exceedingly complex situation.

Although **testosterone** is present in measurable amounts

NATURAL

Testosterone   Progesterone   Pregnandiol

SYNTHETIC

17-Hydroxyprogesterone derivatives

17-Hydroxyprogesterone   17 Hydroxyprogesterone caproate (delalutin)

Medroxy progesterone acetate (provera)   Chlormadinone acetate (lormin)

Testosterone and 19-Nortestosterone derivatives

Ethisterone (pranone, lutocylol)   Norethindrone (norlutin)   Norethynodrel

Fig. 98-4. The structural formulas of some important progestogens and allied compounds.

in the circulation of the human female, the ovarian contribution, as measured in the venous effluent, is negligible. It would appear that such androgen precursors as androstenedione and dehydroepiandrosterone, which are secreted to a small extent by the ovaries and to a greater extent by the adrenal cortex, are converted to active androgens in the peripheral tissues. According to one view, the function of androstenedione and dehydroepiandrosterone may be to serve as prehormones (endocrine secretions which possess little or no inherent biologic activity but which, after peripheral conversion to more active compounds, contribute significantly to the overall biologic effect). Peripheral conversion could be by any tissues, including those of the target organs. This arrangement would enable effective concentrations of an active product (e.g., testosterone or dihydrotestosterone) to be achieved locally in regions such as the clitoris without the high circulating levels of androgen which would virilize a female subject.

Androstenedione is thought to be converted in the liver to testosterone and to undergo intrahepatic conjugation with glucuronic acid without mixing with the plasma testosterone. Thus, testosterone glucosiduronate is not a unique metabolite of testosterone. A proportion of plasma testosterone is reduced by the liver to the weakly androgenic compound, androsterone, and its inactive isomer, 5_β-androsterone, and these compounds are rendered water-soluble by conjugation with glucuronic and sulfuric acid.

Levels in Body Fluids

ESTROGENS. Colorimetric and fluorimetric methods are available for measurement of the natural estrogens in urine. During the menstrual cycle, two peaks of estrogen excretion are generally noted, one in midcycle immediately prior to ovulation, and the other during the midluteal phase. During the midcycle peak, the "total" estrogen excretion (estradiol plus estrone and estriol) does not normally exceed 100 μg per 24 hr. In the fifth decade of life, the urinary estrogen levels of women commence a steady decline. The urinary estrogen level of postmenopausal women is low and is thought to be derived, in large part, from the adrenal cortex.

Urinary levels of endogenous estrogen in patients with liver disease are variable, with only a proportion displaying the increased levels that might be anticipated.

Urinary estrogen determinations are sometimes helpful in detecting granulosa cell or theca cell tumors in postmenopausal women. The adrenogenital syndrome and occasional adrenocortical tumors are also associated with elevated levels of urinary estrogen.

Levels of "free" estrone and estradiol have been measured throughout the menstrual cycle by fluorimetric and isotopic techniques. The range of normal concentration of both compounds is 0.01 to 0.03 μg per 100 ml plasma during the follicular and luteal phases of the cycle, with increases in the levels to 0.1 μg per 100 ml during midcycle.

PROGESTOGENS. *Pregnanediol*, the most important re-

duction product of progesterone, is excreted in the urine as the glucosiduronate and is measurable by gravimetric, colorimetric, and gas chromatographic techniques. Although pregnanediol is not a unique metabolite of progesterone, there is a rough correlation between the rate of pregnanediol excretion and the rate of progesterone secretion. Low and relatively constant levels of urinary pregnanediol (in the vicinity of 1 mg per 24 hr) are detected during the follicular phase of the cycle; higher levels, with a range of 2 to 8 mg per 24 hr, are found during the luteal phase. The urine of children, adult males, and postmenopausal women also contains pregnanediol in low concentrations; in these subjects and in women during the follicular phase of the cycle, the adrenal cortex is presumed to be the source. Since progesterone can be secreted by a luteinized theca interna as well as by a corpus luteum, elevated levels of urinary pregnanediol do not necessarily connote the prior occurrence of ovulation.

Progesterone concentrations in the plasma are low because of the rapidity with which the secreted hormone disappears from the circulation. Plasma levels are measurable in nonpregnant subjects by isotope derivative methods, electron-capture gas-liquid chromatography, and competitive protein-binding assays. In normal women, follicular phase values of the order of 0.05 μg per 100 ml and luteal phase values of 1.5 μg per 100 ml have been obtained.

ANDROGENS. Testosterone glucosiduronate is measurable in the urine by isotopic and gas chromatographic methods. The levels tend to be several times higher in men than in women, and in the latter they are higher during midcycle and the luteal phase than during the follicular phase of the menstrual cycle.

Testosterone, androstenedione, and dehydroepiandrosterone are measurable in the blood by double isotope dilution methods.

For the reasons set out earlier, these androgen measurements are difficult to interpret, and until various biochemical complexities have been resolved they are of limited clinical usefulness.

Actions

ESTROGENS. The name estrogen does scant justice to the diversity of physiologic effects produced by the estrogenic hormones. Their primary role is the development and maintenance of the female sex organs, and perhaps their most general effect is to promote tissue growth. At puberty the tubes, uterus, and vagina enlarge in response to increased estrogen stimulation, and the appearance of the external genitalia changes in consequence of fat deposition in the mons pubis and labia majora. The vaginal epithelium thickens during the follicular phase of the menstrual cycle, with shedding of large numbers of cornified epithelial cells containing pyknotic nuclei. The cervix is stimulated to secrete mucus of low viscosity and high permeability to spermatozoa. The uterine and tubal mucosa and their vasculature proliferate, and their musculature becomes contractile.

The estrogens exert direct effects on the ovary as well as indirect effects via the hypothalamic-pituitary system. Small amounts of estrogen promote the growth of vesicular follicles and increase their responsiveness to FSH. Puberal estrogen secretion causes the breasts to enlarge because of increased fat deposition, development of the supporting stroma, and ductal growth. The increased melanin pigmentation of the nipples and perineum is due, at least in part, to estrogen. There is a widespread deposition of fat in the subcutaneous tissues, particularly in the buttocks and thighs, leading to the characteristic rounding of the female figure.

The estrogens stimulate cell division in the deeper layers of the skin and gingivae, and in the mucosae of the oral cavity, nose, and urethra, causing a more rapid replacement of the outer cornified layers. Bone metabolism is significantly affected with increased osteoblastic activity, a positive calcium and phosphorus balance, widening of the pelvic outlet, and accelerated epiphyseal closure. The composition of the circulating lipids is altered, with a fall in total cholesterol and an increase in the α-lipoprotein fraction over the β fraction. Estrogens increase the levels of serum thyroxine-binding globulin, corticosteroid-binding globulin, ceruloplasmin, total copper, prothrombin, and AC-globulin. Antithrombin activity is decreased by estrogens.

PROGESTOGENS. Although secreted in far greater amounts than estrogen, progesterone exerts only negligible effects on the general body economy. It produces few specific changes when present alone, acting ordinarily in conjunction with estrogen. Progesterone tends to encourage tissue differentiation, rather than growth. Its most important function is to induce secretory changes in the lining of the tubes and uterus, the endometrium being thereby adapted for the implantation of the fertilized ovum. The viscosity of the cervical mucus is increased during the postovulatory phase, rendering it impermeable to spermatozoa, and ferning disappears. Tubal and uterine contractility are altered to favor transport of the fertilized ovum and to prevent its expulsion from the uterus. Lobuloalveolar proliferation of the breast is stimulated. Progesterone exerts a thermogenic action, the basal body temperature increasing by approximately 1° in midcycle and remaining elevated during the luteal phase. A slightly negative nitrogen balance is induced by progesterone, and by antagonism to aldosterone, a negative balance of sodium, chloride, and water is favored. Progesterone acts as a mild respiratory stimulant, increasing minute ventilation while decreasing alveolar and arterial CO_2 tension and the respiratory quotient.

ANDROGENS. The physiologic role of the androgens in the human female has not been clearly delineated. However, it is probable that they act to promote a positive nitrogen balance and to increase libido and muscular strength. Experimental evidence suggests that by local action within the ovary small amounts of androgen hasten antrum formation by separating the granulosa cells; larger amounts cause destruction of ova and granulosa cell atrophy. It may be that atresia of those follicles not destined to ovulate is promoted by androgens. In excess,

these compounds may blight the follicles of the ovary in the Stein-Leventhal syndrome, contributing to its polycystic structure.

ENDOCRINE DISORDERS OF THE OVARY

Diseases of the ovary may be classified as endocrine and nonendocrine, depending on the presence or absence of disturbances in hormonal secretion. Endocrine diseases of the ovary, because of the prominence of their systemic manifestations, are of concern to the internist as well as the gynecologist and will be considered here. Nonendocrine diseases, which comprise such entities as endometriosis, infections, and nonfunctioning tumors of the ovary, tend to produce localized effects and will not be treated in this chapter. The endocrine disorders of the ovary may be classified as (1) hypo-hyper-, or dysfunctional, (2) primarily ovarian in origin or secondary to disturbances elsewhere, and (3) congenital or acquired. Some disorders, particularly those secondary to disturbances of hypothalamic or pituitary secretion, are general in that they affect follicular, luteal, and interstitial function. Others are compartmental in that they involve only one or two of the major subunits of the ovary (Table 98-1). Methodologic difficulties are responsible for the

Table 98-1. A CLASSIFICATION OF THE ENDOCRINE DISORDERS OF THE OVARY

I. Ovarian hypofunction
  A. Primary
    1. General
    2. Gonadal dysgenesis (Turner's syndrome)
    3. Menopause
  B. Secondary
    1. General
      a. Hypothalamic disorders
      b. Hypopituitarism
      c. Constitutional and metabolic disturbances
    2. Compartmental
      a. Anovulatory bleeding
      b. Inadequate luteal phase
II. Ovarian hyperfunction
  A. Primary
    1. Feminizing tumors
    2. Masculinizing tumors
  B. Secondary
    1. General: true precocious puberty
    2. Compartmental
      a. Persistent follicle cyst
      b. Corpus luteum cyst
      c. Stein-Leventhal syndrome and hyperthecosis
III. Ovarian dysfunction
  A. Choriocarcinoma
  B. Struma ovarii
  C. Carcinoid

meager documentation of many ovarian syndromes. However, as these are overcome, a rational biochemical schema for classification is emerging.

Because of the specialized role of the ovary as an **organ of reproduction,** its disturbances tend to give rise to more restricted symptoms than do those of many other endocrine organs. Unless the influence of a feminizing tumor, for example, is projected against the barren sexual background of childhood or the postmenopausal years, the manifestations may be so inconspicuous as to escape notice. Disorders heralded by infrequent menstruation, staining, or the disappearance of cramps may be trivial in systemic terms and yet have profound reproductive consequences. This is attributable to the fact that except during periods of temporary dissociation, such as adolescence and lactation, the exocrine and endocrine activities of the ovary are firmly integrated. Any deficiency in either results in impaired reproductive function.

OVARIAN HYPOFUNCTION

Although the suspension of established ovarian function is readily recognizable as pathologic, it may be less easy to determine whether delayed sexual maturation in a child reflects hypofunction of clinical significance. The menarche presently occurs at a mean age of 13.5 ± 5 years; since its timing is significantly influenced by genetic factors, the family history as regards menarcheal age should be investigated. The menarche is ordinarily preceded by breast development, a spurt in skeletal growth, and the appearance of pubic hair (axillary hair tends to appear almost simultaneously with the menarche). The presence of any of the secondary sex characters, or of superficial cells in the vaginal smear or urinary sediment, constitutes presumptive evidence of incipient ovarian activation.

Gonadal Dysgenesis (Turner's Syndrome)

Upon gaining the germinal ridges, the primordial germ cells may, for obscure reasons, degenerate without undergoing transformation into primordial follicles. A "streak gonad," incapable not only of ovulation but of estrogen secretion, is thereby formed. In rare instances, the medullary stroma and hilus cells of such gonads secrete sufficient androgen to induce mild virilization.

In patients with this genetic disorder, the breasts fail to develop, sex hair growth is sparse, and the titers of FSH and LH early rise to menopausal levels. Although amenorrhea is the rule, the germ cell endowment is occasionally sufficient to permit menstruation for a few years, and one well-documented instance of pregnancy has been reported. The key genetic defect is an abnormality of the second X chromosome in some or all of the cells of the patient. Approximately one-half of the patients have a 45-X chromosome constitution, one-third have mosaicism (most frequently 45-X-46-XX), and a small proportion have a structural defect of the 1-X chromosome with the loss of a proportion of its genetic material. The presence of other congenital anomalies such as short stature, webbing of the neck, short metacarpals, and coarctation of the aorta often suggests the diagnosis during the prepuberal years.

Cyclic replacement therapy is indicated to prevent osteoporosis, premature aging of the skin, and other consequences of estrogen deficiency. Diethylstilbestrol 0.5 to 2.0 mg, or the equivalent dosage of other estrogenic preparations, should be given daily during the first 3 weeks of each month. Once withdrawal bleeding has begun to occur, medroxyprogesterone acetate 5 to 10 mg, or the equivalent dosage of other progestational agents, should be added during the last 5 to 10 days of each course to effect secretory differentiation of the endometrium, thereby preventing cumulative hyperplasia and functional bleeding. "Sequential" antiovulatory preparations are a convenient form of therapy.

Menopause

The menopause, or final cessation of menses, occurs at a mean age of approximately forty-eight years and is frequently delayed until the early fifties. Termination of menstrual function before the age of forty may be considered premature. A small proportion of patients experiencing a precocious menopause have sex chromosomal mosaicism. Additional patients exhibit an unusual propensity to autoimmune disease, which may conceivably affect the ovaries. In the majority of instances, no explanation is available. The cause of the normally timed climacteric is also somewhat obscure. It appears to reflect an unduly rapid depletion of the oocytes, with the loss of their inductive effect upon the granulosa and theca cells. With a diminution of the steroid feedback influence upon the hypothalamus, the gonadotropin titer rises and the release of FSH and LH is no longer coordinated. Eventually, the stroma remains as the only functioning compartment.

The menopause is usually heralded by a period of menstrual irregularity. Amenorrhea tends to alternate with scanty periods or with bleeding which may be disconcertingly profuse. Hot flashes, the classic symptom of the climacteric, may begin at an early stage but tend to become more frequent after the periods have entirely ceased. They occur in approximately 85 percent of menopausal women and are brief in duration, lasting only a few minutes. The sensation of warmth is confined to the chest, neck, and face and may be accompanied by diffuse or patchy flushing of the skin and sweating. Hot flashes occur most frequently when heat production is increased (e.g., after meals or emotional stress) or when the dissipation of heat is impaired by bedclothes or by high ambient temperatures and humidity. Fatigue, arthralgias, insomnia, and emotional instability are common complaints in middle life; whether they are integral components of the climacteric or are only temporally related is in dispute. The rate at which involution of the ovary takes place affects the severity of menopausal symptoms. In women experiencing a sudden (not necessarily surgical) loss of ovarian function, hot flashes are likely to be severe and dyspareunia due to atrophy of the vagina may be troublesome. In women experiencing a gradual decline of ovarian activity, amenorrhea may be the sole symptom.

Treatment of the menopause comprises (1) the exclusion of organic causes of any associated menorrhagia, (2) explanation of the physiologic changes wrought by the climacteric, ventilation of the patient's anxieties, and reassurance, and (3) hormonal replacement. Estrogen therapy not only suppresses hot flashes, diminishes arthralgia, and relieves dyspareunia but also helps to prevent osteoporosis and may delay the onset of coronary arteriosclerotic heart disease. Sex steroid treatment should be administered indefinitely, as described in the section on gonadal dysgenesis. After a number of years, withdrawal bleeding will no longer occur and the progestational component can be omitted. Mild sedatives, such as phenobarbital 15 mg several times daily, are helpful in diminishing tension. Regular periodic examinations of the breasts and pelvis are essential, as are vaginal smears. The latter serve as a screening test for malignancy, particularly of the cervix. Smears are less reliable for the detection of carcinoma of the endometrium and, in the event of bleeding which is abnormal in timing or quantity, should be supplemented with endometrial biopsy and curettage. The maturation index obtainable from vaginal smears is useful for regulating estrogen dosage. If estrogen is given in amounts sufficient to maintain the superficial cells at a level of 10 percent, dyspareunia can be prevented.

Hypothalamic Disorders

Ovarian hypofunction associated with congenital disorders affecting the hypothalamus, such as the **Laurence-Moon-Biedl syndrome**, has been described elsewhere (see Chap. 87).

Destructive lesions of the hypothalamus, such as those resulting from the expansion of tumors and cysts, may induce ovarian hypofunction. The **Frommel-Chiari syndrome** of continued lactation and genital atrophy following childbirth appears to be due to a lesion which somehow impairs the secretion of the prolactin-inhibiting factor and that of the FSH- and LH-releasing factors. In a high proportion of such patients, ovulation can be induced by treatment with clomiphene citrate (Clomid) in 5-day courses at a dosage of 50 to 100 mg per day (Fig. 98-5). This agent, a congener of the synthetic estrogen trichloranisene, evokes the release of FSH and LH from the pituitary.

Emotional strain which alters the afferent neural input to the hypothalamic centers controlling the secretion of the FSH- and LH-releasing factors is perhaps the commonest cause of amenorrhea, apart from pregnancy. The vulnerability of girls in the ten- to twenty-year age group to such stresses as attending school away from home has given rise to the term "boarding school amenorrhea." In older women the menstrual cycle is more resistant to disturbance, and either exceptional stress or frank emotional illness, such as depression, is required to suspend ovarian function. Treatment with Clomid will sometimes bring about ovulation, but in severe cases, psychotherapy may be needed to restore normal cyclicity.

Fig. 98-5. The structural formula of Clomid.

Hypopituitarism

In early life, the commonest pituitary cause of sexual infantilism is a **craniopharyngioma**; in adult life, **chromophobe** or **eosinophil adenomas of the pituitary** and **necrosis resulting from postpartum hemorrhage (Sheehan's syndrome)** are the most frequent pituitary lesions resulting in ovarian insufficiency (Chap. 87). **Granulomatous diseases** (Hand-Schüller-Christian syndrome, sarcoid) and metastatic tumors or neoplasms arising in surrounding structures (meningioma) may diminish pituitary function at any age.

Headache, visual disturbances, or impaired growth suggest the possibility of a pituitary disorder in prepuberal girls, although failure of the menses to begin (primary amenorrhea) may be the sole manifestation. In adults, the cessation of menses previously present (secondary amenorrhea) and the coupling of lactation with amenorrhea should suggest the possibility of a chromophobe or acidophil tumor of the pituitary. X-ray visualization of the sella turcica is an essential component of the investigation of all patients with obscure amenorrheas. Sequential treatment with preparations of human menopausal urinary gonadotropin (as a source of FSH) and of human chorionic gonadotropin (as a source of LH-like activity) has, in occasional cases, resulted in ovulation.

Constitutional and Metabolic Disturbances

Severe constitutional illnesses such as **congenital heart disease, chronic renal disease,** or **rheumatoid arthritis** may delay the menarche and, in adult life, may cause amenorrhea and sterility. Injudicious dieting with too-rapid weight loss, anorexia nervosa, poorly controlled diabetes mellitus, and hyperthyroidism may also impair reproductive function. The point of impact of these different disorders upon the hypothalamic-pituitary-ovarian chain is poorly defined. A recovery of ovarian function generally follows successful treatment of the primary condition.

The adrenogenital syndrome (Chap. 92), a severe metabolic disorder commonly due to adrenocortical hyperplasia, is associated with pseudohermaphroditism and sexual infantilism. The adrenal cortex secretes estrogens as well as the "adrenal androgens" in greatly increased amounts, and the former, in particular, impair the hypothalamic control of FSH and LH release. Suppression of adrenal estrogen secretion by the administration of corticosteroids is speedily followed by sexual maturation and menstruation.

"Postcontraceptive amenorrhea" (i.e., that ensuing

upon the suspension of a program of cyclic sex steroid treatment) is a not uncommon iatrogenic state. Its pathologic physiology bears some resemblance to that of the adrenogenital syndrome, in that elevated levels of the circulating sex steroids appear to disturb the hypothalamic regulation of FSH and LH secretion. Omission of the contraceptive preparation is generally followed promptly by a return of menstrual function (i.e., within a period of a year or less). In some instances prolonged amenorrhea can be aborted by the administration of Clomid.

Anovulatory (Functional) Bleeding

Puberty and the premenopausal years are epochs during which the sluggish waxing and waning of the ovarian follicles, with an abnormally prolonged secretion of estrogen and an absence of ovulation, are particularly likely to occur. A teetering level of circulating estrogen results and is likely to be accompanied by painless menorrhagia (excessive menstrual bleeding), metrorrhagia (intermenstrual bleeding), or both, interspersed with long periods of amenorrhea. Anovulatory (functional) uterine bleeding, or "metropathia hemorrhagica," is so common at the two extremes of reproductive life as to be virtually physiologic. During the postmenarcheal and adult years, the condition is traceable to an absence of the midcycle LH surge with abnormally low levels of estrogen in the circulation and an absence of progesterone.

On rare occasions, a persistent follicle cyst is large enough to be outlined on bimanual examination. However, the diagnosis must ordinarily be made by exclusion. The disorders requiring differentiation vary according to the age of the patient (Table 98.2).

Table 98.2. SOME IMPORTANT CAUSES OF VAGINAL BLEEDING DURING DIFFERENT EPOCHS OF REPRODUCTIVE LIFE

1. Adolescence
   a. Functional uterine bleeding
   b. Blood dyscrasias
2. Maturity
   a. Complications of pregnancy
   b. Benign tumors (fibromyomas of the uterus, polyps of the endometrium and cervix)
   c. Malignant tumors of the cervix and corpus of the uterus
   d. Pelvic inflammatory disease
3. Premenopause
   a. Functional uterine bleeding
   b. Benign and malignant tumors of the uterus
4. Senescence
   a. Estrogen treatment
   b. Senile vaginitis
   c. Malignant tumors of the uterus
   d. Feminizing tumors of the ovary

Functional uterine bleeding is rarely fatal, but anemia is frequent and requires replacement treatment with iron. In younger patients, the oral progestational agents, fortified with estrogen, are exceedingly effective hemostatic agents. Doses of, for example, 5 to 30 mg daily of

norethynodrel with mestranol (Enovid) may be given for a period of 3 weeks and then withdrawn to permit a "medical curettage." When the bleeding has been checked and the hemoglobin level restored, normal ovulatory menstrual function may resume spontaneously. If this does not occur, intermittent treatment with Clomid may establish a normal feedback mechanism, with cyclic release of the gonadotropic hormones. In older patients, pelvic examination under anesthesia and curettage are required to exclude organic lesions.

Inadequate Luteal Phase

A clinically inconspicuous syndrome characterized by somewhat abbreviated menstrual cycles, infertility, and tendency to abortion is the so-called "inadequate luteal phase." In this disorder, the secretory activity of the corpus luteum is deficient and its term of activity is abbreviated.

A short luteal phase is physiologic (1) in the later phases of the postmenarcheal period, when it is an important cause of "adolescent sterility" (anovulation is the proximate cause of infertility during the immediately postmenarcheal years), and (2) in the puerperium, when menstrual periodicity is gradually being regained. At other times it is pathologic.

The diagnosis may be suspected from the character of the basal body temperature pattern, which is characterized by a slow rise to the luteal level and abbreviation of the luteal plateau. Confirmatory evidence may be obtained by histologic dating of appropriately timed endometrial biopsies. In some patients, the LH-like action of chorionic gonadotropin administered during the postovulatory phase has resulted in the formation of a mature endometrium which can support a conceptus. It would thus appear that in certain instances, at least, the disorder reflects the midcycle release of LH in amounts insufficient to form a corpus luteum capable of normal secretory activity.

OVARIAN HYPERFUNCTION

Ovarian hyperfunction may be relative or absolute. Thus, the elaboration of estrogen in amounts which are supraphysiologic for the reproductive age of the subject constitutes hyperfunction, even though the quantity secreted is less than that characteristic of mature reproductive life.

Feminizing Tumors

Granulosa and theca cell tumors and, on occasion, certain other ovarian neoplasms may secrete estrogen. The stromal elements of tumors in the latter category (e.g., cystadenofibroma and primary adenocarcinoma of the ovary) may resemble those of the thecoma or may contain elements resembling theca-lutein or stroma-lutein cells. The histogenesis of these tumors is uncertain. However, it would appear that granulosa and theca cell tumors arise from the stroma or its follicular wall derivatives and recapitulate the elements of the follicular wall. Approximately 5 percent of the reported granulosa cell tumors arise before puberty, 55 percent during the period of reproductive life, and 40 percent after the menopause. Theca cell tumors tend to occur in a slightly older age group.

The **symptoms** depend on the age of the patient. Precocious pseudopuberty and intermittent uterine bleeding result from the function of such tumors during the premenarcheal years; irregular uterine bleeding, frequently alternating with periods of amenorrhea, is common during active reproductive life; bleeding is the characteristic manifestation of these tumors during the postmenopausal years.

Granulosa cell tumors comprise approximately 10 percent of all primary ovarian carcinomas and are the most common hormone-secreting tumors of the ovary. From 10 to 15 percent of granulosa cell tumors exhibit a low degree of malignancy, in contradistinction to theca cell tumors, which are rarely, if ever, malignant. Both are almost invariably unilateral and tend at times to produce ascites. The Meigs syndrome of ascites and hydrothorax has been observed, especially with the theca cell tumor. Endometrial hyperplasia is a frequent concomitant, and the incidence of uterine leiomyoma, adenomyosis, and adenocarcinoma is increased.

The **diagnosis** is sometimes suggested by an unexpectedly high proportion of superficial cells in the vaginal smear. Urinary estrogen levels tend to be somewhat increased, and gonadotropin levels are occasionally depressed for age. Surgical removal is the treatment of choice.

Masculinizing Tumors

The **arrhenoblastoma** and the **hilus cell tumor of the ovary** are rare androgen-secreting lesions, the histogenesis of which is uncertain. The majority of arrhenoblastomas tend to occur in comparatively young women, while the hilus cell tumor is characteristically a neoplasm of the late reproductive or postmenopausal years. Both are ordinarily unilateral and benign. The clinical course is one of defeminization followed by masculinization. The 17-ketosteroid excretion tends to be normal or only slightly increased and to be refractory to dexamethasone suppression. Plasma testosterone levels are often elevated. The treatment is surgical.

The so-called **"lipoid cell tumor" of the ovary** is a lesion with an uncertain histogenesis, although in certain instances it appears to arise from the ovarian stroma. The large rounded polyhedral cells of which the tumor consists lack the pathognomonic crystalloids of Reinke but are otherwise identical with Leydig cells. The syndrome of masculinization resulting from the secretion of this tumor may be clinically indistinguishable from that produced by the arrhenoblastoma. The 17-ketosteroid excretion may assist in the differentiation in that it is generally elevated, sometimes to a marked degree. Both premenarcheal and postmenopausal cases have been reported, but twice as many tumors have occurred in premenopausal as in postmenopausal women.

True Precocious Puberty

Sexual precocity associated with pituitary activation of graafian follicles is generally idiopathic or "constitutional" in origin. Constitutional precocity is presumed to be due to preternaturally early maturation of the hypothalamus, which escapes from the inhibition exerted by the small but physiologically significant amounts of estrogen secreted by the infantile ovary. Gonadotropin secretion can be materially reduced, with regression of the secondary sexual characteristics and protection from the hazard of pregnancy, by intramuscular injections of medroxyprogesterone acetate. The dosage is easily monitored by periodic determinations of the maturation index, either from vaginal smears or from the sediment of freshly voided urine.

Sexual precocity is a cardinal feature of **Albright's syndrome** of **polyostotic fibrous dysplasia** (Chap. 384). There is no clear indication of the pathogenesis, and a genetic basis for the precocity has been postulated. In rare instances, the ovary is activated prematurely by gonadotropic hormones released in consequence of hypothalamic stimulation by cysts or tumors, and by postencephalitic or postmeningitic lesions.

An unusual form of precocity is that associated with **hypothyroidism,** which increases ovarian sensitivity to endogenous gonadotropins. The precocity can be reversed by the administration of desiccated thyroid in doses sufficient to provide physiologic replacement. These observations contrast with the effects of hypothyroidism on adult women, who commonly experience a failure of ovulation, with a tendency to functional bleeding.

Persistent Follicle Cysts

Follicle cysts which persist during the climacteric tend to differ from those of puberty and the reproductive years in that, because of the hypersecretion of FSH and LH, they are likely to secrete estrogen in amounts which exceed those which are physiologic during mature reproductive life. Massive estrogen treatment designed to inhibit the gonadotropic support of a palpable mass presumed to be a cystic follicle is warranted and is sometimes successful. However, because of the impossibility of distinguishing benign cysts from malignant tumors by palpation, the length of such trials should be carefully limited.

Corpus Luteum Cysts

The classic instance of physiologic luteal hyperfunction is the first trimester of pregnancy. In response to stimulation by chorionic gonadotropin, the corpus luteum of pregnancy secretes estrogen and, to a lesser extent, progesterone in amounts which exceed those characteristic of the luteal phase of the menstrual cycle.

A biochemically similar, but pathologic, state results from the formation of corpus luteum cysts. These may arise spontaneously or iatrogenically as a result of the **administration of Clomid.** Those occurring in Clomid-treated patients may be multiple, giving rise to a several-fold enlargement of the ovary; those occurring spontaneously tend to be single, seldom exceeding a walnut in size.

The presenting complaint of patients with spontaneous cysts is often that of **sudden amenorrhea.** Such cases are frequently mistaken for ectopic pregnancy because of the adnexal enlargement, hyperemia of the vagina and cervix, and the swelling and tenderness of the breasts. The cysts are sensitive to touch, with fragile walls which are likely to rupture. The suspicion of ectopic pregnancy is therefore likely to be compounded by the occurrence of acute abdominal pain. So difficult is the clinical diagnosis that many patients are, in fact, operated upon to exclude the possibility of ectopic pregnancy.

The cysts resulting from Clomid treatment may enlarge with sufficient rapidity to induce lower abdominal discomfort. They are less fragile than the spontaneous variety and ordinarily regress spontaneously after the drug is discontinued.

Stein-Leventhal Syndrome and Hyperthecosis of the Ovary

These uncommon but important conditions reflect hypersecretion of androgens by the ovarian stroma and perhaps by the hyperplastic and lutenized theca interna enveloping the subcapsular cysts and atretic follicles. **Plasma levels of androstenedione** and **dehydroepiandrosterone,** which may be converted peripherally to **testosterone,** are elevated, as, on occasion, are plasma levels of testosterone itself. The history is one of **irregular menstrual cycles,** generally experienced from puberty onward, and sometimes interspersed with long periods of amenorrhea and abnormal bleeding. Perhaps in consequence of erratic bursts of LH secretion (with an absence of the normal midcycle surge), the ovaries become polycystic, and, since ovulation occurs only rarely, there is associated sterility. Over a period of time the patients tend to develop hirsutism and, in occasional cases, frank virilism.

If the stroma contains nests of lipid-laden lutein cells, the term **hyperthecosis** is applied. Whether the Stein-Leventhal syndrome and hyperthecosis represent a pathologic continuum or distinct entities is uncertain. Hyperthecosis generally evolves in a manner similar to that described for the Stein-Leventhal syndrome. Occasionally, however, there is an abrupt onset in older women (sometimes after pregnancy), and there may be associated hypertension and impaired glucose tolerance.

There is much to suggest that an abnormal hypothalamic-ovarian feedback mechanism is responsible for the disorder. Prior to the introduction of Clomid treatment, **wedge resection of a substantial amount of ovarian tissue** was the treatment of choice for the induction of ovulation. It is still of value in those patients who prove to be refractory to Clomid. Because of the characteristic hyperresponsiveness of the polycystic ovary, **Clomid is best administered initially** in a dose of 25 to 50 mg daily for 3 to 5 days, which is somewhat lower than that ordinarily effective in patients with persistent anovulation due to other causes. Neither Clomid treatment nor wedge resection ameliorates the hirsutism, except in rare instances.

In a proportion of patients with menstrual irregularities, hirsutism and a high normal or slightly elevated 17-ketosteroid excretion, differentiation of mild adrenocortical hyperplasia from the Stein-Leventhal syndrome may be difficult (Chap. 92). Patients with this complex of findings should be given the benefit of a suppression test with small doses of a glucocorticoid, such as prednisone 2.5 mg three times a day.

OVARIAN DYSFUNCTION

In rare instances, bizarre dysfunction results from the presence of **ovarian teratomas. Choriocarcinoma,** a highly malignant tumor which secretes chorionic gonadotropin, may arise in the ovary of a prepuberal girl and induce sexual precocity. **Struma ovarii,** which is generally a benign neoplasm, may secrete thyroid hormone at any age. Occasionally, the rate of secretion is so rapid as to induce thyrotoxicosis. **Carcinoid tumors** are sometimes found in dermoid cysts containing intestinal or bronchial epithelium. They may induce the characteristic "carcinoid flush," together with cyanosis and diarrhea, and may, in rare instances, exhibit metastatic spread.

REFERENCES

Baird, D., R. Horton, C. Longcope, and J. F. Tait: Steroid Prehormones, Perspect. Biol. Med., 11:384, 1968.
Grady, H. G., and D. E. Smith (Eds.): "The Ovary," Baltimore, The Williams & Wilkins Company, 1963.
Morris, J. M., and R. E. Scully: "Endocrine Pathology of the Ovary," St. Louis, The C. V. Mosby Company, 1958.
Richardson, G. S.: "Ovarian Physiology," Boston, Little, Brown & Company, 1967.
Rogers, J.: "Endocrine and Metabolic Aspects of Gynecology," Philadelphia, W. B. Saunders Company, 1963.
Savard, K., J. M. Marsh, and B. F. Rice: Gonadotropins and Ovarian Steroidogenesis, Recent Progr. Hormone Res. 21:285, 1965.
Zuckerman, S. (Ed.): "The Ovary," vols. I and II, New York, Academic Press, Inc., 1962.

99 DISEASES OF THE BREAST
Kendall Emerson, Jr.

History

The earliest description of cancer of the breast, and probably of cancer in any form, is credited to the Egyptian physician Imhotep in 3000 B.C. and is recorded in the Edwin Smith Surgical Papyrus under Case number 39, "Bulging Tumor of the Breast." The gross anatomy of the lactating breast must have been familiar to the author of the Song of Solomon in the year 1014 B.C., who likened it to "a cluster of grapes." Aside from its obvious function of lactation, however, little was known about the mammary gland, and interest in it throughout the ages has been more esthetic and symbolic than scientific until the studies of Sir Astley Cooper in 1845 provided us with an adequate morphologic description of this organ and the first suggestion of its possible relationship to menstrual dysfunction. In the latter half of the nineteenth century the German investigators discovered that normal breast development in animals depended upon intact ovarian function, and in 1896 Sir George Beatson first demonstrated the inhibition of the growth of mammary cancer by oophorectomy in human beings. The role of the corpus luteum and pituitary in the development of the breasts has been brought to light during the present century by the works of L. Loeb, Gardner, Riddle, Corner, Turner, and many others.

Congenital Anomalies

The occurrence of aberrant breast tissue (polymastia) and supernumerary nipples (polythelia) situated along the so-called "milk line" extending from the midclavicle to the inguinal ligament has been noted in art and legend since recorded time. One wonders if these anomalies may not have been more common when man was closer in evolution to his multiparous animal forebears, since the number of breasts allotted to each member of the animal kingdom is in proportion to the average size of its litter. Absence of one or both breasts (amastia) occurs very rarely but was recorded long ago by the aforementioned author of the Song of Solomon.

Endocrine Relationships

The most comprehensive recent studies of the endocrine factors determining the growth and function of the mammary glands are those of Lyons in rats, which are very briefly summarized here because they seem to support most of the observations in human beings. The development of the normal nonlactating breast is directly dependent upon the synergistic action of three major hormones: estrogens, pituitary growth hormone, and adrenal cortical steroids. Growth hormone alone will cause some growth of mammary ducts, whereas estrogens and adrenal hormones have no effect by themselves. Prolactin (luteotropic hormone, LTH) and progesterone are essential for the functional development of the alveolar lobules and the secretion of milk, whereas in the adult gland estrogens inhibit lactation by suppression of LTH activity. Prolactin with adrenal steroids can induce lactation in the absence of progesterone. Persistent lactation may occur in association with hyperplasia or with prolactin-producing tumors of the pituitary with acromegaly or without (Argonez-del Castillo and Forbes-Albright syndromes); following pregnancy by chronic stimulation of the nipple or in association with amenorrhea, low urinary FSH, and hypothyroidism (Chiari-Frommel syndrome); and occasionally during the administration of certain drugs such as the phenothiazines, methyl DOPA, and reserpine.

The hormones of greatest clinical importance in relation to the breast in man are the estrogens. Engorgement of the breasts may be seen as a transient phenomenon in newborn infants due to the high level of circulating estrogens of placental origin. The normal development of the female breast at puberty, which is sometimes accompanied by intermittent tenderness and edema, results from the rising levels of circulating estrogens secreted by the maturing ovarian follicles just prior to the menarche. Precocious breast development may occur as a result of inherited or constitutional factors; of abnormal pituitary, ovarian, or adrenal activity associated with functional tumors or hyperplasia of these organs; or of locally irritating lesions such as tumors of the pineal or fourth ventricle, fibrous dysplasia of the bones of the base of the skull, as occurs in Albrights' disease (polyostotic fibrous dysplasia), or rarely following viral encephalitis.

Gynecomastia

Gynecomastia occurs physiologically in normal males at puberty and may persist through adolescence. (In some animals such as the bat, the function of lactation is retained by the male who may assist his partner in suckling their young.) This breast enlargement usually subsides spontaneously, but if it presents a sufficiently serious psychologic problem simple mastectomy with preservation of the nipples is justified since any hormonal treatment is ineffective. Gynecomastia should always raise the suspicion of seminiferous tubule dysgenesis with fibrosis, a variant of Klinefelter's syndrome, in which there is usually an elevated urinary excretion of follicle-stimulating hormone and a female pattern of sex chromatin (see Chap. 97).

Marked degrees of breast development in adolescent males or the onset of gynecomastia in later life may indicate the presence of an estrogen-secreting tumor of the adrenal. These tumors are usually associated with an elevation of the urinary 17-ketosteroids, the excretion of which is not further stimulated by ACTH or suppressed by adrenal steroids. Every effort should be made to locate such tumors by radiographic means and to remove them surgically because, though rare, a high percentage, if not all, are malignant.

Choriogenic tumors and, more rarely, interstitial cell and granulosa cell tumors of the testes, may produce gynecomastia. This condition is also seen in males with cirrhosis of the liver and in states of severe malnutrition, presumably in both instances due to failure of inactivation of circulating estrogens. It regularly follows iatrogenic administration of estrogenic compounds in the treatment of carcinoma of the prostate and even occasionally occurs during testosterone therapy in eunuchoidism. Transient gynecomastia occurs as a normal physiologic phenomenon in elderly men and may be associated with the administration of common therapeutic agents having a basic steroid structure such as digitalis and spironolactone.

Infections of the Breast

Acute pyogenic infections of the breast are largely confined to the first 2 months of lactation and usually involve the staphylococcus, less often a beta streptococcus. They should be prevented by proper hygiene and treated with appropriate antibiotics. Very rarely an acute mastitis may occur during the course of paratyphoid or typhoid fever, brucellosis, or mumps, unassociated with lactation.

Chronic tuberculous mastitis is a rarity today. It usually results from the extension of tuberculosis of the underlying bone into the breast tissue and should be suspected from the presence of multiple sinus tracts and the finding of active tuberculosis elsewhere.

Inflammatory Lesions

Mammary duct ectasia (Haagensen) is a benign condition usually seen in elderly women with atrophic breasts wherein the mammary ducts in or just beneath the nipple become dilated and filled with cellular debris and lipid-containing material. Intermittent pain and local inflammatory changes may be present, and because a discharge, at times bloody, and retraction of the nipple may occur, this condition must be differentiated from carcinoma. Excision of the nipple is usually indicated.

Fat necrosis is a common occurrence following trauma, which may be so slight as not to have been noticed. It presents as a painful lump usually associated with some ecchymosis and may be followed by local atrophy and dimpling of the skin, at which stage biopsy must be performed to distinguish it from carcinoma.

Thrombosis of the thoracoepigastric veins and sclerosing subcutaneous phlebitis (Mondor's disease) occur after trauma or for no apparent reason and are manifest by the appearance of long cordlike structures, initially tender, in the outer half of the breast, frequently extending up into the axilla or down toward the epigastrium. They may persist up to a year, but no treatment is indicated.

Sarcoid may very rarely involve the skin of the chest. Eosinophilic granuloma may occur in the submammary folds.

It must not be forgotten that carcinoma of the breast may rarely present as a subacute red, warm, indurated mass, resembling a bacterial cellulitis, the so-called "inflammatory carcinoma." This lesion may be suspected when the skin over it presents the characteristic *peau d'orange* appearance.

Fibrocystic Disease

With each menstrual cycle there is a recurring biphasic stimulation first of proliferation of breast tissue by estrogens, then of alveolar secretory activity by progesterone, followed by a period of involution. In most women these changes are of such slight degree as to cause few if any clinical symptoms. Not infrequently, however, well-marked inflammatory changes may occur preceding each menses, with tenderness, engorgement, and increasing nodularity of the breasts. This is more often seen in nulliparous women and may subside after childbearing and lactation. Methyl testosterone, 5 mg daily for 7 to 10 days before each menstrual period, will often provide relief.

In the later years of reproductive life the continued recurrent stimulation and involution of the breasts in the course of each menstrual cycle may result in diffuse and nodular fibrosis and the formation of cysts of varying sizes, so-called "chronic cystic mastitis." This condition can simulate carcinoma but is usually distinguishable by the fact that it is intermittently painful and may subside to some extent following menstruation. Nevertheless, carcinoma may coexist and be masked by the diffuse nodularity of the cystic disease. Moreover, the incidence of mammary carcinoma is greater in patients with fibrocystic disease of the breasts, and it is unwise to delay biopsy of suspicious areas in the hope that they may subside by the end of the next menstrual cycle. In severe cases simple mastectomy is fully justified.

Tumors of the Breast

Benign fibroadenomas of the breast may occur at any age but are more common in women under the age of thirty. They may be distinguished from carcinomas by their mobility and well-defined margins, but biopsy is nonetheless imperative.

Benign intraductal papillomas may occur and cause a bloody discharge from the nipple. They are usually small and difficult to feel but may be located by noting that area of the breast on which pressure causes the bleeding. Excision is always advisable.

Sarcomas of all types make up less than 3 percent of all breast tumors. Fibrosarcomas are the most frequent; lymphosarcomas occasionally originate in the breast. Liposarcomas and hemangiosarcomas have been reported rarely. Cystosarcoma phyllodes is a curious, very large, relatively rapidly appearing tumor arising usually from a preexisting fibroadenoma. It presents as a tender, warm, cystic mass often replacing the whole breast. The skin over it is thinned, and the superficial veins are dilated. The tumor consists of fibrous cords covered with epithelium arising from the duct system. The cords are separated by cystic areas which become filled with leaflike (phyllodes) projections of epithelial tissue. Although these tumors are usually benign, blood-borne metastases have been reported and surgical removal of the tumor is always indicated.

CARCINOMA OF THE BREAST

In western civilization carcinoma of the breast is the most frequent malignant tumor to which the human female is subject and accounts for a greater number of deaths than any other single form of cancer in women. It occurs with increasing frequency from the age of twenty up to the menopause, when its incidence levels off until a second rise in frequency occurs after the age of sixty-five. For reasons as yet not entirely clear, breast cancer is very much less common in Japan and other oriental countries.

ETIOLOGY. In common with most forms of malignant disease, the etiology of breast cancer is not known. A few factors affecting its incidence are, however, reasonably well established. The very strong hereditary influence seen in mice can be carried over, though in a much smaller degree, to human beings. A two- to sevenfold increase in the familial incidence of the disease is reported.

The role of the estrogenic hormones in the genesis of breast cancer in human beings is still controversial. The incidence of mammary cancer appears to be directly related to the duration of the period of ovarian activity. It is more common in childless women with a late menopause and less frequent in women with multiple pregnancies and a history of prolonged nursing during which ovarian estrogen production is suppressed. The view most widely accepted at the present time is that estrogens do not initiate the cancer but may, nevertheless, hasten its development in genetically susceptible individuals. The prolonged use of these hormones, especially at or beyond the menopause in patients with a family history of cancer, should be discouraged.

Recent observations on the epidemiology of breast cancer suggest that environmental influences may play a role. The disease is more common in Japanese women living in the United States than in Japan, in the women of Denmark than in their Scandinavian sisters in Finland, and in fat women than in thin. Wynder has gone so far as to speculate that one common variable, the quantity of saturated fat in the diet, might affect the growth of mammary cancer directly by providing precursors for the synthesis and/or a vehicle for the storage of the fat-soluble estrogens. Of particular interest is the high incidence of both breast cancer and polycystic ovaries among the Parsis in Bombay, more than twice that of the general population in India. This ancient religious sect comprises a closely interrelated and affluent community having access to a relatively rich diet, thus combining both genetic and environmental factors which might favor the growth of mammary cancer.

PATHOLOGY. The primary site is usually in the ducts, less often in the alveoli. Multicentric origins are a frequent occurrence, and all gradations of differentiation may be observed. It is common to see a marked proliferation of dense connective tissue surrounding groups of malignant cells, whether primary or metastatic, the so-called "scirrhous carcinoma." Unfortunately all degrees of differentiation may be found in different portions of the same tumor and little prognostic value can be attached to the histologic appearance of any one area of such a malignancy.

Mammary carcinoma is prone to metastasize relatively early to the regional lymph nodes—axillary and supraclavicular if the primary site is in the outer half of the breast, the internal mammary chain if the disease arises in the inner quadrants of breast tissue. From thence spread occurs primarily to bone, lungs, liver, skin, and subcutaneous tissues generally, less frequently to the brain. Blood-borne metastases may occur even before lymphatic spread is clinically evident. It is interesting that there is a predilection for metastases to occur in the ovaries, adrenals, and pituitary—areas rich in the hormones stimulating the growth of this type of epithelial cell.

DIAGNOSIS. The diagnosis of breast cancer is facilitated by the fact that it is possible to palpate directly this type of neoplasm, a procedure which should be done gently because of the possibility of spreading the disease. Unfortunately, the diffuse nodularity of the adult female breast makes it difficult to detect early lesions. As a rule the physician must depend on such evidence as hardness, fixation to underlying structures, or dimpling of the overlying skin to distinguish a malignant mass from a benign nodule of breast tissue, and by the time these distinguishing signs have become apparent the cancer has all too often metastasized. Direct exposure of the breasts to irradiation with low-voltage x-rays in order to bring out contrasts in soft tissue densities, so-called "mammography," has been of great value in screening for breast cancer and in eliciting small lesions in large, fatty breasts. When secretions are obtainable from the nipple, cytologic examination may be helpful. The majority of patients with breast cancer suggest the diagnosis themselves because of their ready detection of abnormal lumps or masses during self-examination. Although the procedure of periodic self-examination of the breast may be decried as tending to encourage neuroticism and cancerphobia, it is the only practical way by which we can succeed in reducing the death rate from cancer of the breast until a final cure for cancer has been found.

TREATMENT. Total *surgical excision* provides the only permanent cure for carcinoma of the breast, and x-ray therapy the best palliation for localized disease. The technical details of the surgical and radiologic treatment of breast cancer are beyond the scope of this chapter, as is the controversy over radical versus simple mastectomy with extensive local irradiation, as advocated by McWhirter and others. Because of the susceptibility of breast cancer to changes in its endocrine environment, however, every physician should be cognizant of the remarkable palliative effect which can be achieved in inoperable mammary cancer by intelligent hormonal manipulations.

The two most important factors governing the prognosis of disseminated breast cancer and the success of its treatment or palliation are first, the age of the patient and second, the length of the free interval between the discovery of the primary tumor and the appearance of metastases. In common with neoplasia in general the younger the age at which it occurs, the more rapid and malignant is its growth. The only exceptions to this rule are the rare cases of juvenile breast cancer reported in patients from three to fifteen years of age, which appear to have a more benign course. The length of the free interval is a rough measure of the balance between the biologic activity, or turnover rate, of tumor cells and the poorly understood factors of host resistance.

The rationale of the *endocrine treatment of breast*

cancer is predicated on the assumption that in the total population of malignant cells some portion retain their metabolic dependency for growth upon estrogens for variable lengths of time before ultimately becoming autonomous. The first aim of therapy, therefore, is to remove all sources of estrogen from the afflicted subject. There is increasing evidence, but not universal agreement, that prophylactic oophorectomy and prednisone suppression of adrenal estrogen precursors at the time of initial mastectomy may significantly prolong the free interval, if not the total survival time of those patients with metastases ostensibly confined to axillary lymph nodes. Surgical or adequate x-ray castration will induce subjective and/or objective remissions in approximately 40 percent of patients with demonstrable metastases up to 10 years or even longer after the menopause, the incidence of favorable responses tending to vary directly with age.

A very high incidence of ovarian stromal hyperplasia, which is considered to be evidence of persistence of estrogen synthesis beyond the period of ovulation, has been observed among postmenopausal patients with mammary cancer. Such estrogen activity may be most easily detected by demonstrating the presence of more than 10 percent of cornified cells in the vaginal smear stained by the Papanicolaou method. When this activity is present, oophorectomy is indicated and may produce dramatic remissions even in patients over the age of seventy years.

With cessation of ovarian activity the adrenal cortex takes over the function of supplying precursors for estrogen production, and *bilateral adrenalectomy* will then bring about a further remission in approximately 50 percent of subjects. The remissions following these procedures may last anywhere from 6 months to 5 years or longer. Although no statistics are currently available, some investigators believe that oophorectomy and adrenalectomy carried out simultaneously will bring about a more prolonged remission in a larger percentage of patients than when adrenalectomy is deferred until the remission following oophorectomy is ended or fails to occur. In particular, when the metastatic disease is far advanced, the condition of the patient may preclude the performance of a second operation.

Surgical hypophysectomy, or pituitary stalk section, induces a functional ovarian and adrenal ablation and results in a remission rate equal to but no greater than the surgical extirpation of these target organs. The technical problems involved in total removal of the hypophysis and the degree of morbidity rising therefrom have tended to discourage this procedure. Pituitary ablation by roentgen or nuclear bombardment is too gradual to be of value in retarding the progress of a rapidly growing neoplasm.

Functional suppression of estrogen production by the ovaries may be achieved by the administration of depot progesterone, 200 mg intramuscularly, at monthly intervals, and simultaneously, the production of adrenal estrogen precursors can be inhibited by prednisone, 5 mg at 8-hr intervals daily. Such measures may be successful in retarding mammary cancer growth when surgical procedures are unavailable or unwarranted, but they are less certain and suppression is rarely as complete.

As yet, no reliable means has been found to select beforehand those individuals who will respond favorably to endocrine ablative procedures. A marked stimulation of tumor growth by estrogen administration usually implies a favorable response to oophorectomy, and similarly, a suppression of growth by prednisone indicates that adrenalectomy will have a good effect. The converse is not always true, however, and even lack of response to oophorectomy does not necessarily preclude a favorable response to subsequent adrenalectomy. Bullbrook and associates have presented statistical evidence indicating that in women under sixty five who excrete a low ratio of androgens (11-deoxy-17-ketosteroids) to 17-hydroxy-corticosteroids in their urine, breast cancer has a poorer prognosis in terms of recurrence rate, 3-year survival, and response to adrenalectomy than in women of similar age with a higher androgen excretion rate. Moore and coworkers have noted a tendency for patients who respond favorably to adrenalectomy to show a greater rise in the urinary excretion of 17-keto- and 11-17-hydroxysteroids following ACTH stimulation than those who fail to respond. Statistical discriminants based on data derived from such urinary hormone measurements have been advocated for the preselection of patients for adrenalectomy, but have not yet found general applicability. The length of the free interval is still a much more reliable predictor of response. As a rule of thumb, a free interval of less than 12 months indicates a poor prognosis.

Developments in *cancer chemotherapy*, however, have changed strikingly these predictions. The combination of ovarian and adrenal extirpation followed immediately by 5-Fluoro-uracil (5-FU), 15 mg per kg body weight given as a daily intravenous infusion over 4 to 6 hr for 5 to 7 days has sharply increased the remission rate and extended it to include many patients with a free interval less than 12 months. The 5-FU is well tolerated on this dosage schedule and should be continued as a single weekly intravenous injection as long as the remission lasts, provided no evidence of bone marrow suppression intervenes. Many patients too sick for surgical procedures may show striking improvement for 1 to 2 years following combined administration of prednisone 20 to 40 mg daily and 5-FU in the aforementioned dosage schedule. Undoubtedly other chemotherapeutic agents will be found which are equally or more effective but, hitherto, no agent has been shown to be effective in more than 20 percent of patients unless combined with simultaneous manipulation of the endocrine environment of the cancer cell.

In older patients, 15 years or more past the menopause, *large doses of estrogens* may provide remarkable palliation, and this is the treatment of choice. This paradoxic effect of estrogens, first clearly described by Nathanson, has never been fully explained.

The place of *androgens and estrogens* in the treatment of metastatic breast cancer has been well defined by the recent report of the American Medical Association's

Council on Drugs, based on a 10-year nationwide cooperative study. In summary, androgens produced objective remissions in approximately 20 percent of patients both before and after the menopause. Estrogens, which should not be used before the menopause, will induce remissions in about 36 percent of patients during the first 8 postmenopausal years and in more than 38 percent in later years. Estrogens have a greater relative effect on soft tissue and visceral metastases than on bone but equal or exceed the effect of androgens on all types of tissue. It should be emphasized that estrogens must be employed in large doses to achieve these results, such as stilbestrol, 15 mg, or ethinyl estradiol, 3 mg daily. Smaller amounts may adversely affect the tumor. Nausea and vomiting may occur at the onset of treatment but can be controlled by antiemetic agents and will disappear in time. Uterine bleeding may be troublesome but can usually be controlled by the cyclic administration of progesterone or methyl testosterone.

The optimum dose of *androgens* has been found to be equivalent to 100 mg of testosterone propionate given intramuscularly three times weekly. Recent experience indicates that the newer anabolic androgens such as fluoxymestrone in oral doses of 20 mg daily may be equally effective with much less tendency to produce the undesirable masculinizing side effects of testosterone.

All patients, but especially those within the first 8 postmenopausal years, should be observed carefully during the first few days and weeks of treatment because both androgens and estrogens may cause an exacerbation of their disease, estrogens by a direct stimulating effect and androgens presumably by being converted in small but effective amounts to estrogens. One of the most serious complications produced by administration of these hormones in patients who exhibit extensive skeletal metastases is calcium intoxication. This is presumed to result from the sudden stimulation of growth of the bony metastases by the hormone, with correspondingly rapid destruction of bone and flooding of the circulation with calcium. There is a marked increase in urine calcium excretion, and the serum calcium level may rise to as high as 15 to 20 mg per 100 ml, and drowsiness, coma, convulsions, and death from renal failure may ensue. It is important to distinguish this condition from cerebral or liver metastases or the terminal effects of widespread cancer because it can be reversed by forcing fluids, withdrawal of the offending hormone, and administration of large amounts of hydrocortisone, 200 mg daily by slow intravenous drip or in divided oral doses daily, until symptoms subside. The administration of neutral phosphate salts, in doses equivalent to 1.5 Gm phosphorus daily, may be of great value presumably by redirecting the flow of calcium away from the kidneys back into bone.

Hypercalcemia may, of course, occur spontaneously in far advanced autonomously growing malignancy with widespread skeletal metastases but can still usually be controlled with the above measures plus the addition of a chemotherapeutic agent. Occasionally hypercalcemia

may be found in the absence of demonstrable bony involvement. It has also been reported that a "calcium-mobilizing" steroid may be elaborated by breast tumors.

Carcinoma occurs in the *male breast* at least one hundred times less frequently than in the female. Otherwise it behaves in exactly the same manner. The treatment is the same except that orchiectomy replaces oophorectomy. Prednisone and hypophysectomy have both been shown to induce remissions when the primary disease has metastasized, and progestational compounds may be of value.

REFERENCES

Barnes, A. B.: "Current Concepts: Diagnosis and Treatment of Abnormal Breast Secretions," New Engl. J. Med., 275: 1184, 1966.
Bulbrook, R. D., J. L. Hayward, and B. S. Thomas: "The Relation between the Urinary 17-Hydroxy Corticosteroids and 11-Deoxy-17-Oxysteroids and the Fate of Patients after Mastectomy," Lancet, 1:945, 1964.
Haagensen, C. D.: "Diseases of the Breast," Philadelphia, W. B. Saunders Company, 1956.
Lyons, W. R., C. H. Li, and R. E. Johnson: "Hormonal Control of Mammary Growth and Lactation," Recent Prog. Hormone Res., 14:219, 1958.
Moore, F. D., S. I. Woodrow, M. A. Aliapoulios, and R. E. Wilson: "Carcinoma of the Breast, A Decade of New Results with Old Concepts," New Engl. J. Med., 277:293, 343, 411, 460, 1967.
Wynder, E. L., L. Hyams, and T. Shigematsu: "Correlation of International Cancer Death Rates, An Epidemiological Exercise," Cancer, 20:113, 1967.

100 DISEASES OF THE PINEAL GLAND

Richard J. Wurtman

INTRODUCTION

The past decade has witnessed a great increase in knowledge about the pineal gland. Only a short time ago it was widely believed that this organ was vestigial in mammals, that the pineal had once been a photoreceptor (the "third eye") in amphibians, but with evolution had lost even this function and bore the stigma of calcification. Since the discovery of melatonin in 1958, compelling evidence has accumulated that the mammalian pineal is not a vestige but an important component of a neuroendocrine control system. This organ has been shown to function as a neuroendocrine transducer: it receives a cyclic input of sympathetic nervous "information" which is generated by retinal effects of environmental lighting. In response to this input, the pineal secretes a hormone, melatonin, into the bloodstream, much as the adrenal medulla releases epinephrine in response to cholinergic nervous stimulation. The synthesis and secretion of melatonin vary with a 24 hr periodicity, thereby providing the body with a circulating "clock" apparatus. Largely because of technical difficulties, few attempts have been made to exploit this new knowledge of pineal function in clinical medicine. Hence, the principal circumstance which forces the clinician to think about the pineal continues to be the rare case of a disorder with evidence of a pineal neoplasm. It can be anticipated that as information about pineal physiology increases, more situations will suggest themselves in which pineal malfunction might be a factor in causing a disease.

ANATOMY AND BIOCHEMISTRY OF THE PINEAL

The human pineal gland is a flattened, conical organ which lies beneath the posterior border of the corpus callosum and between the superior colliculi. It originates embryologically as an evagination of the ependyma which lines the roof of the third ventricle, and remains connected to this region by the pineal stalk. The adult gland weighs about 120 mg; its dimensions are 5 to 9 mm in length, 3 to 6 mm in width, and 3 to 5 mm in thickness. Most of the pineal is enveloped by pia mater, from which blood vessels, unmyelinated nerve fibers, and septums of connective tissue penetrate the gland, thereby dividing it into lobules. The pineal glandular or parenchymal cells on the periphery of the lobule are elongated; those in the central zone are ovoid. They contain numerous granular bodies (which might represent a stored secretion), and give rise to processes that terminate adjacent to the capillary endothelium.

For many years it was assumed that the pineal gland was innervated by fibers which originated in the epithalamus, most likely in the habenula or posterior commissure. The pineal was known to share a common embryonic origin with these structures, and tracts were demonstrable

in lower vertebrates (e.g., the frog) that ran from pineal photoreceptors to the epithalamus. Moreover, nerve bundles from the brain clearly could be shown to enter the pineal stalk in most mammals. In 1960, however, Kappers made the important discovery that the primary innervation of the mammalian pineal originates not within the brain but rather from sympathetic cell bodies in the superior cervical ganglions. Subsequent studies using the electron microscope revealed that the sympathetic nerve endings terminate directly on pineal parenchymal cells in an anatomic relationship that resembles the synapse. The sympathetic innervation of pineal glandular cells appears to be a new evolutionary adaptation. Such a parenchymal innervation may be unique in the body, and itself invalidates the vestige theory of pineal function.

In 1917, McCord and Allen showed that the pineal gland of the cow contained a factor which caused amphibian skin to blanch. When pineal homogenates were fed to tadpoles, the melanin granules within dermal melanophores aggregated around the cell nuclei, thereby lightening the skin. (This effect is opposite to that produced by the melanocyte-stimulating hormone, MSH, which is secreted by the pars intermedia of the pituitary gland.) Four decades later, Lerner and his colleagues identified this pineal factor as melatonin (5-methoxy-N-acetyltryptamine) (Fig. 100-1). Melatonin appears to have no effect on the melanocytes which are responsible for normal skin pigmentation in human beings.

Melatonin was shown to be a derivative of serotonin (Fig. 100-1), a widely distributed indole stored in very large quantities in mammalian pineals. It differs from all indoles previously identified in mammals in that it contains a methoxy- group. The enzyme which catalyzes this methoxylation reaction (hydroxyindole-O-methyl transferase, HIOMT) was shown to be highly localized

Fig. 100-1. Synthesis of melatonin in the pineal gland. The pineal takes up tryptophan from the circulation; the amino acid is hydroxylated to form 5-hydroxytryptophan; this is then converted to the amine serotonin (5-hydroxytryptamine) by the enzyme aromatic L-amino acid decarboxylase. Most of the serotonin formed in the pineal and elsewhere is destroyed by oxidative deamination, forming 5-hydroxyindole acetic acid. However, the pineal has the unique capacity to acetylate serotonin and to O-methylate the product to form the hormone melatonin.

within the pineal gland in mammals. All pineals contain this enzyme, and no other mammalian tissues appear capable of making melatonin. (The enzyme is not as highly localized in lower vertebrates; it is present in the eye and brain of the frog, in which species melatonin may function as a neurotransmitter.) The extreme localization of HIOMT has recently been used as a "marker" to differentiate true pinealomas from pineal tumors of glial or other origin.

PHYSIOLOGY OF THE MAMMALIAN PINEAL

Environmental lighting conditions exert several important effects on the mammalian neuroendocrine apparatus. Light acts as an "inducer" that modifies the rate of sexual maturation; girls who have been deprived of light perception from birth may show early pubescence. The sequence of day and night also acts to generate certain 24-hr biologic rhythms, or to synchronize similar rhythms which are produced by signals arising from within the body. There is evidence that one function of the mammalian pineal might be to mediate some of these endocrine effects of light. When rats are placed in continuous light for 2 or 3 days, a significant reduction in pineal weight occurs, accompanied by a marked decrease in the ability of the pineal to make melatonin. Continuous darkness has opposite effects. The effects produced by artificial lighting environments appear simply to be an exaggeration of the changes in pineal metabolism accompanying the normal cycle of day and night. This effect of light on the pineal is indirect and is initiated by the retinal response to light. The "information" about light travels to the pineal by a route which involves (1) the inferior accessory optic tract, (2) centers in the brain and spinal cord that regulate the sympathetic nervous system, and (3) the sympathetic nerves to the pineal which originate in the superior cervical ganglions. The diurnal variation in pineal melatonin secretion provides the body with a circulating "clock" which is under the direct control of the lighting environment.

Less is known about which organs take cues from the pineal "clock" than about the mechanism responsible for its rhythmic changes. It seems likely that melatonin exerts physiologic inhibitory effects on gonadal and thyroid function and also modifies behavior and electroencephalographic activity. For example, when rats are treated with small doses of the indole, the uptake of radioactive iodine by the thyroid is depressed, ovarian growth is inhibited, and the cyclicity of ovulation is disturbed. Circulating melatonin releases MSH from the rat pituitary and inhibits the spontaneous and serotonin-induced contractility of bronchial and gastrointestinal smooth muscle. It is possible that all the endocrine effects of melatonin operate via a common mechanism which involves an action on the brain. When tiny amounts of melatonin are implanted in the median eminence of the hypothalamus or the midbrain reticular formation, the increase in pituitary luteinizing hormone (LH) content which normally follows castration is blocked.

It had been suggested that the mammalian pineal secretes a hormone, "adrenoglomerulotropin," which acts on the adrenal cortex to stimulate the release of aldosterone. This hormone was tentatively identified as 1,methyl-6-methoxy1,2,3,4-tetrahydro-2-carboline; however, subsequent studies failed to demonstrate that the pineal is capable of synthesizing this compound, or that its administration invariably produces a rise in aldosterone secretion. 5-Methoxytryptophol, another indole closely related to melatonin, has been identified in rat and bovine pineals, and may exert effects on gonad function similar to those of melatonin.

PINEAL PATHOLOGY

Two pineal lesions have been of interest to the clinician: pineal calcification, which is a universal autopsy finding, and pineal tumors, which are best known for their endocrine sequelae. In rare instances, pineal glands have also contained cancer metastases, gummas, tuberculous granulomas, or isolated segments of skeletal muscle.

Pineal calcification often first becomes visible on skull roentgenograms around the time of puberty, and it has been suggested that the gland degenerates at this time of life, and then becomes calcified. However, recent studies have not supported this hypothesis. If pineals are examined by appropriate microscopic techniques, evidence of calcification often is seen in patients who died long before the age of puberty. A ground substance believed to serve as the matrix for calcification was seen in 8 of 28 pineals taken from children under one year of age. Moreover, studies of pineal function have failed to show any differences between heavily calcified glands taken from aged subjects and pineals from young subjects with no gross evidence of calcification. The functional significance of pineal calcification remains entirely unexplained. The chemical identity of the calcified material appears to be hydroxyapatite; crystals of this compound taken from human pineals are similar to those prepared from bone or tooth.

Pineal tumors may be divided into several distinct categories by their microscopic appearance. Somewhat more than half of all pineal tumors may be classified as true pinealomas. These tumors contain clusters of two distinct types of cells: large, spheroidal, epithelial cells, and small, dark-staining cells with little cytoplasm and an ultrastructure indistinguishable from that of the lymphocyte. About 10 to 15 percent of all reported pineal tumors have been teratomas; these may contain mucus-secreting columnar epithelial cells, adenocarcinoma tissue, and areas resembling thyroid, muscle, cartilage, bone, and nerve. Like other midline teratomas, they are often malignant. The remainder of pineal tumors have been of vascular or glial origin.

Several theories have been propounded to explain the existence of two distinct cell types in the classical parenchymal pinealoma. Globus and Silbert suggested that the pinealoma arises from an embryonic rest and that consequently its appearance is similar to that of the normal gland during one phase of its prenatal development. Late in prenatal life the human pineal contains two types of cells arranged in a mosaic pattern which superficially resembles that seen in true pinealomas. Pineal embryonic rests without evidence of neoplastic degeneration have, in fact, been observed in normal brains. Russell held that the two-cell types are actually a single cell, and that most tumor specimens classified as parenchymal pinealomas are really only segments of pineal teratomas. Marshall and Dayan have proposed that the presence of cells resembling lymphocytes in pinealomas (and in seminomas, dysgerminomas, and certain mediastinal tumors) results from an immune reaction on the part of the host: all four tumors may release unidentified antigens, and the immunologic responses to these antigens may serve to retard tumor growth. Few data are available on the general immunologic status of patients who have pinealomas.

Confirmation of pineal origin of the large pinealoma cells has been hampered by the lack of a specific pineal function which could be measured in these cells (such as the uptake of 131 iodine by thyroidal cells in follicular adenomas). However, recent studies suggest that assays for the melatonin-forming enzyme (HIOMT) may provide such a "marker." Two pineal tumors containing this enzyme have been described; one was a metastasis from a parenchymal pinealoma, and the other, a specimen from an ectopic pinealoma. Both tumors had the characteristic histologic appearance of the parenchymal pinealoma.

The natural history of a pineal tumor is related to its size and its histologic appearance. Tumors which originate within the pineal gland usually become clinically manifest because of symptoms which arise from their location (e.g., internal hydrocephalus, elevated cerebrospinal fluid pressure, and oculomotor signs such as paralysis of upward gaze, or Parinaud's syndrome); less frequently, the patient's family initially seeks medical attention because of the development of precocious puberty. About one-third of all boys below the normal age of sexual maturation who have pineal tumors develop precocious puberty. This neoplasm accounts for about 10 to 15 percent of all precocious sexual development in males. For unexplained reasons, pineal tumors are much less common among girls and are not associated with precocious menarche. Some investigators have suggested that the precocious sexual development in pinealoma patients is a nonspecific consequence of the pressure that these tumors exert on surrounding brain tissue. Kitay and others have summarized the evidence against this "pressure hypothesis": (1) Pineal tumors may produce precocious puberty, no gonadal signs, or even delayed pubescence. The endocrine effects of a particular tumor appear to be unrelated to its size. (2) Most cases of precocious puberty develop in patients with nonparenchymal tumors (frequently teratomas). An occasional parenchymal tumor leads to gonadal enlargement, but more commonly these neoplasms are associated with delayed pubescence or with

Fig. 100-2. Metastases of parenchymal pinealoma to lung, and response to chemotherapy. Roentgenogram at right was taken 3 weeks after patient received methotrexate, cytoxan, and actinomycin D. (*Photograph courtesy of Dr. Rudolf Toch, Massachusetts General Hospital, Boston.*)

secondary gonadal failure. (3) Gonadal abnormalities have been observed in a large number of pinealoma patients whose tumors had neither produced signs of a chronic elevation in cerebrospinal fluid pressure nor invaded other brain areas. The demonstration that a pineal hormone, melatonin, influences normal sexual maturation in rats supports the hypothesis that precocious puberty develops in pinealoma patients because the damaged pineal fails to release an inhibitory hormone. It has not been possible to test this hypothesis directly, because no assay is available which can be used to measure the level of melatonin or its metabolic products in blood or urine. It is noteworthy, perhaps, that both patients described above whose tumors contained melatonin-forming activity showed evidence of depressed sexual function.

Parenchymal pinealomas frequently show a good, if temporary, clinical remission following irradiation. Patients generally receive 3,000 to 5,000 rads; radiation is administered over a wide portal because pinealomas not infrequently metastasize throughout the ventricles and the subdural space. Japanese surgeons have reported encouraging results following the surgical extirpation of pinealomas; however, this method is complicated by the relative inaccessibility of the pineal, and consequently is used rarely in the United States. A patient with metastatic parenchymal pinealoma has been repeatedly treated during an 8-year period with x-ray and chemotherapeutic agents; each time an objective decrease in tumor mass occurred (Fig. 100-2).

A small number of tumors with the histologic appearance of pinealomas originate elsewhere in the brain at some distance from the normal pineal gland. These "ectopic pinealomas" generally arise in the hypothalamus in the region of the infundibulum. Hence, patients usually present a picture similar to that seen with craniopharyngioma with a clinical triad of bitemporal hemianopsia, hypopituitarism, and diabetes insipidus. Most ectopic pinealomas show a good clinical response to irradiation.

REFERENCES

Kappers, J. A.: Survey of the Innervation of the Epiphysis Cerebri and the Accessory Pineal Organs of Vertebrates, Progr. Brain Res., 10:87, 1965.

Kelly, D. E.: Pineal Organs: Photoreception, Secretion, and Development, Am. Sci., 50:597, 1962.

Kitay, J. I., and M. D. Altschule: "The Pineal Gland: A Review of the Physiologic Literature," Cambridge, Mass., Harvard University Press, 1954.

Ramsey, H. J.: Ultrastructure of a Pineal Tumor, Cancer, 18:1014, 1965.

Scharenberg, K., and L. Liss: The Histologic Structure of the Human Pineal Body, Progr. Brain Res., 10:193, 1965.

Wurtman, R. J.: The Pineal Gland, p. 117 in "Endocrine Pathology," J. M. B. Bloodworth (Ed.), Baltimore, The Williams & Wilkins Company, 1968.

——: Effects of Light and Visual Stimuli on Endocrine Function, p. 20 in "Neuroendocrinology," vol. 2, L. Martini and W. F. Ganong (Eds.), New York, Academic Press, Inc., 1967.

Section 4

Errors of Metabolism

101 ## INTRODUCTION

Lloyd H. Smith, Jr.

Few diseases are either wholly genetic or environmental in their pathogenesis. The degree to which "environment" (microbiologic, physical, psychologic, chemical) is injurious depends on the genetic legacy of the host. This may represent a specific genetic defect phenotypically expressed as altered structure and function or inappropriate amount of a given protein, a group of disorders still often designated by Garrod's term as "inborn errors of metabolism." Perhaps more often the genetic propensity toward disease represents polymeric gene action, the summation of a number of genic expressions which can now be described only by statistical approaches. A number of factors have contributed to recent interest in genetic diseases: (1) With improved control of environment, disease is increasingly endogenous rather than exogenous. (2) Advances in molecular biology have elucidated the mechanisms of transmission and expression of genetic information, allowing the definition of certain diseases with increased precision. (3) Although genetic diseases cannot be cured in the host, knowledge of the resulting biochemical derangements often allows rational means of treatment to be devised.

In this section major attention will be directed to individual genetic diseases rather than to broader topics in population genetics or molecular biology. It is not clear just how many inborn errors of metabolism there are. By the use of current estimates of the number of different kinds of proteins in the body, the average number of amino acids per protein, and the possibility that at a given point any one of 20 amino acids might be substituted, it may be estimated that the possibilities for variation in structural genes alone are $>10^{10}$. Many factors reduce the number of diseases which are recognized.

Certain variations are trivial, lead to no biologic disadvantage, and merely constitute the chemical basis of individuality. Other defects are intrinsically lethal and contribute to the high incidence of spontaneous abortions. Variations may occur not only among diseases but also within diseases, depending on the site of alteration in the protein and the degree of resulting dysfunction. More than 50 types of abnormal hemoglobins have been described. It may well be, by analogy, that there are more than 50 types of galactosemia or phenylketonuria. Individual genetic diseases vary widely in frequency, from diabetes mellitus (3 to 5 percent of the population) to sulfituria (a single case description). The variables in frequency—mutation rate and the balance of biologic advantage and disadvantage—are now the subject of considerable interest in human genetics.

The usual **inborn error** of **metabolism** results from the absence or severe reduction in catalytic activity of an enzyme, whether the protein is physically missing or is present but altered in a fashion which impairs its function. In microorganisms genetic disorders of too much enzyme activity occur. The recent description of increased activity of Δ-aminolevulinic acid synthetase in acute intermittent porphyria suggests that this type of activity may also occur in human disease. In the latter case, however, the process may be a biochemical epiphenomenon rather than the basic defect productive of the neurologic complications. **Genetic disorders** usually produce disease by the **accumulation** of **the substate** of **the enzyme and/or some** of **its by-products** or **by absence or reduced availability of the product of the reaction** normally catalyzed by the defective enzyme. This concept is illustrated simply in diagrammatic form first introduced by Charles Dent:

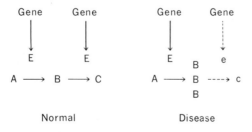

The accumulation of substrate *B* is the most frequently encountered abnormality productive of disease. This may be related to the fact that most genetic disorders so far discovered have dealt with degradative pathways of metabolism. Some examples of substrate (and substrate by-product) toxicity are described in greater detail in subsequent chapters: phenylalanine and its by-products in phenylketonuria, galactose 1-phosphate in galactosemia, oxalate in primary hyperoxaluria, homogentisic acid and its pigment polymer in alcaptonuria. Such defects may result in storage diseases such as the lipidoses, cystinosis, glycogen storage diseases, etc. The accumulated precursor may inhibit other metabolic pathways or interfere with amino acid transport into cells. Often the biochemical mechanism of injury is obscure.

Genetic disorders may lead to disease because of **absence** or **reduced availability** of **the product** rather than through accumulation of the precursor. Most of the recognized examples lie in defects in plasma protein synthesis or in the sequence of hormone synthesis, described elsewhere in this book. For example, deficiency of circulating thyroxine and triiodothyronine is the major defect in the various specific genetic forms of familial cretinism (Chap. 89), producing damage to the developing central nervous system, delayed maturation of the skeleton, hypometabolism, and failure of inhibition of TSH (thyroid-stimulating hormone) release, with resulting goiter. Similarly, deficiency of hydrocortisone in congenital adrenal virilism (Chap. 92) is the ultimate cause of adrenocortical hyperplasia (via ACTH) and of the excessive synthesis of steroidal precursors into adrenal androgens. A large number of genetic disorders of the synthesis of circulating proteins which participate in hemostasis have been described. In fact these proteins have been largely discovered in the study of patients with a hemorrhagic diathesis. The ultimate deficiency common to these disorders is that of appropriate formation of cross-linked fibrin polymer. The multiple types of genetic blocks in glycolysis associated with chronic nonshperocytic hemolytic anemia probably share a common deficiency of erythrocytic ATP (adenosinetriphosphate). The defect in albinism is absence of melanin; and a major defect in the von Gierke form of glycogen storage disease is deficiency of circulating glucose secondary to loss of glucose 1-phosphatase activity. In hereditary orotic aciduria, uridine becomes an essential metabolite. In a sense these disorders represent analogs of auxotrophism in bacteria.

A number of *genetic diseases* have now been described in which there is a **defect** in **the active transport of metabolites across membranes,** as summarized in Chap. 104. Occasionally the physical properties of the abnormal protein may constitute the mechanism of disease, as in the propensity toward stacking and tactoid formation in sickle-cell anemia and the heritable disorders of connective tissue. Pharmacogenetics refers to inherited alterations in drug metabolism, sensitivity of response, and toxicity. As an example, pseudocholinesterase deficiency is innocuous except during the use of certain muscle relaxants in anesthesia, when prolonged paralysis may result. Immunogenetics refers not only to immunologic markers in gamma-globulins but also to the inherited basis of antigenic (chemical) individuality. It is apparent that genetic alterations may be productive of disease through a variety of mechanisms, both subtle and direct.

Genetic diseases cannot be cured in the host. Knowledge of the mechanism of disease, however, often allows effective palliative measures to be instituted. Many of these are illustrated in the discussion of specific diseases in the chapters of this section. The approaches which have been used may be summarized briefly:

1. *Replace the enzyme.* This could be done phenotypically or, in theory, genotypically. The latter would clearly be preferable if genotypic replacement, augmen-

tation, or repair becomes feasible in multicellular organisms. Replacement now is largely limited to extracellular proteins such as coagulation factors, gamma-globulins, or hormones, of transient value only. Homotransplantation raises the possibility of localized extirpation and "cure" of genetic disease. The cystinuric kidney has been replaced. Drugs may alter the expression of genetic information. Phenobarbital has been used successfully to cause marked proliferation of the smooth-surfaced membranes of the endoplasmic reticulum in liver cells and thereby enhance pathways of bilirubin metabolism in certain cases of congenital hyperbilirubinemia.

2. *Reduce the accumulation of substrate.* This is usually carried out by dietary therapy, such as galactose-free diets in galactosemia or phenylalanine-restricted diets in phenylketonuria. The accumulation may be that of a by-product, such as uric acid or oxalate. In these cases new approaches to drug management are being pursued to inhibit the by-product formation or increase its excretion.

3. *Supply the product.* At the present time this approach is rarely employed except in endocrine replacement therapy, e.g., administration of a glucocorticoid in congenital adrenal hyperplasia or of thyroxin in the various forms of familial cretinism. The requirement for uridine in hereditary orotic aciduria is an exception, since this is replacement of an intermediate on a specific biosynthetic pathway.

4. *Miscellaneous.* A number of miscellaneous approaches have been successfully employed to compensate for errors of metabolism. Phlebotomy removes the excess iron of hemochromatosis, and D-penicillamine removes the excess copper of Wilson's disease. D-penicillamine forms a more soluble mixed disulfide of cystine in cystinuria. Chlorothiazide reduces the diuresis of vasopressin-resistant diabetes insipidus. Other examples could be cited. In summary, the treatment of genetic diseases is a challenging and often rewarding category of therapeutics.

Garrod wrote in 1908, "The existence of chemical individuality follows of necessity from chemical specificity, but we should expect the differences between individuals to be still more subtle and difficult of detection." The molecular biology of genetic transmission and expression is perhaps the most important area of scientific advance in the past two decades. Application of these advances in man has elucidated a large number of genetic errors of metabolism, some of which are described in specific detail in the following chapters.

REFERENCES

Harris, H.: "Garrod's Inborn Errors of Metabolism," New York, Oxford University Press, 1963.

Stanbury, J. B., J. B. Wyngaarden, and D. S. Fredrickson (Eds.): "The Metabolic Basis of Inherited Diseases," 2d ed., New York, McGraw-Hill Book Company, 1966.

Crow, J. F., and J. V. Neel (Eds.): "Proceedings of the Third International Congress of Human Genetics," Baltimore, The Johns Hopkins Press, 1967.

102 ERRORS OF METABOLISM ASSOCIATED WITH MENTAL DEFICIENCY

Lloyd H. Smith, Jr.

The biochemistry of cerebral function is not well understood, but is now the subject of extensive investigation. The brain shares with other specialized tissues many common pathways of biosynthesis and catabolism of cell constituents and of energy metabolism. Some biochemical reactions are found uniquely in nervous tissue; and some of its common pathways are catalyzed by isozymes under separate genetic control. Inherited metabolic disorders which affect cerebral function may be considered to be in two general categories: those with abnormal genetic expression in the brain itself (in the synthesis or control of synthesis of proteins) and those in which a metabolic abnormality elsewhere in the body indirectly affects cerebral function (accumulation of a toxic product, deficiency of required metabolite). It is not always possible to distinguish clearly between these categories. No attempt will be made to present all the genetic disorders which could be considered in the classification of this chapter. Phenylketonuria, homocystinuria, and maple syrup urine disease will be reviewed. Some of the other disorders have been summarized in Table 102-1, with reference to review articles. Since almost any disorder which affects general health may influence cerebral function, the selection of disorders included has been an arbitrary one. As an example, chromosomal disorders associated with mental deficiency, such as mongolism, have been excluded. The reader should refer to Chap. 363 for discussion of other metabolic diseases and to Chap. 31 and 365 for a more complete account of the neurologic effects thereof.

PHENYLKETONURIA

Definition

Phenylketonuria, first described by Folling in 1934, is a metabolic disorder secondary to an inherited deficiency of phenylalanine hydroxylase. This results in the accumulation of phenylalanine and some of its metabolites (notably phenylpyruvate, phenyllactate, phenylacetate and O-hydroxyphenylacetate) and a syndrome of mental deficiency. Other neurologic deficits, epileptic seizures, and reduced pigmentation may also occur.

Genetics and Pathogenesis

Phenylketonuria is transmitted as an autosomal recessive trait, occurring in its clinical (homozygous) form with a frequency of about 1 in 10,000 to 15,000 births in the United States. About 0.7 percent of the inmates in institutions for the mentally defective are patients with homozygous phenylketonuria. Heterozygotes (at least 1 percent of the population) usually exhibit slightly elevated fasting levels of plasma phenylalanine and reduced rates of plasma clearance of phenylalanine after its oral

Table 102-1. ERRORS OF METABOLISM ASSOCIATED WITH MENTAL DEFICIENCY

Disease	Enzyme deficiency	Signs and symptoms	Laboratory abnormalities	Transmission	References
Phenylketonuria	Phenylalanine hydroxylase	Severe mental deficiency, tremors, seizures, muscular hypertonicity, hyperkinesis, reduced pigmentation	Plasma phenylalanine elevated, phenylalanine, phenylpyruvate, phenyllactate, phenylacetate, and O-hydroxy phenylacetate, elevated in urine	Autosomal recessive	W. E. Knox, in J. B. Stanbury et al. (Eds.), "The Metabolic Basis of Inherited Disease," 2d ed., New York, McGraw-Hill, 1966.
Homocystinuria	Cystathionine synthetase	Mild mental deficiency (sometimes absent), ectopia lentis, osteoporosis, thromboembolic complications, skeletal deformities resembling Marfan syndrome	Elevated plasma and urine methionine and homocystine	Autosomal recessive	R. N. Schimke, et al., in W. L. Nyhan (Ed.), "Amino Acid Metabolism and Genetic Variation," New York, McGraw-Hill, 1967.
Maple syrup urine disease (branched chain ketoaciduria)	Oxidases of α-ketoisocaproic acid, α-ketoisovaleric acid, α-keto-β-methylvaleric acid	Progressive deterioration of central nervous system function usually beginning shortly after birth and leading to early death; sweet, maple syruplike odor to urine and sweat	Elevated levels of leucine, isoleucine, valine, and their corresponding keto acids in blood and urine	Autosomal recessive	J. Dancis and M. Levitz, in J. B. Stanbury, et al. (Eds.), "The Metabolic Basis of Inherited Disease," 2d ed., New York, McGraw-Hill, 1966.
Galactosemia	Galactose 1-phosphate uridyl transferase	Vomiting, diarrhea, failure of growth and development, hepatosplenomegaly, cataracts, mental retardation; improvement on omission of milk	Blood galactose elevated, abnormal galactose tolerance test; galactose, amino acids, and protein in urine; enzyme defect demonstrable in RBCs	Autosomal recessive	K. J, Isselbacher, in J. B. Stanbury et al. (Eds.), "The Metabolic Basis of Inherited Disease," 2d ed, New York, McGraw-Hill, 1966.
Cystathioninuria	Cystathionine cleavage enzyme (binding site for pyridoxal phosphate)	Mental deficiency may or may not be present; no other specific clinical picture has emerged	Excessive excretion of cystathionine in urine	Not established; probably autosomal recessive	G. W. Frimpter et al, New Eng. J. Med., 268:333, 1963; T. L. Perry et al., New Engl. J. Med., 278:590, 1968.
Argininosuccinic aciduria	Argininosuccinase	Severe mental retardation, ataxia, seizures, hepatic dysfunction, abnormally friable hair	Elevated plasma and CSF argininosuccinate, citrulline, and sometimes ammonia; argininosuccinate in urine	Autosomal recessive	H. W. Moser et al., Am. J. Med., 42:9, 1967.

Disease	Enzyme	Clinical Features	Biochemical	Genetics	Reference
Hyperlysinemia	Not established. Probably block in saccharopine synthesis.	Mental and physical retardation, impaired sexual development, lax ligaments, occasional convulsions	Hyperlysinemia and hyperlysinuria; one patient had hyperammonemia; ornithine, arginine, and cysteine may be increased in urine because of renal tubular competition	Not established; probably autosomal recessive	H. Ghodimi et al., New Engl. J. Med., 273:723, 1965.
Gaucher's disease (cerebroside lipoidosis)	Glucocerebrosidase	Infantile or cerebral form: hyperextension of head, hypertonicity, strabismus, apathy, seizures, mental retardation, hepatosplenomegaly	Gaucher cells in marrow, high levels of serum acid phosphatase	Probably autosomal recessive	D. S. Fredrickson, in J. B. Stanbury et al. (Eds.), "The Metabolic Basis of Inherited Disease," 2d ed., New York, McGraw-Hill, 1966.
Hyper-β-alaninemia	Not established, probably β-alanine: α-ketoglutarate transaminase	Lethargy, somnolence, hypotonicity, seizures, early death in single described case	β-alanine elevated in plasma; β-alanine, taurine, β-amino-isobutyric acid and γ-aminobutyric acid elevated in urine	Not established	C. R. Scriver et al., New Engl. J. Med., 274:635, 1966.
Methylmalonic aciduria	Probably methylmalonyl CoA isomerase	Developmental retardation, severe metabolic acidosis	Large amounts of methylmalonic acid in urine, long chain ketonuria, intermittent hyperglycinemia	Not established	V. G. Oberholzer et al., Arch. Dis. Child., 42:492, 1967; L. E. Rosenberg et al., New Engl. J. Med., 278:1319, 1968.
Sulfituria	Sulfite oxidase	Severe neurologic abnormalities at birth, deteriorating to an almost decorticate state; ectopia lentis in single described case	Excessive urinary excretion of sulfite, thiosulfate, and S-sulfo-L-cysteine; reduced urine sulfate	Not established	L. Laster et al., J. Clin. Invest., 46:1082, 1967.
Hyperglycinemia (ketotic variant)	Not established	Developmental retardation, periodic ketosis, with vomiting, neutropenia, thrombocytopenia, lethargy, coma, seizures, osteoporosis	Glycine elevated in plasma and urine; alanine, serine, leucine, isoleucine, and valine variably elevated in plasma	Not established; probably autosomal recessive	W. L. Nyhan et al., in W. L. Nyhan (Ed.), "Amino Acid Metabolism and Genetic Variation," New York, McGraw-Hill, 1967.
Hyperglycinemia (nonketotic variant)	Not established; possibly glycine oxidase	Developmental retardation, spastic paraplegia, opisthotonos, seizures	Glycine elevated in plasma and urine; urine oxalate lowered	Not established	T. Gerritsen et al., Pediatrics, 36:882, 1965.

Table 102-1. ERRORS OF METABOLISM ASSOCIATED WITH MENTAL DEFICIENCY (*Continued*)

Disease	Enzyme deficiency	Signs and symptoms	Laboratory abnormalities	Transmission	References
Lowe's syndrome (oculo-cerebro-renal syndrome)	Not established	Mental and somatic retardation, cataracts, buphthalmos, corneal clouding, epicanthal folds, typical or atypical Fanconi syndrome, sometimes with rickets	Generalized aminoaciduria (except for valine, leucine, and isoleucine), phosphaturia, and tubular acidosis	X-linked recessive	E. J. Schoen and G. Young, Am. J. Med., 27:781, 1959.
Hypervalinemia	Valine-α-ketoglutarate transaminase	Mental and somatic retardation, nystagmus, hypotonicity, unresponsiveness, vomiting	Valine elevated in plasma and urine	Presumed autosomal recessive	J. Dancis et al., Pediatrics, 39:813, 1967.
Hydroxyprolinemia	Hydroxyproline oxidase	Severe mental retardation; single case	Free L-hydroxyproline elevated in plasma and urine; bound hydroxyproline normal	Not established	M. L. Efron et al., New Engl. J. Med., 272:1299, 1965.
Niemann-Pick disease (sphingomyelin lipoidosis)	Sphingomyelinase	Physical and mental retardation, cherry-red spots in eyes, massive hepatosplenomegaly, foam cells in marrow, early death	Foam cells in marrow; sphingomyelin storage	Probably autosomal recessive	D. S. Fredrickson, in J. B. Stanbury et al. (Eds.), "The Metabolic Basis of Inherited Disease," 2d ed., New York, McGraw-Hill, 1966.
Tay-Sachs disease (ganglioside lipoidosis)	Not established	Progressive retardation, paralysis, dementia, blindness beginning by age 4–6 months, and progressing to death by age 4 years	Accumulation of a monosialoganglioside in ganglion and glial cells of the CNS	Autosomal recessive	D. S. Fredrickson and E. G. Trams, in J. B. Stanbury et al. (Eds.), "The Metabolic Basis of Inherited Disease," 2d ed., New York, McGraw-Hill, 1966.
Metachromatic leukodystrophy (sulfatide lipoidosis)	Cerebroside sulfatase	Progressive generalized neurologic deterioration, beginning about age 12–18 months and leading to death in a few years in the typical late infantile form	Metachromatic granules of sulfatides in white matter; excess sulfatide excreted in the urine	Probably autosomal recessive	H. W. Moser and M. Lees, in J. B. Stanbury et al. (Eds.), "The Metabolic Basis of Inherited Disease," 2d ed., New York, McGraw-Hill, 1966.
Lesch-Nyhan syndrome	Hypoxanthine guanine phosphoribosyltransferase	Mental deficiency, choreoathetosis, self-mutilation, gout	Severe hyperuricemia with hyperuricosuria	X-linked recessive	M. Lesch and W. L. Nyhan, Am. J. Med., 36:561, 1964; W. N. Kelley et al., Proc. Nat. Acad. Sci., 57:1735, 1967.

Disease	Enzyme defect	Clinical features	Biochemical findings	Inheritance	References
Histidinemia	Histidase (histidine α-deaminase)	Variable mental retardation	Increased histidine in blood and urine; increased excretion of imidazole pyruvate, imidazolelactate, and imidazoleacetate; low plasma glutamate; high blood and urine alanine	Autosomal recessive	H. Ghadimi and R. Zischka, in W. L. Nyhan (Ed.), "Amino Acid Metabolism and Genetic Variation," New York, McGraw-Hill, 1967.
Citrullinemia	Argininosuccinic acid synthetase	Mental retardation, nausea, vomiting, tremors, hypotonicity, intermittent hyperammonemia	Citrulline elevated in blood and urine; blood NH_3 elevated postprandially; urea normal	Not established; probably autosomal recessive	W. C. McMurray et al., Pediatrics, 32:347, 1963.
Hyperammonemia	Ornithine transcarbamylase and carbamyl phosphate synthetase	Chronic ammonia intoxication with mental retardation, lethargy, stupor, usually early death	High blood and CSF ammonia; mild general aminoaciduria; glutamine elevated in CSF	Not established	B. Levin, Am. J. Dis. Child., 113:142, 1967; A. Russel et al., Lancet, 2:699, 1962.
Isovaleric acidemia	Probably isovaleryl-CoA dehydrogenase	Mild psychomotor retardation, intention tremor, attacks of acidosis, stupor, and coma; "sweaty-foot smell" of breath	Elevated plasma isovaleric acid	Not established; probably autosomal recessive	M. A. Budd et al., New Engl. J. Med., 277:321, 1967.
Carnosinemia	Probably carnosinase	Mental deterioration in early life, somnolence, seizures; flaccid muscles, myoclonic jerks	Excessive plasma and urine carnosine, increased homocarnosine in CSF	Not established; probably autosomal recessive	T. L. Perry et al., New Engl. J. Med., 277:1219, 1967.

administration. Although some studies have suggested an increased incidence of mental deficiency or psychiatric disturbances in families of patients with phenylketonuria, the heterozygous state has not been demonstrated to be injurious.

Phenylalanine is normally hydroxylated in the para position to form tyrosine, involving a complex biochemical reaction catalyzed by phenylalanine hydroxylase. This enzyme is restricted to liver, where it exhibits increasing activity in the first few weeks after birth. Active enzyme fails to appear in the phenylketonuric infant. This results in accumulation of dietary phenylalanine in the plasma and presumably in cells, with secondary diversion (by transamination) into phenylpyruvate, phenyllactate, phenylacetate, and O-hydroxyphenylacetate, all four of these phenyl acids being excreted together with phenylalanine in the urine. Phenylalanine is a competitive inhibitor of tyrosinase on the pathway of melanin synthesis, which explains the decreased pigmentation of hair, eyes, and skin. High levels of phenylalanine in body fluids inhibit transport of amino acids into cells. The resulting deprivation of essential amino acids in the developing brain may be the immediate cause of cerebral damage, although this has not been established. Other explanations relate to altered patterns of synthesis of pharmacodynamic amines (serotonin, norepinephrine, phenylethylamine, etc.).

Clinical Presentation and Diagnosis

Retardation of mental development, usually of severe degree, is the major manifestation of phenylketonuria. Since the mental defect is stationary and not progressive in older children or adults, the brain injury appears to be limited to a particularly sensitive stage in brain development. Other neurologic abnormalities sometimes found are tremors, seizures, muscular hypertonicity, hyperkinesis, and EEG abnormalities. As noted, there tends to be reduced pigmentation of skin, hair, and eyes. Eczema has been commonly described.

Early diagnosis is essential for successful treatment since the neurologic abnormalities, once established, are largely irreversible. Diagnosis before one month of age requires the demonstration of grossly elevated levels of plasma phenylalanine. The excretion of the associated metabolites may not be remarkable at this time. Testing by screening for phenylketonuria of all newborn infants and of all infants of thirty days and under when admitted to another hospital is now mandatory in 37 states. This routine blood testing can be carried out quite simply using the bacterial inhibition assay (Guthrie) or a fluorometric procedure. Positive tests must be carefully followed up with quantitative measurements of plasma phenylalanine and study of urinary metabolites to differentiate the disease from transient hyperphenylalaninemia related to prematurity, tyrosinemia, or heterozygosity. This is important because restrictive diets may be injurious in patients other than those with phenylketonuria. The ferric chloride test, a transient blue or olive-green color appearing on the addition of a few drops of 5%

$FeCl_3$ to 5 ml urine, is still useful for screening older children or adults and is usually positive in infants.

Treatment

The biochemical abnormalities can be corrected by preventing the accumulation of phenylalanine. This is done by a special diet in which protein is replaced by an amino acid mixture low in phenylalanine (Ketonil, Lofenolac). Supplementary foods are given to supply only the amount of L-phenylalanine needed for body growth. The program should attempt to maintain normal weight gain and near normal plasma phenylalanine levels and should be continued until the child is at least four years of age. The results of dietary treatment are still being assessed. Normal development has been obtained in some patients treated from early infancy. Little permanent improvement can be achieved by treatment begun later, the main effect being that of prevention of further intellectual deterioration.

HOMOCYSTINURIA

Definition

Homocystinuria is a genetic disease resulting from absence of cystathionine synthetase, an enzyme which catalyzes an important step in the transsulfuration pathway converting methionine to cysteine. It is characterized clinically by ectopia lentis, osteoporosis, thromboembolic phenomena, and mental retardation, and chemically by excessive urinary excretion of homocystine. It was described initially in 1962, and approximately 100 cases have been reported.

Genetics and Pathogenesis

Homocystinuria is transmitted as an autosomal recessive trait. Heterozygotes have no stigmata of the disease and have no detectable plasma homocystine and no elevation of plasma methionine. They sometimes exhibit delayed plasma clearance of methionine loads given orally or intravenously. Assays of liver biopsy material from parents of homocystinurics (presumed heterozygotes) have revealed cystathionine synthetase activities intermediate between those of patients and controls. Homozygotes exhibit virtual absence of this enzyme activity in liver and brain.

In the absence of cystathionine synthetase, homocystine and methionine accumulate and cysteine (or cystine) becomes an essential amino acid. There is no clear information about how these chemical derangements result in the diverse structural and functional manifestations of the disease. It has been suggested that the ability of homocystine to form mixed disulfides may inactivate critical sulfhydryl groups of enzymes or impair disulfide cross linkages in structural proteins. No role of cysteine deficiency has been established. Current studies are directed to other sulfur-containing metabolites in urine, such as the recent demonstration of 5-amino-4-imidazole-carboxamide-5'-S-homocysteinyl-riboside.

Clinical Presentation and Diagnosis

Patients with homocystinuria often exhibit a superficial resemblance to the Marfan syndrome (Chap. 395). Some of the skeletal and connective tissue abnormalities which have been described are ectopia lentis, severe juvenile osteoporosis, kyphosis, scoliosis, genu valgum, deformities of the sternum such as pectus excavatum and pectus carinatum, abnormalities of the palate, and arachnodactyly. Mental deficiency is common, but may be absent; when present, it is not usually as severe as that of phenylketonuria. Recurrent arterial and venous thromboses may complicate the course and lead to early death from pulmonary embolism or coronary or carotid occlusion. Patients with homocystinuria tend to resemble one another with their skeletal deformities, light-colored hair, and coarse skin with malar flush and livido reticularis. Diagnosis is established by finding homocystine in the urine using paper or ion exchange column chromatography. As a disulfide, homocystine will also give a positive nitroprusside reaction in urine, but must then be differentiated from cysteine by chromatographic techniques. Plasma methionine is also elevated.

Treatment

In the absence of clear evidence of the mechanism by which loss of cystathionine synthetase activity is injurious, therapy has been attempted with low methionine, cystine-supplemented diets. Early reported results have been encouraging but difficult to evaluate in view of the variability of the clinical course. Some patients have been maintained on coumadin anticoagulation.

MAPLE SYRUP URINE DISEASE
(Branched Chain Ketoaciduria)

Definition

Maple syrup urine disease, so named because of the characteristic odor of the urine and sweat of affected patients, is a rare genetic disorder of the metabolism of branched chain amino acids and their corresponding keto acids. It is associated with severe neurologic damage and mental retardation occurring in the early neonatal period, usually leading to early death. A few atypical milder cases have been described in older children. Approximately 25 to 30 cases have been reported since its initial description in 1954.

Genetics and Pathogenesis

Leucine, isoleucine, and valine are normally metabolized to their corresponding ketoacids (α-ketoisocaproic acid, α-keto-β-methylvaleric acid, and α-ketoisovaleric acid, respectively). These keto acids then undergo oxidative decarboxylation in complex reactions comparable to those catalyzed by pyruvate and α-ketoglutarate oxidases, each keto acid having a specific oxidase. In maple syrup urine disease the activities of all three keto acid oxidases are markedly reduced or virtually absent in brain, kidney, liver, and peripheral leukocytes. The loss of activity of three analogous but distinct enzymes suggests that this disease is caused by the mutation of an operator gene (if this hypothesis is applicable to mammalian genetics) or of a gene controlling a common enzyme subunit. The disease is transmitted as an autosomal mendelian recessive trait. Presumed heterozygotes have reduced activities of the keto acids oxidases in their leukocytes, but otherwise exhibit no clinical or chemical stigmata of the disease. The metabolic block in these parallel degradative pathways leads to the accumulation of three branched chain keto acids and the corresponding amino acids in blood and their excessive excretion in urine. The mechanism of neurologic damage has not been established, although several hypotheses have been advanced. The keto acid derivatives of leucine and valine inhibit the activity of L-glutamic dehydrogenase in brain homogenates. Another suggestion relates to the inhibition of transfer of other essential amino acids into the central nervous system in the presence of elevated plasma levels of the branched chain amino acids.

Clinical Presentation and Diagnosis

Infants with maple syrup urine disease are normal at birth but begin within a few days to exhibit progressive deterioration with lethargy, poor feeding, diminished awareness, hypertonicity alternating with flaccidity, and convulsions. The characteristic urine odor from which the name derives is present. Death generally occurs within the first few weeks of life from severe neurologic damage with respiratory disturbances. If death is delayed, mental retardation becomes apparent. The diagnosis is usually first suggested from the odor of the urine, described as sweet, caramel-like, or like maple syrup. The urine gives a positive ferric chloride test and dinitrophenylhydrazine reaction for keto acids. The diagnosis is best established by ion exchange column chromatography of plasma to demonstrate elevated levels of leucine, isoleucine, and valine. Methods for demonstrating the enzyme defect in circulating leukocytes have been described.

Treatment

The treatment of maple syrup urine disease, like that of phenylketonuria, is based on the use of a diet restricted in the corresponding amino acids beginning early in life before the onset of permanent neurologic damage. In practice this has been very difficult because of the necessity to balance three different amino acids, the ubiquitous distribution of the branched chained amino acids in foods, and the large number of plasma chromatographic analyses required. A few encouraging results have been reported using strict dietary therapy. It is not clear whether such treatment can be omitted in later life.

REFERENCES

Auerbach, V. H., A. M. DiGeorge, and G. G. Carpenter: Phenylalaninemia, p. 5 in W. L. Nyhan (Ed.), "Amino Acid Metabolism and Genetic Variation," New York, McGraw-Hill Book Company, 1967.

Carson, N. A. J., D. C. Cusworth, C. E. Dent, C. M. B. Field, D. W. Neill, and R. G. Westall: Homocystinuria: A New Inborn Error of Metabolism Associated with Mental Deficiency, Arch. Dis. Child., 38:425, 1963.

Dancis, J., and M. Levitz: Maple Syrup Urine Disease (Branched Chain Ketonuria), p. 353 in J. B. Stanbury, J. B. Wyngaarden, and D. S. Fredrickson (Eds.), "The Metabolic Basis of Inherited Disease," 2d ed., New York, McGraw-Hill Book Company, 1966.

Jervis, G. A.: Phenylketonuria, p. 5 in W. L. Nyhan (Ed.), "Amino Acid Metabolism and Genetic Variation," New York, McGraw-Hill Book Company, 1967.

Knox, W. E.: Phenylketonuria, p. 258 in J. B. Stanbury, J. B. Wyngaarden, and D. S. Fredrickson (Eds.), "The Metabolic Basis of Inherited Disease," 2d ed., New York, McGraw-Hill Book Company, 1966.

Menkes, J. H.: The Pathogenesis of Mental Retardation in Phenylketonuria and Other Inborn Errors of Amino Acid Metabolism, Pediatrics, 39:297, 1967.

——, P. L. Hurst, and J. M. Craig: A New Syndrome: Progressive Familial Cerebral Dysfunction with an Unusual Urinary Substance, Pediatrics, 14:462, 1954.

Mudd, S. H., J. D. Finkelstein, F. Irreverre, and L. Laster: Homocystinuria: An Enzymatic Defect, Science, 143:1443, 1964.

Schimke, R. N., V. A. McKusick, and R. G. Weilbaecher: Homocystinuria, p. 297 in W. L. Nyhan (Ed.), "Amino Acid Metabolism and Genetic Variation," New York, McGraw-Hill Book Company, 1967.

Snyderman, S. E.: Maple Syrup Urine Disease, p. 171 in W. L. Nyhan (Ed.), "Amino Acid Metabolism and Genetic Variation," New York, McGraw-Hill Book Company, 1967.

103 STORAGE DISEASES. ALCAPTONURIA AND OCHRONOSIS, PRIMARY HYPEROXALURIA WITH OXALOSIS, AND CYSTINE STORAGE DISEASE

Lloyd H. Smith, Jr.

A number of genetic diseases are characterized by excessive storage of metabolites in the host. Most often these represent blocks in degradative pathways. Examples may be cited in the glycogen storage disease (Chap. 111), the lipidoses (Gaucher's disease, Fabry's disease, Niemann-Pick disease, Tay-Sachs disease, Tangier disease, metachromatic leukodystrophy) (Chap. 113), certain amino acid degradative diseases (primary hyperoxaluria with oxalosis, alcaptonuria with ochronosis, possibly cystine storage disease), and possibly in some

disorders of connective tissues (Hurler's syndrome) (Chap. 399). In addition excessive retention of dietary minerals may occur, as in hemochromatosis (Chap. 107) and Wilson's disease (Chap. 110). Tophaceous gout represents a special case, with excessive production and/or renal retention of a metabolic end product, uric acid (Chap. 106). Most of the above disorders have been described elsewhere in this book. This chapter will be concerned only with certain storage diseases of amino acid metabolism.

ALCAPTONURIA AND OCHRONOSIS

Definition

Alcaptonuria, one of the original inborn errors of metabolism studied by Garrod, is a rare disorder in the degradative pathway of phenylalanine and tyrosine metabolism. The genetic defect in the activity of the enzyme homogentisic acid oxidase leads to the accumulation and excessive urinary excretion of homogentisic acid. There is an associated deposition of dark pigment in connective tissues (ochronosis) and a particular form of degenerative arthritis. Over 600 cases have been reported.

Genetics and Pathogenesis

Homogentisic acid, a normal intermediate in the metabolism of phenylalanine and tyrosine, is oxidized with opening of the phenyl ring to form maleylacetoacetic acid. The enzyme homogentisic acid oxidase, which catalyzes this step, has been found to be missing in activity in liver and kidney from patients with alcaptonuria. The disease seems to be transmitted as an autosomal mendelian trait, with a frequency of about one in 200,000 births. No biochemical method for detection of presumed heterozygotes has been devised, nor do they exhibit any of the clinical features of the disease. The renal excretion of excessive homogentisic acid (3 to 7 Gm per day) fully accounts for the reducing properties of urine, gentisic acid being the only other metabolite excreted in excess. At neutral pH or above, homogentisic acid is rapidly oxidized to a brown or black polymer, with darkening of the urine on standing and with staining of wet diapers or linen. The slower accumulation in the body of a similar polymer bound to cartilage and other connective tissues is presumably the origin of ochronosis. Recently an enzyme has been described in skin and cartilage which oxidizes homogentisic acid to a melanin-like polymer. The mechanism by which this oxidation produces cartilagenous degeneration and arthritis is not clear.

Clinical Presentation and Diagnosis

Alcaptonuria is a benign disorder until middle life, when degenerative joint changes begin in the majority of cases. Prior to this time the darkening of urine is often unnoticed, although a positive but atypical Benedict's test for urine glucose may call it to one's attention. The increasing use of the glucose oxidase test will diminish this method of discovery. With the onset of arthritis, the large joints and the spine are affected with pain and stiffness, interspersed with periods of acute inflammation, which may resemble rheumatoid arthritis. Limitation of motion of the joints and ankylosis of the lumbosacral spine often occur later in the course. The roentgenogram of the spine is often almost pathognomonic, with degeneration and dense calcification of the intervertebral disks and resulting narrowing of the spaces. Ochronotic pigmentation may often be seen in the transmitted blueness of cartilages of the ear, nose, and costochondral junctions, and in brown areas in the sclerae, most frequently located at the insertions of the lateral rectus muscles. A high incidence of degenerative cardiovascular disease has been described in older ochronotic patients, but a cause-and-effect relationship has not been firmly established. The diagnosis is usually made from the triad of *arthritis, ochronotic pigmentation,* and *urine which darkens* on the addition of strong alkali. As noted, the urine reduces alkaline copper solutions, but since it turns black in the process, the erroneous diagnosis of glucosuria can be avoided. Homogentisic aciduria can be further identified by the ability of the urine to blacken undeveloped photographic film exposed to light. It may be conclusively demonstrated by chemical tests, chromatographic characteristics, or a specific enzymatic assay. Reversible acquired ochronosis has been described in the past after the prolonged use of carbolic acid dressings for cutaneous ulcers.

Treatment

Alcaptonuria carries with it no metabolic disadvantage other than the deposition of polymerized pigment in connective tissues and the associated degenerative changes. Ascorbic acid, as a strong reducing agent, will impede the oxidation and polymerization of homogentisic acid in vitro. Its use in large doses has been suggested as a possible means of preventing pigment formation and deposition in ochronotics, but its efficacy has not been demonstrated. The long and relatively benign course of the illness discourages attempts at rigid control of phenylalanine or tyrosine in the diet. Symptomatic treatment is similar to that of osteoarthritis (Chap. 387).

PRIMARY HYPEROXALURIA AND OXALOSIS

Definition

Primary hyperoxaluria is a genetic disorder characterized biochemically by continued excessive urinary excretion of oxalic acid and clinically by calcium oxalate nephrolithiasis and nephrocalcinosis. At postmortem examination calcium oxalate is usually found to be widely deposited in the tissues, a condition called oxalosis. In its typical form primary hyperoxaluria generally leads to uremia and early death. A few milder cases have been described in adult life with recurrent calcium oxalate kidney stones.

Genetics and Pathogenesis

Primary hyperoxaluria has been shown to represent two distinct genetic disorders, associated with glycolic aciduria and L-glyceric aciduria, respectively. They are described here together, since both diseases have similar levels of urinary oxalate and are indistinguishable clinically. The excessive synthesis of oxalate results from a block in an alternate route of metabolism of its precursor, glyoxylic acid. In glycolic aciduria the activity of the enzyme α-ketoglutarate:glyoxylate carboligase, which catalyzes the synthesis of α-hydroxy-β-keto adipic acid, has been found to be markedly reduced in liver, spleen, and kidney preparations. The resulting expansion of the glyoxylate pool behind the site of the metabolic block leads to its excessive oxidation to oxalic acid and reduction to glycolic acid. All three of these 2-carbon acids are excreted in increased amounts in the urine. The disease seems most likely to be transmitted as an autosomal Mendelian recessive trait, but no means of detecting presumed heterozygotes has been found. In L-glyceric aciduria there is absent activity of D-glyceric dehydrogenase (demonstrated in leukocytes), an enzyme which catalyzes the reduction of hydroxypyruvic acid in the catabolic pathway of serine metabolism. The accumulated hydroxypyruvate is reduced by lactic dehydrogenase to the unnatural L isomer of glyceric acid, which is excreted in the urine. D-Glyceric dehydrogenase appears to be the same enzyme as glyoxylate reductase which is an explanation for the accompanying excessive synthesis and excretion of oxalic acid. L-Glyceric aciduria is transmitted as an autosomal recessive trait and partial reductions in D-glyceric dehydrogenase activity are found in heterozygotes. The pathogenesis of stone formation, nephrocalcinosis, and oxalosis seems to relate directly to the insolubility of calcium oxalate. The disease can be simulated in animals, and in man, by pyridoxine deficiency, which presumably inhibits the transamination of glyoxylate to glycine. Glycolic acid and L-glyceric acid have no known toxic effects.

Clinical Presentation and Diagnosis

Primary hyperoxaluria usually presents in childhood with recurrent kidney stones, with or without radiographically demonstrable nephrocalcinosis (Chap. 307). Rarely renal failure secondary to nephrocalcinosis may be the initial finding. The course of the childhood form of the disease is usually that of progressive renal failure leading to death from uremia. In adults kidney stones are frequent and occasionally mild nephrocalcinosis is found, but renal function is usually well preserved. The diagnosis is established by demonstrating excessive excretion of oxalic acid in the absence of pyridoxine deficiency. The normal child or adult excretes less than 60 mg oxalic acid/$1.73m^2$/24 hr. Patients with primary hyperoxaluria usually excrete at least two or three times that amount. The differential diagnosis of the glycolic aciduria (most frequent) and L-glyceric aciduria subvariants depends on specific measurements of those metabolites in urine.

Treatment

There is no specific treatment for primary hyperoxaluria at this time. Large doses of pyridoxine (100 mg per day) may reduce urine oxalate, but the effect is not striking. Measures which may reduce the risk of stone formation are of use, such as forcing fluids, the use of a high phosphate regimen, and oral magnesium oxide (Chap. 307). Because of the seriousness of the disorder, attempts are being made to develop an inhibitor of oxalate synthesis, comparable to the use of allopurinol in gout.

CYSTINOSIS AND FANCONI'S SYNDROME

Definition

Cystine storage disease, or cystinosis (Lignac-de Toni-Fanconi syndrome), is a rare genetic disorder, usually found in childhood in association with Fanconi's syndrome. Rarely, ocular and systemic cystine storage occurs in an adult form in the absence of renal disease. Fanconi's syndrome is a descriptive phrase for a group of physiologic abnormalities which occur with proximal renal tubular dysfunction, notably glucosuria, generalized aminoaciduria, phosphaturia, and renal tubular acidosis. Cystinosis is only one of many diseases which may be associated with Fanconi's syndrome, a classification of which is given in Table 103-1.

Table 103-1. CLASSIFICATIONS OF FANCONI'S SYNDROME

I. Idiopathic
   A. Sporadic
   B. Familial
II. As part of a genetic disease
   A. Cystinosis
   B. Wilson's disease
   C. Tyrosinemia
   D. Lowe's syndrome
   E. Hereditary fructose intolerance (with fructose)
III. Medullary cystic disease
IV. Acquired
   A. Abnormality of protein metabolism
      1. Nephrotic syndrome
      2. Multiple myeloma
      3. Sjögren's syndrome
      4. Amyloidosis
   B. Drugs
      1. Outdated tetracycline
      2. 6-Mercaptopurine
      3. Isophthalanilide
   C. Heavy metals
      1. Mercury
      2. Uranium
      3. Cadmium
   D. Malignancy
V. Experimental (animals)
   A. Maleic acid
   B. Malonic acid

SOURCE: After R. C. Morris, Jr., The Clinical Spectrum of Fanconi's Syndrome, Calif. Med., 108:225, 1968.

Genetics and Pathogenesis

The metabolic defect resulting in cystine storage has not yet been discovered. A number of enzymes in cystine metabolism have been assayed without finding any consistent abnormality, and earlier claims of reduced levels of blood cystine reductase have not been confirmed. Marked increases in cystine have been found in circulating leukocytes and in fibroblasts grown in tissue culture from patients with cystinosis. The free cystine is compartmentalized within the "granular" fraction of the cell. The disease seems to be transmitted as an autosomal recessive trait, with heterozygotes demonstrating intermediate levels of intracellular cystine. Plasma cystine levels are usually normal or slightly elevated only. The biochemical link between cystine storage and proximal renal tubular dysfunction is obscure in the childhood form of the disease and missing in adults. Cystine has the ability to form mixed disulfides with sulfhydryl groups. It has been suggested that the injurious effect of cystine storage may result from inhibition of sulfhydryl-containing enzymes by the formation of half-cystine residues on the proteins.

As outlined in Table 103-1, Fanconi's syndrome may be of diverse origins, both inherited and acquired. It represents a nonspecific pattern of failure of proximal renal tubular absorptive function, varying greatly in the degree of severity and the spectrum of functions impaired. The individual disease processes will not be discussed here. In idiopathic Fanconi's syndrome and that associated with cystinosis, microdissection studies have demonstrated a consistent structural change in the proximal tubule, the so-called "swan neck deformity." The proximal tubule is shortened and exhibits atrophy with flattened epithelium in the region adjacent to a normal-appearing glomerulus.

Clinical Presentation and Diagnosis

Cystine storage disease with Fanconi's syndrome is a serious disorder which usually leads to death from uremia by the age of ten. Failure to thrive and severe resistant rickets with stunting of growth develop in the first few months of life. Rickets results from several derangements: (1) failure of tubular reabsorption of phosphate with hypophosphatemia, (2) proximal renal tubular acidosis with bicarbonate wastage and chronic systemic acidosis, (3) hypercalcuria secondary to acidosis, and (4) the inhibition of osteoid calcification (vitamin D resistance) produced by azotemia. A more complete description of rickets and osteomalacia is presented elsewhere in this book (Chap. 83). Secondary hyperparathyroidism is a frequent complication. Glucosuria may be scanty and intermittent or profuse and constant at a normal blood glucose level; it is sometimes sufficient to produce ketosis and contribute to further exacerbation of acidosis. Excessive urinary loss of potassium associated with renal tubular acidosis may lead to hypokalemia with muscle weakness or paralysis. Potassium depletion may produce "clear-cell nephropathy" with further deterioration of renal tubular function, especially a renal tubular concentration defect productive of polyuria. Generalized aminoaciduria occurs, with a nonspecific pattern. Although cystine is usually excreted in excess, the urinary concentration is not sufficient to lead to cystine kidney stones. Hypouricemia may result from failure of reabsorption of uric acid.

It has been recently found that patients with Fanconi's syndrome excrete lysozyme in the urine as well. Pyelonephritis is frequent and may contribute, along with interstitial fibrosis, to the onset of renal failure. The idiopathic Fanconi's syndrome may occur in an identical clinical and pathologic combination except for the absence of cystine storage. Individual patients may exhibit some but not all of the proximal tubular defects. The clinical presentation may be dominated by other manifestations of the primary disease productive of Fanconi's syndrome (Table 103-1). Rarely, cystinosis may occur in the adult in the absence of renal dysfunction (Cogan's syndrome). Crystalline rods or plates of cystine are found in the cornea and conjunctiva as the only manifestation of adult cystinosis. Similar ocular cystinosis occurs in the infantile form of cystinosis.

The diagnosis of Fanconi's syndrome depends on the demonstration of the characteristic pattern of proximal renal tubular defects, of which the most important are phosphaturia, generalized aminoaciduria, glucosuria, and renal tubular acidosis of the proximal (bicarbonate flooding) type. All these defects may be found individually or in various combinations, and may even vary with time in a given patient. It is therefore most useful to describe the actual physiologic derangements rather than to take refuge in the eponym. Cystinosis as cystine crystals may be demonstrated by slit-lamp examination of the eye, or may be found in bone marrow or circulating leukocytes. Cystinotic leukocytes have very high levels of cystine by chemical analysis, even in the absence of demonstrable crystals.

Treatment

Treatment would logically be directed toward the disease resulting in Fanconi's syndrome and toward replacement therapy to compensate for renal dysfunction. Some of the diseases listed in Table 103-1 can be treated (Wilson's disease, hereditary fructose intolerance, etc.); others cannot. In the absence of specific information about its biochemical defect, attempts to treat cystinosis have generally been unrewarding. The use of D-penicillamine or dimercaptopropanol has been advocated in an attempt to regenerate active sulfhydryl groups on enzymes (see Wilson's disease, Chap. 110). Further information will be required to evaluate the hypothesis on which this form of treatment is based, as well as its efficacy. Cystine is synthesized from the essential amino acid methionine, so that specific dietary treatment has not been vigorously pursued. Treatment of the secondary physiologic derangements has been more successful and has been directed toward replacement of calcium, phosphate, sodium, and potassium to reverse chronic acidosis, rickets (osteomalacia in the adult), and hypokalemia. Large amounts of vitamin D are required (usually 50,000 to 400,000 IU daily) to promote normal calcification of bone. It has been reported that vitamin D may improve certain parameters of tubular function as well, reducing aminoaciduria, glucosuria, and bicarbonate wasting. Shohl's solution (98 Gm sodium citrate and 140 Gm citric acid per liter) is a suitable source of buffer base for chronic treatment of acidosis. Chronic potassium supplementation is not usually required after its initial repletion and the correction of acidosis. Improved healing of rickets may occur with supplemental phosphate if phosphaturia is severe. Despite considerable symptomatic improvement and healing of rickets, progressive renal damage in cystinosis leads to early death from uremia. Adult cystinosis is a benign disorder which does not require treatment. The treatment of adult Fanconi's syndrome is similar to that described for the infantile form, but the prognosis is much better (for detailed therapy see Chap. 104, pp. 592 to 593).

REFERENCES

Cogan, D. G., T. Kuwabara, and C. S. Hurlbut, Jr.: Further Observations on Cystinosis in the Adult, J.A.M.A., 160: 1725, 1958.

Hockaday, T. D. R., J. E. Clayton, E. W. Frederick, and L. H. Smith, Jr.: Primary Hyperoxaluria, Medicine, 43:315, 1964.

La Du, B. N.: Alcaptonuria, p. 303 in "The Metabolic Basis of Inherited Disease," 2d ed., J. B. Stanbury, J. B. Wyngaarden, and D. S. Fredrickson (Eds.), New York, McGraw-Hill Book Company, 1966.

Leaf, A.: The Syndrome of Osteomalacia, Renal Glycosuria, Aminoaciduria, and Increased Phosphorus Clearance (the Fanconi Syndrome), p. 1205 in "The Metabolic Basis of Inherited Disease," 2d ed., J. B. Stanbury, J. B. Wyngaarden, and D. S. Fredrickson (Eds.), New York, McGraw-Hill Book Company, 1966.

Morris, R. C., Jr.: The Clinical Spectrum of Fanconi's Syndrome, Calif. Med., 108:225, 1968.

O'Brien, W. M., B. N. La Du, and J. J. Bunim: Biochemical, Pathologic, and Clinical Aspects of Alcaptonuria, Ochronosis, and Ochronotic Arthropathy, Am. J. Med., 34:813, 1963.

Schneider, J. A., F. M. Rosenbloom, K. H. Bradley, and J. E. Seegmiller: Increased Free-cystine Content of Fibroblasts Cultured from Patients with Cystinosis, Biochem. Biophys. Res. Commun., 29:527, 1967.

Williams, H. E., and L. H. Smith, Jr.: L-Glyceric Aciduria: New Genetic Variant of Primary Hyperoxaluria, New Engl. J. Med., 278:233, 1968.

—— and ——: Disorders of Oxalate Metabolism, Am. J. Med., 45:715, 1968.

Wyngaarden, J. B., and T. D. Elder: Primary Hyperoxaluria and Oxalosis, p. 189 in "The Metabolic Basis of Inherited Disease," 2d ed., J. B. Stanbury, J. B. Wyngaarden, and D. S. Fredrickson (Eds.), New York, McGraw-Hill Book Company, 1966.

104 ERRORS IN MEMBRANE TRANSPORT

Lloyd H. Smith, Jr.

The transfer of metabolites across cell membranes is usually an active energy-requiring process of considerable specificity. The enzymology of these processes and the required structural characteristics of cell membranes are poorly understood, although this now represents an important area of biochemical and biophysical investigation. A number of diseases in man are best described as genetic defects in active transport of specific substances across epithelial cell membranes. In none of them has a specific enzymatic or structural defect been identified, other than in the description of the functional derangement. It is possible that defects may occur in the active transport of metabolites among the specific compartments or organelles within cells.

Some of the genetic diseases which might be classified as errors in membrane transport are cystinuria; Hartnup disease; hereditary renal tubular acidosis; renal glycosuria, familial renal gout; vasopressin—resistant diabetes insipidus; congenital hemolytic anemia with high sodium, low potassium in the red cells; familial goiter with iodide transport defect; methionine malabsorption syndrome; isolated tryptophan malabsorption (blue diaper syndrome); glucose and galactose malabsorption disease; congenital alkalosis with diarrhea (chloridorrhea); and hereditary intestinal malabsorption of vitamin B_{12}. Hemochromatosis might qualify in this category as an error of excessive transport of iron. There are data which suggest that vitamin D–resistant rickets ("phosphate diabetes") represents a defect in vitamin D metabolism rather than a primary transport defect. Similarly cystinosis with the Fanconi syndrome seems to represent a disorder in cystine metabolism rather than a primary renal tubular defect. This section will be limited to brief presentations of cystinuria, Hartnup disease, renal glycosuria, and hereditary renal tubular acidosis.

CYSTINURIA

Definition

Cystinuria is a genetic disorder (or group of closely related disorders) characterized by continued excessive excretion of the dibasic amino acids cystine, lysine, arginine, and ornithine. This results from a transport defect for these amino acids in the renal tubule. Similar transport defects occur in the intestinal mucosa. The sole clinical manifestations are those of recurrent cystine kidney stones and their sequelae. Patients tend to be of short stature, which has been attributed, without supporting evidence, to lysine deficiency.

Genetics and Pathogenesis

Cystinuria has been known to be a familial disease for almost a century. It was one of the four original "inborn errors of metabolism" studied by Sir Archibald Garrod, who demonstrated its transmission in a pattern consistent with autosomal recessive inheritance. Further advances awaited the application of modern methods of amino acid analysis and the study of transport in kidney and in gut mucosal biopsies in vitro. In approximately two-thirds of the family (parents and children) of affected patients, the presumed heterozygotes have normal levels of urinary dibasic amino acid excretion. In the remaining families heterozygotes excrete increased amounts of cystine and lysine. At least one additional phenotype can be identified on the basis of intestinal transport studies. Several families have been studied with different genetic types in conjugal heterozygotes of cystinuria. The resulting patterns of double heterozygote defects have been interpreted as evidence for multiple allelic mutations. The incidence of homozygous cystinuria is approximately 1:20,000.

For many years cystinuria was attributed to a defect in cystine metabolism and was often confused with cystine storage disease (cystinosis). Dent and Rose first demonstrated by clearance techniques that impaired renal tubular reabsorption of the specific amino acids cystine, lysine, and arginine was the explanation of aminoaciduria. Subsequent studies indicated similar defects in tubular reabsorption of ornithine and more recently homocysteine, the mixed disulfide of cysteine. Clearance of cystine may significantly exceed glomerular filtration rate, indicating net tubular secretion of this amino acid. Plasma levels of the four amino acids are reduced. A common mechanism in the kidney has been confirmed by competition of the amino acids for transport during infusion in vitro and in part in tissue slice preparations of kidney in vitro. It has not been possible to demonstrate a defect in cystine transport in vitro in renal biopsies from patients with cystinuria.

The transport defect for dibasic amino acids in cystinuria is also found in the gut. This was first demonstrated by oral tolerance tests. It has been clearly confirmed in studies of active transport in jejunal mucosal biopsy specimens in vitro. With impaired absorption, lysine and ornithine are decarboxylated by intestinal bacteria to cadaverine and putrescine, respectively. These diamines are partially metabolized to pyrrolidine and piperidine, and all these compounds are excreted in increased amounts in cystinuric urine. No impairment of amino acid transport has been found in tissues other than the renal tubules and the gut mucosa in cystinuria.

Normal urinary excretion of cystine varies with size and diet, but has an upper normal range of about 18 mg per Gm creatinine. In homozygous cystinuria cystine excretion usually varies between 0.4 to 1.0 Gm per day, although values as high as 3.0 Gm per day have been found. The solubility of cystine in urine is approximately 350 to 400 mg per liter. Supersaturation and crystallization readily occur, particularly during nocturnal concentration of the urine. The accretion of such crystals as stones, with the resulting complications of obstruction and infection, is the direct cause of disability in cystinuria.

Diagnosis

The clinical manifestations of cystine kidney stones are indistinguishable from those of other kidney stones: flank pain, colic, hematuria, obstructive uropathy, infection. Cystine stones are as densely radiopaque as calcium-containing kidney stones. In overall incidence they constitute approximately 1 to 2 percent of all kidney stones. It is important to establish the composition of kidney stones in order to institute rational programs of stone prophylaxis (Chap. 307).

The most direct diagnostic procedure is that of stone analysis because cystine stones occur only in the genetic disorder cystinuria. The appearance of cystine crystals in the sediment of concentrated, acidified (addition of glacial acetic acid to pH 4.5), chilled urine specimens usually indicates a cystine concentration of greater than 200 to 250 mg per liter. The crystals are hexagonal plates resembling the formula of a benzene ring. The nitroprusside test for cystine is a nonspecific reaction for sulfhydryl groups after reduction of disulfides by sodium cyanide. It can be made semiquantitative for cystine in the absence of other sulfhydryl compounds.

The specific aminoaciduria of cystine, lysine, arginine, and ornithine can be directly demonstrated by paper or ion exchange column chromatography of urine. This pattern is diagnostic of genetic cystinuria. The urinary amino acid pattern of cystinuria may sometimes be found in the rare disorder of familial pancreatitis.

Treatment

As a genetic disease cystinuria cannot be "cured" in the host (except by renal homotransplantation). In order to prevent formation and growth of stones, attempts are made to reduce the concentration of cystine in urine and to increase the solubility of cystine at a given urine concentration. Urinary excretion of cystine can sometimes be minimized by a diet low in methionine, the most important cystine precursor. Of greater practicality, cystine concentration can be reduced by increasing urine volume by forcing fluids, especially at night. Some increase in cystine solubility is obtained by alkalinizing the urine, but the solubility curve rises steeply only at pHs higher than 7.2.

A promising new approach is that of forming mixed disulfides of cysteine with other sulfhydryl compounds with enhancement of solubility. The use of D-penicillamine (1.0 to 2.0 Gm daily) leads to the excretion of a soluble cysteine-penicillamine disulfide (solubility fifty times greater than cystine) with reduction of cystine excretion below saturation concentrations. The toxicity of D-penicillamine has stimulated current attempts to find more suitable compounds with similar properties.

HARTNUP DISEASE

Hartnup disease (also called H disease) is a genetic disorder of the transport of a group of monoamino-monocarboxylic acids which share a common transport mechanism in the renal tubule and in the gut mucosa. The disease, so far described in about 25 patients, seems to be the homozygous manifestation of an autosomal recessive trait; the heterozygous state is not detectable by current techniques. Hartnup disease is characterized by massive aminoaciduria of alanine, serine, threonine, asparagin, glutamine, valine, leucine, isoleucine, phenylalanine, tyrosine, tryptophan, histidine, and citrulline. In contrast to cystinuria, the associated gut defect is more

important in producing the symptoms of the disease—intermittent pellagra-like rash appearing after exposure to sunlight, attacks of cerebellar ataxia often accompanying the skin manifestations, and psychiatric changes varying from emotional instability to dementia. Impaired absorption allows for bacterial degradation of amino acids which may (1) lead to nicotinamide deficiency from loss of precursor tryptophan, thereby producing pellagra, and (2) allow for the production and absorption of toxic metabolic products injurious to the central nervous system. The specific amino acid metabolites responsible for the signs and symptoms of cerebral and cerebellar dysfunction have not been identified. The diagnosis can be established by the pattern of urinary amino acids, measured by paper or ion exchange chromatography. Most patients respond well to maintenance treatment with oral nicotinamide (50 to 200 mg per day). A high protein diet is also recommended to counter the amino acid loss in the gut and in the urine.

RENAL GLYCOSURIA
Definition

Renal glycosuria is a genetic disorder in which glucose is excreted in the urine at normal concentrations of blood glucose. In order to avoid confusion with other conditions associated with melituria, Marble's strict criteria should be followed (Chap. 95): (1) glycosuria occurs in the absence of hyperglycemia; (2) all specimens of urine should contain glucose with relatively little fluctuation in glycosuria related to diet; (3) the oral glucose tolerance test is normal (sometimes slightly flat); (4) the reducing substance is specifically identified as glucose, ruling out other meliturias such as pentosuria, fructosuria, galactosuria, sucrosuria, maltosuria, mannoheptulosuria; (5) the storage and utilization of carbohydrates are normal. By these criteria, including the absence of other disorders of proximal renal tubular function, renal glycosuria can be identified as a rare (94 cases in 50,000 cases of melituria at the Joslin Clinic) isolated transport defect. Use of the more liberal criteria proposed by Lawrence, i.e., glycosuria which occurs with a normal glucose tolerance test, will detect many more abnormalities.

Genetics and Pathogenesis

Current information is most consistent with the transmission of renal glycosuria as a mendelian dominant characteristic, although the suggestion has been made that the defect may be expressed in heterozygotes with homozygotes representing severer forms of the disease. Diabetes mellitus is frequently found in the families of patients with renal glycosuria; whether renal glycosuria defined by the strict Marble criteria is a precursor of diabetes is disputed. Many patients with renal glycosuria by the Lawrence criteria will develop clinical diabetes mellitus within a few years of diagnosis.

No consistent structural alteration has been demonstrated in the renal tubule by light or electron microscopy. Most studies of the renal defect have been carried out by classical clearance techniques. Plasma glucose is completely filterable in the glomerulus and is reabsorbed by an active process in the proximal tubule. The biochemical basis of active reabsorption of glucose has not been demonstrated; specifically, no intermediary product has been found. Reabsorption exhibits saturation kinetics with a transfer maximum (TM) of about 250 to 325 mg glucose per min in the normal adult. Clearance studies in renal glycosuria have failed to yield a consistent pattern. In some patients a low TM for glucose has been found; in others the TM has been normal but there has been an increased splay in the curve describing the relationship of glucose reabsorbed to that filtered. Renal glycosuria could result from any one of the following defects: decrease in the anatomic mass of the proximal tubule in relation to its glomerulus (glomerulotubular imbalance), abnormal distribution of the transport system relative to glomerular filtration whether on a functional or anatomic basis, an abnormality in the presumed enzymatic step or steps (permeability, hypothetical membrane carrier, energy-yielding reactions) which constitute the active transport process. It is likely that there may be different genetic and pathogenetic forms of the disease.

Diagnosis and Clinical Implications

The criteria for diagnosis have been included in the definition. It is important to identify the reducing substance as glucose (by glucose oxidase, for example) and also to rule out other primary or secondary renal tubular defects (aminoaciduria, phosphaturia, renal tubular acidosis, etc.) The recently described disorder of glucose and galactose malabsorption is characterized by impaired intestinal absorption of these monosaccharides and renal glycosuria. The prognosis of renal glycosuria appears to be excellent except insofar as it may herald subsequent clinical diabetes. No treatment is required.

RENAL TUBULAR ACIDOSIS

Definition

Renal tubular acidosis (RTA) is a clinical disorder characterized by inability of the kidney to excrete an appropriately acid urine. This results in a persistent metabolic acidosis with hyperchloremia, and may be complicated by potassium depletion and/or hypercalcuria. RTA may occur as an isolated tubular defect or as one component of more extensive tubular dysfunction (such as in the De Toni-Fanconi syndrome). It has been described in association with glycogenosis, cystinosis, galactosemia, Wilson's disease, Lowe's syndrome, hereditary fructose intolerance, thyrotoxicosis, cadmium poisoning, and in a variety of disorders associated with hypergammaglobulinemia. The syndrome of RTA may be closely simulated by the chronic administration of potent carbonic anhydrase inhibitors. Its extracellular fluid pattern of hyperchloremic acidosis may be found following bilateral ureterosigmoid transplantations, during the in-

gestion of large amounts of ammonium chloride, or in some patients with chronic pyelonephritis.

Genetics and Pathogenesis

Although often secondary to other metabolic disorders, RTA may occur with otherwise normal or nearly normal renal function and in the absence of associated diseases. Some of these cases have appeared to be sporadic; others have exhibited definite familial aggregation. The pattern of inheritance, including transmission in three successive generations, is consistent with a mendelian dominant trait. It seems unlikely that the transient infantile form of RTA, with a negative family history, represents the same disorder.

A complete discussion of the pathogenesis of RTA would demand a full treatment of the role of the kidney in the defense of acid-base balance. In brief, the kidney serves this homeostatic function in several closely related ways: by excretion of certain anionic products of metabolism (phosphate, sulfate), by conservation of filtered bicarbonate, by tubular secretion of hydrogen ions in exchange for sodium, and by tubular synthesis and excretion of ammonia. In RTA phosphate and sulfate excretions are not impaired in the absence of secondary renal failure. Normally the filtered bicarbonate is reclaimed in the proximal renal tubule by hydrogen ion secretion, and the TM for bicarbonate reabsorption is normal. The excretion of ammonia is often reduced, but only in proportion to the reduced urine acidity. The most plausible mechanism for RTA is that of inability of the distal renal tubule to develop a steep H+ gradient between extracellular fluid and tubular urine. This transport defect or "gradient defect" for H+ in the distal tubule results in reduced urine titratable acidity and ammonia, increased urinary loss of sodium and potassium (due to increased tubular exchange of potassium in lieu of H+ for sodium), and systemic acidosis. Sustained acidosis results in mobilization of calcium from bone and hypercalcuria. A few patients have been described with "proximal RTA," i.e., a partial failure of bicarbonate reabsorption with flooding of the normal distal tubular acidification mechanism.

Diagnosis and Clinical Implications

The diagnosis of RTA depends upon demonstration of impaired acidification of the urine in the face of systemic acidosis and in the absence of uremia. In mild cases this may require a further acid challenge (0.1 Gm ammonium chloride per kg body weight). The serum chloride is usually elevated commensurate with the reduction in serum bicarbonate. Other disorders noted above which may lead to secondary impairment of renal tubular acidification must be excluded. The most important complications of RTA are potassium depletion (weakness, paralysis, secondary renal tubular dysfunction), hypercalcuria (nephrocalcinosis, nephrolithiasis, osteomalacia, or rickets), pyelonephritis, and renal failure secondary to these factors.

Treatment

Acidosis, hypercalcuria, and potassium wasting are usually corrected by the oral administration of 1.0 to 1.5 mEq/kg/day of sodium bicarbonate, given in three divided doses. Alkali replacement may be better tolerated as Shohl's solution (140 Gm citric acid and 98 Gm hydrated crystals of sodium citrate per liter), given in a dosage of 50 to 100 ml per day in divided doses. The amount of alkali given should be sufficient to return the serum bicarbonate and pH to a normal range. Supplementary potassium and/or calcium and vitamin D may be required temporarily until body stores of these minerals have been repleted.

REFERENCES

Barron, D. N., C. E. Dent, H. Harris, E. W. Hart, and J. B. Jepson: Hereditary Pellagra-like Skin Rash with Temporary Cerebellar Ataxia, Constant Renal Amino-Aciduria and Other Bizarre Biochemical Features, Lancet, 2:421, 1956.

Bartter, F. C., M. Lotz, S. Thier, L. E. Rosenberg, and J. T. Potts: Cystinuria, Combined Clinical Staff Conference at the National Institutes of Health, Ann. Intern. Med., 62:796, 1965.

Crawhall, J. C., and R. W. E. Watts: Cystinuria, Am. J. Med., 45:736, 1968.

Gill, J. R., Jr., N. H. Bell, and F. C. Bartter: Impaired Conservation of Sodium and Potassium in Renal Tubular Acidosis and Its Correction by Buffer Anions, Clin. Sci., 33:577, 1967.

Jepson, J. B.: Hartnup Disease, p. 1283 in J. B. Stanbury, J. B. Wyngaarden, and D. S. Fredrickson (Eds.), "The Metabolic Basis of Inherited Disease," 2d ed., New York, McGraw-Hill Book Company, 1966.

Krane, S. M.: Renal Glycosuria, p. 1221 in J. B. Stanbury, J. B. Wyngaarden, and D. S. Fredrickson (Eds.), "The Metabolic Basis of Inherited Disease," 2d ed., New York, McGraw-Hill Book Company, 1966.

Lawrence, R. D.: Symptomless Glycosurias: Differentiation by Sugar Tolerance Tests, Med. Clin. N. Am., 31:289, 1947.

Marble, A.: Non-Diabetic Melituria, in E. P. Joslin, H. F. Root, P. White, and A. Marble (Eds.), "The Treatment of Diabetes Mellitus," Philadelphia, Lea & Febiger, 1959.

Milne, M. D., A. M. Asatoor, K. D. G. Edwards, and L. W. Loughridge: The Intestinal Absorption Defect in Cystinuria, Gut, 2:323, 1961.

Morris, R. C., Jr.: Renal Tubular Acidosis: Mechanisms, Classification and Implications; New Engl. J. Med., 281:1405, 1969.

Relman, A. S.: Renal Acidosis and Renal Excretion of Acid in Health and Disease, Advances Intern. Med., 12:295, 1964.

Seldin, D. W., and J. D. Wilson: Renal Tubular Acidosis, p. 1230 in J. B. Stanbury, J. B. Wyngaarden, and D. S. Fredrickson (Eds.): "The Metabolic Basis of Inherited Disease," 2d ed., New York, McGraw-Hill Book Company, 1966.

105 THE CARCINOID SYNDROME
John A. Oates

The association of carcinoid tumors with cutaneous flushes, telangiectasia, diarrhea, cardiac valvular lesions, and bronchial constriction eluded recognition until 1953. Once this connection was established by Thorson, Biörk, Björkman, and Waldenström, and independently by Isler and Hedinger, it was clear that the syndrome was mediated by release of one or more biologically active agents by the tumor. Serotonin was the first such agent to be discovered, and overproduction of this amine is the most consistent biochemical indicator of the carcinoid syndrome. Serotonin, however, is not the sole mediator of the clinical syndrome. These tumors vary in their metabolism of indoles and may elaborate chemically unrelated agents such as bradykinin, histamine, and adrenocorticotropic hormone (ACTH). Furthermore, there is evidence suggesting that an additional unidentified substance participates in the production of flushing. Within the broad classification of carcinoid tumors there is great diversity in the production of biologically active substances and in the mechanisms for their storage and release. Accordingly, there is a varied spectrum of clinical manifestations.

Pathologic Anatomy of the Tumor

Carcinoid tumors are slowly growing neoplasms of enterochromaffin cells. The metastatic tumors associated with carcinoid syndrome usually arise from small primary tumors in the ileum. The syndrome is also produced by neoplasms arising from the remainder of the small intestine, from organs derived from the embryonic foregut (e.g., bronchus, stomach, pancreas, and thyroid), and from ovarian or testicular teratomas.

Carcinoid tumors have an unusual proclivity for metastasis to the liver and may involve this organ extensively with minimal metastatic disease elsewhere. Extrahepatic metastases occur in bone, where they are often osteoblastic, and in lung, pancreas, spleen, ovaries, adrenals, and other organs.

Primary carcinoid tumors of the appendix neither metastasize nor produce carcinoid syndrome. Those from the large bowel may metastasize but do not exhibit an endocrine function.

The usual carcinoid tumor arising from the ileum has the classical histologic pattern of dense nests of cells with uniform size and nuclear appearance. Histochemically, they typically exhibit an argentaffin reaction in which the cells convert a silver salt to metallic silver. A positive argentaffin reaction is not required for the diagnosis, however, and carcinoid tumors arising from organs of the embryonic foregut do not usually contain many argentaffin cells. Tumors from these organs also have a broad histologic spectrum, which in the lung ranges from typical bronchial carcinoid to a form indistinguishable from oat cell carcinoma.

Clinical Features

Unlike most metastatic neoplasms, carcinoid tumors have an unusually slow rate of growth; most patients survive for 5 to 10 years after the disease is recognized. For much of the duration of the illness, morbidity may result largely from the endocrine function of the tumor. Death results from hepatic or cardiac failure and from complications associated with tumor growth.

VASOMOTOR PAROXYSMS. The most common clinical feature is cutaneous flushing. The typical flush is erythematous and involves the head and neck (blush area). Some patients exhibit vivid color changes from red to violaceous to pallor during its course. Prolonged flushing attacks may be associated with lacrimation and periorbital edema. The systemic effects of the flush are variable. It may be accompanied by tachycardia, and the blood pressure usually falls or does not change. A rise in

Fig. 105-1. Metabolic pathway of serotonin.

blood pressure during flushing is rare, and carcinoid syndrome is not a cause of sustained hypertension.

Flushing may be provoked by excitement, exertion, eating, ethanol, and epinephrine.

TELANGIECTASIA. In addition to paroxysms of cutaneous vasodilation, some patients also develop purple telangiectasia, primarily on the face and neck and most marked in the malar area.

GASTROINTESTINAL SYMPTOMS. Intestinal hypermotility with borborygmi, cramping, and explosive diarrhea may accompany the episodic flushes. Chronic hypermotility with diarrhea is more common. When this is severe, malabsorption can occur.

CARDIAC MANIFESTATIONS. There is a unique deposition of fibrous tissue on the endocardium of the valvular cusps and cardiac chambers. It occurs primarily in the right heart, but may involve the left side to a minimal degree. The fibrous deposition does not penetrate the internal elastic membrane. Distortion of the valve cusps, chordae tendineae, and papillary muscles interferes with valvular function in the right heart and may lead to regurgitation, stenosis, or combined functional lesions. There is, however, a tendency for the fibrosing process to produce incompetence at the tricuspid valve and stenosis of the smaller pulmonary orifice, a deleterious hemodynamic combination. The vasomotor changes in carcinoid syndrome may lead to a high cardiac output, with its attendant imposition on cardiac function.

PULMONARY SYMPTOMS. Bronchoconstriction is a less common feature of the syndrome, but it may be severe. It is usually most pronounced during flushing attacks.

GENERAL. In addition to the endocrine effects, the tumors themselves may cause intestinal obstruction or bleeding. Necrosis of intestinal or hepatic tumor masses may produce abdominal pain, tenderness, fever, and leukocytosis. Hepatomegaly from the metastatic disease is usually present with the syndrome. Extensive metastatic involvement of the liver by these slowly growing tumors may occur before the liver function tests become abnormal.

Endocrine Function of the Tumors

SEROTONIN. The most constant biochemical characteristic of carcinoid tumors is the presence of tryptophan hydroxylase, which catalyzes the formation of 5-hydroxytryptophan (5-HTP) from tryptophan (Fig. 105-1). Most tumors also contain the enzyme aromatic L-amino hydroxylase, which catalyzes the formation of 5-hydroxytryptamine (serotonin). Carcinoids from the stomach and from other organs derived from the embryonic foregut, however, are frequently deficient in this decarboxylase and release 5-HTP from the tumor.

Following its release from the tumor, serotonin is inactivated primarily by the enzyme monoamine oxidase; uptake into platelets also contributes to this inactivation. Monamine oxidase oxidizes serotonin to 5-hydroxyindoleacetaldehyde, which is rapidly converted to 5-hydroxyindoleacetic acid (5HIAA) by aldehyde dehydrogenase.

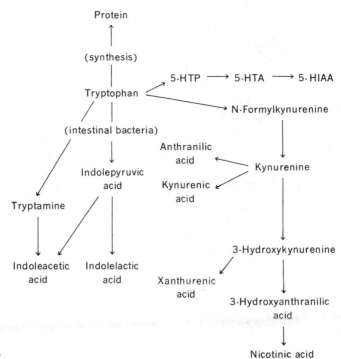

Fig. 105-2. Metabolic pathways of tryptophan.

This acid is rapidly excreted in the urine, and almost all circulating serotonin can be accounted for as urinary 5HIAA.

Carcinoid tumors vary widely in their capacity to store serotonin, with concentrations of the amine in tumors ranging from a few micrograms per gram to 3 mg per Gm. The concentration in the tumor appears unrelated to the rate of synthesis of serotonin as reflected by urinary 5HIAA. Generally, tumors from the ileum have a much higher storage capacity for serotonin than do tumors from organs of the embryonic foregut.

BRADYKININ. A potent vasodilator, bradykinin is released during flushes in some cases of carcinoid syndrome. In a few of these, excessive amounts continue to be released between flushes. Bradykinin and related kinins are formed by the action of a group of enzymes (kallikreins) which split these peptides from kininogen, a plasma globulin. It is thought that bradykinin formation in carcinoid syndrome results from release of a kallikrein from the tumor by catecholamines and possibly other stimuli. In the plasma, this kallikrein then acts on kininogen to form lysyl-bradykinin (a decapeptide), which is rapidly converted to bradykinin (a nonapeptide).

OTHER BIOLOGICALLY ACTIVE SUBSTANCES. Some carcinoid tumors, particularly those of gastric origin, produce and release excessive amounts of histamine. This can be detected by an increased excretion of this amine in the urine.

Carcinoid syndrome has been associated with hyperadrenocorticism in a number of instances. This results from ectopic production of an adrenocorticotropic hormone by the tumors which usually originate from sites other than the ileum (bronchus, pancreas, ovary, and stomach).

In a few cases, "multiple endocrine adenomas" have been seen in conjunction with carcinoids arising from organs of the embryonic foregut. The associated tumors have included parathyroid adenomas and pancreatic tumors producing Zollinger-Ellison syndrome.

Pathophysiology

Serotonin can account for those aspects of the syndrome related to intestinal hypermotility, and there is evidence that the fibrous deposits on the endocardium also result from increased levels of circulating serotonin.

A secondary effect of serotonin overproduction occurs when more than half of dietary tryptophan is shunted into the hydroxylation pathway (Fig. 105-2). This leaves less tryptophan available for the formation of nicotinic acid and protein; when urinary excretion of 5HIAA exceeds 200 to 300 mg daily, low levels of plasma tryptophan and evidence of nicotinamide deficiency are seen.

MECHANISM OF THE FLUSH. The mechanism of the flush is unclear. Release of the flush-provoking substance(s) can be triggered by the catecholamines, and this probably accounts for the association of flushing with excitement and emotional stimuli. For experimental induction of flushing, injection of isoproterenol in amounts as little as 0.5 μg may be effective. Serotonin was originally thought to be the mediator of flushes, but injection of this amine does not mimic the carcinoid flush and patients may exhibit flushes without increased levels of plasma serotonin. Bradykinin is a potent vasodilator, and its injection will simulate one type of carcinoid flush which is characterized by erythema in association with tachycardia and hypotension. Release of this peptide, however, could not be detected in a number of patients during flushing. While bradykinin, serotonin, and histamine may contribute to the varied types of flushes observed in the carcinoid syndrome, there appears to be an additional flush substance which has not yet been identified.

Diagnosis

With its full constellation of clinical features, carcinoid syndrome is easily recognized. The diagnosis also must be considered when any one of its features is present.

The diagnostic hallmark of carcinoid syndrome is *over-production of 5-hydroxyindoles* with *increased urinary excretion of 5-hydroxyindoleacetic acid.* Normally, excretion of 5HIAA does not exceed 9 mg daily. Ingestion of foods containing serotonin may complicate the biochemical diagnosis of carcinoid syndrome; both walnuts and bananas contain enough serotonin to produce abnormally elevated urinary excretion of 5HIAA after their ingestion. Some drugs also interfere with the analysis of urinary 5HIAA; cough syrups containing guaicolate cause falsely elevated values, and phenothiazines interfere with the colorimetric test. When dietary 5-hydroxyindoles are excluded, a urinary excretion of more than 25 mg of 5HIAA daily is diagnostic of carcinoid. Elevations in the range of 9 to 25 mg can be seen with either carcinoid syndrome, nontropical sprue, or acute intestinal obstruction.

Measurement of *serotonin in blood* or platelets is of interest, but has less diagnostic value than assay of the major metabolite of serotonin in the urine.

Measurement of an increased concentration of *serotonin in tumor tissue* is a useful and sometimes necessary supplement to histologic examination. A portion of suspected tumor should always be frozen for serotonin analysis.

Variants of the Syndrome: Relations to Sites of Tumor Origin

The origin of the tumor influences the biologically active substances produced and their storage and release. Carcinoid tumors arising from organs derived from the embryonic foregut (bronchus, stomach, and pancreas) tend to differ from those arising distal to the mid-duodenum (midgut). The typical carcinoid syndrome usually results from tumors of midgut origin, which almost invariably secrete serotonin and rarely release 5-HTP. Tumor serotonin content is likely to be high, and the tumor usually contains dense nests of argentaffin positive cells. Metastasis to bone and skin is infrequent.

In contrast, tumors arising from the embryonic foregut contain fewer argentaffin cells, have lower serotonin content, and may secrete 5-HTP. Hyperadrenocorticism and multiple endocrine adenomas are more likely to be associated with this group, and metastasis to bone and skin is more frequent.

In addition to the general characteristics of the foregut group, certain clinical and biochemical features have been associated with gastric and bronchial carcinoids. Patients with gastric carcinoids frequently exhibit unique flushing which begins as a bright-red patchy erythema with sharply delineated serpentine borders; these patches tend to coalesce as the blush heightens. Food ingestion is especially prone to produce flushes. The tumors usually are deficient in decarboxylase enzyme and secrete 5-HTP; histamine secretion is also common as is a high incidence of peptic ulceration. Diarrhea and heart lesions are not prominent features in the patients who secrete largely 5-HTP from the tumor without much preformed serotonin.

When the carcinoid tumor arises from the bronchus, attacks of flushing tend to be prolonged and severe and may be associated with periorbital edema, excessive lacrimation and salivation, hypotension, tachycardia, anxiety, and tremulousness. Nausea, vomiting, explosive diarrhea, and bronchoconstriction may progress to a severe degree. This group is therapeutically unique in that the severe flushes often can be prevented by corticosteroids, and chlorpromazine may be helpful in relieving the symptomatology.

Treatment

Recognition of the carcinoid syndrome has led to the complete surgical cure of a few patients with tumors arising in ovarian or testicular teratomas or in the bronchus; by releasing their secretions directly into the systemic circulation, tumors from these locations can produce the syndrome before metastatic disease occurs. Because the humoral substances released by tumors draining into the portal circulation are largely metabolized by the liver, tumors arising in this location do not produce the syndrome until hepatic metastases occur. Resection of large isolated hepatic metastases has led to amelioration of symptoms in certain cases.

Pharmacologic therapy directed at the humoral mediators of the syndrome is of benefit in some cases. Methysergide, a serotonin antagonist, will improve the diarrhea, but prolonged therapy with this agent can produce retroperitoneal fibrosis. Blockade of serotonin synthesis with the tryptophan hydroxylase inhibitor *p*-chlorophenylalanine also ameliorates the diarrhea. Nicotinic acid should be given to those patients who shunt a large fraction of dietary tryptophan into the hydroxyindole pathway. The prevention of severe flushing by corticosteroids and amelioration of the syndrome by phenothiazines are limited largely to patients with tumors arising from the bronchus and other organs derived from the embryonic foregut.

Hypotensive episodes should not be treated with catecholamines; by stimulating the release of vasoactive substances from the tumor, norepinephrine and other agents with β adrenergic activity can exaggerate and prolong the circulatory disturbance. If pressor agents must be used, angiotensin or methoxamine are preferred. Of the numerous approaches to chemotherapy of the tumor, the most promising appears to be regional arterial perfusion with agents such as 5-fluorouracil.

REFERENCES

Oates, J. A., and T. C. Butler: Pharmacologic and Endocrine Aspects of Carcinoid Syndrome, Advances Pharmacol., 5:109, 1967.

Robertson, J. I. S., W. S. Pearl, and T. M. Andrews: The Mechanism of Facial Flushing in the Carcinoid Syndrome, Quart. J. Med., 31:103, 1962.

Sjoerdsma, A., H. Weissbach, and S. Undenfriend: A Clinical, Physiologic and Biochemical Study of Patients with Malignant Carcinoid, Am. J. Med., 20:520, 1956.

Thorson, Å., G. Biörck, G. Björkman, and J. Waldenström: Malignant Carcinoid of the Small Intestine with Metastases to the Liver, Valvular Disease of the Right Side of the Heart (Pulmonary Stenosis and Tricuspid Regurgitation without Septal Defects), Peripheral Vasomotor Symptoms, Bronchoconstriction and an Unusual Type of Cyanosis, Am. Heart J., 47:795, 1954.

106   GOUT AND OTHER DISORDERS OF URIC ACID METABOLISM

James B. Wyngaarden

Primary gout is an inborn metabolic disorder manifested by hyperuricemia, recurrent attacks of a characteristic acute arthritis, and tophaceous deposits of sodium urate. Nephrolithiasis and parenchymatous renal disease commonly develop during the course of the illness. Gout is not a single disease, but rather a syndrome resulting from different biochemical abnormalities which lead to hyperuricemia. Secondary gout is an acquired form of the disease which supervenes in the course of a number of disorders in which hyperuricemia occurs.

A classification of gout is presented in Table 106-1.

History

In the fifth century B.C., gout was described as podagra, cheiagra, or gonogra by Hippocrates, depending on whether the big toe, wrist, or knee was involved. Tophi were first described by Galen. The term *gout* is derived from the Latin *gutta*, a drop, and reflects an early belief that the disease was caused by a poison, falling drop by drop into the joint. A drug, probably identical with colchicine, was described in the Ebers Papyrus (1500 B.C.). The agent was known to Byzantine physicians in the fifth century A.D., and was brought to this country from Europe by Benjamin Franklin, who was himself a sufferer from gout. An astonishing list of men of royalty and genius have been afflicted with gout.

The modern clinical history of gout began with Thomas Sydenham, whose surpassing description of the disease (1683), based on 34 years of personal affliction, first clearly differentiated gout from other articular dis-

orders. Uric acid was discovered in a kidney stone by Scheele in 1776. Twenty years later Wollaston and Pearson demonstrated urate in the tophi of patients with gout. Hyperuricemia was discovered by A. B. Garrod in 1848.

When the structure of uric acid was established by Emil Fischer in 1898, its relationship to the purine bases of nucleic acids was at once apparent. The pathways of enzymatic synthesis of purine compounds were elucidated by Buchanan, Greenberg, and others during the 1950s. The first specific enzymatic defect responsible for one subtype of adult primary gout was discovered by Seegmiller and associates in 1966.

Prevalence and Incidence

The prevalence of gout varies from about 0.3 percent in Europe and the United States to 8 percent in adult male Maori of New Zealand. During World Wars I and II acute gouty arthritis was uncommon in Europe. When protein again became plentiful, the incidence returned to prewar levels. Although traditionally considered a disease of middle and upper social classes, gout involves all nationalities and income groups.

Primarily gout is a disease of the adult male. In large series, only 3 to 7 percent of cases of primary gout are found in women, and these are chiefly in the postmenopausal group. Gout is very rare in prepubertal children and, when it occurs, may represent a specific form of gout associated with choreoathetosis, self-mutilation, and mental deficiency (Lesch-Nyhan syndrome), or with glycogen storage disease, type I (von Gierke's disease, Chap. 111).

Secondary gout comprises 5 to 10 percent of cases of gout, and, especially in those instances complicating myeloproliferative disorders or hypertensive cardiovascular disease may involve women in as many as 30 percent of cases.

Inheritance

The familial incidence of gout is generally reported as 6 to 18 percent in the United States, but may be much higher as reflected in figures ranging up to 75 percent in English series. The incidence of hyperuricemia among asymptomatic blood relatives of gouty subjects is about 25 percent. The genetic determinants of hyperuricemia are now thought to be multifactorial. Population studies have suggested that some are autosomal dominant and others are sex-linked dominant factors. The latter postulate is of particular interest, since it is now known that hypoxanthine-guanine phosphoribosyltransferase, an enzyme missing or defective in certain types of gout, is controlled by a gene on the X chromosome. The metabolic and genetic heterogeneity of gout underscores the need for definition of specific subtypes so that genetic patterns of transmission of each may be determined. In addition, it is known that serum urate values are positively correlated with surface area and obesity, and that environmental factors such as age, sex, diet, and drugs,

Table 106-1. CLASSIFICATION OF GOUT

Type	Metabolic Disturbance	Specific Defect	Inheritance

Primary gout:
  Adult primary gout:
    Normal excreter of uric acid (75–80% of primary gout)
	Overproduction of uric acid Underexcretion of uric acid often both in same subject	Undefined	Polygenic ? Autosomal dominant forms

Overexcreter of uric acid (20–25% of primary gout)	Overproduction of uric acid	1. Hypoxanthine-guanine phosphoribosyltransferase: defective enzyme of low activity (rare) 2. Glutamine-PRPP amidotransferase: feedback resistance (rare) 3. Others undefined	X-linked Unknown Unknown
Childhood or juvenile gout: Associated with glycogen storage disease, type I (von Giercke's disease)	Overproduction of uric acid, plus underexcretion of uric acid; excessive deposition of glycogen and lipids; hypoglycemia	Glucose 6-phosphatase: deficiency or absence	Autosomal recessive
Associated with cerebral palsy, mental deficiency, and self mutilation. (Lesch-Nyhan syndrome)	Overproduction of uric acid	Hx-G phosphoribosyltransferase: deficiency or absence	X-linked

Secondary gout:
  Hematologic disorders:
    Myeloproliferative diseases; chronic hemolytic anemia
	Excessive production of uric acid	Accelerated turnover of nucleic acids	

Chronic renal diseases Glomerulonephritis, pyelonephritis, polycystic kidney disease	Reduced excretion of uric acid	Reduced renal functional mass.	
Lead nephropathy	,, ,,		
Hypertensive cardiovascular disease	,, ,,	? Role of hyperlacticacidemia in suppression of tubular secretion of urate	
Hyperuricacidemogenic drugs	Reduced excretion of uric acid	? Suppression of tubular secretion of urate by drug or metabolite	
Starvation, especially in treatment of obesity	Reduced excretion of uric acid	Suppression of renal tubular secretion of urate by β-hydroxy butyric acid and other ketone bodies	

operate in conjunction with genetic factors in determining hyperuricemia.

Pathogenesis of Hyperuricemia

The concentration of uric acid in body fluids will be determined by the balance achieved between rates of production and rates of elimination of urate. Uric acid is formed by oxidation of purine bases, which are of both exogenous (dietary) and endogenous (biosynthetic) origins. The latter source is quantitatively the more important in man, except under unusual dietary circumstances. Normally, the body contains about 1200 mg uric acid and turns over about 700 mg per day. Two-thirds of this amount is excreted in the urine, whereas one-third enters the gastrointestinal tract in bile, gastric, and intestinal secretions, where it is destroyed by bacterial action. The accumulation of excessive quantities of urate in the gouty subject could theoretically result from increased dietary absorption of purines, endogenous overproduction, diminished renal or gastrointestinal excretion, or diminished endogenous destruction of urate, or a combination of these factors. Abnormalities of absorption or of intestinal uricolysis have been excluded, and endogenous uricolysis is not a significant process in human tissues because they lack uricase. In contrast, *abnormalities* of *endogenous purine production* and of *urate excretion* are important in the pathogenesis of hyperuricemia of both primary and secondary gout. The normal range of uric acid excretion in American males is about 250 to 600 mg per day on a low purine diet. About 20 or 25 percent of gouty subjects consistently excrete excessive amounts of uric acid and may be assumed to manufacture abnormally large quantities of purines. Tracer studies of the rate of turnover of the urate pool or of incorporation of labeled precursors, such as glycine, into urinary uric acid have confirmed this. Such studies have also indicated excessive purine production in one-half to two-thirds of gouty subjects who excrete normal amounts of urinary uric acid. However, a significant minority remains in whom present methods of study do not disclose excessive purine synthesis.

The structure of the purine ring and the metabolic precursors of individual atoms are shown in Fig. 106-1, and the major intermediates of nucleotide synthesis and uric acid production in Fig. 106-2. The key reaction in

Fig. 106-1. Metabolic donors of atoms of the purine ring.

purine biosynthesis is the initial step in which L-glutamine and α-phosphoribosyl pyrophosphate interact irreversibly to form β-phosphoribosylamine, the first specific purine precursor.

Purine biosynthesis and catabolism

Fig. 106-2. Purine Biosynthesis and Catabolism. The first reaction of the pathway is under inhibitory control of adenosine and guanosine 5'-phosphates. Key enzymes are indicated in parentheses.

L-glutamine $+$ α-PP-ribose-P $+$ $H_2O \rightarrow$
  β-phosphoribosylamine $+$ L-glutamic acid $+$ PP

This reaction is thought to be rate-limiting for the entire pathway, and it is the site of a feedback regulatory process operated by the nucleotide products of the pathway. The amidotransferase catalyzing this first reaction has special inhibitor sites that are sensitive to levels of adenylic and guanylic acids. Accelerated purine biosynthesis must involve an accelerated rate of this reaction. The rate will depend upon (1) the availability of substrates, especially glutamine and phosphoribosylpyrophosphate, (2) the activity of the first enzyme, and integrity of its regulatory mechanisms and (3) the concentrations of regulatory nucleotides at the enzyme sites.

In gouty subjects, excessive incorporation of ^{15}N from glycine into N-3 and N-9 of urate has been observed, and has been interpreted as signifying an abnormality of glutamine metabolism in gout. In glucose-6-phosphatase deficiency glycogen storage disease, excessive conversion of G-6-P to PP-ribose-P is postulated as leading to excessive purine and uric acid synthesis. PP-ribose-P turnover is accelerated in gouty overexcreters but not in normal excreters. Abnormalities of feedback control, involving either a quantitative or qualitative change in activity of the first purine enzyme, or a disturbance of regulation of AMP or GMP levels have been detected in preliminary studies on two gouty subjects.

In a small number of adult gouty subjects with flamboyant overproduction of uric acid, the responsible metabolic defect is a remarkable deficiency of activity of the enzyme which catalyzes the reconversion of hypoxanthine and guanine to their respective ribonucleotide forms by condensation with phosphoribosylpyrophosphate.

Hypoxanthine $+$ PP-ribose-P $\rightarrow$ Inosinic Acid $+$ PP
  Guanine $+$ PP-ribose-P $\rightarrow$ Guanylic Acid $+$ PP

Hypoxanthine-guanine phosphoribosyltransferase is the same enzyme in which activity is even more severely reduced or absent in children with the Lesch-Nyhan syndrome. In the adult gouty subject the enzyme is apparently structurally abnormal and retains only 2 to 10 percent of normal activity against hypoxanthine and guanine, but in different ratios in different patients. Other adult gouty subjects with equally accelerated rates of purine production and urate excretion (1,200 to 1,500 mg per day) have shown normal activity values of this enzyme, as assayed in erythrocytes. Deficiency of H-G-PRTase presumably allows the continuous escape of hypoxanthine and guanine from tissues and their conversion to uric acid in the liver or small intestinal mucosa, the only human tissues that contain xanthine oxidase. Simultaneously, purine synthesis is "compensatorily" accelerated, either because of reduced levels of intracellular regulators, AMP or GMP, or because PP-ribose-P not used in the salvage pathway is now available for *de novo* purine synthesis, or both. Evidence obtained in tissue culture studies of skin fibroblasts favors the latter explanation.

As pointed out above, evidence for overproduction of uric acid is lacking or equivocal in a substantial percentage of "normal-excreter" gouty subjects. These are the subjects whose urate excretion data often suggest most strongly the existence of a specific tubular defect in handling of urate in gout. Fig. 106-3 illustrates the tendency of gouty subjects to require a plasma urate value of 2 or 3 mg per 100 ml greater than the nongouty subject in order to achieve a given rate of urate excretion. This tendency is least evident in the flamboyant overexcreter, if at all, and most prominent in the gouty subject with normal turnover of the urate pool or normal values of incorporation of purine precursors into uric acid.

The pathophysiologic basis of this putative tubular defect is unknown. Among the possibilities are changes in renal tubular blood flow, in rate of transfer of urate into renal cells, or abnormalities of the secretory transport system itself. The latter mechanism for a transport defect has not been defined at the molecular level, but presumably requires both a specific carrier and an energy generating system. A number of chemical substances are known to inhibit urate excretion, presumably by blocking tubular secretion of urate.

A satisfactory definition of hyperuricemia is difficult to offer, as serum urate values form a continuous distribution from low to high values. Statistical definitions depend on the populations examined and methods employed. In the United States normal ranges (mean $\pm$ 2 SD) in males are approximately 2.2 to 7.5 mg per 100 ml and in females, 2.1 to 6.6 mg per 100 ml. In epi-

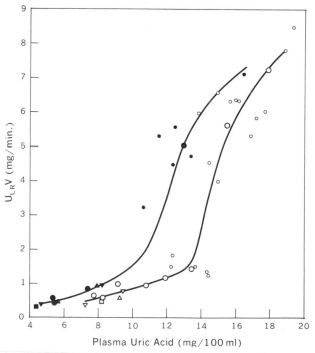

Fig. 106-3. Rates of excretion of uric acid at various plasma urate levels in control and gouty subjects. The urate levels have been raised in both groups by feeding of RNA or by infusion of lithium urate. The gouty group includes asymptomatic hyperuricemic, normal excreter, and overexcreter subjects.

demiologic surveys, values of 7.0 and 6.0 mg per 100 ml respectively are often used as discriminants. The physicochemical solubility of uric acid in body fluids is about 6.4 mg per 100 ml. Only a rare gouty subject will have serum urate values of less than 7 mg per 100 ml when reliable methods, such as the uricase differential spectrophotometric method, are employed.

Pathology

The pathognomonic lesion of gout is the *tophus,* a urate deposit surrounded by tissue exhibiting an inflammatory and foreign body reaction. Because urate crystals are water-soluble, nonaqueous fixatives are necessary to preserve urate deposits in histologic sections. Urate crystals are brilliantly anisotropic when viewed with polarized light under the microscope. In gout, urates tend to deposit in cartilage, epiphyseal bone, periarticular structures, and kidneys. The deposits produce local necrosis and (unless the tissue is avascular) an ensuing foreign body reaction with proliferation of fibrous tissue.

Tophi commonly occur in the helix or antihelix of the ear, the olecranon and patellar bursae, and tendons. Less commonly, they occur in skin of fingertips, palms, or soles, the tarsal plates of the eyelids, the nasal cartilages, in the cornea or sclerotic coats of the eye, or along nerves, causing compression syndromes. Rarely they develop in the myocardium, aortic or mitral valves, vocal cords, and arytenoid cartilages.

In the joint cartilaginous degeneration, synovial proliferation and pannus, destruction of subchondral bone, proliferation of marginal bone, and sometimes fibrous or bony ankylosis may develop. In vertebral bodies, urate deposits are found in marrow spaces adjacent to intervertebral disks, as well as in disk tissue itself. The punched-out lesions of bones commonly seen in roentgenograms of gouty patients represent marrow tophus deposits, which in most instances communicate with the urate crust on the articular surface through erosions and defects in articular cartilage (Fig. 106-4).

The only distinctive histologic feature of the *gouty kidney* is the presence of urate crystals in the medulla or pyramids and surrounding giant-cell reaction. These may be associated with pyelonephritic or vascular changes or both. The pyelonephritic changes are both acute and chronic; the vascular changes include arterial and arteriolar sclerosis.

The traditional view has been that the renal lesions stem from deposition of urates in collecting tubules with resultant obstruction, atrophy of the more proximal tubules, and secondary necrosis and fibrosis. The associated interstitial inflammatory process has been attributed to complicating pyelonephritis. More recent studies have shown that the earliest structural abnormality in the kidney is tubular damage associated with interstitial reaction. There is a distinctive glomerulosclerosis, with uniform fibrillar thickening of glomerular capillary basement membranes, different from that of nephrosclerosis or diabetic glomerulosclerosis. The Henle loops show early atrophy and dilatation, occasionally

Fig. 106-4. Advanced chronic gouty arthritis of the hands, showing extensive destruction of bone by urate deposits and large asymmetrical soft-tissue tophi.

associated with brown pigment degeneration of epithelium. The interstitial reaction is maximal in the region near the changes in the Henle loops. In kidneys without tophi this reaction tends to spare the medulla and juxtamedullary cortex. The changes of chronic pyelonephritis may therefore not be of infectious origin. The vessels, both arteries and arterioles, show increased basophilia and degenerative changes which are out of proportion to the parenchymal changes.

Clinical Manifestations

The natural history of primary gout consists of three phases: asymptomatic hyperuricemia, acute gouty arthritis (which is characteristically recurrent with asymptomatic intervals), and chronic gouty arthritis.

ASYMPTOMATIC HYPERURICEMIA. This phase begins as an accentuation of the normal rise in serum uric acid value that occurs at puberty in the male and at the menopause in the female. Only a limited number of hyperuricemic subjects develops symptomatic gout, urolithiasis, or renal or vascular injury. The majority live their lifetimes with no detectable ill effects of this biochemical abnormality.

In the population study in Framingham, Mass., the cumulative incidence of gouty arthritis in men with serum uric acids of 7.0 mg per 100 ml or above was 2 percent at mean age thirty-four years and 23 percent at mean age fifty-eight years. The likelihood of developing gout increased with the degree of hyperuricemia. With levels of 10.0 mg per 100 ml or greater, the probability approached 50 percent. The peak age of onset of acute gout is about forty years, although first attacks have occurred in men eighty years or older.

ACUTE GOUTY ARTHRITIS. When gout finally becomes clinically manifest, it usually appears abruptly, as fulminating arthritis of a peripheral joint. It is difficult to improve on Sydenham's description of the acute attack:

The victim goes to bed and sleeps in good health. About two o'clock in the morning he is awakened by a severe pain in the great toe; more rarely in the heel, ankle or instep. This pain is like that of a dislocation, and yet the parts feel as if cold water were poured over them. Then follow chills and shivers, and a little fever. The pain, which was at first moderate, becomes more intense. With its intensity the chills and shivers increase. After a time this comes to its height, accommodating itself to the bones and ligaments of the tarsus and metatarsus. Now it is a violent stretching and tearing of the ligaments—now it is a gnawing pain and now a pressure and tightening. So exquisite and lively meanwhile is the feeling of the part affected, that it cannot bear the weight of the bedclothes nor the jar of a person walking in the room. The night is passed in torture, sleeplessness, turning of the part affected, and perpetual change of posture; the tossing about of the body being worse as the fit comes on. Hence the vain effort, by change of posture, both in the body and the limb affected, to obtain an abatement of the pain.

The initial attack usually subsides spontaneously in a few days to a few weeks, and recovery is generally complete. About 50 percent of initial attacks involve the great toe (podagra), and occasionally the initial attack is bilateral. Ninety percent of gouty patients experience podagra during the course of their disease. Next as sites of initial involvement are the instep, ankle, heel, knee, and wrist. Recurring bursitis of shoulder or elbow may be a manifestation of gout. Hench has emphasized that the more distal the site of involvement, the more typical is the character of the attack.

There are no characteristic changes of plasma uric acid levels that precede, accompany, or follow an acute attack of gouty arthritis. There may be an elevation of urinary uric acid excretion values during the acute attack, perhaps mediated by the uricosuric action of corticosteroids secreted during the stress of gouty inflammation. This sequence could explain the normal serum uric acid values occasionally observed during acute attacks. Garrod proposed in 1876 that the acute gouty paroxysm was triggered by precipitation of sodium urate crystals in the joint or neighboring tissues. In 1899, Freudweiler reproduced acute gouty attacks by injection of microcrystals of sodium urate, hypoxanthine, or xanthine. These observations have been confirmed by others with both purine and nonpurine microcrystals. A proposed pathogenetic mechanism involves crystallization of sodium urate from supersaturated body fluids, activation of Hageman factor by crystal surfaces, production of vasoactive kinin-like peptides in synovial fluid, induction of an inflammatory response involving leukotaxic factors,

Fig. 106-5. Crystals of sodium urate monohydrate in leucocytes of synovial fluid in acute gouty arthritis, as viewed under partially polarized light. (*Courtesy, Dr. Daniel J. McCarty, Jr.*)

leukocytosis, ingestion of microcrystals by leukocytes, enhanced production of lactate as a product of anaerobic glycolysis of leukocytes resulting in a drop of local pH and a tendency toward further crystal formation (Fig. 106-5).

The events leading to the initial crystallization of monosodium urate from the supersaturated fluid, after an average of 30 years of asymptomatic hyperuricemia, are poorly understood. Attacks may be precipitated by stress of many kinds, dietary, physical, and emotional. One patient may indict fatiguing travel, another unusual walking or hiking (e.g. "pheasant hunter's gout"), or celebrations such as holiday dinners or alcoholic sprees. Operative procedures are particularly prone to induce acute gout in hyperuricemic individuals, generally on the third to seventh postoperative day.

INTERVAL GOUT. The asymptomatic phase following the acute attack may last from a few weeks to many years. Generally in 6 months to 2 years the patient will suffer another episode in the same or another joint. With time, attacks tend to recur with increasing frequency. Later attacks are often polyarticular, more severe, longer, and accompanied by fever. Roentgenographic changes may develop, and the attacks may abate more gradually than before, but the joints may recover complete function.

CHRONIC GOUTY ARTHRITIS. Before effective control of hyperuricemia became possible, 50 to 60 percent of gouty patients developed visible tophi, permanent joint changes, or chronicity of symptoms. The incidence of tophi now ranges from 13 to 25 percent in various studies. Development of tophi is correlated with height of serum uric acid concentration, severity of renal involvement, and duration of the disease. The time from the initial attack to the beginning of chronic symptomatic or visible tophaceous involvement is usually many years, and ranged from 3 to 42 years in one large series, with an average of 11.6 years (Hench).

Chronic gouty arthritis is a consequence of the progressive inability, in some patients, to dispose of urate as rapidly as they produce it. The urate pool expands and crystalline deposits of urate appear in articular cartilage, synovial membranes, tendons, soft tissues, and elsewhere. In 1 or 2 percent of patients, tophi may be present at the time of the initial acute attack. At later stages, tophaceous enlargement of Achilles tendons, or saccular distensions of olecranon bursae are common and characteristic. Eventually the tophaceous deposits may produce irregular asymmetrical, moderately discrete tumescences over joints, requiring larger shoes or gloves. The classic gouty shoe is one with a window cut out to accommodate an irregularly prominant joint, usually the first metatarsophalangeal.

The process of tophaceous deposition advances slowly and insidiously, and although the tophi themselves are relatively painless, frequently there is progressive stiffness and persistent aching of affected joints. Eventually extensive destruction of joints and large subcutaneous tophi lead to progressive crippling, particularly of hands and feet, and to grotesque deformities (Fig. 106-4). The tense, shiny thin skin overlying the tophus may ulcerate and extrude white chalky or pasty material composed of myriads of fine, needlelike crystals.

Not uncommonly as chronic gouty changes advance, there is a tendency for acute attacks to occur less frequently; those that occur may be superimposed upon the indolent soreness of an involved joint, or may seek out new locations of previously uninvolved sites.

No joint is exempt from chronic gouty involvement, although those of the lower extremity and hand are most commonly involved. The hip and spinal joints are rarely involved in the absence of extensive tophaceous disease elsewhere.

UROLITHIASIS. The incidence of renal stone is about a thousandfold higher in gouty subjects than in the general population. Approximately 20 percent of gouty patients with normal urinary uric acid excretion values and 40 percent of those with elevated excretion values develop stones. Of those who pass stones about 20 percent have had their first episode of urolithiasis before the onset of gouty arthritis. The stones are composed of uric acid, not sodium urate, but in about 80 percent of instances they are mixed and contain in addition calcium phosphate, oxalate, or rarely, carbonate. Such stones are radiopaque, whereas pure uric acid stones are radiolucent. Some gouty subjects pass uric acid sludge, gravel, or sand, occasionally almost daily.

Several factors are at play in the pathogenesis of stones. In 20 to 25 percent of gouty patients, urinary uric acid excretion values are excessive. Also, as a group, gouty subjects tend to produce acid urines, and do not show normal postprandial alkaline tides. Renal ammonia production is subnormal in response to a given acid load. The deficit in ammonia is compensated by an increase in titratable acidity.

RENAL DISEASE IN GOUT. Many gouty subjects show evidence of renal disease. Also, 20 to 40 percent show albuminuria, which is rarely heavy in quantity and is often intermittent. Hypertension is frequent and is usually benign. Concentrating ability may be impaired. Mild degrees of nitrogen retention are common and often stable or only slowly progressive. Renal dysfunction does not shorten life expectancy in the average gouty subject, even though uremia is reported to be the eventual cause of death in 22 to 25 percent of gouty subjects. The majority of gouty patients die of cardiac or cerebral vascular disease, or malignancies, which occur in about the same incidence and at about the same time of life as in nongouty American males.

SECONDARY GOUT. Any acquired hyperuricemic state may be complicated by secondary gout. This disorder occurs in 5 to 9 percent of patients with polycythemia vera, especially those cases merging into the phase of myeloid metaplasia, occasionally in secondary polycythemia complicating congenital heart disease or chronic pulmonary disease, in chronic myelogenous leukemia, acute leukemia, multiple myeloma, or chronic hemolytic anemias. In such instances the mean age of onset is later, women are more commonly involved, and both serum and urinary uric acid values tend to be higher

than in primary gout. Acute gouty arthritis may occasionally antedate evidence of the myeloproliferative disorder by many months.

In all the instances mentioned above, hyperuricemia appears to result from an increased turnover of nucleic acid. Hyperuricemia may also result from reduced renal excretion of urate, either because of chemical interference with tubular secretion of urate or because of reduced renal mass due to parenchymal disease.

Typical gouty attacks may occur in patients receiving such drugs as hydrochlorothiazide or pyrazinamide, which interfere with urate excretion. Extreme obesity may be associated with renal hyperuricemia. Total caloric restriction may result in extreme hyperuricemia, which is correlated with serum levels of β-hydroxybutyric acid and is not infrequently associated with severe attacks of acute gouty arthritis involving especially the knees and ankles. In patients with hyperlipoproteinemias there is a direct correlation between serum triglyceride and uric acid levels.

Chronic renal disease is a frequent cause of hyperuricemia, but apparently few patients with glomerulonephritis, pyelonephritis, or polycystic renal disease live long enough to develop gout. The number may increase with chronic dialysis programs, and acute gouty arthritis has complicated the course of patients so managed. Gout continues to be found in patients who survive lead exposure early in life and go on to develop the slowly progressive vascular nephritis of plumbism.

Hyperuricemia complicates benign essential and renal hypertension in 40 percent of cases, and malignant hypertension in 65 percent of cases and has been attributed provisionally to renal anoxia and local lactic acid excess. Gout occurs in 10 percent or more of patients previously subjected to sympathectomy or adrenalectomy for hypertension. In the absence of family data it may be difficult to distinguish between sporadic primary gout and gout secondary to hypertensive renal disease.

CHILDHOOD AND JUVENILE GOUT. Hyperuricemia is found in patients with glycogen storage disease due to glucose-6-phosphatase deficiency, and those children who survive the early hazards of hypoglycemia may be counted upon to develop severe tophaceous gouty arthritis. The hyperuricemia is of mixed origin: these children overproduce uric acid and also underexcrete it because of the persistent hyperlacticacidemia and triglyceridemia that characterize the disease. The condition is inherited as an autosomal recessive disorder.

Recently a new disease, characterized by cerebral palsy, choreoathetosis, self-mutilation, and mental deficiency associated with extreme hyperuricemia, uricosuria, and gout, has been described by Lesch and Nyhan. Milder variants of this syndrome have been recognized in which self-mutilation is absent, mental deficiency is mild, and the patient has been thought to have a cerebral palsy until gout supervenes. All reported patients are males, although some abnormalities of purine metabolism may be present in the mothers. The disease obeys the laws of X-linked transmission with full expression only in the hemizygous state. The purine abnormalities are attributable to the complete absence or severe deficiency of hypoxanthine-guanine phosphoribosyltransferase.

Diagnosis

Acute gouty arthritis is readily diagnosed by its typical explosive onset, the characteristic severity of involvement of the peripheral joint, the presence of hyperuricemia, and the rapid response to treatment with colchicine. Less typical presentations may be difficult to distinguish from other arthritides on clinical grounds. If present, tophi or typical roentgenologic findings of punched-out, destructive lesions will suggest the correct diagnosis. In patients lacking such lesions, the only pathognomonic finding is the presence in the leukocytes of the synovial fluid, of urate crystals which are needle-like and birefringent under polarized light (Fig. 106-5). Valuable clues in the diagnosis are a history of renal stones or of antecedent mild trauma or surgery in the patient or a history of gout, arthritis, or renal stones in the family.

Chronic gouty arthritis may be diagnosed by the presence of urate deposits in or near the affected joints or bursae or of soft-tissue deposits in the helix of the ear, the finger tips, the Achilles tendon, or other locations. The diagnosis may be confirmed by removal of the chalky contents of a tophus, microscopic identification of sodium urate crystals by optical means, or chemical identification by the murexide test or, preferably, by ultraviolet spectrophotometry and degradation by uricase.

Differential Diagnosis

Acute gout must be differentiated from acute rheumatic fever, rheumatoid arthritis, traumatic arthritis, osteoarthritis, pyogenic arthritis, sarcoid arthritis, cellulitis, bursitis, tendonitis, and thrombophlebitis. *Reiter's syndrome* in men and *palindromic arthritis* in women may present similar clinical manifestations of episodes of acute arthritis followed by periods of complete remission, but hyperuricemia will not generally be present, joint fluid will not contain urate crystals, and colchicine is ineffective. *Pseudogout*, which is chiefly a disorder of elderly persons and is manifested by acute attacks of arthritis of knees and other joints, is always accompanied by calcification of joint cartilage; and the synovial fluid contains nonurate crystals of calcium pyrophosphate or apatite. The patients are not usually hyperuricemic.

Chronic gouty arthritis must be differentiated from all other chronic arthritides which cause deformities of joints, chiefly rheumatoid arthritis, osteoarthritis, traumatic arthritis, and residua of pyogenic arthritis. The history of onset, of progression, of response to colchicine and demonstration of hyperuricemia, of asymmetrical tumescences, typical roentgenographic changes, of tophi or of crystals of urate in synovial fluid and leukocytes, should establish the diagnosis.

Treatment

The therapeutic aims in gout are (1) to terminate the acute gouty attack as promptly as possible; (2) to prevent recurrences of acute gouty arthritis; (3) to prevent or reverse complications of the disease resulting from deposition of sodium urate in joints and kidneys; and (4) to prevent formation of uric acid kidney stones. Treatment depends on the stage at which the patient is seen.

ACUTE ATTACK. Colchicine is the only treatment for acute gout of specific diagnostic value. It should be given as soon as the diagnosis is suspected. The initial dose of 0.5 to 1.2 mg colchicine is followed by 0.5 or 0.6 mg every hour for 8 hr, then every 2 hr until pain is relieved or until nausea, vomiting, cramping, or diarrhea develops. Maximum tolerated doses range from 4 to 10 mg. In most patients dramatic relief of pain and gastrointestinal side effects occur simultaneously. The diarrhea may be treated with paregoric, 4 cc, or kaopectate, 30 cc, after each loose stool. Colchicine should be discontinued until gastrointestinal symptoms subside. Since the effective dose of colchicine varies, each patient should learn his own tolerance dose and stop treatment just short of this in treatment of subsequent attacks. Colchicine usually affords relief within 24 to 48 hr; a second full therapeutic dose should not be repeated sooner than 72 hr.

Colchicine may also be given intravenously. The usual initial dose is 1 to 2 mg in 20 ml saline solution given slowly, and if a single dose is not effective, the injection may be repeated once in 4 to 5 hr (maximum intravenous dose, 3 to 4 mg). Gastrointestinal symptoms are uncommon with intravenous administration.

Phenylbutazone is also effective in acute gouty arthritis, and may be preferred when the gouty attack has proceeded for some time, or when the attack does not abate completely with colchicine. The initial dose is 400 mg orally, followed by 100 mg every 4 to 8 hr for 2 to 3 days. Oxyphenbutazone, a metabolite of phenylbutazone, is also effective in acute gout. The dose is the same as that of phenylbutazone, and the same precautions should be taken.

Patients who recognize prodromal symptoms may abort acute attacks by prompt institution of colchicine or phenylbutazone therapy and frequently require only a few tablets to achieve success.

Indomethacin is sometimes dramatically effective in acute gout. It is given orally in doses of 100 to 150 mg every 6 hours. Larger doses may cause severe headache and a transient depersonalization reaction.

If full doses of colchicine or phenylbutazone are contraindicated, or ineffective, ACTH gel may be employed. Doses of 40 to 80 USP units are given intramuscularly every 6 to 8 hr for 2 to 3 days, rarely longer, following which the doses are reduced in stepwise fashion and discontinued. To avoid rebound attacks of gout after ACTH therapy, 0.6 mg colchicine should be given two or three times daily during and after administration of ACTH for at least 7 days.

Hydrocortisone in a dose of 25 to 50 mg injected intraarticularly into the involved joint is useful in treating acute gout limited to a single joint or bursa, and relief from pain is usually prompt and complete within 24 to 36 hr. Steroid hormones are not recommended for parenteral use in acute gout, as the effects are inconsistent and rebound attacks frequent.

During the acute attack, bearing weight on the involved joints should be avoided. In severe attacks the patient will invariably immobilize himself voluntarily, but in milder attacks it is necessary for the physician to insist on this. Mobilization is permitted as soon as the joint is no longer painful.

INTERVAL PHASE. The patient with gout should avoid high purine foods so as to lessen the burden of uric acid excretion. A severe limitation of purine-containing foods is rarely indicated, unless renal function and the ability to excrete urate are reduced significantly. Many gouty patients are overweight, and gradual weight reduction is indicated. Sudden weight reduction may precipitate gouty attacks and should be avoided. In general, diets of moderate protein content, somewhat low in fat, are preferred.

A high fluid intake is advisable to maintain a urinary output of 2,000 ml per day. Urate excretion is thus promoted, and the dangers of crystal formation in the kidney or ureter are reduced. Alcoholic beverages, especially beer, ale, and wine, should be avoided if possible, as they may precipitate attacks. Distilled alcoholic beverages, in moderation, generally have little influence on the gouty process.

The daily ingestion of 0.6 to 1.8 mg colchicine is generally effective in reducing the number of acute gouty attacks in patients who are subject to frequent episodes. Maintenance colchicine therapy is particularly important during the first year or two after institution of uricosuric drugs.

CHRONIC GOUTY ARTHRITIS. Use of a drug to lower the serum level of uric acid to 6 mg per 100 ml or less is indicated in all gouty patients with visible tophi, with roentgenographic evidence of urate deposits, with serum uric acid levels above 8.5 mg per 100 ml, or with a history of four or more major attacks of acute gouty arthritis per year. The drug of choice is allopurinol, but uricosuric agents may be used. None of these agents is of any value in the immediate treatment of the acute attack. With both types the number of acute gouty attacks may be increased during the first 6 months unless maintenance colchicine therapy is given, whereas after 12 to 18 months the number may be decidedly reduced. Uricosuric drugs block tubular reabsorption of filtered urate. Those of use in gout are probenecid, sulfinpyrazone, and salicylates.

Probenecid is given in doses of 0.5 to 3 Gm daily in two or three evenly spaced doses (average dose, 1 to 1.5 Gm). This drug may produce gastrointestinal upsets, headaches, or skin rash.

Sulfinpyrazone may be given in doses of 100 to 600 mg daily in three or four divided doses (average dose, 300 mg). This drug is related to phenylbutazone and can cause untoward reactions, but is generally somewhat better tolerated than probenecid.

Salicylates block the uricosuric action of both probenecid and sulfinpyrazone and must not be used concurrently. Salicylates are uricosuric when given in high doses (4 to 6 Gm daily), but few patients can tolerate these quantities.

With all uricosuric agents the doses should be low initially, so as to avoid sudden mobilization of large quantities of urate. Fluids should be forced so as to prevent formation of concentrated urine, especially during the late hours of the night. During the first days or weeks of therapy the urine should be alkalinized; this may be difficult to achieve, as gouty patients tend to produce acid urine. In patients who are mobilizing urate, and especially those who form urate gravel, alkalinization during the night, when fluid intake is reduced, is important. A single 250 mg tablet of acetazolamide (Diamox) taken at bedtime will serve to keep the urine alkaline and dilute throughout the night.

A second approach toward controlling serum urate levels is that of regulating production of uric acid, rather than (or in addition to) augmenting its excretion. Allopurinol is a potent inhibitor of xanthine oxidase, which prevents the conversion of hypoxanthine and xanthine to uric acid and permits these uric acid precursors to be excreted instead. Its use results in reduction of levels of uric acid in serum *and in urine*. The drug is effective even in the presence of renal failure, when uricosuric agents are generally ineffective. Its action is not blocked by salicylates. The usual dose is 100 mg, given orally three or four times a day. It is usually well tolerated, but rarely may cause gastric irritation, diarrhea, or skin rash, or induce an attack of gout. Uricosuric agents may be used concurrently to hasten mobilization of urate deposits. Since allopurinol decreases uric acid excretion, it is also very useful in controlling uric acid stone formation, especially in patients who are overproducers of uric acid, but also in nongouty subjects.

In selected patients surgical removal of large extraarticular urate deposits, such as those in olecranon bursae, may be advisable. Occasionally amputation of irreparably damaged digits, especially those containing draining sinuses, is indicated. Physical therapy and appropriate self-help devices are indicated in patients who are partially disabled.

ASYMPTOMATIC HYPERURICEMIA. Asymptomatic hyperuricemia is frequently encountered in family members of patients with gout and in the general population. One must exclude hyperuricemia as a manifestation of reduced renal function or of action of certain drugs. Asymptomatic hyperuricemia generally requires no therapy, as only about one-third of patients will ever develop articular attacks, and adequate therapy can be instituted when these supervene. However, exceptions do exist, as in patients with serum levels of uric acid above 8.5 or 9 mg per 100 ml, especially if the urinary excretion levels are low and there is a family history of tophaceous involvement. In such circumstances the asymptomatic subject should be treated with allopurinol before articular or renal complications develop. It is essential that frequent close observation of the patient by the physician be maintained.

SECONDARY GOUT. Treatment of gouty arthritis occurring secondary to hematopoietic disturbances is the same as for primary gout except that one must be especially alert to potential renal and ureteral complications. The basal uric acid excretion may be high, and use of uricosuric agents may intensify the risk of urate crystalluria and of tubular or ureteral blockade. High fluid intake and alkalinization become of great importance. The drug of choice for control of hyperuricemia is allopurinol.

REFERENCES

Gonick, H. C., M. E. Rubini, I. O. Gleason, and S. C. Sommers: The Renal Lesion in Gout, Ann. Intern. Med., 62: 667, 1965.

McCarty, D. J., Jr.: Crystal-induced Inflammation; Syndromes of Gout and Pseudogout, Geriatrics, 18:467, 1963.

Rosenbloom, F. M., J. F. Henderson, I. C. Caldwell, W. N. Kelley, and J. E. Seegmiller: Biochemical Bases of Accelerated Purine Biosynthesis *de novo* in Human Fibroblasts Lacking Hypoxanthine-Guanine Phosphoribosyltransferase, J. Biol. Chem., 243:1166, 1968.

Rundles, R. W., H. R. Silberman, G. H. Hitchings, and G. B. Elion: Effects of Xanthine Oxidase Inhibitor on Clinical Manifestations and Purine Metabolism in Gout, Ann. Intern. Med., 60:717, 1964.

Seegmiller, J. E., F. M. Rosenbloom, and W. N. Kelley: An Enzyme Defect Associated with an X-linked Human Neurological Disorder and Excessive Purine Synthesis, Science, 155:1682, 1967.

Wyngaarden, J. B.: Gout, in "The Metabolic Basis of Inherited Disease," 2d ed., J. B. Stanbury, J. B. Wyngaarden, and D. S. Fredrickson (Eds.), New York, McGraw-Hill Book Company, 1966.

——, R. W. Rundles, and E. N. Metz: Allopurinol in the Treatment of Gout, Ann. Intern. Med., 62:842, 1965.

Yu, T. F., and A. B. Gutman: Uric Acid Nephrolithiasis in Gout. Predisposing Factors, Ann. Intern. Med., 67:1133, 1967.

107 HEMOCHROMATOSIS
George E. Cartwright

Definition

Idiopathic hemochromatosis (bronze diabetes, pigment cirrhosis) is characterized pathologically by excessive deposits of iron in the body and clinically by hepatomegaly with eventual liver insufficiency, pigmentation of the skin, diabetes mellitus, and frequently cardiac failure.

History

The first clinical description of the disease was given by Trousseau in 1865. In 1889 von Recklinghausen named the disease *hemochromatosis* and described the iron-containing pigment, hemosiderin. Sheldon, in a now classic monograph, reviewed the world's literature in 1935. Finch and Finch in 1955 reviewed the literature since 1935 and added 80 cases of their own. More recently, MacDonald has made important contributions by emphasizing the role of excessive dietary iron and preexisting portal cirrhosis in the pathogenesis of acquired hemochromatosis.

Incidence

Hemochromatosis is a rare disease, recognized in approximately 1 in 20,000 hospital admissions, and 1 in 7,000 hospital deaths. It is observed ten times as frequently in males as in females. Nearly 70 percent of all patients with this disease develop their first symptoms between the ages of forty and sixty years. Hemochromatosis is rarely recognized below the age of twenty years.

Pathogenesis

One of the earliest measurable alterations in iron metabolism in hemochromatosis is the elevation of the plasma iron and saturation of the plasma iron-binding protein, transferrin. As the disease progresses, the amount of storage iron increases. In advanced disease, the tissues contain over 20 Gm of iron; total body iron in normal persons is in the range of 3 to 5 Gm. The excess iron is deposited primarily in parenchymal cells in the form of ferritin and hemosiderin. Increased amounts of iron are found in almost all body tissues, especially those in which there is organ dysfunction. Iron in the liver and pancreas is increased fifty to one hundred times; in the heart, ten to fifteen times; in the spleen, kidney, and skin, about five times.

Since iron is not excreted from the body in appreciable amounts even in normal persons, the conclusion that iron absorption is increased in idiopathic hemochromatosis is inescapable. There are two quite differing explanations as to why this occurs. The classical concept is that idiopathic hemochromatosis is due to an inherited inborn error in metabolism in which the basic abnormality is the increased absorption of iron. According to this view the excessive deposition of iron is the cause of the tissue damage. The other point of view is that hemochromatosis is a variant of portal cirrhosis of the liver. A high incidence (30 to 85 percent) of alcoholism has been observed in patients with idiopathic hemochromatosis, and it has been noted that the iron content of alcoholic beverages, particularly various wines, is high.

Hemochromatosis has been observed (1) as a familial occurrence without apparent cause other than an inherited inborn error of metabolism; (2) in alcoholic subjects with a high dietary intake of iron; (3) in malnourished

Bantu subjects in South Africa secondary to long-term iron overload ("Bantu siderosis"); (4) in isolated instances of parenchymal iron overload following intake of medicinal doses of iron over many years; (5) in association with various types of refractory anemia; and (6) in a few patients given 100 or more transfusions of blood. Therefore, it would seem that hemochromatosis is a syndrome with several possible causes. The common denominator in all cases is the presence of excessive iron in parenchymal tissues.

Pathology

At autopsy the enlarged, nodular liver and pancreas present a striking ochre color. Histologically, hemosiderin is deposited in many organs, particularly the liver and pancreas. The liver shows considerable fibrosis. Testicular atrophy is frequently present, both grossly and histologically. There are hemosiderin deposits in the myocardium, and they may be associated with myocardial edema, fibrosis, and necrosis. The epidermis of the skin is thin, and melanin pigment is found in the cells of the basal layer. Hemosiderin is deposited almost entirely in the corium.

Clinical Manifestations

The symptoms and signs of hemochromatosis are related to the *skin pigmentation, diabetes, liver impairment, and cardiac disease.* Of these the cirrhosis of the liver is the most constant abnormality.

The initial symptoms most frequently encountered are related to the onset of *diabetes.* Weakness, lassitude, weight loss, change in skin color, abdominal pain, dyspnea, edema, ascites, loss of libido, and peripheral neuritis are also frequent initial symptoms. Hepatomegaly, pigmentation, spider angiomas, splenomegaly, ascites, evidences of congestive failure or cardiac arrhythmias, loss of body hair, testicular atrophy, jaundice, and hypertension are the most prominent physical signs, given in decreasing order of frequency.

The liver is the first tissue known to be damaged, and hepatomegaly is present in about 93 percent of symptomatic cases. Hepatic enlargement may exist in the absence of symptoms or in the presence of normal liver function tests. Indeed, over half the patients with symptomatic hemochromatosis have little or no laboratory evidence of functional impairment of the liver in spite of hepatomegaly and proved fibrosis. Loss of body hair, palmar erythema, testicular atrophy, gynecomastia, spider angioma, and, particularly, loss of libido are often seen and are related to the severity of the liver damage. Manifestations of portal hypertension and esophageal varices may occur but are less commonly observed than in Laennec's cirrhosis. A nontender, slightly enlarged spleen is present in approximately half the cases. Primary carcinoma of the liver develops in about 14 percent. The incidence of this last complication increases greatly with age.

Excessive *skin pigmentation* is present in about 90 percent of the patients at the time the diagnosis is established. Pigmentation may be due to deposition of melanin or iron or both. In general, melanin deposition gives rise to bronzing, iron deposition to a metallic gray hue. Pigmentation usually is diffuse and generalized, but frequently it is deeper on the face, neck, extensor aspects of the lower forearms, dorsae of the hands, lower legs, genital regions, and in scars. In only 10 to 15 percent of cases is there demonstrable pigmentation of the oral mucosa.

About 82 percent of all patients develop *diabetes mellitus* and symptoms therefrom. The diabetes may appear rapidly, and insulin requirements may increase rapidly. About 72 percent of the patients require insulin for the control of the diabetes. In some instances severe insulin resistance develops, in others there may be sensitivity to insulin. In most instances, the diabetes is controlled with little difficulty. Since the diabetes is usually present for less than a decade, the late degenerative sequelae of this complication are not prominent.

Approximately one-third of patients with idiopathic hemochromatosis die of *cardiac failure.* The heart disease is extremely common in young adults, and symptoms may develop suddenly, with rapid progression to death. The most important manifestations of heart disease are congestive failure and cardiac arrhythmias, particularly ventricular extrasystoles and paroxysmal atrial tachycardia. Other arrhythmias may occur as well.

Diagnosis

The classical *triad of skin pigmentation, diabetes mellitus, and hepatomegaly,* especially in the presence of heart disease and evidence of hypogonadism, should always suggest the diagnosis. Confirmation of the presence of liver, pancreatic, heart, and gonadal disease should then be obtained by customary tests of the functions of these organs. It then remains to demonstrate that there is excessive storage iron.

The diagnosis is enhanced considerably if the plasma iron level is found to be elevated (above 150 μg per 100 ml) and the iron-binding protein of the plasma is 75 to 100 percent saturated. However, the only definitive test is liver biopsy. Other procedures which indicate an excess of body iron stores are bone marrow aspiration for hemosiderin, examination of the urine sediment for hemosiderin, skin biopsy, and gastric mucosal biopsy.

Finch and Finch state that there are no unique features in idiopathic hemochromatosis by which it may be distinguished pathologically from the terminal stage of other iron-storage diseases, such as dietary or transfusion hemochromatosis. They define *hemosiderosis* as a focal increase in tissue iron or a general increase in iron stores without associated tissue damage, and *hemochromatosis* as a general increase in body iron stores with resultant tissue damage. From these definitions, the differentiation of hemosiderosis from hemochromatosis can be easily made by the presence or absence of organ dysfunction. Dietary and transfusion hemochromatosis can be differentiated from idiopathic hemochromatosis on the basis of a history of excessive iron intake by mouth, by injection, or intravenously in the form of blood. In evaluating dietary iron exposure, the dietary iron content, type of diet, type of cooking utensils, intake of medicinal iron, and iron content of the drinking water or other beverages must be considered.

Prognosis

The life expectancy of patients after signs of clinical hemochromatosis have become manifest averages 4.4 years, but several instances have been recorded of patients living up to 20 or 30 years after manifestation of signs. The average duration of life after diabetes has developed is 3 years. The principal causes of death are cardiac failure (30 percent), hepatic coma (15 percent), hematemesis (14 percent), hepatoma (14 percent), and pneumonia (12 percent). The most recent advance in the therapy of this disease, the introduction of methods for the removal of iron, is expected to increase life expectancy further.

Treatment

The therapy of idiopathic hemochromatosis involves removal of the excess body iron by phlebotomy and supportive treatment of damaged organs. The management of the hepatic failure, cardiac failure, and diabetes differs little from the conventional management of these conditions. Loss of libido and change in secondary sex characteristics are relieved by testosterone therapy. Iron is best removed from the body by a weekly or twice weekly phlebotomy of 500 ml. Since the average amount of iron in a patient with hemochromatosis is approximately 25 Gm, about 2 years of weekly bleeding will be required to deplete the iron stores. Chelating agents such as EDTA and desferrioxamine are of little or no practical value in the management of hemochromatosis.

REFERENCES

Bothwell, T. H., and C. A. Finch: "Iron Metabolism," Boston, Little, Brown and Company, 1962.

Charlton, R. W., and T. H. Bothwell: Hemochromatosis: Dietary and Genetic Aspects, in E. B. Brown and C. V. Moore (Eds.), "Progress in Hematology," vol. 5, p. 298, New York, Grune and Stratton, Inc., 1966.

Finch, S. C., and C. A. Finch: Idiopathic Hemochromatosis: An Iron Storage Disease, Medicine, 34:381, 1955.

MacDonald, R. A.: "Hemochromatosis and Hemosiderosis," Springfield, Ill., Charles C Thomas, Publisher, 1964.

————: Primary Hemochromatosis: Inherited or Acquired?, in E. B. Brown and C. V. Moore (Eds.), "Progress in Hematology," vol. 5, p. 324, New York, Grune and Stratton, Inc., 1966.

Sheldon, J. H.: "Hemochromatosis," Fairlawn, N. J., Oxford University Press, 1935.

108 DISORDERS OF PORPHYRIN METABOLISM

George E. Cartwright

DEFINITIONS

Porphyrins are pigments that possess a basic structure of four pyrrole rings linked by methene ($=CH—$) bridges (Fig. 108-1). The individual porphyrins differ from each other according to the nature of the eight possible side chains. Each porphyrin has a number of stereoisomers. *Porphyrinogens* are colorless compounds (reduced porphyrins) with a basic structure of four pyrrole rings linked by methane ($—CH_2—$) bridges.

Porphyrin pigments are widely distributed throughout the plant and animal worlds in chlorophyll, hemoglobin, catalase, and a number of cytochrome and peroxidase enzymes.

The term *porphyrinuria* refers to excessive excretion of porphyrins in the urine. *Coproporphyrinuria*, the excretion of increased amounts of coproporphyrin, is not uncommon and occurs in a variety of conditions. The term *porphyria* embraces a group of diseases, each with unusual and characteristic manifestations, which have in common the excessive excretion of one or more of the porphyrins, porphyrinogens, and/or porphyrin precursors (Δ-aminolevulinic acid and porphobilinogen) in the urine and/or feces.

HISTORY

Congenital porphyria was first described by Günther in 1911. Much of the knowledge of the chemistry of the porphyrins came from Hans Fischer and his school in Munich. In 1915, these workers described, named, and isolated in crystalline form the uroporphyrins and coproporphyrins from the urine of the patient in their famous case of congenital porphyria (Petry). Shemin and Granick and their groups in New York have made substantial contributions to knowledge of the biosynthesis of the porphyrins. Contributions to the understanding of the types and manifestations of porphyria have come from Waldenström in Sweden, Rimington in England, Barnes and Dean in South Africa, and Watson, Schwartz, and Schmid in the United States.

BIOSYNTHESIS

The rather complex porphyrin molecule is synthesized in the body from two simple precursors, acetate and glycine (Fig. 108-2). Acetate enters the Krebs tricarboxylic acid cycle (Chap. 75) and is converted into succinate. Succinyl CoA (active succinate) is then formed in the presence of Mg^{++} ion, adenosine triphosphate (ATP), and coenzyme A (CoA). The activated form of succinate condenses with a pyridoxal phosphate-glycine enzyme (glycine-PE) to form the 5-carbon compound, Δ-aminolevulinic acid (Δ-ALA), and carbon dioxide by the decarboxylation of glycine. This step is enzymatically controlled (ALA synthetase), and several intermediate compounds have been suggested. Two molecules of Δ-aminolevulinic acid, in the presence of glutathione (GSH) and an enzyme, Δ-aminolevulinic acid dehydrase (Δ-ALA DH), condense to form a substituted monopyrrole, porphobilinogen, which contains acetic acid (A) and propionic acid (P) side chains. In the next step in heme synthesis, four molecules of porphobilinogen condense to form the reduced tetrapyrrolic structure, uroporphyrinogen. This step is catalyzed by at least two enzymes, porphobilinogen deaminase (PD) and uroporphyrinogen isomerase (UI). Details of the action of these enzymes and the sequence of reactions leading from porphobilinogen to uroporphyrinogen types I and III are not known. Uroporphyrin III is not in the direct pathway of heme synthesis, as was formerly assumed, but is a by-product. Uroporphyrinogen III (reduced uroporphyrin) is converted to coproporphyrinogen by the enzyme, uroporphyrinogen decarboxylase (UD). Coproporphyrinogen III is then converted to protoporphyrin III in the presence of the enzyme coproporphyrinogen oxidase. Coproporphyrin III is a by-product, whereas the available evidence suggests that protoporphyrin III is in the direct pathway of heme synthesis. Protoporphyrin III is converted to hemoglobin in the presence of iron, glutathione, globin, and the enzyme heme synthetase (HS). The intermediate steps between protoporphyrin and hemoglobin have not been identified. It is not known whether heme or a porphyrin-globin compound is an intermediate in this reaction, although the former possibility seems more likely.

METABOLISM

The most important of the naturally occurring porphyrins are uroporphyrin (isomer types I and III), coproporphyrin (types I and III), and protoporphyrin (type III).

Protoporphyrin III is present in hemoglobin and is, therefore, the most important of the porphyrins from the physiologic standpoint. It is absent from urine. The concentration of fecal protoporphyrin is related to the amount of blood in the gastrointestinal tract, the rate of liberation of protoporphyrin from hemoglobin by fecal bacteria, and the excretion of protoporphyrin by the liver.

Coproporphyrin is the predominant porphyrin in urine and feces under normal circumstances. Coproporphyrinuria occurs in a variety of clinical conditions, such as lead poisoning, poliomyelitis, liver disease, acute alcoholism, hemolytic anemia, and Hodgkin's disease. In all these disorders the increased coproporphyrinuria accompanies the underlying disease, and it is unlikely that the abnormality in porphyrin metabolism contributes significantly to the clinical picture. Coproporphyrinuria is also found in patients with certain types of porphyria. Abnormally high fecal coproporphyrin values are found in patients with hemolytic anemia, and low values occur in patients with liver disease.

Uroporphyrin is normally excreted in urine in only

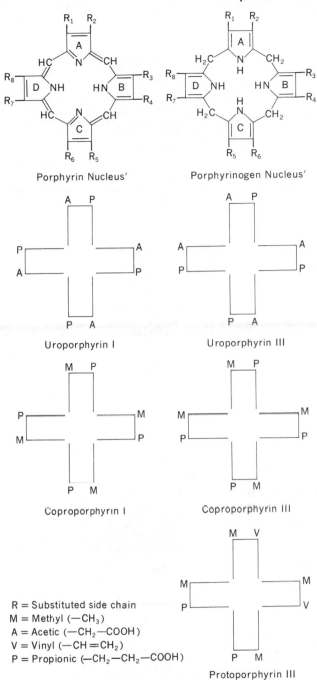

R = Substituted side chain
M = Methyl (—CH₃)
A = Acetic (—CH₂—COOH)
V = Vinyl (—CH=CH₂)
P = Propionic (—CH₂—CH₂—COOH)

Fig. 108-1. The structural formulas of the porphyrin and porphyrinogen nuclei and diagrammatic formulas of the important naturally occurring porphyrins.

trace amounts. The urinary excretion of this porphyrin is moderately increased in lead poisoning and is greatly increased in patients with certain types of porphyria.

PORPHYRIA

Porphyria may be divided into two general groups (Table 108-1). In erythropoietic porphyria, excessive

Fig. 108-2. The biosynthesis of the porphyrins from acetate and glycine and the biosynthetic pathway of hemoglobin. CoA, coenzyme A; ATP, adenosine triphosphate; PE, pyridoxal phosphate enzyme (ALA synthetase); Δ-ALA, delta-aminolevulinic acid; Δ-ALA DH, delta-aminolevulinic acid dehydrase; GSH, glutathione; PD, porphobilinogen deaminase; UI, uroporphyrinogen isomerase; UD, uroporphyrinogen decarboxylase; CO, coproporphyrinogen oxidase; HS, heme synthetase; A, acetic; P, propionic.

quantities of porphyrins accumulate in the normoblasts and erythrocytes. Under these circumstances, red fluorescence may be observed when the cells are exposed to ultraviolet light. The predominant porphyrin synthesized in erythropoietic uroporphyria (congenital porphyria) is uroporphyrin; in erythropoietic protoporphyria, protoporphyrin; and in erythropoietic coproporphyria, coproporphyrin. In porphyria hepatica, excessive porphyrin production occurs in the liver. Hepatic porphyria may be subdivided further into at least four different types: acute intermittent porphyria, porphyria cutanea tarda hereditaria (mixed porphyria, porphyria variegata, South African Caucasian porphyria, protocoproporphyria), porphyria cutanea tarda symptomatica, and hereditary coproporphyria. Not all patients with hepatic porphyria can be so classified and there is some degree of overlapping. It is quite possible that more than a single entity is included in each subtype of hepatic porphyria.

PORPHYRIA ERYTHROPOIETICA
Erythropoietic Uroporphyria

This is a very rare disorder, inherited probably as a recessive mendelian characteristic. The clinical manifestations occur very early in life, sometimes even a few days after birth, but often they are not observed until after an interval of a year of two. *The disease is characterized by the excessive deposition of porphyrin in the tissues, leading to pronounced photosensitization.* The early lesions of photodynamic origin are the blisters of hydroa estivale (hydroa vacciniforme) on skin surfaces exposed to light, especially of the face and hands. In time, scarring and mutilation occur. After years of continued photosensitivity, the mutilation becomes extensive, with loss of fingers, portions of the nose, ears, scarring of the cheeks and about the mouth, ectropion, or symblepharon. Skin not exposed to light remains unaffected. Hemolytic anemia and splenomegaly are an integral part of the disease. Erythrodontia may be observed in those cases in which sufficient porphyrin has been deposited in the teeth to make them grossly red or reddish brown. Teeth which do not show erythrodontia in ordinary light may exhibit red fluorescence in Wood's light. Red fluorescence may be seen in the phalangeal bones if a strong source of ultraviolet light is allowed to shine through the fingers. There is no marked disturbance of the nervous system, nor is there abdominal colic.

Because of the demonstration of large quantities of *uroporphyrin* and *coproporphyrin* in the normoblasts in the bone marrow, it has been suggested that in this type

Table 108-1. DISTINGUISHING FEATURES OF THE SEVERAL TYPES OF PORPHYRIA

Characteristics	Erythropoietic			Hepatic						
	Uro-porphyria	Proto-porphyria	Copro-porphyria	Acute inter-mittent		Cutanea tarda hereditaria		Cutanea tarda sympto-matica	Hereditary coproporphyria	
Inheritance	Recessive	Dominant	Dominant	Dominant		Dominant		Acquired	Dominant	
Sex	Both	Both	....	Both		Both		Both	Both	
Age of onset, years ..	0–5	0–5	....	15–40		10–30		Any age	Any age	
Phase of disease	....	....	....	*latent*	*acute*	*latent*	*acute*	....	*latent*	*acute*
Photosensitivity and cutaneous lesions ..	++++	++	++	0	0	0	+ or 0	++	0	0 or +
Abdominal, psychic, and/or neurologic symptoms	0	0	0	0	++	0	+	0	0	+
RBC:										
Uroporphyrin	++++	++	++	N	N	N	N	N	N	N
Coproporphyrin ...	+++	++	++++	N	N	N	N	N	N	N
Protoporphyrin ...	++	++++	+	N	N	N	N	N	N	N
Urine:										
Color	Red	N	N	N*	Red	N*	N or red	Red	N	N or red
Δ-ALA.†	N	N	N	+	++	N	++	N	+	++
PBG.‡	N	N	N	++	++++	N	++	N	+	++
Uroporphyrin	++++	N	N	++	++	N	+++	++++	N	++
Coproporphyrin ...	++	N	N	++	++	N	+++	++	N or +	+++
Feces:										
Coproporphyrin ...	++	N	N	N	+	++++	+++	+++	++	++++
Protoporphyrin ...	++	N to ++	N	N	+	++++	+++	++	N	+

0, absent; N, normal; +, increased; ++++, greatly increased.

* Freshly voided. On standing, the urine may become deep brownish-red or black.

† Δ-aminolevulinic acid.

‡ Porphobilinogen.

of porphyria the excessive quantities of uroporphyrin are formed in the marrow. It is for this reason that the disease had been called *erythropoietic uroporphyria* rather than congenital porphyria.

The color of the urine varies from pink to red. Uroporphyrin I and coproporphyrin I are the predominant porphyrins excreted. If the concentration of uroporphyrin is sufficiently great, the urine, on the addition of hydrochloric acid, exhibits an intense band at about 552 mμ and a weaker band at 596 mμ when viewed in a hand spectroscope. The excretion of porphyrin precursors, Δ-aminolevulinic acid and porphobilinogen, is not increased.

The disease is slowly progressive, and death is usually due to an intercurrent infection or severe hemolytic anemia. At autopsy there is extensive deposition of porphyrins in the skeleton and tissues. This may be so pronounced as to color the bones red. Erythroid hyperplasia of the bone marrow and splenomegaly are additional pathologic features.

TREATMENT. Exposure to sunlight should be avoided. The harmful and disfiguring effects of light may be ameliorated by the use of quinine cream. Splenectomy is indicated if there is evidence of increased erythrocyte destruc-tion. Splenectomy may be associated not only with amelioration of the hemolytic anemia but also with a reduction in photosensitivity and porphyrin excretion.

Erythropoietic Protoporphyria

Erythropoietic protoporphyria, the most common form of erythropoietic porphyria, is transmitted as an autosomal dominant characteristic. The disease usually becomes manifest in childhood and is characterized clinically by *skin photosensitivity with intense, painful itching, edema, and erythema of the exposed parts.* Chronic skin changes may develop on the dorsa of the hands, especially over the knuckles, but may also be observed on the nose, cheeks, and lips. Biochemically, the disorder is characterized by an increase in the *protoporphyrin content of the normoblasts and erythrocytes,* an increased level of plasma protoporphyrin, and an increased excretion of protoporphyrin in the feces. The urinary excretion of Δ-ALA, porphobilinogen, coproporphyrin, and uroporphyrin is not increased. However, several patterns of chemical abnormality have been demonstrated in patients with the disease and in members of their families. Elevation of free erythrocyte protoporphyrin may occur with no increase in plasma or fecal protoporphyrin. Fecal protoporphyrin may be increased with no abnormalities of plasma or erythrocyte protoporphyrin. The complete biochemical stigmata of the disease have been observed in the absence of skin photosensitivity.

Erythropoietic Coproporphyria

This disorder is less well defined than the two previous disorders, having been described in only two members of one family. Swelling of the skin and itching after exposure to sunlight were the only clinical manifestations in the propositus. The erythrocytes contained large amounts of coproporphyrin III, a moderate increase in protoporphyrin, and a relatively marked increase in uroporphyrin, in comparison with the normal. Urine and fecal porphyrin concentrations were within normal limits and the excretion of porphyrin precursors was not increased.

PORPHYRIA HEPATICA
Acute Intermittent Porphyria

This is an uncommon but not a rare disease which affects both sexes, with a slight predilection for the female. Young adults or the middle-aged are most frequently affected. Acute porphyria is extremely rare below the age of fifteen and after the age of sixty. The familial occurrence of the disease is marked. It is probably transmitted as a mendelian dominant characteristic. The disease is characterized clinically by (1) periodic attacks of intense abdominal colic, usually accompanied by nausea and vomiting; (2) obstinate constipation; (3) neurotic or even psychotic behavior; and (4) neuromuscular disturbances. The mortality rate is high.

Abdominal pain is frequently the presenting complaint. The pain is usually colicky in nature and may be extremely severe and associated with spasm without localizing signs but with fever, tachycardia, and leukocytosis. The abdominal signs may be, and frequently are, mistaken for manifestations of renal colic, acute appendicitis, cholelithiasis, or pancreatitis. It is not uncommon for patients with porphyria to have multiple surgical scars on the abdomen. The neurologic manifestations are quite varied and may include neuritic pain in the extremities, areas of hypoesthesia and paraesthesia, and foot and wrist drop. Paraplegia or a complete flaccid quadriplegia may ensue and may be followed by bulbar paralysis and death. Except for pain in the extremities, sensory changes are usually not prominent and signs of upper motor neurone changes are usually absent. The neurologic manifestations may simulate a wide variety of conditions, including poliomyelitis, encephalitis, and arsenic or lead poisoning. A true ascending paralysis of the Landry type is not observed.

The patients frequently have many vague "neurotic" complaints, even when in remission from an attack. With an attack they may become confused or even psychotic. Hypertension may accompany an attack, there may be temporary loss of vision, and convulsions have been described.

The course of the disease is extraordinarily variable. Recurrent abdominal crises may be present for years, or the patient may die in the first attack. It is not at all uncommon to find in one parent or in several siblings of a patient with porphyria that porphobilinogen, the diagnostic feature of porphyria, is present in the urine, even though they have never had active symptoms of the disease. This condition is called *latent porphyria*. In general, the neuromuscular and psychotic symptoms are late manifestations, and with their appearance the prognosis becomes more grave. Between attacks there may be no symptoms. The mechanism by which the latent disease is converted to manifest disease, i.e., an attack of acute porphyria, is unknown, but it is known quite definitely that attacks may be provoked by the administration of certain drugs, particularly barbiturates. Menstruation, pregnancy, infection, alcohol, or lead may be the precipitating factor in a few patients.

The freshly voided urine is frequently normal in color and on standing in the sunlight turns to a Burgundy wine color or even black. This color change can be hastened by adding a small amount of acid to the urine and boiling for 30 min. The explanation for these color changes is that porphobilinogen (colorless) and not uroporphyrin (red) is excreted in the urine. Heating of porphobilinogen in an acid medium results in the nonenzymatic formation of uroporphyrin, together with a dark-brown or reddish-brown nonporphyrin pigment.

In acute intermittent porphyria during relapse the presence of porphobilinogen is a constant feature. During remission the porphobilinogen reaction is usually positive, but a negative test does not exclude the diagnosis of this type of porphyria. The qualitative determination of porphobilinogen by the Watson-Schwartz modification of the Ehrlich reaction is, therefore, a simple and valuable screening procedure. In this test 5 ml freshly voided urine is mixed with 5 ml Ehrlich's reagent (0.7 Gm paradimethylaminobenzaldehyde, 150 ml concentrated hydrochloric acid, and 100 ml water). After mixing, 10 ml aqueous saturated sodium acetate is added. The solution is then extracted successively with 10 ml chloroform and 10 ml n-butanol. A positive test for porphobilinogen gives an intense red color remaining in the aqueous layer. This test is quite specific for acute intermittent porphyria. The test is negative in erythropoietic porphyria and in porphyria cutanea tarda symptomatica. It is positive in patients with porphyria cutanea tarda hereditaria during acute attacks but is negative in the interval between such episodes.

In addition to porphobilinogen, patients with acute intermittent porphyria excrete excessive quantities of uroporphyrin (types I and III), coproporphyrin (types I and III), and other as yet unidentified porphyrins. As mentioned previously, the porphyrins are formed in the renal tubules by the nonenzymatic transformation of porphobilinogen into uroporphyrin at an acid pH. Examination of the tissues of such patients, in contrast to the findings in erythropoietic porphyria, has revealed that the porphorin content of the bone marrow is normal. The liver, on the contrary, regularly exhibits increased quantities of porphyrin, especially porphyrin precursors. For this reason, acute intermittent porphyria is classified among the hepatic porphyrias.

ALA synthetase has now been shown to be an inducible enzyme in both man and animals. Induction can be augmented by barbiturates, estrogens, certain 5β-H steroid metabolites, and a variety of chemical compounds. Induction can be inhibited by high carbohydrate intake. Thus, the major chemical manifestations of acute intermittent porphyria are best explained as resulting from overproduction of porphyrin precursors, secondary to induction of hepatic ALA synthetase. The genetic lesion in acute intermittent porphyria is most likely in the operator gene mechanism for ALA synthetase.

TREATMENT. Drugs such as barbiturates and estrogens which induce Δ-ALA synthetase must be avoided. There is a theoretical basis for recommending a high carbohydrate intake. In acute attacks, opiates such as meperidine (Demerol) or ganglioplegics such as tetraethylammonium may be used for relief of pain. Chloralhydrate or paraldehyde may be used for sedation. Neostigmine may be of value in treating severe constipation. Chlorpromazine, in doses of 50 to 100 mg, may affect rapid relief of acute symptoms, but without change in the underlying process. Hyponatremia and hypochloremia secondary to inappropriate secretion of antidiuretic hormone may occur in some patients during acute attacks and require therapy. Respiratory support may be needed in some patients. ACTH and corticosteroids and chelating agents such as BAL (2, 3-dimercaptopropanol), EDTA (disodium ethylenediaminetetraacetate), and penicillamine have not been shown definitely to be of value.

Porphyria Cutanea Tarda Hereditaria

Porphyria cutanea tarda hereditaria is characterized clinically by cutaneous lesions or acute attacks of abdominal colic and not infrequently by both. The disease is inherited as a non-sex-linked mendelian dominant. The onset of symptoms is usually between the ages of ten and thirty years. The outstanding biochemical feature of the disorder is the increased excretion of coproporphyrin and protoporphyrin in the feces *at all times* in the course of the disease.

During the latent phase of the disease the patients are entirely asymptomatic. Porphyrinuria is usually absent and the porphyrin precursors, Δ-aminolevulinic acid and porphobilinogen, are not excreted in increased amounts. The disease can be diagnosed only during the latent phase by examination of the stools for porphyrins. A simple screening test can be done by obtaining a small specimen of stool on a glove. The specimen is extracted with about 2 ml of solvent containing equal parts of glacial acetic acid, amyl alcohol, and ether. The supernatant solution is then extracted with 1.5 N HCl and viewed in a Wood's lamp. Red fluorescence in the acid layer is proportional to the porphyrin content.

In a number of patients, particularly males, the skin is unusually sensitive to light and blisters and abrades easily. Healed depigmented scars may be present over the exposed surfaces, particularly the hands. Hyperpigmentation of the skin may occur, and hirsutism has been observed in females. The photosensitivity and cutaneous deformities are not so great as in erythropoietic porphyria.

Acute attacks of jaundice and abdominal colic accompanied in some cases by psychotic manifestations and motor paralysis may intervene in the course of the disease. Indeed, any or all of the manifestations of acute intermittent porphyria may make their appearance. As in acute intermittent porphyria, death or recovery may occur. During the acute attacks the excretion of porphyrins in the feces frequently decreases and the excretion of coproporphyrin and uroporphyrin in the urine increases. Both Δ-aminolevulinic acid and porphobilinogen are usually excreted in increased amounts in the urine during acute attacks. It has been suggested that the disease remains asymptomatic as long as the liver is capable of excreting the porphyrins in the bile (latent phase); when this capacity is impaired bilirubinemia, porphyrinemia, porphyrinuria, and cutaneous lesions appear (cutaneous phase); and finally when porphyrin metabolism is greatly disturbed, Δ-aminolevulinic acid and porphobilinogen appear in the urine and all the manifestations of acute intermittent porphyria may develop (acute phase). Porphyria cutanea tarda hereditaria is not an entirely suitable name for this disorder since not all patients develop cutaneous lesions. It is for this reason that the designation *porphyria variegata* has been suggested.

Porphyria Cutanea Tarda Symptomatica

This type of porphyria is characterized clinically by cutaneous lesions, hyperpigmentation of the skin, evidences of liver disease, and hypertrichosis; and chemically by the excretion of large amounts of uroporphyrin and lesser amounts of coproporphyrin in the urine. Abdominal pain and neurologic complications are conspicuously absent. The urine does not contain increased quantities of Δ-aminolevulinic acid or porphobilinogen. The excretion of protoporphyrin in the feces is normal; the excretion of coproporphyrin in the feces is usually increased.

The skin lesions are indistinguishable from those observed in porphyria cutanea tarda hereditaria. The skin is usually sensitive both to light and to mechanical trauma. Blisters appear on the exposed skin areas, frequently ulcerate, and finally lead to scar formation. The photosensitivity is similar to that in erythropoietic porphyria but not as marked.

This disorder has been described (1) in male subjects, forty to seventy years of age, with alcoholic cirrhosis of the liver; (2) in Bantu subjects in South Africa with nutritional cirrhosis of the liver; (3) in children and adults in Turkey who have ingested the fungicide hexachlorobenzene; (4) in three elderly subjects with a tumor of the liver; and (5) in an occasional young adult without a history of alcoholism or drug exposure. Porphyria cutanea tarda symptomatica is probably acquired, but constitutional factors may be involved in some cases.

Hereditary Coproporphyria

The unique feature of this disease is an increased excretion of coproporphyrin, isomer type III. In the latent phase, the patients are asymptomatic and the only abnormality usually detectable is an increased excretion of coproporphyrin III in the urine and feces, particularly the latter. Urinary Δ-ALA and porphobilinogen may be normal or slightly increased. Acute attacks, similar to those which occur in acute intermittent porphyria, can be provoked by the ingestion of barbiturates and possibly by certain tranquilizers and anticonvulsants. During these attacks there is an excessive excretion of Δ-ALA and porphobilinogen in the urine, in addition to a massive excretion of coproporphyrin in both urine and stool. About 30 cases of this disorder have been reported. Psychiatric symptoms may be present without other clinical manifestations of porphyria. Skin photosensitivity has been described in one case. The disease is inherited as a dominant characteristic and occurs in both sexes. The neurologic and psychiatric aspects of porphyria are discussed further in Chaps. 354 and 30 respectively.

REFERENCES

Donaldson, E. M., A. D. Donaldson, and C. Rimington: Erythropoietic Protoporphyria: A Family Study, Brit. Med. J., 1:659, 1967.

Goldberg, A., and C. Rimington: "Diseases of Porphyrin Metabolism," Springfield, Ill., Charles C Thomas, Publisher, 1962.

——, C. Rimington, and A. C. Lochhead: Hereditary Coproporphyria, Lancet, 1:632, 1967.

Heilmeyer, L., and R. Clotten: Congenital Erythropoietic Coproporphyria, Ger. Med. Mon., 9:1, 1964.

Kappas, A., and S. Granick: Steroid Induction of Porphyrin Synthesis in Liver Cell Culture, J. Biol. Chem., 243:346, 1968.

Tschudy, D. P.: Biochemical Lesions in Porphyria, J.A.M.A., 191:718, 1965.

Watson, C. J., L. Taddeini, and I. Bossenmaier: Present Status of the Ehrlich Aldehyde Reaction for Urinary Porphobilinogen, J.A.M.A., 190:501, 1964.

109 DISORDERS OF MELANIN METABOLISM

Thomas B. Fitzpatrick

DEFINITION OF MELANIN

Melanin is the principal basis of the coloration of human skin, hair, and eyes. In man, it functions primarily as a screen that shields the dermis from the deleterious effects of solar radiation. Since the amount and distribution of melanin in skin and hair are changed in a number of diseases, a detailed study of the irregularities of pigmentation may provide important diagnostic clues to diseases in other organs.

The term *melanin* is derived from the Greek word *melas,* black, and is the name given to a biochrome of high molecular weight formed by enzymatic oxidation of the phenol tyrosine, by the action of tyrosinase. The biochrome is therefore often referred to as *tyrosine melanin.* Tyrosine melanin is the product of unique unicellular glands, *melanocytes,* that secrete melanin particles into epidermal cells. The exact chemical nature of melanin has not been determined, because tyrosine melanin (both natural and synthetic) is so extremely insoluble that all attempts to degrade it into identifiable fragments have failed until now. However, it is now known that all animal melanins are "indole" in type and are composed basically of indole-5,6-quinone units, in contrast with melanins of plant origin, which are "catechol" in type. Also, studies using radioactive dopa (dihydroxyphenylalanine) have revealed that melanin appears to be a copolymer of dopa-quinone, indole-5,6-quinone, and indole-5,6-quinone-2-carboxylic acid in the ratio of 3:2:1.

BIOSYNTHESIS OF MELANIN

Melanocytes are situated at the dermoepidermal interface, in the hair bulb, the uveal tract, retinal pigment epithelium, and the leptomeninges. These scattered groups of cells are known as the *melanocyte system.* They may be considered to constitute a unit, because the melanocytes in all these locations are derived from the neural crest (Fig. 109-1) and can hydroxylate tyrosine to dopa and, ultimately, to the pigment, tyrosine melanin. The melanocyte system is analogous, but not known to be related, to the chromaffin system. Like melanocytes, the cells of the chromaffin system are derived from the neural crest and possess biochemical mechanisms for the hydroxylation of tyrosine to dopa, but by the action of tyrosine hydroxylase, not tyrosinase; unlike melanocytes, they convert dopa to adrenochrome and not to tyrosine melanin. Benign and malignant neoplasms arise in all parts of the melanocyte system except the retinal pigment epithelium and the hair bulbs.

The melanocytes present at the dermoepidermal interface form a horizontal network that is closely connected to the epidermal cells by means of numerous cytoplasmic processes, or dendrites. This intimate relationship permitting cytocrine transfer of melanin particles (melanosomes —see definition below) from melanocytes to malpighian cells has been clearly demonstrated by electron microscopy in a study of the fine structure of cortical cells and hair melanocytes and by tissue culture studies of human epidermis.

It has been possible to demonstrate by electron microscopy that melanocytes contain specialized organelles with a distinctive internal structure. These organelles, known as *melanosomes,* contain tyrosinase, the melanin-synthesizing enzyme. Under normal conditions, melanin is progressively formed and deposited on the surface of melanosomes until they become amorphous particles without detectable tyrosinase activity (Fig. 109-2). Melanosomes are believed to originate in the Golgi area, appearing first as unmelanized vesicles that gradually increase in size and become dark in color and increasingly dense.

Tyrosinase is one of a large group of copper-containing aerobic oxidases that catalyze the oxidation of both mono-hydroxy and o-dihydroxy phenols to orthoquinones. In man and other mammals, this oxidase catalyzes the hydroxylation of the melanin precursor tyrosine to dopa and dopa-quinone (Fig. 109-3). Tyrosinase is required only for the first step in the biosynthesis of tyrosine melanin, i.e., the orthohydroxylation of tyrosine. It is noteworthy that zinc ions catalyze the conversion of dopa-chrome to 5,6-dihydroxyindole and that melanosomes have been shown to contain zinc in high concentration.

In the hair and skin of the various races, characteristic coloration is thought to be determined not by variations in the number of melanocytes present but by variations in the number and type of melanosomes produced by existing melanocytes. The amount of pigment present in individual melanosomes is related to their tyrosinase content; for example, melanosomes that lack tyrosinase remain unpigmented, as in some types of albinism.

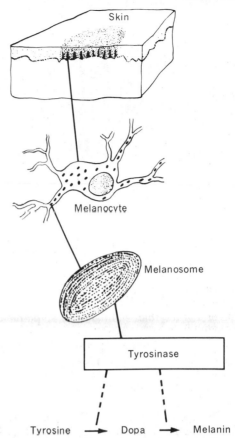

Fig. 109-2. Melanogenesis in human skin, as seen in the light microscope and the electron microscope and at the molecular level.

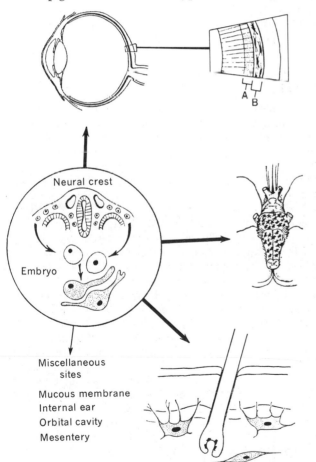

Fig. 109-1. Diagram showing the embryonic origin, dispersal, and developmental fate of melanocytes in man. (*By permission, from J. B. Stanbury et al. (Eds.), "The Metabolic Basis of Inherited Disease," 2d ed., New York, McGraw-Hill Book Company, 1966.*)

PATHOGENESIS OF PIGMENTARY DISORDERS

To explain the pathogenesis of a disturbance of melanin pigmentation, it is necessary to evaluate the rate at which tyrosinase is synthesized on the ribosomes, to determine the rate at which melanosomes progress through successive stages to full melanization, to understand the role played by factors that regulate the biosynthesis of melanin, and to examine the transfer of melanosomes to epidermal cells.

Availability of free tyrosine is essential for the biosynthesis of melanin. Tyrosine that is bound in a peptide linkage cannot act as a substrate if the amino group is blocked.

Aggregation and dispersion of melanosomes probably play no part in the pigmentary anomalies of man. Such movement has thus far been observed only in specialized effector cells, *melanophores,* present only in vertebrates below mammals in the phylogenetic scale.

DIAGNOSIS OF PIGMENTARY DISORDERS

Disorders of melanin pigmentation that involve the melanocyte system may be classed as *hypomelanoses* and *hypermelanoses.* On a morphologic basis, these disorders

Fig. 109-3. Biosynthesis of tyrosine melanin.

can be divided into three main categories: (1) hypomelanosis, in which paucity or absence of pigment renders the skin white or lighter than normal; (2) hypermelanosis (brown), in which excess pigment produces a brown-black color; and (3) hypermelanosis (blue), in which excess pigment produces a blue, slate, or gray hue. Pigmentary disorders with similar etiology may also be grouped together. Table 109-1 incorporates these various methods of classification. Hypomelanosis (decreased pigmentation) may result from loss of melanocytes, as in thermal burns, or from absence or paucity of melanin. In the disorders listed under the heading of Brown Hypermelanosis in Table 109-1, the brown pigmentation results, in most instances, from an increase in the *activity* of epidermal melanocytes and not from an increase in the number of these cells. Gray, slate, or blue hypermelanosis results from the presence of melanin within dermal phagocytes or ectopic dermal melanocytes. The blue, slate, or gray hue is related to the Tyndall light-scattering phenomenon.

Recognition of hypomelanosis and of gray, slate, or blue hypermelanosis is usually not difficult. When the degree of hypomelanosis is very slight, diagnosis may be facilitated by the use of black light. Differentiation between abnormal diffuse brown hyperpigmentation and normal pigmentation frequently poses a problem because there is such a wide range of coloration in different individuals. It is usually possible, however, to determine whether the patient has observed an unusual or progressive change in coloration that has had no obvious cause. A summer tan may not have faded, or the patient's associates may have detected a gradual deepening of his skin color. The degree of brown hypermelanosis that develops appears to be related to the basic skin color of the patient. For example, a patient of Mediterranean extraction (Italian, French, Spanish) may become intensely pigmented with the onset of primary adrenocortical in-

sufficiency, whereas a light-skinned patient will have only a minimal degree of hypermelanosis that may or may not be detectable. Localized pigmentation that develops newly in the mucous membranes and in specific areas, such as the axillas and palmar creases, is usually easier to identify as a pathologic change than is generalized hyperpigmentation.[1]

CLINICAL DISORDERS
Genetic

ALBINISM. Albinism, a mendelian autosomal recessive trait, is characterized by paucity or absence of melanin in affected areas of the body. In this disorder, whatever tyrosinase may be synthesized by the melanocytes is functionally defective and unable to catalyze the oxidation of tyrosine to melanin. The formation of melanosomes is interrupted in the early stages; few or no mature melanosomes are present in albinotic skin or hair. Albinism is diagnosed and classified on the basis of ocular and cutaneous findings.[2] The same ocular abnormalities, e.g., hypopigmentation of the fundus oculi, translucency of the irides, and nystagmus, are found in both the oculocutaneous and the ocular types of the disorder. In *oculocutaneous* albinism, these ocular changes are associated with total, unpatterned hypopigmentation of the skin; in *ocular* albinism, pigmentation of the skin is normal. The deficiency of melanin in oculocutaneous albinism has two disturbing consequences for man: decreased visual acuity and an abnormal degree of intolerance to sunlight. The sensitivity of human albinos to ultraviolet light leads to the development of carcinoma in exposed areas of the skin, especially in albinos living in the tropics.

PHENYLKETONURIA. In phenylketonuria, there is a single metabolic block in the conversion of phenylalanine to tyrosine. The condition is associated with subnormal

---

[1] Pigmentation of the gums, tongue, and buccal mucosa is a normal finding in Asiatics, American Indians, and Negroes and often in East Indians.

[2] Two types of oculocutaneous albinism, with separate gene loci, are now described, based on the presence of tyrosinase, which causes darkening, when plucked hair follicles are incubated in tyrosine. "Tyrosinase-positive" indicates darkening; "tyrosinase-negative," no darkening.

Table 109-1. DISTURBANCES OF HUMAN MELANIN PIGMENTATION[1]

Causative factors	Classification		
	Hypomelanosis (white) *in association with*	Brown hypermelanosis *in association with*	Gray, slate, or blue hypermelanosis[2] *in association with*
Genetic disorders	Piebaldism Waardenburg's syndrome Vitiligo[3] Albinism, oculocutaneous[4] Albinism, ocular Hypomelanotic macules in tuberous sclerosis[5] Phenylketonuria[6,7]	*Café au lait* macules in neurofibromatosis Melanotic macules in polyostotic fibrous dysplasia (Albright's syndrome) Lentigines with cardiac arrhythmias Neurocutaneous melanosis Xeroderma pigmentosum Acanthosis nigricans, juvenile type Peutz-Jeghers syndrome	Oculodermal melanocytosis (nevus of Ota) Dermal melanocytosis (Mongolian spot)
Metabolic diseases		Hemochromatosis[4] Hepatolenticular disease (Wilson's disease)[4] Porphyria (congenital erythropoietica and porphyria variegata and cutanea tarda) Gaucher's disease[4] Niemann-Pick disease	Hemochromatosis[4]
Endocrine disorders	Hypopituitarism[4] Addison's disease Hyperthyroidism	ACTH-producing and MSH-producing pituitary and other tumors[4] ACTH therapy[4] Pregnancy[9] Addison's disease[4] Estrogen therapy[10] Melasma[11]	
Nutritional disorders	Chronic protein deficiency or loss, as in kwashiorkor, nephrosis, ulcerative colitis, malabsorption syndrome; the hair is gray or reddish[6] Vitamin B_{12} deficiency[6]	Kwashiorkor Pellagra[12] Sprue[12] Vitamin B_{12} deficiency[6]	Chronic nutritional insufficiency
Chemical and pharmacologic agents	Monobenzyl ether of hydroquinone Chloroquine and hydroxychloroquine[6] Arsenical intoxication	Arsenical intoxication[4] Busulfan administration[4] Photochemical agents (topical or systemic drugs, tar) Dibromomannitol administration[4]	
Physical agents	Burns: Thermal, ultraviolet, ionizing radiation[8] Trauma	Ultraviolet light Heat Alpha, beta, and gamma radiation Trauma (e.g., chronic pruritus)	
Inflammations and infectious diseases	Pinta Leprosy[5] Fungous infections (tinea versicolor)[5] Miscellaneous dermatoses: Psoriasis Lupus erythematosus, discoid	Postinflammation pigmentation (exanthems, drug eruptions) Miscellaneous dermatoses: Lupus erythematosus, discoid Lichen simplex chronicus Atopic dermatitis[4] Psoriasis	Pinta in exposed areas
Neoplasms	In sites of melanoma after disappearance (therapeutic or spontaneous) of tumor	Mastocytosis (urticaria pigmentosa) Adenocarcinoma with acanthosis nigricans	Dermal-pigmentation syndrome with metastatic melanoma and melanogenuria[4]
Miscellaneous disorders	Vogt-Koyanagi syndrome Scleroderma, circumscribed or systemic Horner's syndrome, congenital and acquired[7]	Scleroderma, systemic[4] Chronic hepatic insufficiency[4] Whipple's syndrome[4] Melasma (chloasma) Lentigo, senile ("liver spots")	

[1] This classification includes disorders of interest to physicians in general; many pigmentary disorders not listed are of special interest to dermatologists.
[2] Gray, slate, or blue color results from the presence of *dermal* melanocytes or phagocytized melanin in the dermis.
[3] Total loss of pigment in the skin and hair may occur.
[4] Pigment change is diffuse, not circumscribed, and there are no identifiable borders.
[5] Loss of pigmentation is usually partial; viewed with Wood's light, the lesions are not snow-white, as in vitiligo.
[6] Pigment is decreased in the hair.
[7] Pigment is decreased in the iris.
[8] There is a loss of melanocytes.
[9] Pigment change may be diffuse or circumscribed.
[10] Nipples are affected.
[11] Idiopathic or due to progestational agents.
[12] May be diffuse.
SOURCE: 1968 revision of table from T. B. Fitzpatrick, in T. R. Harrison et al., *"Principles of Internal Medicine,"* 5th ed., Chap. 102, p. 565, New York, McGraw-Hill Book Company, 1966.

pigmentation of the hair and the iris. The hair of patients with phenylketonuria ranges in color from light blond to dark brown, and it is only by comparison with the hair of siblings that the characteristic dilution of color becomes evident. The diminution of melanin formation results from the fact that the large amounts of phenylalanine and its metabolites present in serum and extracellular fluid act as competitive inhibitors of tyrosinase activity, thus blocking melanin synthesis (Chap. 102).

PIEBALDISM. Piebaldism, an autosomal dominant trait, involves the skin and the hair only. In piebaldism, there are hypomelanotic patterned areas on the extremities and anterior surface of the thorax, and there is commonly a white forelock. The melanin content of the eyes, however, usually remains normal. Piebaldism is associated with congenital deafness in a syndrome known as Waardenburg's. Electron microscopic studies have revealed that the areas of skin lacking in pigment lack melanocytes, as in vitiligo (see below).

VITILIGO. Vitiligo may be localized or generalized. When localized, the hypomelanosis of the skin and hair may be restricted to one region, such as the genitalia or perianal area or scalp area. When generalized, the pattern of hypomelanosis is quite typical, with lesions particularly on the face, axillas, neck, and extremities, and with loss of pigment in the hair. Idiopathic vitiligo is fairly common, affecting 1 percent of the population. The lesions are completely lacking in pigment, and this snow-whiteness is distinctive and serves to differentiate vitiligo from other hypomelanoses. Vitiligo is inherited as an autosomal dominant trait with irregular penetrance. In the majority of cases, the vitiligo is idiopathic, but typical vitiligo, as just described, is known to occur with a variety of diseases, such as Addison's disease, hyperthyroidism, hypo-

parathyroidism, pernicious anemia, and alopecia areata. Electron microscopic studies of vitiligo of the skin reveal a severe reduction or, more commonly, a total absence of melanocytes so that the hypomelanosis is the result of a structural defect, rather than a metabolic change, in the existing melanocytes.

TUBEROUS SCLEROSIS. (See Chap. 365.) Tuberous sclerosis, a serious autosomal dominant trait usually causing mental retardation and convulsions, is associated with characteristic white macules in 67 percent of the patients. These white macules are present at birth and therefore constitute an important sign that permits the physician to establish an early diagnosis in an infant and to forewarn the parents about a possible genetic defect in any other children that they might have. These white macules are present when other diagnostic skin signs of tuberous sclerosis are not evident, because the typical facial lesions do not appear until the second to the sixth year after birth. The lesions are not snow-white, as in vitiligo, but are off-white. The white lesions are usually larger than 1 cm in diameter and are more easily detected with the aid of a black or Wood's light, especially in fair-skinned infants. Although the predominant outline of the lesion is similar to that of a mountain-ash leaflet, from which it takes its name (Fig. 109-4), other configurations occur, such as round or oval; sometimes the distribution follows a dermatomal pattern. The ash-leaf spots vary in number from 3 to 100, and may be present on any part of the skin surface, but are more common on the trunk and lower extremities. Histochemical and electron microscopic studies reveal that there is not an absence of melanocytes, as in vitiligo, but a marked reduction of melanin deposition on the melanosomes within the melanocytes present in the affected areas, with resultant hypomelanosis.

NEUROFIBROMATOSIS (VON RECKLINGHAUSEN'S DISEASE). This condition is inherited as a dominant trait. It is characterized by the presence, primarily on the trunk but also on the extremities, of numerous pale yellow-brown macules, so-called *café au lait* spots, that vary in diameter from less than 1 to more than 15 cm. Spotty generalized pigmentation may also be present, especially in the axillas. Often, but not always, a few or myriads of soft, rounded, cone-shaped or pendulous cutaneous tumors covered by normal skin are seen. Nerve sheath tumors may occur.

The presence of six or more *café au lait* spots with a diameter greater than 1.5 cm is diagnostic of neurofibromatosis even when there is no familial history of the condition. In *polyostotic fibrous dysplasia*, there are rarely more than three or four macules, unilaterally distributed usually on the buttocks or cervical area (Chap. 384). Clinically, the single large isolated *café au lait* spot of neurofibromatosis resembles the pigmented macule of *polyostotic fibrous dysplasia (Albright's disease)*. It is possible, however, to detect peculiar large extracellular globules of melanin in whole mounts of epidermis prepared from the *café au lait* macules of neurofibromatosis; these extracellular melanin globules are not found in the macular pigmented areas present in polyostotic fibrous dysplasia.

Fig. 109-4. A 4-cm lesion showing the typical configuration of a leaf from a mountain-ash tree. A projected outline of an actual leaf is shown next to the lesion.

Metabolic

Generalized brown hypermelanosis of the skin is a characteristic manifestation of *hemochromatosis* and *cutaneous porphyria (porphyria cutanea tarda)* (Chap. 108). The hyperpigmentation observed in hemochromatosis (Chap. 107) may have a grayish-brown hue or be indistinguishable from that of Addison's disease (Chap. 92). The diagnosis of hemochromatosis is established by the presence of hemosiderin in the sweat glands of the skin. Porphyria may be recognized by the abnormally large amounts of *uroporphyrin* in the urine, stools, and plasma and by other characteristic clinical features, such as the presence of bullae, atrophic scars, and milia on the exposed surfaces of the face and hands.

Nutritional

CHRONIC PROTEIN DEFICIENCY. Chronic protein deficiency, as, for example, in kwashiorkor, chronic nephrosis, ulcerative colitis, and malabsorption syndrome, is sometimes associated with a change in hair color, first to a reddish-brown and eventually to gray. In chronic nutritional insufficiency, splotches of dirty-brown hyperpigmentation appear, especially on the trunk. In *sprue,* brown hypermelanosis may be generalized. In *pellagra,* hypermelanosis is limited to areas of skin that have been exposed to light. *Vitamin B$_{12}$ deficiency* leads to loss of hair color and intense brown hypermelanosis around the small joints and a generalized Addisonian type of hypermelanosis.

Endocrine

Diffuse brown hypermelanosis is a striking feature of primary adrenocortical insufficiency (Chap. 92). Although this hypermelanosis is diffuse, there is marked accentuation of pigmentation in certain areas, namely, on the pressure points (vertebras, knuckles, elbows, knees), and in the body folds, the palmar creases, and the gingival mucous membrane. An identical type of diffuse hyperpigmentation has also been reported to follow adrenalectomy in patients with Cushing's disease. In these patients, there are usually signs and symptoms of pituitary tumors; all the tumors recorded have been chromophobe adenomas. A third example of the Addison type of melanosis described above has been reported in patients with tumors of organs other than the adrenal or pituitary glands. The generalized brown hypermelanosis found in all these conditions results from overproduction of two hormones: alpha-melanocyte-stimulating hormone (MSH) and ACTH. Both peptides, MSH and ACTH, share common peptide sequences. It appears that an excess of alpha-melanocyte-stimulating hormone plays the dominant role in the pigmentation that occurs in adrenocortical insufficiency. Both MSH and ACTH are increased as a result of the decreased output of hydrocortisone by the adrenals. Hypermelanosis of the Addison type can be produced in adrenalectomized human subjects by administering large amounts of homogeneous ACTH and alpha-MSH.

Chemical

Chemicals can induce both hypomelanosis and hypermelanosis. Hydroquinone and 4-isopropylcatechol prevent the formation of melanin and are of therapeutic value in treating hypermelanosis. Striking generalized Addisonian hypermelanosis of the skin follows busulfan therapy; the mechanism of action of this drug is not known. Inorganic trivalent arsenicals produce both generalized Addisonian hypermelanosis and scattered macular hypomelanosis, as well as punctate keratoses on the palms and soles.

Physical

Mechanical trauma, as well as burns caused by heat, ultraviolet light, or alpha-, beta-, and gamma-radiation, can lead to hypomelanosis or hypermelanosis. The effect of these physical agents on pigmentation is determined by the intensity and duration of exposure and is limited to the site of injury. The hypomelanosis results from destruction of melanocytes.

Chronic pruritus, such as that associated with chronic biliary-tract disease and lymphoma, may lead to generalized brown hypermelanosis.

Inflammatory and Infectious

Circumscribed hypomelanosis is a characteristic feature of tuberculoid leprosy. It occurs in areas of anesthesia, and the degree of pigment loss is only partial; the lesions are lighter in color than the areas of surrounding skin but are not snow-white as in vitiligo. Generalized spotty hyperpigmentation not uncommonly follows *exanthems* and *eruptions due to drugs;* it usually disappears spontaneously within 2 or 3 months.

Neoplastic

Hypomelanosis is seen in rare instances at the site of a primary or a metastatic *malignant melanoma* that has undergone remission spontaneously or as the result of chemotherapy. During the terminal stages of malignant melanoma, striking generalized blue hypermelanosis sometimes develops, and large amounts of a conjugated derivative of 5,6-dihydroxyindole are excreted in the urine ("melanogenuria"). This intermediate in the metabolic pathway from tyrosine to melanin can be oxidized to melanin in the absence of tyrosinase, and therefore melanin can be synthesized at almost any site in which oxidation can take place. Consequently, diffuse black pigmentation may develop in the peritoneum, liver, heart, muscle, and dermis of patients during the late stages of malignant melanoma. The brown melanin present in the dermal phagocytes appears as blue in the skin, because of the Tyndall light-scattering phenomenon.

The multiple, irregular, round or oval, yellow-brown-to-red-brown macules and papules characteristic of *urticaria pigmentosa* are related to the presence in the dermis of clusters of mast cells. Urticarial wheals develop when the individual lesions are stroked vigorously. In rare instances (*systemic mastocytosis*), mast cells infiltrate diffusely into the liver, spleen, gastrointestinal system, and bones, as well as into the skin.

Miscellaneous

Generalized brown hypermelanosis of the type seen in Addison's disease is not infrequently associated with *systemic scleroderma* and may appear very early in the course of the disorder. Generalized hyperpigmentation occasionally develops in patients with *chronic hepatic insufficiency,* especially that due to portal cirrhosis. The pathogenesis of the pigmentation in both these conditions is unknown.

Melasma (chloasma) is seen most commonly in pregnant women, but it also occurs in men and in nonpregnant women. The lesions consist of large macules with irregular borders on the exposed areas of the face and vary in color from yellow-brown to red-brown and very dark brown. Melasma is sometimes observed in women receiving oral progestational agents.

REFERENCES

Della Porta, G., and O. Mühlbock (Eds.): "Symposium on Structure and Control of the Melanocyte: Proceedings of the International Pigment Cell Conference," sponsored by the International Union against Cancer, Sofia, Bulgaria, May 1965, Berlin, Springer-Verlag, 1966.

Fitzpatrick, T. B., M. Miyamoto, and K. Ishikawa: The Evolution of Concepts of Melanin Biology, pp. 1–30 in W. Montanga and F. Hu (Eds.), "Advances in Biology of Skin: Volume VIII: The Pigmentary System," Oxford, Pergamon Press, 1967.

—— and W. C. Quevedo, Jr.: Albinism, in "The Metabolic Basis of Inherited Disease," 2d ed., J. B. Stanbury, J. B. Wyngaarden, and D. S. Fredrickson (Eds.), New York, McGraw-Hill Book Company, 1966.

——, M. Seiji, and A. D. McGugan: Melanin Pigmentation, New Engl. J. Med., 265:328, 374, 430, 1961.

Jeghers, H., and H. Mescon: Pigmentation of the Skin, in C. M. MacBryde (Ed.), "Signs and Symptoms: Applied Pathologic Physiology and Clinical Interpretation," 4th ed., Philadelphia, J. B. Lippincott Company, 1964.

Lerner, A. B.: Melanin Pigmentation, Am. J. Med., 19:902, 1955.

—— and J. S. McGuire: Melanocyte-stimulating Hormone and Adrenocorticotrophic Hormone; Their Relation to Pigmentation, New Engl. J. Med., 270:539, 1964.

Riley, V., and J. G. Fortner (Eds.): The Pigment Cell: Molecular, Biological and Clinical Aspects, Ann. N. Y. Acad. Sci., 100, pts. I and II, February, 1963.

110 HEPATOLENTICULAR DEGENERATION (Wilson's Disease)

George E. Cartwright

Definition

Hepatolenticular degeneration (progressive lenticular degeneration, Wilson's disease, pseudosclerosis of Westphal and Strümpell, tetanoid chorea of Gowers) is an uncommon, familial, progressive, fatal disease which becomes manifest usually in the first three decades of life and is characterized by the triad of basal ganglion degeneration, cirrhosis of the liver, and a ring of brown pigment at the corneal margins known as the Kayser-Fleischer ring.

History

Kinnier Wilson, in 1912, in his classic monograph "Progressive Lenticular Degeneration," first clearly defined the disease entity to which his name is now affixed. A similar condition had previously been described in 1883 by Westphal and later by Strümpell. The symptoms resembled those of multiple sclerosis, but no demyelinative plaques were observed. For that reason it was called *pseudosclerosis.* The cirrhosis of the liver was overlooked until Spielmeyer reexamined the cases many years later. His studies and the clinical observations of Hall left little doubt that hepatolenticular degeneration and pseudosclerosis were the same disease. The corneal ring was described in 1902 by Kayser in a case diagnosed as "multiple sclerosis," but to Fleischer is due the credit for appreciating its significance in relation to the disease as it is now known.

A marked increase in the copper content of both the brain and the liver was demonstrated by Haurowitz in 1930 and was later confirmed by Glazebrook and Cummings. Mandelbrote and his associates in 1948 observed by chance that the urinary output of copper was high and that this output is increased by the administration of BAL (British antilewisite). In the same year Uzman and Denny-Brown found that a persistent aminoaciduria is associated with the disease. Ceruloplasmin deficiency was recognized as a feature of the disease by Scheinberg and Gitlin in 1952. An effective treatment of the disease was introduced by Walshe in 1956.

Inheritance

The condition is inherited as an autosomal recessive trait, the affected individuals inheriting the gene from both parents who, while phenotypically normal, are heterozygous for the abnormal allele. Since the frequency of the abnormal gene is low in the general population, affected individuals may be expected to be, most often, the products of consanguineous marriages. This has proved to be the case.

Pathogenesis

Two different types of metabolic disturbance have been described, namely (1) abnormalities in the metabolism of copper and (2) impairment in renal tubular reabsorption.

A number of alterations in the metabolism of copper has been described (Table 110-1). The amount of copper in the tissues, particularly in the liver and brain, is increased about tenfold above the normal. The golden-

Table 110-1. BIOCHEMICAL ALTERATIONS IN
WILSON'S DISEASE

Determination	Normal subjects*	Wilson's disease
Total plasma copper, μg/100 ml	114 (81–147)	60 (19–103)
Direct-reacting plasma copper, μg/100 ml	7 (0–20)	26 (12–40)
Ceruloplasmin, mg/100 ml	33 (25–43)	9 (0–19)
Urine copper, μg/24 hr	15 (5–25)	522 (95–1,300)†
Liver copper, μg/Gm wet tissue	5 (3–10)	79 (53–100)†
Urine α-amino nitrogen, mg/day	164 (118–204)	337 (90–519)

* The figures in parentheses refer to ±2 standard deviations.
† Determined range.

brown pigment of the Kayser-Fleischer ring contains copper. The amount of copper excreted in the urine is increased. The specific copper protein of plasma, ceruloplasmin, is almost invariably decreased. On the other hand, the "direct-reacting" fraction of plasma copper, the copper which is probably loosely bound to albumin, is increased. Since there is a greater reduction in ceruloplasmin copper than there is increase in direct-reacting copper, the net effect on the total plasma copper is such that there is usually hypocupremia. In an occasional patient the total plasma copper concentration may be as high as 116 μg per 100 ml. Patients with this disease retain more than the normal amount of copper in the body. This is apparently because of an increased rate of absorption of copper from the gastrointestinal tract. Whether or not copper is excreted by the liver into the bile at the normal rate has not yet been determined with certainty. There may be a normal copper content in the bile, but this is not normal when the total copper content of the liver is considered.

Renal dysfunction which is present in many, but not all, patients includes abnormalities in tubular reabsorption manifested by aminoaciduria, peptiduria, proteinuria, glucosuria, uricosuria, or phosphaturia. The aminoaciduria involves most of the amino acids found in normal urine and, in addition, proline and citrulline. Taurine, aspartic acid, isoleucine, methyl histidine, and arginine are excreted in amounts close to the normal range. The urinary amino acid pattern and the severity of the aminoaciduria depend in part on the amount and type of protein ingested and vary considerably from patient to patient without relation to the type, duration, or stage of disease. The aminoaciduria is not accompanied by any significant elevation in the blood α-amino nitrogen level. The uricosuria may be associated with a diminished level of uric acid in the serum. The phosphaturia may result in hypophosphatemia and eventually in osseous changes.

The pathogenesis of the metabolic and pathologic changes is not fully understood. Because of the excessive deposition of copper in the tissues of patients with Wilson's disease, it has been suggested that the lesions in the liver and in the lenticular nuclei are the consequence of the excessive deposition of copper in these tissues and that the accumulation of copper in the kidney causes a functional impairment in the reabsorption of amino acids, peptides, and other substances. In support of this concept is the observation that excessive deposition of copper in the liver precedes the development of significant parenchymal damage. Furthermore, in most patients with the disease, the mobilization of copper from the body is associated with dramatic improvement in the clinical state of the patient.

Copper absorbed from the gastrointestinal tract enters first into the direct-reacting fraction of plasma copper. Therefore, the increase in this fraction reflects the increased turnover of copper between the gastrointestinal tract, the tissues, and the excretory routes. The copper in this fraction is easily dissociable from the albumin, and the increase in the direct-reacting fraction probably accounts for the increased excretion of copper by the kidneys.

The most widely held concept of the disease is that the inherited defect is an inability to synthesize ceruloplasmin. However, some individuals heterozygous for the gene may have as low a ceruloplasmin concentration as some patients with the disease. Furthermore, there is a poor correlation between the ceruloplasmin level and the severity or duration of the disease. An additional difficulty with this theory is that a mechanism whereby a deficiency of ceruloplasmin can lead to excessive tissue deposits of copper is not known.

Another theory which has been proposed is that the genetically determined abnormality in protein metabolism results in the formation of abnormal tissue proteins which have a high avidity for copper. The difficulty with this theory is that it does not explain the low concentrations of the plasma copper protein, ceruloplasmin.

Pathology

The characteristic pathologic findings are in the liver and the brain. The liver is usually small, firm, and coarsely nodular. It may or may not be bile-stained. Nodules of regenerating liver cells are separated by trabeculae of fibrous connective tissue. The picture is that of healed subacute yellow atrophy or the nonalcoholic variety of Laennec's cirrhosis. The most striking gross finding in the brain is cavitation of the putamen on each side and rarely of cerebral cortex and white matter. In many cases, probably more than half, the putamen and caudate nuclei are atrophic and of light grayish-brown color, and there is no evidence of cavitation. Microscopic examination almost invariably reveals a remarkable hyperplasia of protoplasmic astrocytes in the cerebral cortex, lenticular and caudate nuclei, subthalamic nuclei of Luys, substantia nigra, dentate and red nuclei. Nerve cell loss is widespread but is most pronounced in the lenticular and dentate nuclei and cerebral cortex. The protoplasmic astrocytosis does not differ from that observed in hepatic coma. Splenomegaly is a common finding.

Clinical Manifestations

The disease usually begins in adolescence, but it may appear as early as the age of four or as late as age forty. The mode of onset is somewhat variable. In a few cases the first manifestation is related to liver insufficiency, i.e., jaundice, ascites, or splenomegaly. More often the initial symptom is related to the neurologic system: tremor, dysarthria, ataxia, incoordination, or personality change. The disease may run an acute course of several months' duration associated with fever, rapid emaciation, and mental deterioration, or an extremely chronic afebrile course of 30 or 40 years' duration. The usual course in the untreated patient is 5 to 10 years.

The clinical picture of a well-developed case is quite characteristic. *Tremor* of one or both of the upper extremities is an outstanding as well as an early manifestation. The tremor consists of regular, rhythmic, alternating contractions and may occur in the earliest stages only on movement of the extremity. Later it is also present when the arm is maintained in an attitude of repose. It is accentuated by excitement or by attention being drawn to it. One of the most certain ways of demonstrating the tremor is by having the patient extend the arms in front of the body. In this position "flapping" or "wingbeating" may be noted. The tremor may also increase during fine volitional movements, taking a form that resembles intention tremor. Indeed, in some cases cerebellar ataxia and tremor are the principal neurologic manifestations. In severe cases a tremor of the mandible or even of the entire head is present. *Abnormal movements* of choreic or choreoathetoid type are present in some patients but are not frequent. *Rigidity* of the skeletal muscles, often reaching an extreme degree, is another characteristic. The rigidity may be intermittent or constant, and the resulting clinical state may vary from transient spasms in the acute cases to permanent *contractures* and *deformities* in the chronic. In the late stages of the disease the facial muscles become set in a stiff, vacuous smile, the neck and trunk become rigid, the upper extremities are held rigidly in flexion at the elbow, wrist, and metacarpal joints, and the lower extremities are held in a position of extension. *Dysarthria* or even anarthria in advanced cases is an almost constant finding. *Cachexia* and muscular wasting may be extreme. Some form of *mental disturbance* is common, and in severely affected patients changes in character and personality and terminally marked mental deterioration may be present. The sensory system is intact, and the reflexes are essentially normal. Pyramidal signs are usually absent.

The clinical course of the liver disease is extremely variable. In many patients signs of liver insufficiency are completely lacking, even though the liver function tests are abnormal and cirrhosis can be demonstrated by needle biopsy. In other patients the signs of liver insufficiency, such as splenomegaly, ascites, jaundice, hepatomegaly, hematemesis, and spider angiomas, dominate the clinical picture. When liver function is markedly impaired, anemia, leukopenia, and thrombocytopenia may be found to accompany the splenomegaly.

The most remarkable, unique, and consistent feature of the disease is the Kayser-Fleischer ring (see Chap. 401), a golden-brown or greenish-brown ring of pigment located at the periphery of the cornea in Descemet's membrane. The pigment usually goes completely around the cornea; occasionally there may be only a crescent-shaped distribution. Although the rings are frequently visible in ordinary light, in the early stages of the disease or in patients in whom the color of the iris is brown, it may be necessary to use a slit lamp to visualize the rings. Under slit-lamp examination, the ring is seen to be composed of a multitude of granular specks. The rings are pathognomonic of the disease and are present in all patients with neurologic manifestations. Failure of an experienced observer to demonstrate rings by slit-lamp examination of a patient with neurologic abnormalities virtually rules out Wilson's disease. Although the rings may be present in some patients long before the appearance of other clinical abnormalities, they are usually absent in asymptomatic subjects. They are occasionally absent in children whose only manifestations of Wilson's disease are those of hepatic involvement.

Skeletal abnormality, manifested by roentgenographic evidences of osteomalacia, cartilage injury, or bone fragmentation, is a frequent finding in the disease. Azure lunulas, bluish crescent areas at the nail bases, have been observed in several patients.

Diagnosis

The triad of Kayser-Fleischer rings, cirrhosis of the liver, and signs of basal ganglion disease is pathognomonic of this condition.

The various clinical findings combine to form several different clinical pictures, the most frequent of which is Parkinson's syndrome. Occasionally cerebellar ataxia, chorea, choreoathetosis, or dystonia predominates. If signs of liver insufficiency are not evident from physical examination, liver function studies or needle biopsy of the liver will demonstrate the presence of liver disease. Rubeanic acid stain may be used to demonstrate the excessive deposition of copper. In young patients in whom neurologic disease is not manifest and the signs of liver disease are marked, the condition has been confused with "juvenile" or "familial" cirrhosis.

The presence of hypocupremia, hypoceruloplasminemia, hypercupruria, and hyperaminoaciduria confirms the diagnosis, although it is rarely necessary to perform the difficult laboratory examinations in order to establish the diagnosis. In a rare patient with the disease, hypocupremia and hypoceruloplasminemia may not be present. Hypocupremia and hypoceruloplasminemia may be present in some normal individuals who are heterozygous for the gene. These two biochemical alterations are also present in all normal newborn infants and in at least some patients with kwashiorkor, sprue, celiac disease, and the nephrotic syndrome. Hypercupruria may be present only in the last condition mentioned. Hypercupruria may be present in patients with alcoholic cirrhosis of the liver, but the copper excreted rarely exceeds 200 µg per day; in this condition the concentration of copper and ceruloplasmin in the plasma is either normal or increased.

Prognosis

The disease is progressive and invariably fatal if untreated; death usually results from hepatic failure or intercurrent infection. There is now little doubt but that the early, continuous, and energetic therapy outlined below is associated with prolongation of life.

Treatment

The therapy of Wilson's disease is directed toward (1) the prevention of the continued accumulation of copper in the body and (2) the removal of copper already deposited.

Potassium sulfide (potash sulfurated technical, 20 mg three times daily with meals) prevents the absorption of copper by the formation of insoluble unabsorbable copper sulfide in the gut. This therapy is continued for 6 to 12 months and then discontinued. No undesirable side effects have been observed when such therapy has been given continuously for periods up to 5 years.

The administration of the copper chelating agent, penicillamine (β,β-dimethyl cysteine), results in the mobilization of copper from the tissues and an increase in its excretion in the urine. Therapy is started with 2 to 4 Gm daily in four divided doses on an empty stomach. Acute "sensitivity" reactions manifested by fever, skin rash, adenopathy, severe leukopenia, or thrombocytopenia develop in about one-third of patients. Desensitization, sometimes with corticosteroids, is required in such cases. Maintenance therapy with 1.5 Gm D-penicillamine daily should be given for the lifetime of the patient. Chronic administration of less than 2 Gm D-penicillamine is rarely associated with toxicity other than minor skin changes. Reversible optic neuritis and the nephrotic syndrome have followed the administration of the DL isomer but not the D isomer.

Therapy as outlined above results in clinical improvement beginning in several months and continuing for 6 to 12 months when stabilization occurs. If mental changes are present, they may revert toward normal, while the tremors and rigidity become less pronounced, sometimes to a remarkable degree. Liver function may improve and the Kayser-Fleischer rings diminish in intensity, but the plasma copper aberrations remain unchanged.

REFERENCES

Scheinberg, I. H., and I. Sternlieb: The Pathogenesis and Clinical Significance of the Liver Disease in Hepatolenticular Degeneration (Wilson's Disease), Med. Clin. N. Am., 44:665, 1960.

——— and I. Sternlieb: Wilson's Disease, Annual Rev. Med., 16:119, 1965.

Sternlieb, I., and I. H. Scheinberg: Penicillamine Therapy for Hepatolenticular Degeneration, J.A.M.A., 189:748, 1964.

Walshe, J. M., and J. N. Cumings: "Wilson's Disease: Some Current Concepts," Oxford, Blackwell Scientific Publications, Ltd., 1961.

Wilson, S. A. K.: Progressive Lenticular Degeneration: A Familial Nervous Disease Associated with Cirrhosis of the Liver, Brain, 34:395, 1912.

111 DISORDERS OF GLYCOGEN SYNTHESIS AND MOBILIZATION

Richard A. Field

The glycogen deposition diseases occupy a noteworthy place in the evolution of the conceptual approaches to the modern methods of study of disease. In 1952, Dr. Gerty T. Cori demonstrated by specific enzymatic studies of tissue from patients that von Gierke's disease is due to the loss of activity of a single tissue enzyme, and thus she provided a prototype for the study of genetically determined metabolic aberrations. Since the points of enzymatic abnormality of most of the syndromes to be discussed in this chapter concern the steps of synthesis and degradation between glucose 6-phosphate and glycogen, a working schema of these pathways is presented in Fig. 111-1. The Cori classification of glycogen deposition diseases is shown in Table 111-1.

Glucose 6-Phosphatase Deficiency Hepatorenal Glycogenosis

First described pathologically by von Gierke in 1929, this condition, characterized by enlargement of liver and kidneys and bouts of severe hypoglycemia, is probably the most frequent form of glycogenosis. Symptoms and recognizable clinical signs usually appear in the first year of life, and hepatomegaly may be detectable at birth. The disorder is transmitted as an autosomal mendelian recessive characteristic.

PATHOLOGIC PHYSIOLOGY. Under normal conditions hepatic glycogen serves as the main reservoir compound in the overall economy of blood glucose homeostasis. During and after ingestion of carbohydrate foods, a major portion of the glucose arriving in the liver via the portal system is phosphorylated and, by several intermediary steps, is stored as the regularly branched polysaccharide, glycogen (Chap. 75). During the postcibal period, peripheral utilization of glucose depletes circulating glucose, with the result that liver glycogen is depolymerized and free glucose is released into the hepatic vein (Chap. 75). The overall intracellular reactions in this process are called glycogenolysis, and the final enzymatic step is the hydrolytic dephosphorylation by the specific enzyme, hepatic glucose 6-phosphatase (Fig.

Fig. 111-1. Pathways of glycogen synthesis and breakdown.

111-1). Absence or marked reduction of this enzyme activity can be demonstrated by direct tissue assay in hepatorenal glycogenosis and accounts for most, if not all, of the metabolic disturbances noted in patients with this condition. The central feature of this limitation of hepatic glucose release is hypoglycemia, and it follows that little or no elevation of blood glucose concentration occurs following the injection of glucagon or epinephrine. Likewise, the normal expected rise in blood glucose level is not observed in patients with this hepatic enzyme deficiency following the intravenous administration of fructose or galactose. For all intents and purposes, these hexoses are metabolized solely by the liver and ultimately are converted intracellularly to glucose 6-phosphate, which, like the molecules of the same compound derived from glycogen depolymerization, cannot be dephos-

phorylated in the absence of glucose 6-phosphatase so as to appear in the bloodstream as free glucose. Apparently large quantities of glucose 6-phosphate are disposed of by increasing the amounts carried through the steps of anaerobic glycolysis resulting in an increased production and release of lactic and pyruvic acids; thus, hyperlacticacidemia is a characteristic finding in the syndrome and can be strikingly augmented by the administration of glucagon or other stimuli of hepatic glycogenolysis. Although ketonemia, lipemia, and ketonuria are frequently observed, because of the relative unavailability of glycogen stores and the resultant hypoglycemia which triggers mobilization of fat to meet energy requirements, marked and dangerous lacticacidosis is also frequent and may supervene precipitously. It is believed that the chronic hyperlacticacidemia is respon-

Table 111-1. DISORDERS OF GLYCOGEN DEPOSITION AND MOBILIZATION

Cori type	Enzyme defect	Organ	Glycogen structure	Eponymic name	Suggested clinical name
1	Glucose 6-phospha-tase	Liver, kidney, intestine (?)	Normal	von Gierke's disease	Glucose 6-phospha-tase deficiency hepatorenal glycogenosis
2	α-Glucosidase (maltase)	Generalized	Normal	Pompe's disease	α-Glucosidase defi-ciency generalized glycogenosis
3	Amylo-1,6-glucosidase (debrancher)	Liver, heart, muscle, leukocytes	Abnormal; missing or very short outer chains	Forbes's disease	Debrancher deficiency limit dextrinosis
4	Amylo-(1,4:1,6) transglucosidase (brancher)	Liver, probably other organs	Abnormal; very long inner and outer un-branched chains	Andersen's disease	Brancher deficiency amylopectinosis
5	Muscle phosphorylase	Skeletal and cardiac muscle	Normal	McArdle-Schmid-Pearson disease	Myophosphorylase deficiency glyco-genosis
6	Liver phosphorylase	Liver	Normal	Hers's disease	Hepatophosphorylase deficiency glyco-genosis

sible for disturbance in renal clearance of water and accounts for the hyperuricemia seen in this condition. Chronic acidosis on a cellular level may play a role in the generally retarded growth, mild normochromic un-responsive anemia, hypophosphatemia, and generalized decreased bone density with mushrooming of the meta physes and frequent fractures observed in these patients. Glycosuria and nonspecific aminoaciduria without amino-acidemia also occur and may be striking. It has been suggested that these findings correlate with the severity of glycogen infiltration and the hypothetically intra-cellular accumulation of phosphorylated hexoses in the renal tubular cells; but other impairments of renal func-tion are not prominent.

PATHOLOGY. The liver is markedly enlarged, smooth, firm, and brownish in color. Microscopic study shows the liver cells to be enlarged up to three times the normal size and to be filled with glycogen and at times excessive amounts of fat. In the kidneys, which are usually at least double normal size, intracellular excess of glycogen is found in the cells of the proximal tubules. That the excess of glycogen persists in these organs long after death is not surprising when the nature of the biochemi-cal defect is recalled.

CLINICAL PICTURE. The child is pale and undersized, with a fat face and neck and a markedly distended abdomen containing a huge, easily palpable liver with-out associated ascites or splenomegaly. Xanthomas with prominent lipemia may be a feature. Occasionally, epi-leptiform seizures and vomiting occur; however, more often the gravity and prevalence of the low blood sugar level are not appreciated until serious central nervous system deterioration has resulted.

LABORATORY EXAMINATIONS. These examinations re-veal fasting hypoglycemia, hyperlipidemia, hyperlactic-acidemia, anemia, and, at times, ketonemia and ketonuria. After glucose ingestion or infusion, the fall of blood levels may be delayed, yielding a pseudodiabetic curve. This may be explained as impaired capacity to increase the already superabundant stores of liver glycogen, rather than as a failure to utilize glucose at a normal rate in peripheral tissues. There is hypersensitivity to insulin, and severe prolonged hypoglycemia may follow its administration. Suspicion of this disorder is warranted when typical clinical characteristics are present and consonant results with glucagon or epinephrine challenge tests and of galactose or fructose infusion have been obtained. Final diagnosis, as with all glycogenoses, rests on biochemical assay of enzyme activity in biopsy material, in this instance, liver. In typical cases, liver glucose 6-phosphatase activity is found to be absent or reduced to less than 10 percent of normal. There is no ready explanation for the three cases reported in which glucose 6-phosphatase activity was either normal or only moderately reduced despite the careful characterization of the cases as clinically and pathophysiologically entirely consistent with the diagnosis.

DIFFERENTIAL DIAGNOSIS. The sporadic reports of cases of liver glycogenosis in which multiple enzymatic abnormalities in the glycogen pathways can be demon-strated and other cases in which members of the same kinship have distinctly different enzymatic lesions have given rise to both diagnostic and conceptual confusion. At present, it is not clear whether such cases result from secondarily induced adaptations, a close relationship of chromosomal genetic loci for determining and controlling the formation of the different enzymes, or from the influences of environmental factors. Until further investigations clarify these situations or augment the details of pathways of glycogen metabolism, the nonrestrictive labeling of cases that do not fit, either biochemically or functionally, into the classical groupings as simply "liver glycogen disease" seems wise.

TREATMENT. Although no means of increasing tissue activity levels of glucose 6-phosphatase in typical cases is available, earlier diagnosis, combined with recognition of hypoglycemia, acidosis, and intercurrent infection as the causes of morbidity and mortality, has markedly improved the life expectancy in this disease. The observation that the disturbances in metabolism and function in patients who survive beyond the fifth year tend to ameliorate provokes inquiry into the biochemical mechanisms by which such could occur and points to the necessity for assiduous care of the afflicted infant. It appears that in cases with prolonged survival the hyperuricemia and urate deposition which result, especially in the kidneys, become the major causes of difficulties. For this the daily administration of 0.5 to 2.0 Gm probenecid (Benemid) may be employed (Chap. 106).

The use of allopurinol, an inhibitor of urate formation, can also be recommended when secondary complications of hyperuricemia are manifested.

In a small number of cases, surgical transposition of the vena cava and the portal vein has been performed with clinical improvement in hypoglycemia. Diazoxide, a thiazide compound with capability of inhibiting insulin release, has been shown to improve hypoglycemia in one case.

α–Glucosidase Deficiency Generalized Glycogenosis

This disorder, the most devastating form of glycogenosis, causes death within the first 2 years of life. It is marked by a generalized deposition of glycogen and by striking cardiomegaly. Symptoms and signs appear within 1 or 2 months after birth and quickly produce an infant with marked muscular hypotonia, enlarged tongue, cretinoid appearance, cardiomegaly, and neurologic deficits. Increased susceptibility to recurrent respiratory infections is based on poor ventilative and tussive efforts.

The structure of isolated glycogen is normal, and hyperglycemia promptly follows glucagon or epinephrine administration or the infusion of galactose or fructose. Glycogen accumulation in vacuoles located in the cytoplasm of almost all body cells occurs to a variable degree and is a process in which the leukocytes participate. The principal mechanisms of death are cardiac failure and aspiration pneumonitis. The disease is familial in occurrence, and the mode of inheritance appears to be through a single recessive autosomal gene.

Hers has demonstrated in the tissues of five affected infants the absence of a normally ubiquitous α-$(1 \to 4)$ glucosidase which has optimum activity in the acid range.

The enzyme characteristically hydrolyzes maltose and glycogen to glucose and can catalyze the transglucosylation from maltose to glycogen. Present hypotheses regarding glycogen metabolism do not provide a locus of influence at which this enzyme could effect glycogen deposition. Furthermore, spontaneous glycogenolysis occurs in excised tissues. Hers emphasizes the possible lysosomal nature of the enzyme and suggests that the polysaccharide accumulation is the result of a failure of physiologic digestion of areas of cytoplasm by the defective lysosomes. This interpretation is in agreement with the clinical observations of an absence of hypoglycemia, ketosis, and hyperlipidemia and the concept that the manifestations are the result of disruption of muscle fibers by the progressive glycogen accumulation. Although the clinical picture is highly characteristic, diagnosis depends on the demonstration of the absence of the acid α-$(1 \to 4)$ glucosidase in biopsy material.

Electron microscopic studies have demonstrated two forms of cytoplasmic glycogen aggregates, a monogranular and a multigranular. The ensacculated membrane-limited vacuoles found only in this condition probably represent lysosomes which have autophaged large amounts of monogranular glycogen and are unable to digest it because of their deficiency of acid maltase.

Treatment is unavailing, although chemotherapy of intercurrent bacterial respiratory infections appears to prolong life.

Debrancher Enzyme Deficiency (Limit Dextrinosis) and Brancher Enzyme Deficiency (Amylopectinosis)

These two conditions are the result of defects of the enzymes concerned with the formation and the disengagement of the branch points of the typically arborized glycogen molecule (3 and 4 in Table 111-1). In the first instance, there is a deficiency of the specific enzyme required for cleavage of the branch point bond, and therefore glycogenolysis is interrupted as the first branch point is reached and a glycogen of abnormal structure with excessively frequent branch points and shortened inner and outer chains results. When the branching enzyme is deficient, an unusually structured glycogen which possesses excessively lengthened inner and outer chains and a paucity of branch points is produced. Apparently, this structure formation, which resembles that of plant starch, gives the polysaccharide the physical characteristics which lead to its sequestration within the cells, where it acts as an irritative nidus, producing a characteristic increase in periportal connective tissue.

Limit dextrinosis is a relatively frequent type of glycogenosis; amylopectinosis is exceedingly rare, only two cases having been recognized. Since the clinical picture of the debrancher deficiency disturbance (limit dextrinosis) so closely resembles a mild form of the glucose 6-phosphatase deficiency, many cases of the former were mistakenly diagnosed as the latter before precise enzymatic assay techniques were available. The confusion need no longer arise even on clinical grounds or on the basis of functional tests, for in limit dextrinosis infusions of galactose lead to prompt intrahepatic conversion to glucose, with prompt hyperglycemia, there being no impediment to dephosphorylation and release. In the differential diagnosis in cases with equivocal hyperglycemic responses to glucagon or epinephrine and in which hepatomegaly, growth retardation, and a tendency to hypoglycemia and ketonuria contribute uncertainty, a liver biopsy need not be done, since it has been demonstrated that the debrancher enzyme is also absent in leukocytes, muscle, and erythrocytes. Furthermore, fasting levels of lactate and pyruvate are likely to be normal, in contrast to the situation with the type I case (glucose 6-phosphatase deficiency), where they are distinctly elevated. In the type III case, erythrocyte glycogen content is elevated, but again this is not so in the type I individual.

Prognosis for the type III defect appears to be relatively good, and at least two patients with this condition have reached the fifth decade of life. Logical treatment consists of a high protein, relatively low fat diet, with frequent feedings, prompt treatment of intercurrent infections, and prohibition of strenuous exercise, cardiodepressant drugs, and anesthetics, since the myocardium is involved.

Glycogen Deposition Syndromes Due to Deficiencies of Glycogen Phosphorylases

Glycogen phosphorylase (5, Table 111-1) catalyzes glycogen depolymerization by phosphorylytic cleavage to yield glucose 1 phosphate and thus mediates the major initiating step in making the glucose moieties available for metabolism. In the liver the bulk of the glucose derived from the action of this enzyme ultimately defends the level of blood sugar and maintains an adequate supply for the peripheral tissues, while in the muscle the phosphorylase-produced hexose phosphate provides an immediate fuel source for the energy demanded by quick, sharp increases in contractile activity. Muscle and liver phosphorylase are distinctly different proteins immunologically, structurally, and functionally, and it appears that each has its own genetic determinant. Both enzyme activities are enhanced by epinephrine, while only liver phosphorylase responds in vivo to injections of glucagon.

Myophosphorylase Deficiency Glycogenosis (McArdle)

A group of patients consisting of members of several unrelated families have been shown to be lacking in muscle phosphorylase activity. None has any growth retardation, disturbance in carbohydrate economy, or abnormality of response to glucagon or epinephrine administration. However, they have in common an incapacity to perform prolonged or strenuous muscle work and are excessively sensitive to ischemic conditions in this regard because of the occurrence of weakness, pain, and spasm of the exercised muscle. The demonstration of the isolated absence of muscle phosphorylase adequately explains the clinical phenomena when the importance of brisk glycogenolysis in supplying substrate for anaerobic glycolysis during ischemic muscle work is recalled. The impediment limiting the acceleration and augmentation of anaerobic glycolysis thus curtails increased lactate production. The failure to detect a significant rise in lactate concentration in the venous return from a muscle working under imposed ischemic conditions is a useful diagnostic test. A modest excess of glycogen in the muscles has been described, and in some cases prolonged exercise may cause breakdown of muscle cells and myoglobinuria. Although it has been shown that cardiac muscle shares the defect, no cardiac disturbance on this account has been described.

Since liver phosphorylase is normal in amount and activity, patients do quite well provided they accept limitations in excertion, protect themselves from tight garments that produce muscle ischemia, and fortify themselves with exogenous carbohydrates before attempting unusual physical tasks.

Hepatophosphorylase Deficiency Glycogenosis (Hers)

Isolated development of hepatomegaly in infancy or childhood with a tendency to fasting hypoglycemia due to excessive accumulation of hepatic glycogen of normal structure characterizes this condition. Little in the way of other metabolic or developmental disturbance accrues as a consequence of the sluggish glycogenolysis which results from the absent or markedly reduced hepatophosphorylase activity. The deficiency of the enzyme can be demonstrated biochemically in hepatic tissue or in leukocytes. A possibly contingent deficiency of glucose 6-phosphate dehydrogenase has been described in some cases. No therapy beyond avoidance of prolonged fasting and the administration of a high protein diet with frequent feedings appears to be necessary. The mechanism of failure of hyperglycemic response to glucagon or epinephrine is obvious, and the normal response to galactose infusion as well as the normal serum lactate level and lack of hyperlipemia allows easy differentiation of this disease from the more devastating glucose 6-phosphatase deficiency. Transmission appears to be by means of an autosomal recessive gene.

REFERENCES

Cori, G. T.: Glycogen Structure and Enzyme Deficiencies in Glycogen Storage Disease, Harvey Lectures, 48:145, 1952–1953.

——: "Glycogen Metabolism," Ciba Symposium, Boston, Little, Brown and Company, 1964.

Hers, H. G.: Glycogen Storage Disease, in "Advances in Metabolic Disorders," Vol. 1, Academic Press Inc., New York, 1964.

Stanbury, J. B., J. B. Wyngaarden, and D. S. Fredrickson: "The Metabolic Basis of Inherited Disease," 2d ed., New York, McGraw-Hill Book Company, 1966.

Van Creveld, S.: Glycogen Disease, Arch. Dis. Child., 34:298, 1959.

112 GALACTOSEMIA
Kurt J. Isselbacher

Galactosemia is an inborn error of metabolism associated with an impairment in the conversion of galactose to glucose and its derivatives. The disease is due to a congenital absence of a specific enzyme, galactose 1-phosphate uridyl transferase.

Clinical Features

The disease manifests itself shortly after birth when the afflicted infant is exposed to galactose (in the form of lactose) in cow's milk or breast milk. Vomiting and diarrhea occur, and as a result there is an impairment in nutrition or failure to thrive. Jaundice may then become evident, together with enlargement of the liver and spleen. The clinical picture at this point may readily be confused with that of hepatitis. If the dietary ingestion of milk or galactose continues, cataracts are likely to form, followed by the development of mental retardation. Cataracts may be evident at three or four weeks of age; several months may elapse before mental retardation is recognized. When blood galactose levels are very high, episodes of hypoglucosemia may occur and may be associated with convulsions.

If the infant is examined shortly after the ingestion of milk, galactose will be found in the blood as well as in the urine. The urine will also show an increase in amino acids (predominantly of the neutral type), and occasionally albuminuria is observed. It must be remembered that if, because of vomiting, no milk has been ingested, galactosuria will probably not be found.

All the clinical features except for mental retardation may regress completely when galactose is removed from the diet. The jaundice will readily subside, together with a diminution of the hepatosplenomegaly. Although cirrhosis of the liver may occur in the untreated galactosemic patient, only a residual fibrosis may remain in later years in patients who have been treated. Cataracts may improve greatly and, in fact, have been known to disappear completely on a galactose-free diet. Unfortunately, mental retardation is a lifelong feature, and once it has developed it is not reversible.

Pathologic Physiology

Both breast milk and cow's milk have as their sole content of carbohydrate the disaccharide lactose. This sugar is split within the intestinal epithelial cell into its component monosaccharides, namely, galactose and glu-cose. The infant with galactosemia has difficulty in converting the galactose that is liberated to glucose and its derivatives. The main enzymes and the reactions involved in galactose utilization by the mammalian organism are as follows:

1. Galactokinase:
   Galactose + ATP → galactose 1-phosphate + ADP
2. Galactose 1-phosphate uridyl transferase:
   Galactose 1-phosphate + UDP-glucose →
   UDP-galactose + glucose 1-phosphate
3. UDP-galactose-4-epimerase:
   $$DPN$$
   UDP-galactose ⇌ UDP-glucose
4. UDP-galactose-pyrophosphorylase:
   UTP + galactose 1-phosphate ⇌ UDP-galactose
   + pyrophosphate
5. Direct oxidation of galactose:
   Galactose → galactonolactone → galactonate →
   → β-keto-galactonic acid → xylulose + CO_2

It is seen from these reactions that the first step in galactose utilization consists in its conversion to galactose 1-phosphate by the enzyme galactokinase. The galactose 1-phosphate must then be converted to glucose 1-phosphate; this is accomplished by the second reaction, catalyzed by the enzyme galactose 1-phosphate uridyl transferase. It is this enzyme and this reaction which are deficient in galactosemia. As a consequence, galactose 1-phosphate accumulates in the tissues. The epimerase serves to interconvert UDP-galactose and UDP-glucose and is a mechanism whereby normally in a galactosemic individual, galactose-containing substances, especially those found in brain lipids, may be synthesized from glucose even in the absence of dietary galactose. The fourth enzyme occurs mostly in liver, and it will be observed that it allows for some conversion of galactose 1-phosphate to UDP-galactose by a mechanism other than the transferase reaction. A fifth enzyme system has also been shown whereby galactose is directly oxidized by galactose dehydrogenase leading eventually to the liberation of CO_2 and xylulose. It has been suggested that one or both of these latter two pathways may account for the partial oxidation of galactose in patients with galactosemia and perhaps in part for the improved galactose tolerance which occurs in some of these patients with increasing age.

The present evidence indicates that a number of the toxic symptoms found in galactosemia may be related to the accumulation of galactose 1-phosphate in the tissues. This sugar accumulates in lens, liver, and red cells and has been shown to inhibit the enzyme phosphoglucomutase. However, the mechanism whereby this accumulation and subsequent enzyme inhibition lead to changes such as hepatic fibrosis and central nervous system damage has not yet been determined. One observation suggests that cataract formation may be related to the accumulation of a nonphosphorylated derivative of galactose (galactitol) in the lens. The reduction in blood glucose levels in association with elevated galactose levels in the blood appears to be due to a decreased hepatic output of glucose. The basis for the aminoaciduria is not completely understood, but in animal studies (with intestine and kidney slices) it has been observed that sugars such as galactose tend to inhibit the transport of certain groups of amino acids.

Diagnosis

The usual clue to the diagnosis consists of the clinical picture described above, together with the finding of a reducing sugar in the urine. Such a urine will give a positive reaction to Benedict's test (copper reduction) but a negative glucose oxidase test. If the urine is chromatographed, it shows predominantly galactose rather than glucose. If these initial screening tests suggest the diagnosis of galactosemia, then more specific tests are necessary.

In the past galactose tolerance tests have been performed which typically show a delayed clearance of galactose from the bloodstream when the sugar was given by mouth or intravenously. However, because of the toxicity of this sugar in the patient with galactosemia and because of the availability of more specific tests, this procedure is no longer recommended. The specific diagnostic test for this disease consists in the demonstration of the absence of galactose 1-phosphate uridyl transferase in the patient's red blood cells. In this test, the cells are incubated together with the two substrates, galactose 1-phosphate and UDP glucose. After a period of incubation, the amount of uridine diphosphate glucose remaining is determined. In the normal individual the UDP-glucose disappears, because of the presence of the transferase in the red cells, but in galactosemia no utilization of UDP-glucose occurs when it is incubated in the presence of galactose 1-phosphate.

It is also possible to measure the transferase deficiency indirectly by a number of other procedures. For example, one may incubate red cells with galactose and demonstrate either enzymatically or chromatographically that galactose 1-phosphate accumulates. One may also incubate red cells or whole blood with radioactive galactose. Normal cells will oxidize the galactose, and, thus, radioactive carbon dioxide (CO_2) will be produced, but in the galactosemic cells, very little of any radioactive CO_2 will be liberated because of the defect in the oxidation of galactose.

Differential Diagnosis

The most important condition from which galactosemia needs to be differentiated in the neonatal period is primary liver disease, either acute or chronic. It must be recalled that in the presence of decreased liver function, galactose removal from the bloodstream is impaired, and as a consequence, both elevated blood galactose levels and galactosuria may be found. However, in liver disease (either hepatitis or cirrhosis) normal levels of red cell transferase are found and galactose utilization and oxidation by red cells or whole blood are completely normal.

Since these patients are often seen when nausea, vomiting, and diarrhea have developed and therefore dietary intake of galactose may be minimal, it must be emphasized that neither elevated blood nor urine galactose levels will be found in the absence of recent dietary intake of this sugar. Hence, an analysis of the blood and urine at these times may be misleading.

Treatment

The treatment of this disease consists in the exclusion of galactose and galactose-containing foods from the diet. In early infancy this involves the elimination of lactose as well as galactose. The milk substitutes which have been used effectively are Dextri-Maltose and Nutramigen. Soybean preparations have been used in the past, but they possess galactose-containing polysaccharides and should be avoided. As indicated above, fairly dramatic improvement will occur when the infant is placed on a galactose-free diet, and all symptoms except for the mental retardation may improve completely. These patients must remain on very restricted galactose diets until they have reached adequate physical and neurologic development.

Genetics

Abundant evidence has been obtained to indicate that this is a disorder transmitted by an autosomal recessive gene. Specific enzyme studies have demonstrated both parents to be heterozygous with respect to galactose 1-phosphate uridyl transferase activities in their red cells. The exact incidence of this disease has not been determined, but the most recent data indicate that cases may be as frequent as 1 in 18,000 births. The occurrence of the carrier state is believed to be 1 out of 130 individuals.

REFERENCES

Hansen, R. G., R. K. Bretthauer, J. Mayes, and J. H. Nordin: Estimation of Frequency of Occurrence of Galactosemia in the Population, Proc. Soc. Exp. Biol. Med., 115:560, 1964.

Isselbacher, K. J.: Galactosemia, pp. 178–188 in J. B. Stanbury, J. B. Wyngaarden, and D. S. Fredrickson (Eds.), "The Metabolic Basis of Inherited Disease," 2d ed., New York, McGraw-Hill Book Company, 1966.

Kalckar, H. M., E. P. Anderson, and K. J. Isselbacher: Galactosemia: Congenital Defect in a Nucleotide Transferase, Biochim. Biophys. Acta, 20:262, 1956.

113 DISORDERS OF LIPID METABOLISM AND XANTHOMATOSIS

Donald S. Fredrickson

Lipidosis is a general term applied to disorders characterized by abnormal concentrations of lipids in tissues

Table 113-1. LIPIDOSES AND XANTHOMATOSES

I. Abnormal plasma lipoprotein concentrations (dyslipoproteinemias)
  A. Hyperlipoproteinemia
    1. Type I (hyperchylomicronemia; exogenous hyperglyceridemia)
      a. Familial lipoprotein lipase deficiency
      b. Acquired with dysproteinemias
    2. Type II (hyperbetalipoproteinemia; hypercholesterolemia)
      a. Familial (familial hypercholesterolemia)
      b. Acquired
    3. Type III (beta-lipoproteins of abnormal density)
      a. Familial ("broad beta disease;" "xanthoma tuberosum")
      b. Acquired
    4. Type IV (hyperprebetalipoproteinemia; endogenous hyperglyceridemia)
      a. Familial
      b. Acquired
    5. Type V (hyperchylomicronemia and hyperprebetalipoproteinemia; mixed hyperglyceridemia)
      a. Familial
      b. Acquired
    6. Other (including hyperlipidemia of obstructive jaundice)
  B. Hypolipoproteinemia
    1. Abetalipoproteinemia (familial absence of low-density lipoproteins)
    2. Hypobetalipoproteinemia
      a. Familial
      b. Acquired
    3. Tangier disease (familial alpha-lipoprotein deficiency)
    4. Familial deficiency of lecithin: cholesterol acyltransferase (with alpha-lipoprotein deficiency)
II. Primary tissue lipid storage diseases
  A. Sphingolipidoses
    1. Glucosylceramidoses
      a. Gangliosidoses ("familial amaurotic idiocies")
        1) G_{M1} gangliosidosis (generalized gangliosidosis)
        2) G_{M2} gangliosidosis (Tay-Sachs disease)
        3) G_{M3} gangliosidosis
      b. Glucosylcerebrosidoses (Gaucher's disease)
        1) Infantile (CNS involvement)
        2) Juvenile (CNS involvement)
        3) Adult (no CNS involvement)
      c. Trihexosidosis (Fabry's disease; angiokeratoma corporis diffusum)
    2. Galactosylceramidoses
      a. Galactosylsulfatidosis (metachromatic leukodystrophy; Scholz's disease; Greenfield's disease)
      b. Galactosylcerebrosidosis (Krabbe's disease)
    3. Phosphorylceramidoses (sphingomyelin lipidoses)
      a. Sphingomyelinase deficient
        1) Classical infantile form (Niemann-Pick disease)
        2) Visceral form without CNS involvement
      b. Sphingomyelinase present
        1) Late CNS involvement
        2) Nova Scotia variant
  B. Storage of less polar lipids
    1. Phytanic oxidase deficiency (storage of 3,7,11,15-tetramethyl hexanoic acid; Refsum's disease)
    2. Cholesterol ester and triglyceride storage with adrenal calcification (Wolman's disease)
    3. Hepatic cholesterol ester storage disease
    4. Ceroid storage
III. Granulomatous diseases with lipid storage
  A. Histiocytosis X (xanthoma disseminatum, eosinophilic granuloma, Hand-Schüller-Christian disease, Letterer-Siwe disease)
  B. Lipoid proteinosis (Urbach-Wiethe disease)
  C. Lipoid dermatoarthritis
  D. Disseminated lipogranulomatosis (Farber's disease)
  E. Hereditary tendinous and tuberous xanthomatosis without hyperlipidemia
  F. Cerebrotendinous xanthomatosis
IV. Xanthomas
  A. Simple (xanthelasma, juvenile xanthoma)
  B. Associated with trauma and chronic infections
V. Adipose tissue disorders
  A. Relapsing panniculitis (Weber-Christian disease)
  B. Lipodystrophy
    1. Lipomas
    2. Adiposis dolorosa (Dercum's disease)
    3. Insulin lipodystrophy
  C. Lipoatrophy
    1. Partial (progressive lipodystrophy)
    2. Total (lipoatrophic diabetes mellitus)

or in extracellular fluid. Sometimes it is restricted to only those abnormalities of lipid metabolism that are inheritable. *Xanthomatosis* is a morphologic term referring to lipid accumulation in tissues in association with large "foam cells." The list of lipidoses and xanthomatoses in Table 113-1 encompasses most of the *primary* disturbances in lipid metabolism and includes some disorders in which secondary lipid storage is prominent and some of the disorders of adipose tissue. Omitted are several disorders in which lipids accumulate concomitant with primary abnormalities in metabolism of other substances. Noteworthy among these are mucopolysaccharidoses (gargoylism) and the glycogen storage diseases.

PLASMA LIPOPROTEIN ABNORMALITIES

The commonest of the lipidoses are those associated with primary alterations in concentrations of the plasma lipids. These can be better understood when considered in terms of lipoproteins, the form in which nearly all lipids, except for free fatty acids, are present in plasma. Both selective increases or severe deficiency and absence of some of the groups or classes of lipoproteins can occur. Abnormalities in the lipoproteins themselves may characterize a few disorders.

HYPERLIPOPROTEINEMIA

Increased concentrations of plasma lipids and lipoproteins represent metabolic problems that are difficult both to classify and to treat. Diagnosis requires two major steps: (1) Reasonable delineation of the dominant abnormality in the lipoprotein pattern. This may usually be estimated from measurement of plasma cholesterol *and* triglyceride concentrations; further qualitative information about the four major lipoprotein classes (Table 113-2) may be required and obtained by either electrophoresis or ultracentrifugation. The former is more practical, the latter more quantitative. (2) Separation of secondary (acquired) from primary (mainly, inheritable or familial) hyperlipoproteinemia. For this purpose evidence of familial involvement and a careful examination of skin and tendons for xanthomas are essential. Helpful ancillary information can also be gained by a careful history of diet, estimates of glucose tolerance, response of lipoproteins to controlled diets, and measurements of plasma postheparin lipolytic activity (PHLA).

The classification of hyperlipoproteinemia is undergoing rapid evolution. At present a useful method is based on five major types of abnormal lipoprotein patterns (Table 113-1).

These patterns usually do not represent specific diseases and require modifiers for proper diagnostic use, e.g., "type I hyperlipoproteinemia, familial"; "type II hyperlipoproteinemia, familial, heterozygote with xanthoma tendinosum"; or "type V hyperlipoproteinemia, secondary to diabetes mellitus." Each major type is associated with particular clinical manifestations and responds to different forms of therapy. The index lipoprotein patterns described below are those obtained in the postabsorptive state (12 to 14 hr after the last meal) and while the patient is eating a normal diet (approximately 20, 40, and 40 percent of calories coming from protein, fat, and carbohydrate, respectively).

Type I Hyperlipoproteinemia

DEFINITION. Normally, chylomicrons are not visible on paper electrophoresis in the postabsorptive state and less than 30 mg per 100 ml are obtained by ultracentrifugation. In the type I pattern there is marked hyperchylomicronemia and a decrease in all other lipoproteins. The plasma is milky and, after standing overnight at 4° centigrade, contains a cream layer over a clear infranatant layer. The triglyceride concentration ranges between 1,500 to 15,000 mg per 100 ml; cholesterol is abnormally high when the glycerides exceed 1,000. The ratio of cholesterol to glyceride concentrations is very low, <0.15. Within 3 to 5 days after institution of a fat-free diet, chylomicrons disappear, a modest increase in prebeta lipoproteins occurs, and beta- and alpha-lipoproteins increase but remain low; the plasma clears, glycerides are in the range of 200 to 400, and cholesterol is <150. Classical type I is seen under two conditions: one, a familial syndrome; the other, in association with dysglobulinemia.

FAMILIAL TYPE I. Hyperlipemia (lactescent plasma or serum due to hyperglyceridemia) dependent upon dietary fat intake was first reported in a child by Bürger and Grütz in 1932; and familial incidence was recorded by Holt, Aylward, and Timbres shortly thereafter. About 100 cases have since been discovered. This exogenous, or *fat-induced, hyperlipemia* is due to an inherited defect in removal of chylomicrons from plasma. The enzyme lipoprotein lipase probably plays an important role in this process in adipose tissue and perhaps at the endothelial wall in other tissues. The enzyme is "released" into plasma by heparin, and patients with this syndrome have uniquely low postheparin lipolytic activity and low levels of lipoprotein lipase in adipose tissue. The metabolic defect in the disease must still be demonstrated precisely, but all examples thus far appear to be homozygous for a relatively rare mutant gene.

Clinical picture. The disease is usually detected within the first decade, although sometimes not until early adulthood, usually when marked hyperlipemia is discovered during work-up for either sudden appearance of eruptive xanthomas, moderate hepatosplenomegaly, or bouts of se-

Table 113-2. CLASSIFICATION OF LIPOPROTEINS

Lipoproteins*	Synonyms	Component lipids† Cholesterol phospholipids triglyceride		
Chylomicrons	Exogenous glyceride in particles of $S\hat{f} > 400$; primary and secondary particles	+	+	++++
β-lipoprotein	Low-density lipoproteins (LDL) of $S\hat{f}$ 0–20; density 1.006–1.063	++++	+++	+
Pre-β-lipoprotein	Very low-density lipoproteins (VLDL) of $S\hat{f}$ 20–400; density < 1.006; α_2-lipoprotein; "hyperlipemic" particles of endogenous origin	++	++	+++
α_1-lipoprotein	High-density lipoproteins (HDL); density 1.063–1.21	+++	++++	+

* As defined by paper electrophoresis according to technique of Lees and Hatch (J. Lab. Clin. Med., 61:518, 1963).

† Indicating the relative degree to which the concentrations of plasma lipids will be altered by an increase in the species of lipoproteins.

vere abdominal pain. These abnormalities are only suggestive and not diagnostic for this type of hyperlipemia. The episodic abdominal pain usually follows a period of high fat intake. It is usually epigastric or midabdominal, rarely radiates to the back, and can be associated with signs of peritoneal irritation and fever, mimicking a number of "acute abdominal emergencies." Pancreatitis may develop, although, when associated with chronic pancreatitis, hyperlipemia may often be the result rather than the cause. There is no evidence that familial hyperchylomicronemia is associated with accelerated vascular disease, and the major hazard appears to be accumulation of fat in reticuloendothelial tissues and the precipitation of abdominal crises. Glucose tolerance is usually normal.

Diagnosis. The typical lipid and lipoprotein pattern and other manifestations in an otherwise healthy child or young adult provide a presumptive diagnosis if the acquired form has been specifically excluded. A fat-free diet should be administered for 1 week; the predicted changes in lipoproteins should occur rapidly. A *modest reduction* of hyperlipemia, which occurs in many patients on low-fat diets, is not diagnostic of this particular syndrome. Postheparin lipolytic activity should be demonstrated to be deficient by one of several in vitro tests. Parents will have low normal PHLA and usually normal plasma lipids. One or more siblings may have the type I pattern and low PHLA. The full-blown disease occurs in either sex.

Treatment. To avoid the crippling attacks of abdominal pain, pancreatitis, and foam cell accumulation in liver, spleen, and bone marrow seen in most cases, it is recommended that the daily intake of fat not represent more than 25 percent of calories, or 50 Gm fat per day. Both saturated and unsaturated fats are cleared poorly. Commercial preparations of medium chain glycerides, such as Protagen, offer means of occasionally satisfying craving for fat without inducing chylomicronemia, since these glycerides go directly to the liver in the portal vein.

ACQUIRED TYPE I. The typical lipoprotein pattern and other manifestations have been found in patients with systemic lupus erythematosus, myeloma, macroglobulinemia, lymphomas, or other diseases in which there are abnormal circulating globulins or other proteins. Heparin resistance, possibly due to heparin binding by the abnormal protein, is manifested by decreased prolongation of thrombin time. PHLA is abnormally low unless the usual test dose of 10 units per kg is greatly increased. The hyperlipoproteinemia fluctuates with changes in the plasma protein abnormality. Treatment is directed toward the underlying disease.

Type II Hyperlipoproteinemia

DEFINITION. This common pattern is characterized by increased concentrations of beta-lipoproteins. Both S_f 0 to 12 and 12 to 20 classes may be increased. Plasma cholesterol is elevated, and usually the plasma is quite clear. Particularly in familial cases there may be accompanying modest increases in prebeta-lipoproteins with associated elevation in plasma triglycerides, usually not above 300 mg per 100 ml. In the latter event the plasma may be slightly turbid. The C/T ratio is nearly always > 1 and can sometimes be > 10. Lipoprotein and lipid levels are relatively constant. The influence of dietary cholesterol, saturated fat (S), and polyunsaturated fat (P) upon plasma cholesterol concentrations is mainly expressed in changes in beta-lipoproteins. The definition of hypercholesterolemia or hyperbetalipoproteinemia is arbitrary due to the spread of usual lipoprotein levels in Americans. In young men, cholesterol concentrations > 260 mg per 100 ml are clearly associated with increased incidence of premature atherosclerosis.

FAMILIAL TYPE II (Familial Hypercholesterolemia). History and Clinical Picture. This syndrome was first described in the latter half of the nineteenth century in terms of its usual xanthomatous and atheromatous manifestations. Once called *xanthoma tendinosum* and sometimes termed *essential hypercholesterolemia,* it appears to represent the expression of a highly penetrant mutant at an autosomal locus primarily regulating plasma beta-lipoprotein concentrations. The heterozygote may have normal cholesterol concentrations in cord blood and during the first year. By age one the type II pattern is evident. In the first or second decade, xanthomas may begin in the Achilles or extensor tendons of the hands. Later these may involve plantar or other tendons and tibial tuberosities, and tuberous xanthomas may appear on the elbows. Ankles, knees, toes, or other joints involved with xanthomas may become tender and inflamed. The attacks usually last a few days, regress spontaneously, and can be confused with gout. Xanthelasma or arcus cornea is common. Some heterozygous patients never have xanthomas. The homozygous abnormal patient generally has higher beta-lipoprotein and cholesterol concentrations (> 500 mg per 100 ml) and will usually develop xanthomas between birth and age ten. These are generally florid and often include chamois-colored skin xanthomas on the hands, plantar, or (rarely) palmar surfaces, in the popliteal space, and on the buttocks. Homozygotes particularly are prone to premature ischemic heart disease, aortic stenosis, and atherosclerosis in peripheral and cerebral vessels. Abnormal glucose tolerance and hyperuricemia are not distinguishing features. The genetic expression varies considerably, xanthomatosis and the degree of hyperbetalipoproteinemia tending to be more similar within than between affected families.

Diagnosis. There is no absolute test for phenotype, but diagnosis can be fairly precise. All possible acquired causes must first be excluded. The heterozygote usually has a cholesterol concentration between 300 and 500 mg per 100 ml (>250 before age ten) and beta-lipoprotein cholesterols are usually >250. Diagnosis requires the type II pattern plus either (1) typical xanthomas or (2) the type II pattern in at least one parent or sibling. The homozygote usually has about double the lipoprotein abnormality of the heterozygote; at present ascertainment of this genotype requires demonstration of type II in both parents or, at least, both parental lines. The association of increased prebeta-lipoproteins and triglycerides in some patients varies in the same sibship and does not now constitute evidence of a different disease.

It may be due to concomitant presence of other genes, particularly that for diabetes.

Treatment. The first step in treatment of any primary hyperlipoproteinemia is diet. Reduction to ideal body weight does not influence familial type II patterns; it is nevertheless advisable, considering the increased hazard for vascular disease. A diet designed to increase polyunsaturated fatty acids and decrease saturated fatty acids and cholesterol to the maximum practical extent should be rigorously followed. It is most effective in children, will decrease lipoprotein levels in nearly all patients, but rarely, if ever, normalizes them. The total amount of fat or carbohydrate in the diet does not have a significant relationship to lipoprotein levels in most familial type II patients. Following achievement of maximum effect by diet, a drug may be used. The agent of choice is cholestyramine given in three divided doses to a total of 24 to 48 Gm per day (adult dose). If the chief but uncommon side effects, nausea, constipation, or steatorrhea, prove unmanageable, clofibrate (2.0 Gm per day) or d-thyroxin (4 to 8 mg per day) may be substituted. Failure of a drug to lower cholesterol concentrations by less than 15 percent in 4 to 6 weeks is an indication for its discontinuance. Exceptions are younger xanthomatous patients who may be mobilizing tissue lipid stores without changes in plasma lipid levels. In these cases drugs may be maintained if xanthomas appear to be softening.

ACQUIRED TYPE II. Acquired type II hyperbetalipoproteinemia may reach levels seen in heterozygotes for the familial disorder, but usually the plasma cholesterol levels are below 300 mg per 100 ml. Xanthelasma may be seen in patients with normolipoproteinemia, but tendon and tuberous xanthomas usually occur only in familial hyperlipoproteinemia. The diagnosis of acquired type II requires the elimination of familial involvement. If both parents are clearly normal, familial type II is excluded. The acquired pattern must then be differentiated into primary or secondary forms. The type II lipoprotein pattern can be seen in hypothyroidism, the nephrotic syndrome, some dysproteinemias including macroglobulinemia, diabetes mellitus, and possibly other diseases. The commonest cause of primary nonfamilial type II is dietary excess. Many Americans normally eat twice the average intake of 600 mg of cholesterol per day, associated with high amounts of saturated fats. A prompt fall to normal cholesterol levels on a diet restricted in cholesterol and saturated fats and high in polyunsaturated fats is both a good diagnostic test and adequate therapy (Table 275-6). It has not yet been proved that hypolipidemic agents are useful or necessary in treatment of acquired type II.

Type III Hyperlipoproteinemia

DEFINITION. This pattern is characterized by a heavy broad beta-lipoprotein band on electrophoresis. The unique feature is the presence of beta-migrating lipoproteins of density < 1.006, a test which requires preparative ultracentrifugation. The profile in the analytical ultracentrifuge is characterized by a bizarre increase in lipoproteins from about S_f 12 to 70. There are usually increased prebeta-lipoproteins and often very modest hyperchylomicronemia. The cholesterol and glyceride concentrations fluctuate considerably and often are very similar, lying usually between 200 and 1,000 mg per 100 ml. Type III hyperlipoproteinemia is almost always due to a familial disorder, apparently a recessive gene, requiring the homozygous phenotype for clinical expression. It has only recently been established as a disease, the first cases being described as *xanthoma tuberosum* by Gofman and co-workers in 1954.

FAMILIAL TYPE III. Clinical Picture. The disorder is usually detected after age twenty, earlier in men than in women. In addition to the typical lipoprotein pattern, two-thirds of patients have peculiar raised yellow plaques (plane xanthomas) in the palmar creases or on the fingers. Most of these also have soft, reddish-yellow, single or confluent xanthomas on the elbows. Some have pedunculated xanthomas on the buttocks, elsewhere on the limbs, and a few have tendon xanthomas. The majority of patients have intermittent claudication and evidence of decreased blood flow in the lower extremities; some have premature ischemic heart and cerebrovascular disease. The majority of patients have glucose intolerance, many are hypersecretors of insulin. Practically all are abnormally "carbohydrate-inducible," in terms of an exaggerated rise of plasma glycerides on high carbohydrate feeding. Hyperuricemia may be present.

Etiology. The basis for the disorder is not known. Triglycerides appear to associate with beta-lipoproteins in such a way that their efflux from plasma is retarded, and abnormal very low density lipoproteins with a peculiarly high cholesterol content persist in plasma. The beta-lipoproteins appear to be identical in immunochemical behavior to those in normals or other types of hyperlipoproteinemia.

Diagnosis. The ascertainment of the anomalous lipoprotein pattern is necessary for absolute diagnosis. However, the lipid pattern combined with other clinical features, particularly palmar xanthomas and the response to therapy, allow a presumptive diagnosis, and this is enhanced if a parent, sibling, or adult offspring can be demonstrated to have the same abnormalities. Due to the recessive character or low penetrance, both parents are usually normal, as are the majority of other first-degree relatives. The frequency of type IV patterns is also abnormally high in affected families. Familial types II and III have not been observed in the same kindreds.

Treatment. The lipoprotein pattern and plasma lipids can usually be returned to normal in type III with appropriate treatment. The skin xanthomas also disappear, allowing a presumption that treatment may desirably affect the hazard for premature vascular disease. Treatment consists sequentially of (1) reduction to ideal weight; (2) institution of a rigorous diet, with special attention to keeping carbohydrate intake below 5 Gm per kg per day by increasing the intake of polyunsaturated fat if necessary; and (3) clofibrate, 2 Gm per day. The therapeutic effect of these steps is additive. Lipids should be monitored not less than every 3 to 6 months and even closer surveillance maintained for side effects of clofibrate, including muscle pain and creatine phosphokinase elevations. Nicotinic acid, 3 Gm per day, or *d*-thyroxin may be tried in place of clofibrate; the latter is the drug of choice.

ACQUIRED TYPE III. Transient lipoprotein abnormalities of the same type have been seen in diabetes mellitus during recovery from coma. The anomalous flotation of beta-lipoproteins is also seen in Tangier disease, but in this instance alpha-lipoproteins are absent, and the differential diagnosis is no problem.

Type IV Hyperlipoproteinemia (Endogenous Hyperglyceridemia)

DEFINITION. Excessive endogenous glycerides, synthesized mainly in the liver, cause an increase in prebetalipoproteins. All but 30 to 50 mg per 100 ml of plasma glycerides circulate in pre-beta or very low-density lipoproteins, small amounts of which are normally present. Since an excess of chylomicrons (mainly exogenous glyceride) is relatively uncommon, hyperglyceridemia usually signifies hyperprebetalipoproteinemia. Glyceride elevations between 180 and 300 mg per 100 ml occur with normal cholesterol concentrations. The plasma is not usually turbid until glycerides exceed 300, when they are also accompanied by hypercholesterolemia. Type IV hyperlipoproteinemia is not a specific disease; it is a sign of a variety of metabolic defects, some related to abnormal carbohydrate metabolism. When all well-defined diseases have been excluded, there remain many patients with unexplained type IV; frequently, screening of the families reveals more adults with the same lipoprotein abnormality.

ETIOLOGY. Many, but not all, cases of endogenous hyperglyceridemia are probably related to exaggerated *carbohydrate induction*. This is the conversion of excess starches or sugars to glyceride in amounts that maintain a higher than normal plasma glyceride level. Sometimes the rate limit may be in removal rather than overproduction. All normal subjects have transient rises in glycerides in switching from a regular diet to one in which 60 percent or more of calories comes from carbohydrate. Some patients who have type IV patterns on regular diets, particularly those who are overweight and have abnormal glucose tolerance with abnormally low or high insulin responses to glucose, over-respond to high carbohydrate feeding. If possible, such exaggerated carbohydrate induction should be sought for by dietary trials. If this cannot be excluded as an etiologic factor, patients with type IV are arbitrarily restricted to 40 percent or less of calories from carbohydrate. Other mechanisms include chonic increases in free fatty acid concentrations, sometimes related to stress or poor management of diabetes, and excess alcohol intake.

FAMILIAL TYPE IV. When all secondary causes have been eliminated, type IV should be looked for in adult relatives. Frequently one parent and half the siblings may have the same pattern, suggesting that one or more dominant genes may be involved. Children in such families below age twenty are usually normal, indicating factors associated with adulthood that determine expression. These include caloric excess and maturity onset diabetes, common in affected adults. Insulin secretion may be low, normal, or high. Primary type IV hyperlipoproteinemia has been found in a high percentage of patients with premature ischemic heart disease and is considered an important risk factor for atherosclerosis in young adults. PHLA is normal in familial Type IV.

ACQUIRED TYPE IV. This lipoprotein pattern may be seen with dysglobulinemias such as myeloma or macroglobulinemia, hypothyroidism, nephrotic syndrome, idiopathic hypercalcemia, Werner's syndrome, glycogen storage disease, and other disorders, as well as during administration of progestational hormones for contraception. The latter may enhance a familial abnormality.

TREATMENT. Management of primary type IV consists of (1) reduction to ideal weight, (2) maintenance of a diet generally high in P/S ratio and low in cholesterol with care to maintain carbohydrate between 30 and 40 percent of calories; then, if response is inadequate, (3) use of one of several drugs. Clofibrate or nicotinic acid may be effective in helping to lower glycerides, but in some patients there is little response. In patients with mild or minimal diabetes, tolbutamide (0.5 to 1.5 Gm) may help control both hyperglycemia and hyperglyceridemia. Drug or diet therapy must be followed initially by weekly glyceride measurements to establish effectiveness of regimen. Discontinue a drug if no response is obtained in 4 weeks, provided diet is followed carefully.

Type V Hyperlipoproteinemia

DEFINITION. This is mixed hyperlipemia in which chylomicrons and prebeta-lipoproteins are in excess. The plasma is turbid and, after standing overnight in the cold, contains a creamy layer over a milky infranatant layer. Triglycerides are usually between 500 to 5,000 mg per 100 ml, and cholesterol between 200 and 1,000, the C/T ratio usually lying between 0.2 and 0.4. The type V pattern occurs in many disorders and implies defective metabolism of glycerides that are either synthesized in the body or eaten. Some patients who usually have the type IV pattern will also accumulate chylomicrons when levels of endogenous hyperglyceridemia become very high. The resulting Type V pattern is thus a function of diet and the degree of saturation of glyceride-clearing mechanisms. Transient type V patterns occur in temporary deficiency of PHLA associated with insulin-deficient diabetes, acute or chronic pancreatitis, and alcoholism. The mechanisms are vague, but recognition of the pattern has clinical value, for it is commonly associated with a predictable constellation of signs and symptoms.

CLINICAL PICTURE. Usually type V hyperlipoproteinemia occurs in adults, many of whom are overweight and have glucose intolerance or a family history of diabetes. The presenting symptom is frequently bouts of abdominal pain indistinguishable from that seen in type I except that transient amylase elevations are more common. Lipemia retinalis, eruptive xanthomas, and hepatosplenomegaly may be present; and there are frequent complaints of paresthesias or painful extremities. Recurrent abdominal attacks frequently lead to laparotomy, when milky peritoneal fluid and sometimes chalky deposits on the pancreas may be found. Hyperuricemia is common especially if heavy alcoholic excess has preceded the attack.

DIAGNOSIS. Type V is both acquired and familial. After establishment of the typical pattern, insulin-deficient diabetes, acute pancreatitis, and dysglobulinemia must be excluded as well as other disorders commonly associated with hyperlipemia. Adult family members must then be examined; more than half may have type IV or type V patterns. Relationship to mutants causing type IV hyperlipoproteinemia is not clear; and type V may be the expression of one or more aberrant genes, possibly related to both diabetes and hyperlipoproteinemia. Glucose tolerance should always be examined; test of response to high carbohydrate feeding is useful; high fat test diets must be tried cautiously, for they often precipitate abdominal crises.

TREATMENT. The prognosis of type V hyperlipoproteinemia depends on the cause. The primary forms probably carry a hazard for accelerated atherogenesis, but pancreatitis and abdominal pain are the more immediate threats. The sequence of treatment is (1) reduction to ideal body weight, (2) adjustment of diet empirically by response of plasma glycerides, generally using the highest practical protein intake to avoid excesses of either carbohydrate or fat, and severe restriction of alcohol; and, if necessary, (3) trial of drugs. Clofibrate or nicotinic acid will usually effect some reduction in glycerides in type V. Tolbutamide may be helpful, especially if insulinopenia is present. Their use must be accompanied by close followup of plasma lipids. The acute abdominal crises are usually adequately managed by parenteral fluids for 24 to 48 hr. The high protein diet is then cautiously resumed.

Other Hyperlipoproteinemias

All hyperlipidemia is not encompassed in the five major lipoprotein patterns. A notable exception is hypercholesterolemia and massive hyperphospholipidemia associated with obstructive liver disease. This is usually accompanied by marked increase of alpha-lipoproteins with both unusual electrophoretic mobility and abnormally low density. This is best detected by the combination of jaundice, hypercholesterolemia, and a great increase in *unesterified* plasma cholesterol. In otherwise normal subjects, high doses of estrogens may also raise alpha lipoproteins sufficiently to cause modest hypercholesterolemia.

HYPOLIPOPROTEINEMIA
Beta (Low Density) Lipoprotein Deficiency

ABETALIPOPROTEINEMIA. Abetalipoproteinemia is a rare familial disease, uniquely characterized by complete absence of beta-lipoproteins. The plasma contains only alpha-lipoproteins; no chylomicrons or prebeta (very low density)lipoproteins are present. The syndrome follows a fairly uniform course, beginning before the age of one year, with *malnutrition* and growth retardation, lordosis, abdominal distension, and steatorrhea. *Ataxia*, nystagmus, weakness and areflexia, and other signs of progressive neurologic dysfunction, particularly involving the posterolateral columns and spinocerebellar tracts, then appear. *Pigmentary retinal degeneration* develops during adolescence. The erythrocytes have a crenated appearance (*acanthocytosis*). The esterified lipids of these cells and of the plasma are deficient in both lecithin and linoleic acid. Dietary fat is assimilated but is held up in the intestinal mucosal cells, creating a pathognomonic picture detectable by peroral biopsy. Some fat is absorbed, possibly by direct passage through the portal system into the liver.

The disease may occur in siblings and is likely due to a double dose of a mutant autosomal gene, since the consanguinity rate in affected families is high. Most relatives have normal concentrations of plasma lipoproteins. Whether the primary defect is related to formation of beta-apoprotein, beta-lipoprotein, or some other aspect of fat absorption is not known. The prognosis is guarded; patients may succumb relatively young, sometimes from cardiac arrhythmias. Familial instances of acanthocytosis and neurologic abnormalities without abetalipoproteinemia have also been reported.

Diagnosis. The diagnosis is suspected when a plasma cholesterol concentration less than 100 mg per 100 ml is associated with the above clinical picture. It must be confirmed by immunochemical evidence of the absence of plasma beta-lipoprotein.

Treatment. There is no definitive therapy. Medium-chain triglycerides may help provide some fat intake in the absence of chylomicron formation, and low vitamin A levels have been increased with supplements.

HYPOBETALIPOPROTEINEMIA. Abnormally low cholesterol and glyceride concentrations with decreased, but not absent, beta- and very low density lipoproteins are common in malnutrition or malabsorption due to a variety of causes. Remissions are promptly associated with a rise in cholesterol and beta-lipoproteins. There are also *heritable* forms of hypobetalipoproteinemia, at least one due to a dominant gene.

Alpha (High Density) Lipoprotein Deficiency and LCAT Deficiency

Familial high density lipoprotein deficiency is also called *Tangier disease*, after the island home of the first cases. The disease has been detected in other children and adults and must be suspected when hypocholesterolemia is associated with orange or yellowish-gray discoloration of the tonsils and pharyngeal or rectal mucosa or *enlargement* of *spleen, liver,* or *lymph nodes.* Reticuloendothelial tissues are infiltrated with *foam cells* containing large amounts of cholesterol esters. In adults *corneal infiltration,* hypersplenism, papular skin lesions containing foam cells, peripheral neuropathy with loss of tendon reflexes and abnormal electromyograms, and possibly premature coronary artery disease have been seen as complications.

Parents and other relatives of patients with Tangier disease have lower than normal amounts of plasma high-density (alpha$_1$) lipoprotein. The propositi are probably homozygous for a mutant gene that normally governs the synthesis of this lipoprotein.

DIAGNOSIS. Diagnosis is suspected when plasma cholesterol is between 50 and 125 mg per 100 ml with normal or slightly elevated glycerides. It is established by immunochemical evidence that the alpha-polypeptide characteristic of plasma high-density lipoprotein is present in only trace amounts and as an immunochemically different form. Carriers also have similar amounts of the abnormal alpha lipoprotein in plasma. Splenectomy may be required for hypersplenism. There is no definitive therapy.

Deficient Plasma Lecithin: Cholesterol Acyltransferase

LCAT is a familial disorder discovered in a Norwegian family. The clinical manifestations include proteinuria, anemia, and arcus cornea. Plasma alpha lipoproteins are severely deficient, although total cholesterol and glyceride concentrations may be normal or elevated. *Diagnosis is suspected when the clinical picture is accompanied by absence of esterified cholesterol in plasma.* Assay of the enzyme is required for confirmation.

LIPID STORAGE DISEASES

The Sphingolipidoses

There are other storage diseases characterized more by tissue rather than plasma lipid abnormalities. *In all it is exceedingly important that specimens of tissues obtained for diagnostic purposes be retained frozen without fixatives for chemical and enzymatic analyses. Histochemical diagnosis is usually not definitive.* The sphingolipidoses represent one group of these disorders and are so called because they have in common the accumulation of a different derivative (—R) of ceramide (acyl-sphingosine).

$$CH_3(CH_2)_{13}CH=CH-C-C-C-O-R$$

$$CH_3-(CH_2)_n-CO-NH$$

Ceramide

These are all inheritable disorders; each may involve the nervous system. Most occur in several clinical forms or syndromes, possibly reflecting mutations at different loci. Specific enzyme deficiencies have now been identified in some and probably represent the genetically-determined defects.

Glucosylceramidoses (Gangliosidoses, Gaucher's Disease, Fabry's Disease

GANGLIOSIDOSES. (See Chap. 364). *Gangliosidoses (amaurotic family idiocy)* is a generic term for several familial neurologic disorders associated with varying degrees of blindness and dementia. Three of these diseases have been identified as characterized by accumulation, and presumably defective metabolism, of a different ganglioside, the major lipid in gray matter. G_{M_1}-*gangliosidosis,* or *generalized gangliosidosis,* or *pseudo-Hurler's disease,* involves both brain and viscera. The tissues contain abnormal amounts of galactosyl-galactosaminyl-(N-acetylneuraminido) galactosyl-glucosylceramide. A galactosidase attacking the terminal glycosidic bond is deficient. G_{M_2}-*gangliosidosis* is classical *Tay-Sachs disease,* which fatally involves only the central nervous system. The excess ganglioside is N-acetylgalactosaminyl-(N-acetylneuraminido)galactosyl-glucosylceramide. A G_{M_3}-*gangliosidosis* has also recently been identified. Other forms of amaurotic idiocy, such as Batten's disease (Vogt-Spielmeyer or juvenile amaurotic idiocy), and the Bieloschowsky, Kufs, or Hallevorden types have not been chemically differentiated as lipidoses.

GLUCOSYLCEREBROSIDOSIS (see Chap. 350) (Gaucher's Disease). First described by Gaucher in 1882, these disorders represent storage of glucocerebrosides (ceramide-glucose) in reticuloendothelial cells, producing marked splenomegaly and hepatomegaly. In adults there are often bone lesions, associated skin pigmentation, and characteristic pingueculas of the scleras. In infants progressive neurologic disturbances usually occur and are associated with a rapidly fatal course. There is also a juvenile form. Deficient glucocerebrosidase has been found in spleen, liver, and white cells of patients with infantile and adult varieties.

GLUCOSYLCERAMIDETRIHEXOSIDOSIS (see Chap. 347) (Fabry's disease). In this sex-linked disorder, the manifestations are usually only seen in males and are due to deposition of glycolipids, mainly a trihexoside (ceramide-glucose-galactose-galactose), in blood vessels and nerves. Galactosyl-galactosylceramide also accumulates. The disease is also known by its unusual skin manifestations, *angiokeratoma corporis diffusum.* Deficient galactosidase which normally cleaves the terminal galactose from the trihexoside has been detected in this disease.

Galactosylceramidoses (see Chap 364)

GALACTOSYLSULFATIDOSIS. Galactosylsulfatidosis, or *metachromatic leukodystrophy* is a disorder of children in which abnormal amounts of cerebroside-sulfatide (ceramide-galactose-SO_3H) accumulate in the brain and kidney. The material is also excreted in bile, causing fibrosis of the gallbladder, and in urine, where it may be detected as an aid to diagnosis. Deficiency of an arylsulfatase appears to be the genetic abnormality.

Galactosylcerebrosides accumulate in the brain in *Krabbe's disease*, although this disorder is not yet proved to be a genetically determined lipidosis.

Phosphorylceramidoses (see Chap 350) (Niemann-Pick Disease)

Accumulation of massive amounts of sphingomyelin and cholesterol characterize lipidoses that take several forms. They may be partially distinguished by measurement of sphingomyelin-cleavage enzyme in liver, spleen, or fibroblasts in tissue culture. The enzyme is deficient in both the classical infantile form or Niemann-Pick disease and in older children with visceral but not CNS involvement. The enzyme has been normal or low normal in tissues examined from most of the older patients with late CNS involvement or those with the so-called "Nova Scotia" variant. Sphingomyelin lipidoses appear to result from several mutations.

OTHER RARE TISSUE LIPID STORAGE DISEASES
Phytanic Oxidase Deficiency

In addition to the sphingolipidoses, there are other rare disorders in which less polar lipids pile up in tissues apparently because of enzymatic defects. In *Refsum's disease* there is accumulation of phytanic acid (3,7,11,15-tetramethyl hexadecanoic acid) in the esterified lipids present in both tissues and plasma. This familial disease is characterized by ataxic neuropathy, anosmia, retinitis pigmentosa, dry skin, skeletal deformities, and ichthyosis and is commonest in children or young adults of Scandinavian ancestry. Parents may have high levels of phytanic acid in plasma without other abnormalities. The prognosis is guarded, with the symptoms sometimes progressing to complete blindness and deafness, but often waxing and waning, relapses being irregular correlated with the degree of increase in CSF protein. Phytanic acid, which may make up 10 to 30 percent of total plasma fatty acids in the patients, is normally present only in very small amounts. It is derived from dietary phytols, and present therapy consists of a low-phytol diet. The inherited defects include a block in the alpha oxidation of the phytanic acid derived from phytols. The relationship of phytanate accumulation to the nervous disorders is unknown. Diagnosis is usually made by chromatographic analysis of plasma.

Familial Xanthomatosis with Adrenal Calcification (Wolman's Disease)

This disease resembles Niemann-Pick disease in the presence of hepatosplenomegaly, foam cell deposition in tissues, and death in early childhood. The stored lipids are mainly triglycerides and cholesterol, much of it esterified. The etiology and effective treatment are unknown.

Hepatic Cholesterol Ester Storage Disease

This is a disorder seen in siblings in which the liver is selectively enlarged, butter-yellow in color, shows slight cirrhosis, and has a very high content of cholesteryl esters, predominantly cholesteryl oleate. Plasma lipids are not altered in a diagnostic fashion and the diagnosis must be made by liver biopsy. The parenchyma stains very deeply with Oil-Red-O and the Schultz technique; lipid analyses must also be made. The ultimate prognosis and treatment are not established.

Ceroid Storage Disease

Ceroid storage disease, or the accumulation of ceroid, a pigmented lipid of unknown chemical composition, may also include sufficient organ involvement to produce a clinical picture similar to severe Niemann-Pick disease. It may also be associated with cirrhosis of the liver and intestinal malabsorption. Ceroid may be identified histochemically by the combination of red periodic acid-Schiff stain, acid-fastness, and fluorescence. Deposition of this material has also been seen in aorta, liver, intestinal musculature, and other tissues in a variety of conditions, including tocopherol deficiency. The biochemical basis for ceroid formation and storage is not known.

GRANULOMATOUS DISEASES WITH LIPID STORAGE

Frequently considered among the lipid storage diseases are certain tissue proliferative disorders sometimes accompanied by lipid deposition.

Histiocytosis X

Histiocytosis X (see Chap. 350) is the generic term for a group of disorders that affect the reticuloendothelial system and which may be either different stages or forms of the same disease. *Letterer-Siwe disease* and *xanthoma disseminatum* may be the two extremes of such abnormalities, with *eosinophilic granuloma* and *Hand-Schuller-Christian disease* representing intermediate and special forms. The usual order of progression of the pathologic lesions is reticuloendothelial cell proliferation and hyperplasia, granulomatous changes featuring eosinophils and giant cells, conversion of reticulum cells and histiocytes to foam cells or xanthomas, and finally, fibrosis. These disorders do not appear to be hereditary.

Several other uncommon diseases are associated with proliferation of histiocytes and deposition of material considered to represent both lipid and carbohydrate because it stains by both the Sudan and periodic acid-Schiff techniques. The chemical composition of the lesions has not been characterized. It is likely that any faulty metabolism of lipid is secondary to some other processes, perhaps involving mucopolysaccharide metabolism.

Lipoid Proteinosis

In *lipoid - proteinosis* (cutaneous-mucosal hyalinosis; Urbach-Wiethe disease) the lesions share enough histologic features of *histiocytosis X* to suggest an etiologic relationship. The skin and mucous membranes of the pharynx and larynx are infiltrated by extracellular deposits of hyaline material. Clinical manifestations include hoarseness or aphonia, widely distributed skin papules, dental anomalies, and symmetric calcifications in the region of the sella turcica as seen by x-ray. The disease is not incompatible with long life. This disorder may be inheritable.

Lipoid Dermatoarthritis

In *lipoid dermatoarthritis* polyarthritis is associated with multiple nodular or papular skin lesions. In both skin and synovial tissues there is an infiltration of histiocytes, eosinophils, lymphocytes, red blood cells, and multinucleated giant cells. The joint changes may be extremely destructive, producing *arthritis mutilans,* or the "opera-glass hand." Serologic reactions for rheumatoid arthritis are negative. Familial occurrence has not been reported.

Disseminated Lipogranulomatosis (Farber's Disease)

This is a rare disease that appears in infancy as generalized nodular periarticular swelling and dysphonia. There is progressive systemic involvement with widespread proliferation of histiocytes and neuronal abnormalities. Storage cells appear containing both mucopolysaccharide and lipids. The basic disorder probably involves the metabolism of certain acid mucopolysaccharides similar to those in Hurler's disease (Chap. 399).

Hereditary Tendinous and Tuberous Xanthomatosis without Hyperlipidemia

This disorder has been reported in siblings who had multiple xanthomas of the Achilles tendons and subcutaneously over the knee, elbow, and shoulder, and diffuse pulmonary infiltration. Giant cells but no eosinophils are present.

Cerebrotendinous Xanthomatosis

The preceding disorder bears an uncertain resemblance to cerebrotendinous xanthomatosis, which is a familial disease in which cholesterol deposits in tendons, pulmonary parenchyma, and the cerebellum and other areas in the brain are associated with progressive spastic ataxia, large xanthomas, and sometimes, dementia and cataracts. Hyperlipidemia may or may not be present. The proper etiologic classification of these two disorders is not established.

XANTHOMAS

Many chronic infections, particularly accompanied by exudates, and other proliferative processes, such as osteitis fibrosa cystica or traumatic lesions, may be associated with collections of foam cells (*xanthomas*) and sometimes crystals of cholesterol. Most skin xanthomas are secondary to hyperlipoproteinemia, but *juvenile xanthomas* (nevoxanthoepithelioma) are benign skin lesions that can appear without abnormal plasma lipids. *Xanthelasmas* need not always be associated with hyperlipoproteinemia and sometimes occur in family members who are normolipoproteinemic.

ADIPOSE TISSUE DISORDERS

Adipose tissue can be a site of expression of many disorders including those of connective tissue, lipid, and carbohydrate metabolism. There is therefore no simple classification of the adipose tissue diseases.

Relapsing Panniculitis (Weber-Christian Disease)

This classification may represent several diseases that share similar but rather nonspecific histologic changes (see Chap. 394).

Lipodystrophy

Although the term *lipodystrophy* is sometimes used to describe *lipoathrophy,* it also has a generic meaning that allows it to encompass several disorders in which adipose tissue is abnormal but not necessarily absent. Several abnormalities may properly be considered forms of lipodystrophy.

LIPOMAS. These are benign mesenchymal tumors consisting of circumscribed masses of adipose tissue. There is usually a capsule, but the cells are histologically indistinguishable from ordinary fat. They may occur nearly anywhere in the body, singly or as multiple fatty growths (lipomatosis), most commonly in subcutaneous tissues. They also arise in retroperitoneal or peritoneal areas, in breast, mesentery, and mediastinum, and in other body cavities and organs. Lipomas have caused intestinal obstruction or dyspnea by superior mediastinal obstruction and may embarrass the function of other vital tissues. Rarely they may calcify, and it has been presumed that they may on occasion give rise to liposarcomas or other malignant tumors, but there is no general agreement on this. Multiple lipomas may be symmetrically placed and may run in families. The therapy is surgical excision; occasionally they will recur in the same site.

ADIPOSIS DOLOROSA (Dercum's Disease). *Adiposis dolorosa* refers to a poorly defined disorder in which painful subcutaneous lipomas, often widely and symmetrically situated, are sometimes associated with asthenia, decreased cutaneous sensation, motor weakness, or other evidence of peripheral neuropathy. Some patients have also had adenomas in the pituitary, thyroid, or adrenal glands. There may or may not be accompanying generalized obesity. Siblings may be similarly involved. The interstitial neuritis observed in the original adipose tissue nodules by Dercum has not been seen in many subsequent cases. There is no specific therapy.

INSULIN LIPODYSTROPHY. This term refers to changes in subcutaneous fat at the site of insulin injection (see Chap. 94) and may involve either localized hypertrophy or atrophy of adipose tissue.

Lipoatrophy

Lipoatrophy may be partial or complete.

PARTIAL LIPOATROPHY. Also called *progressive lipodystrophy*, partial lipodystrophy is characterized by the absence of subcutaneous fat over wide, symmetric areas of the body. The remaining parts of the body have normal or sometimes increased subcutaneous fat deposits. It occurs predominantly in females and often begins in childhood. The onset is usually insidious and may begin with loss of subcutaneous fat in the face and subsequently involve that of the upper extremities and upper trunk. In other instances the disorder may begin at the level of the iliac crest and extend downward. There are no subjective symptoms. The cause is unknown. There is no known therapy.

TOTAL LIPOATROPHY. In total lipoatrophy (lipoatrophic diabetes mellitus), generalized atrophy of body fat occurs gradually. In addition to subcutaneous fat deposits, nearly all other body fat, excepting that in the breasts, may disappear. This is usually but not always associated with diabetes, which may precede or follow the onset of lipoatrophy. There is also hyperlipoproteinemia with types IV or V patterns, decreased postheparin lipolytic activity, hepatomegaly, and sometimes acanthosis nigricans; serious nephropathy, including both nephritic and nephrotic manifestations, may occur whether the patient has diabetes or not. Some patients may also have hypermetabolism, others have features suggestive of "leprechaunism," and the syndrome undoubtedly results from several different causes. The diabetes is associated with high plasma insulin levels and may be very difficult to control. The course of the disease may be either indolent or rapidly progressive. No therapy is known.

REFERENCES

Abul-Haj, S. K., D. G. Martz, W. F. Douglas, and L. J. Geppert: Farber's Disease, J. Pediat., 61:221, 1962.

Bortz, A. I., and M. Vincent: Lipoid Dermato-arthritis and Arthritis Mutilans, Am. J. Med., 30:951, 1961.

Brady, R. O., Jr.: The Sphingolipidoses, New Engl. J. Med., 275:312, 1966.

Fredrickson, D. S., R. I. Levy, and R. S. Lees: Fat Transport in Lipoproteins—An Integrated Approach to Mechanisms and Disorders, New Engl. J. Med., 276:34, 94, 148, 215, 273, 1967.

Harlan, W. R., Jr., and W. J. S. Still: Hereditary Tendinous and Tuberous Xanthomatosis without Hyperlipidemia, New Engl. J. Med., 278:416, 1968.

McCusker, J. J., and R. M. Caplan: Lipoid Proteinosis (Lipoglycoproteinosis), Am. J. Pathol., 40:599, 1962.

Norum, K. R.: Biochemical Study of New Familial Syndrome Characterized by a Marked Reduction of Esterified Cholesterol in Serum, Scand. J. Clin. Lab. Invest., 19 (suppl. 100):102, 1967.

Oppenheimer, E. H., and E. C. Andrews, Jr.: Ceroid Storage Disease in Childhood, Pediatrics, 23:1091, 1959.

Schiff, L., W. K. Schubert, A. J. McAdams, E. L. Spiegel, and J. F. O'Donnell: Hepatic Cholesterol Ester Storage Disease, A Familial Disorder, Am. J. Med., 44:538, 1968.

Schimschock, J. R., E. C. Alvord, Jr., and P. D. Swanson: Cerebrotendinous Xanthomatosis, Arch. Neurol., 18:688, 1968.

Schwartz, R., I. A. Schafer, and A. E. Renold: Generalized Lipoatrophy, Hepatic Cirrhosis, Disturbed Carbohydrate Metabolism and Accelerated Growth (Lipoatrophic Diabetes), Am. J. Med., 28:973, 1960.

Senior, B., and S. S. Gellis: The Syndromes of Total Lipodystrophy and of Partial Lipodystrophy, Pediatrics, 33:593, 1964.

Stanbury, J. B., J. B. Wyngaarden, and D. S. Fredrickson (Eds.): "The Metabolic Basis of Inherited Disease," 2d ed., chaps. 22–29, New York, McGraw-Hill Book Company, 1966.

Tedeschi, C. G., and W. H. Lyon: Fat Tissue Growths, J. Mt. Sinai Hosp., 24:1272, 1957.

Wolman, M., V. V. Sterk, S. Gatt, and M. Frenkel: Primary Familial Xanthomatosis with Involvement and Calcification of the Adrenals, Pediatrics, 28:742, 1961.

114 AMYLOIDOSIS
Evan Calkins

Introduction

Although amyloidosis has been recognized as a clinical and pathologic entity for over 100 years, our knowledge about the nature, pathogenesis, distribution, and possible clinical importance of amyloid is still in a state of evolution.

The hyaline, apparently amorphous, eosinophilic material known as *amyloid* was named by Virchow because of its affinity to iodine, a property which suggested a resemblance to starch. Although amyloid was at first recognized in association with tuberculosis, and other prolonged septic processes, it soon became apparent that material indistinguishable from amyloid could be identified in the myocardium and other tissues of certain individuals who had never had chronic infections. Although this group of patients has been considered relatively infrequent, there is evidence that, at least in elderly patients, the incidence of *primary amyloidosis* may be frequent.

Sensitive histologic techniques, utilizing polarization and fluorescence microscopy, have detected what appears to be amyloid in a high percentage of people over sixty; and in a recent study amyloid was detected in the meningeal vessels and brain substance (senile plaques) in one-half of the patients over sixty and in 63 percent of the patients over seventy years of age. Cardiac amyloid deposits were present in 30 percent of patients over sixty and aortic deposits in over 39 percent of patients in the same age group. Pancreatic islet hyalin, commonly attributed to diabetes mellitus, is also common in elderly patients. Recent studies have indicated that this islet deposition is similar if not identical to amyloid.

Further studies utilizing electron microscopy and immunochemistry will be required before senile amyloid can be considered identical with the more classical form of amyloid. Electron microscopy of pancreatic hyalin and senile cardiac amyloid has, however, shown the presence of the fibrillar component which has been regarded as specific for amyloid. The clinical implications of this sort of amyloid infiltration are not yet clear. The close association of this connective tissue change with atherosclerotic plaques raised the possibility, as yet unproved, of a relationship between amyloidosis and atherosclerosis. The association with hyalin or amyloid infiltration of the pancreatic islets with diabetes mellitus has long been recognized. Preliminary studies have also indicated a relationship between amyloid infiltration of the brain and behavioral abnormalities in elderly patients without otherwise demonstrable cerebral pathology.

The concept that amyloid accumulation is an age-related process has strong support from studies in experimental animals. It has been shown that certain animal species and certain strains within a given species have a greatly enhanced predilection for developing senile amyloidosis.

These findings provide increasing support for the hypothesis that amyloidosis may represent a nonspecific phenomenon of ageing. According to this hypothesis, genetic factors and certain diseases (prolonged infections, neoplasms, etc.) enhance the development of an apparently common biologic process which results in the disease state of *secondary amyloidosis* and the various syndromes of primary amyloidosis (see below).

Physical and Chemical Characteristics

Amyloid has been shown to consist of a relatively amorphous ground substance, containing a high concentration of fibrils. The characteristics of these fibrils have been fairly well defined by electron microscopy. They are long, ranging from 300 to 100,000 Å in length, non-branching, and undulant as opposed to straight. Their diameter appears to range from 70 to 100 Å, and they may occur singularly or in bundles of varying number. They appear irregularly beaded at intervals of 35 to 100 Å. The fibrils are predominantly protein. The content of amino acids and carbohydrate components has been well defined. By all criteria amyloid fibrils are distinct from collagen, elastin, fibrin, and other known body fibers. It has been shown that the fibrils themselves do not contain gamma-globulin. On the other hand, gamma-globulin (IgG), several components of complement (C'1, C'3, and C'4), fibrinogen, and a component of normal tissue protein appear to be adsorbed onto or closely associated with amyloid fibriles.

The nature of amyloid ground substance has not been well defined. Extracts of amyloid have shown, in addition to the fibrils, a relatively small concentration of a second, apparently unique globular component, 80 to 100 Å in diameter, resembling and referred to as "doughnuts." The relationship of this component, if any, to the amyloid fibril is not known. Preliminary analyses indicate that it has a somewhat different chemical composition from the fibril.

The precise events which lead to the accumulation of amyloid are not known. It is not known with certainty, for example, whether the formation of the amyloid fibril represents the initiating process or whether the fibril is synthesized in response to a primary change in the ground substance. It has been suggested that the amyloid fibril is synthesized by mesenchymal cells in a fashion analogous to the synthesis of collagen fibers. Immunochemical studies have failed to disclose any component of amyloid, including the fibril and doughnut, which is clearly abnormal. It seems probable that amyloidosis represents excessive accumulation of normal components.

Clinical Classification

It appears from the above discussion that amyloidosis, defined most broadly, is the tissue accumulation of detectable amounts of extracellular hyaline material which has certain rather unique tinctorial characteristics and contains characteristic fibrils which can be identified by electron microscopy. Using this definition, the incidence of amyloidosis is probably extremely high, and may be almost universal in the ageing human population.

A more practical clinical definition is that amyloidosis is the accumulation of amyloid in amounts that result in interference with normal bodily function. According to this definition the entity is probably quite rare, except in certain countries, such as Israel and Turkey, in which there appears to be a striking genetic predisposition. The remainder of this discussion will focus on amyloidosis as defined in this more restricted clinical sense.

SECONDARY AMYLOIDOSIS

Secondary amyloidosis is that which may accompany prolonged inflammatory or infectious diseases. Histologic evidence of amyloidosis is seen in approximately 25 percent of all patients with rheumatoid arthritis, dying of any cause. It becomes clinically manifest in only a small percentage of these cases however. Secondary amyloidosis is a common cause of death in paraplegics who have developed decubitus ulcers and urinary tract infections. It is seen in approximately one-third of patients with leprosy at the U.S. Public Health Service Hospital in Carville, La., and is one of the chief causes of death at that hospital. Secondary amyloidosis is manifested chiefly by nephrosis and subsequent azotemia; hepatomegaly and splenomegaly may also be seen. At autopsy the predominant sites of involvement are the kidney, spleen, liver, and adrenal glands. Microscopic traces of amyloid may be widely distributed, especially in blood vessel walls.

AMYLOIDOSIS ASSOCIATED WITH MULTIPLE MYELOMA

A second category of amyloidosis is that which accompanies multiple myeloma. Between 10 and 20 percent of patients with multiple myeloma are known to develop this complication. Clinical involvement may resemble that seen in secondary amyloidosis. More widespread manifestations, such as neuropathy of the ulnar nerve resulting in the carpal tunnel syndrome, may also be seen. The manifestations may be indistinguishable from those of primary amyloidosis (see below).

PRIMARY AMYLOIDOSIS

In the third and probably most common category of amyloidosis seen today the disease develops without any known predisposing disease. Recent studies have provided increasing evidence that this so-called "primary" form of amyloidosis is, in turn, comprised of a number of relatively discrete syndromes, each with characteristic clinical expression and pattern of occurrence.

In several of these entities the involvement resembles that seen in the secondary form. One example is the amyloidosis which often occurs in association with *familial Mediterranean fever* (FMF), primarily in members of the Sephardic and Iraqui Jewish races. The two disorders appear to be inherited as independent recessive traits; amyloidosis may be seen in members of a family who do not have FMF and vice versa (Chap. 256).

Other varieties of primary amyloidosis are manifested by more widespread evidence of the disease. One example is the primary familial amyloidosis described by Andrade. In this entity, which occurs predominantly in individuals of Portuguese ancestry, severe impairment of the sensory function of the peripheral nerves, as well as less severe impairment of motor function is encountered. This is often accompanied by involvement of the sympathetic ganglions, with postural hypotension, impotence, absence of sweating, and intestinal hypermotility and malabsorption. Adie's pupil is apt to be present. The patients usually die from severe malnutrition and inanition. Another example of primary amyloidosis occurring in families is that described by Rukavina et al. in a family of Swiss ancestry. Although some members of the family resembled the patients described by Andrade, others exhibited a variety of different clinical manifestations. Other family constellations, yielding a variety of syndromes, have also been described.

Despite the increasing awareness of the familial incidence of amyloidosis, many patients who develop the disease, without known predisposing cause, do not appear to have any genetic or familial predisposition. In some of these cases the distribution of the amyloid resembles that seen in the secondary form of the disease; others exhibit diffuse involvement, especially of the skin or the heart. In many patients the accumulation may be localized to a single area, such as the respiratory passages, without evidence of widespread involvement.

Clinical Manifestations

The clinical manifestations of amyloidosis depend on the organ or system involved. Since the symptoms may resemble those of a variety of other disorders, amyloidosis must frequently be considered in differential diagnosis.

Amyloidosis of the skin is most typically characterized by hyaline plaques, occurring chiefly in or near the folds of the skin, as in the inguinal regions. Occasionally, the disease results in widespread purpura.

Although in most cases this purpura is thought to be due to involvement of the walls of small blood vessels, other mechanisms may be involved. These may include thrombocytopenia, deficiencies of several different clotting factors, and increased plasmin activity. As a result of the defects in hemostasis, prolonged bleeding may follow such minor surgical procedures as a gingival biopsy. Other parameters of coagulation are usually within normal limits. The bleeding time may be prolonged, presumably because of increased rigidity of small blood vessels.

Ocular involvement may consist of diffuse infiltrates in the posterior chamber, discrete deposits of amyloid beneath the bulbar conjunctiva, and an Adie pupil.

Amyloid infiltration of the heart classically results in enlargement, which is due to an increased thickness of the myocardial wall, without change in intracardiac volume. The resultant syndrome, due to a stiffened myocardium, may yield results on cardiac catheterization which closely resemble those seen in constrictive pericarditis. In other cases, the clinical picture may more nearly resemble that seen in diffuse arteriosclerotic heart disease, with an enlarged and inefficient myocardium. Electrocardiogram often reveals low voltage in the QRS complex. Arteriovenous block and arrhythmias may also be seen. Amyloidosis is one of a group of conditions which may cause cardiac failure, without detectable murmurs. Unfortunately, it is very seldom correctly diagnosed ante mortem.

Amyloid involvement of the liver is characterized primarily by hepatomegaly. Clinical evidence of hepatic dysfunction and jaundice is rare. Liver function tests characteristically show minimal abnormalities, which are usually suggestive of biliary obstruction. Although liver biopsy has been recommended and often yields diagnostic information, it has been followed in a few instances by intractable bleeding and/or rupture of the liver. For this reason liver biopsy should probably be avoided when amyloidosis is suspected.

Renal amyloidosis is manifested predominantly by the nephrotic syndrome. The appearance of progressively severe proteinuria in patients with chronic inflammatory diseases such as rheumatoid arthritis should always lead to a suspicion of amyloidosis. In attempting to differentiate renal amyloidosis from chronic pyelonephritis, the size of the kidneys, as seen on x-ray, may be helpful. In pyelonephritis the kidneys are usually reduced in size; amyloid-laden kidneys are likely to be normal in size or may be enlarged. Hypertension is not commonly observed in amyloidosis. Azotemia is a very late manifestation. Kidney biopsy is a satisfactory method of confirming the diagnosis of renal amyloidosis in cases in which the clinical syndrome, plus rectal or gingival biopsy, has not already led to a definite diagnosis.

Amyloidosis may result in a variety of *neurologic lesions.* Diffuse motor and sensory neuropathy, together with interference with function of the sympathetic nervous system, is characteristic of the primary familial amyloidosis of Andrade. Sensory involvement may also be seen in amyloidosis secondary to multiple myeloma, because of diffuse involvement of the sheaths of the peripheral nerves.

Accumulations of *amyloid* in the *trachea* or bronchi may result in serious obstruction to the respiratory passages. Local excision, often with epithelial grafting, is the preferred form of treatment. Recurrences are frequent but by no means invariable.

Amyloid may infiltrate any portion of the *gastrointestinal tract,* resulting in a variety of syndromes, ranging from esophageal obstruction to malabsorption syndrome. Infiltration of the endocrine organs may also ensue. This rarely results in insufficiency of function of the involved gland, however.

Diagnosis

Confirmation of the diagnosis is best obtained by biopsy. Gingival biopsy has been helpful, permitting confirmation of the diagnosis in between one-half and two-thirds of the cases. In the experience of Sohar and his associates, the rectal biopsy has proved even more sensitive. Skin biopsy may be positive in patients with primary or secondary amyloidosis even in the absence of clinical evidence of dermatologic involvement. Renal and hepatic biopsy carry a higher risk of bleeding, and consideration should be given to this when such diagnostic studies are contemplated.

Histologic examination of biopsy specimens must be conducted with great care. Traces of amyloid should be sought in the walls of small blood vessels. In specimens of skin, deposits may also be seen in sweat glands, sebaceous glands, and surrounding the fat cells in the subcutaneous tissue (amyloid rings). Tissue should be fixed in formalin and stained with hematoxylin and eosin, crystal violet, Congo red (preferably the alkaline Congo red method of Puchtler) and thioflavine T or S. Sections should be examined under regular, ultraviolet, and polarized light. The appearance of traces of brilliant greenish-yellow fluorescence with thioflavine T or S permits identification of areas for further study, but is not, in itself, specific for amyloid. On a section stained with Congo red, the appearance of areas exhibiting a characteristic green color, together with dichroism, provides what is, in all probability, specific histologic evidence for the presence of amyloid. Definitive confirmation of this diagnosis, however, requires electron microscopy.

The Congo red test has been almost entirely abandoned as an aid in the diagnosis of amyloidosis due to occasional incidence of severe toxic reactions and greatly improved sensitivity and specificity of histologic methods.

Course and Treatment

The course of amyloidosis is usually progressively downhill, especially if the organs involved include the kidneys, heart, or gastrointestinal tract. Of the fifty odd cases studied by the author, none has exhibited a remission, except for those cases of localized amyloidosis in which surgical extirpation has been possible. The course may be prolonged, however, lasting for periods of many years. Treatment with large doses of ascorbic acid (1,000 mg per day) or of lightly seared liver (¼ lb per day) has been attempted, chiefly on empirical grounds, but there is no sound clinical evidence, to date, to support this program. If amyloidosis accompanies other inflammatory conditions, vigorous efforts to treat the underlying condition should be initiated. If these efforts are successful, remission of the amyloidosis may ensue. This outcome is rarely seen, however, chiefly because potentially treatable chronic inflammatory conditions usually receive treatment prior to the onset of amyloidosis.

REFERENCES

Bladen, H. A., M. U. Nylen, and G. G. Glenner: The Ultrastructure of Human Amyloid as Revealed by the Negative Staining Techniques, J. Ultrastruct. Res., 14: 449, 1966.

Cohen, A. S.: Amyloidosis, New Engl. J. Med., 277:522, 1967.

———: Constitution and Genesis of Amyloid, pp. 159–243 in G. W. Richter and M. A. Epstein (Eds.), "International Review of Experimental Pathology," Vol. 4, New York, Academic Press, 1965.

Heller, H., E. Sohar, J. Gafni, and J. Heller: Amyloidosis in Familial Mediterranean Fever: An Independent Genetically Determined Characteristic, Arch. Intern. Med., 107:539, 1961.

Kenney, J. D., and E. Calkins: Clinical Aspects of Amyloidosis, in A. St. J. Dixon (Ed.), "Progress in Clinical Rheumatology," London, J. and A. Churchill, Ltd., 1965.

Wright, J. R., E. Calkins, W. Breen, G. Stolte, and R. T. Schultz: Relationship of Amyloid to Aging, Medicine, 48:39, 1969.

Part Six
Disorders due to Chemical and Physical Agents

Section 1
Chemical Intoxications

115 GENERAL CONSIDERATIONS AND PRINCIPLES OF MANAGEMENT

Jan Koch-Weser

Poisoning by chemical agents is a common and serious medical problem. In the United States accidental poisonings cause at least 4,000 deaths each year. Suicides by chemical agents annually number more than 6,000. Malicious poisoning has become less common since the development of scientific toxicology, but toxic chemicals administered by homicides and abortionists are responsible for more deaths than is generally appreciated. In addition to fatal poisonings there is a much greater number of persons who are made seriously ill by chemical agents but recover after appropriate therapy. Unfortunately, some such victims are left with permanent sequelae of their intoxication. Finally, chemical agents impair the health of very many people by mechanisms not generally thought of as intoxications. Chemical carcinogenesis and mutagenesis, chronic pulmonary disease due to common inhalants, chronic alcoholic liver disease, allergic reactions, and chemical addiction and withdrawal syndromes are the most important examples.

Accidental poisonings may occur in the home or through industrial exposure. The former are far more frequent and usually acute; industrial intoxication is ordinarily the result of chronic exposure. Accidental poisoning is most commonly due to ingestion of toxic substances and involves children in the majority of cases. Each year 1 to 2 million American children accidentally swallow toxic materials, and approximately 1 ingestion in 1,000 is fatal. Aspirin is involved in 25 percent of all ingestions, other medicines in another 25 percent. Cleaning and polishing agents are ingested by 15 percent, while cosmetics, pesticides, petroleum products, and turpentine paints account for 6 percent each. Younger children tend to ingest household products, older children are more likely to choose drugs.

The frequency of accidental poisonings reflects the enormous number of toxic substances found in the American home. Many such accidents could be avoided by simple preventive measures. Physicians can play an effective role in safety education. All toxic substances must be kept out of the reach of small children. Household chemicals and medicines should be kept in the original containers, and all such containers should be labelled. Before taking or administering any medicine the label should be checked carefully.

Despite all precautions, accidental, suicidal, and criminal poisonings will remain an important problem which every physician must be prepared to treat promptly and effectively. Besides their immediate therapeutic responsibilities, physicians have legal obligations in cases of attempted suicide, homicide, or criminal abortion and of industrial exposure. The physician should also obtain psychiatric care for any patient who has attempted suicide by poison.

DIAGNOSIS OF CHEMICAL POISONING

Optimal management of the poisoned patient requires a correct diagnosis. Unfortunately, in many such patients poisoning is initially not even considered as a possible cause of the clinical picture. The patient may be unaware of exposure to poison or, as after attempted suicide or abortion, he may be unwilling to admit it. Although the toxic effects of some chemical substances are quite characteristic, most poisoning syndromes can simulate other diseases.

Poisoning is usually included in the differential diagnosis of coma, convulsions, acute psychosis, acute hepatic or renal insufficiency, and bone marrow depression. It may not be considered when the major manifestation is a mild psychiatric disturbance or neurologic disorder, abdominal pain, bleeding, fever, hypotension, pulmonary congestion, or skin eruption. Chronic, insidious intoxications are much more frequently missed than acute poisonings whose symptoms appear suddenly and may be immediately related to a specific event. Physicians should always remember the variegated manifestations of poisoning and maintain a high index of suspicion.

In every case of poisoning identification of the toxic agent should be attempted. Specific antidotal therapy is obviously impossible without such identification. In cases of homicide, suicide, or criminal abortion the identity of the poison may be of legal importance. When poisoning results from industrial exposure or therapeutic mishap, accurate knowledge of the responsible agents is essential for future prevention.

In acute accidental poisoning the offending substance may be known to the patient. In many other cases information can be obtained from relatives or acquaintances, by a search for containers at the scene of the poisoning, or by questioning the patient's physician or pharmacist. Frequently such procedures yield only the trade name of a product, which gives no clue to its component chemicals. A number of books which identify the active ingredients of household products, agricultural compounds, proprietary medicines, and poisonous plants are listed in the references to this chapter. A small handbook of this type should be carried in every physician's bag. Poison control centers and manufacturers' representatives are other useful sources of such information. When poisoning is chronic, rapid identification of the toxic agent from the history is frequently impossible. It is therefore fortunate that the lesser therapeutic urgency of such cases usually permits the required painstaking exploration of the patient's habits and environment.

Some poisons can produce clinical features characteristic enough to strongly suggest the diagnosis. Careful examination of the patient may reveal the unmistakable odor of cyanide; the cherry-colored flush of carboxyhemoglobin in skin and mucous membranes; the pupillary constriction, salivation, and gastrointestinal hyperactivity produced by cholinesterase-inhibitor insecticides; or the lead line and extensor paralyses of chronic lead poisoning. Unfortunately, these features are not always present, and in any case telltales are the exception in chemical poisonings.

Chemical analysis of body fluids provides the most definite identification of the intoxicating agent. Some common poisons, such as aspirin, bromides, and barbiturates, can be identified and even quantitated by relatively simple laboratory procedures. Others require more complex toxicologic techniques, such as gas chromatography or bioassay, which are performed only in specialized laboratories. Furthermore, the results of toxicologic determinations are rarely available in time to guide the initial treatment of acute poisoning. Nevertheless, specimens of vomitus, gastric aspirate, blood, urine and feces should always be saved for toxicologic study if diagnostic or legal questions are likely to arise. Chemical analyses of body fluids or tissues are of particular value in the diagnosis and evaluation of chronic intoxications. Finally, they are useful in following the success of some forms of therapy.

TREATMENT OF CHEMICAL POISONING

Although the physician should always try to identify the poison, such attempts must never delay vital therapeutic measures. Most poisons do not have specific antidotes. Essential supportive care must be given as indicated by the patient's clinical state and does not require knowledge of the toxic agent. Symptomatic treatment of circulatory, respiratory, neurologic, and renal function should be immediately administered as to any other seriously ill patient.

Correct treatment of the poisoned patients thus requires knowledge both of the general principles of management and of the details of therapy for specific poisons. Treatment may be divided into four approaches: (1) prevention of further absorption of the poison, (2) removal of absorbed poison from the body, (3) symptomatic or supportive therapy, and (4) administration of systemic antidotes (Table 115-1). The first three ap-

Table 115-1. TREATMENT OF ACUTE CHEMICAL POISONING

I. Prevention of further absorption of poison
   A. Poisoning by ingestion
      1. Emptying the stomach
         a. Induction of vomiting
         b. Gastric lavage
      2. Minimizing gastrointestinal absorption
         a. Neutralization and precipitation
         b. Adsorption
         c. Catharsis
   B. Poisoning by other routes
II. Removal of absorbed poisons from body
   A. Detoxification—enzyme induction?
   B. Biliary excretion—interruption of enterohepatic circulation
   C. Urinary excretion
      1. Osmotic diuresis
      2. Alteration of urinary pH
   D. Dialysis
      1. Peritoneal dialysis
      2. Hemodialysis
   E. Exchange transfusion
   F. Chelation and chemical binding
III. Supportive therapy
IV. Administration of systemic antidotes
   A. Chemical agents
   B. Pharmacologic antagonists

proaches are applicable to most types of poisoning, the fourth can be used only when the toxic agent is known and a specific antidote is available. Success often depends upon speed of treatment and, when indicated by the clinical situation, several approaches should be used simultaneously.

Prevention of Absorption of Ingested Poisons

If appreciable amounts of a poison have been ingested, one should always attempt to minimize its absorption from the gastrointestinal tract. The success of such endeavors depends upon the time elapsed since ingestion and upon the site and speed of absorption of the poison. Prompt action is essential, and it is better to proceed with makeshifts than to waste time while waiting for special equipment or drugs. Conversely, it is unwise to temporize with unpredictable remedies when reliable and effective methods for removal of poison from the gastrointestinal tract are available. When skillfully applied, these methods do not lead to such complications as pulmonary aspiration, gastrointestinal perforation, or convulsions.

EVACUATION OF THE STOMACH. Attempts to empty the stomach are always worthwhile unless specifically contraindicated. They may be highly successful if made soon after ingestion. Significant amounts of poison may be recovered from the stomach hours after ingestion because gastric emptying may be delayed by gastric atony or pylorospasm.

Emesis occurs spontaneously after the ingestion of many poisons. It may be induced in the home by mechanical stimulation of the posterior pharynx or by administration of gastric irritants such as a strong solution of salt or mustard. The emetic action of syrup of ipecac (not the fourteen times more concentrated fluid extract) in 10 to 20 ml dosage is more effective and is safe enough for home use. Regrettably its action has an average latent period of 20 min and depends in part on gastrointestinal absorption, so that it cannot be used in conjunction with other measures intended to minimize absorption of the poison. Apomorphine, 0.06 mg per kg intramuscularly, acts within 5 min but may cause prolonged vomiting. When given intravenously in doses of 0.01 mg per kg, apomorphine tends to produce almost immediate vomiting which is not followed by any other central nervous system effects. All attempts to induce emesis are more often successful if large amounts of fluid have been administered, but these may also hasten passage of the poison through the pylorus. Fluids with high fat content are preferable, since they enter the duodenum more slowly. Not uncommonly it is impossible to induce vomiting, and valuable time should not be lost with hopeful waiting. Induction of vomiting should not be attempted after ingestion of antiemetic drugs, in severely depressed or convulsing patients, or, because of the danger of gastroesophageal perforation or tracheal aspiration of vomitus, in patients who have ingested strong caustics or liquid hydrocarbons which are potent lung irritants (e.g., kerosene, furniture polish).

Unlike emesis, *gastric lavage* is predictably and immediately effective in removing poison from the stomach. Furthermore, it can be employed in unconscious patients, and removal of gastric contents reduces the risk of aspiration of vomitus in such patients. It is, however, contraindicated after the ingestion of strong corrosives because of danger of perforating injured tissues. When properly performed, gastric lavage carries little risk of aspiration of gastric contents into the lungs. The patient should be prone with head and shoulders lowered. A mouth gag is placed and a gastric tube of sufficient diameter to permit withdrawal of particulate matter (size 30) is passed into the stomach. If central nervous system function is depressed and introduction of the tube produces retching, or if pulmonary irritants have been ingested, it is wise to place a *cuffed endotracheal tube* before lavaging. Gastric contents are withdrawn with a large syringe and usually contain most of the poison that will be removed. Thereafter 200 ml (less in children) of warm water or other lavaging solution are alternately instilled and withdrawn until the aspirate becomes clear.

INTERFERENCE WITH GASTROINTESTINAL ABSORPTION. Since neither emesis nor gastric lavage empty the stomach completely, one should also minimize absorption by administering substances which inactivate or trap ingested poisons. If mineral acids, alkalis, or other corrosives have been swallowed, water, milk, or a neutralizer (aluminum hydroxide, milk of magnesia, dilute vinegar) is given. Some toxic alkaloids can be precipitated and rendered insoluble by the administration of sulfate. Many other poisons are effectively adsorbed by powdered, activated charcoal. A good grade of activated charcoal can rapidly adsorb as much as half its weight of many common poisons. It is more effective than the so-called "universal antidote" which should be relegated to oblivion. Administration of 100 to 200 ml of a slurry of activated charcoal should be alternated with evacuation of the stomach.

Adsorption by charcoal is reversible, and the effectiveness of adsorption of many poisons varies with the pH. Acidic substances are adsorbed better in acid solutions and may therefore be released in the small intestine. It is desirable to speed the charcoal with its adsorbed poison through the intestine as quickly as possible. This will also decrease intestinal absorption of any unadsorbed poison which has passed beyond the pylorus. It is best accomplished by oral or gastric administration of an osmotic cathartic. Sodium sulfate in 10 to 30 Gm dosage is the cathartic of choice, since, unlike magnesium sulfate, it produces no symptoms after systemic absorption. Cathartics are generally contraindicated after the ingestion of strong corrosives.

Prevention of Absorption of Poison from Other Sites

Most topically applied poisons can be removed by copious flushing with water. In certain instances weak acids or bases or appropriate organic solvents are more effective, but rapid and voluminous washing with water should always proceed while they are being obtained. Chemical antidotes can be hazardous because tissue injury may result from the heat of the chemical reaction.

The systemic distribution of injected poisons can be slowed by the application of cold to the injection site or by the proximal application of a tourniquet. Cruciate incision and suction is generally ineffective except after poisonous bites.

Following inhalation of toxic gases, vapors, or dusts, the victim should be removed into clean air and adequate ventilation maintained. If the patient cannot be moved, a protective mask should be applied.

Removal of Absorbed Poison from the Body

Unlike prevention or retardation of absorption, measures to speed removal of the toxic agent from the body rarely have much influence on the peak poison concentration. However, they can significantly abbreviate the time during which the concentration of many poisons remains above any given level and thereby greatly reduce morbidity, avoid complications, and save lives. In judging the need for such measures one must consider the patient's clinical state, the properties and metabolic fate of the poison, and the amount absorbed as judged by the history and the blood level. Removal of some poisons can be accelerated by several methods; selection depends on the clinical urgency, the amount in the body, and the skills and equipment available.

DETOXIFICATION. Since many poisons are metabolically inactivated in the body, it is regrettable that no clinically effective measures to accelerate detoxification are known. Induction of hepatic enzymes would seem to hold some promise in the treatment of poisonings by certain long-acting drugs whose inactivation depends on the activity of inducible enzymes. The clinical usefulness of this approach remains to be shown. At present, therefore, one must rely on measures capable of accelerating excretion of the poison.

BILIARY EXCRETION. Certain organic acids and active drugs are secreted into the bile against large concentration gradients. Again, this process cannot presently be accelerated. However, the intestinal resorption of substances already secreted into the bile can be decreased by duodenal suction or osmotic catharsis. These procedures are useful in poisonings by substances such as glutethimide and chlortetracycline, the action of which is significantly prolonged by their enterohepatic circulation.

URINARY EXCRETION. Acceleration of renal excretion is applicable to a much larger number of poisons. Renal excretion of toxic substances depends on glomerular filtration, active tubular secretion, and passive tubular resorption. The first two processes should be protected by maintenance of adequate circulation and renal function, but for practical purposes they cannot be accelerated. On the other hand, passive tubular resorption of many poisons plays an important role in the prolongation of their action and can frequently be decreased by readily available methods.

Passive resorption of most filtered poisons occurs largely in the proximal tubules because their concentration in the filtrate increases as salt and water are reabsorbed. It can be partly prevented by inhibiting water resorption at this site. This is best accomplished by the administration of osmotic diuretics such as mannitol or urea. By infusing 10 to 20 Gm per hour of mannitol or urea after a loading dose of 25 to 50 Gm, urine volumes up to 1 liter per hour can be achieved. Great care must be used to supply water and electrolyte needs at the same time. Osmotic diuretics should not be used in the presence of congestive heart failure, shock, or renal failure. The effectiveness of osmotic diuretic therapy in increasing renal excretion has been demonstrated for salicylates, barbiturates, meprobamate, and glutethimide but is potentially applicable to all ultrafiltered poisons which are passively reabsorbed.

Alteration of the urinary pH can also inhibit passive back-diffusion of some poisons and increase their renal clearance. The renal tubular epithelium is more permeable to uncharged molecules than to ionized solutes. Weak organic acids and bases readily diffuse out of the tubular fluid in their unionized form but are trapped in it when ionized. Acidic poisons are largely ionized only at pHs above their pK_a. Alkalinization of the urine greatly increases the ionization in the tubular fluid of such organic acids as phenobarbital and salicylate. In contrast, the pK_a of pentobarbital (8.1) and secobarbital (8.0) is so high that renal clearance is not greatly increased by raising the urinary pH into the physiologic alkaline range. Alkalinization of the urine is achieved by the infusion of sodium bicarbonate, sodium lactate, or tromethamine (which also acts as an osmotic diuretic) at a rate determined by the urinary and blood pH. Excessive systemic alkalosis or electrolyte disturbances must be carefully prevented. A combination of osmotic diuresis and alkalinization of the urine can raise the renal clearance of some acidic poisons tenfold or more and has been found highly effective in poisoning by salicylate and phenobarbital. The full range of its clinical applicability is undoubtedly much wider but remains to be established. Depression of the urinary pH beyond its usual range may increase the renal clearance of some weakly basic poisons, but clinical data are lacking.

Finally, the renal excretion of certain poisons can be increased in a highly specific fashion. An example is the removal of bromide by administration of chloride and chloriuretics. Such methods will be discussed with the individual poisons.

DIALYSIS. The relative effectiveness of osmotic diuresis at favorable urinary pH and of dialysis must differ widely among drugs but has been established for very few. For barbiturates and some other poisons which are not actively secreted by the renal tubules, maximal clearance rates during extracorporeal dialysis are considerably greater than during peritoneal dialysis or forced diuresis. The latter two maneuvers appear about equally effective. Of course, a skilled team can proceed simultaneously with dialysis and solute diuresis. Dialysis has been found effective in the removal of barbiturates, borate, bromide, chlorate, dimercaprol, diphenylhydantoin, ethanol, ethinamate, glutethimide, glycols, isoniazid, methanol, salicylate, sulfonamides, and thiocyanate. Beyond these, it should theoretically accelerate the removal from the body of any dialyzable toxin which is not irreversibly bound to tissues.

Peritoneal dialysis can be easily performed in any hospital and may be continued for long periods. It is particularly valuable for the removal of poisons if renal function is impaired. Obviously, its effectiveness does not extend to large-molecule, nondialyzable poisons and is decreased by a high degree of protein binding or lipid solubility of the toxic substance. Peritoneal clearance can be increased if the dialyzed poison can be trapped chemically in the dialysis fluid so that a high gradient of the dialyzable portion is maintained from blood to peritoneal cavity between fluid changes. A percent concentration of albumin in the dialysis solution acts as an effective ligand during the dialysis of salicylate and should be similarly useful for the removal of other albumin-bound poisons. Another approach to prevent back-diffusion consists of making the pH of dialysis fluid sufficiently greater or less than 7.4 to ionize poisons which are dialyzable only in the undissociated form. Finally, the addition of various drugs to the dialysis fluid can increase peritoneal dialysis, presumably by increasing peritoneal blood flow or mesothelial permeability. The clinical value of this approach has not yet been defined.

Hemodialysis is unquestionably the most effective procedure for removing large amounts of dialyzable poisons. For barbiturates dialysance rates of 50 to 100 ml per min have been achieved, a removal rate two to five times faster than during peritoneal dialysis or osmotic diuresis. Dialysis against solutions containing albumin or lipids or perfusion of the blood through activated charcoal further speed removal of certain poisons. Extracorporeal dialysis is clearly the procedure of choice for the rapid removal of dialyzable poisons from patients who have absorbed amounts which make survival unlikely even under the best supportive care. Since the required equipment and skilled personnel are available only in a few hospitals, the possibility of transfer of such patients to one of these institutions should be considered.

EXCHANGE TRANSFUSION. Withdrawal and replacement of blood is an effective procedure for the removal of those poisons which are not highly tissue-bound or lipid-soluble and therefore remain in the blood in appreciable concentration. It has obvious advantages in poisoning by nondiffusible and particularly by highly albumin-bound toxins. While it requires little specialized equipment, its applicability to adults is limited by the requirement of large amounts of blood.

CHELATION AND CHEMICAL BINDING. The removal of some poisons is accelerated by chemical interaction with other substances followed by renal excretion. These substances are usually considered specific antidotes and will be discussed with the individual poisons.

Supportive Therapy

Most chemical poisonings are reversible and self-limited disease states. Skillful supportive therapy can keep many seriously poisoned patients alive and their detoxifying and excretory mechanisms functioning until the concentration of poison in the body has fallen to safe levels. Symptomatic measures are especially important when the poison is one of the many compounds for which no specific antidote is known. Even when an antidote is available, disturbances of vital functions must be prevented or controlled by appropriate supportive care.

The poisoned patient may suffer a variety of physiologic disturbances. Most of these are not peculiar to chemical intoxications, and their therapeutic management is described elsewhere in this text. Only those aspects of supportive therapy specially relevant to poisonings are briefly discussed here.

CENTRAL NERVOUS SYSTEM DEPRESSION. Specific therapy directed against the depressant effects of poisons on the central nervous system is usually both unnecessary and difficult. Most poisoned patients will emerge from coma as from a prolonged anesthesia. During the period of unconsciousness meticulous nursing care and close observation are essential. If depression of medullary centers results in circulatory or respiratory failure, these vital functions must be immediately and vigorously supported by chemical or mechanical means.

The use of analeptics in the treatment of poison-induced central nervous system depression is being increasingly abandoned. First, their effect is unpredictable and their use in intoxicated patients produces an abnormal pattern of nervous activity in which paroxysmal excitation and convulsions may be superimposed on depression. Secondly, the availability of artificial ventilation and of effective measures to support the circulation has lessened the need for rapid restoration of normal medullary function. It is doubtful that analeptics shorten the duration of coma sufficiently to justify their risks, and they have not been shown to improve prognosis. Certainly these agents should never be employed to restore consciousness, but under some circumstances their use to hasten the restoration of spontaneous breathing and active reflexes may be justified. Picrotoxin, pentylenetetrazol, bemegride, and ethamivan are the most useful analeptics.

CONVULSIONS. Many poisons (e.g., chlorinated hydrocarbons, insecticides, strychnine) cause convulsions by their specific excitatory effects. Poisoned patients may also convulse because of hypoxia, hypoglycemia, cerebral edema, or metabolic disturbances. In such cases these abnormalities should be corrected as far as possible. Regardless of the cause of the convulsions, anticonvulsant drugs are often required. Short-acting compounds, such as intravenously administered thiopental or amobarbital, are preferable, because in poisoned patients profound depression may accompany or quickly follow convulsions.

CEREBRAL EDEMA. Intracranial hypertension due to cerebral edema is also a characteristic effect of some poisons and a nonspecific result of other chemical intoxications. Cerebral edema is characteristically seen in poisoning by lead, carbon monoxide, and methanol. Symptomatic treatment consists of adrenocortical steroids and, when necessary, the intravenous administration of hypertonic solutions of mannitol or urea.

HYPOTENSION. The causes of hypotension and shock in the poisoned patient are legion, and often several of them coexist. Poisons can depress the medullary vasomotor centers, block autonomic ganglia or adrenergic receptors, directly depress the tone of arterial or venous smooth muscle, reduce myocardial contractility, or induce cardiac arrhythmias. Less specifically, the poisoned patient may be in shock because of tissue hypoxia, extensive tissue destruction from corrosives, loss of blood or fluids, or metabolic disturbances. When possible, these abnormalities should be promptly corrected. Vasopressor drugs are helpful and often essential in the hypotensive poisoned patient, particularly in shock resulting from central depression. As in shock of other etiologies, choice of the most appropriate agent requires an analysis of the hemodynamic disturbance which goes beyond determination of the arterial pressure.

CARDIAC ARRHYTHMIAS. Disturbances of cardiac impulse generation or conduction in the poisoned patient arise from the effects of certain poisons on the electrical properties of cardiac fibers or from myocardial hypoxia or metabolic disturbances. The latter should be corrected and antiarrhythmic agents administered as indicated by the nature of the arrhythmia.

PULMONARY EDEMA. The poisoned patient may develop pulmonary edema because of depressed myocardial contractility or because of alveolar injury from irritant gases or aspirated fluids. The latter type is less responsive to treatment and may be associated with laryngeal edema. Therapeutic measures include suctioning, high concentrations of oxygen under positive pressure, aerosols of surface-active agents, bronchodilators, and adrenocortical steroids.

HYPOXIA. Poisoning may cause tissue hypoxia by various mechanisms, and several of these may operate in one patient. Inadequate ventilation can result from central respiratory depression, from muscular paralysis, or from airway obstruction by retained secretions, laryngeal edema, or bronchospasm. Alveolar-capillary diffusion may be impaired by pulmonary edema. Anemia, methemoglobinemia, carboxyhemoglobinemia, or shock can interfere with oxygen transport. Cellular oxidation may be inhibited by cyanide, fluoroacetate, or general protoplasmic poisons. The highest priority in treatment must be given to maintenance of an adequate airway. The clinical situation and the site of obstruction may indicate frequent suctioning, insertion of an oropharyngeal airway or of an endotracheal tube, or a tracheotomy. If despite a clear airway ventilation remains inadequate as judged by clinical appearance or by measurement of minute volume or blood gases, artificial ventilation by appropriate mechanical means is imperative. Administration of high concentrations of oxygen is indicated whenever tissue hypoxia occurs. When the central nervous system is severely depressed, oxygen administration often results in apnea and must be combined with artifical ventilation. Hyperbaric oxygen may be helpful in some situations. The treatment of methemoglobinemia, carboxyhemoglobinemia, and inhibition of cellular oxidation is discussed under the specific poisons which produce these changes.

ACUTE RENAL INSUFFICIENCY. Renal failure with oliguria or anuria may occur in the poisoned patient because of shock, dehydration, or electrolyte disturbances. More specifically, it may be due to the nephrotoxic potential of poisons (e.g., mercury, phosphorus, carbon tetrachloride, bromate) many of which are concentrated and excreted by the kidney. Renal damage due to poisons is usually reversible. The management of acute renal insufficiency is outlined in Chap. 300.

ELECTROLYTE AND WATER DISTURBANCES. Imbalance of fluid and electrolytes are common features of chemical poisoning. They may result from vomiting, diarrhea, renal insufficiency, or from therapeutic maneuvers such as catharsis, osmotic diuresis, or dialysis. These disturbances are corrected or ideally prevented by appropriate therapy. Certain poisons produce more specific defects such as metabolic acidosis (e.g., methanol, phenol, salicylate) or hypocalcemia (e.g., fluoride, oxalate). These abnormalities and any specific treatment will be described under the individual poisons.

ACUTE HEPATIC INSUFFICIENCY. The primary manifestation of some poisonings (e.g., chlorinated hydrocarbons, phosphorus, cinchophen, certain mushrooms) is acute hepatic failure. Its management is described in Chap. 326.

Administration of Systemic Antidotes

Specific antidotal therapy is available for only a few poisons. Some systemic antidotes are chemicals which exert their therapeutic effect by reducing the concentration of the toxic substance. They may do this by combining with the poison (e.g., ethylene diaminetetraacetate with lead, dimercaprol with mercury) or by increasing its excretion (e.g., chloride or mercurial diuretics in bromide poisoning). Other systemic antidotes compete with the poison for its receptor site (e.g., atropine with muscarine, nallorphine with morphine, vitamin K_1 with coumarins). Specific antidotes will be discussed with the individual poisons.

REFERENCES

General

Arena, J. M.: "Poisoning," 2nd ed., Springfield, Ill., Charles C Thomas Publisher, 1969.

Coleman, A. B.: Accidental Poisoning, New Engl. J. Med., 277:1135, 1967.

Corby, D. G., R. C. Lisciandro, R. H. Lehman, and W. J. Decker: The Efficiency of Methods Used to Evacuate the Stomach after Acute Ingestions, Pediatrics, 40:871, 1967.

Dabbous, I. A., A. B. Bergman, and W. O. Robertson: The Ineffectiveness of Mechanically Induced Vomiting, J. Pediat., 66:952, 1965.

Deichmann, W. B., and H. W. Gerarde: "Symptomatology and Therapy of Toxicological Emergencies," New York, Academic Press, Inc., 1964.

De Myttenaere, M. H., J. F. Maher, and C. E. Schreiner: Hemoperfusion through a Charcoal Column for Glutethimide Poisoning, Trans. Am. Soc. Artificial Internal Organs, 13:190, 1967.

Done, A. K.: Clinical Pharmacology of Systemic Antidotes, Clin. Pharmacol. Therap., 2:750, 1961.

Dreisbach, R. H.: "Handbook of Poisoning, Diagnosis and Treatment," 6th ed., Los Altos, Calif., Lange Medical Publications, 1969.

Gosselin, R. E., and R. P. Smith: Trends in the Therapy of Acute Poisonings, Clin. Pharmacol. Therap., 7:279, 1966.

Holt, L. E., Jr., and P. H. Holz: The Black Bottle, a Consideration of the Role of Charcoal in the Treatment of Poisoning in Children, J. Pediat., 63:306, 1963.

Maher, J. F., and G. E. Schreiner: Current Status of Dialysis of Poisons and Drugs, Trans. Am. Soc. Artificial Internal Organs, 15:461, 1969.

Matthew, H., and A. A. H. Lawson: "Treatment of Common Acute Poisonings," Edinburgh, E. & S. Livingstone Ltd., 1967.

Milne, M. D.: Potentiation of Excretion of Drugs, Proc. Roy. Soc. Med., 57:809, 1964.

Myschetzky, A., and N. A. Lassen: Urea-induced Osmotic Diuresis and Alkalinization of Urine in Acute Barbiturate Intoxication, J. Amer. Med. Ass., 185:936, 1963.

Picchioni, A. L.: Activated Charcoal versus "Universal Antidote" as an Antidote for Poisons, Toxicol. Appl. Pharmacol., 8:447, 1966.

Shinaberger, J. H., L. Shear, L. E. Clayton, K. G. Barry, M. Knowlton, and L. R. Goldbaum: Dialysis for Intoxication with Lipid Soluble Drugs, Enhancement of Glutethimide Extraction with Lipid Dialysate, Trans. Am. Soc. Artificial Internal Organs, 11:173, 1965.

Shirkey, H. C.: Ipecac Syrup, Its Use as an Emetic in Poison Control, J. Pediat., 69:139, 1966.

Strickler, J. C.: Forced Diuresis in the Management of Barbiturate Intoxication, Clin. Pharmacol. Therap., 6:693, 1965.

Thienes, C. H., and T. J. Haley: "Clinical Toxicology," 4th ed., Philadelphia, Lea & Febiger, 1964.

Verhulst, H. L., and J. J. Crotty: Childhood Poisoning Accidents, J.A.M.A., 203:1049, 1968.

Toxic Product Information

Adams, W. C.: Poison Control Centers: Their Purpose and Operation, Clin. Pharmacol. Therap., 4:293, 1963.

Brown, R. L.: "Pesticides in Clinical Practice," Springfield, Ill., Charles C Thomas, Publisher, 1966.

Directory, Poison Control Centers, U.S. Public Health Service, Publ. No. 1278, 1967.

Gleason, M. N., R. E. Gosselin, H. C. Hodge, and R. P. Smith: "Clinical Toxicology of Commercial Products," 3d ed., Baltimore, The Williams & Wilkins Company, 1969.

Goodman, L. S., and A. Gilman: "The Pharmacological Basis of Therapeutics," 3d ed., New York, The Macmillan Company, 1965.

Kingsbury, J. M.: "Poisonous Plants of the United States and Canada," Englewood Cliffs, N.J., Prentice-Hall, Inc., 1964.

"The Merck Index," 8th ed., Rahway, N.J., Merck & Co., Inc., 1968.

Sax, N. I.: "Dangerous Properties of Industrial Materials," 3d ed., New York, Reinhold Book Corporation, 1968.

"Toxicants Occurring Naturally in Foods," Washington, National Academy of Sciences, Publication No. 1354, 1966.

Wilson, C. O., and T. E. Jones: "American Drug Index," Philadelphia, J. B. Lippincott Company, 1969.

116 COMMON POISONS
Jan Koch-Weser

The poisons discussed in this chapter are those which are encountered by the general population such as commonly used drugs, household products, solvents, pesticides, and poisonous plants. It has been necessary to disregard many uncommon toxic materials as well as products to which exposure occurs only in specialized industrial environments. Details concerning poisoning by such compounds may be found in some of the references following Chap. 115. Toxic effects of many drugs are considered throughout this text in conjunction with their therapeutic use. Manifestations of hypersensitivity to chemicals are described in Chap. 73. The following discussions of specific poisons stress those details of their action which are pertinent to the recognition or treatment of clinical poisoning.

ACIDS

Corrosive acids are used widely in industry and laboratories. Ingestion is almost always with suicidal intent. Death has occurred after an oral dose of 1 ml of a corrosive acid.

Toxic effects of corrosive acids are largely due to their direct chemical action. They convert tissue protein to acid proteinate which is soluble in the acid. Irritation, bleeding, sloughing, and perforation of the esophagus and stomach are common. Mouth and pharynx are brownish-black and may have a charred appearance. Yellow staining is seen after ingestion of nitric and picric acids. Severe pain in mouth, pharynx, chest, and abdomen is the rule and is soon followed by vomiting and diarrhea of coffee grounds appearance. Frequently profound shock develops. About half of those who ingest significant amounts of acid die from its immediate effects. The survivors often develop mediastinitis or peritonitis from esophageal or gastric perforation. Delayed perforation of the esophagus or stomach also occurs. Recovery from acid ingestion is often associated with esophageal stricture.

Ingested acid must be immediately diluted a hundred fold by water or milk or neutralized with weak alkali. Milk of magnesia or magnesium and aluminum antacids are excellent for the purpose. Sodium bicarbonate should be avoided because the evolved carbon dioxide may rupture an eroded viscus. The danger of perforation also contraindicates the use of emesis or gastric lavage except during the first 30 min after ingestion. Following the emergency measures, appropriate supportive therapy is administered for the relief of pain and the treatment of shock, perforation, and infection.

Certain gases found in industry may combine with water in the lungs to form corrosive acids. During rapid decomposition of plant material in silos, oxides of nitrogen are released which form nitric acid in the lungs. Inhalation of such gases causes coughing and choking sensations which are followed after a latent period of 6 to 8 hr by pulmonary edema. Treatment is supportive. Symptoms of dyspnea and hemoptysis may be prolonged and frequent relapses may occur.

ALKALIS

Strong alkalis such as ammonium hydroxide, potassium hydroxide (potash), potassium carbonate, sodium hydroxide (lye), and sodium carbonate (washing soda) are widely used in industry and in cleansers and drain cleaners. Sodium and potassium phosphates find use as water softeners. Strong alkalis form soaps with fats and proteinates with proteins, resulting in penetrating necrosis of tissues. Fatalities have occurred from the ingestion of 5 to 30 Gm of such compounds.

The toxic effects of alkalis are almost entirely due to irritation and destruction of local tissues. Ingestion is followed by severe pain in mouth, pharynx, chest, and abdomen. Vomiting of blood and sloughed mucosa and diarrhea are common. Reflex loss of vascular tone frequently leads to profound shock. Perforation of the esophagus or stomach may be immediate or delayed for several days. Mouth and pharynx show erythema and gelatinous necrotic areas. After ingestion of water softeners profound reduction in serum calcium may be seen and lead to tetany and hypotension. Ingestion of strong alkali is rapidly fatal in about 25 percent of cases. Survivors usually suffer from esophageal strictures.

Treatment consists of immediate administration of large amounts of water, milk, fruit juices, or 10 percent vinegar. The volume of liquids should exceed that of the ingested alkali a hundred fold. Vomiting should be allowed to occur and gastric lavage may be performed during the first half hour after ingestion. Because of the danger of perforation both are contraindicated thereafter. After the ingestion of water softeners (phosphates), calcium gluconate should be administered intravenously as needed. Treatment is otherwise symptomatic and directed at the relief of pain, respiratory obstruction due to edema of the hypopharynx, fluid loss, and shock.

Inhalation of ammonia, which is used as a refrigerant, results in irritation of the upper and lower respiratory tract. Laryngeal and pulmonary edema may occur and must be treated symptomatically.

ANILINE

This substance is used in printing and cloth-marking inks, crayons, paints, and paint removers. Both aniline and its derivatives, such as toluidine, nitroaniline, and nitrobenzene, are widely used in industrial synthesis. Aniline is absorbed from the gastrointestinal tract and through the lungs or skin. Ingestion of 1 Gm aniline has been fatal. Methemoglobinemia is the most important manifestation. Headache, dizziness, hypotension, convulsions, and coma may occur. If the acute period is survived, jaundice and anemia may appear. Treatment consists of correction of methemoglobinemia (see Chap. 344) and supportive measures.

ANTIHISTAMINES

The common and unprescribed use of antihistamines makes them readily available for accidental overdosage and suicidal attempts. There is wide variation from patient to patient in tolerance to these drugs and in the manifestations of poisoning. A dose of 200 mg diphenhydramine has been fatal in one adult, whereas another tolerated 2 Gm. Manifestations of poisoning are central nervous system excitement or depression. In children the

usual toxic manifestations are excitement, hyperthermia, hyperreflexia, tremors, and convulsions, followed by central nervous system depression. In adults depressive manifestations with drowsiness, stupor, and coma predominate, but convulsions followed by further depression may occur.

Treatment is supportive and directed toward removal of the unabsorbed drug and maintenance of vital functions. Stimulants should be avoided. Convulsions may be controlled with short-acting barbiturates, ether, or succinylcholine. Some antihistamines have prominent atropine-like properties. Patients poisoned with these drugs may show manifestations of atropine poisoning and are treated correspondingly.

ANTIMUSCARINIC COMPOUNDS

Atropine, related belladonna alkaloids (hyoscyamine, scopolamine), and synthetic substitutes (e.g., benztropine, cyclopentolate, homatropine, methantheline, propantheline) are widely prescribed drugs and occur in many proprietary mixtures used in the treatment of gastrointestinal and upper respiratory diseases, asthma, and parkinsonism. Poisoning, especially in children, may also occur from the excessive use of ophthalmic solutions containing such compounds. Finally, children may be intoxicated by eating plants containing up to 0.5 percent of atropine or related alkaloids. Such plants are *Atropa belladonna* (deadly nightshade), *Hioscyamus niger* (henbane), and *Datura stramonium* (Jamestown or Jimson weed).

Individual sensitivity to the toxic effects of belladonna alkaloids varies widely: fatalities have occurred from as little as 10 mg atropine, but doses of 500 mg have been survived. Young children are particularly susceptible to poisoning with belladonna alkaloids. Old people appear to be more sensitive to the central nervous system effects of these drugs. Since atropine is both hydrolyzed in the liver and excreted unchanged in the urine, insufficiency of hepatic or renal function may lead to poisoning on therapeutic dosage.

The most characteristic manifestations of atropine poisoning are those of parasympathetic blockade: dryness of mucous membranes, thirst, dysphagia, hoarseness, xerophthalmia, dilated pupils, blurring of vision, rise in intraocular tension, flushing, dryness and increased temperature of the skin, fever, tachycardia, hypertension, urinary retention, and abdominal distension. This widespread parasympatholysis is almost diagnostic of belladonna poisoning, but the diagnosis can be further confirmed by the absence of any parasympathomimetic effects following the intramuscular injection of 10 mg methacholine.

Central nervous system symptoms are also very common during belladonna intoxication. Atropine and scopolamine produce similar toxic psychoses. Restlessness, excitation, confusion, and incoordination precede mania, hallucinations, and delirium. Patients intoxicated by scopolamine not infrequently show lethargy and somnolence rather than excitement. In severe intoxication with belladonna alkaloids central nervous system depression and coma are the rule. Death occurs due to circulatory collapse and respiratory failure.

In the treatment of belladonna poisoning gastric lavage with an aqueous slurry of activated charcoal should be initiated quickly. Symptomatic treatment is directed at the reduction of body temperature, the moistening of mucous membranes, and, when necessary, urethral catheterization. Excitement, convulsions, or depression may require appropriate pharmacotherapy. Parasympathomimetic agents, such as methacholine or pilocarpine, are of little value, since they cannot be given in concentrations sufficient to overcome the peripheral cholinergic blockade. Furthermore, they have no effect on the potentially lethal central nervous system toxicity of the belladonna alkaloids.

Death occurs in fewer than 1 percent of cases of atropine or scopolamine poisoning. No permanent sequelae have been observed, but manifestations may persist for several days.

BARIUM

Poisoning may be due to the ingestion of rodenticides which contain soluble barium salts or of depilatories that contain barium sulfide. Intoxication may also occur in industry or from the accidental use of a soluble barium salt as a radiopaque contrast medium. Barium is extremely toxic, producing intense stimulation of muscles of all types. Its action on the gastrointestinal musculature causes vomiting, colic, and diarrhea. Skeletal muscle tremors and spasm are commonly seen. Arteriolar spasm results in marked hypertension. Cardiac arrhythmias may proceed to ventricular fibrillation. Anxiety, weakness, and convulsions may occur. Death is usually due to cardiac arrhythmia or respiratory arrest.

Treatment consists of the oral administration of 250 ml of 10% sodium sulfate or 5% magnesium sulfate. This will precipitate and remove any unabsorbed barium in the gastrointestinal tract. A dose of 10 ml of a 10% solution of sodium sulfate should be slowly administered intravenously every 30 min until symptoms subside. Procainamide may be used to reduce the danger of fatal cardiac arrhythmias. If necessary, pain should be relieved and artificial ventilation with oxygen administered.

BENZENE, TOLUENE

These solvents are used in paint removers, dry-cleaning solutions, and rubber or plastic cements. Benzene is also present, to some extent, in most gasolines. Poisoning may result from ingestion or from the breathing of concentrated vapors. Toluene is the major ingredient in the cement used by teen-age glue sniffers.

Acute poisoning by these compounds causes central nervous system manifestations. With sufficient exposure, symptoms progress from an initial period of restlessness, excitement, euphoria, and dizziness to coma, convulsions, and respiratory failure. Ventricular arrhythmias may occur.

Chronic poisoning by benzene or toluene results from repeated exposure to their vapors in low concentration. Central nervous system symptoms include irritability, insomnia, headache, tremors, and paresthesias. Anorexia and nausea are also common. Fatty degeneration of the heart, liver, and kidneys may occur. By far the most important manifestation of chronic exposure to benzene is bone marrow depression, which may progress to aplastic anemia and complete aplasia of the bone marrow. Individual susceptibility to this effect varies greatly and may not become apparent for months after the initial exposure to the poison.

Treatment of both acute and chronic poisoning is symptomatic. After ingestion emesis must not be induced, and gastric lavage should await placement of an endotracheal tube with an inflatable cuff. Neurologic, pulmonary, or cardiovascular problems are treated as in poisoning by petroleum distillates.

BLEACHES

Clorox, Purex, Sanichlor, and other bleaching solutions contain 3 to 6 percent sodium hypochlorite. Their corrosive action in mouth, pharynx, and esophagus is similar to that of sodium hydroxide. Acid gastric juice releases hypochlorous acid from such solutions. This compound is very irritating to mucous membranes, and inhalation of its fumes causes severe pulmonary irritation and pulmonary edema. However, the systemic toxicity of hypochlorous acid is low. Perforation and stricture formation is rare after the ingestion of bleaching solutions. The fatal dose is approximately 30 ml.

Treatment consists of emesis or gastric lavage with water, milk, milk of magnesia, aluminum hydroxide, or sodium bicarbonate solution. Acid antidotes should not be used. If available, 200 ml of a 5% solution of sodium thiosulfate should be administered by mouth, since this will immediately reduce hypochlorite to nontoxic products. Supportive measures may be needed as in alkali poisoning.

BORIC ACID

This compound is a very weak germicide and has been widely employed in powders, lotions, solutions, and ointments. While not highly toxic, boric acid is not nearly as benign as widely assumed. The lethal dose is approximately 15 Gm in adults and 5 Gm in infants. Such amounts can be easily absorbed through abraded skin, from serous cavities, and after ingestion. Furthermore, accumulation of the compound occurs because of slow renal excretion.

Regardless of the route of administration, the first symptoms of poisoning are nausea, vomiting, and diarrhea. This is followed by headache, weakness, restlessness, and an erythematous rash which may progress to desquamation of skin and mucous membranes. Renal toxicity and shock are common, and more than 100 fatalities have occurred. Treatment is entirely supportive. Boric acid should always be labeled as a poison and must not be applied to extensive skin lesions.

BROMATES

These compounds are used as neutralizers in cold wave preparations. They produce widespread tissue injury, particularly in central nervous system and kidneys. The fatal oral dose of bromates is approximately 5 Gm. On contact of bromate with gastric acid, hydrogen bromate, an irritating acid, is formed. Ingestion of bromates is followed by vomiting, diarrhea, abdominal pain, drowsiness, coma, convulsions, hypotension, hematuria, oliguria, anuria, and hemolysis.

Treatment consists of emesis or gastric lavage with sodium bicarbonate solution followed by catharsis. A dose of 250 ml of a 1% sodium thiosulfate solution should be administered intravenously. Peritoneal dialysis or hemodialysis effectively removes bromate from the body. Appropriate supportive therapy should be given.

CANTHARIDIN

This active principle of Cantharis vesicatoria (Spanish fly) is not a useful therapeutic agent. Poisoning is due to the unfortunate and wishful reputation of cantharidin as an abortifacient or aphrodisiac. The compound is a very potent irritant to all tissues, and ingestion of 10 mg may be fatal. Initial symptoms after ingestion are severe burning pain in the upper gastrointestinal tract, hematemesis, and bloody diarrhea. This is rapidly followed by burning urethral pain, priapism, hematuria, oliguria, anuria, uremia, hepatic failure, myocarditis, shock, delirium, and coma. Death may occur within a few hours or up to 1 week after poisoning. Treatment is entirely symptomatic and supportive.

CARBON MONOXIDE

Carbon monoxide is a colorless, odorless, tasteless and nonirritating gas produced by the incomplete combustion of carbonaceous materials. Almost any flame or combustion device emits carbon monoxide. The gas is present in the exhaust of internal combustion engines in a concentration of 3 to 7 percent. Much higher concentrations are present in most illuminating and heating gases, but not in natural gas. Carbon monoxide is annually responsible for hundreds of accidental and suicidal deaths.

The toxic effects of carbon monoxide are the result of tissue hypoxia. Carbon monoxide combines with hemoglobin to form carboxyhemoglobin. Since carbon monoxide and oxygen react with the same group in the hemoglobin molecule, carboxyhemoglobin is incapable of carrying oxygen. The affinity of hemoglobin for carbon monoxide is two hundred times greater than for oxygen, and at equilibrium 1 part of carbon monoxide in 1,500 parts of air will result in 50 percent conversion of hemoglobin into carboxyhemoglobin. Carboxyhemoglobin also interferes with the release of oxygen from oxyhemoglobin. This further reduces the amount of oxygen available to the tissues and explains why tissue anoxia appears in the carbon monoxide poisoned individual at levels of ar-

terial oxyhemoglobin concentration well tolerated by the anemic patient.

The extent of saturation of hemoglobin with carbon monoxide depends on the concentration of the gas in inspired air and on the time of exposure. The severity of hypoxic symptoms depends further on the state of activity of the individual, his tissue oxygen needs, and his hemoglobin concentration. As a general rule, no symptoms will develop at a concentration of 0.01 percent carbon monoxide in inspired air, since this will not raise blood saturation above 10 percent. Exposure to 0.05 percent for 1 hr during light activity will produce a blood concentration of 20 percent carboxyhemoglobin and result in a mild or throbbing headache. Greater activity or longer exposure to the same concentration causes a blood saturation of 30 to 50 percent. At this point headache, irritability, confusion, dizziness, visual disturbances, nausea, vomiting, and fainting on exertion may be observed. After exposure for 1 hr to concentrations of 0.1 percent in inspired air the blood will contain 50 to 80 percent carboxyhemoglobin, which results in coma, convulsions, respiratory failure, and death. On inhalation of high concentrations of carbon monoxide, saturation of the blood proceeds so rapidly that unconsciousness may occur suddenly and without warning symptoms. When poisoning is more gradual, the individual may notice decreased exercise tolerance and dyspnea on exertion or even at rest. Excessive sweating, fever, hepatomegaly, skin lesions, leukocytosis, bleeding diathesis, albuminuria, and glycosuria have also been described. Cerebral edema and intracranial hypertension may result from the increased permeability of hypoxic capillaries. Myocardial hypoxia is reflected by electrocardiographic abnormalities.

The most characteristic sign of carbon monoxide poisoning is the cherry color of skin and mucous membranes, which is due to the bright red carboxyhemoglobin. If the characteristic flush is not present, 5 ml of 40% sodium hydroxide may be added to 5 ml of a 5% solution of blood in water. An oxyhemoglobin solution will turn brown, but a carboxyhemoglobin solution remains red.

Treatment of carbon monoxide poisoning requires effective ventilation in the presence of high oxygen tensions and in the absence of carbon monoxide. If necessary, ventilation should be supported artificially. Pure oxygen should be administered. This will result not only in the replacement of carbon monoxide by oxygen in the hemoglobin molecule but also in the partial relief of tissue hypoxia by oxygen dissolved in the plasma. For the same reasons hyperbaric oxygen is helpful in seriously poisoned patients. Transfusion of blood or packed cells is also of value. In order to reduce tissue needs for oxygen the patient must be kept absolutely quiet. The induction of hypothermia may further reduce oxygen requirements.

During the recovery from carbon monoxide poisoning symptoms regress gradually. If severe tissue hypoxia has obtained too long, neurologic symptoms such as tremors, mental deterioration, and psychotic behavior may persist.

Histologic changes characteristic of hypoxia may be observed in cerebral cortex, medulla, myocardium, and other organs.

CASTOR BEANS

The castor bean plant (*Ricinus communis*) is grown for commercial and ornamental purposes. The beans contain ricin, an extremely toxic albumin, which causes agglutination and hemolysis of red cells and injury to all other cells. After a delay of several hours to 2 days following ingestion abdominal pain, vomiting, and profuse diarrhea appear and produce severe dehydration. Extreme weakness, drowsiness, disorientation, stupor, coma, convulsions, respiratory depression, and circulatory collapse may develop. Intravascular clotting and hemolysis have been observed. If the patient survives the acute symptoms, oliguria may progress to anuria and uremia, with death after several days. Treatment consists of fluid replacement, alkalinization of the urine with sodium bicarbonate to prevent precipitation of hemoglobin in the kidneys, and supportive measures.

CATHARTIC RESINS

Colocynth, croton oil, gamboge, and podophyllum are drastic cathartics due to their content of highly irritating plant resins. These compounds have no therapeutic use; poisoning is usually the work of ignorant pranksters. Oral administration of 1 Gm of these substances has been fatal. Symptoms are burning pain in mouth, esophagus, and stomach, hematemesis, watery or bloody diarrhea, dehydration, shock, coma, and death. Treatment consists of removal of the irritant from the gastrointestinal tract and supportive measures. Large amounts of parenteral fluids, blood replacement, and morphine and atropine to quiet the bowel may be required.

CHLORATES

Sodium and potassium chlorates are strong oxidizing agents and are found in gargles, mouthwashes, matches, and weed killers. After oral ingestion, 2 Gm has been fatal for children and 10 Gm for adults. Chlorate ion acts as a catalyst in the production of methemoglobinemia, and absorption of a small amount can result in a high methemoglobin concentration. The symptoms of chlorate ingestion are those of local mucosal irritation and of methemoglobinemia (see Chap. 344). Renal toxicity is common. Treatment is directed at the methemoglobinemia and is otherwise supportive.

CHLORINATED INSECTICIDES

These compounds are common ingredients of dusts, sprays, and solutions used as insecticides. The great majority of these compounds are chlorinated diphenyls (e.g., DDT, TDE, DFDT, DMC, Neotran) or chlorinated polycyclic compounds (e.g., Aldrin, Chlordane, Dieldrin, Endrin, Heptachlor). Lindane is a hexachlorbenzene. The toxic effects of all these agents are similar. The chlorinated insecticides are soluble in lipid and organic solvents but not in water. They are poorly absorbed unless dissolved in a vehicle such as kerosene, petroleum distillates, or other organic solvents. Under these circumstances they readily enter the body through the skin, lungs, or gastrointestinal tract. These compounds vary considerably in toxicity, and the toxicity of the dissolving vehicle must also be considered. The effects of the solvent may overshadow or modify those of the insecticide.

The initial symptoms of acute poisoning are nausea, vomiting, headache, dizziness, apprehension, excitement, and muscular tremors and weakness. These symptoms progress to generalized central nervous system hyperexcitability with delirium and clonic or tonic convulsions. This stage is in turn followed by progressive depression with paralysis, coma, and death. In chronically poisoned patients cerebellar symptoms and evidence of liver damage may develop. Hepatic toxicity is particularly prominent in poisoning by hexachlorbenzene. Treatment consists of gastric lavage and catharsis, anticonvulsive therapy with short-acting barbiturates, artificial ventilation, and other supportive measures. Sympathomimetic compounds should be avoided, since chlorinated insecticides apparently increase susceptibility to ventricular fibrillation.

CHOLINESTERASE INHIBITOR INSECTICIDES

Many substances used in agriculture for control of soft-bodied insects are potent inhibitors of cholinesterase. Most of these compounds are organic phosphates (e.g., Parathion, Malathion, Systox, TEPP, HETP, OMPA), others are carbamates (e.g., Dimetan, Matacil). The toxicity of these compounds varies widely. They are usually prepared for use by dilution with powders, organic solvents, or water. Formulations containing 1 to 95 percent of the active ingredient are available. The cholinesterase inhibitor insecticides are rapidly absorbed through the intact skin and after inhalation or ingestion.

The organic phosphate esters act by combining with and inactivating acetylcholinesterase. Since this enzyme normally breaks down the acetylcholine liberated by the central nervous system, autonomic ganglia, parasympathetic nerve endings, and motor nerve endings, its inactivation allows the accumulation of large amounts of acetylcholine at these sites. In the central nervous system initial stimulation is followed by depression of cells, resulting in convulsions followed by coma and respiratory depression. Initial stimulation and later blockade of autonomic ganglia results in multiple and variable dysfunctions of structures innervated by the autonomic nervous system. Accumulation of acetylcholine at parasympathetic nerve endings produces pupillary constriction and blurring of vision; stimulation of intestinal muscle resulting in abdominal cramps, vomiting, and diarrhea; stimulation of secretory glands causing rhinorrhea, salivation, sweating, and bronchorrhea; constriction of the bronchial musculature with symptoms of respiratory distress; depression of the cardiac sinus pacemaker activity; and impairment of atrioventricular conduction. Persistence of acetylcholine at the neuromuscular junction results in muscular tremors, cramps, and fasciculations which are followed by neuromuscular block and flaccid paralysis. Other important clinical manifestations of these poisons are cyanosis, and pulmonary edema.

Management consists of emesis or lavage, catharsis, and washing of contaminated skin with soap and water. Atropine should be given immediately to block the parasympathetic and central nervous system effects. A dose of 2 mg is injected intramuscularly and repeated every 10 min until parasympathetic manifestations are controlled and signs of atropinization appear. The same dosage must be repeated frequently to maintain xerostomia and mild tachycardia. Fatal respiratory failure or pulmonary edema may occur quickly upon cessation of atropine therapy. Atropine is virtually ineffective against the autonomic ganglionic actions of acetylcholine and against the peripheral neuromuscular paralysis. Certain oximes act as cholinesterase reactivators. Pralidoxime is useful in the treatment of organic phosphate cholinesterase inhibition but should not be used if the inhibition is due to a carbamate. A dose of 1 Gm pralidoxime in aqueous solution is administered intravenously over a 5 min period and may be repeated twice each day. Supportive therapy includes administration of oxygen with artificial ventilation if necessary, removal of pulmonary secretions by suction, and treatment of convulsions with short-acting barbiturates. Energetic therapy with artificial ventilation, atropine, and pralidoxime allows survival of doses of organic phosphate esters vastly exceeding the usual fatal dose.

CYANIDE

The cyanide ion is an exceedingly potent and rapid acting poison, but one for which specific and effective antidotal therapy is available. Cyanide poisoning may result from the inhalation of hydrocyanic acid and from the ingestion of soluble inorganic cyanide salts or cyanide-releasing substances such as cyanamide, cyanogen chloride, and nitroprusside. Parts of many plants also contain substances such as amygdalin which release cyanide on digestion. Among these are the seeds of certain stone fruits (choke cherry, pin cherry, wild black cherry, peach, apricot, bitter almond), cassava roots, the berries of the jet berry bush, the leaves and shoots of elderberry, and all parts of hydrangea. Cyanides are widely used in industry and for fumigation and may reach the home in photographic chemicals or silver polishes. As little as 300 mg potassium cyanide may cause death.

The extreme toxicity of cyanide is due to its ready reaction with the trivalent iron of cytochrome oxidase. The role of the enzyme in cellular oxygen utilization is inhibited by the formation of the cytochrome oxidase-cyanide complex. The resultant cytotoxic hypoxia leads to cellular dysfunction and death.

Inhalation of hydrogen cyanide may cause death within a minute. Oral doses act more slowly, requiring several minutes for the appearance of symptoms and up to several hours for death. The first effect is an increase in ventilation because of the blockade of oxidative metabolism in the chemoreceptor cells. As more cyanide is absorbed, there is headache, dizziness, nausea, drowsiness, hypotension, profound dyspnea, characteristic electrocardiographic changes, coma, and convulsions. Death always occurs within 4 hr.

Cyanide poisoning is a true medical emergency. Treatment is highly effective if given rapidly. The chemical antidotes should be immediately available wherever emergency medical care is dispensed. The diagnosis may be made by the characteristic "bitter almond" odor on the breath of the victim, and physicians should familiarize themselves with this smell. Since the saturation of hemoglobin is not disturbed by cyanide, cyanosis is not seen until respiratory depression supervenes. The objective of treatment is the production of methemoglobin by the administration of nitrite. The trivalent iron of methemoglobin competes with cytochrome oxidase for the cyanide ion. The cytochrome oxidase-cyanide complex dissociates and enzymatic function and cell respiration are restored. Further detoxification is then achieved by the administration of thiosulfate. Under the influence of the tissue enzyme rhodanese thiosulfate reacts with cyanide liberated by the dissociation of cyanmethemoglobin to form thiocyanate. This substance is relatively nontoxic and readily excreted in the urine.

Since speed is of the essence, nitrite should be immediately administered by inhalation of amyl nitrite perles, one every 2 min unless blood pressure is below 80 mm. This is followed as soon as possible by the intravenous injection of 10 ml of 3% sodium nitrite over a 3-min period. An intravenous infusion of norepinephrine may be necessary to maintain blood pressure during this injection period. After the administration of sodium nitrite, 50 ml of 25% sodium thiosulfate should be administered intravenously over a 10-min period. Supportive measures, especially artificial respiration with 100% oxygen, should be instituted as soon as possible, but, unless methemoglobinemia is produced promptly, other forms of treatment are of no value. Administration of sodium nitrite and sodium thiosulfate may have to be repeated. If the patient survives 4 hr, recovery is likely but residual cerebral symptoms may persist.

DETERGENTS AND SOAPS

These substances fall into the three groups of anionic, nonionic, and cationic detergents. The first group contains common soaps and household detergents. They may cause vomiting and diarrhea but have no serious effects, and no treatment is required. However, some laundry compounds contain phosphate water softeners whose ingestion may cause hypocalcemia. The ingestion of nonionic detergents is harmless and requires no treatment.

Cationic detergents, such as benzalkonium chloride (Zephiran) and many others, are commonly used for bacteriocidal purposes in hospitals and homes. These compounds are well absorbed from the gastrointestinal tract and interfere with cellular functions. The fatal oral dose is approximately 3 Gm. Ingestion produces nausea and vomiting, and shock, coma, convulsions, and death may occur in a few hours. Treatment consists of minimizing gastrointestinal absorption by emesis or gastric lavage with ordinary soap solution, which rapidly inactivates cationic detergents. If significant absorption has occurred, intensive supportive therapy may be required.

ERGOT

This fungus (*Claviceps purpurea*) grows on rye and contains a number of highly toxic alkaloids (e.g., ergotamine, ergonovine) which are used in the treatment of migraine or as uterine stimulants. Poisoning may be due to therapeutic overdosage, particularly in patients with severe infections or liver disease, but more commonly results from the use of ergot as an abortifacient. The epidemic form of chronic ergot poisoning due to the ingestion of contaminated grain is now rarely seen. Ingestion of 1 Gm ergot has been fatal, ergotamine has caused gangrene in doses of 10 mg per day. Symptoms of acute or chronic ergot poisoning are vomiting, diarrhea, burning abdominal pain, severe muscle pains, ischemic peripheral gangrene, headache, psychotic behavior, muscle tremors, convulsions, and coma. Circulatory disturbances are due both to prolonged vasoconstriction and to intimal hyperplasia and thrombosis. Treatment of ergot poisoning is symptomatic. Vigorous vasodilator and analgesic therapy should be employed.

FLUORIDES

Fluoride salts are widely used in insecticides. The gases fluorine and hydrogen fluoride are used in industry. The latter is a strong corrosive. Fluorine and fluorides are cellular poisons which block the glycolytic degradation of glucose. Fluorides also form an insoluble precipitate with calcium and cause hypocalcemia. Finally, in an acid medium fluorides form the corrosive hydrofluoric acid. Ingestion of 1 to 2 Gm sodium fluoride may be fatal.

Inhalation of fluorine or hydrogen fluoride produces coughing and choking. After an asymptomatic period of a day or two, fever, cough, cyanosis, and pulmonary edema may develop. Ingestion of fluoride salts is followed by nausea, vomiting productive of corroded tissues, diarrhea, and abdominal pain. Consequent to the decrease in serum calcium the victim develops muscular hyperirritability, fasciculations, tremors, spasms, and convulsions. Death is due to respiratory paralysis or circulatory collapse. If the patient survives the acute period, jaundice and oliguria may appear. Chronic fluoride poisoning (fluorosis) is characterized by weight loss, weakness, anemia, brittle bones, and stiff joints. Mottling of teeth is seen when exposure occurs during enamel formation.

Acute fluoride poisoning is treated by immediate administration of milk, lime water, calcium gluconate, or calcium lactate solution. Following lavage or emesis 10 Gm calcium gluconate and 30 Gm sodium sulfate should be administered to precipitate and remove fluoride from the intestine. Then 10% calcium gluconate or 1% calcium chloride should be slowly injected intravenously and repeated as needed to prevent a positive Chvostek sign. Symptomatic and supportive therapy is administered as indicated.

FORMALDEHYDE

This gas is available as a 40% solution (Formalin) which is used as a disinfectant, fumigant, or deodorant. Poisoning by Formalin may be diagnosed by the characteristic odor of formaldehyde. Formaldehyde reacts chemically with cellular constituents, depresses cellular functions, and causes cell death. The fatal dose of Formalin is about 60 ml.

Ingestion of Formalin immediately causes severe abdominal pain, nausea, vomiting, and diarrhea. This may be followed by collapse, coma, severe metabolic acidosis, and anuria. Death is usually due to circulatory failure.

Treatment consists of immediate administration of activated charcoal followed by emesis and gastric lavage with a solution containing 1% ammonium carbonate and 2% sodium bicarbonate. Parenteral administration of sodium bicarbonate is indicated to combat acidosis. The treatment is otherwise supportive.

GLYCOLS

Ethylene glycol and diethylene glycol are commonly used in antifreeze solutions. The more than 50 annual deaths from these compounds usually result from intentional drinking of antifreeze by alcoholics. The fatal dose of ethylene glycol is about 100 Gm, that of diethylene glycol somewhat lower. Both compounds are metabolized to oxalate in the body.

The initial symptoms of acute poisoning by these glycols resemble alcoholic intoxication. They may progress to vomiting, stupor, coma with absent reflexes and anisocoria, and convulsions. Tachypnea, bradycardia, and hypothermia are commonly seen. After massive ingestion death may occur from respiratory failure within a few hours or from pulmonary edema within a day or two. If the patient survives the acute stage, hepatic and renal necroses manifest themselves with jaundice, anuria, and uremia.

Treatment is largely supportive. The administration of ethyl alcohol and of intravenous calcium gluconate may be helpful by slowing the oxidation to oxalic acid and by precipitating the acid. However, the effectiveness of these procedures has not been definitely established. Dialysis is highly successful in the removal of ethylene and diethylene glycol from the body.

HALOGENATED HYDROCARBONS

Halogenated hydrocarbons (carbon tetrachloride, ethylene chlorohydrin, ethylene dichloride, methyl halides, tetrachloroethane, trichloroethylene) find wide industrial use as solvents, refrigerants, fumigants, and in chemical synthesis. They enter the home in household cleaners, floor waxes, fire extinguishers, and rubber or plastic cements. These compounds are highly fat-soluble and produce cell damage either directly or after conversion in the body to other compounds. Individual halogenated hydrocarbons differ considerably in the degree and the exact manifestations of their toxicity, but in sufficient concentration all these compounds are capable of inducing central nervous system depression and varying amounts of hepatic and renal toxicity. Myocardial depression, vascular damage, and pulmonary edema may also occur.

The most important halogenated hydrocarbon is carbon tetrachloride, widely employed as a nonflammable solvent and fire extinguisher fluid. Poisoning may occur from inhalation of the vapor, ingestion, or, rarely, percutaneous absorption. An oral dose of as little as 4 ml may be fatal. Absorption from the gastrointestinal tract is slow and unpredictable but is increased by the presence of fats and alcohol. Abdominal pain, hematemesis, and hepatic damage are more common and severe after ingestion than when the poison is inhaled. Inhalation may lead to irritation of the upper respiratory tract.

Acute systemic absorption of carbon tetrachloride results in nausea, dizziness, confusion, and headache within a few minutes. Depending upon the quantity absorbed, the symptoms may quickly progress to stupor, coma, convulsions, respiratory failure, hypotension, or ventricular fibrillation. The patient may recover from these immediate manifestations until evidence of hepatic or renal toxicity appears several hours to several days after the exposure. Liver and kidney damage may also occur in the absence of any severe early central nervous system effects. Initially tender hepatomegaly may be present, jaundice may be rapidly progressive, and death due to severe centrilobular necrosis may occur within days. The renal lesion has the characteristics of acute tubular necrosis and manifests itself by proteinuria, hematuria, oliguria, or anuria. Uremia, acidosis, hypertension, and pulmonary edema may develop as complications of renal failure. Optic neuritis, pancreatitis, and adrenal cortical necrosis are less common manifestations of carbon tetrachloride intoxication.

Chronic poisoning may occur after repeated exposures to low concentrations of carbon tetrachloride and may also lead to liver or kidney damage. More usually it manifests itself by vague symptoms of fatigue, weakness, mental confusion, abdominal pain, anorexia, nausea, blurring of vision, and paresthesias.

Treatment of acute poisoning by halogenated hydrocarbons includes vigorous effects at minimizing gastrointestinal absorption by lavage or emesis and catharsis. Treatment is otherwise symptomatic. Sympathometic drugs should be avoided because of the danger of inducing ventricular arrhythmias in the sensitized myocardium. Acute renal and hepatic failure must be carefully managed. Hemodialysis is often required and may be lifesaving until kidney function returns 3 or more weeks after poisoning.

IODINE

The traditional antiseptic Iodine Tincture is an alcoholic solution of 2% iodine and 2% sodium iodide. Strong Iodine Solution (Lugol's solution) is an aqueous solution of 5% iodine and 10% potassium iodide. Tincture of iodine is often taken for suicidal purposes. The fatal dose of iodine is approximately 2 Gm. Iodides are very much less toxic and no fatalities have been reported.

The diagnosis of iodine poisoning is suggested by the brown staining of the oral mucous membranes. The effects are largely due to the corrosive effects of the compound on the gastrointestinal tract. Burning abdominal pain, nausea, vomiting, and bloody diarrhea may occur soon after ingestion. If the stomach contained starch, the vomitus is blue or black. Tissue trauma from corrosive gastroenteritis and fluid loss by vomiting and diarrhea may result in shock. Severe edema of the glottis, fever, delirium, stupor, and anuria have also been observed.

Treatment consists of gastric lavage with a starch solution made by adding 15 Gm flour or cornstarch to 500 ml water. Thereafter, catharsis should be induced, and milk should be given orally to relieve gastric irritation. Sodium thiosulfate will reduce iodine to less toxic iodide; 100 ml of a 5% solution should be given orally and 10 ml of a 10% solution intravenously every 4 hr. With appropriate treatment most patients poisoned by iodine survive, but esophageal strictures may complicate their recovery.

IPECAC, EMETINE

Emetine is the major alkaloid of ipecac (dried roots or rhizomes of *Cephaelis ipecacuanha*) and is used for the treatment of amebiasis. Syrup of ipecac is used as an emetic or expectorant. Poisoning may be accidental or suicidal but most commonly results from overdosage during therapy, at times due to the erroneous substitution of the much more potent fluid extract of ipecac for syrup of ipecac. Emetine and other alkaloids of ipecac have serious toxic gastrointestinal, central nervous, and myocardial effects. The fatal oral dose of emetine is about 1 Gm.

Manifestations of poisoning begin with nausea, vomiting, diarrhea, and abdominal pain. Cardiac effects are heralded by electrocardiographic changes, and the depression of myocardial contractility leads to dyspnea, tachycardia, shock, and congestive heart failure. Coma and convulsions may occur, but death is usually due to heart failure. Treatment is symptomatic. Administration of digitalis may be of value.

IRON SALTS

Ferrous or ferric salts produce gastrointestinal corrosive damage. Following mucosal damage, large amounts of iron may be absorbed, particularly in children. The fatal oral dose in children is 5 to 10 Gm.

Very soon after ingestion nausea, vomiting, diarrhea, and abdominal pain appear. Systemic effects include acidosis, shock, drowsiness, coma, and respiratory failure.

These initial symptoms may partially clear but then recur with increased severity. In the later stages signs of hepatic and renal toxicity may appear.

The absorption of ingested iron should be minimized by the usual measures. Gastric lavage with a 10% sodium bicarbonate solution will precipitate the ferrous ion. Edetate calcium disodium 30 mg per kg daily in divided doses should be administered intravenously or orally. Deferoxamine methane sulfonate (Desferal) is even more effective as an iron chelating agent than edetate. Use of chelating agents is guided by determinations of serum iron and iron-binding capacity. Peritoneal dialysis and hemodialysis effectively remove iron from the body. Acidosis, shock, and renal or hepatic toxicity must be treated supportively.

ISOPROPYL ALCOHOL

This compound is used as a sterilizing agent or as rubbing alcohol. Ingestion produces gastric irritation and raises the danger of vomiting with aspiration. The systemic effects of isopropyl alcohol are similar to those of ethyl alcohol, but it is approximately twice as potent as the latter. Coma is readily produced but rarely lasts longer than 12 hr. Isopropyl alcohol is oxidized to acetone in the body, and transient acetonuria is common, but significant acidosis does not occur. Gastric lavage should always be performed to minimize the danger of aspiration following vomiting in the unconscious patient. Supportive therapy is required only after ingestion of massive amounts, and there are no sequelae other than transient gastritis.

MAGNESIUM

Magnesium sulfate is used intravenously as a hypotensive agent and orally as a cathartic. The magnesium ion is a profound depressant of the central nervous system and of neuromuscular transmission. Poisoning after oral or rectal administration is unlikely in the presence of normal renal function, because the kidney removes magnesium more rapidly than it is absorbed by the gastrointestinal tract. In the presence of impaired renal function an oral dose of 30 Gm may be fatal. Symptoms begin at a serum magnesium level of 4 mEq per liter and concentrations of over 12 mEq per liter may be fatal. Oral ingestion of concentrated solutions may cause gastrointestinal irritation. Manifestations of systemic poisoning are depression of reflexes, flaccid paralysis, hypotension, hypothermia, coma, and respiratory failure. Respiratory death usually precedes significant myocardial depression. The actions of magnesium on neurologic and neuromuscular function are antagonized by calcium. Treatment of magnesium poisoning therefore includes the intravenous administration of 10 ml of a 10% solution of calcium gluconate, which may be repeated as necessary.

METHYL ALCOHOL

This simplest of the alcohols, also called wood alcohol or methanol, is used as a solvent, antifreeze, paint remover, and as a denaturant in ethyl alcohol. Denatured ethyl alcohol preparations, such as Sterno or Solox, contain 5 to 15 percent methyl alcohol as well as other denaturants. Methyl alcohol poisoning is due almost entirely to its ingestion as a substitute for ethanol or to the drinking of denatured ethyl alcohol. The toxic dose is very variable: death has occurred after a dose of 20 ml but 250 ml have been ingested with survival. As little as 15 ml of methanol has caused permanent blindness.

Methanol is less inebriating than ethyl alcohol, and inebriation is not a prominent symptom of methyl alcohol intoxication. Methanol is oxidized in the body to formaldehyde and to formic acid. The rate of its metabolism is independent of the concentration in the body and is only 15 percent that of ethanol. The enzyme alcohol dehydrogenase appears to be responsible for the first step in oxidation. The enzyme system will preferentially utilize ethyl alcohol if this compound is also available. Thus ethyl alcohol may depress the rate of metabolism of methanol. The manifestations of methanol poisoning are largely due to the accumulation of its toxic metabolites. These products, especially formaldehyde, have toxic actions on many cells, and the retina and optic nerve are specifically damaged. The toxic metabolites of methyl alcohol are also responsible for the severe acidosis, which is the most prominent feature of methyl alcohol poisoning. This acidosis is partly due to the accumulation of formic acid, but formate also appears to exert an inhibitory effect upon enzymes involved in the oxidation of carbohydrate with consequent accumulation of acid intermediates.

Symptoms of methanol poisoning usually do not appear until 12 to 24 hr after ingestion, when sufficient toxic metabolites have accumulated. Manifestations consist of headache, dizziness, nausea, vomiting, severe abdominal and back pain probably due to pancreatitis, vasomotor disturbances, central nervous system depression, and respiratory failure. Visual disturbance is almost universal and ranges from mild blurring of vision to total blindness. Impairment of vision may be transient, but permanent blindness may follow survival of the acute intoxication. The pupils are dilated and nonreactive and there is hyperemia of the optic disc and retinal edema. Severe abdominal tenderness and spasm or nuchal rigidity may be present. Acidosis is commonly severe, but Kussmaul respiration is absent in many severely acidotic patients (plasma carbon dioxide–combining power below 20 mEq per liter).

In the treatment of methyl alcohol intoxication gastric lavage is of use only during the first hour or two. The mainstay of treatment is intravenous administration of large amounts of sodium bicarbonate. Return of acidosis is frequent after initial correction, and additional alkali must be administered as indicated by close observation of the patient and laboratory determinations. Peritoneal dialysis and hemodialysis effectively remove methanol from the body and are useful in view of its slow oxidation. The administration of 0.5 ml per kg of ethyl alcohol every 2 hr may inhibit the metabolism of methyl alcohol and is useful in conjunction with dialysis. Supportive therapy must be administered as required by the patient's clinical state.

MUSHROOMS

There are many species of poisonous mushrooms, but in the United States most poisoning is due to *Amanita muscaria* (fly agaric) or *Amanita phalloides* (destroying angel). More than 100 deaths result each year from consumption of wild poisonous mushrooms, 90 percent are due to *A. phalloides*. Fatalities have occurred after ingestion of only part of one mushroom.

Amanita muscaria contains the parasympathomimetic alkaloid muscarine, as well as variable amounts of a substance active on the central nervous system and a parasympatholytic alkaloid. Symptoms are largely those of parasympathetic stimulation: lacrimation, pupillary constriction, perspiration, salivation, nausea, vomiting, diarrhea, abdominal pain, bronchorrhea, wheezing, dyspnea, bradycardia, and hypotension. Muscular tremors, confusion, excitement, and delirium are common in severe poisoning. Very rarely symptoms of atropine poisoning have predominated. After ingestion of *A. muscaria* symptoms appear within minutes to 2 hr. The patient may die within a few hours, but with appropriate therapy complete recovery in 24 hr is the rule

Amanita phalloides, some other *Amanita* species, and *Galerina venenata* contain heat-stable polypeptide cytotoxins which are rapidly bound to tissues. Severe cell damage and fatty degeneration may occur in liver, kidneys, striated muscle, and brain. Ingestion of these dangerous mushrooms is followed by a latent period of 6 to 20 hr. Manifestations of cytotoxicity may then appear suddenly and consist of severe nausea, violent abdominal pain, bloody vomiting and diarrhea, and cardiovascular collapse. Headache, mental confusion, coma, or convulsions are common. Painful and tender hepatomegaly, jaundice, hypoglycemia, dehydration, and oliguria or anuria frequently arise on the first or second day after ingestion. The victim may die from acute yellow atrophy within 4 days. About one-half of all poisonings with *A. phalloides* have a fatal outcome in 5 to 8 days. Recovery tends to be slow.

Ingestion of other poisonous mushrooms may cause gastrointestinal symptoms, visual disturbances, ataxia, disorientation, convulsions, coma, fever, hemolysis, and methemoglobinemia.

Treatment of mushroom poisoning depends upon the species ingested. If parasympathomimetic manifestations are prominent, atropine in doses of 1 to 2 mg is given intramuscularly and repeated every 30 min until symptoms are controlled. Poisoning by cytotoxic mushrooms can only be treated symptomatically. Fluid and electrolyte balance must be carefully maintained. Hypoglycemia should be avoided, and large quantities of carbohydrate may exert some protective effect on the liver. Excitement, convulsions, pain, hypotension, and fever may need symptomatic therapy. Hemodialysis is of no value in removing the toxin but may be required to maintain renal function until recovery occurs.

NAPHTHALENE

Poisoning by this substance is almost always due to ingestion of moth repellents. An oral dose of 2 Gm has been fatal. Nausea, vomiting, and diarrhea are the initial symptoms. Larger doses may produce hepatic damage with jaundice and renal toxicity which may progress to hematuria, oliguria, or anuria. Depending upon the amount ingested, central nervous system manifestations may range from headache, mental confusion, and excitement to coma and convulsions. In individuals with glucose 6-phosphate dehydrogenase–deficient red cells the ingestion of naphthalene will produce hemolysis. Treatment consists of emesis or gastric lavage and catharsis and supportive measures.

NICOTINE

This alkaloid is an exceedingly potent and rapidly acting poison. It is a component of many insecticides. Nicotine is readily absorbed from the oral and gastrointestinal mucosa, from the respiratory tract, and through the skin. The lethal dose for an adult is approximately 50 mg, the quantity contained in two cigarettes. However, tobacco is much less toxic than would be anticipated on the basis of its nicotine content. Nicotine is poorly absorbed from ingested tobacco, and on smoking, most of the nicotine is burned. Nicotine acts on chemoreceptors, on synapses in the central nervous system and in autonomic ganglia, on the adrenal medulla, and on neuroeffector junctions. Furthermore, its initial stimulant effects are followed by a depressant phase of action. It is not surprising that the manifestations of nicotine poisoning are highly complex and somewhat unpredictable.

Small doses of nicotine produce nausea, vomiting, diarrhea, headache, dizziness, and neurologic stimulation manifested by tachycardia, hypertension, hyperpnea, tachypnea, sweating, and salivation. Larger doses also cause cortical irritability progressing to convulsions, and myocardial arrhythmias. Finally coma, respiratory depression and arrest, and cardiac arrest or fibrillation may supervene. Severe poisoning may cause death within a few minutes.

Treatment consists of gastric lavage with activated charcoal or with a 1:10,000 solution of potassium permanganate, which oxidizes nicotine. Atropine, 2 mg, and phentolamine, 5 mg, may be given intramuscularly or intravenously and repeated as often as required to control signs and symptoms of parasympathetic or sympathetic hyperactivity. These compounds are ineffective in preventing paralysis of the respiratory muscles and disturbances in cardiac rhythm. Careful attention must be given to artificial ventilation with oxygen and to therapy of active, catecholamine-induced cardiac arrhythmias. Propranolol is probably the drug of choice for the latter purpose. Nicotine is rapidly detoxified in the liver and recovery will be prompt if the patient can be tided over the initial period.

NITRITES

Poisoning by the nitrite ion may result from the ingestion of large amounts of drugs such as amyl nitrite or sodium nitrite. Nitrites are also used to preserve the color of meat, and amounts in excess of the allowable residue of 0.01 percent may appear in food. Ingested nitrates may be reduced to nitrite by intestinal bacteria, especially *E. coli*. Except after the ingestion of very large amounts adults usually absorb all nitrate before this reduction takes place. However, in children nitrite poisoning may result from the ingestion of nitrates or nitrate containing well water. Fatalities have occurred from the oral ingestion of 2 to 4 Gm of nitrites.

Acute nitrite poisoning may lead to severe headache, flushing, dizziness, hypotension, and syncope. Usually the patient need only be positioned to facilitate venous return to the heart. Pressor agents are seldom required. The most important toxic effect of the nitrite ion is its ability to oxidize hemoglobin to methemoglobin (Chap. 344).

OXALIC ACID

This acid is found in ink eradicators and stain removers. It is corrosive and combines with calcium to form insoluble calcium oxalate. Ingestion causes irritation and corrosion of mouth, esophagus, and stomach followed by vomiting and abdominal pain. After absorption the reduction in serum calcium leads to muscular tremors, tetany, convulsions, and cardiovascular collapse. Ingestion of 5 Gm may cause death within minutes. Following recovery from the acute episode there may be renal failure due to blockage of renal tubules by calcium oxalate crystals.

Treatment consists of induction of emesis or gastric lavage with milk, limewater, chalk, or calcium salts. A dose of 10 ml of 10% calcium gluconate should be given intravenously and repeated as required to maintain normal serum calcium and prevent tetany. In supportive therapy the maintenance of a high urine output is essential.

PETROLEUM DISTILLATES

Petroleum distillates (diesel oil, gasoline, kerosene, paint thinner, solvent distillate) are liquids with a boiling point between 50 and 325°C. They contain variable amounts of branched or straight-chain aliphatic and aromatic hydrocarbons. Kerosene is widely used as a fuel and as a vehicle for cleaning agents, furniture polishes, insecticides, and paint thinners. Not surprisingly, each year petroleum distillates cause about 100 accidental deaths in the United States, 90 percent of these in young children. Furthermore, these products are annually responsible for almost 20,000 hospitalizations. Ingestion of 10 ml kerosene has been fatal, but adults have recovered from as much as 250 ml. Petroleum distillates are central nervous system depressants and damage cells by dissolving cellular lipids. Pulmonary damage manifested by pulmonary edema or pneumonitis is a common and serious complication.

Inhalation of gasoline or kerosene vapors induces a state resembling alcoholic intoxication. Headache, nausea, tinnitus, and a burning sensation in the chest may also be present. When aliphatic hydrocarbons are inhaled, these symptoms may progress to profound drowsiness or coma with absence of deep reflexes. If the distillate contains a high proportion of aromatic hydrocarbons, the coma is characterized by tremors, muscle jactitations, hyperactive reflexes, and convulsions. Death is usually due to respiratory depression, rarely to ventricular fibrillation.

The oral ingestion of petroleum distillates causes irritation of the mucous membranes of the upper intestinal tract. When large amounts have been ingested, the same manifestations as after inhalation may appear. Frequently eructation or vomiting results in aspiration of petroleum distillates into the trachea. Because of their low surface tension, minute amounts of these substances may then spread widely throughout the lungs and produce pulmonary edema and pneumonitis. Pulmonary damage may also arise due to absorption of ingested petroleum distillates from the gastrointestinal tract. However, kerosene is at least one hundred times more toxic by the intratracheal route than when ingested.

In the treatment of poisoning by petroleum distillates extreme care must be used to prevent aspiration. When large amounts have been ingested, gastric lavage should be performed but only after insertion of an endotracheal tube with an inflatable cuff. A vegetable oil and a saline cathartic may be administered to decrease the absorption of the poison. All cases of kerosene poisoning should be hospitalized for at least 24 hr for observation. If signs or symptoms of pulmonary irritation appear, adrenal steroids, oxygen under positive pressure, and antibiotics to prevent bacterial pneumonia are often of value. Symptomatic therapy for central nervous system depression or convulsions may be necessary. Sympathomimetic amines should be avoided because of the danger of inducing ventricular fibrillation in the hydrocarbon-sensitized heart.

PHENOL

Phenol and related compounds (creosote, cresols, hexachlorophene, hydroquinone, Lysol, resorcinol, tannic acid) are widely used as antiseptics, caustics, and preservatives. These substances poison all cells by denaturing and precipitating cellular proteins. The approximate fatal oral dose ranges from 2 ml for phenol and cresols to 20 ml for tannic acid.

Ingestion of phenolic compounds produces erosion of mucosa from mouth to stomach. The corroded areas may have a characteristic dead-white appearance. Hematemesis and bloody diarrhea may occur. After an initial phase of hyperpnea due to stimulation of the respiratory center, stupor, coma, convulsions, pulmonary edema, and shock are seen. The initial respiratory alkalosis is soon followed by a profound acidosis. The latter results from the renal excretion of base during the alkalotic stage, from the acidic nature of the phenolic radical, and from disturbances in carbohydrate metabolism presumably due to defects in enzymatic function. If the patient survives the acute stage, acute tubular necrosis may lead to oliguria or anuria and hepatic toxicity to jaundice.

Poisoning by phenolic compounds may often be diagnosed by their characteristic odor. Development of a violet or blue color of the urine after addition of a few drops of ferric chloride indicates the presence of a phenolic compound.

Treatment is directed at decreasing the absorption of ingested poison by administration of water, milk, or activated charcoal slurry and their removal by emesis or gastric lavage. Olive oil or castor oil dissolve phenol and retard its absorption. Supportive therapy consists of correction of the acidosis, the control of shock and convulsions, and the maintenance of a patent airway in the face of glottal edema by intubation or tracheotomy.

PHOSPHORUS

Phosphorus occurs in two forms: a red, nonpoisonous form and a yellow, fat-soluble, highly toxic form. The latter is used in rodent and insect poisons and in fireworks. Yellow phosphorus and phosphides cause fatty degeneration and necrosis of tissues, particularly of the liver. The lethal ingested dose of yellow phosphorus is approximately 50 mg.

Ingestion of yellow phosphorus is followed within 1 hr by burning pain in the upper gastrointestinal tract, vomiting, diarrhea, and a garlic odor of the breath and excreta. The patient may die in coma during the first day or two, or symptoms may subside after a few hours. Then, 1 to 2 days later, the victim may develop tender hepatomegaly, jaundice, hypocalcemia, hypotension, oliguria, and die following convulsions and coma. Death from acute yellow atrophy may occur in a few days.

Treatment consists of vigorous and repeated induction of emesis or gastric lavage. Calcium gluconate is given intravenously to maintain serum calcium. Treatment is otherwise supportive and a protective regimen for the liver should be instituted.

SALICYLATES

Each year 30 million pounds of aspirin are consumed in the United States, and salicylates can probably be found in every American household. It is therefore not surprising that salicylates (aspirin, methyl salicylate, salicylic acid, sodium salicylate) are more commonly involved in poisonings than any other agent. Aspirin is found in almost all compound analgesic tablets. Methyl salicylate (oil of wintergreen) is present in most skin liniments, and salicylic acid is used in ointments and corn plasters. The ingestion of 10 to 30 Gm aspirin or sodium salicylate may be fatal to adults, but survival has been reported after an oral dose of 130 Gm aspirin. On the other hand 3 Gm salicylate in a teaspoon of methyl salicylate has been fatal in children.

Salicylate intoxication may result from the cumulative effect of therapeutic administration of high doses. There is considerable individual variation: toxic symptoms may begin at dosages of 3 Gm per day or may not appear when 10 Gm per day are given. Toxic symptoms are also poorly correlated with the serum salicylate concentration, but few patients become intoxicated at levels less than 15 mg per 100 ml and most at levels over 35 mg per 100 ml. Therapeutic salicylate intoxication is usually mild and is called "salicylism." The earliest symptoms are vertigo, tinnitus, and impairment of hearing. Further overdosage causes nausea, vomiting, sweating, diarrhea, fever, drowsiness, headache, dimness of vision, and mental aberrations. The latter may be characterized by confusion, excitement, restlessness, and talkativeness; this "salicylate jag" resembles alcoholic intoxication without the euphoria. The central nervous system effects may progress to hallucinations, convulsions, and coma. Toxic doses of salicylates also have a direct stimulant effect on the respiratory center resulting in hyperventilation, loss of carbon dioxide, and respiratory alkalosis. Renal excretion of bicarbonate may partially compensate for this.

In acute salicylate poisoning due to accidental or suicidal ingestion of massive amounts, the same manifestations may be seen in more rapid succession. However, they are usually overshadowed by severe disturbances in the acid-base balance which follow a definite sequence. Early in the course of intoxication there may be only hyperpnea, and the seriousness of the poisoning may not be appreciated at that time. The hyperventilation causes a fall in blood P_{CO_2} and an increase in pH. Renal excretion of bicarbonate, sodium, and potassium will bring the pH back toward normal and produce a compensated respiratory alkalosis. At that point the buffering capacity of the extracellular fluid will have been significantly decreased. In young children and after large doses in adults further developments may then produce a combination of respiratory acidosis and metabolic acidosis which stem from a number of factors. High concentrations of salicylate depress the respiratory center and cause CO_2 retention. Renal function becomes impaired because of dehydration and hypotension, and inorganic, metabolic acids accumulate. Furthermore, salicylic acid derivatives may displace several mEq of blood bicarbonate. Finally, salicylates impair carbohydrate metabolism and cause accumulation of acetoacetic, lactic, and pyruvic acids. Severe acidosis and disturbances in electrolyte balance are most commonly seen in febrile young children.

Blood salicylate levels are of value in the estimation of the severity of poisoning. Serious poisoning is rare at levels less than 50 mg per 100 ml but usual at levels between 50 and 100 mg per 100 ml. Levels above 100 mg per 100 ml during the first 6 hr after poisoning signify severe intoxication and may be fatal. Excretion of salicylates is renal, and in the presence of normal renal function about 50 percent will be excreted in 24 hr. Addition of a few drops of ferric chloride solution to 5 ml of boiled acidified urine containing salicylate yields a violet color and may aid in diagnosis.

Treatment of salicylate poisoning is largely supportive. In order to decrease absorption, activated charcoal is administered and emesis is induced or lavage with sodium bicarbonate solution is performed. Disturbances of acid base or electrolyte balance and hypoglycemia are corrected by the intravenous administration of appropriate solutions. Respiratory depression may require artificial ventilation with oxygen. Convulsions may best be treated by the administration of succinylcholine and artificial ventilation with oxygen. Central nervous system–depressant agents should not be used. In order to increase renal excretion of salicylate, osmotic diuresis is induced and the urine is alkalinized. Peritoneal dialysis and hemodialysis are also highly effective in removing salicylate from seriously poisoned patients.

SMOKE

Poisoning by smoke is usually due to carbon monoxide inhalation. However, burning material may also release irritant fumes. Many irritant gases combine with water to form corrosive acids or alkalis and cause chemical burns of exposed skin and of the upper respiratory tract. Such gases (and the corrosives formed) are: ammonia (ammonium hydroxide), nitrogen oxide (nitric acid), sulfur dioxide (sulfurous acid), and sulfur trioxide (sulfuric acid). These irritating gases as well as hydrogen sulfide may also be present in smog. Another highly toxic gas which may be inhaled by firefighters or victims is phosgene. This compound is formed by the high-temperature decomposition of chlorinated hydrocarbons and is released when carbon tetrachloride from fire extinguishers comes into contact with hot surfaces.

After inhalation of irritant gases the victim may notice burning pain in throat and chest and severe coughing. These symptoms may subside completely, but from several hours to a day after exposure dyspnea and cyanosis may appear and progress rapidly to severe pulmonary edema and death from respiratory and circulatory failure. Treatment consists of administration of oxygen and adrenal steroids and appropriate therapy of pulmonary edema should that develop.

In many localities the term *smoke* is used to describe paint removers, lacquer thinners, antifreezes, and other solvent mixtures which are ingested for their supposed alcohol content. The toxicity of these compounds depends on their ingredients. Some such materials have caused profound hypoglycemia by a poorly understood mechanism. This possibility should be considered in the differential diagnosis of what appears to be alcoholic coma. Intravenous administration of glucose as a therapeutic test may be indicated.

SULFIDES

Hydrogen sulfide is a gas released by the decomposition of organic sulfur compounds and is widely used in industry. Carbon disulfide is an industrial solvent. Other sulfides have industrial uses and release hydrogen sulfide in contact with water or acids. Significant concentrations of hydrogen sulfide may be present in smoke or smog. Inhalation of hydrogen sulfide in concentrations above 50 ppm (50 times the minimum detectable by smell) causes conjunctivitis, headache, nausea, soreness of the upper respiratory passages, pulmonary edema, and drowsiness. Concentrations in excess of 300 ppm may cause coma, respiratory depression, and death. Ingestion of carbon disulfide or soluble sulfides is followed by vomiting, headache, hypotension, respiratory depression, tremors, coma, convulsions, and death. The fatal oral dose of carbon disulfide is approximately 1 Gm. Treatment of sulfide intoxication is supportive. Administration of sodium nitrite may promote the binding of sulfide in sulfmethemoglobin.

VOLATILE OILS

The volatile or essential oils (citronella oil, eucalyptus oil, menthol, pine oil, turpentine) are colorless liquids which irritate all tissues. Poisoning may result from occupational exposure (painters) and accidental or suicidal ingestion. Unfortunately, some volatile oils also have an undeserved reputation as abortifacients. Absorption occurs from skin, intestine, or lungs; the less volatile oils are more slowly absorbed. Ingestion of 15 Gm turpentine has been fatal.

Ingestion is rapidly followed by abdominal burning, nausea, vomiting, and diarrhea. Inhalation produces severe bronchial irritation and may be followed by delirium, coma, and convulsions. If the patient survives the acute stage of poisoning, evidence of renal damage may appear and progress to acute tubular necrosis with anuria.

Treatment is entirely supportive. When gastric lavage is undertaken, aspiration must be prevented with extreme care. Since the renal lesion is reversible, treatment for renal failure should be vigorous and include dialysis if necessary.

REFERENCES

Antimuscarinic Compounds

Hoefnagel, D.: Toxic Effects of Atropine and Homatropine Eyedrops in Children, New Engl. J. Med., 264:168, 1961.

Weintraub, S.: Stramonium Poisoning, Postgrad. Med., 28: 364, 1960.

Barium

Dean, G.: Seven Cases of Barium Carbonate Poisoning, Brit. Med. J., II:817, 1950.

Benzene, Toluene

Browning, E.: Toxic Solvents: A Review, Brit. J. Indust. Med., 16:23, 1959.

Brozovsky, M., and E. M. Winkler: Glue Sniffing in Children and Adolescents, N.Y. J. Med., 65:1984, 1965.

Glaser, H. H., and O. N. Massengale: "Glue-Sniffing" in Children. Deliberate Inhalation of Vaporized Plastic Cements, J.A.M.A., 181:300, 1962.

Boric Acid

Rosen, F. S., and R. J. Haggerty: Fatal Poisoning from Topical Use of Boric Acid Powder, New Engl. J. Med., 255:530, 1956.

Valdes-Dapena, M. A., and J. B. Arey: Boric Acid Poisoning, J. Pediat., 61:531, 1962.

Cantharidin

Oaks, W. W., J. F. DiTunno, T. Magnani, H. A. Levy, and L. C. Mills: Cantharidin Poisoning, A.M.A. Arch. Intern. Med., 105:574, 1960.

Carbon Monoxide

Anderson, R. F., D. C. Allenworth, and W. J. DeGroot: Myocardial Toxicity from Carbon Monoxide Poisoning, Ann. Intern. Med., 67:1172, 1967.

Cosby, R. S., and M. Bergeron: Electrocardiographic Changes in Carbon Monoxide Poisoning, Am. J. Cardiol., 11:93, 1963.

Craig, T. V., W. Hunt, and R. Atkinson: Hypothermia. Its Use in Severe Carbon Monoxide Poisoning, New Engl. J. Med., 261:854, 1959.

Lilienthal, J. L., Jr.: Cabon Monoxide, Pharmacol. Rev., 2:324, 1950.

Meigs, J. W., and J. P. W. Hughes: Acute Carbon Monoxide Poisoning. An Analysis of 105 Cases, A.M.A. Arch. Ind. Hyg., 1:90, 1950.

Smith, G., I. M. Ledingham, G. R. Sharp, J. N. Norman, and E. H. Bates: Treatment of Coal Gas Poisoning with Oxygen at 2 Atmospheres Pressure, Lancet, I:816, 1962.

Castor Bean

Brugsch, H. G.: The Castor Bean, New Engl. J. Med., 262:1039, 1960.

Caustics

Haller, J. A., and K. Bachman: The Comparative Effect of Current Therapy on Experimental Caustic Burns of the Esophagus, Pediatrics, 34:236, 1964.

Yarington, C. T., Jr.: Ingestion of Caustic; a Pediatric Problem, J. Pediat., 67:674, 1965.

Chlorinated Insecticides

Finley, A. H., and R. J. Haggerty: Toxic Hazards, Insecticides. Chlorinated Hydrocarbons, New Engl. J. Med., 258:812, 1958.

Zavon, M. R.: Chlorinated Hydrocarbon Insecticides, J.A.M.A., 190:595, 1964.

Cholinesterase Inhibitor Insecticides

Heath, D. F.: "Organophosphorus Poisons," Oxford, Pergamon Press, 1961.

Hobbiger, F.: Reactivation of Phosphorylated Acetylcholinesterase, in "Cholinesterases and Anticholinesterase Agents," Handb. Exp. Pharmak., Suppl. 15:921, 1963.

Mann, J. B.: Diagnostic Aids in Organophosphate Poisoning, Ann. Intern. Med., 67:905, 1967.

Quinby, G. E.: Further Therapeutic Experience with Pralidoximes in Organic Phosphorus Poisoning, J.A.M.A., 187:202, 1964.

Wyckoff, D. W., J. E. Davies, A. Barquet, and J. H. Davis: Diagnostic and Therapeutic Problems of Parathion Poisonings, Ann. Intern. Med., 68:875, 1968.

Cyanide

Chen, K. K., and C. L. Rose: Treatment of Acute Cyanide Poisoning, J.A.M.A., 162:1154, 1956.

Cope, C.: The Importance of Oxygen in the Treatment of Cyanide Poisoning, J.A.M.A., 175:1061, 1961.

Pijoan, M.: Cyanide Poisoning from Choke Cherry Seed, Am. J. Med. Sci., 204:550, 1942.

Detergents

Arena, J. M.: Poisonings and Other Health Hazards Associated with Use of Detergents, J.A.M.A., 190:56, 1964.

Cann, H. M., and H. L. Verhulst: Toxicity of Household Soap and Detergents and Treatment of their Ingestion, Am. J. Dis. Child., 100:287, 1960.

Fluorides

Peters, J. H.: Therapy of Acute Fluoride Poisoning, Am. J. Med. Sci., 216:278, 1948.

Glycols

Haggerty, R. J.: Toxic Hazards, Deaths from Permanent Anti-freeze Ingestion, New Engl. J. Med., 261:1296, 1959.

Peterson, D. I., J. E. Peterson, M. G. Hardinge, and W. E. C. Wacker: Experimental Treatment of Ethylene Glycol Poisoning, J. Am. Med. Ass., 186:965, 1963.

Pons, C. A., and R. P. Custer: Acute Ethylene Glycol Poisoning: A Clinicopathologic Report of Eighteen Fatal Cases, Am. J. Med. Sci., 211:544, 1946.

Halogenated Hydrocarbons

Browning, E.: Toxicology of Organic Compounds of Industrial Importance, Ann. Rev. Pharmacol., 1:397, 1961.

Myatt, A. V., and J. A. Salmons: Carbon Tetrachloride Poisoning, Arch. Ind. Hyg. Occup. Med., 6:74, 1952.

Oettingen, W. F. von: "The Halogenated Hydrocarbons of Industrial and Toxicological Importance," Amsterdam, Elsevier Publishing Company, 1964.

Ipecac, Emetine

Smith, R. P., and D. M. Smith: Acute Ipecac Poisoning, New Engl. J. Med., 265:523, 1961.

Welchman, J. M.: The Cardiac Toxicity of Emetine, J. Trop. Med. Hyg., 60:296, 1957.

Iron Salts

Covey, T. J.: Ferrous Sulfate Poisoning: Review, Case Summaries and Therapeutic Regimen, J. Pediat., 64:218, 1964.

Jacobs, J., H. Greene, and B. R. Gendel: Acute Iron Intoxication, New Engl. J. Med., 273:1124, 1965.

Leikin, S.: Deferoxamine as a Chelating Agent, J. Pediat., 72:148, 1968.

Isopropyl Alcohol

Freireich, A. W., T. J. Cinque, G. Xanthaky, and D. Landau: Hemodialysis for Isopropanol Poisoning, New Engl. J. Med., 277:699, 1967.

Methyl Alcohol

Bennett, I. L., Jr., F. H. Cary, G. L. Mitchell, Jr., and M. N. Cooper: Acute Methyl Alcohol Poisoning: A Review Based on Experiences in an Outbreak of 323 Cases, Medicine, 32:431, 1953.

Cooper, J. R., and M. M. Kini: Biochemical Aspects of Methanol Poisoning, Biochem. Pharmacol., 11:405, 1962.

Setter, J. G., R. Singh, N. C. Brackett, Jr., and R. E. Randall, Jr.: Studies on the Dialysis of Methanol, Trans. Am. Soc. Artificial Internal Organs, 13:178, 1967.

Smith, M. E.: Interrelations in Ethanol and Methanol Metabolism, J. Pharmacol., 134:233, 1961.

Mushrooms

Buck, R. W.: Mushroom Toxins—A Brief Review of the Literature, New Engl. J. Med., 265:681, 1961.

Grossman, C. M., and B. Malbin: Mushroom Poisoning: A Review of the Literature and Report of Two Cases Caused by a Previously Undescribed Species, Ann. Intern. Med., 40:249, 1954.

Naphthalene

Haggerty, R. J.: Naphthalene Poisoning, New Engl. J. Med., 255:919, 1956.

Nicotine

Oberst, B. B., and R. A. McIntyre: Acute Nicotine Poisoning, Pediatrics, 11:338, 1953.

Nitrites

Bucklin, R., and M. K. Myint: Fatal Methemoglobinemia due to Well Water Nitrates, Ann. Intern. Med., 52:703, 1960.

Petroleum Distillates

Browning, E.: "Toxicity and Metabolism of Industrial Solvents," Amsterdam, Elsevier Publishing Company, 1965.

Jacobziner, H., and H. W. Raybin: Kerosene and Other Petroleum Distillate Poisonings, N.Y. J. Med., 63:3428, 1963.

Lawton, J. J., Jr., and C. P. Malmquist: Gasoline Addiction in Children, Psychiat. Quart., 35:555, 1961.

Mayock, R. L., N. Bozorgnia, and H. F. Zinsser: Kerosene Pneumonitis Treated with Adrenal Steroids, Ann. Intern. Med., 54:559, 1961.

Subcommittee on Accidental Poisoning: Cooperative Kerosene Poisoning Study, Pediatrics, 29:648, 1962.

Phosphorus

Arena, J. M.: Phosphorus Poisoning, Clin. Ped., 2:132, 1963.

Diaz-Rivera, R. S., P. J. Collazo, E. R. Pons, and M. V. Torregrosa: Acute Phosphorus Poisoning in Man; a Study of 56 Cases, Medicine, 29:269, 1950.

Fletcher, G. F., and J. T. Galambos: Phosphorus Poisoning in Humans, Arch. Intern. Med., 112:846, 1963.

Salicylates

Done, A. K.: Salicylate Intoxication; Significance of Measurements of Salicylate in Blood in Cases of Acute Ingestions, Pediatrics, 26:800, 1960.

——: Salicylate Poisoning, J.A.M.A., 192:770, 1965.

——: Treatment of Salicylate Poisoning, Mod. Treatment, 4:648, 1967.

Dukes, D. C., J. D. Bainey, G. Cumming, and G. Widdowson: Treatment of Severe Aspirin Poisoning, Lancet, II:329, 1963.

Segar, W. E., and M. A. Holliday: Physiologic Abnormalities of Salicylate Intoxication, New Engl. J. Med., 259:1191, 1958.

Singer, R. B.: The Acid-Base Disturbance in Salicylate Intoxication, Medicine, 33:1, 1954.

Summitt, R. L., and J. N. Etteldorf: Salicylate Intoxication in Children. Experience with Peritoneal Dialysis and Alkalinization of the Urine, J. Pediat., 64:803, 1964.

117 HEAVY METALS

Ivan L. Bennett, Jr. and David C. Poskanzer

Three highly effective chemicals, BAL, Versene, and penicillamine, are now available for treatment of systemic poisoning with heavy metals by forming nontoxic, stable cyclic compounds with polyvalent metallic ions, thus permitting the offending material to be excreted safely in the urine.

The first to be developed was BAL (British antilewisite, 2,3-dimercaptopropanol, dimercaprol), which was originally intended as an antidote against the arsenical war gas, lewisite. Its tendency to combine with certain metallic ions such as arsenic, mercury, cobalt, nickel, antimony, and gold is so great that it can remove them from combination with the enzymes whose function they impair in the body. BAL is not useful in the treatment of lead poisoning. Because the effectiveness of BAL depends to some extent upon the speed with which its administration is begun, every attempt should be made to avoid delay in its use. For serious systemic intoxications, BAL should be given in doses of 4 mg per kg body weight intramuscularly as a 10% solution in oil and 20% benzyl benzoate. No single dose should exceed 300 mg. This dose should be repeated every 4 hr on the first day and every 6 hr on the second day. Thereafter, it should be given three times daily for several days; doses should then be tapered and discontinued about 10 days after acute poisoning. When the dose of poison has been relatively small, the schedule of BAL administration may be reduced by one-third. Because BAL is excreted in part by the kidneys, it can accumulate to toxic concentrations in anuric patients. Overdosage results in nervousness, hyperactivity, muscle twitching, and hyperreflexia. Large doses may produce convulsions. The presence of the material in tears sometimes causes blepharospasm. In patients with anuria or oliguria, therefore, BAL should be administered with caution and at a lower dosage than outlined above. If too much is given, sedatives should be administered.

The second antidote to metal poisons is the chelating agent Versene (ethylenediaminetetraacetate, EDTA), which forms cyclic, stable, soluble, nontoxic compounds with most metals. Because Versene reacts with calcium in the same way as with other metals, it must be given as the calcium salt (Calcium Disodium Versenate; calcium disodiumedetate) to avoid hypocalcemia. The material has been used with notable success in the treatment of lead poisoning.

It is given in a dosage of 500 mg in 250 ml of 5% glucose IV every 12 hr for 5 days. After a pause to allow for further solution of metal from body stores a second and even a third course may be given.

Penicillamine (cuprimine, beta, beta-dimethylcysteine) is an excellent chelating agent for copper, mercury, and lead, promotes their excretion in the urine, and has the additional advantage of being well absorbed from the gastrointestinal tract. It may be given orally, while BAL and Versene require systemic injection. N-acetyl-*dl*-penicillamine is even more effective than penicillamine in protecting against the effects of mercury, probably because it is more resistant to metabolic degradation and is less toxic. Penicillamine is administered orally in a dose of 1 to 4 Gm daily on an empty stomach to avoid chelation of dietary metals. It has much lower toxicity compared to BAL, the only other agent which is effective in the treatment of Wilson's disease (hepatolenticular degeneration), in which toxic amounts of copper are deposited in various tissues, but has the disadvantage of acute sensitivity reactions. It has also been shown to be useful in lead poisoning, but the excretion of urinary lead may not be as high after oral penicillamine as after intravenous Calcium Disodium Versenate.

N-acetyl-*dl*-penicillamine, though still an investigational drug, has been demonstrated to be effective in mercury poisoning and has the advantage of allowing much higher doses with fewer toxic effects. It has less effect on copper levels than penicillamine and is therefore used in the treatment of mercury poisoning when one would wish to maintain copper levels. Courses of 10 days of 1 to 2 Gm daily in divided doses have been employed in patients with good results.

ANTIMONY

Symptoms of poisoning after the ingestion of antimony may occur when an acid food is allowed to stand in cheap enamelware or "graniteware" for a sufficient time to allow solution of antimony, which is used in the manufacture of these products. The symptoms are similar to those produced by arsenic, except that antimony causes a more rapid onset of gastrointestinal symptoms. Treatment is the same as for arsenic, including BAL. Circulatory collapse occurs early and requires vigorous supportive treatment. The therapeutic injection of antimony (tartar emetic, etc.) may result in severe coughing, muscle and joint pains, or bradycardia. The last is an indication for stopping medication (See Chap. 267).

ARSENIC

Arsenic poisoning is usually the result of accidental or suicidal ingestion of insecticides or rodenticides containing Paris green (copper acetoarsenate) or calcium or lead arsenate. Pesticides containing arsenic are a frequent source of poisoning in rural areas of the United States. Medications such as Fowler's solution (potassium arsenite) and the organic arsenicals (arsphenamines and arsenoxides) were once common causes of intoxication.

The toxic dose of inorganic arsenic varies considerably and seems to depend upon individual susceptibility. Orchardists have been found to ingest as much as 6.8 mg arsenic a day without any signs of intoxication. On the other hand, as little as 30 mg arsenic trioxide has been fatal. Arsenic has a predilection for keratin, and the concentration of arsenic in the hair and nails is higher than that in other tissues. Arsenic reacts with the —SH groups in certain tissue proteins and thus interferes with a number of enzyme systems essential to cellular metabolism. Pathologic changes in fatal inorganic arsenical poisoning are fatty degeneration of the liver, hyperemia and hemorrhages of the gut, and renal tubular necrosis. The peripheral nerves often show fragmentation and resorption of myelin with disintegration of axis cylinders.

The symptoms of acute poisoning by the oral route are nausea, vomiting, diarrhea, severe burning of the mouth and throat, and agonizing abdominal pains. The vomitus often contains blood. Circulatory collapse is frequent, and death may ensue within a few hours. With chronic exposure, the first signs of poisoning are usually weakness, prostration, muscular aching, or nervous system involvement; gastrointestinal symptoms are minimal. In patients exposed to arsine gas (hydrogen arsenide), the outstanding features are hemolysis, chills, fever, and hemoglobinuria.

Patients who recover from acute poisoning and those with chronic intoxication usually develop skin and mucosal changes, peripheral neuropathy, and linear pigmentations in the fingernails (see Chap. 354). The *cutaneous manifestations* appear within 1 to 4 weeks and consist of a diffuse, dry, scaly desquamation, occasionally with hyperpigmentation, over the trunk and extremities. Hyperkeratoses of the palms and soles and edema of the face and extremities may also occur. The mucous membranes also show evidence of irritation, with conjunctivitis, photophobia, pharyngitis, or irritating cough. About 5 weeks after exposure to arsenic, a transverse white stria, 1 to 2 mm in width, appears above the lunula of each fingernail (*Mees lines*). Patients with more than one exposure to arsenic may show double lines several millimeters apart.

Symptoms of headache, drowsiness, confusion, and convulsions are seen in both acute and chronic intoxication. Evidence of peripheral neuropathy usually appears 1 to 3 weeks after exposure. There are numbness, tingling, and burning of the feet and hands followed by muscular weakness. The extremities show a decrease in touch, pain, and temperature sensations, in a symmetrical "stocking-glove" distribution, and distal weakness with inability to walk or stand, weakness of grip, and wrist drop. Tendon reflexes are absent or diminished, and atrophy of the affected muscles develops rapidly.

The laboratory findings usually consist of moderate anemia and a leukopenia of 2,000 to 5,000 white blood cells with mild eosinophilia. There is slight proteinuria, and liver function tests show mild abnormalities. The spinal fluid is normal.

None of the clinical or laboratory manifestations of arsenic poisoning is specific, and the diagnosis depends upon analysis of the hair and urine for arsenic. Normal individuals have an average concentration of 0.05 mg arsenic per 100 mg of hair, with a range of 0.025 to 0.088 mg. Concentrations of arsenic greater than 0.1 mg per 100 mg of hair are indicative of poisoning. The minimal level of arsenic in the urine indicating intoxication is difficult to establish. Normal persons have been found to excrete between 0.01 and 0.06 mg of arsenic per liter, and a few individuals as much as 0.2 mg per liter. Although there is considerable overlap, most patients with evidence of arsenic intoxication will be found to excrete more than 0.1 mg per liter; soon after acute exposure, many will show levels greater than 1 mg per liter.

The treatment for acute ingestion is gastric lavage (see Chap. 115). Replacement of lost fluids and elevation of blood pressure by vasopressor agents is often indicated. Immediate treatment with BAL should be instituted. Patients with peripheral neuropathy rarely show significant improvement with BAL and continue to have sensory disturbances and weakness for many months. Dramatic responses, however, have been observed with the use of BAL in the treatment of exfoliative dermatitis, bone marrow depression, and encephalopathy caused by the arsphenamines and the organic arsenicals. BAL is of little value in the treatment of the hemolysis caused by inhalation of arsine.

BISMUTH

Poisoning by bismuth is almost entirely a complication of antisyphilitic therapy. Toxic manifestations may appear in the mouth (gingivitis, followed by stomatitis), the kidneys (albuminuria and nephrotic syndrome), or the skin (exfoliative dermatitis), requiring immediate interruption of bismuth injections. The development of a bluish stippled line of pigmentation just at the margin of the gums is not dangerous but suggests that oral hygiene should be improved. Bismuth subnitrate occasionally gives rise to methemoglobinemia (Chap. 344).

CADMIUM

Poisoning is likely to occur after ingestion of an acid food prepared in a cadmium-lined vessel. The classic example is lemonade served from metal cans. Symptoms of nausea, vomiting, diarrhea, and prostration usually develop within 10 min after ingestion. Treatment is symptomatic, and symptoms ordinarily subside within 24 hr. The short incubation and the typical circumstances suggest the diagnosis. Inhalation of cadmium fumes in industry produces an acute, extremely severe pneumonitis (Chap. 288). The use of BAL is not recommended for cadmium intoxication, as the BAL-cadmium complex dissociates in the kidneys and cadmium is nephrotoxic.

COPPER

Acute poisoning due to ingestion of copper salts is rare. Copper sulfate (blue vitriol) is the chief offender, in which case the vomitus has a characteristic blue color. Manifestations are nausea, vomiting, bloody diarrhea, headache, severe thirst, and tachycardia. In fatal cases, death is preceded by convulsions. Treatment consists of gastric lavage with 1% solution of potassium ferrocyanide, fluid replacement, and control of pain and diarrhea with opiates.

GOLD

Because practically all cases of poisoning by gold are associated with its use in the treatment of arthritis, diagnosis is usually easy. Manifestations are skin rashes of various types, bone marrow depression, icterus, oliguria, nausea, vomiting, and gastrointestinal bleeding. Treatment consists of symptomatic relief of discomfort and the use of BAL, an effective antidote.

LEAD

Poisoning results from ingestion of lead-containing materials such as paint or water which has stood in lead pipes or from inhalation of fumes from burning storage batteries, solder, etc. Illicit whiskey contaminated by lead solder in the pipes of stills has been responsible for many cases of poisoning. Bullets or buckshot containing lead can cause poisoning years after becoming embedded in a serous cavity. Absorption is slow by any route, and prolonged exposure is required for the development of symptoms. Lead is a cumulative poison, excreted slowly. Acute poisoning is virtually nonexistent, although it was observed when lead was used for the treatment of malignant disease. Symptoms may develop suddenly after chronic exposure. Most of the absorbed lead is deposited in the bones; blood, urine, and feces contain only small amounts.

Manifestations of poisoning are colic, encephalopathy, peripheral neuritis, and anemia.

Lead colic, or painter's cramps, is characterized by agonizing, wandering, poorly localized abdominal pain, often with spasm and rigidity of the musculature of the abdominal wall. There is no fever or leukocytosis. Needless surgery has been carried out in these patients for supposed perforation of peptic ulcer or other catastrophe. Morphine has surprisingly little effect upon the pain; intravenous injection of calcium salts affords relief within a short time, although pain may recur. Attacks of colic seem to be brought on by intercurrent infection or alcoholic overindulgence.

Encephalopathy occurs chiefly in children and is manifested by convulsions, somnolence, mania, delirium, or coma. Mortality is high when convulsive seizures and coma occur. Mental enfeeblement is a common sequel.

Peripheral neuritis with paralysis, characteristically involving the muscles most used (e.g., wrist drop in painters, etc.), occurs in patients exposed to lead, often in the absence of other symptoms. It is rare in children. (See Chap. 354.)

Mild anemia, probably the result of increased brittleness of the erythrocytes as well as of a defect in cell maturation, is common. Pallor is out of proportion to anemia in patients with chronic plumbism and is attributed to spasm of small vessels in the skin. Anemia is almost never severe and is characterized by the presence of large numbers of erythrocytes with basophilic stippling. This is seen in other hematologic disorders, but a smear showing stippling should arouse suspicion of lead poisoning. In patients with poor oral hygiene a "lead line" of black lead sulfide may develop along the gingival margins. This is not seen in edentulous persons and is rare in children.

Patients with lead poisoning excrete increased amounts of coproporphyrin III in the urine (see Chap. 108). This is so consistent that examination of a urine specimen for porphyrin is the best screening test in suspected cases. A few milliliters of urine should be acidified with acetic acid and shaken with an equal volume of ether. Exposure of a specimen prepared in this manner under a Woods lamp will reveal reddish fluorescence of the ether layer if coproporphyrin is present. A positive test is strongly in favor of lead intoxication. Urinary lead determinations are of aid in confirming the diagnosis; a level of 0.2 mg per liter or more is usually regarded as significant, although interpretations vary.

Lead encephalopathy occurs chiefly in children, has a significant mortality, and causes severe permanent brain damage in 25 percent of survivors. Encephalopathy in adults is rare and usually results from consumption of lead-contaminated illicit liquor (moonshine). Once minor symptoms of poisoning are present, acute encephalopathy can develop with unpredictable rapidity. Any child with symptoms suggestive of lead poisoning should be considered a medical emergency and hospitalized immediately. The onset of encephalopathy is signaled by the development of gross ataxia, persistent vomiting, and intermittent lethargy and stupor. These symptoms are followed by convulsions, mania, and coma.

The most important single feature of treatment is removal of the patient from further exposure to lead. Once abnormal absorption is terminated, virtually all the lead in the body is shifted into bone. Chelating agents do not remove significant quantities of lead from bone. It takes approximately twice as long to excrete a given burden of lead as it does to accumulate it. As long as significant quantities of lead remain in bone any intercurrent illness which causes demineralization can cause mobilization of toxic quantities of lead into soft tissues and exacerbate plumbism.

The treatment of lead encephalopathy is begun once adequate urine flow is established. A combination of BAL and Calcium Sodium Versenate is employed, and the Versene therapy continued for 5 to 7 days. If Calcium Disodium Versenate is given alone in the presence of very high tissue concentrations of lead, some of the toxic effects may be intensified. Acute symptoms usually subside within 48 to 72 hr after Versene is begun. Within 2 weeks urinary excretion of copro-porphyrin ceases, and there is sometimes a dramatic improvement in neuritis.

Symptoms of acute increased intracranial pressure are best treated with repeated doses of mannitol intravenously. Evidence for the use of high potency steroids to relieve cerebral edema in patients with lead encephalopathy is incomplete. Treatment of increased intracranial pressure by surgical decompression is no longer indicated.

In adults combined therapy with BAL and Calcium Disodium Versenate followed by oral penicillamine is probably indicated whenever blood levels exceed 100 mg lead per 100 Cm blood even in the absence of symptoms. Evidence of lead toxicity is usually present at this level, and the risk of symptomatic episodes is considerable. The use of oral penicillamine alone in a dose of 1 to 1.5 Gm daily for 3 to 5 days in mildly symptomatic cases has been suggested and has the advantage of easy administration and the avoidance of painful injections.

MERCURY

Poisoning occurs chiefly as a result of the acute ingestion of a soluble salt, usually mercuric chloride (bichloride of mercury). Toxic symptoms may occur with 0.1 Gm, and 0.5 Gm is almost always fatal unless immediate treatment is instituted. The mercuric ion is corrosive and produces severe local inflammation. Oral, pharyngeal, and laryngeal pain are severe; abdominal cramps with nausea and vomiting occur within 15 min. As mercury is absorbed, it is concentrated in the kidneys, where it poisons the tubular cells, producing a tendency to diuresis within the first 2 to 3 hr. The combination of vomiting, dehydration, shock, and progressive tubular damage, however, soon leads to anuria and uremia. The poison is also excreted into the colon and produces severe enteritis with bloody diarrhea and tenesmus. Death is usually from uremia. The chief objectives of treatment are to prevent the shock of dehydration and to remove mercury from the body. Early in treatment, copious quantities of fluid should be infused intravenously to prevent dehydration and to reduce the concentration of mercuric ion in the renal tubules. That the patient is anuric early is often simply the result of dehydration and shock. In such instances, forcing fluids is advisable. However, the gradual development of oliguria and anuria in a hydrated patient indicates renal damage by mercury, and at this stage a regimen for acute renal shutdown should be instituted (Chap. 300).

Chronic poisoning from metallic mercury vapor occurs in individuals exposed to large amounts of the metal in laboratories or in industry and occasionally as a result of prolonged therapeutic use, as in vaginal douches. Manifestations may be those of subacute poisoning, with salivation, stomatitis, and diarrhea or primary neurologic signs, including tremors of the extremities, tongue, and lips, ataxia and dysarthria, erethism, a state of easy embarrassment, irritability, apprehension, withdrawal, and depression.

Some poison can be removed from the body by gastric

lavage, but more important in treatment is the binding of the mercuric ion in a harmless compound by BAL. The therapeutic usefulness of BAL depends on its immediate administration. In chronic mercury poisoning, N-acetyl-*dl*-penicillamine may well be the drug of choice. It can be administered orally and appears to selectively chelate mercury with considerably less effect on copper, which is essential to many metabolic processes.

SILVER

Most poisoning by silver involves silver nitrate, a caustic salt. There are intense nausea, vomiting, and diarrhea after swallowing nitrate (lunar caustic), and death from shock may occur within a few hours. The mouth is usually deeply stained by silver nitrate. Treatment is entirely supportive, with fluid replacement and control of pain.

Chronic exposure (usually to nose drops) produces a peculiar bluish skin discoloration (argyria).

THALLIUM

Thallium is a component of certain rodenticides and depilatories, and clinical poisoning is usually a result of accidental ingestion of these materials. The fatal dose is approximately 1.0 Gm. Manifestations are vomiting, diarrhea, and leg pains, followed by weakness and paralysis of the legs. There may be visual and mental disturbances. About 3 weeks after poisoning, the patient's hair falls out, providing a strong diagnostic clue if the cause has not previously been determined. Treatment is symptomatic. The alopecia is temporary if the patient recovers.

REFERENCES

Levine, W. G.: Heavy-Metal Antagonists, pp. 929–942 in *The Pharmacological Basis of Therapeutics*, 3d ed., Louis S. Goodman and Alfred Gilman (Eds.), New York: The Macmillan Company, 1965.

Arsenic

Jenkins, R. B.: Inorganic Arsenic and the Nervous System, Brain, 89:479, 1966.
Keusler, C. J., J. C. Abels, and C. P. Rhoads: Arsine Poisoning, Mode of Action and Treatment, J. Pharmacol. Exp. Therap., 88:99, 1946.
Longcope, W. T., and J. A. Luetscher: The Use of BAL (British Antilewisite) in the Treatment of the Injurious Effects of Arsenic, Mercury, and Other Metallic Poisons, Ann. Intern. Med., 31:545, 1949.

Bismuth

Heyman, A.: Systemic Manifestations of Bismuth Toxicity; Observations on 4 Patients with Pre-existent Kidney Disease, Am. J. Syph., Gonor., Vener. Dis., 28:721, 1944.

Cadmium

Ross, P.: Cadmium Poisoning, Brit. Med. J., 1:252, 1944.

Gold

Strauss, J. F., Sr., R. M. Barrett, and E. F. Rosenberg: BAL Treatment of Toxic Reactions to Gold: A Review of the Literature and Report of Two Cases, Ann. Intern. Med., 37:323, 1952.

Lead

Aub, J. C., L. T. Fairhall, A. S. Minot, and P. Reznikoff: Lead Poisoning, Medicine, 4:1, 1925.
Chisolm, J. J., Jr.: Treatment of Lead Poisoning, Mod. Treatment, 4:710, 1967.

Mercury

Arena, J. M.: Treatment of Mercury Poisoning, Mod. Treatment, 4:734, 1967.
Doolan, P. D., W. C. Hess, and L. R. Kyle: Acute Renal Insufficiency Due to Dichloride of Mercury: Observations on Gastrointestinal Hemorrhage and BAL Therapy, New Engl. J. Med., 249:273, 1953.
Hirschman, S. Z., M. Feingold, and G. Boylen: Mercury in House Paint as a Cause of Acrodynia, New Engl. J. Med., 269:889, 1963.

Thallium

Munch, J. C.: Human Thallotoxicosis, J.A.M.A., 102:1929, 1934.

118   ALCOHOL
Maurice Victor and Raymond D. Adams

Intemperance creates many problems in modern society, the importance of which can be judged by the repeated emphasis they receive in contemporary writings, both literary and scientific, as well as from health, social, and religious agencies. These problems may be divided into three categories—psychologic, medical, and sociologic. The main psychologic problem is why a person drinks excessively, often with full knowledge that such action will result in physical injury to himself and irreparable harm to his family. The medical problem embraces all the diseases which relate to overindulgence in alcohol. The sociologic problem comprises the effects of sustained inebriety on the family and community.

The various problems raised by excessive drinking cannot be separated from one another, and the physician must therefore be conversant with all aspects of the subject. He may be asked to help the patient conquer his alcoholic tendency or to diagnose and to treat the numerous diseases to which he is subject; often he must admit or commit the patient to a general or mental hospital, according to the nature of the presenting clinical disorder; and lastly, he may be required to enlist the aid of available social agencies when their services are needed by either the patient or his family.

Alcoholism has been defined as both a chronic disease and a disorder of behavior, characterized in either context by the repeated drinking of alcoholic beverages to an extent that exceeds customary dietary use or surpasses the social drinking customs of the community and that interferes with the drinker's health, interpersonal relations, or economic functioning. Stated more succinctly, it is alcoholic addiction. The precise number of such individuals, commonly known as alcoholics, in the United States is not known. The estimate is 5 million—approximately 4 percent of the total adult population. It requires little projection of the imagination to conceive the havoc wrought by alcohol in terms of decreased productivity, accidents, crime, mental and physical disease, and disruption of family life.

PHARMACOLOGY AND METABOLISM OF ALCOHOL

Ethyl alcohol, or ethanol, is the active ingredient in beer, wine, whiskey, gin, brandy, and other less common alcoholic beverages. In addition, the stronger spirits contain enanthic ethers, which give the flavor but have no important pharmacologic properties, and impurities such as amyl alcohol (fusel oil) and acetaldehyde, which act like alcohol but are more toxic. Contrary to prevailing opinion, the content of B vitamins in American beer and other liquors is so low as to offer little or no protection against avitaminosis.

Alcohol is absorbed unaltered from the gastrointestinal tract, about 80 percent from the intestine and the remainder from the stomach. Its presence may be detected in the blood within 5 min after ingestion, and the maximum concentration is reached in ½ to 2 hr. The ingestion of milk and fatty foods impedes and water facilitates its absorption. In habituated persons the blood alcohol concentration rises somewhat faster and reaches a higher maximum than in abstainers.

Alcohol is carried chiefly in the plasma and enters the various organs of the body, as well as the spinal fluid, urine, and pulmonary alveolar air, in concentrations which bear a constant relationship to that in the blood. Elimination of alcohol is accomplished chiefly by oxidation, 5 percent or less being excreted chemically unchanged in the urine, sweat, and breath. The energy liberated by the oxidation of alcohol (7 Cal per Gm) can be utilized as completely as that of fats, sugars, and proteins, which it replaces isodynamically. It should be emphasized that alcohol cannot be stored in the body or used in the replacement of destroyed tissue. Unless, therefore, the protein intake is adequate, a state of negative nitrogen balance will develop, a common finding in chronic alcoholics.

The first step in the metabolism of alcohol is accomplished mainly in the liver, where alcohol dehydrogenase oxidizes alcohol to acetaldehyde. The latter substance may be further metabolized in the liver or carried to other tissues, where it is converted, possibly via the stage of free acetate, to acetyl coenzyme A, of which the acetate portion can be oxidized completely to carbon dioxide and water.

For all practical purposes it may be accepted that once absorption is ended and an equilibrium established with the tissues, ethyl alcohol is oxidized at a constant rate, independent of its concentration in the blood. Actually, slightly more alcohol is burned per hour when the initial concentrations are very high, but this increment is of little clinical significance. On the other hand, the rate of oxidation of acetaldehyde does depend on its concentration in the tissues. This fact is of importance in connection with the drug disulfiram (Antabuse), which increases the tissue concentration necessary to metabolize a certain amount of acetaldehyde per unit of time. The patient taking both Antabuse and alcohol will accumulate an inordinate amount of acetaldehyde, resulting in nausea, vomiting, and hypotension, sometimes pronounced and even fatal in degree. This pharmacologic principle underlies the treatment of alcoholism with Antabuse.

Very few factors capable of increasing the rate of alcohol metabolism are known. There is some evidence that repeated ingestion induces an increased rate of metabolism of alcohol, and this holds true for both normal and alcoholic subjects. The rate of alcohol metabolism may also be increased by the administration of insulin and perhaps amino acids, but neither of these has proved to make a significant difference in the treatment of intoxication. On the other hand, starvation slows the rate of alcohol metabolism in the liver, although this varies greatly in degree from one individual to another.

PHYSIOLOGIC AND PSYCHOLOGIC EFFECTS OF ALCOHOL

The immediate effects of alcohol on organs other than the central nervous system are relatively unimportant. There appears to be a direct action on the excitability and contractility of heart muscle. With intoxicating doses there is a rise in cardiac rate and output, systolic and pulse pressures, and there is cutaneous vasodilatation at the expense of splanchnic constriction. Prolonged intoxication has led on occasion to cardiac and skeletal myopathy, a degeneration of fibers due, it is said, to suppression of myophosphorylase activity. Increased sweating and vasodilatation cause a loss of body heat and a fall in temperature. In low concentrations, by whatever route it is administered, alcohol is capable of stimulating the gastric glands to produce acid, apparently by causing the tissues to form or release histamine. With the ingestion of alcohol in concentrations of over 10 to 15 percent the secretion of mucus is increased, the stomach mucosa becomes congested and hyperemic, and the secretion of acid then becomes depressed. This is a state of acute gastritis, from which recovery is relatively rapid. The increase in appetite following ingestion of alcohol is due to the stimulation of the end organs of taste and to a general sense of well-being. Similarly, the reviving effect of alcohol in fatigue states is a cerebral one, not due to a direct stimulating effect on muscle or other organs.

Alcohol has an effect on intermediary metabolism in the liver cells, particularly lipid metabolism (see Chap.

323), and also exerts a distinct effect on the renal excretion of water and electrolytes. The ingestion of 4 oz 100 proof bourbon whiskey, for example, results in a diuresis qualitatively indistinguishable from that which follows the drinking of large amounts of water. This diuresis is most likely due to the transient suppression of the release of antidiuretic hormone (ADH) from the neurohypophysis, since a relatively small amount of alcohol injected directly into a carotid artery evokes a prompt diuresis without a detectable rise in the concentration of alcohol in the systemic blood. The exact locus of action within the supraopticohypophyseal system is unknown. Alcohol does not alter the sensitivity of the kidney tubules to endogenous or exogenous ADH (Pitressin) and has no discernible effect on renal hemodynamic function in normal persons. The degree of diuresis seems to be more closely related to the duration of the rising blood alcohol level than to the rate of increase or the absolute level attained. In recumbent persons, the water diuresis following the ingestion of alcohol is associated with a diminished excretion of electrolytes (Na, K, Cl), presumably because of vasodilatation and the consequent redistribution of the circulating blood volume. There is also an increased urinary excretion of ammonium and titratable acidity following alcohol, owing to a mild degree of both metabolic and respiratory acidosis. The former is presumably due to an accumulation of acid metabolites and the latter to the direct action of alcohol on the respiratory center.

If the period of alcohol intoxication is sustained, the effects are somewhat different. Diuresis occurs only during the initial phase of alcohol administration and does not persist during prolonged drinking. However, hematocrit levels decrease and serum osmolality and sodium levels rise, even if dietary and vitamin intake is adequate. These derangements tend to resolve spontaneously after cessation of drinking and cannot be explained by the known diuretic or hormonal changes induced by ethanol ingestion.

Apart from the derangements noted above, the obvious effects of acute, nonlethal doses of alcohol are those exerted on the nervous system, constituting the characteristic symptoms and signs of alcohol intoxication. A large body of data has accumulated regarding the psychomotor effects of alcohol, the nature of tolerance, and the relation of blood alcohol levels to various manifestations of intoxication. Only the most pertinent data are presented here.

It is now generally accepted that alcohol is not a stimulant of the central nervous system, but a depressant. Some of the early effects of alcohol, manifested by garrulousness, aggressiveness, excessive activity and increased electrical excitability of the cerebral cortex, suggest a state of stimulation. There is evidence, however, that the initial action of alcohol is to depress certain subcortical structures (?high brainstem reticular formation) which ordinarily modulate or inhibit cerebral cortical activity. Similarly, the initial hyperactivity of tendon reflexes may represent a transitory escape of spinal motor neurones from higher inhibitory centers.

With increasing amounts of alcohol, however, the depressant action spreads to involve the cerebral cortical neurones directly, as well as other cerebral and spinal neurones.

All manner of motor performance, whether simply the maintenance of a standing posture, the control of speech and eye movements, or highly organized and complex motor skills are adversely affected by alcohol. The movements involved in these acts are not only slower than normal, but more inaccurate and random in character and therefore less well adapted to the accomplishment of specific ends.

Alcohol also impairs the efficiency of mental function by interfering with the learning process, which is slowed and rendered less effective. The faculty of forming associations, whether in the form of words or of figures, tends to be hampered, and the power of attention and concentration is reduced. The individual is not as versatile as usual in directing thought along new lines appropriate to the problems at hand. Finally, alcohol impairs the faculties of judgment and discrimination and all in all the ability to think and reason clearly.

A scale relating the various degrees of clinical intoxication to the blood alcohol level in nonhabituated persons has been constructed by Miles. He found that at blood alcohol levels of 30 mg per 100 ml, a mild euphoria was detectable, and at 50 mg per 100 ml, a mild incoordination. At 100 mg per 100 ml, ataxia was obvious; at 300 mg per 100 ml, the patient was stuporous; and a level of 400 mg per 100 ml was accompanied by deep anesthesia and could prove fatal. These figures are valid, provided that the alcohol content rises steadily over a 2-hr period.

It should be emphasized that such a scale has virtually no value in the chronic alcoholic patient, for it does not take into account the adjustment which the organism makes to alcohol, i.e., the phenomenon of tolerance. It is common knowledge that a habituated individual can drink more and show fewer effects than the moderate drinker or abstainer. Talland studied a series of alcoholic subjects during a period of sustained inebriation, when they were ingesting between 30 and 40 oz 86 proof alcohol per day, and found practically no decrement in the performance of tasks designed to measure attention, motor skills, and reaction time to visual or auditory stimuli; the blood alcohol levels, at the time of testing of these subjects, ranged from 60 to 200 mg per 100 ml.

This phenomenon of tolerance accounts for the surprisingly large amounts of alcohol that can be consumed by the chronic inebriate without significant signs of drunkenness. Three patients studied at the Addiction Research Center in Lexington, Ky., for example, consumed 397 to 466 ml of 94 percent alcohol per day without showing any significant amounts of alcohol in the blood or clinical evidence of intoxication. In these patients, there was a very narrow margin between the doses associated with low blood alcohol levels and sobriety and the doses (430 to 479 ml daily) associated with high blood levels and drunkenness. Observations such as these would tend to invalidate the use of a single estimation of alcohol concentration as a reliable index of drunkenness. The organism is capable of adapting itself to the presence of alcohol after a very short exposure. If the alcohol concentration in the blood is raised very slowly, no symptoms appear, even at quite high levels. It would appear that the important factor in this rapid adaptability is not so much the rate of increment or the height of the blood alcohol level, but the length of time the alcohol had been present in the body. It has also been shown that, if the dosage of alcohol which just causes blood levels to be high is held constant, the blood alcohol concentration falls and clinical evidence of intoxication disappears. The cause of this fall in alcohol concentration is not clear. This type of tolerance has been referred to as "metabolic" in contrast to "tissue tolerance," which refers to the adjustments made by the nervous system to long-continued exposure to alcohol. The latter seems to depend on an altered nervous tissue response, i.e., a biochemical adaptation of the habituated individual enabling him to function more effectively at a given alcohol concentration. The precise nature of the adaptation is still a matter of conjecture. Undoubtedly some inborn factor plays a part in determining relative susceptibility. It is also conceivable that there is a psychologic adjustment to high concentrations of alcohol in nervous tissues. The habituated individual may learn to compensate for his lack of coordination and the removal of his inhibitions in a manner that would be impossible for the abstainer.

CLINICAL MANIFESTATIONS OF ALCOHOLISM

The clinical effects of alcohol are mainly on the digestive organs and on the nervous system. Each of these will now be considered.

EFFECT OF ALCOHOL ON THE DIGESTIVE ORGANS. Symptoms of disordered gastrointestinal function are particularly common in alcoholics, and of these the most distinctive are morning nausea and vomiting. Characteristically, the patient can suppress these symptoms by taking a drink or two, after which he is able to consume large quantities of alcohol without recurrence of nausea and vomiting, until the following morning. Since sufficient alcohol actually relieves these symptoms, they are probably not due to the local effects of alcohol on the stomach. Indeed, gastroscopic studies indicate that they are not related to gastritis but instead probably have a "central" origin and represent the mildest manifestations of the withdrawal syndrome (see below).

Other complaints referable to the gastrointestinal system are abdominal distension, epigastric distress, belching, typical or atypical ulcer symptoms, and hematemesis. The most common pathologic basis for these symptoms is a superficial gastritis which is an almost invariable sequel to prolonged drinking. Most instances of gastritis are benign, and the symptoms subside in a matter of days, but more severe forms are associated with mucosal erosions or ulcerations and may be the source of serious bleeding. The incidence of peptic ulcer is exceptionally high in the alcoholic population. A less frequent but serious cause of hematemesis is the so-called "Mallory-Weiss syndrome," which is characterized by lacerations of the gastric mucosa, occurring at or just below the gastroesophageal junction. In many of these cases bleeding is preceded by an episode of forceful vomiting or protracted retching; in others, the presence of a hiatus hernia or mucosal atrophy appears to be the predisposing factor. The typical lesions have been produced experimentally, in the cadaver, by occluding the esophagus and antrum and raising the intragastric pressure to 100 to 150 mm Hg, i.e., to the range of pressure attained by normal subjects during a period of induced straining and retching.

Patients admitted to the hospital following a period of prolonged drinking and severe dietary depletion almost invariably show enlargement of the liver due to infiltration of the parenchymal cells with fat. *Fatty hepatosis,* as this is called, is essentially a reversible state, providing the patient remains abstinent and receives a nutritious diet. About 10 percent of patients with severe alcoholism develop a permanent form of liver disease, i.e., *cirrhosis,* in which a diffuse proliferation of fibrous tissue destroys the normal lobular architecture of the organ. The alcoholic variety of cirrhosis (also referred to as *Laennec's* or *portal cirrhosis*); its complications and possible relationship to fatty liver are discussed in Chap. 328.

The excessive use of alcohol is also a significant factor in the causation of *pancreatitis*. The mildest form of this disorder may be attributed to gastritis or may go unnoticed, unless detected by a transient elevation of the serum amylase. Sometimes pancreatitis presents as an acute abdominal catastrophe, i.e., with epigastric pain, vomiting, and rigidity of the upper abdominal muscles. These symptoms closely simulate those of perforated peptic ulcer, so that an operation may be performed needlessly. In these circumstances the pancreas appears tense and edematous, often with a serosanguineous exudation of fluid on its surface. The most severe form of acute pancreatitis is characterized by widespread necrosis and hemorrhage (see Chap. 334).

It is generally believed that acute pancreatitis is caused by the activation of proteolytic enzymes with consequent autodigestion of the pancreatic tissue. Two factors are probably important in the pathogenesis: (1) the powerful stimulating effect of alcohol on the gastric acidity, which stimulates the production of secretin and which in turn provokes an increase in the formation of pancreatic enzymes; (2) obstruction to the flow of pancreatic enzymes, the result of inflammatory changes in the duodenum with edema and spasm of the sphincter of Oddi.

Alcoholics are also likely to develop a *chronic relapsing form of pancreatitis*. The type associated with irregular calcification of the pancreas is practically always associated with alcoholism. The etiology of this disorder is obscure, but the occurrence of chronic pancreatic changes in human nutritional disease (Kwashiorkor), as well as in certain experimental animals (rats given a methionine-deficient diet), suggests that it may be a deficiency disease. This subject is discussed further in Chap. 333.

THE EFFECT OF ALCOHOL ON THE NERVOUS SYSTEM. A large number of neurologic disorders are associated with alcoholism. The factor common to all of them, of course, is the abuse of alcohol, but the mechanism by which alcohol produces its effects is quite different from one group of disorders to another. The classification which follows is based on these mechanisms, insofar as they are known.

    I. Alcohol intoxication—drunkenness, coma, excitement ("pathologic intoxication")

    II. The abstinence or withdrawal syndrome—tremulousness, hallucinosis, "rum fits," delirium tremens and auditory hallucinosis

    III. Nutritional diseases of the nervous system secondary to alcoholism
        A. Wernicke-Korsakoff syndrome
        B. Polyneuropathy
        C. Retrobulbar neuropathy ("tobacco-alcohol amblyopia")
        D. Pellagra

    IV. Diseases of uncertain pathogenesis, associated with alcoholism
        A. Cerebellar degeneration
        B. Marchiafava-Bignami disease
        C. Central pontine myelinolysis
        D. Cerebral atrophy
        E. "Alcoholic" cardiomyopathy and myopathy

    V. Neurologic disorders consequent upon Laennec's cirrhosis and portal-systemic shunts
        A. Hepatic stupor and coma
        B. Chronic hepatocerebral degeneration

ALCOHOLIC INTOXICATION. Drunkenness is such a common phenomenon that its psychologic and physical manifestations require little elaboration. The signs consist of varying degrees of exhilaration and excitement, loss of restraint, irregularity of behavior, loquacity, slurred speech, incoordination of movement and gait, irritability, drowsiness, and, in advanced cases, stupor and coma. On rare occasions acute intoxication is characterized by an outburst of irrational, combative and destructive behavior, a state referred to as "pathologic intoxication" or "acute alcoholic paranoid state." Allegedly the latter reaction may follow the ingestion of small amounts of alcohol, and it has been variously ascribed to constitutional differences in susceptibility to alcohol, previous cerebral injury, and "an underlying epileptic predisposition." However, there are no critical data to support any of these contentions. An analogy may be drawn between this state of alcoholic excitement and a similar reaction which occasionally complicates the administration of barbiturates.

The symptoms of intoxication are caused by the depressant action of alcohol on nerve cells, acting in a manner akin to that of the general anesthetics. Unlike the general anesthetics, however, the margin between the dose of alcohol that produces surgical anesthesia and that which dangerously depresses respiration is very narrow, a fact which accounts for the occasional fatality in cases of alcoholic narcosis.

The signs of alcohol intoxication are quite distinctive and as a rule present no problem in diagnosis or management. On the other hand, coma due to alcohol may present difficulties in differential diagnosis. It should be stressed that the diagnosis of alcoholic coma is made not merely on the basis of a flushed face, stupor, and the odor of alcohol, but only after the careful exclusion of all other causes of coma (see Chap. 26). Furthermore, alcoholic coma is not always benign, as are the more common manifestations of intoxication. Serious depression of respiration, heralded by a loss of corneal and pupillary reflexes, calls for the use of respiratory stimulants and the treatment of peripheral vascular collapse, if this should manifest itself.

THE ABSTINENCE OR WITHDRAWAL SYNDROME

Of more serious consequence than the states of intoxication are the tremulous, hallucinatory, epileptic, and delirious states. Although a sustained period of chronic intoxication is the underlying factor in these illnesses, the symptoms become manifest only after a period of relative or absolute abstinence from alcohol—hence the designation *abstinence or withdrawal syndrome.* Each of the major manifestations of the withdrawal syndrome may occur distinct from the others and will be so described; more frequently, however, they occur in various combinations. The prototype of the patients afflicted with these symptoms is the spree or periodic drinker, although the steady drinker is not immune if, for some reason, alcohol is withdrawn.

TREMULOUSNESS. By far the most common manifestation of the abstinence syndrome is a state of tremulousness, commonly referred to as "the shakes" or "the jitters," combined with general irritability and gastrointestinal symptoms, particularly nausea and vomiting. The symptoms first show themselves after several days of drinking, in the morning, after the short period of abstinence that occurs during sleep. The patient needs to "quiet his nerves" by a few drinks; his symptoms are in fact relieved by alcohol, only to return on successive mornings with increasing persistence and severity. The usual spree lasts about 2 weeks, but the duration varies greatly. It is terminated not only because of recurrent tremor and vomiting, but for one or more other reasons such as lack of funds, weakness, self-disgust, or collapse. The symptoms then become greatly augmented, reaching their peak intensity 24 to 36 hr after the complete cessation of drinking.

At this stage, the patient presents a distinctive clinical picture. He is alert and startles easily. His face is deeply flushed, the conjunctivas are injected, and there is usually a tachycardia. Anorexia, nausea, and retching are always in evidence. He may complain of insomnia and craves rest and sleep. He is preoccupied with his misery, inattentive, and disinclined to answer questions; or he may respond in a rude or perfunctory manner. The patient may be mildly disoriented in time and have a poor memory for events of the last few days of his drinking spree but shows no serious confusion, being generally aware of his surroundings and the nature of his illness.

Generalized tremor is an outstanding feature of this illness. It fluctuates widely in severity, being hardly recognizable when the patient is calm, becoming gross and irregular upon attempted activity and during periods of emotional stress. The tremor may be so violent that the patient cannot stand without help, speak clearly, or feed himself. Sometimes there is little objective evidence of tremor, and the patient complains only of being "shaky inside."

Although the flushed facies, anorexia, tachycardia, and tremor subside to a large extent within a few days, the patient does not regain his full composure for a much longer time. The overalertness, tendency to startle easily, and jerkiness of movement may persist for a week or longer; the curious feeling of uneasiness may not leave the patient completely for 10 or 14 days, and only at the end of this time is he able to sleep undisturbed, without sedation. An attempt should be made to keep the patient in hospital for this length of time; to discharge him after a few days increases the likelihood that he will turn to alcohol to suppress his still-present tenseness and sleeplessness.

HALLUCINOSIS. Symptoms of disorder perception occur in about one-quarter of the tremulous patients. The patient may complain of "bad dreams"—nightmarish episodes associated with disturbed sleep, which are difficult to separate from real experience. Sounds and shadows may be misinterpreted, or familiar objects may be distorted and assume unreal forms. Although these are not hallucinations in the strict sense of the term, they represent the most common forms of disordered sense perception in the alcoholic. Hallucinations may be purely visual or auditory in type, mixed visual and auditory, and occasionally tactile or olfactory. There is little evidence to support the popular belief that certain visual hallucinations are specific to alcoholism. They are more commonly animated than inanimate and may comprise various forms of human, animal, or insect life. They may occur singly or in panoramas; they may appear shrunken or enlarged; they may be natural in appearance or take distorted and hideous forms (see Chap. 30).

ACUTE AND CHRONIC AUDITORY HALLUCINOSIS. This phenomenon merits separate consideration. For many years, an alcoholic psychosis has been recognized in which vivid auditory hallucinations are the major abnormality. Kraepelin referred to this as the *hallucinatory insanity of drunkards* or *alcoholic mania,* and Wernicke, as the *acute hallucinosis of drunkards.* The central feature of the illness, in the beginning, is the occurrence of auditory hallucinations in the face of an otherwise clear sensorium, i.e., the patients are not confused, disoriented, or obtunded and have an intact memory. The hallucinations are almost always vocal in nature, although there may be other auditory phenomena, such as the sound of running motors, buzzing, music, ringing of telephones, or dogs barking. When the voices can be identified, they are attributed to the patient's family, friends, or neighbors, rarely to God, radio, or radar. The voices may be

addressed directly to the patient, but more frequently they discuss him in the third person. In the majority of cases the voices are maligning, reproachful, or threatening in nature and are disturbing to the patient; a significant proportion, however, are not unpleasant and leave the patient undisturbed. The voices are intensely real and vivid, and they tend to be exteriorized; i.e., they come from behind the door, from the corridor, or through the floor. Another quality of these hallucinations (and of visual ones) is the appropriateness of the patient's emotional response to the hallucinatory content. He may call on the police for protection or barricade himself against invaders; even more dramatically, he may attempt suicide to avoid what the voices threaten. The hallucinations are most prominent during the night, and their duration varies greatly—they may be momentary or they may recur intermittently for days on end and, in exceptional instances, for weeks or months.

Most patients, while hallucinating, have no appreciation of the unreality of their hallucinations. As improvement occurs, the patient begins to doubt their reality, is reluctant to talk about them, and may even question whether he had been sane during the episode. Full recovery is characterized by the realization that the voices were imaginary and by the ability to recall, sometimes with remarkable clarity, the abnormal thought content of parts of the psychotic episode.

A unique feature of this psychosis is the evolution of a chronic auditory hallucinosis in a small proportion of the patients. At the outset, these patients show the characteristics of the more transient form of the illness, but after a variable period of time (as short as 1 week) the patient becomes quiet and resigned, despite the fact that the hallucinations remain threatening and derogatory. Ideas of reference and influence and other poorly systematized paranoid delusions become prominent. At this stage these patients show many of the symptoms of schizophrenia—illogical thinking, vagueness, tangential associations, and a dissociation of affect and of thought content. There is some evidence that repeated attacks of acute auditory hallucinosis render the patient more vulnerable to this chronic form of the illness. Despite the similarities to schizophrenia, there are also points of difference. In the alcoholic illness there is no family history, the age of onset is considerably beyond that of "classic" schizophrenia; the past history reveals no evidence of schizophrenia or "schizoid" personality traits, and the symptoms develop in close temporal relationship to a drinking bout.

ALCOHOLIC EPILEPSY. In this particular setting (i.e., where relative or absolute abstinence follows a period of chronic inebriation) there is a marked liability to develop convulsive seizures. Characteristically, these seizures occupy a discrete period (usually 12 to 48 hr) following the cessation of drinking, after which the patient remains free of seizures until the next cycle of drinking and abstinence. During the period of seizure activity of electroencephalogram may be abnormal, particularly in response to stroboscopic stimulation and other activating procedures, but it reverts to normal in a matter of days, even though the patient may go on to develop delirium tremens.

Seizures occurring in the abstinence period have a number of other distinctive features. There may be only a single seizure, but in the majority of cases they occur in short bursts of two to six, or even more, and an occasional patient develops status epilepticus. The seizures are grand mal in type, i.e., major generalized convulsions with loss of consciousness. If they are focal in nature, then it is likely that a focal lesion (usually traumatic) will be found in addition to the factor of alcohol. Almost one-third of the patients with generalized seizure activity go on to develop delirium tremens, in which case the seizures invariably precede the delirium. The postictal confusional state may blend imperceptibly with the onset of the delirium, or there may be a clearing of the postictal state, over several hours or even a day or two, before the delirium sets in. Seizures of this type occur in patients who have been drinking for many years, so that they have to be distinguished from other forms of epilepsy beginning in adult life.

It is suggested that the term *rum fits,* i.e., the words used by the alcoholic himself, be reserved for seizures which possess the attributes described above. This would serve to distinguish this form of seizure activity, which occurs only in the immediate abstinence period, from that which occurs in the interdrinking period, long after withdrawal has been accomplished. This is not to deny that the "idiopathic" or posttraumatic forms of epilepsy may be influenced by alcohol; indeed, it has been shown that the incidence of both these types of epilepsy is increased if the patient drinks. In patients with idiopathic or posttraumatic epilepsy, a seizure or seizures may be precipitated by only a short period of drinking (e.g., a weekend, or even one evening of heavy social drinking); interestingly, in these circumstances, the seizures occur not when the patient is intoxicated, but usually the morning after, in the "sobering-up" period.

Electroencephalographic (EEG) findings in alcoholic subjects with "rum fits" do not support the notion that the seizures merely represent latent epilepsy made manifest by alcohol, or that alcohol precipitates convulsive attacks in patients who are subject or constitutionally predisposed to seizures. Instead, the EEG reflects a sequence of changes engendered by alcohol itself—a decrease in the frequency of brain waves during the period of chronic intoxication; a rapid return of the EEG to normal immediately after cessation of drinking; the occurrence of a brief period of dysrhythmia (sharp waves and paroxysmal changes) which coincides with the flurry of convulsive activity; and again, a rapid return of the EEG to normal. Except for the transient dysrhythmia in the withdrawal period, the incidence of EEG abnormalities in patients who have had "rum fits" is not greater than in the normal population, in sharp contrast to patients who are indeed subject to seizures (see Chap. 353).

DELIRIUM TREMENS. This is the most dramatic and grave of all the alcoholic complications. It is characterized by a state of profound confusion, delusions, vivid hallucinations, tremor, agitation, and sleeplessness, as well as by increased activity of the autonomic nervous system, i.e., dilated pupils, fever, tachycardia, and profuse perspiration. The clinical features of delirium have been presented in detail in Chap. 30; only those features peculiar to the alcoholic variety (delirium tremens) are considered here. Delirium tremens develops in one of several settings. The patient, an excessive and steady drinker of many years' duration, may have been admitted to the hospital for an unrelated illness, accident, or operation, and 3 to 4 four days later becomes delirious. Or, following a prolonged spree, he may have already experienced several days of tremulousness and hallucinosis, or one or more seizures, and may even be recovering from these symptoms, when he suddenly develops delirium tremens.

In the majority of cases delirium tremens is benign and short-lived, ending as abruptly as it begins. Consumed by the relentless activity and wakefulness of several days' duration, the patient falls into a deep sleep; he awakens lucid, quiet, hungry, and exhausted, with virtually no memory for the events of the delirious period. Less commonly, the delirious state subsides gradually; more rarely still, there may be one or more relapses, several discrete episodes of delirium being separated by lucidity, the entire process lasting for as little as several days or as long as 4 or 5 weeks. The recurrent type presents the most confusing picture of all, for the delirious periods may be of varying severity and duration, and the lucid intervals of varying degrees of completeness. Where the delirium occurs as a single episode, the duration is 72 hr or less in over 80 percent of the cases.

About 15 percent of cases of delirium tremens end fatally. In many of these there is an associated infectious illness or injury, but in others there is no discernible complicating illness. Frequently, these patients die in a state of hyperthermia or peripheral circulatory collapse; in some, death comes so suddenly that the terminal events cannot be discerned.

Closely related to typical delirium tremens and about as common are the *atypical delirious-hallucinatory states,* in which one facet of the delirium tremens complex assumes prominence to the practical exclusion of the other symptoms. The patient may simply exhibit a transient state of quiet confusion, agitation, and peculiar behavior, or he may become violent and disturbed. Other patients present a vivid delusional state and abnormal behavior, consistent with their false beliefs. Such a patient may relate a loosely connected and fantastic tale of fighting pitched battles, participation in the Indian wars or bank robberies, or the like, although he may be superficially oriented and may later recall his delusions to some extent. Several of these symptoms may be combined, and these states blend imperceptibly with fully developed delirium tremens. Unlike typical delirium tremens, the atypical states always present as a single circumscribed episode without recurrences, are only rarely preceded by epilepsy, and do not end fatally. This may be another way of saying that they are a partial or less severe form of the disease.

Pathologic examination is singularly unrevealing in patients with delirium tremens. Edema and brain swelling have been absent in the authors' pathologic material except when there was shock, terminal hypoxia, or electrolyte imbalance, and there have not been any significant microscopic changes in the brain. Abnormalities of the blood nonprotein nitrogen, carbon dioxide, spinal fluid, serum sodium, chloride, sugar, potassium, and magnesium occur unpredictably. The electroencephalographic findings have been discussed in relation to alcoholic epilepsy.

The *pathogenesis* of the tremulous-hallucinatory-delirious state has been a matter of considerable controversy. The idea that it simply represents the most severe form of alcohol intoxication is not tenable. The symptoms of toxicity, consisting of slurred speech, uninhibited behavior, staggering gait, stupor, and coma are distinctive and different from the symptom complex of tremor, hallucinations, fits, and delirium. The former symptoms are associated with an elevated blood alcohol level, whereas the latter become evident only when the blood alcohol is reduced. Finally, the toxic symptoms increase in severity as more alcohol is consumed, whereas tremor and hallucinosis and even full-blown delirium tremens may be nullified by the administration of alcohol.

A specific adrenal deficiency has been postulated as the cause of delirium tremens and its variants, but it is now clear, from several critical studies, that the administration of ACTH or adrenal corticosteroids does not alter the course of the illness in any way that could not be accounted for by its natural history. Since many alcoholics eat poorly, nutritional deficiency has been invoked as a cause, but this factor is not of fundamental importance, since delirium tremens may develop in patients taking a normal diet, and it may subside uneventfully, even though the patient is denied all food and vitamins.

As has been indicated, the tremulous-hallucinatory-epileptic-delirious states depend not only on chronic intoxication but on the relative or absolute withdrawal of alcohol. The mildest degree of this syndrome, tremor and nausea, may arise after only a few days of drinking and after a relatively short period of abstinence. These symptoms may be controlled by reestablishing the blood alcohol level. The most severe form of this syndrome, delirium tremens, requires a background of months of inebriation and becomes manifest only after several days of abstinence. Any given patient may show one or all of the symptoms of abstinence, but in the latter instance they become manifest in a predictable sequence—first tremulousness and hallucinosis (and/or seizures), followed by delirium tremens.

That withdrawal of alcohol, following chronic intoxication, is an essential factor in the genesis of this syndrome has been confirmed by experimental observations in human volunteers as well as in dogs and monkeys. The exact mechanisms involved in the production of withdrawal symptoms are poorly understood. Recently it has been shown that the early phase of alcohol withdrawal (beginning 7–8 hr after cessation of drinking) is regularly attended by a drop in serum magnesium levels and a rise in arterial pH values, on the basis of respiratory alkalosis. It is possible that the compounded effect of these two factors, both of which are associated with nervous system hyperexcitability, may be responsible for seizures and perhaps other symptoms which characterize the early phase of withdrawal. Probably neither of these factors is important in the causation of delirium tremens, since the hypomagnesemia and alkalemia are transient, and frequently have been restored to normal before the onset of delirium tremens.

NUTRITIONAL DISEASES OF THE NERVOUS SYSTEM

Nutritional diseases of the nervous system comprise a relatively small but serious group of illnesses in chronic alcoholics. In contrast to the abstinence syndrome, the role of alcohol is purely secondary, serving mainly to displace food in the diet. These illnesses and the role of alcohol in their production are discussed in Chap. 363, Metabolic and Nutritional Disorders of the Brain, and Chap. 354, Diseases of Peripheral Nervous System.

ALCOHOLIC DISEASES IN WHICH THE PATHOGENESIS IS UNCERTAIN

Included in this category are several diverse disorders which are practically always encountered in alcoholic patients. The relationship of these disorders to the excessive use of alcohol is not fully understood and probably not crucial, since all of them have been described in nonalcoholic patients. There is a considerable amount of indirect evidence that these disorders are nutritional in origin, but as yet this etiology must be regarded as unproved.

ALCOHOLIC CEREBELLAR DEGENERATION. This term is applied to a nonfamilial type of cerebellar ataxia which occurs in adult life against a background of prolonged ingestion of alcohol. The symptoms may progress slowly over a long period, but more frequently they evolve in a subacute fashion (several weeks or months), after which they remain stationary for many years. The signs are those of cerebellar dysfunction, affecting stance and gait predominantly. The legs are involved more frequently and severely than the arms, and nystagmus and speech disturbances are rare. Once established, the signs change very little, although some improvement of gait (due mainly to recovery from complicating polyneuropathy) may follow cessation of drinking. The essential pathologic changes consist of degeneration of varying severity of all the neurocellular elements of the cerebellar cortex, particularly the Purkinje cells, with a striking topographic restriction to the anterior and superior aspects of the vermis, and hemispheres. The disorder of stance and gait seems to be related to the vermis lesion, and the ataxia of the limbs to the hemispheral involvement. A similar clinical syndrome has been observed in a few nutritionally depleted nonalcoholic patients.

MARCHIAFAVA-BIGNAMI DISEASE (Primary Degeneration of the Corpus Callosum). This is a rare complication of alcoholism originally described in Italian men addicted to crude red wine. The symptoms are diverse and include psychic and emotional disorders, delirium and intellectual deterioration, convulsive seizures, and varying degrees of tremor, rigidity, paralysis, apraxia, aphasia, and sucking and grasping reflexes. The duration is variable, from several weeks to months, and recovery is possible. The pathologic picture is more constant than the clinical one. It consists of symmetrically placed areas of demyelination in the corpus callosum, particularly the middle lamina, and less consistently of the anterior commissure and other parts of the white matter. Axis cylinders are better preserved than medullated fibers in these areas, and there are appropriate reactions in the macrophages and astrocytes. Various degrees of recovery may occur if alcoholic abstinence and good nutrition are established and maintained.

PONTINE MYELINOLYSIS. This term refers to a unique pathologic change affecting the center of the basis pontis, in which the medullated fibers are destroyed in a single symmetric focus of varying size. In contrast, the axis cylinders, nerve cells, and blood vessels are relatively well preserved. The disease may manifest itself by pseudobulbar palsy and quadriplegia, but usually the lesion is so small that it causes no symptoms and is found only at postmortem examination. The relationship of this condition to either alcoholism or malnutrition is obscure, but most of the cases have occurred in patients with prolonged and severe nutritional depletion.

CEREBRAL ATROPHY. The pathologic examination of relatively young alcoholic patients not infrequently discloses an unexpected degree of convolutional atrophy, most prominent in the frontal lobes, and a symmetric enlargement of the lateral and third ventricles. The ventricular enlargement may also be found on pneumoen cephalography. In some patients these findings are associated with overt complications of alcoholism, such as the Wernicke-Korsakoff syndrome, but in many of them no other abnormalities can be found, and the history discloses no symptoms of neurologic disease. The nature of this disorder is quite unclear.

"ALCOHOLIC" MYOPATHY. In recent years attention has been drawn to several disorders of skeletal and cardiac muscle, apparently primary in nature, in association with chronic alcoholism. One type of myopathic syndrome, which may be generalized or focal, is characterized by the acute onset of severe pain, tenderness and edema of muscles, accompanied by myoglobinuria, renal damage and hyperpotassemia in severe cases. Another type is characterized by the subacute development of weakness and atrophy of the proximal limb and girdle muscles, without local pain or edema and without evidence of polyneuropathy, and by myopathic changes in the electromyogram and serum enzymes. Muscle power is slowly restored in these patients following abstinence from alcohol and improvement in nutrition. "Alcoholic cardiomyopathy" is the name given to a nonspecific affection of cardiac muscle, which allegedly has a higher incidence in patients with chronic alcoholism than in the nonalcoholic population. The role of alcohol or malnutrition, or some hitherto unsuspected factor in the genesis of these disorders, is not known, and the structural and biochem-

ical basis of these syndromes requires further study (see Chap. 373).

THE NEUROLOGIC DISORDERS CONSEQUENT UPON CIRRHOSIS AND PORTAL-SYSTEMIC SHUNTS

Hepatic coma refers to an episodic disorder of consciousness which frequently complicates (or terminates) advanced liver disease and/or portal systemic shunts. It is associated with typical electroencephalographic abnormalities and a peculiar intermittency of sustained muscular contraction which presents as an irregular flapping movement of the outstretched limbs (asterixis). Patients dying in hepatic coma consistently show an increase in the number and size of the protoplasmic astrocytes throughout the central nervous system, but particularly in the deep layers of the cerebral and cerebellar cortex, the basal ganglia and dentate nuclei.

Less frequently, cirrhosis is complicated by a chronic and largely irreversible form of hepatocerebral disease, the main symptoms of which are dementia, dysarthria, ataxia, and athetosis. The brain in such cases shows not only an astrocytic hyperplasia but also a degeneration of nerve cells and fibers, the distribution of the destructive lesions following closely that of the astrocytic changes. Both hepatic coma and the chronic form of hepatocerebral disease are characterized by hyperammonemia, which is probably important in their pathogenesis. Ammonium is derived from the bacterial action on intestinal proteins and normally is converted to urea in the liver. A failure to metabolize ammonium, or perhaps some other substance absorbed from the bowel, may be the result of either hepatocellular disease or of shunting of blood around the liver. Presumably, the acute and rapidly developing effect of this toxin on the brain is episodic stupor or coma, which is reflected pathologically by a diffuse astrocytic hyperplasia; a prolongation of this effect may lead to irreversible neurological symptoms and parenchymal lesions.

The treatment of recurrent hepatic stupor and coma consists essentially of the use of a low protein diet and neomycin. Intractable cases of coma and protein intolerance, as well as the chronic form hepatocerebral disease cannot, as a rule, be controlled by these medical means alone; such cases have been improved by surgical means, either by colectomy or by exclusion of the colon. However, the number of patients treated in this way is still small, and the precise indications and effectiveness of the surgical measures remain to be determined. The neurologic complications of liver disease are considered further in Chaps. 328 and 363.

MANAGEMENT OF THE ALCOHOLIC PATIENT

The management of the various gastrointestinal complications of alcoholism is considered in the section dealing with these diseases. The management of the neurologic complications, coma, delirium tremens, and status epilepticus is discussed in Chaps. 26 and 368. Here a few remarks will be made about alcohol habituation. This presents quite a different and often a more difficult problem in management than the medical or neurologic illnesses associated with alcoholism. The patient may not have any disease that requires admission to a hospital but may nevertheless be seriously disabled in his marital, social, and economic life.

The problem of excessive drinking is a formidable one, as every physician knows. However, it is not necessarily hopeless, and an attitude of complete pessimism is not justified. It is also a common misconception among physicians that specialized training in psychiatry and an inordinately large amount of time are required to deal with the addictive drinker. Actually, a successful program treatment can be initiated by any physician with an interest in this problem, using the standard techniques of history-taking, establishing rapport with the patient, and seeing the patient frequently, though not necessarily for prolonged periods. A useful point at which to undertake this task is during convalescence of the patient from a serious medical or neurological complication of alcoholism or in relation to loss of employment, arrest, or threatened divorce. Such a crisis may help convince the patient, better than any argument presented by family or physician, that his alcoholism has attained serious proportions and that his drinking does indeed constitute a serious problem.

A number of premises about alcoholism and the alcoholic are generally accepted as prerequisites for successful treatment. The most important one is total abstinence from alcohol, and for all practical purposes, this represents the only permanent solution to the problem. It is generally agreed that any attempts to curb the drinking habit will fail if the patient continues to drink. There are said to be cases in which the patient has been able to reduce his intake of alcohol and eventually to drink in moderation, but such instances must be extremely rare.

A number of other commonly held notions about the treatment of alcoholism require qualification. It is frequently stated that the patient must recognize that he is an alcoholic, i.e., that his drinking is beyond his control, and he must express willingness to be helped. Undoubtedly there is truth in both of these statements, but they should not be interpreted to mean that the patient must gain this recognition and willingness entirely on his own initiative and that he will be helped only after he does so. Actually, the physician, or for that matter, any other interested person, can do a great deal to help the patient understand the nature of his problem and thus to motivate him to accept treatment. Every device of logic and reasoning must be used to convince the patient that abstinence is preferable to chronic inebriety. The patient must be made fully aware of the medical and social consequences of continued drinking and must also be made to understand that because of some constitutional peculiarity (like the diabetic who cannot handle sugar) he is incapable of drinking in moderation. These facts should be presented in a forthright manner, in much the same

way as one would explain the essential features of any other disease. There is nothing to be gained from adopting a punitive or moralizing attitude; nor should the patient be given the idea that he is in no way blameworthy for his illness. There appears to be an advantage in making the patient feel that he is responsible for doing something about his drinking.

The prevalent belief that an alcoholic will not stop drinking under duress also requires qualification. In fact, one of the few careful studies of this matter disclosed that relatively few patients would have sought help unless pressure had been exerted by family or employer; furthermore, patients who came to the clinic under duress of this sort did just as well as those who came voluntarily.

If an earnest and sustained effort by the physician fails to convince the patient that alcohol offers a problem, it is usually impossible to modify his alcoholic tendency. The only way to make such an individual discontinue drinking is to commit him to a psychiatric hospital or special institution for the management of alcoholism in the hope that with forced abstinence and improvement in his physical state he will gain insight and later accept psychiatric or other forms of therapy.

On the other hand, if the patient comes to realize that his drinking is beyond control and that he needs to do something about it, his chances of being helped are considerable. Indeed, under these circumstances, many individuals stop drinking of their own volition. Some of these patients, despite the best of intentions, will relapse. However, this should not serve as an excuse to abandon the therapeutic program, and there are many examples of patients who have attained a state of prolonged sobriety after several false starts. A number of methods have proved valuable in the long-term management of these patients. The most important of these are the use of Antabuse, aversion treatment, psychotherapy, and the participation in social organizations for combating alcoholism.

Antabuse (tetraethylthiuram disulfide, disulfiram) interferes with the metabolism of alcohol, so that a patient who takes both alcohol and Antabuse accumulates an inordinate amount of acetaldehyde in the tissues, resulting in nausea, vomiting, and hypotension, sometimes pronounced in degree. It is no longer considered necessary to demonstrate these effects to the patient; it is sufficient to warn him of the severe reactions that may result if he drinks while he has the drug in his body. Treatment with Antabuse is instituted only after the patient has been sober for several days, preferably longer. It should never be given to patients with cardiac or liver disease. The drug is taken each morning, or at another suitable time daily, in a dosage of 0.5 Gm, preferably under supervision. This form of treatment is of particular value in the spree or periodical drinker, in whom relapse from abstinence usually represents an impulsive rather than a carefully planned or premeditated act. The patient taking Antabuse, aware of the dangers of mixing liquor and the drug, is "protected" against the impulse to drink, and this protection can be renewed every 24 hr by the simple expedient of taking a pill. The willingness with which the patient accepts this form of treatment also serves as a rough index of his motivation. Should the patient drink when he is taking Antabuse, the ensuing reaction is usually severe enough to require medical attention, and a protracted spree can thus be prevented. Antabuse may lead to a mild polyneuropathy if continued over a long period of time (months or years).

The aversion treatment consists of the simultaneous administration of a drink of alcohol and an injection of emetin. The violent nausea and vomiting which ensue are intended to create in the patient a strong revulsion for alcohol. This form of treatment as well as other types of conditioned reflex treatment have been successfully employed in special clinics, but have not gained widespread popularity.

Alcoholics Anonymous (AA), an informal fellowship of former alcoholics, has proved to be the single most effective force in the rehabilitation of alcoholic patients. The philosophy of this organization is embodied in their so-called "twelve steps," a series of propositions about alcohol and alcoholism which guide the patient to recovery. The AA philosophy stresses in particular the practice of making restitution, the necessity to help other alcoholics, trust in God, the group confessional, and the belief that the alcoholic is powerless over alcohol. AA philosophy also embodies the 24-hr plan, in which the alcoholic strives for but 24 hr of abstinence (a concept inspired by the Sermon on the Mount) as a means of facilitating the maintenance of sobriety. Although accurate statistics are lacking, it is stated that about half of the members who express more than a passing interest in the program have no relapses, and that a significant additional number relapse, but eventually recover.

The methods used by AA are not suited to every patient, and some prefer the more personalized approach offered by special clinics and centers for the treatment of alcoholism. The physician should, therefore, be fully aware of all the community resources which are available for the management of this problem, and should be prepared to take advantage of them in appropriate cases.

It is not possible, within the confines of this chapter, to discuss the numerous theories of the etiology of alcohol addiction, and the various forms of treatment based on these theories. Alcoholism has been attributed to endocrine or other biochemical abnormalities, a biologic predisposition, special types of personality structures or racial and sociocultural factors, and an infinite number of psychologic defects. The multiplicity of theories in itself suggests that no single one of them adequately explains why some people become addicted to alcohol. There is no conclusive evidence that a difference in personality or any other factor distinguishes the alcoholic from the nonalcoholic, or that any particular form of psychotherapy accomplishes more than a regimen which utilizes the principles of therapy outlined above. In a certain proportion of alcoholic patients (the exact proportion has not been determined) drinking is symptomatic of manic-depressive disease; in such patients, treatment must be directed to the latter disorder.

REFERENCES

Alcohol and Alcoholism, U.S.P.H.S. Publ. No. 1640, Washington, D.C.

Isbell, H., H. F. Fraser, A. Wikler, R. E. Belleville, and A. J. Eisenman: An Experimental Study of the Etiology of "Rum Fits" and Delirium Tremens, Quart. J. Stud. Alc., 16:1, 1955.

Victor, M.: The Pathophysiology of Alcoholic Epilepsy, in "The Addictive States," Res. Publ. Assoc. Res. Nervous Mental Disease, 46:431, 1968.

Victor, M., and R. D. Adams: The Effect of Alcohol on the Nervous System, in "Metabolic and Toxic Diseases of the Nervous System," Res. Publ. Assoc. Res. Nervous Mental Disease, 32:526, 1953.

——, and J. Hope: The Phenomenon of Auditory Hallucinations in Chronic Alcoholism, J. Nervous Mental Disease, 126 (Nos. 5 and 6):451, 1958.

——, R. D. Adams, and E. L. Mancall: A Restricted Form of Cerebellar Cortical Degeneration Occurring in Alcoholic Patients, A.M.A. Arch. Neurol., 1:579, 1959.

——, and R. D. Adams: On the Etiology of the Alcoholic Neurologic Diseases: With Special Reference to the Role of Nutrition, Am. J. Clin. Nutrition, 9:379, 1961.

119 OPIATES AND OTHER SYNTHETIC ANALGESIC DRUGS

*Maurice Victor and
Raymond D. Adams*

The drugs included in this category are morphine, opium, heroin (diacetylmorphine), Dilaudid (dihydromorphinone), codeine (methylmorphine), Pantopon, dihydrocodeinone (Hycodan), dihydroxycodeinone (Eucodal), and 14-hydroxydihydromorphinone (Numorphan). The synthetic analgesics meperidine (Demerol), the meparidine derivatives anileridine and alphaprodine (Nisentil), methadone (Dolophine or amidone), metopon (methyl-dihydromorphinone), racemorphan (Dromoran), levorphan (*l*-Dromoran), *d*-propoxyphene (Darvon), diphenoxylate (Lomotil), and phenazocine (Prinadol) should also be listed here, since they are similar to the opiates both in their pharmacologic effects and in the patterns of abuse, the differences being mainly quantitative. In fact, *d*-propoxyphene and diphenoxylate have such low addiction liabilities that they are not controlled by the Federal Narcotic Laws. A knowledge of the properties of these analgesic agents is important for the prevention of medical addiction, which is a lesser problem than social addiction, but far from negligible.

Like alcohol and the barbiturates, the opiates may suitably be considered from two points of view: (1) acute poisoning, and (2) addiction.

OPIATE POISONING

Severe poisoning with morphine or related alkaloids is not a frequent accident, but moderate degrees are relatively common, the result of ingestion with suicidal intent, errors in the calculation of dosage, or unusual sensitivity. In children as well as in adults with myxedema, Addison's disease, chronic liver disease, or pneumonia, there may be an increased susceptibility to opiates, and relatively small doses may prove toxic. Acute poisoning may occur in addicts who are unaware that tolerance for opiates declines quickly after the withdrawal of the drug and who resume the habit at a formerly well-tolerated dose.

The clinical manifestations of acute poisoning are varying degrees of unresponsiveness, shallow respirations, miosis, bradycardia, and hypothermia. Mild intoxication is manifested by anorexia, nausea, vomiting, constipation, and loss of sexual interest. In the most severe degrees of intoxication, the pupils are dilated and cyanosis and circulatory collapse occur. The immediate cause of death is usually respiratory depression, with consequent asphyxia.

Treatment consists of gastric lavage if the drug was taken orally. This procedure may be efficacious many hours after ingestion, since one of the toxic effects of opiates is severe pylorospasm, which may cause much of the drug to be retained in the stomach. Other measures are directed toward the maintenance of an adequate airway and oxygenation, as described in the section dealing with barbiturate intoxication. If the patient does not respond rapidly to these measures, N-allylnormorphine (Nalline) should be administered. This is a specific antidote to the opiates and also to the synthetic analgesics. It is given in doses of 5 to 10 mg subcutaneously or intravenously. The improvement of circulation and respiration is usually dramatic; in fact, failure of Nalline to produce a striking improvement in respiration should cast doubt on the diagnosis of opiate intoxication. Nalline does little to restore consciousness, however, and the patient may remain drowsy for many hours. This is not harmful, provided that respiration is well maintained. Since the duration of action of Nalline is shorter than that of all the analgesics except Dilaudid and meperidine, respirations may again become depressed an hour or so after the administration of the antidote. It should then be given a second time, in smaller dosage.

Once the patient regains consciousness, usually in about 8 hr, other complaints such as severe pruritus, sneezing, persistent obstipation, and urinary retention may necessitate symptomatic treatment. Nausea and severe abdominal pain, due presumably to pancreatitis resulting from spasm of the sphincter of Oddi, are other troublesome symptoms. Nalline must be used with great caution in the case of an addict who has taken an overdose of opiate because in this circumstance the withdrawal symptoms may be particularly severe.

OPIATE ADDICTION

It is estimated that there are about 60,000 persons addicted to narcotic drugs in the United States, apart from patients who are addicted because of hopeless medical illnesses. This is a relatively small number, considering the numbers who abuse barbiturates and alcohol. Nevertheless, the problem of narcotic addiction is important for several reasons. To the patient and his family it is a tragedy which often brings about complete physical, social, and economic ruin. The physician must be constantly alert to the dangers of the long-term use of narcotic drugs and the synthetic analgesics and aware of the methods of legal control and treatment of addiction. Without the restraining influence of public health measures, addiction could conceivably assume epidemic proportions.

ETIOLOGY AND PATHOGENESIS. A number of factors, socioeconomic, psychologic, and pharmacologic, all contribute to the genesis of opiate addiction. In our culture, the most susceptible subjects are young men or delinquent youths living in the economically depressed areas of certain large cities—New York, Chicago, Los Angeles, Washington, D.C., and Detroit. A disproportionately large number of addicts are American Negroes and persons of Puerto Rican or Mexican descent. Most of these individuals show psychiatric disorders, psychoneurosis and psychopathy being the most common. However, the precise "personality" factor which renders them vulnerable to addiction has not been defined. Association with addicts is the chief reason for beginning addiction. A relatively small proportion of all addicts are introduced to drugs by physicians in the course of an illness. Judging from the studies at the Addiction Research Center, Lexington, Ky., only a few of these "medical" or "accidental" addicts can be regarded as normal, well-adjusted persons. The majority have psychologic abnormalities similar to those of the "social" addicts, the only difference being the original mode of contact with the drug.

According to Wikler, the abuse of opiate drugs evolves in three successive phases: (1) episodic intoxication, or euphoria, (2) pharmacogenic dependence, or addiction, and (3) the propensity to "relapse after cure," or habituation.

Some of the symptoms of opiate intoxication have already been considered. Of equal importance are the symptoms designated as *morphine euphoria*, a term which refers to the pain- and anxiety-reducing abilities of this drug, as well as to the state of elation or sense of unusual well being which it produces and which is especially prized by psychopathic thrill seekers. Individuals who take opiates for their euphoria-producing effects quickly discover the need to increase the dose in order to obtain an effect which approaches that of the original dose. Although the intensity of the initial "euphoria" is not fully recaptured, the progressively increasing dose of drug does ablate the discomfort which arises as the effects of each injection wear off. In this way the use of opiates becomes self-perpetuating and a marked degree of tolerance is produced, so that enormous amounts of drugs, e.g., 5,000 mg morphine daily, have been administered without the development of toxic symptoms. The mechanism of tolerance is not understood. There is some experimental evidence that during addiction there is a progressive decrease in the capacity of the liver to N-demethylate morphine and other opiates.

With the continued administration of the drug, an

altered physiologic state develops, such that if administration of the drug is suddenly terminated, a drug-specific illness develops, termed the *abstinence syndrome*. This, strictly speaking, is the definition of *addiction*, alternate terms being *physical* or *pharmacologic dependence*. This definition distinguishes between "addicting" drugs (opiates, alcohol, barbiturates) and "habit-forming" drugs (bromides, amphetamine, cocaine, and marijuana), since no abstinence symptoms follow the discontinuation of the latter group, even after prolonged exposure. Stated in another way, all addicting drugs are habit-forming, but the opposite is not true.

The intensity of the abstinence syndrome depends mainly on the dose of the drug and duration of addiction, but also on individual factors. In respect to morphine it has been found that the majority of individuals receiving 240 mg daily for 30 days or more will show moderately severe abstinence symptoms following withdrawal, whereas mild grades of abstinence may be detected following as little as 80 mg daily for a similar period.

The abstinence syndrome which occurs in the morphine addict may be taken as the prototype of the opiate group. The first 8 to 16 hr of abstinence usually pass asymptomatically. At the end of this period yawning, rhinorrhea, sweating, and lacrimation become manifest. These symptoms are at first mild, but they increase in severity over a period of several hours and then remain constant for several days. The patient may be able to sleep during this early period but is restless, and thereafter insomnia remains a prominent feature. Dilatation of the pupils, recurring waves of gooseflesh, and twitchings of the muscles appear. The patient complains of severe aches in the back, abdomen, and legs and of hot and cold "flashes," so that he covers himself with blankets. By the end of about 36 hr the restlessness becomes more extreme, and nausea, vomiting, and diarrhea usually develop. The temperature, respiration, and blood pressure are slightly elevated. All these symptoms reach their peak intensity 48 to 72 hr after withdrawal, and then gradually decline. After 7 to 10 days, all objective signs of abstinence have disappeared, although the patient may complain of insomnia, nervousness, weakness, and muscle aches for several more weeks.

Wikler speaks of two types of abstinence changes— "nonpurposive" and "purposive." The former comprise the various automatic and neuromuscular signs and are relatively transient in nature. That these symptoms represent an altered physiologic state and are not psychic in origin has been clearly demonstrated experimentally; physical dependence on morphine and other opiate drugs develops even in the isolated segment of the spinal cord in chronic spinal and in chronic decorticated dogs. The flexor and crossed extensor spinal reflexes are depressed or abolished during continued administration of opiate and become remarkably hyperirritable when the drug is withdrawn. The purposive changes refer to the patient's craving for the drug and the manipulative activity directed toward obtaining it. These symptoms may persist indefinitely and are important in relation to that characteristic of addiction referred to as *habituation, emo-*

tional dependence, or *psychologic dependence.* These terms are used interchangeably and refer to the substitution of drug-seeking activities for all other aims and objects in life. Habituation is regarded by psychiatrists as the most important quality of addiction, since it is this feature which governs the initial use of the drug and relapse following apparent cure of addiction. An individual takes drugs initially not because he needs the drug to prevent withdrawal symptoms but because of its euphoria-producing effect, i.e., the relief of pain and emotional discomfort. Similarly, relapse to the use of the drug may occur long after the nonpurposive abstinence changes seem to have disappeared. The cause for relapse is imperfectly understood. It has been theorized by Wikler that fragments of the abstinence syndrome may remain as a conditioned response, and that these abstinence signs may be evoked by the appropriate environmental stimuli. Thus, when a "cured" addict finds himself in a situation where narcotic drugs are readily available, or in circumstances that were responsible for the initial use of drugs, the incompletely extinguished drug-seeking behavior reasserts itself.

The characteristics of addiction and of abstinence are qualitatively similar with all the drugs of the opiate group as well as the related synthetic analgesics. The differences are mainly quantitative and are related to the differences in potency and length of action. Heroin is two to three times more potent than morphine but otherwise the same. Dilaudid and metopon are more potent than morphine and have a shorter duration of action; hence the addict requires more doses per day, and the abstinence syndrome comes on and subsides more rapidly. The length of action of Dromoran is somewhat longer than that of morphine, but withdrawal phenomena are similar to those of morphine in temporal course and intensity. Abstinence symptoms from codeine, while very definite, are less intense than those from morphine. The addiction liabilities of Darvon are even less than those of codeine. Abstinence symptoms from methadone are less intense than those from morphine and do not become evident until 3 or 4 days after withdrawal; furthermore, this drug is qualitatively different from morphine insofar as autonomic signs are less severe in the abstinence period. For these reasons methadone is used in the treatment of morphine addiction. Demerol addiction is of particular importance because of the high incidence among doctors and nurses and because there is still a widespread belief that this drug is nonaddicting. Tolerance to the toxic effects of Demerol is not complete, so that the addict may show tremors, twitching of the muscles, confusion, hallucinations, and at times convulsions. Signs of abstinence appear 3 to 4 hr after the last dose and reach maximum intensity in 8 to 12 hr, at which time they may be worse than those of morphine abstinence.

DIAGNOSIS. This is usually made by the patient's statement that he is addicted to and needs drugs. If the patient conceals his addiction, the diagnosis may be difficult. Miosis, needle marks, emaciation, or abscess scars are suggestive but not specific signs. Demerol addicts are likely to show dilated pupils and twitching of muscles. Test procedures for opiates in the urine are difficult and usually unavailable. Formerly it was necessary to isolate questionable cases and to observe the patient over a period of at least two days for signs of abstinence. By using the specific antagonist N-allylnormorphine (Nalline) a diagnosis of addiction to opiates and related analgesic drugs can be made within an hour.

Nalline should be administered only in the presence of another physician or nurse, with the full understanding and permission of the patient. A dose of 3 mg of the antidote is given subcutaneously, and if no signs of abstinence have appeared in 20 min, an additional 5 mg is given. If no signs have appeared in another 20 min, a final dose of 8 mg is given. Provided that the patient has taken more than occasional doses of the drug within a week of the test, the administration of Nalline will precipitate symptoms of abstinence. These become evident within 5 min of the first injection, reach their peak intensity in 20 min, begin to decline in 60 min, and disappear after 3 hr. Curiously, Nalline does not precipitate abstinence symptoms in Demerol addiction, unless the patient has been taking more than 1,600 mg daily.

The diagnosis of drug addiction or the suspicion of this diagnosis should always prompt a search for infectious complications, which are due to the frequent contamination of illegally procured drugs by various organisms and to the unsterile practices of the addict in taking drugs. The usual forms of infection in the addict are abscesses at injection sites and hepatitis; occasionally tetanus and bacterial or mycotic endocarditis occur.

MANAGEMENT AND AVOIDANCE OF ADDICTION. The ambulatory treatment of addiction never succeeds and should therefore not be undertaken. Addicts who are refused opiates may ask for methadone, Demerol, or Dromoran, on the grounds that these drugs are synthetic and nonaddicting. These drugs are addicting and have been legally defined as opiates. The physician should also be aware that he is breaking both the letter and the spirit of the regulations if he prescribes narcotics for an addict, merely for the purpose of preventing abstinence changes. Occasional exceptions may be made in cases of seriously ill addicts who are awaiting hospital treatment, or in patients who are suffering from incurable painful disease.

Treatment of the hospitalized patient consists of the administration of morphine in doses just sufficient to prevent nonpurposive abstinence changes. Usually 30 mg four times daily suffices. After 3 days on this dosage, the drug is withdrawn by the so-called "rapid reduction" method, in which successively smaller doses are administered over a 5- to 10-day period. A much longer time is required in the presence of serious medical disease. Flow baths, aspirin, intravenous fluids, and the cautious use of barbiturates help to control the abstinence symptoms.

An alternate method, once the patient has been stabilized on morphine, is to substitute methadone for morphine, in the ratio of 1 to 3 mg. After a period of a week, in which the patient receives 10 mg methadone two to four times daily, the drug is rapidly withdrawn. With this method the abstinence symptoms are relatively mild but long-lasting, so that some patients prefer the first method.

Regardless of the method of drug withdrawal employed, treatment is best carried out in an institution with proper facilities for postwithdrawal rehabilitation in a drug-free environment. If such institutional facilities are not available locally (private, municipal, or state), the patient may apply to the U.S. Attorney in his community for commitment to a Federal institution (Lexington, Ky. or Fort Worth, Texas) under the Narcotic Addict Rehabilitation Act ("NARA") of 1966. Acceptance of the patient under the provisions of this act entails institutional treatment for up to 6 months after admission, followed by after-care in the patient's community for 3 years.

In recent years, attention has centered on the use of drugs in the ambulatory treatment of narcotic addiction. One of these is the narcotic antagonist, cyclazocine, which effectively blocks the pharmacologic effects of opiates and which may serve, if taken for prolonged periods, to extinguish the addict's drug-seeking behavior. In other patients, an impressive degree of social adjustment has been achieved by the oral administration of methadone (80 to 120 mg orally, once daily), which blocks the action of heroin through cross-tolerance. Both of these therapeutic methods are promising but experimental in nature, and their ultimate utility in the long-term management of the narcotic addict remains to be determined.

The physician must be constantly alert to the dangers of addiction, particularly in susceptible individuals, i.e., in those with psychoneurosis, psychopathic personality, or alcoholism. The use of opiates should be limited to cases where pain is the chief problem; they should not be used primarily as sedatives, or for the relief of asthma, or even in chronic pain until all other measures have been exhausted. It follows that it is most important to make a precise diagnosis of the cause or causes of pain, since in some cases measures other than opiates will suffice, while in others, such as hysteria and depression, narcotics are contraindicated.

If narcotics have to be used for the relief of pain, then consideration should be given to the choice of the appropriate drug and to the mode of administration. Morphine is still the drug of choice for most patients requiring relief of severe pain for short periods. Demerol may be useful in patients who cannot tolerate morphine. Patients with chronic pain should be managed with the least potent and smallest dosage of drug that will do the job; doses should be spaced as far apart as possible and discontinued as soon as the need for pain relief has passed. In general, the opiates should be administered orally whenever possible and the intravenous route should be avoided, since the latter method produces maximum euphoria and, hence, the greatest danger of addiction. The oral administration of codeine and aspirin is a useful way to begin treatment of the patient with chronic pain. If these drugs fail to control the pain, the parenteral administration of codeine should be tried. If more potent opiates are needed, methadone and levorphan should be used, because of their effectiveness by the oral route and the relatively slow development of tolerance. Should long-continued injections of morphine or meperidine become necessary, it should be kept in mind that maximum analgesic effect is obtained with 10 mg morphine rather than with 15 mg, as is often prescribed, and with 60 to 70 mg rather than with 100 mg of meperidine. In these cases, the use of the new narcotic antagonist, pentazocine (Talwin) might be considered. This drug, administered parenterally in doses of 40 to 60 mg, is said to have analgesic effects comparable to morphine and other opiates, but less of the addicting properties, features which are still under investigation. However, the respiratory depression produced by pentazocine is not counteracted by Nalline, a serious disadvantage in some patients.

REFERENCES

Dole, V. P., and M. E. Nyswander: Methadone Maintenance and Its Implication for Theories of Narcotic Addiction, Res. Publ. Assoc. Res. Nervous Mental Disease, 46:359, 1968.

Isbell, H.: Perspectives in Research on Opiate Addiction, Brit. J. Addict., 57:17, 1961.

———, and W. M. White: Clinical Characteristics of Addiction, Am. J. Med., 14:558, 1953.

Martin, W. R.: The Basis and Possible Utility of the Use of Opioid Antagonists in the Ambulatory Treatment of the Addict, Res. Publ. Assoc. Res. Nervous Mental Disease, 46:367, 1968.

Wikler, A.: Narcotics: The Effect of Pharmacologic Agents on the Nervous System, Res. Publ. Assoc. Res. Nervous Mental Disease, 37:334, 1959.

———: Drug Addictions, in F. Tice (Ed.), "Practice of Medicine," Hagerstown, Md., W. F. Prior Co., 1962.

120 BARBITURATES AND OTHER NONBARBITURATE HYPNOTIC-SEDATIVE DRUGS

Maurice Victor and Raymond D. Adams

The high incidence of addiction, suicides, and accidental deaths attributable to the improper use of the barbiturate drugs is a matter of continuing concern to the medical profession. The production of barbiturates greatly exceeds the amount needed for therapeutic purposes. It is estimated that barbiturates account for 20 percent of acute poisonings admitted to general hospitals and that they are responsible for 6 percent of suicides and 18 percent of accidental deaths, figures exceeded by no other single poison. Despite an estimated mortality rate of only 8 percent of hospitalized cases, barbiturates reportedly cause about 1,500 deaths annually in the United States. This figure is probably a gross underestimation, since in 1964 there were over 2,200 registered deaths in Great Britain due to barbiturate poisoning.

About fifty barbiturates have been marketed for clinical use, but only the following are encountered with any frequency: barbital (Veronal), phenobarbital (Luminal), diallylbarbituric acid (Dial), amobarbital (Amytal), aprobarbital (Alurate), pentobarbital (Nembutal), secobarbital (Seconal), and thiopental (Pentothal). In the United States, pentobarbital, secobarbital, and amobarbital are the most commonly abused barbiturates. These drugs are similar pharmacologically and differ only in their speed of onset and duration of action.

In addition to the barbiturates, a number of nonbarbiturate sedative and hypnotic drugs have to be considered, since they have been shown to possess very much the same intoxicating and addicting properties as the barbiturates.

The clinical problems posed by the barbiturates differ considerably, however, depending on whether the intoxication is acute or chronic, and these two types will be treated separately.

ACUTE BARBITURATE INTOXICATION

Acute barbiturate intoxication results from the ingestion of large amounts of the drug either accidentally or with suicidal intent, the incidence of the two types being about equal. An uncommon form of accidental poisoning occurs in individuals who are intoxicated with barbiturates or with alcohol and who, being confused, ingest more of the drug. This type of poisoning has been termed *involuntary suicide* or *automatism*.

The ingestion of barbiturates with suicidal intent is most frequently the act of a depressed person. An individual with hysteria or psychopathic personality may take an overdose as a suicidal gesture and sometimes become seriously intoxicated because of a miscalculation or ignorance of the toxic dosage. At times, no psychiatric disease is present, the drug being taken impulsively or while the patient is inebriated. The combination of alcohol and barbiturate intoxication is frequent and particularly dangerous, since these drugs have an additive effect.

SITE AND MODE OF ACTION OF BARBITURATES. Barbiturates decrease the excitability of nerve cells, although the mechanism is not fully understood. Attempts have been made to localize the action of barbiturates to certain anatomic regions, or even to specific nuclei within the nervous system, but it would appear that all parts are to some extent sensitive to the drug. Nevertheless, the reticular formation of the thalami and midbrain are particularly susceptible. There is little experimental evidence to support the clinical impression that with the administration of barbiturates the cerebral cortex is affected first and that lower centers are then successively affected. Reflex and other activity of the nervous system are probably depressed at all levels simultaneously and progressively, although in the early stages of poisoning, spinal reflexes may be accentuated.

SYMPTOMS AND SIGNS. The symptoms and signs of acute barbiturate intoxication vary with the type and the amount of drug, as well as with the length of time that has elapsed since it was ingested. Pentobarbital and secobarbital produce their effects quickly, and recovery is relatively rapid. Phenobarbital induces coma more slowly, and its effects tend to be prolonged. The duration of action of these drugs can be judged from the hypnotic effect of an average oral dose. In the case of the long-acting barbiturates, such as phenobarbital, barbital, and diallylbarbituric acid, it lasts 6 hr or more; with the intermediate-acting drugs, amobarbital and aprobarbital, 3 to 6 hr; with the short-acting drugs, secobarbital and pentobarbital, less than 3 hr.

In general, much larger doses of long-acting barbiturates are required to produce a depth of unconsciousness comparable to that produced by the short-acting ones. The ingestion by adults of more than 3.0 Gm secobarbital, pentobarbital, amobarbital, or diallybarbituric acid at one time may be fatal unless intensive and skillful treatment is applied promptly; in series of cases, it has been estimated, the usual intake of drug is 6.0 to 9.0 Gm phenobarbital, 5.0 to 20.0 Gm barbital, and 15.0 Gm aprobarbital. Because of the serious complications of prolonged coma, the fatalities are greater with the long-acting than with the short-acting drugs.

Clinically, it is useful to recognize three grades of severity of acute barbiturate intoxication, particularly in regard to prognosis and treatment. Mild intoxication follows the ingestion of approximately 0.6 Gm pentobarbital or its equivalent. The patient is drowsy or asleep, a state from which he is readily roused by calling his name loudly or by shaking him. The symptoms resemble those of alcoholic inebriation, except that the face is not flushed, the conjunctivas are not suffused, and there is no odor of alcohol. The patient thinks slowly, and there may be mild disorientation, lability of mood, impairment of judgment, slurred speech, drunken gait, and nystagmus. Reflex activity and vital signs are not affected.

Moderate intoxication follows the ingestion of five to ten times the oral hypnotic dose. Here the state of consciousness is more severely depressed and is usually accompanied by depressed or absent deep reflexes and slow but not shallow respiration. Corneal reflexes are retained, with occasional exceptions. At times the patient can be roused by vigorous manual stimulation; when awakened, he is confused and dysarthric, and after a few moments he drifts back into coma. At other times the patient cannot be roused by this means. In the latter cases the depth of coma and seriousness of the respiratory depression may be roughly judged by the response of respiration to painful stimulation such as the application of firm pressure to the sternum or supraorbital ridge, or to the inhalation of 10% carbon dioxide. If these stimuli cause an increase in the depth and rate of respiration, the outlook for recovery is good, and only symptomatic treatment is indicated.

Severe intoxication occurs with the ingestion of fifteen to twenty times the oral hypnotic dose. The patient cannot be roused by any of the means indicated. Respiration is slow and shallow or irregular, and pulmonary edema and cyanosis may be present. The deep tendon reflexes are usually but not invariably absent. Most often, the patients show no response to plantar stimulation, but in those who do, the plantar responses are extensor. In the most advanced cases the corneal and gag reflexes may also be abolished. Ordinarily the pupillary light reflex is retained in severe intoxication and is lost only if the patient is asphyxiated. In the early hours of coma, there may be a phase of rigidity of the limbs, hyperactive reflexes, ankle clonus, extensor plantar signs, and decerebrate posturing; persistence of these signs indicates a severe degree of anoxia. The temperature may be subnormal, the pulse thready and rapid, and the blood pressure at shock levels.

DIAGNOSIS. The diagnosis of barbiturate intoxication is made from the history and physical findings. If a reasonable suspicion of the diagnosis exists, then a careful search for drugs or their containers may be rewarding. One should also examine the mouth and gastric contents for any characteristically colored capsules. Acute barbiturate intoxication which presents as a state of coma must be distinguished from other forms of coma by the method outlined in Chap. 26, Coma and Related Disturbances of Consciousness. Actually there are few conditions other than barbiturate intoxication which cause a flaccid coma with reactive pupils, hypothermia, and hypotension. Glutethimide poisoning may produce an identical clinical picture, excepting that the pupils are fixed (a parasympathomimetic action). In the differential diagnosis, hysteria presents the main problem.

Reliable methods are now available for the *estimation of amount of barbiturates in the blood.* The ultraviolet spectrophotometric method of Goldbaum is most widely used. The major virtue of this test is in identifying the cause of coma, when this is in question. The blood level also helps to identify the drug as long- or short-acting, thus giving information as to whether the therapeutic problem will be short or prolonged. A blood barbiturate level of 2 mg per 100 ml in a *comatose* patient is usually due to poisoning with secobarbital or pentobarbital; although the immediate mortality is high in such instances, the therapeutic problem will be short. A level of 11.5 to 12.0 mg per 100 ml is usually due to poisoning with barbital or phenobarbital, and the comatose state will be prolonged. Because of the potentiating effects of alcohol, a patient who has ingested both drugs may be comatose with relatively low blood barbiturate levels. For this reason, and also because of differences in individual tolerance, the correlation between blood barbiturate levels and depth of coma is not entirely dependable.

The *electroencephalogram* may also be useful in diagnosis, since characteristic patterns accompany barbiturate intoxication. In mild intoxication, the normal activity is replaced by fast activity, in the range of 20 to 30 per sec, most prominent in the frontal regions. In more severe intoxication, the fast waves become less regular and interspersed with 3- to 4-per-sec slow activity. In the most advanced cases, there are short periods of suppression of all activity, separated by bursts of slow (delta) waves of variable frequency.

MANAGEMENT. The management of acute barbiturate intoxication depends on its severity. In mild or moderate intoxication, recovery is the rule and no vigorous treatment is required. The mildly intoxicated patient should be watched closely for signs of deepening coma, and analeptics such as coffee or parenteral caffeine sodium benzoate may be used. If the patient is unresponsive, special attention should be given to maintaining respiration and urinary excretion and to the prevention of infection. It is most important to maintain a patent airway, at first usually by the insertion of an endotracheal tube; suctioning should be used when necessary, and the patient should be turned frequently. Tracheotomy and bronchoscopic suctioning should be resorted to if atelectasis becomes manifest, or if intubation must be maintained for longer than 48 hr. If there is any risk of respiratory depression or underventilation, it is advisable to treat the patient with a positive pressure ventilator, so as to provide adequate oxygenation and minimize the risk of atelectasis.

Cases of severe respiratory depression, with cyanosis and pupillary dilatation, represent a serious medical emergency. A clear airway should be secured immediately and artificial respiration begun, preferably utilizing an automatic intermittent positive-pressure respirator. If the patient is in shock, the foot of the bed should be elevated, and norepinephrine and whole blood or plasma administered. Catheterization is required to determine the adequacy of urinary output, to obtain samples for laboratory examination, and to prevent distension of the bladder. Since the amount of barbiturate cleared by the kidney is directly proportional to the amount of urine formed, 8 to 10 liters of 5% glucose in saline solution should be given daily. Forced diuresis is also important because toxic amounts of barbiturate have an antidiuretic effect. Coma of any significant duration requires the administration of other electrolytes as well, the amounts being governed by their serum and urinary values. The occurrence of pulmonary and urinary infections calls for the use of appropriate antibiotic treatment.

If ingestion has been recent, gastric lavage may be a therapeutic as well as a diagnostic measure. It must be performed within several hours of ingestion of the drug, since barbiturates are absorbed rapidly and completely. Laryngospasm may complicate this procedure but can be avoided by preliminary endotracheal intubation; the stomach must be entirely emptied to prevent aspiration.

Dialysis of the blood by means of the artificial kidney has proved to be an effective form of therapy. This measure should be reserved for cases of profound intoxication due to long-acting barbiturates, in which a trial of symptomatic measures has failed, and in which uremia or anuria develops.

The treatment of severe barbiturate intoxication with analeptic drugs (metrazol, picritosin, Megimide), which enjoyed a brief period of popularity, has been generally abandoned. These drugs are antagonistic to barbiturates only insofar as they are powerful cortical stimulants as well as overall nervous system excitants; they do not affect the rate of metabolism or excretion of barbiturate. Their effectiveness could never be substantiated, since there was no precise way of quantitating the depth of central nervous system depression in any particular patient, and hence no way of predicting whether or not recovery would have occurred without analeptic therapy. Because of this uncertainty, as well as the danger of convulsions with the use of these stimulants, clinicians now agree that therapy should consist of constant attention to and support of respiration, circulation, and excretion, and the prevention of infection. The mortality has been greatly reduced by the use of such methods alone. The use of nonconvulsive electrical stimulation also has no proven value in the severely intoxicated patient. Recent reports have stressed the value of alkalinization of the blood, by the use of large amounts of bicarbonate solution, as a means of mobilizing the barbiturate and increasing its rate of excretion. This method of therapy does seem to be useful, particularly where phenobarbital is the responsible agent.

Occasionally, in the case of a barbiturate addict who has taken an overdose of the drug, recovery from coma is followed by the development of an abstinence syndrome, which has to be managed by the methods outlined below.

CHRONIC BARBITURATE INTOXICATION
(Barbiturate Addiction)

The problem of chronic barbiturate intoxication is quite different from that of acute intoxication, for it embraces the phenomena of tolerance and addiction as well as the effects of ultimate withdrawal of the drugs. In these respects there is a remarkable similarity to the problem of chronic alcoholism. This concept of chronic barbiturate intoxication has gained credence only in recent years, mainly through the work of Isbell and his associates at the Addiction Research Center in Lexington, Ky. The following remarks are based largely on their studies.

Chronic barbiturate intoxication, like other addictions, usually develops on a background of some psychiatric disorder, most commonly psychoneurosis with symptoms of anxiety and insomnia, or a so-called "character disorder." The patients with symptoms of anxiety and insomnia are originally given the drug by their physicians; and as the desired sleep-producing effect of the barbiturate is lost, the dose is slowly increased until the patient is taking an amount sufficient to produce symptoms when it is withdrawn. Individuals with character disorders are usually introduced to the drug by associates; since the drug is taken for its intoxicating effect, the dose tends to be increased rapidly. Addiction to alcohol or to opiates may predispose to barbiturate addiction. Alcoholics find that barbiturates effectively relieve their nervousness and tremor and then may continue to take both alcohol and barbiturates, or the barbiturate may replace the alcohol. Morphine addicts may turn to barbiturates when they are unable to obtain opiates. As with other addicting drugs, the incidence of barbiturism is particularly high in individuals with ready access to drugs, such as physicians, pharmacists, and nurses.

The symptoms and signs of chronic barbiturate intoxication may be described in relation to (1) the toxic effects of the drug, (2) the development of tolerance, and (3) the effects of sudden withdrawal of the drug after a period of prolonged intoxication.

The toxic symptoms of chronic barbiturism are much the same as those of mild acute intoxication or of alcoholic inebriation. The barbiturate addict thinks slowly, shows an increased emotional lability, and becomes untidy in his dress and personal habits. The neurologic signs are quite characteristic and include dysarthria, nystagmus, and cerebellar incoordination. Both the mental and neurologic signs fluctuate greatly in the same individual, being more severe if the drug is taken in the fasting state and tending to increase during the day as more of the drug is ingested. If the dosage is elevated rapidly, the signs of moderate or severe intoxication become manifest.

A characteristic feature of chronic barbiturate intoxication is the development of tolerance, sometimes striking in degree. The average addict will ingest about 1.5 Gm daily of a potent barbiturate and will not develop signs of severe intoxication unless this amount is exceeded. Individual variations in the degree of tolerance make it difficult to state precisely the minimal amount of drug which must be ingested before the resulting condition is designated as chronic barbiturate intoxication. Most persons can ingest 0.4 Gm daily for years without developing major withdrawal signs (seizures or delirium), although epileptic patients accustomed to this dosage may develop continuous seizures when the drug is withdrawn. With a dosage of 0.8 Gm daily, the efficiency at all tasks is greatly reduced, and after a period of 2 months on this dosage, abrupt withdrawal will result in serious symptoms in the majority of patients. Even after 2 weeks of this dosage some patients will show mild withdrawal symptoms and paroxysmal electroencephalogram changes with photic stimulation. Individuals taking 0.4 to 0.7 Gm daily fall into an intermediate category; practically all show some mental dulling, and occasionally severe withdrawal symptoms may occur.

THE ABSTINENCE OR WITHDRAWAL SYNDROME. Following the withdrawal of barbiturates from addicted individuals, characteristic symptoms occur. Immediately following withdrawal the patient seemingly improves, as he loses the symptoms of intoxication over 8 to 12 hr. After this short period a new group of symptoms appears, consisting of nervousness, tremor, and weakness. Generalized seizures, with loss of consciousness, may then occur, usually between the second and fourth days of abstinence, occasionally as long as 6 or 7 days after withdrawal. There may be a single seizure, or several, or rarely status epilepticus. A varying degree of improvement follows the convulsive phase, to be followed by a delusional-hallucinatory state or a full-blown delirium,

indistinguishable from delirium tremens. Death has been reported under these circumstances. The abstinence syndrome may occur in varying degrees of completeness; some patients have seizures and recover without developing delirium and others have a delirium without preceding seizures. The abrupt onset of seizures or an acute psychosis in adult life should always raise the suspicion of addiction to barbiturates or other sedative-hypnotic drugs.

The *electroencephalogram* shows a number of changes in chronic barbiturate intoxication and following withdrawal. During chronic intoxication, the predominant pattern is that of fast activity of moderate voltage, interspersed with short bursts of high-voltage 6- to 8-per-sec rhythms, chiefly in the frontal and parietal regions. The electroencephalogram does not correlate closely with the degree of intoxication, nor does it reflect the development of tolerance. On withdrawal of barbiturates the fast activity diminishes. Also in the first few days of abstinence, paroxysmal bursts of mixed spike and slow waves or 4-per-sec spike and dome paroxysmal discharges occur, and these may or may not be associated with seizures. These changes disappear after 4 or 5 days, the record returning to a normal pattern. The most characteristic electroencephalogram findings which follow the withdrawal of barbiturates, according to Wulff, are paroxysmal changes evoked by photic stimulation.

INTOXICATING AND ADDICTING EFFECTS OF OTHER SEDATIVE-HYPNOTIC DRUGS. In recent years a large number of nonbarbiturate sedative-hypnotic drugs have been introduced into medical practice. At least seven of them have the same intoxicating and addicting effects as barbiturates. These drugs are meprobamate (Miltown, Equanil), glutethimide (Doriden), ethinamate (Valmid), ethchlorvynol (Placidyl), methyprylon (Noludar), chlorodiazepoxide (Librium), and diazepam (Valium). Like the barbiturates, each of these drugs can cause slurred speech, nystagmus, ataxic gait, drowsiness, confusion, and coma. Furthermore, if the daily dose exceeds a minimal safe range, a state of physical dependence develops, so that withdrawal of excessive dosages can result in abstinence symptoms. These include hallucinations, seizures, and delirium, and closely resemble those observed with barbiturates and alcohol. The seriousness of the abstinence syndrome in these cases is emphasized by reports of death following withdrawal of meprobamate and methyprylon. In view of these observations, physicians might well be skeptical of the new sedative drugs which are continually being introduced and which are said to possess no addicting or habit-forming properties. Treatment of the symptoms which result from withdrawal of the nonbarbiturate sedative drugs requires barbiturate substitution, followed by its gradual withdrawal at a rate not to exceed 0.1 Gm daily. It should be noted that diphenylhydantoin (Dilantin) and phenothiazine derivatives are not effective against the abstinence convulsions.

TREATMENT OF CHRONIC BARBITURATE INTOXICATION. This should always be carried out in the hospital. If the diagnosis of addiction is made before signs of abstinence have appeared, the first step in treatment should be the determination of the "stabilization dosage." This is the amount of short-acting barbiturate required to produce mild symptoms of intoxication (nystagmus, slight ataxia, and dysarthria). Usually 0.2 Gm pentobarbital given orally every 6 hr is sufficient for this purpose. The patient is examined 1 hr after each dose. If the signs of intoxication are severe, the next scheduled dose is reduced or omitted. If, instead, tremulousness and postural tachycardia appear, an additional 0.1 Gm of pentobarbital is given and the next scheduled dose is increased. This method is preferable to a blind reduction of dosage, since patients frequently underestimate the amount of drug taken. In such patients, establishment of the "stabilization dosage" may have diagnostic as well as therapeutic value. A patient who can take 0.8 Gm or more of pentobarbital daily, without developing signs of intoxication, is probably physically dependent on drugs of this type. Then a gradual withdrawal of the drug is undertaken, 0.1 Gm daily, the reduction being stopped for several days if abstinence symptoms appear. In this way a severely addicted person can be withdrawn in 14 to 21 days. Patients undergoing withdrawal treatment require careful observation for symptoms of abstinence, and special precautions have to be taken to prevent the smuggling or concealment of drugs.

If the patient comes to the physician with severe symptoms of abstinence, such as seizures, he should be given 0.3 to 0.5 Gm sodium Luminal intramuscularly and then enough to maintain mild intoxication. Most anticonvulsant medicines have been shown, both in animals and in man, to be ineffective against barbiturate withdrawal convulsions. Withdrawal should then be carried out as indicated above. If the abstinence symptoms are not severe, it is not necessary to reintoxicate the patient, but treatment can proceed along the lines laid down for the delirious and confused patient (Chap. 30).

The same principles of treatment apply to patients who are addicted to nonbarbiturate hypnotic-sedative drugs. Thus, if the drug and its dosage can be determined, it should be withdrawn at the rate of one therapeutic dose per day. Should abstinence symptoms appear, the reduction in dosage is stopped for several days. If the offending drug cannot be identified, a barbiturate such as Seconal can be administered to the point of mild intoxication and then withdrawn, in the manner indicated above.

After recovery has taken place, whether from the symptoms of chronic intoxication or of abstinence or from acute intoxication due to attempted suicide, the psychiatric problem requires evaluation and an appropriate plan of therapy. Many of the considerations in the management of alcoholism are equally applicable to the patient addicted to barbiturate or nonbarbiturate hypnotic drugs (Chap. 118, Alcohol).

BARBITURATE PROVOCATION OF OTHER DISEASES. At times the administration of one of the barbiturates may induce an attack of another disease. The most striking example of this is hereditary porphyria where a severe and sometimes fatal outbreak of abdominal pain, psychosis, and polyneuropathy may follow the ingestion of a few capsules of Seconal (see Chap. 101). With severe liver disease detoxification of barbiturates may be impaired, as will be discussed in Chap. 323.

REFERENCES

Clemmesen, C., and E. Nilsson: Therapeutic Trends in the Treatment of Barbiturate Poisoning: The Scandinavian Method, Clin. Pharmacol. Therap., 2:220, 1961.

Essig, C.: Sedative Drugs that Can Cause States of Intoxication and Dependence of Barbiturate Type, J.A.M.A., 196:714–717, 1966.

Fraser, H. F., A. Wikler, C. F. Essig, and H. Isbell: Degree of Physical Dependence Induced by Decobarbital or Pentobarbital, J.A.M.A. 166:127–129, 1958.

Plum, F., and A. C. Swanson: Barbiturate Poisoning Treated by Physiological Methods, J.A.M.A., 163:827, 1957.

Wulff, M. H.: "The Barbiturate Withdrawal Syndrome," Copenhagen, Ejnar Munksgaard, 1959; Suppl. No. 14, Electroencephalography Clinical Neurophysiology, 1959.

121 DEPRESSANTS, STIMULANTS, AND PSYCHOTOGENIC DRUGS

Maurice Victor and Raymond D. Adams

DEPRESSANT DRUGS

These drugs may be divided into two main classes, according to the pattern of the sedative and hypnotic responses when the dose of drug is progressively increased. One class, which may be designated *general depressants*, is exemplified by the barbiturates; these drugs cause a more or less progressive depression of central nervous system excitability in response to increasing dosage, until death ensues. A second class of *special depressants*, generally referred to as tranquilizers, is exemplified by chlorpromazine, chlordiazepoxide, and meprobamate. These drugs also reduce hyperexcitability of the nervous system, but the sedative-hypnotic effects fail to keep pace with the increase in dosage, and excitability may remain at relatively normal levels over a wide range of dosages. Thus, the special depressants have the capacity to suppress symptoms of anxiety, irritability, and so forth, leaving the patient alert enough to work and function in an acceptable manner. An added advantage of these drugs is that large single doses, ingested with suicidal intent, may cause no serious depression of nervous system function.

General Depressants

The most important members of this group, the barbiturates, have been fully discussed in the preceding chapter. Other general depressants of clinical importance are the bromides, paraldehyde, and chloral hydrate.

Bromides are seldom prescribed by physicians at the present time, but are contained in many "nerve tonics" and proprietary headache remedies (such as Bromo-Seltzer), so that cases of bromide intoxication are encountered with some regularity. Acute poisoning with bromide is rare because large doses of the drug are irritating to the gastric mucosa and vomiting prevents the attainment of significant blood levels. Taken in smaller doses, however, bromide tends to accumulate in the body because of its slow excretion by the kidney, and toxic symptoms may appear in a matter of weeks. These symptoms are caused by the bromide ion itself and do not simply reflect a decrease in chloride, caused by displacement of the chloride by the bromide ion.

The symptoms of chronic bromide intoxication are predominantly in the mental sphere and range from dizziness, drowsiness, irritability, and emotional lability to a quiet confusional state, with impairment of thinking and memory, and in severe cases, to delirium and mania or to stupor and coma. Skin manifestations are associated in many cases, taking the form usually of an acnelike eruption and less frequently of proliferative nodular lesions, resembling those of tertiary syphilis. Headache, mild conjunctivitis, gastric distress, anorexia, and constipation may be associated as well. The blood bromide levels and the severity of toxic symptoms do not necessarily correspond. As a general rule, levels of 75 mg per 100 ml (9 mEq per liter) or more are considered abnormal and diagnostic of bromism, if the clinical picture suggests it. However, higher levels are sometimes well tolerated, and symptoms of bromism may persist even after the blood levels have been reduced to normal or near normal levels.

Treatment consists of removing the source of the bromide and administration of sodium chloride (at least 6 Gm daily, in divided doses). Ammonium chloride may be substituted if an accumulation of sodium is to be avoided and if there is no danger of an uncompensated acidosis. Confused or delirious patients require sedation, paraldehyde being the drug of choice, and the anorectic and emaciated patients need careful nursing care and special attention to diet. The administration of a mercurial or thiazide diuretic serves to promote a bromide diuresis. Hemodialysis is an effective means of removing bromide and should be utilized in the most severe cases of intoxication.

Chloral Hydrate is the oldest and at the same time one of the safest, most effective, and cheapest of the sedative-hypnotic drugs. After oral administration, chloral is reduced rapidly to trichloroethanol, which is the agent responsible for the depressant effects on the central nervous system. A significant portion of the trichloroethanol is excreted in the urine as the glucuronide, which may give a false positive test for glucose.

In large doses chloral is toxic to the heart, kidneys, and liver, but only in the presence of preexisting disease in these organs. Chloral is a strong gastric irritant, so that it should be diluted sufficiently and not taken on an empty stomach. Tolerance and addiction to chloral develop only rarely, and for these reasons it is an appropriate medication for the management of insomnia, particularly the type which is associated with the alcohol

withdrawal syndrome and depression. Poisoning with chloral is a rare occurrence and resembles acute barbiturate intoxication, except for the finding of miosis, which is said to characterize the former. Death from poisoning is due to respiratory depression and hypotension, and patients who survive these events may show signs of liver and kidney disease.

Paraldehyde is also an effective and safe hypnotic, providing that certain precautions are taken in its preparation and administration. On exposure to light paraldehyde decomposes to acetaldehyde, which is very toxic, and oxidizes to acetic acid. It must be freshly prepared, therefore, and stored in tightly stoppered, amber-colored bottles. Paraldehyde is unique in that a significant proportion is excreted unchanged through the lungs; the remainder is detoxified in the liver, so that it should be used cautiously in patients with liver disease.

Paraldehyde has a wide margin of safety when administered orally (or rectally) and even three or four times the usual dose (8 to 10 ml) causes no more than prolonged sleep or mild stupor. Intramuscular and intravenous use of the drug should be avoided because of its propensity to produce sterile abscesses and to damage the sciatic nerve and because of its unpredictable effects on respiration. The main objections to this drug are its bitter taste (this can be obviated by diluting in fruit juice) and its lingering, unpleasant odor.

Paraldehyde has its greatest value in the treatment of the alcoholic patient, following a period of prolonged intoxication. It is very effective in suppressing the tremulousness, restlessness, and insomnia that characterize the early phases (6 to 72 hr) of the withdrawal period. It remains to be proved, however, that the administration of paraldehyde (or any other depressant drug) can prevent delirium tremens or reduce the duration of or the mortality from this disorder.

The use of paraldehyde in the alcoholic patient allegedly carries the risk of replacing an addiction to alcohol with one to paraldehyde. Patients with symptoms of alcohol withdrawal do make repeated demands for the drug, which is not surprising, in view of the pharmacologic similarities between paraldehyde and alcohol and the effectiveness of both drugs in suppressing withdrawal symptoms. This does not present a problem in management, however, if the need for the drug is determined before each dose is given and the drug is withdrawn as soon as the agitation and tremor are under control. Should a relapse from abstinence then occur, some patients are said to substitute paraldehyde for alcohol, but such an occurrence must be extremely rare.

Special Depressants

Since the mid-1950s, a large new series of pharmacologic agents, generally referred to as tranquilizers, has come into prominent use, mainly for the control of nervousness, agitation, apprehension, anxiety, and depression. Their application in medical practice, which has been on an enormous scale, is fraught with difficulty. Since the symptoms for which they are prescribed are manifestations of many conditions, some of them being normal reactions to trying environmental circumstances and others being symptoms of a disease state such as anxiety neurosis or depression, the physician should be certain of the diagnosis before using them. These drugs are not curative, but only suppress or partially alleviate the symptoms, and they should not serve as a substitute for or divert the physician from the use of other measures for the relief of the abnormal mental state. They are so toxic and expensive that they should not be used indefinitely.

At the time of writing this chapter, more than 50 of these tranquilizing agents are on the market. No attempt will be made here to describe or even list all of them. Some have had only an evanescent popularity and others have yet to prove their value. Chemically these compounds form a heterogeneous group, four categories of which are of particular clinical importance: (1) the ethylamine group of drugs (including the phenothiazines), (2) the rauwolfia alkaloids, (3) the bensodiazepine compounds, and (4) the carbonic acid or urea derivatives.

The *phenothiazines* comprise some of the most widely used tranquilizers, such as chlorpromazine (Thorazine), prochlorperazine (Compazine), perphenazine (Trifalon), fluphenazine (Permatil), and thioridazine (Mellaril). In addition to sedative effects, this group of drugs has a number of other actions, so that congeners of these compounds are used as conduction anesthetics (procaine), cardiodepressants (procaine amide), antiemetics (prochlorperazine), and antihistaminics (promethazine).

The phenothiazines have had their widest application in the treatment of the psychoses. Under the influence of these drugs, many patients who would otherwise be hospitalized are able to live at home and even work productively and the hospital care of hyperactive and combative patients has been greatly facilitated.

Side effects of the phenothiazines are frequent and often serious. All of them may cause a cholestatic type of jaundice, agranulocytosis, convulsive seizures, orthostatic hypotension, skin sensitivity reactions, mental depression, and disorders of the extrapyramidal motor system. Jaundice and blood dyscrasias have occurred less often with prochlorperazine, perphenazine, and fluphenazine than with other members of the group, but the extrapyramidal side effects have been relatively more pronounced. Several types of extrapyramidal symptoms have been noted: (1) A parkinsonian syndrome—masklike facies, tremor, generalized rigidity, shuffling gait, and slowness of movement. These symptoms usually appear after several weeks of drug therapy. (2) Muscle spasms and dystonia, taking the form of involuntary protrusion of the tongue, dysphagia, torticollis and retrocollis, oculogyric crises, and tonic spasms of a limb; these complications usually occur early in the administration of the drug, sometimes after the initial dose, and often can be improved dramatically by the intravenous administration of diphenhydramine hydrochloride (Benadryl). (3) An inability to sit still and an inner restlessness or turmoil, so that the patient paces the floor constantly

(*akathisia*); involuntary movements of a choreathetotic type may be added.

These reactions must be recognized at once and the medication discontinued, but even then the extrapyramidal disorder may persist for weeks or months, *and exceptionally, even for years*. Administration of antiparkinsonian drugs (trihexyphenidyl, procyclidine, benztropine) hastens recovery. Chlorprothixene (Taractin), a thioxanthene drug with effects similar to the phenothiazines, and thioridazine (Mellaril), although not the best tranquilizing agents, are favored by some because of their lesser tendency to produce symptoms of extrapyramidal motor disorder. The latter drug, however, if given in large doses over a period of time, may cause retinal deposits with resulting visual impairment.

Reserpine is the prototype of the rauwolfia alkaloids; these drugs, so effective in controlling hypertension, are no longer to be recommended as tranquilizing agents. When given in doses adequate to attain this effect, they often provoke a parkinsonian syndrome or a serious depression of mood, which may prove more troublesome than the anxiety for which they were prescribed.

Two agents of the *benzodiazepine* group, chlordiazepoxide (Librium) and diazepam (Valium), have been used extensively to control anxiety, overactivity, destructive behaviour in children, and the symptoms of alcohol withdrawal. These drugs possess anticonvulsant properties, and the intravenous use of diazepam is a very effective means of controlling status epilepticus. In addition, diazepam has been used with moderate success in the treatment of extrapyramidal movement disorders and dystonic spasms. The benzodiazepine drugs, while comparatively safe in the recommended dosages, frequently cause unsteadiness of gait and drowsiness and at times hypotension and syncope, particularly in the elderly. In severely disturbed schizophrenic patients, rage, hostility, uncontrollable excitement, confusion, and depersonalization may develop. Nausea, diminished libido, headache, skin rashes, leukopenia, eosinophilia, agranulocytosis, and enhancement of the effects of alcohol have all been reported but are rare. Additional central nervous disorders are slurred speech, dysphagia, ataxia, confusion, and faulty memory.

The *carbonic acid or urea derivatives* are capable of modest depressant action and are appropriate for relieving mild degrees of nervousness, anxiety, and muscle tension. Maximal action occurs with reatively small doses of these drugs. Ataxia, drowsiness, autonomic and extrapyramidal effects are singularly absent with therapeutic doses. *Meprobamate* (Equanil, Miltown) is the best known but a somewhat anomalous member of this group; in its pharmacologic actions it resembles the barbiturates much more than the other special depressants. With average doses (400 mg, three or four times a day) the patient is able to function quite effectively; large doses cause drowsiness, stupor, coma, and vasomotor collapse. Hypersensitivity reactions in the form of fever, pruritis, and erythematous, maculopapular and occasionally urticarial or bullous eruptions have been reported. Cutaneous petechiae or ecchymoses may also occur without thrombocytopenia. Diplopia, syncope, menstrual irregularities, angioneurotic edema, peripheral edema, leucopenia, thrombocytopenia, and pancytopenia are other rare complications.

It is important to note that addiction to meprobamate does occur and if four or more times the daily recommended dose is administered over a period of weeks to months, withdrawal symptoms (including convulsions) may appear, resembling those which follow withdrawal of barbiturate in a chronically intoxicated patient. Several other special depressant drugs, described in the preceding chapter, have the same liability.

It hardly need be pointed out that the tranquilizing drugs have been much abused. This would be suspected just from the frequency with which they are being prescribed (it is stated that in the past decade 50 million patients have received chlorpromazine alone). Often these toxic and expensive agents are prescribed when safer and less expensive drugs, such as phenobarbital, in small sedating doses would accomplish the same purpose.

STIMULANTS

Drugs that act primarily as stimulants of the central nervous system can be divided into two general groups, based on differences in their pharmacologic actions and clinical use. (1) The first group is exemplified by analeptics such as picritoxin, which produce a prompt and short-lived effect on the nervous system and a grossly recognizable increase in motor and electrical activity, often taking the form of convulsive seizures. The effects of these drugs can be readily reproduced in animals and have been of great interest to pharmacologists and physiologists but of little clinical value. (2) The monoamine oxidase inhibitors and dibenzazepine compounds, which comprise the second group of stimulant drugs, have considerable clinical usefulness, mainly in elevating mood and ameliorating the symptoms and signs of mental depression. The effects of these drugs on the nervous system, in contrast to the more direct acting stimulants, are slow to appear, persist for long periods after their administration has been stopped, and cannot be assessed in animals.

Such a division, though clinically useful, is far from absolute. Certain of the direct acting stimulants, e.g., amphetamine, may have a beneficial effect on mental depression. Also, certain drugs that are useful in the treatment of depression (e.g., amobarbital) are not central nervous system stimulants, but depressants. In the latter case, a depressant acts as an antidepressant. These commonly used terms must not be confused—the former referring to a drug that reduces nervous system excitability and the latter to the capacity of the drug to ameliorate the symptoms of mental depression.

Direct-acting Stimulants

Amphetamine (benzedrine) and its *d*-isomer, *dextroamphetamine,* are powerful analeptics and in addition have significant hypertensive, respiratory stimulant, and appetite depressant effects. These drugs are useful in the management of narcolepsy, but they are much more widely and indiscriminately used for the control of obesity and the abolition of fatigue. Undoubtedly they are able to reverse fatigue, postpone the need for sleep, and elevate mood, but these effects are not entirely predictable and certainly not indefinite, and the user must pay for the period of wakefulness with even greater fatigue and often with depression. Because of the popularity of the amphetamines and ease with which they can be procured, instances of acute and chronic intoxication are observed frequently. The toxic signs are essentially an exaggeration of the analeptic effects—restlessness, speech and motor overactivity, tremor, and insomnia. In severe cases, a schizophrenia-like picture may occur, with hallucinations, delusions, and changes in affect and thought processes. Treatment consists of removal of the offending drug and the administration of barbiturates. Nitrites may be useful if the blood pressure is markedly elevated.

Picritoxin is a powerful nervous system excitant, the main effects of which are to produce convulsive seizures and to reverse respiratory depression induced by drugs, particularly by barbiturates. However, the modern treatment of barbiturate intoxication does not include the use of picritoxin or other analeptics, because of their epileptogenic properties and because barbiturate intoxication can be managed successfully by other means (see Chap. 120).

It has been shown by Eccles and his colleagues that picritoxin increases neuronal activity by blocking presynaptic inhibition, i.e., blocking the action of inhibitory fibres that synapse with the presynaptic terminals of excitatory fibres. *Strychnine,* on the other hand, increases neuronal excitability by interfering with postsynaptic inhibition. The therapeutic value of strychnine is negligible, but in children accidental poisoning may occur from ingestion of "A.S. & B." cathartic pills or "rat biscuits." Very rarely, strychnine is taken with suicidal intent. After a period of heightened irritability and muscle twitching, tonic seizures occur, characterized by opisthotonus, rigid extension of the legs, facial tetanus, and apnea due to spasm of the muscles of respiration. Death from anoxia may follow several seizures.

The immediate need, in the treatment of strychnine poisoning, is to control the convulsions. This calls for the intravenous administration of a short-acting barbiturate or the application of inhalation anesthesia if the appropriate drug is not immediately available; endotracheal intubation is an important safeguard. The patient must then be observed carefully, and if any signs of irritability recur, more sedative should be given. During this period, supportive care is indicated, as for any comatose patient. Morphine, which is a medullary depressant but a spinal cord stimulant, is contraindicated.

Pentylenetetrazol (metrazal, cardiazol) is a potent stimulant of all parts of the nervous system. For a number of years it served as the convulsive agent in the "shock treatment" of depression and schizophrenia but was abandoned in favor of less dangerous and more effective forms of convulsive therapy. The use of this drug to activate latent epileptogenic foci or to reproduce convulsions, with the purpose of studying the underlying cerebral mechanisms, is restricted to a few clinical centres.

The actions of *bemegride* and *nikethamide* (Coramine) are much like those of pentylenetetrazol. For many years it was common clinical practice to administer nikethamide as a final therapeutic gesture in patients dying of cardiac and respiratory failure, but there is little evidence that this drug has a significant stimulant effect on either heart or respiration. Poisoning with these drugs, which is usually due to parenteral overdosage, is best treated with barbiturates.

Caffeine and other xanthine derivatives do have therapeutic value, by virtue of their diuretic effects and their ability to stimulate the heart and nervous system. The major use of these agents is to abolish fatigue and maintain wakefulness, and the usual mode of administration is in coffee, a cup of which contains 100 to 150 mg caffeine. Overdosage leads to insomnia, mild delirium, tinnitus, tachycardia, prominent diuresis, and cardiac arrhythmias. The excitatory effects are easily controlled with barbiturates, and fatalities due to caffeine poisoning are extremely rare.

Camphor (camphorated oil) was formerly a popular stimulant, but is now rarely used therapeutically; however, occasional cases of poisoning are still seen as a result of ingestion of liniment or moth flakes. The manifestations of poisoning are headache, sensation of warmth, confusion, clonic convulsions, and terminal respiratory depression; the characteristic odor of camphor facilitates the diagnosis. Treatment consists of supportive care and the cautious use of barbiturates to combat convulsions.

Indirect-acting Stimulants

MONOAMINE OXIDASE (MAO) INHIBITORS. The observation that iproniazid, an inhibitor of monoamine oxidase (MAO), had a mood-elevating effect in tuberculous patients initiated a great deal of interest in compounds of this type, and led to their quick exploitation in the treatment of depression. Iproniazid (Marsilid) proved exceedingly toxic and was taken off the market, as have several more recently developed MAO inhibitors; but other drugs, much better tolerated, have become available. These include isocarboxazid (Marplan), nialamide (Niamid), phenelzine (Nardil), and tranylcypromine (Parnate), the latter two being the most frequently used. Tranylcypromine has proved to be the most potent of these agents, but it has also produced the most serious toxic effects.

The exact mode of action of the MAO inhibitors has not been determined. They have in common the ability to block the oxidative deamination of naturally occurring amines (norepinephrine, epinephrine, and serotonin), and it has been suggested that the accumulation of these neurohormonal substances is responsible for the antidepressant effect. However, these drugs inhibit many enzymes other than monoamine oxidases and have numerous actions unrelated to enzyme inhibition. Furthermore, many agents with antidepressant effects like those of the

monoamine oxidase inhibitors do not inhibit this enzyme. At the present time, one cannot assume that the therapeutic effect of these drugs has a direct relationship to the property of MAO inhibitors.

These drugs must be dispensed with great caution and a constant awareness of their potentially serious side effects. Patients taking the drugs must be warned against the use of sympathomimetic amines and tyramine, for this may induce a severe hypertensive episode and cerebral vascular accident, headache, atrial and ventricular arrhythmia, pulmonary edema, and even death. Orthostatic hypotension of a serious degree may also develop. Sympathomimetic amines are taken in the form of nasal sprays, nose drops, and in so-called "coryza" tablets and the common tyramine-containing compounds are cheeses, yogurt, beer, and wine.

The MAO inhibitors may at times cause excitement, restlessness, agitation, insomnia, and anxiety, and occasionally, with the usual dose and more often with an overdose, mania and convulsions may occur (especially in epileptic patients). Other side effects are increased neuromuscular activity in the form of muscle twitching and involuntary movement of an extremity, urinary retention, skin rashes, tachycardia, hepatic disturbance, jaundice, visual impairment, enhancement of glaucoma, impotence, sweating, muscle spasms, and a variety of parasthesias.

Since the MAO inhibitors have such widespread possibilities of causing toxic effects and potentiating the effect of other drugs, it is wise not to give them concurrently with other medications. In particular, the phenothiazines and other powerful central nervous system stimulants should not be used with the MAO inhibitors, since occasional fatalities and severe reactions have followed their concomitant use. Exaggerated responses to the usual dose of meperidine (Demerol) and other narcotic drugs have also been observed; respiratory function may be depressed to a serious degree, and hyperpyrexia, agitation, and pronounced hypotension also may occur, sometimes with fatal issue. Unpredictable side effects may also accompany the simultaneous administration of barbiturates, alcohol, anesthetics, and insulin.

DIBENZAZEPINE DERIVATIVES. Soon after the first convincing successes in the treatment of depression with MAO inhibitors, a new class of antidepressant compounds appeared. The first of this group was imipramine (Tofranil), which was soon followed by amitriptyline (Elavil), and more recently by desipramine (Norpramine) and nortryptyline (Aventyl). The first two members of this group have proved to be the most popular.

The exact mode of action of these agents is unknown, but they produce a central stimulating effect. In the absence of other considerations, they are presently the most effective drugs for the treatment of depressive illnesses that are associated with anxiety and agitation. Persistence of their pharmacologic effects after the drug is stopped is very short in comparison with the MAO inhibitors, and their side effects are far less frequent and serious.

All of the dibenzazepine compounds are capable of

causing orthostatic hypotension, urinary bladder weakness, dizziness, and occasionally, ataxia and blood dyscrasias. They may produce central nervous system excitement, leading to insomnia, agitation, and restlessness, but usually these effects are controlled readily by the use of phenothiazines or chlordiazepoxide given concurrently or in the evenings. The dibenzazepine drugs should never be given with an MAO inhibitor, since the reactions which may occur are frequently serious; hypertensive seizures and lethal hyperpyrexia have been reported. These reactions have allegedly occurred when small doses of imipramine were given to patients who had discontinued the MAO inhibitor one week previously.

PSYCHOTOGENIC DRUGS

Included in this category are a heterogeneous group of drugs, the primary effect of which is to alter perception, mood, and thinking out of proportion to other aspects of cognitive function and consciousness. Tolerance to these drugs and addiction (i.e., the occurrence of abstinence symptoms when the drug is withdrawn) do not develop, although users may become dependent upon them for emotional support. This group of drugs comprises lysergic acid derivatives, e.g., lysergic acid diethylamide (LSD); phenylethylamine derivatives (mescaline or peyote); psilocybin; certain indolic derivatives, cannabis (marihuana), and a number of less important compounds. They are also referred to as psychotomimetic drugs, hallucinogens and psychedelics but none of these names is entirely suitable.

LSD, mescaline, and psilocybin produce much the same clinical effects if given in comparable amounts. The somatic symptoms consist of dizziness, nausea, drowsiness, paresthesias and blurring of vision. The perceptual abnormalities are the most dramatic—the user describes vivid visual hallucinations, alterations in the shape and color of objects, unusual dreams, and feelings of depersonalization. An increase in auditory acuity has been described but auditory hallucinations are rare. Cognitive functions are difficult to assess because of inattention, drowsiness, and inability to concentrate and to cooperate in mental testing. Sympathomimetic effects—pupillary dilatation, piloerection, hyperthermia, and tachycardia are prominent, and the user may also show hyperreflexia, incoordination of the limbs, and ataxia.

The effects of *marihuana*, when taken by inhaling the smoke from cigarettes, are prompt in onset and evanescent. In low doses the symptoms are like those of mild intoxication with alcohol. With increasing amounts of drug, the effects are similar to those of LSD, mescaline,

and psilocybin, and they may be quite disabling for many hours. Very large doses result in severe depression and stupor, but death is unusual.

The fact that small quantities of these drugs can produce gross mental aberrations has stimulated the search for similar endogenous substances that may be responsible for schizophrenia and other psychoses. The mechanisms involved in producing and antagonizing the "psychotomimetic" effects are also being studied intensively, in the hope of elucidating the mechanisms of the psychoses and finding improved psychotherapeutic agents. Doubtless these studies are adding greatly to our knowledge of abnormal behavior, but the fundamental problems remain to be solved.

Numerous claims have been made that LSD and related drugs are effective in the treatment of mental disease and a wide variety of social ills and that they have the capacity to increase one's intellectual performance, creativity, and self-understanding. At this time, there are no acceptable studies that validate any of these claims.

LSD is not yet an approved drug, and marihuana falls under the federal narcotic laws. Nevertheless, these drugs are very widely used. They are taken by narcotic addicts as a temporary substitute for more potent drugs, by "drug heads," i.e., individuals who use literally any agent that alters consciousness, and by many college and high school students, for reasons that are not easy to define.

The unsupervised use of these drugs is attended by a number of serious adverse reactions, taking the form of acute panic attacks, long-lasting psychotic states resembling paranoid schizophrenia, or serious physical injury, consequent upon impairment of the user's critical faculties. Recent reports have suggested that LSD may cause chromosomal damage. A discussion of the legal implications of the illicit use of these drugs and their social impact is beyond the scope of this chapter.

REFERENCES

Hollister, L. E.: "Chemical Psychoses. LSD and Related Drugs," Springfield, Ill., Charles C Thomas, Publisher, 1968.

———: Symposium on adverse drug reactions. Psychopharmacological drugs, J.A.M.A. 196:411–413, 1966.

Jarvik, M. E.: Drugs used in the treatment of psychiatric disorders, pp. 159–214 in "Pharmacological Basis of Therapeutics," 3d ed., L. S. Goodman and Alfred Gilman (Eds.), New York, The MacMillan Company, 1965.

"Psychopharmacology. A Review of Progress, 1957–1967." U.S.P.H.S. Pub. No. 1836. Washington, D.C., 1968.

Section 2

Disorders Caused by Venoms, Bites, and Stings

122 SNAKE AND LIZARD BITES
Ivan L. Bennett, Jr.

SNAKE BITES

Fewer than one-tenth of the nearly 2,500 known species of snakes are venomous. These poisonous varieties belong to five families or subfamilies: Elapidae (cobras, kraits, coral snakes), found in all parts of the world but Europe; Viperinae (true vipers), found in all parts of the world but the Americas; Hydrophidae (sea snakes); Crotalinae (pit vipers), found in Asia and the Americas; and Colubridae, represented by a few rear-fanged species of Africa. The poisonous varieties of the United States, with the single exception of the coral snake of the Elapidae, are pit vipers and include the rattlesnakes, the water moccasin, and the copperhead. This discussion will center around these species, but the therapeutic measures outlined are applicable to snake bites in all parts of the world.

The number of individuals bitten by poisonous snakes in the United States is estimated at 2,000 to 3,000 per year; deaths are not reported separately but are undoubtedly rare, numbering fewer than 20 per year. In many European countries, deaths from snake bite have averaged only one every 3 to 5 years for the last half-century. In contrast, the estimate of annual deaths from snake bite in Brazil is 2,000 (4 per 100,000 population), and 2,000 in Burma (15.4 per 100,000).

ETIOLOGY. The coral snake is found in the Southern states from Florida to Arizona. It is marked by alternating red and black bands separated by yellow rings. Coral snakes are nocturnal and placid and rarely bite man. The fangs are short and permanently erect; the highly toxic venom is injected into multiple puncture wounds produced by a series of chewing movements.

The pit vipers are so named because of a small pit between the eye and the nostril. Large venom glands in the temporal region give the head a triangular appearance. They are generally aggressive and likely to strike if disturbed. The fangs are long and hinged, folding posteriorly when the mouth is closed. Pit vipers strike suddenly with a forward thrust of the head, and the instant that the erect fangs make contact, venom is expressed by sudden muscular contraction.

The rattlesnakes, recognized by the horny rattle on the tail which buzzes when the snake is disturbed, are widely distributed. The diamondbacks (*Crotalus adamanteus* in the Southeast and *C. atrox* in the Southwest) are the largest and most dangerous snakes in this country. Others include the prairie rattler (*C. confluentus*), the timber rattler (*C. horridus*), and the pigmy rattlers.

The water moccasin, or cottonmouth (*Agkistrodon piscivorus*), is found in swampy areas or along the banks of streams. It is a strong swimmer and can bite under water. This snake is notorious for inflicting severe facial bites when disturbed in the branches of small trees. The copperhead, or highland moccasin (*A. mokasen*), is a closely related species. Its bite is painful but rarely fatal.

PATHOGENESIS. Snake Venoms. The venoms of many species have been analyzed; invariably each proves to be a mixture of several toxic proteins and enzymes. As an example, the venom of the Indian cobra (*Naja naja*) contains these distinct and separate substances: a neurotoxin, a hemolysin, a cardiotoxin, a cholinesterase, at least three phosphatases, a nucleotidase, and a potent inhibitor of cytochrome oxidase. Several venoms, including those of the pit vipers, contain hyaluronidase and numerous proteolytic enzymes. Although opinions differ about the exact role of these components in toxicity, the action of the venom of a given species is usually predominantly *neurotoxic* or *necrotizing;* frequently associated changes are hemolysis and changes in blood coagulation. The venom of elapids, including the coral snake, is neurotoxic, and death results from respiratory paralysis, probably caused by damage to brain centers, and a curariform interference with transmission at the neuromuscular junction. The venom of crotalid snakes produces local tissue injury, hemorrhage, and hemolysis; death is preceded by circulatory collapse, the mechanism of which is poorly understood. Systemic absorption of venom occurs through lymphatics, and therapeutic measures designed to reduce lymphatic function are helpful in controlling symptoms. On rare occasions, when venom is discharged directly into a blood vessel, death occurs in less than 10 min.

Factors Affecting Severity. Several factors affect the outcome of snake bite:

1. The age, size, and health of the patient. Envenomation in children is usually serious and a fatal outcome more likely.

2. Bites on extremities or into adipose tissues are less dangerous than those on the trunk or face or penetrating a vessel. A direct stroke of the fangs is more dangerous than a scratch, a glancing blow, or one hitting a bone. The discharge orifice of the fang is well above its tip, and the point of the fang can penetrate the skin without envenomation. Even a thin layer of clothing may afford great protection.

3. The size of the snake, the extent of its anger or fear (if hurt it may inject a large dose of venom), the condition of the venom glands (recently discharged or full), and the condition of the fangs (broken, recently renewed) are all important.

4. The presence of various bacteria in the mouth of the snake or on the skin of the victim (especially clostridia) may lead to serious infection in the necrotic tissues at the local site.

5. Exercise or exertion, such as running, immediately after the bite speeds sytemic absorption of toxin.

MANIFESTATIONS. The bite of a pit viper produces severe pain at the local site within a few minutes. There is rapid swelling; ecchymoses and bullae appear over the involved areas, and as the edema spreads, serosanguineous fluid oozes from the puncture wounds. Systemic effects include circulatory collapse with hypotension, clammy skin, tachycardia, intense thirst, nausea, hematemesis, bloody diarrhea, icterus (rarely intense), hemorrhages from the nose and into the skin, and convulsions. Death may occur after 6 to 48 hr. Survival may be attended by massive local tissue loss from gangrene and secondary infection; amputation of an extremity is sometimes necessary. Fever with a temperature of 101 to 104°F, polymorphonuclear leukocytosis of 20,000 to 30,000, and albuminuria appear within a few hours in severe cases.

The bite of a coral snake causes little pain, and local swelling is slight. There are usually multiple fang marks. Numbness and weakness begin in the region of the bite within 10 to 15 min and are followed by ataxia, ptosis, pupillary dilatation and loss of reaction to light and accommodation, palatal and pharyngeal palsies, slurring of speech, salivation, and, occasionally, nausea and vomiting. The patient becomes comatose, respirations falter, there are convulsions, and death occurs within 8 to 72 hr.

Cobra bites are painful, and, in general, the clinical picture is a combination of neurotoxic and hemolytic manifestations.

TREATMENT. An attempt should be made to determine with certainty that the patient has been bitten by a poisonous snake. Absence of distinct fang punctures and failure of local pain, edema, numbness, or weakness to appear within 20 min are strong evidence against a bite's having been inflicted by a venomous species.

Treatment consists of immobilization, application of a tourniquet, incision and suction, antivenin, local hypothermia, measures to combat infection, and general support. All patients should be transported to a hospital as quickly as possible.

Local Measures. A tourniquet, preferably flat, should be placed a few centimeters above the bite (if anatomically feasible) and made tight enough to allow one finger to pass beneath it with difficulty. The purpose is to impede lymph flow, and it is not necessary to obstruct venous return; the tourniquet should be loosened and moved proximally at hourly intervals when local swelling causes it to tighten. Using whatever antisepsis is available, 1-cm linear (*not cruciate*) incisions about 0.5 cm deep should be made through each fang mark and suction applied for

at least 30 min. A rubber bulb for this purpose is contained in first-aid kits, but a breast pump, funnel attached to a vacuum line, or heated jar can be used. Mouth suction is permissible if no oral lesions are present. Suction should be carried out for 15 min every hour, then every 2 hr, as long as fluid is obtainable. As the swelling progresses, successive rings of radiating, linear, shallow incisions at the advancing edge of the edema are useful; such cuts will be expanded by the progressive swelling. Once a patient has been hospitalized, a pavex boot is a convenient means of applying suction to an extremity. Extensive or deep slashes over the area are unnecessary. Incision and suction are extremely important and should be carried out diligently in every poisonous snake bite. Antivenin is not a substitute for them and should not be relied on alone.

Immobilization of the affected part during transportation is important in controlling lymph flow; splinting is useful in achieving this. The application of ice packs to the affected area reduces inflammation and swelling, slows drainage by lymphatics, relieves pain, and curtails local necrosis. Care should be taken to avoid freezing the tissues.

Antivenin. Many of the components of venom are antigenic, and effective antiserum can be prepared by inoculation of horses with graded doses. In the United States, polyvalent antivenin, effective against all American pit vipers, is available commercially. Kits contain lyophilized antivenin (reconstituted with distilled water to 10 ml per ampul), syringe, normal horse serum for prior sensitivity testing of the patient, and detailed instructions. The initial dose for a serious bite should be 5 ampuls intramuscularly or intravenously. It is not advisable to infiltrate antivenin at the local site. Further antivenin can be given as indicated by progression of swelling or systemic symptoms.

No antivenin for other snakes is manufactured in the United States, but antiserum of various types is usually kept on hand at large zoos all over the world.

Other Measures. The maintenance of respiration by manual or mechanical aids is important in patients bitten by the elapine snakes. It has been suggested that the cholinesterase of cobra and coral venom is responsible for much of the neurotoxicity and that neostigmine and atropine given as for myasthenia gravis might help. This has not been tested clinically.

Tetanus toxoid or antiserum should be given. If pyogenic infection develops, antibiotics should be used.

Alcohol has no place in the treatment of snake bite. Opiates are contraindicated. Relief of pain with salicylates or Demerol, sedation, maintenance of fluid intake, measures to combat shock, and appropriate management of coma or convulsions are all important.

Limited trials of ACTH and adrenal steroids have not shown any great usefulness of these hormones in lessening local necrosis or systemic intoxication.

PREVENTION. In snake-infested regions, long trousers, high shoes, boots or leggings, and gloves should be worn. Most important of all is to look where one steps or reaches. A sharp knife or lancet, tourniquet, suction bulb, and antiseptic suffice for an emergency kit, and in inaccessible areas, antivenin also should be carried.

GILA MONSTER BITE

The Gila monsters include the large orange and black lizard (*Heloderma suspectum*) of the arid Southwest and *H. horridum,* a closely related Mexican species. These reptiles are not aggressive, and virtually every instance of their attacking man has involved teasing or handling the animals in captivity. The venom is elaborated in eight glands in the floor of the mouth and secreted directly into the oral cavity, where it bathes the teeth, which are grooved posteriorly. The lizard clings tenaciously and is often dislodged only after considerable effort; envenomation occurs by contamination of the wound. The venom contains a potent neurotoxin which is undoubtedly responsible for its lethal effect in experimental animals. Death in man has been reported as occurring within a few hours (in one case, 30 min) after a bite. The venom also produces local tissue injury, excruciating pain, massive edema, and patchy erythema. In recovered patients, acute symptoms have lasted for 3 to 4 days and include nausea, vomiting, hematemesis, blurred vision, dyspnea, dysphonia, and profound weakness. Intense hyperesthesia of the bitten extremity may persist for several weeks. There is no antivenin available. Treatment should consist of tourniquet, incision, suction, refrigeration of the bitten area, measures to prevent or combat infection, including tetanus, and supportive measures. Because Demerol has been shown to potentiate the venom's action in animals, some other analgesic should be used to relieve pain.

REFERENCES

Buckley, E. E., and N. Porges (Eds.): "Symposium on Venoms," Am. Assoc. Advan. Sci., Publ. 44, Washington, 1956.

Ellis, E. F., and R. T. Smith: Systemic Anaphylaxis after Rattlesnake Bite, J.A.M.A., 193:401, 401, 1965.

Klauber, L. M.: "Rattlesnakes, Their Habits, Life History and Influence on Mankind," vol. 2, Berkeley, University of California Press, 1956.

Lockhart, W. E.: Treatment of Snakebite, J.A.M.A., 193: 336, 1965.

National Research Council: Ad Hoc Committee on Snakebite Report, Toxicon, 1:81, 1963.

Russell, F. E., and R. S. Scharffenberg: "Bibliography of Snake Venoms and Venomous Snakes," Oxford, Pergamon Press, 1965.

Shannon, F. A.: Case Reports of Two Gila Monster Bites, Herpetology, 9:127, 1953.

123 SPIDERS, SCORPIONS, INSECTS, AND OTHER ARTHROPODS

Ivan L. Bennett, Jr.

The bite of many spiders is locally irritating, and several species can cause severe, even fatal systemic poisoning in man. The most numerous and important of the venomous spiders are members of the genus *Latrodectus,* widely distributed throughout the world. In the United States and Canada, *Lat. mactans,* the black widow or shoe-button spider, causes a majority of clinically significant arachnidism. In Florida, *Lat. bishopi,* the red-legged widow spider, has been reported to produce human poisoning resembling mild black widow bite. From the Southern and Midwestern states, there are increasing numbers of reports of poisoning from the bite of common brown spiders, including *Loxosceles reclusa* and *Lox. unicolor.* These are characterized by pain, local necrosis, and, occasionally, a hemolytic syndrome, which can be fatal.

The symptoms and mortality from bites of large, hairy spiders, the tarantulas, such as *Lycosa raptoria* and *Phoneutria fera* in Brazil or *Glyptocranium gastereanthoides* in Peru, and of such spiders as *Loxosceles laeta* in Chile are similar, with severe ulceration, necrosis, and hemolysis. Neurotoxic manifestations of the type produced by *Latrodectus* are sometimes admixed with local necrosis and hemolysis.

It is the female *Lat. mactans,* the black widow, that bites man. She is glossy black with a body 1 cm in diameter, a leg span of 5 cm, and a characteristic red "hourglass" mark on her abdomen. She spins her web in wood-piles, sheds, basements, or outdoor privies, is very aggressive, and will bite on slight provocation. The venom produces diffuse central and peripheral nervous excitement, autonomic activity, muscle spasm, hypertension, and vasoconstriction.

In the United States, most spider bites occur between April and October, and many patients are males bitten on the genitalia or buttocks while using a privy. After a momentary sharp pain at the site, there is cramping pain that begins locally within 15 to 60 min and gradually spreads. It may involve all extremities and the trunk. The abdomen is boardlike, and the waves of pain become excruciating, causing the patient to turn, toss, and cry out. Respirations are often labored and grunting. There are also nausea, vomiting, headache, sweating, salivation, hyperactive reflexes, twitching, tremor, paresthesias of hands and feet, and, occasionally, systolic hypertension. A mild polymorphonuclear leukocytosis is usual, and many patients have slight fever. After several hours, the pains subside, although mild recurrences for 2 or 3 days are common. It may be a week before well-being is restored. Deaths have occurred, mostly in children and the aged. In an analysis of nearly 1,300 cases from the United States and Canada, the mortality rate was found to vary from 2.4 to 6.0 percent. This is higher than is usually stated.

Because the bite itself is not prominent, patients are often thought to have some abdominal catastrophe such as perforated ulcer, pancreatitis, or volvulus. Renal colic, coronary occlusion, tetanus, strychnine poisoning, tabetic crisis, lead colic, and porphyria are other conditions to be ruled out. The abdomen is not tender to palpation in arachnidism, and pains in the extremities are not typical of most of these other disorders.

TREATMENT. This consists of antiserum and measures to relieve pain. A single intramuscular injection of 1 ampul (2.5 ml) of reconstituted antiserum is all that is needed in most cases; relief is gradual. Hot baths alleviate pain temporarily, and intravenous calcium gluconate or magnesium sulfate usually produces dramatic, but transient, cessation of cramps. Opiates are sometimes necessary. Neostigmine, epinephrine, ACTH, and adrenal steroids have all been reported to give relief in isolated cases and are worth trying.

SCORPION STING

Scorpions are eight-legged arthropods. Glands in the terminal segment produce venom, which is injected into the victim by a stinger located on the tip of the tail. Scorpions often enter dwellings. During the day they retreat into crevices; emerging at night, they often get into shoes and clothing and even into bedding. They do not deliberately attack man, but accidental contact results in a sting.

Of about 650 species, roughly 40 occur in the United States, distributed over three-fourths of the nation. They are most numerous in the South from Florida to California, but the only two lethal species, *Centruroides sculpturatus* and *C. gertschi,* are limited to Arizona and portions of neighboring states.

Dangerous species found in the United States, *C. sculpturatus* and *C. gertschi,* reach a maximal length of about 7 cm. Their sting may be fatal to young children or old people, but seldom to a healthy adult. In the years 1929 to 1948, 68 deaths from scorpion sting were reported from the state of Arizona.

Most of the nonlethal species of scorpions in the United States cause only minor reactions, like a bee sting. Some in the Southwest, however, produce local edema and ecchymosis, with burning pain. In contrast, many species whose venom has potentially dangerous systemic effects, including the Arizona *Centruroides,* evoke little or no visible reaction at the site of the sting. There is an immediate burning sensation followed by local paresthesia ("pins and needles"), hyperesthesia, or numbness. These sensations spread to involve the whole extremity, and within an hour or two, malaise, restlessness, lacrimation, rhinorrhea, salivation, perspiration, nausea, and vomiting appear. Transient hypertension, glucosuria, premature ventricular contractions, and feeble pulse may be noted, or there may be bradycardia and irregular or Cheyne-Stokes breathing. Pulmonary edema develops terminally. The patient passes from an agitated state with hyperactive reflexes into coma; convulsions follow. Death usually occurs within 12 hr, but sometimes as late as 2 days after the sting.

TREATMENT. This consists of immediately placing a tight ligature on the extremity just proximal to the sting, followed by application of ice and, as soon as possible, immersion of the involved member above the ligature in ice water. The ligature must be removed in 5 to 10 min, but the limb is kept refrigerated for at least 2 hr.

After this time, if treatment has been applied promptly, it is said that no serious effects are experienced following the sting of *C. sculpturatus* or *C. gertschi.* If the sting is on the head, trunk, or genitalia, of course, the ligature cannot be used, but the area may be chilled with an ice pack.

Although tourniquet, incision, and suction as in the treatment of snake bite have been recommended, the amount of venom is minute; it produces no local necrotizing effect and is absorbed very rapidly.

Supportive therapy is directed at combating shock and dehydration. Barbiturates in large doses are useful in reducing restlessness.

PREVENTION. This depends upon alertness in avoiding contact with scorpions in infested areas. Clothing and shoes should be well shaken before being put on in the morning. Towels and bedclothes should be inspected. A house infested with scorpions can in time be rid of them by closing all obvious ways of ingress; picking up debris in the environment, such as piles of brush, logs, stones; introducing a mixture of fuel oil or kerosene, containing a small amount of creosote, between the earth and the house foundation; and spraying with a mixture of 2 percent Chlordane, 10 percent DDT, and 0.2 percent pyrethrins in an oil base.

BEES, WASPS, AND ANTS

Bee or wasp venom is hemolytic and neurotoxic and has a histamine-like action. Multiple stings in man cause pain and discomfort, but only in enormous numbers (500 to 1,000) can they cause death. Apiarists often become immune to the venom and can sustain many stings without effect.

The usual reaction to a single bee or wasp sting is sharp pain, local wheal and erythema, intense itching, and, in loose tissues such as the eyelid or genitalia, considerable edema which subsides in a few hours. Only in the rare case when a bee is inhaled or swallowed and edema of the laryngopharynx or glottis develops is there danger. A sting directly into a peripheral nerve may destroy its function for a time, much as does an injection of alcohol. Bell's palsy has followed a sting into the trunk of the facial nerve.

In hypersensitive individuals, a single sting may produce serious anaphylaxis with urticaria, nausea, abdominal cramps, asthma, massive edema of the face and glottis, dyspnea, cyanosis, hypotension, coma, and death. Sensitization is usually a result of previous stings. Beekeepers who develop allergic rhinitis followed by asthma when near bees or objects that have been in contact with bees are likely to have serious reactions to a sting.

Many ants can produce stinging bites with local redness and swelling, including the notorious "fire ant" whose bite may result in vesiculation.

The usual sting is treated by local cool applications and antipruritic lotions or oral antihistaminics. Epinephrine, 0.3 to 0.5 ml of 1:1,000 aqueous solution subcutaneously, repeated every 20 to 30 min, may be lifesaving in patients allergic to bees and/or wasps. This drug may be given as 1:100 solution in oil intramuscularly. Oxygen, antihistaminic drugs, and other supportive measures should be used. Desensitization by injections of extracts of whole bees and wasps is effective. If this is not practical, contact with these insects should be avoided and, if exposure seems likely, epinephrine or sublingual Isuprel tablets should be kept on hand.

TICK BITE AND TICK PARALYSIS

The local reaction to the bite of a tick may be nothing more than an itching papule which subsides within a few days unless there is secondary bacterial infection. However, incomplete removal of a tick, with retention of the mouthparts may result in the local formation of a nodule which continues to grow and is sometimes annoyingly pruritic. The definitive treatment is surgical excision of the nodule. Histologically, the nodule is a granuloma, but the inflammatory response is sometimes so bizarre and changes in the overlying epithelium are so striking that, in the absence of a history of tick bite, a mistaken diagnosis of malignant tumor may be made.

Removal of a tick by steady pulling is preferable to crushing. Touching with a glowing cigarette, freezing, or application of a drop of oil facilitates removal without leaving embedded remnants.

TICK PARALYSIS. Tick paralysis is a reversible disorder of the nervous system which sometimes develops in the host while a tick is engorging. It occurs in man and animals. The disease has been reported from many countries and has long been recognized in the northwestern United States and western Canada, where the wood tick, *Dermacentor andersoni* Stiles, is responsible. The dog tick, *D. variabilis* Say, has been identified in a number of cases occurring in the Eastern states. *Amblyomma americanum*, the lone star tick, and *A. maculatum*, the Gulf Coast tick, have also been incriminated.

While engorging, the tick apparently injects a neurotoxin which acts upon the spinal cord and bulbar nuclei, causing incoordination, weakness, and paralysis. It has been shown in animals that there is failure of neuromuscular transmission and striking impairment of stretch reflexes. The toxin appears to be destroyed or excreted rapidly, for when the tick is removed the nerve cells soon regain normal function.

Tick paralysis has been produced in experimental animals only with gravid female ticks, suggesting that the toxin might be elaborated by the ova. However, injection of extracts prepared from tick eggs has failed to reproduce the clinical picture in convincing fashion.

The tick must feed for several days before symptoms develop. Female ticks commonly remain attached for 7 to 9 days or longer. Paralysis is seen in experimental animals after 5 to 7 days of engorgement. Male ticks feed for a shorter period, a fact which may explain why they are less likely to cause paralysis.

Experimental confirmation of the hypothesis that the toxin is produced in tick salivary glands is also lacking. It has been found that not all gravid female ticks of incriminated species cause paralysis. In short, the nature, site of production, and mode of action of the toxin are still unknown.

Most human cases occur in children, generally in young girls. The tick is usually attached to the scalp and hidden by the hair, but may be found on any part of the body, especially the ear, axilla, groin, vulva, or popliteal region.

The patient may be irritable and have mild diarrhea for 24 hr before frank motor involvement appears. There are weakness and poor control of the legs, the tendon reflexes in the legs are diminished or absent, and the Romberg sign is positive. Temporary improvement may occur, and if the tick is removed at this stage, true paralysis may never develop. Otherwise the symptoms recur within 24 hr, with flaccid paralysis which extends in 24 to 48 hr to involve the trunk, arms, neck, tongue, and pharynx. Sensory changes are usually absent, but there may be paresthesia and hyperesthesia in the affected extremities. Nystagmus, strabismus, and facial paralysis are sometimes noted. The respirations become shallow, rapid, and irregular. The patient sinks into stupor, cyanosis appears, and death results from respiratory paralysis or from obstruction of the airway by aspirated material.

There is little or no fever unless a secondary infection is present. The leukocyte count is usually not elevated, but moderate leukocytosis may occur. The spinal fluid is almost always normal.

Tick paralysis is apt to be confused with poliomyelitis, the more so because ticks are active in warm weather when poliomyelitis is most prevalent.

Among other diseases which might be considered in differential diagnosis are polyneuritis, transverse myelitis, and infectious neuronitis (Guillain-Barré syndrome).

Definitive treatment is removal of the tick. Mouthparts retained in the skin should be promptly excised. The patient's body should be searched for other ticks. There is striking improvement within a few hours after removal of ticks.

If the tick is removed before bulbar involvement develops, the paralysis subsides, and recovery is complete in a few days, sometimes within 24 hr. The patient should be observed until the recovery trend is established, because if other ticks or retained mouthparts have been overlooked, the paralysis may progress. When bulbar or respiratory paralysis is present, death may occur if the tick is not removed in time. Other treatment is supportive.

OTHER ARTHROPODS

FLEA BITE. There are many fleas that attack man, including *Pulex irritans* and chicken fleas. In sensitive individuals, the salivary secretion of these bloodsuckers produces large, itching papules. Treatment is symptomatic only. Elimination of fleas in an environment may be very difficult, but persistent treatment of animals and of premises with appropriate insecticides is usually successful.

CENTIPEDE BITE. Local irritation is the usual reaction to centipede venom, although extensive necrosis and systemic illness have followed severe poisoning by tropical species. Treatment is purely symptomatic.

CATERPILLAR URTICARIA. Contact with hairy caterpillars of many species produces irritation of skin or mucous membranes. The type of venom involved is not known, but severe pain, erythema, urticaria, and even blister formation may come on rapidly after direct contact with caterpillars, after handling cocoons, or on being exposed to windblown fuzz. There are often a regional lymphangitis and transient eosinophilic leukocytosis. The discomfort subsides within 24 hr, but local soaks, oral antihistaminics, and when pain is severe, oral codeine are often indicated.

BEDBUG BITE. Members of the genus *Cimex* inflict bites that leave reactions varying from a simple puncture to large urticarial lesions, apparently depending on the sensitivity of the bitten individual. There is no specific treatment.

CHIGGERS OR REDBUGS. These are tiny mites which are commonly found in foliage, grass, etc., in many parts of the world. In the United States, the larval form of *Eutrobicula alfreddugesi* attacks the skin by secreting a substance which digests tissue, creating a red papule that itches intensely. The tiny reddish larva can be seen in the center of the lesion. Treatment is palliative with antipruritic applications. There is no better example of the virtues of prevention than this annoying affliction. The use of insect repellents, appropriate protective clothing, and prompt bathing after exposure reduce the risk of infestation considerably.

MYIASIS. There are, generally speaking, three ways in which human tissues may become infested by maggots. Species of flies which usually deposit eggs in carrion, feces, or garbage may lay eggs in an open wound or ulcer, usually a lesion that is necrotic and suppurating. When the larvae hatch, they feed upon the dead tissue, and despite the unesthetic aspects, the deliberate introduction of maggots has been used to supplement surgical debridement.

Occasionally, food containing fly eggs will be ingested, and when the larvae hatch, *intestinal myiasis* can result in nausea, cramps, and diarrhea. The larvae are passed in the feces.

Finally the larvae of many flies, including the sheep fly and horsefly, will attack living, viable tissue. If eggs are laid in the eyes, nose, ears, mouth, or vagina, an event that usually occurs in sleeping infants, the larvae hatch out and can produce extensive destructive lesions; indeed, fatalities have been reported.

The treatment for maggot infestation is surgical removal by irrigation and mechanical extraction. Obviously, control of fly populations by appropriate sanitary precautions is the important step in prevention. Protection of infants by screening and of wounds by bandaging is indicated in infested areas.

REFERENCES

Bee Sting

Helm, S.: Severe Anaphylactic Reaction to a Bee or Wasp Sting, Mil. Surg., 92:64, 1943.
Perlman, F.: Desensitization to Wasp Sting, J.A.M.A., 156:1470, 1954.

Caterpillar Urticaria

McMillan, C. W., and W. R. Purcell: Health Hazard from Caterpillars, New Eng. J. Med., 271:147, 1964.

Scorpion Sting

De Magalhaes, O.: Scorpionism, J. Trop. Med. Hyg., 41:393, 1938.
Essex, H. E.: Animal Venoms and Their Physiologic Action, Physiol. Rev., 25:150, 1945.
Waterman, J. A.: Some Notes on Scorpion Poisoning in Trinidad, Trans. Roy. Soc. Trop. Med. Hyg., 31:607, 1938.

Spider Bite

Dillaha, C. J., et al.: North American Loxoscelism. Necrotic Bite of the Brown Recluse Spider, J.A.M.A., 188:33, 1964.
Nance, W. E.: Hemolytic Anemia of Necrotic Arachnidism, Am. J. Med., 31:801, 1961.
Thorpe, R. W., and W. D. Woodson: "The Black Widow: America's Most Poisonous Spider," Chapel Hill, N.C., University of North Carolina Press, 1945.

Tick Paralysis

Ransmeier, J. C.: Tick Paralysis in the Eastern United States, J. Pediat., 34:299, 1949.
Stanbury, J. B., and J. H. Huyck: Tick Paralysis: A Critical Review, Medicine, 24:219, 1945.

124 MARINE ANIMALS
Ivan L. Bennett, Jr.

The elaboration of substances that are poisonous for man is by no means an exclusive property of reptiles and arthropods. Several plant and animal products that are toxic when ingested are described in Chap. 116. Here, discussion will center around venoms of marine animals known definitely to cause illness in man after injection or inoculation under naturally occurring conditions. Information about these toxins is limited, a few isolated clinical observations being the only data available about some of them. An excellent compilation and bibliography will be found in the reviews listed at the end of the chapter.

SEA ANEMONE STING (SPONGE DIVER'S DISEASE). Contact with certain sea anemones (especially *Sargatia elegans*) in Mediterranean and African waters produces extensive dermatitis with chronic ulceration. Occasionally, especially during August and September, systemic symptoms of headache, sneezing, nausea, chills, fever, and collapse are noted. Rare fatalities have occurred. No specific therapy is known; the skin lesions have been thought to benefit from local x-ray irradiation. The disease confers no immunity.

SPONGE POISONING. Direct contact with several species of sponge results in a painful dermatitis. It is known that extracts of the sponges are lethal for mice. Dilute acetic acid ameliorates local pain strikingly, and alkali will intensify it. The lesions are self-limited.

PORTUGUESE MAN–O–WAR AND JELLYFISH STINGS. The burning discomfort induced by contact with "sea nettles" or jellyfish is familiar to most surf bathers. Contact with the tentacles of the colorful Portuguese man-o-war (*Physalia* species) or more toxic jellyfish (*Chiropsalmus* of the Indian Ocean and *Rhizostoma* of the Atlantic) is followed by severe pain, swelling, and erythema. Muscle pain, weakness, abdominal cramps, nausea, dyspnea, cyanosis, and collapse may persist for several days, and fatalities have occurred, sometimes within hours after contact.

Treatment consists of local application of ammonia, alcohol, or calamine, oral or parenteral antihistaminics, and systemic support. Cortisone has been thought to help in a few cases.

CONE SHELL POISONING. The colorful cone shells are highly prized by collectors. Many species in the Pacific are venomous, a great danger to unwary hobbyists who pick them up. The poison is delivered into a wound inflicted by pointed hollow teeth resembling darts in the long proboscis of the animal. Local manifestations include sudden intense pain, swelling, and cyanosis followed by numbness. The venom is apparently a neurotoxin and produces muscular incoordination, weakness, confusion, tachycardia, and dyspnea. Death may occur within 3 to 5 hr, but recovery within 24 hr is the rule. Recommended treatment is the use of tourniquet, incision, and suction (as for snake bite) and supportive measures which may include artificial respiration and administration oxygen.

SEA URCHIN STING. Contact with the spines of some species of sea urchin results in painful erythema and ulceration with or without neurotoxic symptoms of weakness and frank paralysis of lips, tongue, and face lasting for several hours. Treatment is purely symptomatic and supportive. The toxins isolated from sea urchins have produced paralysis in animals and are notably resistant to heat. Deaths from paralysis and drowning have been reported.

FISH STINGS. The dorsal fins or spines of bullhead sharks, dogfish (the familiar *Squalus acanthias* of biology classes), and ratfish and the dorsal and other fins of the scorpion fish, weeverfish, toadfish, and catfish are grooved, and at their bases are found venom glands. Injury by these spines results in severe pain and swelling and, in some instances, neurotoxic manifestations. Local gangrene with extensive tissue loss is a complication of catfish stings that may prolong convalescence. Little or nothing is known of the venoms involved. Suction and hot applications are advocated immediately after injury. Tetanus toxoid or antitoxin should be given also. Narcotics are often required to control the pain. Secondary pyogenic infection is a frequent complication.

Probably the most frequent type of venomous fish injury in the United States is that produced by the lashing tail of the stingray of the California coast (*Urobatis halleri*). The bony spine is encased in a sheath of epithelial cells containing venom which is expressed into the puncture wound. The wound may be several centimeters deep; portions of the bony spine may break off in it, or, more often, the integumentary sheath remains in the wound. The venom is a circulatory depressant in animals, but local injury predominates in man. There are immediately severe pain and cyanosis followed by erythema and edema. Weakness, rarely, convulsions, and death may ensue. Treatment consists of application of a tourniquet (the vast majority of these injuries occur on the legs) and copious syringing of the wound with salt water to remove fragments of sheath followed by immersion in water as hot as the patient can stand for 1 hr. The venom is heat-labile, and extensive trials have indicated the usefulness of this last procedure. Tetanus toxoid or antiserum is indicated; as with other fish stings, pyogenic infection is a frequent complication.

REFERENCES

Abbott, R. T.: "Mollusks and Medicine in World War II," Smithsonian Annual Report for 1947, p. 325, Washington, 1948.

Halstead, B. W.: Animal Phyla Known to Contain Poisonous Marine Animals, p. 9 in Symposium on Venoms, American Association for the Advancement of Science, Washington, 1956.

Keegan, H. L., and W. V. Macfarlane (Eds.): "Venomous and Poisonous Animals and Noxious Plants of the Pacific Region," Oxford, Pergamon Press, 1965.

Russell, F. E.: Marine Toxins and Venomous and Poisonous Marine Animals, Advance. Marine Biol., 3:255, 1965.

Section 3
Physical Agents

125 DISORDERS DUE TO ENVIRONMENTAL TEMPERATURES

John H. Talbott

Three clinical syndromes are associated with high environmental temperature: heat cramps, heat exhaustion, and heat pyrexia. Although each entity may be identified clinically, there is considerable overlapping of the internal changes produced by a high environmental temperature, sequelae of excessive or prolonged physiologic responses. The alterations are especially prevalent during the first days of a heat wave before effective acclimatization. Prophylaxis, by augmented sodium chloride intake prior to exposure or by restoration of the physiologic balance prior to the onset of overt morbidity, is helpful in preventing dire consequences. The child and the older person are more susceptible to heat stress. Strenuous physical activity or the presence of an acute or chronic disease may hasten the development of any one of the morbid states.

Acclimatization

The basic mechanism remains obscure, although more is known of acclimatization of man to heat than to cold. The threshold for onset of sweating is not increased. Sweating is the most effective natural means of combating heat stress with little or no change in the core temperature of the body. As long as sweating continues, provided water and salt are replaced, man can withstand remarkably high temperatures. Two, three, or more liters of sweat may be lost per day. Water and sodium chloride are the most important physiologic constituents of sweat. The concentration of sodium chloride may be low; at other times, it may approach that of interstitial body fluid. Since the sodium chloride concentration of sweat is less than that of body fluid, the excess salt must be retained in the body during the initial stages of sweating. Studies reveal the skin to be the repository. Dilatation of the peripheral blood vessels is a well-known phenomenon in high environmental temperatures. Histamine and histidine in the sweat may participate in the vasodilatation. Other alterations include a decrease in total circulating blood volume, a decrease in renal blood flow, and an increase of the antidiuretic substance in the urine (ADH). Aldosterone, the most potent mineralocorticoid, has been detected in increased quantities in the urine following

exposure. Vasodilatation, with an increased circulation in the blood vessels of the skin, permits dissipation of heat. The cardiac output is increased initially. As the stress persists, there is diminished venous return with the peripheral type of forward failure. Failure of dissipation of heat with persistence of environmental temperatures greater than the temperature of the body leads to retention of heat and development of hyperpyrexia.

Heat Cramps

"Miner's cramps" and "stoker's cramps" describe the heat syndrome associated with painful spasms of the voluntary musculature following strenuous exercise. Only persons in good physical condition are victims. External temperatures need not exceed the body temperature. Direct exposure to the sun is not necessary. Muscle cramps have been observed following excessive sweating, precipitated by strenuous exercise in cold environments in untrained persons heavily clothed. Muscles of the extremities bear the brunt of physical activity and show the highest incidence of cramps. Excruciating pain accompanies the spasms and subsides with cessation of cramps. Physical examination is essentially normal between the paroxysms. Examination of the blood reveals a concentration of the formed elements and a decreased concentration of total base, especially sodium. A diminished excretion of sodium chloride in the urine is characteristic. Cessation of cramps with *replacement of sodium chloride and water* is striking and supports the hypothesis that the cause of heat cramps is associated with body depletion of these essential electrolytes.

Heat Exhaustion

Heat prostration, or heat collapse, is probably the most common heat syndrome. Weakness, vertigo, headache, nausea, anorexia, and faintness may precede collapse or participate as predisposing factors. The physically active as well as the sedentary person is susceptible. Onset may be sudden and the duration of collapse brief. During the acute stage, evidence of peripheral vascular failure and poor venous return may be detected from the ashen-gray appearance. The skin is cold and clammy. The pupils are dilated. The blood pressure may be decreased, with a significant increase in the pulse pressure. Since prostration develops before exposure is prolonged, body temperature is subnormal or normal. The duration of exposure and the extent of sweat loss determine the degree of hemoconcentration. *Treatment* embraces supporting measures and removal to a cool area. Intravenous administration of saline solution or whole blood usually is not necessary. Although the pathogenetic mechanism of prostration is not primarily a depletion of water and salt, there are theoretical and practical reasons for maintaining optimal concentration of these essential body constituents in persons exposed to high temperatures.

Heat Pyrexia

Heat hyperpyrexia, heat stroke, or sunstroke is most common in the person with a preexisting acute or chronic malady. Direct exposure to the sun is not a necessary prerequisite. A high relative humidity is an important predisposing factor. Heat pyrexia may develop during any period of hot weather, but the incidence in temperate climates increases with the prolongation of a heat wave. A diminution or cessation of sweating before onset of acute symptoms may be observed and is indicative of a breakdown of the heat regulatory mechanism. The exact cause of the cessation of sweating is not known. Persons mildly afflicted may reveal no premonitory symptoms. Others may complain of headache, vertigo, faintness, or abdominal distress. Delirium may develop in the severely afflicted patient.

Pyrexia and prostration are significant findings on physical examination. A rectal temperature greater than 106°F is a grave prognostic sign. Internal body temperatures as high as 110°F have been observed. The skin is hot and dry, and sweating is absent. The pulse rate is increased, and respirations are rapid and weak. Systolic blood pressure may be elevated. The tendon reflexes may be diminished. Clinical evidence of circulatory collapse may be observed. Examination of the blood and urine may show few alterations from the normal. A leukocytosis is characteristic. A temporary retention of nitrogenous products with albumin and casts in the urine may be noted, as well as a decrease of total body potassium. The electrocardiogram may show, in addition to tachycardia and sinus arrhythmia, flattening and subsequent inversion of the 'T' wave and depression of the S-T segment. The roentgenogram may show a detectable decrease in the size of the cardiac silhouette. Venous pressures more than double the control level have been noted in normal persons exposed to high temperatures. The extent to which such elevations are due to increase venous return to the heart, or to early failure of this organ, or to a combination has not been clearly defined. It has been suggested that the elevation of venous pressure may be responsible for the diminished sweating, but proof for this concept is lacking.

If the patient survives 24 or 48 hr of pyrexia, and acute renal failure does not develop, recovery may be anticipated. One attack of heat pyrexia renders a person susceptible to future attacks. Extensive parenchymal damage to various organs, either from hyperpyrexia per se or from petechial hemorrhages, may complicate recovery. The brain, heart, kidneys, and liver have been the sites of petechial hemorrhages. Shibolet et al. reported increased fibrinolysis, afibrinogenemia, and especially brain damage in fatal cases of heat stroke which showed multiple hemorrhages. Low prothrombin values have been observed by several investigators.

MANAGEMENT. Heat pyrexia requires heroic emergency measures. Time is most important. The patient should be placed in a cool place with adequate circulation of fresh air and with most of the clothing removed. Since the pathogenesis of the condition involves a failure of the heat-regulating mechanism with cessation of sweating, external means of heat dissipation must be substituted for those temporarily absent. An ice water bath is drastic treatment for an acutely ill person, but there is no effective substitute. Immersion in ice water does not induce shock or stimulate significant cutaneous vasoconstriction. An ice tub bath should be given with a minimum of delay. The patient should be watched constantly by a nurse or physician, and the rectal temperature should be taken repeatedly. The bath may be discontinued when the core temperature falls below 103°F. The treatment should be resumed if it recrudesces. Ice water sponge baths, rubbing with ice, wet sheets, and an electric fan are ineffective substitutes. Following the bath the patient should be placed in a cool, well-ventilated room. Massage of the skin aids in the acceleration of heat loss and stimulates return of the cool peripheral blood to the overheated brain and viscera. Stimulants such as epinephrine and narcotics are contraindicated. Intravenous saline solution may be recommended if the patient is not in cardiac failure and if the prepyrexic clinical state does not contraindicate it. Fresh blood, fibrinogen solutions, and possibly glucocorticoids should be prescribed (without waiting for laboratory confirmation) if afibrinogenemia is suspected. Several days of convalescence may be required after such an insult.

Although most patients die or recover completely, occasionally survivors have severe and permanent brain damage.

REFERENCES

Clinicopathologic Conference: A Sixty-Five-Year-Old Woman with Heat Stroke, Am. J. Med., 43:113, 1967.

Collins, K. J., and J. S. Weiner: Endocrinological Aspects of Exposure to High Environmental Temperatures, Physiol. Rev., 48:785, 1968.

Knochel, J. P., W. R. Beisel, E. G. Herndon, Jr., E. S. Gerad, and K. G. Barry: The Renal, Cardiovascular, Hematologic and Serum Electrolyte Abnormalities of Heat Stroke, Am. J. Med., 30.299, 1961.

Leithead, C.: Prevention of the Disorders Due to Heat, Roy. Soc. Trop. Med. Hygiene, 61:739, 1967.

Menard, D.: Evaluation of Heat Stress under Working Conditions, Industry and Tropical Health VI: Proc. of the Sixth Conference of the Industrial Council for Tropical Health, Oct. 25–27, 1966, Boston, Harvard School of Public Health, 1967.

Shibolet, S., S. Fisher, T. Gilat, H. Bank, and H. Heller: Fibrinolysis and Hemorrhages in Fatal Heatstroke, New Engl. J. Med., 266:169, 1962.

Yoshimura, H., K. Ogata, and S. Itoh (Eds.): "Essential Problems in Climatic Physiology: A Tribute to Professor Yaskuno," Kyoto, Nandodo, 1960.

126 COLD INJURY AND HYPOTHERMIA

*Albert R. Behnke and
Ralph W. Brauer*

COLD INJURY

In warfare, cold has been of prime concern as the most disabling environmental stress. In Korea during the winter of 1950–1951, there were approximately 8,000 injuries due to cold; about two-thirds of these were evacuated to Japan and the United States for continued treatment. Exposure to both wet and dry cold, not only of ground troops but also of aviators and shipwreck survivors, emphasizes the importance of protection, particularly of hands and feet, and of acclimatization.

In biology and medicine, dynamic progress has been made in cryobiology and in applications of hypothermia in surgery and in therapy. Hypothermia combined with hyperbaric oxygenation shows promise of eliminating complications arising from hypoxia.

The temperature ranges of concern are (1) very low temperatures, often associated with freezing of some water in tissues, (2) hypothermic temperatures which are in the range of a few degrees above freezing to a level below deep body temperature, and (3) reduced temperatures which are compensated for by physiologic adjustments. At freezing and hypothermic levels, cold injury embraces frostbite and immersion foot.

Local Cold Injury

DIRECT AND INDIRECT MECHANISMS OF INJURY. Frostbite and other lesions due to cold have been intensively studied in man and animals but the results of these investigations have not resolved controversies in regard to underlying pathology and therapeutic measures. Mechanisms of freezing injury can be separated into phenomena which affect cells and extracellular fluids (direct effects) and those which disrupt the function of organized tissues and integrity of circulation (indirect effects).

Certain *direct effects* have been delineated with unequivocal clarity. When tissue freezes, ice crystals form, and concomitantly, solutes in the residual liquid become concentrated. It is clear from a study of a histologic section of tissue fixed while frozen to preserve distortion by ice crystals that the physical dislocation during slow freezing is extreme. Ice crystals many times the size of individual cells form, but only in the extracellular spaces. There is ample evidence that large ice crystals can develop between cells in soft tissue without producing irreversible injury as long as the percentage of water frozen does not exceed a critical amount. In hamster experiments it has been demonstrated that freezing at temperatures as low as −6°C for periods up to 1 hr and the presence of large quantities of ice crystals in the skin and subcutaneous tissue are compatible with full recovery and absence of peripheral lesions. Of prime importance clinically is the observation that trauma induced by bending a frozen extremity resulted in lesions which grossly and microscopically resemble frostbite in man.

A major source of damage to living cells during freezing and thawing appears to be the deleterious effect of strong salt solutions which develop during formation and dissolution of ice; changes in the proportions of lipids and phospholipids in the cell membrane are also of great importance. The discovery of the protective value of such substances as glycerol and dimethylsulfoxide, which enter cells and prevent freezing injury during comparatively slow cooling to and rewarming from low temperatures, represents a significant advance. This method has been used extensively in banking spermatoza for subsequent artificial insemination in the bovine species. It has not been possible, however, to protect organs in this manner since the protective substance must be delivered to all cells.

Turning now to the *indirect effects* of cold on organized tissue, vascular stasis and ensuing derangements appear to be the major cause of tissue injury. There is abundant experimental evidence that the fulminating vascular reaction and stasis which supervene are associated with production of histaminelike substances which increase the permeability of the capillary bed. Within blood vessels, cellular elements aggregate. Irreversible occlusion of small blood vessels by cell masses has been demonstrated in thawed tissue following freezing injury. Structural damage of the frozen tissue simulates damage produced by burns.

CLINICAL CONSIDERATIONS. Local cold injury may be divided into freezing (frostbite) and nonfreezing (immersion foot) injuries. The two types may be observed in the same extremity or in different extremities in the same individual, e.g., trench foot, freezing of the hands and nonfreezing of the feet of shipwreck survivors. It is important to recognize differences in clinical appearance, signs and symptoms; underlying pathologic derangements; and sequelae of the two entities which may require divergent courses of therapy. The diagnosis of freezing versus nonfreezing injury can be made generally on the basis of history and clinical manifestations.

Immersion Foot

In this entity, observed in shipwreck survivors or in soldiers (trench foot) whose feet have been wet but not freezing cold for prolonged periods, there is primarily injury to nerve and muscle tissue, with no gross or irreparable pathologic changes in blood vessels and skin. The clinical picture reflects primary hypoxic trauma giving rise to three clearly recognizable conditions: (1) *ischemia*, denoted by a pale pulseless extremity; (2) *hyperemia*, characterized by a bounding pulsatile circulation in red swollen painful feet; and (3) *posthyperemic* recovery period. The initial cold-induced vasoconstriction, increased blood viscosity, and impaired oxygen transport in the ischemic state are aggravated by such factors as undernutrition, general hypothermia, dehydration, and trauma from relatively fixed, pendant extremities. The problem of rewarming is critical in these patients during the stage of ischemia, when overheating of tissue may lead to gangrene. In the state of hyperemia, the red swollen feet require judicious cooling. Severe cases may show muscular weakness, atrophy, ulceration, and gangrene of superficial areas. The sequelae of even milder injuries are sensitivity to cold and pain on weight bearing, which may be severe and last for many years.

Frostbite

In true frostbite, in contrast with immersion foot, the blood vessels may be severely or irreparably injured, the circulation of blood ceases, and the vascular beds of the frozen tissues are occluded by agglutinated cell aggregates and thrombi. The cutaneous injury consists in part of separation of the epidermal-dermal interface. There is a distinction between direct injury to cells and the subsequent fulminating vascular reaction and stasis which precede tissue necrosis. In the early postthawing stage much of the intravascular clumping is reversible. However, with the passage of time, clumped red cells within vessels in injured tissue lose their morphologic identity and take on the appearance of a homogeneous, hyalinaceous plug. It has been shown experimentally that much of the intravascular aggregation following freezing injury can be reversed, and microcirculatory perfusion improved when low molecular weight dextran is given intravenously shortly after injury.

The discouraging clinical aspects of cold injury, which present a myriad of pathologic derangements, stem from its origin. In the military, cold injury is often the badge of depression, demoralization, and defeat. It afflicts isolated scattered units with their heavy toll of wounded. Lack of food, equipment, shelter, and warmth make inevitable the disastrous injury inflicted by cold. Civilians, apart from persons who engage in expeditions which take them into snow and ice and to hypoxic altitudes, are frequently victims of circumstances associated with vagrancy and alcoholism. In both military and civilian life the physician will be confronted with tissues not frozen, but in a thawed, macerated condition. The manner of rewarming, slow or rapid, generally may be irrelevant. If thawing becomes necessary, the consensus is to use well-stirred water at about 40°C (104°F) until flushing extends to the distal parts but no longer. The rationale that led to immersion at above body temperature was based on experimental work with animals in which the conditions of the tests were not those which usually pertain to freezing in man. German experience in World War II and Swiss experience in treatment of Alpine cold exposure placed emphasis on warming the "core" of the body before treating the local area of frostbite. Heat was applied to the trunk of the body and subsequently the frozen part was placed in water at 10 to 15°C, then increased 5°C every 5 min up to 40°C but no higher.

Sympathectomy is a specific measure for the treatment of frostbite. Shumacker believes that operative sympathetic denervation is indicated as soon after injury as is possible in any good-risk patient who has sustained frostbite of such severity as to indicate likely development of gangrene and loss of tissue. For the late sequelae of frostbite, the benefits of sympathectomy are well established.

SEQUELAE OF FROSTBITE INJURY. A follow-up of 100 Korean cold-injury casualties revealed that both after 4 and after 13 years, there was excessive sweating, pain, cold feet, numbness, abnormal color, and joint symptomatology. Symptoms were more severe during the winter months or on exposure to cold. Characteristic physical findings (after 4 years) were tissue loss and scarring, abnormal nails, discoloration and depigmentation, hyperhydrosis, and on x-ray, osteoporosis and cystic defects in bone near joint surfaces. Patients who had had sympathectomy were almost free of complaints.

Prevention of Cold Injury

Assiduous effort has been made to develop protective equipment and to indoctrinate personnel by "hardening" in cold environment. Although a period of several generations is perhaps required to confer a "Patagonian" ability to exist with little protection in subzero weather, nevertheless, a degree of acclimatization is possible over a period of months to graded exposure to cold which should render individuals resistant who otherwise might become casualties.

COLD ACCLIMATIZATION. Cold acclimatization represents a state of increased resistance to cold injury and is the result of exposure to a cold but tolerable environment. Adaptive responses are *circulatory adjustments* protecting the temperatures of exposed portions of the body; *metabolic adaptation* results in greater heat production to compensate for increased heat loss; and *behavioral and neural adaptations* which minimize either the actual cold stress or the discomfort resulting from physiologically tolerable hypothermia. In contrast with heat acclimatization, it is not possible to delineate adaptive physiologic changes to cold. Nevertheless, primitive peoples live at zero temperatures wearing little or no clothing; pain perception is less in persons who work periodically with their hands in ice water such as fishermen; and military personnel shiver less during test cold exposure after training in the arctic. Comparison of temperature patterns and incidence of shivering during sleep show two distinct adaptive responses. In one, displayed by cold-acclimatized young Norwegian subjects, relatively high skin temperatures are maintained at the expense of intense shivering throughout the night, but ability develops to sleep despite bouts of shivering. The second response, displayed in extreme degree by Australian aborigines, entails marked temperature drop of the body as a whole accompanied by minimal shivering. For restoration, the natives depend upon heat absorption in the morning; hence, a tendency to welcome or worship the sun.

HYPOTHERMIA

Levels of Hypothermia and Metabolism

The moderate range of hypothermia, useful in general surgery and relatively safe, is about 28 to 34°C; deep or profound hypothermia is in the range below 28°C to about 0°C, which is compatible with survival of small mammals for limited periods of time. In man, not until cooling has reduced deep body temperature to less than 30°C is contact with the environment lost. Lowering the body temperature decreases oxygen consumption without jeopardizing vital functions. For every degree of centigrade reduction in body temperature, metabolism decreases 6.5 percent. Thus at 30°C, oxygen consumption is about 50 percent of normal, and at this temperature complete circulatory arrest can be maintained for as long as 8 to 10 min. In man, there is a high incidence of ventricular fibrillation at temperatures below 28°C. It is possible that the heart with its high extraction requirement for ozygen may be inadequately supplied by cold oxygen-bound hemoglobin. There is some evidence that hyperbaric oxygen greatly reduces the tendency of the hypothermic heart to fibrillate.

Immersion Hypothermia

Responses to cold water immersion may be classified as (1) stimulatory, deep body temperature normal to 35°C (95°F); (2) depressant, deep body temperature 35 to 30°C; and (3) critical, deep body temperature 30 to 25°C (86 to 77°F).

CARDIOVASCULAR RESPONSES. The long-distance swimmer is able to maintain a normal deep body temperature for periods of 15 to 25 hr or more under conditions in which water and skin temperatures (15°C, 59°F, or lower) are some 38°F less than deep body temperature. Such data lend support to the useful concept of a body core insulated by a body shell, which in the case of the distance swimmer consists of a substantial thickness of fat. With vasoconstriction operative in cold water, there is a virtual cutoff of peripheral circulation, which greatly reduces heat loss. There is great individual variability in heat loss when the body is immersed in cold water. The relatively obese swimmer may maintain a normal rectal temperature for 2 hr without shivering in 16°C water. A lean man under the same conditions, despite violent shivering, may experience a fall in rectal temperature of several degrees and become incapacitated from rigor. In hypersensitive persons, immersion in cold water may be followed by vascular spasm, vomiting, and syncope—a histamine-type reaction.

In tests of volunteers immersed to the neck in cold water (5 to 15°C), there was initial vasoconstriction and slight rise of rectal temperature, blood pressure, and pulse rate. The heart rate then decreases, presumably an effect of lowered temperature on the pacemaker. In contrast with bradycardia associated with inhalation of oxygen at normal and high pressures, bradycardia in the cold bath is not abolished by atropine or vagotomy. At a rectal temperature of 30°C (86°F), arrhythmias may appear, and atrial fibrillation is observed. In the dog, when deep body temperature declines to about 25°C (77°F), blood pressure may fall sharply, and at 22°C, ventricular fibrillation brings about death.

REWARMING. In contrast to the equivocal procedure of rapid rewarming of a frozen extremity in man is the mandatory (which may be lifesaving) measure of rapid rewarming in water (45°C, 113°F) of persons removed from cold water. Otherwise, a precipitous fall in deep body temperature of several degrees may follow return of blood flow through the cold peripheral tissues. It was observed, for example, that a volunteer removed from a cold bath and warmed in air on a hot Washington summer day shivered for a period of about 2 hr. An individual rewarmed in the bath, however, must be removed prior to return of deep body temperature to normal, in order to forestall circulatory collapse from vasodilatation and excessive diversion of cardiac output to peripheral tissues.

Clinical Uses of Low Temperatures

LOCALIZED APPLICATION. Extensive application of low temperatures has been made in recent years, notably in preservation of viability and banking of cells and tissues. Two basic uses of cryogenic temperatures encompass selective destruction by freezing in cryosurgery as well as preservation of biologic material. A system, for example, for cryogenic surgery has been developed which can be applied to any part of the body. Practical advantages are safety and hemostasis; the results in therapeutic management of tumors have been encouraging. If blood is cooled ultra-rapidly to the temperature of liquid nitrogen and then rapidly thawed, only a few cells are hemolyzed. This technique has been employed routinely on Naval hospital ships serving the battlefield. Mention has been made of the notable discovery that glycerol protects certain cells from freezing. This has made possible preservation of red blood cells, spermatozoa, and other viable materials in their native condition.

Hypothermia combined with hyperbaric oxygenation has been employed with notable success in harvesting, preserving, and transplanting organs, chiefly the kidney.

Local gastric hypothermia has been used effectively to control upper gastrointestinal bleeding from esophageal varices, hemorrhagic gastritis, and gastric and duodenal ulcers. This form of treatment is primarily useful in patients for whom definitive surgery must be delayed or avoided.

Medical Problems Relating to the Use of Hypothermia in Surgery

Periods of ischemia sufficient to permit surgical intervention can be tolerated by critical organs such as the brain and heart, provided that tissue temperature has been lowered to reduce metabolism before blood supply is interrupted. Hypothermia can be induced with light anesthesia and surface cooling or, more effectively, by means of pump-oxygenators to provide extracorporeal circulation. Prior to the introduction of this technique, surgical hypothermia was limited to temperatures of about 28°C; temperatures below 25°C were dangerous. At present, extracorporeal circulation has extended the application of hypothermia to temperatures of 10°C or lower. The principal medical problem arises from disturbances in acid-base balance. One aspect of this complicated problem, apart from large fluctuations in dissolved CO_2 in relation to temperature change, is an oxygen debt incurred by some tissues and an excess lactic acid production. The oxygen debt is present not only during induction of hypothermia but even more so during the period of recovery when cardiac function is less than optimal. The body's buffer mechanisms may be wholly inadequate to regulate pH. Intravenously administered buffers of the amine type (Tris or THAM) have given encouraging results. Coupling of these methods for the induction and maintenance of hypothermia with hyperbaric oxygenation may not only correct the difficulties of pH control, but enhance as well the period during which ischemia may be safely maintained.

With surface cooling the high incidence of ventricular fibrillation at temperatures below 28°C is the most serious complication of hypothermia. A contributing factor is the use of citrated blood; with heparinized blood irreversible ventricular fibrillation is not a problem. In view of the effectiveness of hyperbaric oxygenation in controlling ligature-induced ventricular fibrillation in dogs, it would appear that this modality may well diminish hypothermic cardiac irritability related to tissue hypoxia. With employment of the pump-oxygenator, however, the problem of ventricular fibrillation appears to have been circumvented.

Gastric hemorrhage occurs in animals cooled to low temperatures, and this condition may occur in man. In the rabbit, massive hemorrhage occurs from the fundus of the stomach. A similar hemorrhagic lesion is induced in rabbits at normal temperature after injection of posterior pituitary extract. It is due to intense gastric vasoconstriction and resultant reduction in volume and increase in acidity of gastric juice secreted. *It can be prevented by neutralizing gastric contents.*

Lastly, at temperatures around 10°C, with circulatory arrest, conditions favor intravascular clumping of cellular elements, which was mentioned earlier in connection with freezing injury. Cellular aggregates as part of a "sludging" phenomenon may deprive the brain of blood supply and lead to neurologic damage and possibly death.

REFERENCES

Brown, I. W., Jr., and B. G. Cox (Eds.): "Hyperbaric Medicine," Third Internat. Congress, Publ. 1404, Nat. Acad. Sci. Nat. Res. Council, Washington, 1966.

Burton, A. C., and O. G. Edholm: "Man in a Cold Environment," London, Edward Arnold & Co., 1955.

Hart, J. S. (Ed.): Proceeding of the International Symposium on Altitude and Cold, Federation Proceedings, 28:933–1321, 1969.

Taylor, A. C. (Ed.): Hypothermia, Ann. N.Y. Acad. Sci., 80:285–550, 1959.

Viereck, E. (Ed.): IV. Frostbite. Proc. Symposia Arctic Med. and Biol., Arctic Aeromedical Lab, Fort Wainwright, Alaska, 1964.

127 DISORDERS DUE TO ALTERATIONS IN BAROMETRIC PRESSURE

Albert R. Behnke

Introduction

Since 1958, man has landed on the moon, orbited the earth in excursions as long as 2 weeks, explored the ocean floor to depths of 650 ft (20.7 atm), and extended his ability to work effectively in the dry, pressurized environment to simulated depths of 1,000 ft (31.3 atm). The hyperbaric oxygen environment is being exploited in medicine through operation of numerous single- and multiple-unit pressure chambers. Pressurized tunneling is required routinely for the construction of sewage conduits, vehicular tunnels, and underground rapid transit systems. The recreational and exploratory aspects of *scuba* diving (self-contained underwater breathing apparatus) claimed the interest of several million enthusiasts. These dynamic developments make it necessary for the physician to be aware of the physiologic problems, hazards, and therapeutic measures connected with alterations in barometric pressure in the effort to control potential accidents.

Injury arises from too rapid ascent (aeroembolism, decompression sickness); indirectly from cold, hypoxia, nitrogen narcosis, hyperventilation tetany, and overexertion; and in closed breathing systems from oxygen toxicity and carbon dioxide excess. Mishaps are caused by logistic failure (the empty gas bottle); equipment deficiencies, notably lack of recompression chambers; and casual organization. Always in imminent danger of drowning, the scuba diver (breathing unnaturally through a mouthpiece and with head surrounded by water) often complicates the environmental hazard with his obsession to establish new records with diving gear which for the novice should be restricted to "free ascent" depths (without need for recompression). The practice, particularly among adolescents, of breath holding underwater is conducive to hypoxic heart failure, especially during the course of heavy exertion required in swimming. Too rapid ascent of scuba divers may overexpand the lungs and give rise to air embolism, pneumothorax, and subcutaneous emphysema. "Squeeze" effects may involve the eye, middle ear and mastoid cells, and paranasal sinuses, and occasionally produce minute gas aggregates in pulp of diseased teeth. Rapid decompression after sojourn at diving depths, and even following rapid ascent to simulated or actual high altitude, may initiate bubble evolution and decompression sickness. Diving tables evolved on an empirical basis, for the most part from fragmentary tests, afford high (96 to 99 percent) but not complete protection against decompression sickness. In carefully supervised decompressions of personnel attending a hospital hyperbaric chamber, the complication of scotoma was observed in 3 out of 1,000 otherwise uneventful decompressions. Oxygen inhalation during at least part of the decompression period provides adequate safeguard.

Experience with work in compressed air dictates the likelihood that all decompressions (not employing oxygen inhalation) conducted in accord with current diving tables are attended by some degree of nascent bubble evolution in circulating blood. Of importance to hospital personnel is the abrupt onset of post-decompression malaise, which may be related to liberation of painless "silent bubbles" but which nevertheless may induce hypoxic liberation into the circulation of such substances as proteolytic enzymes, peptides, and potassium ions. In rapidly decompressed animals, and occasionally in man at autopsy, fat emboli and even bone marrow cells are seen in the lungs and brain.

Advances in recompression therapy emphasize the value of oxygen inhalation at tolerance pressures (27 psi) without resorting to high air or helium-oxygen atmospheres except in unusual circumstances. Dramatic recoveries have occurred when prompt treatment has been accorded seemingly moribund divers. Even divers rendered paraplegic as a result of delay in treatment due to lack of on-site pressure chambers nevertheless may recover motor function following prolonged pressurization and appropriate follow-up hospital therapy. Promising advances in treatment relate to the value of fluid (dextran) administration to counteract hemoconcentration frequently observed in serious cases, notably in aviation personnel who have not been recompressed to hyperbaric atmospheres. Further, success in promoting survival of rapidly decompressed animals has followed inhalation of aerosols which incorporate heparin and antispasmolytic drugs.

It is essential that the physician have available a schedule of emergency procedures when calls are received to care for injured divers. Despite the absence of "on-the-spot" recompression chambers, it may be lifesaving to administer oxygen immediately and fluids at the first sign of hemoconcentration. Some benefit may accrue from a lowered head position to minimize brain embolization and from the recumbent position to ensure rest in the effort to minimize growth of bubbles.

Hyperbaric Chambers

Catastrophic fires have occurred in oxygen-enriched atmospheres at normal and even hypobaric pressures, but the hazard is compounded in the hyperbaric chamber. In a fire costing two lives, the pressurized chamber (3.9 atm, 95 ft) contained 36 percent helium, 36 percent nitrogen, and *28 percent oxygen*. To remove carbon dioxide, a scrubber system utilizing an electric motor was employed to circulate an oxygen-enriched atmosphere. Spontaneous combustion occurred in the scrubber filter and within 15 sec the chamber was enveloped in flame; within 1 min the pressure had increased to 7.9 atm (260 ft) due to the intense heat. *In an oxygen-enriched atmosphere in contrast with air atmospheres, there are no immediately effective measures to quench a fire.* In large chambers in which attending personnel are present, it

is mandatory that oxygen be administered to patients by means of closed systems which cannot enrich the ambient air. There is danger of implosion if sealed capsules or containers are brought into the pressurized chamber.

With reference to the physical examination, it is essential that personnel be free from pulmonary pathology (cysts, chronic bronchiolitis) conducive to aeroembolism. To ensure symptom-free decompression, oxygen inhalation is effective. The National Research Council brochure provides guidelines for safe operation of hyperbaric chambers, but indoctrination at successfully operating installations is strongly recommended.

PRIMARY PRESSURE PHENOMENA

Effect of Pressure per se and of Barotrauma

Normally some tissues of the body are subjected to compressive or distending pressure (the arteries, vertebras, and lower extremities) of the order of 100 to 200 mm Hg (1 to 2 psi). Pressure gradients may also exist in an individual who is immersed in water up to his neck. By contrast, the pressure of the atmosphere (sea level, 760 mm Hg, 14.7 psi, equivalent to 33 ft of seawater) can be increased to more than 30 atm in the hyperbaric chamber without gross signs of impairment. Some individuals, however, may experience *compression* joint pain, which subsides with slower application of pressure. Initially during rapid compression when equilibration is incomplete between inert gas in blood and tissue, there may be an "osmotic" effect affecting hydration of joint cartilage which may account for compression pain in susceptible individuals. At extreme pressures (31.3 to 37.5 atm, 1,000 to 1,200 ft) compression of protoplasm (pressure per se) may be responsible for tremors and somnolence reported in human tests, which are not attributable to narcosis. Small animals tolerate much higher pressures (100 atm) without gross impairment.

Density of inhaled gas increases linearly with pressure, but the work of breathing is roughly proportional to the square root of pressure. Compared with air, the equivalent pressure breathing helium-oxygen is reduced by a factor of 7. Respiratory impairment is not a limiting factor at deep depths. Test data show that man can spend long periods of time at the depths of the continental shelves and perform moderate work.

In air (3 atm) despite the increased density, emphysematous patients may report improvement during and following sojourn under pressure. However, respiration conducted with valvular systems may cause respiratory distress. Hence, it is mandatory *that there be physician-technician trial of all respiratory equipment prior to patient usage at all pressures.*

In contrast to innocuous application of great external forces, equally distributed over the body, is the small pressure difference (50 to 100 mm Hg) which serves to distend blood vessels and induce edema in occluded sinal (aerosinustis) and aural (aerotitis media) spaces.

Following hyperbaric oxygen therapy, patients may experience this cupping effect during sleep, when the auditory tubes are not opened periodically by swallowing. The most frequent cause of blockage of auditory tubes (which usually is only relative in relation to rate of pressure application) is acute and chronic infection of the nasopharynx. At any one time as many as one-third of submarine personnel may show varying grades of barotrauma. A convenient classification employed in the U.S. Navy is *grade* O (normal), 1 (redness of Shrapnell's membrane and along the manubrium), 2 (redness of entire membrane), 3 (same as grade 2 plus fluid or fluid and bubbles in the middle ear), and 4 (blood in the middle ear, perforation of the tympanic membrane or both). These changes are clearly apparent on routine otoscopic inspection. Remarkably there is no residual impairment of auditory acuity in the speech range incurred by this type of trauma. Deafness for higher tones is frequent in divers and implicates noise as the etiologic factor. *Specific therapy is not required for barotrauma;* healing in the author's experience is spontaneous and rarely complicated by secondary infection. In grade 4 (blood in middle ear) the otologist should be consulted.

Complications Arising from Overinflation of the Lungs

If a diver holds his breath on ascent to the surface, the intrapulmonic pressure tends to increase relative to hydrostatic pressure. Excess pressures of 80 mm Hg or higher overinflate the lungs, rupture blood vessels, and force gas along dissecting planes. With the first inhalation of air by the diver on reaching the surface, gas is aspirated into pulmonary veins and disseminated to the central nervous system to bring about collapse. This type of accident has occurred 23 times in 150,000 submarine training escapes. In one instance death followed a too rapid ascent from the shallow depth of 15 ft. It is not an uncommon accident in scuba diving. Acute collapse during decompression has been reported in tunnel workers. The signs and symptoms were those of aeroembolism, not decompression sickness. In several of the patients lung cysts were identified. Treatment of aeroembolism calls for immediate recompression with oxygen inhalation. This disability can be prevented by physical examination to exclude pulmonary pathology (cysts, costophrenic adhesions, bronchiolitis) and by proper training. Routine free ascents can be made from depths of 100 ft if exhalation is continuous. The practice, however, is not encouraged.

SECONDARY PRESSURE PHENOMENA RELATED TO INCREASED PARTIAL PRESSURE OF GASES

Narcotic Action of Nitrogen

When the air pressure in a chamber is raised above 3 atm, the increased partial pressure of nitrogen is associated with changes in mood, notably euphoria, and impaired judgment and motor performance. The effects are similar to those induced by intoxicants, such as alcohol. Although all individuals are in varying degrees narcotized at diving depths, emotionally stable persons react to the stress by compensatory effort and are able to carry out an assigned task (slowly at high pressures) until consciousness is lost. The unstable person is incapable of purposeful effort and gives way to emotional aberrations characteristic of some alcoholics. Sophisticated studies have provided quantitative assessment of the impairment. If, for example, the electroencephalogram is recorded at normal pressure when a subject is attempting to solve an arithmetical problem, there is a blocking of occipital alpha rhythm which at increased pressure ("nitrogen threshold") disappears after a latent period. The period of latency is inversely proportional to the square of the pressure. Of interest is the fact that at relatively low pressures (2.5 atm, 50 ft) not associated with overt impairment, a nitrogen effect on the brain may be detected. The nitrogen narcotic phenomenon, as an innocuous stress without residual impairment, may be applied in psychic evaluation of individuals. The lack of narcotic effect of helium makes diving to depths of 1,000 ft feasible.

Oxygen Poisoning

Although inhalation of oxygen at high pressures (OHP) may give rise to limiting pulmonary and CNS alterations, it has been breathed routinely up to 3 atm during decompression of divers, in the treatment of decompression sickness, and in hyperbaric chambers in hospitals. Oxygen (OHP) therapy is possible because there is a latent period preceding overt signs and symptoms, during which cardiac function is not impaired, and initial untoward reactions are reversible when air breathing is resumed. Tolerance time for inhalation of oxygen at higher pressures is greatly extended by short intervals of air inhalation in accord with the outline in Table 127-1.

Table 127-1. GUIDE FOR ADMINISTRATION OF HYPERBARIC OXYGEN DURING DECOMPRESSION AND IN RECOMPRESSION THERAPY
Based on U.S. Navy experience

Pressure, psi	Unit exposure (U.E.) intervals, min		No. of U.E. for routine inhalation*
	Oxygen	Air	
27	20	5	1, 2, 3
27 to 13	40	...	1
13	20	5	1, 2, 3
13 to 0	40	...	1

* Depending upon duration of previous hyperbaric air exposure (decompression), or the condition of the patient during recompression.

Subjectively, inhalation of oxygen (OHP) is stimulating and may be similar to an adrenergic response. Adrenal, thyroid, and pituitary hormones, exercise, increased CO_2 tensions, elevated metabolism, and apprehension shorten the latent period of comparative well-being. On the other hand, individuals *at rest*, following overnight fast, and phlegmatic in disposition have tolerated the inhalation of oxygen (99 percent) for periods of 30 min at the usually convulsive level of 4 atm. Of clinical importance are experimental data which support a durable impression that hypoxemic patients tolerate unusually high pulmonary oxygen tensions. Venous admixture of arterial blood of dogs produced by surgical shunt, for example, prevented the pulmonary damage observed in control animals (Winter et al.). Pulmonary injury (OHP) may not be a direct (phosgene) effect but a response mediated by the same endocrine factors which augment neurotoxic reactions. Notably, cardiac function is not impaired as is respiration, despite the inhibitory action of OHP on many enzyme systems, particularly those containing essential sulfhydryl groups. Thus the heart in anesthetized dogs may beat for periods of 1 hr or longer following respiratory paralysis, and succumbs only after asphyxial concentrations of CO_2 ($+100$ to 200 mm Hg) have accumulated in the lungs.

Limitations to OHP therapy pertain to toxic pulmonary effects and striking CNS response. A serious drawback is not only lack of knowledge of the specific etiology, but also the variability of individual response and unpredictability of tissue oxygen tensions. At 3 atm (oxygen) arterial blood may contain 6 vol percent of oxygen in solution (pO_2: $2,000$ mm Hg). As a result of vasoconstriction (a direct oxygen effect) or vasodilation (a CO_2 effect), there may be widely fluctuating tensions (70 to 1,400 mm Hg) of oxygen in mixed venous blood withdrawn from the right ventricle. The inference is that O_2 tensions at the cellular level also fluctuate widely.

In man, pulmonary (and tracheal) irritation is elicited at lower pressure levels (0.6 to 2 atm), while neurotoxic effects are observed at higher pressures. In carefully monitored studies, it was found that healthy men could breathe oxygen (2 atm) for about 8 hr before significant (5 to 10 percent) decreases in vital capacity occurred. After 8 to 12 hr of inhalation, the symptoms, progressive in intensity, were burning sensation on deep inspiration, carinal irritation, cough, and dyspnea. At higher pressures, the pulmonary limit for oxygen inhalation has not been determined. In earlier tests there were no pulmonary symptoms at the end of 4 hr of oxygen inhalation at 3 atm (Behnke).

Neurotoxic effects terminate the relatively benign latent period after about 2 hr of oxygen inhalation at 3 atm. Untoward responses at from 3 to 4 atm are twitching or tremors of facial muscles (notably lips and eyebrows), restlessness, anxiety, periodic waves of nausea, occasional vomiting, diminished visual acuity, narrowing of visual fields, numbness of fingers and toes, reversal of pulse rate, sharp rise in diastolic pressure, auditory hallucinations and other aura, fainting (occasionally), and violent convulsive seizures. Residual effects following seizures have not been observed in man. In small animals (which have severe limitations for comparative studies, e.g., high metabolic rates, chronic pulmonary disease), neuromuscular impairment and brain lesions have been reported following extreme exposures.

Physical examination of persons subjected to OHP should include tests of visual and pulmonary function, EEG, and for monitoring purposes, pulse rate and blood pressure.

Alteration of Carbon Dioxide Tension

Carbon dioxide not only enhances the toxicity of oxygen (a specific CO_2 effect independent of the lowering of pH), but the narcotic effect of nitrogen and other inert gases as well. An elementary assessment of this phenomenon relates CO_2 enhancement to increased cerebral blood flow. During rapid descent in deep sea diving, momentary vertigo and confusion are in part attributed to inadequate exhalation of CO_2 as a result of rapid compression. The effective CO_2 percentage should not exceed 1.5 percent, although percentages of CO_2 up to 5, are fairly well tolerated in submarines for at least 60 hr. There are no reliable data for extended periods of inhalation of high concentrations of CO_2 ($+3$ percent).

In the presence of elevated concentrations of CO_2 during inhalation of oxygen at 1 atm or higher pressures, consciousness may be lost suddenly (oxygen blackout) without onset of dyspnea. Divers working in air at high pressures have tolerated some remarkably high pCO_2 levels (e.g., 57 mm Hg) in arterial blood without distress when using breathing apparatus which prevented adequate pulmonary ventilation. A critical consideration is that warning signs of CO_2 excess at normal pressures may be absent in the pressurized environment. Hyperventilation may induce respiratory alkalosis and tetany. The danger of hypoxemia is greatly enhanced when hyperventilation in air removes the CO_2 stimulus during breath holding.

Uptake of Nitrogen at Increased Pressure

At atmospheric pressure (pN_2: 570 mm Hg) about 9 ml of nitrogen is dissolved per kg of body fluid, and about 55 ml per kg of body fat. In a lean, 70-kg man (7 kg fat) about 400 ml of nitrogen is in body fluids, 100 ml in bone and spinal cord, and 400 ml in fat. About 5.2 liters of blood per min perfuses the nonlipid cellular mass, and only about 0.7 liter of blood perfuses bone and adipose tissue. The half-time for N_2 uptake of various nonlipid tissues varies from 2 to 20 min (98.5 percent saturation in 12 to 120 min), and for organs containing large amounts of lipid (adipose tissue, long bones, spinal cord), half-time uptake may vary from 60 to 120 min (1 to 2 hr) in a lean man. In the United States, the duration of stay of personnel in diving and tunnel operations in air is such that nitrogen uptake is restricted mainly to nonlipid, rapidly saturating tissues. This is not the case in England where operational schedules are more rigorous.

Decompression Procedures

It is evident that decompression time following prolonged exposures will be greatly influenced in air dives by the amount of fat in the body. If exposures are of short duration, the amount of fat is not important as a decompression hazard. Haldane's ratio principle applies to short exposures in compressed air, and it is relatively safe to halve the absolute pressure to permit rapid ascent to the first stop. However, after prolonged (saturation) exposures in the hyperbaric environment, it is becoming increasingly evident that the ratio principle does not apply to *successive stages* of decompression and that only a small pressure head (ΔP) governs inert gas transport from tissues to lungs. In accord with the isobaric ("oxygen window") principle of decompression, ΔP is the difference between arterial and venous oxygen pressures. Hence safe decompression following helium-oxygen saturation exposures at deep depths requires from 10 to 15 min per ft of ascent. The time required for decompression is measured not in hours, but in days. Based on the hypothesis that ΔP can be appreciably elevated above isobaric tissue levels (i.e., inert gas pressure in tissue is never allowed to exceed ambient pressure during decompression), diving tables become in effect "treatment" tables applicable to a state of gas transport not in solution but, in part at least, in bubble form.

Factors Affecting Bubble Formation

After exposure to high pressure or high altitudes (in chambers, unpressurized aircraft), factors conducive to decompression sickness fall into two groups. In the first are conditions which increase gas content of tissues, namely, the amount of fat, degree and duration of exposure, intensity of work, and, in rapid ascent to high altitudes, exercise, which expands the gaseous reservoir with CO_2 accretion and facilitates cavitation. In the second group are variables affecting tissue perfusion and diffusion of gas in transport from tissue as well as surface tension and other biophysical factors affecting blood. Thus age, time of day, disruption of circadian rhythms, dehydration, fright, injury, and postalcoholic residuum seemingly affect gas transport.

Acclimatization

Divers subjected to older decompression schedules for tunnel workers developed a high incidence of bends. It appears that men who expose themselves regularly to compressed air day after day become less susceptible to attacks of decompression sickness. About 14 days are required for maximal effect. Acclimatization is gradually lost when men cease to work in compressed air. The recognition of this phenomenon by Paton and Walder is of practical importance.

DECOMPRESSION SICKNESS

Etiology

The preponderance of experimental data implicates intravascular bubbles as the initiating causal agent. In rapidly decompressed animals circulating bubbles can be observed in arteries and veins; subsequently sequestered bubbles accumulate in veins. Secondary phenomena complicate the simple etiology. Thus fat particles may enter the bloodstream from gas-distended adipose tissue, bone marrow, or even fatty liver cells when present as in alcoholics. The hypothesis has been mentioned that hypoxic cellular destruction may explain such symptoms as malaise or give rise to delayed febrile response.

Signs and Symptoms

Sequestration of nascent gas bubbles in vascular beds of tissues and organs gives rise to a remarkable array of dissimilar syndromes (Table 127-2). In British classifica-

Table 127-2. SIGNS AND SYMPTOMS OF DECOMPRESSION SICKNESS

Central nervous system	Cardiorespiratory	Extremities	Skin; systemic
Loss of consciousness	substernal distress	pain	pruritus
Scintillating scotomata	paroxysmal coughing	paresthesia	mottling
Mèniére's syndrome	tachypnea	numbness	rash
Vertigo, aphasia	asphyxia (chokes)	weakness	pallor
Staggering gait	shock	bone necrosis	
Spastic paralysis	hemoconcentration	cartilage destruction	lowered temperature
Sensory loss		edema	fever, sweating malaise
Bladder, bowel paralysis			

tion, pain in the region of joints (bends) is designated Type I (mild); respiratory, cardiovascular, and neurologic involvement is designated Type II (serious), which includes *aeroembolism* arising as explained previously from gas introduced extraneously into the circulation. Type I cases may progress to Type II. The chief problem concerns the early recognition of signs and symptoms and application of recompression therapy.

BENDS. The bends may be described as an aching, radiating type of pain, occasionally synchronous with pulse beat, of gradual onset, progressive in intensity, and felt in the joints, muscles, and bones of the extremities. Response to recompression therapy is immediate (occasionally there is exacerbation of pain if pressure is applied too rapidly), and there is no residual disability with the reservation that the relationship of bends to aseptic bone necrosis remains to be clarified.

CHOKES AND THE SHOCK SYNDROME. A type of asphyxia referred to by early workers as "chokes" may be preceded by several hours of well-being following decompression. An early symptom is a sensation of substernal soreness elicited by deep inspiration which may provoke paroxysmal coughing. Inhalation of cigarette smoke aggravates the untoward reaction. Hemoconcentration and classical signs of circulatory shock are associated with this disability, particularly if onset is gradual.

NEUROLOGIC INVOLVEMENT (CNS). Scintillating scotomata and transient episodes of vertigo and dizziness are not uncommon. The staggering gait and slurred speech simulate drunkenness, and recompression must be resorted to for differential diagnosis. Ménière's syndrome, presumably resulting from infraction of blood supply to the inner ear, was not uncommon in early tunnel workers. In recent decompressions following saturation dives, nerve deafness has been reported. Aeroembolism usually can be recognized as distinct from the neurologic sign of decompression sickness, by abrupt onset, unconsciousness with convulsion, usually focal, and independence of duration of exposure.

Paralysis of spinal cord origin, manifest as a spastic monoplegia or paraplegia, is usually confined to the lower extremities. Areas of hypersensitivity are present above the site of the cord lesion, and paresthesia of sensory paralysis occurs below. *An early premonitory sign is numbness*, which should alert the physician to anticipate a Type II condition rather than bends. There is incontinence of urine and feces following involvement of the lower part of the spinal cord. The imperative requirement to catheterize the bladder in the acute condition may be overlooked. Recovery or at least considerable improvement may occur following prolonged recompression with oxygen, even though many hours may elapse between onset of disability and recompression therapy. Prognosis for ultimate restoration of function cannot be made early since improvement may continue over a 2-year period following injury. Gas bubbles impair blood supply but do not transect the spinal cord!

BONE LESIONS. A serious complication associated with work in pressurized tunnel operations is aseptic bone necrosis, and as many as 75 percent of oldtime workmen show radiographic bone pathology. Frank lesions have not been observed in our Navy divers but have been reported occasionally in divers from other countries. Aseptic bone necrosis is related to the number of times a man has been decompressed, to the pressure level at which he has worked, and to the number of reported bends. Accepted decompression procedures in England, where hours of work are relatively long, are not adequate to prevent bone lesions. Innovations in decompression practice as incorporated into Washington State Tables (1963) greatly extend decompression time by stage rather than uniform decompression. There is good reason to believe that the extended decompression time and *shorter daily exposures* will prevent occurrence of crippling lesions.

Crippling lesions which are the result of juxtaarticular infarction and subsequent deformity and destruction of the joint surface are confined to shoulder and hip joints. By contrast, the knee joint, which is the most common site of bends, is not disabled. *A prime consideration is that the lesions are asymptomatic unless joint surfaces are involved.* The vivid x-ray-visualized lesions in the medullary shaft of long bones are innocuous. An impediment in diagnosis is a latent period of a year or longer before pathologic change becomes manifest. Our lack of definitive knowledge of aseptic bone necrosis is reflected by inability to explain why similar workmen in the same environment remain free from joint and medullary lesions. An essential part of the physical examination *prior to work in compressed air* and at yearly intervals during work in compressed air is radiologic survey of the long bones.

Recompression Treatment of Decompression Sickness and Air Embolism

The value of oxygen therapy without the need for higher air or oxygen pressures has been confirmed for Type I cases (bends), and shows promise also in management of Type II cases including aeroembolism. However, with availability of proper gas mixtures, in the author's opinion, high pressures should be utilized for treatment of serious cases. The outline of oxygen decompression and recompression procedures (Table 127-1), adapted from earlier and current U.S. Navy experience, is a guide for employment of hyperbaric oxygen inhalation. Recompression procedure in the U.S. Navy Diving Manual is to be regarded as standard practice. Occasionally long periods of time measured in days are required for compression therapy to be fully effective. Patients can be kept for weeks (if necessary) at 2.52 atm (50 ft) if there is indication that pressure decrement will cause further deterioration. Occasionally a puzzling relapse may occur during the course of treatment which is not responsive to additional pressure (occasionally to 10 atm). Errors in treatment relate to (1) inadequate time spent at peak pressure when patients are seriously ill—*the condition of the patient must regulate decompression therapy,* (2) failure to apply the compression test to doubtful cases, (3) inadequate medical monitoring during the recompression period, and (4) failure to keep the treated patient near the recompression for a 24-hr period.

ADJUVANTS TO RECOMPRESSION. Oral administration of fluid in the recompression chamber may be followed by return of blood hematocrit to normal. Intravenous fluids may be required to prevent onset of shock. The guidelines by Malette and coworkers (1962) have proved effective in restoration of normal rheology in serious cases of altitude dysbarism which are remarkable often for the many hours that patients have survived during a state of shock. For reasons unknown, heart failure does not occur even when gas embolization is extensive, and aviation patients apparently in extremis have responded quickly to recompression therapy. Follow-up investigations of Cockett have demonstrated the effectiveness of dextran in promoting recovery of rapidly decompressed dogs who otherwise would die.

An emergency tray should provide catheters, tracheal airways, instruments for myringotomy and for relief of pneumothorax, sedative drugs, and needles and syringes (see National Research Council brochure).

Special Problems

SCUBA AND SKIN DIVING. The problems are chiefly administrative, not medical, and require a "tightly-run ship." Instructors should be trained to administer resuscitation in water and to give oxygen. They should be delegated the authority to disqualify the obviously unfit. Under the initial supervision of the physician, the instructors should administer timed pulmonary function and step-up tests of not more than 5-min duration and record the results to provide evaluation of fitness on an individual basis. Divers must be good swimmers ("fit to swim, fit to dive"). Apart from the hazard of drowning, there is the matter of air purity, which is not always easy to ensure if "smog" is compressed. Maximum permissible levels of noxious substances must be reduced proportionately to pressure. Thus carbon monoxide is restricted to 20 ppm, which is one fifth of the permissible level for an 8-hr exposure in vehicular tunnels.

The skin diver must rely upon breath holding. As he descends to depths, the volume of the thorax is diminished. At 100 ft (4 atm) oxygen and nitrogen pressures have increased about threefold and elevated alveolar pO_2 (200 mm Hg) permits extended bottom time. On ascent to the surface the expansion of the thorax reduces the oxygen tension precipitously to hypoxic levels of 25 to 35 mm Hg, and the diver faces imminent collapse. *Competitive breath holding and swimming underwater are dangerous.* Man shows the bradycardic response during apneic underwater diving, which is not prevented by vigorous exercise, and serious arrhythmias have been recorded in healthy men.

MONITORING OF PRESSURIZED TUNNEL WORKERS. Medical monitoring of rugged independent workers who build tunnels is feasible if a small group of men (sometimes no more than three per shift) will report weekly to the physician for definitive but brief tests of fitness (similar to the physical evaluation for divers) and for systematic survey of compression and postcompression responses. These should include the deep inspiratory test and inhalation of cigarette smoke, examination of the skin to detect mottling, and questioning about postpressure malaise in the effort to ascertain presence of "silent" bubbles and adequacy of decompression.

DERANGEMENTS AT HIGH ALTITUDE
Physiologic Considerations

Altitudes of 3,500 to 7,000 ft are noted for salubrious climate. At higher altitudes the decreased partial pressure of oxygen gives rise to arterial hypoxemia. In response to hypoxic stimulation of aortic and carotid chemoreceptors, hyperventilation lowers alveolar CO_2 and brings about respiratory alkalosis. The newcomer to high altitude is thus affected by both hypoxia and alkalosis, which account for typical symptoms and signs of dyspnea, tachycardia, malaise, headache, and insomnia. Maximal heart rate in response to strenuous exertion decreases and pulmonary arterial pressure increases, and these changes are correlated with altitude level.

Acclimatization

The symptoms of acute mountain sickness usually disappear within 3 to 10 days, and their amelioration is hastened by graded exercise. The mountain climber may acclimatize sufficiently during a period of 1 to 3 months at intermediate altitudes so as to enable him to climb Mt. Everest (29,002 ft) with the aid of supplemental oxygen, and Nanga Parbat (26,660 ft) without added oxygen. These feats represent the exceptional acclimatization, but it is limited to about 10 days since rapid deterioration ensues after longer periods at elevations above 25,000 ft. Despite extreme difficulties, physicians and physiologists have spent more than 5 months conducting cardiopulmonary tests at altitudes of 19,000 ft and higher. In regard to permanent residence man cannot live above 18,000 ft. However, Andeans are well adapted to perform strenuous work and to engage in football games for recreation in the hypoxic atmosphere of 15,000 ft.

Characteristics of the Andean

Hurtado and Hultgren and Grover have enumerated morphologic and functional characteristics of the resident reared at high altitudes, namely, (1) decreased weight relative to stature; (2) increased vital capacity and pulmonary ventilation; (3) hypertrophy of the free wall of the right ventricle, increased thickness of the muscle mass of smaller pulmonary vessels, and sustained, hypoxic arteriolar vasoconstriction; (4) increased blood volume, hematocrit, and myoglobin; and (5) greatly increased tissue vascularization. In the above-listed adaptations, attention focuses on the unique properties of the pulmonary circulation. "The vascular wall or 'the container' of the arterial side of the pulmonary circulation is less compliant than that of sea level dwellers. . . . A rigid, fluid-filled system is more responsive to alterations in blood volume, blood flow, and vascular tone in terms of changes in intravascular pressure than is a more compliant system such as the normal pulmonary circulation of the sea level resident."

The Andean descended from generations of inhabitants living continuously at high altitude has attained nearly complete adaptation to a lowered alveolar oxygen tension of 45 mm Hg. He is able to perform strenuous physical labor as exemplified by the incredible cultivation of the slopes of the Andes. Despite the arduous life and deprivations, it is uncommon to find peripheral hypertension, coronary thrombosis, myocardial infarction, or peripheral arteriosclerosis. Blood viscosity associated with the hematocrit range of 40 to 60 percent does not significantly affect blood flow or coagulation. The erythrocytosis is stabilized and differs from the erythremia and attendant thrombocytosis of polycythemia vera. The hypoxic stimulus, specifically erythropoietin, affects strictly erythropoiesis. General myeloid hyperplasia has not been reported.

Chronic Mountain Sickness (Soroche, Monge's Disease)

The Andean, however, is affected by a clinical condition which represents a breakdown in compensation and adaptation to low oxygen tension. Loss of tolerance to the altitude environment, as pointed out by Monge in 1928, may be observed in the striking accentuation of the "normal" erythrocytosis. Hurtado has reported in detail derangements associated with this pathologic condition. In comparison with values (N) characteristic of the healthy native resident at high altitude, hemoglobin values increase to 25 Gm/100 ml (N 21 Gm), and blood hematocrit to 80 (N 60). Blood volume is increased about 50 percent chiefly as a result of erythrocytosis. Plasma volume however is decreased. There is hyperplasia and hyperactivity of bone marrow erythroid cells and increased red cell destruction, but no derangements in leukocytogenesis. The severely impaired ability to work is associated with cyanosis, hypoventilation, lowered alveolar pO_2 and pCO_2, increased cardiac output, and greater pulmonary hypertension and lower systolic blood pressure than are found in the healthy residents. Electrocardiographic findings are consistent with a diagnosis of cor pulmonale.

The features of Monge's disease have much in common with Ayerza's syndrome, or cardiaco negro (erythrocytosis, hyperplasia of bone marrow, cyanosis, dyspnea, and notably pulmonary arterial and arteriolar sclerosis). This entity appears to have a multiple etiology. Of extrinsic interest is similarity of vascular pathology (with pulmonary hypertension) in chronic oxygen poisoning affecting rats exposed to 4 atm air (0.83 atm O_2) for 3 months.

High-altitude Pulmonary Edema

Pulmonary edema occurs in persons who travel within a day or two to elevations of over 9,000 ft and also in acclimatized mountain residents who visit a low altitude for 1 to 3 weeks and then return to a higher elevation. Symptoms usually occur 6 to 36 hr after arrival and consist of dry cough, dyspnea, and a feeling of pain in the lower substernal area. X-rays of the chest in severe cases demonstrate confluent or nodular densities throughout all lung fields. Altitude pulmonary edema is distinct from acute mountain sickness in which symptoms appear promptly on reaching altitude, and do not include cough, dyspnea, or rhonchal respiration. Treatment includes rapid removal to a lower elevation if transportation is available, or hospitalization with bed rest and oxygen therapy. Prevention consists in taking adequate time for altitude ascent, and upon reaching altitude, it is important to avoid overexertion, which may precipitate pulmonary edema in well-acclimatized persons.

CONCLUDING NOTE. The studies of man and lower animals at high altitude present many challenging problems. The remarkable physical feats of the Andean, who subsists largely on a diet of vegetable protein and carbohydrate and does not get peripheral vascular disease despite the stress of heavy work, have no precedent in a European population at sea level. An intriguing problem is whether or not acclimatization (one generation) is associated with the same degree of tissue vascularization conferred by adaptation (several generations).

REFERENCES

Bennett, P. B.: "The Aetiology of Compressed Air Intoxication and Inert Gas Narcosis," New York, Pergamon Press, 1966.

Brown, I. W., Jr., and B. G. Cox (Eds.): "Hyperbaric Medicine," Third Internat. Congress, Publ. 1404, Nat. Acad. Sci. Nat. Res. Council, Washington, 1966.

Cockett, A. T. K., R. M. Nakamura, and J. J. Franks: Recent Findings in the Pathogenesis of Decompression Sickness (Dysbarism), Surgery, 58:384, 1965.

Hart, J. S. (Ed.): Proceedings of the International Symposium on Altitude and Cold, Federation Proceedings, 28:933–1321, 1969.

Hultgren, H. N., and R. F. Grover: Circulatory Adaptation to High Altitude, Annual Rev. Med., 19:119, 1968.

Lambertsen, C. J. (Ed.): "Underwater Physiology," Third Symposium, Baltimore, The Williams & Wilkins Company, 1967. See J. M. Clark and C. J. Lambertsen, p. 439; P. B. Bennett, p. 327; E. E. P. Barnard, p. 156; and M. W. Goodman, p. 165.

Lanphier, E. H., and H. W. Gillen: Management of Sports Diving Accidents, New York J. Med., 63:667, 1963.

McCallum, R. I. (Ed.): "Decompression of Compressed Air Workers in Civil Engineering," Newcastle upon Tyne, Oriel Press, Ltd., 1967.

Malette, W. G., J. B. Fitzgerald, and A. T. K. Cockett: Dysbarism, A Review of Thirty-five Cases with Suggestion for Therapy, Aerospace Med., 33:1132, 1962.

Miles, S.: "Underwater Medicine," 2d ed., Philadelphia, J. B. Lippincott Company, 1966.

Nat. Acad. of Sci. Nat. Res. Council: "Fundamentals of Hyperbaric Medicine," Washington.

U. S. Navy Diving Manual, NAVSHIPS 250–538, Navy Dept., Washington.

128 PROBLEMS OF AIR AND SPACE TRAVEL

Stuart Bondurant

Ordinary air travel imposes so little physiologic stress that most patients who can be moved at all can be moved by air if proper equipment and attendants are available.

Medical problems unique to air travel may be caused by unusual environmental conditions which may be encountered because of limitations of equipment or abnormal operating circumstances.

Many modern aircraft fly at altitudes of 20,000 to 40,000 ft, with cabins pressurized to maintain an effective cabin altitude of less than 7,500 ft (jets) or 9,000 ft (reciprocating engines). Unusual accelerations may be encountered and the normal metabolic diurnal rhythm may be disturbed by rapid movement between time zones.

Altitude

An increase in altitude is equivalent to a decrease in barometric pressure. There is a consequent reduction in the partial pressure of oxygen and an increase in the volume of any gas trapped within the body (Table 128-1).

Table 128-1.   REPRESENTATIVE VALUES OF ARTERIAL OXYGEN AND THE RELATIVE VOLUME OF GAS AT VARIOUS ALTITUDES

Altitude, ft	Pressure, mm Hg	Arterial blood		Relative volume of gas
		Oxygen tension, mm Hg	Oxygen saturation, %	
0	760	94	98	1.0
5,000	632	66	92	1.2
8,000	564	60	89	1.25
10,000	523	53	86	1.5
14,000	446	44	79	1.7
18,000	379	36	71	2.0
37,500 with 100% O_2	159	74	94	4.8
44,000 with 100% O_2	116	36	72	6.5

The normal person acclimatized to sea level tolerates oxygen tension equivalent to that at altitudes of 10,000 to 12,000 ft with little change in arterial oxygen saturation. At altitudes above 12,000 ft, hypoxia becomes more marked and supplementary oxygen is usually used. By breathing 100 percent oxygen, one can maintain normal oxygen saturation at altitudes of 30,000 to 35,000 ft. An ascent of 5,000 ft or more may be followed by a period of lethargy, sleepiness, and headache. These symptoms usually subside within 24 hr.

A second consequence of decreased barometric pressure is expansion of gas trapped in body cavities. In the normal person, intestinal gas is passed as it expands and middle-ear and sinus air escapes without difficulty during ascent. Gas which cannot escape (pneumothorax, pneumoperitoneum) may cause pain, injury, or death. Patients with trapped gas in body cavities should not be exposed to a significant decrease in barometric pressure.

Acceleration

Acceleration is the instantaneous rate of change of velocity. The unit of acceleration *g* is the acceleration of a body which is falling freely *in vacuo* due to earth's gravity. It represents a change in velocity of 32.2 ft per sec each second. Most of the physiologic consequences of acceleration are due to the force (inertia) which is equal in magnitude but opposite in direction to that causing the acceleration. Thus, headward acceleration causes footward displacement of soft tissues and blood. Duration, magnitude, direction, and rate of onset of acceleration determine the physiologic effects. In general, the longer and greater the acceleration, the less well it is tolerated. Prolonged forward or backward acceleration is tolerated better (approximately 14 to 20*g*, limited by apnea) than headward acceleration (4 to 7*g*, limited by blackout and cerebral ischemia); footward acceleration (3 to 5*g*, limited by asystole and conjunctival and mucous membrane bleeding) is tolerated least well. Brief headward accelerations of 25*g* and backward accelerations of 40*g* are tolerated by normal subjects when well positioned and supported. In ordinary flight, linear accelerations greater than 1*g* are not encountered. Turbulent flight may cause brief linear accelerations of 10 to 12*g*, which are great enough to cause fractures in persons who are not restrained. Angular accelerations of turn and the linear-angular accelerations of turbulent flight are important causes of motion sickness.

Diurnal Rhythms

A dissociation between metabolic diurnal rhythms and actual local time may occur following longitudinal flight or flight over the poles in high-speed aircraft. From 3 to 5 days may be required for diurnal metabolic rhythms to come into phase with the new local time. There are no proved adverse clinical or physiologic effects of changing the diurnal rhythm. However, the management of diseases with diurnal manifestations, such as peptic ulcer, and the scheduling of all important medications should be carefully planned in preparation for a trip to another time zone.

Miscellaneous

Some fuels and lubricants and their combustion products are toxic and may, with equipment failure, become concentrated in closed cabins. Reciprocating engines produce large quantities of carbon monoxide. Jet engines use fuels which are vesicants, with fumes that may cause nausea, vomiting, and headache. Pyrolysis of lubricating oils produces fumes which cause conjunctival irritation. Ozone has not accumulated in toxic quantities.

Flight line personnel develop hearing loss after prolonged exposure to jet noise unless protected by position or by mechanical devices. Noise levels inside aircraft are very low, and those in terminals and around airfields are apparently insufficient to cause hearing loss.

Supersonic Transport

Supersonic transports cruise at speeds of Mach 2 to Mach 3 (1,300 to 1,800 mph) at altitudes of 50,000 to 70,000 ft. Flight characteristics are well known from extensive experience in military aircraft. Cabin pressure, oxygen content, and temperature will be similar to those of current jet aircraft. There are two environmental hazards which are not present in ordinary subsonic air travel: ozone and radiation.

Ozone is present in the toxic concentration of 6 to 9 ppm at the operational altitude of the supersonic transport. For this reason, the cabin atmosphere control system includes thermal or catalytic devices for the dissociation of ozone to maintain concentrations below 0.2 ppm.

Passengers and crew will be exposed to galactic cosmic radiation and to solar flare radiation. Under the most adverse ordinary circumstances galactic cosmic radiation, composed of protons, alpha particles, and a few heavy nuclei, will be less than 2 millirem per hr or approximately 6 millirem for a single intercontinental flight. The aircrew may receive 2 rem per year from this source. Solar flares produce protons and heavy nuclei. During a major solar flare, the dose rate for a passenger may reach 2 millirads per hr. For this reason, the aircraft will carry radiation monitoring equipment and will descend to lower altitudes when major solar flares occur.

The supersonic transport will cause a sonic boom, or wave of overpressure, of approximately 2.0 lb per sq ft at ground level along a corridor of 25 miles on each side of the flight path. Overpressure of this magnitude will not cause physical or physiologic damage but does cause psychological reactions.

Aircrew Selection

Physical requirements for aircrews are described in appropriate governmental and airlines literature. Absence of circulatory, pulmonary, neurologic, visual, and auditory defects is of particular importance.

Air Transportation of Patients

Since it is now possible to fly without experiencing physiologically significant departure from the usual environmental conditions, there are no absolute medical contraindications to moving patients by air. However, in many instances patients should not be moved at all, and in others, adequate aircraft with pressurized cabin and attending personnel may not be available. Commercial airlines will carry many patients subject to the discretion of the airline medical director. In addition to the condition of the patient, the comfort and convenience of other passengers must be a major factor in the decision of the commercial airlines. The following points apply to air transportation in general. Specific advice concern-

ing commercial air transportation should be obtained from the appropriate airline medical director.

CIRCULATORY DISEASE. The lower partial pressure of oxygen which may be encountered constitutes the major deterrent to flight for patients with circulatory diseases. With oxygen breathing, normal arterial oxygen saturation can be maintained at all altitudes encountered in routine flight (Table 128-1). There is no evidence that ordinary flying is associated with an increased incidence of angina, myocardial infarction, or cerebral vascular accidents. Coronary artery disease manifested by occasional angina or old myocardial infarction, minimal cerebral or peripheral vascular disease, hypertension, and compensated congenital or rheumatic heart disease appear to entail no added risk in flying. Patients with angina related to emotional stress may benefit from preflight sedation.

Patients with severe or frequent angina, severe hypertension, recent vascular accidents, or cardiac decompensation at rest or with moderate exercise should fly only when a pressurized aircraft or supplementary oxygen is available to maintain ambient oxygen tension at levels of 150 mm Hg (sea level equivalent) or more. It is probably preferable to forego unnecessary flying for 6 weeks after a myocardial infarction or a cerebral vascular accident.

PULMONARY DISEASE. Persons with pulmonary decompensation at rest or with very mild exercise should fly only if ambient oxygen tension is maintained at levels of 150 mm Hg or more and facilities and personnel are available to treat acute decompensation. Persons with pulmonary decompensation with moderate (two flights of stairs) or severe exercise usually fly without difficulty to altitudes of 10,000 ft. Asthmatic patients who do not respond well to self-administered treatment should not fly unattended during acute episodes. The likelihood of rupture of an emphysematous bleb does not appear to be increased by ordinary flight. Because of the increase in volume of bullae as altitude increases (Table 128-1), patients with marked bullous emphysema are not advised to fly above 6,000 ft. Individuals with pneumothorax should not fly unless the cabin pressure is maintained at ground-level equivalent. Expansion of the trapped gas causes, in effect, a tension pneumothorax. Several patients with therapeutic pneumothorax have died in flight.

HEMATOLOGIC DISEASE. In the absence of cardiopulmonary disease, patients with a hemoglobin of 7 to 9 Gm per 100 ml usually tolerate flight at 4,000 to 6,000 ft without difficulty. If greater cabin altitudes are to be encountered, hemoglobin should be above 10 Gm per 100 ml.

Hypoxia causes increased sickling of erythrocytes containing hemoglobin S. There have been many well-documented reports of splenic infarction in patients with hemoglobin S during flights which usually exceeded 10,000 ft and lasted for several hours. Two patients with SC hemoglobin have had splenic infarctions during flights which did not exceed 6,000 ft. If ambient oxygen tension cannot be maintained at 150 mm Hg, flying is contraindicated for patients with SS (sickle-cell anemia) and

SC hemoglobin and for those with SA (sickle-cell trait) who have large quantities of hemoglobin S. Others with hemoglobin S should be restricted to cabin altitudes below 10,000 ft. Symptoms of splenic infarction, nausea, vomiting, left upper quadrant pain, and shock should be treated with supplemental oxygen and immediate return to ground level.

PREGNANCY. A large amount of experience has accumulated which suggests that ordinary flying has no adverse effects on the normal pregnant woman or fetus. Pregnant women should sit, when possible, facing the rear of the plane and should place the seat belt over the upper thighs and hips rather than around the abdomen. When pregnancy is complicated by preeclampsia or cardiopulmonary or hematologic disease, considerations similar to those discussed above for the nonpregnant patient apply.

EAR, NOSE, AND THROAT DISEASE. Acute infections of the upper part of the respiratory tract and chronic sinusitis may obstruct the eustachian tubes or sinus ducts with barotitis or barosinusitis resulting when external pressure is increased during descent. If flight is necessary, use of a nasal spray [½ percent phenylephrine (Neo-Synephrine)] 6, 3, and ½ hr before flight and ½ hr before descent may help to maintain patency of the ducts. A swallow or a Valsalva maneuver with the nose occluded will usually open the ducts. Children may be fed during descent to encourage swallowing. The treatment of barotrauma depends on its severity and the underlying cause. Intubation of the eustachian tubes is not advised. In most instances, conservative treatment with decongestants will suffice. Severe barotitis may be associated with hemorrhage into the middle ear, requiring myringotomy and aspiration of blood to prevent ossicular ankylosis. Plastic repair of the ducts may be required to prevent recurrence.

METABOLIC DISEASE. Control of diabetes may be complicated by rapid movement from one time zone to another and by motion sickness. Careful planning of the flight in terms of elapsed rather than local time, with consideration of the meals to be served and appropriate management of motion sickness, should enable the patient with well-controlled diabetes to fly without difficulty. Patients in diabetic acidosis may be transported after treatment is started if in-flight medical facilities are adequate.

COMMUNICABLE DISEASE. Persons known to have a communicable disease may not enter a state or nation without the consent of the local health department.

POSTOPERATIVE CONDITIONS. Because of the expansion of abdominal gas with decrease in barometric pressure, it is generally considered preferable to forego flying for 10 days after abdominal or other major surgery. However, experience with air evacuation of military casualties suggests that, with proper facilities and personnel, practically all patients whose condition is stable can be moved by air if necessary. Most persons with fractures are flown without difficulty. Fracture of the mandible, particularly when the mandible is immobilized, constitutes a special problem because of the possibility of vomiting

and aspiration. A quick-release wire support has been designed for in-flight use.

EPILEPSY. Most patients with well-controlled epilepsy fly to altitudes of 10,000 ft without difficulty. Flight to greater altitude in unpressurized aircraft may precipitate seizures.

Motion Sickness

The use of modern aircraft has considerably reduced the incidence of motion sickness. The problem remains because of occasional turbulent flights and persons who are extremely susceptible to motion sickness. Such persons should sit over the wings of the aircraft where motion is least. Cyclizine (Marezine) 50 mg, meclizine (Bonine) 25 mg, and dimenhydrinate (Dramamine) 50 mg are effective prophylactic agents.

Space Travel

The medical problems of space flight relate in part to the design of spacecraft and propulsion systems and in part to the characteristics of the space environment.

With design and engineering improvements it will be possible to build spacecraft which require only a small departure from man's ordinary environment. For example, the accelerations of launch and reentery which are of the order of 4 to 8g in present systems could be reduced to a fraction of a g by prolonging the time of acceleration. Present Soviet manned space systems operate with a cabin atmosphere which is very near to that at sea level or earth. To avoid the effects of weightlessness, an acceleration equivalent to that of the earth's gravity can be produced by rotating the spacecraft if this should prove necessary. Radiation shielding can be provided, albeit with a weight penalty. Present space systems represent a series of engineering compromises which are necessary largely because of the limitations of the propulsion systems.

During the flights of the Mercury and Gemini series, several adaptations were observed. Human performance, eating, drinking, urination and defecation, respiration, heart rate, and blood pressure showed no important changes. Weight loss occurred predominantly during the first few days of orbital flight. It was related in part, at least, to negative water balance associated with decreased fluid intake. Several astronauts have had leukocytosis of 20,000 to 30,000 upon return to earth, presumably due to stress and immobilization. There is evidence that red blood cell mass was reduced during orbital flight, possibly related in part to the high ambient oxygen tension. Astronauts manifest orthostatic hypotension after return to a gravitational field. This may be due to reduced blood volume as well as impaired cardiovascular response to gravity. Weightlessness is expected to be associated with a negative calcium balance. There is limited evidence that negative calcium balance and bone demineralization occur, but the effect has not been important in flights of less than 2 weeks' duration.

REFERENCES

Armstrong, H. B.: "Aerospace Medicine," Baltimore, The Williams & Wilkins Company, 1960.

Gauer, O. H., and G. W. Zuidema: "Gravitational Stress in Aerospace Medicine," Boston, Little, Brown and Company, 1961.

Gerathewohl, S. J.: Aeromedical Aspects of the Supersonic Transport, Aerospace Med., 38:1225, 1967.

Gullett, C. C.: Aeromedical Aspects of Turbo-jet Commercial Aircraft, Aerospace Med., 32:818, 1961.

Lafontaine, E., J. Lavernhe, J. Courillon, M. Medvedeff, and J. Ghata: Influence of Air Travel on Circadian Rhythms, Aerospace Med., 38:944, 1967.

129 RADIATION INJURY
Eugene P. Cronkite

Types of Radiation

The types of ionizing radiation most often causing injury are x-rays, gamma rays, alpha and beta rays, protons, and neutrons. X-rays and gamma rays are identical; a separate name was given because of their difference in origin. The former are produced by x-ray machines and as secondary emissions from particle accelerators or electron tubes. The latter are produced by radioactive decay. In general, gamma radiations are more energetic than x-rays; however, the energy spectrum of x-rays is continuous. Beta rays are electrons. Ordinary electrons originate from the shells surounding the atomic nucleus, and beta rays originate only from within the nucleus. Alpha rays are the stripped nuclei of the helium atom with a mass of 4 and a charge of 2+. Protons are stripped nuclei of hydrogen atoms with a mass of 1 and a charge of 1+. Protons are becoming of more interest because of their common use as primary particles in accelerators and their prevalence as an extraterrestial space radiation as described by Van Allen. Protons are of additional interest since they are usually the secondary damaging particle produced by neutron interaction with tissue or other materials. Neutrons have a mass of 1 and charge of 0. Biologic injury is produced primarily by ionization from secondary charged particles. Neutrons produce the secondary charged particles in diverse ways. Fast neutrons react principally with the hydrogen atoms, and as a result of the collision a portion of the energy is imparted to the hydrogen atom and a proton is ejected which does the damage. With thermal or slow neutrons the damage is done by actual capture of the neutrons and a secondary emission of ionizing radiation as the transmuted hydrogen, nitrogen, or other substance in tissue decays and emits radioactivity. These are the basic types of radiation with which a physician may be concerned.

Mechanism of Action

Historically the theories and concepts for mechanism of action of ionizing radiation on living things are dis-cussed in the classic volume by Lea. The concepts of direct hits on the target molecules versus the indirect action mediated through products of reaction with the protoplasmic solvent water are analyzed lucidly. The most acceptable current view to account for a major part of the biologic effects of radiation may be divided into three interlinked steps. First, photons, or particles, penetrate the protoplasm, interacting to produce ion pairs. This reaction takes of the order of 10^{-13} sec. The second step is a primary radiochemical reaction of these ions primarily with water, producing free radicals such as H and OH. These reactions take about 10^{-9} sec. These free radicals produce a further chain of reactions with themselves and tissue water to produce further reactive forms such as H_2O_2 and HO_2. These products persist for microseconds or in part a few seconds. The last reaction is between these products and critical protoplasmic molecules. The nature of this last reaction is not known, but since the actual amount of energy imparted to the system is small, it is generally thought that the damage must involve substances of low concentration but major importance to the living system, for example, nucleic acids or enzymes. It is of interest that the amount of energy deposited to produce 100 percent mortality in animals will raise the body temperature only 0.001°C. Whatever the mechanism may be, it sets into motion a series of observable histologic or chemical lesions that unfold with time. In addition to the effects observable within days, "bad invisible information" may be stored in the proliferative or nonproliferative cells, presumably in DNA, that may not be manifested as a disease process for several years.

Dose Units

In pharmacology, standardization of drugs becomes scientific only when the structure is known and one can measure the drug in an appropriate unit such as a milligram. With ionizing radiation one is concerned not with the mass of the agent administered but with the *amount* and the distribution of energy that has been absorbed by tissue at the *point of interest* (tumor, tissue essential for life, gonads, etc.).

Two dose units are essential for the understanding of the quantitative effects of radiation. The *roentgen* (R), a measure of total dose in air, is defined as the quantity of x-ray or gamma radiation such that the associated corpuscular emission per 0.001293 Gm of air at standard conditions produces in air ions carrying one electrostatic unit of either sign. For energy to be deposited, there must be an interaction with matter. Hence, with x-rays passing through a vacuum, no radiation dose is delivered. In practice we are interested in the energy imparted to various tissues from a number of different types of radiation, and it is therefore essential to have a second unit of radiation which overcomes the limitation of the roentgen. This second unit, the *rad,* is a unit of absorbed dose equal to 100 ergs per Gm of absorbed energy which applies to any type of radiation in any tissue. For small pieces of tissue in an x-ray beam of 1 r per min, the absorbed dose is very close to 1 rad per min. However, as irradiated objects become larger and change in composition, one must consider the diminution in intensity due to the interaction of radiation with matter (buildup and then exponential attenuation) and the changing types of interaction (photoelectric effect, Compton effect, etc.). In tissue of uniform density this leads to a decreasing absorbed dose at successive levels after equilibrium is attained. However, at interfaces such as soft tissue and bone, the absorbed dose may sharply increase. Thus, in addition to the exposure dose in roentgens and the absorbed dose in rads, one must be concerned with the distribution of the absorbed dose in the areas of interest. For example, if there is sufficient protection of bone marrow by shielding of one's own tissues to permit marrow regeneration and survival from what is considered an otherwise fatal *exposure dose*, one may ascribe incorrectly some great benefit to a procedure used therapeutically. Unfortunately, failure to consider the critical influence of the distribution of absorbed dose at the site of interest on the outcome of radiation injury has resulted in ascribing therapeutic benefit to various agents of no value at all.

The *density of ionization* in tissue varies with the energy and type of radiation as well as the tissue composition. The density of ionization is referred to as *specific ionization* (ions per unit track length) or as *linear energy transfer* (LET, kiloelectron volts deposited per unit track length). Among other factors, the density of ionization influences the biologic effect for equivalent amounts of energy deposited, in general the effect being greater with more densely ionizing radiation. This leads to consideration of the relative biologic effectiveness (RBE), which is defined as the ratio of the dose in rads of standard radiation (usually x-ray or gamma radiation of 250 to 400 kv energy) to produce a given degree of biologic effect, to the dose in rads of an unknown radiation to produce the same degree of biologic effect. For example, if the LD-50 dose of x-rays is 600 rads and for neutrons 300 rads, the RBE will be 2. The RBE may vary with the biologic response or the conditions of irradiation. For example, when the same radiations are used, a different value may be obtained for mortality, cataract, or tumor development. Another useful unit is the rem, which stands for roentgen equivalent mammal. Numerically, rem = rads × RBE.

Also of importance is the *dose rate*. In general, the lower the dose rate, the less will be the acute somatic effect. In a crude sense, dose rates in excess of approximately 5 r per min give essentially the same result. However, as the dose rate falls below 5 r per min, the effect per unit of radiation becomes less. In the past, genetic effects were believed independent of dose rate. This implies that all increments of radiation received by the gonads, irrespective of when or how, would add up directly as mutations, to give a total effect ultimately to be measured as detectable effects in succeeding generations. However, it is now known that there is a dose-rate dependence in respect to the production of mutations by irradiation of spermatogonia in mice and also for leukemogenesis in mice, which is considered to be a somatic genetic effect of bone marrow irradiation.

If the dose of radiation is sufficiently high, actual death of any living cell can be observed promptly in terms of classical pathologic criteria of cell necrosis. However, after lower doses of radiation (precise values vary with the tissue), only disturbances in cell proliferation are seen. The rate at which cells divide is decreased. DNA synthesis is impaired in two manners: (1) the rate of synthesis is slower; (2) cells may continue DNA synthesis and become polyploid. It is reasonably certain that radiation has effects other than the outright killing of cells and the interference with mitosis and DNA synthesis. Among the less well understood manifestations of radiation exposure are those dealing with the effects of rather small doses of radiation on the nondividing central nervous system. This work, pioneered by the Russians, has in recent years received more attention from Western radiobiologists. However, it is still not completley understood.

The diminution in the production of new cells in these tissues that are undergoing continual renewal (mucosa, blood, gonads, etc.) results in a progressive hypoplasia to total atrophy, depending on dose. Some cells still capable of mitosis that are not killed outright may be so injured that they will go through one or two generative cycles, producing abnormal progeny, such as giant metamyelocytes and hypersegmented neutrophils, before dying. The atrophy of these steady-state cell renewal systems and direct injury of other tissues produce clearly defined clinical syndromes.

Clinical Phenomena in Relation to Dose and Time after Exposure

Human experience is based on the effects of atomic bombs; accidental exposure to fallout from a hydrogen bomb; laboratory and reactor accidents in the United States, U.S.S.R., and Yugoslavia; and on *whole-body* clinical radiotherapy. After any radiation accident close cooperation of the physician and health physicist is essential to obtain the best estimate of the radiation dose and to evaluate its probable effect in terms of the likely *distribution of the absorbed dose* in rads. However, clinical signs and symptoms remain paramount in the management of human disease and injury. Physical estimates of dose never substitute for clinical judgment and experience.

For teaching purposes three acute radiation syndromes may be classified generally as *cerebral, gastrointestinal,* and *hematopoietic*.

The *cerebral* syndrome is produced by extremely high doses of radiation, i.e., following exposure to several thousand roentgens. It is always fatal, whether the radiation is delivered to the brain alone or to the whole body. Three processes have been described: a prodromal phase of nausea and vomiting; then listlessness and drowsiness ranging from apathy to prostration (probably traceable to nonbacterial inflammatory foci in the brain); and finally, a more generalized component characterized by tremors, convulsions, ataxia, and death. This sequence was observed in an industrial accident, death occurring 36 hr after exposure.

The *gastrointestinal* syndrome occurs when the dose of radiation is lower, in the range of 600 to 1,500 r. It is characterized by intractable nausea, vomiting, and diarrhea; these lead to severe dehydration, diminished plasma volume, vascular collapse, and death. The syndrome is initiated by a pronounced "intoxication," arising presumably from diffuse necrosis of tissue throughout the body; it is extended by severe injury to the gastrointestinal tract. The latter development is caused by two factors: direct killing of a fraction of the crypt cells and inhibition of mitosis. The mature epithelial cells continue to migrate out on to the villus in an orderly fashion, eventually being lost from the tip of the villi; this produces a progressive diminution in the number of cells covering the villi. The epithelial cells progressively become cuboidal and then squamous in appearance and ultimately the intestinal villi become denuded, with massive loss of bloody plasma into the intestine. The usual 3- to 4-day death from the gastrointestinal syndrome can be prevented by massive plasma replacement during the first 4 to 6 days after irradiation. After doses greater than circa, 1,300 r, regeneration is poor and slow. After doses below roughly 1,300 r, regeneration commences around the sixth day with complete restoration of the gastrointestinal epithelium. However, the respite is only temporary, since hematopoietic failure will ensue, commencing within 2 to 3 weeks.

The *hematopoietic syndrome* which occurs following whole-body exposure in the midlethal range is accompanied by temporary anorexia, nausea, and vomiting which is maximal between 6 and 12 hr after exposure to doses of radiation between 600 and 800 r. Thereafter, the gastrointestinal symptoms rapidly subside so that within 24 to 36 hr after exposure the subject is usually asymptomatic. These symptoms have been correlated with a period of rapid necrosis of radiosensitive tissues. The prodromes must be distinguished from the gastrointestinal syndrome described earlier and from that which occurs later on. After subsidence of the prodromes, a period of relative well-being is experienced, during which atrophy of lymph nodes, spleen, and bone marrow progresses, leading to a pancytopenia. This atrophy is the result of two clearly defined processes—direct killing of radiosensitive cells and inhibition of new cell production. In the peripheral blood, lymphopenia commences immediately, becoming maximal within 24 to 36 hr. Thereafter, the lymphocytes remain at low levels for weeks and recover over several months. Within a few hours after irradiation a neutrophilic leukocytosis appears. Following this an oscillation in the neutrophil count occurs, the rate at which it falls to the minimum being a function of the dose of radiation. After sublethal and low lethal doses, the minimal values occur in 4 to 6 weeks; after high lethal doses granulocytes

diminish more rapidly and minimal values approaching zero appear within 7 to 10 days.

Thrombopenia and its relation to radiation bleeding have been studied exhaustively. After single doses of radiation a close correlation with the decrease in the platelet count and the tendency to bleed is evident. In animals and after various accidents, significant purpura was seen only when the platelet counts fell below 20,000 per cu mm. The platelets remain steady or increase for 2 to 3 days after irradiation and thereafter diminish more or less linearly with time, the ultimate minimum and the rate attained being dose-dependent. After about 200 rads, it takes about 30 days for minimum platelet levels to develop. After 600 to 800 rads, minimal levels were observed within 10 to 12 days. Earlier observations in which bleeding in radiation injury was attributed primarily to hyperheparinemia have been refuted. Today there is no evidence of hyperheparinemia; consequently the use of antiheparin agents in the therapy of bleeding induced by radiation is not indicated. Fresh viable platelet transfusions will stop bleeding, and maintenance of platelet levels by platelet transfusions will prevent development of bleeding in animals.

Decreases in the red blood cell count are prominent only after large doses of radiation that significantly interfere with new cell production and produce bleeding.

Studies of *decreased resistance to infection* have resulted in the conclusion that there are (1) a dose-dependent decrease in circulating granulocytes and lymphocytes; (2) a dose-dependent impairment of antibody production; (3) impairment of granulocyte migration and phagocytosis; (4) decreased ability of the reticulo-endothelial system to kill phagocytized bacteria; (5) diminished resistance to diffusion in subcutaneous tissues; and (6) hemorrhagic areas of the skin and bowel that present foci for entrance and growth of bacteria. Obviously an increased susceptibility to infection by both commensals and pathogens must be present.

The preceding syndromes may be produced when the whole body is uniformly exposed to radiation or if there is a substantial inhomogeneous exposure of the whole body. An expression of the lethal dose range for man is desirable to assist in the management of casualties. In the case of inhomogeneous exposure, one can see how misleading any single air or exposure dose may be. There is a hierarchy of effects that vary with time, dose, and organs involved. Although 10,000 rads to the brain will be fatal, 10,000 rads to a hand may only necessitate amputation. Since the bone marrow is somewhat more sensitive than other tissues, ultimate survival is determined in large part by the dose to this tissue. For uniform whole-body exposure *without therapy* it has been estimated that the lethal dose curve will commence at about 200 rads and that survivals will be rare after doses in excess of 800 rads. Between these limits the percentage mortality dose curve is sigmoid. Even if the dose to an individual is known with precision, the prognosis must remain probable because one can never predict whether an individual belongs on the sensitive or resistant portion of the curve.

Inhomogeneous Exposure to Radiation

The preceding description of radiation injury was based primarily on human clinical experience and animal experimentation in which the distribution of dose absorbed by tissues was relatively uniform. However, in actuality, conditions of exposure may be such that there are marked inhomogeneities in absorbed dose. For example, the geometry of an exposure may result in almost no exposure to the lower part of the body and very heavy exposure to the abdomen and hands, resulting in extensive necrosis of the skin of these areas in addition to the fatal injury to deeper tissues. In one accident, the direction of the beam resulted in severe exposure to the head, but the low energy permitted marked attenuation of the beam within the head, so that the absorbed dose through the brain decreased markedly from the side closest to the beam to the side farthest from it. The superficial layers of the brain were injured badly, but death did not ensue because vital centers were not destroyed. In evaluating any radiation accident, one must reconstruct the geometry and consider the probable distribution of absorbed dose within the body. What may initially appear as a fatal accident in terms of air exposure dose may turn out to be sublethal when effects of distribution of the absorbed dose are considered.

Management of Acute Human Radiation Injury

Presumptive evidence of exposure to radiation and signs or symptoms described earlier must be recognized before there need be cause for concern. No therapy is available for the cerebral form of radiation injury after uniform brain exposure. Whereas a small percentage of persons with the gastrointestinal syndrome may be kept alive until the affected tract regenerates, they must also face the hematopoietic syndrome; hence that is the real therapeutic problem. Therapy rests on the control of the sequelae of marrow aplasia and thus is similar to management of drug-induced and idiopathic marrow aplasia, suggesting that combined use of antibacterials and transfusions would be useful. The spontaneous course of radiation injury in man has clearly shown that signs and symptoms develop at different times in different subjects after identical doses of radiation. Accordingly, the time of institution and type of therapy should be individualized. The following general therapeutic regimen is outlined.

1. *Maintain rigid asepsis* until one is confident that a sublethal exposure to radiation has been experienced. All medical staff involved in the care of irradiated individuals must have negative cultures of the nasopharynx for pathogenic organisms. Physicians and nursing staff with any evidence of respiratory or other infections are forbidden entrance to the rooms of irradiated patients. If at all possible, reverse isolation should be instituted to prevent introduction of pathogens into the environment of the patient. This requires either the use of plastic rooms in which the patient is placed or the sterilization of a room and the institution of laminar flow air barriers and appropriate ultraviolet light sources to prevent the introduction of pathogens into the patient's environment.

2. Observe *fluid and electrolyte balance* closely and restore as necessary with appropriate replacement solutions.

3. *Provide sterile, bland diet* prepared in the patient's room.

4. Administer *nonabsorbable intestinal antibiotics* such as neomycin to sterilize the gastrointestinal tract and minimize the probability of invasion by commensal organisms in the gastrointestinal tract.

5. *Treat infection* when it develops or relapses, using various antibiotics sequentially in doses two to three times the usual size. Use sulfonamides when antibiotics are exhausted. One is fighting for additional time to permit spontaneous regeneration.

6. *Use fresh whole blood* to control bleeding and/or to restore adequate red cell levels. Fresh blood is defined as that which has been taken from the donor not more than 1 hr previously and placed in plastic bags with Na_2EDTA. When the hematocrit is returned to normal range, to control bleeding use fresh platelet-rich plasma as clinically indicated, not on an inflexible schedule. Despite many claims concerning the value of lyophilized and frozen platelets, radiation bleeding has been successfully managed to date only by the use of fresh viable platelets that circulate in adequate numbers.

The preceding therapy has increased the survival rate of animals. Unless infection or serious hemorrhage develops, therapy is not needed. Prophylactic therapy other than the use of nonabsorbable intestinal antibiotics is believed to be contraindicated. Many human beings with epilation, severe pancytopenia, and purpura have recovered without therapy from doses of radiation ranging from 200 to 300 r. Recently individuals who received 400 to 500 r inhomogeneous irradiation have recovered when treated in accordance with this therapeutic regimen despite near-zero granulocyte and platelet counts.

Syngenesious and autologous bone marrow transplantation will prevent death in almost all otherwise fatally irradiated animals up to doses of about 1,200 r. In fatally irradiated animals saved by allogenic bone marrow transplantation, the transplanted marrow may eventually produce a reaction (presumably against the host) of immunologic nature, resulting in a severe late degenerative disease of the skin, kidneys, liver, and lymph nodes. A similar late fatal effect has been observed in children treated for leukemia with extensive chemotherapy and whole-body irradiation in whom allogeneic marrow transplantation was successful.

Although marrow transplantation has been widely acclaimed as the solution to fatal whole-body radiation, the results in human beings so far do not warrant optimism. This author believes it should be reserved for patients in whom there is a progressive deterioration of the hematopoietic system with granulocytes falling below 500 per cu mm in the first 2 weeks after exposure and an early rapid decline in the platelet count. The profile scoring method of Thomas and Wald may be useful on a day-to-day basis of evaluating the severity and may give some indication as to when one may be forced to resort to allogeneic marrow transplantation. In the rare case in which there is an identical twin, bone marrow transplantation should be lifesaving following fatal radiation injury up to a maximum exposure of about 1,200 r. Rigid rules cannot be formulated in advance. Decisions can be made only at the bedside.

Prevention

Nothing can substitute for prevention. Shielding, distance, and limiting of exposure time are the only effective preventive measures against exposures from radiation sources, whether in industry, medical practice, military action, or civil defense. A series of drugs, primarily sulfhydryl groups, that will protect against radiation by an effective dose reduction up to 50 percent are available. However, these must be administered within minutes preceding exposure. Accidents and warfare are not predictable. The severe toxic effects of these drugs prevent continuous prophylactic administration.

Long-term Effects

Radiation alters the "information system" of proliferating somatic and germ cells. Thus the perpetuating cells of the blood, gastrointestinal tract, skin, lens, gonads, and other areas pass on either "bad or inadequate information," presumably in altered DNA, to their progeny, resulting in late somatic disease, e.g., cancer, cataracts, degenerative disorders, or nonspecific shortening of life. Leukemia yield from radiation in human groups has been quantified. It is asserted, but not proved, that there is no threshold and that the yield of leukemia increases with dose. However, the greatest exposure of the American public comes from the medical uses of diverse types of radiation (predominantly diagnostic x-rays). If the assumption of no threshold dose for leukemia is correct, the medical uses of radiation are producing their small toll in an additional burden of leukemia and probably other disease also. Therefore, it behooves the practitioner to be exceedingly cautious and to expose patients to radiation only when it is clearly indicated and needed for diagnosis.

Radiation can produce mutation of genes, the information and transmission centers for heredity. Of this there is no doubt. Not all mutations are harmful, but the chances are overwhelming that a change will be detrimental to the species. Not all mutations produce visible immediately detectable effects. The concern is not only with an increase in the number of obvious freaks or cripples but with changes that will lead to such undesirable characteristics as lowered life expectancy, decreased fertility, a general increase in physical and mental disease, and an increase in fetal or neonatal death rates. It is the less obvious changes that are of the greatest importance. The more obvious changes usually lead to early death in the individual and reduced fertility in those that survive. Thus the harmful mutant is relatively quickly deleted from the population. The more subtle changes, however,

are propagated longer and affect a very large number of persons. The mutation may be dominant or recessive. Most dominant mutations are also lethal, and many such mutations may be missed because the fertilized egg never develops far enough to be recognized as a new individual. If the mutation is recessive, the mutant will not become evident unless both parents of the individual have the same mutant genes and transfer these to the individual concerned. It is extremely difficult to quantify these considerations. If the mutation rate were increased by a single exposure of the population to radiation, the effects would be spread through many generations. Half the total damage produced would not be observed until some 30 to 50 generations had been born. These are the practical considerations that make the problem particularly difficult to analyze. Damage that is inflicted now cannot be detected now and will only become evident many generations hence. These considerations also indicate why it is not possible to take negative evidence in populations that have been exposed to date as an indication that the degree of genetic damage is small. If, for instance, an effect was already obvious in the children born of individuals irradiated in Japan by the atom bombs, it would mean that the total genetic effect would be great indeed. These are sobering considerations for thoughtful persons. Since exposure to irradiation cannot be avoided in our modern industrial society and in the practice of medicine and because of the uncertainty about the quantitative effect in producing somatic or genetic effects, it is mandatory that exposure be minimal and rigidly controlled in order to protect the present generations from somatic effects and future generations from genetic effects.

Radium Poisoning

Today it appears strange that radium water was used as a therapeutic agent only three decades ago and resulted in poisoning. In addition, radium watch dial painters were poisoned during World War I. The radium (often mesothorium) is deposited primarily on the surface of the bones, and its distribution changes with the slow rebuilding of the osseous structure. Histologically one sees Havarsian systems plugged with highly calcified material; gross regions of resorption; and osteocyte death as evidenced by empty and highly calcified lacunae. Autoradiographs show both a "diffuse" distribution and "hot spots" of radioactivity. Pathologists consider the characteristic bony injury almost pathognomic of chronic radium poisoning. Many of the effects are due to direct radiation injury; some are secondary to vascular injury. Bone necrosis and interference with normal processes of internal reconstruction of bone result in the formation of small and large cavities, which give the characteristic radiolucency in radiographs of bone. Fibrosis of the bone is a constant feature, usually limited to the endosteal surfaces of cortical and trabecular bone. The marrow may be spottily fibrotic. The disturbed structure of bone may so weaken it as to permit pathologic fractures. The long-term irradiation is carcinogenic. Malignant bone tumors arise. The induction time is long—greater than 10 years, with an average of about 20 years. The types of tumors are not different from human bone tumors in general. In addition to bone tumors, carcinomas of the sinuses and nasopharynx have been seen in greatly increased numbers over the rare expected incidence. Leukemias have been conspicuous by their almost total absence. Aplastic anemia has also been observed as a cause of death. There is no satisfactory treatment of early or late radium poisoning. Prevention is the cure. Although these cases are mainly of historical interest, many elderly persons are still alive with significant body burdens of radium from therapy and employment in the watch dial industry. It is not possible to construct a dose-effect curve for radium poisoning. An estimate of the numerator of the incidence ratio is possible, since the diseases are brought to the attention of physicians. However, the denominator is sadly lacking since those who did not develop a disease that necessitated medical care are absent from most serious studies of the problem.

Microwaves

Microwave frequency extends from 300 to 200,000 megacycles, with wavelengths from about 1 to 50 cm.

Microwaves are the output of radars; they are used to accelerate nuclear particles in accelerators, for cooking, for industrial heating problems, and in medical diathermy for local heating of tissue. A common diathermy today utilizes a magnetron tube which operates at 2,450 megacycles and 12 cm wavelength. Numerous applicators are available for heating surfaces, within the rectum, vagina, etc. Medically the local heating of tissue at depths apparently increases blood flow and promotes more rapid healing of traumatized or inflamed areas.

Harmful effects are produced from deposition of energy too rapidly, producing excessive local heating of tissue. Deposition of energy varies with the type of tissue and the reflection from interfaces. Experimentally, bone growth has been impaired, testicles have been destroyed, and cataracts have been produced. Very high intensity radar exposure for 1 min 10 ft from the antenna resulted in sufficient injury to the bowel to produce an acute abdominal emergency, necessitating laparotomy and followed later by intestinal perforations, peritonitis, and death. Presumably the bowel was "cooked" in part. A few servicemen looked down the wave guide of a radar and later developed cataracts. Cataracts also developed in an employee who worked near an operating microwave antenna. A hazard is known to exist. Injuries can be avoided by educating those who work near and plan the propagation of microwaves so that the beam is directed away from human beings.

Ultrasound

Ultrasound consists of sound waves from a few hundred kilocycles per second to many megacycles per second. The passage of the sound wave through tissue produces successive positive and negative pressures which increase molecular motion and then generate heat via frictional forces. With large intensities (greater than 1 watt per sq cm), cavities are produced during the negative phase which become filled with gas dissolved in the medium. Cavitation produces large local temperatures, electrical discharges, and intense mechanical movement. Chemical reactions involving "free radicals" produced by the electrical discharges may occur, depending on the chemical nature of dissolved gases which may enhance or suppress the free radicals.

Ultrasound can kill cells, disrupt bacteria, etc., but local heat may inactivate enzymes and disturb subsequent chemical studies.

Ultrasound has been used in therapy, with some success, to produce local heating, as in diathermy for the treatment of arthritis, painful neuromas, and myositis. There is little danger since destruction of tissue takes about fifty times as much energy as production of pain; hence there is a built-in physiologic safeguard.

Unique ingenious multiple-port focusing devices have been built to focus ultrasonic energy in distinctly circumscribed volumes to destroy tissue. Such devices are being developed for neurosurgical work. Bone overlying the area at which the sound is focused must be removed. It is possible to destroy all neural components in a specific region without interrupting the capillary network. Ultrasonic neurosurgery is being evaluated in the treatment and relief of the hyperkinetic, hypertonic, and intractable pain disorders. It has also been used for prefrontal lobotomy instead of the usual surgical approach.

Ultrasound can also be used to localize foreign bodies and some tumors.

See Chap. 59. Sunlight and Photosensitivity Reactions.

REFERENCES

Bond, V. P., T. M. Fliedner, and J. Archambeau: "Mammalian Radiation Lethality," New York, Academic Press Inc., 1965.

Casarett, A. P.: "Radiation Biology," Englewood Cliffs, N.J., Prentice-Hall, Inc., 1968.

Cronkite, E. P., and V. P. Bond: "Radiation Injury in Man," Springfield, Ill., Charles C Thomas, Publisher, 1960.

——, W. C. Moloney, and V. P. Bond: Radiation Leukemogenesis, Am. J. Med., 28:673, 1960.

Elkind, M. M., and G. P. Whitmore: "The Radiobiology of Cultured Mammalian Cells," New York, Gordon and Breach, Science Publishers, Inc., 1967.

Hempelmann, L. H., H. Lisco, and J. G. Hoffman: The Acute Radiation Syndrome: A Study of 9 Cases and a Review, Ann. Intern. Med., 36:279, 1952.

Knauff, G. M.: Biological Effects of Microwave Radiation on Air Force Personnel, A.M.A. Arch. Indust. Health, 17:48, 1958.

Lea, D. E.: "Actions of Radiation on Living Cells," New York, The Macmillan Company, 1947.

McLaughlin, J. T.: Tissue Destruction and Death from Microwave Radiation (Radar), Calif. Med., 86:336, 1957.

Report of U.N. Scientific Committee on the Effects of Atomic Radiation, 19th Session, Suppl. 14 (A/5814), Chap. 3: Radiation Carcinogenesis in Man, 1964.

Rubin, P. R., and G. W. Casarett: "Clinical Radiation Pathology," Philadelphia, W. B. Saunders Company, 1968.

Schwan, H. P.: Biophysics of Diathermy, p. 55 in S. Licht (Ed.), "Therapeutic Heat," New Haven, Conn., S. Licht Publisher, 1958.

130 ELECTRICAL INJURIES

Ivan L. Bennett, Jr.

The first human fatality from accidental electrocution occurred in 1879 and was produced by an alternating current of 250 v. Since that time, continuing increase in household and commercial uses of electrical power has made accidents almost inevitable. Injury and death from lightning have occurred, of course, since time immemorial.

ETIOLOGY AND PATHOGENESIS. The end result of passage of an electrical current through the human body is unpredictable in the individual case. Certain generalizations are possible, however, and many of the factors that influence severity of injury by electricity are known. *Alternating currents* tend to produce tetanization of muscles and sweating (which lowers skin resistance), and *direct currents* produce electrolytic changes in the tissues. It has been estimated that alternating is about four or five times as dangerous as direct current; fatal electrocution from exposure to household circuits of 115 v at 60 cycles is relatively common.

The conductivity of tissues parallels their water content; consequently, the vascular system and musculature are good conductors, whereas bones, peripheral nerves, and skin offer high resistance. The resistance of normal skin is lowered by *moisture,* and this factor alone may convert what might ordinarily be a mild injury to fatal shock. The *grounding* of the body at the time of contact is important. It is well known that a person in water or on a wet surface is more susceptible to electrical injury. The *pathway of the current* through the body is crucial. Obviously, an accident involving passage of current between a point of contact on the leg and the ground is likely to be less injurious than one in which the poles of the circuit are the head and a foot. The *duration of contact* influences the outcome. Because, as mentioned, an electrical current can stimulate skeletal muscle to contract, a victim who has grasped an uninsulated wire may be unable to release it; this is far more likely with alternating than with direct currents and accounts in part for the greater danger of alternating circuits. Sudden convulsive contraction of muscles can result in fractures of bone; sometimes, however, it throws the individual clear of contact. This may lead to additional mechanical trauma if the victim is thrown from a high place.

In traversing the skin, energy of high-tension currents is converted to heat. When one considers that electric arcs with temperatures as high as 8000°C may be generated, it is not surprising that fourth or fifth degree burns often result. The term *electrical necrosis* is probably more appropriate than *burn* for this injury. It has been suggested that the immediate damage is aggravated by vasospasm in adjacent tissues.

The systemic effects of electricity are incompletely understood, but, in general, low voltage produces ventricular fibrillation and death from circulatory failure, and high voltage produces respiratory arrest. High-tension currents produce cardiac standstill, but ventricular function resumes when the current stops, and death is presumably attributable to injury of medullary centers. Whether this neurologic damage results from vasospasm, increase in temperature of the brain, or direct injury to neurones is not known.

A lightning flash is a rush of electrical energy (about 1 billion v and 20,000 amp) along a path more than a mile long and 18 to 20 ft in diameter. The duration of the current is about 0.001 sec. When the bolt reaches the earth, secondary flashes occur and objects within a radius of 100 ft may be struck. Direct contact usually results in immediate death. Persons nearby may be injured by the electrical current, by burning from heated air, or by the concussive force of compressed air.

If patients die immediately, autopsy findings are limited to burns and generalized petechial hemorrhage. If patients survive for a period of days or longer, postmortem examination reveals focal necroses of nerve, spinal cord, or brain, involving both neurones and white matter, with appropriate glial and vascular reactions. Acute renal failure is an occasional complication if tissue destruction is extensive, as from high-tension accidents.

MANIFESTATIONS. Immediately after severe shock, patients are usually comatose and apneic, although the heart may continue to beat until anoxia leads to circulatory failure. Surviving this stage, patients are often disoriented and combative; convulsions are frequent. Blackened, charred areas at the points of entrance and exit of the current may appear to be relatively small and well localized. After a few days, however, huge sloughs, often involving major blood vessels, reveal the true extent of the destruction. A frequent finding in victims of lightning is a characteristic, lacy network of superficial "arborescent burns," or "lightning prints," on the skin. These fade within 24 to 48 hr. Late effects include various neurologic disabilities, visual disturbances, and, of course, the residual damage left by burns. A curious finding in many victims of lightning is temporary flaccid paralysis of the lower extremities with loss of sensation, so-called "keraunoparalysis," which passes off in 12 to 24 hr. This condition is often accompanied by blanching and coldness of the legs and is believed to be a result of severe vasoconstriction. Hemoglobinuria, oliguria, and acute renal failure may complicate massive injury to soft tissues. Injuries to the nervous system can leave symptoms resembling peripheral neuritis or multiple sclerosis. The development of cataracts has been reported as a late complication.

As many as 50 percent of persons who survive severe electrical accidents may develop a "post-electric shock syndrome," characterized by dull pain in the shoulders and chest, unrelated to exertion but aggravated by moving the arms or by deep breathing. This apparently results from traumatic myositis after severe muscular contraction during exposure to the electric current. It may produce considerable apprehension and concern about heart disease in tense or nervous individuals.

The use of electrical shock in psychiatric treatment has led to occasional accidents of two types. Sudden death, attributed to ventricular fibrillation, has been observed in elderly patients. Fracture of vertebral bodies during the convulsion has occurred; this is preventable by use of relaxant drugs.

LABORATORY FINDINGS. Leukocytosis with many large, immature granulocytes in the peripheral blood is common after severe electrical shock. Albuminuria is the rule; hemoglobinuria has been reported in many cases, probably secondary to severe burns. Although elevation of cerebrospinal fluid pressure is often mentioned in electrical shock, it is an inconstant finding; bloody spinal fluid occurs in some cases as a result of widespread vascular injury.

MANAGEMENT. Immediate *removal of the victim from contact* with the current is obviously important; this should always be preceded by cutting off the source of the current, when possible. Rescuers should be insulated by rubber gloves or a thick layer of dry cloth or newspapers. Many needless deaths have followed ill-planned attempts to rescue the body of a person already dead from electrical shock.

Artificial respiration should be instituted immediately if the victim is not breathing. The importance of this maneuver cannot be overemphasized. In one series of 700 cases of electrical injury (Maclachlan), there were 479 with respiratory arrest, of which 323 responded to artificial respiration. Most patients who respond do so within 20 min, but recovery after longer periods is frequent enough that manual or mechanical respiration should be continued for a minimum of 4 hr. It has been estimated that a delay of 6 min in the institution of resuscitative measures increases the death rate by 80 percent. External cardiac massage, coupled with defibrillation, if indicated, is extremely important in emergency management.

Other treatment is supportive. Stimulants should be used with caution during the first few hours because of the tendency of many patients toward convulsions. There is no evidence that the frequently advocated procedure of cerebrospinal fluid drainage is beneficial. Survivors of the acute episode often require extensive treatment for burns, infection, and hemorrhage as the devitalized tissues slough. If acute renal failure occurs, it should be managed as described in Chap. 300.

PREVENTION. Proper insulation of appliances, grounding of telephone lines and radio or television aerials, and the use of rubber gloves and dry shoes when working with circuits should be routine.

In a thunderstorm, the safest shelter is a closed house; an automobile, cave, or ditch is relatively secure. Hilltops, riverbanks, hedges, and wire fences should be avoided.

Ventricular fibrillation in patients undergoing elec-

trocardiography, cardiac catheterization, angiocardiography, pacemaking, etc., has been reported often enough to indicate the need for stringent precautions as electronic equipment is used with increasing frequency in hospitals. Almost all accidents have involved a leakage of 60-cycle "house" current through the patient. Personnel should be aware of the hazards involved, the wiring of apparatus including oxygen machines and electrically operated beds should be checked carefully, and equipment should always be grounded *before* a patient is connected to an instrument.

REFERENCES

Fischer, H.: Pathologic Effects and Sequelae of Electrical Accidents, J. Occup. Med., 7:564, 1965.

Jude, J. R., W. B. Kouwenhoven, and G. G. Knickerbocker: Cardiac Arrest, J.A.M.A., 178:1063, 1961.

LaJoie, R. J.: Post-electroshock Syndrome, Indust. Med. Surg., 31:051, 1962.

Lightning Injuries, Lancet, I:351, 1946.

Maclachlan, W.: Electrical Injuries, J. Indust. Hyg., 16:52, 1934.

Ravitch, M. M., R. Lane, P. Safar, F. M. Steichen, and P. Knowles: Lightning Stroke, New Engl. J. Med., 264:36, 1961.,

131 IMMERSION INJURY AND DROWNING

Russell S. Fisher

About 7,000 deaths by drowning occur in the United States each year. This represents about one-fifteenth of the total number of fatal accidents.

Diagnosis

The term *drowning* is used to categorize a series of related phenomena resulting from submersion in a liquid medium that is per se innocuous. It, therefore, includes asphyxial changes as well as complex acute hemodynamic alterations and disturbances of the biochemical equilibrium of the blood.

Pathogenesis

Knowledge of the sequence of phenomena that occur in drowning is based upon a number of observations on humans and on experimental drowning in animals. Submersion is usually followed by an intensive and panicky struggle in an effort to reach the surface. Breath holding for varying lengths of time has been recorded to occur in the next stage, possibly lasting until the accumulating CO_2 in blood and tissues stimulates the respiratory center sufficiently to lead to an inevitable inhalation of considerable volumes of water. Swallowing of water, coughing and vomiting, loss of consciousness, and terminal gasping with flooding of the lungs and death then take place in rapid succession. When the process is interrupted before terminal gasping has set in, spontaneous recovery sometimes occurs. It has commonly been asserted that drowning essentially involves asphyxia resulting from obstruction of the airway by the drowning fluid. More recent investigations, however, show that asphyxial death in drowning is limited to between 10 and 15 percent of all cases and is due to laryngospasm and closure of the glottis. Moreover comparative enzymologic studies in rats of fresh and salt water drowning and asphyxia by exclusion of air indicate significant statistical differences between test and control groups. This seems to further stress the distinction between the mode of death in asphyxia versus that of drowning. In the majority of fatalities, death results from complex pathophysiologic events differing widely according to the chemical composition of the submersion liquid. For purposes of illustration, drowning in fresh water and sea water may be considered as separate entities.

Drowning in Fresh Water

Large amounts of water enter the lungs and due to the hypotonicity of fresh water, rapid absorption into the circulating bloodstream takes place. This results in a sudden and violent increase in blood volume with hemodilution and hypervolemia. Using deuterium oxide in the water as a tracer, Swann and Spafford have demonstrated that after 2 min submersion, a dog's blood may be diluted by as much as 51 percent of its original volume. This hemodilution is associated with massive hemolysis and an inevitable upset of the normal balance of the blood constituents. Sodium, chloride, calcium, proteins, and hemoglobin are all diluted, and the level of potassium rises. Ventricular fibrillation is often considered to be a characteristic feature of fresh water drowning. When it occurs, expulsive heartbeats are arrested at once. Ventricular fibrillation is believed to be directly related to the dilution of the blood electrolytes, in particular sodium. It cannot, however, be produced experimentally by injecting large volumes of water intravenously. The precedent condition is anoxia; the animal must be anoxic for an experimental hydremic plethora to cause fibrillation. The original hypothesis, based upon animal experiments, of "potassium intoxication" secondary to massive hemolysis as the underlying factor causing ventricular fibrillation has proved erroneous. The main intracellular cation in dog erythrocytes is not potassium as in man, but sodium, and fresh water drowning and hemolysis in the dog does not release a flood of potassium ions. The slight increase observed in plasma potassium after fresh water drowning may be accounted for by prolonged anoxia, as described by Fenn. These speculations do not answer the question of whether ventricular fibrillation occurs in fresh water drowning in man, but it would appear desirable to include defibrillation in the emergency treatment of a drowning victim.

Drowning in Sea Water

Sea water is strongly hypertonic. Its salt concentration, mainly sodium chloride, is over 3.0 percent. Submersion in sea water results in a rapid diffusion of salts into the bloodstream. The concentration of sodium, chloride, magnesium, etc., in the plasma rise conspicuously, while water moves from the circulation into the pulmonary alveoli—thus reestablishing the osmotic equilbrium. The consequences are marked hemoconcentration and fulminant pulmonary edema. Hypotension and hypovolemia accompanied by considerable bradycardia develop, and death supervenes within a few minutes. Ventricular fibrillation is not usually observed in experimental salt water drowning in spite of the adverse prevailing electrolyte environment, probably because the plasma sodium level is elevated rather than low.

Death Associated with Diving

(Refer also to Chap. 127.) In the case of divers, death is often the result of underwater asphyxia following hyperventilation; the latter leads to a sharp fall in blood carbon dioxide and to vasconstriction, which in turn brings about a decrease of the cerebral circulation. Diminished cerebral blood flow is followed by loss of consciousness, which leads to inhalation of water. Involuntary exhalation against a closed glottis resulting in hypotension and diminished cardiac output further aggravate the condition. In diving with a scuba (self-contained underwater breathing apparatus) the cause of death is usually closely associated with the overconfidence of the diver in his breathing machine. *Nitrogen narcosis* occurs commonly, resulting from the increase of nitrogen concentration in the tissues as evident from Henry's law, according to which the solubility of a gas is directly proportional to the absolute pressure upon it. There is an increase of 1 atm of pressure for each 33 ft of water depth. Barotrauma and air embolism are second in frequency and occur during the ascent of the diver, when the air inhaled from the scuba expands proportionately as the pressure decreases (Boyle's law). An ascent, for instance, from 33 ft results in a twofold increase in volume due to the decrease in pressure from 2 to 1 atm. At this point any interference with expiration prevents release of this increased volume and results in acute pulmonary emphysema with tears in the lungs, hemoptysis, hemothorax, air embolism, and often death.

Resuscitation from Drowning

The main objective of adequate resuscitation in drowning is to institute such measures before circulatory failure sets in. Resuscitative procedures currently employed consist of clearing the airway by postural drainage, suction, etc., and giving artificial respiration, supplemented by closed-chest cardiac massage if no heart sounds are obtainable and the pulse is absent. Intermittent positive-pressure breathing with air, or preferably with oxygen, should be employed when such is available, and external electrical defibrillation should be carried out as soon as feasible after the condition arises. Plasma infusion to correct hemoconcentration is often thought to be of great value in salt water drowning, while in fresh water drowning it may be expected that an exchange transfusion, which in itself is a relatively harmless procedure, will be effective in reestablishing a normal circulating blood volume and in correcting an upset electrolyte balance. So-called "semi-" or "near drowning" in which death occurs suddenly several hours or longer after submersion has been repeatedly reported, but the mechanism of death in such cases remains obscure. Treatment should be directed to maintaining high cerebral oxygen supply and preventing pneumonia. Lower nephron nephrosis may also be anticipated in survivors of fresh water submersion due to hemoglobinemia; if oliguria or anuria develops, appropriate therapy should be initiated.

REFERENCES

Denny, M. K., and R. C. Read: Scuba-diving Deaths in Michigan, J.A.M.A., 192:220, 1965.

Kvittingen, T. D., and A. Naess: Recovery from Drowning in Fresh Water, Brit. Med. J., 1:1315, 1963.

Spitz, W. U.: Recovery from Drowning, Brit. Med. J., 1:1678, 1963.

Swann, H. G.: Mechanism of Circulatory Failure in Fresh and Sea Water Drowning, Circ. Res., 4:241, 1956.

Part Seven

Disorders Caused by Biologic Agents

Section 1

Basic Considerations

132 AN APPROACH TO INFECTIOUS DISEASES

Ivan L. Bennett, Jr., and
Robert G. Petersdorf

The vast majority of human and animal diseases of known etiology are produced by biologic agents, viruses, rickettsias, bacteria, mycoplasma, fungi, protozoa, or nematodes. No small part of the past and present importance of infectious diseases in medical practice is attributable to their enormous frequency and the public health implications of the contagiousness of many of them. However, development in sanitary engineering, vector control, techniques of immunization, and specific chemotherapy have modified the situation favorably. Although important exceptions remain, infectious diseases as a class are more easily prevented and more easily cured than any other major group of disorders. Despite the virtual elimination of certain infectious diseases and profound reduction in the morbidity and mortality of many, man is by no means free of infection. In fact, the *total human load of disease produced by microbial parasites has been only moderately, if at all, decreased.* As certain specific microbial infections have been controlled, others have emerged as troublesome therapeutic and epidemiologic problems. With the introduction of cytotoxic drugs in the treatment of malignant diseases and of immunosuppressive agents to control the rejection of transplanted organs, infections due to organisms previously considered saprophytic or commensal have increased. As Dubos has pointed out, microbial infections appear to form an inherent part of human life.

Because better environmental sanitation and other measures now prevent contact with many microbial agents and the development of acquired immunity early in childhood, certain infections have been seen more frequently in adults. For example, as contact with poliomyelitis virus in childhood declined in many countries, paralytic poliomyelitis became more common in young adults. Similarly, decreasing infection with the tubercle bacillus raises questions about the status of antituberculous immunity in adults.

As antimicrobial agents reduce the mortality associated with certain common infections, other microbes emerge as important causes of human disease. It is relatively unusual nowadays for patients to die of uncomplicated pneumococcal pneumonia—a disease readily handled with available antimicrobials. However, it is common to see serious disease produced by microorganisms which form part of man's normal microbial flora. These include infections produced by staphylococci, enteric bacilli, and fungi.

THE PARASITE AND THE HOST

The complex interaction between microorganism and man that results in infection and disease has been subjected to extensive study. Much has been learned about the initiation of the process, the ways in which microbes produce tissue injury, the influence of specific immunity and "nonspecific" resistance of the host, and mechanisms of recovery. Unfortunately, it is not yet possible to transfer in any specific way much of the information that has been acquired to the individual patient with an infection. In a textbook of medicine, therefore, it seems appropriate to emphasize those general aspects of the host-parasite relationship that form a basis for diagnostic procedures, that are of importance in deriving therapeutic principles, or that help explain the epidemiology of infection. This necessitates omitting from these pages discussion of many highly significant and interesting experimental studies, controversial issues, and theoretical or incompletely established concepts. The bibliography at the end of the chapter contains excellent reviews of these important subjects.

Infection and Clinical Disease

It is well known that microorganisms of different species or different strains of the same species vary widely in their capacity to produce disease and that human beings are not equally susceptible to the disease caused by a given bacterium or virus. Furthermore, while a specific infectious disease will not occur in the absence of the causative organism, the mere presence of the organism in the human body does not lead invariably to clinical illness. Indeed, the production of symptoms in man by many parasites is an exception rather than the rule, and a *subclinical infection* or the "carrier state" is the usual host-parasite relationship. *Disease* in a clinical sense is not synonymous with the presence of the organism or *infection* in a microbiologic sense. The ratio of subclinical infection to overt clinical disease varies widely for different microbial species. For example, subclinical infections with the agent causing infectious hepatitis are the rule. By contrast, active human infection with the rabies virus probably always produces progressive fatal disease and subclinical infections with rabies have not been observed.

Mechanisms of Injury

It is customary to refer to bacteria or other microorganisms that are capable of producing disease as *pathogenic*. *Virulence*, the *degree* of pathogenicity, should be distinguished from *invasiveness*, the ability to spread and disseminate in the body. For example, *Clostridium tetani* is pathogenic and, by virtue of its exotoxin, highly virulent, but it is almost completely lacking in invasiveness. These distinctions are valuable in microbiology and experimental pathology, but they often mean relatively little at a clinical level. Under certain circumstances and in certain anatomic locations, mildly "pathogenic" organisms can produce fatal disease, or highly "pathogenic" species can dwell and multiply without producing any harmful effect.

A few parasites produce *toxins* that account for the tissue damage and physiologic alterations of infection. *Hypersensitivity* to components of the parasite is demonstrable in several infections to account for the manifestations of disease. For many pathogenic agents, an explanation of their damaging effects upon the host is incomplete or wholly lacking. Generally, therefore, the aim of therapy is to stop multiplication or to kill the parasites with appropriate drugs; in diseases caused by toxin-producing organisms, the use of antiserum (as in tetanus or diphtheria) is the definitive procedure and chemotherapy is secondary.

The tendency of certain pathogenic organisms to *localize in certain cells or organs* and to produce damage is also unexplained in most instances. Clinically, however, the presence of disease in a specific anatomic site or a combination of symptoms referable to certain organs often suggests the identity of the causative organism. For example, the pneumococcus usually causes infection in the lung but almost never in the kidney, and *Hemophilus influenzae* infections are confined almost solely to the respiratory tract and meninges. Similarly, in the presence of disease known to be caused by a given agent, complicating involvement of other tissues can be anticipated or predicted. Examples include the multiple lung abscesses which are so characteristic of hematogenously disseminated staphylococcal disease and metastatic skin lesions which complicate *Pseudomonas* bacteremia.

Frequently, the proper management of infectious disease involves the use of techniques completely unrelated to microbiology or chemotherapy, in an effort to support the function of damaged organs. Survival in poliomyelitis may depend upon treatment of respiratory failure, the management of heart failure in endocarditis is sometimes a greater problem than the eradication of the causative organism, and in epidemic hemorrhagic fever, or Weil's disease, maintenance of fluid and electrolyte balance, with peritoneal dialysis or hemodialysis during the stage of acute renal failure is the important therapeutic objective.

Resistance and Susceptibility

Many so called "host factors" are known to influence the likelihood that disease will occur if organisms enter the tissues or, if infection becomes established, to play a determining role in the outcome of infection—recovery or death. These include natural antibodies, interferon, phagocytic activity, and the level of the general inflammatory response.

In experimental animals, *sex, strain, age, route of infection,* the presence of *specific antibody, other diseases, nutritional state,* and the use of such procedures as exposure to ionizing radiation or high environmental temperature or administration of mucin, nitrogen mustard, adrenal steroids, epinephrine, xerosin, and metabolic analogues can be shown to exert a profound effect upon infection by bacteria, viruses, and other agents.

In man, these factors are no less impressive, although controlled studies are lacking for many. Alcoholism; diabetes; deficiency or absence of immunoglobulins (Chap. 69); defects in cellular immunity (Chap. 69); malnutrition; chronic administration of adrenal hormones; chronic lymphedema, ischemia; the presence of foreign bodies such as bullets, calculi, or bone fragments; obstruction of a bronchus, the urethra, or any hollow tube; agranulocytosis; various blood dyscrasias, and many other circumstances influence susceptibility to systemic or local infection. Furthermore, in those instances where the extenuating condition is remediable, the probability of recovery is enhanced.

Racial differences in susceptibility, such as the poor resistance of dark-skinned people to tuberculosis, their predilection for developing disseminated coccidioidomycosis, and the resistance of Negroes to malaria caused by *Plasmodium vivax*, are well established in several infections. Resistance to infection may be determined genetically, at least in part. The relationship of sickle-cell trait to malaria is one example. The increased frequency and severity of some infections in children, others in pregnant women, and still others in the aged are familiar clinical facts.

Prior contact with an organism or its products, whether by active infection or by artificial immunization, increases resistance to some infections, such as measles, diphtheria, and pertussis by stimulating antibody production, but seems to have little influence on resistance to others, such as gonorrhea.

Present knowledge of the factors involved in human

resistance and susceptibility is incomplete. Explanations such as changes in physical or chemical activity of phagocytes; antibacterial substances such as lysozyme, phagocytin, or lysozomal enzymes; qualitative or quantitative alterations in serum proteins; disordered metabolism at the cellular level; "products of tissue injury" that influence vascular permeability, and the effects of tissue pressure remain to a considerable extent in the realm of hypothesis.

The profound influence of host factors upon the infectious process makes it clear, however, that if understanding them ever reaches a point that permits their control in predictable fashion, a new era in the management and control of infectious disease will be at hand. There is no more important and fertile field for investigation in medicine.

PATHOGENESIS OF INFECTION

With relatively minor variations, the development of an infectious disease follows a consistent pattern. The parasites enter the body through the skin, nasopharynx, lung, intestine, urethra, or other portal, and a regular sequence ensues. Once established in the host, the organisms can multiply and, in so doing, establish a *local* or *primary lesion*. From this site, there may be *local spread* along fascial planes or tubular structures, such as a bronchus or ureter. The next step is *systemic spread* of the microorganisms by the circulating blood, which they reach by direct invasion of vessels (a relatively unusual occurrence) or by the common method of being borne in lymph to the thoracic duct and entering the venous system. In the bloodstream, they spread to other tissues and can produce *distant,* or *secondary, lesions*. In infections such as tetanus and diphtheria, distant lesions are produced by toxins elaborated at the primary lesion without systemic spread of the parasites. The infectious process may terminate in recovery or death at any stage: the local lesion, systemic spread, or distant lesion.

The apparent inconsistency of this pattern in clinical medicine is attributable to the fact that the infection has been recognized as a *clinical entity* only at the stage when symptoms are most likely to appear. For example, pneumococcal pneumonia is a local lesion, and the distant lesion, pneumococcal meningitis, is referred to clinically as a *complication*. In meningococcal infections, the local lesion, a nasopharyngitis, is rarely symptomatic and has no status as a clinical entity, but the stage of spread, meningococcemia, and the commonest distant lesion, meningitis, are clinical entities. A rarer distant lesion, arthritis, is called a complication. In a patient who has osteomyelitis, a clinical entity, a recent furuncle may be referred to as a *predisposing factor*. In another patient with extensive furunculosis who develops osteomyelitis, the infection in bone may be regarded by the clinician as a complication of the superficial infection. The stages mentioned are in no way limited to bacterial diseases; the primary lesion of poliomyelitis is intestinal, viremia may occur without neurologic involvement, or a distant lesion, the classic "infantile paralysis," may be established.

Because of established clinical usage and terminology based upon the symptomatic illness that leads patients to seek medical aid, the consistency of this general sequence in the pathogenesis of infection is often not recognized. However, the concept is useful to the clinician and offers some basis for systematizing what may otherwise seem to be a miscellaneous collection of unrelated clinical signs and symptoms.

CLINICAL MANIFESTATIONS OF INFECTIONS

So varied are the disorders attributable to infection or infestation of man by lower organisms that generalization about them is difficult. The clinical manifestations of infection can duplicate those of diseases of any other etiology. Certain clinical features are highly suggestive of infection, including abrupt onset, fever, chills, myalgia, photophobia, pharyngitis, acute lymphadenopathy or splenomegaly, gastroenteritis, and leukocytosis or leukopenia. It is obvious that the presence of one, several, or all of these features does not constitute proof of the microbial origin of illness in a given patient. Conversely, serious, even fatal, infectious disease may exist in the absence of fever or the other signs and symptoms mentioned.

Although there is no infallible clinical criterion of infection, it is still possible to recognize accurately many specific infectious diseases from information obtained by *history, physical examination, blood count,* and *urinalysis*. The importance of interrogation about past illness, predisposing factors such as alcoholism, familial disease, exposure to ill persons, contact with animals or insects, ingestion of contaminated food, type and order of onset of symptoms, and recent or remote residence in endemic areas is discussed in subsequent chapters for specific diseases and etiologic agents. Cardinal physical signs are also described for each entity.

It is fitting to acknowledge ignorance of the mechanisms that produce most of the signs and symptoms of human infection. As discussed in Chap. 16 the pathogenesis of fever is understood incompletely. The physiologic alterations underlying "malaise," "postinfectious asthenia," "toxicity," and other common complaints are completely mysterious. The factors responsible for the leukocytoses or leukopenias that characterize certain infections are only partially understood (Chap. 64). Why the rash of typhus begins on the trunk while that of another rickettsiosis, Rocky Mountain spotted fever, begins on the extremities is unanswered. It cannot be said that failure to understand the production of these manifestations impairs their clinical usefulness in differential diagnosis, but it is probable that understanding would bring with it clues to more accurate diagnosis and better management.

DIAGNOSTIC PROCEDURES

When dealing with diseases produced by living agents, it is soon evident that confirmation of a presumptive diagnosis, or sometimes the first suggestion as to the etiology of illness, depends upon laboratory procedures. The availability of a multitude of laboratory tests in the modern hospital has not made it possible to substitute a "routine lab work-up" for history, physical examination, and observation of a patient's course. Indeed, the information derived from these procedures is the only reasonable basis for selecting the tests to be performed by the laboratory.

The importance of roentgenographic changes, alterations in chemical constituents of the blood, and tests of the functional capacity of organs such as the liver and kidney is as great in infectious disease as in illnesses of other etiologies and needs no discussion here.

The specific procedures for the diagnosis of infectious disease involve *direct demonstration of the causative organism* or *proof of its presence by indirect means.*

Demonstration of the Organism

In bacterial diseases, it is often possible to find the causative organism by *microscopic examination of properly stained preparations of sputum, spinal fluid, and other body fluids.* This simple procedure is often neglected as an unnecessary bother when material is being sent for bacteriologic culture, but it is a most valuable source of immediate information. In many diseases, the etiologic agent cannot be cultured (bartonellosis), and in others, isolation is time-consuming (tuberculosis, blastomycosis). The diagnosis of meningococcal infection by finding the organism in fluid from skin lesions or in the buffy coat or the finding of *H. influenzae* in stained smears of cerebrospinal fluid enables the clinician to initiate specific chemotherapy immediately with assurance that the regimen is the proper one.

Direct examination of bone marrow is a useful method for demonstrating organisms in some diseases, kala-azar, histoplasmosis, and tuberculosis being examples. In protozoan (amebiasis, malaria) and parasitic diseases (schistosomiasis, filariasis), *direct examination of blood, feces, or urine* is the only feasible method for establishing a diagnosis.

There are also infections in which the *detection of characteristic cytologic changes or the causative organism itself in smears or histologic sections of biopsy material* may be the quickest method for diagnosis. Tubercles and tubercle bacilli in lymph nodes or liver biopsy material, leprosy bacilli in skin or nasal scrapings, inclusion bodies in the skin lesions of varicella or variola and the exudate of inclusion blenorrhea, "Warthin" cells from the nasal mucosa in measles, schistosome ova in pinch biopsies of rectal mucosa, and the Councilman bodies of yellow fever in liver are examples. In addition, characteristic histologic changes make it feasible to identify the lesions of chancroid, syphilis, lymphogranuloma venereum, or viral hepatitis in biopsy specimens. Indeed, even in diseases where other reliable tests are available, diagnosis by histologic examination is sometimes the most rapid method, an example being the characteristic muscle lesion of Weil's disease (Chap. 181).

Special Microscopic Techniques

Dark-field examination of material from genital lesions for the spirochete of syphilis is a well-known but often neglected procedure. In several other spirochetal diseases, including leptospirosis, the dark-field technique can be useful, but experience in recognition of the organisms is necessary for correct interpretation of findings.

Fluorescence microscopy, in which the causative organisms can be recognized and identified rapidly by the use of fluorescent-antibody preparations (the Coons technique) is being applied increasingly in the diagnosis of streptococcal pharyngitis, gonorrhea, and pertussis. With continuing refinement and simplification, it may be expected to be extended to other infections including those viruses which carry specific antigens.

Culture and Animal Inoculation

Specimens for bacteriologic culture should be collected before the *initiation of chemotherapy.* The material to be cultured—sputum, pus, blood, or bone marrow—should be selected on the basis of the suspected infections, and the precise cultural techniques employed—media, CO_2 incubation, anaerobic incubation, etc.—must be decided upon in a similar fashion. New developments in tissue culture techniques have facilitated the isolation and identification of a wide range of viruses, and refinements in these techniques are increasing the value of tissue culture in clinical diagnosis.

In several infections, including Weil's disease, rat-bite fever, certain mycoses, tuberculosis, and the rickettsioses, the etiologic organism can be isolated by *inoculation of appropriate material into mice or guinea pigs.* This is a cumbersome procedure for routine use, but should be employed in selected instances. Many viruses can also be isolated by inoculation of appropriate animals. This is rarely feasible for ordinary clinical diagnosis and, for several agents, is hazardous.

Blood Cultures and Bacteremia

Because of the peculiar clinical importance of demonstrating bacteria in the bloodstream and because there are varying opinions about optimal timing and sites of sampling for blood cultures, it is of practical importance to understand something about the mechanisms of bacteremia.

Excepting intravascular infections (bacterial endocarditis or endarteritis, mycotic aneurysm, suppurative thrombophlebitis), bacteria enter the circulation almost invariably through the lymphatic system. Consequently, when bacteria multiply at a site of local infection in the tissues, the likelihood of bacteremia parallels the occurrence of local conditions that favor drainage of lymph from the area to the thoracic duct and eventually, the venous blood. These factors include the number and anatomic arrangement of local lymph vessels, accumulation of fluid and increase in tissue pressure, and manipulation of the part.

Once bacteria enter the blood, they are removed rapidly by the fixed phagocytes of the reticuloendothelial system in the liver and spleen and by engulfment in polymorphonuclear leukocytes in capillaries, especially those of the lung.

Clinically, bacteremia can be transient, intermittent, or continuous. Many transient bacteremias result from manipulation of infected or contaminated tissues, common examples being instrumentation of the genitourinary tract, tonsillectomy, dental procedures, and massage or surgical incision of furuncles or abscesses. In the vast majority of instances, the sudden discharge of bacteria into the blood produces no symptoms or, at most, a rigor and brief fever, and the organisms are promptly dealt with by the removal of mechanisms already mentioned. The great danger of these "man-made" bacteremias is their role in producing bacterial endocarditis in patients with endocardial damage.

Transient bacteremia accompanies the early phase of many infections. In pneumococcal pneumonia, the typical rigor at onset is a result of transient bacteremia. In most cases, with localization of the pulmonary lesion, blood cultures rapidly revert to negative. The poor prognosis of patients with pneumonia who continue to have positive blood cultures is not based on the danger from the mere presence of organisms in the blood as much as it is on bacteremia as a reflection of spreading infection in the lung itself.

A sudden single influx of microorganisms into the bloodstream may be followed by a shaking chill and fever. However, there is a "lag period" of 30 to 90 min before the febrile response (Chap. 16). During this delay, the bacteria are usually promptly removed from the circulation by phagocytosis and, consequently, a blood culture taken at the time of the rigor may be negative.

Continuous bacteremia is a feature of the first several days of typhoid fever, of brucellosis, and of intravascular infections such as endocarditis.

Blood cultures should be taken at frequent intervals in patients with febrile disease of unknown cause; in general, an attempt should be made to obtain blood *before* an expected rise in fever or chill. When a patient is suspected of bacterial endocarditis, or another of the diseases in which bacteremia is constant, two to four cultures daily for 2 to 3 days are more than sufficient to establish diagnosis, and treatment in such cases should not be withheld for a longer period.

There is no evidence that arterial blood possesses any advantage over blood from the antecubital veins for culture. Suspected bacteremia is sometimes mentioned as a contraindication to diagnostic lumbar puncture because of the possible development of meningitis, but clinical evidence does not support this idea. Culture of bone marrow is occasionally superior to peripheral blood for recovery of organisms in typhoid, brucellosis, and rare cases of subacute bacterial endocarditis. While it is common practice to make pour plates of blood and to quantify bacteremia in terms of a certain number of colonies per milliliter of blood, the results of this rather cumbersome procedure have no diagnostic or prognostic significance. Colony counts may be useful, however, to distinguish contaminating organisms. When blood cultures are taken for diagnostic purposes, some should be incubated in carbon dioxide, and a sample of blood should also be cultured in thioglycollate broth or some other anaerobic medium. Anaerobic cultures are especially important in women with puerperal or postabortal infections.

Immunologic Methods

These diagnostic methods are intended to supply evidence of past or present infection by demonstrating antibodies in serum or other body fluids, by showing changed reactivity of the host (hypersensitivity, allergy) to products of the organism, or rarely, to detect components of the causative organism in the body (Chaps. 68 to 70). Emphasis here is directed toward the interpretation of immunologic tests commonly used for clinical diagnosis.

SEROLOGIC TESTS. The finding on a single occasion that a patient's serum contains antibody that reacts with a certain antigen merely indicates that the patient has had previous contact with the antigen or a closely related substance. For this reason, with rare exceptions, the clinical interpretation of serologic tests depends on serial determinations. If the antibody titer is found to *rise or fall significantly*, it is likely that the response is a result of recent contact with the antigen. In subsequent chapters, the need for serologic testing of acute phase and convalescent serum is emphasized repeatedly. *In any patient with a puzzling illness, a sterile specimen of serum should be preserved in a frozen state so that it can, if necessary, be studied and compared with serum collected at a later date.*

Prior contact with an antigen may be the result of past artificial immunization with vaccines; interpretation of serum agglutinin titers for typhoid bacilli is often made difficult by prior immunization. The so-called "anamnestic reaction," a nonspecific stimulation of antibody formation by an acute illness (e.g., a rise in brucella agglutinins in a patient with acute tularemia), occurs only when the two organisms are antigenically related and rarely presents a serious problem.

The methods employed for detecting antibody rises in various infections have been selected empirically on the basis of the ease of performing the test and careful study to correlate the results of the test with other diagnostic criteria in patients. Therefore, the fact that antibodies against one agent are detected by a precipitin technique, another by agglutination of whole organisms or the production of capsular swelling, another by indirect fluorescent-antibody methods, and still another by complement fixation is a practical matter and bears no necessary relationship to the agent, the type of infection, or its pathogenesis. By coating some particulate material, such as erythrocytes or latex with antigen derived from a certain organism, antibody can sometimes be demonstrated by an agglutination test rather than by some more complex method.

Particular properties of the causative organism can sometimes be utilized to devise a simplified clinical test for antibody. Two striking instances of this are widely used. The ability of influenza and related viruses to clump erythrocytes makes possible the demonstration of antibody to virus by merely testing the capacity of a patient's serum to prevent the agglutination of red cells by suspensions of virus, the so-called "hemagglutination-inhibition" reaction. Similarly, because many microorganisms possess hemolytic components or toxins, the assay of a patient's serum for capacity to prevent lysis of red cells is a convenient and simple clinical test for antibody. The antistreptolysin O test in group A beta-hemolytic streptococcal infections is an example of this.

In a few infections, predominantly those caused by viruses, the only reliable serologic test is a *neutralization or protection* test, an assay of the protection afforded by the patient's serum against active infection in tissue culture or in experimental animals. This technique is time-consuming and is usually performed only in diagnostic virology laboratories.

Some mention of "nonspecific" serologic changes may serve to emphasize again that clinical laboratory tests have come into use *only because they have been found to correlate reasonably well with clinical findings*. In several diseases, it has been found, often accidentally, that serum antibody develops that will react with antigens derived from sources other than the etiologic agent (which may actually be unknown). Common examples are heterophil agglutinins in infectious mononucleosis, cold agglutinins in some forms of nonbacterial pneumonia, and the agglutination of certain strains of proteus bacilli by serum of patients with rickettsial diseases. The Wassermann test for syphilis and related flocculation tests are performed with antigens derived from sources completely unrelated to *Treponema pallidum*.

The results of serologic tests must be interpreted in the light of other information about the patient, including such factors as previous immunizations and illnesses, the possibility of exposure to chemically but etiologically unrelated antigens, and the importance of a changing titer in serial tests as opposed to a single isolated observation.

SKIN TESTS. Exposure to antigens of certain types, by various routes, and under circumstances not completely understood often results in the development of *immediate (anaphylactic, atopic) hypersensitivity* or *delayed (bacterial, tuberculin) hypersensitivity*.

Active infection with some, but not all, bacteria and viruses results in delayed hypersensitivity to the infecting agent in some, but not all, individuals. Clinically, this allergic state is detected by intradermal injection of the organisms or some component of them; in a sensitive person, induration and erythema will appear at the local site within 24 to 48 hr. If an individual is highly sensitive or if the amount of antigen injected is excessive, there may be extensive local inflammation with necrosis, vesicle formation, edema, regional lymphadenopathy, and

even malaise and fever. Antigens prepared in concentrations unlikely to provoke severe reactions are generally available for intradermal testing for tuberculosis, leprosy, mumps, lymphogranuloma venereum, cat-scratch disease, chancroid, brucellosis, tularemia, glanders, toxoplasmosis, blastomycosis, histoplasmosis, coccidioidomycosis, and many other infections. The "immune reaction" to vaccination (Chap. 223) is also an example of delayed dermal hypersensitivity.

The reliability, specificity, and usefulness of the individual tests differ and are discussed in the chapters on specific infections. However, certain general principles apply to their use and interpretation:

1. They are highly useful in epidemiologic surveys as indicators of the incidence of infection in a population.

2. In most individuals, dermal reactivity persists for many years or for life. A single positive test means only that at some past time the individual was exposed to the organism (or a closely related one). Unless supplementary information in the form of clinical findings, cultural studies, or more specific serologic data bear out the presence of active infection, a diagnosis of the disease is not justified.

3. The appearance of a positive dermal reaction in an individual known to have been nonreactive a short time before is good evidence of recent infection; this is a useful method for detecting tuberculosis.

4. A *negative intradermal test does not rule out past or present infection.* For unknown reasons, patients with measles, Hodgkin's disease, or sarcoidosis often develop a state of "anergy," or inability to react to intradermally injected antigens. In several diseases, dermal sensitivity develops after weeks or months of infection; an important example of this is acute histoplasmosis, in which patients can be ill for many weeks without showing a positive skin test. The skin test to coccidioidin is always negative in disseminated coccidioidomycosis, and in far-advanced or miliary tuberculosis in elderly patients, failure to react to intradermal tuberculin in the usual amounts employed for testing occurs in as many as 10 to 15 percent of the cases.

Intradermal injection of antigens derived from sources other than microorganisms usually produces an immediate "wheal and erythema" reaction which subsides promptly. The greatest clinical usefulness of this type of reaction is in the detection of allergy to foreign serums, pollens, and animal dander (Chap. 72). The skin tests for demonstrating infestation with helminths (trichinosis, filariasis) produce reactions of the immediate type in allergic individuals, but many of the antigens employed are so nonspecific that they are of little use in diagnosis.

THE IMPORTANCE OF SPECIFIC DIAGNOSIS IN INFECTIOUS DISEASES

Medicine and Microbiology

The diagnostic procedures employed for infectious diseases are no more absolute than those in other diseases; they cannot be blindly equated with the science of microbiology. The responsibility for interpreting the facts supplied by the bacteriologist, immunologist, and virologist in the total context of a patient's illness remains that of the physician. A positive tuberculin skin test certainly does not indicate that a patient has active tuberculosis. The finding of *Candida albicans* (monilia) in a stool culture does not necessarily mean that a patient's diarrhea is caused by intestinal moniliasis. The presence of staphylococci in nasal cultures from a patient with headaches does not establish a diagnosis of staphylococcal sinusitis. A throat culture containing beta-hemolytic streptococci does not rule out diphtheria; nor does such a culture establish that a febrile illness in a patient with mitral stenosis is a recurrence of acute rheumatic fever rather than bacterial endocarditis. A positive serologic test for syphilis, which measures Wassermann-type antibodies, may be the first sign of incipient lupus erythematosus.

The Etiologic Agent

From a practical point of view, two important steps are vital to the correct diagnosis of infection: (1) The organ(s) or organ systems involved must be found; (2) the etiologic agents causing the infections must be identified precisely. A previous section has dealt with the diagnostic approaches that are available and the following three chapters describe some important problems in infectious diseases, namely, complicated infections, which, by and large, occur in debilitated patients in the hospital, endotoxin shock, and antimicrobial therapy. The remaining chapters take up the specific bacteria, spirochetes, fungi, rickettsias, viruses, mycoplasma, and protozoa which cause infections. The common syndromes caused by these agents are described in the individual chapters. For example, bacterial pneumonia is discussed in detail in the chapter on pneumococcal infections

Table 132-1. THE SYNDROMIC APPROACH TO INFECTION

Type of infection	Etiologic agents		
	Common	Relatively common	Unusual but important
Skin and subcutaneous tissue	*Staphylococcus aureus*	Group A streptococcus, *candida* and superficial fungi	Gram-negative bacilli (burns, wounds)
Sinusitis	*S. aureus*	Group A streptococcus, *Diplococcus pneumoniae*	Mucor
Pharyngitis	Respiratory viruses, Group A streptococcus	*Hemophilus influenzae* (children), fusiform bacilli	*Corynebacterium diphtheriae*
Otitis, mastoiditis	*D. pneumoniae*, *H. influenzae* (children)	*S. aureus*, Group A streptococcus	*Pseudomonas*, *Proteus*
Pneumonitis	*D. pneumoniae*, *Mycoplasma pneumoniae*, *Mycobacterium tuberculosis*	*S. aureus*, *Klebsiella*, respiratory viruses	Group A streptococcus, gram-negative enteric bacilli, psittacosis, systemic mycoses, pneumocystis
Empyema and lung abscess	*S. aureus*, anaerobic streptococcus, *Bacteroides*	*Klebsiella* (abscess)	
Bacterial endocarditis	*Streptococcus viridans*, *S. aureus*, enterococcus	*D. pneumoniae*, anaerobic streptococcus	Gram-negative bacilli, *Candida*
Gastroenteritis	Enteroviruses, *Salmonella*, *Shigella*	*S. aureus*, *Escherichia coli* (infants), *Clostridia*	*Pseudomonas*, *Endamoeba histolytica*
Peritonitis, cholangitis, intraabdominal abscess	*E. coli*, enterococcus, *Bacteroides*	*Klebsiella-Aerobacter*, *Proteus* species, paracolon, anaerobic streptococcus	*Clostridia*, *S. aureus*
Urinary infection (cystitis, pyelonephritis)	*E. coli*, *Klebsiella-Aerobacter*, paracolon, *Proteus*, enterococcus	*Pseudomonas*	*S. aureus*
Urethritis	Gonococcus, ?*Mycoplasma*, ?*Mima-Herellea*	*Treponema pallidum*	
Pelvic inflammatory disease	Gonococcus, *E. coli*	*Klebsiella-Aerobacter*, *Bacteroides*, anaerobic streptococcus, enterococcus	*Clostridia*, *S. aureus*
Bones (osteomyelitis)	*S. aureus*	*Salmonella*	Group A streptococcus
Joints	*S. aureus*, gonococcus, *D. pneumoniae*	Group A streptococcus, *Neisseria meningitidis*	*E. coli*, *Proteus*, *Pseudomonas*
Meninges	*D. pneumoniae*, *H. influenzae* (children), *N. meningitidis*, ECHO and mumps viruses	*E. coli*, *Klebsiella-Aerobacter*, *Proteus*, *Pseudomonas*	Group A streptococcus, *M. tuberculosis*, *Cryptococcus*, *S. aureus*, *Listeria monocytogenes*

(Chap. 138), osteomyelitis is described with staphylococcal infections (Chap. 139), the manifestations of bacteriuria are described in Chap. 144 and 303, and those of meningitis in Chap. 142, 360, and 361. Nevertheless, when confronted with specific organ involvement, it is important to know the most common pathogens which cause disease in the involved organ. Table 132-1 provides a listing of these pathogens. Used in conjunction with the individual chapters dealing with specific agents and the summary of chemotherapy (Chap. 135), the table should provide a rational guide to treatment which often must be instituted before the results of antimicrobial sensitivity tests are available.

Chemotherapy

The impact of chemotherapy upon mortality and morbidity from infection and upon epidemic disease is now a matter of historical record. These therapeutic agents, however, have in no way lessened the importance of specific diagnosis; indeed their availability has increased the need for obtaining exact etiologic information. It requires but a moment's reflection to realize that the substitution of a prescription for a broad-spectrum antibiotic or a quick injection of penicillin for the systematic collection of facts and thoughtful consideration of diagnostic possibilities is a fallacious, unwise, and dangerous practice. Numerous antibiotics with overlapping spectrums are now available, dosages for different infections vary widely, the drugs themselves are potentially dangerous, and their administration entails considerable expense. They should never be prescribed as placebos, antipyretics, or substitutes for diagnosis. In the vast majority of instances in which this is done, patients recover just as they would if no "therapy" had been given and the drugs are wasted. More important, inadequate dosage or the wrong agent may suppress symptoms temporarily without curing, make isolation of the etiologic agent difficult, delay the recognition of the true nature of an illness, and postpone the institution of curative treatment. Furthermore, antibiotics may select out resistant variants or facilitate spread of infection by conferring resistance to bacteria due to R factors with subsequent hazard that these resistant organisms may spread to others. Finally, to expose a patient to the risk of drug reaction without proper indication is inexcusable, whether the drug is an antibiotic, a sedative, a laxative, or a narcotic.

Epidemiologic and Other Considerations

Just as the decision to administer antibiotics to a patient with a febrile illness of presumed infectious etiology must be made on an individual basis, the selection of cases in which extensive cultural and serologic testing is required is a matter of judgment. The majority of common "grippelike" illnesses subsides spontaneously, and symptomatic treatment is sufficient. However, because of this tendency toward spontaneous recovery and also because the results of serologic tests may not be available until a patient is convalescent, there are many who regard continued effort to determine the specific etiology of illness as an impractical, "academic" procedure. Such an attitude fails to recognize that the responsibility of the physician extends beyond the individual patient to include the community. For example, a patient recently recovered from "viral pneumonitis" may feel that his physician has cared for him competently and well. The doctor himself may feel that he has discharged his professional duties properly and that his having refrained from giving the patient antibiotics for what was clinically a virus disease and therefore unlikely to benefit from chemotherapy was a laudable act of forbearance. However, if a serologic test is reported a few days later as showing that the patient's serum has shown a rise in complement-fixing antibody against psittacosis, the situation might change. The patient himself would continue to be well, but a search for the source of the disease, such as the patient's pet parakeet, would certainly be indicated, and further illnesses in others might be prevented.

Despite the fact that pursuing diagnosis of obscure, often self-limited, illnesses may be academic, this approach has led to clarification of some important etiologic relationships. For example, the syndrome of infectious mononucleosis has been linked with development of antibody to a herpeslike virus, the EB virus, as well as cytomegalovirus (Chap. 255); some cases of erythema multiforme may be due to herpes simplex virus; several patients with encephalitis have been found to have central nervous system infections with myxoviruses. Some congenital anomalies have been related to prenatal viral infections; the relationship of subendocardial fibroelastosis to mumps is just one example (Chap. 231). The finding of bacterialike bodies in the intestinal mucosa of patients with Whipples disease and the improvement of these patients with tetracycline therapy provides another example of an entity of unknown etiology entering the realm of infectious diseases. Finally, the possibility has been raised that the Chediak-Higashi syndrome, a rare familial disorder characterized by albinism, photophobia, nystagmus, anomalous cellular granules, marked susceptibility to infection, and development of lymphoma, is caused by a virus. This association, among others, relates the field of infection to that of oncogenesis.

These discoveries clearly are the result of academic procedures which might have little immediate applicability to infection in a particular patient, yet few can question the fundamental biologic importance of these observations; moreover, it is conceivable that they will assume practical importance in the future.

REFERENCES

Bennett, I. L., Jr., and P. B. Beeson: Bacteremia: A Consideration of Some Experimental and Clinical Aspects, Yale J. Biol. Med., 26:241, 1954.

Burnet, M.: "Natural History of Infectious Disease," New York, Cambridge University Press, 1953.

Davis, B. D., R. Dulbecco, H. Eisen, H. S. Ginsberg, and W.

B. Wood, Jr.: "Microbiology" New York, Harper and Row, Publishers, Incorporated, 1968.

Dubos, R. J.: "Biochemical Determinants of Microbial Diseases," Cambridge, Mass., Harvard University Press, 1954.

——: The Evolution of Microbial Diseases, p. 20 in "Bacterial and Mycotic Diseases of Man," 4th ed., Philadelphia, J. B. Lippincott Company, 1965.

Horsfall, F. L., Jr.: Cancer and Viruses, Bull. N.Y. Acad. Med., 42:167, 1966.

—— and I. Tamm (Eds.): "Viral and Rickettsial Diseases of Man," 4th ed., Philadelphia, J. B. Lippincott Company, 1965.

MacLeod, C. M., and L. E. Cluff (Eds.): Symposium on Non-specific Resistance to Infection, Bacteriol. Rev., 24:1, 1960.

Rich, A. R.: "The Pathogenesis of Tuberculosis," 2d ed., Springfield, Ill., Charles C Thomas, Publisher, 1951.

Rogers, D. E.: The Changing Pattern of Life-threatening Microbial Disease, New Eng. J. Med., 261:677, 1959.

White, J. G.: Virus-like Particles in the Peripheral Blood Cells of Two Patients with Chediak-Higashi Syndrome, Cancer, 19:877, 1966.

Wilson, G. S., and A. A. Miles: "Topley and Wilson's Principles of Bacteriology and Immunity," 5th ed., Baltimore, The Williams and Wilkins Company, 1965.

Wood, W. B., Jr.: Studies on the Cellular Immunology of Acute Bacterial Infections, Harvey Lectures, 47:72, 1951–1952.

133 COMPLICATING INFECTIONS
Robert G. Petersdorf

A complicating infection is defined here as an infection occurring in a patient with a defect in host resistance or one which develops during hospitalization. Most of this chapter will deal with *hospital-acquired* (nosocomial) infections, because numerically they represent the most significant problem. Infections occurring in the host whose resistance has been altered by another disease or drug will be listed briefly.

EPIDEMIOLOGY. Hospital-acquired infections occur in 4 to 5 percent of all patients admitted to a general hospital. Moreover, at any one time approximately 5 percent of all patients in a general hospital will have such an infection, and among patients in the hospital with infections, fully one-third will have acquired their infection while in the hospital. The most common nosocomial infections encountered are postoperative infections, urinary tract infections, pneumonia, septic thrombophlebitis, and bacteremia.

PREDISPOSING FACTORS. Defects in Host Resistance. Certain infections occur with increased frequency with particular diseases. For example, patients with diabetes mellitus are prone to development of cutaneous infections, bacteriuria, tuberculosis, moniliasis, and, when ketoacidosis is uncontrolled, mucormycosis. Monilia infections have a predilection for patients with hypopara-

thyroidism; nocardiosis is more common in alveolar proteinosis; salmonella infections are more prevalent in patients with sickle-cell disease, schistosomiasis, malaria, and bartonellosis; pneumococcal infections occur often in very young children who have undergone splenectomy, in individuals with hypogammaglobulinemia (Chap. 69), and in association with multiple myeloma; cryptococcosis tends to infect patients with Hodgkin's disease and sarcoidosis; and a variety of bacterial infections complicates diseases associated with granulocytopenia. The reasons for the coexistence of these infections and the underlying diseases are largely unknown. In a sense, however, these associations represent peculiar experiments of nature and are overshadowed by infections resulting from the iatrogenic alterations in host resistance that follow the use of corticosteroids, antimetabolites, and radiomimetic, immunosuppressive, and antimicrobial drugs. Corticosteroids not only favor acquisition of new infections but may result in reactivation and dissemination of latent disease. Why these hormones increase susceptibility to infection is unknown; perhaps they depress the reticuloendothelial system, impair the development of immunity by decreasing antibody formation, and stabilize lysozomal membranes. Usually steroids produce infections in patients with those underlying diseases for which they were given, but because of their antiinflammatory effects, the hormones may mask the signs and symptoms of the complicating infections until they are relatively far advanced. The increased incidence of infection following cytotoxic drugs is probably a consequence of these agents' ability to produce granulocytopenia and lymphopenia and to decrease antibody production (Chap. 71).

Superinfections. Superinfections may be defined as infections which occur when antimicrobial therapy is administered for both therapeutic and prophylactic purposes. Their incidence is approximately 2 percent of all patients treated with antibiotics, and they are more common when such drugs are given in large doses, when several antimicrobials are administered concurrently, or when broad-spectrum agents are employed.

Clinical superinfections must be distinguished from the normal ecologic change in bacterial flora which accompanies all antimicrobial therapy. Most antibiotics lower the number of resident microorganisms and occasionally eradicate them entirely; the normal flora is then replaced by resistant exogenous or endogenous bacteria. In the vast majority of instances the number of bacteria replacing those eradicated by the drug is small and clinical disease does not take place. However, when the concentration of the superinfecting organisms is high, a clinical superinfection is more likely to occur.

Superinfections are particularly common with certain drugs; the tendency for *Pseudomonas* to colonize and infect patients receiving one of the cephalosporins is a notable example. Clinically significant superinfections usually appear 4 to 5 days after chemotherapy is instituted and must be watched for especially in patients being treated for pneumonia, chronic obstructive lung disease, otitis, and urinary tract infection, when a urethral catheter is in place. They often complicate the course of patients with respiratory viral diseases who are given antibiotics to prevent bacterial complications.

As a rule, they are caused by organisms that are resistant to the drug the patient is receiving, and penicillinase-producing staphylococci, gram-negative enteric bacilli, and fungi are the most common superinfecting microorganisms. The usual clinical manifestations include recrudescence of fever and other signs and symptoms at the site of the initial infection.

Other Diagnostic and Therapeutic Measures Resulting in Infections. The hospitalized patient is subjected to a variety of diagnostic and therapeutic procedures which predispose to infection. These include insertion of intravenous catheters and urethral catheterization, particularly if an indwelling catheter is left in place; uncommonly injections, thoracenteses, paracenteses, aspiration of joints, lumbar punctures, and tissue biopsies may be incriminated. At least 2 to 3 percent of operative procedures are complicated by infections; the rates vary with the type of operation. Infections are common in association with the use of equipment for inhalation therapy, and may be spread in the hospital by a variety of inanimate vehicles. The risk of complicating infections depends on the number and complexity of therapeutic or diagnostic manipulations and is enhanced by the concomitant indiscriminate use of antibiotics.

ETIOLOGY. The bacteria usually responsible for complicating infections are penicillinase-producing staphylococci (Chap. 139), *Escherichia coli* (Chap. 144), *Klebsiella-Aerobacter* (Chap. 148), *Proteus* (Chap. 145), *Pseudomonas* (Chap. 146), *Mima-Herellea* (Chap. 160), and less commonly, group D streptococci, enterococci (Chap. 141), and *Clostridia* (Chap. 172). Among the fungi, monilia (Chap. 190), mucor (Chap. 191), and aspergillus (Chap. 193) are frequent pathogens implicated in secondary infections. Cytomegalovirus (Chap. 232) and pneumocystis (Chap. 245) are common causes of complicating infections in patients with depressed host resistance.

MANIFESTATIONS. Obviously, the clinical picture of a complicating infection will vary with its site and, to a lesser extent, the microorganisms causing it. In most instances, the major sign is fever, which usually occurs after patients have been in the hospital 4 to 5 days or longer. However, in some patients the diagnosis rests only on signs of local inflammation such as phlebitis, cellulitis, or evidence of a deep-seated infection. Sometimes a complicating infection may be heralded by no more than unexplained hyperventilation, confusion, or disorientation. Specific types of infection will be considered below.

Postoperative Infections. These consist primarily of wound infections or collections of pus which form in and around the operative site. Although urinary tract infections and pneumonia are common in patients who have undergone surgery, postoperative infections are usually related to the surgical locus rather than an unrelated organ system.

Relatively few surgical procedures are responsible for the majority of wound infections, and these infections are particularly likely to occur when operations are long or require extensive resection and when contamination is unavoidable. Abdominal perineal resections, wounds involving arterial bypass grafts, insertion of cardiac prostheses, and portacaval shunts are associated with a relatively high rate of complicating infections. Most postoperative wound infections are caused by staphylococci and gram-negative enteric bacteria. Although group A streptococcal infections are averted with most chemoprophylactic regimens, wound infections which develop in patients receiving postoperative chemoprophylaxis usually are caused by organisms resistant to the drug being given. In general, chemoprophylaxis has not been successful in preventing wound infections, although the regimen which involves the administration of 10 million units of penicillin G at 2-hr intervals beginning immediately prior to and continuing throughout the operation has been shown to reduce postoperative wound sepsis.

Cutaneous, Subcutaneous, and Soft-tissue Infections. While wound sepsis comprises the major part of superficial infections, other sites are involved. These include abscesses in the skin, subcutaneous tissues and muscle, cellulitis, decubitus ulcers, vascular stasis ulcers, and lesions secondary to diminished arterial blood supply. Most often staphylococci are the causative organisms, but group A and anaerobic streptococci, gram-negative enteric bacilli, and even clostridia may be pathogenic under these circumstances. These infections may follow subcutaneous or intramuscular injections or extravasation of intravenous infusions. Although the infections usually remain localized, they may involve contiguous structures and may produce bacteremia. Gas in soft tissues should call to mind infection with *E. coli* (Chap. 144) as well as anaerobic organisms. Antimicrobial therapy should be directed at the specific organism. Staphylococcal infections should be treated with a penicillinase-resistant penicillin until the organism is shown to be sensitive to penicillin G. Surgical drainage and debridement are often essential to recovery.

Burns regularly become infected secondarily. Most of these patients are receiving systemic or local chemoprophylaxis, and usually infection develops after the gram-positive flora has been replaced by gram-negative organisms, particularly *Pseudomonas*. These organisms are usually acquired from the environment and have been shown to survive on the floors, walls, and equipment used on burn wards. The sudden development of shock in a patient with a burn is almost certain evidence that pseudomonas bacteremia is present. Treatment is discussed in Chaps. 134 and 146.

Urinary Tract Infections. Urinary tract infections usually are associated with instrumentation of the urethra, bladder, or ureters, and most often are due to insertion of an indwelling urethral catheter, which permits entry of bacteria from the external environment into the bladder. Nosocomial urinary infections do not occur without predisposing instrumentation. The organisms are usually *E. coli, Klebsiella-Aerobacter*, paracolon, *Proteus, Pseudomonas*, and enterococci and tend to be resistant to one or several antibiotics. Epidemics of *Klebsiella-Aerobacter* and *Pseudomonas* urinary infections following spread of bacteria from contaminated equipment have been reported. Most patients with hospital-acquired bacteriuria are asymptomatic, some have cystitis, and others have clear-cut evidence of pyelonephritis which may be associated with bacteremia. Treatment should be reserved for patients with symptoms and for those suspected of bacteremia. Patients with indwelling catheters who have asymptomatic bacteriuria should not receive antibiotics because it is unlikely that the organisms will be eradicated; instead, superinfections will develop.

Considerable progress has been made in preventing hospital-acquired urinary infections by maintaining a system of closed drainage. In this fashion, the urine can be kept sterile for 5 to 7 days after insertion of the catheter. Failure to maintain closed drainage will result in infection in almost all patients within 48 hr after catheter drainage is instituted.

Pneumonia. Pulmonary infections are common events in hospitalized patients with a variety of severe medical or surgical diseases. They may follow aspiration from any cause, atelectasis, heart failure, tracheostomy, and therapy with drugs that depress respiration. In a general hospital, pneumonia occurs commonly as a complication of cardiac or neurosurgery, but these infections are also seen in debilitated general medical patients, particularly when respiratory assistance devices have been employed. Mainstream reservoir nebulizers containing saline solutions are often heavily contaminated with *Pseudomonas,* flavobacteria, *Herellea,* and *Achromobacter* and are capable of producing severe pulmonary infections when nebulized directly into the tracheobronchial tree. This risk can be reduced sharply by bubbling a 0.25 percent acetic acid solution through the nebulizing equipment for 5 min prior to use. Gram-negative enteric bacteria usually are implicated in complicating pulmonary infections, particularly when patients have received antimicrobials. Although tracheostomies are often necessary to maintain adequate ventilation, they are almost invariably associated with infections. These infections can only be prevented by meticulous aseptic technique during suctioning and the use of sterile suction catheters. The major therapeutic problem in many patients with complicating infections of the lung is mechanical; positive pressure breathing, postural drainage, frequent suctioning, and sometimes bronchoscopy are at least as important in the treatment of these infections as appropriate antibiotics.

Bacterial Endocarditis. Patients undergoing open-heart surgery have a relatively high incidence of wound, urinary, and pulmonary infections, but the most dreaded complication of open-heart surgery is endocarditis on a prosthetic valve. It occurs predominantly in patients whose operation is conducted on cardiopulmonary bypass, and surgery on the aortic valve is complicated by endocarditis much more frequently than surgery on the mitral valve. *Staphylococcus aureus* and *S. albus* are the most common pathogens. Clinical signs of endocarditis are often absent, and fever during the first 4 postoperative weeks provides the best clue to infections which follow in the wake of surgery. However, in some instances

the prosthetic valve becomes infected years after its insertion, emphasizing the importance of preventing bacteremia in the patients. The prophylactic regimens for preventing endocarditis are detailed in Chap. 137.

The diagnosis depends upon isolation of the organism in blood cultures. Treatment of endocarditis on intracardiac prostheses have been notoriously unsuccessful, and although the infection may be suppressed with antibiotics, reoperation, which often eventuates fatally, is usually necessary. Therefore, to prevent endocarditis, antimicrobial administration to patients undergoing open-heart surgery has become routine practice. It is clear that administration of a penicillinase-resistant penicillin will prevent postoperative pneumococcal endocarditis, but the efficacy of these drugs in preventing endocarditis with other organisms, including staphylococci, is less certain.

Bacteremia. Invasion of the bloodstream can occur in any nosocomial infection, and among the various foci, the urinary tract predominates. However, the indwelling venous catheter is fast becoming the most common source of bacteremia in hospitalized patients, particularly when it is left in place longer than 48 hr. Many of these patients develop phlebitis before bacteremia, and the catheter should be removed from all patients with inflammation at the catheter site. Staphylococci are implicated most often in catheter-associated infections, but *Mima-herellea* and other gram-negative organisms have been cultured from both the local site and the bloodstream.

Treatment of catheter-induced bacteremia requires removal of the catheter and systemic antimicrobial therapy; the treatment of staphylococcal bacteremia is discussed in Chap. 139 and that of gram-negative sepsis in Chap. 134. These infections can be prevented by (1) use of the catheter only when absolutely necessary; (2) strict aseptic technique during placement of the catheter; (3) application of bacitracin-neomycin-polymyxin ointment to the catheter site; and (4) removal of the catheter within 48 hr, or sooner if phlebitis or cellulitis is present.

Miscellaneous Complicating Infections. *Staphylococcal parotitis* is common in debilitated patients with a variety of medical diseases; it often follows in the wake of dehydration (Chap. 231). *Septic arthritis* is not uncommon in patients with antecedent rheumatoid or degenerative joint disease who are subjected to diagnostic aspiration of the joint or who are treated with intraarticular drugs, usually corticosteroids. Pneumococcus, group A streptococcus, and staphylococcus are the most common pathogens. *Iatrogenic meningitis* is a rare complication of spinal anesthesia, epidural block, injection of the stellate ganglion, diagnostic lumbar puncture, and myelography. Pneumococcus, staphylococcus, and pseudomonas have been cultured from these patients. Staphylococcal enterocolitis occurs primarily in patients who have had gastrointestinal surgery and who were given antibiotics preoperatively. It is also common in patients with liver disease who are treated with neomycin to reduce ammonia production by the bowel flora. Oral vancomycin (0.5 Gm every 6 to 12 hr for four doses) or systemic penicillinase-resistant penicillins or cephalosporins are all effective modes of treatment.

Infections Occurring During Organ Transplantation. Aside from host versus graft reactions (Chap. 71), infections pose the most serious threat to patients undergoing organ transplantation. These patients all receive immunosuppressive drugs and large quantities of adrenal cortical hormones and have readily available portals of entry for a variety of microorganisms. Multiple infections are common. Coagulase-positive staphylococci are the most common bacteria isolated, but pseudomonas, gram-negative enteric bacilli, and streptococci other than group A are also cultured. The organisms are often present in the nasopharynx or on the skin of patients prior to transplantation, and for this reason, it is recommended by some authorities that all staphylococcal carriers be treated with a penicillinase-resistant penicillin for several days prior to the procedure and afterward until the wound has healed. Likewise, bacteriuria should be eradicated before surgery. When transplantation is performed for pyelonephritis, the ureters should be excised in their entirety along with the kidneys.

Patients who have undergone transplantation are particularly susceptible to fatal pulmonary infections which may produce few symptoms and signs. In addition to the bacteria mentioned above, cytomegalovirus (Chap. 232), monilia (Chap. 190), aspergillus (Chap. 193), and pneumocystis (Chap. 245) are found at autopsy. These infections are characterized by little in the way of an inflammatory response, and the fungi, in particular, tend to produce a necrotizing reaction. Although no definitive information is available, it is likely that pulmonary superinfections with fungi or cytomegalovirus in these patients have an almost uniformly fatal prognosis.

LABORATORY FINDINGS. Cultures of pus, appropriate body fluids, and blood form the cornerstone of treatment and always should be obtained, even in patients receiving chemotherapy. Antimicrobial sensitivity tests should be performed when indicated. Gram stains of pus or secretions are helpful when only one or two types of bacteria are present in large numbers, but may be misleading and should be interpreted with caution. Superinfections usually are accompanied by leukocytosis, but granulocytopenia may be seen because of previous drug therapy or underlying disease. Moreover, many patients have a leukocytosis to begin with, and an elevated leukocyte count is of value as a clue to a complicating infection only if it was normal previously.

THERAPEUTIC CONSIDERATIONS. Because most complicating infections are caused by bacteria, treatment depends upon identification of the organism but must not be delayed until the results of cultures and sensitivity tests are at hand. Hence, the antibiotic must be chosen on the basis of previous cultures, the gram-stained smear, and the clinical picture. For example, patients with subcutaneous and soft-tissue infections should be treated with a penicillinase-resistant penicillin and those with bacteriuria with a drug active against enteric bacteria or enterococci. Patients with pneumonia or sepsis may require treatment with several drugs pending identification of the pathogen. The appropriate regimens are found in chapters dealing with the specific organisms and in the chapter on chemotherapy (Chap. 135). A general approach to therapy of undiagnosed bacteremia is provided in Chap. 134. Removal of the mechanical factors which are often the basis for complicating infections is as important as chemotherapy. This may involve withdrawing intravenous or urethral catheters, drainage of pus, debridement of a burn eschar, removal of sutures, aspiration of bronchial secretions, a change in inhalation equipment, and even, occasionally, removal of a cardiac prosthesis.

CHEMOPROPHYLAXIS AND COMPLICATING INFECTIONS. Most patients who develop a complicating infection are receiving antibiotics, providing *prima facie* evidence that these drugs are not successful in preventing these infections. The experience with chemoprophylaxis in many clinical situations is summarized in Chap. 135. With a few notable exceptions, antibiotics have been incapable of preventing infection in patients with depressed host resistance and have usually been the primary factors leading to infections by resistant organisms.

PROGNOSIS. Most complicating infections occur in patients being treated for another disease which is often chronic, disabling, and potentially fatal. While these secondary infections demand vigorous treatment, they may be only incidental to the patient's primary problem. For example, a patient with disseminated carcinomatosis will die even if his complicating infection is contained; and conversely, a complicating infection often will not respond to therapy unless a remission is produced in the underlying disease.

REFERENCES

Barrett, F. F., J. I. Casey, and M. Finland: Infections and Antibiotic Use among Patients at Boston City Hospital, February, 1967, New Engl. J. Med., 278:5, 1968.

Beaty, H. N., and R. C. Petersdorf: Iatrogenic Factors in Infectious Disease, Ann. Intern. Med., 65:641, 1966.

Bentley, D. W., and M. H. Lepper: Septicemia Related to Indwelling Venous Catheter, J.A.M.A., 206:1749, 1968.

Goodman, J. S., W. Schaffner, H. A. Collins, E. J. Battersby, and M. G. Koenig: Infection after Cardiovascular Surgery: Clinical Study Including Examination of Antimicrobial Prophylaxis, New Engl. J. Med., 278:117, 1968.

Kunin, C. M., and R. C. McCormack: Prevention of Catheter-induced Urinary Tract Infections by Sterile Closed Drainage, New Engl. J. Med., 274:1155, 1966.

Moser, R. H.: "Diseases of Medical Progress," Springfield, Ill., Charles C Thomas, Publisher, 1969.

Petersdorf, R. G.: "The Prophylaxis of Infection," London, Pergamon Press, 1964.

Reinarz, J. A., A. K. Pierce, B. B. Mays, and J. P. Sanford: Potential Role of Inhalation Therapy Equipment in Nosocomial Pulmonary Infection, J. Clin. Invest., 44:831, 1965.

Rifkind, D., T. L. Marchioro, W. R. Waddell, and T. E. Starzl: Infectious Diseases Associated with Renal Homotransplantation, J.A.M.A., 189:397, 1964.

Thoburn, R., F. R. Fekety, Jr., L. E. Cluff, and V. B. Melvin:

Infections Acquired by Hospitalized Patients, Arch. Intern Med., 121:1, 1968.

Weinstein, L.: Superinfection: Complication of Antimicrobial Therapy and Prophylaxis, Am. J. Surg., 107:704, 1964.

134 SEPTIC SHOCK

Robert G. Petersdorf

DEFINITION. Septic shock is characterized by inadequate tissue perfusion, usually following bacteremia with gram-negative enteric bacilli. This circulatory insufficiency is a consequence of increased peripheral vascular resistance, pooling of blood in the microcirculation, diminished cardiac output, and tissue anoxia.

ETIOLOGY. Shock is sometimes associated with gram-positive infections, in which there are usually hypotension, peripheral vasodilatation, normovolemia, and normal cardiac output—so-called "warm shock" that is readily corrected with fluids and appropriate antibiotics. For practical purposes, septic shock follows bacteremia with gram-negative enteric bacilli: *E. coli* (Chap. 144), paracolon species, *Klebsiella-Enterobacter* (Chap. 148), *Proteus* species (Chap. 145), *Pseudomonas* (Chap. 146), and *Mima-Herellea* species (Chap. 160). Furthermore, the vasoactive phenomena collectively termed septic shock are probably not due to bacteremia per se but are related to release into the circulation of endotoxin, the lipopolysaccharide moiety of the organisms' cell walls.

EPIDEMIOLOGY. Gram-negative bacteremia and endotoxin shock occur primarily in hospitalized patients who usually have an underlying disease which renders them susceptible to bloodstream invasion. Predisposing factors include diabetes mellitus; cirrhosis; leukemia, lymphoma, or disseminated carcinoma; childbirth; and a variety of surgical procedures and antecedent infections in the urinary, biliary, or gastrointestinal tracts. Most adults with gram-negative sepsis are elderly males, but neonates are also prone to develop endotoxin shock. There has been an appreciable increase in the prevalence of serious gram-negative infections among hospitalized patients since 1935. Moreover, concurrent with the introduction and widespread use of antibiotics, cytotoxic agents, adrenal steroids, intravenous catheters, humidifiers, and other hospital equipment (Chap. 133) and the increasing longevity of patients with chronic diseases, this upward trend has gained momentum and in most hospitals gram-negative are now more common than gram-positive bacteremias.

PATHOGENESIS AND PATHOLOGY. With the exception of *Pseudomonas* and *Mima-Herellea*, which are ubiquitous in the hospital environment, most of the bacteria causing gram-negative sepsis are normal commensals in the gastrointestinal tract. From there they may spread to contiguous structures, as in peritonitis following appendiceal perforation, or migrate from the perineum into the urethra or bladder. Gram-negative bacteremia follows infection in a primary focus, usually in the genitourinary tract, biliary tree, gastrointestinal tract, and adjoining structures, or lungs and, less commonly, the skin, bones, and joints. In many patients, however, particularly those with chronic disease, cirrhosis, and tumors of the reticuloendothelial system, no primary focus is apparent. When bacteremia is followed by metastatic lesions in distant sites, classical abscess formation occurs. More often, however, the autopsy findings in gram-negative sepsis are scanty or nonspecific and reflect primarily the infection at the primary locus. This lack of concrete morphologic data has led some investigators to question the role of endotoxin in gram-negative shock in man. On the other hand, damage to the endothelial lining of capillary walls has been demonstrated early in experimental endotoxin shock, and many patients who die with gram-negative shock have been treated intensively, which would tend to obfuscate the pathologic findings that are often clear-cut in experimental animals.

PATHOPHYSIOLOGY. General Considerations. Endotoxin exerts its major effects on small blood vessels with sympathetic (alpha-receptor) innervation. The toxin causes intense arteriolar and venous spasm leading to significant immobilization of blood in the pulmonary, splanchnic, and renal capillaries and to stagnant anoxia in these tissues. Local acidosis develops and promotes relaxation of the arteriolar sphincter while the venule remains constricted. Blood pools in the capillary bed, and the increased hydrostatic pressure results in leakage of plasma into the interstitial fluid. This, in turn, causes a sharp decrease in effective circulating blood volume, lowered cardiac output, and systemic arterial hypotension. These result in stimulation of the baroreceptors, further sympathetic activity, vasoconstriction, and selective reduction of blood flow to visceral organs and skin. If ineffective perfusion of vital organs is permitted to continue, metabolic acidosis and severe parenchymal damage ensue and shock is then irreversible. In man, the kidneys and lungs are the organs particularly susceptible to endotoxin; oliguria as well as tachypnea and, in some instances, pulmonary edema, develops early. On the other hand, the heart and brain are spared in the early stages of shock; myocardial failure and coma are late and often terminal manifestations of the shock syndrome.

Hemodynamic Alterations in Man. Many of the observations dealing with the pathophysiology of endotoxin shock were made in animals, and the hemodynamic data often varied according to the species studied and the dose of endotoxin administered. The establishment of centers for the study of shock has permitted detailed pathophysiologic studies in man, and several hemodynamic patterns have appeared:

1. Shock characterized by a normal cardiac output, normal blood volume, normal circulation time, normal or high central venous pressure, normal or high pH, and *reduced* peripheral resistance. These patients have warm dry skin and may have bacteremia with both gram-positive as well as gram-negative organisms; many have cirrhosis; their prognosis is generally good. Hypotension, oliguria, and lactic acidemia are present. Shock in this

group has been attributed to shunting of blood through arteriovenous communications, making it unavailable for perfusion of vital organs.

2. Shock characterized by normal blood volume, high central venous pressure, normal or high cardiac output, reduced peripheral resistance, but *marked metabolic acidosis,* oliguria, and very high blood lactate indicating ineffective tissue perfusion or impaired oxygen utilization. These patients generally have bacteremia with gram-negative organisms, and despite the presence of warm dry extremities, their prognosis is extremely poor.

3. Patients with low blood volume, low central venous pressure, high hematocrit, increased peripheral resistance, low cardiac output, hypotension, oliguria, but only a moderate elevation of blood lactate and normal or slightly high pH. These patients may be hypovolemic prior to bacteremia, and their prognosis is reasonably good provided blood volume is restored, bacteremia is treated with appropriate antibiotics, septic foci are removed or drained, and vasoactive drugs are given.

4. Shock characterized by low blood volume, low central venous pressure, low cardiac output, marked decompensated metabolic acidosis, and lactic acidemia. In these patients the extremities are cool and cyanotic, and all forms of therapy fail to reverse shock.

Although these observations suggest that there are various forms of septic shock, for the most part the data are consistent with the hypothesis that the basic abnormality in endotoxin shock is *vasoconstriction, reduction in cardiac output, hypotension,* and *oliguria.* When peripheral resistance is low and cardiac output is normal or high, other explanations are available to explain these deviations from the more typical findings. For example, arteriovenous shunts occur in cirrhosis or in the inflamed peritoneum or lung and prevent perfusion and oxygenation of vital organs. Sometimes, seemingly high cardiac output is insufficient to meet the needs of the body, and occasionally, because of cell death, oxygen utilization at the cellular level does not occur despite minor alterations in blood volume.

Coagulation Defects in Shock. In most patients with septic shock there is a deficiency in several clotting factors, probably due to consumption of these factors by disseminated intravascular coagulation. Usually, there is no clinical bleeding, although hemorrhagic phenomena due to thrombocytopenia or deficiency in clotting factors occur occasionally. A more important effect of disseminated intravascular coagulation is development of capillary thrombi, particularly in the lung. Unless there is bleeding, the coagulopathy requires no therapy and disappears spontaneously as shock is treated.

The Lung in Septic Shock. Respiratory failure is the most important cause of death in patients with shock, particularly after the hemodynamic aberrations have been corrected. The respiratory lesion has been called the "shock lung" and is characterized by pulmonary congestion, hemorrhage, atelectasis, edema, and formation of capillary thrombi. This lesion may develop and progress even as other abnormalities return to normal. Pulmonary surfactant decreases, and pO_2 progressively falls.

Renal Failure. Oliguria occurs early in shock and is probably due to inadequate perfusion of renal capillaries. If renal perfusion remains inadequate, acute tubular necrosis develops.

CLINICAL MANIFESTATIONS. Usually gram-negative bacteremia begins abruptly with chills, fever, nausea, vomiting, diarrhea, and prostration. When septic shock develops, there are, in addition, tachycardia, tachypnea; hypotension; cool, pale extremities, often with peripheral cyanosis; mental obtundation; and oliguria. When present in its full-blown form, gram-negative shock is detected readily, but occasionally the findings are quite subtle, particularly in old debilitated patients or in infants. Unexplained hypotension, increasing confusion and disorientation, and hyperventilation may be the only clues to gram-negative shock. Jaundice occurs occasionally and signifies infection in the biliary tree or intravascular hemolysis. As shock progresses, oliguria persists, and heart failure, respiratory insufficiency, and coma supervene. Death usually occurs from pulmonary edema, generalized anoxemia secondary to respiratory insufficiency, cardiac arrhythmia, disseminated intravascular coagulation with bleeding, cerebral anoxia, or a combination of these factors.

LABORATORY FINDINGS. The laboratory data in septic shock vary greatly and depend in many instances on the cause of the shock syndrome and on the stage of shock. The volume of packed red cells is often elevated and falls to below normal as the volume deficit is repaired. There usually is *leukocytosis* of between 15,000 and 30,000 with a shift to the left. However, the white blood cell count may be normal, and some patients have leukopenia. The *platelet count* is usually decreased, and a variety of *clotting factor defects* is present.

The *urinalysis* shows no specific abnormalities. Initially, the specific gravity is high; as oliguria persists, isosthenuria develops. The *blood urea nitrogen* and *creatinine* are elevated, and creatinine clearance is reduced. Electrolyte patterns vary considerably, but there is a tendency to *hyponatremia* and hypochloremia. The serum potassium may be high, low, or normal. The *bicarbonate concentration* is usually low, and *blood lactate* is elevated.

Early in endotoxin shock there is *respiratory alkalosis* manifested by a low pCO_2 and high arterial pH—probably an attempt to blow off CO_2 to compensate for developing lactic acidemia and because of progressive anoxemia. As shock progresses, *metabolic acidosis* develops. There often is striking *anoxemia,* and pO_2 values below 70 mm Hg are common. Hemodynamic measurements usually show a low *central venous pressure, low cardiac output* and cardiac index, high *peripheral resistance,* and slow circulation time. *Blood volume* is usually low, but this determination is notoriously unreliable in septic shock and should not be trusted. The *electrocardiogram* generally shows depression of the S-T segment, inversion of the T waves, and a variety of arrhythmias, and may mistakenly suggest the diagnosis of myocardial infarction.

In untreated gram-negative shock, the blood cultures should reveal the causative pathogens, but bacteremia is often intermittent and the blood cultures may be negative. Furthermore, many patients will have received antimicrobial agents when they are first seen, masking the bacteriologic diagnosis. *A negative blood culture does not exclude the diagnosis of septic shock.* Culture of the primary septic focus may aid in the diagnosis, but the bacteriology may have been altered by prior chemotherapy.

DIAGNOSIS. The diagnosis of septic shock is not difficult in the presence of chills, fever, and an overt focus of infection. However, none of the obvious clues may be present. Elderly debilitated patients, in particular, may have severe infections in the absence of fever. Unexplained confusion and disorientation and hyperventilation without abnormal chest x-rays should call the diagnosis to mind. Pulmonary embolism, myocardial infarction, cardiac tamponade, aortic dissection, and silent hemorrhage are entities often confused with septic shock.

COURSE. The rational treatment of septic shock depends upon careful monitoring of patients. Specifically, four parameters need to be followed at the bedside:

1. The *central venous pressure* (CVP) should be measured. Insertion of a catheter into the great veins or right atrium provides an accurate index of the relationship between right ventricular competence and effective blood volume and should be used as a guide to fluid replacement therapy. When the CVP exceeds 10 to 12 cm of water, there is some danger of overloading the circulation and precipitating pulmonary edema. It is important to be sure that the flow through the catheter is free and that the catheter is not in the right ventricle. *The CVP is the cornerstone of managing shock and should be measured in every patient.*

2. The *pulse pressure* serves as an estimate of stroke volume.

3. *Cutaneous vasoconstriction* provides a clue to peripheral resistance although it does not reflect accurately blood flow to kidney, brain, or gut.

4. Hourly *urine output* should be used to monitor splanchnic blood flow and visceral perfusion. Usually this requires placement of an indwelling urethral catheter.

With these four measurements the patient with shock can be followed carefully and managed intelligently. Arterial blood pressure does not provide an accurate picture of the hemodynamic situation, and perfusion of vital organs may be adequate in patients with hypotension; conversely, some patients with normal blood pressures may have marked pooling and inadequate visceral blood flow.

In units organized for treatment of shock, frequent measurements of pulmonary artery and systemic pressures, arterial and venous pH, blood gases, blood lactate, renal function tests, and electrolytes are performed.

TREATMENT. Support of Respiration. In many patients with septic shock arterial pO_2 is markedly depressed. It is essential to establish an airway at the outset and to administer oxygen nasally or by mask. Tracheal intubation or tracheostomy and use of respiratory assistance devices usually are necessary.

Volume Replacement. Using the CVP as a guide, blood volume should be replaced with blood (if anemia is present), plasma, dextran (molecular weight 70,000 or 40,000), human serum albumin, and appropriate electrolyte solutions, primarily dextrose-saline and bicarbonate (which is preferable to lactate for treating the acidosis). The quantity of fluid required is often far in excess of "normal blood volume" and may amount to 8 to 12 liters in only a few hours. Large quantities may be required even when the cardiac index is normal. *Oliguria in the presence of hypotension is not a contraindication to continued vigorous fluid therapy.* Some investigators feel that the pulmonary artery pressure is the best indicator of incipient pulmonary edema and that a sharp rise in it calls for a reduction in fluid administration.

Antibiotics. Blood cultures and cultures of relevant body fluids or exudates should be taken before instituting antimicrobial therapy. Drugs should be given intravenously and bactericidal agents used when possible. When the results of blood cultures and sensitivities are known, one of the appropriate drugs recommended in the chapters dealing with the specific infections and discussed in Chap. 135 should be given. Usually cultures and sensitivities are not at hand at the onset of shock and the etiologic diagnosis entails an educated guess based upon culture from the primary focus—urine, bile, pus, or sputum; or on the setting in which the infection occurs. For example, a young woman with dysuria, chills and flank pain, and septic shock is likely to have *E. coli* bacteremia, while gram-negative sepsis in a burn patient is probably caused by *Pseudomonas*. The drugs of choice for gram-negative bacteremia are:

E. coli:	ampicillin
Klebsiella-Enterobacter:	kanamycin or gentamicin
Proteus mirabilis:	ampicillin
Proteus rettgeri, Pr.	
morganii, or *Pr. vulgaris:*	kanamycin or gentamicin
Mima-Herellea:	kanamycin
Pseudomonas:	polymyxin B or E
	(colistin) or gentamicin

The dosages and routes of administration for these agents are detailed in Chap 135. Cephalothin can be substituted for ampicillin in patients with a history of penicillin allergy. Because of its ototoxicity, kanamycin should be given cautiously to oliguric patients; a single dose of 1.0 Gm achieves blood levels which should suffice throughout the period of oliguria. The central nervous system toxicity of the polymyxins also is accentuated in patients with poor renal function. A new drug, Gentamicin, has been effective in *Proteus* and *Pseudomonas* bacteremia.

When the cause of septic shock is unknown, therapy should be initiated with both kanamycin and a polymyxin, or gentamicin; and if the possibility of gram-positive sepsis cannot be ruled out, a penicillinase-resistant penicillin or cephalothin should be given in addition. As soon as culture results become available, the agents which are unnecessary should be deleted from the regimen.

Surgical Intervention. Many patients with septic shock have an abscess, an infarcted or necrotic bowel, an inflamed gallbladder, an infected uterus, pyonephrosis, or other local situations which lend themselves to surgical drainage or excision. As a rule, successful treatment of shock requires surgical intervention even if the patient is desperately ill. Operations should not be postponed "to get the patient in shape" because these patients' condition will continue to deteriorate unless the septic focus is removed or drained.

Vasoactive Drugs. Septic shock is accompanied by maximal stimulation of alpha-adrenergic receptors, and pressor agents which act by stimulating these receptors such as norepinephrine, levarterenol, and metaraminol are contraindicated. The two groups of drugs which have been of value in septic shock are alpha-receptor blocking agents, exemplified by phenoxybenzamine, and beta-receptor stimulants, notably isoproterenol. *Phenoxybenzamine* (dibenzylene), an adrenolytic agent, effects a central phlebotomy by reducing resistance and increasing intravascular capacity. Hence, there is a redistribution of blood. Blood leaves the lungs, relieving pulmonary edema and enhancing gas exchange. Central venous pressure and left ventricular end-diastolic pressure fall, cardiac output rises, and peripheral venous constriction regresses. The recommended dose is 0.2 to 2.0 mg per kg intravenously. Small doses can be injected instantaneously and large doses over a period of 40 to 60 min. Fluids must be given simultaneously to compensate for the increment in venous capacitance; failure to do so aggravates shock. *Chlorpromazine* in multiple small doses of 2.5 to 5 mg also relieves vasoconstriction through its direct adrenolytic effect and by ganglionic blockade.

Isoproterenol (Isuprel) counteracts arteriolar and venous constriction in the microcirculation by its direct vasodilating effect. In addition, the drug exerts a direct inotropic effect on the heart. Cardiac output is increased by stimulating the myocardium and by reducing cardiac work as peripheral resistance decreases. The dose of isoproterenol is 2 to 8 μg per min for the average adult. Ventricular arrhythmias may result from this drug and shock may be made worse if fluid administration does not keep pace with relieved vasoconstriction.

Digitalis. A rapidly acting preparation of digoxin or Cedilanid (lanatoside C) should be given when the CVP or pulmonary artery pressures remain high in the face of systemic hypotension.

Adrenal Cortical Hormones. In large doses these agents overcome peripheral resistance and mitigate the cellular injury evoked by endotoxin. Although their use has been controversial, it seems reasonable to institute therapy with these drugs when the CVP has reached 10 to 12 cm of water and hypotension persists. Hydrocortisone in dosage of 50 mg per kg should be given intravenously in the first 12 hr. This dose may be repeated during the next 24 hr, but often shock is reversed with a single course.

Other Measures. In some patients with oliguria and a high CVP, infusions of mannitol or administration of ethacrynic acid has initiated diuresis; more often than not these maneuvers have failed. Hemorrhage as a consequence of clotting-factor deficiencies has been controlled with fresh frozen plasma, but when thrombocytopenia is the cause of bleeding, whole-blood transfusions must be given. Hyperbaric oxygen has been tried in gram-negative bacteremia with indifferent results.

PROGNOSIS. The measures described above usually will resuscitate most patients, at least temporarily. The ultimate outcome is dependent upon several factors:

1. Ability to eliminate the source of infection with surgery or antibiotics. The prognosis of urinary tract infections, septic abortion, abdominal abscess, gastrointestinal or biliary fistula, and subcutaneous or anorectal abscesses is better than that of primary foci in the skin or lungs.

2. Previous contact with the organism. Patients with chronic urinary tract infections who develop bacteremia rarely have severe gram-negative shock, perhaps because they have become tolerant to the endotoxin.

3. Underlying disease. Patients with lymphoma or leukemia who develop endotoxemia while their hematologic disease is out of control rarely recover; conversely, if hematologic remission is achieved, the shock is more likely to respond to therapy.

4. Metabolic status. The development of severe metabolic acidosis and lactic acidemia—irrespective of cardiac output—is associated with a poor prognosis.

5. Development of pulmonary insufficiency even after the hemodynamic abnormalities have been corrected.

The overall mortality of septic shock has been between 50 and 90 percent.

PREVENTION. The poor results in the treatment of septic shock are not due to lack of potent antibiotics or vasoactive agents. Rather, *failure to institute therapy sufficiently early* is a major roadblock to success. Septic shock usually is recognized too late, all too often after irreversible changes have taken place. Because many patients who are likely to develop septic shock are in the hospital *before* signs and symptoms of shock appear, it is essential to watch patients who are candidates for development of shock assiduously, to treat their infections vigorously and early, and to perform appropriate surgery before catastrophic complications occur.

REFERENCES

Clauss, R. H., and J. F. R. Ray: Pharmacologic Assistance to the Failing Circulation, Surg. Gynecol. Obstet., 126:611, 1968.

Hardaway, R. M., P. M. James, R. W. Anderson, C. E. Bredenberg, and R. L. West: Intensive Study and Treatment of Shock in Man, J.A.M.A., 199:799, 1967.

Lillehei, R. C., R. H. Dietzman, S. Movsas, and J. H. Bloch: Treatment of Septic Shock, Modern Treatment, 4:321, 1967.

MacLean, L. D., W. G. Mulligan, A. P. H. McLean, and J. H. Duff: Patterns of Septic Shock in Man: A Detailed Study of 56 Patients, Ann. Surg., 166:543, 1967.

Maiztegui, J. I., J. Z. Biegeleisen, W. B. Cherry, and E. H. Kass: Bacteremia Due to Gram-negative Rods: Clinical, Bacteriologic, Serological and Immunofluorescent Study, New Engl. J. Med., 272:222, 1965.

Petersdorf, R. G., and H. N. Beaty: The Role of Antibiotics,

Vasoactive Drugs and Steroids in Gram-negative Bacteremia, Ann. N. Y. Acad. Sci. 145:319, 1967.

Udhoji, V. S., and M. H. Weil: Hemodynamic and Metabolic Studies on Shock Associated with Bacteremia: Observations on 16 Patients, Ann. Intern. Med., 62:966, 1965.

Waisbren, B. A., and J. Arena: Shock Associated with Bacteremia Due to Gram-negative Bacilli: Autopsy Findings, Arch. Intern. Med., 116:336, 1965.

135 CHEMOTHERAPY OF INFECTION

Louis Weinstein

The use of substances elaborated by one organism to kill or inhibit the growth of another is centuries old. Over 2,500 years ago, the Chinese treated carbuncles, boils, and similar infections by applying moldy curd of soybean to such lesions. The clinical possibilities of this phenomenon were first clearly recognized in 1877 by Pasteur and Joubert, who noted that the anthrax bacillus grew well in sterile urine but failed to multiply when other bacteria were present in the urine. Similar results were observed in animals, leading them to suggest that this observation held "great promise for therapeutics."

Although numerous attempts were made over the years to develop agents that might exert a beneficial effect in bacterial, mycotic, and rickettsial infections, the era of effective chemotherapy of such disease began with the discovery and first application of the sulfonamides in 1936. The "golden age" of antimicrobial therapy was initiated by the commercial production of penicillin, an agent first discovered in 1929. Since then, the number of drugs of value in the management of a variety of infections has multiplied rapidly. The agents now available are of three types: (1) biosynthetic compounds of which penicillin G is an example; (2) semisynthetic substances such as some of the more recently developed penicillin derivatives; (3) purely synthetic agents such as the sulfonamides and some of the tuberculostatic drugs. Those derived in part or as a whole from the fermentative activity of microorganisms are classified as *antibiotics*.

THE CHEMOTHERAPEUTIC AGENTS

To be of practical value in the therapy of infection, an antimicrobial agent must exert its effect on the invading organism without seriously damaging the cells of the host. It is remarkable that so many compounds with these characteristics have been developed. As far as is known, all these drugs are effective because they act directly on the parasite and not because they enhance the natural defenses of the host. The principal result of their activity is retardation of bacterial growth. Some of them are bactericidal while others exert only a bacteriostatic effect in vitro. When these substances are administered in large doses, especially in the course of some infections, depression, delay, or abolition of the immune response to the invading microorganism may follow.

Sulfonamides

The sulfonamide compounds have been used in clinical medicine since 1937. The important members of this group are sulfadiazine, sulfisoxazole (Gantrisin), succinylsulfathiazole (Sulfasuxidine), and phthalylsulfathiazole (Sulfathalidine).

Despite the availability of newer antimicrobial agents, the sulfonamides are still very valuable in the management of some infections. Although they have been the drugs of choice for the therapy of meningococcal infections in the past, the isolation of sulfonamide-resistant strains of *Neisseria meningitidis* has decreased the universal applicability of these drugs (Chap. 142). Some but not all cases of bacillary dysentery respond to treatment with sulfonamides (Chap. 151). These compounds are very useful in uncomplicated urinary tract infections, especially those due to *Escherichia coli* and those in which instrumentation and obstruction are not problems. They also can be employed for the prophylaxis of recurrences of rheumatic fever.

The sulfonamide compounds presently employed to treat systemic infections are readily absorbed from the gastrointestinal tract and are probably best administered by this route to conscious patients. Sodium salts for either intramuscular or intravenous use are also available. Liquid preparations made palatable by the addition of flavoring materials are useful in treating young children. For most of the infectious diseases in which the sulfonamides are of value, the duration of therapy should be no less than 1 week.

When the rapidly absorbed and excreted sulfonamides (sulfadiazine or sulfisoxazole) are administered orally to adults, a "loading" dose of 4 Gm is given; this is followed by 1 Gm every 4 hr. The loading dose for parenteral injection of sodium sulfadiazine or sulfisoxazole is 5 Gm; 1 Gm may be given subcutaneously thereafter every 4 to 6 hr. As soon as patients are able to take drugs by mouth, the parenteral route need no longer be employed. Determinations of sulfonamide blood levels are of little or no value in estimating therapeutic effects; they are helpful in indicating excessive and potentially dangerous blood levels or in establishing that the drug is being taken by a patient.

Most of the sulfonamide compounds are widely distributed in the body. After absorption, the major metabolic alteration is acetylation of the primary amino group. Sulfonamides are excreted by the kidney, chiefly by glomerular filtration. Derivatives not firmly bound to plasma or tissue proteins tend to be distributed evenly in total body water and thus reach high concentrations in cells, whereas those with a tendency to be bound are concentrated in the plasma.

The bacteriostatic activity of the sulfonamides is dependent upon their antimetabolic action. Para-aminobenzoic acid (PABA), which impairs the antibacterial effect of most of these drugs, is an essential metabolite of many bacteria and is part of the molecule of folic acid. It has been suggested that sulfonamides prevent the incorporation of PABA into folic acid, but it is probable that they inhibit several steps in enzymatic activity. The principal toxic effects are hypersensitivity reactions and renal injury. These may develop any time after the first week of therapy, or even earlier in patients who have received the drugs previously. Sensitivity to one type of compound frequently confers sensitivity to others. Crystallization of the drug in the renal tubules is most likely to occur when an inadequate quantity of fluid has been ingested or when the reaction of the urine is acid, since the solubility of both acetylated and free forms is considerably greater in neutral or alkaline medium. The best method of avoiding renal injury is to maintain a copious urine output—at least 1,200 ml per day. Another method of preventing precipitation of sulfonamide crystals in the urinary tract is to administer two or three sulfonamides concomitantly because the solubility of each is independent of the presence of the others. Among other reactions observed with sulfonamides are hemolytic and aplastic anemia, thrombopenia, vascular lesions resembling those of polyarteritis nodosa, erythema multiforme including the Stevens-Johnson syndrome, Behçet's syndrome, contact dermatitis, serum sickness, hepatitis, arthritis, insomnia, confusion, vertigo, ataxia, tinnitus, peripheral neuritis, anorexia, nausea, vomiting, and hypersensitivity myocarditis (sulfamethoxypyridazine).

Sulfadiazine (2-sulfanilamidopyrimidine) is absorbed from the gastrointestinal tract slowly and incompletely, and renal excretion is relatively slow. The tissue concentration is 60 to 75 percent of that in the plasma. Sulfadiazine appears in the urine in both free and acetylated forms; neither is very soluble, and crystalluria is common. For most systemic infections in adults, sulfadiazine is administered in a dosage of 4 to 6 Gm per day after an initial dose of 4 Gm. In young children, 0.065 to 0.1 Gm/lb body weight/24 hr usually produces an adequate effect; the initial dose should be about one-half this quantity.

Sulfisoxazole (3,4-dimethyl-5-sulfanilamidoisoxazole) is more soluble than sulfadiazine. The administration of the same quantity of drug will yield a plasma concentration of sulfisoxazole three times that for sulfanilamide and about twice that for sulfadiazine and sulfamerazine. The dosage and clinical effectiveness of sulfisoxazole are of the same order as those of sulfadiazine.

Succinylsulfathiazole (2-N⁴-succinylsulfanilamidothiazole) and *phthalylsulfathiazole* [2-(N⁴-phthalylsulfanilamido)thiazole] are absorbed poorly from the intestinal tract and are used primarily to suppress bacterial growth in the intestine.

ANTIBIOTICS

The development of antibiotics for the treatment of infections represents one of the most important developments in modern medicine. The presently available agents of this class may be classified into several groups on the basis of their mechanism of action, as follows: (1) *Agents acting on bacterial cell wall synthesis*—penicillins, cephalosporin derivatives, vancomycin, and bacitracin. (2) *Agents affecting cell membranes and exerting a detergent effect*—polymyxin, colistin, novobiocin, and the polyene antifungal drugs nystatin and amphotericin. (3) *Agents producing suppression or abnormalities of protein synthesis*—chloramphenicol, tetracyclines, kanamycin, neomycin, streptomycin, and the macrolide antibiotic erythromycin. Although these mechanisms of action appear valid as of 1968, continued study may modify these concepts. Secondary changes in the anatomy or metabolism of the bacterial cell often follow the primary effect of an antimicrobial drug; the two may be easily confused. Some agents may have more than one primary site or mode of action, especially when present in high concentration. The antibiotics are classified, for clinical purposes, on the basis of the "spectrum" of organisms against which they act. For example, penicillin G is considered to have a narrow spectrum because, in conventional doses, it affects primarily gram-positive bacteria and *Neisseria*. On the other hand, antibiotics such as the tetracyclines and chloramphenicol are classified as broad-spectrum agents because they inhibit the growth of gram-positive and -negative organisms, rickettsia, Tric (TRachoma and Inclusion Conjunctivitis) agents, the psittacosis-lymphogranuloma group (*Bedsonia*), and some *Mycoplasma*.

Testing Organisms for Sensitivity to Antibiotics

The sensitivities of bacteria to chemotherapeutic agents are usually determined by bacteriologic techniques. The most accurate method for routine use involves inoculation of the organism into serial dilutions of the drug. After a suitable period of incubation, the lowest concentration of antibiotic that inhibits growth of the bacteria is expressed as the "sensitivity." A more rapid method utilizes filter paper disks impregnated with a known quantity of drug; these are applied to the surface of agar plates over which the organism is heavily streaked. The smallest quantity of antibiotic around which a given zone of inhibition of growth is present is the level of sensitivity of the bacteria. This procedure is relatively crude, but it is useful in clinical practice for the rapid determination of relative sensitivities. These tests are not necessary in all cases, but, if performed correctly, there is a good correlation between clinical response to drug and the test. Often the procedure is invaluable in indicating which therapeutic agent to employ.

Resistance of Bacteria to Antibiotics

All antibiotics are not effective against all microorganisms. The spectrum of activity of each drug is probably related to several factors among which are the availability of appropriate binding sites on the organism, the presence of essential microbial enzyme systems that can be inhibited by the drug, and the elaboration of substances, either intra- or extracellular, that inactivate the antimicrobial agent. Drug resistance is not universal, and even after 25 years, no significant degree of resistance to penicillin G has developed in group A *Streptococcus pyogenes* or *Diplococcus pneumoniae*. On the other hand, shortly after this antibiotic came into use, it became apparent that an increasing number of strains of *Staphylococcus aureus* insensitive to it were being recovered from human infections. In some instances, species of bacteria isolated prior to the availability of an antimicrobial compound have been found to be resistant, while in others the resistance seems to have become prominent only after the drug had been used for a varying period of time. Resistance of bacteria to antibiotics is, therefore, of two types—*naturally occurring* and *acquired.*

Naturally occurring drug resistance may be due to one of three mechanisms.

1. *Spontaneous mutation.* Some species of organisms, many strains of which are sensitive to a specific antimicrobial agent, may mutate spontaneously and become resistant. This is not due to exposure to the drug. When mutation occurs during therapy, it may be misinterpreted as induction of resistance because of activity of the antibiotic. This is not the case, however. The action of the antimicrobial agent is merely to *select* out the resistant mutant, as it eliminates the sensitive clones. The spontaneous mutants resist the activity of the antibiotic either by elaborating substances which degrade it or by developing alternate pathways of essential metabolic activity. An example is strains of *S. aureus* resistant to penicillin G, which produce penicillinase, a β-lactamase which inactivates the antibiotic by splitting its β-lactam ring.

2. *Failure of an antibiotic to affect essential enzyme systems.* This is the probable explanation for the selective activity of antibiotics. Some species of organisms possess enzyme systems necessary for growth and multiplication that are totally insensitive to the effects of certain drugs but not those of others. This determines the spectrum of activity of an antibiotic in many cases.

3. *Absence of appropriate binding sites* may be responsible for failure of an antimicrobial agent to inhibit microbial growth despite the fact that sensitive essential enzyme systems may be present in the organism.

Acquired drug resistance may appear in several ways.

1. Organisms cultured in vitro in media containing increasing concentrations of an antibiotic frequently become resistant to the drug either by a one-step process or gradually. The mechanisms responsible for this phenomenon are not clear, but the possibility that alternate but inactive metabolic pathways, unaffected by the antimicrobial agent, become active and take over for suppressed ones during exposure to increasing quantities of the drug, seems likely. "One-step" resistance is exemplified by streptomycin. This agent causes misreading of the genetic code leading to the production of abnormal proteins lethal to the organism. The development of resistance to the drug involves a mutation that results in a second misreading of the genetic code and the synthesis of new proteins compatible with cell life. That the mechanism involved in resistance developing as a result of spontaneous mutation is not the same as that operating when bacteria are made insensitive in vitro is illustrated

by *S. aureus*. Spontaneous mutants of this organism elaborate penicillinase, while those made penicillin-resistant in the laboratory do not produce this enzyme.

2. *Transduction* is another mechanism involved in the acquisition of acquired drug resistance. In this instance, a piece of DNA carrying a gene for resistance to a specific antibiotic is enclosed within the coat of bacteriophage and passed from the resistant organism to a sensitive one which then becomes insusceptible to the antibiotic.

3. *Episome transfer* has recently been demonstrated to be an important mechanism in the development of bacterial drug resistance. This phenomenon involves only gram-negative bacilli, primarily the *Enterobacteriaceae*. Episomes may be part of and replicate with chromosomes, or be separate from them and replicate autonomously. This genetic material is transferred from one organism to another in the process of conjugation. The resistance factor (R) consists of 2 parts, (*a*) resistance transfer factor (RTF) and (*b*) attached genes for drug resistance (R genes). In addition to transmitting other characteristics, resistance to one or more antibiotics may be transferred from the insensitive organism to the sensitive one as they come in contact with each other either in the test tube or in the intestinal tract. Insensitivity to more than one antibiotic may be induced simultaneously. Resistance to streptomycin, sulfonamides, tetracycline, and chloramphenicol may develop after a single contact. Insensitivity to ampicillin and other antimicrobial compounds may also be initiated by this mechanism. Episomal transfer occurs between organisms of the same or unrelated species. A relatively common phenomenon of considerable therapeutic importance is the development of chloramphenicol or ampicillin resistance or both in strains of *Shigella* or *Salmonella* as they become the recipients of episomes carrying such R genes from *E. coli* with which they come in contact and conjugate in the human intestinal tract.

The isolation of a sensitive organism prior to the initiation of chemotherapy, followed by the appearance during treatment of the same species now insensitive to the drug, may be interpreted erroneously as representing selection of a resistant mutant. This may be due to the implantation of a new strain of the same species, usually from the external environment, that is drug-resistant. For example, it has been demonstrated occasionally that relapse of wound infection due to penicillin G–sensitive *S. aureus* during treatment with this drug is due to invasion by a strain of different bacteriophage type of an entirely different range of sensitivity than the one recovered initially.

The general problem of bacterial drug resistance continues to be important. Solutions to it, achieved by the development of new and effective antimicrobial agents, are often only temporary. Staphylococci resistant to the penicillinase-resistant semisynthetic penicillins and the cephalosporin derivatives are presently being recovered from infections. Such strains were present prior to the development of these drugs, but the use of these agents appears to have selected out the resistant mutants. Usually *S. aureus* insensitive to methicillin is also not inhibited by oxacillin, nafcillin, and cloxacillin; a varying number are not suppressed by cephalothin or cephaloridine.

As a rule, organisms insensitive to a particular antibiotic tend to be resistant to all other chemically related antimicrobial agents. Bacteria unaffected by tetracycline are usually unresponsive to chlortetracycline, oxytetracycline, and demethylchlortetracycline. Some strains of *Pseudomonas* are an exception and are sensitive only to oxytetracycline, while being resistant to tetracycline, chlortetracycline, and other congeners. Occasionally, cross resistance may involve two agents that are chemically dissimilar; erythromycin and oleandomycin are examples. These agents have unrelated molecular structures; despite this, some erythromycin-resistant staphylococci are also insensitive to oleandomycin. In addition to inducing resistance, streptomycin may be an essential growth factor for some organisms (streptomycin dependence).

Combinations of antimicrobial agents may diminish the speed with which bacterial resistance to any of the drugs in the mixture develops. Resistance of the tubercle bacillus to a single tuberculostatic compound, such as isoniazid, is appreciably delayed when this drug is given together with another effective agent such as streptomycin or para-aminosalicylic acid (Chap. 174).

Penicillins

Penicillin is an antibacterial substance produced by various strains of *Penicillium*. Although this mold elaborates several penicillins closely related in chemical and biologic activity, the one used most extensively in clinical practice at the present time is penicillin G, or benzylpenicillin. Several modifications of the drug have been produced primarily for the purpose of prolonging the duration of antibacterial activity or increasing resistance of the drug to gastric acidity; these include the procaine ester dibenzylethylenediamine dipenicillin (Bicillin), and phenoxymethyl penicillin (penicillin V).

Penicillin G is highly effective in vitro against many but not all gram-positive and -negative cocci. Among the streptococci, groups A, C, G, H, L, and M are highly sensitive; groups B, E, F, K, and N are moderately resistant; enterococci are the least susceptible. From 85 to 90 percent of S. *aureus* isolated from infections are resistant to penicillin in ordinary dosage (600,000 to 1,200,000 units per day). Although gonococci are still relatively susceptible to penicillin, they are less sensitive than they were when this antibiotic first came into use. Pneumococci and meningococci remain highly susceptible to the drug. Most but not all strains of C. *diphtheriae*, *B. anthracis*, *Clostridia*, *Actinomyces*, *Streptobacillus* (*Haverhillia*), *Leptospira*, and *Listeria* are inhibited. One of the most exquisitely sensitive organisms is *Treponema pallidum*. Although many species of gram-negative bacilli are resistant to relatively low concentrations of penicillin G, some strains of E. *coli*, *Proteus mirabilis*, *Salmonella*, *Shigella*, *Aerobacter*, and *Alcaligenes* are suppressed in the presence of the high blood levels that follow the administration of large doses of the antibiotic (20 to 80 million units per day).

Several semisynthetic penicillins, which are compounds made up of the basic nucleus (6-aminopenicillanic acid) to which a variety of side chains have been attached, are available. Among these are methicillin (2,6-dimethoxybenzamido penicillanate), oxacillin (5-methyl-3-phenyl-4-isoxazolylpenicillin), cloxacillin (5-methyl-3-o-chlorophenyl-4-isoxazolylpenicillin), dicloxacillin [3-(2, 6-dichlorphenyl)-5-methyl-4-isoxazolylpenicillin sodium monohydrate], nafcillin [6-(2-ethoxy-1-napthamido) penicillanic acid], and ampicillin (alpha-aminobenzylpenicillin). Some of these are resistant to penicillinase (methicillin, oxacillin, nafcillin, cloxacillin, dicloxacillin), some are acid-stable (oxacillin, nafcillin, cloxacillin, dicloxacillin, ampicillin), and one has a broad spectrum of activity but is penicillinase-sensitive (ampicillin).

Penicillin in low concentrations is bacteriostatic; large quantities are bactericidal. Organisms are killed only if they are exposed to the drug while in an active phase of multiplication. The mode of action of the antibiotic is interference with the formation of bacterial cell walls by inhibiting the incorporation of a compound containing a uridine nucleotide, an acetyl amino sugar, and a peptide of three amino acids (DL-alanine, D-glutamate, and lysine) that is an intermediate in cell wall production.

BIOSYNTHETIC PENICILLINS

Penicillin G can be administered by several routes: orally, intramuscularly, subcutaneously, or intravenously. It has also been applied topically. Application to the skin is to be avoided wherever possible, because the degree of sensitization to the drug produced by this type of therapy is very high. The procaine salt of the antibiotic is an extensively used preparation because absorption is slowed and detectable blood levels may be present for as long as 24 hr. The addition of aluminum monostearate to procaine penicillin may allow detectable blood levels to be maintained for as long as 48 to 72 hr.

Benzathine penicillin (Bicillin) may be administered either orally or parenterally. When given by mouth, however, the absorption of this agent is more erratic than that of buffered penicillin G, which yields three to six times the penicillin activity of Bicillin. Intramuscular injection of Bicillin has the advantage over penicillin G of prolonging blood levels; the administration of 1.2 to 2.4 million units may produce a detectable concentration of antibiotic in the blood for as long as 4.5 weeks. The free acid and potassium salt of phenoxymethyl penicillin (penicillin V) are more stable and less soluble at the pH of gastric juice than is penicillin G. It is rapidly dissolved in alkaline solution and is readily absorbed from the upper small intestine. Taken by mouth, penicillin V produces higher and more prolonged blood levels than the same quantity of penicillin G. It produces adequate blood levels even when taken shortly after a meal.

Much larger doses of penicillin G are needed for oral than for parenteral therapy. When penicillin is injected subcutaneously or intramuscularly, it causes little local irritation and is absorbed rapidly into the bloodstream. Normally, only minute amounts penetrate into the cerebrospinal fluid, but in the presence of meningeal inflammation, appreciable levels of the drug may be obtained.

Penicillin G is excreted by the kidneys with great rapidity, mainly by a tubular mechanism. Renal excretion is delayed by concurrent administration of substances that compete for available tubular excretory structures. Benemid [probenecid, *p*-(di-*n*-propylsulfamyl)-benzoic acid] appears to be the most effective in reducing the rapidity of excretion of penicillin; the dose is 0.5 Gm four times a day.

SEMISYNTHETIC PENICILLINS

Dimethoxyphenyl penicillin (Methicillin) is effective both in vitro and in vivo against most strains of penicillinase-producing *S. aureus*. The drug, is, however, only one-twentieth to one-fortieth as active against group A beta-hemolytic streptococci and *Neisseria* and about one-tenth as active against *D. pneumoniae* and *Streptococcus viridans* as penicillin G. It is inactive against gram-negative bacilli, even those moderately sensitive to penicillin, and only slightly inhibitory for *H. influenzae*. It is at least fifty times more active than benzylpenicillin for penicillinase-elaborating straphylococci, but probably only one-fiftieth as effective for strains that do not produce this enzyme. A few methicillin-resistant strains of *S. aureus* have recently been recovered from human infections. Dimethoxyphenyl penicillin is little, if at all, inactivated by staphylococcal penicillinase, but it is inhibited by the penicillinases of *Bacillus licheniformis* and *B. cereus* (Neutrapen).

The recommended dose for adults is 1 Gm every 3 to 4 hr, and for children, 100 mg/kg body weight/day in equally divided quantities. The agent must be given parenterally; intramuscular or intravenous injection leads to rapid excretion, adequate blood levels being demonstrable for 4 hr when the intramuscular and for 3 hr when the intravenous routes are employed.

Because methicillin is acid-labile, it should *not* be given as a slow drip dissolved in large volumes of physiologic saline or dextrose in water. The pH of both of these solutions is acid. The drug is best administered by dissolving each dose in 30 to 40 ml of either of these solutions and infusing into a vein over a period of 20 to 30 min. Methicillin is excreted very rapidly; Benemid retards the rate of loss in the urine. Large quantities must be administered before the antibiotic will diffuse into the cerebrospinal fluid.

Oxacillin is less active in vitro against pneumococci, staphylococci, and streptococci than penicillin V or penicillin G. Its minimal inhibitory concentration for these organisms is considerably lower than that of methicillin. The drug is penicillinase-resistant. Penicillinase-producing staphylococci are more susceptible, in general, to oxacillin than to methicillin. Oxacillin is acid-stable and may be administered orally or parenterally. About 80 percent of the drug is bound to serum protein. A dose of 0.5 Gm intramuscularly yields plasma concentrations

equivalent to those produced by 1 Gm administered orally. Benemid blocks the renal excretion of oxacillin. The daily dose in adults is 2.0 to 4.0 Gm.

Cloxacillin has a range of antibacterial activity similar to that of oxacillin. It is equally effective against penicillinase-producing staphylococci and strains that do not elaborate this enzyme. It possesses a greater degree of antistaphylococcal activity than methicillin. Plasma concentrations of cloxacillin after oral administration are higher than those that develop after an equal dose of oxacillin. The drug is not available in parenteral form.

Dicloxacillin, like oxacillin and dicloxacillin, is acid-stable and penicillinase-resistant. It appears to be more active against staphylococci than the other agents of the group. Methicillin-resistant *S. aureus* are generally resistant to dicloxacillin as well. This drug is ineffective against enterococci and gram-negative bacilli. It appears to be more active than cloxacillin but less inhibitory than oxacillin for pneumococci. It has the same degree of suppressive effect as the other isoxazolyl penicillins against group A streptococci. Patterns of blood levels of dicloxacillin after oral administration differ little from those that result from intramuscular injection of the drug. Serum concentrations are four times higher than those produced by oxacillin and twice as high as those following cloxacillin, when equal doses of all these agents are administered by mouth. Protein binding is approximately the same for all these drugs, 80 to 85 percent. About 65 to 75 percent of an administered dose is excreted in the urine in 24 hr. The recommended oral dose of dicloxacillin for adults with mild to moderate infections is 250 mg every 6 hr; for more serious disease, this should be increased to 500 mg every 6 hr. Children should receive 50 mg/kg/day divided into equal doses every 6 hr. Larger quantities may be required for severe infections. Children weighing more than 20 kg are treated with the adult dose.

Nafcillin, acid-stable and insensitive to penicillinase, is highly active against penicillinase-producing staphylococci. It is more effective than methicillin against such organisms but is not as potent as penicillin G for staphylococci sensitive to this agent. Its antistaphylococcal effects approximate those of oxacillin. In general, the antibacterial spectrum of nafcillin for other organisms is similar to that of penicillin G. Orally administered nafcillin yields lower plasma concentrations than an equivalent dose of cloxacillin; however, on a weight-for-weight basis, nafcillin is more active than cloxacillin against streptococci, pneumococci, and staphylococci. Only about 10 percent of an oral dose of nafcillin is excreted by the kidney, and about 90 percent of a single intravenous injection is excreted in the bile and reabsorbed from the intestine; the enterohepatic circulation of the drug probably accounts for its persistence in the body. Benemid also retards the excretion of nafcillin.

Ampicillin is termed broad spectrum in its antimicrobial activity because it inhibits a number of both gram-positive and -negative bacteria. It is destroyed by contact with penicillinase and is, therefore, ineffective against penicillin G–resistant staphylococci and all gram-negative species that elaborate this enzyme. Ampicillin is somewhat less inhibitory than penicillin G for gram-positive cocci highly sensitive to this agent. It is highly effective for *H. influenzae* and enterococci, moderately active against *E. coli*, mildly active against most strains of *Aerobacter* and *Alcaligenes fecalis*, and inactive against *Pseudomonas* and indole-producing strains of *Proteus*. Indole-negative *Proteus* are highly susceptible to the drug as are most *Salmonella* and *Shigella*. The incidence of drug-resistant strains of *Salmonella*, *Shigella*, *E. coli*, and *Aerobacter* has been increasing. Ampicillin is acid-stable; it is absorbed after oral administration to about the same extent as phenoxymethyl penicillin (penicillin V). Food appears to retard absorption of the drug. Higher and more rapidly attained blood levels follow intramuscular administration. The renal excretion of the drug is retarded by probenecid. The drug appears in active form in the bile, in concentrations very much higher (approximately 30 times) than those concurrently present in the serum. Ampicillin diffuses poorly into cerebrospinal fluid in normal individuals, but appreciable quantities can be attained in meningitis. About 20 percent of the agent is bound to plasma protein. The dose of ampicillin varies with the severity of the infection; 100 to 200 mg per kg has been employed for serious disease in children; 2 to 10 or 12 Gm per day has been administered to adults.

The penicillins are responsible for a number of untoward effects. Some result from sensitization, others are related to toxic and irritative properties, and still others are induced by the development of biologic alterations in the host other than allergy or toxicity. Among the reactions that have been observed in patients receiving the penicillins are skin eruptions including morbilliform, scarlatiniform, urticarial, and purpuric lesions; fever; angioedema; contact dermatitis; erythema multiforme, including the Stevens-Johnson syndrome; anaphylaxis, with death in some instances; glossitis; brown or black discoloration of the tongue; cheilosis; eosinophilia; Arthus' phenomenon; allergic vasculitis; pain at site of injection and sterile or infected abscesses in muscles in which the drug is injected; arachnoiditis and encephalopathy when excessive doses are injected intrathecally; thrombophlebitis following intravenous infusion; Herxheimer reactions in the early therapy of syphilis; and superinfection (discussed below). Hematuria, albuminuria, pyuria, renal cell casts, increase in serum creatinine, and oliguria have been observed rarely in patients receiving methicillin. This agent has also been responsible for a few instances of bone marrow depression.

The clinical uses and dosage schedules of the penicillins are discussed in detail in the chapters dealing with the management of specific infections.

Streptomycin

Streptomycin, an antibiotic produced by *Streptomyces griseus*, is active against the tubercle bacillus and both gram-positive and gram-negative bacteria. For antibacterial activity to be present, the exposed organisms must be metabolically active but do not have to be growing. The drug causes misreading of the genetic code, resulting in the formation of abnormal proteins which are lethal for bacteria.

Streptomycin is poorly absorbed from the gastrointestinal tract but when given parenterally is well absorbed and distributed evenly in extracellular fluids. It penetrates the blood–spinal fluid barrier poorly unless meningeal inflammation is present. Renal excretion is largely by filtration, and 80 percent of the antibiotic appears in the urine over a period of 24 hr.

The main route of administration of streptomycin is intramuscular. When a local effect in the intestinal tract is desired, the drug is given orally. The infections in which streptomycin is of value are those produced by *H. influenzae*, *Pasteurella tularensis*, some strains of *E. coli*, *A. aerogenes*, the tubercle bacillus, and some strains of enterococci (together with penicillin). The usual dose for adults is 1 to 2 Gm per day in equally spaced and divided quantities; in tuberculosis, the entire daily dose may be given as a single injection; administration of 1 Gm twice a week is common practice in this disease.

The reactions that accompany the use of streptomycin may include various types of skin eruptions, fever, eosinophilia, angioedema, exfoliative dermatitis, stomatitis, anaphylaxis, contact dermatitis, lymphadenopathy, neutropenia, agranulocytosis, aplastic anemia, thrombopenia, pain at sites of injection, nausea, vomiting, diarrhea (oral therapy), labyrinthine damage, deafness, scotomas, peripheral neuritis, paresthesias, acute encephalopathy (intrathecal injection), neuromuscular paralysis with cessation of respiration (parenteral or intraperitoneal instillation), renal irritation, and superinfection.

Specific indications for the use of streptomycin in various diseases are discussed in other chapters.

The Tetracyclines

CHLORTETRACYCLINE (AUREOMYCIN)

This antibiotic, a product of *S. aureofaciens*, has a wide range of activity, encompassing not only many gram-positive and gram-negative bacteria but also the *Rickettsia*, *Mycoplasma*, and *Bedsonia*. Many strains of *S. aureus* and some of the gram-negative bacteria such as *Proteus vulgaris* and *Pseudomonas* may become rapidly resistant to the drug. After a single oral dose, the antibiotic can be demonstrated in the urine for as long as 24 hr, but only a small proportion of a parenteral dose of the drug can be demonstrated in the urine. Aureomycin diffuses into the spinal fluid in smaller amounts than into the plasma. Subcutaneous and intramuscular injections are not practical because of local irritation. When the drug is given by mouth, nausea and vomiting occur occasionally. Attempts to overcome this gastric irritation by the administration of magnesium salts, aluminum hydroxide, or milk lead to a reduction of the serum concentration. Mild diarrhea, with bulky stools, may be caused by local irritation or alteration in the bacterial flora of the intestinal tract due to the antibiotic.

The oral dose of Aureomycin is 1 to 2 Gm per day,

given in divided doses at 6-hr intervals. No more than 2 Gm per day should be given intravenously because of the risk of "toxic" hepatitis.

OXYTETRACYCLINE (TERRAMYCIN)

Terramycin, an antibiotic produced by *Streptomyces rimosus,* is very closely related chemically to Aureomycin. It may be administered orally or intravenously. Intravenous injection of this antibiotic should be reserved for instances of severe illness or for cases in which it cannot be taken by mouth. Solutions of Terramycin must be properly buffered. A single oral dose may produce detectable concentration in the blood for as long as 24 hr. When 250 mg of the drug is given at 6-hr intervals, blood levels are usually in the range of 5 to 10 μg per ml.

The clinical applications of Terramycin are practically the same as those of Aureomycin, except for an occasional case of *Pseudomonas* (see above).

TETRACYCLINE (ACHROMYCIN)

Achromycin is closely related chemically to both Aureomycin and Terramycin. It contains the skeleton structure of these two antibiotics and is prepared synthetically. The biologic activity of Achromycin is equal to that of Aureomycin and Terramycin. Achromycin is useful in the same infections that are known to respond favorably to either of the other tetracyclines. The incidence of side reactions, such as nausea, vomiting, and diarrhea, is said to be lower following Achromycin than has been observed with the other related drugs.

Intravenous therapy should be employed only in patients who are unable to take medication by mouth. The average adult dose is 500 mg intravenously at 12-hr intervals. For oral treatment, 1 to 2 Gm, divided into four doses per day, is usually adequate.

DEMETHYLCHLORTETRACYCLINE (DECLOMYCIN)

Demethylchlortetracycline is a fermentation product of a mutant strain of *S. aureofaciens.* It differs from chlortetracycline in the absence of a methyl group. Declomycin is very stable and is about twice as active as Achromycin against most organisms. The rate of renal excretion is less than half that of Achromycin. Smaller doses of Declomycin are required than of Achromycin to obtain the same clinical result. The demethylated compound needs to be given less frequently; two doses per day are said to suffice.

METHACYCLINE (RONDOMYCIN)

Methacycline (6-methylene-5-hydroxy tetracycline) is a semisynthetic compound derived from oxytetracycline. Its antibacterial spectrum approximates that of the other tetracyclines except for somewhat greater potency. With some methods of assaying antimicrobial activity, no differences between this drug and tetracycline, chlortetracycline, and oxytetracycline can be detected. Equivalent doses of methacycline and demethylchlortetracycline produce approximately the same serum concentrations. The administration of 150 mg of methacycline orally every 6 hr leads to the development of lower blood levels than those that result from giving 250 mg of tetracycline at the same interval. Because of its prolonged half-life, the recommended dose of methacycline is 150 mg every 6 hr or 300 mg every 12 hr; therapeutic activity may be demonstrable in the blood for 24 to 36 hr after treatment is stopped.

DOXYCYCLINE (VIBRAMYCIN)

Doxycycline (6-deoxy-5-hydroxytetracycline) is a synthetic derivative of methacycline. Its activity against group A streptococci and staphylococci is the same as that of demethylchlortetracycline. The drug appears to be better absorbed than the other tetracyclines when administered orally. Its activity is decreased to a much lesser degree than that of demethylchlortetracycline by the ingestion of food or dairy products. Because of its prolonged half-life, the daily and total dose requirements are lower than those for other tetracyclines. The administration of 100 mg of doxycycline produces serum concentrations only slightly lower than those attainable with 300 mg of demethylchlortetracycline. The urinary excretion of doxycycline is slower than that of demethylchlortetracycline. The urinary excretion of both agents, in percentage of the dose given, is the same during a 72-hr period. About 90 percent of the drug is bound to serum protein. The recommended dose of doxycycline for adults is 200 mg the first day (100 mg every 12 hr), followed by 100 mg per day (single dose or 50 mg every 12 hr). In severe infections, the administration of 100 mg every 12 hr has been suggested. The administration of aluminum hydroxide decreases absorption of the drug, leading to decreased blood and tissue fluid levels.

REACTION TO THE TETRACYCLINES

With few exceptions, all the tetracycline compounds produce the same untoward effects. Because they resemble each other very closely chemically, hypersensitivity reactions initiated by one may appear when another tetracycline is used at a later date. Organisms resistant to one of these compounds are usually resistant to the others. Among the reactions that have been observed in patients receiving tetracyclines are various rashes; exfoliative dermatitis; angioedema; anaphylaxis; cheilosis and discoloration of the tongue; glossitis; proctitis; pruritus ani or vulvae; fever; gastrointestinal irritation with nausea, vomiting, or diarrhea; thrombophlebitis (intravenous infusions); leukocytosis; leukopenia; atypical lymphocytes in the peripheral blood; photosensitivity (primarily demethylchlortetracycline); onycholysis (demethylchlortetracycline); liver damage (cases of renal insufficiency and pregnancy); increased intracranial pressure in young infants; discoloration of the teeth when the drugs are given to babies or to women in the early months of pregnancy; superinfections; and a variant of the Fanconi syndrome (administration of outdated drug).

Chloramphenicol (Chloromycetin)

Chloramphenicol, a fermentation product of *Streptomyces venezuelae,* has been isolated in pure crystalline form and synthesized. There is no difference in the antibacterial activity of the synthetic and the natural products. The drug inhibits protein synthesis in sensitive organisms.

Chloramphenicol is administered orally or by intravenous injection. The maximal plasma concentration after an oral dose occurs at the end of 2 hr, but some activity remains after 16 or 24 hr. About 80 percent of an oral dose can be demonstrated in the urine; however, only about 15 percent is biologically active.

Many organisms are susceptible to chloramphenicol. Although it is active against some types of gram-positive bacteria, it is most effective against the rickettsias and gram-negative organisms. *Staphylococcus aureus,* coliform bacilli, and other enteric organisms are known to become resistant to this antibiotic.

The most serious reaction produced by chloramphenicol is depression of the bone marrow, with agranulocytosis or pancytopenia. This phenomenon is not dose-related and may be an allergic response to the drug. It is observed most frequently when therapy is given over an extended period or repeated exposure to the antibiotic takes place. It is imperative that all patients receiving chloramphenicol have a white blood count and differential determination carried out every 48 hr during the entire course of treatment and for several days after it is discontinued. Decrease of the total number of white blood cells below 4,000 per cu mm or a fall in the percentage of neutrophils below 40 makes cessation of therapy mandatory; exercise of this precaution prevents the development of serious and potentially lethal bone marrow depression. Anemia with failure of reticulocyte response is common in individuals receiving chloramphenicol. This reaction is dose-related and usually disappears within a short time after treatment is stopped; it is not an indication for withdrawing the drug unless the anemia becomes severe.

Another potentially fatal reaction to the drug is observed in neonates, especially premature infants. This is the so-called "gray syndrome," characterized by weakness, listlessness, pallor, hypotension, and death; an inadequate quantity of glucuronyl transferase, the enzyme involved in conjugation of the antibiotic with glucuronic acid, is thought to be responsible for this reaction. Treatment with quantities no larger than 25 mg/kg/day in this age group avoids this reaction. Among other untoward effects observed with chloramphenicol are skin eruptions, fever, atrophic glossitis, Herxheimer reaction, nausea, vomiting, diarrhea, optic neuritis, blurred vision, digital paresthesias, decrease in prothrombin, superinfections, inhibition of mitosis in phytohemagglutinin-stimulated lymphocytes, and chromosome breaks.

Erythromycin

Erythromycin is an antibiotic elaborated by *Streptomyces erythreus.* The usual route of administration is by mouth. Peak serum concentrations appear 1 to 2 hr after ingestion of a dose and decline rapidly over 4 to 6 hr.

Gram-positive organisms, including many strains of *S. aureus,* are highly sensitive to erythromycin and are inhibited by concentrations of less than 1 μg per ml.

In clinical practice, the use of erythromycin should be restricted to infections due to sensitive staphylococci or other penicillin-resistant gram-positive organisms that occur in patients allergic to penicillin and cephalosporin derivatives. It is of value in the treatment of pneumococcal and group A beta-hemolytic streptococcal infections. The drug is therapeutically effective in pulmonary infection due to *Mycoplasma pneumoniae.* It is also active against some species of atypical *Mycobacteria.*

Bacteria exposed to erythromycin either in vitro or vivo may become resistant to the drug.

Erythromycin administration is accompanied by a small risk of untoward effects. Among the commonest reactions are skin eruptions, fever, and eosinophilia. Epigastric burning is common when the drug is taken orally in moderate amounts. The intramuscular injection of the antibiotic is so irritating that quantities larger than 100 mg should not be given. Intravenous infusion is frequently accompanied by venous irritation or thrombophlebitis. Erythromycin estolate may produce cholestatic hepatitis in some patients; this reaction does not appear to be induced by the antibiotic itself but seems to be associated with the administration of this particular ester. Superinfections by organisms resistant to erythromycin may occur.

Novobiocin

Novobiocin is an antibiotic derived from *Streptomyces niveus* and *S. spheroides.* It has an antimicrobial spectrum very similar to that of penicillin G and erythromycin; *S. aureus* and pneumococci are the most sensitive organisms. Group A *S. pyogenes, S. viridans, H. influenzae, H. pertussis,* and *N. meningitidis* are sensitive to the drug. Although a few strains of *Proteus* are susceptible to novobiocin, the majority are resistant.

Novobiocin is well absorbed from the gastrointestinal tract; peak plasma concentrations are reached at about 2 hr after an oral dose, and blood levels are higher when the drug is given in the fasting state.

The incidence of reactions to novobiocin is relatively high; commonest are extensive skin erruptions (12 percent) and fever (1 percent). Among other untoward effects are leukopenia, eosinophilia, pancytopenia, allergic pneumonitis, myocarditis, angioedema, exudative erythema multiforme, serum sickness, nausea, vomiting, diarrhea, jaundice, alopecia, intestinal hemorrhage, and superinfections. Yellow discoloration of the skin, plasma, and scleras, due in most instances to a circulating lipochrome pigment that is a degradation product of the antibiotic, is commonly present.

The oral dose of novobiocin for adults is 0.5 Gm every 6 hr; in severe infections, this may be increased to 1 Gm every 6 hr. The quantity recommended for intravenous or intramuscular injection is 1 to 2 Gm per day; intramuscular administration is usually painful.

Lincomycin (Lincocin)

Lincomycin, a fermentation product of *Streptomyces lincolnensis*, is a monobasic substance that differs chemically from all other antibiotics available for clinical use. The majority of strains of *S. aureus* are sensitive to the drug. *Diplococcus pneumoniae*, group A. *S. pyogenes*, *S. viridans*, *Bacillus anthracis*, *C. diphtheriae*, and *Clostrisium welchii* are highly susceptible to the antibiotic. Most enterococci are resistant. Gram-negative bacteria, fungi, and viruses are not inhibited by lincomycin. Some but not all erythromycin-resistant strains of staphylococci are also insensitive to lincomycin.

Plasma concentrations are maintained at higher levels than the minimal inhibitory quantities for most grampositive organisms for 6 to 8 hr after oral ingestion of a single dose of 0.5 Gm; detectable antibacterial activity is demonstrable for 12 to 24 hr when 1 Gm is given by mouth. Intramuscular injection produces peak plasma concentrations in about ½ hr. Intravenous infusion yields levels in the therapeutic range for about 14 hr.

Diarrhea may occur in 10 to 20 percent of patients. Nausea, vomiting, abdominal pain, urticaria, skin eruptions, generalized pruritus, rectal irritation, vaginitis, transient jaundice, and neutropenia have also been noted.

The recommended oral dose of lincomycin for adults is 500 mg every 6 to 8 hr; for children, it is 30 to 60 mg/kg/day given in three or four equal doses. The intramuscular dose for adults is 600 mg every 12 to 24 hr. Intravenous therapy requires the infusion of 600 mg (in 250 ml of 5 percent dextrose or 0.85 percent saline solution) every 8 to 12 hr.

Cephalothin (Keflin)

Cephalothin is a semisynthetic derivative of cephalosporin C, a fermentation product of *Cephalosporium*. Group A *S. pyogenes*, *S. viridans*, *D. pneumoniae*, penicillin G–sensitive and –resistant *S. aureus*, *Cl. welchii*, *N. gonorrheae*, *N. meningitidis*, *C. diphtheriae*, and *Actinomyces* are highly sensitive to the agent. Gramnegative organisms are, in general, less susceptible, but most strains of *Salmonella, Shigella*, all *Proteus mirabilis*, 70 percent of *E. coli*, and many strains of *H. influenzae* are inhibited by concentrations readily produced by conventional doses of the drug. *Proteus vulgaris, Pseudomonas, Herellea*, and enterococci are resistant to the antibiotic. Cephalothin is not inactivated by penicillinase. Its activity is destroyed in vitro by cephalosporinase, an enzyme elaborated by some gram-negative bacteria and by enterococci; production of cephalosporinase is not always associated with resistance to cephalothin.

Cephalothin is not absorbed when given orally. It is rapidly absorbed after intramuscular injection and reaches peak plasma levels in about ½ hr. Therapeutic levels of the drug are present in cerebrospinal fluid. Cephalothin may accumulate in the blood of patients with poor renal function.

Among the untoward effects that have been related to the administration of cephalothin are fever, eosinophilia, neutropenia, hemolytic anemia, urticaria, anaphylactic reactions, and serum sickness and pain on injection. Superinfections have occurred in some patients.

The dose of cephalothin for adults is from 6 to 12 Gm per day administered intramuscularly or intravenously in equal-sized and -spaced doses.

Cephaloridine (Loridine)

Cephaloridine [7-(2-thenyl acetamido)-3-pyridylmethyl cephalosporanic acid] is another semisynthetic derivative of cephalosporin C. Its activity against penicillin G–sensitive and –resistant strains of *S. aureus* is about the same as that of cephalothin. *Diplococcus pneumoniae*, *S. viridans*, group A streptococci are organisms which are highly sensitive to the drug. Enterococci are not inhibited. Sensitivity to cephaloridine and cephalothin distinguishes *Klebsiella*, which is sensitive, from *Aerobacter* which is resistant. Among other gram-negative organisms susceptible to cephaloridine are indole-negative *Proteus*, most *E. coli*, and *Salmonella*. Many strains of *H. influenzae* are moderately sensitive. Indole-positive *Proteus* and *Pseudomonas* are totally resistant. The minimal inhibitory and bactericidal concentrations for both grampositive and -negative bacteria are, with few exceptions, approximately the same. The intramuscular injection of 0.6 Gm of cephaloridine leads to peak blood levels within ½ hr; small but detectable amounts are present in most instances after 8 hr. The administration of probenecid together with the antibiotic produces higher maximal serum concentrations and longer persistence of antibacterial activity. Cephaloridine is excreted primarily by the kidneys; 70 percent appears in the urine within 24 hr after a single dose. The recommended dose is 1 Gm every 6 hr for adults. Doses above 4.0 Gm per day in adults have been associated with both tubular and glomerular damage and are contraindicated. Intramuscular injection produces much less discomfort than does cephalothin.

Polymyxin (Aerosporin)

Polymyxin is a polypeptide antibiotic obtained from *B. polymyxa*. The principal effect is upon gram-negative bacilli, for which it is one of the most potent chemotherapeutic agents; strains of *Proteus* are, however, resistant. The drug can be administered intramuscularly at intervals of 8 to 12 hr with a total daily dose no larger than 2.5 mg per kg. It is not absorbed from the bowel, but eliminates sensitive organisms from the intestinal flora when given orally. It does not pass into the cerebrospinal fluid and cannot be detected in the bile or in the urine in biologically active form. Although highly effective against many species of gram-negative bacteria, polymyxin is most useful for the management of infections due to *Ps. aeruginosa*, practically all strains of which are sensitive to the agent. The untoward effects of this agent are similar to those of colistin and are described below.

Colistin

Colistin, and antibiotic produced by *B. colistinus,* is a basic polypeptide, the salts of which are water-soluble. The antimicrobial spectra of colistin and polymyxin B are very similar; there is complete cross resistance between these compounds.

Colistin is not absorbed from the gastrointestinal tract. After parenteral injection, peak plasma concentration develops at about 1 hr; at 3 hr, the blood level is about 25 percent of peak. Patients with renal insufficiency excrete this antibiotic poorly and exhibit high and sustained antimicrobial activity in the circulation. Colistin does not appear in significant quantities in cerebrospinal fluid.

Among the untoward effects associated with the administration of colistin are skin eruptions, pruritus, transient paresthesias, dizziness, speech abnormalities, fever, apnea, leukopenia, ataxia, partial deafness, gastrointestinal disturbances, superinfection, and reduction of renal function. The renal effects are usually transient and disappear when therapy is discontinued.

The parenteral dose of sodium colistimethate for the treatment of urinary tract infections is 2 to 3 mg per kg divided into four equal injections. For disease involving other organs, doses of 5 mg per kg for adults and 7 to 10 mg/kg/day for children may be given when the kidneys are normal. Great care must be exercised in the parenteral use of colistin when renal insufficiency is present and in older adults in whom kidney function appears to be normal.

Neomycin

Neomycin, an antibiotic derived from a strain of *Streptomyces* closely related to *S. fradia,* is bactericidal for many gram-negative and gram-positive organisms. Absorption from the intestinal tract is relatively poor. The usual oral dose of neomycin is 4 to 8 Gm in divided doses per day. The antibiotic may also be administered intramuscularly; the daily dose is 1 to 2 Gm.

The usefulness of neomycin is sharply limited by high toxicity when it is given parenterally. Kidney and eighth nerve damage occur in a significant number of patients. In view of these untoward effects, neomycin should never be the first drug employed in the treatment of any infection. It should be reserved for those diseases in which no other antibiotic is effective and in which the infection threatens life. This agent is used only infrequently by the parenteral route. Two other significant reactions may be produced by neomycin. When the drug is instilled into the peritoneal cavity, especially in anesthetized patients who have been given a muscle-relaxing agent such as succinyl choline, a curarelike reaction may ensue and paralyze respiration; the same phenomenon occurs rarely when the antibiotic is administered parenterally. Neostigmine reverses the reaction rapidly. Individuals who receive neomycin orally for prolonged periods may develop steatorrhea and a sprue-like syndrome. Acute staphylococcal enterocolitis has occurred in patients receiving this agent to "prepare" the bowel for surgery. In cases of renal insufficiency, enough of the antibiotic may be absorbed from the intestine to cause accumulation of concentrations in the blood that may be harmful to the ears and kidneys.

Kanamycin (Kantrex)

Kanamycin is a fermentation product of *Streptomyces kanamyceticus.* It is distinct from but related closely to neomycin and has a lesser relationship to streptomycin. It is active against gram-negative bacteria such as *E. coli, A. aerogenes, Salmonella;* gram-positive organisms such as *S. aureus;* and the tubercle bacillus. It is ineffective against streptococci, *D. pneumoniae,* and *Clostridia.* In high concentrations the drug is bactericidal.

Kanamycin has been shown to be of use in urinary tract infections, shigellosis, bacteremia due to gram-negative bacteria, peritonitis, and systemic staphylococcal infections. Although kanamycin is called a broad-spectrum antibiotic, it is not a substitute for all other antimicrobial agents; it should be reserved for the management of infections due to organisms not susceptible to those antibiotics which are potentially less toxic. In particular, there are many better antistaphylococcal agents than kanamycin; thus, it should rarely be used in staphylococcal infections.

For the treatment of systemic infection in adults, the recommended dose of kanamycin is 0.5 Gm every 6 to 8 hr intramuscularly. When this antibiotic is given orally, the suggested dose is 4 to 12 Gm per day. Intramuscular injection of the drug yields peak blood levels at 1 to 2 hr. The total dose administered should not exceed 15 Gm.

The two most dangerous side effects of treatment with kanamycin are damage to the eighth nerve, with permanent deafness, and nephrotoxicity, which varies from abnormalities of urine sediment to severe kidney involvement with renal failure and death. The drug should be used with caution in individuals with any degree of renal insufficiency. Other untoward effects that have been observed include various rashes, pruritus, pain at sites of injection, stomatitis, diarrhea, proctitis, and paresthesias. Like neomycin, kanamycin may produce myoneural junction dysfunction with paralysis of respiration when given intraperitoneally or parenterally.

Gentamicin (Garamycin)

This aminoglycoside antibiotic is derived from a species of the genus *Micromonospora,* and is closely related to streptomycin, neomycin, and kanamycin. It has a wide antibacterial spectrum, including staphylococci and many gram-negative bacteria such as *E. coli, Klebsiella-Enterobacter, Proteus mirabilis,* and, in particular, indole-positive species of *Proteus* and *Pseudomonas.* The drug has been useful in urinary tract infections, gram-negative pneumonia and bacteremias, and some have suggested that it will become the drug of choice in gram-negative sepsis. The recommended dose is 3.0 to 5.0 mg/kg/day given intramuscularly at 6 to 8 hr intervals in patients with normal renal function. Inasmuch as the drug is excreted by the kidneys, the dose should be reduced in patients with renal failure. The major toxic effect of gentamicin is on the vestibular portion of the eighth nerve, although hearing loss occurs occasionally. Careful adjustment of the dose, particularly in patients with impaired renal function, can minimize these side effects.

Vancomycin (Vancocin)

Vancomycin, a water-soluble antibiotic elaborated by *Streptococcus orientalis*, is active mainly against group A beta-hemolytic streptococcus, *S. fecalis*, *D. pneumoniae*, *N. gonorrheae*, *C. diphtheriae*, *Cl. tetani*, and staphylococcus, including strains resistant to semisynthetic penicillins; it is ineffective against all gram-negative bacilli.

The drug is not absorbed from the gastrointestinal tract and must be administered intravenously. The administration of 500 mg intravenously every 6 hr is recommended for the treatment of staphylococcal bacteremia. This is increased to 1 Gm every 6 hr in cases of endocarditis or meningitis.

Pain at the site of intravenous injection of vancomycin is relatively frequent. Thrombophlebitis is common. Skin eruptions may result from sensitization to the drug. Most patients receiving vancomycin show hyaline and granular casts and albumin in the urine; nitrogen retention can occur. Among other reactions induced by the antibiotic are nerve deafness, chills, fever, a shocklike state, and superinfections.

Paromomycin (Humatin)

Paromomycin, an oral antibiotic produced by a strain of *Streptomyces*, is employed to reduce the number of bacteria in the intestinal tract and to treat intestinal infections due to *Salmonella*, *Shigella*, and *Endamoeba histolytica*. The drug is effective in vitro against gram-positive organisms including *C. diphtheriae*, *S. aureus*, and *S. fecalis* and gram-negative bacilli such as *E. coli*, *A. aerogenes*, paracolon bacillus, *Klebsiella pneumoniae*, *Pasteurella multocida*, *Brucella* and some species of *Proteus*. It is also active both in vitro and in vivo against the tubercle bacillus. *Pseudomonas aeruginosa* is not affected. The drug can also be administered orally in cases of hepatic coma, for preparation of the bowel for surgery, for the treatment of Salmonella and Shigella carrier states, and in amebic colitis. The dose is 0.5 Gm every 6 hr; a parenteral dosage form is not available. Outside of bulky soft stools, there are no major toxic reactions. Paromomycin is not absorbed from the intestinal tract except in very tiny quantities. Nevertheless, it should be given with care to patients with significant renal insufficiency in whom it may produce damage to the ears and kidneys.

Nystatin (Mycostatin)

Nystatin is elaborated by *Streptomyces noursei*. It is poorly absorbed from the gastrointestinal tract. High blood levels follow intravenous injection. This antimycotic agent is employed for local application in the form of ointments, solutions, powders, suppositories, and gels. Topical use in the treatment of *Candida* infections of the skin and vagina has been reported to be successful.

The usual oral dose of nystatin is 150 mg (500,000 units) three times a day. Although an occasional case of disseminated mycotic infection has been treated parenterally with nystatin with reported good results, the place of this agent in the therapy of deep-seated mycoses is questionable.

When nystatin is administered orally, nausea and vomiting may occur. Local application may be irritating to skin and mucous membranes.

Amphotericin B (Fungizone)

Amphotericin B is the best agent available for the treatment of deep-seated mycotic infections. It produces cure in many cases of cryptococcosis, histoplasmosis, blastomycosis, disseminated candidiasis, and coccidiomycosis; it may have a beneficial effect in some instances of aspergillosis and mucormycosis. Amphotericin B is usually administered intravenously, dissolved in 5 percent dextrose. It should not be dissolved in saline because it precipitates in this medium. Fresh solutions should be prepared for each dose. The recommended dose for intravenous administration is 0.25 mg per kg the first day, followed by an increase of 0.25 mg per kg each succeeding day. When 1 mg/kg/day is reached, this dose is continued for the rest of the treatment period. Infusion of the drug should be carried out over a period of 6 hr.

After the maximal dose has been reached, an alternative regimen is to give 1.5 mg per kg every other day. Another method is to administer 1 mg of amphotericin B dissolved in 250 ml of 5 percent dextrose solution on the first day and increase this to 5 mg (in 500 ml of 5 percent dextrose) on the second day and 10 mg (in 1,000 ml of 5 percent dextrose) on the third day; the dose is then increased by 5 to 10 mg each day until 1 mg per kg is being administered daily. At this point, the dose may be changed to 1.5 mg per kg every other day. Treatment is continued for 6 weeks to 3 to 4 months, depending on the nature and severity of the infection.

The intravenous infusion of amphotericin B is often accompanied by chills, fever, vomiting, and headache; the frequency and intensity of these manifestations may be reduced by prior administration of an antipyretic or an antihistamine. A procedure that may control these reactions in some instances is the infusion of 25 mg hydrocortisone sodium succinate directly into the tubing of the intravenous set immediately after injection of the antibiotic has been started.

Among other untoward effects that may follow the systemic administration of amphotericin are phlebitis, hepatitis, anaphylaxis, thrombopenia, flushing, hypokalemia, hypomagnesemia, electrocardiographic abnormalities, and superinfections.

Nitrofurantoin (Furadantin)

Nitrofurantoin [N-(5-nitro-2-furfurylidene)-1-aminohydantoin] is an antibacterial agent of value primarily in the treatment of some types of urinary tract infection. It is poorly soluble in water. The drug is most active against *E. coli* (bactericidal), of intermediate effectiveness against *A. aerogenes*, and without effect against *Pseudomonas*. The activity of the drug against *Proteus* is variable, although many strains are quite sensitive. *Staphylococcus aureus* and enterococci are inhibited by low concentrations.

Nitrofurantoin is administered orally, usually in a dose of 7 to 10 mg per kg body weight (100 to 200 mg four times a day). Useful blood levels cannot be produced. The drug is excreted in the urine. Within 4 to 6 hr after a maximal dose, the concentration in the urine is 25 to 50 mg per 100 ml; 8 hr after a dose, the levels are low. With highly alkaline urine, the effect of nitrofurantoin appears to be depressed, for this reason, the simultaneous administration of an acidifying agent has been suggested. The development of bacterial resistance to the drug has not been noted.

The infections of the urinary tract that respond most favorably to therapy with nitrofurantoin are the acute and uncomplicated ones produced by *E. coli*.

Nitrofurantoin is relatively nontoxic. Nausea, with or without vomiting, is the commonest untoward reaction. Various types of rashes have been described. Leukopenia occurs rarely. A syndrome resembling acute pulmonary edema has been reported.

Nalidixic Acid (Neggram)

Nalidixic acid is a naphthyridine derivative active against many gram-negative bacilli including *E. coli*, *Aerobacter*, *Klebsiella*, and *Proteus*, organisms commonly involved in infections of the urinary tract. *Pseudomonas* is resistant to the drug. The drug is administered orally. Blood levels are inadequate for the control of systemic infections. Sensitive bacteria may become resistant rapidly, sometimes in as short a period as 5 days after exposure. For this reason, follow-up urine cultures should be obtained within a few days after instituting therapy. Organisms developing resistance to nalidixic acid remain sensitive to other agents. Side reactions include nausea, vomiting, skin eruptions, and in a few instances, convulsive seizures. The dose recommended for adults is 4 Gm daily in divided doses for 1 to 2 weeks, followed by 2 Gm per day.

TUBERCULOSTATIC DRUGS

Although streptomycin is effective in the treatment of tuberculosis, the use of this agent alone leaves much to be desired in the way of maximal antibacterial effect as well as in preventing the emergence of drug-resistant strains of *Mycobacterium tuberculosis*. For these reasons, attempts have been made to develop other compounds possessing tuberculostatic activity that might be given concurrently with streptomycin. Among such agents are para-aminosalicylic acid (PAS), isonicotinic acid hydrazide (INH), cycloserine, pyrazinamide, ethambutol, and ethionamide.

Para-aminosalicylic Acids (PAS)

Para-aminosalicylic acid, a white crystalline powder, is sparingly soluble in water but easily dissolved in the form of its sodium salt. This agent has a bacteriostatic effect in vitro against many strains of *M. tuberculosis*, even those which have become streptomycin-resistant.

Para-aminosalicylic acid and its sodium salt, when given orally, are rapidly absorbed and quickly excreted. A single dose produces maximal serum concentration within 30 to 60 min of administration; thereafter, there is a gradual fall, with disappearance in 2 to 3 hr.

Para-aminosalicylic acid is usually given orally, but preparations for intravenous use are also available; these should be reserved for patients in whom severe gastric distress prohibits oral use or for those in coma. The daily dose of the drug is 8 to 12 Gm. Among the untoward effects of this drug are gastrointestinal irritation with anorexia, nausea, vomiting, abdominal distress, and increased frequency of bowel evacuation. Epigastric burning and pain are common. Hypersensitivity phenomena include fever, joint pain, lymphadenopathy, various skin eruptions and, eosinophilia. Other reactions that have been noted are peptic ulceration, renal irritation, meningitis, myeloradiculoneuritis, hepatic necrosis, a clinical picture resembling infectious mononucleosis (atypical lymphocytes, negative heterophile agglutination), acute hemolytic anemia, leukopenia, agranulocytosis, perifocal infiltrations in the lungs, and Loeffler's syndrome.

Isonicotinic Acid Hydrazide

Of all the tuberculostatic agents, isonicotinic acid hydrazide has the highest activity in vitro. It is not effective against organisms other than *Mycobacteria*. The drug is administered orally, as a rule, and is almost completely absorbed from the digestive tract. Peak serum concentrations may occur 1 to 3 hr after administration, and minimal detectable concentrations persist for 6 to 24 hr.

Cultures of tubercle bacilli readily acquire resistance to isonicotinic acid hydrazide. Resistant strains are recovered from some patients who receive this drug alone. There is no cross resistance between isonicotinic acid hydrazide and streptomycin or PAS.

Isonicotinic acid hydrazide should be given in combination with streptomycin, PAS, or another tuberculostatic agent.

There is a great deal of variation in the metabolism of isonicotinic acid hydrazide in man. Some individuals inactivate the drug slowly, others rapidly. Individuals who inactivate the drug slowly are autosomal homozygous recessives; rapid inactivators are heterozygotes or homozygous dominants. The process of inactivation is enzyme-mediated and consists in facilitation of or speeding in acetylation of the drug. The development of poly-neuritis and the reversal of infectiousness are more frequent and occur earlier in slow than rapid inactivators. There is no association between the type of isonicotinic acid hydrazide inactivator and the appearance of drug resistance in tubercle bacilli.

The incidence of reactions to isoniazid varies with the dose. When 3 mg/kg/day are given, untoward effects occur in less than 1 percent of cases; with 10 mg/kg/day, these may develop in 15 percent or more of cases. Some of the reactions are the result of sensitization to the drug. These include fever, various types of skin eruptions, eosinophilia, and hepatitis. The toxic effects are manifested primarily by nervous system abnormalities among which are peripheral neuritis, muscle twitching, convulsions, dizziness, ataxia, paresthesias, stupor, toxic encephalopathy, euphoria, transient loss of memory, separation of ideas and reality, loss of self-control, florid psychosis, and optic neuritis. Dry mouth, epigastric distress, urinary retention in men, methemoglobinemia, agranulocytosis, jaundice, pellagra, vasculitis, and pyridoxine deficiency have also been noted in persons taking this agent. The nervous system difficulties are largely prevented by the administration of 100 mg pyridoxine per day. All the reactions tend to be more frequent in slow inactivators of INH.

Cycloserine

Cycloserine is an antibiotic produced by *Streptomyces orchidaceus*. It is active against *M. tuberculosis*, including strains resistant to other tuberculostatic agents. In vivo, the drug is effective in infections due to enterococci, strains of paracolon bacilli, *E. coli*, *S. aureus*, and agents of the psittacosis-ornithosis-lymphogranuloma venereum group. Cycloserine is rapidly absorbed from the stomach and small intestine. Peak blood levels are reached within 3 to 4 hr after a single dose. Multiple doses lead to accumulation of the drug in the circulation after 3 days. Cycloserine is highly diffusible and is distributed throughout the body fluids and tissues. Cerebrospinal fluid levels in patients with normal or inflamed meninges are approximately the same as in the blood. About 50 percent of a parenteral dose of this antibiotic is excreted in unchanged form in the urine in the first 12 hr; a total of 65 percent is recoverable in urine over a period of 72 hr. Urine concentrations are high. Excessive blood levels develop in patients with decreased renal function.

Reactions to cycloserine tend to appear in the first 2 weeks of therapy and involve the central nervous system primarily. Among these are somnolence, headache, tremor, dysarthria, vertigo, confusional and other abnormal behavioral states, paresis, acute psychotic episodes, and seizures. The oral dose of the drug is 250 mg twice a day.

Pyrazinamide

Pyrazinamide (pyrazine-2-carboxyamide), a synthetic agent, is more active against the tubercle bacillus than para-aminosalicylic acid or cycloserine but less effective than streptomycin or isonicotinic acid hydrazide. Bacterial resistance to pyrazinamide develops in 6 to 8 weeks in patients treated with this agent alone. When given with another tuberculostatic agent, good therapeutic results are produced. The drug is well absorbed from the gastrointestinal tract. Peak plasma levels are reached about 2 hr after oral administration. Excretion is primarily by the kidneys. The dose for adults is 25 to 35 mg/kg/day given in 3 or 4 equally divided and equally spaced doses. A total quantity of 3 Gm per day must not be exceeded.

Injury to the liver is the most common and serious side effect of pyrazinamide; elevations of SGOT and SGPT are the earliest abnormalities. With a dose of 3 Gm per day, manifestations of liver disease develop in about 15 percent of patients; jaundice appears in 2 to 3 percent and death from hepatic necrosis results rarely. All individuals receiving this agent must have studies of liver function carried out before and during therapy. Among other untoward effects of the drug are arthralgia, anorexia, nausea, vomiting, dysuria, malaise, and fever.

Ethambutol

Ethambutol (ethylene diamino-di-1-butanol dihydrochloride) is active in low concentrations against most strains of *M. tuberculosis*. Bovine tubercle bacilli and group I atypical *Mycobacteria* (photochromogens, *M. batteyi*) are also highly sensitive to the drug. However, *M. avium* as well as scotochromogens and nonchromogenic *Mycobacteria* are less predictably affected. Ethambutol suppresses the growth of isoniazid-and streptomycin-resistant tubercle bacilli. Bacterial resistance develops in vivo when the compound is given alone. About 75 to 80 percent of an orally administered dose of ethambutol is absorbed from the gastrointestinal tract. Plasma levels are maximal 2 to 4 hr after the drug is taken orally. About 50 percent of the peak concentration is present in the blood at 8 hr and less than 10 percent at 24 hr after a dose. From 80 to 95 percent of an oral dose of ethambutol is excreted in the urine and feces within 1 to 4 hr after it is administered. In 24 hr, 50 percent of the ingested drug is present in the urine; 8 to 15 percent is excreted in the form of two metabolic products, an intermediary aldehyde and a terminal butyric acid derivative. The oral dose of ethambutol is 25 to 50 mg per kg once a day.

Loss of vision is the outstanding untoward effect produced by ethambutol. It occurs in about 10 percent of patients receiving 25 to 50 mg/kg/day of the drug. Evidence of visual difficulty first appears 1 to 7 months after therapy is started. The intensity of visual loss is related to the duration of treatment after decrease in visual activity becomes apparent. Recovery occurs when ethambutol is withdrawn; the time required is a function of the degree of visual impairment present when therapy is stopped.

Ethionamide

Ethionamide (2-ethylthioisonicotinamide), a derivative of isonicotinic acid, suppresses the growth of *M. tuberculosis* and is effective against strains resistant to streptomycin, para-aminosalicylic acid, isonicotinic acid hydrazide, and cycloserine. About 75 percent of photochromogenic *Mycobacteria* are suppressed by a concentration of 10 mg per ml or less; the scotochromogens are more resistant.

The oral administration of 1 Gm of ethionamide yields peak plasma levels of about 20 mg per ml in 3 hr. Slightly higher and more sustained levels follow rectal instillation of the drug, although absorption from this site may be delayed. Ethionamide is present in significant quantities in the cerebrospinal fluid.

Among the commonest reactions to ethionamide are anorexia, nausea, and vomiting. Manifestations resembling those resulting of ganglionic blockade—severe postural hypotension, mental depression, drowsiness, and asthenia—are common. Among other untoward effects are convulsions, peripheral neuropathy, allergic skin rashes, purpura, stomatitis, gynecomastia, impotence, menorrhagia, and difficulty in control of diabetes mellitus. Hepatitis may occur in diabetics but disappears when therapy is stopped.

The initial dose of ethionamide for adults is 250 mg orally twice a day. This is increased by 125 mg per day every 5 days until 1 Gm is being given daily; this dose must not be exceeded.

Ethionamide should not be used alone to treat tuberculosis. In various combinations with para-aminosalicylic acid, isoniazid, streptomycin, cycloserine, and pyrazinamide, ethionamide has produced good results.

SELECTION OF A CHEMOTHERAPEUTIC AGENT

When faced with the necessity of treating an infection, the physician finds that an ever-increasing number of antibacterial drugs is available. Bacterial cultures are desirable in most infections, but are not always practicable. In many instances, the etiology can be inferred from the mode of onset, the clinical features, and the epidemiologic background of the disease. Nevertheless, there are situations in which careful bacteriologic studies are essential to proper treatment.

Even when the etiology of an infectious process is determined, selection of an appropriate drug does not follow automatically, because there may be wide variations in susceptibility among organisms of the same or related species. The cost of the different drugs also has to be considered at times, since there are enormous differences. In addition, the nature of the illness may affect the choice of agent; for example, an orally administered drug may be unsatisfactory in a patient who is vomiting. In critically ill patients, it is sometimes safest to give a combination of drugs until cultural and sensitivity studies reveal which agent is specifically indicated.

In such cases, cultures should always be taken *before initiation of therapy*. If an individual has previously shown hypersensitivity or any other serious reaction to a drug, or if he develops a reaction during therapy, a different agent should be used, if possible. Therapy of specific infections is discussed in other parts of this book, where the agents of primary and secondary value in treatment are indicated.

COMBINATIONS OF ANTIBACTERIAL AGENTS

TREATMENT OF MIXED BACTERIAL INFECTIONS. In bronchiectasis, peritonitis, and some cases of acute or chronic otitis media and urinary tract infection, two or more organisms may sometimes be involved. In some instances, the responsible bacteria although of different species, are sensitive to a single antimicrobial agent; in others they have distinctly different drug susceptibilities. This emphasizes the need to determine the drug sensitivity of each of the components of a mixed flora individually before therapy is initiated. The antibiotics to be given are selected on the basis of these studies and administered in *full doses*. In some cases, it may be unnecessary and even dangerous to delay initiation of treatment until definitive bacteriologic data are available. Peritonitis is an outstanding example. Because both gram-positive and gram-negative organisms may be acting synergistically to produce this disease and because delay in therapy may result in a rapidly fatal outcome, treatment should be started immediately with maximal quantities of the antibiotics known to be most effective against these bacteria.

DELAY IN RATE OF EMERGENCE OF RESISTANCE. The emergence of antibiotic resistance is delayed by combinations of antimicrobial drugs in some but not in all infections. For example, the concomitant administration of two or more drugs suppresses strikingly the development of resistance in the tubercle bacillus. Tuberculosis is best treated, therefore, with at least two, and in some instances (miliary tuberculosis and tuberculous meningitis), three, tuberculostatic agents simultaneously.

"FIXED-DOSE" COMBINATIONS. These encourage inadequate treatment, because there is an inevitable tendency to use the same total dose of the combination as of the single agent, which does not provide the expected effective quantity of either, particularly of the inferior drug. Fixed-dose combinations provide a false sense of security because they are alleged to offer wider coverage, when in fact, they provide a narrower effective spectrum by substituting less active agents and smaller amounts of individual agents than would be the case if most active antibiotics were used in the proper dosage individually. If combined therapy is necessary at all, each of the drugs should be selected on the basis of its activity and the results of sensitivity tests and should be given in full dosage.

THERAPY OF SEVERE INFECTIONS IN WHICH SPECIFIC ETIOLOGY IS UNKNOWN. The commonest use of antibiotic combinations is for the therapy of infections in which the etiology is not immediately apparent, but where the possibility that bacterial infection is present is sufficiently great to make chemotherapy necessary. Because the exact cause cannot be immediately determined, more than one agent is given in the hope that this will "cover" the situation; fixed-dose mixtures are used all too often. In a large number of cases, the infectious process is viral and an antimicrobial agent is not indicated.

When full-dose combinations are given in the absence of a specific bacteriologic diagnosis, it must be determined, on the basis of the clinical features of the disease, a detailed history, and laboratory investigations (including examination of stained preparations, if possible), not only that a patient has a bacterial infection but also what type of organism is most likely to be involved. *Under no circumstances should chemotherapy be initiated until all the necessary bacteriologic investigations have been started.* However, in many instances, treatment need not and should not be delayed until the results of these studies become available.

ALTERATION OF ANTIBACTERIAL ACTIVITY BY COMBINING ANTIBIOTICS. A number of studies indicate that the antimicrobial activity of antibiotic combinations may be unpredictable and that in vitro activity may be unrelated to therapeutic effectiveness in vivo. Enhancement, depression, or no change in activity of the combination, when compared with single drugs, have been demonstrated. However, antibiotic combinations usually have a broad-spectrum effect in vivo if the organisms being treated are sensitive to the compounds. Clinical experience has indicated those infections in which combined therapy appears to be more effective as well as those in which such treatment produces inferior results. Enterococcal infections appear to respond better when treated with a combination of penicillin and streptomycin than with either of these antibiotics alone (Chaps. 137 and 141). Combined treatment also seems to be superior to the use of single drugs in *K. pneumoniae* pneumonia (chloramphenicol and streptomycin—Chap. 148), tuberculosis (two or sometimes three effective tuberculostatic agents—Chap. 174), and brucellosis (tetracycline and streptomycin—Chap. 154). On the other hand, the use of tetracycline plus penicillin in pneumococcal meningitis produces a much lower recovery rate than does penicillin alone. This is probably also true for the treatment of this disease with a combination of chloramphenicol and penicillin. The results of therapy for streptococcal pharyngitis are better with penicillin than with erythromycin, and intermediate when these antibiotics are given together.

HOST DETERMINANTS OF RESPONSE TO ANTIMICROBIAL AGENTS

The nature of an infection determines to a great degree the kind of antimicrobial therapy to be employed. However, innate host factors, completely unrelated to the acute disorder, are often the prime determinants not only of the type of antibiotic selected but also of its dose, route of administration, risk and nature of untoward effects, and therapeutic effectiveness. Among such factors are age, genetic factors, pregnancy, metabolic abnormalities, atopic allergy, nervous system disorders, indigenous microbial flora, hepatic function, renal function, electrolyte balance, and host defense mechanisms.

AGE. Although the dose of many commonly used antibiotics may be calculated on the basis of body weight or surface area, that of others, especially those excreted in unchanged form by the kidney, exemplified by the penicillins, is determined almost entirely by the state of renal function. In addition to dose of antibiotics, age also plays an important role in conditioning the risks of some types of reactions, route of administration, and therapeutic activity.

Renal function is relatively poor in newborn children, especially premature infants, and in older persons. Although renal function increases markedly from birth, complete maturity is probably not reached until the age of one year. With advancing age, glomerular function, effective blood flow, and tubular excretion diminish. Because of these renal changes, the dose of a number of antimicrobial agents, especially those excreted in biologically active form by the kidney, needs to be relatively low in the first month of life, particularly in premature babies, considerably higher in young children, and reduced considerably in individuals over the age of fifty, even when BUN and serum creatinine are within the normal range. Among these drugs are penicillin G, methicillin, oxacillin, ampicillin, cephalothin, streptomycin, tetracycline, and kanamycin. Although the dose of colistin does not vary in children of different ages, its excretion is relatively slow in the elderly and necessitates the administration of smaller than conventional quantities despite normal BUN and creatinine.

Because the level of gastric acidity is relatively low during the first month of life and with advancing age (one-third of individuals aged sixty to sixty-nine years have achlorhydria), adequate blood levels of penicillin may follow oral administration of this antibiotic in these age groups.

The type of reaction to an antimicrobial agent is determined by age, in some instances. The livers of newborn babies produce only small quantities of glucuronyl transferase, the enzyme involved in the inactivation of chloramphenicol by conjugation with UDP glucuronic acid. Because of this, these children develop excessively high circulating levels of unconjugated biologically active drug which is toxic. This is responsible for the "gray syndrome" (abdominal distension, progressive pallor and cyanosis, vasomotor collapse, and death) which may appear when a dose in excess of 25 mg/kg/day is given. The immaturity of the acetylation process in the newborn liver also may expose babies to high blood levels of sulfonamides. Sulfisoxazole predisposes to the development of kernicterus when administered to very young infants. This drug competes effectively with bilirubin for binding sites on albumin and displaces the bile pigment. The central nervous system lesion is due to exposure to excessive concentrations of bilirubin. The teeth of young children may exhibit discoloration and enamel hypoplasia when treated with tetracycline compounds between the ages of two months and two years when the permanent dentition is undergoing calcification. Disturbances in bone growth may also be produced in youngsters receiving this group of antibiotics.

GENETIC FACTORS. The rate at which isonicotinic acid hydrazide is inactivated in the liver by conjugation with acetyl radical is genetically determined. About 50 percent of Americans are rapid inactivators; the other half are slow inactivators. This varies with race; about 95 percent of Eskimos are rapid inactivators. There is no good evidence that rapid acetylation of the drug is responsible for therapeutic failure when standard doses are employed. However, standard doses of the drug have been shown to produce toxic reactions to INH more often in persons who acetylate it slowly.

Acute hemolysis may develop in individuals given some antimicrobial compounds in the presence of glucose 6-phosphate dehydrogenase (G-6-PD) deficiency. Although common in Negro males, the defect may be expressed more actively in white people in whom the incidence is lower. The drugs which have provoked episodes of hemolytic anemia in such individuals are sulfanilamide, sulfacetamide, sulfamethoxypyridazine, sulfamethoxypyrimidine (Madribon), sulfisoxazole, chloramphenicol, salicylazosulfapyridine (Azulfidine), nitrofuration, and diaminodiphenyl sulfone (dapsone). Patients with hemoglobin Zurich and hemoglobin H may also develop hemolysis when given some of these agents.

PREGNANCY. Pregnancy imposes an increased risk of reactions to some antimicrobial agents on both the mother and the fetus. The drugs that cross the placental barrier include penicillin G, streptomycin, chloramphenicol, methicillin, oxacillin, ampicillin, cephalothin, sulfonamides, and tetracyclines. The embryo may be exposed to some degree of hearing loss when streptomycin is given to its mother. Sulfonamides and INH have produced fetal injury when administered during pregnancy. The tetracyclines pose a special danger to pregnant women. The developing teeth of the embryo may be injured if one of these compounds is given from midpregnancy on, the period when the crowns of the teeth are being formed. The pregnant patient with pyelonephritis who is treated with a tetracycline, especially if it is given intravenously in a dose of more than 2 Gm a day, may develop fatal hepatic toxicity. Pancreatitis also has been noted even when only 1 to 2 Gm per day is administered parenterally. These problems are greatest in the presence of significant renal insufficiency.

METABOLIC ABNORMALITIES. Penicillin G and sulfonamides are absorbed from intramuscular and subcutaneous sites to a lesser degree in persons with *diabetes mellitus* than in those who do not have this metabolic defect. This results in lower maximal serum concentrations than is the case in normal individuals. Poor response to treatment with vitamin B_{12} has been noted in patients with *pernicious anemia* and to iron administra-

tion in those with *iron-deficiency anemia* when they are receiving chloramphenicol simultaneously.

ATOPIC ALLERGY. Persons with a history of atopic allergy are highly susceptible to the development of hypersensitivity to antimicrobial agents whether or not they have been exposed to them previously (Chap. 73).

NERVOUS SYSTEM DISORDERS. Patients with either localized or diffuse central nervous system disease are more prone to the development of seizures than are normal individuals when treated with "massive" doses (40 to 80 million units per day) of penicillin G. These are more apt to occur when the antibiotic is administered as a continuous drip than when it is given as multiple single injections. Penetration of chloramphenicol into cerebrospinal fluid is impaired by the presence of hydrocephalus. Streptomycin, kanamycin, neomycin, polymyxin, and colistin may cause respiratory arrest in anesthetized patients, especially if they have received a muscle relaxant such as succinylcholine. This reaction also may occur in patients with myasthenia gravis and is a special problem in the presence of renal failure.

INDIGENOUS MICROBIAL FLORA. The organisms responsible for superinfections are, for the most part, members of the normal microbial flora that inhabit various areas of the body such as the intestinal and upper respiratory tracts. In some cases, the organisms are derived from the external environment and become part of the indigenous microflora. Exposure to antimicrobial agents allows the members of the bacterial population that are resistant to the drug being given to flourish and, in some instances, to produce disease. The normal microflora may condition response to treatment in special situations. Therapeutic failure or relapse of S. *pyogenes* pharyngitis treated with penicillin G may be due to the presence of penicillinase-producing S *aureus*, E. *coli*, Ps. *aeruginosa* or *Klebsiella* in the throat.

HEPATIC FUNCTION. Antimicrobial agents metabolized by, inactivated by, or concentrated in the liver may behave abnormally when administered to persons with impaired hepatic function. For example, blood levels of chloramphenicol are elevated in such patients, and toxic reactions may supervene. Persons with cirrhosis or chronic or convalescent hepatitis may develop untoward effects when given 2 Gm of tetracycline orally per day. The half-life of lincomycin is almost doubled in the presence of hepatic dysfunction. Antibiotics concentrated in the liver (methicillin, ampicillin, and nafcillin) may be absent or present only in reduced quantities in the bile in the face of hepatic disease. Erythromycin and novobiocin must be used with caution when liver dysfunction is a problem.

RENAL FUNCTION. Renal function is one of the most important determinants of response to antimicrobial agents. It not only is a major consideration in the choice of a drug, but also influences selection of dose and the risk of reactions involving the kidney and other organs. The extent to which elimination of an antibiotic is affected by the presence of kidney disease depends on whether it is cleared by this organ, the rate at which this is accomplished, clearance or inactivation by other mechanisms, and the degree of renal impairment. The drugs that are removed entirely by the kidney include penicillin, streptomycin, cephalothin, kanamycin, vancomycin, and polymyxin. The renal excretion of other commonly used agents is as follows: tetracycline, 20 to 60 percent; oxytetracycline, 10 to 35 percent; chlortetracycline, 10 to 15 percent after oral and 60 percent in 12 hr after intravenous administration. The clearance of demethylchlortetracycline is about one-half that of tetracycline. Some antibiotics are excreted in only low concentrations in the urine; erythromycin, 2 to 5 percent of an oral and 12 to 15 percent of an intravenous dose; lincomycin, 4 percent when the drug is given by mouth and 15 percent when it is administered parenterally. The kidney excretes 80 percent of para-aminosalicylic acid and 50 to 70 percent of isonicotinic acid hydrazide. Retention of oxacillin, methicillin, cephalothin, and colistimethate sodium occurs in the presence of decreased renal function. Chloramphenicol and erythromycin present no important problems in patients with impaired activity of the kidneys. Lincomycin, however, may produce elevated serum concentrations when renal disease is present. It is clear that antimicrobial agents excreted to a significant degree by the kidney must be given cautiously to patients with dysfunction of this organ and, in some cases, must be avoided completely. On the other hand, those drugs which are not handled by renal mechanisms may, with few exceptions, be given in conventional doses even when the kidneys are virtually functionless. A very important aspect of penicillin G therapy that is often overlooked and that may be responsible for serious difficulty and even death is the fact that most commercially available compounds are in the form of potassium salts. Extreme care must be exercised, therefore, in the use of this drug in the presence of renal impairment, particularly if hyperkalemia is present. It is important that the status of renal function be determined not only before but also during the entire period of treatment, if serious or even lethal effects are to be avoided when potentially toxic antibiotics, especially those which may injure the kidney, are administered. Even when BUN and creatinine are normal, older individuals may accumulate antibiotics and show toxic reactions if the agents are excreted mainly by the kidney.

HOST DEFENSE MECHANISMS. Probably the most important determinant of the therapeutic effectiveness of antimicrobial agents is the functional state of the defense mechanisms of the host. Both humoral and cellular phenomena are involved. Inadequacy of type, quantity and quality of the immunoglobulins (Chap. 70), alterations in delayed hypersensitivity, and ineffective phagocytosis, acting independently or in varying combination, may result in therapeutic failure despite use of a potent antibiotic to treat an infection produced by a highly sensitive organism. This may occur in Hodgkins' disease, lymphoma, leukemia, cancer of various types, uremia, vasculitis, and granulomatous disease of childhood, which are all disorders in which immunosuppression, abnormal activity of immunoglobulins, or inadequate phagocytosis are problems. In addition, some of the drugs commonly employed to treat these disorders (cytotoxic agents, antimetabolites, and corticosteroids) as well as to prevent rejection of transplanted organs, may add to the difficulty because they are immunosuppressive (Chap. 71).

That the normal activity of defense mechanisms is a requirement for the therapeutic effectiveness of all antimicrobial agents is frequently overlooked. The tetracyclines, sulfonamides, and chloramphenicol, which are all bacteriostatic, should, by definition, never completely eradicate sensitive organisms. However, *cure* of some infectious diseases is accomplished by these drugs, and relapse does not occur when treatment is stopped. This is strong evidence for the role of effective host defenses, which, acting on microorganisms after they have been injured by one of these compounds, are finally responsible for the eradication of infection. Clinical experience suggests that even bactericidal antibiotics probably require the adjunct activity of cellular and humoral defenses to dispose of bacteria.

THE PROPHYLAXIS OF INFECTION

The available chemotherapeutic agents offer an excellent means of prophylaxis in some but not all infectious diseases. Chemoprophylaxis has been used primarily for four purposes: (1) to protect healthy individuals, whether singly or in groups of varying size, against invasion by specific microorganisms; (2) to prevent bacterial infection in individuals acutely ill with diseases, often of viral origin, for which antimicrobial agents are not effective; (3) to reduce the risk of infection in patients with various types of chronic illness; and (4) to inhibit the spread of disease from areas of localized infection or to prevent infection, in general, in persons who have been subjected to accidental or surgical trauma. Experience has indicated the areas in which chemoprophylaxis is of value and those in which it is ineffective and may, in fact, increase the risk of infection. There still remain, however, instances in which opinion concerning the efficacy of antimicrobial agents in preventing bacterial invasion is unsettled. In general, when chemoprophylaxis is used to prevent implantation or to eradicate a single specific organism by the use of a single potent drug, it has had a high degree of success. If, on the other hand, the purpose is to prevent implantation of any or all bacteria that happen to be in the patient's internal or external environment, failure is the rule.

Table 135-1 lists the diseases or situations in which chemoprophylaxis is of proved or unsettled value and those in which experience has indicated lack of success. The antibiotics listed are not necessarily the ones recommended, but merely indicate that some success in preventing infection with them has been reported. In some instances, for example, shigellosis and meningococcal infections, many strains are resistant to sulfonamides, and prophylaxis with these agents is no longer effective. The dosage and methods of administration for each drug are discussed in the sections dealing with the specific diseases.

DANGERS OF CHEMOPROPHYLAXIS. It is important to point out that the same untoward effects that occur when

Table 135-1. VALUE OF CHEMOPROPHYLAXIS

I. Chemoprophylaxis of proved value
   A. Streptococcal (group A) infections and rheumatic fever recurrences: sulfonamides, various forms of penicillin, erythromycin
   B. Bacillary dysentery: sulfonamides, chloramphenicol, ampicillin
   C. Diarrhea due to enteropathogenic *E. coli:* neomycin orally
   D. Gonorrhea, acute urethritis, and ophthalmia: penicillin
   E. Congenital syphilis (treatment of mother): penicillin
   F. Meningococcal infections: sulfonamides in selected cases (Chap. 142)
   G. Dental extraction in presence of heart disease: penicillin, vancomycin
   H. Mucoviscidosis: tetracycline compounds
   I. Hepatic coma: neomycin or paromomycin orally
   J. Contaminated or infected wound surgery: penicillin plus streptomycin, ampicillin, tetracyclines
   K. Labor when membranes ruptured over 24 to 48 hr: penicillin plus streptomycin, ampicillin, tetracyclines
   L. Steroid therapy in patients with high risk of tuberculosis: tuberculostatic drugs

II. Chemoprophylaxis of no value
   A. Viral infections of upper respiratory tract including common cold, influenza, and rhinovirus, ECHO, Coxsackie, and adenovirus infections
   B. Childhood viral diseases: mumps, measles, rubella, chickenpox, vaccinia
   C. Poliomyelitis
   D. Infectious mononucleosis
   E. Smallpox
   F. "Clean" surgical and obstetric procedures
   G. Pertussis
   H. Burns
   I. Shock
   J. Coma
   K. Cardiac failure
   L. Catheterization or other instrumentation of urinary tract
   M. Premature infants
   N. X-ray irradiation
   O. Administration of steroids, except in instances with high risk of tuberculosis

III. Chemoprophylaxis of unsettled value
   A. Surgical procedures on heart or urinary tract in presence of valvular heart disease
   B. Acute diffuse glomerulonephritis
   C. Syphilis—venereal contact
   D. Chronic nontuberculous pulmonary disease
   E. Tuberculin-negative contacts of active case of tuberculosis
   F. Staphylococcus carrier state
   G. Transmission of *S. aureus* in nurseries and other hospital areas
   H. Reduction of number of intestinal bacteria before bowel resection
   I. Cardiac catheterization
   J. Exchange transfusion

antibiotic agents are used for therapeutic purposes are observed when patients who have no active infection are given these drugs. The risk of reactions as well as the cost of the drug must always be taken into consideration in planning a program of chemoprophylaxis. When there is no evidence that chemoprophylaxis will be effective, it should not be used.

SUPERINFECTIONS

These occur with all chemotherapeutic agents and are due to invasion by normal endogenous flora or by organisms acquired by contact with other patients or attendants. They may result from the accidental introduction of bacteria during injection of the drug; in all instances, the new infections are produced by strains of organisms insensitive to the antibiotic being administered at the time they first appear. Infections due to organisms of the genus *Candida (Monilia)* may also occur during chemotherapy; they may involve the mouth, pharynx, or lung, or they may spread systemically. This type of superinfection is being reported more frequently and is particularly important because systemic candidiosis is difficult to treat.

Superinfections occur in about 2 percent of patients who receive a chemotherapeutic agent. The organs involved in the secondary infection are most frequently those affected by the primary disease. The organisms responsible for superinfections are often difficult to treat with the presently available antibacterial drugs. The factors that predispose to the development of superinfection are (1) age of three years or less, (2) primary disease of the lower respiratory tract, (3) infection of the middle ear, and (4) the use of a drug or combination of antibiotic agents which tend to have a broad antibacterial effect; the wider the antimicrobial spectrum, the greater the danger of secondary bacterial invasion. Superinfections appear most frequently on the fourth or fifth day after initiation of chemotherapy and may convert a benign self-limited disease into a serious, prolonged, or even fatal one. It is essential to carry out frequent bacteriologic studies, whenever possible, to determine changes in bacterial flora that may subsequently be responsible for a secondary infection, and to treat this infection promptly when it appears (Chap. 133).

MISUSES OF CHEMOTHERAPY

There is little doubt that the antimicrobial agents are used in many situations in which they are not required and that, even when they are indicated, failure to utilize them properly may lead to poor clinical results. Listed below are the commonest misuses of the chemotherapeutic compounds.

1. Treatment of fever of obscure origin
2. Choice of ineffective antibiotic
3. Inadequate or excessive doses
4. Improper route of administration
5. Continuation of therapy with drug to which bacterial resistance develops
6. Failure to stop treatment in presence of serious toxic or allergic reaction
7. Failure to alter therapy when superinfection occurs

8. Prophylaxis of unpreventable secondary bacterial infection (see above)
9. Therapy of insusceptible infections—infections produced by true viruses
10. Use of combinations of drugs when not specifically indicated
11. Reliance on chemotherapy or prophylaxis to the exclusion of necessary surgical intervention, e.g., drainage of localized areas of infection

Probably the most frequent misuse of antimicrobial drugs is in the therapy of fever of unknown origin. The mere presence of fever, in the absence of localizing signs, does not necessarily indicate an infectious process (Chap. 16). In the absence of strong clinical evidence that a febrile episode is infectious in origin, particularly when there is no detectable focus, chemotherapy should be delayed until adequate clinical and laboratory studies have been performed.

REFERENCES

Abraham, E. P.: The Cephalosporins, Pharmacol. Rev., 14:473, 1962.

Anderson, K. N., R. P. Kennedy, J. J. Plorde, J. A. Shulman, and R. G. Petersdorf: Effectiveness of Ampicillin against Gram-negative Bacteria, J.A.M.A., 187:555, 1964.

Andriole, V. T., and H. M. Kravetz: The Use of Amphotericin B in Man, J.A.M.A., 180:269, 1962.

Chang, T. W., and L. Weinstein: A Comparison of the in Vitro and in Vivo Activity of Methacycline and Other Tetracycline Compounds, Antibiot. Chemotherap., 12:671, 1962.

Coles, H. M. T., B. McNamara, L. Mutch, R. J. Holt, and G. T. Stewart: Paromomycin in the Treatment of Shigella and Salmonella Infections in Children, Lancet, II:944, 1960.

Dowling, H. F.: "Tetracycline," New York, Medical Encyclopedia, Inc., 1955.

Feingold, D. S.: Antimicrobial Therapeutic Agents: The Nature of Their Action and Selective Toxicity, New Engl. J. Med., 269:900, 957, 1964.

Finland, M.: Chemoprophylaxis of Infectious Disease, Disease-a-Month, Chicago, Year Book Publishers, Inc., December, 1959, July, 1960, September, 1960.

——: The Symposium on Gentamicin, J. Infec. Dis., 119:537, 1969.

——and L. P. Garrod: Demethylchlortetracycline, Lancet, II:959, 1960.

—— and R. L. Nichols: Novobiocin, Practitioner, 179:84, 1957.

—— and L. Weinstein: Complications Induced by Antimicrobial Agents, New Engl. J. Med., 248:220, 1953.

Gale, E. F.: Mechanism of Antibiotic Action, Pharmacol. Rev., 15:481, 1963.

Gravenkemper, C. F., J. V. Bennett, J. L. Brodie and W. M. M. Kirby: Dicloxacillin: In Vitro and Pharmacologic Comparisons with Oxacillin and Cloxacillin, A.M.A. Arch. Intern. Med., 116:340, 1965.

Herrell, W. E.: "Erythromycin," New York, Medical Encyclopedia, Inc., 1955.

Hirsh, L. H., and L. E. Putman: "Penicillin," New York, Medical Encyclopedia, Inc., 1956.

Jawetz, E.: "Polymyxin, Neomycin, Bacitracin," New York, Medical Encyclopedia, Inc., 1956.

Kaplan, K., B. E. Reisberg, and L. Weinstein. Cephaloridine: Antimicrobial Activity and Pharmacologic Behavior, Am. J. Med. Sci., 253:667, 1967.

—— and L. Weinstein: Lincomycin, Pediat. Clin. N. Am., 15:131, 1968.

Klein, J. O., and M. Finland: The New Penicillins, New Engl. J. Med., 269:1019, 1963.

Kunin, C. M., and M. Finland: Restrictions Imposed on Antibiotic Therapy by Renal Failure, A.M.A. Arch. Intern. Med., 104:1030, 1959.

Lepper, M. H.: "Aureomycin (Chlortetracycline)," New York, Medical Encyclopedia, Inc., 1956.

Musselman, M. M.: "Terramycin (Oxytetracycline)," New York, Medical Encyclopedia, Inc., 1956.

Nord, N. M., and P. D. Hoeprich: Polymyxin B and Colistin: A Critical Comparison, New Engl. J. Med., 270:1030, 1964.

Place, V. A., and J. P. Thomas: Clinical Pharmacology of Ethambutol, Am. Rev. Resp. Dis., 87:901, 1963.

Richards, W. A., E. Riss, E. H. Kass, and M. Finland: Nitrofurantoin: Clinical and Laboratory Studies in Urinary Tract Infection, A.M.A. Arch. Intern. Med., 96:437, 1955.

Robson, J. F., and F. M. Sullivan: Antituberculous Drugs, Pharamacol. Rev., 15:169, 1963.

Utz, J. P.: Chemotherapeutic Agents for the Systemic Mycoses, New Engl. J. Med., 268:928, 1963.

Weinstein, L.: The Chemoprophylaxis of Infection, Ann. Intern. Med., 43:287, 1955.

——: A Clinical Evaluation of the Therapeutic Application of Antibiotic Combinations, Conn. State Med. J., 24:87, 1960.

——: Sulfonamides, Antibiotics and Other Antimicrobial Agents, in L. S. Goodman and A. Gilman (Eds.), "The Pharmacological Basis of Therapeutics," New York, The Macmillan Company, 1965.

—— and A. C. Dalton: Host Determinants of Response to Antimicrobial Agents, New Engl. J. Med., 279:467, 524, 580, 1968.

—— and N. J. Ehrenkranz: "Streptomycin and Dihydrostreptomycin," New York, Medical Encyclopedia, Inc., 1958.

——, M. Goldfield, and T. W. Chang: Infections Occurring during Chemotherapy: A Study of Their Frequency, Type and Predisposing Factors, New Engl. J. Med., 251:247, 1954.

——, K. Kaplan, and T. W. Chang: Treatment of Infections in Man with Cephalothin, J.A.M.A., 189:829, 1964.

——, M. A. Madoff, and C. M. Samet: The Sulfonamides, New Engl. J. Med., 263:793, 842, 900, 952, 1960.

——, C. A Samet, and R. H. Meade, III: Effect of Paromycin on the Bacterial Flora of the Human Intestine, J.A.M.A., 178:891, 1961.

Wolinsky, E.: Modern Drug Treatment of Mycobacterial Diseases, Med. Clin. N. Am., 47:1271, 1963.

Woodward, T. E., and C. L. Wisseman, Jr.: "Chloromycetin (Chloramphenicol)," New York, Medical Encyclopedia, Inc., 1958.

Section 2

Infections of Specific Tissues and Anatomic Sites

INTRODUCTION

Ivan L. Bennett, Jr.

It is traditional and convenient to classify bacterial diseases in terms of etiologic agents. This is adequate for those that follow more or less consistent patterns as do typhoid, anthrax, brucellosis, tularemia, or tetanus, but there are other important disorders that lend themselves poorly to this categorization. Because many microbial agents are able to invade and to localize in almost any tissue, they are not regularly associated with a single symptom complex. Furthermore, infection of an anatomic site such as the urinary tract or the meninges by any one of a wide variety of unrelated bacterial species produces essentially the same symptoms and clinical signs. Recognition of the basic pathologic process by the clinician is, in most instances, independent of microbiologic techniques, although specific identification of infecting bacteria is the basis for choosing the appropriate antimicrobial drugs.

In this section, many clinical entities are described. Several are more likely to be caused by certain microorganisms than others, but all can be produced by many species. Most of them can be recognized in their typical forms by history, physical examination, and clinical tests of blood and urine. Final identification of the infecting agent may depend on time-consuming bacteriologic tests, but a knowledge of the likely pathogens often enables the physician to initiate appropriate therapy before this information is available. Surgical drainage is an essential part of proper management for several of the disorders; indeed, surgery may be an emergency procedure for many of them, necessitated not by the species of the infecting organisms but by the anatomic location of the infection.

For these reasons, it seems logical to describe these diseases in terms of their manifestations in the patient. Cross references to other sections of the book have been given where specific causative organisms are mentioned or where descriptions of related entities have been included under an organ system. Pyelonephritis and cystitis are described in Chap. 303, and suppurative disorders of the central nervous system are covered in Chap. 360.

136 LOCALIZED INFECTIONS AND ABSCESSES

Ivan L. Bennett, Jr., and
Robert G. Petersdorf

Localized pyogenic infection can develop in any region or organ of the body, and may be initiated by *trauma* and secondary bacterial contamination, by some *alteration in local conditions* that renders a tissue susceptible to organisms already present as part of the "normal flora" to which it is ordinarily immune, by *contiguous spread* from a nearby lesion, or by *metastatic implantation* of microorganisms carried in blood or lymph.

The definitive treatment of many circumscribed infections, particularly if abscess formation occurs, is primarily surgical. Most often, however, infections are complications of diseases that are ordinarily cared for by the internist, and their treatment calls for careful integration of medical and surgical measures. It is important, therefore, to recognize the major types of localized suppurative disease and know something of the principles of their management.

ETIOLOGY. Under appropriate conditions of lowered tissue resistance, almost any of the common bacteria can initiate an infectious process. Cultures from open lesions such as those of the skin or from intraabdominal foci arising from perforations of the gastrointestinal tract frequently contain several bacterial species; as might be expected, the organisms found most frequently are the "normal flora" of these regions.

Infection in some areas is more likely to be caused by certain organisms (e.g., staphylococci in the skin and coliform bacteria in the urinary tract), and special features of the tissue reaction produced by some bacterial species make it possible to recognize infection by them with considerable accuracy. The *staphylococci* produce rapid necrosis and early suppuration with large amounts of creamy yellow pus (Chap. 139). Group A beta-hemolytic streptococcal infections (Chap. 140) tend to spread rapidly through tissues, causing intense edema and erythema but relatively little necrosis and thin, serum-like exudates; anaerobic streptococci (Chap. 141) and members of the *Bacteroides* group (Chap. 147) produce necrosis and profuse, brownish, foul-smelling pus. *Pseudomonas* infections (Chap. 146) are often rather indolent, and their thick, bluish green exudate is familiar to most clinicians; the *pneumococcus* (Chap. 138) stimulates the production of viscid greenish pus containing large plaques of fibrin and denatured protein.

The causative agents of many other diseases are capable of producing localized infection in tissues that are not usually involved in the specific "clinical entities" ascribed to them. Examples include the typhoid bacillus, *Corynebacterium diphtheriae* (cutaneous ulcers), the *brucellas*, and *Pasteurella tularensis*.

The identification of infecting organisms is important in the choice of local or systemic chemotherapy. However, when infection occurs in an area where there is constant exposure to the microflora, as in sputum, paranasal sinusitis, and cutaneous ulcers, it is unlikely that the site will ever become *sterile*, and serial cultures during therapy must be interpreted in the light of this knowledge.

PATHOGENESIS. Factors predisposing to the initiation and persistence of infection in a tissue include trauma, obstruction of normal drainage (sweat glands, biliary tract, bronchial tree, urinary tract), ischemia (infarction, gangrene), chemical irritants (gastric contents, bile, intramuscularly injected drugs), hematoma formation, accumulation of fluid (lymphatic obstruction, cardiac edema), foreign bodies (bullets, splinters, sutures), and others such as the occurrence of turbulence in the vascular system.

Infection in soft tissue usually begins as a *cellulitis*, a diffuse acute inflammation with hyperemia, edema, and leukocytic infiltration but little or no necrosis and suppuration. With some organisms, this is followed by necrosis, liquefaction, accumulation of leukocytes and debris, suppuration, loculation and walling off of the pus, and formation of one or more *abscesses*. Abscess formation is particularly likely to follow infection in a preexisting space or cavity, examples being the fallopian tubes, lung cysts, and renal pelvis (*pyonephrosis*).

The local spread of infection generally follows the path of least resistance along fascial planes; proper surgical treatment is based upon a knowledge of these routes, which will be described for specific infections later in this chapter. Lymphatic spread may lead to lymphangitis, lymphadenitis, or, if the regional nodes suppurate, to the formation of a *bubo*. Involvement of local venules or large veins may lead to infective thrombophlebitis with resulting bacteremia, septic embolization, and systemic dissemination of infection. Staphylococci, streptococci, and bacteroides are notorious for the frequency with which they produce vascular lesions of this type.

Depending upon the infecting organism and the anatomy of the affected region, a small abscess may subside completely, there may be gradual encapsulation of the accumulated pus and persistence of the focus in a quiescent state, or the lesion may "point" and rupture into adjacent tissues or to the outside surface of the body, as usually happens with furuncles. Spontaneous drainage ordinarily leads to subsidence and healing of a superficially situated suppurative focus. However, if the abscess is deeply situated and well encapsulated, there are often persistence of a fistulous tract and the formation of a chronic, draining sinus. *The development of persistent sinuses over an area of suppuration produced by ordinary pyogenic bacteria should always suggest involvement of underlying bone or the presence of a foreign body.* Fistulas that open onto the skin are, of course, soon colonized by microorganisms from the external environment. Ordinary bacterial cultures of drainage fluid almost invariably show a mixed flora and should never be relied upon for the etiologic diagnosis of the underlying disease. This is particularly important in disorders that characteristically lead to persistent sinus formation: tuberculosis, mycotic infection (actinomycosis,

blastomycosis), melioidosis, glanders, tularemia, and, rarely, amebic abscess of the liver or cecum.

THERAPEUTIC CONSIDERATIONS. Recognition of the striking symptomatic improvement that follows spontaneous evacuation of a suppurative focus led long ago to the adoption of *surgical incision* for the treatment of abscesses. The exact reasons for the amelioration of local and constitutional manifestations that results from drainage of pus are unknown, but, clinically, the benefits of adequate incision and drainage are unequivocal.

Incision of infected tissue before the stage of liquefaction and accumulation of pus is often deleterious and fails to relieve discomfort. Premature incision may even at times facilitate spread of infection. For this reason, it is sometimes necessary to wait until an abscess "ripens," i.e., localizes and "comes to a head." The *application of heat* to an area of inflammation will relieve pain and often speed the subsidence of cellulitis without suppuration. If necrosis of tissue is already under way, hot applications appear to facilitate localization of the process and accumulation of pus, making incision and drainage feasible at an earlier time. Another procedure that aids in reduction of swelling and relief of pain is *elevation of the affected part.*

The availability of specific chemotherapeutic drugs has modified the need for heat, elevation, and incision surprisingly little. The early administration of chemotherapeutics has reduced the incidence of suppurative complications in many disorders, but once suppuration has appeared, antimicrobial drugs become remarkably incapable of eradicating the infecting organisms, although they may mask the classical clinical features of abscess formation.

Antibiotics can be demonstrated in vitro to retain their antibacterial activity in the presence of pus and necrotic tissue, and failure of the drug to penetrate into an area of suppuration is rarely the reason for therapeutic failure. Although this possibility exists in some infections, such as osteomyelitis, it is usually overcome by increasing dosage. Because direct instillation of the antibiotic into an infected area is not, by itself, a curative procedure, other factors are probably more important than faulty diffusion of the agent into the focus. Nevertheless, in some infection such as empyema or pyarthrosis, and with some agents which provide poor tissue levels, such as the polymyxins, direct instillation of an antimicrobial into an area of suppuration is distinctly worthwhile.

The experiments of Eagle and Wood have shown clearly that an established inflammatory exudate is a relatively poor environment for bacterial multiplication. Because the bactericidal action of penicillin is exerted only against multiplying organisms, it is believed that failure of this antibiotic to eradicate bacteria in an abscess is related to their inactive metabolic state. Bacteriostatic agents such as tetracycline or chloramphenicol also are incapable of eradicating bacteria in the static phase of growth. Furthermore, by definition, these drugs are capable only of inhibiting multiplication of bacteria and usually exert no direct lethal action; the death of organisms in any infection treated with bacteriostatic agents is dependent on other mechanisms. For most pyogenic bacteria, phagocytosis is one of the most important of these mechanisms (although there must be others that have not been studied so carefully), and it is known that in the absence of phagocytes or in circumstances which inhibit their activity, bacteriostatic drugs are relatively ineffective. In fluid-filled cavities, particularly in the metabolically unfavorable milieu of an abscess, phagocytosis is greatly reduced. Consequently, despite inhibition of bacterial multiplication, organisms can remain dormant and survive for long periods of time. It is probably a combination of these two circumstances, decreased multiplication of bacteria and decreased phagocytosis, that makes infection on the heart valves, in the kidney, or in the meninges so relatively resistant to antimicrobial therapy. Large doses of bactericidal drugs for long periods are needed to achieve cure.

Antimicrobial drugs may be expected to prevent suppuration if given early or to prevent spread of an existing abscess, but cannot be substituted for surgical drainage. Indeed, their use in the face of a lesion requiring evacuation of pus is one of the most common serious errors in treating infections.

In empyema, suppurative pericarditis, or pyarthrosis, excellent therapeutic results are sometimes achieved by aspiration of pus and instillation of antibiotics into the infected area. The success of this procedure, however, is fully as dependent on the adequacy of drainage as it is upon the instillation of the antibiotic, and if there is loculation or the exudate becomes too viscid to allow removal, surgical incision becomes mandatory.

In the presence of infective thrombophlebitis, surgical interruption of the veins by ligation or, in certain instances, by total excision of an infected segment is often indicated to prevent seeding of other organs by infected emboli.

MANIFESTATIONS. Secondary infection of wounds and cutaneous ulcers is usually recognizable by inspection. Infections of the skin and subcutaneous tissues almost invariably produce the classic manifestations, *redness, tenderness, heat,* and *swelling*. Reddish streaks extending proximally and associated with tender enlargement of regional lymph nodes indicate lymphangitis. Systemic symptoms may be absent or mild, or there may be fever, malaise, prostration, and leukocytosis.

Infection and suppuration in deeper tissues or in body cavities are often manifested by local pain and tenderness, but the task of locating and determining the exact nature of the lesion may be difficult. The palpation of a tender mass is helpful, but muscle spasm and intervening structures often interfere. Abdominal or pelvic examination under anesthesia is sometimes useful in these circumstances.

Auscultation may reveal a friction rub over an abdominal viscus, the pleura, or the pericardium. The rapid development of an effusion in the pericardium, pleura, abdomen, or a joint should suggest infection. Similarly,

fluid detected by transillumination of paranasal sinuses or inspection of the tympanic membrane may be the first sign of infection.

Depending on the location of an abscess, symptoms and signs referable to encroachment upon adjacent structures may dominate the picture. Respiratory obstruction may be the first sign of mediastinal abscess; dysphagia often first calls attention to peritonsillar or retropharyngeal abscesses; and tamponade is sometimes the initial clue to pericardial infection. Localizing signs of dysfunction are especially striking and important with brain and spinal cord abscesses, although brain abscesses may be clinically silent (Chap. 360).

Local pain and tenderness or signs of dysfunction are mild or equivocal in some patients, and fever, prostration, and weight loss dominate the picture. The fever may be low-grade but is often hectic, with repeated rigors and drenching night sweats. Fatigue and anemia are frequent, and weight loss may be so rapid as to result in emaciation within a few weeks. A patient with these symptoms and signs may have chronic subphrenic, perinephric, or other abscess in the complete absence of any detectable physical sign pointing to the location of a large accumulation of pus.

Fluctuation of a mass on palpation is a reliable sign that it contains fluid, perhaps pus, but failure to detect this sign when deeper structures are examined is no guarantee that suppuration is absent and should not be taken by itself to indicate that the mass is noninfectious in origin or that drainage is not required.

LABORATORY FINDINGS. Peripheral polymorphonuclear leukocytosis is frequent with abscesses, and unexplained elevation of the white blood cell count in any patient should lead to a search for localized suppuration. Depending on the severity and duration of infection, there may be a chronic normocytic, normochromic anemia. Mild albuminuria, occasionally noted in febrile patients, has no diagnostic import.

Pus or fluid obtained by needle aspiration or incision of a suspected lesion should *always* be stained and examined directly in addition to being cultured aerobically and anaerobically. Pus is a poor metabolic substrate, and bacteria may fail to grow in cultures from an abscess of long standing. In such instances, the findings on microscopic examination may be the only guide in choosing proper chemotherapy. Failure to gram-stain exudates is the single greatest deterrent to appropriate antimicrobial therapy; it is the responsibility of the internist as well as the surgeon to see that this procedure is performed.

Blood cultures are often positive in intravascular infections such as endocarditis (Chap. 137), and in pyogenic infections in which localized abscesses are metastatic, as in staphylococcal, streptococcal, and salmonella bacteremias. Moreover, manipulation, including surgical incision, of any localized infection may be followed by transient bacteremia.

X-ray examinations are of great help in detecting localized collections of pus, primarily because they show atypical collections of gas, displacement of organs, and tissue densities in abnormal locations. Angiography of visceral organs and scintiscans using radioactive materials are also helpful in localizing abscesses.

CLINICAL FEATURES OF INFECTIONS IN VARIOUS REGIONS

The pathogenesis, diagnosis, and treatment of several important infections in specific anatomic sites and organs are discussed in detail in other parts of this book. These include lung abscess (Chap. 291), mediastinitis (Chap. 293), bacterial endocarditis (Chap. 137), pericarditis (Chap. 272), infections of the brain and spinal cord (Chap. 360), osteomyelitis (Chap. 139), pyelonephritis (Chap. 303), appendicitis and appendiceal abscess (Chap. 319), pyelophlebitis and hepatic abscess (Chap. 330), pancreatic abscess (Chap. 334), and diverticulitis (Chap. 320).

The remainder of this chapter is devoted to some features of dermal infection, chronic ulcerations, and a number of other regional infections.

Skin and Subcutaneous Tissues

Impetigo is a superficial infection caused by hemolytic staphylococci and group A hemolytic streptococci. It is primarily a disease of children, common in warm weather, characterized by multiple erythematous lesions which vesiculate and are intensely pruritic. Local spread occurs through scratching and release of infected vesicle fluid. Serious complications are metastatic abscesses and hemorrhagic nephritis. Treatment consists of local and general cleansing of the skin, application of bacitracin-neomycin ointment, covering with a loose dressing to prevent further contamination, and appropriate systemic antibiotics.

Deeper infections of the skin are almost invariably staphylococcal in origin and are described in Chap. 139. Erysipelas, a characteristic dermal lesion produced by group A streptococci, is described in Chap. 140.

Lymphadenitis with or without suppuration may complicate any pyogenic skin lesion and is often striking with superficial streptococcal infections. Specific diseases characterized by suppurative regional lymphadenitis include lymphogranuloma venereum (Chap. 229), cat-scratch disease (Chap. 230), tularemia (Chap. 155), and bubonic plague (Chap. 156).

Infections of the Hand

These are almost invariably secondary to trauma and are very common. Because of the rapidity with which infection can spread through the complex fascial spaces of the hand, wrist, and forearm, with the production of irreparable functional damage, *any deep infection in this area should receive expert surgical attention immediately.* The importance of such care has in no way been lessened by the availability of antibiotics.

The ordinary *paronychia,* or "run-around," is a superficial infection of the epithelium lateral to a nail, usually a result of tearing a "hangnail" and most frequently caused by the staphylococcus. Hot applications will lead to subsidence of paronychial cellulitis, but often a superficial blister of pus appears or the infection burrows beneath the nail to form a painful *subungual abscess.* Incision and drainage with partial or complete removal of the nail are then necessary. Recurrence is common, especially in nail biters, and this seemingly trivial infection can cause painful disability. Chronic paronychial inflammation produced by various fungi occurs in diabetics, and a similar lesion is seen in psoriasis and some types of pemphigus.

What appears to be a small furuncle of the webs of the fingers sometimes produces a *collar-button abscess,* consisting of a superficial and a deep compartment connected by a narrow tract. Evacuation of the shallow pocket without emptying the deeper abscess can lead to puzzling persistence of infection. Sometimes a foreign-body granuloma forms in the skin of the digital webs. This is most common in barbers, in whom a hair is the core of the foreign-body granuloma, the "barber's interdigital pilonidal sinus."

Infection of the distal phalanx of a finger, usually acquired by pinprick, thorn prick, etc., may lead to the formation of a *felon* or *whitlow.* This is a suppurative infection in the tightly enclosed fibrous compartments of the finger pulp (the "anterior closed space") which can compromise the distal blood supply by compression of the digital arteries, with consequent necrosis of bone and the development of osteomyelitis. The manifestations are swelling, extreme pain, and tenderness of the palmar surface of the finger tip. The treatment is immediate incision, using a lateral approach and cutting all the fibrous septums that radiate from the periosteum to the subcutaneous fascia.

Suppurative tenosynovitis, usually a complication of a puncture wound, is an even more serious infection of the hand from the point of view of functional damage; early diagnosis and treatment are mandatory to prevent permanent disability from destruction of the tendon or its sheath. The three cardinal manifestations of tenosynovitis are (1) exquisite tenderness limited to the course of the sheath; (2) the fingers held in flexion; and (3) extension of the involved finger, producing excruciating pain, most marked at the base of the digit. *Immediate incision* of the sheath is indicated, not only to prevent damage to the tendon itself but to avoid proximal extension of the process into the major fascial spaces of the hand or forearm. Vigorous antibiotic treatment should accompany surgery. The definitive treatment of any serious infection of the hand is a matter for a skilled surgeon, but the early recognition of the need for surgery often falls to other physicians.

Human bites are very important hand infections, which, if neglected almost invariably produce a highly destructive, necrotizing lesion contaminated by a mixture of aerobic and anaerobic organisms. A deliberately inflicted bite on the hand or elsewere is usually recognized as dangerously contaminated, but wounds on the knuckles produced by striking an opponent's teeth with the fists may not be recognized as potentially dangerous. In general, bite wounds should be cleaned thoroughly and not sutured. Patients should be given prophylaxis for tetanus and antibiotics, preferably a penicillinase-resistant penicillin.

Chronic Cutaneous Ulcers

A partial list of the causes of chronic ulcers of the skin includes circulatory disturbances such as varicose veins and obliterative arterial disease, extensive injury from frost bite or burns, trophic changes accompanying many neurologic disorders, bedsores, or decubiti, systemic diseases such as sicklemia and myxedema, neoplasms, and various infections. No matter what the underlying disease, secondary infection is very likely to occur and to interfere with healing, complicate grafting or other restorative procedures, or produce extension of the process.

The management of secondary bacterial infection in skin ulcers associated with obliterative arterial disease, a common problem in diabetics, is especially important, because infection is frequently the factor that precipitates spreading gangrene and makes amputation necessary.

Studies of the microflora of chronic cutaneous ulcers have almost invariably shown bacteria of many species, including staphylococci, aerobic and anaerobic streptococci, coliform bacilli, and members of the *Proteus* and *Pseudomonas* groups. Depending on the patient's environment and on systemically or locally administered antimicrobial drugs, the predominating bacterial species show great variation when lesions are cultured serially. Particularly noteworthy is the replacement of sensitive organisms by resistant strains or species during the course of chemotherapy.

Treatment of chronic dermal ulcers should be directed toward the underlying disorder but should also include *local debridement* and *chemotherapy*. Debridement by surgical excision is often needed, but the local application of proteolytic enzymes such as Varidase, a mixture of streptokinase and streptodornase, or trypsin, so-called "chemical or medical debridement," is sometimes sufficient. Intensive systemic administration of antibiotics should be carried out only in conjunction with definitive surgical procedures or when infection can be controlled in no other way, but the prevention of infection by "prophylactic" administration of antimicrobial drugs is futile because it results in the development of a flora resistant to the drugs being used. The *local application of antibiotics* is sometimes highly effective, and it is in the management of chronic mixed infections of this type that several potent but toxic antibiotics have great value. An ointment or solution containing neomycin, bacitracin, and polymyxin exerts a bactericidal effect against a wide variety of organisms and will sometimes temporarily sterilize a chronic lesion. Other useful topical medications are Furacin and 3 percent acetic acid, which is especially helpful in pseudomonas infections.

Diphtheritic ulcer of the skin is discussed in Chap. 169.

Infections of the Head and Neck

Pustules of the nose and upper lip may be particularly dangerous because they are likely to extend intracranially through the angular vein to the cavernous sinus. These lesions should be treated conservatively, manipulation or incision should be avoided if possible, and systemic antibiotics should be used if local swelling or redness appears.

Suppurative parotitis, which is usually a complication of chronic debilitating disease or blockage of Stensen's duct by a calculus, is largely avoidable by maintenance of hydration and oral hygiene. Its onset is heralded by local pain and swelling; fever and chills are frequent. Frank pus can sometimes be expressed from the duct, and the gland itself is firm and tender, often with pitting edema of the overlying skin and facial palsy. Most cases of suppurative parotitis are caused by hemolytic *Staphylococcus aureus.* Treatment consists of removal of obstructing calculi, but its mainstay is antimicrobial therapy with a penicillinase-resistant penicillin, cephalothin or vancomycin. Incision and drainage of a septate gland such as the parotid has not been particularly effective. Despite chemotherapy and drainage, the mortality rate of suppurative parotitis is 30 to 50 percent, perhaps because this infection occurs in patients with debilitating disease.

The use of penicillin and other antibiotics has reduced the incidence of many formerly common suppurative complications of streptococcal pharyngitis. However, as a result of streptococcal sore throat, bacteroides infections of the pharynx, or introduction of infection by trauma to the floor of the mouth or the pharyngeal wall, abscesses of the deep cervical structures still occur. *Suppurative cervical adenitis,* once an all-too-common sequel to streptococcal pharyngitis in children, is now rare. *Peritonsillar abscess,* or *quinsy,* is manifested by fever, sore throat, unilateral pain radiating to the ear on swallowing, and enlargement of the tonsil with redness and swelling of the adjacent soft palate. Treatment with penicillin and irrigations of warm saline solution sometimes lead to subsidence of the process, but if digital palpation reveals fluctuation, surgical drainage with or without tonsillectomy is indicated.

The course of *deep cervical infections* is fully as dependent upon the anatomic arrangement of fascial planes as is that of infections of the hand. Infection in this area is serious and is attended by fever, prostration, and leukocytosis. A tender mass may be palpated, but *surgical evacuation of such an infection should not be delayed because of failure to detect fluctuation,* which is usually absent because of the dense fascial layers.

Infection of the *sublingual space,* so-called "Ludwig's angina," is characterized by brawny induration of the submaxillary region, edema of the floor of the mouth, and elevation of the tongue. There are severe pain, dysphagia, and, within hours, dyspnea from respiratory obstruction. The usual causative organism is the streptococcus. Mortality was formerly about 50 percent. *Treatment* consists of large doses of penicillin and careful observation. If there is significant progression of obstruction during the 4 to 6 hr after treatment is instituted, wide incision is indicated and tracheostomy may need to be performed.

The retropharyngeal space lies between the muscles anterior to the cervical vertebrae and the pharyngeal mucosa. *Retropharyngeal abscess,* formerly common in children, is manifested by dysphagia, progressive stridor, pain, and fever. The bulging mass is easily seen and can completely occlude the airway within hours. Incision and drainage are mandatory; spontaneous rupture may lead to death by aspiration. Tuberculous abscess, secondary to spinal disease, occasionally appears in the retropharyngeal space; it is painless, and relief of obstruction follows surgical incision. Suppuration in the submastoid space, *Bezold's abscess,* is usually secondary to otitis and produces nuchal rigidity, which may lead to a mistaken diagnosis of otogenous meningitis. Infection can extend down the carotid sheath to the mediastinum. A suppurative thrombophlebitis of the jugular vein usually accompanies this infection, and the vessel is easily felt as a tender cord. Bacteremia and systemic spread of infection are common, and the involved venous segment may need to be excised. Spontaneous rupture of the carotid artery with rapid death from exsanguination is a rare complication.

Splenic Abscess

Splenic abscess occurs by several mechanisms: (1) dissemination via the bloodstream during bacteremia; primary foci include the endocardium, lung (lung abscess or pneumonia), pleural cavity (empyema), skin and soft tissues, ear and nasopharyngeal structures, and pelvis (pelvic inflammatory disease and septic abortion); (2) infection in a spleen damaged by bland infarcts (sickle-cell disease, leukemia) or more rarely other diseases such as malaria, typhoid, hydatid or dermoid cysts, and ameboma and trauma (following subcapsular hematoma formation); (3) extension from a perforated or diseased stomach, colon, or tail of the pancreas, as in carcinoma; and (4) rarely, without apparent cause. Onset is sudden, with chills, fever, and left upper quadrant pain. There are tenderness and muscle spasm, and the skin and subcutaneous tissues overlying the spleen may be edematous. Involvement of the upper pole commonly leads to left pleuritic pain, radiating to the shoulder, with elevation of the diaphragm or left pleural effusion. Lower pole abscess gives signs of tender splenomegaly and peritoneal inflammation. Splenic friction rub is often audible. Disorders to be considered in differential diagnosis are subphrenic abscess, infection of the left lung, bland infarction of the spleen, pancreatic pseudocyst, pyelonephritis, and abscess secondary to perforation of the transverse colon. X-ray examinations are an important adjunct in the diagnosis. Abnormal radiographic findings include (1) soft-tissue mass in left upper quadrant; (2) extraintestinal gas, which may occur even in the absence of gas-forming bacteria; (3) downward displacement of the splenic flexure of the colon; (4) inferior displacement of the left kidney, best visualized on an intravenous pyelogram; (5) displacement of the stomach bubble medially; (6) elevation of the left hemidiaphragm; and (7) left pleural effusion. Spleen scan is also of great value in localizing the mass.

Treatment consists of administering antibiotics and performing splenectomy. The splenic artery and vein should be ligated prior to splenectomy. Small or multiple abscesses during bacteremia may subside with antibiotics alone, and abscess in a very ill patient may require splenotomy and drainage, with more definitive surgery at a later time. Splenic abscess is particularly common in patients with sickle-cell disease, but splenic infarction in subacute bacterial endocarditis caused by *Streptococcus viridans* almost never suppurates. Infected splenic infarcts are a rare cause of continued bacteremia in the face of massive chemotherapy, and splenectomy may then be necessary to achieve the final eradication of the organism.

Subphrenic Abscess

Peritoneal infections show a striking tendency to localize the upper part of the abdomen between the transverse colon and the diaphragm. True subphrenic abscesses are located between the liver and diaphragm on the left or right; and many so-called subphrenic infections are, in fact, subhepatic. Most of these infections are related to perforations of a disease in the gastrointestinal or biliary tracts, and over half of them follow operations on the gallbladder, duodenum, or stomach. Subphrenic abscesses following perforated appendicitis occur rarely nowadays. Closed blunt trauma following laceration of the liver is an important cause, and a few abscesses occur without predisposing neighborhood infection. These may occur on the left and may be caused by *Salmonella.* The most common organisms are *Escherichia coli,* non-group A streptococci, and staphylococci; mixed infections are common. Most abscesses occur on the right and are more common in males and elderly patients, who often have a debilitating disease such as cancer. *Any patient with persistent fever and a history of recent intraabdominal sepsis should be suspected of having a subphrenic abscess.*

The *manifestations* include fever, upper quadrant pain, and tenderness, usually along the costal margin. Shoulder pain, dyspnea, dullness, and rales at the lung base are more common than abdominal signs and symptoms, and emphasize the location of a true abscess between the liver and the diaphragm. Foul sputum connotes perforation of the abscess into the lung. The localizing signs are by no means striking in all cases, however. The widespread practice of "covering" postoperative patients with antibiotics prophylactically can attenuate subphrenic infection without eradicating it, and may result in an insidiously progressive illness with weight loss and low-grade fever beginning weeks or months after a laparotomy. Roentgenograms may show gas, sometimes with an air-fluid level beneath the diaphragm. The gas is usually from a perforated viscus or enters through an external sinus; it is only rarely the result of bacterial multiplication.

Other radiographic findings include pleural effusion, which is usually sterile, basilar infiltrates, and elevation —but not necessarily fixation—of the diaphragm. Combined lung-liver scintiscan is a considerable advance in the diagnosis of subphrenic abscess. Pneumoperitoneum may be helpful occasionally.

The outlook in subphrenic abscess is poor because so many patients have cancer as an underlying cause. Even with surgical drainage, the mortality rate approaches 40 percent; without it, nearly 80 percent of patients die. Drainage should be extraperitoneal, usually through the bed of the twelfth rib. Appropriate antibiotics should be given, both locally and systemically.

Retroperitoneal Infections

Strictly speaking, all perinephric and many subphrenic abscesses are located outside the peritoneum, but the term *retroperitoneal abscess* usually refers to infection in the lumbar and iliac regions. Suppuration in these areas is relatively rare, but the importance of recognizing its existence in patients with fever and low-back pain is great. In one series, the average duration of illness in 65 patients before diagnosis was approximately 1 month.

Infection in the retroperitoneal space may arise as a complication of staphylococcal bacteremia, but more often it reflects extension from posterior perforations of the appendix or colon, renal or spinal infections, and suppurative lymphadenitis in the iliac area, usually secondary to streptococcal infections of the lower extremities in children.

In *lumbar abscess,* there are tenderness and spasm of the back muscles on the affected side, and a mass is usually palpable in the lumbar region, or there may be a prominent, tender abdominal mass without lumbar pain or spasm. Flexion of the hip (psoas sign) occurs in a few cases but is more often present with infections lower in the retroperitoneal area. *Fever, leukocytosis,* and *lumbar spasm* should suggest the diagnosis. The absence of a palpable mass may lead to protracted observation, and it is in these instances that palpation under anesthesia is often helpful.

In *iliac abscess,* there is abdominal pain in the iliac or inguinal region and, particularly when the psoas muscle is involved, severe pain may be referred to the hip, thigh, or knee. Careful palpation of the lower part of the abdomen usually reveals a mass, and fullness and tenderness on rectal examination are common. Hip spasm (psoas sign) is often present.

Roentgenograms may delineate the inflammatory mass; pyelography shows displacement of the kidney or ureter in some cases, and scoliosis with concavity on the side of the infection and blurring of the psoas shadow are also useful findings.

Treatment consists of surgical drainage and appropriate antibiotic therapy.

Renal Abscess

Single or multiple abscesses of the renal *cortex* are almost invariably the result of metastatic implantation of staphylococci from another focus. There is no relationship to previous renal disease; the infection occurs in younger individuals, is usually unilateral, and occurs on the right side oftener than on the left. Many patients give a history of recent skin infection such as furuncle. Although acute pyelonephritis is a diffuse disease with foci of cellular infiltrates in the interstitium of the renal medulla, these inflammatory foci may coalesce to form a distinct abscess cavity. This situation probably ensues more frequently than is generally appreciated.

The onset of renal abscess is abrupt, with chill and fever, followed by costovertebral pain and tenderness. If the abscess is cortical, the urine contains *no white blood cells;* medullary abscesses are usually accompanied by pyuria. The stained urinary sediment will show myriads of gram-positive cocci in cortical abscesses, and gram-negative organisms in medullary abscesses. Transient gross or microscopic hematuria may occur at the onset. The white blood cell count is usually elevated and may exceed 30,000 cells per cu mm. Physical signs are usually localized to the region of the kidney, but abdominal spasm may lead to confusion with appendicitis, cholecystitis, or pancreatitis. Early in the disease, ureteral calculus or acute hydronephrosis may be considered as possible diagnoses. Sudden onset of *fever, leukocytosis, and renal pain in the absence of pyuria* should suggest the diagnosis of kidney abscess, especially in a patient with infection elsewhere. Obstruction of the ureter by pus or cellular debris may also yield a urine sediment sparse in white blood cells and bacteria. *Treatment* consists of appropriate antibiotics, adequate fluids, and relief of pain. An abscess may suddenly discharge into the renal pelvis, with relief of pain and the passage of cloudy urine containing enormous numbers of leukocytes and bacteria. *Complications* include formation of a thick-walled chronic renal "carbuncle," requiring surgical removal, rupture into the perirenal space, and secondary pyelonephritis, usually produced by coliform bacilli. Recovery is ordinarily prompt, and chronic sequelae are rare.

In the past, *perinephric abscess* was most often due to hematogenous dissemination during streptococcal or staphylococcal infection, but at present it more often follows calculi in the ureter and hydronephroses, noncalculous renal infection, tuberculosis, and actinomycosis. Diabetics are particularly susceptible. The causative organisms are those which are primarily responsible in acute pyelonephritis—*E. coli, Proteus* species, and *Klebsiella aerogenes.* Flank pain with radiation to the upper part of the abdomen, back, or even the shoulder, nausea, vomiting, fever, malaise, leukocytosis, tenderness with spasm of flank and upper abdominal muscles, and a palpable mass which moves with respiration are the main manifestations. Symptoms referable to the urinary tract are present when perinephric abscess is associated with pyelonephritis or stone. In a few patients, elevation of the diaphragm on the diseased side occurs and leads to confusion with subphrenic infection. The psoas muscle is involved by the inflammatory process, and patients are frequently more comfortable with the thigh held in flexion. The roentgenogram occasionally will reveal a mass; there is usually blurring of the kidney silhouette; and the psoas shadow is indistinct on the involved side. There may also be scoliosis to the side of the lesion, fixation of the kidney, anterior displacement of the organ on lateral pyelograms, and gas formation within the perinephric mass, or total nonvisualization of the kidney. Chest roentgenograms often show basal infiltrates and pleural effusions. Complications include perforation into adjacent organs, particularly the colon. *Treatment* by surgical drainage and systemic administration of antibiotics (*not* urinary antiseptics) is usually followed by dramatic subsidence of pain and fever, and unless intrinsic renal disease is present, recovery is complete. Nevertheless, the overall outcome is poor, in part because the diagnosis is often made too late or is missed altogether, and also because of the generally poor condition of many of these patients.

Rectal Abscess

Suppurations of the anorectal region have been classified anatomically in several ways, most of the classifications being based on the surgical approaches required for drainage. Infection in the apocrine glands (hidradenitis) or folliculitis in the perianal region, extension of cryptitis or obstructions in the "anal glands" which open into the crypts of Morgagni, and contamination of submucosal hematomas, sclerosed hemorrhoids, or anal fissures may lead to abscess formation. These are usually painful, easily palpable, often visible on inspection. Superficial rectal abscesses also may be confused with Bartholin's cysts, sebaceous cysts, tuberculosis, actinomycosis, urethroperineal fistulas, carcinoma of the anus, foreign body, and pilonidal sinus. Treatment is application of heat and appropriate drainage or excision. Antibiotics may be indicated in some instances.

Difficulties in diagnosis are more likely to arise with infections higher in the rectum, especially those above the pelvic diaphragm, the so-called *supralevator abscess.* Patients with this type of infection often have fever, malaise, and leukocytosis for several days or even weeks before any symptoms referable to the rectum develop. There is vague pelvic discomfort, relieved by defecation, and constipation punctuated by short episodes of diarrhea is common. In males, the inflammation often involves the base of the bladder, and urinary urgency or retention is not infrequent, falsely centering attention on the urinary tract as the source of fever and malaise. Eventually, the abscess produces severe pain, chills, and fever; palpation and instrumentation will reveal the swelling in the rectal ampulla. Such an abscess may surround the rectum and produce narrowing that is differentiated from that caused by neoplasm by the fact that the mucosa remains intact. A useful sign of deep rectal abscess is eliciting of severe pain by pressure in the region between the anus and the coccyx. The supralevator space is continuous with the ischiorectal space, with both the gluteal and obturator regions, and with the retroperitoneal space. In neglected cases, the abscess may drain through the skin of the perineum, the groin, or the buttock or may extend as high as the perirenal areas. Rectal abscesses are not uncommon in patients with diabetes, and infections in this area are also peculiarly frequent in patients with monocytic leukemia. Because the clinical picture may be that of "fever of unknown origin" for a long period, it is important that thorough digital and endoscopic examination of the rectum be carried out in febrile patients. A rectal examination should be made in all patients with diabetes, especially if ketosis is present; failure to observe this rule has more than once led to delay in detecting the infection responsible for diabetic ketosis or coma.

Rectal abscesses may be a forerunner of both ulcerative colitis and regional enteritis, and may occur months and even years before other overt manifestations of these diseases. For this reason, proctosigmoidoscopy, barium enema, and, often upper gastrointestinal roentgenograms, are indicated in nonhealing rectal lesions.

Treatment of high rectal abscesses consists of incision and drainage, hot sitz baths, analgesics, and antibiotics as indicated by culture of the exudate.

REFERENCES

General

Bunnell, S.: "Surgery of the Hand," 4th ed., T. H. Boyes (Ed.), Philadelphia, J. B. Lippincott Company, 1964.

Eagle, H.: Experimental Approach to the Problem of Treatment Failure with Penicillin: I. Group A Streptococcal Infection in Mice, Am. J. Med., 13:389, 1952.

Plorde, J. J., D. Hovland, M. Garcia, and R. G. Petersdorf: Studies on the Pathogenesis of Meningitis: V. Action of Penicillin in Experimental Pneumococcal Meningitis, J. Lab. Clin. Med., 65:71, 1965.

Smith, M. R., and W. B. Wood, Jr.: An Experimental Analysis of the Curative Action of Penicillin in Acute Bacterial Infections: III. The Effect of Suppuration upon the Antibacterial Action of the Drug, J. Exp. Med., 103:509, 1956.

Specific Infections

Barnhill, J. F.: Deep Abscess of the Neck: Surgical Treatment, Am. J. Surg., 42:207, 1938.

Burger, R. H., J. N. Ward, and J. W. Draper: Perinephric Abscess with Gas Formation, Am. Surgeon, 30:302, 1964.

Curreri, W. P., J. A. Coller, and H. MacVaugh, III: Subphrenic Abscess Secondary to Salmonellosis, Arch. Surg., 95:189, 1967.

Eisenhammer, S.: The Internal Anal Sphincter and the Anorectal Abscess, Surg. Gynecol. Obstet., 103:501, 1956.

Frankel, A., H. Ashikari, D. A. Dreiling, and A. E. Kark: Splenic Abscess, J. Mt. Sinai Hosp., 33:404, 1966.

Gaston, E. A., and L. O. Warren: Supralevator Abscess, New Engl. J. Med., 229:613, 1943.

Janke, W. H., and M. A. Block: Chronic Retroperitoneal Pelvic Abscesses, Arch. Surg., 90:389, 1965.

Magilligan, D. J., Jr.: Suprahepatic Abscess, Arch. Surg., 96:14, 1968.

Neuhof, H., and E. E. Arnheim: Acute Retroperitoneal Abscess and Phlegmon: A Study of Sixty-five Cases, Ann. Surg., 119:741, 1944.

Ozeran, R. S.: Subdiaphragmatic Abscess, Am. Surgeon, 33:64, 1967.

Petersdorf, R. G., B. A. Forsythe, and A. D. Bernanke: Staphylococcal Parotitis, New Engl. J. Med., 259:1259, 1958.

Richards, L.: Retropharyngeal Abscess, New Engl. J. Med., 215:1120, 1936.

Salvatierra, O., Jr., W. B. Bucklew, and J. W. Morrow: Perinephric Abscess, J. Urol., 98:296, 1967.

Vicher, E. E., J. W. Soska, and G. G. Jackson: Microbiologic Flora of Chronic Cutaneous Ulcers: In Vitro Sensitivity of Microbiologic Flora to Three Antibiotics—Penicillin, Streptomycin, and Bacitracin, A.M.A. Arch. Surg., 66:283, 1953.

137 BACTERIAL ENDOCARDITIS

Leighton E. Cluff and F. Robert Fekety

DEFINITION. Bacterial endocarditis is a microbial infection of the heart valves or of the endocardium in proximity to congenital or acquired cardiac defects. A similar clinical illness develops when there is infection of arteriovenous fistulas or aneurysms. The infection may develop abruptly or insidiously, may pursue a fulminant or prolonged course, and is fatal unless treated. The infection caused by indigenous microorganisms with low pathogenicity is ordinarily subacute, whereas infection by microorganisms with high pathogenicity is often acute. Fever, cardiac murmurs, splenomegaly, anemia, hematuria, mucocutaneous petechiae, and embolic manifestations are characteristic of the disease. *Streptococcus viridans* is the commonest cause of bacterial endocarditis when superimposed upon congenital or acquired endocardial lesions and usually is associated with a subacute course.

ETIOLOGY AND EPIDEMIOLOGY. *Acute bacterial endocarditis* is caused by relatively pathogenic microorganisms, exemplified by *Staphylococcus aureus*, pneumococcus, group A streptococcus, gonococcus, and less often *Histoplasma capsulatum*, *Brucella*, and *Listeria*. Endocarditis attributed to these organisms usually follows dissemination from an infected focus, which is often insignificant. Gonococcal, staphylococcal, and monilial endocarditis has been described frequently in narcotic addicts. Staphylococcal, monilial, and coliform bacilli infection of the heart resembling endocarditis has become a serious complication of surgery in which sutures or prostheses are placed in the heart or peripheral arteries. Endocarditis is sometimes observed in association with pneumococcal meningitis and bacteremia (Chap. 138). Staphylococcal endocarditis can result from bacteremia associated with septic thrombophlebitis or complicating a cutaneous, bone, or pulmonary infection. Group A streptococcal endocarditis is probably never a complication of septic sore throat, but it may follow the bacteremia of streptococcal skin or puerperal infection.

Subacute bacterial endocarditis develops usually in persons with acquired valvular or congenital cardiac lesions. It is most commonly caused by S. *viridans*, which is part of the normal upper respiratory bacterial flora. *Streptococcus faecalis* (enterococcus), indigenous to the fecal and perineal flora, is also an important cause of subacute bacterial endocarditis, particularly in elderly men, and often occurs in association with prostatism or other genitourinary conditions. *Staphylococcus aureus* may produce subacute as well as acute bacterial endocarditis. Suppuration, cellulitis, or other infected foci may precede subacute bacterial endocarditis but are recognized infrequently. *Streptococcus viridans* is commonly found in the blood immediately after dental extractions. Tonsillectomy is also occasionally associated with transient bacteremia. Chewing of food may result in bacteremia in patients with gingival disease or dental infection. Transient bacteremia of this sort is probably an important initiating factor in subacute bacterial endocarditis.

PATHOGENESIS. Subacute bacterial endocarditis occurs most frequently in persons with preexisting heart disease in the absence of congestive cardiac failure or chronic atrial fibrillation. Valvular stenosis without insufficiency is infrequently associated with bacterial endocarditis. Infection most commonly involves the left side of the heart. The mitral valve, aortic valve, pulmonary valve, and tricuspid valve may be involved, in the order of frequency as listed. Valves damaged by rheumatic fever are most commonly involved, but valves damaged by syphilis and arteriosclerosis are also susceptible to bacterial endocarditis. Enterococcal endocarditis in elderly men is associated with involvement of the aortic valve, and frequently results rapidly in marked valvular damage. Subacute bacterial endocarditis rarely involves interatrial septal defects. Infection in patients with interventricular septal defects often involves the endocardium opposite the septal defect in the direction of the shunt. Infection associated with patent ductus arteriosus develops in the pulmonary side of the ductus when the shunt is from the aorta to the pulmonary artery, but is on the aortic side of the ductus when the shunt is reversed. Valvular infection in association with rheumatic heart disease is usually on the valve edge along the line of closure.

Hemodynamic events are important in the pathogenesis of the disease. Alterations in blood flow can cause marked changes in vascular endothelium. It has been demonstrated experimentally that bacteria are deposited on the endothelium in areas of high flow with decreased lateral pressure. These factors are undoubtedly important in determining the situations and location where bacterial endocarditis develops. Infection in the heart is most often at a site of a structural change or abnormality. Thrombi developing on endocardial irregularities have been implicated as foci for bacterial implantation, and infection has been shown in thrombotic endocardial lesions. It seems unlikely, however, that endocardial thrombi are commonly involved in the pathogenesis of bacterial endocarditis, except as a feature of the infection.

Serum antibody in high titer against the infecting microorganism is often found in patients with bacterial endocarditis. Pneumococci found in the blood during pneumococcal endocarditis usually show pronounced capsular swelling attributable to serum antibody and intravenous injection of pneumococci into hyperimmunized horses can result in bacterial endocarditis. Immunity to the bacteria may facilitate localization of infection in the endocardium, but whether this mechanism plays a role in bacterial endocarditis of man is not known.

Bacterial endocarditis leads to deposition of fibrin and platelets at the site of infection, producing a *vegetation*. Highly pathogenic microorganisms often cause valvular destruction and ulceration. Less pathogenic microorganisms usually cause less valvular destruction or ulceration but can lead to development of large polypoid vegetations. The infection may extend from the valve to the mural endocardium. Involvement of chordae tendineae may lead to rupture and profound valvular insufficiency. Acute bacterial endocarditis, particularly when caused by S. *aureus*, often is associated with abscesses in the valve ring. Vascularization of involved valves may increase during endocarditis but rarely extends into the area of infection. Phagocytes are not prominent in the area of bacterial growth, which may explain why infection by microorganisms of low pathogenicity progresses uncontrolled without bactericidal antimicrobial therapy. The lack of vascularization of the granulation tissue in the vegetation also may account for ineffectiveness of host defenses and the requirement for intensive and prolonged treatment of the infection.

The bacteremia of bacterial endocarditis is ordinarily continuous. For this reason very few blood cultures are required to demonstrate the microorganisms. The microorganisms are primarily cleared from the blood by the reticuloendothelial cells of liver and spleen. There is no obvious reduction in the number of bacteria in the blood during circulation through the extremities. Arterial blood cultures, therefore, are no more likely to show bacteremia than are venous blood cultures.

Embolization is a characteristic feature of bacterial endocarditis. The friable fibrin vegetations may separate from the site of infection and be propelled as emboli into the systemic or pulmonary circulation, depending on whether the endocarditis involves the left or right side of the heart. Emboli vary in size but may involve the brain, spleen, kidney, gastrointestinal tract, or extremities. Pulmonary infarction is common in right-sided endocarditis. Septic infarction is uncommon in subacute bacterial endocarditis caused by microorganisms of low pathogenicity, and suppurative complications are rarely seen at these sites when S. *viridans* is the offending agent. Osteomyelitis has been described, however, as an embolic complication of endocarditis due to S. *viridans* and enterococci. Septic infarction is common in acute bacterial endocarditis attributable to bacteria of high pathogenicity as are metastatic abscesses. Involvement of vasa vasorum in major arteries by emboli produces mycotic aneurysms, which may rupture. Myocardial infarction may develop after coronary embolization. In addition, focal myocarditis is common in subacute bacterial endocarditis and may be embolic.

The spleen is almost always enlarged, particularly in subacute cases. Three types of renal lesions may be produced. When large emboli find their way into the kidney, infarction may develop. Smaller emboli may produce a focal glomerulitis. In some instances there is a diffuse glomerulonephritis that is difficult to distinguish from that seen after streptococcal infection. Petechial skin lesions, characterized histologically by acute vasculitis, are probably not embolic and may be immunologic in origin. Other skin lesions associated with pain, tenderness, and cellulitis, however, may be embolic.

MANIFESTATIONS. Subacute Bacterial Endocarditis. Patients ordinarily cannot date the onset of the infection. Symptoms begin insidiously, and gradually the illness becomes apparent. In some individuals, however, the onset of infection can be related to a recent dental extraction, urethral instrumentation, tonsillectomy, acute respiratory infection, or abortion.

Weakness, fatigability, weight loss, feverishness, night sweats, anorexia, and arthralgia are the usual symptoms of subacute bacterial endocarditis. Emboli may produce paralysis, chest pain, acute vascular insufficiency with pain in the extremities, hematuria, acute abdominal pain, or sudden blindness. Painful fingers or toes and painful skin lesions may also be important symptoms. Chills are not common.

Physical examination may reveal a variety of findings, none of which alone is pathognomonic of subacute bacterial endocarditis. The association of the different manifestations, however, usually provides a characteristic picture of the disease. The patient usually appears chronically ill and pale and has an elevated temperature. The fever is most often remittent, with afternoon or evening peaks. The pulse is usually rapid, and if cardiac failure complicates the infection, it may be greater than expected with the degree of fever.

Mucocutaneous lesions are common and vary in type. Petechiae are most frequent and may be found in the mucosa of the mouth, pharynx, or conjunctivas. These small red hemorrhagic-appearing lesions do not blanch

Fig. 137-1. White-centered conjunctival petechia in a patient with subacute bacterial endocarditis. (*Courtesy Dr. John Wedgwood, Cambridge, England.*)

on pressure and are not tender or painful. On the mucous membranes or conjunctivas these petechiae may have a pale center (Fig. 137-1). Small, occasionally flame-shaped, hemorrhages are found in the retina, and may also have pale centers (*Roth's spots*). Petechiae may be found anywhere on the skin and are frequently difficult to distinguish from angiomas, but they gradually become brownish and disappear. Frequently, petechiae continue to appear, even during convalescence. Linear hemorrhages (splinter hemorrhages) may be found under the nails, but these are difficult to differentiate from traumatic lesions, particularly in manual laborers. These muco-cutaneous lesions are not specific for bacterial endocarditis but may be found in patients with other diseases such as profound anemia, leukemia, trichinosis, and sepsis without endocarditis.

The pulp of the fingers may show tender subcutaneous papules which are purplish or erythematous (*Osler's nodes*). Larger erythematous, painful, and tender nodules may develop on the palms of the hands or soles of the feet. These are probably embolic lesions. Emboli to larger peripheral arteries may result in gangrene of fingers, toes, or larger portions of the extremities.

Clubbing of the fingers is uncommon but is observed in long-standing or prolonged bacterial endocarditis. Mild jaundice is found occasionally.

Findings in the heart are usually those of the underlying heart disease. Major changes in cardiac murmurs may be attributable to ulceration of a valve, dilatation of the heart or valve ring, rupture of chordae tendineae, or development of a very large vegetation. In rare instances, no cardiac murmurs are detected. In this situation, right-sided endocarditis or an infected pulmonary or peripheral arteriovenous fistula should be suspected.

Splenomegaly is common in subacute bacterial endocarditis. Rarely is the spleen tender, but a friction rub may be heard over it when there is infarction. Hepatomegaly is not characteristic unless heart failure develops.

Arthralgia is relatively common, and arthritis resembling acute rheumatic fever may occur.

Embolic phenomena may precipitate awareness of the infection. Sudden development of hemiplegia, flank pain with hematuria, abdominal pain with melena, pleuritic pain and hemoptysis, left upper abdominal pain with splenic friction rub, blindness, or monoplegia in a patient with fever and cardiac murmurs makes bacterial endocarditis suspect. Pulmonary emboli in right-sided endocarditis may be confused with pneumonia.

Acute Bacterial Endocarditis. Infectious endocarditis caused by highly pathogenic microorganisms usually begins abruptly. Suppurative infection commonly antedates the onset of endocarditis. For example, infection of the heart may develop as a complication of pneumococcal meningitis, septic thrombophlebitis, group A streptococcal cellulitis, or staphylococcal abscesses. The source of cardiovascular infection, therefore, is often evident.

Acute bacterial endocarditis often involves the normal heart, in contrast to the subacute infection, which almost invariably involves the abnormal heart. The acute infection is fulminant and pursues a rapid course. Fever is

often greater, may be intermittent, and in certain instances (as in gonococcal endocarditis) may be characterized by a double quotidian temperature curve. Chills are common. Petechiae may be numerous, and embolic phenomena are prominent. Osler's nodes and painful erythematous nodules of palms and soles are uncommon. Hematuria is seen with embolic lesions of the kidney, but diffuse glomerulonephritis is less common than in subacute bacterial endocarditis. Destruction of the cardiac valves can be complicated by rupture of chordae tendineae or perforation of cusps, leading to rapidly progressing cardiac failure. Metastatic abscesses are frequent following septic emboli.

Because of the abrupt onset of acute bacterial endocarditis, anemia and weight loss are absent when the illness is first recognized. These changes, however, develop rapidly.

LABORATORY FINDINGS. Leukocytosis with neutrophilia is the rule but is by no means an invariable finding. Macrophages (histiocytes) may be found in the blood, particularly in the first drop of blood obtained from the earlobe. Normocytic, normochromic anemia is almost always found in subacute bacterial endocarditis, but it may not be present early in acute bacterial endocarditis. The erythrocyte sedimentation rate is increased, and the C-reactive protein test is markedly positive. Serum immunoglobulins are increased but return to normal during convalescence. The anti-gamma-globulin latex fixation test is commonly positive, and the Rose-Waaler test is negative. The thymol turbidity and cephalin flocculation tests are usually abnormal, and mild bilirubinemia is detected occasionally. Proteinuria is common, and microscopic hematuria is frequent.

Blood cultures are positive in the majority (85 percent) of cases. Three to five cultures of 10 ml blood taken at short or long intervals, depending on the patient's clinical status, are usually adequate to demonstrate the bacteremia, if it is demonstrable at all. Blood cultures may not become positive for seven or more days, however, in patients who have been receiving penicillin prophylactically for rheumatic heart disease. Similarly, the cultures may be temporarily negative or growth may be delayed in patients who have received antibiotics prior to the time when cultures are obtained. Failure to demonstrate bacteremia also may be attributable to infection by an unusual microorganism such as *H. capsulatum, Brucella,* or anaerobic streptococci which require special nutrient media or culture methods. Endocarditis of the right side of the heart seems to be as likely to produce bacteremia as endocarditis involving the left side of the heart.

DIFFERENTIAL DIAGNOSIS. When several of the manifestations of bacterial endocarditis occur together, the diagnosis is not difficult. In particular, the presence of fever, petechiae, splenomegaly, microscopic hematuria, and anemia in a patient with cardiac murmurs is most suggestive of the cardiovascular infection. When few manifestations are present, however, the diagnosis is not simple. Prolonged fever in the patient with rheumatic heart disease is particularly troublesome, but the diagnosis of bacterial endocarditis should be considered in every patient with fever and a heart murmur. The diagnosis becomes even more difficult when blood cultures show no growth.

Acute rheumatic fever with carditis is often difficult to distinguish from bacterial endocarditis, and in a few instances, active rheumatic fever has been found to coexist with the valvular infection. The diagnosis of rheumatic carditis hinges on a combination of clinical and laboratory criteria (Chap. 269).

Subacute bacterial endocarditis is a common cause of "fever of undetermined origin" (Chap. 16). It may be mistaken for a hidden neoplasm, systemic lupus erythematosus, periarteritis nodosa, poststreptococcal glomerulonephiritis, and intracardiac tumors such as myxoma of the atrium. Dissecting aneurysms with acute aortic insufficiency also may mimic bacterial endocarditis. Drug fever may be erroneously diagnosed as bacterial endocarditis.

Development of fever, anemia, and leukocytosis after cardiovascular surgery may indicate development of intracardiac infection about a suture or prosthesis. This infection is identical to that of bacterial endocarditis but usually cannot be controlled unless the foreign body is removed. In these postoperative patients, the various postthoracotomy and postcardiotomy syndromes must also be considered.

PROGNOSIS. Recovery from untreated bacterial endocarditis is rare. With appropriate antibiotic therapy, however, over 70 percent of patients survive the infection. The infection has a poor prognosis when complicated by congestive heart failure, when unassociated with demonstrable bacteremia, when produced by antibiotic-resistant microorganisms, or when therapy is delayed. Acute bacterial endocarditis is associated with the poorest prognosis.

The commonest cause of death in treated endocarditis is congestive heart failure, attributable either to valve destruction or myocardial damage. Additionally, death may be precipitated by embolization to vital organs, by renal insufficiency, or by rupture of a mycotic aneurysm. Many patients recover completely without apparent worsening of the underlying cardiovascular disease. When recurrent endocarditis develops, it usually involves the same valve and is due to failure to kill microorganisms in an environment of suboptimal host resistance.

PROPHYLAXIS. Patients with congenital, syphilitic, arteriosclerotic, and rheumatic valvular heart disease should be given antibiotics before and immediately after dental manipulation, urethral catheterization, or other forms of intubation. Procaine penicillin G, in a dosage of 600,000 units 1 hr before dental manipulation and 12 and 24 hr later, is preferred, although erythromycin, tetracycline, and other antibiotics may be used to prevent infection by S. viridans. Penicillin in the same dosage plus streptomycin (1.0 Gm), or ampicillin, might be used similarly before and after urethral or pelvic manipulation so as to prevent infection by S. faecalis. *The prophylactic doses of penicillin used to prevent group A streptococcal infection and recurrent rheumatic fever will not prevent*

bacterial endocarditis. Furthermore, these doses of penicillin (200,000 units once or twice daily) do not predispose to bacterial endocarditis caused by penicillin-resistant microorganisms.

TREATMENT. Successful therapy of bacterial endocarditis is assured when treatment is begun early in the illness, when an effective *bactericidal* antimicrobial is selected, and when treatment is continued over a long period of time.

Selection of the most effective antibiotic for treatment of bacterial endocarditis depends on the sensitivity of the infecting microorganism. When bacteremia is not demonstrated, selection of the therapeutic agent depends on understanding the probable infecting bacteria and their probable antibiotic sensitivity.

Administration of penicillin G in dosage of 12 to 20 million units per day plus streptomycin 1.0 Gm daily is the treatment of choice in most instances, and should be continued for at least 4 weeks.

Bacterial endocarditis in young persons with rheumatic or congenital heart disease is most often due to S. viridans. These microorganisms are usually very sensitive to penicillin G. Administration of 2.4 to 6 million units of penicillin daily to these patients is usually effective in eliminating the infection when therapy is continued for 4 weeks. The penicillin should be given parenterally, either intramuscularly or intravenously. There is a synergistic effect of streptomycin with penicillin on S. viridans, and it has been suggested that streptomycin in a dose of 0.5 Gm twice a day should be administered in addition to penicillin. The superiority of this regimen over penicillin alone, however, has not been demonstrated. When patients with S. viridans endocarditis respond promptly, some authorities recommend that parenteral therapy be discontinued after 2 weeks; an additional 2-week course of an oral acid-resistant penicillin (phenethicillin, or V-cillin) may be given with safety.

Bacterial endocarditis in older men and in women after abortion or endometritis is often due to S. faecalis (enterococci). These microorganisms are either resistant to penicillin alone or acquire resistance during penicillin treatment. The combination of penicillin with streptomycin is synergistic against these bacteria, however, and administration of these two antibiotics together is the treatment of choice in the infection. Penicillin G should be given parenterally in a dose of 6 to 20 million units a day, together with streptomycin in a dose of 0.5 to 1.0 Gm twice a day. Ampicillin in dosage of 6 to 12 Gm a day may be substituted for penicillin G. Treatment must be continued for a minimum of 4 weeks.

Penicillin G, 3 to 6 million units a day given parenterally, is satisfactory for treatment of pneumococcal and group A streptococcal endocarditis. Treatment should be continued for 4 weeks. Penicillinase-resistant penicillin analogs are preferred initially in treating staphylococcal endocarditis, because of the possibility that the infection is due to a penicillin-resistant organism. Methicillin should be given parenterally in a dose of 12 Gm per day, intramuscularly in divided doses or intravenously. If injected intravenously, the antibiotic should be given in divided doses in 50-ml volumes injected over 5 to 10 min. Methicillin is unstable in acid solutions and should not be given by continuous intravenous drip unless the suspending medium is brought to pH 7.0. Oxacillin, nafcillin, and cephalothin may be administered in lieu of methicillin. If the staphylococcus is found to be sensitive to penicillin G, this antibiotic should be given rather than methicillin, in a dose of 6 to 10 million units per day. Treatment should be continued for at least 4 weeks. In staphylococcal endocarditis, in particular, attention must be given to possible metastatic abscesses requiring surgical drainage.

In patients allergic to penicillin, cephalothin, erythromycin, vancomycin, and lincomycin are alternative drugs. If an allergic reaction to penicillin develops during the course of therapy, suppressant drugs such as antihistamines may be used to alleviate the manifestations of the reaction. In several instances, corticosteroids have been employed to suppress allergic drug reactions during treatment of bacterial endocarditis without deleterious consequences, as long as an effective antimicrobial drug is used to treat the infection.

At times, Probenecid in dosage of 0.5 Gm twice daily, may be given with penicillin or its analogs to slow renal excretion of the antibiotic and to increase blood levels. This regimen may be employed to provide a margin of safety but should not be substituted for adequate doses of the antibiotic.

Fever begins to disappear usually within 3 to 7 days after beginning treatment of bacterial endocarditis. Embolic complications of the disease, heart failure, and infection by insusceptible microorganisms, however, may delay defervescence. Drug fever may occasionally supervene and complicate the febrile course. Cessation of all therapy for 72 hr is not hazardous and may identify such a drug reaction readily.

Some patients with arteriovenous fistulas and infected cardiac prostheses may require surgical intervention before the infection can be controlled. In addition, early corrective surgery should be considered in patients who develop marked valvular damage (particularly aortic regurgitation) as a consequence of bacterial endocarditis. Valve replacement has been lifesaving and must be effected before intractable heart failure ensues.

When bacterial endocarditis recurs, it usually develops within 4 weeks after treatment stops. Reinstitution of antibiotic therapy will be required, but the sensitivity of the microorganism to the antibiotic must be reevaluated. Relapse may indicate inadequate or inappropriate therapy. If bacterial endocarditis develops more than 6 weeks after cessation of treatment, it usually is a new infection.

REFERENCES

Bashour, F. A., and C. P. Winchell: Right-sided Bacterial Endocarditis, Am. J. Med. Sci., 240:411, 1960.

Braniff, B. A., N. E. Shumway, and D. C. Harrison: Valve Replacement in Active Bacterial Endocarditis, New Engl. J. Med., 276:1464, 1967.

Goodman, J. S., W. Schaffner, H. A. Collins, E. J. Battersby, and M. G. Koenig: Infection after Cardiovascular Surgery: Clinical Study Including Examination of Antimicrobial Prophylaxis, New Engl. J. Med., 278:117, 1968.

Green, G. R., G. A. Peters, and J. E. Geraci: Treatment of Bacterial Endocarditis in Patients with Penicillin Hypersensitivity, Ann. Intern. Med., 67:235, 1967.

Hook, E. W., and D. Kaye: Prophylaxis of Bacterial Endocarditis, J. Chronic Dis., 15:635, 1962.

Kerr, A. J., Jr.: "Subacute Bacterial Endocarditis," Springfield, Ill., Charles C Thomas, Publisher, 1955.

Lord, J. W., A. M. Imparato, A. Hackel, and E. F. Doyle: Endocarditis Complicating Open-heart Surgery, Circulation, 23:489, 1961.

Section 3

Diseases Caused by Gram-positive Cocci

138 PNEUMOCOCCAL INFECTIONS

Robert Austrian and Ivan L. Bennett, Jr.

ETIOLOGY. The pneumococcus is a gram-positive encapsulated coccus that usually grows in pairs or short chains. In the diplococcal form, the adjacent margins are rounded and the opposite ends slightly pointed, giving the organisms a "lancet" shape. In stained preparations of exudate, gram-negative forms are sometimes present. Because pneumococci produce greenish discoloration of blood agar, they are sometimes confused with alpha-hemolytic streptococci to which they are closely related. The two organisms can be distinguished by the bile solubility and mouse virulence of the pneumococcus or by serologic typing. Another method, utilizing inhibition of pneumococci by Optochin-impregnated paper disks, is less cumbersome and very effective.

The capsular substances are complex polysaccharides and are the basis for dividing pneumococci into serotypes. Organisms exposed to type-specific antiserum show a positive capsular precipitin reaction, the *Neufeld quellung reaction;* by this means, 82 serotypes have been identified. All are pathogenic for man, but types 1, 3, 4, 7, 8, and 12 are encountered most frequently in clinical practice. Types 6, 14, and 19 often cause pneumonia in children but are less common in adults.

Specific typing of pneumococci remains of great clinical importance if pneumococcus is to be identified with regularity, but has been largely abandoned since the introduction of sulfonamides and antibiotics which are effective against pneumococci of all types. Recognition of pneumococcus has decreased significantly since the abandonment of pneumococcal typing by many clinical laboratories.

EPIDEMIOLOGY. Pneumococci are normal inhabitants of the human upper respiratory tract in 5 to 60 percent of the population, depending upon the season. Pneumococcal infection occurs predominantly during the winter and early spring; the ratio of infection in males and females is 3:2, and morbidity and mortality are higher for Negroes than whites. Person-to-person transmission by droplets is undoubtedly common, but true epidemics of pneumococcal pneumonia are rare, even in closed populations. Patients with pneumococcal infection need not be isolated because the risk of cross infection is relatively small.

PATHOGENESIS. The mechanism by which pneumococci damage tissue is obscure. It is conceivable that toxic substances may be elaborated, but no such toxin has been demonstrated. It has been suggested that rapid growth of pneumococci interferes with essential metabolic processes in the host, but this hypothesis is not supported by firm evidence. The capsular substances, though nontoxic, are known to be necessary factors in virulence, and protect the organism to a certain extent from engulfment by phagocytes.

Invasion of the tissues of the nasopharynx rarely, if ever, occurs, and "pneumococcal pharyngitis" is a doubtful entity. The organisms multiply readily in vivo, however, and may produce acute inflammation in the lungs, serous cavities, and the endocardium.

The normal human respiratory tract is provided with a variety of mechanisms which act to protect the lungs from infection. The lower respiratory tract is protected by the glottis and larynx and material passing these barriers stimulates the expulsive cough reflex. Removal of small particles impinging on the walls of the trachea and bronchi is facilitated by their mucociliary lining; and growth of bacteria reaching normal alveoli is inhibited by their relative dryness and by the phagocytic activity of alveolar macrophages. Any anatomic or physiologic derangement of these coordinated defenses tends to augment the susceptibility of the lungs to infection. Anesthesia, alcoholic intoxication, convulsions and disturbed innervation of the larynx depress cough reflex and may permit aspiration of infected material. Alterations in the tracheobronchial tree leading to anatomic changes in the epithelial lining or to localized obstruction increase the vulnerability of the lungs to infection. Pulmonary edema, local or generalized, resulting from viral infection, inhalation of irritant gases, cardiac failure, or contusion of the chest wall, provides a fluid menstruum in the alveoli for the growth of bacteria and their spread to adjacent areas of the lung. Viral infection of the respiratory epithelium with concomitant disruption of its component cells interferes significantly with the clearance of bacteria from the lungs, an observation in accord with the high incidence of pneumococcal pneumonia during epidemics of viral influenza and its frequent clinical association with sporadic viral respiratory infections.

Pneumonia begins usually in the right lower, right middle, or left lower lobe, those areas to which gravity is most likely to carry upper respiratory secretions aspirated during sleep. Bronchial embolization with infected mucinous secretions during the course of an upper respiratory infection appears to be the initiating factor in many cases of pneumococcal pneumonia. Protected initially from phagocytosis by mucinous material, the bacteria multiply and, in infected alveoli, evoke the outpouring of proteinaceous fluid which serves both as a nutrient and as a vehicle for spread to adjacent alveoli. Soon thereafter, polymorphonuclear leukocytes migrate from the pulmonary capillaries to phagocytize a part of the pneumococcal population before the appearance of detectable antibody. Delay in the polymorphonuclear leukocytic response occurs during alcoholic intoxication and certain forms of anesthesia, permitting spread of infection. Adrenocortical steroids and their congeners may also interfere with leukocyte migration. Later, as the pneumonic lesion evolves, macrophages appear in the exudate and remove the debris of fibrin and cells. It is probable that antibody to the capsular polysaccharide of the invading pneumococcus makes its appearance locally in the lung before being detectable in the circulation. Such antibody increases the efficiency of phagocytosis approximately twofold and causes agglutination of the organisms and their adherence to alveolar walls, thereby slowing their dissemination in the lung. The outcome of infection depends, therefore, on the rate at which bacteria can multiply in the edema fluid and spread and the host's ability to immobilize and destroy them by phagocytosis. Individuals with hypogammaglobulinemia and patients with multiple myeloma incapable of producing anticapsular antibody are prone to recurrent attacks of pneumococcal pneumonia. Repeated infection with the same pneumococcal type should always prompt a search for dysgammaglobulinemia.

Failure of local defense mechanisms in the lung results in lymphatic spread of pneumococci to the hilar lymph nodes. In the sinusoids of these organs, a sequence of events not unlike that in the lung ensues. If infection is not checked in this secondary line of defense, organisms find their way into the thoracic duct and then into the circulation. Although transient bacteremia may occur at the onset of many cases of pneumococcal pneumonia, it is detectable in only 25 to 30 percent of cases. Bacteremia, which reflects the body's inability to localize the pulmonary infection, is a poor prognostic sign and carries with it the danger of metastatic infection. The mortality of treated or untreated bacteremic pneumococcal pneumonia is four times that resulting from comparably managed nonbacteremic infections. Metastatic infection secondary to bacteremia may occur in the meninges, joints, or peritoneum or on the endocardium. Direct spread from the infected lung may give rise to pleural empyema or to pericarditis.

Natural recovery from pneumococcal infection coincides usually, but not invariably, with the appearance of detectable type-specific antibody in the circulation and is often accompanied by a dramatic and abrupt fall in temperature, the so-called "crisis." Antibody aids recovery by increasing the efficiency of phagocytosis and by limiting dissemination of the organisms. Bacteriostatic drugs, such as sulfonamides, facilitate control of the infection by limiting the size of the pneumococcal population, but the host's defense mechanisms are still required for the elimination of the bacteria. Bactericidal agents, such as penicillin, cause the death of pneumococci in the lung and are effective when some of the host's defense mechanisms are inoperable. With the arrest of infection, the alveolar exudate undergoes liquefaction, the inflammatory debris is removed by expectoration and via the lymphatic channels, and the lung is restored to its normal state. Necrosis of pulmonary tissue as a result of pneumococcal infection is distinctly uncommon. Primary pneumococcal lung abscess is a rare clinical entity, although the diagnosis is mistakenly made at times when pneumococcal infection complicates lung abscess of other origins.

In addition to causing pneumonia and its metastatic sequelae, pneumococcus can extend from the nasopharynx to its adjacent structures, giving rise to otitis media, mastoiditis, paranasal sinusitis, or conjunctivitis.

PNEUMOCOCCAL PNEUMONIA

Pneumococcal pneumonia is a disease remarkable for its uniformity, in contrast to other infections such as typhoid fever and tuberculosis. The diseases produced by different pneumococcal serotypes show little variation in severity or in clinical manifestations. The prognosis in type 3 pneumococcal pneumonia is usually regarded as poor, probably because type 3 infections occur frequently in the aged and in patients with other debilitating diseases such as diabetes and congestive heart failure. The type 3 pneumococcus possesses, however, an unusually large capsule, is especially difficult for neutrophils to engulf, and is most likely to produce abscesses in the lungs of man and experimental animals, suggesting that its virulence is partly intrinsic and not wholly the result of its attacking susceptible hosts. It is customary to classify pneumococcal pneumonias as *lobar*, when the process involves one or more large segments or lobes of the lung, or as *bronchopneumonia*, in which there is patchy involvement, often of both lungs. This distinction has little clinical importance; the treatment is the same for both types, and the prognosis depends upon other factors. The usual lesion in adults is lobar in distribution, but in children and the aged, bronchopneumonia is frequent.

MANIFESTATIONS. Pneumonia is often preceded for a few days by coryza or some other form of common respiratory disease. The onset is usually so abrupt that patients frequently can state the exact hour that illness began. There is a sudden *shaking chill* in more than 80 percent of the cases, a rapid rise in temperature, and a corresponding tachycardia. Most patients with pneumococcal pneumonia have a single rigor unless antipyretic drugs are administered, and repeated chills should suggest another etiologic agent.

About 75 percent of patients develop severe *pleuritic pain* and *cough*, productive of pinkish or "rusty" mucoid sputum within a few hours. The chest pain is agonizing, and respirations become rapid, shallow, and grunting as the patient tries to splint the affected side. Many patients are mildly cyanotic as a result of reduced alveolar ventilation, which accompanies altered respiration, and show dilatation of the alae nasae when first seen. Patients appear acutely ill; but nausea, headache, and malaise are not prominent, and most individuals are alert. Pleuritic pain and dyspnea are the dominant complaints.

In the untreated disease, there are sustained fever of 102.5 to 105°F, continued pleuritic pain, cough, and expectoration; and *abdominal distension* is frequent. *Herpes labialis* is a common complication. After 7 to 10 days, there are diaphoresis, abrupt defervescence, and dramatic improvement in well-being, the "crisis."

In cases which terminate fatally, there is usually extensive pulmonary involvement, and dyspnea, cyanosis, and tachycardia are prominent. Circulatory collapse or a picture resembling heart failure is common. Death in a few patients is associated with empyema or some other suppurative complication such as meningitis or endocarditis.

Physical examination reveals restricted motion of the affected hemithorax. Tactile fremitus may be decreased during the initial day of illness but is usually increased when consolidation is fully established. Deviation of the trachea away from the affected lung suggests pleural effusion or empyema. The percussion note is dull, and if the lesion is in an upper lobe, impaired motion of the diaphragm can be detected on the affected side. Very early in the course of infection, breath sounds are diminished, but as the lesion evolves, they become tubular or bronchial in quality and bronchophony and whispered pectoriloquy can be elicited. These findings are accompanied by fine crepitant rales.

EFFECT OF SPECIFIC CHEMOTHERAPY. Pneumococcal pneumonia usually improves promptly when an appropriate antimicrobial drug is given. Within 12 to 36 hr after initiation of treatment with penicillin, temperature, pulse, and respiration begin to fall and may reach normal values in that period, pleuritic pain subsides, and the spread of the inflammatory process is halted. The temperature of approximately half the patients so treated, however, requires 4 days or longer to become normal, and failure of the patient's temperature to reach normal in 24 to 48 hr should not prompt a change in antibacterial therapy in the absence of other indications.

COMPLICATIONS. The typical course of pneumococcal pneumonia can be modified by the development of one or more local or distant complications:

In the Lung. Atelectasis. Atelectasis of all or part of a lobe may occur during the active stage of pneumonia or after treatment has been instituted. The patient may complain of sudden recurrence of pleuritic pain and show rapid respirations. Small areas of atelectasis are often detected by x-ray in the absence of symptoms. These areas usually clear with coughing and deep breathing, but bronchoscopic aspiration is occasionally necessary. If atelectasis is allowed to persist, the affected area becomes fibrotic and functionless.

Delayed Resolution. The removal of exudate from the lung following pneumococcal infection is usually complete within 2 to 3 weeks, at which time the x-ray of the chest appears normal; but, occasionally, especially in elderly individuals and in alcoholics, consolidation persists for longer periods. Sometimes the involved area never becomes reaerated, and fibrosis results.

Abscess. Lung abscess is a rare sequel to pneumococcal infection, although pneumococcal pneumonia is a not uncommon complication of lung abscess of other origins. It is manifested by continued fever and profuse expectoration of purulent sputum. X-ray shows one or more cavities. This complication is exceedingly rare in patients who receive penicillin therapy and is most likely to follow infection with pneumococcus type 3.

In Adjacent Structures. **Pleural Effusion.** Pleural effusion occurs in about 5 percent of patients with pneumococcal pneumonia, even with specific therapy. The amount of fluid is usually not sufficient to cause obvious displacement of mediastinal structures. Usually the effusion is sterile and is reabsorbed spontaneously within a week or two. Sometimes, however, the effusion is large and becomes loculated. In these instances it should be aspirated by needle and occasionally tube drainage must be used.

Empyema. Prior to the introduction of effective chemotherapy, empyema occurred in 5 to 8 percent of patients with pneumococcal pneumonia; it is now observed in less than 1 percent of treated cases. It is manifested by persistent fever or pleuritic pain, together with signs of pleural effusion. In the early stages, the gross appearance of infected fluid may not differ from that of a sterile pleural effusion; later, there is a profuse outpouring of polymorphonuclear leukocytes and fibrin, resulting in an exudate of thick greenish pus containing large clots of fibrin. The quantity of exudate may become large enough to displace mediastinal structures. In neglected cases, this process leads to extensive pleural scarring, with limitation of thoracic movement. Rupture and drainage through the chest wall (*empyema necessitatis*) occurs but is rare. Metastatic *brain abscess* is an occasional complication of chronic empyema. This lesion is caused by passage of septic thrombi through the intercostal and vertebral veins.

Pericarditis. A particularly serious complication is spread of infection to the pericardial sac. This lesion is characterized by pain in the precordial region, a friction rub synchronous with the heartbeat, and distension of cervical veins, although one or all of these findings is not always present. The possibility of coexisting purulent pericarditis should be considered whenever a very ill patient with pneumonia develops empyema.

Metastatic Infections. *Arthritis* occurs more often in children than in adults. The affected joint is swollen, red, and painful, with a purulent effusion. It usually subsides promptly with systemic administration of penicillin, although intraarticular injection of penicillin may be necessary in adults.

Acute bacterial endocarditis complicates pneumococcal pneumonia in less than 0.5 percent of cases. Its manifestations and treatment are discussed below. *Meningitis,*

another complication of pneumococcal pneumonia, is also discussed subsequently.

Paralytic Ileus. Gaseous abdominal distension is commonly present and in severely ill patients may assume such serious proportions that the term *paralytic ileus* is justified. This complication further impairs respiratory movement by elevation of the diaphragm and constitutes a difficult problem in management. A rarer and more serious gastrointestinal complication is acute gastric dilatation.

Impaired Liver Function. Alterations in liver function are very common during the course of pneumococcal pneumonia, and mild jaundice is not at all rare. The pathogenesis of the jaundice is not entirely clear.

LABORATORY FINDINGS. X-ray of the chest reveals a homogeneous density in the affected area of lung. In well-established cases, the density may occupy one or more entire lobes. The white blood count usually shows a polymorphonuclear *leukocytosis* ranging from 12,000 to 25,000 cells per cu mm. A normal leukocyte count or leukopenia is sometimes observed in patients with overwhelming infection and bacteremia, in the aged, and in alcoholics. The *blood culture* is positive for pneumococci during the first 3 or 4 days of the untreated illness in 20 to 25 percent of cases. The *sputum,* when stained by Gram's method, shows polymorphonuclear leukocytes and variable numbers of gram-positive cocci, singly and in pairs. These can be typed directly, by the Neufeld quellung, or capsular precipitin reaction technique, and this procedure should be employed to facilitate diagnosis whenever possible.

DIFFERENTIAL DIAGNOSIS OF PNEUMONIA

Fever, cough, and pulmonary consolidation on physical or x-ray examination form a symptom complex that can be produced by many diseases of infectious, toxic, or other etiology.

Staphylococcal Pneumonia (Chap. 139). Staphylococcal pneumonia is likely to be encountered in children, in adults during or after an epidemic of influenza, and in debilitated elderly individuals as a nosocomial infection. The clinical picture is less uniform than that of pneumococcal pneumonia, varying from bronchitis with few systemic symptoms to a fulminating infection. Multiple chills, hectic fever, early formation of lung abscesses, empyema, and in infants, pneumatoceles or pyopneumothorax, suggest the diagnosis. The sputum is often grossly bloody or purulent and contains myriads of staphylococci readily detectable in stained smears of sputum. Culture of sputum and blood confirms the diagnosis.

Hemolytic Streptococcal Pneumonia (Chap. 140). Hemolytic streptococcal pneumonia can also occur in association with influenza or as a complication of measles. The clinical picture closely resembles that of pneumococcal pneumonia, but multiple chills, hectic fever, early prostration, and rapid pleural involvement with accumulation of fluid, or associated streptococcal pharyngitis, are distinctive signs. The diagnosis can be made by blood and sputum culture or, inferentially, by finding a rise in anti-streptolysin 0 titer in convalescent serum.

Friedländer's Bacillus (Klebsiella) Pneumonia (Chap. 148). Klebsiella is commonest in adult men, especially alcoholics, although 50 percent of these infections occur in those who do not use alcohol to excess. The patients are usually severely ill, and the sputum tends to be thick and tenacious. Physical findings in the chest are often surprisingly scanty despite massive consolidation by x-ray; nausea, diarrhea, jaundice, and delirium are more frequent than in pneumococcal infections, and large numbers of gram-negative bacilli are usually present in stained smears of sputum.

Tularemia. (Chap. 155). Tularemia is often accompanied by pulmonary lesions. There may be no respiratory symptoms and a paucity of physical signs, or pleurisy, hemoptysis, and consolidation may dominate the clinical picture. Patients are usually very ill, often delirious, with temperatures of 104 to 106°F. The disease does not respond to penicillin but does to streptomycin. Agglutinins for the organism may not appear until the third week. A history of contact with wild rabbits, ticks, or deer flies or the finding of a cutaneous ulcer and regional lymphadenitis is helpful in diagnosis.

Other Bacterial Pneumonias. Infection by other bacteria can produce pneumonia. Pulmonary involvement is frequent in patients with salmonella bacteremia, especially in *Salmonella choleraesuis* infections (Chap. 150). Pneumonia caused by other enterobacteria (*Escherichia coli, Proteus* species, *Pseudomonas*) occurs usually in the debilitated and the aged, in alcoholics, and in those with deranged defenses against infection. In most instances these patients have received antimicrobials for other infections. Necrotizing pneumonia caused by one of the several species of the anaerobic genus *Bacteroides* is seen occasionally. *Hemophilus influenzae* is a common cause of pulmonary disease in children; in adults it occasionally produces a necrotizing bronchiolitis or lobar pneumonia, and in elderly patients with chronic lung disease, it may produce bronchopneumonia (Chap. 152). The diagnosis is usually made only by culture of sputum. Pulmonary lesions with cough and hemoptysis can be prominent in Weil's disease (Chap. 181), and the plague bacillus can cause an overwhelming and rapidly fatal pneumonia, especially when plague becomes epidemic (Chap. 156).

Mycoplasma Pneumoniae Infection (Chap. 207). This infection is usually more insidious in onset than bacterial pneumonia. Chills are infrequent, fever is usually lower and falls by lysis, pleuritic pain and effusions are unusual, headache and malaise are prominent, and the cough is hacking, irritating, and productive of small amounts of mucoid sputum. Physical signs are scanty in comparison with x-ray changes. Herpes labialis is unusual.

Viral Pneumonias (Chap. 206). Viral pneumonias may result from infection with a variety of agents including myxoviruses, respiratory syncytial virus, adenoviruses, Coxsackie, ECHO, and reoviruses and those of measles and varicella. Although many of these illnesses are mild and resemble that caused by *Mycoplasma pneumoniae*, occasional infections caused by influenza virus may be difficult to distinguish from bacterial pneumonia. Secondary bacterial pneumonia is a not uncommon complication of influenza viral infection and of severe measles.

Psittacosis (Ornithosis) (Chap. 209). Psittacosis is characterized by systemic symptoms of headache, fever, lethargy, and malaise for several days before pulmonary lesions develop. The pulse is usually slow in proportion to fever, and patients are sometimes suspected of having typhoid. The leukocyte count may be normal or moderately elevated.

Q Fever (Chap. 201). Q fever is characterized by severe headache, sustained fever, and, usually, minimal symptoms of respiratory disease, although a large proportion of patients show roentgenographic evidence of patchy pulmonary involvement.

Tuberculosis. *Acute tuberculous pneumonia* (Chap. 174) may be difficult to recognize because, early in the disease, tubercle bacilli may not be demonstrable in the sputum; the first consolidation is often the result of an inflammatory response to discharge of tuberculin-containing material into the lung. Fever is usually remittent or intermittent, and the temperature may not exceed 102°F. Many patients with tuberculous pneumonia feel surprisingly well, despite consolidation of an entire lobe. *Pleurisy with effusion* is seldom abrupt in onset, its course is prolonged, and physical and x-ray findings are those of accumulating pleural fluid rather than parenchymal consolidation. Cough is usually nonproductive. The leukocyte count is frequently normal. Herpes labialis is rare in tuberculosis.

Mycotic Infections. *Blastomycosis* (Chap. 186) can produce acute lobar or bronchopneumonia, with high fever, pleuritic pain, dyspnea, and pleural fluid. The organisms usually are found easily in the sputum, and cavitation develops early in the illness. The usual course of pulmonary blastomycosis is less acute than that of bacterial pneumonia, with low-grade fever and slow evolution of the pulmonary findings. *Actinomycosis* of the lung (Chap. 184) is usually a more chronic disease than bacterial pneumonia and is more likely to be confused with tuberculosis or lung tumors. Other mycotic infections of the lung include *primary histoplasmosis* (Chap. 188), which can produce an acute illness that lasts for several weeks with fever, cough, and multiple nodular pulmonary densities; and primary coccidioidomycosis (Chap. 187), distinguishable in endemic areas by pulmonary infiltration, fever, eosinophilia, and, often erythema nodosum.

Lung Abscess (Chap. 291). Lung abscess may have an abrupt onset, with chill, fever, and pleuritic pain and can be confused with acute pneumonias. Pneumococcal pneumonia at the site of the lesion may complicate the course of any stage prior to treatment. The development of cavitation in a well-circumscribed pulmonary density and profuse, purulent, often foul-smelling sputum make the diagnosis clear. In individuals with chronic abscess, weight loss is prominent and cavitation readily apparent. There is usually intermittent or remittent fever. A history of epilepsy, alcoholic intoxication, anesthesia, dental extraction, tonsillectomy, or aspiration of a foreign body may be elicited. Abscess may be the first sign of bronchogenic carcinoma.

Atelectasis (Chap. 291). Atelectasis may occur in patients confined to bed, especially if respiratory motion is limited (as after an abdominal operation) or when the cough reflex is depressed by drugs or central nervous system disease. Infection of the collapsed pulmonary segment leads to fever, pleuritic pain, and purulent sputum. There is often a shift of the mediastinum toward the affected side. Tumor, enlarged hilar nodes, and foreign body are important causes of persistent collapse, although plugging of bronchi by inspissated mucus is by far the most frequent cause.

Neoplasms (Chap. 292).

Pulmonary Adenomatosis (Chap. 292). Pulmonary adenomatosis, a diffuse neoplastic disease, can be accompanied by fever, profuse glairy sputum, and hemoptysis, with various x-ray findings, and is sometimes mistaken at first for acute bacterial pneumonia. Much more commonly a bronchogenic carcinoma, at or near the hilum, presents as pneumonia. Failure of any "lobar pneumonia" to resolve should lead to vigorous search for malignant disease.

Pulmonary Infarction (Chap. 285). Pulmonary infarction is especially frequent in patients with congestive heart failure and after surgical procedures. Prostatic surgery and pelvic infections in women as well as delivery are particularly likely to lead to embolization from the pelvic veins. Pulmonary embolization may be asymptomatic, but in many patients, there are sudden pleuritic pain, dyspnea, anxiety, transient hypotension, and hemoptysis. Fever is common, but true chills are rare. Icterus may accompany pulmonary infarcts in individuals with congestive heart failure. Signs of consolidation and pleural fluid are common, and often evidence of phlebothrombosis can be detected in the legs. In women, *septic pulmonary infarcts* with abscess formation and cavitation should always suggest puerperal sepsis or infected abortions with pelvic thrombophlebitis. For reasons that are obscure, phlebothrombosis and pulmonary infarction are relatively frequent complications of convalescence from psittacosis.

Other Differential Diagnostic Points. The lungs of patients with *uremia* sometimes show x-ray changes consisting of infiltrations that flare toward the periphery from both hilar areas. Roentgenographically, the changes in the lungs of patients with *acute pulmonary edema* and *heart failure* are sometimes surprisingly well localized to a segment or lobe of one lung.

The inhalation of *noxious materials or irritants* (Chap. 116), including smoke, chlorine, phosgene, cadmium fumes, bagasse fibers, and other organic dusts, can lead to bronchitis, bronchiolitis, patchy or even lobar infiltration in the lung, dyspnea, and low-grade fever. The diagnosis is usually made by eliciting a history of exposure. The ingestion of gasoline or kerosene is almost invariably complicated by severe chemical bronchopneumonia. A more benign and chronic pneumonia known as *lipoid pneumonia* may follow the nocturnal ingestion of mineral oil or the use of nose drops containing oil.

Pneumonitis is detectable by physical examination or x-ray in some patients with erythema multiforme, lupus erythematosus, rheumatic fever, or intestinal helminthiasis. Infectious mononucleosis and lymphocytic choriomeningitis are sometimes accompanied by pulmonary infiltrations and, occasionally, by signs of respiratory irritation with cough and sputum. Pulmonary lesions, usually in the form of scattered nodular densities, with accompanying cough, dyspnea, and cyanosis, occur in a small proportion of patients with smallpox, chickenpox, or measles; the involvement in these diseases is believed to be caused by the virus rather than by secondary bacterial invaders. Rupture of amebic abscess into the pleural cavity can be mistaken for acute pneumonia, and in a few patients with estivo-autumnal malaria, blockage of pulmonary capillaries by parasites can lead to confusion with respiratory infections.

PNEUMOCOCCAL MENINGITIS

The pneumococcus is second only to the meningococcus as a cause of purulent meningitis in adults; in children, meningitis caused by *Hemophilus influenzae* is also more frequent than pneumococcal infection.

Pneumococcal meningitis can develop as a "primary" disease without preceding signs of infection elsewhere; as a complication of pneumococcal pneumonia; by extension from otitis, mastoiditis, or sinusitis; or following a skull fracture which creates an opening between the subarachnoid space and the nasal cavity or paranasal sinuses. Patients with pneumococcal endocarditis frequently develop meningeal infection. Patients with multiple myeloma seem to be prone to pneumococcal infection of the meninges, just as they are to pneumonia.

The *manifestations* are those of any acute pyogenic meningitis (Chap. 360) and include chills, fever, headache, nuchal rigidity, Kernig's and Brudzinski's signs, delirium, and cranial nerve palsies. Evidence of otitis, sinusitis, or pneumonia should be carefully sought by physical and roentgenographic examination in all patients.

The *spinal fluid* is under increased pressure, appears cloudy, often with a greenish tint, and shows a high protein and low glucose content. Stained smears usually reveal gram-positive diplococci and polymorphonuclear leukocytes; in some patients, the number of cells in the spinal fluid is surprisingly small, and much of the cloudiness is produced by the bacterial content. The diagnosis can be established rapidly by identification of pneumococci in the spinal fluid by Gram stain and by direct typing with the Neufeld quellung reaction.

With appropriate chemotherapy, recovery can be expected in 50 to 70 percent of cases; the prognosis is better in children than in infants or in adults. Before penicillin was available, the mortality rate exceeded 95 percent, and sulfonamides did little to reduce it. Relapse may occur but is unusual if adequate treatment is carried out. Subarachnoid block, the result of accumulation of large amounts of thick exudate in the meningeal space and at the base of the brain, is now an unusual complication.

PNEUMOCOCCAL ENDOCARDITIS

Endocarditis is usually a complication of pneumonia or meningitis. The clinical picture is that of acute bacterial endocarditis (Chap. 137), with remittent fever, splenomegaly, and metastatic infection of the lungs, meninges, joints, eye, and other tissues. Petechiae are uncommon. The infection can attack normal valves and is particularly likely to occur on the aortic valve. The valvular infection is destructive, and loud murmurs and heart failure develop rapidly. Rupture or perforation of cusps or even rupture of the aorta may occur. The blood culture is consistently positive for the pneumococcus in the absence of treatment with antimicrobial drugs; yet at the same time antibodies to the infecting organism may be demonstrable in the blood, a combination of findings seldom observed except in endocarditis or brucellosis. Although the infection is relatively easy to cure with penicillin, damage to valve leaflets, especially to the cusps of the aortic valve, may be followed by rapidly progressive heart failure. Surgical repair or replacement of damaged valvular structures should be carried out early, before heart failure becomes intractable.

PNEUMOCOCCAL PERITONITIS

Pneumococcal peritonitis is a rare disease which occurs in young girls; presumably the vagina and fallopian tubes are the portal of entry. Symptoms are fever, pain, abdominal distension, vomiting, and accumulation of peritoneal fluid. The diagnosis is made by examination of the purulent ascitic fluid; blood cultures are often positive, and a polymorphonuclear leukocytosis is the rule. In adults, the disease may occur in association with cirrhosis or with carcinoma of the liver. Peritonitis used to be a common complication of the nephrotic syndrome, particularly in children, but is rare nowadays.

TREATMENT

SPECIFIC ANTIMICROBIAL THERAPY. Penicillin G (benzathine penicillin) is the drug of choice for all pneumococcal infections. The minimum curative dose for *pneumonia* is less than 60,000 units daily, and a total dose of 600,000 units daily provides a good margin of safety for bacteremic and nonbacteremic infections in adults in the absence of an extrapulmonary focus of infection. Treatment may be administered at 12-hr intervals in doses of 300,000 units aqueous crystalline penicillin G or procaine penicillin. Therapy should be continued until the patient has been afebrile for 48 to 72 hr. The response is usually dramatic, and relapse is extremely uncommon. Pneumococcal pneumonia can be treated adequately with oral penicillin (preferably one of the drugs resistant to gastric acid, see Chap. 135) in dosage of 1.2 to 2.4 million units daily. *Peritonitis* usually responds within 36 to 48 hr to 2 to 4 million units of penicillin daily.

Pneumococcal *meningitis* should be treated with 12 to 20 million units aqueous penicillin G daily intrave-nously in adults. In many clinics, even larger amounts are used, though care must be taken to avoid neurotoxicity from excessive dosage. Intrathecal administration of penicillin is of no value. The addition of sulfadiazine to this regimen affords no advantage, and supplementary administration of chlortetracycline (and presumably, of other broad-spectrum drugs) actually exerts a deleterious effect. In the presence of sinusitis, otitis, or mastoiditis, surgical drainage should be carried out as soon as is feasible. The response of meningitis is usually less dramatic than that of pneumonia; patients often remain febrile and disoriented, and signs of meningeal irritation may persist for several days, but improvement becomes gradually evident with continued treatment.

Large doses are required in pneumococcal endocarditis also—12 to 20 million units daily by intravenous injection. Rapidly developing heart failure in these patients and the tendency to form myocardial abscess, however, often lead to a fatal outcome despite large doses of antibiotics. Surgical repair or replacement of damaged heart valves should be considered when cardiac failure develops.

Sulfonamides are effective in pneumococcal pneumonia but less so than antibiotics, and their action is not as prompt or dramatic as that of penicillin. They are useless in meningitis and endocarditis. The *tetracyclines* in doses of 1.0 to 2.0 Gm daily, *erythromycin* in doses of 1.6 Gm daily, and *Lincomycin* in doses of 1.2 Gm daily are effective treatment of pneumococcal pneumonia, but are recommended only for patients who have had untoward reactions to penicillin. Mutants of pneumococcus resistant to each of these antibiotics have been isolated from man; and, if one of these drugs is to be employed, it is essential that the organism be sensitive to the agent administered. Despite its efficacy, chloramphenicol should not be used to treat pneumococcal infections, except when unusual circumstances exist.

Pneumococcal arthritis responds to systemic penicillin, but aspiration and intraarticular instillation of the drug may be necessary.

Empyema should be detected and treated as early as possible. When an effusion is found, the fluid should be examined for organisms; and if they are present, 50,000 to 200,000 units of penicillin G should be injected intrapleurally. In addition, the same antibiotic should be administered systemically in doses of 6 to 8 million units a day. Aspiration of fluid and instillation of penicillin should be carried out at 1- to 2-day intervals until cultures are persistently negative and fever disappears. Fluoroscopic guidance may be needed for aspiration of small empyema pockets. If the exudate is especially thick or viscid, streptokinase-streptodornase (Varidase) may facilitate its withdrawal. When definite improvement is not evident in 4 to 6 days or when the empyema is of long duration, a large-lumen intercostal tube should be placed in the pleural cavity to facilitate drainage. Failure to effect prompt cure of empyema may be followed by pleural fibrosis and necessitate subsequent surgical decortication of the lung to restore pulmonary function. Aspiration of exudate and instillation of penicillin may also be used to treat *pericarditis*, but when cardiac tamponade is present, pericardiotomy may be preferable. Although medical treatment of emypema and of pericarditis is successful in some patients, there should be no hesitation in employing surgical drainage when rapid and steady improvement is not observed.

OTHER MEASURES. *Oxygen* should be used to treat intense cyanosis in pneumonia but may aggravate abdominal distension. Codeine, 30 to 60 mg every few hours, will usually control cough and mild *pleuritic pain.* A chest binder may diminish pain but may also increase the likelihood of atelectasis. When pain is severe, intercostal nerve block by injection of 2.0 ml of 1 percent procaine beneath the rib margins proximal to the site of pain is usually effective and is not technically difficult or dangerous. Other methods of relieving pleuritic pain are usually transient in their effect but are sometimes worth trying; they include ethyl chloride spray over the painful area and intravenous injection of calcium gluconate.

PROGNOSIS

With proper antimicrobial therapy, the mortality from all cases of pneumococcal pneumonia has fallen to approximately 5 percent, but that of patients with bacteremic infections is 17 percent. The recovery rate in meningitis is 50 to 70 percent; the prognosis is better in childhood. Pneumococcal endocarditis is still fatal in at least half the cases; death results from valvular damage and cardiac failure more often than from infection.

Signs of poor prognosis in pneumonia include leukopenia, bacteremia, multilobar involvement, any extrapulmonary focus of pneumococcal infection, presence of preexisting systemic disease, circulatory collapse, and occurrence of the infection in the first year of life or after the age of fifty-five. Infection with pneumococcus type 3 has a higher mortality than that caused by other pneumococcal types.

REFERENCES

Austrian, R.: Pneumococcal Endocarditis, Meningitis, and Rupture of Aortic Valve, A.M.A. Arch. Intern. Med., 99:539, 1957.

———, and J. Gold: Pneumococcal Bacteremia with Especial Reference to Bacteremic Pneumococcal Pneumonia, Ann. Intern. Med., 60:759, 1964.

Dowling, H. F., and M. H. Lepper: The Effect of Antibiotics (Penicillin, Aureomycin, and Terramycin) on the Fatality Rate and Incidence of Complications in Pneumococcic Pneumonia, Am. J. Med. Sci., 222:396, 1951.

Finland, M., and H. I. L. Lovernd: Massive Atelectatic Collapse of the Lung Complicating Pneumococcus Pneumonia, Ann. Intern. Med., 10:1828, 1937.

Heffron, R.: "Pneumonia with Special Reference to Pneumococcus Lobar Pneumonia," New York, The Commonwealth Fund, 1939.

Lepper, M. H., and H. F. Dowling: Treatment of Pneumococcic Meningitis with Penicillin Compared with Penicillin plus Aureomycin, A.M.A. Arch. Intern. Med., 88: 489, 1951.

Shulman, J. A., L. A. Phillips, and R. G. Petersdorf: Errors and Hazards in the Diagnosis and Treatment of Bacterial Pneumonias, Ann. Intern. Med., 62:41, 1965.

Wood, W. Barry, Jr.: Studies on the Mechanism of Recovery in Pneumococcal Pneumonia: I. The Action of Type Specific Antibody upon the Pulmonary Lesion of Experimental Pneumonia, J. Exp. Med., 73:201, 1941.

Zimmerman, H. J., and L. J. Thomas: The Liver in Pneumococcal Pneumonia: Observations in 94 Cases on Liver Function and Jaundice in Pneumonia, J. Lab. Clin. Med., 35:556, 1950.

Zinneman, H. H., and W. H. Hall: Recurrent Pneumonia in Multiple Myeloma, Ann. Intern. Med., 41:1152, 1954.

139 STAFFYLOCOCCAL INFECTIONS
David E. Rogers

Staphylococci cause most superficial suppurative infections in man. They also produce certain serious infections of the lungs, pleural space, endocardium, myocardium, long bones, kidneys, and surgical wounds.

While serious staphylococcal infections have always produced problems in hospitalized patients, they have much greater clinical importance since the development of antibiotics. The majority of life-threatening staphylococcal infections now arise within hospitals. Certain characteristics of staphylococci appear to have led to this situation: (1) the frequency of potentially pathogenic strains as part of man's normal flora, (2) the maintenance of staphylococci resistant to many antimicrobials in wide use in hospitals and hospital personnel, (3) the tendency of staphylococci to produce disease in debilitated patients, and (4) the rapid tissue destruction, abscess formation, and sluggish response of staphylococcal disease to antibacterial therapy.

BACTERIOLOGY. Staphylococci are members of the genus *Micrococcus*. This genus includes many morphologically similar saprophytic microorganisms which do not cause human infection. The parasitic micrococci of primary concern in medicine are grouped in the species *Micrococcus pyogenes*. Through established usage, these pathogenic micrococci are termed *staphylococci*.

Staphylococci are spherical gram-positive cells which grow abundantly in the usual meat extract or infusion media. On solid agar media, staphylococcal colonies develop characteristic pigmentation by which three species can be differentiated: *M. pyogenes* var. *aureus* (*Staphylococcus aureus*), golden yellow; *M. pyogenes* var. *albus* (*S. albus*), ivory white; and *M. citreus*, lemon yellow. Most human infections are caused by *S. aureus*, a few by *S. albus*. The name staphylococcus derives from the characteristic grapelike clusters of organisms seen in stained smears prepared from colonies on solid media (Greek *staphule* = "grape"). In stained smears obtained from pus, smaller clusters, diploids, and short chains are seen. In such preparations, staphylococci characteristically retain their uniform round shape, in contrast to the boat-like forms assumed by pneumococci. Staphylococci may be seen within the cytoplasm of polymorphonuclear cells in pus, a finding not common in other gram-positive coccal infections.

In general, pathogenic strains possess a broader complement of biochemical activity than do nonpathogenic strains. Most staphylococci isolated from human infections produce yellow pigment and hemolyze rabbit, sheep, and human red blood cells in blood agar plates. The ability to produce coagulase, a substance which clots the plasma of certain animals and man, the elaboration of *alpha toxin*, the fermentation of *mannite*, and the hydrolysis of *phenolphthalein phosphate* are characteristics of infection-producing strains. The ability of a given strain to produce coagulase is generally considered the best evidence of pathogenicity.

Different strains of pathogenic staphylococci can be recognized by the patterns of lysis produced by staphylococcal bacteriophages. Although the technique is cumbersome, phage typing of staphylococci has allowed more precise strain characterization and is commonly used in studies of intrahospital disease and epidemics of staphylococcal infection.

PATHOGENESIS. Little is known of the events which allow staphylococci to invade host tissues. While strains of staphylococci capable of producing infection are common skin and mucous membrane inhabitants, an enormous number of bacteria must be used to establish experimental infections in animals or man. Over 50 percent of serious staphylococcal infections of deep tissues arise from cutaneous foci. A lesser number of staphylococcal infections originate in the respiratory or genitourinary tract.

Staphylococcal disease appears more common in patients with *diabetes, liver disease, renal failure,* under circumstances of severe *debilitation* and/or *malnutrition,* or when skin continuity is broken. *Abrasions, wounds, burns,* and skin areas denuded by *exfoliative dermatitis* are commonly infected with staphylococci. Individuals who work with greasy skin irritants have a greater incidence of superficial staphylococcal infections. *Influenza, measles,* and *mucoviscoidosis* appear to predispose to primary staphylococcal invasion of the lung. Patients receiving *broad-spectrum antimicrobial therapy* also appear to have a higher incidence of staphylococcal disease.

Staphylococci invade the integument via hair follicles and sebaceous glands. When skin continuity has been breached, local microbial multiplication is accompanied by inflammation and tissue necrosis at the site of infection. Polymorphonuclear leukocytes rapidly enter the area and ingest large numbers of staphylococci. Thrombosis of surrounding capillaries occurs, fibrin is deposited about the periphery, and later, fibroblasts create a relatively avascular wall about the area. The fully developed staphylococcal lesion consists of a central core of dead and dying leukocytes and bacteria which gradually liquefies to form characteristic thick creamy staphylococcal pus, surrounded by a fibroblastic wall, the *pyogenic membrane.*

When host mechanisms fail to contain the cutaneous or subcutaneous infection, staphylococci may enter the bloodstream. Common sites of metastatic seeding are the diaphyseal ends of long bones in children, lungs, kidneys, endocardium, myocardium, liver, spleen, and brain.

Certain biologic properties of staphylococci appear to contribute to pathogenicity. Many pathogenic strains elaborate an *exotoxin* (alpha toxin) capable of causing dermal necrosis in animals. Fever, tachycardia, cyanosis, shock, and death ensue when exotoxin is administered to experimental animals, a picture similar to that seen occasionally in certain fulminating cases of staphylococcal bacteremia in man.

The high correlation between *coagulase* production and virulence suggests that this substance is important in the pathogenesis of staphylococcal infections. Coagulase has been said to protect staphylococci from phagocytosis by polymorphonuclear leukocytes, to promote abscess formation in man and animal species who have coagulable plasmas, or to protect staphylococci from bacteriostatic substances present in normal serum. However, none of these postulates has proven that coagulase per se is a determinant of pathogenicity, and its precise role has not been established.

Certain pathogenic staphylococci produce a *leukocidin* which destroys human and rabbit leukocytes in vitro. Some strains elaborate *hyaluronidase.* Many staphylococci produce an *enterotoxin* which produces nausea, vomiting, and diarrhea in certain experimental animals and man.

In vitro and in vivo studies have indicated that pathogenic staphylococci can survive within human leukocytes while nonpathogenic strains do not. Such intracellular survival may be a means of transporting staphylococci and spreading them to distant tissues.

IMMUNITY. Some degree of resistance to staphylococcal infections develops with age and the host's experience with staphylococci. Primary staphylococcal pneumonia is common in infants, but rare in adults. Acute staphylococcal osteomyelitis is almost exclusively a disease of children. Abscess formation appears less common and bacteremia more frequent in infants than in adults.

Coagulase-positive staphylococci have a characteristic cell wall teichoic acid which may be antiphagocytic. Certain unusual strains possess a definite capsular structure which impedes phagocytosis, and specific opsonizing antibody is required for the ingestion of these unusual strains. A number of antistaphylococcal antibodies have been shown to pass from mother to fetus, and the incidence of a variety of antibodies rapidly rises with age. Virtually 100 percent of adults possess antibodies to several staphylococcal antigens in their serum. Nevertheless, the role of humoral immunity in modifying or protecting against staphylococcal infection is uncertain. Immunization of animals with alpha toxin, toxoids, coagulase, or whole staphylococci may prolong experimental staphylococcal infection, but does not protect against eventual death. At present there has been no satisfactory demonstration that human staphylococcal disease is followed by immunity or that infection can be modified significantly by vaccination.

EPIDEMIOLOGY. Pathogenic strains of staphylococci reside in the anterior nares and upon the skin of 20 to

60 percent of humans. Hospital patients and personnel have significantly higher staphylococcal carrier rates than the general population. Over 90 percent of newborns acquire staphylococci within the anterior nares within 2 weeks. These infants are commonly colonized by the same staphylococcal phage types carried by nursery personnel.

While staphylococci remain viable for long periods in dust, blankets, or clothing, and viable staphylococci are often demonstrable in the environment by air-sampling techniques, the significance of airborne transmission remains uncertain, and the best evidence suggests that direct person-to-person contact is the most important means of transmission of staphylococci. Active staphylococcal infections are probably a more serious source of cross infection than the simple carrier state.

Certain phage types of staphylococci cause the majority of intrahospital infections. Some strains, particularly antibiotic-resistant strains in phage group III, appear to have greater "epidemic virulence" than other staphylococci. In specific hospitals, one phage type often emerges to prominence and may cause most of the serious intrahospital infections. Such "epidemic strains" have shifted from time to time and vary from hospital to hospital. The high incidence of active staphylococcal disease in carriers of certain strains (for example, the 80/81 strains) suggests that some staphylococci may possess higher virulence for humans than others.

ANTIMICROBIAL RESISTANCE. The introduction of new antibiotics active against staphylococci has generally been followed by the appearance of staphylococci specifically resistant to that agent. When penicillin was first introduced, less than 10 percent of staphylococcal strains isolated from patients or carriers were resistant to penicillin. Now 60 to 90 percent of staphylococci isolated from hospitalized patients throughout the Western world are resistant to penicillin G and the incidence of infection due to penicillinase-producing strains in nonhospitalized individuals is almost as high as in hospitalized patients. The incidence of resistance to a specific antimicrobial has correlated closely with the frequency of its administration, and the emegence of resistant strains has followed the use of streptomycin, the tetracyclines, chloramphenicol, erythromycin, oleandomycin, novobiocin, and kanamycin. Vancomycin, first employed in 1958, and the penicillinase-resistant penicillins and the cephalosporins, both introduced in the 1960s, have been exceptions to this rule. Although some strains of S. aureus resistant to the penicillinase-resistant penicillins have produced infections in England, France, and the United States, such strains have been unusual and, in general, all these agents have retained a high degree of activity against both penicillin-sensitive and penicillin-resistant staphylococci.

Most observations on the incidence of antimicrobial-resistant strains have been made within hospitals where antimicrobial use is heaviest. It has been shown that drug-susceptible strains carried by patients may be replaced by drug-resistant phage group III staphylococci present in the hospital environment during antimicrobial treatment. These strains are in turn acquired by hospital personnel who serve as reservoirs of potentially pathogenic, antimicrobial-resistant strains. Staphylococci isolated from population groups outside the hospital have shown a slower increase in the incidence of antimicrobial-resistant strains, but in many communities the incidence of extra-hospital infections caused by penicillin-resistant strains is now similar to that found in hospitalized patients.

SUPERFICIAL INFECTIONS

Simple infection of hair follicles manifested by a minute erythematous nodule without involvement of the surrounding skin or deeper tissues is termed *folliculitis*. Chronic recurrent folliculitis of the beard area is termed *sycosis barbae*.

A more extensive and invasive follicular or sebaceous gland infection with some involvement of subcutaneous tissues is termed a *furuncle* or *boil*. Itching and mild pain are followed by progressive local swelling and erythema. The overlying skin becomes thin, tense, shiny, and exquisitely painful on pressure or motion. Relief of pain occurs promptly after spontaneous or surgical drainage.

Furuncles occur most commonly on the face, neck, axillas, forearms, buttocks, thighs, breasts, upper back, and labia. The acne of adolescence is frequently complicated by secondary furunculosis. Staphylococcal infection may involve the sweat glands in the axillas (*hidradenitis suppurativa*). These infections may be deep-seated, slow to localize and drain, and are prone to recurrence and scarring.

Staphylococcal infections within the thick, fibrous, inelastic skin of the back of the neck and upper back lead to formation of a *carbuncle*. The relative thickness and impermeability of the overlying skin leads to lateral extension and loculation, and a large indurated, painful lesion with multiple ineffective drainage sites results. Carbuncles produce fever, leukocytosis, extreme pain, and prostration. Bacteremia is common.

OSTEOMYELITIS

Staphylococci are responsible for the majority of cases of *acute osteomyelitis*. This infection occurs almost exclusively in children under the age of twelve and has dropped sharply in incidence since the introduction of antibiotics. Men are affected more commonly than women. Approximately 50 percent of patients give a history of a furuncle or superficial staphylococcal infection preceding osteomyelitis. Bone involvement follows hematogenous dissemination of bacteria. The frequent localization in the diaphyseal end of long bones is thought to be due to the endarterial circulation of the diaphysis. Many patients give a history of preceding trauma to the involved area.

Once established, infection spreads through the newly formed juxtaepiphyseal bone to the periosteum or along the marrow cavity. If the infection reaches the subperiosteal space, the periosteum is lifted, a subperiosteal abscess forms, and rupture with infection of the subcutaneous tissues may occur. Rarely, the joint capsule is penetrated producing a pyogenic arthritis. There is death of bone producing a *sequestrum* followed by new bone formation (the *involucrum*).

Occasionally indolent staphylococcal infections of bone remain localized within dense granulation tissue about a central necrotic cavity. Such a local infection may persist for years as a so-called "Brodie's abscess."

Osteomyelitis in children usually begins abruptly with chills, high fever, nausea, vomiting, and progressive pain at the site of bony involvement. Muscle spasm about the affected bone is a common early sign of osteomyelitis, and the child may refuse to move the affected limb. Leukocytosis is the rule. Blood cultures are positive for staphylococci in 50 to 60 percent of cases early in the disease. The tissues overlying the involved bone become edematous and warm, and the skin becomes erythematous and shiny. Anemia develops during the course of untreated disease. Roentgenograms are usually normal during the first week. Bony rarefaction, local periosteal elevation, and new bone formation can frequently be seen during the second week.

DIAGNOSIS. Osteomyelitis should be suspected in any child with fever, limb pain, and leukocytosis. History of a preceding cutaneous infection, local tenderness over the end of a long bone, and the finding of S. *aureus* in blood cultures are confirmatory. In early stages, osteomyelitis must be differentiated from acute rheumatic fever, poliomyelitis, pyogenic arthritis, scurvy, and syphilitic periostitis.

PROGNOSIS. Prior to the advent of antimicrobials, the overall mortality was approximately 25 percent. Death was more common in individuals with demonstrable bacteremia. Chronic osteomyelitis with recurrent activation and metastatic foci in other bones was common. Today acute staphylococcal osteomyelitis is declining in incidence, death is rare, and chronic osteomyelitis is disappearing.

STAPHYLOCOCCAL PNEUMONIA

Staphylococci are the cause of 1 to 5 percent of bacterial pneumonias. This disease occurs sporadically except during epidemics of influenza when staphylococcal pneumonia is more common.

Primary staphylococcal pneumonia in infants and young children is a frequent cause of pyopneumothorax. This complication occurs early and should suggest S. *aureus* infection. In older children and adults, primary staphylococcal pneumonia is usually secondary to influenza or measles. More recently, staphylococcal pneumonia has been seen with increasing frequency in hospitalized patients with mucoviscidosis, leukemia, diffuse collagen disease, or other chronic debilitating disease.

In healthy adults, staphylococcal pneumonia is generally preceded by an influenza-like respiratory infection. Onset of staphylococcal involvement is abrupt with chills, high fever, progressive dyspnea, cyanosis, cough, and pleural pain. Early peripheral vascular collapse is common, and examination frequently reveals a patient who seems sicker than his physical findings would suggest.

Sputum in the early phases is not characteristic, but may be bloody or frankly purulent. Admixture with blood may produce a thick, creamy pink sputum.

Staphylococcal pneumonia arising in hospitalized patients is a common problem. This illness usually begins more insidiously. Increasing fever, tachycardia, and an elevated respiratory rate may be the only indications of infection. Typical pneumonic symptoms may be absent. This is also true when metastatic pulmonary involvement occurs during the course of staphylococcal bacteremia. Staphylococci generally produce patchy, centrally located areas of pneumonia. Pleural involvement and empyema are common.

Because of the central pulmonary involvement, chest findings are variable. Signs of frank consolidation are rare. Scattered fine to coarse rales and rhonchi may be heard over the involved areas. Empyema produces typical signs of pleural fluid. Signs of abscess may appear late in the course of the disease. Bacteremia is unusual (less than 20 percent of patients), and *its presence should suggest that the pneumonic involvement is metastatic and secondary to foci of infection elsewhere.* Chest x-rays commonly reveal a patchy pneumonic process about the hilar area and may show early evidence of pleural fluid accumulation.

The course of staphylococcal pneumonia may be stormy despite adequate antimicrobial therapy. Gradual defervescence starting 48 to 72 hr after the initiation of therapy is the rule. Pulmonary abscesses or empyema cavities may require local surgical treatment.

DIAGNOSIS. Staphylococcal pneumonia must be differentiated from other pneumonias. The preceding influenza-like illness, rapid onset of pleural pain, cyanosis, and prostration out of proportion to physical findings should suggest primary staphylococcal pneumonia. The finding of masses of polymorphonuclear leukocytes and gram-positive intraleukocytic cocci strongly suggests the diagnosis. The blood leukocyte count is generally above 15,000. The sudden or insidious development of pneumonia with higher fever, tachycardia, and leukocytosis in debilitated hospitalized patients receiving antimicrobials should be considered to be staphylococcal in origin.

PROGNOSIS. Prior to 1942, mortality ranged from 50 to 95 percent. The presence of bacteremia was almost invariably associated with a fatal outcome. The prognosis has improved with the use of antimicrobials but continues to range from 15 to 20 percent in primary staphylococcal pneumonia. Higher mortality is seen in debilitated individuals acquiring staphylococcal pneumonia in the hospital. Abscess formation and pleural involvement often prolong convalescence.

STAPHYLOCOCCAL BACTEREMIA

Staphylococcal bacteremia may arise from any local staphylococcal infection. Infections of the skin (including infections about inlying venous cutdowns or catheters), respiratory tract, long bones, or genitourinary tract precede bacteremia in descending order of frequency. Trauma to local lesions, such as pinching, or surgical drainage before adequate localization may precipitate bacteremia.

Rarely, patients with bacteremia die in 12 to 24 hr, with high fever, tachycardia, cyanosis, gastrointestinal symptoms, and vascular collapse. More commonly, the disease is slower, with hectic fever and metastatic abscess formation in the skin, bones, kidneys, brain, myocardium, spleen, or other tissues. *Meningitis* is an occasional complication.

Endocarditis occurs in 20 to 60 percent of patients with protracted bacteremia. Normal heart valves are frequently involved. Typically, staphylococcal endocarditis runs an acute course with high fever, progressive anemia, and metastatic abscesses in the skin and deeper structures. Rupture of the valve leaflets and valve ring abscesses are common. Specific diagnosis of endocardial involvement is difficult and because of its frequency, should be assumed to be present in patients with staphylococcal bacteremia with demonstrable cutaneous lesions (petechiae or cutaneous pustules) and a significant heart murmur. Both coagulase-positive and coagulase-negative staphylococci have been a major cause of endocarditis in patients undergoing cardiac surgical procedures, particularly valve replacement, and both coagulase-positive and coagulase-negative staphylococci occasionally produce a subacute endocarditis indistinguishable from that produced by *Streptococcus viridans*. Persistent *Staphylococcus albus* bacteremia has also been common after ventriculoatriostomy. These clinical settings should be remembered when blood cultures are reported as "contaminated" with S. *albus* strains.

Staphylococcal bacteremia is generally accompanied by a polymorphonuclear leukocytosis of 12 to 20,000, but a normal leukocyte count or leukopenia is occasionally seen. Anemia develops rapidly during the course of the illness.

PROGNOSIS. Staphylococcal bacteremia is an extremely serious disease. Prior to the development of antimicrobials, over 80 percent of individuals died, the majority within 10 days of the onset of illness. The development of endocarditis or meningitis during bacteremia was almost invariably fatal. The sulfonamides produced little alteration in this mortality. With the administration of effective antibiotics and appropriate surgical treatment of local sites of infection, 50 to 70 percent of patients survive. However, when staphylococcal endocarditis has occurred on a prosthetic cardiac valve, the outcome has been almost invariably fatal.

STAPHYLOCOCCAL FOOD POISONING

Certain strains of staphylococci produce an enterotoxin which is responsible for many outbreaks of acute gastroenteritis. Foods are commonly contaminated from superficial infections in food handlers or by nasal droplets containing pathogenic staphylococci. Cream-filled pastries, custards, cottage cheese, milk products, or meats subjected to improper refrigeration allowing staphylococcal multiplication are the common offenders.

Symptoms typically appear 1 to 6 hr after ingestion of enterotoxin—contaminated food. Onset is usually abrupt, with severe nausea, vomiting, cramping abdominal pain, diarrhea, and prostration. The disease is brief and requires only rest and sedation. Rare fatalities have occurred in the aged. The diagnosis is based on the short incubation period, the epidemic nature of the disease, the short duration of symptoms, and the lack of fever. The etiology can be established only if specimens of ingested food can be shown to contain large numbers of enterotoxin-producing staphylococci.

STAPHYLOCOCCAL ENTERITIS

Staphylococcal enteritis, a true infection of the gut that sometimes complicates antimicrobial therapy, is described in Chap. 133 and 320.

MISCELLANEOUS INFECTIONS

Staphylococci may cause otitis, sinusitis, or mastoid infections. Certain strains elaborate on erythrogenic toxin that results in a rash indistinguishable from streptococcal scarlet fever. Epidemics of staphylococcal pyoderma in newborn infants and maternal breast abscesses are a recurring problem in maternity units.

THE CURRENT PATTERN OF STAPHYLOCOCCAL INFECTIONS

In prolonging the life span of many patients with serious illnesses, a group of individuals with increased susceptibility to many infections has emerged. These individuals are congregated in the modern hospital. The adrenal steroids, corticotropins, nitrogen mustards, or other cytotoxic chemotherapeutic agents appear to alter host defense mechanisms. Many surgical procedures create portals of entry for microorganisms. The use of broad-spectrum antimicrobials often alters normal host flora, and hospital staff have higher carrier rates of antimicrobial-resistant microorganisms. In this setting, staphylococcal infections (along with gram-negative bacillary infections and certain fungal infections) have become an increasing problem.

Staphylococcal infections now fall into two relatively distinct groups. Individuals who develop infections *outside* the hospital commonly present with the typical acute staphylococcal syndromes already discussed. Individuals who acquire staphylococcal infections *inside* hospitals often develop atypical disease. Staphylococcal pneumonia, formerly rare, now occurs as a terminal complication of many diseases. Postoperative wound infections due to staphylococci have continued to plague major hospital centers. Staphylococcal bacteremia is a common problem, staphylococcal endocarditis is a much-feared complication of cardiac surgery when prostheses are inserted, and staphylococcal enteritis is almost exclusively a hospital disease.

There is little to suggest that staphylococcal strains resistant to antimicrobials are any more invasive than those which have always been prevalent. Nevertheless, the disease states in which staphylococcal infections commonly arise are themselves so severe that staphylococcal infections in these situations continue to have a high mortality.

TREATMENT

FEATURES OF STAPHYLOCOCCAL INFECTION WHICH INFLUENCE THERAPY. While the development of penicillinase-resistant penicillins, cephalosporins, and vancomycin has simplified treatment, certain characteristics of staphylococcal disease should be borne in mind in designing therapy.

1. The host setting in which infection occurs. Acute staphylococcal infections arising outside the hospital in otherwise healthy adults have a better prognosis than intrahospital infections arising in sick individuals with compromised host defense mechanisms.

2. The rapid necrosis of tissues produced by staphylococci. Delays in effective therapy may allow a progressing infection to advance to frank abscess formation. While many antimicrobials reach abscess cavities in adequate concentrations, the physiologic insusceptibility of microorganisms residing in areas of extensive necrosis or suppuration render antibiotic therapy quite ineffective in this situation. Surgical drainage of such lesions is often required.

3. The sluggish response to therapy. Staphylococci are killed slowly by antimicrobials and relapses are frequent. Hence antimicrobial therapy must be continued longer than in many bacterial infections.

4. The problem of antimicrobial resistance. While treatment must be initiated empirically when serious staphylococcal infection is suspected, rational therapy requires that the antibiotic susceptibility of the infecting strain be known.

5. Bactericidal versus bacteriostatic antimicrobials. It is generally believed that the so-called "bactericidal" antimicrobials (the penicillins, cephalosporins, vancomycin, bacitracin) are more effective than the "bacteriostatic" agents (erythromycin, lincomycin, novobiocin, chloramphenicol) in treating serious staphylococcal disease.

TREATMENT OF SERIOUS STAPHYLOCOCCAL INFECTIONS. The increasing incidence of penicillin-resistant strains as a cause of extrahospital infections, coupled with the effectiveness of the penicillinase-resistant penicillins, makes it reasonable to use one regimen for initial therapy for all life-threatening staphylococcal disease no matter where it arises. Two methods of initiating treatment when serious staphylococcal disease is suspected have been proposed.

1. Following appropriate cultures, treatment with large doses of both aqueous penicillin *and* methicillin (or parenteral oxacillin or nafcillin) should be instituted immediately. In adults, aqueous penicillin, 20 million units, should be given by continuous intravenous drip. The companion penicillinase-resistant penicillin can be given intravenously or intramuscularly. Methicillin is rapidly eliminated from the body, and initial doses of at least 2 Gm every 4 hr are indicated. When given intravenously,

this drug should be diluted in 50 to 100 ml of 5 percent dextrose and water and given over a 10- to 30-min period because of its tendency to deteriorate when left in intravenous infusion bottles. Parenteral oxacillin or nafcillin in doses of 1 or 2 Gm every 4 hr can be substituted for methicillin.

If in vitro sensitivity studies show the infecting strain to be sensitive to penicillin G, therapy with methicillin can be discontinued and treatment maintained with aqueous penicillin alone. If the strain is penicillin-resistant, the penicillinase-resistant penicillins alone should be continued, and, if necessary, doses as high as 30 Gm per day can be employed.

The above regimen may be advantageous because penicillin-sensitive strains of staphylococci are twenty- to fiftyfold more susceptible to penicillin G than to methicillin, and it seems reasonable to obtain this advantage from the outset in treating penicillin G–susceptible staphylococcal disease.

2. The other alternative is to use a penicillinase-resistant penicillin alone. All strains of staphylococci are susceptible to penicillinase-resistant penicillins, and because of the high incidence of penicillinase-producing staphylococci as causes of infection, some authorities initiate treatment with methicillin, oxacillin, or nafcillin alone, shifting to aqueous penicillin G if the strain is subsequently proven to be susceptible to that drug.

Despite differences in structure, the major allergenic properties of the penicillins reside in the basic 6-aminopenicillanic acid molecule. There is significant cross allergenicity between penicillins, and patients who have had well-established allergic reactions to penicillin G should not receive penicillinase-resistant penicillins. Further, there is increasing evidence that a significant number of these individuals may be allergic to the cephalosporin derivatives as well. These agents, which are good antistaphylococcal drugs, have a 7-aminocephalosporanic acid nucleus quite similar to that of penicillins.

In dealing with such allergic patients, two courses of action are open. If the use of a penicillin or cephalosporin is deemed imperative, skin testing can be performed with cephalothin and the major and minor penicillin antigens. If the skin tests are negative, therapy can be instituted. If skin tests to the agent of choice are positive, desensitization can be attempted. This procedure is not of established value, however, and the use of vancomycin, an agent which has produced therapeutic results quite comparable to the penicillins, seems preferable.

Cephalothin and cephaloridine are semisynthetic derivatives of cephalosporin C. Cephalothin is highly active against both penicillin-sensitive and penicillin-resistant strains. Cephaloridine appears more susceptible to staphylococcal penicillinase and should not be used in treatment of infections by penicillin-resistant strains unless the organism is shown to be sensitive to it. Intramuscular or intravenous doses of 1.0 to 2.0 Gm cephalothin every 4 hr are recommended; the dose of cephaloridine is limited to 1.0 Gm every 6 hr by regulation.

Vancomycin is uniformly active against coagulase-positive staphylococci regardless of their sensitivity to penicillin. It should be given intravenously in doses of 1.0 to 1.5 Gm over a 30- to 40-min period every 12 hr.

The development of these new agents has relegated several antibiotics formerly used in treatment to minor or secondary roles. These include bacitracin and kanamycin, both bactericidal drugs with good antistaphylococcal activity, and the bacteriostatic drugs erythromycin, chloramphenicol and novobiocin. Despite the fact that many strains of staphylococci remain susceptible to these agents, they appear less effective in treating serious staphylococcal disease.

CHANGES IN THERAPY. Established staphylococcal infections respond slowly even to the most effective antimicrobial regimens, making it difficult to know when therapy should be considered inadequate. Characteristically, 24 to 48 hr elapse before a decline in fever is noted, and recovery is accompanied by slow return of the temperature to normal in 7 to 10 days. If the infection shows evidence of rapid progression during the first 24 to 48 hr of treatment, or if fever remains high for over 96 hr in the absence of detectable abscess formation, dosage levels of the penicillins should be increased. Other antimicrobials may be added, but there is little evidence that this practice is helpful. Treatment should be continued for a minimum of 4 to 6 weeks. If the response appears inadequate or staphylococcal endocarditis is suspected, treatment should be prolonged to 8 weeks to 4 months.

Special Therapeutic Situations

ASYMPTOMATIC NASAL CARRIER STATE. The role of asymptomatic carriers in hospital transmission of infection remains controversial. However, it is generally agreed that hospital personnel who harbor in their anterior nares strains of coagulase-positive staphylococci which are producing intrahospital disease must be removed from nursery units, operating theaters, delivery rooms, and surgical floors. Although no method of treatment has been uniformly satisfactory, the following regimens have had limited success in treatment of nasal carriers.

1. Simple removal from the hospital environment for 3 to 4 weeks

2. Frequent baths with germicidal soaps

3. The use of topical antibiotics of low sensitizing potential in a water soluble base (i.e., bacitracin, neomycin, or a combination of these agents) four to five times daily for 2 weeks.

If the carrier state returns, a second course of treatment is indicated. In infants, colonization with disease-producing strains may be prevented by deliberate implantation of a staphylococcal strain of low virulence. This approach has been applied to adult carriers in a limited way, but evidence regarding its efficacy is not yet available.

SUPERFICIAL INFECTIONS. Superficial infections frequently do not require the use of antibiotics. There is no adequate therapy for recurrent furunculosis, but if the disease is severe, antimicrobial treatment may be attempted. Antibiotics to which the strain is susceptible should be administered systemically for a minimum of 10 to 14 days. Local moist heat, immobilization of the infected part, and incision and drainage should be utilized. The surrounding skin should be protected with a coating of zinc oxide to prevent maceration. Treatment of the nasal carrier state by the local application of topical antibiotics (see above) may be advisable. Careful daily baths with germicidal soaps, attention to personal and family hygiene, and the passage of time appear to be measures most likely to interrupt the process. Attempts to prevent recurrence by autogenous or other vaccines have not proved effective.

EMPYEMA. Empyema should be treated by aspiration. In penicillin G–sensitive infections the installation of 200,000 to 500,000 units of penicillin may be worthwhile. Local instillation of methicillin or oxacillin may be utilized in penicillin G–resistant infection. Loculation and thick exudate may prevent adequate needle drainage. While the local instillation of proteolytic enzymes may occasionally aid in liquefying the exudate, surgical drainage is generally necessary and should be performed promptly.

OSTEOMYELITIS. The initial regimen already outlined for other serious infections is recommended and treatment should be continued for 14 to 28 days. Local drainage of abscess cavities in soft tissues or bones should be considered in all patients in whom therapy is initiated after the third day, when severe pain persists, or when response to antimicrobials is inadequate. If sequestration occurs, devitalized bone should be removed. Lincomycin has been reported to be superior to other agents in the treatment of chronic osteomyelitis, but the evidence for this is not convincing.

NURSERY EPIDEMICS. The hazards of epidemic staphylococcal disease in newborn nurseries are well recognized. Pediatric texts should be consulted for full discussion of the special techniques employed in prevention and management of nursery infections. The use of deliberate colonization of newborns with a staphylococcus of low disease potential to prevent colonization with more pathogenic strains has important biologic implications.

REFERENCES

Elek, S. D.: "Staphylococcus Pyogenes," Edinburgh, E. & S. Livingstone, Ltd., 1959.

Koenig, M. G.: Staphylococcal Infections: Treatment and Control, Disease-a-Month, April, 1968.

Morse, S. L.: The Staphylococci and Other Micrococci, chap. 17 in "Bacterial and Mycotic Infections of Man," 4th ed., R. Dubos & J. Hirsch (Eds.), Philadelphia, J. B. Lippincott Company, 1965.

Nahmias, A. J., and T. C. Eickhoff: Staphylococcal Infections in Hospitals, New Engl. J. Med., 265:74–81, 120–128, 177–182, 1962.

Rogers, D. E.: Staphylococcal Infections, Disease-a-Month, pp. 1–48, April, 1958.

Shinefield, H. R., J. C. Ribble, M. Boris, and H. Eichenwald: Bacterial Interference: Its Effect on Nursery Acquired Infection with *Staphylococcus Aureus*, Am. J. Dis. Child., 105:646, 1963.

Whipple, H. E. (Ed.): The Staphylococci: Ecologic Perspectives, Ann. N.Y. Acad. Sci., 128:1–456, 1965.

140 HEMOLYTIC STREPTOCOCCAL INFECTIONS

Charles H. Rammelkamp, Jr.

Aerobic streptococci, as a group, are among the most important bacterial pathogens of man. They can invade any tissue or organ and, depending on the site of invasion and the parasite-host relationship, produce different clinical syndromes. Streptococcal infections may be divided into two large groups. The acute and often dramatic illnesses, such as sore throat, scarlet fever, erysipelas, puerperal fever, and lymphangitis, are included in the first group. These infections occur frequently and are characterized by certain toxic, septic, or suppurative features. The second group of diseases have been called the late, nonsuppurative complications of streptococcal infections. These illnesses, which include acute glomerulonephritis and acute rheumatic fever, commonly become manifest 2 and 3 weeks, respectively, after an acute streptococcal infection. They assume major importance because they may be followed by chronic valvular heart disease or possibly by chronic nephritis. Acute glomerulonephritis is covered in Chap. 304, and rheumatic fever in Chap. 269.

HISTORY. Although scarlet fever was recognized in 1676 by Sydenham, rheumatic fever and acute nephritis were not well described until 1805 and 1836, respectively. The role of the streptococcus as the inciting agent of scarlet fever was established in 1924. With the realization that rheumatic fever and nephritis were related to streptococcal infections, methods for the control and management of these complications developed rapidly.

BACTERIOLOGY. Streptococci are gram-positive and tend to form chains. When grown on a sheep blood agar plate, they can be divided into three groups. *Alpha* colonies show a zone of incomplete or green hemolysis; *beta* streptococci exhibit a clear zone of complete hemolysis; and *gamma* streptococci produce no hemolysis. Streaking a culture on a blood agar plate is sufficient to indicate the important pathogenic streptococci, because those exhibiting beta hemolysis are responsible for the majority of infections in man.

On the basis of a specific carbohydrate, 12 groups of streptococci have been identified and designated Lancefield groups A through N. Respiratory infections are caused by group A and only rarely by groups C and G streptococci. Group D streptococcus, previously referred to as *Streptococcus faecalis* or enterococcus, inhabits the gastrointestinal tract and is responsible for infections of the abdominal cavity and the urinary tract.

Group A comprises at least 40 specific types. Typing is determined either by an agglutinin reaction based on the T-substance or by the precipitin test, for which the M-substance is the type-specific antigen.

By grouping and typing streptococci, considerable information has been accumulated concerning streptococcal infections. The carbohydrate responsible for the group characteristics is nontoxic and unassociated with virulence or immunity. In contrast, the M-protein is probably responsible in part for the virulence of the organism as well as for type-specific immunity. Glossy forms of group A streptococci which contain no M-substance are avirulent whereas virulent organisms always contain this specific protein. The T-substance is not related to virulence.

Several substances produced during the growth serve to differentiate these organisms from other streptococci, as well as to explain, in part, their pathogenic effects. The type of hemolysis has been used for classification of these bacteria. Of the various hemolysins produced by streptococci, at least two types have been recognized and termed *streptolysin O* and *streptolysin S*. They are produced by streptococci of Lancefield groups A, C, and G, the three organisms which cause the majority of human infections. The role of these hemolysins in infections in man is not known. Approximately 85 percent of patients develop antistreptolysin O antibody during the second to third week of convalescence, and the determination of the antistreptolysin titers of acute and convalescent serums may establish the diagnosis of a streptococcal infection.

Another filtrable toxin produced by group A streptococci is the erythrogenic or *scarlatinal toxin*, which causes a scarlatiniform rash when injected into man and, if sufficient quantities are given, fever and nausea. That this toxin is responsible for the rash and toxic features of scarlet fever is well established. Trask and Blake were able to demonstrate a toxin in the circulating blood of patients with scarlet fever and showed that it was neutralized by specific antitoxin. Using the erythrogenic toxin as an antigen, a skin test for susceptibility to scarlet fever was developed by the Dicks. When one skin test dose is injected intradermally, persons susceptible to the erythrogenic toxin respond with an area of erythema which reaches its maximum within 24 hr. Persons in whom this skin reaction is positive are susceptible to scarlatiniform rashes when infected by streptococci which produce erythrogenic toxin. The occasional occurrence of second attacks of scarlet fever may be explained by the fact that there are at least two types of immunologically distinct erythrogenic toxins.

In 1933, it was observed that hemolytic streptococci rapidly liquefied human fibrin. The extracellular substance responsible for this action is termed *streptokinase*. Streptokinase does not lyse fibrin directly but activates a serum enzyme, plasminogen, which in turn lyses the clot. Streptokinase is produced by strains of Lancefield groups A, C, and G, and only occasionally in small amounts by groups B and F. The spreading nature of streptococcal infections has been thought to be due to streptokinase which breaks down the fibrin barrier.

Following infection in man by a strain of group A streptococcus which produces large amounts of streptokinase, antibody usually develops which specifically prevents the lysis of fibrin. Measurement of antistreptokinase may aid in diagnosis, but this serologic test is not as useful as the antistreptolysin test because not all group A streptococci produce sufficient streptokinase to stimulate antibody formation.

Streptodornase (deoxyribonuclease) is an enzyme produced by several groups of streptococci. Group A organisms produce three (A, B, and C) immunologically distinct deoxyribonucleases which depolymerize deoxyribonucleoprotein and deoxyribonucleic acid, the two substances which account for the high viscosity of exudates. A preparation of streptokinase-streptodornase (SK-SD) is available for injection into body cavities containing pus or blood and may result in liquefaction of fibrin and cellular debris.

Other substances produced by streptococci are leukocidin, hyaluronidase, and streptococcal proteinase. Leukocidin, which is probably identical with streptolysin O, is able to inhibit phagocytosis in vitro. The enzyme hyaluronidase, or spreading factor, facilitates the spread of bacteria by increasing tissue permeability. It is produced in large quantities by types 4 and 22 of group A streptococci.

ACUTE STREPTOCOCCAL INFECTIONS

Epidemiology

Aerobic streptococcal infections are observed in all races, in both sexes, and at all ages and occur during any season of the year throughout the world. The *incidence* and the *clinical manifestations* are altered by certain of the above factors. For example, streptococcal respiratory infections, including scarlet fever, are encountered especially during the colder months of the year. Scarlet fever is rare in the tropics. Under the age of three months, streptococcal infections are rare and, when they occur, are associated with a high mortality. Between the ages of six months and ten years, scarlet fever occurs frequently. Tonsillitis and pharyngitis are especially prevalent throughout childhood and early adult life. In women during the childbearing period, puerperal infections caused by streptococci occur occasionally. Finally, erysipelas, which may occur at any age, appears to be more prevalent in infants and the older age groups.

Soon after birth, alpha streptococci appear in the upper part of the respiratory tract and may be isolated therefrom throughout life. Streptococci of Lancefield groups C and G and, more rarely, organisms of groups other than A may be isolated from the oropharynx of 5 percent or more of the normal population. Occasionally group C and G streptococci cause tonsillitis.

The group A flora of the oropharynx is made up of many different specific types, but usually several types predominate. In general, at least 5 percent of the people of any community harbor group A streptococci. The prevalance varies and depends upon the cultural methods used as well as upon environmental, host, and bacterial factors. Persons under twenty years of age are most likely to harbor group A streptococci, especially if the tonsils are present.

Following either apparent or inapparent infection, the carrier state usually persists for several months and occasionally for longer periods. Throat cultures, which are inoculated directly on blood agar plates during the first, fourth, eighth, and eleventh weeks following infection,

show 10 or more colonies of streptococci in 90, 65, 25, and 10 percent of patients, respectively. Carriers of non-group A streptococci usually show only a few colonies on culture. In addition, as the carrier state progresses, the streptococci lose their ability to produce M-protein, so that by the eleventh week, about 40 percent of strains cannot be typed. Thus, quantitative examination of cultures and typing provide important data regarding the possible duration of the carrier state, and this information is valuable in determining whether or not therapy should be instituted.

Ability to spread disease appears to be an attribute of individuals who have been infected recently. Whether such persons harbor numerous streptococci in the nose and throat or whether the organisms are especially capable of parasitizing another person cannot be determined from the available evidence. It is established that nasal carriers of group A streptococci are likely to spread disease. The spread of streptococci in any population group is related to the degree of exposure, and, during the winter months when people are confined to enclosed areas, and under crowded conditions, dissemination of bacteria is especially likely to occur.

Group A streptococci naturally deposited in dust and on blankets will not produce respiratory infections in man. The evidence implicates the direct mode of transfer as primarily responsible for dissemination of such infections.

Outbreaks of streptococcal infection occasionally occur following the contamination of food. These outbreaks are dramatic because a large number of persons are affected almost simultaneously. Formerly this type of infection was termed *septic sore throat;* except that the infection is caused by a single type of streptococcus, it varies clinically in no way from other streptococcal epidemics.

Primary infection of the upper part of the respiratory tract is undoubtedly the most common form of streptococcal infection in man. It is doubtful whether anyone in the United States escapes one or more of these infections. The disease occurs especially in individuals between the ages of one and twenty years, but it may develop at any age. It is especially prevalent in the temperate zones during the winter and early spring seasons. In most areas the disease is endemic. Epidemics are usually due to one or, at the most, several types of group A streptococci, while many different types are responsible for cases of pharyngitis and tonsillitis occurring sporadically.

Tonsillitis and pharyngitis due to the beta streptococcus are characterized by an acute sore throat which may or may not be accompanied by a cutaneous rash. If a rash is observed, a diagnosis of *scarlet fever* is made. The incidence of scarlet fever has not changed significantly in the past 30 years, but there has been a spectacular decline in mortality. Top reports a fatality rate in Detroit of 2.7 in 1920, 1.3 in 1930, and 0.3 in 1940. The reason for the apparent decreasing severity of scarlet fever is not entirely clear.

Infections of the *paranasal sinuses* and middle ear often develop following infection of the tonsils or pharynx. Not only may they occur as a complication of streptococcal sore throat, but they are also commonly seen following measles, influenza, pertusis, and other respiratory infections.

Bacterial pneumonia caused by aerobic streptococci accounts for less than 5 percent of all cases of pneumonia. The disease is almost invariably caused by group A streptococci and may arise secondarily to an infection of the upper respiratory tract. Epidemics have been observed following influenza and measles. Streptococcal empyema, a complication of pneumonia in most instances, is observed most frequently in patients under thirty years of age.

Formerly it was thought that *erysipelas* was caused by a specific strain of beta-hemolytic streptococcus, but it is now known that group A, C, or G streptococci may be isolated from the skin lesions. Group A organisms are responsible for the majority of infections, and the organisms may belong to any of the various types in this group. Erysipelas tends to occur in the older age groups, especially in those individuals with chronic disabling diseases. Immunity does not develop; in fact, individuals who have had one attack are more susceptible than the normal population. In some of the recurrences, however, the organisms cannot be isolated from the skin lesions but may be found in the oropharynx. In these instances the disease may be due to absorption of some streptococcal toxin, which, in turn, causes the local inflammatory lesion in the skin that has altered its reactivity.

Wounds may be infected by droplet contamination at the time of dressing. *Lymphangitis* may arise from a minute abrasion.

Numerous studies have indicated that either aerobic or anaerobic streptococci cause *puerperal sepsis*, but approximately 70 percent of fatal cases are due to beta-hemolytic streptococci, usually group A. Because the group A streptococcus is rarely isolated from the genital tract either before or after labor, infection probably is contracted from an outside source and occasionally from the respiratory tract of the patient herself.

Pathogenesis

Streptococci gain entrance to the body primarily through the upper respiratory tract. The organisms lodge on the mucous membranes or on other tissues and probably remain viable for relatively short periods unless they actually invade the tissues. They usually gain entrance through the lymphoid tissues of the throat, especially the tonsils. Occasionally the primary infection may be in the paranasal sinuses.

Multiple factors determine whether an infection follows exposure to the organism. The *dosage*, or number of streptococci, is apparently decisive; infection usually results when there is exposure to large numbers of group A streptococci, as occurs in food-borne outbreaks. A second factor is the *virulence* of the organism. Streptococci of groups other than A may be considered relatively avirulent when implanted in the lymphoid tissues of the throat. Whether there is variation in the virulence of group A streptococci according to the specific type is not known, nor is there much evidence that rapid passage of a given type from man to man increases the virulence of the organisms.

Perhaps as important as the organism itself is the susceptibility of the host. It is stated that a recent or simultaneous infection with one of the common respiratory viruses renders the host more susceptible to bacterial invasion. Experience during World War I indicates that influenza does indeed increase susceptibility to bacterial infections. Whether the common cold or acute respiratory disease acts in a similar fashion is not known.

Whether the group A streptococcus gains a foothold in the tissues is also governed by the immune status of the host, and the presence of type-specific antibodies undoubtedly protects him against infection.

The organisms may invade the bloodstream if the local defense mechanism is not functioning adequately and cause either metastatic infections, such as meningitis, brain abscess, and endocarditis, or a generalized infection, which without treatment almost invariably results in death. In fulminating streptococcal infections the streptococci may be seen in blood vessels throughout the body, as well as in the endothelial cells of the endocardium and in the perivascular areas. There is little cellular reaction around the organisms, but their distribution is similar to that of lesions observed in patients dying several days after onset of the infection, in whom foci of lymphocytes, plasma cells, and histiocytes commonly are found in the heart, especially just under the surface endothelium, and endocardium. Occasionally some of the foci show polymorphonuclear leukocytes. In the kidneys, there are focal areas of round-cell infiltration in the tissue surrounding the tubules, glomeruli, and blood vessels. Similar lesions may be observed in other organs.

Most streptococcal infections are of short duration, and the acute phase ends within 5 to 7 days. The exact mechanism for recovery at this time has not been defined, but, as in other bacterial infections, it is assumed that antibodies develop which aid in the destruction of the organism.

Acute Tonsillitis, Pharyngitis, and Scarlet Fever

The terminology used to classify streptococcal infections of the upper respiratory tract was introduced before it was realized that *scarlet fever, septic sore throat, acute tonsillitis,* and *pharyngitis* with or without exudate were all caused by any of the numerous types of group A streptococci. In these diseases the organism establishes itself in the lymphoid tissue; *streptococcal lymphoiditis* might well be substituted for the above names.

SYMPTOMS. The incubation period varies from 1 to 10 days but is usually 3 to 5 days. The illness begins abruptly with symptoms of feverishness, chilliness, headache, and sore throat. Nausea and vomiting are especially common in children. A few patients complain of diarrhea. Within a period of 24 to 48 hr the disease reaches its maximum intensity. Chilliness is a constant symptom, but true rigors are rare. Approximately 75 percent or more of the patients complain of headache, malaise, and loss of appetite.

Sore throat is almost constantly present within 24 hr of onset. The soreness is aggravated by swallowing and may be referred to the neck, so that even turning of the head is accompanied by pain. Nasal obstruction and discharge are minor complaints but occur in 60 percent of patients. About half the patients develop very mild symptoms referable to the lower part of the respiratory tract, including cough and hoarseness. The cough is not productive and is rarely associated with chest pain. Loss of voice due to laryngitis does not occur. Earache is common and may last a few hours to several days. Occasionally, epistaxis is observed.

During the period of maximum temperature there may be a diffuse blush of the skin. In some cases it becomes more pronounced, and a diagnosis of *scarlet fever* is made. The rash appears 1 to 5 days after onset of illness and is first noticed over the neck and upper part of the chest. It spreads rapidly to include the skin over the abdomen and upper and lower extremities. The face appears flushed, and circumoral pallor is prominent. Itching occasionally occurs but is rarely severe.

PHYSICAL SIGNS. The degree of prostration varies, but the majority of patients appear mildly or moderately ill. The temperature is usually elevated to 102 to 104°F; occasionally it may be as high as 106°F. A few patients

have no fever. In children the pulse rate is between 140 and 160, in adults between 120 and 140 per min.

Various degrees of diffuse redness of the mucous membranes of the posterior pharynx, faucial tonsils, and soft palate are invariably present. The uvula is frequently edematous, as are the tonsils and pharynx. Lymphoid hyperplasia and edema give the posterior pharynx a cobblestone appearance. Characteristically there is discrete to confluent exudate on the tonsils, and variable numbers of pinhead-size areas of exudate appear on the pharynx. In severely ill patients these are seldom seen, because nasal secretions cover the posterior wall. The exudate is often yellow, sometimes gray or white, and is relatively easily removed by swabbing. In about 20 percent of adults, and more frequently in infants, exudative lesions on the mucous membranes do not develop. If sinusitis and rhinitis are present there is a thick mucopurulent nasal discharge which may be tinged with blood. In children the nares may be excoriated. The cervical lymph nodes are swollen and frequently tender. The lymph nodes just below the angle of the jaw are the first to enlarge; rarely they attain such size that the head is thrown back. Marked adenopathy is frequently followed by suppuration.

In those patients with *scarlet fever* the signs include both an enanthem and an exanthem. The appearance of the throat is similar to that seen in tonsillitis and pharyngitis without rash, except that diffuse redness is more intense and has been described as "boiled-lobster" red. There may be punctate redness of the soft and hard palate. The buccal mucous membranes appear red and swollen, as do the lips. About the second to fifth day, small milk-white patches may be seen on the buccal mucous membranes. They represent desquamation of the epithelium and are easily peeled off.

Early in the course of the infection the tongue is heavily coated and grayish. Soon the tip and edges become an angry red. Fungiform papillae become swollen and emerge through the gray surface of the tongue. By the fourth to fifth day there is complete lingual desquamation, which leaves multiple papillary elevations, the so-called "strawberry tongue."

The color of the exanthem varies and has been described as scarlet, bright red, rose-colored, or dull, dusky red. At a distance there appears to be a uniform blush, but upon close inspection innumerable small reddish points are seen. Because of pinpoint elevations at the site of the hair follicles, the skin may feel like sandpaper. This sign is of special importance in races where the skin is heavily pigmented. When the eruption is intense, there may be many small miliary vesicles over the chest and abdomen. The face may be free of rash, but ordinarily the temples and cheeks are deep red, leaving an area of pallor around the mouth and nose. The rash is due to hyperemia, and pressure causes it to fade. In some areas there may be punctate hemorrhages which do not fade; these are commonly seen in the creases at the elbow flexure (Pastia's sign), groin, and axillary folds.

COURSE OF ILLNESS (Fig. 140-1). The majority of upper respiratory illnesses caused by group A streptococci are

Avg.
WBC. 14,500 14,250 12,300 10,700

Fig. 140-1. The natural course of group A streptococcal tonsillitis.

self-limited. In adults the temperature usually returns to normal by the third to fourth day; in children fever may persist for 5 to 9 days. The temperature curve is not characteristic, although there is usually a slight morning remission. In patients with scarlet fever the temperature remains elevated until the rash has reached its maximum intensity. Fever may last for several weeks, but in such instances it is well to search for some suppurative complications. The constitutional symptoms, as well as the localizing symptom of sore throat, usually disappear shortly after the fever subsides.

The edema, redness, and exudate disappear rapidly, and except for a few small isolated spots of exudate and a slight degree of redness, the throat appears normal shortly after the fever subsides. The lymphoid tissues of the posterior pharynx as well as the tonsils decrease in size and by the third to sixth week appear to be normal. The lymph nodes may not return to normal size for 6 weeks.

When rash does occur, it usually makes its appearance on the second day, reaches its maximum intensity shortly thereafter, and then begins to fade. The exfoliation of the epithelium begins during the decline of the eruption and is seen first in those areas where the rash originally appeared. By the sixth to seventh day it is more or less generalized. On the hands and feet the skin sheds in flakes or, more rarely, as an entire cast of the hand or foot. The skin in these areas becomes dry, hard, and wrinkled. The most typical form of desquamation is seen beneath the free edge of the fingernails. A fissure appears under the edge of the nail and then widens, revealing the soft, pinkish underlying skin.

LABORATORY FINDINGS. In 80 percent of patients the total leukocyte count is increased. During the first 2 days of disease the average count is 14,000, and as the illness progresses, it returns to normal values. If the number of leukocytes remains elevated after 1 week, evidence of a complication may be found. During the first 2 days of illness eosinophils are rarely seen, but convalescence is characterized by an increase of these cells. Patients with scarlet fever are especially likely to have eosinophilia. Not frequently a trace of albumin may be found in the urine during the acute phase of the illness, and rarely, such specimens show a few red cells or casts. Proteinuria during the first 5 days of illness is transient and is not attended by serious sequelae.

DIAGNOSIS. Important features in the diagnosis of streptococcal pharyngitis and tonsillitis are the history of an acute onset of soreness on swallowing, associated with feverishness and other constitutional symptoms. The physical signs of diffuse redness and edema of the mucous membranes of the oropharynx, tonsils, and soft palate, the presence of discrete to confluent exudate, and the enlargement and tenderness of the lymph nodes at the angle of the jaw are especially helpful. These findings, together with a leukocyte count of at least 12,000, suggest a streptococcal infection. If the culture of the local lesion shows a predominant growth of beta streptococci, the diagnosis is established with certainty. When only a few colonies grow on the blood agar plate, it is

impossible to be sure whether the patient is a carrier or actually has an infection due to the streptococcus. In such cases it is of considerable help to obtain acute and convalescent blood specimens for determination of antistreptolysin titers.

When a rash is associated with the above clinical and laboratory findings, the diagnosis is scarlet fever. Confirmation is obtained if the skin desquamates.

DIFFERENTIAL DIAGNOSIS OF SORE THROAT. *Nonbacterial exudative tonsillitis and pharyngitis* must be differentiated from streptococcal infections of the oropharynx (Chap. 206). Adenoviruses will produce respiratory infections associated with exudate lesions, and in some outbreaks there is involvement of the conjunctiva. In general the onset of illness is not rapid, sore throat is seldom marked, and constitutional symptoms are mild. Hoarseness and cough are likely to occur several days after the onset. The exudate is rarely confluent. The lymph nodes may be slightly enlarged, but are not remarkably tender. The leukocyte count is usually normal, although in a few cases it may be slightly elevated. Cultures of the throat fail to show beta-hemolytic streptococci. Occasionally a few streptococci are recovered, but these organisms usually belong to groups other than A and occur only in small numbers.

Infectious mononucleosis is most frequently observed in young adults and, because of the local reaction in the throat, is likely to be confused with streptococcal pharyngitis (Chap. 255). The onset may be insidious, and malaise is prominent. Sore throat with exudative lesions of the tonsils is observed in over half the cases. Fever is more prolonged than is usual in streptococcal infections. Lymph node enlargement is more generalized, but suppuration is not observed. The spleen may be palpable. In 10 to 15 percent of cases a fleeting skin rash occurs, which may be identical with that seen in scarlet fever. The blood changes are characteristic, and a positive heterophil antibody test is usually obtained.

Vincent's angina (Chap. 168) is not easily confused with streptococcal infections. The disease is characterized by insidious onset without constitutional symptoms. Fever is rare. The area surrounding the exudate shows little inflammatory reaction, generally only one tonsil is involved, and cervical adenopathy is usually unilateral.

In contrast to streptococcal pharyngitis, the onset of *diphtheria* is rarely sudden and the symptoms are not severe (Chap. 169). Sore throat is not a constant feature of the disease. The exudate is smooth and cream-colored and appears to be incorporated in the mucous membranes. The membrane is removed with difficulty, leaving a bleeding bed. Cutaneous rashes are absent. Cultures show *Corynebacterium diphtheriae*.

In patients with a rash, the disease must be differentiated from *rubella* (Chap. 221) and *rubeola* (Chap. 220). In German measles the posterior cervical lymph node enlargement is helpful, as well as the fact that the rash tends to be macular and discrete. The tongue never peels, and a leukopenia is characteristic. In measles there are prodromal respiratory symptoms, and the maculopapular rash occurs chiefly on the face and neck. The presence of Koplik's spots aids in establishing the diagnosis.

Streptococcal infections without exudate or a cutaneous rash must be differentiated from *influenza virus infection* (Chap. 208) and *common respiratory diseases* (Chap. 206). In general, this differentiation cannot be made on clinical evidence alone, and the leukocyte count, culture studies, and serologic tests must be employed.

Primary *herpes simplex pharyngitis* (Chap. 226) and *herpangina* (Chap. 210) are characterized by vesicles which rupture and produce small ulcers covered with exudate. Herpetic lesions are scattered over all mucous membranes of the mouth, and the kissing ulcer under the tip of the tongue is typical. The ulcers of herpangina, caused by Coxsackie A viruses, are observed on the anterior pillars and the soft palate. In both diseases the leukocyte count is usually normal.

Sinusitis, Otitis Media, Mastoiditis, and Peritonsillar Abscess

Infection of the paranasal sinuses probably occurs to a minor degree in all patients with streptococcal respiratory infections. Sinusitis and otitis media presenting overt clinical signs develop in approximately 3 percent of patients whose tonsils and adenoids are intact. Mastoiditis is observed in less than 1 percent of patients. Peritonsillar cellulitis is observed in 2.5 percent of patients with tonsils, but it rarely occurs in those whose tonsils have been removed or in those patients who receive proper therapy with antibiotics. The diagnosis and management of these suppurative complications are described in Chap. 282.

Pneumonia and Empyema

The natural course of pneumonia caused by Lancefield group A streptococci is extremely variable, probably because in many instances it is secondary to such infections as influenza, tonsillitis, measles, and erysipelas. It may occur as the sole manifestation of streptococcal infection or may arise as a metastatic complication of streptococcal bacteremia. Although it is not a common complication of streptococcal sore throat, about 25 percent of cases follow this infection. Characteristically, this organism produces an interstitial or confluent pneumonia. The reported mortality rate varies from 15 to 60 percent.

The onset of pneumonia may be abrupt, with such constitutional symptoms as chills, feverishness, anorexia, and vomiting. Symptoms include cough, expectoration of purulent sputum, and chest pain. The pulse and respiratory rates are increased, and cyanosis may be prominent. The temperature tends to be high (104°F), and the fever is intermittent. Examination reveals local signs of pneumonia, with scattered fine rales and occasional areas of dullness. Frank signs of lobar consolidation are rare.

The leukocyte count is almost invariably elevated to 20,000 to 30,000, and the sputum is found to contain large numbers of group A organisms. Usually the blood cultures are sterile; when bacteremia occurs, the prognosis is poor.

The untreated disease runs a variable course. In most instances recovery is delayed for several weeks, and lung abscess and bronchiectasis are not uncommon complications. In fatal cases mediastinitis and pericarditis may occur. The most frequent complication is empyema, which occurs in 20 percent of the cases.

Streptococcal *empyema* is usually secondary to pneumonia caused by the same organism, but occasionally arises following other infections of the lung, infarcts, or lung tumors. The mortality rate in untreated cases is high. Early in the disease the pleural fluid may be hemorrhagic, and it becomes thick and purulent slowly, in contrast to the exudate seen in pneumococcal empyema.

Pericarditis, Arthritis, Peritonitis, and Meningitis

Streptococcal infections of the various body cavities result from bacteremia or from extension from a local lesion. *Pericarditis,* a rare complication, is especially likely to occur during the course of pneumonia or empyema. The diagnosis is difficult, because the symptoms arising from pericarditis are overshadowed by the primary disease. The first sign may be a sudden increase in pulse rate and the development of an audible pericardial friction rub.

Suppurative arthritis is secondary to bacteremia or to extension of a local cellulitis. It is a rare complication of streptococcal sore throat. Pain is the most common symptom, and usually only one joint is involved. The pain is first noticed on motion, but within a short period redness, swelling, and tenderness develop and the pain becomes intense. Aspiration reveals a fluid containing polymorphonuclear leukocytes and streptococci. Nonsuppurative arthritis seen in patients with scarlet fever during the first week of illness indicates the onset of rheumatic fever and should not be considered a manifestation of erythrogenic toxin.

Infection of the peritoneum with the hemolytic streptococcus is rare but is especially apt to be associated with such local infections as erysipelas and scarlet fever. In these cases the organism belongs to Lancefield group A. Symptoms develop rapidly, and in addition to fever and other constitutional symptoms, prostration, abdominal pain, and vomiting are prominent. The pulse is rapid and weak. The abdomen is distended, tender, and rigid to palpation.

Streptococcal *meningitis* is usually caused by group A organisms, but occasionally members of other groups may be isolated from the spinal fluid. In most instances the meningitis arises by extension from otitis media, mastoiditis, or petrositis, which are especially likely to develop following infection of the respiratory tract and are seen most frequently in the young. Prior to the introduction of specific therapy these infections were always fatal. The symptoms are not distinguishable from those of other types of bacterial meningitis. All patients, especially infants, with infections of the middle ear should be watched for signs of meningeal irritation.

Wound and Skin Infections, Lymphangitis, Puerperal Fever, and Erysipelas

Wound and skin infections are usually the result of contamination. Children with chickenpox, impetigo, and other skin lesions may become infected with group A and C streptococci. *Impetigo* caused by group A streptococci is sometimes followed by acute nephritis.

Hemolytic streptococci are responsible for the majority of cases of *lymphangitis,* characterized by the rapid development of one or more fine red streaks extending upward from the hand or foot. Usually the process continues up to the axilla or groin, and the lymph nodes in these areas become enlarged and tender. Associated with the spread of the infection in the lymphatics, such symptoms as rigor, fever, malaise, headache, and vomiting occur. Occasionally the bloodstream is invaded. The original site of infection in these cases of lymphangitis may not be apparent. Although these infections may be serious, the course of the illness is usually short, and suppuration along the course of the lymphatics seldom occurs. Within 2 weeks after a streptococcal respiratory infection, some children develop persistent *lymphadenitis.* In children with enlarged cervical nodes 75 percent of the cases are secondary to a streptococcal infection. In these patients aspiration of the node will usually reveal the organism.

Puerperal infections caused by hemolytic streptococci are always serious. Following abortion or delivery, the streptococci invade the endometrium and lymphatics. The infection may spread to the surrounding structures, producing cellulitis, phlebitis, abscess, peritonitis, or bacteremia. The patient develops a high irregular fever associated with rigors. The pulse is rapid. The diagnosis is based on local signs of infection as well as on such laboratory findings as leukocytosis and isolation of streptococci from the bloodstream or from the cervical discharge.

Erysipelas is an acute streptococcal infection of the skin and, to a lesser extent, of the mucous membranes. The onset is usually abrupt, after an incubation period of 1 to 4 days. A history of preceding respiratory infection is sometimes obtained. The initial symptoms include chilliness, feverishness, headache, malaise, anorexia, and vomiting. At the onset the local cutaneous lesion may not be apparent. The skin may itch and feel sore around the point of entry of the organisms. Within a few hours, the cutaneous lesion becomes obvious.

The face is most commonly involved, but any area of the body may be infected. The point of entry may be just anterior to the ear, at the inner canthus of the eye, around the lips and nose, or over the cheeks. From these points the lesion spreads rapidly, reaching its maximum extent within 3 to 6 days. Erysipelas frequently involves the butterfly area of the cheeks and nose. The lesion consists of an advancing border which is raised from the surrounding normal skin and may be purple. Within this border the skin is tense and usually a dark dull red. If the infection occurs in areas where the skin is lax, such as around the eyes, edema is pronounced. The eyelids frequently become so swollen that they cannot be opened. Blebs or necrotic areas may appear as the disease progresses.

At the height of the infection the temperature is usually high (104 to 105°F), although occasionally the febrile response is slight. The bloodstream is not uncommonly invaded during this period. In most instances recovery is apparent by the sixth to seventh day. The local lesion begins to fade in the center, with some desquamation and pigmentation. No scarring results unless abscesses develop.

Before the introduction of chemotherapy, the fatality rate was about 15 percent. During the first 6 months of life approximately 65 percent of patients die, while in older children and young adults the death rate is low. In patients with fatal infections the lesion is likely to involve the trunk.

Bacteremia

Streptococci are a common cause of bacteremia, but in uncomplicated tonsillitis and pharyngitis the organisms rarely invade the bloodstream. Bacteremia occurring under the age of twenty usually is secondary to otitis media, mastoiditis, or thrombosis of the lateral or cavernous sinuses. In adults, invasion of the bloodstream is especially likely to occur in puerperal infections, whereas after the age of forty bacteremia is usually secondary to cellulitis and erysipelas. Metastatic abscesses are infrequent.

The diagnosis of bacteremia is difficult and can be made only by culturing the organisms from the blood. The sudden development of chills and high fever suggests invasion of the bloodstream. There may be arthritis, signs of pneumonia, petechiae, or skin eruptions. In fulminating cases, anemia develops rapidly and jaundice may occur. Without specific therapy the mortality rate is 70 percent.

Treatment

There are now several agents which may be employed in the therapy of aerobic streptococcal infections. The sulfonamides exert a bacteriostatic effect against all Lancefield groups except D. However, some strains of group A streptococci have acquired resistance. Most antibiotics have some antistreptococcal activity, but penicillin clearly is the best antistreptococcal drug because it kills group A organisms. If it is administered for at least 10 days, in most instances all streptococci are eliminated. Therapeutic measures which do not result in the eradication of the infecting organism do not alter the attack rate of rheumatic fever.

The administration of penicillin or other antibiotics

within 24 hr of the onset of streptococcal respiratory infections results in definite improvement of the symptoms and signs. When therapy is instituted after 48 hr, a favorable effect is difficult to demonstrate, but suppurative complications, including sinusitis, otitis media, and peritonsillar cellulitis are prevented. The time that treatment is started is not decisive in the reduction of rheumatic fever; however, early therapy may be important in the prevention of nephritis. In general, proper therapy instituted during the first 24 hr of illness will reduce the predicted rheumatic fever attack rate by 95 to 98 percent. If therapy is started 1, 2, or 3 weeks after the onset of sore throat, the reduction in attack rates is 90, 67, and 42 percent, respectively. Therefore to prevent rheumatic fever, a full course of therapy should be given to those individuals who have recovered from acute phase symptoms and received no therapy even though the onset was 3 weeks previously.

In the average case of streptococcal infection, whether scarlet fever, tonsillitis, or erysipelas, sufficient concentration of antibiotic can be maintained readily by a single injection of 600,000 to 1,200,000 units of benzathine penicillin. In patients with rheumatic heart disease who develop a streptococcal infection, it is advisable to administer 600,000 units of procaine penicillin twice daily for 2 weeks.

Oral therapy may be prescribed, but many patients discontinue the medication when the acute symptoms subside. Under these circumstances, the organism frequently invades the tissues again, and a clinical relapse occurs. More important, the attack rate of the nonsuppurative complications is not altered. All forms of oral medication must be taken in full doses for at least 10 days and preferably for 2 weeks. Oral penicillin G should be given in doses of at least 250,000 units four times daily. Penicillin V in dosage of 1 to 2 Gm daily or phenethicillin may be preferable because these agents resist degradation by gastric acid. Patients sensitive to penicillin may be given erythromycin in doses of 0.25 Gm every 6 hr. Tetracycline drugs should not be employed because of the high prevalence of resistant strains.

The *sulfonamides* should never be employed in the treatment of streptococcal infections because they fail to eliminate the infecting organism and do not alter the subsequent attack rate of rheumatic fever. Penicillin troches or sprays have little effect on the local inflammatory lesion or on the infecting organism. Penicillin appears to decrease the incidence of suppurative complications of tonsillitis and pharyngitis.

Infections of the mastoid and paranasal sinuses should be treated by the parenteral administration of 1.2 to 2.4 million units penicillin G every day. Streptococcal pneumonia should be treated with somewhat larger amounts of penicillin. Empyema, purulent pericarditis, and arthritis are treated best by local instillation of 10,000 to 50,000 units penicillin G every 48 to 72 hr until cultures are sterile. In addition, full doses of parenteral penicillin should be administered. In these infections early treatment is required if surgical drainage is to be avoided.

Prevention

There is no completely adequate method for the prevention of streptococcal infections. A number of procedures will limit the spread of the organism. The problem is exceedingly complicated because group A streptococci occur in the upper part of the respiratory tract of many individuals.

In the past it was customary to isolate all patients with scarlet fever, but this seems unwarranted, particularly because no precautions are taken for sore throat without a rash caused by the same bacterium. Any patient with a streptococcal infection of the upper respiratory tract may be a source of infection. During the acute stage of all such illnesses the patient should be advised against intimate contact with others.

Approximately 90 percent of patients with streptococcal infections continue to carry the organism in the pharynx 3 months after the acute infection. Usually the number of organisms is small. Individuals with suppurative sinusitis are likely to harbor large numbers of streptococci and are a dangerous source of infection. Proper therapy of acute infections with penicillin prevents the development of the carrier state and promptly eliminates the organism.

Individuals or groups can be protected from streptococcal infections by the prophylactic use of sulfonamides. For this purpose 1 Gm sulfadiazine or sulfisoxazole is administered daily. When given to populations already experiencing an epidemic, this prophylactic measure will control the outbreak as long as the drug is administered. When therapy is discontinued, streptococcal infections again occur because of the failure of sulfonamides to eliminate the infecting organism. For this reason, oral penicillin in doses of 250,000 units two or three times daily for 10 days or a single injection of 1,200,000 units of benzathine penicillin is a preferred form of prophylaxis in large groups. Benzathine penicillin in doses of 600,000 and 1,200,000 units will protect the individual from new infections for 3 or 4 to 6 weeks, respectively.

Tonsillectomy has been employed widely as a prophylactic measure against streptococcal infections because tonsillitis cannot occur if the organ is removed. However, no protection is afforded against streptococcal pharyngitis. Indeed, tonsillectomy makes subsequent recognition of the cause of the respiratory illness more difficult.

Many attempts have been made to control respiratory disease by altering certain environmental factors, by using ultraviolet light, aerosols, and various dust-holding procedures, and by treating bed clothing with oils. It has been demonstrated that these methods decrease the contamination of the air, but their effectiveness in preventing infection is slight.

REFERENCES

Dajani, A. S., R. E. Garcia, and E. Wolinsky: Etiology of Cervical Lymphadenitis in Children, New Engl. J. Med., 268:1329, 1963.
Denny, F. W., L. W. Wannamaker, and E. O. Hahn: Com-

parative Effects of Penicillin, Aureomycin and Terramycin on Streptococcal Tonsillitis and Pharyngitis, Pediatrics, 2:7, 1953.

Rammelkamp, C. H., Jr.: Epidemiology of Streptococcal Infections, Harvey Lectures, 51:113, 1957.

—— and B. L. Stolzer: The Latent Period before the Onset of Acute Rheumatic Fever, Yale J. Biol. Med., 34:386, 1961–62.

141 OTHER STREPTOCOCCAL INFECTIONS

Leighton E. Cluff

Group A streptococci account for the majority of streptococcal infections in man. Group C, D, and G streptococci, identifiable by antigenically different cell wall C polysaccharides, have also been identified as occasional causes of human infection. Other streptococci, including *Streptococcus viridans* and *anaerobic streptococci,* not characterized antigenically, also cause infection in human beings. Many of these streptococci are indigenous to the respiratory, genital, or gastrointestinal tract. They are commonly opportunistic and produce infection particularly in patients with reduced natural resistance. Contrasted with group A streptococci, these other streptococcal infections are not followed by late consequences such as rheumatic fever and glomerulonephritis.

Streptococci other than group A may or may not produce hemolysis when cultured on blood agar. Certain strains of *groups C and D* are nonhemolytic; others cause beta or complete hemolysis. Strains of *S. viridans* are usually alpha-hemolytic, producing a green zone about colonies on blood agar. Some strains of *S. viridans,* however, are nonhemolytic (gamma). *Group D streptococci* also may cause alpha hemolysis.

Streptococci of all types characteristically grow in chains, but under certain culture conditions and in clinical specimens they may be found in clusters or pairs of gram-positive cocci.

Group C strains have a low pathogenicity for man. They may be isolated from the normal respiratory tract but have been associated with acute pharyngitis, sinusitis, and rarely bacteremia. *Group G streptococci* also have been isolated from the normal nasopharynx but have produced tonsillitis, endocarditis, and urinary tract infections in man.

The prevalence of streptococci other than group A in the normal oropharynx, genital mucosa, and gastrointestinal tract complicates the problem of relating them specifically to disease. Identification of the organisms in pure culture or from pus, blood, or urine, however, is indicative of their pathogenicity.

STREPTOCOCCUS VIRIDANS. These bacteria are occasionally called alpha, or green, streptococci. Streptococci other than strains belonging to this group, however, may cause alpha, or green, hemolysis on blood agar. *Streptococcus viridans* is most commonly confused on culture with pneumococci. In some instances these bacteria are differentiated into strains referred to as *S. mitis* and *S. salivarius.* For practical purposes, however, these bacteria may be considered the same. *Streptococcus viridans* is important largely as a cause of subacute bacterial endocarditis (Chap. 137), but it has been associated with "mixed" pulmonary infections and sinusitis. It is a part of the normal bacterial population of the oropharynx. These bacteria are usually sensitive to penicillin. Some strains of oropharyngeal *S. viridans* in persons receiving penicillin prophylaxis for rheumatic fever may become resistant to penicillin, but this has not yet presented a serious problem in management of patients with bacterial endocarditis.

GROUP D STREPTOCOCCI. These bacteria possess group-specific C polysaccharide and are frequently designated as *enterococcus* or *Streptococcus faecalis.* These microorganisms are characterized by their ability to grow in 6.5 percent NaCl and to reduce methylene blue. Many strains cause alpha hemolysis and for this reason may be confused with *S. viridans.* Group D streptococci are often resistant to, or acquire resistance to, penicillin. They are of greatest importance as causes of urinary tract infection, purulent infection involving the peritoneal cavity, and bacterial endocarditis. The presence of the bacteria in the normal gastrointestinal tract and on the genitalia is significant in their relationship to both these infections. Bacterial endocarditis due to group D streptococci is commonest in elderly men with prostatism and in women with valvular heart disease following abortion. Urinary tract infection develops usually in persons with recurrent or chronic pyelonephritis or in persons with structurally abnormal urinary tracts. Septic endometritis and parametritis following abortion or prolonged and difficult labor have been associated with group D streptococcal infection, usually in combination with other microorganisms.

Administration of penicillin G or ampicillin combined with streptomycin is the preferred treatment of group D streptococcal infection. However, many strains are sensitive to the tetracyclines, erythromycin, and vancomycin (Chap. 135), and these agents have been effective in many clinical situations.

ANAEROBIC STREPTOCOCCI. Among the body's normal inhabitants are many streptococci that cannot be cultured at atmospheric concentrations of oxygen, although most of them are not obligate anaerobes and are properly termed microaerophilic. They are often found in exudates with other organisms, especially *Bacteroides,* coliform bacilli, and clostridial species.

They infect soft-tissue wounds and compound fractures, sometimes producing a crepitant myositis that resembles clostridial gas gangrene (Chap. 172). Post-abortal and puerperal sepsis with pelvic thrombophlebitis and septic pulmonary infarcts, peritonitis, empyema, abscesses of the lung, liver, and brain, perirectal abscesses, mastoiditis, dental infections, and wounds produced by human bites are the most frequent lesions from which anaerobic streptococci are isolated in pure or mixed cultures.

Certain characteristics of anaerobic streptococcal infections are distinct enough to arouse strong suspicion clinically. They cause the production of copious amounts of brown thin pus. Gas-producing infections in wounds may mimic clostridial gangrene. The pus, lochia in uterine infection, and breath of patients with lung abscess attributable to group D streptococcal infection possess a penetrating, overwhelmingly foul odor. The fetor often ascribed to colon bacillus exudates is a result of the concomitant presence of anaerobic streptococci or *Bacteroides* bacilli. Some strains (*Streptococcus foetidus*) are sometimes recognizable in stained smears by the tendency to grow in parallel chains; others (*S. parvulus*) produce black pigment on agar plates.

Patients with empyema caused by anaerobic streptococci often develop painful areas of cellulitis around the site of thoracentesis needle punctures; this is rare in other empyemas.

Two more or less distinct clinical entities have been attributed to anaerobic streptococci: *burrowing ulcer* and *progressive bacterial synergistic gangrene*. Both are unusual but sufficiently characteristic to be recognized by inspection. Burrowing ulcer occurs on the trunk or extremities and consists of a ragged ulceration from which necrotic sinuses extend subcutaneously, occasionally breaking through to the surface. The process is chronic and is accompanied by pain, fever, and emaciation; occasionally death occurs from necrosis of a major blood vessel. It does not attack muscle, and stops at the fascial layer. Anaerobic streptococci in pure culture are usually obtained from the exudate. Progressive bacterial synergistic gangrene usually complicates surgical operations on the abdomen and consists of progressive spreading ulceration, often around a stay suture. It is caused by a mixture of *Staphylococcus aureus* and anaerobic streptococci. The lesion is discolored, with a gangrenous granulating center.

Surgical drainage and debridement are important in the management of anaerobic streptococcal infections. Penicillin and its analogues in large doses are the drugs of choice; tetracyclines, erythromycin, and vancomycin may be effective in certain cases.

REFERENCES

Evan, A. C., and A. L. Chinn: The Enterococci: With Special Reference to Their Association with Human Disease, J. Bacteriol., 54:495, 1947.

Feingold, D. S., N. L. Stagg, and L. J. Kunz: Extrarespiratory Streptococcal Infections: Importance of the Various Serologic Groups, New Engl. J. Med., 275:356, 1966.

Fisher, A. M., and T. J. Abernathy: Putrid Empyema with Special Reference to Anaerobic Streptococci, Arch. Intern. Med., 54:552, 1934.

Heineman, H. S., and A. I. Braude: Anaerobic Infection of the Brain: Observations on 18 Consecutive Cases of Brain Abscess, Am. J. Med., 35:682, 1963.

Rantz, L. A., and W. M. M. Kirby: Enterococcic Infections, Arch. Intern. Med., 71:516, 1943.

Reinarz, J. A., and J. P. Sanford: Human Infections Caused by Non-group A or D Streptococci, Medicine, 44:81, 1965.

Reynolds, R. C., F. I. Catlin, and L. E. Cluff: Bacteriology and Antibiotic Treatment of Acute Maxillary Sinusitis, Bull. Johns Hopkins Hosp., 114:269, 1964.

Smith, L. D. S.: "Introduction to the Pathogenic Anaerobes," Chicago, University of Chicago Press, 1955.

Section 4

Diseases Caused by Gram-negative Cocci

142 MENINGOCOCCAL INFECTIONS

*Harry N. Beaty and
Robert G. Petersdorf*

DEFINITION. Meningococcal infections are defined as the varied manifestations which result from entry of meningococci into man. Characteristically, these organisms infect the nasopharynx of many individuals, but produce illness in only a few. Serious meningococcal disease occurs when there is invasion of the bloodstream and development of meningitis or fulminating bacteremia with circulatory collapse and death.

ETIOLOGY. The organism responsible for "cerebrospinal fever" was first described by Weichselbaum in 1887. It was subsequently assigned to the genus *Neisseria*, and is now designated by the binomial *Neisseria meningitidis* and the common name meningococcus. In stained smears, meningococci are gram-negative and characteristically appear as single cocci or diplococci with flattened adjacent sides. They grow well on solid or semisolid media containing blood, serum, or ascitic fluid, and thrive best at temperatures between 35 and 37°C in an atmosphere reduced in oxygen and containing 5 to 10 percent CO_2. The organism is recovered readily from biologic fluids when fresh specimens are inoculated on warm chocolate agar plates which are incubated 18 to 24 hr in a candle jar or in a more sophisticated apparatus which provides a suitable environment.

The biochemical reactions of the *Neisseria* are relatively limited, but they do contain cytochrome oxidase, which is responsible for the positive "oxidase" test, and clinically significant species usually are differentiated by their ability to produce acid in glucose, maltose, and sucrose. Although the typical meningococcus ferments glucose and maltose and the gonococcus ferments only glucose, the value of fermentation reactions for the identification of the pathogenic *Neisseria* has become limited because naturally occurring maltose-negative meningococci are being recovered with increasing frequency, probably because of the organism's progressive development of resistance to sulfonamides.

Meningococci can be divided into serologic groups on the basis of agglutination reactions with immune serum. The present classification into groups, A, B, C, and D was agreed upon in 1950, but since 1960, increasing numbers of nontypable strains have been recovered, and grouping sera X, Y, Z, and Boshard have been developed as additional serologic markers.

EPIDEMIOLOGY. The natural habitat of meningococci is the nasopharynx of man, and no other reservoir or vector has been recognized. The principal means of spread is through inhalation of droplets of infected nasopharyngeal secretions, and it is unlikely that the disease is spread by contact with contaminated fomites. Meningococci cause either epidemic or sporadic disease, and there is a cyclic variation in the prevalence of meningococcal infection, with peaks of increased frequency occurring every 8 to 12 years and lasting 4 to 6 years. The most recent upward trend of this cycle began in 1962; early in 1968, the attack rate was 2.23 per 100,000. The prevalence of meningococcal infection is also subject to seasonal influences; the lowest attack rate occurs in midsummer and the highest in late winter and early spring. This seasonal variation follows that of other bacterial and viral respiratory infections and probably reflects crowded living conditions encountered during the winter months.

Meningococcal disease occurs most frequently in children and adolescents. There is no clear-cut tendency for racial or sexual predominance, but presumably because of an increased opportunity to acquire infection, males develop meningitis and meningococcemia more frequently than females. Military recruits are particularly susceptible, and worldwide epidemics of meningococcal disease have occurred during most major wars. The military is not the major source of meningococcal infection, however, because epidemiologic studies indicate that outbreaks among military personnel usually parallel less apparent trends in the civilian population.

Since 1915, most epidemics of meningococcal disease have been caused by group A meningococci, and strains of groups B and C have been associated with sporadic, interepidemic infections. However, in the outbreaks of 1963 and 1964 a major shift in the pattern of meningococcal infection became apparent as group B meningococci were isolated from the majority of clinical infections in both civilian and military populations. In 1967, over 70 percent of meningococci isolated were group B. However, early in 1968, another shift in serogroup occurred, and 43 percent of the meningococcal strains submitted to the National Communicable Disease Center were group C. The significance of these epidemiologic shifts is enhanced by the fact that a high proportion of the meningococci in groups B and C are resistant to 1 mg per 100 ml sulfadiazine, and prophylaxis with this drug, which was successful in aborting epidemics during World War II, has been relatively ineffective since 1960. Group A meningococci recovered in this country have retained their sensitivity to sulfonamides, but in Africa, sulfonamide-resistant strains have been isolated.

Carriers. Between epidemics, 2 to 5 percent of the individuals in urban centers harbor meningococci in the nasopharynx. When sporadic cases of meningococcal disease occur, the carrier rate in close contacts may rise to 25 percent, and in closed populations or during epidemics, it may be as high as 40 to 90 percent. Although some individuals harbor meningococci for months or years, nasopharyngeal infection is usually transient, and in 75 percent of carriers, the organism disappears within 2 weeks. The relationship between the proportion of carriers in a population and the occurrence of meningococcal disease is unclear. Case to case transmission of infection is documented rarely, and carriers, not patients, are the foci from which disease is spread. It appears that the prevalence of meningococcal disease can be attributed to the prevailing carrier rate only in a general way, and that the occurrence of clinical disease is most dependent on unknown circumstances within the host which lead to spread of infection beyond the nasopharynx. Factors which may promote dissemination include (1) failure of nasopharyngeal infection to confer immunity; (2) in vivo development of invasive mutants; (3) concomitant viral infection of the upper respiratory tract.

Immunity. The role of acquired immunity in recovery from illness or protection against infection is not known. Some degree of immunity must develop because the attack rate of meningococcal infection is much higher in young children than it is in adults. However, antibody formed during clinical infection or the asymptomatic carrier state does not provide lifelong protection against reinfection.

PATHOGENESIS. Meningococci usually enter the body through the upper respiratory tract and infect the nasopharynx. In most instances, this infection is subclinical, but occasionally, localized inflammation occurs and mild symptoms develop. Dissemination of meningococci from the nasopharynx occurs via the bloodstream and generally is followed by clinical manifestations of meningococcal disease. Purulent meningitis is the most common form of metastatic infection and is either associated with signs and symptoms of meningococcemia or constitutes the predominant clinical expression of illness. Organisms in the meninges induce an acute inflammatory reaction, and purulent exudate spreads across the surface of the brain. Rarely, a more extensive inflammatory reaction in the brain produces an acute diffuse encephalitic syndrome.

Although the mechanisms responsible for the pathologic changes associated with meningococcal infection have not been explained entirely, early investigations indicated that the tissue injury observed in laboratory animals was caused by a toxic substance liberated from dead bacteria. This substance is presumed to be an endotoxin that has not been characterized biochemically, but which produces physiologic effects similar to endotoxins of other gram-negative bacteria. It may be responsible for hypotension and vascular collapse observed in fulminant meningococcemia and may also play a role in the pathogenesis of the purpura and visceral hemorhages associated with meningococcal bacteremia. Thrombosis of dermal venules, adrenal sinusoids, and renal glomerular capillaries is commonly seen in patients who die of fulminant meningococcemia and is strikingly similar to the pathologic changes observed in experimental Shwartzman reactions (Chap. 74). It is postulated that endotoxin either induces a Shwartzman reaction directly or effects the release of clotting factors which initiate intravascular coagulation and produce these characteristic pathologic changes.

CLINICAL MANIFESTATIONS. Of patients with meningococcal disease, 90 to 95 percent have meningococcemia and/or meningitis.

Meningococcemia. Of those patients who develop overt disease, 30 to 50 percent have meningococcemia without meningitis. The onset of clinical illness may be abrupt, but patients usually have nonspecific prodromal symptoms of cough, headache, and sore throat followed by the sudden development of spiking fever, chills, arthralgia, and muscle pains which may be particularly severe in the lower extremities and back. Patients usually appear acutely ill, with an inordinate degree of prostration. In addition to high fever, tachycardia, and tachypnea, mild hypotension may be present. However, clinical shock does not occur unless fulminant meningococcemia supervenes. In the course of meningococcal bacteremia, about three-fourths of the patients develop a characteristic petechial rash. Lesions are frequently sparse, and the axillas, flanks, wrists, and ankles are the most commonly involved sites. Typically, lesions are 1 to 3 mm in diameter, deep red in color, and do not blanch with pressure. Often, petechiae are located in the center of lighter colored macules, and they may become nodular as the disease progresses. The diagnosis of meningococcemia occasionally can be established by demonstrating gram-negative diplococci in scrapings from these nodular petechiae. In severe cases, purpuric spots or large ecchymoses develop, and a widespread petechial or purpuric eruption suggests fulminating disease. However, the absence of rash does not necessarily indicate that the illness will be mild.

Fulminant meningococcemia. Also known as the Waterhouse-Friderichsen Syndrome, this is meningococcemia associated with vasomotor collapse and shock. It occurs in 10 to 20 percent of patients with generalized meningococcal infection and is associated with a high fatality rate. The onset is abrupt, and profound prostration frequently occurs within a few hours. Petechiae and purpuric lesions enlarge rapidly, and hemorrhage into the skin may be extensive. Early in the preshock stage, there is generalized vasoconstriction; patients are alert and pale, with cir-

cumoral cyanosis and cold extremities. Upon entering the shock stage, however, coma develops, the cardiac output decreases, and the blood pressure drops. Unless incipient shock is recognized and appropriate therapy instituted early, death from cardiac and/or respiratory failure almost invariably occurs. Patients who recover may have extensive sloughing of skin lesions and even loss of digits because of gangrene.

Chronic meningococcemia. This is a rare form of meningococcal infection which lasts for weeks or months and is characterized by fever, rash, and arthritis or arthralgia. Typically, the fever is intermittent, and during afebrile periods, which may last several days, patients appear remarkably well. The usual rash is a maculopapular or polymorphous eruption which waxes and wanes with the fever, but petechial or nodular lesions may be seen. Joint involvement is present in two-thirds of the patients, and splenomegaly is detected in about 20 percent. If the diagnosis is not suspected or treatment is otherwise delayed, complications such as meningitis, carditis, or nephritis may occur.

Meningitis. Meningitis is a common form of meningococcal disease which occurs primarily in adolescents and children over six months of age. Fever, vomiting, headache, and confusion or lethargy are the commonest symptoms; in about one-fourth of the patients, they begin abruptly and rapidly increase in severity. The more typical patient, however, has symptoms of an upper respiratory tract infection followed by an illness which progresses over several days. Because 20 to 40 percent of patients have meningitis without clinical evidence of meningococcemia, the diagnosis depends upon bacteriologic examination of the cerebrospinal fluid. However, when meningitis occurs in association with a petechial or purpuric rash, a presumptive diagnosis of meningococcal disease is warranted, since this pattern of illness is seen only rarely in other infections.

Rarer Manifestations. The meningococcus is a rare cause of purulent conjunctivitis or sinusitis, and it has been reported to cause lobar or bronchopneumonia in patients without evidence of meningitis or meningococcemia. Bacterial endocarditis also has been reported.

LABORATORY FINDINGS. Aside from bacteriologic data, laboratory studies are of little value in establishing the diagnosis of meningococcal infection. Polymorphonuclear leukocyte counts usually range from 12,000 to 40,000 cells per cu mm, but in meningococcemia, normal or low leukocyte counts may be encountered. Anemia is uncommon, and levels of serum electrolytes and blood urea nitrogen are normal unless shock develops. Patients with prominent hemorrhagic manifestations may have low platelet counts and decreased levels of circulating clotting factors as a result of intravascular coagulation. In meningitis, the cerebrospinal fluid pressure is increased, and the fluid usually contains from 100 to 40,000 polymorphonuclear leukocytes per cu mm. The protein content of the fluid is increased, and the concentration of glucose is almost always less than 35 mg per 100 ml and often is between 0 and 10 mg per 100 ml.

Meningococci can be recovered readily from cultures

of blood or spinal fluid, and on occasion, material aspirated from skin lesions or joints yields the organism. In addition, gram-negative diplococci may be seen in stains of nodular petechiae or the buffy coat of blood from patients with meningococcemia. In meningococcal meningitis, a smear of the spinal fluid is diagnostic in about half the patients but often shows only a few intracellular bacteria which are located with difficulty.

COMPLICATIONS. *Herpes labialis* occurs in 5 to 20 percent of patients with meningococcal disease. Other complications, which result from neurologic damage or secondary foci of infection, are uncommon following appropriate treatment and are often transient. Seizures or deafness occur in 10 to 20 percent of patients during the acute stages of meningitis, but postmeningitic epilepsy is rare and the frequency of permanent eighth-nerve damage is probably less than 5 percent. Peripheral neuropathy, cranial nerve palsies, and hemiplegia are seen occasionally, but usually clear completely within 2 to 4 months. Hydrocephalus and thrombosis of venous sinuses, once frequent sequelae of meningococcal meningitis, are encountered rarely. A number of patients complain of recurrent headache, emotional lability, insomnia, backache, memory loss, and difficulty in concentrating for months after an episode of meningitis. The organic basis for these symptoms is obscure, but they usually disappear a year or two after the infection.

Arthritis is a common metastatic complication of meningococcemia and occurs in 2 to 10 percent of patients. As a rule, multiple joints are involved, and signs and symptoms of joint involvement may not appear until after treatment of meningitis or meningococcemia has been instituted. Joint fluid usually contains many granulocytes, but meningococci are recovered infrequently. Antibiotic therapy does not appear to influence the course of the arthritis, and permanent joint changes are rare. Other purulent complications have become extremely uncommon since antibiotics have gained widespread use. Pneumonia occurs occasionally, but it is uncertain whether it is caused by the meningococcus or coexistent infection with other bacteria. Bacterial endocarditis is quite rare, but a high proportion of patients who die of meningococcal infection have myocarditis. The etiology of these myocardial changes is uncertain, but cardiac failure may be an important factor in the pathogenesis of the shock syndrome in meningococcemia.

DIAGNOSIS. The diagnosis of meningococcal disease depends upon recovering *N. meningitidis* from cultures of blood, spinal fluid, or petechial scrapings from patients with a typical clinical picture. Recovery of meningococci from the nasopharynx does not, in itself, establish the diagnosis of meningococcal disease.

Few diseases need to be seriously considered in the differential diagnosis of meningococcal infection. If meningococcal meningitis is not accompanied by manifestations of bacteremia, it is indistinguishable from meningitis caused by other common pathogens. Occasionally, the common viral exanthems, certain rickettsial infections, particularly Rocky Mountain Spotted Fever (Chap. 195), and vascular purpuras (Chap. 345) may be confused with meningococcemia, and their differentiation depends upon demonstration of the organism and knowledge of the epidemiology and clinical manifestations of each disease.

TREATMENT. Antimicrobial therapy of suspected or documented meningococcal disease should be instituted as early as possible. Penicillin G is the drug of choice, and should be administered intravenously. The dosage for the treatment of meningitis in adults is 12 to 24 million units per day, and in the pediatric age group, 16 million units/sq m/day. Meningococcemia can be treated with 5 to 10 million units a day because it is not necessary to achieve high levels of antibiotic in the spinal fluid. If treatment with these doses is continued for a minimum of 7 days, or 4 to 5 days after the patient becomes afebrile, relapse is extremely rare. Ampicillin in doses of 200 mg/kg/day is as effective as penicillin G, and it has been recommended for initial treatment of meningitis in children because it is effective against *H. influenzae.* Meningococci are susceptible to other antimicrobial agents such as chloramphenicol and tetracycline, but they should not be used unless a patient is allergic to penicillin. Under these circumstances, chloramphenicol hemisuccinate 4.0 to 6.0 Gm per day in divided doses (in adults) is an acceptable regimen. Because a significant proportion of meningococci isolated are resistant to sulfonamides, these drugs should not be used in the treatment of meningococcal infections. The combination of sulfonamides with penicillin offers no advantage and should not be used.

Patients with meningococcal infections require supportive treatment as well as antimicrobial therapy. Maintenance of fluid and electrolyte balance and prevention of respiratory complications in comatose patients are of primary concern. When shock occurs, visceral perfusion must be improved by maintenance of an adequate intravascular volume, treatment of heart failure when it is present, and support of the blood pressure. Vasopressors may produce temporary improvement, but agents which block alpha adrenergic receptors (Dibenzylene) or which stimulate beta receptors (isoproterenol) have been promising, and deserve further trial (Chap. 134). If central venous pressure is elevated, digitalis should be given, and when intravascular coagulation is recognized, treatment with heparin, whole blood, or fibrinogen is indicated. Adrenal cortical steroids are often used, but are of uncertain value, and dramatic results should not be expected.

PREVENTION. There is little likelihood that meningococcal infections can be prevented entirely. Effective chemoprophylaxis depends upon first treating an entire population at risk with a drug capable of eradicating the carrier state and then isolating the group to prevent further introduction of meningococci. This is not only impractical when applied to the general public, but the majority of carriers now harbor strains which are resistant to sulfonamides, and other drugs do not eradicate the carrier state permanently. Nevertheless, under certain circumstances, such as epidemic outbreaks in military populations, these measures may have to be instituted.

Treatment of contacts of sporadic cases with a 2-day course of a sulfonamide (on the assumption that the organism is sensitive) or a 7-day course of oral penicillin has been advocated, but the usefulness of this practice has not been documented. Attempts at development of a meningococcal vaccine are under way, but no trials have been reported in man.

PROGNOSIS. Before the introduction of antibiotics, meningococcal meningitis, and meningococcemia were almost invariably fatal. With prompt and appropriate chemotherapy, the mortality rate of meningitis without fulminant meningococcemia has dropped to less than 10 percent in the United States, and neurologic sequelae are rare. The mortality of fulminant infection remains high primarily because patients are often in irreversible shock when treatment is instituted. Chronic meningococcemia is cured readily if the disease is recognized.

REFERENCES

Banks, H. S.: Meningococcal Fever, in "Modern Practice in Infectious Fevers," vol. 1, New York, Paul B. Hoeber, Inc., 1951.

Benoit, F. L.: Chronic Meningococcemia, Am. J. Med., 35:103, 1963.

Eickhoff, T. C., and M. Finland: Changing Susceptibility of Meningococci to Antimicrobial Agents, New Engl. J. Med., 272:395, 1965.

Feldman, H. A.: Recent Developments in the Therapy and Control of Meningococcal Infections, Disease-a-Month, February, 1966.

Levin, S., and M. B. Painter: The Treatment of Acute Meningococcal Infection in Adults, Ann. Intern. Med., 64:1049, 1966.

Pinals, R. S., and M. Ropes: Arthritis in Meningococcal Infection, Arthritis Rheum., 7:241, 1964.

143 GONOCOCCAL INFECTIONS

Harry N. Beaty and
Robert G. Petersdorf

INTRODUCTION. Gonorrhea, an infection of columnar and transitional epithelium of the genitourinary tract, is the principal infection caused by the gonococcus. It is transmitted almost exclusively by direct sexual contact and is the commonest venereal disease of man. Most other clinical manifestations of gonococcal infection are relatively uncommon today and develop as a result of contamination with infected secretions or as a complication of venereal infection.

ETIOLOGY. *Neisseria gonorrhoeae,* or the gonococcus, is a gram-negative spherical organism which closely resembles the meningococcus in its morphology and growth requirements. In stained preparations of infected secretions, gonococci appear as reniform diplococci which often are located within granulocytes. Their recovery from infected genitourinary sites is facilitated if a selective medium containing 25 units per ml polymyxin B and 10 μg per ml ristocetin is used for initial cultures.

The biochemical reactions of these organisms are limited, but they are "oxidase positive" and usually can be distinguished from other species of *Neisseria* by their ability to ferment only glucose. Confusion arises when an occasional gonococcus which produces acid very slowly in glucose is mistaken for *N. catarrhalis,* or when a sulfonamide-resistant meningococcus is classified as a gonococcus because it fails to ferment maltose. Final identification of these strains can be accomplished with immunofluorescent techniques.

Gonococci are a heterogeneous group of organisms, and at least four morphologically distinct colonial types have been recognized. Type 1 cells are recovered only from the purulent exudate of acute gonorrhea, but on subculture, other types appear. After passage in vitro, certain of these types lose their virulence, but type 1 cells always retain their ability to infect male volunteers. Serologic heterogeneity has also been documented, but classification of gonococci on the basis of agglutination reactions is not practical.

EPIDEMIOLOGY. Man is the only host in whom infection with *N. gonorrhoeae* occurs naturally; the major reservoir is the asymptomatic female. With the exception of ophthalmia neonatorum, which results from contamination of the conjunctiva during parturition, gonococcal infection is transmitted almost exclusively by sexual contact. Gonorrhea is worldwide in distribution, and most countries reporting to the World Health Organization have documented a progressive increase in the disease rate since 1960. In the United States, it is estimated that 1.5 to 2 million new cases occur annually, but only 10 to 20 percent of these cases are reported, and approximately 70 percent are treated outside of public clinics. The disease is most common in lower socioeconomic groups, but susceptibility to infection is quite general, with no recognizable predilection for either race or sex. The highest incidence of infection is in the twenty to twenty-four-year-old age group, but the frequency of gonorrhea among teen-agers has reached alarming proportions.

Many females harbor asymptomatic infection for weeks to months, but a more prolonged true carrier state is relatively uncommon. Not all males exposed to a female with gonorrhea become infected, but those who do almost always develop acute urethritis. This is usually a self-limited infection and although asymptomatic male carriers have been recognized, they are distinctly uncommon. Individuals of either sex with asymptomatic infection can transmit the disease for months or years unless they receive effective therapy.

One of the major factors which has prevented successful control of gonorrhea is the lack of natural or acquired resistance to infection. The antibody response to acute gonorrhea is minimal and provides no significant protection against reinfection. To date, immunologic studies of this disease have had little practical value. However, attempts to develop a skin test or serologic reaction which will identify patients with active infection continue because these tests would have great epidemiologic importance.

PATHOGENESIS. Gonococci cannot penetrate stratified squamous epithelium, but they are able to infect columnar or transitional cells. Three to four days after organisms come in contact with susceptible epithelium, bacteria can be identified in subepithelial spaces. Leukocytes accumulate in these regions, and soon, granulocytes containing organisms migrate into the urethral lumen and form a purulent exudate. In males, the urethral glands are usually involved, and prostatitis or epididymitis may develop as a result of direct extension or lymphatic spread of infection. Urethritis is usually transient in females, but infection of Skene's or Bartholin's glands is common. The epithelium and glands of the endocervix also are involved frequently, and as infection spreads along the endometrium, it causes congestion, edema, and formation of a purulent exudate. The disease may continue to spread to the endosalpinx where plicae become swollen, hyperemic, and heavily infiltrated with leukocytes. Extension of the infection through the mucosa to involve the muscularis sometimes leads to abscess formation or pelvic peritonitis. Proctitis is present in about 40 percent of women with gonococcal infection of the urogenital tract, and occasionally may be recognized in males. It is likely that transient subclinical gonococcemia occurs in many patients with either acute or asymptomatic urogenital infections, but the mechanisms responsible for dissemination are unknown.

Untreated gonococcal infections tend to heal with the formation of dense scar tissue. Urethral strictures and sterility, resulting from stenosis of the epididymis or fallopian tubes, were fairly common sequelae of gonorrhea before the availability of effective antimicrobial agents.

CLINICAL MANIFESTATIONS. Genital infections and the clinical manifestations of associated bacteremia are the most likely forms of gonococcal disease to be encountered. Metastatic infections such as visceral abscesses, meningitis, endocarditis, and purulent myocarditis or pericarditis are extremely rare.

Gonorrhea in the Male ("Clap" or "Strain"). The incubation period of naturally acquired infection is 2 to 8 days, but in experimental infection of humans it has been as long as 31 days. The onset of symptoms is usually abrupt, and patients complain of urinary frequency and urgency, dysuria, and a profuse mucopurulent urethral discharge. Urinary retention, perineal pain, and hematuria may be seen occasionally. Acute prostatitis and seminal vesiculitis are uncommon, but if treatment is delayed, unilateral epididymitis complicates 5 to 10 percent of cases. In these patients, systemic manifestations such as fever and chills may occur. Untreated disease usually subsides within 6 weeks, and with rare exception, organisms cannot be recovered from the urogenital tract. Occasionally, however, gonococci persist despite apparently adequate therapy, presumably because they are sequestered in mucosal folds or the prostate. Urethral dilatation or prostatic massage may activate latent gonorrhea in these patients. A significant proportion of individuals have either pyuria or a slight urethral discharge for weeks to months after the successful treatment of gonorrhea. This postgonococcal urethritis (PGU, "gleet") may be due to latent or coexistent mycoplasma infection and can be eradicated with tetracycline. Urethral stricture is a common sequel of genital gonococcal disease if treatment is inadequate or a patient has repeated infections.

Gonorrhea in the Female. Women with acute gonorrhea are often completely asymptomatic and first come to attention as contacts of males with venereal infections. Transient urethritis may cause mild urinary symptoms, and involvement of the cervix often produces a copious, irritating vaginal discharge. If the infection spreads to the endosalpinx and produces acute salpingitis or pelvic peritonitis (pelvic inflammatory disease, PID), patients may complain of chills, fever, malaise, myalgia, anorexia, nausea, vomiting, and lower abdominal pain. Depending on the extent of the infection, the physical examination may be negative or nonspecific. However, if there is an abscess of Skene's or Bartholin's glands, or if there is pain on movement of the cervix, with or without signs of peritoneal irritation, gonococcal infection should be suspected. Proctitis, often manifested by tenesmus and bloody mucoid stools, may be caused by the gonococcus, and persistence of the organisms in this site may be responsible for treatment failures.

Prior to the availability of antimicrobials, conception after bilateral gonorrheal salpingitis was exceptional. Today, approximately 80 percent of patients have at least one patent tube after effective therapy. The duration of the infection prior to treatment is of major importance in determining the outcome.

Unlike the situation in adults, gonococcal infection of prepubescent females usually causes vulvovaginitis. The exterior cervix may be infected, but salpingitis and pelvic peritonitis are rare. The reason for this unusual expression of gonococcal disease in children is probably due to anatomic and biochemical factors, but acquisition of infection still seems to be the result of voluntary or involuntary sexual contact.

Arthritis. Arthritis occurs as a manifestation of gonococcemia in about 1 percent of patients with genital infection. In the past it occurred primarily in males and frequently destroyed the involved joints; today, it is seen predominately in females and male homosexuals, responds well to antibiotics, and leaves no residual joint damage. Symptoms usually develop after acute gonorrhea, but particularly in females, may follow exacerbation of an indolent or subclinical infection. The onset is often abrupt, and the clinical picture consists of fever, arthralgia, and painful arthritis. About 50 percent of patients develop a sparse rash which is most commonly seen over the distal portion of the extremities. The typical lesion is an erythematous papule with a hemorrhagic or vesiculopustular center. Although gonococcal arthritis has been characterized as monoarticular, it is actually polyarticular in 80 percent of cases. The knee is the most frequently involved joint, followed in order of frequency by wrists, ankles, hands, elbows, hips, and shoulders. Tenosynovitis occurs in 50 to 75 percent of cases, and should call attention to the possibility of gonococcal infection.

Patients usually have a mild leukocytosis, and fluid aspirated from involved joints may contain only a few granulocytes or may be frankly purulent. Careful bacteriologic study of joint fluid fails to reveal gonococci in the majority of cases, particularly if patients are seen relatively early in the course of their illness. Joint symptoms usually begin to improve a few days after treatment is started, and complete recovery occurs within 1 to 2 weeks. In an occasional patient, however, the response to treatment may be less dramatic and symptoms will persist for much longer.

Ophthalmitis. Gonococcal keratoconjunctivitis is rare in adults, but is one of the commonest forms of gonococcal infection in children. *Ophthalmia neonatorum,* ophthalmitis in the newborn, formerly was responsible for 12 percent of all blindness, but with the advent of effective prophylaxis, this figure has been reduced to less than 0.3 percent. Infection occurs when the conjunctiva is contaminated during birth or by the hands of infected adults with poor personal hygiene. Three to four days after the gonococcus comes in contact with the corneal epithelium, acute purulent conjunctivitis develops. It usually begins unilaterally, but soon becomes bilateral, and if untreated, most cases rapidly progress to corneal ulceration, perforation, and scarring. Gonococci are readily apparent on a gram stain of the purulent exudate, and if treatment is instituted early, results are satisfactory. The best agent for prophylaxis has not been determined, but a 1 percent silver nitrate solution may be superior to penicillin G, which, however, is also highly effective.

Perihepatitis (Fitzhugh-Curtis Syndrome). This is an unusual complication of genital infection in the female. It occurs when gonococci spread from the fallopian tube and produce a localized peritonitis. Any area of the peritoneal cavity can be involved, but the right upper quadrant is the commonest site. Patients usually present with fever and abdominal pain and have signs of peritonitis on physical examination. A friction rub is heard over the liver in some patients. Usually, liver function studies are normal, but jaundice and other mild abnormalities have been reported. Liver biopsies have been normal in most cases, but thickening of the capsule and mild subcapsular hepatitis may be seen occasionally. Perihepatitis is often confused with acute cholecystitis because of its clinical presentation and the fact that the gallbladder may not be visualized on cholecystograms until after the inflammation subsides. Specific therapy results in prompt improvement, but even without treatment, symptoms usually disappear within 2 weeks. Untreated, this form of gonococcal infection leads to the formation of "violin-string" adhesions between the liver and the anterior abdominal wall.

Gonococcemia and Endocarditis. Very rarely, gonococcemia produces a febrile illness which is so similar to meningococcemia that differentiation on clinical grounds is not possible. Otherwise, the manifestations of gonococcal bacteremia are those discussed in the section on arthritis.

Endocarditis due to the gonococcus has virtually disappeared with the availability of effective treatment of gonorrhea. Gonococci usually attack normal valves, but the course of the infection borders between acute and subacute. Left-sided endocarditis, with involvement of the aortic valve, is the commonest form of this infection, but the gonococcus is one organism which is particularly likely to infect the tricuspid or pulmonic valve. In addition to petechiae, glomerulonephritis, embolic phenomena, anemia, and splenomegaly, two clinical features of gonococcal endocarditis may suggest the diagnosis. Jaundice, presumably due to "toxic" hepatitis, is very common, and a majority of patients have two distinct spikes of fever during a 24-hr period (the double quotidian pattern).

DIAGNOSIS. A definitive diagnosis of gonococcal infection is established by demonstrating *N. gonorrhoeae* in cultures of infected secretions or biologic fluids. In males, a presumptive diagnosis of gonorrhea can be made if typical organisms are seen on gram stain of the urethral discharge. However, a negative smear does not rule out gonococcal disease, and false-positive results may be due to infection with *Mima polymorpha*. The bacillary nature of these organisms can quickly be determined, however, by culture on eosin-methylene blue or meat-broth media. The diagnosis of gonorrhea in the female often has been difficult to establish because demonstration of the gonococcus on routine smears or cultures has been inconsistent. However, use of the selective Thayer-Martin medium or the delayed fluorescent-antibody technique has simplified the task of diagnosis. Carefully obtained cultures also can be used to assess the effectiveness of therapy, but since nonviable gonococci fluoresce, the fluorescent antibody test is not a good measure of successful treatment.

The diagnosis of gonococcal arthritis often must be made on the basis of clinical data alone. Blood cultures are positive in only 10 to 20 percent of patients with presumed gonococcemia, and bacteriologic study of fluid from involved joints often fails to reveal organisms. The presence of tenosynovitis in patients with evidence of gonorrheal infection and arthritis which responds promptly to penicillin should suggest the diagnosis.

TREATMENT. Despite the fact that surveillance studies of *N. gonorrhoeae* sensitivity have revealed a steady increase in resistance in vitro to penicillin, this drug remains the preferred choice for management of gonococcal infections. However, the dose required to produce acceptable results has required repeated upward adjustments, and it is possible that sometime in the future, further increases will be impractical.

In males, gonorrhea should be treated with a single injection of 2.4 million units of procaine penicillin. Gonorrhea in females requires more drug, 4.8 million units in one dose, to achieve an 85 to 90 percent cure rate. Treatment failure may occur when organisms are sequestered in a site where antibiotics cannot reach them, when there is a concommitant infection with penicillinase-producing organisms, or when the infecting gonococcus is relatively resistant to penicillin. Only the last possibility is of major clinical significance. A variety of drugs, including kanamycin, chloramphenicol, erythromycin, ampicillin, and the cephalosporins, have been used effectively in the treatment of gonorrhea, but tetracycline seems to provide a particularly good alternative to penicillin therapy and it reduces the incidence of postgonococcal urethritis.

Gonococcal arthritis should be treated with 2 to 4 million units of penicillin per day parenterally for 10 to 14 days. Intraarticular penicillin is not recommended. Endocarditis should be treated with 4 to 10 million units of penicillin daily for 4 to 6 weeks. Pelvic inflammatory disease and perihepatitis usually respond to 1.2 million units of penicillin a day for 7 days. Ophthalmitis is best managed with topical penicillin G plus parenteral drug.

Simultaneous acquisition of gonorrhea and syphilis occurs in about 3 percent of patients. The gonococcal infection usually becomes evident first, and therapy for that alone may abort the clinical manifestations of syphilis without effectively treating the disease. Therefore, all patients with gonorrhea should have serologic tests for syphilis before treatment and at intervals for 6 months. The onset of fever and chills in a patient given penicillin for gonorrhea is highly suggestive of a syphilitic Herxheimer reaction.

PREVENTION AND CONTROL. Effective prophylaxis against infection can be achieved with a single 250-mg tablet of penicillin G taken just before or just after exposure. A condom also provides protection against gonorrhea because it prevents contact of organisms with susceptible epithelium. In women, mechanical cleansing may help prevent infection.

Control of gonorrhea as a public health problem can-not be accomplished so readily. Thayer and Garson pointed out four principles necessary for the control of contagion: quarantine, immunization, eradication of animal reservoirs or vectors, and specific therapy. When applied to gonorrhea, it is apparent that *quarantine* is out of the question. Artificial *immunization* is not available, and more important, an attack of gonorrhea confers no significant resistance to reinfection. Man is the only *reservoir*, so the end result of *specific treatment* is the return of nonimmune susceptibles to the population within a few days. These patients can be reinfected almost immediately, which makes evaluation of treatment very difficult, and the disease maintains itself in the population. There is probably no more striking illustration than gonorrhea of the failure of specific treatment alone to eradicate a communicable disease.

REFERENCES

Ashamalla, G., N. B. Walters, and M. Crohon: Recent Clinical laboratory Observations in the Treatment of Acute Gonococcal Urethritis in Men, J.A.M.A., 195:1115, 1966.

Keiser, H., F. L. Ruben, E. Wolinsky, and I. Kushner: Clinical Forms of Gonococcal Arthritis, New Engl. J. Med., 279:234, 1968.

Lucas, J. B., E. V. Price, J. D. Thayer, and A. Schroeter: Diagnosis and Treatment of Gonorrhea in the Female, New Engl. J. Med., 276:1454, 1967.

Thayer, J. D., and W. Garson: The Gonococcus, p. 451 in "Bacterial and Mycotic Infections of Man," 4th ed., Philadelphia, J. B. Lippincott Company, 1965.

Vickers, F. N., and P. J. Maloney: Gonococcic Perihepatitis: Report of Three Cases with Comments on Diagnosis and Treatment, Arch. Intern. Med., 114:120, 1964.

Section 5

Diseases Caused by Enteric Gram-negative Bacilli

144 COLIFORM BACTERIAL INFECTIONS
(*Escherichia coli* Infections)

Marvin Turck and
Robert G. Petersdorf

ETIOLOGY. The most important "coliforms" medically, are *Escherichia coli* and organisms of the *Klebsiella-Aerobacter* group (Chap. 148). The coliforms do not constitute a distinct nosologic entity and are a group of gram-negative nonsporing rods which belong to the tribe *Enterobacteriaceae*. Coliforms generally ferment lactose, as opposed to the medically significant non-lactose-fermenting organisms, *Salmonella*, *Shigella*, and *Proteus*. The so-called "paracolon" bacilli are organisms which ferment lactose late, irregularly, or not at all, and on more careful biochemical and antigenic testing are found to belong to one or another of the genera of the tribe *Enterobacteriaceae*, which is comprised of *Salmonella*, *Arizona*, *Citrobacter*, *Shigella*, *Escherichia*, *Klebsiella*, *Aerobacter*, *Hafnia*, *Serratia*, *Proteus*, and *Providence*. All of these organisms are readily culturable on ordinary media and are aerobic and facultatively anaerobic. All species ferment glucose, reduce nitrates to nitrites, and are oxidase-negative and catalase-positive. They are differentiated among members of their own tribe by biochemical and serologic tests. It is important to make this differentiation, not only from the point of view of taxonomy, but also because of epidemiologic and therapeutic implications.

PATHOGENESIS. *Escherichia coli* is regarded generally as a normal commensal in the gastrointestinal tract, from which it may spread to infect contiguous structures if normal anatomic barriers are interrupted, as occurs in appendiceal perforation. It is believed that the urinary tract is infected from without via urethral contamination, but direct hematogenous or, rarely, lymphatic spread accounts for renal infection. Once infection has occurred in a primary focus, further spread to distant organs occurs via the bloodstream. There is experimental and clinical evidence that *E. coli* tends to settle in avascular or necrotic tissue. In more than 50 percent of *E. coli* infections the urinary tract is the portal of entry; infections of the hepatobiliary tree, peritoneal cavity, skin, and lung are not uncommon. A number of patients with *E. coli* bacteremia have no demonstrable portal of entry; they often have neoplastic and hematologic diseases, and *E. coli* is considered an "opportunistic" invader. There may be other defects in host resistance, including diabetes mellitus, cirrhosis, and sickle-cell anemia, or recent administration of irradiation, cytotoxic drugs, adrenal steroids, or antibiotics. Morphologically the lesions produced in various tissues show typical acute inflammation with pus and abscess formation. There is a common misconception that *E. coli* bacterial infections are characterized by a foul-smelling, feculent exudate. Such an odor is caused by anaerobic streptococci or *Bacteroides* species, which are often associated with coliform bacteria in mixed infections. In fact, organisms of the genus *Bacteroides* frequently far outnumber *E. coli* as the most prevalent gram-negative flora in the intestine.

EPIDEMIOLOGY. Strains of *E. coli* are characterized by their somatic (O), flagellar (H), and capsular (K or B) antigens, and there are hundreds of different serologic varieties. Any of the strains is capable of causing disease. Clinical and epidemiologic studies have demonstrated that certain specific *E. coli* serotypes are more frequently incriminated in diarrheal disease of the infant and newborn, i.e., 026:B6, 055:B5, 0111:B4, and 0127:B8. It is less clear whether certain strains are also more commonly associated with nonenteric infections.

Some epidemiologic studies performed between 1960 and 1965 suggested that *E. coli* 04, 06, and 075 were responsible for most *E. coli* infections other than infantile diarrhea. In particular, these strains appeared to colonize more avidly and more commonly infect hospital patients. With the passage of time the epidemiologic virulence of these organisms may have become attenuated, and they are no more likely to cause infections than other strains. A similar ecologic change has been observed with staphylococci of phage type 80/81.

Strains incriminated in infantile diarrhea probably are disseminated within nurseries by symptomatic or asymptomatic infant carriers, mothers, and nurses. Although fecal contamination is the usual mode of spread, airborne contamination of the environment and fomite spread may also occur.

MANIFESTATIONS. Urinary tract infections. *Escherichia coli* account for well over 75 percent of urinary tract infections, including cystitis, pyelitis, pyelonephritis, and asymptomatic bacteriuria. Strains cultured from patients with acute, uncomplicated urinary tract infections are almost invariably *E. coli*, whereas other *Enterobacteriaceae* and strains of *Pseudomonas* become prevalent among patients with chronic infection. Urinary tract infections are discussed in Chap. 303.

Peritoneal and Biliary Infections. *Escherichia coli* can usually be cultured from a perforated or inflamed appendix or abscesses secondary to perforated diverticuli, peptic ulcers, subphrenic or lesser sac abscesses, mesenteric infarction, etc. Often, other organisms, including anaerobic streptococci, clostridia, and bacteroides, are found along with *E. coli*. Acute cholecystitis with gangrene and perforation is often associated with *E. coli* infection. An air-fluid level associated with stones or a circumferential layer of gas in the wall of the gallbladder may be detectable by x-ray and is characteristic of acute emphysematous cholecystitis. From the gallbladder, infection may ascend via the biliary tree to produce cholangitis and multiple liver abscesses. More rarely *E. coli* infection in the peritoneal cavity may produce a septic thrombophlebitis of the portal vein (pylephlebitis), which in turn is followed by liver abscesses.

BACTEREMIA. Invasion of the bloodstream is the most serious manifestation of *E. coli* infection; it is characterized usually by the sudden onset of fever and chills, but sometimes only by mental confusion, dyspnea, or unexplained hypotension. It is most common in patients with urinary tract infection and biliary or intraperitoneal sepsis, and following abortions or pelvic surgery. In some patients no portal of entry is evident. Most cases occur in elderly males, presumably because of the high incidence of urethral instrumentation and catheterization in this group. Fever ranges between 100 and 106°F and is higher in younger patients. Hyperventilation may be an early sign. Hypotension may be present from the onset but usually occurs within 12 to 16 hr after bacteremia, if it is persistent; it is accompanied by oliguria and often by mental confusion, stupor, and coma. The skin is warm and dry initially, but most patients develop some evidence of peripheral vasoconstriction characterized by cold and cyanotic extremities. Fortunately hypotension is transient and self-limited in most patients with *E. coli* bacteremia and is absent altogether in some. However, about 25 percent of patients with bacteremia develop more prolonged hypotension, a syndrome known as gram-negative or endotoxin shock, which is discussed in Chap. 134.

Occasionally *E. coli* bacteremia develops in patients with cirrhosis without an overt portal of entry. This has been variably attributed to portosystemic shunts, impaired reticuloendothelial function, and diminution in humoral defense mechanisms.

Other Manifestations. *Escherichia coli* may produce abscesses anywhere in the body. Subcutaneous infections are common at the site of insulin administration in diabetics, in extremities with ischemic gangrene, or in surgical wounds. Perirectal phlegmons are not uncommon in patients with leukemia. Subcutaneous abscesses are often characterized by formation of gas in tissues, which may be detected by crepitation or by x-ray and which must be differentiated from clostridial infection. From 5 to 10 percent of patients with *E. coli* bacteremia develop metastatic infection in bone, brain, liver, and lung. *Escherichia coli* rarely causes pneumonia *de novo*, although coliform bacilli are often cultured from sputum in pulmonary superinfections.

Neonatal infection. Neonates, particularly premature infants, often develop *E. coli* bacteremia associated with meningitis and blood-borne pyelonephritis. Fecal soiling and absence of maternal IgM antibody are two of the factors which render this group particularly susceptible to coliform infections.

Gastroenteritis. Children under two years of age develop gastroenteritis, typified by nausea, vomiting, and diarrhea. Most outbreaks have occurred in nurseries and have been due to specific strains of enteropathogenic *E. coli* (EPEC). Fluorescent antibody techniques have been most useful in the rapid identification of these organisms. The rapid dehydration, with its attendant high mortality, demands prompt recognition of this condition, isolation of the infants, and treatment of both patients and contacts with the appropriate antibiotic. *Escherichia coli* per se has not been incriminated in diarrheal disease in adults, although certain strains of Arizona have presumably been responsible for benign outbreaks of gastroenteritis.

LABORATORY FINDINGS. There are no characteristic laboratory abnormalities. The white blood cell count is usually elevated, and there is a preponderance of granulocytes. At times, however, the white count is normal or low. When *E. coli* infection occurs in previously healthy individuals, anemia is absent, but more commonly there is anemia which is usually related to the patient's underlying disease. *Escherichia coli* grows readily in a variety of bacteriologic media and should be cultured from appropriate secretions and blood. In the presence of gram-negative shock, there are often profound metabolic derangements, including azotemia, metabolic acidosis, hypokalemia, and hyperkalemia, as well as a variety of coagulation defects (Chap. 134).

DIAGNOSIS. *Escherichia coli* cannot be differentiated from most other gram-negative bacteria on gram stain, and culture followed by appropriate biochemical characterization is necessary to identify the organism precisely. Flourescent antibody techniques are valuable for identifying EPEC. Serologic typing is of no value in individual patients, although it is essential for gathering epidemiologic data.

TREATMENT. As with other infections, drainage of pus and removal of foreign bodies are essential. If *E. coli* is suspected as the etiologic agent in a particular infection, choice of an appropriate antimicrobial will depend upon the site and type of infection as well as upon its severity. Often the outcome of the infection depends upon the status of the associated disease, rather than on eradication of bacteria. For example, in acute uncomplicated urinary tract infection in females, the disease is frequently self-limited even without antimicrobial therapy, and there is no evidence that antibiotics are superior to

sulfonamides. Conversely, *E. coli* bacteremia in a patient with leukemia may not respond to antimicrobials unless a hematologic remission is achieved simultaneously.

In most situations, antibiotics should be selected, when possible, on the basis of their in vitro sensitivity tests. Although no drug is uniformly active against all strains of *E. coli*, a number of agents are effective against the majority of clinical isolates. If average obtainable plasma concentrations become the criteria for in vitro susceptibility, approximately 75 percent of *E. coli* strains is likely to be sensitive to the tetracyclines, 85 percent, to chloramphenicol or ampicillin, and 90 percent, to kanamycin, polymyxin B, or colistin; 50 percent of *E. coli* isolated from hospitalized patients will be inhibited by streptomycin, and 65 percent by cephalothin. Many strains of *E. coli* are sensitive to high concentrations of penicillin G (50 to 100 μg) and this drug may be used in dosage of 10 to 40 million units intravenously daily, particularly if probenecid is given concomitantly. This regimen has been largely superseded by ampicillin, 2 to 4 Gm per day intravenously or intramuscularly; in some instances the dose can be raised to 6 to 12 Gm per day. The antibacterial spectrum of ampicillin against *E. coli* is probably identical to that achieved with very high concentrations of penicillin G, and to the spectrum covered by the tetracyclines or chloramphenicol. However, the bactericidal properties of ampicillin may be a distinct advantage over these two drugs, particularly in deep seated, gram-negative infections. Kanamycin sulfate is most useful for the initial treatment of serious *E. coli* infections. Severe urinary tract infections refractory to other antimicrobials have responded to 15 mg/kg/day, intramuscularly, in divided doses every 12 hr. In life-threatening infections, kanamycin can probably be used for 24 to 48 hr with little hazard of ototoxicity or nephrotoxicity, even in patients with concomitant renal impairment, pending results of in vitro sensitivity tests. However, some recent isolations of specific serologic strains of hospital-derived *E. coli* from newborn with diarrheal disease have been resistant to kanamycin and neomycin. Cephalothin in concentration of 25 μg per ml is effective against many *E. coli* strains. This serum concentration can be obtained only with 1.5 to 2.0 gm dosages at 3- to 4-hr intervals. Although cephalothin is highly effective against many common pathogens, peak serum concentrations after standard doses barely reach or may fall short of requirements for *E. coli*. Another cephalosporin antibiotic, cephaloridine, has become available for the treatment of *E. coli* infections. This agent yields higher and more sustained levels than does a comparable amount of cephalothin and is more active against *E. coli* in vitro. However, because of potential nephrotoxicity, the total daily dose of cephaloridine is limited to 4.0 Gm per day by law. Tetracyclines and chloramphenicol are still widely used in the treatment of *E. coli* infection, but better drugs are now available. Polymyxin B and colistin are also highly effective in vitro against the majority of *E. coli*. However, it is difficult to obtain adequate tissue and serum concentrations with these agents, and they should probably not be used for treatment of systemic *E. coli* infections. Although combinations of antimicrobials, i.e., streptomycin and tetracycline or streptomycin and chloramphenicol, have been recommended, there is little need to employ more than one agent in most situations. Nitrofurantoin (400 mg) and nalidixic acid (2 to 4 Gm) are reserved for treating patients with *E. coli* bacteriuria, and are not employed when infection is suspected outside of the urinary tract.

PREVENTION. Isolation and antimicrobial therapy of infants and contacts are essential to abort epidemic infantile diarrhea. In adults, many *E. coli* infections are hospital associated, and their incidence can be reduced by limiting use of indwelling urinary catheters, careful surgical aseptic technique, appropriate isolation of infection-prone patients, and judicious use of antibiotics, steroids, and cytotoxic agents. There is mounting evidence that the promiscuous employment of antibiotics may propagate the transfer of resistance factors among intestinal *E. coli*. These organisms may in turn transmit their resistance to other virulent *Enterobactericae*, such as, *Salmonella*.

REFERENCES

Kennedy, R. P., J. J. Plorde, and R. G. Petersdorf: Studies in the Epidemiology of *Escherichia coli* Infections: IV. Evidence for a Nosocomial Flora, J. Clin. Invest., 44: 193, 1965.

McCabe, W. R., and G. G. Jackson: Gram-negative Bacteremia, A.M.A. Arch. Intern. Med., 110:847, 856, 1962.

Marshall, T. F., and D. C. Hartzog, Jr.: Acute Emphysematous Cholecystitis, Ann. Surg., 159:1011, 1964.

Neter, E.: Enteropathogenic *Escherichia coli* Enteritis, Pediat. Clin. N. Am., 7:1015, 1960.

Studdiford, W. E., and G. W. Douglas: Placental Bacteremia: A Significant Finding in Septic Abortion Accompanied by Vascular Collapse, Am. J. Obstet. Gynecol., 71:842, 1956.

Sweet, A. Y., and E. Wolinsky: An Outbreak of Urinary and Other Infections Due to *E. coli*, Pediatrics, 33:865, 1964.

Tisdale, W. A.: Spontaneous Colon Bacillus Bacteremia in Laennec's Cirrhosis, Gastroenterology, 40:141, 1961.

145 PROTEUS INFECTIONS

Marvin Turck and
Robert G. Petersdorf

ETIOLOGY. The genus *Proteus* consists of gram-negative bacilli which do not ferment lactose and are characterized by their active motility and spreading growth on solid media. There are four pathogenic species: *P. mirabilis, P. vulgaris, P. morganii,* and *P. rettgeri. Proteus mirabilis* causes 75 to 90 percent of human infections and is distinguishable from the other three species by its inability to form indole. All four split urea, with production of ammonia. Some strains of *P. vulgaris* share a common antigen with certain rickettsia, accounting for the appearance of antibodies against proteus organisms (Weil-Felix reaction) in typhus, scrub typhus, and Rocky Mountain spotted fever. The Providence group of organisms resembles those of the genus *Proteus* closely except that it fails to produce a urease.

EPIDEMIOLOGY AND PATHOGENESIS. Members of the genus *Proteus* are normally found in soil, water, and sewage and are part of the normal fecal flora. Occasionally, they have been implicated as a cause of epidemic diarrhea in infants, but the evidence for this is inconclusive. The organism is frequently cultured from superficial wounds, draining ears, and sputum, particularly in patients who have received antibiotics, and replaces the more susceptible flora eradicated by these drugs. Proteus organisms often localize in already damaged tissues, where they produce a typical exudative inflammatory reaction.

MANIFESTATIONS. Proteus organisms are rarely primary invaders but produce disease in locations previously infected by other organisms. These locations include the skin, ears and mastoid sinuses, eyes, peritoneal cavity, urinary tract, meninges, lung, and bloodstream.

Cutaneous Infections. Proteus organisms are frequently isolated from surgical wounds, particularly following antimicrobial therapy, but they do not interfere with normal wound healing provided that the tissues are viable and foreign bodies are not present. Burns, varicose ulcers, and decubiti may become contaminated with proteus organisms, often in company with other gram-negative organisms or staphylococci.

Infections of the Ears and Mastoid Sinuses. Otitis media and mastoiditis in which proteus organisms are present can result in extensive destruction of the middle ear and mastoid sinuses. Fetid otorrhea, cholesteatoma, and granulation tissue constitute a chronic focus of infection in the middle and inner ears and mastoid, and deafness ensues. Paralysis of the facial nerve is an occasional complication. The great danger of these infections lies in intracranial extension, leading to thrombosis of the lateral sinus, meningitis, brain abscess, and bacteremia.

Ocular Infections. Proteus infection may cause corneal ulcers, usually following trauma to the eye, which occasionally terminate in panophthalmitis and destruction of the eyeball.

Peritonitis. Being part of the normal intestinal flora, proteus organisms may be isolated from the peritoneal cavity following perforation of viscera or mesenteric infarction.

Urinary Tract Infections. Proteus organisms are a common cause of urinary tract infections, usually in patients with chronic bacteriuria, many of whom have had obstructive uropathy, a history of instrumentation of the bladder, and repeated courses of chemotherapy. The organism is rarely a pathogen in anatomically normal urinary tracts except occasionally in patients with diabetes mellitus. Proteus organisms are also often cultured from bacteriuric patients with renal or bladder calculi. This may be related to the ammoniagenic property of this organism, which renders the urine alkaline and provides a fertile medium for formation of ammonium-magnesium-phosphate stones.

Bacteremia. Bloodstream invasion is the most serious

manifestation of infection with this organism. In 75 percent of cases, the urinary tract serves as the portal of entry; in the remainder, the biliary tree, gastrointestinal tract, ears and sinuses, and skin are the primary foci. Proteus bacteremia is frequently preceded by cystoscopy, urethral catheterization, transurethral prostatic resection, or other operative procedures. Clinically, the signs, symptoms, and laboratory findings of proteus sepsis—high fever, chills, shock, metastatic abscesses, leukocytosis, and rarely thrombocytopenia—are indistinguishable from those of bloodstream infections with other gram-negative bacteria (Chaps. 134 and 144).

DIAGNOSIS. The diagnosis of proteus infection depends on culture of the organism from blood, urine, or exudate and its identification by appropriate biochemical tests. It is especially important to separate *P. mirabilis*, the indole-negative species, from *P. morganii, rettgeri,* and *vulgaris,* which are indole-positive, because only *P. mirabilis* is susceptible to the action of penicillin and most other antibiotics. Proteus organisms are often present in mixed infections with other pathogens. Particular care should be exercised in the isolation of other organisms growing in the same medium with members of the genus *Proteus* lest they be masked by its spreading growth. The spreading character of this organism may also make antibiotic sensitivity tests difficult to interpret.

TREATMENT. Most strains of *P. mirabilis* are sensitive to penicillin in high concentration (10 units per ml or greater), ampicillin, kanamycin, cephalothin, and chloramphenicol. Proteus bacteriuria can be readily eradicated with any of these drugs during treatment; ampicillin in dosage of 0.5 Gm every 4 to 6 hr is highly effective. In severe infection, therapy should be parenteral: 6 to 12 Gm ampicillin or 20,000,000 units of penicillin G plus kanamycin 1.5 to 2.0 Gm per day, if renal function is adequate. There is good evidence that kanamycin is synergistic with ampicillin and penicillin G in proteus infections, and that chloramphenicol may be ineffective despite the results of in vitro tests. In view of the numerous more effective agents, there is no reason to use chloramphenicol in proteus infections. In general, all strains of *P. mirabilis* are resistant to tetracycline. Most strains other than *P. mirabilis* and Providence bacilli are sensitive only to kanamycin. A newer agent, gentamycin, appears to be very effective against indole-positive proteus organisms in vitro and in vivo. In addition, although ampicillin and penicillin G alone are ineffective against indole-positive proteus, a combination of either drug and kanamycin or gentamycin displays synergism. Carbenicillin is also effective against the majority of indole-positive proteus species. As with all other gram-negative infections, appropriate attention must be given to drainage of pus, maintenance of fluid and electrolyte status, and treatment of circulatory collapse.

REFERENCES

Anderson, K. N., R. P. Kennedy, J. J. Plorde, J. A. Shulman, and R. G. Petersdorf: In Vitro and in Vivo Activity of Ampicillin in Gram-negative Infections, J.A.M.A., 187: 555, 1964.

Chin, V. S. W., and P. D. Hoeprich: Susceptibility of Proteus and Providence Bacilli to 10 Antibacterial Agents, Am. J. Med. Sci., 242:309, 1961.

Kaye, D., M. G. Koenig, and E. W. Hook: The Action of Certain Antibiotics and Antibiotic Combinations against *Proteus mirabilis* with Demonstration of in Vitro Synergism and Antagonism, Am. J. Med. Sci., 242:321, 1961.

McCabe, W. R., and G. G. Jackson: Gram-negative Bacteremia, A.M.A. Arch. Intern. Med., 110:847, 856, 1962.

Tillotson, J. R., and A. M. Lerner: Characteristics of Pneumonias Caused by Bacillus Proteus, Ann. Intern. Med., 68:287, 1968.

146 PSEUDOMONAS INFECTIONS

Marvin Turck and
Robert G. Petersdorf

ETIOLOGY. *Pseudomonas aeruginosa* is a gram-negative motile rod which generally is not encapsulated and forms no spores. It grows readily in all ordinary culture media, and on agar it forms irregular, soft, irridescent colonies which usually have a fluorescent yellow-green color because of diffusion into the medium of two pigments, pyocyanin and fluorescin. *Pseudomonas* produces acid but no gas in glucose, and it is proteolytic. It is oxidase-positive and produces ammonia from arginine. A number of different strains have been identified by immunofluorescent techniques or bacteriophage typing. There is no evidence that these strains vary in their virulence for man.

EPIDEMIOLOGY. Pseudomonas organisms are present on the skin of some normal persons, particularly in the axilla and anogenital regions. They are uncommon in the stools of adults not receiving antibiotics. In the majority of instances, pseudomonas organisms are cultured as avirulent secondary contaminants in superficial wounds, or from the sputum of patients treated with antibiotics. Ordinarily this is of little consequence because the organisms merely fill the bacteriologic vacuum left by the elimination of more sensitive bacteria. Occasionally, however, superinfections with pseudomonas organisms occur in the ear, lung, skin, or urinary tract of patients whose primary pathogen has been eradicated by antibiotics. Serious infections are almost invariably associated with damage to local tissue or with diminished host resistance. Premature infants; children with congenital anomalies, patients with leukemia, usually receiving antibiotics, adrenal steroids, or antimetabolites; patients with burns; and geriatric patients with debilitating diseases are likely to develop pseudomonas infections. Most often these infections occur in the hospital environment, and the organisms have been cultured from a variety of sources in hospitals, including water from laboratory sinks and washbasins, antiseptic solutions, including benzalkonium chloride (Zephiran) and hexachlorophene soap, ophthalmic fluorescein and contact lens solution, saline, penicillin, procaine, and a variety of other medications. Other sources are incubators, humidifying equipment, air-cooling systems, forceps, and syringes. The organism is prevalent in urine receptacles and catheters, and on the hands of orderlies, nurses, and surgeons on urologic wards; in several outbreaks, pseudomonas urinary tract infections have presumably been transmitted from patient to patient by human carriers. Similar epidemics have been reported in nurseries among premature infants, and cross infection on burn wards is also common.

PATHOGENESIS. The portal of entry of pseudomonas organisms varies with the patient's age and underlying disease. In infancy and childhood, the skin, umbilical cord, and gastrointestinal tract predominate; in old age, the urinary tract is more often the primary focus. Often the infections remain localized in the skin or subcutaneous tissues. In burns the region below the eschar may become massively infiltrated with bacteria and inflammatory cells, and usually serves as the focus for bacteremia, the single most lethal complication. Hematogenous dissemination is characterized by hemorrhagic nodules in many areas, including the skin, heart, lungs, kidneys, and meninges. The histologic picture is one of necrosis and hemorrhage. Typically the walls of arterioles are heavily infiltrated with bacteria and the vessels are partially or wholly thrombosed.

MANIFESTATIONS. Pseudomonas infections occur in many locations, including the skin, subcutaneous tissue, bone and joints, eyes, ears, mastoid and paranasal sinuses, meninges, and heart valves. Bacteremia without a detectable primary focus may also occur.

Infections of the Skin and Subcutaneous Tissues. Pseudomonas organisms are frequently cultured from surgical wounds, varicose and decubitus ulcers, and burns, particularly following antibiotic therapy. Draining tuberculous or osteomyelitic sinuses may become secondarily infected. The mere presence of pseudomonas in these sites is of little significance provided that bacterial multiplication deep in subcutaneous tissues does not occur and bacteremia does not ensue. Cutaneous infections usually heal following removal or slough of devitalized tissue. Pseudomonas organisms may be responsible for green nails in persons whose hands are excessively exposed to water, soap, and detergents, who have onychomycosis, or whose hands are subject to mechanical trauma. The organism can usually be cultured from the nail plate.

Infections of the Ear, Mastoid, and Paranasal Sinuses. Otitis externa is the most common form of pseudomonas infection involving the ear. It is particularly troublesome in tropical climates and is characterized by chronic serosanguineous and purulent drainage from the external auditory canal. Otitis media or mastoiditis usually occurs as a superinfection following eradication of pneumococci, streptococci, or staphylococci by antimicrobial agents. Frequently pseudomonas organisms are present in association with other gram-negative or gram-positive organisms.

Infection of the Eye. Corneal ulceration is the most severe form of ocular pseudomonas infection. It usually follows a traumatic abrasion and may terminate in panophthalmitis and destruction of the globe. Purulent conjunctivitis occurs as a manifestation of pseudomonas infection in premature infants. Contamination of contact lenses or lens fluid may be an important means of infecting the eyes with pseudomonas organisms.

Urinary Tract Infections. Pseudomonas organisms are common pathogens in the urinary tract and are usually found in patients with obstructive uropathy who have been subjected to repeated urethral manipulations or to urologic surgery. They are rarely cultured from the urine of patients who have not seen a urologist. At times *Pseudomonas* is one of several pathogenic genuses in the urine, the others being *Escherichia coli, Aerobacter-Klebsiella, Proteus,* and enterococci. Pseudomonas bacteriuria is in no way unique and cannot be distinguished from infection with other organisms on clinical grounds.

Gastrointestinal Tract. Pseudomonas organisms have been implicated as a cause of epidemic diarrhea of infancy. In addition, a number of infants dying from neonatal sepsis have the classical necrotic, avascular ulcers of pseudomonas bacteremia in the bowel at autopsy. A "typhoidal" form of pseudomonas infection characterized by fever, myalgia, and diarrhea occurs predominantly in the Tropics. This illness, also called *13-day fever* or *Shanghai fever,* is self-limited, and the prognosis is good.

Respiratory Tract. Primary pseudomonas pneumonia is infrequent, and culture of this organism from the sputum usually is indicative of aspiration of gastric contents with secondary infection or of superinfection following eradication of a more sensitive flora with antibiotics. Pulmonary infection is often associated with microabscesses. The organism is often isolated from the sputum of patients with bronchiectasis, chronic bronchitis, or cystic fibrosis who have lingering infections punctuated by multiple courses of chemotherapy. Pseudomonas bronchitis and bronchiolitis may be the terminal event in cystic fibrosis.

Meningitis. Spontaneous pseudomonas meningitis is most unusual, but the bacilli may be introduced into the subarachnoid space by lumbar puncture, spinal anesthesia, intrathecal medication, or head trauma. Ventriculomastoid or ventriculoatrial shunts performed for hydrocephalus may become contaminated with pseudomonas organisms. Usually revision or removal of the shunt offers the best hope of cure. Meningitis may be a terminal phenomenon in pseudomonas bacteremia and in this instance represents a metastatic infection in the meninges.

Bacteremia. Bloodstream invasion tends to occur in debilitated patients, premature infants, children with congenital defects, patients with lymphomas, leukemias, or other malignant tumors, and elderly patients who have undergone surgery or instrumentation of the biliary or urinary tracts. Pseudomonas bacteremia is an important cause of death in patients with severe burns. In adults, pseudomonas bacteremia is indistinguishable from bloodstream infection with other bacterial species except for two findings (1) *ecthyma gangrenosum,* the classical skin lesion, often located in the anogenital region as a round, indurated, purple-black area about 1 cm in diameter with an ulcerated center and a surrounding zone of erythema; and (2) the passage of green urine, presumably due to the hemoglobin pigment, verdoglobin. Other features of pseudomonas sepsis include hectic fever, shaking chills, hyperventilation, confusion, delirium, and circulatory collapse. Hypothermia, leukopenia, and thrombocytopenia are more common in pseudomonas bacteremia than in other gram-negative bacteremias but are often related to an underlying blood dyscrasia. In addition to ecthyma gangrenosum, other skin lesions consist of hemorrhagic cellulitis and macular lesions on the trunk similar to "rose spots." Organisms usually can be cultured from cutaneous lesions and may provide an early clue to the diagnosis. Pseudomonas organisms may be in the bloodstream concomitantly with other organisms, notably *Enterobacteriaceae* or staphylococci. More often, however, pseudomonas bacteremia follows staphylococcal sepsis in patients with burns.

Bacterial Endocarditis. A number of cases of pseudomonas subacute bacterial endocarditis have followed open-heart surgery. Usually the organisms become implanted on a silk suture or a synthetic patch employed for closure of septal defects. Reoperation with removal of the vegetation and foreign bodies offers the best hope of cure. Pseudomonas endocarditis has been found on normal heart valves in patients with burns; it has been postulated that staphylococcal endocarditis develops first and that the vegetation is secondarily infected with pseudomonas organisms. Metastatic abscesses in bone, joints, brain, adrenal glands, and lungs are frequent consequences of pseudomonas endocarditis.

TREATMENT. Localized infections should be treated by irrigation with 1 percent acetic acid or topical therapy with colistin or polymyxin B. The administration of colistin subconjunctivally has been of value in ocular infections. Drainage of purulent material and removal of devitalized tissues are essential. The outcome of pseudomonas bacteremia is more dependent on the underlying disease than on the chemotherapy. For example, in patients with leukemia, remission must be attained before sepsis can be controlled. In burns, wound infection must be eradicated before the bloodstream can be cleared of organisms. Most strains of *Pseudomonas* are sensitive to polymyxin B and colistin, and a number of strains respond to oxytetracycline. These drugs should be used in full dosage of 30 to 50 mg every 6 hr for polymyxin B (in adults) and 75 to 100 mg every 6 hr (in adults) for colistin in life-threatening pseudomonas bacteremia. Both drugs are excellent for eradicating bacteriuria, but because blood levels exceed minimal inhibitory concentrations only two- or threefold, the results in bacteremia are inconsistent. Gentamycin, an aminoglycoside antibiotic, inhibits a number of strains of *Pseudomonas*. Carbenicillin, a new semisynthetic penicillin, is also active against many isolates and may be useful. Further experience with these drugs is necessary. Asymptomatic bacteriuria, particularly when confined to the bladder, should be treated with the least toxic and least painful agent, which, at times, may be a sulfonamide.

The prognosis has been improved in burned patients with pseudomonas sepsis as well as in a few other patients with endocarditis and with necrotizing papillitis by the use of large doses of hyperimmune γ-globulin in addition to antimicrobials.

PROPHYLAXIS. Pseudomonas cross infections in hospitals can be reduced by careful attention to aseptic techniques, particularly in nurseries for premature infants, operating rooms, and urologic wards; avoidance of cold sterilization procedures wherever possible; and scrupulous attention to clean plumbing fixtures, humidifying equipment, etc. Judicious use of antibiotics, steroids, and cytotoxic agents should also diminish the incidence of pseudomonas infections. Systemic antibiotic prophylaxis aimed at preventing colonization and infection with pseudomonas organisms has been notoriously unsuccessful and should be interdicted.

PROGNOSIS. The mortality rate in pseudomonas bacteremia is 75 percent and is highest in patients with shock or severe associated disease such as massive third degree burns, leukemia, or prematurity. When bacteremia originates in the urinary tract and is not accompanied by shock, the prognosis is considerably better. Localized pseudomonas infections do not present a threat to life unless hematogenous dissemination occurs.

REFERENCES

Curtin, J. A., R. G. Petersdrof, and I. L. Bennett, Jr.: Pseudomonas Bacteremia. Review of 91 Cases, Ann. Intern. Med., 54:1077, 1961.

Fierer, J., P. M. Taylor, and H. M. Gezon: *Pseudomonas Aeruginosa* Epidemic Traced to Delivery-Room Resuscitators, New Engl. J. Med., 276:991, 1967.

Forkner, C. E.: *Pseudomonas Aeruginosa* Infections, Modern Medical Monographs, No. 22, New York, Grune & Stratton, Inc., 1960.

——, E. Frei, III, J. H. Edgcomb, and J. P. Utz: Pseudomonas Septicemia, Am. J. Med., 25:877, 1958.

Rabin, E. R., C. D. Graber, E. H. Vogel, Jr., R. A. Finkelstein, and W. A. Turnbush: Fatal Pseudomonas Infection in Burned Patients, New Engl. J. Med., 265:1225, 1961.

Tillotson, J. R., and A. M. Lerner: Characteristics of Nonbacteremic Pseudomonas Pneumonia, Ann. Intern. Med., 68:295, 1968.

147 BACTEROIDES INFECTIONS
Edward W. Hook

ETIOLOGY. The genus *Bacteroides* includes a group of gram-negative, non-spore-forming, strictly anaerobic bacilli that are normal inhabitants of the mouth, intestinal tract, and vagina. These organisms are found in large numbers in human feces in an average concentration of about 10^9 viable units per gram, and often outnumber coliform bacilli by one-hundredfold.

Bacteroides funduliformis (*B. necrophorus*), *B. fragilis*, and *B. nigrescens* (*B. melaninogenicus*) are the species usually responsible for local or systemic infection of man.

PATHOGENESIS. Species of bacteroides are not highly invasive microorganisms, and infection is usually secondary to an underlying disease, a surgical procedure, or drug or radiation therapy which impairs the normal defenses of the host. The initial reaction to infection results in a localized suppurative lesion characterized by the formation of fetid pus. Infection usually remains localized, but bloodstream invasion may occur. In instances of bacteremia, suppurative thrombophlebitis adjacent to the site of initial infection is a frequent occurrence, and emboli harboring viable bacilli may be dislodged, resulting in septic pulmonary infarction. Organisms of the genus *Bacteroides* elaborate a heparinase, but the role of this enzyme in the formation of thrombi is unknown. Localization of blood-borne organisms at distant sites is not unusual and may result in abscess formation in brain, lung, liver, joints, kidneys, or other organs.

Although bacteroides may be isolated in pure culture from infected tissue or pus, other organisms are present in the majority of cases, usually anaerobic or aerobic streptococci, coliform species, or staphylococci. Bacteroides and anaerobic streptococci have been shown to act synergistically in the induction of abscesses in mice.

CLINICAL MANIFESTATIONS. Local Infections. Species of bacteroides are frequently isolated from local suppurative lesions of any tissue liable to contamination with the flora of the mouth, intestinal tract, or vagina. For example, members of this genus have been isolated from peritonsillar, appendiceal, ischiorectal, or pelvic abscesses, and from infected Skene's or Bartholin's glands. These organisms may be associated with sinusitis and otitis media, and can also be cultured from the surfaces of acutely inflamed appendices, from exudate in localized or generalized peritonitis, and from purulent discharge in patients with endometritis. Surgical wounds of the gastrointestinal or genitourinary tract may be complicated by bacteroides infection.

Local infection is usually manifested by pain and tenderness, and the course and outcome depend on the site of involvement and extent of infection. Necrosis of blood vessels in an abscess cavity occasionally results in severe hemorrhage.

Systemic infection. Invasion of the bloodstream by bacteroides is usually secondary to local infection of the tonsils, female genital tract, or peritoneum. The initial manifestations are determined by the portal of entry and may be those of peritonsillar abscess, endometritis, or appendicitis. When bloodstream invasion occurs, the patient becomes extremely ill. Severe chills, hectic fever ranging from 101 to 106°F, and severe diaphoresis are common. When bacteremia complicates tonsillar infection, the internal jugular vein may be the site of suppurative thrombophlebitis, and in pelvic infections the iliac and femoral veins may be involved. Palpation along the course of an involved vein, such as the internal jugular, may disclose a firm, tender cord, indicating the presence of a thrombus. Emboli may be dislodged, resulting in multiple septic pulmonary infarcts manifested by râles, dyspnea, cough, hemoptysis, pleurisy, and roentgenographic evidence of consolidation. Lung abscess and empyema often complicate pulmonary infection. Metastatic infection at other sites is not unusual, and may be manifested as brain abscess, liver abscess, or septic arthritis. A diffuse hepatitis may develop, leading to en-

largement and tenderness of the liver and jaundice. The prognosis in systemic bacteroides infection is grave, and death may occur in a few days.

The genus *Bacteroides* has also been implicated in certain other serious systemic infections. Meningitis or brain abscess occasionally results from direct extension of infection from the middle ear or sinuses. Aspiration of secretions harboring bacteroides may lead to pneumonia, lung abscess formation, or empyema. Transient bacteroides bacteremia may occur after dental extraction, and a few cases of subacute bacterial endocarditis have been described. These organisms occasionally cause infection of the urinary tract.

LABORATORY FINDINGS. Leukocytosis of 12,000 to 25,000 cells per cu mm may occur in localized bacteroides infections and is almost always present in systemic infection. Patients with liver abscesses or hepatitis have elevated serum bilirubin values and other aberrations of hepatic function. Gas formation at sites of infection occasionally results in air-fluid levels detectable by roentgenography.

Bacteroides infection should be considered whenever pus with an extremely foul odor is encountered, and anaerobic cultures should be made. A smear of the pus reveals slightly elongated gram-negative bacilli, and often another organism, usually a gram-positive coccus. Definitive diagnosis depends on isolation of the organisms from infected tissue or blood. Bacteroides grow slowly and may be difficult to detect when associated with another organism. Agglutinins against the strain responsible for an infection develop during the second or third week of infection, but because of the variable antigenic composition of these organisms, serologic methods are not of diagnostic aid.

TREATMENT. Surgical drainage of abscess cavities is of prime importance and should be carried out as soon as fluctuation and localization occur. Antimicrobial therapy is indicated when infection is not localized. Tetracycline in dosage of 2 Gm per day is the antibiotic of choice. Penicillin G in doses of 20 million units intravenously per day may be used as an alternative to tetracycline. Species of bacteroides are not highly sensitive to penicillin G, but most strains are inhibited in vitro by concentrations that are achieved in the blood of patients receiving massive penicillin therapy. Ampicillin in doses of 6 gm per day parenterally can be used instead of penicillin G. Chloramphenicol is also active against the majority of isolates from human infections, and cephalothin is inhibitory for some strains. Many strains of *Bacteroides* are highly resistant to the penicillinase-resistant penicillins and practically all isolates are resistant to streptomycin and neomycin.

Anticoagulant therapy and venous ligation should be considered in patients with thrombophlebitis and multiple septic pulmonary infarctions.

REFERENCES

Alston, J. M.: Necrobacillosis in Great Britain, Brit. Med. J., II:1524, 1955.

Bornstein, D. L., A. N. Weinberg, M. N. Swartz, and L. J. Kunz: Anaerobic Infections—Review of Current Experience, Medicine, 43:207, 1964.

Gunn, A. A.: Bacteroides Septicaemia, J. Roy. Coll. Surg. Edinburgh, 2:41, 1956.

Heineman, H. S., and A. I. Braude: Anaerobic Infection of the Brain, Am. J. Med., 35:682, 1963.

Keusch, G. T., and C. J. O'Connell: The Susceptibility of Bacteroides to the Penicillins and Cephalothin, Am. J. Med. Sci., 251:428, 1966.

McHenry, M. C., W. E. Wellman, and W. J. Martin: Bacteremia Due to Bacteroides, Arch. Intern. Med., 107:572, 1961.

Tillotson, J. R., and A. M. Lerner: Bacteroides Pneumonias, Ann. Intern. Med., 68:308, 1968.

Tynes, B. S., and W. B. Frommeyer, Jr.: Bacteroides Septicemia, Cultural, Clinical, and Therapeutic Features in a Series of Twenty-five Patients, Ann. Intern. Med., 56:12, 1962.

148   KLEBSIELLA (Aerobactor) INFECTION

Marvin Turck and
Robert G. Petersdorf

ETIOLOGY. Next to *Escherichia coli*, strains of *Klebsiella-Aerobacter* are the most important enteric organisms infecting man. In many laboratories *Klebsiella-Aerobacter* is not differentiated from *E. coli*. This is potentially a serious error because strains of *Klebsiella-Aerobacter* are, in general, more resistant to antibiotics and their isolation from blood, purulent exudates, and urine is of more serious prognostic significance. The Friedländer bacilli (*Klebsiella pneumoniae*) are encapsulated gram-negative bacilli, found among the normal flora of the mouth and intestinal tracts. *Klebsiella pneumoniae* has been considered to be a virulent respiratory pathogen since first described by Friedländer in 1882. *Klebsiella* is closely related to the genera *Aerobacter* (*Enterobacter**) and *Serratia* and may be differentiated only by certain amino acid decarboxylase tests. The significance of *Aerobacter* and *Serratia* in human infections has been less well clarified than infections secondary to *Klebsiella*, but all are potential pathogens, especially as opportunistic invaders in the compromised host. The strains of *Klebsiella* isolated from respiratory infections usually are nonmotile and form large mucoid colonies on solid media. *Aerobacters* on the other hand, tend to be motile. Klebsiellas are usually sensitive to the antibiotic cephalothin, to which *Aerobacters* are resistant. These characteristics, however, are not invariable enough to differentiate respiratory from intestinal isolates.

Klebsiella rhinoscleromatis, is probably the causative agent of rhinoscleroma, and *Klebsiella ozenae* has been isolated occasionally from the nose of patients with ozena (Chap. 282).

PATHOGENESIS. *Klebsiella*, *Aerobacter*, and *Serratia* are all capable of causing disease in diverse anatomic

* This name is now also acceptable.

sites. However, results of clinical and epidemiologic studies suggest that differences in pathogenicity do exist among these genera and that precise taxonomic identification is of value. Although infections of the respiratory tract with *K. pneumoniae* have been emphasized most in the past, the urinary tract presently accounts for the majority of clinical isolates. In this site clinical manifestations and pathogenesis are similar to infections produced by *E. coli*, but Klebsiellas are more frequently found in patients with complicated and obstructive urinary tract disease. Infections of the biliary tract, the peritoneal cavity, the middle ear, mastoids, paranasal sinuses, and meninges also are not uncommon. In these locations, Klebsiellas are more frequent than either *Aerobacters* or serratias and are more likely to produce an illness of greater severity. The apparent increased frequency of infection by serratias represents an increase primarily due to nosocomial spread of this organism.

MANIFESTATIONS. Symptoms and signs of common infections caused by *Klebsiella-Aerobacter*—namely those involving the urinary tract, biliary tree, peritoneal cavity—are indistinguishable from those caused by *E. coli* (Chap. 144). These infections commonly occur in diabetics and in the form of superinfections in patients who have received antimicrobials to which these organisms are resistant. Klebsiella-aerobacter infection is also an important etiologic factor in septic shock (Chap. 134).

Acute Pneumonia. *Klebsiella* is well recognized as a pulmonary pathogen, but probably accounts for less than 1 percent of all cases of bacterial pneumonia. The disease is most common in men over forty years of age and is more frequently found in alcoholics. Other factors associated with increased susceptibility include diabetes mellitus and chronic bronchopulmonary disease. Aspiration of oropharyngeal secretions containing klebsiella organisms is the likely inciting factor among alcoholic patients. The clinical manifestations are indistinguishable from those of pneumococcal pneumonia (Chap. 138), with sudden onset of chills, fever, productive cough, and severe pleuritic chest pain. Patients are frequently delirious and prostrated, but this may also occur with pneumococcal infection. A "characteristic" clinical feature, which occurs in only 25 to 50 percent of patients, is the dark brown or red currant-jelly sputum which may be so tenacious that the patient has difficulty in expelling it from his mouth and lips. The pulmonary lesion is most frequent in the right upper lobe but often rapidly progresses and if untreated, may spread from lobe to lobe. Cyanosis and dyspnea develop rapidly, and jaundice, vomiting, and diarrhea may be present. Physical findings consist primarily of signs of consolidation unless pleural effusion or necrotizing pneumonitis with rapid cavitation have intervened. The blood leukocyte count may be elevated but is often low, which probably is merely a reflection of severe infection in an alcoholic patient with poor bone marrow reserve. Lung abscess and empyema are much more frequent than in pneumococcal pneumonia and are related to the destructive capabilities of this organism. So-called "characteristic" radiographic features such as bulging fissures and loss of lung volume occur only in varying frequency, and also may be found in pneumococcal infection.

Chronic infection of the lung. Rarely, infection with *Klebsiella* may progress, often in indolent fashion, to a chronic necrotizing pneumonitis resembling tuberculosis. It may follow acute Friedländer pneumonia but is also seen in patients who give no history of acute onset. The principal symptoms are productive cough, weakness, and anemia. Hemoptysis, chronic empyema, or sterile serous effusions are also encountered. Cavitation, frequently with thin walls, occurs primarily in the upper lobes.

DIAGNOSIS. Diagnosis is established by an awareness of the clinical setting in which Klebsiella infections occur and by isolation of the organism. A presumptive diagnosis of klebsiella pneumonia should be made on the basis of gram stain of the sputum which shows a predominance of short, plump, gram-negative bacilli, frequently surrounded by a clear space because of the capsule. Often these gram-negative organisms occur together with gram-positive cocci and because the gram-positives are easier to see, the gram-negative bacteria may be ignored and the diagnosis may be missed, which in turn, may lead to potentially serious delays in instituting therapy. Additional proof of klebsiella-aerobacter infection in the lung is afforded by isolation of the organisms from blood and pleural exudate. In extrapulmonary infections, the organisms are readily seen in and cultured from pus or secretions of involved organs.

TREATMENT. Klebsiellas have variable susceptibility to antimicrobial drugs, but the majority of strains is susceptible to kanamycin, streptomycin, cephalothin, tetracycline, chloramphenicol, or polymyxin B or colistin. The organism does not respond to penicillin and its analogues. A popular regimen employs streptomycin in large doses (2 to 3 Gm daily) with chloramphenicol or a tetracycline. Kanamycin (25 mg/kg/day) is probably more active than streptomycin and has been advocated along with cephalothin (6 to 12 Gm per day). It is of clinical importance that most strains of *K. pneumoniae* are sensitive to cephalothin, but most enterobacter are highly resistant. Because of the relative poor blood and tissue levels achieved with the polymyxins, they should probably not be employed as first line agents in the treatment of klebsiella infections. Regardless of the antimicrobial regimen employed, treatment should be continued for a minimum of 10 to 14 days and prolonged if there is extensive cavitation. Pleural effusion must be drained appropriately; antibiotic therapy alone is not sufficient treatment for closed-space infections of the pleural cavity. At times, rib resection with open drainage may be necessary, and should be considered if effusions recur.

PROGNOSIS. Prior to the introduction of antimicrobials, the fatality rate reported in different clinics varied from 50 to 80 percent and death within 48 hr was not infrequent. Even with antimicrobial treatment the course of the disease is quite variable and the prognosis must be guarded. For the most part, this reflects the age group involved and the frequent association of klebsiella infection

with alcoholism, malnutrition, and severe underlying disease.

REFERENCES

Edmondson, E. G., and J. P. Sanford: The Klebsiella-Enterobacter (Aerobacter)-Serratia Group, Medicine 46:323, 1967.

Eickhoff, T. C., B. W. Steinhauer, and M. Finland: The Klebsiella-Enterobacter-Serratia Division. Biochemical and Serologic Characteristics and Susceptibility to Antibiotics, Ann. Intern. Med., 65:1163, 1966.

Manfredi, F., W. J. Daly, and R. H. Rehnke: Clinical Observations of Acute Friedländer Pneumonia, Ann. Intern Med., 58:642, 1963.

149 TYPHOID FEVER

Richard B. Hornick and Theodore E. Woodward

DEFINITION. Typhoid fever is a systemic infection unique to man. Following ingestion of *Salmonella typhosa* no other animal develops prolonged remittent fever, characteristic rash (rose spots), splenomegaly, lymphadenopathy, or intestinal complications. Predominant symptoms include fever, headache, abdominal pain, disturbances in bowel function, anorexia, and lassitude. Diagnosis is confirmed by isolation of the causative organisms from the blood, feces, or urine and by demonstrating rising titers of agglutinins to the somatic (O) and flagellar (H) antigens of the bacillus.

HISTORY. In 1829, Louis studied 158 cases and described intestinal lesions, enlarged mesenteric lymph glands, splenomegaly, rose spots, and intestinal hemorrhage and perforation. This great clinician first employed the term *typhoide*. The British, however, continued to view the intestinal lesion as an incidental complication of typhus. In 1836 William Gerhard of Philadelphia, a former student of Louis, clearly defined differences between typhus and typhoid based on precise clinical and anatomic findings.

Budd, an English practitioner, in a series of publications from 1856 to 1870, suggested the contagiousness of typhoid and stressed the importance of spread by the bowel discharges of infected persons. His hypothesis was not verified until 1885 when Pfeiffer reported the first stool isolation. The discovery of the organism is credited to Eberth, who in 1880 reported the presence of bacteria in stained smears of mesenteric lymph nodes and spleen. Widal in 1896 described the test for agglutinins in the serum of patients.

EPIDEMIOLOGY. *Salmonella typhosa* resides solely in man and is perpetuated in nature by its transmission to healthy persons from patients or carriers. Water, milk, and food are contaminated from infected feces. It is an epidemiologic axiom that for every outbreak or sporadic case of typhoid fever there must be a carrier that is, an individual who sheds virulent organisms in spite of apparent good health. Once identified, typhoid carriers should be prevented from handling food until they have been freed of S. typhosa.

Flies have been incriminated in the transmission of typhoid fever because of their ability to carry the bacilli from feces to food or liquids.

The incidence of typhoid fever in the United States has declined steadily in the past century. Occupational control of carriers and improvement of water supply and sewage disposal have been the major contributors to this decline. From 1962 to 1966, the annual median number of cases reported in this country was 461. Formerly the majority of cases occurred during the summer months, but seasonal variation has disappeared as the number of carriers has lessened. The disease has not been controlled in some countries, primarily because of crowded living conditions and poor sanitation.

Typhoid fever emerges as a significant cause of disability and death among civilian and military populations during war or following severe natural catastrophes. Major epidemics have occurred in recent years in Switzerland and Great Britain, emphasizing the ability of this disease to spread unexpectedly when defects in sewage disposal or food handling occur.

PATHOGENESIS. As in other enteric infections, causative organisms gain access to the host via the oral cavity. Studies of infectivity in human subjects have failed to confirm that S. typhosa invade via the lymphoid tissue of the pharynx and have also ruled out the respiratory tract as a significant portal of entry. Rather, typhoid bacilli survive the acidity of the stomach, pass on into the small and large intestine, multiply, and invade the mucosal barrier. It is during the critical 24 to 72 hr after ingestion that the outcome of the infection is decided. If the organisms overcome inhibitory influences of commensal bacteria and reproduce in sufficient numbers to overwhelm the phagocytic activities of intestinal mucosa, successful entry can be made into the host. Once the intestinal barrier has been penetrated, stool cultures, which have been positive for S. typhosa for the few days after swallowing the organisms, usually become free of the pathogen. The bacteria probably enter the systemic circulation by way of the mesenteric-thoracic duct lymphatic drainage. From this stage in the incubation period until overt disease occurs, typhoid bacilli reside within the reticuloendothelial system, mainly the liver. Subsequent bacteremia heralds the onset of clinical signs and symptoms of typhoid fever. Shortly thereafter S. typhosa reappears in stool cultures, having escaped from the liver and perhaps local foci in the intestine.

Clinical manifestations and pathologic findings of typhoid fever have been attributed to the effects of circulating endotoxin. Endotoxin of S. typhosa is a lipopolysaccharide-protein complex with toxic activities identical to those of other endotoxins. It is derived from the cell wall and evokes numerous pharmacologic actions. Intravenous infusion of endotoxin in man produces fever, chills,

headache, nausea, backache, and abdominal pain. Volunteers could not differentiate these symptoms from those subsequently produced in the course of induced typhoid fever.

Despite this circumstantial evidence, certain well-known effects of endotoxin are inconsistent with the thesis that attributes the manifestations of typhoid fever to endotoxemia. For example, from three to five daily intravenous infusions of endotoxin result in development of tolerance to its pyrogenicity, i.e., chills and fever are no longer induced unless dosage is markedly increased. This tolerance differs from the sustained febrile course which typifies typhoid fever. Moreover, recent studies indicate that endotoxin tolerance continues to operate effectively in volunteers with induced typhoid fever. In addition, deliberate activation of tolerance either before or during induced typhoid did not mitigate the febrile or toxic course of disease. It appears, therefore, that circulating endotoxin does not play a major role in the pathogenesis of typhoid fever.

PATHOLOGY. Early in the disease, a nonspecific enteritis is present in the jejunum. Mesenteric adenopathy is striking in chimpanzees sacrificed 48 hr after ingestion of typhoid bacilli. Other components of the reticuloendothelial system (RES) are involved during the first few days of disease. Pharyngeal lymphoid tissue and peripheral nodes are enlarged; later the spleen and liver become palpable. Using ^{131}I aggregated albumin in volunteer typhoid subjects, increased phagocytic activity of the RES, coinciding with the overt hypertrophy, was demonstrable by the third to the fifth day of disease.

The Peyer's patches are initially swollen and ultimately undergo necrosis, forming oval-shaped ulcers most numerous in the terminal 24 in. of the ileum. Ulceration may occur in the jejunum and lymphoid follicles of the cecum and colon. Necrosis of these lesions, usually during the third febrile week, leads to the common complications of hemorrhage and perforation. The intestinal ulcer eventually heals without scarring.

Histologic changes in the intestinal lesions are proliferation of large mononuclear cells and edema. Similar alterations occur in mesenteric nodes, spleen, bone marrow, and liver (typhoid nodules). Lymph nodes often exhibit necrosis and marked proliferation of the sinusoidal cells; sinusoids are filled with macrophages. Skin lesions (rose spots) consist of clumps of typhoid bacilli in the dermis, with round-cell infiltration and dilated vascular spaces.

Focal metastatic infection may be responsible for cholecystitis, osteomyelitis, chrondritis, meningitis, endocarditis, or nephritis. The gallbladder is frequently infected, although acute cholecystitis is less common. Bronchitis is not uncommon, and pneumonia due to S. typhosa occasionally occurs.

The intestinal lesions subside ultimately, whereas the infection in the liver and biliary tract may continue indefinitely, characterizing the carrier state. Fully developed, this chronic infection produces no symptoms, and reinfection of the host does not occur despite constant presence in the intestine of millions of typhoid bacilli.

MANIFESTATIONS. Unrecognized and inadequately treated typhoid infection may persist as a continuous or remittent fever for 3 or more weeks, with a prolonged period of convalescence.

The incubation period averages about 10 days, with a range of 3 to 25 days, which probably depends on the infecting dose. In volunteer studies, the largest number of organisms produced illness in the shortest period of time.

Onset of illness in a typical case is gradual, with symptoms appearing and increasing in severity over a 2- to 3-day period. Headache, the most common initial complaint, is generalized and constant, and worsens as the fever rises. Headache, plus the associated malaise, chilly sensations, and fever, cause the patient to take to bed. Intestinal complaints develop rapidly, beginning with continuous abdominal pain, frequently in the lower quadrants. Mild ileus occurs with associated constipation, anorexia, and nausea. Palpation elicits the feeling of gas-liquid-filled loops of intestine being compressed and displaced. Cough and bronchitic symptoms are common. Conjunctival injection occurs early in the febrile course. Sudden and unprovoked epistaxis may occur.

Fever increases in stepwise fashion for 2 to 3 days and then plateaus, with a continuous febrile pattern in the range of 103 to 105°F. It maintains this level for 2 to 3 weeks in untreated cases before abating slowly during the third and fourth weeks of disease. Many patients react to this debilitating febrile course with frank psychosis, delirium, or mania, which complicates management. Chills and sweating are not a regular accompaniment of the fever. As the temperature wanes, symptoms disappear.

The increment in pulse rate is usually inconsistent with the elevated temperature early in the course of typhoid. Etiology of this relative bradycardia has not been ascertained. Myocarditis, a not-infrequent complication, occurs later.

Some patients have diarrhea early in the disease, and in many it is a late manifestation.

Rose spots, the characteristic exanthem of enteric forms of salmonellosis, appear in only 10 percent of cases, and early therapy may reduce the incidence. Rose spots appear on the anterior thorax and abdomen early in the second week as rose-pink hyperemic papules 2 to 4 mm in diameter, that blanch on pressure. They are usually few in number, persist for only 2 to 3 days, and are detected with great difficulty in darkly pigmented patients. As they regress, the reddish color changes to a faint brown discoloration which does not blanch with pressure. Only careful scrutiny utilizing good lighting will reveal this delicate rash.

The spleen is frequently enlarged late in the first week of illness. Occasionally there is splenic tenderness, and rarely a friction rub appears, because of perisplenitis.

COMPLICATIONS. Formerly, numerous complications were associated with the prolonged convalescence of typhoid fever. Appropriate antibiotic and supportive care has eliminated the profound weakness, weight loss, and abnormalities due to nutritional deficiencies. However, patients occasionally will have thrombophlebitis, arthral-

gia, and peripheral neuritis despite adequate nursing and dietary management.

Gastrointestinal Hemorrhage. Gross hemorrhage of typhoidal ulcers occurs in approximately 10 percent of cases; occult bleeding is present in about 20 percent. Characteristically, hemorrhage occurs during the second or third week of disease, either as sudden gross hemorrhage or as continuous slow oozing. Clinical signs indicative of blood loss are apprehension, sweating, pallor, depression of cutaneous temperature, rapid weak pulse, hypotension, and narrow pulse pressure. Chloramphenicol therapy has reduced but not eliminated the incidence of this serious complication.

Intestinal Perforation. Intestinal perforation occurs in about 3 percent of untreated patients and was formerly an important cause of death. Rupture of the intestinal ulcer with peritonitis still occurs, although antibiotics have reduced the number of fatalities sharply. In most instances perforation of an ulcer in the lower ileum occurs early in the third week. Patients manifesting tympanites, diarrhea, and hemorrhage are likely to suffer this complication; it may strike unexpectedly in convalescent patients. Sudden, sharp pain in the right lower quadrant, soon associated with abdominal distension, muscle rigidity, rebound tenderness, and diminished peristalsis, is a characteristic sign. Obliteration of liver flatness on percussion, with excessive tympanites, is a valuable sign of free abdominal air. Pallor, clammy perspiration, tachycardia, and lowered pressure all herald impending shock. At this stage there is hypothermia and the blood leukocyte count ranges from 9,000 to 13,000 cells per cu mm. Perforation may be mistaken for appendicitis, acute cholecystitis, or merely an accentuation of the abdominal pain in the debilitated typhoid patient. Frequent examination and upright abdominal x-ray to demonstrate air under the diaphragm provide very helpful diagnostic clues. Rarely, typhoidal peritonitis may result from rupture of an enlarged softened mesenteric lymph gland.

Other Complications. Bacterial or lobar pneumonia developing at the height of the disease was formerly a serious complication of typhoid fever. Cultures of sputum or consolidated lungs have yielded predominantly pneumococci or occasionally typhoid bacilli. Other pyogenic complications include parotitis, sinusitis, and furunculosis. Folliculitis is a common sequel, despite early chloramphenicol therapy, but tends to be mild and disappears spontaneously within several weeks. Typhoidal meningitis is rare but serious. Chondritis and periostitis are indolent focal infections from which S. *typhosa* may be isolated. Monoarticular and polyarticular arthritis are rare complications. Cholecystitis may occur during the acute disease, creating a confusing diagnostic problem because of physical findings similar to those seen with intestinal perforation. Months or years later there may be chronic cholecystitis with calculi from which viable typhoid bacilli can be isolated. Acute nephritis or pyelonephritis is seen occasionally at the height of the illness or during convalescence. Deafness is common but seldom permanent. Herpes labialis is rare in typhoid patients. Severe hemolytic anemia has occurred during the acute phase of the illness, with patients showing positive Coombs tests or red cells deficient in glucose 6-phosphate dehydrogenase. Whether hemolysis is due to an enzymatic defect in the red cell, drug therapy, or typhoid per se is not clear.

Relapse. The incidence of relapse varies from 5 to 15 percent. Antibiotic therapy appears to have altered the host's recuperative powers adversely in this disease, since relapse rates are greater (20 percent) in groups of patients treated with chloramphenicol. On an average, relapse occurs approximately 15 days after cessation of chemotherapy, regardless of the duration of treatment or the stage at which the antibiotic is first given. Onset of the relapse is usually associated with recurrent bacteremia and symptoms similar to those of the primary disease. As a rule, the manifestations are milder and may abate without specific therapy. The cause of the relapse is not the emergence of chloramphenicol-resistant organisms and does not appear to be correlated with the presence or absence of somatic (O) or flagellar (H) antibodies. Cultivation of typhoid bacilli in tissue culture cells has revealed the persistence of viable, but nonmultiplying, intracellular *S. typhosa* despite presence of antibiotic. Removal of chemotherapeutic agents (3 weeks later) from the medium resulted in reactivation of the tissue culture infection. Persistence of organisms in the hepatic cells of patients treated with therapeutic doses of chloramphenicol may explain the development of relapses as well as carrier states. Reasons for the "microbial indifference" are unknown.

The Typhoid Carrier. Typhoid bacilli persist indefinitely in the bile passages and in the intestines of about 3 percent of patients who recover from the disease. Many carriers have no history of prior infection, and all are in apparent good health. A carrier is defined as one who excretes *S. typhosa* in the stools beyond 1 year following the acute infection. Most typhoid patients will have negative stool cultures after 4 months; persistence beyond this period usually indicates a carrier. The carrier state is three times as common in women as in men. The incidence increases with advancing age, suggesting that the greater frequency of biliary tract disease in older females favors development of a carrier state. Removal of a diseased gallbladder, with or without stones, eradicates the carrier state in a significant number of patients. The gallbladder is not the sole source for this persistent infection, since typhoid bacilli can be isolated from bile obtained from the T tube left in the common duct following cholecystectomy. Cultures of bile and stools usually become negative when the T tube has been removed and complete healing occurs. Typhoid carriers with cholelithiasis should be treated by cholecystectomy and antibiotics. Those without stones can often be cleared with intensive chemotherapeutic regimens. The following schedules have been successful in reported series of treated carriers: (1) Ampicillin 3 to 6 Gm per day for as long as 84 days. (2) Penicillin in a dosage of 12 million units daily, supplemented with Benemid for 14 days. (3) Combined treatment with chloramphenicol (1.0 Gm every 8 hr) and streptomycin (1.0 Gm twice daily) for 3 weeks.

Urinary tract carriers are infrequent and represent a minor health hazard in this country. Chronic bladder scarring, with pseudoabscess and stone formation secondary to *Schistosoma haematobium* infection, predisposes to development of the urinary carrier state following acute typhoid fever.

LABORATORY DIAGNOSIS. One of the distinctive hematologic features of typhoid fever is leukopenia, with cell counts ranging from 4,000 to 6,000 cells per cu mm during the first 2 weeks and 3,000 to 5,000 cells per cu mm during the third and fourth weeks. In the presence of intestinal perforation or pyogenic complications, the leukocyte count rises moderately, to 10,000 to 14,000 cells per cu mm. Normocytic anemia is present in many patients; with blood loss the anemia becomes hypochromic and microcytic. Except for transient albuminuria during the febrile stage, the urine is normal. Occult blood may be present in the feces beginning the second week.

Isolation of *S. typhosa* from the blood and feces is the most dependable diagnostic test. Blood cultures are positive in most cases during the first and early in the second febrile week. Bacteremia is also demonstrable during relapse. Typhoid bacilli are usually present in fecal cultures after the tenth day; the incidence of isolates increases up to the fourth or fifth week. Bone marrow aspirations and culture of rose spots have yielded the organism, but they offer no advantage over blood cultures. Likewise, in a small percentage of patients, *S. typhosa* can be detected in urine during the second or third week of disease.

The readily available Widal test aids in the diagnosis of typhoid fever. Specific agglutinins appear in the serum after 7 to 10 days of illness. The titer rises steadily to a peak during the third to fifth week and falls gradually over several weeks. It does not rise appreciably during relapse. The titer of the flagellar (H) antibody is usually higher than the somatic (O) agglutinin. Measurement of Vi (capsular) antibody by the agglutination of sensitized red cells has been used in conjunction with stool cultures to determine the presence of or the cessation of the carrier state. Many carriers will have elevated Vi hemagglutination titers, but this antibody should not be used as a single criterion to evaluate the activity of the typhoid carrier.

DIFFERENTIAL DIAGNOSIS. No single symptom or clinical feature is pathognomonic at the time of onset. Manifestations such as headache, fever, malaise, weakness, anorexia, cough, and abdominal pain are common to many diseases. These include the major rickettsioses, brucellosis, tularemia, leptospirosis, psittacosis, infectious hepatitis, infectious mononucleosis, primary atypical pneumonia, miliary tuberculosis, malaria, lymphoma (including Hodgkin's disease), and rheumatic fever. The rose spot is the most valuable single sign and, when coupled with fever, splenomegaly, and leukopenia, usually clinches the diagnosis. Differentiation of typhoid fever from diseases which it resembles depends on laboratory confirmation by (1) culture of the blood, feces, and urine, and (2) the demonstration of a positive Widal test. Repeatedly negative cultures of the blood and feces and negative agglutination tests should suggest other illnesses. Rarely are the bacteriologic and serologic tests entirely negative.

MANAGEMENT. The mortality and prolonged morbidity of typhoid fever have been reduced effectively by antibiotics and other supportive measures. In spite of specific therapeutic advances, intestinal hemorrhage and perforation occur in a small percentage of patients. The incidence of relapse has not been significantly reduced and, in fact, may be greater as a result of chloramphenicol therapy. Nonetheless, it is advisable to begin specific therapy as early as possible, with the aim of preventing the development of serious complications.

Specific Treatment. Although many antibiotics show excellent in vitro bacteriostatic action against *S. typhosa*, chloramphenicol gives the most consistent therapeutic results. Ampicillin therapy has been reported to be effective; but the accumulated evidence indicates that patients do not respond as uniformly or as rapidly as with chloramphenicol therapy. The delay in clinical response and the high relapse rate following chloramphenicol treatment stress the need for a more effective antisalmonella drug.

Following institution of chloramphenicol, patients are subjectively improved, with lessened headache and toxemia within 48 hr and normal temperature in less than 4 days. At this stage the patient is more vigorous, appetite has returned, and abdominal pain has abated. Bacteremia is no longer demonstrable several hours after beginning treatment, although stool cultures may be intermittently positive throughout the course.

Failure of typhoid patients to respond to chloramphenicol is unusual. Recommended administration of this drug is as follows: a loading dose comprised of 50 mg per kg of body weight, followed by the same amount divided into three doses daily given at 8-hr intervals. After the patient has become afebrile, the dose can be reduced to 2.0 Gm per day. Chloramphenicol should be continued for a total of 14 days. If nausea and vomiting obviate the oral route, the sodium succinate ester of chloramphenicol can be given intravenously or intramuscularly, on the basis of a daily dose of 25 mg per kg. Daily intravenous doses exceeding 3.0 Gm are not advised, and the oral route is preferred. In the rare situations where chloramphenicol proves to be ineffective, ampicillin can be tried, using 6 to 8 Gm per day and continuing therapy for 2 weeks.

Antitoxemic Effects of Steroids. In severely ill patients 3 to 4 days elapse after institution of chloramphenicol therapy before toxemia and pyrexia disappear. This interval can be shortened appreciably if chloramphenicol is supplemented with steroids.

Cortisone, 200 to 300 mg, or prednisone, 40 to 60 mg, is given daily. Three days of treatment with steroids are sufficient. European investigators have reported a "typhoid shock" syndrome following chloramphenicol treatment, presumably as a result of excessive endotoxin release. Under these conditions steroid treatment may exert a protective effect. Steroids should be reserved for those clinical situations associated with severe typhoidal toxemia.

Supportive Therapy. General supportive care is a vital supplement to antibiotic therapy. Bed rest extending into early convalescence is essential. Ambulation should be gradual, to avoid undue fatigue or exertion. Laxatives and promiscuous use of enemas are ill advised because of the danger of perforation or hemorrhage. Analgesics aid in ameliorating headache, although salicylates should be avoided because of the propensity of typhoid patients to show exaggerated reactions to the antipyretic action of these drugs. Tepid sponge baths are effective in lowering body temperature and should be employed when fever in excess of 104°F appears.

Good nursing care is essential and includes special attention to oral hygiene and adequate bathing. The observations of pulse rate, onset of severe abdominal pain, the presence of tarry or bloody stools, or the occurrence of vomiting are of utmost importance in the early recognition of complications.

A bland or liquid diet is prescribed until the appetite improves. Attention to fluid and electrolyte balance is essential. The judicious transfusion of whole blood given slowly and in small amounts may be lifesaving in severely ill, anemic patients.

Intestinal Hemorrhage. An awareness of this complication and its early detection are essential for proper management. The prevention of shock or its early treatment by blood transfusions is of prime importance. The extent and duration of bleeding should be assessed by frequent determinations of hematocrit and stool guaics. Adequate reserves of blood should be readily available. Strict bed rest should be enforced, and oral alimentation should be restricted. Under these conditions the antibiotics may be given parenterally.

Intestinal Perforation. A severely damaged intestine requires time for healing. Hence the threat of intestinal perforation exists for several days after specific therapy is instituted. The debilitated toxic condition of the patient and the friability of the intestinal lesion make the typhoid patient a poor surgical risk. It is justified to place greater emphasis on medical management, i.e., to combat shock, to decompress the bowel, and to continue antibiotic treatment. Should the process fail to localize, as evidenced by abdominal examination, persistence of shock, continued leukocytosis, and other signs, surgical intervention may be indicated.

Relapses. The greatest incidence of relapse occurs about 2 weeks after the cessation of chloramphenicol therapy. Patients should be followed for 3 weeks after becoming afebrile. Specific treatment should be reinstituted and continued for a week when symptoms and fever persist beyond 24 hr.

CONTROL AND IMMUNIZATION. All typhoid patients should be reported to appropriate health authorities in order that the source of illness and infection among contacts can be investigated. Patients' stools should be cultured frequently during convalescence to determine if *S. typhosa* is being shed. Usually three consecutively negative stool cultures obtained at weekly intervals indicate that a carrier state has not developed. Convalescent carriers continue to have organisms in stool cultures for 3 months, occasionally for a year. These patients and chronic carriers should be carefully controlled to ensure that they do not engage in occupations that would allow dissemination of typhoid bacilli through accidental contamination of food or water. It is perfectly safe with modern plumbing and sewage disposal to discard stools in flush toilets. Typhoid carriers should be instructed in adequate hand-washing techniques.

The patient should be isolated during the acute phase of the disease, and hospital personnel in attendance should be gowned to protect their clothing. Bed pans, urinals, linens, and eating utensils should be sterilized in boiling water or by autoclaving.

The effectiveness of typhoid vaccines has been a debated point and recently their relative efficacy has been quantitated in volunteers. Inactivated vaccines administered to adult males induce significant but not complete resistance to an inoculum of S. *typhosa* which cause disease in 25 percent of a healthy unimmunized population. Larger numbers of organisms overcome vaccine associated immunity. The number of bacteria ingested under natural circumstances can only be estimated with retrospective analysis. It appears likely from such evidence water-borne outbreaks are caused by small numbers of bacteria, while food contaminated by a carrier may contain 10 to 1,000 times as many organisms. In these settings vaccine may cause an individual to be protected against the smaller but not the larger inoculum. The large-scale field trials conducted by the World Health Organization in Yugoslavia, Poland, and British Guiana produced results consistent with this thesis. In these countries the main method of spread of typhoid has been by impure water supply. Population groups in these studies who received typhoid vaccine were protected for as long as 7 years. However, the disease rate was many times greater in the populace that received no vaccine of any sort (including placebo), suggesting that individuals volunteering for the vaccine trials were more careful and had less exposure. Nevertheless, typhoid vaccines can reduce the incidence of disease in endemic areas but prior vaccine administration does not ensure protection.

Currently, TAB (typhoid, paratyphoid A and B) vaccine is commercially available, but it will be replaced by a monovalent preparation containing only typhoid bacilli inactivated by acetone. This preparation is rich in Vi antigen and without the paratyphoid antigens and phenol causes much less systemic and local reactivity. The schedule of vaccine administration should be 0.5 ml for adults given subcutaneously followed in 1 to 2 weeks by a second dose. TAB vaccine can be given in the same fashion. Yearly booster doses are indicated for those persons at great risk because of occupation or travel. Reactions are common with TAB vaccine and somewhat less with the newer monovalent preparation. Pain and/or swelling at site of injection, chills and fever occurring several hours after administration, myalgia, arthralgia, nausea, and occasional vomiting can be anticipated. Salicylatis may ameliorate these reactions.

PROGNOSIS. The mortality rate in typhoid fever in the United States prior to the introduction of antibiotic ther-

apy was about 12 percent. Most deaths occurred from intestinal perforation, hemorrhage, or both. Toxemia, with resultant inanition, was responsible for some fatalities. Despite the therapeutic efficacy of chloramphenicol, 2 to 3 percent of patients now die of typhoid fever. Most deaths are in the aged, in infants, and in malnourished and anemic patients. Early diagnosis and prompt institution of treatment, reduce mortality to nil.

REFERENCES

Freitag, J. L.: Treatment of Chronic Typhoid Carriers by Cholecystectomy, Public Health Rept. U.S., 79:7, 1964.

Greisman, S. E., R. D. Hornick, and T. E. Woodward: On the Role of Endotoxin during Typhoid Fever and Tularemia in Man: III. Hyperreactivity to Endotoxin during Infection, J. Clin. Invest., 43:9, 1964.

McCrae, T.: The Symptoms of Typhoid Fever, chap. 4 in "Modern Medicine," vol. 2, "Infectious Diseases," p. 104, W. Osler and T. McCrae (Eds.), Philadelphia, Lea Bros. and Company, 1907.

Robertson, R. P., M. F. A. Wahab, and F. O. Raasch: Chloramphenicol and Ampicillin in Salmonella Enteric Fever, New Engl. J. Med., 278:171, 1968.

Stuart, B. M., and R. L. Pullen: Typhoid: Clinical Analysis of 360 Cases, Arch. Intern. Med., 78:629, 1946.

Woodward, T. E., J. E. Smadel, R. T. Parker, and C. L. Wisseman, Jr.: Treatment of Typhoid Fever with Antibiotics, Ann. N.Y. Acad. Sci., 55:1043, 1052.

150 OTHER SALMONELLA INFECTIONS
Edward W. Hook

INTRODUCTION. Since the isolation of the first member of the genus *Salmonella* from swine in 1885 by Salmon and Smith, more than 1,200 different serologic types have been identified. Although there is striking variation in the pathogenicity of the various serotypes, almost all are capable of producing human disease. The infections in man are *acute gastroenteritis, enteric* or *paratyphoid fever, bacteremia,* and *localized infections* ranging from osteomyelitis to endocarditis.

ETIOLOGY AND EPIDEMIOLOGY. The salmonellas are motile gram-negative bacilli that do not ferment lactose or sucrose but utilize glucose, maltose, and mannitol. All serotypes produce gas with the exception of S. *typhosa* and S. *gallinarum-pullorum.* These organisms are typed by immunologic methods on the basis of antigenic components in the cell body (O, or somatic antigens) and flagellar (H antigens). Specific serotyping is necessary for epidemiologic studies.

Salmonellas can be isolated from the intestinal tracts of man and many lower animals. The incidence of asymptomatic excretors of these organisms in the general population is about 0.2 percent, but the most important reservoir of infection is in domestic and wild animal species in which infection rates vary from less than 1 to more than 40 percent. An incomplete list of animals from which salmonella species have been isolated includes chickens, turkeys, ducks, pigs, cows, dogs, cats, rats, parakeets, as well as certain cold-blooded animals and insects. Animals sold as pets especially baby chicks, ducks, and turtles, may also harbor salmonella and serve as sources of infection.

Salmonella infection is almost always acquired by the oral route, usually by ingestion of contaminated food or drink. Any food product, especially those of animal origin, is a potential source of human infection. Meat or egg products obtained from animals harboring salmonellas, and food, dried or fresh milk, or water contaminated by excreta of man or animals may serve as vehicles of infection. Salmonellas may survive cooking at low temperature or food may be recontaminated after cooking by organisms from personnel or kitchen equipment.

Salmonella species may also be transmitted directly from man to man or from animals to man without the intervention of contaminated food or drink, but the latter method of spread is not common. Cross infection of this type has been shown to be responsible for a number of outbreaks of salmonellosis among patients in nurseries and hospitals. A few outbreaks apparently have been related to spread of infection by the aerial route.

Fish meal, meat meal, bone meal, and other by-products of the meat-packing industry are often contaminated with salmonella organisms. Their products are incorporated in animal and poultry feeds and apparently play an important role in the spread of infection among domestic animals.

The true incidence of salmonella infection is difficult to determine. The number of reported isolations of salmonellas from humans in the United States from 1964 to 1967 was about 20,000 isolations per year, or about 10 cases per 100,000 population. However, reported cases represent only a small proportion of the actual number of cases because bacteriologic studies are usually performed only on patients with severe or protracted diarrhea, and many outbreaks are not investigated. Although salmonella infection occurs throughout the year, the Salmonella Surveillance Unit of the National Communicable Disease Center has observed a distinct seasonal pattern with the greatest number of isolations reported from July through October for each year.

In the United States the serotypes most often responsible for human infection are S. typhimurium, S. heidelberg, S. enteritidis, S. newport, S. infantis, S. saint-paul, S. blockley, S. thompson, S. oranienburg, S. anatum, S. derby, and S. montevideo. Salmonella typhimurium is the most prevalent type throughout the world and accounts for about 30 percent of isolates from man in the United States. There is a close correlation between the species of Salmonella isolated from man and animals in any specific geographic area.

PATHOGENESIS. The course of events after salmonella organisms have gained access to the gastrointestinal tract is determined by the dose, serotype, and invasive potential of the organism, and by the resistance of the host. Multiplication of ingested organisms in the intestinal tract may be followed by symptoms of gastroenteritis. The

intestinal irritation and inflammation are produced by a true infection of the mucosa; ingestion of billions of dead organisms causes no ill effects. Bloodstream invasion may occur as a complication of gastroenteritis but usually develops without preceding intestinal symptoms. Bacteremia may be transient or prolonged, and may be accompanied by recurrent chills and fever or manifestations of paratyphoid fever. Blood-borne bacteria may localize at any site and lead to suppuration in bone, joints, meninges, pleura, or other tissues.

Studies in volunteers are limited but indicate that large numbers of viable organisms must be ingested to produce clinically apparent disease. However, a transient carrier state can be produced with doses 10 or 100 times smaller than those required to evoke symptoms of infection. The minimal infectious dose varies markedly among different serotypes.

Salmonella serotypes also show marked variation in invasive potential and capacity to produce disease. For example, S. anatum characteristically produces asymptomatic intestinal infection and only rarely invades the bloodstream. In contrast, S. choleraesuis frequently produces bacteremia and metastatic infection.

The bacterial flora of the intestine is apparently important in determining the fate of ingested salmonellas. This suggestion is based on the observation that administration of certain antibiotics to mice results in a 100,000-fold increase in susceptibility to infection with S. enteritidis. The effect of antibiotic therapy may be related to a marked diminution in number of bacteroides organisms which produce butyric and acetic acids that are lethal for salmonellas. Although salmonella enteritis has been reported as a rare complication of antimicrobial therapy in man, adequate clinical documentation of the phenomenon does not exist. Alteration in intestinal flora also has been suggested as a mechanism of the increased susceptibility of patients with previous major gastric surgery, especially gastrectomy and gastroenterostomy, to intestinal infection with salmonellas. However, reduced acidity or rapid emptying time consequent to gastric surgery also may play a role by increasing the number of viable organisms reaching the small intestine.

About one-third of patients who are hospitalized because of salmonellosis have some type of major underlying disease, such as leukemia, lymphoma, lupus erythematosus, or aplastic anemia. This may be coincidence but more often reflects a decrease in resistance to bacterial infection in general. In a few diseases there is evidence to indicate an almost specific predisposition to infection by salmonellas that exceeds susceptibility to other bacterial species. Patients with sickle-cell anemia and other sickle hemoglobinopathies are unusually susceptible to bloodstream invasion by salmonellas. In these patients there is a strong tendency for localization in bone, and salmonellas, not staphylococci, are the most common cause of osteomyelitis in patients with sickle-cell diseases. Salmonella bacteremia is also an unusually frequent complication of the acute hemolytic phase of bartonellosis.

Infants are more susceptible to salmonella infection

and remain convalescent carriers for a longer period of time than adults. The mortality rate from the disease is also higher in infants than in adults.

CLINICAL MANIFESTATIONS. Gastroenteritis. Although gastroenteritis often occurs in large epidemics among individuals who have eaten the same contaminated food, family outbreaks and sporadic cases are even more common. After an incubation period of 8 to 48 hr, there is sudden onset of colicky abdominal pain and loose, watery diarrhea, occasionally with mucus or blood. Nausea and vomiting are frequent but are rarely severe or protracted. Fever of 101 to 102°F is common, and there may be an initial chill. Symptoms usually subside promptly within 2 to 5 days and recovery is uneventful. However, illness is occasionally more protracted, with persistence of diarrhea and low-grade fever for 10 to 14 days. Fatalities rarely exceed 1 percent of the affected population and are limited almost entirely to infants, the aged, and debilitated patients.

The causative organism can often be isolated from the suspected food and from feces during the acute illness. Stool cultures usually become negative for salmonellas within 1 to 4 weeks, but occasional patients continue to excrete organisms for months. The blood leukocyte count is usually normal.

Enteric or Paratyphoid Fever. Certain species can produce an illness which is clinically indistinguishable from typhoid fever, i.e., a prolonged febrile illness with rose spots, splenomegaly, leukopenia, gastrointestinal symptoms, and positive blood and stool cultures (Chap. 149). The organisms most likely to produce this picture are S. *paratyphi A*, S. *paratyphi B* (S. *schottmuelleri*), and S. *choleraesuis* (S. *suipestifer*). Occasionally a typical attack of food poisoning is followed in a few days by manifestations of paratyphoid fever. Generally, paratyphoid fevers tend to be milder than S. *typhosa* infections, but differentiation on clinical grounds alone is not possible in the individual case. Recovery may be followed by continued excretion of the causative organism in the stools for several months, but the chronic carrier state is less frequent than in typhoid fever.

Bacteremia. Salmonella species may produce a syndrome characterized primarily by prolonged fever and positive blood cultures. Although symptoms of gastroenteritis can precede bacteremia, they are usually lacking, and most cases arise sporadically. In many instances, the only manifestations are prolonged fever, sometimes low-grade, but often spiking and accompanied by repeated rigors, sweats, aching, anorexia, and weight loss. The characteristic features of typhoid and paratyphoid fever, such as rose spots, persistent leukopenia, and sustained fever, are absent. Stool cultures are usually negative. In contrast to the constant bacteremia of typhoid fever, discharge of organisms into the bloodstream is intermittent, and repeated blood cultures are often required to demonstrate the causative organism. At some time in the course of the illness, localizing signs of infection appear in about one-fourth of the cases. Pulmonary infection in the form of bronchopneumonia or abscess, pleurisy, empyema, pericarditis, endocarditis, pyelonephritis,

meningitis, osteomyelitis, and arthritis are relatively common. The blood leukocyte count is usually normal, but with the development of focal lesions, polymorphonuclear leukocytosis as high as 20,000 to 25,000 cells per cu mm occurs. Salmonella bacteremia can be a very puzzling disorder, especially before localization takes place, and should be considered in cases of fever of unknown origin.

Local Pyogenic Infections. Salmonella organisms can produce abscesses in almost any anatomic site, and these can occur independently of previous symptoms of gastroenteritis or other systemic illness, or as complications of bacteremias. There is nothing characteristic about the suppurative lesions, and the correct etiologic diagnosis is rarely made on the basis of clinical findings alone. There is a strong tendency for salmonellas to localize in tissues that are the site of preexisting disease. Localization has been described in aneurysms, bone adjacent to aortic aneurysms, hematomas, and many different tumors, including hypernephroma, ovarian cyst, and pheochromocytoma. Meningeal localization of infection is common in newborns and infants, and occasional small outbreaks of salmonella infection in nurseries have consisted almost entirely of meningitis.

DIAGNOSIS. Febrile gastroenteritis produced by presumed viral agents and shigellosis can be distinguished from salmonella gastroenteritis only by appropriate stool cultures, especially in sporadic cases. Staphylococcal food poisoning usually is not associated with fever, and vomiting is a more prominent feature than in most salmonella infections. Systemic manifestations are usually absent in patients with gastroenteritis caused by *Clostridium welchii*. Many toxic agents and drugs can produce diarrhea, nausea, and abdominal pain, but fever is rarely a feature of these disorders, and the diagnosis depends upon a history of exposure or ingestion.

The diagnosis of paratyphoid fever or salmonella bacteremia depends upon isolation of the causative organism. Agglutination tests with acute and convalescent sera as performed in the usual clinical laboratory are not very helpful.

TREATMENT. The treatment of salmonella gastroenteritis is supportive. Dehydration should be corrected by parenteral administration of fluids and electrolytes. Abdominal cramps and diarrhea can be alleviated by small doses of morphine or paregoric and often are much improved if the patient takes nothing by mouth for 8 to 12 hr. There is no convincing evidence that antimicrobial drugs modify the course of salmonella gastroenteritis.

Chloramphenicol in doses of 3 Gm daily in adults is the antibiotic of choice in systemic infections including salmonella bacteremia, metastatic infection, and paratyphoid fever. Response is characteristically slow, and the temperature rarely returns to normal until 3 to 4 days after beginning therapy. Therapy should be continued for at least 2 weeks, but in certain infections, such as osteomyelitis or meningitis, the duration may have to be extended.

Ampicillin is also effective in systemic infections caused by salmonella strains sensitive to the action of this antibiotic. However, a significant proportion of salmonella strains are highly resistant in vitro to ampicillin. For this reason, ampicillin should not be used in therapy of serious infections unless it is known that the causative organism is sensitive. The tetracycline derivatives have sometimes appeared to exert a beneficial effect, but streptomycin, polymyxin, neomycin, kanamycin, and the sulfonamides are generally ineffective.

Antimicrobial therapy is usually not indicated in convalescent or asymptomatic transient carriers of salmonella species. The carrier state will spontaneously cease in 1 to 3 months in the vast majority of individuals.

The chronic carrier state with localization of infection in the gallbladder and positive stool cultures for a period of time exceeding 1 year is rarely caused by salmonella serotypes other than *S. typhosa* and *S. paratyphi A* and *B*. The therapy of the chronic carrier is discussed in Chap. 149.

Surgically accessible suppurative lesions should be drained.

REFERENCES

Bennett, I. L., Jr., and E. W. Hook: Some Aspects of Salmonellosis, Ann. Rev. Med., 10:1, 1959.

Black, P. H., L. J. Kunz, and M. N. Swartz: Salmonellosis—A Review of Some Unusual Aspects, New Engl. J. Med., 262:811, 864, 921, 1960.

Gezon, H. M.: Salmonellosis, Disease-a-Month, July, 1959.

Hook, E. W.: Salmonellosis: Certain Factors Influencing the Interaction of Salmonella and the Human Host, Bull. N.Y. Acad. Med., 37:499, 1961.

Proceedings of the National Conference on Salmonellosis, March 11–13, 1964: Washington, D.C., Public Health Service Publ. No. 1262, 1965.

Prost, E., and H. Riemann: Food-borne Salmonellosis, Ann. Rev. Microbiol. 21:495, 1967.

Robertson, R. P., M. F. A. Wahab, and F. O. Raasch: Chloramphenicol and Ampicillin in Salmonella Enteric Fever, New Engl. J. Med., 278:171, 1968.

van Oye, E. (Ed.): "The World Problem of Salmonellosis," The Hague, Dr. W. Junk Publishers, 1964.

151   SHIGELLOSIS (Bacillary Dysentery)

Harry N. Beaty and Robert G. Petersdorf

DEFINITION. *Shigellosis* is an acute, self-limited, infectious disease of man which is restricted to the intestinal tract and is characterized by diarrhea, fever, and abdominal pain. The disease is usually called *bacillary dysentery*, but the term *shigellosis* is preferred.

ETIOLOGY. The genus *Shigella* includes a group of more or less closely related species which are members of the family *Enterobacteriaceae*. Shigella organisms are nonmotile, nonencapsulated, slender, gram-negative rods which may appear as coccobacilli on initial isolation.

They are aerobes or facultative anaerobes and grow best at 37°C. Nutritional requirements are relatively simple, and the ability of these organisms to grow in the presence of bile salts is used in devising selective media which facilitate their isolation from the intestinal tract. Fermentation of carbohydrates differs according to the species, but all strains produce acid in glucose and either fail to ferment lactose or do so only slowly. The classification of shigellas depends upon a combination of biochemical and antigenic characteristics. The most important species from a clinical viewpoint are *Shigella dysenteriae* (*S. shigae*), *S. flexneri*, (*S. paradysenteriae*), *S. boydii* and *S. sonnei*. Antigenically, the shigellas are extremely complex. Strains of *S. sonnei* are fairly homogeneous, but the other groups contain from 6 to 11 different types which are identified with specific antigens. There is significant serologic overlap between species, and some strains share group antigens with other enteric bacilli.

The somatic antigen of the shigellas is an endotoxin which is chemically and biologically similar to the endotoxins of other gram-negative bacilli. *Shigella dysenteriae* type 1 (Shiga bacillus) also produces an exotoxin which causes neurologic abnormalities when injected into experimental animals. The role of this neurotoxin in the pathogenesis of shigellosis is unknown, and there is no evidence that other species of shigella produce a similar substance.

EPIDEMIOLOGY. The principal habitat of the shigellas is the gastrointestinal tract of higher primates. However, on rare occasions dogs and other mammals have been found to excrete organisms. Natural disease is limited almost entirely to man, and the convalescent or asymptomatic carrier is the only recognized reservoir. Infection is transmitted predominantly by contact with inanimate objects which are contaminated with fecal material containing dysentery bacilli. Waterborne outbreaks are uncommon, but food is readily contaminated by careless personnel or flies which have fed upon infected human feces.

Bacillary dysentery is worldwide in distribution, and is particularly common in countries where effective sanitation is lacking. There are between 10,000 and 15,000 cases reported in the United States each year, but this probably represents only a small fraction of the total number. The common organisms encountered in this country are *S. flexneri* and *S. sonnei*; *S. dysenteriae* type 1 is rarely the cause of infection outside Asia. Shigellosis is extremely rare during the first month of life, but is very common in children over six months of age. In adults, clinical illness occurs in about 50 percent of persons infected. Major epidemics of bacillary dysentery are rare nowadays, but in closed populations, such as mental institutions, jails, and orphanages, outbreaks develop over a period of several weeks. Poor sanitation, low standards of personal hygiene, crowded conditions, and a high proportion of children in a population favor spread of the infection. For the most part, shigella species do not persist in the stool for more than a few days, possibly because they are susceptible to the action of bacteriophage. Organisms may be excreted intermittently during convalescence, but the carrier state rarely persists longer than 3 months.

The role of immunity in the recovery from clinical infection or protection against reinfection is not known. Humoral antibodies appear in response to infection, but there is no evidence that they influence the course of the disease. Coproantibodies are also present, but their significance is unknown. Repeated attacks of bacillary dysentery are not uncommon, but persons living in endemic areas seem to develop immunity to recurrent episodes of clinical disease. Polyvalent shigella vaccines protect mice against intraperitoneal infection, but their effectiveness in man has not been established.

PATHOGENESIS AND PATHOLOGY. The pathogenesis of shigellosis is poorly understood, in part because it is difficult to produce the infection in laboratory animals. Studies in volunteers have shown that it is necessary to ingest very large numbers of bacilli to establish infection in man. Organisms presumably multiply in the lower gastrointestinal tract, where they produce an inflammatory reaction which usually involves the entire colon and may extend into the terminal ileum. The mucosa becomes uniformly inflamed and edematous and often is covered by a fibrinous exudate. Necrosis of the mucosa produces shallow ulcers which bleed readily. Microscopic examination shows that the submucosa and muscularis are infiltrated with bacteria and polymorphonuclear leukocytes. Ulcers are sharply outlined and are not undermined. The mechanisms responsible for these pathologic alterations are unclear. Shigella endotoxin is often implicated, but a variety of enteric bacteria elaborate endotoxins without producing disease.

The systemic manifestations of bacillary dysentery are primarily due to the fluid and electrolyte disturbances consequent to the diarrhea. Bacteremia in shigellosis is rare, and fever is often attributed to "toxins" which presumably are absorbed from the intestinal tract.

CLINICAL MANIFESTATIONS. Shigella infections are characterized by fever, abdominal pain, and diarrhea. However, mild diarrhea alone or asymptomatic infection occurs in a significant proportion of individuals infected. The incubation period is usually 24 to 48 hr, and the first symptom is often colicky abdominal pain, which is followed within an hour by high fever and diarrhea, often accompanied by tenesmus. Other symptoms include nausea, vomiting, headache, convulsions in children, and myalgia. The stools are liquid, greenish in color, contain shreds of mucus, and in 20 to 30 percent of cases contain various amounts of gross blood. Depending upon the severity of diarrhea and the height of fever, patients may become profoundly dehydrated, and circulatory collapse can occur. Lower abdominal tenderness and hyperactive bowel sounds are common, but there is no peritoneal irritation. Splenomegaly has been reported, but is rare. Sigmoidoscopic examination reveals diffuse mucosal inflammation, often with multiple ulcerations.

LABORATORY FINDINGS. Blood leukocyte counts usually range between 5,000 and 15,000 per cu mm, and anemia is uncommon. Microscopic examination of the stool re-

veals shreds of mucus, erythrocytes, and many polymorphonuclear leukocytes. Stool culture is positive, but blood cultures rarely are. Electrolyte abnormalities depend upon the degree of vomiting and diarrhea.

COURSE. Shigellosis is generally a self-limited disease, and patients usually become afebrile within 2 to 3 days. Diarrhea may continue a few days longer, but within a week most patients have recovered and no longer excrete organisms in their stool. In about 10 percent of cases a clinical or bacterologic relapse occurs unless antibiotics are given. In the United States, the overall mortality rate associated with bacillary dysentery is less than 0.1 percent. However, among young children and elderly patients, the illness is often more severe and the prognosis poorer. *Shigella dysenteriae* produces particularly severe infections, and mortality rates of 25 to 50 percent have been recorded in epidemics produced by this species.

Complications of *Shigella* infections are encountered infrequently. Chronic bacillary dysentery occurs in the tropics, particularly after *S. dysenteriae* infections, but is rare in this country. Perforation of the colon is uncommon. Hematogenous dissemination of the shigellas is also rare, but these organisms have been recovered from metastatic foci of infection such as abscesses or meningitis. In some series, bacteremia due to other gram-negative bacilli has been seen in association with shigellosis. An acute, nonsuppurative arthritis involving large, weight-bearing joints, may occur during convalescence, but in patients given chemotherapy this complication is unusual. Conjunctivitis, iritis, and peripheral neuropathy accompany bacillary dysentery on rare occasions.

DIAGNOSIS. A definitive diagnosis of shigellosis can only be established when pathogenic members of the genus *Shigella* are isolated from cultures. These organisms survive for only a short time in feces, and fresh stool specimens or rectal swabs should be cultured promptly. Recovery of the shigellas is facilitated if saline suspensions of the material to be cultured are streaked directly onto selective media such as SS agar or desoxycholate citrate agar. Selenite broth is of limited usefulness in the isolation of the shigellas. Agglutinating antibodies can be detected in the serum of a majority of patients with positive cultures, but serologic tests are of little value in establishing the diagnosis of shigellosis. Immunofluorescent techniques have been developed, however, which allow rapid detection of organisms in the stool.

Shigella infection should be considered in every febrile illness associated with diarrhea. Occasionally, children with infections such as tonsillitis or otitis have diarrhea, but the major differential diagnosis of shigellosis includes viral enteritis, amebic dysentery (Chap. 240), salmonellosis (Chap. 150), and staphylococcal food poisoning (Chap. 139). In viral infections, fever is uncommon, and the stool does not contain gross blood or pus. The onset of amebic colitis is gradual, and the diarrhea is relatively mild. Staphylococcal food poisoning is associated with more nausea and vomiting, and usually is not associated with fever. Salmonella infections can be differentiated with certainty only by bacteriologic studies.

TREATMENT. The treatment of shigellosis is primarily supportive, and the major goal is correction of fluid and electrolyte abnormalities. Antibiotics are of secondary importance and are used chiefly to shorten the duration of illness and to prevent relapse. Sulfonamides formerly were effective in the treatment of bacillary dysentery, but in 1968, almost two-thirds of shigellas isolated are resistant to these drugs. More significantly, since 1955, epidemics of shigellosis in various parts of the world, including the United States, have been caused by organisms resistant to multiple antibiotics. The molecular basis for multiple drug resistance involves the episomal transfer of drug resistance determinants between enteric bacilli.

Although some strains of shigella resistant to ampicillin and tetracycline have been identified, these drugs are preferred for the treatment of bacillary dysentery, and in adults should be given in dosage of 2.0 Gm per day. Chloramphenicol is also likely to be effective, but should be given only in severe cases where other agents cannot be used. Kanamycin, neomycin, and streptomycin are often administered orally for the treatment of shigel-losis, but absorbable agents are probably more effective.

PREVENTION. The most important prophylactic measures are the maintenance of proper sanitation and adequate sewage disposal. The detection and elimination of carriers is difficult and rarely practical. Methods for increasing resistance to infection have not been developed.

REFERENCES

Farrar, W. E., and L. C. Dekle: Transferable Antibiotic Resistance Associated with an Outbreak of Shigellosis, Ann. Intern. Med., 67:1208, 1967.

Garfinkel, B. T., G. M. Martin, J. Watt, F. J. Payne, R. P. Mason, and A. V. Hardy: Antibiotics in Acute Bacillary Dysentery: Observations in 1,408 Cases with Positive Cultures, J.A.M.A., 151:1157, 1953.

Haltalin, K. C., J. D. Nelson, L. U. Hinton, R. W. Kusmiesz, and B. S. Sladoje: Comparison of Orally Absorbable and Nonabsorbable Antibiotics in Shigellosis, J. Pediat., 72:708, 1968.

Morgan, H. R.: The Enteric Bacteria, p. 634 in "Bacterial and Mycotic Infections of Man," 4th ed., Philadelphia, J. B. Lippincott Company, 1965.

Section 6

Diseases Caused by Other Gram-negative Bacilli

152 HEMOPHILUS INFECTIONS
Louis Weinstein

The genus *Hemophilus* consists of nonmotile, gram-negative rods or coccobacilli which require specific growth factors (X and V) for multiplication. The organisms of importance in human disease are *H. influenzae*, *H. pertussis*, *H. ducreyi*, the Koch-Weeks bacillus, and *Moraxella lacunata*. Two other species are found in the pharynges of normal individuals and, rarely, may produce pharyngitis (*H. hemolyticus*) or endocarditis (*H. para-influenzae*). The site invaded most frequently is the respiratory tract, and the organisms responsible for the bulk of infections are *H. influenzae* and *H. pertussis*.

HEMOPHILUS INFLUENZA INFECTIONS

Hemophilus influenzae produces a wide variety of diseases in many organ systems. The organism was first isolated by Pfeiffer during a pandemic of influenza in 1890, and was thought to be the causative agent of this disease. During the 1918 influenza pandemic, extensive bacteriologic investigations revealed a high incidence of *H. influenzae* in the nasopharynges and lungs of patients in many parts of the world.

ETIOLOGY. *Hemophilus influenzae* is a gram-negative, nonsporulating, pleomorphic rod. In exudates, the organisms are usually predominantly coccobacillary and can be mistaken for pneumococci or meningococci. Some strains demonstrate bipolar staining, and bacillary forms that vary from short rods to long filamentous ones occur.

Hemophilus influenzae grows well on chocolate agar and Levinthal's medium, which has the advantage of being transparent. On Levinthal's agar, typical colonies are iridescent when viewed by obliquely transmitted light when they are about 4 to 6 hr old; this property disappears after 24 hr.

Although it had been thought that strains without capsules were nonpathogenic, these strains have been implicated in infections of the respiratory tract. On the basis of specific capsular polysaccharides, *H. influenzae* may be classified into six types. Type B produces about 95 percent of human infections.

EPIDEMIOLOGY. *Hemophilus influenzae* infects only man. It is not ordinarily invasive for any of the smaller animals, although monkeys can be infected experimentally.

The incidence of *H. influenzae* infections is greatest in the winter and early spring. Nose and throat cultures during these seasons reveal the organisms of many asymptomatic individuals. Penicillin therapy increases the incidence of positive throat cultures in a population.

Children in the first 2 months of life have a high level of passively transferred bactericidal antibody. Between the ages of two months and three years, most children show little antibody, but with aging, the levels increase.

PATHOLOGY. The characteristic tissue response to *H. influenzae* is acute suppurative inflammation. Infections of the larynx, trachea, and bronchial tree are characterized by edema of the mucosa and thick exudate, and invasion of the lungs results in a bronchopneumonia. Particularly in young children, a severe, diffuse bronchiolitis can occur. In influenzal meningitis, the vertex of the brain is covered with thick, greenish-yellow exudate.

Microscopic examination of the lesions produced by *H. influenzae* reveals an exudate consisting primarily of polymorphonuclear leukocytes and large numbers of organisms enmeshed in fibrin.

CLINICAL MANIFESTATIONS. Severe *H. influenzae* infections are usually accompanied by high fever, usually without rigors, and generalized malaise. In milder infections, fever is inconstant. The commonest diseases produced by *H. influenzae* are pharyngitis, epiglottitis, laryngotracheitis, pneumonia, bronchitis and bronchiolitis, otitis media, and meningitis. The symptoms and signs of influenzal invasion of the respiratory tract or meninges are similar to those of infection of these areas by other organisms, and differential etiologic diagnosis depends upon epidemiologic background, the age of the patient, and demonstration of the causative agent.

Pharyngitis. *Hemophilus influenzae* is a relatively common cause of pharyngitis in children, and acute influenzal pharyngitis is also observed in adults, where it often occurs as a complication of the chemotherapy of other infections. Examination of the throat usually reveals only marked redness and injection. Very rarely, patches of soft yellow exudate may be present. The pharyngitis tends to persist for many days unless properly treated. Dissociation between the appearance of the pharynx and the intensity of local discomfort is common in adults. The pharyngeal mucosa frequently appears normal or shows only slight diffuse redness at the same time that pain is so severe that swallowing of saliva is difficult and eating impossible.

Epiglottitis. Disease of the upper part of the respiratory tract produced by *H. influenzae* is sometimes limited to the epiglottis, which becomes reddened, swollen, and stiff. Discomfort in the hypopharynx and "croupy" breathing may progress to a point at which tracheotomy becomes necessary. This disease is rare in adults.

Laryngotracheobronchitis. The entire laryngotracheobronchial tree may be the site of infection, with resulting rapidly progressive obstruction of the airway. "Croupy" cough is accompanied by increasing signs of respiratory embarrassment, and tracheotomy is sometimes necessary. Influenzal laryngotracheitis is very rare in adults. The disease can lead to death within 18 to 24 hr.

Pneumonia. Primary pneumonia due to *H. influenzae*, with rare exceptions, is a disease of children. In the adult, it is usually secondary to viral influenza, measles, or bacterial pneumonitis. It may complicate rubeola or pertussis in the young. Bacteremia occurs in approximately one-third of the cases.

Bronchitis and Bronchiolitis. Severe, diffuse bronchiolitis characterized by persistent nonproductive cough, wheezing, and dyspnea occurs in children. Physical examination usually reveals lowering and fixation of the diaphragm, prolonged expirations, and typically asthmatic breathing. Roentgenographic examination of the chest reveals increased radiolucence, and flattening of the diaphragm consistent with emphysema. This is an extremely serious illness and unless promptly recognized and treated may be rapidly fatal.

The factor of infection contributes significantly to the clinical manifestations and progressive deterioration in established chronic bronchitis or "senile emphysema" in adults. Among the bacteria involved, the pneumococcus and *H. influenzae* are the commonest. *Hemophilus influenzae* has been isolated from the respiratory tracts of 80 to 90 percent of patients in some studies.

Otitis Media. *Hemophilus influenzae* is a common cause of suppurative otitis media in children; the infection is uncommon in adults. In some instances, middle ear disease due to this species is indistinguishable from that produced by *Staphylococcus aureus*, *Diplococcus pneumoniae* or group A *Streptococcus pyogenes*. In many cases, however, the appearance is that of serous otitis media and leads to a misdiagnosis of nonbacterial disease. Aspiration of fluid from the middle ear and culture may be necessary to establish the diagnosis of the presence of *H. influenzae* and to dictate appropriate chemotherapy.

Meningitis. The influenza bacillus is the commonest cause of meningitis between the ages of six months and two years and is frequent in later childhood. In adults, it may follow operation on or injury to the head. In rare instances, *H. influenzae* may be responsible for acute meningitis in otherwise healthy adults of any age. Next to pneumococcus, *H. influenzae* is the organism most likely to cause recurrent bacterial meningitis. Of these cases, 95 percent are produced by type B organisms, a few by type A, and a rare one by nonencapsulated strains. About two-thirds of the patients have a preceding infection of the upper respiratory tract, and about one-third have bronchopneumonia. Signs of meningeal irritation are usually prominent, except in very young babies in whom bulging of the fontanels may be the only sign. The diagnosis should be suspected because of the age of the patient and the frequent prodrome of respiratory infection.

Other Diseases. Subacute and acute bacterial endocarditis may be produced by *H. influenzae*, although more infections of the heart valves have been due to *H. parainfluenzae*. The influenza bacillus is a rare cause of suppurative pericarditis. In the winter, acute conjunctivitis may be due to *H. influenzae*. Although no clinical features distinguish it from "pink eye" produced by the Koch-Weeks bacillus, epidemics of conjunctivitis due to this organism are most common in the summer. Although *H. influenzae* and the Koch-Weeks bacillus are antigenically related, they are distinct species. *Moraxella lacunata* is also an occasional cause of acute purulent conjunctivitis. Acute pyogenic arthritis due to *H. influenzae* has been reported. Among other diseases produced by this organism are cystitis, pyelonephritis, osteomyelitis, paranasal sinusitis, appendicitis, cellulitis, and infections of the liver, genital tract, and skin.

LABORATORY FINDINGS. As a rule, infections due to *H. influenzae* are accompanied by polymorphonuclear leukocytosis ranging from 15,000 to 30,000 per cu mm. In young children with severe disease, leukopenia (2,000 to 3,000 leukocytes per cu mm) with a deficiency of polymorphonuclear leukocytes can occur. Bacteremia is rare in influenzal infections of the respiratory tract but is demonstrable in about 50 percent of cases of meningitis.

COURSE AND COMPLICATIONS. The course of *H. influenzae* infections is determined by the location of the disease. Epiglottitis, laryngotracheobronchitis, bronchiolitis, or pneumonia may be fulminating. Some of these patients die because of uncontrolled infection, but in many, the cause of death is obstruction of the airway, which cannot always be relieved by surgical methods, because impediment to flow of air is most marked in the smaller radicles of the bronchial tree. Virtually 100 percent of untreated cases of influenzal meningitis terminate fatally. Internal and external hydrocephalus, brain abscess, subdural empyema, diffuse cortical necrosis, and shock are possible complications. With specific therapy, the incidence of complications is sharply reduced. However, if subdural aspiration is carried out routinely in children with influenzal meningitis which is responding to antibiotics, sterile fluid is demonstrable in about half the cases. Neurologic disturbances from subdural effusions are uncommon. Epileptiform seizures can occur while the disease is responding favorably to chemotherapy.

TREATMENT. *H. influenzae* is susceptible in vitro to several antimicrobial agents including streptomycin, the tetracyclines, chloramphenicol, and the sulfonamides. Most strains are inhibited by 0.6 μg penicillin G or less per ml. All appear to be highly sensitive to ampicillin, a drug which has simplified greatly the management of disease produced by this organism. The dose of ampicillin in *H. influenzae* meningitis is 100 to 200 mg/kg/day, given parenterally in equal sized and spaced quantities; the larger dose is preferred. The management of otitis media or pharyngitis often requires no more than 100 to 150 mg/kg/day given by mouth. For adults respiratory infections, 2 to 4 Gm per day orally for 7 to 10 days usually suffices. Ampicillin therapy may fail in influenzal meningitis when complications, e.g., subdural empyema, supervene. Although the *H. influenzae* organism has been resistant to ampicillin only rarely, continued surveillance of this problem is indicated because of the increasing frequency with which other gram-negative bacilli resistant to this agent are being recovered. Despite the fact that practically all strains of *H. influenzae* are sensitive to very small quantities of penicillin G, the therapeutic effects of this antibiotic are poor, and it must not be used as the sole agent for the treatment of meningitis due to this organism. The results with the tetracyclines are too variable to recommend their use. An alternate regimen is chloramphenicol (50 mg per kg in equal sized and spaced doses per day) intramuscularly plus sulfisoxazole or sulfadiazine (100 mg/kg/day). Regardless of the drug employed, *H. influenzae* meningitis should be treated for 2 weeks. Chloramphenicol alone or a tetracycline is usually sufficient to treat upper respiratory tract infections, pneumonia or otitis media in penicillin-sensitive children or adults allergic to penicillin.

PERTUSSIS

Whooping cough affects about 85 percent of all unimmunized children. It is characterized by an inflammation of the entire respiratory tract which produces paroxysmal cough and the typical inspiratory stridor, or "whoop."

ETIOLOGY. The causative agent is *Hemophilus pertussis* (also called *Bordatella pertussis*), a short or ovoid gram-negative, nonmotile, nonsporulating, facultatively anaerobic bacillus. Bipolar staining is frequent, and encapsulation can be demonstrated by special stains.

The pertussis bacillus requires both the X and V factors for growth, especially for initial isolation, and multiplies best on Bordet-Gengou medium. The organism contains two antigens, the heat-stable O, common to all strains, and the heat-labile specific agglutinogens K (1,2,3,4,5). All strains contain two or more of these antigens. This is of clinical importance because, in some areas of the world, the infecting strain has been found to have different K agglutinogens than those present in the vaccine being used to prevent the disease, resulting in failure of immunization.

Other infectious agents rarely produce the syndrome of whooping cough. Among these are *Bordetella parapertussis, B. bronchisepticus,* and adenovirus type 12, which is responsible for a contagious disease featured by paroxysmal coughing, whooping, lymphocytosis, and eosinophilia.

EPIDEMIOLOGY. Pertussis is worldwide. Where the disease has not been present for several years, it tends to assume epidemic proportions when it reappears. In some locations, the disease is most common during the winter, and in others it is seen with greatest frequency in the late summer and fall. The index of contagion is 80 to 100 percent; about 200,000 cases occur in the United States each year.

Approximately 40 percent of cases of pertussis occur in the first 2 years of life; the same number is observed between the ages of two and five. At least 50 percent of all children have had whooping cough before they reach the age of five and 75 percent by the age of seventeen.

Pertussis is spread by droplets from the respiratory tract. Rarely, the organisms may be transmitted by fomites. Infectivity during the incubation period is questionable; the disease is most contagious during the catarrhal stage. Healthy carriers play no role in dissemination, but mild or missed cases are of great importance.

PATHOLOGY. The initial lesion in whooping cough is hyperplasia of the peribronchial and tracheobronchial lymphoid tissue. The bronchi, trachea, larynx, and nasopharynx are then involved in a necrotizing inflammatory reaction. The organisms are present in large numbers between the cilia of the trachea, and desquamation of the alveolar epithelium occurs.

CLINICAL MANIFESTATIONS. The incubation period of whooping cough averages 12 to 15 days, although it can be as long as 20 days. The first clinical manifestations are slight nasal discharge, conjunctivitis, and mild cough without fever. This catarrhal stage lasts for 7 to 14 days.

The paroxysmal phase of pertussis follows and is characterized by paroxysms of coughing ending in a loud, crowing inspiratory noise (the whoop), the expulsion of varying quantities of thick, mucoid sputum from the respiratory tract, and vomiting. Episodes of cough may be as few as 1 or 2 or as many as 40 to 50 per day. Children under the age of six months frequently do not whoop. The mere presence of a whoop is in itself not diagnostic of pertussis. Rarely, the paroxysms of coughing are replaced completely by sneezing.

Fever does not occur in the paroxysmal phase unless complications are present. Soreness over the trachea and main bronchi is common. Spasm, ulcer, or edema of the glottis sometimes occurs. In cases with severe vomiting and inability to retain food, serious inanition, wasting, and tetany may appear.

There is a bleeding tendency in pertussis. Hemoptysis, epistaxis, purpura, and subconjunctival or intestinal hemorrhages occur but are usually of little clinical significance. The mechanism of bleeding is not known.

Physical examination in pertussis is often entirely normal, but there may be injection of the blood vessels of the nose and pharynx. Although there are usually no abnormal findings in the lungs, fine, crackling, "sticky" râles are sometimes present. There are ulcers of the frenum of the tongue in about 20 percent of cases; these occur only when the lower central incisor teeth are present.

The paroxysmal stage of pertussis usually lasts from 1 to 6 weeks. When coughing persists beyond 6 weeks, it is usually due to the development of a so-called "habit whoop," not to continuation of the disease.

LABORATORY FINDINGS. The total peripheral leukocyte count may be over 100,000 cells per cu mm, and mature lymphocytes may constitute 90 percent of the cells. This helps to distinguish the blood picture from that of acute leukemia but not from acute lymphocytosis. The lymphocytosis appears to be induced by a constituent of the organism; most of the cells are released from lymphoid tissue, including the thymus. Blood cultures are sterile. Cultures of the upper part of the nasopharynx reveal *H. pertussis;* the incidence of positive isolations varies with the stage of the disease. X-ray of the lungs in the uncomplicated case usually reveals only hilar lymphadenopathy and increase in the density of the bronchovascular markings.

COMPLICATIONS. Bronchopneumonia occurs in from 1 to 10 percent of cases; the organisms most frequently involved are the beta-hemolytic streptococcus, *Diplococcus pneumoniae, Staphylococcus aureus, H. influenzae,* and *H. pertussis.* When pneumonitis appears during the course of chemotherapy, the bacteria most often responsible are *Escherichia coli, Proteus* strains, *Aerobacter aerogenes,* or *Pseudomonas aeruginosa.* Another important complication is atelectasis; small areas of collapse are an almost constant finding, but major portions or a whole lung may be involved. Pneumothorax is rare.

The severe coughing of pertussis can lead to several complications. Hemorrhage may appear in the anterior chamber of the eye or in the retina. Detachment of the retina and blindness develop in rare cases. Prolapse of the rectum and inguinal or umbilical hernias have been noted.

Nervous system manifestations are not rare in pertussis. The commonest is convulsions; they often come with the sudden fever of secondary bacterial infection. Other causes of seizures are encephalopathy (1 to 14 percent of cases), multiple petechial or gross hemorrhages of the brain, and cerebral hypoxia due to the combined effect of anoxic anoxia and venous stasis. The encephalopathy is characterized by an increase in the protein and cell content of the spinal fluid. Its etiology is unknown. Hyperreflexia, nuchal rigidity, cranial nerve palsies, areflexia, extensor plantar responses, flaccid hemiplegia, spasticity of the extremities, opisthotonos, difficulty in speaking, twitching, papilledema, nystagmus, blindness, strabismus, and dysphagia can all occur. Some of the more important residua are mental retardation, recurrent convulsions, personality disorders, amnesia, aphasia, diffuse cerebral atrophy, chorea, and athetosis.

DIAGNOSIS. The diagnosis of pertussis can frequently be made on clinical grounds alone. A known contact is helpful, but the appearance of paroxysms of typical coughing and whooping after a short period of upper respiratory symptoms is strongly suggestive. In babies under the age of six months there is usually only paroxysmal coughing, without the characteristic whoop.

An increased lymphocyte count is characteristic.

Isolation of *H. pertussis* from the respiratory tract establishes the diagnosis. Using cough plates and nasopharyngeal swabs, positive cultures can be obtained in 90 percent of patients in the catarrhal stage of the disease. The incidence of positive cultures is lower after paroxysmal coughing appears, and decreases with the duration of symptoms. Serologic studies are of little or no help in establishing the presence of pertussis.

PREVENTION. Active immunization is effective in preventing pertussis in the majority of individuals, and may be started at the age of three months; both antibody production and protection against invasion by *H. pertussis* result. If the procedure is carried out at this early age, a "booster" injection should be administered at the end of the first year of life and again just before the child starts to school. Although it is not commonly practiced, passive immunity can be conferred on the newborn child by active immunization of the mother beginning in the sixth or seventh month of pregnancy. Vaccine should not be given in the presence of the active disease; not only is it useless, but it may provoke serious neurologic reactions. There is evidence that the administration of "quadruple" vaccine—poliomyelitis virus, tetanus and diphtheria toxoid, and *H. pertussis*—leads to some degree of suppression of the response to the pertussis bacillus. For this reason, when poliomyelitis vaccine (formalinized) is used, it should be given separately from the "triple" vaccine.

In children who have been exposed to pertussis but have not been actively immunized, passive protection may be given by the injection of 20 to 30 ml human hyperimmune pertussis antiserum, or 2 ml immune γ-globulin as soon as possible after exposure and again 1 week later. This type of prophylaxis is 75 to 85 percent effective. The use of γ-globulin is preferable because hyperimmune serum has been associated with the subsequent development of infectious hepatitis.

TREATMENT. Although most of the antimicrobial drugs have been employed in the treatment of pertussis, there is no incontrovertible evidence that they are beneficial. Chlortetracycline, chloramphenicol, oxytetracycline, and erythromycin have been used, but the results obtained in controlled studies are not convincing.

There are few controlled studies of serum therapy in whooping cough, but in many clinics it is the practice to administer human hyperimmune serum (20 ml every 48 hr for three doses), or immune γ-globulin (2 ml every 48 hr for three doses) to all children with pertussis under the age of two years.

Most important in therapy is repair of the water and salt loss which follows severe and frequent vomiting. Prompt refeeding is necessary in order to maintain or gain weight.

Early detection and treatment of complications is one of the most important factors in the reduction of mortality in pertussis. The prompt recognition of secondary bacterial infections of the lungs or middle ear and therapy with a properly selected antibiotic agent lead to cure in practically all cases. When atelectasis occurs, correction by tracheal catheter suction or bronchoscopy may be lifesaving. Little can be done to influence the course or outcome of such complications as gross cerebral hemorrhage or encephalopathy.

Proper management of whooping cough has made the outlook for complete recovery excellent.

REFERENCES

Hemophilus Influenzae

Baty, J., and M. Kriedberg: Acute Laryngotracheobronchitis, Med. Clinics N. Am., 37:1279, 1952.

Collier, A. M., J. D. Connor, and W. L. Nykan: Systemic Infection with Hemophilus Influenzae in Very Young Infants, J. Pediat., 70:539, 1967.

Feingold, M., and S. S. Gellis: Cellulitis Due to Hemophilus Influenzae Type B, New Engl. J. Med., 272:788, 1965.

Goldstein, E., A. K. Daly, and C. Seamans: Haemophilus Influenzae as a Cause of Adult Penumonia, Ann. Intern. Med., 66:35, 1967.

Holdaway, M. D., and D. C. Turk: Capsulated Haemophilus Influenzae and Respiratory-tract Disease, Lancet, 1:358, 1967.

Kaplan, N. M., and A. I. Braude: Hemophilus Influenzae Infection in Adults. Observations on the Immune Disturbance, A.M.A. Arch. Intern. Med., 101:515, 1958.

Patterson, R. L., Jr., and D. B. Levine: Hemophilus Influenzae Pyarthrosis in an Adult, J. Bone Joint Surg., 47A:1250, 1965.

Turk, D. C., and J. R. May: Hemophilus Influenzae. Its Clinical Importance, London, English Universities Press, Ltd., 1967.

Walker, S. H.: The Respiratory Manifestations of Systemic Hemophilus Influenzae Infection, J. Pediat., 62:386, 1963.

Wehrle, P. F., A. W. Hathies, J. M. Leedom, and D. Ivler: Bacterial Meningitis, Ann. N.Y. Acad. Sci., 145:488, 1967.

Pertussis

Brooksaler, F., and J. D. Nelson: Pertussis. A Reappraisal and Report of 190 Confirmed Cases, Am. J. Dis. Child., 114:389, 1967.

Eldering, G., C. Hornbeck, and J. Baker: Serological Study of *Bordetella Pertussis* and Related Species, J. Bacteriol., 74:133, 1957.

Morse, S. I.: Studies of the Lymphocytosis Induced in Mice by Bordetella Pertussis, J. Exp. Med., 121:49, 1965.

Preston, N. W.: Type-Specific Immunity Against Whooping Cough, Brit. Med. J., 2:724, 1963.

Weinstein, L., R. Seltser, and C. T. Marrow: The Treatment of Pertussis with Aureomycin, Chloramphenicol and Terramycin, J. Pediat., 39:549, 1951.

White, R., L. Finberg, and A. Tramer: The Modern Morbidity of Pertussis in Infants, Pediatrics, 33:705, 1964.

Wilson, A. T., I. A. Henderson, E. J. H. Moore, and S. N. Heywood: Whooping Cough: Difficulties in Diagnosis and Ineffectiveness of Immunization, Lancet, 2:623, 1965.

153 CHANCROID
Albert Heyman

DEFINITION. Chancroid is an acute, localized, venereal disease caused by the Ducrey bacillus (*Hemophilus ducreyi*). It is characterized by ulceration at the site of inoculation and by enlargement and suppuration of the regional lymph nodes.

ETIOLOGY. The etiologic agent of chancroid, the Ducrey bacillus, is a short, plump, gram-negative organism with rounded ends. When stained by special methods, the bacillus exhibits bipolar staining. In the stained smears of genital lesions the organisms usually appear singly or in small clusters, but they may be arranged in long parallel columns between cells or shreds of mucus. Occasionally, the bacilli are situated intracellularly. The organism can be cultivated in whole defibrinated blood or nutrient broth containing blood. When grown in pure culture in a liquid medium, the Ducrey bacillus appears in long, tangled chains composed of both coccal and bacillary forms.

INCIDENCE. The number of cases of chancroid occurring every year cannot be determined satisfactorily, since accurate diagnosis of this condition is not generally attempted. A diagnosis of chancroid is frequently applied to genital lesions improving with sulfonamide therapy in which the *Treponema pallidum* cannot be demonstrated. The disease is encountered in the West Indies, North

Africa, and the Orient, particularly in the lower economic groups of the population. It is also prevalent in the Southeastern part of the United States and is more frequent in Negroes than in whites. Approximately 950 cases were reported in the United States in 1966; the true incidence is probably considerably higher.

PATHOGENESIS. Chancroid is usually contracted by sexual intercourse, and the lesions are almost always located about the genitalia. The disease can apparently be acquired from sexual partners who show no evidence of an active chancroidal infection. The organism has been cultivated from the smegma and vaginal secretions in patients without clinical manifestations of the disease. Such individuals may be carriers of the Ducrey bacillus. The organism readily produces an infection when inoculated into open or slightly abraded areas of the skin or mucous membranes. Chancroidal ulcerations frequently occur in areas of the genitalia, where minor abrasions may be present (fourchette of the vulva, edge of phimotic prepuce, and frenum). After an incubation period of 3 to 5 days, a localized ulceration appears at the site of inoculation. This may be followed later by inflammation and suppuration of the regional lymph nodes.

Chancroidal infection produces a distinct histologic appearance. The base of the ulcer is a shallow zone made up of polymorphonuclear leukocytes, fibrin, red blood cells, and necrotic tissue. Below this is a fairly wide layer, consisting chiefly of proliferating endothelial cells and newly formed blood vessels, some of which show degeneration of their walls. Finally, there is a deep zone in which a dense infiltration of plasma cells and lymphocytes occurs. This histologic pattern is sufficiently characteristic to permit differentiation from other genital lesions. Biopsy is a valuable diagnostic procedure.

CLINICAL MANIFESTATIONS. The typical chancroidal lesion is a painful, shallow, irregular ulcer with ragged undermined edges, a granular, friable base, and a dirty-yellow exudate. The lesion is characteristically nonindurated and for this reason has been called *soft chancre*. The size of the ulceration varies but seldom exceeds 2 cm in diameter. Multiple lesions resemble a folliculitis or pyogenic infection. Almost any portion of the genitalia may be involved, but extragenital lesions are rare. In about 50 percent of the patients inflammation and suppuration of the inguinal lymph nodes will occur. The term *bubo* is given to this type of lymphadenitis. The chancroidal bubo develops rapidly and becomes a very painful, inflammatory inguinal mass. When suppuration occurs, the mass may become tensely fluctuant and may rupture spontaneously, leaving a large, single, craterlike abscess. Mild constitutional symptoms may accompany the involvement of the inguinal lymph nodes, and the patient may complain of headache, malaise, fever, or anorexia.

DIAGNOSIS. Although the clinical appearance of chancroid is often sufficiently characteristic to suggest the correct diagnosis, laboratory confirmation is desirable. Stained smears or culture of the exudate taken from the undermined edge of the lesion will reveal the Ducrey bacillus in the majority of the early cases. The organism is not easily demonstrated, however, in larger lesions when secondary bacterial contamination has occurred. Biopsy is feasible in such cases and is an efficient method of diagnosis. Attempts to demonstrate the organism in the buboes by either culture or smear usually are not successful. The majority of patients with chancroidal infection will exhibit a positive skin reaction to an intradermal injection of killed Ducrey bacilli. The value of this skin test is limited by the fact that a positive reaction persists for years after exposure to the infection. One cannot be certain, therefore, whether a positive skin test in an individual patient represents the existing chancroidal infection or a previous one. Early syphilis may be present concurrently with chancroid in these patients. Serologic tests and dark-field examination of the lesions and regional lymph nodes should be done to rule out this possibility.

TREATMENT. Sulfisoxazole (Gantrisin) is the drug of choice in the treatment of chancroid; doses of 4 Gm a day for 7 to 12 days are usually curative. Local medication is not necessary, but saline soaks and cleanliness are advised. Although the buboes usually subside with sulfonamide therapy, fluctuation may persist, and the node should be aspirated in order to prevent spontaneous rupture. Streptomycin, chloramphenicol, and the tetracyclines in doses of 2 Gm a day for 7 to 10 days will each produce satisfactory healing of the lesions of chancroid. The use of these agents is rarely necessary because sulfisoxazole is equally effective. The antibiotics with treponomicidal properties should not be used in the treatment of chancroid until repeated dark-field examinations and serologic tests have ruled out the possibility of early syphilis.

REFERENCES

Heyman, A., P. B. Beeson, and W. H. Sheldon: Diagnosis of Chancroid, J.A.M.A., 129:935, 1945.

Sullivan, M.: Chancroid, Am. J. Syph., Gonor., Vener. Dis., 24:482, 1940.

154 BRUCELLOSIS (Undulant Fever)
Wesley W. Spink

DEFINITION. Brucellosis is caused by microorganisms belonging to the genus *Brucella*, and is transmitted to man from lower animals. The acute illness is frequently characterized by fever without localized findings, while the chronic form is featured by fever, weakness, and vague complaints, which may persist for months and years.

HISTORY. The first clear-cut picture of the disease was presented in 1863 by Marston, who, as a British Army surgeon in Malta, detailed his own case and those of others. The etiologic agent was discovered by Bruce in 1886. The outstanding clinical description of the disease is contained in the monograph by Hughes published in 1897. Wright and Semple in 1897 demonstrated agglutinins for brucella in human blood. In the same year, Bang reported that *Bacillus abortus* was the cause of contagious abortion in cattle in Denmark. The Mediterranean Fever Commission Reports of 1905 to 1907 detail the classic studies on epidemiology. The first recognized human case of brucellosis in the United States occurred in a nurse in Washington, D.C., and was described by Craig in 1906. In 1911 brucellosis was found to be endemic in the goats of Texas, and Gentry and Ferenbaugh traced human cases to this source. Traum first identified brucella organisms from aborting sows in 1914, and Evans in 1918 distinguished the difference between *Brucella melitensis* and *Brucella abortus*, and suggested that raw milk from infected cows could be the source of human cases. In 1924 Keefer described the first human case of brucellosis in this country due to organisms other than *B. melitensis*. A new species, *Brucella canis*, was described in 1966, causing abortions in dogs, especially the Beagle breed. In 1956, Spink described the over-all position of brucellosis in the United States.

ETIOLOGY. Human brucellosis is due to one of three species of *Brucella*: *B. melitensis* (goats), *B. suis* (hogs), and *B. abortus* (cattle). Several subtypes have been described under each of these three main categories. Brucellas are small, nonmotile, non-spore-forming rods staining gram-negative. Growth is best supported at 37°C in trypticase soy broth or tryptose phosphate broth having a pH of 6.6 to 6.8. The primary isolation of *B. abortus* requires displacement of 10 percent of the air by carbon dioxide. The differentiation of the three species is dependent upon biochemical and serologic reaction. *Brucella canis* differs from the foregoing species in that the isolates are rough colonies and lack lipopolysaccharide in the cell wall. No recognized human cases have been caused by this species.

EPIDEMIOLOGY. The natural reservoir of brucellosis is in domestic animals, particularly cattle, swine, goats, and sheep. The disease is very rarely transmitted from human to human.

Studies in the United States and elsewhere indicate that the majority of cases are acquired through contact, and fewer and fewer cases are caused by the ingestion of milk or milk products. This trend is due to the enactment of local and state ordinances requiring all milk sold for human consumption to be pasteurized. There is some evidence that brucellosis may be air-borne, with the disease resulting from the inhalation of brucella. Infections caused by *B. abortus* are spread through cow's milk or through dermal contact with brucella. Epidemics of brucellosis traced to raw cow's milk have been caused by *B. suis*. Contact with infected porcine tissue is a common cause of infections due to *B. suis*. It is readily appreciated why brucellosis is primarily a disease of rural areas and why it is considered an occupational disease involving meat-packing plant employees, farmers, veterinarians, and livestock producers.

PATHOGENESIS. Following invasion of the body by brucellas through the oropharynx or through the skin, the organisms tend to localize in tissues of the reticuloendothelial system, such as the bone marrow, lymph nodes, liver, spleen, and also the kidneys. A characteristic but nonspecific reaction of these tissues to the brucella is the appearance of epithelioid cells, giant cells of the foreign body and Langhans' types, and lymphocytes and plasma cells. Necrosis and caseation rarely occur in these granulomatous areas. When caseation is encountered, it is usually caused by *B. suis*. The granulomas are similar to those of sarcoidosis and tuberculosis. Other less frequent sites of localization of brucella organisms are the bones, especially the spine, the endocardium, and the testes. Although the central nervous system and peripheral nerves are commonly affected deleteriously by brucellas, the mechanism whereby this takes place is not known. Like other blood-borne infections, brucellas may on occasion localize in any tissue or organ in the body. Though brucellosis is a common cause of abortions in cattle, swine, and goats, authentic human abortions occur no more frequently with this disease than with other bacteremias. Orchitis in the male is rarely the cause of subsequent sterility.

MANIFESTATIONS. The incubation period varies between 5 and 21 days, though many months may elapse between the time of infection and the first appearance of symptoms. The onset in many instances may be insidious, the patients exhibiting a low-grade fever with no localized findings, and complaining of headache, weakness, insomnia, sweats, anorexia, constipation, pain over the spine, and generalized aches and pains. Less frequently, the disease may be ushered in by chills, high fever, and prostration, but, again, localized abnormal physical findings may be absent. In general, about 50 percent of the patients exhibit enlarged lymph nodes, especially of the cervical region, and splenomegaly is detected in about one-third of the cases. An enlarged and tender spleen is usually associated with the more severe cases. Pain on pressure over the vertebras occurs occasionally. Pain distributed over the course of the peripheral nerves, particularly the sciatic nerve, is encountered. Orchitis appears after several days of illness and, like the orchitis of mumps, is ushered in with a chill or chilliness, high fever, and tender and enlarged testes. Painful and swollen joints are seen occasionally, but persistent and deforming arthritis is not specific for the disease. Signs and symptoms referable to the lungs and pleurae are uncommon. A rare but serious complication is subacute bacterial endocarditis. Ocular disorders are associated with the more chronic forms of the disease.

The initial febrile stage of the illness may endure for only a few days or up to several weeks. The persistence of fever and symptoms is definitely related to physical activity. Rest in bed during the acute illness is frequently associated with prompt improvement. The natural course of the disease in the majority of patients is marked by a permanent remission of fever and symptoms within 3 to 6 months. A small number of patients with bacteriologically proved cases may have an illness that persists longer than 1 year.

The status of chronic brucellosis is extremely difficult to assess. There is no doubt that the infection may persist in a relatively small number of individuals for months and years. Such patients exhibit a state of ill health manifested by weakness, fatigue, mental depression, vague aches and pains, and no abnormal physical findings. Intermittent fever may occur. Of considerable importance in the suspected chronic case is the investigation of possible sites of chronic suppuration manifested by calcified caseating areas in the liver and spleen that can be detected by careful x-ray films of the abdomen. "Abacteric pyuria" should suggest, among other causes, renal suppuration due to brucellas.

LABORATORY FINDINGS. A precise diagnosis of brucellosis is dependent upon the results of laboratory procedures.

Blood. The total leukocyte count is usually normal or slightly reduced but is rarely over 10,000 cells per cu mm. The differential count reveals a relative lymphocytosis. The erythrocyte sedimentation rate is of no specific diagnostic aid, the rates being normal or accelerated.

The most practical method for screening suspected cases of brucellosis is the *agglutination* reaction. Agglutinins usually appear during the second or third week of illness. If proper techniques and antigen are employed, agglutinins are demonstrated in the vast majority of bacteriologically proved cases. Active brucellosis is usually associated with titers of 1:100 or above. On rare occasions, the titer may be depressed by "blocking antibodies" in chronic illness. Only very rarely are agglutinins absent in patients with bacteriologically proved disease. Agglutinins for brucellosis are not always specific, since cross reactions occur with the cholera vibrio and with *Pasteurella tularensis*. Agglutinins may persist in the blood long after the patient has recovered. One of the most critical diagnostic problems in the sporadic case of brucellosis is the interpretation of an agglutination titer of 1 to 100 or lower in the absence of both definitive bacteriologic data and localizing signs. Brucella-agglutinating immunoglobulins in serum consist of both 7S and 19S globulins, but only 7S has been associated with active disease in acute and chronic cases, providing a stimulating dose of antigen (skin test) has not been given prior to obtaining blood from the patient.

At least one *culture* of blood, and preferably more, should be carried out in every suspected case of brucellosis. *Brucella* have been isolated from aspirated sternal bone marrow, when simultaneous blood cultures remained sterile. It is too impractical for routine purposes to attempt to isolate brucellas from the urine, bile, or feces.

The *opsonocytophagic test,* which is a measure of the phagocytosis of brucellas by polymorphonuclear neutrophil leukocytes, is of no diagnostic value.

Intradermal Tests. A positive reaction to brucella antigen has no more significance than that obtained with tuberculin in suspected cases of tuberculosis. A positive reaction indicates previous invasion of the body by brucellas and does not mean that active disease is present. When agglutinins are absent and cultures remain sterile, considerable caution must be exercised before making a diagnosis of brucellosis, even though the skin test is positive.

DIFFERENTIAL DIAGNOSIS. Brucellosis must be differentiated from other acute febrile illnesses such as *influenza* and other *upper respiratory diseases* of doubtful etiology. Brucellosis is not commonly associated with coryza or pharyngitis. Other diseases from which it must be differentiated include *malaria* and *typhoid fever*. Brucellosis may be confused with *infectious mononucleosis,* but the characteristic blood picture and the elevated titer of heterophil antibodies in this disease are helpful differential aids.

Chronic brucellosis simulates *psychoneurosis, anxiety states,* and *chronic nervous exhaustion*. Indeed, a patient with brucellosis may suffer from the foregoing nervous disorders. Some confusion may arise in differentiating it from other diseases, including tuberculosis and lymphoblastoma, especially Hodgkin's disease.

TREATMENT. Patients with acute brucellosis should be reassured that a large majority of those with the disease recover spontaneously. Rest and psychotherapy are important during the febrile illness.

The course of acute brucellosis can be shortened and complications prevented by the prompt use of tetracycline, with an oral dose of 0.5 Gm four times daily for at least 3 weeks. In case of a relapse, this dose schedule can be repeated. Except in rare instances there is no advantage in more than two courses of tetracycline therapy. For the more seriously ill patients some authorities recommend the simultaneous use of streptomycin in dosages of 0.5 Gm twice daily and tetracycline. Tetracycline therapy, with and without streptomycin, is also effective in proved chronic brucellosis.

Febrile patients with either acute or chronic brucellosis can suffer from a severe toxic state with anorexia, depression, and a generalized debilitated condition. Such individuals should receive an adrenocorticoid steroid preparation in addition to antibiotic therapy. Prednisone in oral dosage of 20 mg can be given twice daily for 72 to 96 hr, or 100 mg of hydrocortisone can be administered intravenously followed by 50 mg orally twice daily.

A common therapeutic practice in the more chronic cases is to attempt desensitization to brucella organisms by treating patients with one of the several antigenic preparations, such as heat-killed brucella cells or filtrates of brucella cultures. Although hypersensitivity to brucellas is a factor in the symptomatology, and the use of ascending doses of antigenic material may be sound therapy, the results are difficult to evaluate, and treatment must often be continued for several months. Violent local and systemic reactions often occur, even following the injection of minute amounts of antigen.

For the relief of headache and the generalized aches and pains, salicylates may be prescribed; the occasional use of barbiturates is desirable for the insomnia which is so commonly a part of the disease.

PROGNOSIS. Although brucellosis may be a chronic and disabling disease, the overall mortality rate is not more than 2 percent and is negligible when appropriate antibiotic therapy is promptly employed. The physician today may learn a great deal about the prognosis of this disease by turning back and looking over the rich experience of the Mediterranean Fever Commission, which was recorded in 1905 to 1907. Without the aid of effective drug therapy, only 15 percent of patients had an illness exceeding 3 months.

Over the succeeding years, it has been observed that a relatively small, but important, number of patients will have a protracted illness. Cases of bacteriologically proved brucellosis in which the disease has continued for up to 25 years have been studied at the University of Minnesota Hospitals, but such cases are not commonly encountered. One cannot escape the conviction that so-called "chronic brucellosis" is being mislabeled too often on the basis of procedures of doubtful value, especially the intradermal test with brucella antigen.

Relapses do occur in the more chronic cases of brucellosis. These recurrences are manifested by fever and by mental and physical disability, with generalized aches and pains. But too little attention has been given to the problem of reinfections. Clinical observations in meat-packing plant employees have confirmed studies made with experimentally infected animals, in that the immunity induced by one attack of brucellosis is only relative. Second and third infections do take place. In individuals who continue to be exposed to the disease, it may be quite difficult to differentiate between relapses and reinfections. Furthermore, patients having recovered from brucellosis have an acquired brucella hypersensitivity that may render them extremely susceptible to the effects of contact with brucella antigen. This is particularly applicable to veterinarians who have accidentally injected viable brucella antigen into their skin while immunizing animals. Violent local and systemic febrile reactions follow such an incident within a few hours.

PREVENTION. As long as the reservoir of brucellosis persists in domestic animals, human brucellosis will occur. The only practical means of eliminating the disease in human beings is to eradicate the disease from cattle, hogs, sheep, and goats. Control measures in animals are being worked out in several areas in the United States. Since human brucellosis is contracted through the ingestion of contaminated milk and milk products, it is essential that only properly pasteurized milk be utilized for human consumption. Brucellosis is an occupational disease involving farmers, livestock workers, veterinarians, and those working in meat-packing plants and there is no entirely safe means for immunizing these groups against the disease.

REFERENCES

Carmichael, L. E., and R. M. Kennedy: Canine Abortion Caused by *Brucella canis*, J. Am. Vet. Med. Assn., 152: 605, 1966.

Eyre, J. W. H.: Melitensis Septicemia, Lancet, I:1677, 1747, 1826, 1908.

Hughes, M. L.: "Mediterranean, Malta or Undulant Fever," London, The Macmillan Company, Ltd., 1897.

"Reports of the Commission for the Investigation of Mediterranean Fever," pts. 1 to 7, London, Harrison & Sons, Ltd., 1905–1907.

Reddin, J. L., R. K. Anderson, R. Jenness, and W. W. Spink:

Significance of 7S and Macroglobulin Brucella Agglutinins in Human Brucellosis, New Engl. J. Med., 272:1263, 1965.

Spink, W. W.: "The Nature of Brucellosis," Minneapolis, University of Minnesota Press, 1956.

155 TULAREMIA
Leighton E. Cluff

DEFINITION. Tularemia (rabbit fever, deer-fly fever, Ohara's disease) is an infectious disease of animals transmitted to man by direct contact or by insect vectors. A cutaneous or mucous membrane lesion at the site of inoculation and regional lymph node enlargement are the characteristic manifestations of the disease in man.

HISTORY. The microorganism responsible for tularemia was identified by McCoy and Chapin in 1912 among infected ground squirrels in Tulare County, California. The first description of tularemia in man was by Wherry and Lamb in 1914.

ETIOLOGY. *Pasteurella tularensis* is a pleomorphic, nonsporulating, gram-negative bacillus. It can be cultured only on media containing glucose, cystine, and serum. Thorough cooking renders meat from infected animals safe for consumption, but tularemia can develop in persons handling carcasses that have been frozen for many days. *Pasteurella tularensis* is related antigenically to the causative organisms of brucellosis and plague and possesses an endotoxin similar to those of many other gram-negative bacteria.

EPIDEMIOLOGY AND PATHOGENESIS. Contact with infected animals is the commonest source of tularemia in man, but the disease also may be acquired from insects or by exposure to the organism in the laboratory. A variety of rodents, carnivores, ungulates, birds, and arthropods is naturally infected by *P. tularensis,* including rabbits, squirrels, woodchucks, muskrats, skunks, coyotes, foxes, opossums, mice, rats, quail, chickens, pheasants, snakes, ticks, and flies. The Rocky Mountain tick, western wood tick, eastern dog tick, and the Lone Star tick (*Dermacentor andersoni, D. variabilis, D. occidentalis,* and *Amblyomma americanum*) may act as reservoirs of infection. One species of deer fly (*Chrysops discalis*) and, in Sweden, a mosquito (*Aëdes cinereus*) can transmit tularemia to man. Ticks are an important reservoir of the disease because the microorganism is transferred transovarially from the female to her progeny. Sporadic episodes and epidemic tularemia have occurred following contact with water and fish contaminated by infected animal carcasses. However, human-to-human transmission of infection does not occur. Wild cottontail rabbits are the principal source of tularemia in the United States.

Man is highly susceptible to tularemia; the organism usually invades through the skin, mucous membrane, gastrointestinal tract, or respiratory tract. Hunters, butchers, and housewives are most often affected.

PATHOLOGY. Microscopically, the primary cutaneous lesion shows neutrophilic infiltration, granulomatous reaction, and necrosis. The regional lymph nodes develop similar changes and often suppurate. The granulomatous reaction in tularemia resembles tubercles in liver, spleen, lung, and kidney. *Pasteurella tularensis* has been recovered from lymph nodes many days after apparent subsidence of the disease.

MANIFESTATIONS. The incubation period is 3 to 7 days. Because a typical lesion of skin or mucous membranes is not invariably present, tularemia classically has been separated into several clinical types.

More than 80 percent of infections by *P. tularensis* produce a lesion of the skin or mucous membranes which begins as a reddened papule that may be pruritic and soon ulcerates. The primary lesion in this *ulceroglandular* form of the disease is rarely very painful, is usually present before onset of systemic symptoms, and may not heal until convalescence is well under way. Frequently it is overlooked, or its relationship to severe systemic symptoms is not recognized. Regional lymph node enlargement is usually more prominent than that accompanying infections of similar severity produced by other microorganisms. The involved nodes are often exquisitely tender, fluctuant, hot, and reddened. Drainage can occur spontaneously. Generalized lymphadenopathy is present in some cases, but the regional nodes are most prominently involved. There is considerable variation in the intensity of the systemic symptoms of ulceroglandular tularemia; the patient may be almost asymptomatic or severely prostrated. Clinical and roentgenographic evidence of pneumonitis may accompany this form of the disease, illustrating its disseminated character, but bacteremia is rarely demonstrable.

Localized lymph node enlargement without detectable skin lesion is referred to as *glandular* tularemia. The pathogenesis of this form of the disease is probably identical with that of ulceroglandular tularemia, and the features of the illness are also the same.

Rarely, the portal of entry of the organism is the conjunctiva, where there develops an ulcer, with edema, congestion, lacrimation, photophobia, and pain. In this *oculoglandular* type of tularemia the preauricular, submaxillary, and anterior cervical lymph nodes may enlarge. Corneal ulceration and scarring or perforation of the globe may occur.

Ingestion of contaminated meat or water may result in primary lesions in the *gastrointestinal* tract. This rare form of the disease produces diarrhea, abdominal pain, nausea, vomiting, melena, and hematemesis, but otherwise differs little from tularemia introduced through other portals. Ulcerative lesions are often found in the buccal mucosa, pharynx, or intestine, and the mesenteric or cervical lymph nodes are involved early in the disease.

Tularemia without obvious primary ulcer or localized lymphadenitis is referred to as *typhoidal*. Constitutional symptoms in typhoidal tularemia differ in no way from those in other types of the disease, although there is usually more prostration. In the absence of localized manifestations, the diagnosis of tularemia is more difficult and depends on serologic tests, isolation of the organism, or a strong epidemiologic history.

Pneumonia may accompany tularemia. Involvement of the lung is secondary to hematogenous dissemination, even when infection is acquired by inhalation of the organism (as in bacteriology laboratories). Pneumonitis in tularemia may cause cough, mucoid sputum, hemoptysis, pleuritic pain, dyspnea, and cyanosis, but extensive x-ray evidence of pneumonitis is sometimes present in the absence of any symptoms of pulmonary disease. Physical findings often correlate poorly with the roentgenologic changes, which consist of diffuse patchy or lobar infiltrations and inconstant hilar adenopathy. Pleural effusion may occur, but lung abscess is rare.

Rarely *P. tularensis* causes endocarditis, pericarditis, peritonitis, appendicitis, osteomyelitis, or meningitis.

Fever in tularemia develops abruptly, often with rigors, and in untreated patients may persist with temperatures of 104 to 106°F for as long as 4 weeks. The fever is sustained or mildly remittent, and defervescence is by lysis.

Splenomegaly is detectable in many patients. An evanescent macular or papular *rash* is sometimes present on the trunk and extremities early in the disease.

Convalescence in untreated tularemia is prolonged, and fever, lassitude, fatigability, myalgia, irritability, or anorexia may persist or recur for many months. Recovery is usually prompt if acute tularemia is treated with antibiotics. When therapy is delayed, however, patients are more likely to be left with mild debilitation that is unresponsive to further administration of antimicrobial drugs.

Recovery from tularemia is usually followed by immunity to recurrence of disease. However, immunity is not complete, and several instances of second, even third attacks of tularemia have been recorded. Almost invariably, they have consisted of the development of a local lesion and mild regional adenopathy without systemic symptoms and with little or no fever.

LABORATORY FINDINGS. Serum agglutinins for *P. tularensis* are present after the second week of illness. Cross agglutination may occur with antigens of *Brucella,* but this is not a constant finding.

Pasteurella tularensis can be recovered by appropriate cultures or animal inoculation. It is rarely found in blood but can be isolated from the mucocutaneous ulcer or regional lymph nodes with regularity. The organism has been cultured from the sputum and gastric washings even in patients without roentgenographic evidence of pneumonitis. Accidental infection of personnel in diagnostic laboratories may occur.

Skin test with a diluted suspension of killed *P. tularensis,* or purified antigen, becomes positive during the first week of disease. The cutaneous hypersensitivity response is "delayed" and resembles the tuberculin reaction.

The total blood leukocyte count is usually normal. The erythrocyte sedimentation rate is normal in ulceroglandular or mild disease but is frequently elevated in severe typhoidal tularemia.

DIFFERENTIAL DIAGNOSIS. Brucellosis, typhoid fever, disseminated tuberculosis, the early stage of several rickettsial diseases, and infectious mononucleosis may closely resemble typhoidal tularemia. History of possible contacts is important, and appropriate serologic and cultural studies are usually successful in differentiating these infections. Pneumonic tularemia must be distinguished from viral, mycotic, and other bacterial infections of the lung. The differential diagnosis of pneumonia is discussed in Chap. 138. Oculoglandular syndromes likely to be confused with tularemia are described in Chap. 230.

Ulceroglandular tularemia must be distinguished from a variety of infections in which a *local cutaneous ulcer with regional lymphadenopathy* may occur. Besides pyoderma caused by streptococci or staphylococci, these infections include lymphogranuloma venereum, cat-scratch fever, rat-bite fever, bubonic plague, anthrax, glanders, several rickettsioses of which the important one in this country is rickettsialpox, several viral infections of the skin such as orf and cowpox, and inoculation syphilis or tuberculosis. In all these, with the exception of lymphogranuloma venereum and cat-scratch fever, the regional lymph node involvement is usually proportional to the size of the cutaneous ulcer. Extragenital lymphogranuloma is rare; fever and systemic symptoms in cat-scratch fever are rarely severe for more than a few days.

TREATMENT. Streptomycin is the antibiotic of choice for tularemia. The dosage is 0.5 to 1.0 Gm every 12 hr for 10 days. *Pasteurella tularensis* cannot be recovered from lymph nodes or skin lesions after 24 to 48 hr of therapy. However, the regional lymph nodes may continue to enlarge and suppurate for several days. Pulmonary lesions usually subside rapidly, although the evolution of the cutaneous lesion is not interrupted. The tetracycline antibiotics and chloramphenicol, also are effective, although fever and other manifestations may recur 7 to 14 days after cessation of therapy. Recrudescent illness, however, responds rapidly to readministration of the antibiotic. Aspiration of pus from suppurating nodes rarely is necessary; but if fistulas persist, total surgical removal of the involved tissue can be carried out. Surgery may be followed by transient recurrence of fever despite failure to demonstrate the organism in excised tissues.

PROPHYLAXIS. A killed bacterial vaccine developed by Foshay has been shown to stimulate serum agglutinins and induces positive skin reactions to the bacterial antigens, but it produces little immunity to infection with *P. tularensis*. An attenuated live bacterial vaccine has been developed, however, and is effective in inducing protection against infection.

Antibiotic prophylaxis with streptomycin following exposure to tularemia will protect against infection. Chloramphenicol and tetracycline, however, only prolong the incubation period of the disease and do not prevent its occurrence.

Avoidance of contact with possible sources of infection is important in prevention, and the incidence of tularemia in several localities has fallen sharply with the introduction of laws prohibiting the sale of wild rabbits by butchers.

PROGNOSIS. The mortality rate in untreated tularemia is 6 to 7 percent. With antimicrobial therapy, death is rare.

REFERENCES

Foshay, L.: Treatment of Tularemia with Streptomycin, Am. J. Med., 2:467, 1947.

Francis, E.: Tularemia, in "Oxford Medicine," Fair Lawn, N.J. Oxford University Press, 1948.

McCrumb, F. R., Jr., M. I. Snyder, and T. E. Woodward: Studies on Human Infection with *Pasteurella tularensis*: Comparison of Streptomycin and Chloramphenicol in the Prophylaxis of Clinical Disease, Trans. Assoc. Am. Physicians, 70:74, 1957.

Stuart, B. M., and R. L. Pullen: Tularemic Pneumonia: Review of American Literature and Report of Fifteen Additional Cases, Am. J. Med. Sci., 210:233, 1945.

Woodward, T. E., W. T. Raby, W. Eppes, W. A. Holbrook, and J. A. Hightower: Aureomycin in Treatment of Experimental and Human Tularemia, J.A.M.A., 139:830, 1949.

156 PLAGUE
Joseph E. Johnson, III

DEFINITION. Plague is an infectious disease of animals (principally wild and domestic rodents) which is transmitted to man through the bite of infected ectoparasites (especially the rat flea). Disease in man is usually characterized by the abrupt onset of high fever, lymphadenopathy and suppuration of regional lymph nodes draining the exposure site, bacteremia, and prostration. This clinical form of the disease is known as *bubonic* plague because of the presence of enlarged suppurating lymph nodes, or *buboes*. Secondary pneumonia may occur and lead to direct respiratory transmission by infectious aerosols from man to man. This primary *pneumonic* type of human disease is highly fatal.

HISTORY. Plague was known and feared in ancient times and has been the subject of dread as well as a source of literary stimulation to authors from Dionysius in the third century to Camus in the present. It has undoubtedly been endemic in Asia and Europe for centuries. At least three major pandemics have occurred in which large segments of the population were destroyed. The first authentic pandemic was recorded in the sixth century A.D., and is estimated to have claimed 100 million victims. The second great pandemic occurred in the fourteenth century and was known as the "Black Death," presumably because of the severe cyanosis produced in some of its victims. Fifty million persons, including one-quarter of the population of Europe, died. In subsequent centuries, consecutive outbreaks of plague ravaged Europe and Africa. The last major pandemic originated in China in 1894, spread eventually to all continents, and was first recognized in the United States in 1900. It is likely, however, that the disease was present in the wild rodent population (sylvatic plague) in California long before this. The disease is now well established in wild rodents in many parts of the world, including the western United States. It is present on every continent except

Australia. Human disease is endemic in parts of Asia, Africa, and South America, and sporadic human cases still occur in the United States.

ETIOLOGY. The causative agent, *Pasteurella pestis*, is a gram-negative, nonmotile, and non-spore-forming bacillus which grows both aerobically and anaerobically. It is pleomorphic in exudate or sputum, and may appear bacillary, ovid, or coccal. When stained with Giemsa or Wayson's stain, it displays a bipolar "safety pin" structure. *Pasteurella pestis* grows readily although somewhat slowly on ordinary culture media, forming small, round, transparent colonies which assume a "beaten-copper" appearance after 48 hr. At least two types of toxins have been identified, including a soluble exotoxinlike protein, and an insoluble endotoxic lipopolysaccharide. Although readily killed by sunlight, organisms have been shown to survive in sterile soil for 16 months and in nonsterile soil for as long as 7 months, and it is likely that organisms may be present in rodent burrows in the absence of fleas and rats for long periods.

Pasteurella pestis is generally susceptible to streptomycin, chloramphenicol, and the tetracycline antibiotics. A few streptomycin-resistant strains recently have been isolated in Vietnam, but no therapeutic failures have been attributable to drug-resistance. Drug resistance may pose a threat in the future, however, because transfer of drug-resistance factors (R factors) from *E. Coli* to *P. Pestis* has been demonstrated.

EPIDEMIOLOGY. Plague is firmly entrenched as an enzootic among approximately 200 species of rodents in many parts of the world. While the disease in wild rodents (sylvatic plague) is not usually a direct threat to man, it nevertheless serves as a vast reservoir for infection of domestic rats (murine or rat plague) which, along with their ectoparasites, live in close association with man. The endemic reservoir of sylvatic plague includes wild rats, ground squirrels, mice, marmots, owls, gophers, badgers, rabbits, prairie dogs, and chipmunks; in the Western Hemisphere the disease is firmly entrenched in the wild rodent population of California, Oregon, Washington, Utah, Idaho, Nevada, New Mexico, Texas, Louisiana, Florida, Michigan, Arizona, Colorado, Montana, Wyoming, Kansas, North Dakota, Hawaii, western Mexico, and western Canada. The principal murine hosts are the domestic rats, *Rattus rattus* and *R. norvegicus*, which are found throughout the world. Although ticks, lice, and bedbugs may occasionally serve as vectors, the principal ectoparasite vector is the oriental rat flea, *Xenopsylla cheopis.*

Between epidemics the infection persists as a chronic disease of wild rodents which is maintained by the insect vector. Although occasionally acquired through contact with wild rodents and their parasites, human disease is usually a result of association with domestic rats and occurs in urban areas in the wake of rat epizootics. When the concentration of people and of rats under circumstances of poor sanitation provides opportunity for the migration of fleas from rats to man, an outbreak is likely to occur. Because sylvatic plague appears virtually impossible to eradicate, it will continue to pose a constant threat of extension into urban rat populations and thence to man. Infection of the flea takes place through ingestion of blood of a bacteremic animal. After multiplication in the intestinal tract of the flea, the organisms are regurgitated when the flea attempts to ingest another blood meal. Because rat fleas will attack man if rats are not immediately available, the infection is likely to be transmitted as the rat population decreases and the fleas transfer from dead hosts to human beings. Plague can be acquired by direct contact with the tissues of an infected animal, by its bite, or by scratching of infected material into the skin.

The bubonic form of the disease rarely results in transmission from man to man because bacteremia in human disease is rarely of a level sufficient to allow infection of fleas. The principal mode of spread from man to man is by the pulmonary route, which occurs when a patient with bubonic disease develops secondary plague pneumonia and thereafter excretes large quantities of organisms in the sputum. Airborne infection by droplet nuclei is highly contagious, and primary pneumonic plague is common among those attending such a patient. Although asymptomatic oropharyngeal carriers have been identified among healthy family contacts of bubonic plague patients in Vietnam, the role of these carriers in the transmission of the disease has not been determined.

PATHOGENESIS. In the more common bubonic form of disease, *P. pestis* gains entry into the human host through the bite of an infected flea. Organisms are carried to the local lymphatics, then to the bloodstream and finally are disseminated. The prominent clinical manifestations are usually in the lymphatic system. In bubonic plague, a hemorrhagic zone of edema surrounds an inflamed and suppurating group of regional lymph nodes. The glands are hyperplastic and show multiple areas of necrosis, in which there are swarms of organisms. Metastatic lesions sometimes develop in other lymphatics or in the viscera. Particularly likely is the occurrence of secondary pneumonia, which constitutes a potential source of pneumonic spread. Hemorrhages are numerous, probably as a result of a toxin produced by *P. pestis,* and it is not unusual for individuals given chemotherapy at a late date to die of toxemia when plague bacilli can no longer be cultured from any organ. Primary pneumonic spread occurs through the inhalation of infectious aerosols emanating from another case or, rarely, from infected fomites. It is apparent that the tonsils and/or oropharyngeal mucous membranes may occasionally serve as portals of entry resulting in a cervical bubonic-septicemic form of the disease. Rarely a skin papule forms at the site of entry of the bacillus, and may develop into a pustule or a carbuncle.

Bacteremia is a constant feature of bubonic and pneumonic plague. The precise mechanisms by which the plague bacillus and its toxic factors produce severe tissue injury are not understood completely.

MANIFESTATIONS. After an incubation period of 1 to 12 days (usually 2 to 4 days), the patient develops an acute and often fulminant illness. In the more common *bubonic* variety, symptoms begin abruptly with chills, a rise in temperature to 102 to 105°F, tachycardia, headache, vomiting, uncertain gait, marked prostration, and delirium. The spleen is sometimes palpable. The fleabite at the portal of entry rarely can be seen; if present, it is marked by a papule or vesicle which ultimately becomes pustular. Pain and tenderness are present in the infected regional lymph nodes. Of the buboes, 60 to 75 percent are in the inquinal or femoral regions because the lower extremities are more commonly the site of the initial fleabite. Less often, especially in children, buboes are found in the axillary or cervical regions. Infection may extend to other superficial or deeply situated groups of glands. The bubo consists of a firm, matted group of glands measuring 2 to 5 cm in diameter and is surrounded by a boggy and frequently hemorrhagic zone of edema. It usually suppurates and drains spontaneously after 1 or 2 weeks, although in some instances there is complete resorption.

There is a marked hemorrhagic tendency, presumably because of the effect of plague toxin on blood vessels. Petechiae or ecchymoses occur often. Bleeding may occur into a viscus or a serous cavity, or from the nose and alimentary, respiratory, or urinary tracts.

The course of bubonic plague is marked by an irregular or remittent fever, which often drops at the time of appearance of the bubo, only to rise again. In favorable cases, the temperature falls gradually during the second week concomitant with improvement in the general clinical condition. A rise to hyperpyrexic levels or a precipitous fall to normal or to subnormal, frequently heralds approaching death. Most fatalities occur during the first week of illness. Although bubonic plague is usually severe, mild cases called *pestis minor* are sometimes seen during epidemics.

The "primary septicemic" form of plague is actually a variant of bubonic disease. The patient experiences a sudden and overwhelming systemic illness. There is a marked constitutional reaction, with chills, fever, rapid pulse, severe headache, nausea, vomiting, and delirium. Death ensues within a few days, before localizing lesions become clinically apparent. Nevertheless, autopsy usually reveals inflammation in some part of the lymphatic system.

Plague also may take the form of pneumonia. The initial cases appear in patients with bubonic plague, of whom as many as 5 percent develop secondary lesions in the lungs. These individuals may provide the starting point for a man-to-man epidemiologic cycle of airborne primary pneumonic plague. It is a fulminating infection accompanied by great prostration, cough, dyspnea, and in the later stages, cyanosis. The sputum is abundant, bloodstained, and teeming with *P. pestis*. Often there are no clear-cut pulmonary signs, though scattered râles or areas of dullness may be found. In the absence of specific therapy, plague pneumonia invariably ends fatally within 1 to 5 days.

Infection may localize in other regions of the body. Subcutaneous abscesses and cutaneous ulcerations sometimes occur, and occasionally the meninges are involved.

LABORATORY FINDINGS. Laboratory confirmation of plague is relatively simple, although the disease is often misdiagnosed in the United States because of its rarity. Consideration of epidemiologic and clinical features provide highly characteristic leads, and once a suspicion of plague is entertained, it can readily be verified by smear, culture, and animal inoculation of appropriate specimens. The technique of staining a suspected specimen with fluorescent specific antiserum provides an elegant method for rapid identification of *P. pestis*. If a bubo is present, a small quantity of interstitial fluid should be aspirated from its center. Large numbers of morphologically characteristic bacilli are usually seen in a stained smear. Infected sputum likewise contains many organisms. Bacteremia of varying degrees occurs at some time during the course of the disease in nearly all cases. Pus and sputum should be cultured on blood agar plates, while blood is inoculated into nutrient broth. Organisms are identified by their morphologic and colonial characteristics and by agglutination with specific antiserum. Guinea pig inoculation is the final step in identification. In this animal the gross and microscopic lesions are highly characteristic. Caution should be observed in handling infected materials or animals, because of the great danger of infection to laboratory workers.

Specific antibodies appear in the serum of patients convalescing from the disease and can usually be detected early in the second week by complement fixation, agglutination, passive hemagglutination, or immunoelectrophoretic agar-gel precipitation methods. A passive mouse-protective test serves to indicate the immune status of a convalescent or vaccinated individual.

The white blood cell count is elevated to levels often above 20,000 cells per cu mm, and there is a predominance of polymorphonuclear leukocytes. The red blood cell count usually is normal.

DIAGNOSIS. Early in the acute phase of illness, before the appearance of localizing signs, plague may be confused with severe systemic illnesses such as typhoid, typhus, or malaria. The presence of buboes may suggest other forms of infectious lymphadenitis, including tularemia, syphilis, and lymphogranuloma venereum, as well as lymphadenitis of staphylococcal or streptococcal origin. Pneumonic plague must be distinguished from tularemic, pneumococcal, and other gram-negative pneumonias as well as from anthrax, psittacosis, and mycoplasma pneumonia. The consideration of epidemiologic factors, plus bacteriologic studies, will aid in the differentiation. Serologic diagnosis is of aid only for retrospective confirmation. When plague is suspected, it is imperative to begin treatment as soon as adequate specimens have been taken for culture because early institution of therapy is essential to ensure recovery. To delay treatment may risk toxemic death in the face of a bacteriologic cure.

TREATMENT. When antibiotic treatment is instituted early in the course of the disease, the response is usually dramatic and complete. Even patients with pneumonic or septicemic disease can be cured if treatment is initiated within the first 15 to 20 hr after onset. Streptomycin is the drug of choice and is given in divided doses of 4 Gm daily for 48 hr followed by 1.5 Gm daily for a total of 7 to 10 days or until the patient has been afebrile at least 3 days. Chloramphenicol and tetracyclines are also potent antiplague agents. Chloramphenicol should be given in initial doses of 6 to 8 Gm daily intravenously, and the dose should be reduced to 3 to 4 Gm when improvement occurs. Tetracyclines are given in initial doses of 2 to 3 Gm daily intravenously, and the dose is reduced to 2 Gm daily orally when improvement occurs. Sulfadiazine has been somewhat less effective, particularly in pneumonic plague, but can be used when the other antibiotics are not available. Buboes are treated with hot, moist applications. Incision and drainage should be postponed until the lesion becomes well localized and the patient has been treated with antibiotics.

CONTROL. Prevention of plague must be directed toward elimination of endemic rodent foci, and in endemic urban areas constant vigilance is required in detecting and combating rodent epizootics. Prevention includes extermination of rats, eradication of ectoparasite vectors, and sometimes the immunization of the human population. Rats are attacked by poisoning and trapping, by elimination of harborage areas, and by separating them from their food supplies. Unfortunately, rodent control has proved to be most difficult in the endemic areas because of generally poor living standards. Vector control with DDT has been used with brilliant success in diminishing the flea population infecting both rodents and human beings, but recent studies in southeast Asia unfortunately show a significant incidence of DDT-resistant fleas, but these may yield to other insecticides such as Aldrin, Dieldrin, and Chlordane. The complete elimination of sylvatic plague appears to be impossible in the foreseeable future, and the control program must be aimed at eradicating foci of wild rodent infection around areas of human habitation. In these peripheral zones, the wild and the domestic rodents live commensally, exchange fleas, and threaten the human community.

Patients must be disinfested and carefully isolated, while other intimately exposed persons should be quarantined. Prophylaxis has been achieved effectively in the past by administering sulfadiazine in a dose of 3 Gm per day for 1 week. Recent southeast Asian studies, however, have revealed significant in vitro resistance to sulfadiazine. Alternatively, prophylaxis with streptomycin in a dose of 1 Gm per day is often effective.

Vaccines have been used for many years and apparently provide limited and transitory immunity. Three types of vaccines have been available. A formalin-killed vaccine approved for use in the United States has been advised for all persons traveling to Vietnam, Cambodia, and Laos, for those whose vocations bring them into frequent and regular contact with wild rodents in plague enzootic areas, and for all laboratory personnel working with *P. pestis* or with plague-infected rodents. Although the precise effectiveness of this vaccine has not been measured satisfactorily, it appears to reduce the incidence and severity of the disease. A second promising vaccine is a living attenuated strain of the organism which may be particularly suitable for endemic areas in Asia. Russian studies indicate that the attenuated vaccine administered by the aerosol route may be especially valuable in prevention of pneumonic plague. A third vaccine consisting of a chemical extract has been effective in experimental laboratory infections. Immunity is relative, and protection is not always conferred by the active disease, since a number of reinfections have been described. Although general vaccination may be worthwhile in an area threatened by an epidemic, the results are too slow for immediate prophylaxis. In such epidemic situations, combined use of all available control measures is indicated.

PROGNOSIS. The availability of effective antibiotic therapy has improved the prognosis in this formerly highly fatal disease. In the past the mortality rate of bubonic plague varied from 50 to 90 percent, and the pneumonic, septicemic, and meningitic forms were almost invariably fatal. In treated cases the mortality is 5 to 10 percent and even the gravest varieties of infection respond to chemotherapy if treated early enough.

REFERENCES

Cavanaugh, D. C., H. G. Dangerfield, D. H. Hunter, R. J. T. Joy, J. D. Marshall, D. V. Quy, S. Vivona, and P. E. Winter: Some Observations on the Current Plague Outbreak in the Republic of Vietnam, Am. J. Public Health, 58:742, 1968.

Gilbert, D. N., W. L. Moore, L. L. Hedberg, and J. P. Sanford: Potential Medical Problems in Personnel Returning from Vietnam, Ann. Intern. Med. 68:662, 1968.

Girard, G.: Plague, Ann. Rev. Microbiol., 69:253, 1955.

Hirst, L. F.: "The Conquest of Plague: A Study of the Evolution of Epidemiology," Fair Lawn, N.J., Oxford University Press, 1953.

Kartman, L., F. M. Prince, S. F. Quan, and H. E. Stark: New Knowledge on the Ecology of Sylvatic Plague, Ann. N.Y. Acad. Sci., 70:668, 1958.

Meyer, K. F., S. F. Quan, F. R. McCrumb, and A. Larson: Effective Treatment of Plague, Ann. N.Y. Acad. Sci., 55: 1228, 1952.

Pollitzer, R.: "Plague," World Health Organ. Monograph Series, No. 22, Geneva, 1954.

———: A Review of Recent Literature on Plague. Bull. World Health Organ, no. 23, pp. 313–400, Geneva, 1960.

157 GLANDERS
Jay P. Sanford

DEFINITION: Glanders is a serious infection of equine animals caused by *Malleomyces mallei*, which is transmitted occasionally to other domestic animals and to man.

ETIOLOGY. *Malleomyces mallei* is a small, slender, nonmotile, gram-negative bacillus. When stained with methylene blue, marked irregularities in staining are observed. Organisms grow on most common meat infusion media, but require glycerol for optimum growth.

EPIDEMIOLOGY. Glanders was at one time widespread throughout Europe, but due to the introduction of control measures, its incidence has decreased steadily in most countries. The disease still occurs in Asia, Africa, and South America, but not in the United States. Glanders has never been common in man, but the occasional infection may be very serious. There have been no naturally acquired infections in the United States since 1938, but with increasing international travel, patients with glanders may be encountered.

Glanders is primarily a disease of horses, mules, and donkeys, although goats, sheep, cats, and dogs sometimes naturally contract the disease. Rabbits, guinea pigs, and hamsters are susceptible to experimental infection. Pigs and cattle are said to be absolutely resistant. In horses, the disease may be systemic with prominent pulmonary involvement, *glanders,* or characterized by subcutaneous ulcerative lesions, and lymphatic thickening with nodules, *farcy.* The route of infection in animals remains controversial; inhalation, ingestion, or inoculation through breaks in the skin have been suggested. In man, the disease occurs primarily in individuals with close contact with horses, mules, or donkeys through inoculation or a break in the skin or by exposing the nasal mucosa to contaminated discharges. A number of instances of airborne infection have been reported in laboratory workers.

PATHOLOGY. The acute lesion is characterized by nodules consisting of polymorphonuclear leukocytes surrounded by a zone of congestion. A characteristic histologic feature is a peculiar nuclear degeneration known as chromatotexis which occurs early and is extensive. Small foci of deeply staining detritus within the abscess result from this degeneration. In older nodules, the reaction is characterized by epithelioid cells surrounding an area of central necrosis. Giant cells may be present. Occasionally calcification may occur. Virtually any organ may be involved.

CLINICAL MANIFESTATIONS. The manifestations in man are protean and are determined in part by the route of infection. Nearly 60 percent of patients have been between the ages of twenty and forty years. The disease has been rare in women, probably because of less opportunity for contact. The manifestations which frequently overlap may be categorized as (1) acute localized suppurative infection, (2) acute pulmonary infection, (3) acute septicemic infection, and (4) chronic suppurative infection.

Infection acquired by inoculation through an abrasion or scratch in the skin usually results in a nodule with an area of acute lymphangitis. The incubation period is probably 1 to 5 days. In all types of acute glanders, there is usually fever and extreme generalized malaise and prostration.

Infection of the mucous membranes may result in mucopurulent discharge involving the eye, nose, or lips followed by extensive ulcerating granulomatous lesions which may or may not be associated with systemic reactions. With systemic invasion, a generalized papular eruption which may become pustular is frequent. This septicemic form of disease is usually fatal in 7 to 10 days.

Infection by inhalation is followed by an incubation period of 10 to 14 days. The more common symptoms include fever, occasionally associated with rigors, generalized myalgia, fatigue, headache, and pleuritic chest pain. Other symptoms consist of photophobia, lacrimation, and diarrhea. Examination is usually normal except for fever and occasional lymphadenopathy, especially in the cervical chain, and splenomegaly. Laboratory findings include mild leukocytosis with 60 to 80 percent neutrophilic leukocytes, but leukopenia with relative lymphocytosis has been recorded. In the acute pulmonary form, chest radiographs characteristically reveal circumscribed densities which suggest early lung abscesses. Other findings may include lobar or bronchopneumonia. In the chronic suppurative form of disease, the most frequent finding is multiple subcutaneous and intramuscular abscesses which most often involve the arms or legs. Approximately one-half of the patients will have associated fever, lymphadenopathy, and nasal discharge or ulceration. Pain at sites other than developing foci and skin eruptions occur in one-third. Visceral involvement including pulmonary or pleural, ocular, skeletal, hepatic, splenic, and meningeal or intracranial involvement occurred in one-fourth or less of the 156 patients summarized by Robins.

DIAGNOSIS. Microscopic examination of exudates may reveal small gram-negative bacilli which stain irregularly with methylene blue; however, organisms are generally very scanty and it is often difficult to find them even in acute abscesses. Giemsa or other modifications of the Romanowski stain may be the best way to identify organisms. *Malleomyces mallei* and *Pseudomonas pseudomallei* cannot be distinguished morphologically from one another. Culturing is often avoided because of the hazard to laboratory personnel; however, if cultures are made, growth occurs on most meat infusion nutrient media. The material often is contaminated with other microorganisms and incubation with benzyl penicillin G (1,000 units per ml) prior to culturing may be helpful. Subcutaneous inoculation of material into a guinea pig or hamster affords an alternative means of isolation. Blood cultures are usually negative except in the terminal stages of disease. Serologic tests show a rapidly rising agglutination titer, which reaches levels of 1:640 within 2 weeks. Serum from normal persons has been reported to show agglutination titers in dilutions up to 1:320. The complement fixation test is less sensitive but more specific and usually becomes positive during the third week; it is considered positive in dilutions of 1:20 or greater. The mallein skin test is of help diagnostically; 0.1 ml of a 1:10,000 dilution of commercial mallein is injected intradermally. Erythema exceeding 10 mm in 48 hr is considered to represent a specific test. The test becomes positive in most patients by the third or fourth week of disease and remains positive for years.

TREATMENT. The limited number of infections in man has precluded evaluation of most of the antibiotic agents. Sulfadiazine has been found to be an effective agent in experimental animals and in man. The dosage utilized has been approximately 100 mg per kg administered in divided doses. In experimental infections, 3 weeks of therapy gave better results than 1 week. Benzyl penicillin is ineffective in vitro and in experimental infections. Streptomycin is bacteriostatic in vitro but was ineffective in experimental infections in hamsters. Broad-spectrum antibiotics such as tetracycline, chloramphenicol, and kanamycin have not been evaluated. In the acute infections, appropriate supportive measures are essential, and in the chronic suppurative infections, the usual principles of surgical drainage should be followed.

PROGNOSIS. The prognosis depends upon the type of infection. The acute septicemic form has been uniformly fatal. The localized or chronic forms have a much better prognosis.

PREVENTION. Next to acquisition from diseased horses, the commonest source of natural disease in man has been contact with human glanders. Isolation is indicated.

REFERENCES

Bernstein, J. M., and E. R. Carling: Observations on Human Glanders with a Study of Six Cases and a Discussion of the Methods of Diagnosis, Brit. Med. J., 1:319, 1909.

Howe, C., and W. R. Miller: Human Glanders: Report of Six Cases, Ann. Intern. Med., 26:93, 1947.

Robins, G. D.: A Study of Chronic Glanders in Man with Report of a Case, Studies from Royal Victoria Hospital, Montreal, 2, No. 1, 1906.

158 MELIOIDOSIS
Jay P. Sanford

DEFINITION. Melioidosis is a glanderslike infection of man and animals with a protean clinical spectrum. It was described first by Whitmore and Krishnaswami in 1912. Stanton and Fletcher chose the name *melioidosis*, meaning "a resemblance to distemper of asses." Melioidosis bears a striking resemblance to glanders both clinically and pathologically, but it is epidemiologically dissimilar.

ETIOLOGY. Melioidosis is caused by a gram-negative motile baccillus, *Pseudomonas pseudomallei*, which can be differentiated from *Malleomyces mallei* by bacteriologic and serologic means. *Pseudomonas pseudomallei* (also known as Whitmore's bacillus, *Malleomyces pseudomallei*, or *Pfeifferella whitmori*) is a small gram-negative motile aerobic bacillus with occasional filamentous chains. When stained with methylene blue, Wayson's, or Wright's stain, marked irregularities with a bipolar "safety pin" pattern are observed. It grows well on standard bacteriologic media.

EPIDEMIOLOGY. The disease is endemic in southeast Asia, with the greatest concentration of cases reported from Vietnam, Cambodia, Laos, Thailand, Malaysia, and Burma. Cases in humans have also been reported from adjacent areas including India, Borneo, the Philippines, Guam, Indonesia, Ceylon, New Guinea, and North Queensland. Cases in man or animals have been reported from Madagascar, Chad, and Turkey. Human melioidosis has been described only rarely in the Western Hemisphere, and confirmed melioidosis has occurred in United States or European residents only when they have traveled in endemic areas. Even when fatal, melioidosis is quite rare; in an autopsy series from Malaya the incidence was 1.5 per 1,000 deaths. Since the original report, cases have been reported from southeast Asia, and by 1953 over 300 human cases were described, including approximately 100 cases in French troops in Indochina between 1948 to 1954. From the early 1960s through January 1968, a total of 80 cases of melioidosis including 9 fatalities have been reported in active duty Army personnel in Vietnam. Of particular interest, but not yet explained, is the observation that at least one-fifth of the cases reported in Army personnel have occurred in patients with moderately severe thermal burns; the majority of these had the acute septicemic form of the disease.

Pseudomonas pseudomallei is a natural saprophyte which can be isolated from soil, stagnant streams, ponds, rice paddies, and market produce in endemic areas. Its ubiquitous nature is illustrated by its isolation as a laboratory contaminant. *Pseudomonas pseudomallei* is capable of causing disease in epizootic form among sheep, goats, swine and horses. Occasional isolates have also been reported from cows, rodents, and cats. Although animals are susceptible to the disease, they apparently do not represent a reservoir for human disease. Attempts to culture *P. pseudomallei* from the urine and feces of a large variety of healthy animals have been unsuccessful. Arthropod-borne infection does not occur naturally, although guinea pigs have been infected experimentally by the bite of both the mosquito (*Aëdes aegypti*) and the rat flea (*Xenopsylla cheopis*). French researchers concluded that man contracts melioidosis by soil contamination of skin abrasions. Ingestion, nasal instillation, or inhalation are other possible methods of spread. In contrast to glanders, infections have been rare in laboratory workers. Man to man transmission of melioidosis has not been described.

PATHOLOGY. The gross and microscopic anatomic findings are fairly consistent for the acute and subacute forms of the disease. In acute infections, the majority of lesions occur in the lungs with occasional abscesses in other organs. In subacute infections, lung abscesses tend to be more extensive and lesions are found throughout the body, in the skin, subcutaneous tissue, meninges, brain, eye, heart, liver, kidney, spleen, bone, and lymph nodes. The acute abscesses are characterized by an outer border of hemorrhage, a medial zone heavily infiltrated with polymorphonuclear leukocytes and an inner core of necrotic debris containing large histiocytes with two or three nuclei that have been termed "giant cells." As in glanders, a striking histologic feature has been the marked karyorrhexis. In chronic infections, the lesion consists of a central area of caseation necrosis, mononuclear and plasma cells, and granulation tissue. Calcification does not occur.

CLINICAL MANIFESTATIONS. The clinical manifestations of melioidosis are variable. The illness can present as an acute, subacute, or chronic process. The incubation period has not been defined; however, based upon the development of infection following injury, it may be as short as 2 days. Following a laboratory accident, an incubation period of 3 days ensued. Clinically inapparent infections may remain latent for a number of years after an individual leaves an endemic area before disease appears. Males are more often affected than women, which is thought to represent occupational exposure. Melioidosis may be recognized as inapparent infection, asymptomatic pulmonary infiltration, acute localized suppurative infection, acute pulmonary infection, acute septicemic infection, or chronic suppurative infection.

Inapparent Infection. Using the complement fixation test, 8.3 percent of apparently healthy adult Thai males gave positive reactions, while only 1 percent of Thai women had positive reactions. None of the sera from a control group from the United States was positive. The incidence of inapparent infections in United States personnel is unknown, but in a recent study, 1.3 percent of a group of patients evacuated for other medical conditions had a significant hemagglutination titer for melioidosis. Occasionally, asymptomatic infections have been discovered by routine chest x-ray.

Acute Localized Suppurative Infection. Infection by inoculation of a break in the skin usually results in a nodule with an area of acute lymphangitis and regional lymphadenitis. There is usually fever and generalized malaise. This form of infection may rapidly progress to the acute septicemic form.

Acute Pulmonary Infection. The most common form of the disease has been pulmonary infection, which may represent a primary pneumonitis or hematogenous spread. The acute pulmonary infection can vary in severity from a mild bronchitis to overwhelming necrotizing pneumonia. The onset may be abrupt without prodromal symptoms or more gradual with headache, anorexia, and generalized myalgia. Fever occurs in almost all patients, is often in excess of 102°F, and may be associated with rigors. Dull or pleuritic chest pain is common. Cough, with or without sputum, occurs. There may be mild pharyngitis. Tachypnea may be out of proportion to the fever and findings on physical or x-ray examination. Chest findings may be minimal but usually consist of râles in the area of pneumonitis. In the absence of dissemination, the spleen and liver are not palpable. Laboratory findings include total leukocyte counts ranging from normal to 20,000 per cu mm. Mild normochromic, normocytic anemia may appear during the illness. The pneumonia usually involves the upper lobes with the radiographic appearance of consolidation. Cavitation frequently occurs. Without specific therapy, the temperature may become normal within a few days; however, the upper lobe cavitation persists, resulting in a radiographic appearance of tuberculosis. In some instances there is progressive pulmonary spread or hematogenous dissemination with the development of septicemic manifestations.

Acute Septicemic Infection. This is the form originally described by Whitmore primarily among narcotic addicts. Subsequent reports, however, have not shown a predilection for debilitated patients. The onset may be abrupt with the dominant symptoms depending upon site of major involvement. In individuals with bacteremia complicating pneumonitis, symptoms may include disorientation, extreme dyspnea, severe headache, pharyngitis, diarrhea, and development of cutaneous pustular lesions on the head, trunk, or extremities. There is high fever, extreme tachypnea, a flushed skin, and cyanosis. Muscle tenderness may be striking. On examination of the chest, signs may be absent or râles, rhonchi, and pleural rubs may be heard. The liver and spleen may be palpable. Signs of arthritis or meningitis may appear. Patients with the septicemic form usually have a rapidly progressive fatal course which in some instances may be too fulminant to affect with therapy. The leukocyte count may be normal or slightly increased. Chest radiographs most commonly show irregular nodular densities 4 to 10 mm in diameter disseminated throughout the lungs. These enlarge, coalesce, and often undergo cavitation as the disease progresses. Pleural effusion is rare. Other radiographic patterns include unilateral irregular mottled densities which became confluent.

Chronic Suppurative Infection. In some patients secondary abscesses develop which dominate the clinical picture. Organs involved include skin, brain, lung, myocardium, liver, spleen, bones, joints, lymph nodes, and even the eye. Such patients may be afebrile.

DIAGNOSIS. Melioidosis should be considered in the differential diagnosis of any febrile illness in an individual who has been in an endemic area, especially if the presenting features are those of fulminant respiratory failure, if multiple pustular or necrotic skin or subcutaneous lesions develop, or if there is a radiographic pattern of tuberculosis in a patient from whom tubercle bacilli cannot be isolated.

Microscopic examination of exudates will reveal poorly staining small gram-negative bacilli which show the characteristic staining irregularities and "safety pin" bipolar staining with methylene blue or Wright's stain. For rapid screening of suspected specimens the direct fluorescent antibody technique is the procedure of choice. *Pseudomonas pseudomallei* will grow on most laboratory media, including eosin-methylene blue agar (EMB) or MacConkey's agar, in 24 to 48 hr. The organisms can be readily differentiated from *M. mallei* and *P. aeruginosa* by standard bacteriologic procedures, which include the hanging drop test for motility. The characteristic wrinkling of the colonies may require 72 hr or longer. The hemagglutination, direct agglutination test, and complement fixation tests are an aid in diagnosis if a fourfold or greater rise in titer is demonstrated in paired sera. Single low titers are difficult to interpret because of nonspecific responses. The complement fixation test is said to be specific with titers above 1:8 during the acute illness, but may cross-react with *M. mallei*. A negative complement fixation test does not exclude disease. The hemagglutination and agglutination tests show more cross-reactions. Titers of 1:40 or more suggest infection.

TREATMENT. The treatment regimen should vary with the form of the disease. Individuals with low titer positive serologic tests, but with no clinical evidence of infection do not require therapy. The choice of antibiotics in active infection should be based upon sensitivity studies, and therapy should be given for a minimum of 30 days. *Pseudomonas pseudomallei* is usually sensitive in vitro to the tetracyclines, chloramphenicol, novobiocin, kanamycin, and sulfadiazine or sulfisoxazole, and in most instances is resistant to benzyl penicillin G, ampicillin, streptomycin, and colistin. In patients with pneumonitis or chronic suppurative lesions who are not too ill, effective therapy has included tetracycline, 2 to 3 Gm daily (40 mg per kg); chloramphenicol, 3 Gm daily (40 mg per kg); or sulfisoxazole, 4 Gm daily (70 mg per kg). If the patient is severely ill, two of these antimicrobials in combination have been recommended for 30 days followed by another 30 to 60 days of tetracycline alone. In patients with extrapulmonary suppurative lesions, prolonged therapy for 6 months to 1 year should be considered. In addition, the usual principles of surgical drainage should be followed. In desperately ill patients with severe pneumonitis or the septicemic form of melioidosis, multiple antibiotics should be administered by the parenteral route. One such regimen has included the use of chloramphenicol, 12 Gm per day; novobiocin, 6 Gm per day; and kanamycin, 4 Gm per day (Chap. 135). In view of the severe potential toxicity of this regimen, its use should be considered only in extremely ill patients, and then only on a short-term basis. Current recommendations for antibiotics in the septicemic form of melioidosis are tetracycline, 4 to 6 Gm per day (80 mg/kg); chloramphenicol, 4 to 6 Gm per day (80 mg/kg); and one of the following: sulfisoxazole (140 mg/kg); or kanamycin (30 mg/kg); or novobiocin (60 mg/kg). The dosage should be tapered rapidly as clinical improvement occurs.

PROGNOSIS. Prior to antimicrobials, the mortality of apparent infection was 95 percent. French experience in Indochina indicated that with chloramphenicol therapy the mortality was 20 percent. With better diagnosis and more prolonged appropriate therapy, the mortality in all except the septicemic form is low. Even with vigorous appropriate antibiotics and supportive therapy, the mortality rate in patients with melioidosis septicemia is greater than 50 percent. Very few patients have had long-term follow-up, and the incidence of late relapses cannot be predicted.

PREVENTION. There is no means of active immunization. In endemic areas, vigorous cleansing of abrasions and lacerations is recommended.

REFERENCES

Brundage, W. G., C. J. Thus, Jr., and D. C. Walden: Four Fatal Cases of Melioidosis in U.S. Soldiers in Vietnam, Am. J. Trop. Med. Hyg., 17:183, 1968.

Gilbert, D. N., W. L. Moore, Jr., C. L. Hedberg, and J. P. Sanford: Potential Medical Problems in Personnel Returning from Vietnam, Ann. Intern. Med., 68:662, 1968.

Nigg, C.: Serologic Studies on Subclinical Melioidosis, J. Immunol., 91:18, 1963.

Prevatt, A. L., and J. S. Hunt: Chronic Systemic Melioidosis, Am. J. Med., 23:810, 1957.

Rubin, H. L., A. D. Alexander, and R. H. Yager: Melioidosis

—A Military Medical Problem?, Mil. Med., 128:538, 1963.

Spotnitz, M., J. Rudnitsky, and J. J. Rambaud: Melioidosis Pneumonitis, J.A.M.A., 202:950, 1967.

159 VIBRIO FETUS INFECTIONS

Robert G. Petersdorf and Marvin Turck

DEFINITION. *Vibrio fetus* infection is economically the most important cause of infectious abortion in cattle. In man, this organism may be associated with obscure febrile illnesses, subacute bacterial endocarditis, meningoencephalitis, and perhaps, abortion.

ETIOLOGY. *Vibrio fetus* is a motile, comma-shaped or spirillar, gram-negative rod with a single unipolar flagellum. It is best identified by its appearance in smears made from cultured material. The organism is slow-growing and microaerophilic, and grows best in liquid media incubated under increased CO_2 tension. Several serotypes have been isolated by agglutination with antiserums from human and bovine strains. Cross agglutination reactions occur with other bacterial species, particularly *Brucella abortus*.

EPIDEMIOLOGY AND PATHOGENESIS. Vibriosis is a venereal infection of cattle, sheep, and goats; when transmitted to gravid heifers or ewes, it results in abortion. The male acts as an asymptomatic carrier of the infection, and the organism has been isolated from the genitalia and semen of bulls. Although vibriosis has been thought to occur only rarely in man, reports of this disease are appearing with increasing frequency. Vibriosis in man may result from direct contact with the organism, as happens in laboratory-acquired infection, or from direct contact with infected cattle. Food and water have been implicated, without convincing evidence, as vehicles for infection. The mouth has been postulated as a portal of entry because cases of *V. fetus* endocarditis have followed dental extractions. Because *V. fetus* has been isolated from several aborted fetuses and has been the cause of neonatal meningitis, a venereal route of infection has been postulated. It is presumed that, as in cattle, the male acts as an asymptomatic carrier who transmits the infection to a pregnant partner. The relationship of *V. fetus* to prematurity, abortion, and neonatal meningitis requires further documentation. In most instances of vibriosis, the portal of entry is not known.

MANIFESTATIONS. Fever is the only characteristic sign of vibriosis in adults, and may be relapsing in character. Thrombophlebitis involving both arms and legs is not uncommon. The disease may also present as classical subacute bacterial endocarditis; septic arthritis; chronic, indolent meningoencephalitis; and fever and abortion in pregnant women. A number of patients have had coexisting disease, including cirrhosis, cardiac amyloidosis, and chronic lymphatic leukemia, or antecedent gastric surgery. Several neonates with a fulminating, lethal meningoencephalitis have been reported. It has been postulated that infection was transmitted to these infants via the placenta. A mild, self-limited diarrheal disease in which vibrios closely related but not identical to *V. fetus* have been isolated from the stool has also been reported in infants.

DIAGNOSIS. Lack of awareness of vibriosis by both the bacteriologist and the clinician has resulted in mistaken diagnosis in most instances. The organisms have been erroneously described as "fastidious strains of *Hemophilus*." Recovery of spirillar organisms in blood cultures should suggest the diagnosis because other spirochetes causing relapsing fever usually do not grow in artificial media. Failure to incubate blood cultures under increased CO_2 tension may delay growth. Identification of the organisms in smears of cultures is the only definitive method of making the diagnosis, which should then be confirmed by agglutinating the vibrios with specific antiserums. Complement-fixing antibody may be present in high titers in the active phase of the disease. Clinically, vibriosis should be suspected in obscure febrile illnesses associated with thrombophlebitis or abortion and premature delivery in pregnant women.

TREATMENT. There are few reports of antibiotic sensitivity of the organisms and various antibiotics, alone or in combination, have been used. A 10-day course of tetracycline or chloramphenicol in dosage of 2.0 Gm per day, alone or coupled with streptomycin, 1.0 Gm per day should eradicate the organisms in most instances. In cases of endocarditis antimicrobial therapy should be extended to 6 weeks. Kanamycin and erythromycin have also been effective in vitro. Penicillin, novobiocin, vancomycin, and polymyxin B are ineffective.

REFERENCES

Collins, H. S., A. Blevins, and E. Benter: Protracted Bacteremia and Meningitis Due to *Vibrio fetus*, A.M.A. Arch. Intern. Med., 113:361, 1964.

Jackson, J. F., P. Hinton, and F. Allison, Jr.: Human Vibriosis, Am. J. Med., 28:986, 1960.

Kahler, R. L., and H. Sheldon: *Vibrio fetus* Infection in Man, New Engl. J. Med., 262:1218, 1960.

Lawrence, G. D., R. D. Biggs, Jr., and T. E. Woodward: Infection Caused by Vibrio Fetus, Arch. Intern. Med., 120: 459, 1967.

White, W. D.: Human Vibriosis: Indigenous Cases in England, Brit. Med. J., II:283, 1967.

160 MIMA-HERELLEA INFECTIONS
Robert G. Petersdorf and Marvin Turck

DEFINITION. Organisms of the tribe *Mimae* are pleomorphic, gram-negative bacilli which are easily confused with members of the genus *Neisseria*. Severe infections with these organisms, including meningitis, bacterial endocarditis, pneumonia, and bacteremia, are being described with increasing frequency.

ETIOLOGY. *Mima polymorpha*, described by DeBord in 1939, is one of two well-characterized species within the tribe Mimae, the other being *Herellea vaginicola*. Organisms formerly described as *Bacterium anitratum* and B5W are synonymous with *H. vaginicola*. These organisms are pleomorphic, gram-negative, encapsulated, and nonmotile. They grow well on ordinary media, forming white, convex, smooth colonies. Diplococcal forms predominate in colonies grown on solid media; rods and filamentous forms are more common in liquid media. The species can be differentiated from the Enterobacteriaceae by their negative nitrate reaction and from members of the genus *Neisseria*, which they may resemble morphologically, by their simple growth requirements, their bacillary form in liquid media, and their usually negative oxidase reaction. *Herellea vaginicola* may be distinguished from *M. polymorpha* by its capacity to ferment 10 percent lactose.

EPIDEMIOLOGY AND PATHOGENESIS. Mimae are ubiquitous and have been cultured from a variety of human sources, including urethral, vaginal, and conjunctival secretions, sputum, pleural fluid, blood, cerebrospinal fluid, feces, cutaneous ulcers, abscesses, chancroid lesions, joint fluid, ascitic fluid, and bone marrow. In addition, these organisms have been found in river water, humidifiers, and oxygen tents. Recent observations indicate that 25 percent of normal subjects are skin carriers of *H. vaginicola*, and 10 percent of *M. polymorpha*. The striking association of mima-herellea bacteremia with cutdowns or indwelling intravenous catheters favors the skin as a major portal of entry in man. The increasing incidence of mima-herellea pneumonia, both as a primary infection and as a superinfection, also points to the respiratory tract as an important portal of entry. It is most likely that the mima organisms are normal human commensals of relatively low virulence which produce serious infections under conditions of decreased host resistance, or in the presence of local tissue trauma, and in this way resemble the Enterobacteriaceae. Although members of the mima tribe have been implicated as an important cause of penicillin-resistant venereal urethritis, the evidence for this relationship is not convincing. Similarly, the role of these organisms as a cause of conjunctivitis and vaginitis requires documentation.

MANIFESTATIONS. Serious infections caused by mima organisms include (1) meningitis, (2) subacute and acute bacterial endocarditis, (3) pneumonia, (4) urinary tract infections, and (5) bacteremia. Usually, the signs and symptoms associated with infections in these sites are no different from those produced by other pathogens. For example, subacute bacterial endocarditis has usually been reported in patients with congenital or rheumatic heart disease and pursues an indolent course, while urinary tract infections may be manifested by asymptomatic bacteriuria, cystitis, or pyelonephritis. Pneumonia often occurs in the form of a superinfection in patients who have received antibiotics, but occasionally herelleae may be primary pathogens in the lung. Occasionally, *M. polymorpha* may be the cause of a fulminating bacteremia, with high fever, vascular collapse, petechiae, and ecchymoses, indistinguishable from fulminant meningococcemia (Chap. 142). More often, however, bacteremia is associated with an overt portal of entry, such as infected cutdowns or indwelling intravenous catheters, surgical wounds, or burns, or it may follow urethral or other surgical instrumentation. These patients usually have severe debilitating disease or have undergone surgery. Many times they have received antibiotics, adrenal cortical hormones, irradiation, or tumor chemotherapy and have had infections with other organisms, usually gram-positive, prior to development of sepsis with mimae. The clinical picture presented by these patients is dominated by endotoxemia (Chap. 134), and the prognosis is very poor.

DIAGNOSIS. The diagnosis of herellosis is usually missed because the clinical bacteriology laboratory is unfamiliar with these organisms and reports them incorrectly or because they are considered contaminants. The confusion attending the taxonomic classification of these organisms has not simplified matters. For practical purposes, isolation of mimae-herelleae (or their synonyms, *B. anitratum*, B5W, *Diplococcus mucosus*, or *Neisseria winogradskyi*) from blood, spinal fluid, sputum, urine, or pus should be considered significant unless there is no evidence of infection on clinical grounds. Since mimae are resistant to penicillin and members of the genus *Neisseria* are sensitive, differentiation of these organisms is of obvious importance.

TREATMENT. Antibiotic sensitivities of *Mima* and *Herellea* strains vary, but most strains are inhibited by kanamycin, colistin, or polymyxin B. Sensitivity to the tetracyclines is unpredictable and most strains are also resistant to penicillin, ampicillin, cephalothin, erythromycin, and chloramphenicol. For serious systemic infections, kanamycin should be administered in doses of 0.5 Gm intramuscularly every 8 to 12 hr (in adults). Since these organisms may produce localized abscesses, surgical drainage may be necessary.

REFERENCES

Daly, A. K., B. Postic, and E. H. Kass: Infections Due to Organisms with the Genus *Herellea*, A.M.A. Arch. Intern. Med., 110:86, 1962.

King, O. H., Jr., G. D. Copeland, and W. M. Berton: Cardiovascular Lesions of Mimae Organisms, Am. J. Med., 35: 241, 1963.

Reinarz, J. A., B. B. Mays, and J. P. Sanford: In Vitro Sensitivity Determinations on *Herellea* and *Flavobacterium* Species, Antimicrob. Agents Chemo., 4:451, 1964.

Reynolds, R. C., and L. E. Cluff: Infections of Man with Mimae, Ann. Intern. Med., 58:759, 1963.

161   *PASTEURELLA MULTOCIDA INFECTION*

Leighton E. Cluff

DEFINITION. *Pasteurella multocida* (*Pasteurella septica*) is a gram-negative, nonsporulating bacillus belonging to the same genus as *Pasteurella pestis*. *Pasteurella multocida*, however, differs in its cultural characteristics, antibiotic sensitivity, antigenicity, and pattern of animal parasitism. All strains are sensitive to penicillin. *Pasteurella multocida* is a respiratory or intestinal commensal in several animals, including cattle, horses, swine, sheep, fowl, dogs, cats, and rats. The bacteria produce fatal disease, so-called "hemorrhagic septicemia," in animals with lowered resistance to infection. Chronic pulmonary infection also may develop. *Pasteurella multocida* is not a common human pathogen but has been isolated from the blood of patients with bronchopulmonary disease. The source of infection in human beings is not clearly identified, but in some instances it has been related to animal contact.

MANIFESTATIONS. Localized infection with cellulitis, suppuration, and adenitis has been described after dog and cat bites. Osteomyelitis has followed such infections. Chronic pulmonary infection has been demonstrated, particularly in patients with bronchiectasis. The respiratory tract may be infected by *P. multocida* alone or in company with other pathogens. Rarely, empyema has been caused by the bacillus. The microorganism has been isolated from the nasal sinuses, but its relationship to infection of the upper part of the respiratory tract is not clear. Veterinarians and other animal handlers have been found to harbor *P. multocida* in the upper part of the respiratory tract without disease. Bacteremia with fever and chills may develop after an animal bite, occasionally without an apparent local lesion. Meningitis, brain abscess, pyogenic arthritis, endocarditis, and pyelonephritis may occasionally complicate the bacteremia.

Not all *P. multocida* infections follow documented animal bites or animal contact. The source of these infections remains unidentified.

DIAGNOSIS. There is nothing specific about the characteristics of infection by *P. multocida*, other than its relationship to animal, particularly cat, bites. Involvement of joints, brain, meninges, and pleural space is associated with abscess formation. The local skin lesion with adenitis may be confused clinically with cat-scratch fever, tularemia, or staphylococcal or streptococcal infection. Leukocytosis is the rule in *P. multocida* infection but is uncommon in tularemia and cat-scratch fever.

Gram stain of infected material shows pleomorphic gram-negative bacilli, usually extracellular. The bacteria may have bipolar staining and can be mistaken for gram-negative diplococci. *Hemophilus influenzae* and neisseria and mimae organisms are most often confused with *P. multocida* but are easily differentiated by cultural characteristics, fermentation reaction, and serology.

TREATMENT. *Pasteurella multocida* is invariably sensitive to penicillin, and administration of this antibiotic in a dosage of 600,000 to 1,200,000 units daily is the preferred regimen. The microorganism is also sensitive to many other antibiotics, however, which can be substituted effectively for penicillin. The variation in sensitivity to antibiotics other than penicillin makes it desirable to test the organism in vitro if other drugs are to be used.

REFERENCES

Bearn, A. G., K. Jacobs, and M. McCarty: *Pasteurella multocida* Septicemia in Man, Am. J. Med., 18:167, 1955.

Morris, A. J., G. B. Heckler, I. G. Schaub, and E. G. Scott: *Pasteurella multocida and* Bronchiectasis, Bull. Johns Hopkins Hosp., 91:174, 1952.

Olsen, A. M., and G. M. Medham: *Pasteurella multocida* in Suppurative Diseases of the Respiratory Tract, Am. J. Med. Sci., 224:77, 1952.

Swartz, M. N., and L. J. Kunz: *Pasteurella multocida* Infections in Man: Report of Two Cases—Meningitis and Infected Cat Bite, New Engl. J. Med., 261:888, 1959.

162 STREPTOBACILLUS MONILIFORMIS INFECTION

Edward W. Hook

Streptobacillus moniliformis causes an acute febrile disease characterized by skin rash and arthritis. Infection is usually transmitted to man through the bite of a rat, and the disease acquired in this manner is termed *rat-bite fever*. Infection is occasionally acquired by ingestion of food or drink contaminated with the streptobacillus. *Spirillum minus* is also responsible for certain cases of rat-bite fever, and the clinical manifestations of S. *moniliformis* and S. *minus* infections (Chap. 183) are sometimes indistinguishable.

ETIOLOGY. *Streptobacillus moniliformis* is a microaerophilic, pleomorphic, gram-negative bacterium that grows in artificial media as tangled chains of bacilli of variable length with beaded or fusiform swellings. Long filamentous forms in interwoven masses may be observed. Primary isolation is best achieved in a fluid medium such as tryptose phosphate broth enriched with 10 to 20 percent blood, serum, or ascitic fluid. In blood cultures, growth usually appears after 48 hr as minute "fluff balls" on the surface of sedimented red blood cells.

A pleuropneumonia-like L (L = Lister Institute) variant can be isolated from the bacterial phase of most strains of S. *moniliformis*. The L form can be maintained in pure culture and transformed back to the bacterial phase. The L variant has been isolated from the blood of man as long as 10 weeks after onset of S. *moniliformis* infection.

The organism is highly pathogenic for mice and for chick embryos, and in these hosts shows a striking affinity for joints and periarticular tissues. Abortion and arrested pregnancy have also been described in mice with streptobacillus infection.

EPIDEMIOLOGY. *Streptobacillus moniliformis* is a normal inhabitant of the nasopharynx of wild or laboratory rats; the carrier rate sometimes exceeds 50 percent. Although most sporadic cases of streptobacillus infection follow the bite of a wild rat, infection may be transmitted by the bite of a laboratory rat, mouse, squirrel, cat, or weasel. Frequently there is no history of rodent bite or direct animal contact. Infection with this organism occurs primarily in infants and children and in men and women whose occupations involve exposure to rats or rat-infested areas. The incidence of the disease is highest in urban areas with poor sanitation and large populations of rats.

Streptobacillus moniliformis infection may occur in an epidemic form related to ingestion of contaminated food or milk. The outbreak in Haverhill, Mass., in 1926 involved 86 persons and was apparently caused by streptobacillus in raw unpasteurized milk or ice cream. The names *Haverhill fever* and *erythema arthriticum epidemicum* have been applied to cases in which there is no history of rodent bite.

CLINICAL MANIFESTATIONS. The incubation period is short, usually 1 to 3 days, although extremes of a few hours to 22 days have been described. The onset of the disease is sudden, with fever, headache, myalgia, and malaise. Chills occur in about 60 percent of patients. A healing puncture wound or ulcerative lesion may be observed at the site of the rat bite, which is usually on an extremity, the face, or tongue. Regional lymphadenopathy may be present but is usually not a prominent feature. A discrete macular rash which fades on pressure develops 1 to 3 days after onset of symptoms in 75 to 80 percent of the patients. The rash is most marked on the extremities, sometimes involves the palms or soles, and may be generalized. The cutaneous lesions may occasionally become confluent, papular, pustular, or petechial. Arthritis of multiple joints appears in about 50 percent of patients during the first week of disease. Large joints are usually involved, but small joints such as those of the fingers and toes may also be affected. The joints are swollen, hot, and tender, and effusions may occur, especially in the knee joints.

Manifestations of disease usually subside after about 1 to 2 weeks, although in the absence of antimicrobial therapy convalescence may be prolonged because of arthritis and recurrent fever.

Bacterial endocarditis and abscess formation in brain, myocardium, or other tissues are rare but serious complications.

The clinical manifestations of food-borne infection are similar to those after rat bite except for the absence of a local lesion.

LABORATORY FINDINGS. The blood leukocyte count ranges from 6,000 to 30,000 cells per cu mm, but the average count is about 12,000. Differential leukocyte count may reveal an increase in the proportion of neutrophils. *Streptobacillus moniliformis* can usually be isolated from blood, joint fluid, or pus during the acute febrile phase of the disease and occasionally for 1 to 2 weeks after subsidence of fever. Agglutinins against the organism develop during the second or third week of illness and are of diagnostic importance if an increasing titer is demonstrated. A false positive serologic test for syphilis occurs in about 15 percent of the cases.

DIFFERENTIAL DIAGNOSIS. *Streptobacillus moniliformis* and S. *minus* infections both occur after rat bite and present remarkably similar manifestations. Differentiation on the basis of clinical data is difficult, sometimes impossible. However, *S. moniliformis* infection is characterized by an incubation period that is usually less than 10 days, prompt healing of the primary lesion without flare-up at the onset of systemic symptoms, a high incidence (50 percent) of arthritis, and a low incidence (15 percent) of false positive serologic tests for syphilis. In contrast, *S. minus* infection is distinguished by an incubation period of 1 to 4 weeks, recurrence of pain, induration, or ulceration at the site of the bite during the acute phase of illness, a very low incidence of arthritis, and a high incidence (50 percent) of false positive tests for syphilis. A relapsing febrile course is typical of *S. minus* infection and is observed only occasionally in streptobacillus infection.

Streptobacillus moniliformis infection must also be differentiated from other forms of acute infectious arthritis, rheumatic fever, meningococcemia, and many other processes characterized by macular eruption and fever.

TREATMENT. *Streptobacillus moniliformis* infections usually respond promptly to therapy with penicillin in moderate doses. A suitable schedule for an adult is procaine penicillin, 600,000 units intramuscularly twice daily for 7 to 10 days. The organism is also sensitive to most of the other commonly used antimicrobials, and erythromycin can be substituted if penicillin is contraindicated. Therapy of endocarditis should be with penicillin, or perhaps penicillin in combination with streptomycin, in dosages similar to that given for streptococcal endocarditis (Chap. 137).

PROGNOSIS. The mortality rate in sporadic cases prior to the advent of effective antimicrobial therapy was about 10 percent. Death was usually related to the presence of bacterial endocarditis, and occasionally to myocarditis, myocardial abscesses, or bronchopneumonia. In patients treated with penicillin or other effective antibiotics the mortality rate approaches zero.

REFERENCES

Brown, T. McP., and J. C. Nunemaker: Rat-bite Fever: A Review of the American Cases with Re-evaluation of Etiology, Bull. Johns Hopkins Hosp., 70:201, 1942.

Dolman, C. E., D. E. Kerr, H. Chang, and A. R. Shearer: Two Cases of Rat-bite Fever Due to *Streptobacillus moniliformis,* Can. J. Public Health, 42:228, 1951.

Hamburger, M., and H. C. Knowles: *Streptobacillus moniliformis* Infection Complicated by Acute Bacterial Endocarditis, A.M.A. Arch. Intern. Med., 92:216, 1953.

Levine, B., and W. H. Civin: *Streptobacillus moniliformis* Bacteremia with Minor Clinical Manifestations, A.M.A. Arch. Intern. Med., 80:53, 1947.

McCormack, R. C., D. Kaye, and E. W. Hook: Endocarditis Due to *Streptobacillus moniliformis.* A Report of Two Cases and Review of the Literature, J.A.M.A., 200:77, 1967.

Roughgarden, J. W.: Antimicrobial Therapy of Rat-bite Fever. A Review, A.M.A. Arch. Intern. Med., 116:39, 1965.

Watkins, C. F.: Rat-bite Fever, J. Pediat., 28:429, 1946.

163 BARTONELLOSIS
Ivan L. Bennett, Jr., and Robert G. Petersdorf

DEFINITION. Bartonellosis (Carrion's disease) is an infection with *Bartonella bacilliformis.* Two well-defined clinical types may develop—an acute febrile anemia of rapid onset and high mortality, designated *Oroya fever;* and a benign eruptive form with chronic cutaneous lesions, called *verruga peruana.* Either of these types may be mild, and asymptomatic cases constitute the greatest epidemiologic hazard.

ETIOLOGY. *Bartonella bacilliformis* is a small, motile, pleomorphic, gram-negative bacillus which stains reddish violet with Giemsa's stain. It can be cultured on enriched media and chick embryos. The organisms are sensitive to several antibiotics in vitro.

EPIDEMIOLOGY. The disease is limited to certain valleys in the Andes Mountains comprising parts of Peru, Ecuador, and Colombia. It occurs in regions between the altitudes of 2,400 and 8,000 ft where the sandfly vector, *Phlebotomus,* propagates. The reservoir of infection in nature is not known, but certain plants and lower animals have been suspected because the disease is often contracted in regions which are practically uninhabited. Epidemics occur more frequently during the rainy season and often coincide with immigration of workers from uninfected areas. In 1966 an acute febrile anemia associated with bartonella-like erythrocytic structures was reported from northern Thailand, the first time this disease has been demonstrated outside western South America. The organisms were similar but not identical to bartonella.

MANIFESTATIONS. The incubation period is approximately 3 weeks but may be longer. The initial symptoms are fever and pains in the bones, joints, and muscles. In the early stages, the disease often resembles influenza or malaria, but blood cultures are positive even in the absence of anemia. Following this initial stage, the patient develops one of the two classic types of the infection.

Oroya Fever. This type is characterized by sudden onset of high fever, extreme pallor, weakness, and a precipitous drop in the number of red blood cells. The count may fall from normal to 1 million per cu mm within 4 or 5 days. The anemia is characterized by normochromic macrocytes in the peripheral blood, striking polychromasia and polychromatophilia, nucleated red cells, Howell-Jolly bodies, Cabot rings, and basophilic stippling. There is also leukocytosis with a shift to the left. Organisms are numerous in the blood, and stained smears may show 90 percent of the erythrocytes heavily invaded. They are also present in the circulating monocytes and fixed phagocytes of the reticuloendothelial system. Secondary infection with salmonellas is an important factor in fatal cases. Neither hemolysins nor agglutinins for bartonellas are found in the serum of patients.

Muscle and joint pain and headache are severe, and insomnia, delirium, and coma are the terminal manifestations. Death can occur within 10 days to 4 weeks. With treatment, or sometimes spontaneously, recovery results if the organisms decrease and fever abates. The red cell count stabilizes, then approaches normal values in about 6 weeks, when convalescence begins.

Verruga Peruana. This form of the disease, characterized by a profuse skin eruption, may follow the anemic form or may occur in patients without previous symptoms. The verrugas vary in color from red to purple. They may be miliary, nodular, or eroding, and they range in size from 2 to 10 mm up to 3 or 4 cm in diameter. The three types of verrugas may occur together, since eruption takes place in successive crops; verrugas of all types and in all stages of development may be found on the same patient. The chief sites involved are the limbs and face, and less frequently the genitalia, scalp, and mucosa of the mouth and pharynx. They may persist for 1 month to 2 years. The eruption is accompanied by pain, fever, and moderate anemia. Bartonellas may be demonstrated in the lesions and cultured from the blood.

TREATMENT. Chloramphenicol, orally or intravenously, is highly effective, particularly when salmonella infection is also present.

REFERENCES

Cuadra, M. C.: Salmonellosis Complication in Human Bartonellosis, Texas Rep. Biol. Med., 14:97, 1956.

Ricketts, W. E.: Clinical Manifestations of Carrion's Disease, A.M.A. Arch. Intern. Med., 84:751, 1949.

Schultz, M. G.: Daniel Carrion's Experiment, New Engl. J. Med., 278:1323, 1968.

Ureteaga, O. B., and E. H. Payne: Treatment of the Acute Febrile Phase of Carrion's Disease with Chloramphenicol, Am. J. Trop. Med. Hyg., 4:507, 1955.

164 GRANULOMA INGUINALE
Albert Heyman

DEFINITION. Granuloma inguinale is a chronic, ulcerative granulomatous disease, usually confined to the skin and mucous membranes of the genitoinguinal area but occasionally appearing in other portions of the body.

ETIOLOGY. The etiologic agent of this disease is the Donovan body (*Donovania granulomatis*), a nonmotile, gram-negative bacillus. In stained smears of the lesions the organisms appear as encapsulated, bipolar bodies situated within large mononuclear cells. In chick embryo cultures, the morphology of the organism is variable and may consist of bipolar forms, curved rods, chains, or unencapsulated bodies. The organism is not pathogenic for laboratory animals and can be cultivated only in artificial media containing yolk material.

INCIDENCE. Granuloma inguinale was once regarded as occurring only in tropical or subtropical areas, but it has been shown to exist in almost every country and climate. The majority of the cases in the United States are found in the Southeastern section, usually among Negroes. The incidence of the disease has decreased significantly in this country during recent years. Approximately 165 cases were reported in 1966.

PATHOGENESIS. Granuloma inguinale is generally believed to be acquired by sexual intercourse. The disease is apparently not highly infectious, however, since it is frequently not transmitted to sexual partners. The factors predisposing to invasion of the organism are not definitely known, but the disease is found most frequently among sexually promiscuous individuals and in association with other venereal diseases. The incubation period varies from 3 to 40 days. Although the majority of infections appear on or near the external genitalia, lesions about the face, hands, and neck are not uncommon. Systemic complications of granuloma inguinale (such as invasion of the bones, joints, and viscera) have also been noted, suggesting that the infecting agent can spread throughout the body by way of the bloodstream.

CLINICAL MANIFESTATIONS. The lesion of granuloma inguinale usually is a painless, sharply demarcated ulcer having an exuberant, red, granulating base which bleeds easily on trauma. The disease is extremely chronic, and the ulcers slowly enlarge and coalesce. Secondary infection frequently is present and produces a foul-smelling, seropurulent discharge. Interference with lymphatic drainage may occur, leading to swelling and elephantiasis of the genitalia, similar to that caused by lymphogranuloma venereum. When healing occurs, further scarring and deformity may appear. Lesions of the cervix of the uterus are frequent and sometimes are mistaken for carcinoma. Lesions about the perianal area closely resemble condylomata lata of secondary syphilis, and dark-field examinations and serologic tests for syphilis are often necessary to differentiate the two conditions.

The disease occasionally produces widespread manifestations such as arthritis and osteomyelitis. In such instances there may be general debility, anemia, and malnutrition; occasionally, these have resulted in death.

DIAGNOSIS. The diagnosis of granuloma inguinale is based upon demonstration of the presence of Donovan bodies. Impression smears of early lesions stained by Wright's method usually will show Donovan bodies lying within the cytoplasm of large mononuclear cells. The smear is of less value in chronic cases. The diagnosis can also be made by histologic examination of fixed tissues. The microscopic appearance of granuloma inguinale is essentially that of a richly vascularized granulation tissue with marked inflammatory cell infiltration. Polymorphonuclear leukocytes are scattered throughout the tissue and form small microabscesses. Numerous large mononuclear cells are also present and show finely reticulated or vacuolated cytoplasm. Phagocytosis of polymorphonuclear leukocytes and other cellular debris by these cells is common. Intracellular or extracellular Donovan bodies are readily seen in tissue sections, particularly in acute cases. In chronic cases they may be found only after considerable search, but the histologic pattern is sufficiently characteristic to permit a tentative diagnosis, even when organisms are not found. Specific serologic tests (complement fixation) and skin tests have been developed, but their diagnostic value is yet to be determined.

TREATMENT. Healing of granuloma inguinale will usually occur promptly following treatment with streptomycin, chloramphenicol, or the tetracyclines. Streptomycin has the disadvantage of requiring parenteral administration. The other antibiotics seem to be more effective and are given orally in doses of 2 Gm a day for approximately fifteen days. These antibiotics have treponemicidal properties and should not be given until repeated darkfield examinations and serologic tests have excluded the diagnosis of early syphilis.

REFERENCES

Pariser, H., and H. Beerman: Granuloma Inguinale, Am. J. Med. Sci., 208:547, 1944.

Rajam, R. V., and P. N. Rangiah: "Donovaniosis (Granuloma Inguinale and Granuloma Venereum)," World Health Organization Monograph Series, no. 24, 1954.

Sheldon, W. H., B. R. Thebaut, A. Heyman, and M. J. Wall: Osteomyelitis Caused by Granuloma Inguinale, Am. J. Med. Sci., 210:237, 1945.

Stewart, D. B.: The Gynecological Lesions of Lymphogranuloma Venereum and Granuloma Inguinale, Med. Clinics N. Am. 48:773, 1964.

Section 7

Miscellaneous Bacterial Diseases

165 ANTHRAX
Leighton E. Cluff

DEFINITION. Anthrax (malignant pustule, charbon, splenic fever, milzbrand, woolsorters' disease) is a disease of wild and domesticated animals that is transmitted to man by contact with infected animals or their products and, rarely, by insect vectors which act as mechanical carriers of the etiologic organism. The characteristic lesion of human anthrax is a necrotic cutaneous ulcer, the *malignant pustule.*

HISTORY. The anthrax bacillus was identified by Royer and Davaine in sheep in 1849 and was, therefore, the first causative agent of an infectious disease ever demonstrated. The classic studies of Robert Koch in 1877, showing that *Bacillus anthracis* was the cause of anthrax, serve as the prototype for the establishment of causation of infectious diseases.

ETIOLOGY. *Bacillus anthracis* is a large, encapsulated, gram-positive, aerobic, spore-forming microorganism that grows well in most nutrient media. Its pathogenicity for laboratory animals differentiates it from *Bacillus subtilis,* which it closely resembles. The spores are killed by boiling for 10 min but can survive for many years in soil and animal products, an important factor in persistence and spread of the disease. The anthrax bacillus possesses a capsule of glutamyl polypeptide, which interferes with phagocytosis of the microorganism. In addition, it contains an anticomplementary substance and elaborates a "protective" antigen and a toxin which is probably of importance in determining virulence.

EPIDEMIOLOGY. Anthrax is worldwide; repeated outbreaks have occurred in Southern Europe, Africa, Australia, Asia, and on both American continents.

Cattle, horses, sheep, goats, and swine are most commonly infected. There have been outbreaks of anthrax among animals in the United States, centering mostly in South Dakota, Nebraska, Arkansas, Mississippi, Louisiana, Texas, and California. The disease tends to occur in animals in late summer and early fall.

The disease in man is acquired by butchering, skinning, or dissecting infected carcasses or by handling contaminated hides, wool, hair, or other materials. It is seen principally in agricultural and industrial employees. The majority of cases of human anthrax involves workers handling imported and unprocessed wool, hair, or hides. The disease usually follows inoculation of bacilli or spores into the skin, often through a wound or abrasion. Intestinal infection has followed ingestion of contaminated meat, and anthrax may develop after inhalation of spores.

PATHOGENESIS. The malignant pustule which follows cutaneous inoculation of anthrax organisms is characterized by vesiculation, neutrophilic infiltration, gelatinous edema, and necrosis. Suppuration is rare in the absence of secondary pyogenic infection. Spread of the bacilli to the regional lymph nodes may be followed by systemic dissemination. Examination of tissues from fatal human cases reveals masses of the bacteria in blood vessels, lymph nodes, and the parenchyma of various organs. There is scanty or absent cellular exudation at these foci, but hemorrhage and edema are widespread. So-called "anthrax pneumonia" and "anthrax meningitis" are, in all probability, an expression of this generalized hemorrhage and edema.

The blood of fatally infected experimental animals contains a lethal toxin, which can be neutralized by specific antiserum. This toxin has been isolated in vitro, but its exact role in the pathogenesis of the disease requires further study.

MANIFESTATIONS. The malignant pustule of human anthrax begins usually on an exposed body surface, as a painless, pruritic, erythematous papule, which vesiculates and ulcerates to form a black eschar. Tiny satellite vesicles are frequent. The ulcer may be surrounded by extensive edematous swelling, which is nontender, nonpitting, and so characteristic of anthrax that it is a valuable diagnostic sign. After about 5 days the ulcer begins to subside, but edema may persist for many days or weeks. Mild tenderness and enlargement of regional lymph nodes are frequently present. Constitutional symptoms are often absent despite extensive local changes, but there may be mild fever, headache, and malaise. In disseminated anthrax, high fever, prostration, and a rapidly fatal course are seen. So-called "woolsorters' disease," a highly fatal disseminated infection, is characterized by cyanosis, dyspnea, mediastinitis, and hemoptysis and is probably dependent on the pulmonary route of inoculation. Human infection may occur from ingestion of the uncooked meat of infected animals; however, enormous numbers of organisms are probably necessary to produce disease by this route.

LABORATORY FINDINGS. The fluid from the cutaneous lesion frequently contains many bacilli, demonstrable by the Gram stain and culture. Bacilli may be found on direct examination or culture of the blood of patients with bacteremia. The blood leukocyte count is normal in mild cases, but there is polymorphonuclear leukocytosis in severe disease. Similarly, the erythrocyte sedimentation rate may be increased. Patients with meningeal involvement show bloody spinal fluid in which the organisms are easily found by direct examination or culture.

DIAGNOSIS. A serologic agar-gel precipitin inhibition test has been devised which has proved useful in epidemiologic studies of anthrax, showing that subclinical infection may occur in persons exposed to the microorganism in industry and demonstrating increasing serum antibody titers following vaccination. A positive diagnosis of anthrax can be made by isolation of the organism in culture. A history of occupational exposure and characteristic eschar and edema should suggest the proper diagnosis. Pyogenic infections of the skin are usually painful; the malignant pustule is not. In addition, cutaneous anthrax is rarely purulent. The differential diagnosis of other diseases characterized by local ulceration at the portal of entry is discussed in Chap. 155.

TREATMENT AND PROPHYLAXIS. Many antibiotics are effective in the treatment of human anthrax, including penicillin, chloramphenicol, tetracycline, erythromycin, and streptomycin. A dosage of 600,000 units of penicillin should be given once or twice daily until the local edema subsides. The eschar goes through its natural evolution in spite of treatment, and lymph node enlargement may persist for several days. *Bacillus anthracis* cannot be recovered from the skin lesion after 24 to 48 hr of penicillin therapy, but it may persist for a longer period when chloramphenicol or tetracycline is used.

Infection of personnel in industrial plants where contaminated animal products are handled still occurs. An outbreak of inhalation anthrax with a high mortality rate was reported in a goat hair processing mill in the United States in the late 1950s. Sterilization of all raw wool, mohair, etc., would probably remove this hazard but has had only limited use. A vaccine prepared from the "protective" antigen of *B. anthracis* is available and is effective in reducing the incidence of infection in an exposed population. Spore vaccines of various types are used with good effect in domestic animals in endemic areas but are not suitable for use in human beings.

Transmission of anthrax from one human being to another has never been recognized. The cutaneous disease was fatal in 20 to 30 percent of cases before antimicrobial drugs were available. The mortality now is less than 1 percent with proper treatment.

REFERENCES

Brachman, P. S., S. A. Plotkin, F. H. Bumford, and M. A. Atchison: An Epidemic of Inhalation Anthrax: II. Epidemiologic Investigation, Med. J. Hyg., 72:6, 1960.

Gold, H.: Anthrax: Report of 117 Cases, A.M.A. Arch. Intern. Med., 96:387, 1955.

Howe, C.: Anthrax, in "Oxford Medicine," New York, Oxford University Press, 1950.

Norman, P. S., J. G. Ray, P. S. Brachman, S. A. Plotkin, and J. S. Pagano: Serologic Testing for Anthrax Antibodies in Workers in a Goat Hair Processing Mill, Am. J. Hyg., 72:32, 1960.

Smith, H., and J. Keffie: Observations on Experimental Anthrax: Demonstrations of a Specific Lethal Factor Produced *in Vivo* by *Bacillus Anthracis*, Nature, 173:869, 1954.

166 LISTERIA INFECTIONS
Paul D. Hoeprich

Listeria monocytogenes is known to cause infection and/or reside in 34 kinds of mammals (including man) and 17 kinds of birds, as well as ticks and crustaceans. Genital tract involvement of the fertile female with consequent perinatal infection of offspring is the most characteristic of the many clinical syndromes collectively known as *listerosis*.

ETIOLOGY. On isolation from nature, listeria are grampositive, microaerophilic, motile bacilli. Serotypes 1 and 4b account for virtually all listerosis in man. Typing serums are not generally available; however, the definitive, epidemiologically essential aid of typing is provided by reference laboratories (Communicable Disease Center, U.S. Public Health Service, Department of Health, Education, and Welfare, Atlanta, Georgia). The usual clinical laboratory can distinguish between *Listeria* and *Corynebacterium*, *Erysipelothrix*, and *Streptococcus*—the bacteria most often confused with listeria—by testing for motility, ability to reduce 2,3,5-triphenyltetrazolium chloride, and animal pathogenicity. In the classic ocular test of Anton, keratoconjunctivitis develops 3 to 5 days after conjunctival inoculation of listeria into a rabbit or guinea pig. Generalized listerosis in the rabbit is associated with monocytosis, which is maximal 3 to 7 days after inoculation.

EPIDEMIOLOGY AND PATHOGENESIS. Worldwide in distribution, listeria have been isolated not only from a variety of animals but also from stream water, mud, sewage, silage, and dry vegetation. Such broad distribution is at variance with the infrequent occurrence of overt disease. Contact with the fluids of infected animals, ingestion of contaminated milk, and inhalation of infected dust have all been implicated as means for infecting human beings on the basis of a few proved cases of listerosis.

Whatever the route of infection, when the gravid female is infected, listeria infection of her offspring can occur either (1) prepartum, via the placenta, or (2) during parturition. In the former situation, dissemination of listeria within the fetus is assured by bacteremia originating in the infected placenta; the fetus is stillborn or is prematurely ejected, virtually always with lethal listerosis. Intrapartum listeria infections may also be associated with premature delivery, but often do not become clinically manifest for 1 or 2 weeks post partum, and then usually present as a meningitis.

Listerosis in other than pregnant women occurs most commonly in persons debilitated by other diseases. There appears to be a predisposition to listerosis in patients with neoplasia—particularly, when it involves the lymphoreticular system, alcoholism, cardiovascular disease, diabetes mellitus, tuberculosis, and any condition requiring treatment with pharmacologic doses of adrenocorticosteroids, irradiation, or cytotoxic agents. Culturally proved listerosis is preponderantly a disease of individuals under one month (about 38 percent) and over forty years (about 32 percent) of age.

MANIFESTATIONS. *Leptomeningitis* accounts for about three-fourths of the cases verified by culture and is the predominant clinical form of listerosis in the United States. Clinically, meningitis caused by *L. monocytogenes* cannot be distinguished from meningitis caused by other kinds of bacteria.

Listerosis of the newborn, the most nearly unique clinical form of listerosis, ranges from meningitis that is clinically apparent within one month post partum, to diffuse disseminated disease in aborted, premature, and stillborn infants and neonatal children who die within minutes to days after birth. In newborn infants listerosis becomes overt 1 to 4 weeks post partum. They, like children one month to six years of age, generally have listerosis localized in the central nervous system.

Infants born alive with listerosis may or may not have fever; yet these babies are critically ill with cardiorespiratory distress, vomiting, and diarrhea. Dark-red skin papules are frequent, particularly on the lower extremities. Hepatosplenomegaly may be present. This form of listerosis, also known as septic or miliary granulomatosis, granulomatosis infantiseptica, argentophile-rod infection, or pseudotuberculosis, was described as a pathologic entity by Henle in 1893.

The findings at postmortem examination are characteristic and mimic those seen in listerosis of rodents: widely disseminated abscesses varying in size from grossly visible to microscopic, involving (in decreasing frequency)

liver, spleen, adrenal glands, lungs, pharynx, gastrointestinal tract, central nervous system, and skin. Typically, the lesions are abscesses, but classic granuloma formation may be seen, depending principally on the duration of infection before death. Microscopic examination of a gram-stained smear of meconium from the normal newborn infant does not disclose bacteria; fetal listerosis results in meconium laden with gram-positive bacilli. For this reason, examination of meconium by gram-stained smear and by culture should be carried out whenever there is gross soiling of the amniotic liquid with meconium, prematurity, or unexplained fever in the mother before or at the onset of labor. This recommendation is reasonable because listerosis in the pregnant woman may be asymptomatic. At most, a week to a month prepartum there may have been malaise, a shaking chill, perhaps diarrhea, pain in the back or flanks, and itching of the skin. Even when symptomatic, the disease is benign and self-limited in the mother; however, as symptoms subside, decrease or cessation of fetal movement may be noted. Infection of the fetus may occur as early as the fifth month of gestation.

The possibility has been considered that repeated abortion is caused by chronic, asymptomatic genital tract listerosis. However, there has been no support from studies of women who had repeated abortions, and *L. monocytogenes* has not been cultured from currettings, lochia, and cervical swabbings, nor have antilisteria antibodies been found in the serum. Furthermore, following delivery of infants with proved fetal listerosis, cervical cultures are, or soon become, negative for listeria; subsequently, conception, gestation, and delivery of normal offspring are usual.

Oculoglandular listerosis is the rare human analogue of the illness initiated in the rabbit by conjunctival inoculation of listeria. There is a purulent conjunctivitis, which may lead to corneal ulceration. Regional node involvement usually limits the spread from the eye. However, listeria meningitis has been reported as a complication of oculoglandular listerosis.

Other rare syndromes caused by listeria include generalized illness with bacteremia and high fever, endocarditis, polyserositis, and cutaneous infection.

LABORATORY FINDINGS. The major difficulty in the laboratory identification of listeria lies in distinguishing it from diphtheroids. Listerias grow well on the usual laboratory media. However, specimens from sites where many other kinds of bacteria are normally present are best cultured on selective enriched media. If the numbers of listerias in a specimen are likely to be few, greater success in isolation may result when the specimen is kept in glucose broth at 4°C and is subcultured weekly.

Serologic methods, using the patient's serum, are not sufficiently specific to be useful to diagnosis.

Monocytosis is not common in human listerosis. Leukocytosis with neutrophilia, as in any acute bacterial infection, is seen in listeria meningitis, oculoglandular infection, bacteremia, and endocarditis. Other laboratory findings, e.g., cerebrospinal fluid in meningitis, are in keeping with the clinical syndromes.

DIFFERENTIAL DIAGNOSIS. Abortion, premature delivery, stillbirth, and neonatal death are more often due to causes other than listerosis—Rh incompatibility, syphilis, or toxoplasmosis.

In patients with leptomeningitis, conjunctivitis, endocarditis, bacteremia, or polyserositis, reports of isolation of "diphtheroids" or "nonpathogens" must always be challenged with the possibility that these may be listerias.

TREATMENT. *Listeria monocytogenes* is susceptible by in vitro testing to sulfonamides, penicillins (of the two most active penicillins, benzylpenicillin, i.e., penicillin G, is significantly more active than ampicillin), cephalosporins, streptomycin, chloramphenicol, the tetracyclines, erythromycin, kanamycin, and novobiocin in concentrations attainable in the blood of patients. Sulfonamides, penicillin, streptomycin, the tetracyclines, and erythromycin have had most frequent clinical trial. On the basis of potency, bactericidal potential, safety, and cost, a combination of penicillin G and erythromycin appears most reasonable. Extensive clinical experience attests to the value of the tetracycline group of antibiotics. Dosage and duration of therapy should vary according to the kind of infection. In fetal listerosis, where therapy must be rapidly effective to be of value, a successful regimen is yet to be devised, although 150 to 200 mg penicillin G per kg body weight per day, by intravenous infusion, merits trial. For listeria meningitis in adults, 12 to 20 million units potassium benzylpenicillin by continuous intravenous infusion per day plus 3 to 4 Gm erythromycin estolate by mouth (or one-half as much erythromycin by intravenous injection) per day are given for 5 to 7 days beyond defervescence. Alternatively, tetracycline, 2 Gm per day by mouth (or one-third as much by intramuscular or intravenous injection), may be used in combination with erythromycin.

Listerosis in the pregnant female requires prompt effective treatment lest the fetus be infected. Tetracycline, 1 Gm per day, plus erythromycin estolate, 2 Gm per day by mouth, should be given for 2 weeks.

Oculoglandular listerosis warrants less massive therapy: 600,000 units procaine benzylpenicillin by intramuscular injection twice daily plus 2 to 3 Gm erythromycin estolate by mouth per day, for 10 days.

Endocarditis and bacteremia from an unknown site have been infrequently treated but are justification for vigorous therapy: 10 to 20 million units potassium benzylpenicillin by intravenous injection per day plus 2 to 3 Gm erythromycin estolate by mouth per day for 6 weeks.

PROGNOSIS. Prompt antibiotic therapy of the acute forms of listerosis, excepting fetal listerosis, is highly effective. On the basis of agglutinin titers, circulating antibody disappears during the months following cure of listeria infections.

REFERENCES

Gray, M. L. (Ed.): Second Symposium on Listeric Infection, Aug. 29–31, 1962, Bozeman, Mont., Montana State College, 1963.

Hoeprich, P. D.: Infection Due to *Listeria Monocytogenes,* Medicine, 37:142, 1958.

Seeliger, H. P. R.: "Listerosis," Basel, S. Karger AG, 1958.

Simpson, J. F., J. P. Leddy, and J. D. Hare: Listeriosis Complicating Lymphoma: Report of Four Cases and Interpretive Review of Pathogenic Factors, Am. J. Med., 43:39, 1967.

167 ERYSIPELOTHRIX INFECTIONS
Paul D. Hoeprich

The parasitic incursions of *Erysipelothrix insidiosa* (*E. rhusiopathiae*) are more frequently expressed in some 20 species of animals than in man. Clinically, unique cutaneous infection is the most common form of human illness; although endocarditis and arthritis have been described, they are encountered but rarely.

HISTORY. Although isolated from mice by Koch in 1880 and from pigs (swine erysipelas) by Loeffler in 1882, erysipelothrix was first related to human disease in 1884 when Rosenbach cultured the bacillus from the skin lesion of erysipeloid in a patient.

ETIOLOGY. As isolated from human disease, erysipelothrix are gram-positive, microaerophilic, nonmotile bacilli. Confusion with nontoxinogenic bacilli of the genus *Corynebacterium* or *Listeria* is not certainly resolved on morphologic grounds alone. Serologic differentiation is reliable when available. Generally, animal inoculation is required: conjunctival inoculation of erysipelothrix in the rabbit only rarely leads to a conjunctivitis; generalized infection in the rabbit may cause a mild monocytosis—a much less marked reaction than is caused by listeria; intraperitoneal injection in mice leads to death in 2 to 4 days, with purulent conjunctivitis the most notable lesion.

EPIDEMIOLOGY AND PATHOGENESIS. Widespread in nature, erysipelothrix gain a foothold through injuries to the skin. Erysipeloid is the usual result and is virtually restricted to persons who in their occupations handle animals, fish, shellfish, or materials derived from animals. The incidence of erysipeloid parallels the incidence of swine erysipelas, being highest in summer and early fall. Yet, persons who tend pigs, even pigs ill with porcine erysipelas, do not commonly develop erysipeloid. If dermal containment of erysipelothrix is not accomplished, bacteremia in persons with damaged heart valves may result in endocarditis.

MANIFESTATIONS. From 2 to 7 days after injury, which has usually healed, a maculopapular, nonvesiculated, sharply defined, raised, purplish-red zone surrounds the site of entry. An itching, burning, painful irritation may precede, and always accompanies, this typical skin lesion. There is local swelling, and when, as is usual, a finger or the hand is involved, nearby joints may become stiff and painful. Centrifugal spread from the site of inoculation is apparent in a day or so. Movement is slow, ½ in. per 24 hr maximally, and more rapid proximally than distally; involvement of the terminal phalanx of a finger is rare, while spread to other fingers and the hand below the wrist is common. With extension, the original center subsides, without desquamation or suppuration. There are usually no systemic signs or symptoms; regional lymphangitis and lymphadenitis are rarely seen. Untreated, the disease heals within 3 weeks in most patients, although relapse has been observed.

The manifestations of erysipelothrix endocarditis may be either acute or subacute, depending on the virulence of the infecting strain of bacilli and on the state of resistance of the host. Usually there are no classic erysiploid skin lesions to suggest the disease at the time that endocarditis is clinically evident. However, a history of recent erysipeloid, when obtained, may be helpful.

Erysipelothrix arthritis is not clinically characteristic but usually can be related to erysipeloid or erysipelothrix bacteremia. Isolation of erysipelothrix from synovial fluid has not been reported.

LABORATORY FINDINGS. Isolation of erysipelothrix depends primarily on awareness of the possibility of the presence of these bacteria. The usual laboratory culture media are adequate for growth of erysipelothrix, but recognition of their significance on culture requires distinction from diphtheroids and listeria. In erysipeloid, organisms are best recovered by incubating a full-thickness biopsy of skin removed from the advancing edge of a lesion in broth containing glucose. Culture of aspirate obtained after injection of sterile, normal saline solution into the periphery of a lesion may also yield erysipelothrix.

With endocarditis and arthritis, the clinical findings are in keeping with the respective clinical syndromes and are in no way characteristic for *E. insidiosa*.

DIFFERENTIAL DIAGNOSIS. The appearance and location of erysipeloid, its slow and limited spread, the lack of constitutional reaction, the history of occupation and injury all serve to identify this disease. The afflicted skin in erysipelas is very erythematous and the face and scalp are affected; there are regional lymphangitis and lymphadenitis, leukocytosis, fever, and malaise. Eczematous lesions may itch, but they display vesicles and little abnormal color. The various erythemas have a different location and do not usually itch or burn; they are more apt to be chronic and nonmigratory.

TREATMENT. Erysipelothrix are inhibited by penicillin, the tetracyclines, chloramphenicol, erythromycin, and novobiocin. The agent of choice is penicillin G. Erysipeloid is adequately treated by injection of 1,200,000 units benzathine penicillin G. Cure of erysipelothrix endocarditis has followed benzylpenicillin therapy in dosages of 2 to 20 million units per day for 4 to 6 weeks.

PROGNOSIS. Prompt antibiotic therapy is highly effective in eradicating erysipelothrix. Second attacks of erysipeloid have been reported. As with bacterial endocarditis from any cause, the prognosis depends on the extent of valvular dysfunction.

REFERENCES

Nelson, E.: Five Hundred Cases of Erysipeloid, Rocky Mountain Med. J., 52:40, 1955.

Wilson, G. S., and A. A. Miles: "Principles of Bacteriology and Immunology," 5th ed., Baltimore, The Williams & Wilkins Company, 1964.

168 FUSOSPIROCHETAL INFECTIONS
John C. Ribble

Fusospirochetal infections are characterized by gangrenous foul-smelling ulcers containing large numbers of spirochetes and bacteria. The lesions are usually located in the mouth and pharynx but may occur in the respiratory tract, the genitalia, surgical wounds, or human bites.

ETIOLOGY. The term *fusospirochetal infection* has been used to indicate that both fusobacteria and spirochetes are found in the lesions. In addition to these organisms, common mouth bacteria such as bacteroides, anaerobic streptococci, anaerobic vibrios, and spirilla are also present. Smith demonstrated that individual strains of bacteria or spirochetes isolated from mouth ulcers did not produce disease after subcutaneous injection into guinea pigs. However, administration of mixed cultures of spirochetes and bacteria resulted in necrotic lesions resembling those found in human disease, making it probable that fusospirochetal disease results from synergistic action of several organisms.

The bacteria and spirochetes associated with fusospirochetal disease are found as normal flora in the mouths of most adults and grow best under anaerobic conditions. Fusobacteria are gram-negative, unencapsulated, nonmotile, spindle-shaped bacilli. The spirochetes associated with the disease are identifiable by a rapid, characteristic motility and can be cultured in artificial media under strict anaerobiasis.

CLINICAL MANIFESTATIONS. Acute Ulcerative Gingivitis (Trench Mouth, Vincent's Stomatitis). The onset of disease is usually sudden and is associated with tender bleeding gums, fetid breath, and a bad taste. The gingival mucosa, especially the papillae between the teeth, becomes ulcerated and may be covered with gray exudate which is removable with gentle pressure. Although involvement of the gums is usually patchy, the process can extend to most of the gingival tissue. If the ulceration is extensive, there are fever, cervical lymphadenopathy, and leukocytosis. The disease may spread to involve other tissues of the oropharynx; it may become less severe and chronic; or it may subside spontaneously. Recurrent ulceration has been described. Most patients who develop fusospirochetal infection have poor oral hygiene. Tartar deposits and eruption or extraction of teeth may damage the gums and allow for bacterial invasion. Edentulous persons almost never develop the disease. Ulcerative gingivitis is prevalent in wartime when nutritional deficiency, crowding, and emotional upsets are common, but the role of these factors in pathogenesis is not known.

Cancrum oris (Noma). Occasionally, ulcerative gingivitis spreads to involve the buccal mucosa, the cheek, and the mandible or maxilla, resulting in widespread destruction of bone and soft tissue. The first indication of cancrum oris is usually slight inflammation of the skin of the cheek. The destruction of tissue proceeds very rapidly. The teeth may fall out, and large areas of bone, even the whole mandible, may be sloughed. A strong putrid odor is present. The lesions are not usually painful, and children may push their fingers through the necrotic areas. The gangrenous lesions eventually heal, but large disfiguring defects are left. Cancrum oris is seen most commonly in severely malnourished children in under-developed areas of the world.

Fusospirochetal Pharyngitis (Vincent's Angina). Fuso-spirochetal infections of the pharynx may occur alone or in association with ulcerative gingivitis. The main complaints are an extremely sore throat, foul breath, bad taste in the mouth, sensation of choking, and fever. The pharynx in the area of the tonsillar pillars is swollen, red, and ulcerated and is covered with a grayish membrane which peels easily. Lymphadenopathy and leukocytosis are common. The disease may last for only a few days or persist for weeks if not treated. The lesion begins unilaterally but can spread to the other side of the pharynx or to the larynx. Aspiration of infected material may result in lung abscess.

Infections of Human Bites. Gangrenous lesions resulting from human bites commonly contain fusospirochetal flora, and fusobacterial septicemia following an infected human bite has been reported. Human bites are much more likely to become infected than dog bites, possibly because of the large number of bacteria and spirochetes surrounding the teeth of human beings and the relative lack of the organisms in dogs and other animals with widely spaced teeth.

Infection of Genitalia. Gangrenous balanitis and ulcers and gangrene of the vulva have been associated with the fusospirochetal flora.

DIAGNOSIS. The diagnosis can be made with certainty only by demonstrating the typical bacteria and spirochetes in sections of necrotic lesions. In clinical practice the diagnosis is made by the appearance and putrid odor of the lesions. Smears of material from mouth ulcers are not usually helpful because fusospirochetal flora are found in the mouths of healthy persons. Ulcerative gingivitis can be distinguished from herpetic gingivostoma-titis by the absence of vesicles and the tendency to involve mainly the gingival papillae. In suspected cases of fusospirochetal pharyngitis, diphtheria and streptococcal pharyngitis must be excluded by appropriate cultures.

TREATMENT. Treatment of ulcerative gingivitis consists of local measures and antibacterial therapy if the disease is severe and painful. During the acute phase the patient should avoid brushing his teeth or other trauma to the gums. A 3 percent solution of hydrogen peroxide diluted with equal amounts of warm water should be used as a mouthwash several times a day. Tartar and necrotic debris should be removed from the gum margins by a dentist. In severe painful cases of gingivitis 600,000 units procaine penicillin twice a day or 1.0 Gm tetracycline a day should be used until improvement is evident. Metronidazole, a drug with some activity against spirochetes and fusobacteria, administered in dosage of 200 mg three times a day for 3 to 7 days is as effective as penicillin in promoting healing of gingival lesions and is considered by some to be the most satisfactory drug for the treatment of fusospirochetal gingivitis. Patients with fusospirochetal pharyngitis or infections of the genitalia should receive 600,000 units procaine penicillin twice a day or 1.0 Gm per day of tetracycline. The treatment of cancrum oris consists of antibiotic therapy with penicillin or tetracycline, debridement of necrotic tissue, and eventual repair of damaged structures. Human bites should be cleansed thoroughly, and obviously necrotic tissue should be removed. The wounds should not be sutured but should be left open and irrigated frequently. Antibiotic therapy should be given to all patients with human bites.

REFERENCES

Glenwright, H. D., and D. A. Sidaway: The Use of Metronidazole in the Treatment of Acute Ulcerative Gingivitis, Brit. Dental J., 121:175, 1966.

Rosebury, T.: "Microorganisms Indigenous to Man," New York, McGraw-Hill Book Company, 1962.

Smith, D. T.: "Oral Spirochetes and Related Organisms in Fusospirochetal Disease," Baltimore, The Williams & Wilkins Company, 1932.

Uohara, G. I., and M. J. Knapp: Oral Fusospirochetosis and Associated Lesions, Oral Surg. Oral Med. Oral Pathol., 24:113, 1967.

Section 8

Diseases Caused by Toxin-producing Bacteria

169 DIPHTHERIA
Louis Weinstein

DEFINITION. Diphtheria is an acute infectious disease produced by *Corynebacterium diphtheriae*, which is char-acterized by a local inflammatory lesion in the upper part of the respiratory tract and by remote effects resulting from toxin which affects particularly the heart and peripheral nerves.

HISTORY. The earliest precise description of diphtheria

is attributed to Bretonneau, who, in 1821, separated diphtheria from other clinical entities with which it had been grouped together as "the croup." Klebs reported the morphologic appearance of *C. diphtheriae* in 1883, and the next year Loeffler isolated the organism in pure culture. The toxin of diphtheria was defined in 1888 by Roux and Yersin. Diphtheria antitoxin was produced by von Behring in 1890 and was soon followed by application of serotherapy in the human disease. The skin test for susceptibility to diphtheria was developed by Shick in 1913. In 1923 Ramon developed the first diphtheria toxoid.

ETIOLOGY. *Corynebacterium diphtheriae* is a gram-positive, nonsporulating, nonmotile rod. Pseudobranching and "palisade" formations are often seen in stained smears. Characteristically, there is a swelling at one end of the bacillus, which gives it a club shape. Diphtheria bacilli have been classified into mitis, gravis, and intermedius groups on the basis of their colonial appearance on tellurite medium, their fermentation reactions, and their ability to produce hemolysis. Some European workers believe that there is a significant difference in the clinical manifestations and severity of the disease related to the strain; gravis and intermedius infections are thought to be accompanied by more severe toxic manifestations and a higher death rate. In the United States, the gravis strain is comparatively uncommon, and less significance is attached to the relationship of the type of organism to the clinical form of the disease.

Corynebacterium diphtheriae produces a toxin which is responsible for many of the clinical manifestations. This material is a protein; as little as 0.0001 mg is a lethal dose for guinea pigs. Strains of diphtheria bacilli which elaborate exotoxin are lysogenic; i.e., they carry bacteriophage ("prophage"). Absence of lysogeny is associated with lack of toxin formation and virulence. The lysogenic state results in a metabolic alteration manifested by toxin production. In the presence of a cofactor, nicotinamide adenine dinucleotide, diphtheria toxin inactivates soluble transferase II, which results in failure to transfer amino acids from soluble RNA to the growing polypeptide chain. Nicotinamide blocks the inhibitory effect of the toxin. The mechanism thought to be involved in the development of diphtheritic myocarditis is interference with the metabolism of carnitine, leading to a decrease in the rate of oxidation of long-chain fatty acids with accumulation of triglycerides and fatty degeneration of the myocardium.

EPIDEMIOLOGY. Diphtheria occurs primarily in the Temperate Zone and is still very common in Europe and Asia. The number of cases of diphtheria in the United States and the British Isles had been decreasing steadily. In 1959 and 1960, however, this falling trend was reversed and 1,741 cases were recorded from 45 states in the United States. The largest number was observed in the South, and more than 80 percent of the patients had never received primary immunization.

Since 1927, the highest frequency has been in children over six years of age, and adults have been involved with increasing frequency. Another striking change has been a decrease in the incidence of laryngeal involvement.

Diphtheria is acquired by droplet transmission from active cases or carriers. Fomites play little role in spread of the infection, but *C. diphtheriae* may remain alive and virulent in the dust of a darkened room for several weeks.

PATHOGENESIS AND PATHOLOGY. The commonest portal of entry for the diphtheria bacillus is the upper part of the respiratory tract. The skin, genitalia, eye, or middle ear may also be primary sites. Growth of the organism is superficial in most cases, and there is little tendency to invade the lymphatics or bloodstream except in the terminal stages. The exotoxin elaborated in the local lesion is carried by the blood to all parts of the body. Dissemination of toxin with damage to remote areas appears to be greater when the primary lesion is in the nasopharynx, less when it is limited to the larynx, and least when it is confined to the nasal mucous membrane; the most intense intoxication is observed when lesions are present in the pharynx, larynx, trachea, and bronchial tree simultaneously.

The primary lesion of diphtheria is the membrane. It is thick, leathery, and blue-white and is composed of bacteria, necrotic epithelium, phagocytes, and fibrin. The membrane is surrounded by a narrow zone of inflammation and is firmly adherent to the underlying tissues; when it is removed forcibly, bleeding follows. Ulceration is not a regular feature; when it occurs, it is very superficial. Regional lymphadenitis is frequent, especially with gravis infections.

The systemic lesions of diphtheria are primarily in the heart, kidneys, and peripheral nerves. The brain is rarely affected. Cardiac enlargement is frequent and appears to be related to myocarditis and not to myocardial hypertrophy. The kidneys reveal cloudy swelling and interstitial changes; they may be quite enlarged. In some cases, particularly those with laryngeal involvement, there is a bronchopneumonia which may be due to *C. diphtheriae* or to secondary invading organisms. When the pneumonitis is caused by the diphtheria bacillus, membrane is present throughout the bronchial tree. The peripheral nerves may reveal fatty degeneration, breaking up of the medullary sheaths, and involvement of the axis cylinder. Both motor and sensory fibers are affected, but the main impact is on motor innervation. The anterior horn cells and the posterior columns of the spinal cord may be damaged. Other central nervous system involvement includes cerebral hemorrhage, meningitis, and encephalitis. Petechial and purpuric lesions are occasionally present in the kidneys, skin, or adrenals. Bacterial endocarditis due to the diphtheria bacillus is extremely rare.

Death results from respiratory obstruction by membrane or edema or from the action of toxin on the heart, nervous system, or other organs.

IMMUNITY. Susceptibility to diphtheria is determined by the presence or absence of circulating antibody to exotoxin. The *Schick test* yields a rough estimate of the quantity of antitoxin in the circulation. The present method of carrying out this test is as follows: 0.1 ml purified diphtheria toxin ($\frac{1}{50}$ MLD) dissolved in buffered human serum albumin is injected intradermally in the volar surface of the forearm; 0.1 ml purified diphtheria toxoid (0.01 Lf) is injected into the other arm as a control. These areas are examined at 24 and 48 hr and between the fourth and seventh days:

1. When the reaction is positive, the site of toxin injection begins to redden in 24 hr; this increases and reaches a maximum in about a week, at which time the lesion may be as large as 3 cm in diameter and moderately swollen and tender. There is usually a small (1 to 1.5 cm) dark red central zone which gradually turns brown, desquamates, and leaves a pigmented area. The area of toxoid injection shows no reaction. A positive test indicates little or no circulating antitoxin or immunity.

2. In a negative test, there is no reaction at the site of either toxoid or toxin instillation. This is consistent with a blood antitoxin level of $\frac{1}{30}$ to $\frac{1}{100}$ unit and immunity to ordinary exposure.

3. Inflammation at both sites of injection within 12 to 14 hr, which reaches a maximum in 48 to 72 hr and then fades, constitutes a pseudoreaction. This practically always indicates immunity plus hypersensitivity to the toxin or other materials in the solution.

4. The combined reaction begins like the pseudoreaction, but the inflammatory response at the toxin site persists after that in the area of toxoid injection has faded. This type of reaction indicates delayed sensitivity to toxin or other proteins and absent or low circulating antitoxin. Combined reactions probably result from previous unapparent diphtheritic infection; their frequency increases with age and is highest in unimmunized groups living in areas where diphtheria is prevalent.

Individuals with negative Schick tests occasionally contract diphtheria, and some persons with positive Schick reactions do not develop the disease after exposure. Fewer than 50 percent of adults in some parts of the United States have "protective" levels of circulating antitoxin.

Second attacks of diphtheria are very rare despite the fact that only about 90 percent of patients who have had the disease become Schick-negative. This suggests that factors other than antitoxin may play a role in protection against infection. In general, immunized patients have a milder illness than unimmunized ones when the initial clinical picture and level of circulating antitoxin are the same. Early therapy of diphtheria with antibiotics may lead to recurrence of the disease if exposure to fresh infections occurs shortly after discontinuation of treatment, suggesting that the development of antitoxic immunity is suppressed in these instances.

CLINICAL MANIFESTATIONS. The incubation period is 1 to 7 days. The local symptoms vary with the site of the primary lesion. Systemic reactions, in the uncomplicated disease, are usually of only minor to moderate severity. Although fever may be present, it is usually low (100 to 101°F), unless infection with another organism (often the beta-hemolytic streptococcus) supervenes. When toxic manifestations are absent, patients feel well except for varying degrees of discomfort at the site of the local lesion. Pallor, listlessness, tachycardia, and weakness are common in more severe cases. Peripheral vascular collapse often develops in the terminal stages of the disease.

Nasal Diphtheria. Diphtheria is occasionally restricted to the nasal mucosa. The infection is usually localized to one side, and a unilateral serosanguineous discharge is characteristic. Membrane is present on the septum or turbinates in the anterior portion of the nose and may persist for a long time. When the disease is located in the posterior nasal areas, extension to the pharynx is frequent and is followed by absorption of toxin.

Pharyngeal Diphtheria. The very early diphtheritic membrane in the pharynx consists of small areas of soft exudate which wipe off easily and leave no bleeding points. As the disease progresses, these coalesce to form an easily removable thin sheet which spreads to cover tonsils or pharynx, or both. Later, it becomes more dense; is bluish-white, gray, or black, depending on the degree of hemorrhage; and is so firmly attached that when it is taken off bleeding occurs. If infection with organisms such as the beta-hemolytic streptococcus is superimposed, the pharynx is diffusely red and edematous. In the average case of diphtheria sore throat is mild but occasionally discomfort can be severe. There is usually a moderate leukocytosis, 15,000 or fewer white blood cells per cu mm.

Marked local spread of the pharyngeal membrane may take place, and the throat, tonsils, and soft and hard palates may be completely covered. Patients with severe disease may show the picture of so-called "malignant" diphtheria. There is great swelling of the submandibular areas and the anterior neck, giving the characteristic "bull neck" appearance. The breathing is noisy, the tongue protrudes, the breath is foul, and the speech thick. The pharyngeal tissues are red and edematous, and the cervical lmyph nodes are enlarged. The skin is pale and cool. There is marked weakness. Occasionally, purpuric eruptions of the skin may appear, particularly on the neck and anterior chest wall. Drowsiness and delirium are common.

Laryngeal Diphtheria. Involvement of the larynx in the course of diphtheria usually results from extension of membrane from the pharynx. Rarely, however, the infection may begin in and be limited to the larynx or trachea. This possibility should be considered in the differential diagnosis of all cases of "croup"; it can be ruled out only by direct examination of the airway. The clinical features of this type of disease are described below.

Skin Diphtheria. Although skin diphtheria is a problem primarily in tropical areas where it is responsible for some cases of "jungle sore" and may become epidemic, it occurs occasionally in the Temperate Zone. Corynebacterium diphtheriae is unable to penetrate unbroken skin and invades wounds, burns, etc. Although the lesions develop most often on the lower extremities, they may appear at any site, including the perianal region. The typical lesion is a round, deep, "punched-out" ulcer 0.5 cm to several centimeters in diameter. In the early stages, the lesions are covered by a gray, yellow, or gray-brown membrane which strips off easily to reveal a clean hemorrhagic base.

This dries quickly and becomes covered by thin, leathery, dark brown or black, adherent membrane which separates spontaneously 1 to 3 weeks after infection. The margin of the fully developed ulcer is usually slightly undermined, purple, rolled, and sharply defined. Breakdown, either after minor trauma or spontaneously, is frequent, and development of anesthesia, after a few weeks, is characteristic. Healing is usually slow, and scarring is the rule. Myocarditis occurs in about 5 percent and peripheral neuritis in about 20 percent of cases of skin diphtheria; the Guillain-Barré syndrome may develop.

Diphtheria Lesions in Other Areas. Diphtheria may involve the uterine cervix, vagina, vulva, or penis (after circumcision). Diphtheritic cystitis and urethritis have been observed following prostatectomy. These lesions are often secondary to respiratory tract involvement but may be primary. Toxic manifestations are common. The tongue, buccal mucous membrane, gums, and esophagus may also be affected. Infection of the conjunctiva occurs rarely. Otitis media may occur as an isolated syndrome or secondary to diphtheria in the upper part of the respiratory tract; aural discharge from which virulent organisms can be isolated may persist for many months.

COMPLICATIONS OF DIPHTHERIA. The complications of diphtheria are of two types: those which result from spread of the membrane in the respiratory tract and those which are due to the activity of the toxin absorbed from the local lesion.

Extension and Spread of Membrane. The membrane of diphtheria may spread from the fauces over the posterior pharyngeal wall into the nasopharynx and anterior portion of the nose. This usually produces severe illness and is accompanied by a high risk of toxic manifestations. Occlusion of the airway is first manifested by tachypnea and, as obstruction increases, restlessness, use of accessory muscles of respiration, and finally cyanosis and death. This progression of events occurs most frequently in children. In some cases, the membrane extends diffusely into the bronchial tree and produces clinical manifestations of pneumonia. Bronchopulmonary diphtheria is very serious not only because of obstruction but also because of the large surface from which toxin can be absorbed; the death rate is very high. When the pulmonary lesion regresses, pieces of membrane may break off and produce sudden occlusion of the airway; a cast of the bronchial tree may be coughed up. On occasion, pharyngeal membrane has extended into the esophagus and cardia of the stomach.

Toxic Complications of Diphtheria. Studies of the mode of action of diphtheria toxin suggest that it inhibits the transfer of amino acids from soluble RNA to growing polypeptide chains, resulting in failure of the amino acids to be incorporated into the polypeptide; a cofactor, nicotinamide adenine dinucleotide, is required for toxin activity. The effects of the toxin on the myocardium are thought to result from its production of a decrease in the rate of oxidation of long-chain fatty acids by interfering with the metabolism of carnitine. Because of this block, triglycerides accumulate in the myocardium and cause fatty degeneration of muscle.

Myocarditis develops in about two-thirds of patients with diphtheria but is clinically evident in about 10 percent. In these, softening of the heart sounds, systolic murmurs, bundle branch block, incomplete or complete heart block, atrial fibrillation, ventricular premature beats or tachycardia, or both, are detectable. Ventricular fibrillation is a constant threat and is frequently the mechanism responsible for sudden death. Ninety percent of the patients with atrial fibrillation, ventricular tachycardia, or complete heart block die. Frank congestive failure due to diphtheritic myocarditis occurs infrequently. Evidence of failure of the right side of the heart usually develops first, and the most common symptom is pain in the right upper quadrant of the abdomen due to rapid engorgement of the liver. Decompensation of the left side of the heart with dyspnea and rales may appear later. Diphtheritic heart disease is not necessarily "benign," and permanent cardiac damage can occur in survivors. Fibrosis of the myocardium has been observed in patients who have expired several weeks after mild myocarditis was detected by electrocardiographic study; the degree and extent of fibrotic change are often greater than would be predicted from the type of abnormality in the tracing.

Peripheral neuritis can occur at three different times in the course of diphtheria. Paralysis of the soft palate and posterior pharyngeal wall occasionally appears very early in the disease (2 to 3 days). Neuritis develops most frequently during the second to sixth week. At this time, cranial nerve dysfunction is most common; the third, sixth, seventh, ninth, and tenth nerves are involved most often. Loss of accommodation, nasal voice, and difficulty in swallowing are the most frequent manifestations. However, any of the peripheral nerves may be affected, with resulting paralysis of the extremities, diaphragm, or intercostal muscles; death may occur from respiratory failure. The peripheral neuritides which appear in the second to the sixth week of the disease are featured almost completely by motor loss; sensory changes are uncommon and, when present, are minor in degree. Peripheral neuritis may not appear until 2 to 3 months after the onset of diphtheria. In these cases, the clinical picture and course resemble infectious polyneuritis. The outstanding findings are loss of sensation in a "glove and stocking" distribution and albuminocytologic dissociation in the cerebrospinal fluid identical with that observed in the Guillain-Barré syndrome. Motor weakness and areflexia may develop with progression of involvement. Very rarely, a fatal ascending paralysis of the Landry type may develop. Complete recovery is the rule but may take as long as a year.

Encephalitis is a rare toxic complication of diphtheria. Shock, which develops suddenly and without warning, is an occasional cause of rapid death in this disease. In some instances, it may be a consequence of myocarditis; in others, no cause can be discovered.

Other Complications. Cerebral infarction with hemiplegia occurs rarely in diphtheria; it is probably due to embolization from atrial thrombi in patients with myocarditis and cardiac dilatation. Superinfection of the lungs is a risk in all patients with diphtheria who are given antimicrobial agents. Purpuric skin eruptions may be seen in severe cases, especially those with the malignant or "bull neck" form of the disease. Thrombocytopenia is a rare finding. A mild morbilliform rash may be present during the early stage of development of the diphtheritic membrane. Beta-hemolytic streptococcal pharyngitis is uncommon because antibiotics are usually administered from the beginning of the disease to eradicate the carrier state. Serum sickness occasionally follows the use of antitoxin. Relapses of diphtheria may occur when patients given antimicrobial agents are exposed to fresh cases soon after therapy has been discontinued. Bacteremia, endocarditis, and meningitis are rare complications.

COURSE AND PROGNOSIS. The membrane may be present for only 3 to 4 days in mild faucial diphtheria, even when no antitoxin is given; it usually lasts for about a week in cases of moderate severity. It is quite common for the pharyngeal lesion to increase in extent and thickness during the first 24 hr after the administration of antitoxin. As the disease begins to recede, the exudate softens, wipes off easily leaving no bleeding areas, becomes patchy so that it resembles the picture of "follicular" tonsillitis, and finally disappears, leaving normal underlying mucous membrane.

The fatality rate in diphtheria prior to the use of specific antitoxin was about 35 percent in average cases and 90 percent in those with laryngeal involvement. Since specific serotherapy has been employed, mortality has been reduced to a range of 3.5 to 22 percent, but it is still highest when the larynx is affected. The overall death rate in the United States is about 10 percent. Although there is no difference in the distribution of gravis and mitis strains in mild forms of myocarditis, the gravis type is three times as common as mitis in cases with severe myocardial disease and a high death rate. Age influences the outcome of diphtheria, and death is most frequent in the very young and old. Immunization is a factor of great importance in determining prognosis. The fatality rate in immunized individuals is one-tenth that in the unimmunized population. Paralysis is five times and "bull neck" fifteen times less common in immunized patients. As a rule, the longer the delay in the use of serotherapy, the greater the incidence of complications and death.

A white blood cell count higher than 25,000 per cu mm is associated with a higher risk of complications and death. This is possibly related to the fact that this degree of leukocytosis is often present in patients in whom another organism, hemolytic streptococci for example, is producing disease at the same site as the diphtheria bacillus.

DIAGNOSIS. The features of the fully developed diphtheritic membrane, especially in the pharynx, are sufficiently characteristic to suggest the possibility of the disease. However, not much reliance can be placed on the appearance of the pharyngeal exudate in establishing the diagnosis. There are a number of other infections in which pseudomembranes which may be confused with those of diphtheria are present; among these are infectious mononucleosis (Chap. 255), streptococcal pharyn-

gitis (Chap. 140), viral exudative pharyngitis, fusospirochetal angina (Chap. 168), acute moniliasis (Chap. 190), and staphylococcal infections of the pharynx which may follow chemotherapy.

The only positive method of establishing the presence of diphtheria is by demonstrating the typical organisms in stained smears and cultures. With some experience, it is possible to make a positive diagnosis from methylene blue–stained preparations in 75 to 85 percent of cases. These observations require confirmation by isolation of the organisms. Diphtheria bacilli can be recovered from patients who have not been given antibiotic agents in 8 to 12 hr on Loeffler's medium incubated at 37°C; C. diphtheriae also multiplies, but more slowly, on ordinary blood agar. If drugs, especially penicillin or erythromycin, have been administered prior to obtaining material for culture, the organisms may not grow out for as long as 5 days or may fail to grow at all.

Staining of suspected material with fluorescein-labeled diphtheria antitoxin may allow the microbiologic diagnosis of diphtheria to be made rapidly. All strains of the diphtheria bacillus recovered from patients should be examined for toxin production. This can be accomplished in guinea pigs or by an in vitro technique.

TREATMENT. Patients with diphtheria should be isolated and kept at strict bed rest, with reduction of physical effort during the early convalescent stages. Local therapy of the diphtheritic lesion is usually not required. A soft diet is preferred. There is no indication for parenteral feeding if the patient is able to take adequate calories and fluid by mouth.

The only specific treatment for diphtheria is antitoxin. Dosage schedules are somewhat empiric, but experience has suggested the use of certain quantities in the therapy of lesions of varying severity, extent, and location. Antiserum must never be given until the presence of sensitivity to horse serum, using the eye and skin tests, has been determined. Despite a negative test for hypersensitivity, it is probably best to administer antiserum in divided doses to all adults. The following schedule is widely used: When exudate is present on only one tonsil, 5,000 units of antitoxin are given; for lesions covering both tonsils, 10,000 units are administered. When the entire pharyngeal wall and the tonsils are involved, the quantity is increased to 20,000 to 50,000 units. Laryngeal diphtheria is treated with 50,000 to 100,000 units of antitoxin. Because of the length of time required for antibody to reach maximal levels in the blood after intramuscular injection, one-half the calculated dose is given by this route. If no reaction occurs, the rest of the antitoxin is infused slowly by vein. Desensitization should be attempted if the initial skin or eye tests are positive. A rare patient may be sensitive to such a high degree that the antiserum cannot be administered without the risk of death. Nothing is gained by repeated injections of antitoxin.

Antitoxin should be given as early in the course of diphtheria as possible. It has been suggested that larger quantities of antiserum than those recommended above should be used when therapy is given late; because toxin is fixed instantaneously to tissues and then cannot be neutralized by antitoxin, the effectiveness of this practice is questionable. Antimicrobial agents do not alter the course, incidence of complications, or outcome of diphtheria.

Patients with laryngeal obstruction should be watched very carefully. In mild cases, inhalation of warm or cool steam may be beneficial. If advancing signs of airway obstruction develop, intubation or tracheostomy should be performed. These procedures must never be delayed until cyanosis appears, because, at this point, stimulation of the pharynx or trachea can result in sudden cardiac standstill and death. Sedative or hypnotic agents should not be given because they may obscure increasing respiratory difficulty. Intubation is the preferred method of relieving diphtheritic laryngeal obstruction. However, if experienced personnel are not available, tracheostomy is probably the safer measure. Because patients with tracheal tubes in place cannot call for help, special nurses must be on duty at all times to ensure prompt and proper care. Tracheostomy or intubation has to be maintained for at least 3 or 4 days.

The pulse and blood pressure should be determined frequently. Little can be done to alter the course of the myocarditis. Quinidine has been tried to prevent arrhythmias, but with little success. This drug has also been given after abnormal cardiac rhythms have appeared; the results have not been striking, and deleterious effects have been suspected in some instances. Likewise the effectiveness of procaine amide when ventricular premature beats or tachycardia supervene has not been documented. The administration of digitalis when cardiac failure occurs in diphtheria is controversial. Some observers consider this drug completely contraindicated and employ fluid and salt restriction and diuretics. Others feel, however, that careful administration of digitalis is both safe and beneficial. The treatment of shock is discussed in Chap. 134. There is no evidence that corticosteroids or corticotropin are of value in the treatment of diphtheria or of its complications.

Treatment of the Carrier. *Corynebacterium diphtheriae* usually disappears from the upper part of the respiratory tract after 2 to 4 weeks in patients who do not receive antimicrobial drugs; in a small number of individuals the organism may persist for a long time or be present permanently. The most effective treatment of the acute and chronic carrier state is penicillin or erythromycin. The administration of 300,000 to 600,000 units penicillin G in divided doses per day for 10 to 12 days eliminates the diphtheria bacilli in practically all cases. A single injection of 600,000 units of procaine penicillin per day produces about the same results. Erythromycin, 25 to 50 mg per kg body weight per day orally, is also highly effective and is the drug of choice in persons known to be allergic to penicillin. Retreatment is indicated for carriers in whom the organisms are not eradicated after the first trial. This is preferable to tonsillectomy, which may be considered as a last resort should the carrier state persist despite repeated courses of antibiotics.

PREVENTION. Diphtheria is, for the most part, a preventable disease. Immunization at the age of three months should be routine. Diphtheria toxoid is best given together with tetanus toxoid and pertussis vaccine (DPT), because antibody titers are higher with combined immunization. Booster doses should be administered at the age of one year and again just before a child goes to school. Although it has been suggested that Schick testing is not necessary in those who have been immunized, many physicians still carry this out to determine the status of antitoxic immunity. A Schick test acts as a booster. A negative reaction does not indicate absolute protection against diphtheria. The development of highly purified toxoid has made protection possible with little or no risk of untoward sequelae. The usual procedure is to inject 0.1 ml purified toxoid subcutaneously (Moloney test). If there is no reaction in 24 to 48 hr, the regular immunization procedure is carried out.

Unimmunized persons exposed to an active case of diphtheria should be given 2,000 units of antitoxin intramuscularly, after appropriate skin and eye tests. In individuals who have been immunized previously, a booster dose of toxoid is usually sufficient. Patients with diphtheria should be quarantined until three successive cultures of the nose, throat, or other infected areas, taken at 24-hr intervals, are negative. If antibiotics have been administered, cultural studies should not be initiated until at least 24 hr after cessation of therapy.

REFERENCES

Beach, M. W., W. B. Gamble, Jr., C. H. Zemp, Jr., and M. Q. Jenkins: Erythromycin in the Treatment of Diphtheria and Diphtheria Carrier State, Pediatrics, 16:335, 1955.

Boyer, N. H., and L. Weinstein: Diphtheritic Myocarditis, New Engl. J. Med., 239:913, 1948.

Doege, T. C., C. W. Heath, Jr., and I. L. Sherman: Diphtheria in the United States, 1959–1960, Pediatrics, 30:194, 1962.

Goor, R. S., and A. M. Pappenheimer, Jr.: Studies on the Mode of Action of Diphtheria Toxin, J. Exp. Med., 126:899, 913, 923, 1967.

Gore, I.: Myocardial Changes in Fatal Diphtheria: A Summary of Observations in 221 Cases, Am. J. Med. Sci., 219:257, 1948.

Hollander, M. H.: Diphtheria of the Skin, U.S. Air Force Med. J., 2:229, 1951.

Ipsen, J.: Circulating Antitoxin at the Onset of Diphtheria in 425 Patients, Medicine, 251:459, 1954.

——: Immunization of Adults against Diphtheria and Tetanus, New Engl. J. Med., 251:459, 1954.

Naiditch, M. J., and A. G. Bower: Diphtheria: A Study of 1,433 Cases Observed during a Ten-year Period at the Los Angeles County Hospital, Am. J. Med., 17:229, 1954.

Parsons, E. I.: Induction of Toxigenicity in Non-toxigenic Strains of C. Diphtheriae with Bacteriophages Derived from Non-toxigenic Strains, Proc. Soc. Exp. Biol. Med., 90:91, 1955.

——, M. Frobisher, M. More, and M. A. Aiden: Rapid Virulence Test in Diagnosis of Diphtheria, Proc. Soc. Exp. Biol. Med., 88:368, 1955.

Scheid, W.: Diphtherial Paralysis: An Analysis of 2,292 Cases of Diphtheria in Adults Which Included 174 Cases of Polyneuritis, J. Nervous Mental Dis., 116:1095, 1952.

Weinstein, L.: The Treatment of Acute Diphtheria and the Chronic Carrier State with Penicillin, Am. J. Med. Sci., 213:308, 1947.

Witaker, J. A., J. D. Nelson, and C. W. Fink: The Fluorescent Antitoxin Test for the Immediate Diagnosis of Diphtheria, Pediatrics, 27:214, 1961.

Wittels, B., and R. Bressler: Biochemical Lesion of Diphtheria Toxin on the Heart, J. Clin. Invest., 43:630, 1964.

170 TETANUS
Edward S. Miller

DEFINITION. Tetanus is a severe intoxication characterized by generalized hypertonicity of skeletal muscles and convulsive seizures. The disease is caused by an exotoxin produced by *Clostridium tetani*.

HISTORY. Tetanus was described by Hippocrates, and has been documented over the centuries by many authors as a scourge of parturient women, newborn babies, and wounded soldiers. For example, in the eighteenth century, 1 of every 6 infants born in the Rotunda Hospital in Dublin died of tetanus neonatorum. Modern knowledge of this disease had its inception in 1884, when Nicolaier produced tetanus in animals by injecting garden soil. Subsequently, the bacillus was isolated in pure culture and found to produce an exotoxin. In 1890, Von Behring and Kitasato succeeded in immunizing animals by injecting minute amounts of toxin, and found that these animals produced antibodies. Ramon created tetanus toxoid in 1923. These studies permitted the development of immunologic methods for the prevention of the disease.

ETIOLOGY. *Clostridium tetani* is a large, motile, spore-forming, gram-positive bacillus without a capsule. It is an obligate anaerobe. The organism produces spherical terminal spores which, when protected from direct sunlight, can survive for many years. The spores are found in soil and street dust in most of the world and are often present in the intestinal contents of man and animals. Under suitable conditions, the spores germinate to the vegetative forms, which then elaborate a powerful exotoxin. At least 10 antigenic types have been distinguished, but differentiation is of no practical importance, because the exotoxins of all have the same immunologic properties. The vegetative forms and the exotoxin are destroyed in 10 min at 65°C. Spores can be eradicated with certainty only by autoclaving at 115°C for 20 min.

EPIDEMIOLOGY. Tetanus is endemic throughout the world, but has a low incidence in the cold polar regions and occurs with increasing frequency in damp, warm climates. The prevalence is greatest in developing areas of the world and is associated with lack of education, poor hygiene, deficient public health practices, poverty, and unavailability of good medical care. It has been estimated that between 1951 and 1960, 1 million people in the world contracted tetanus, and one-half of them died. The disease has become relatively rare in the United

States; approximately 400 to 500 cases per year are recorded, but it is estimated that only 20 percent of cases are reported. The majority of cases occurs in the Southeast and South Central states, and fatality rates vary from 30 to 70 percent. One-third of these deaths occur in children less than one year of age, chiefly as the result of contamination of the umbilical stump at birth.

PATHOGENESIS. Tetanus organisms gain entrance to the body through wounds. The organism is so ubiquitous in nature that almost any injured part may be contaminated. Many lesions, both large and small, including lacerations, slivers, compound fractures, gunshot wounds, varicose ulcers, tooth extractions, burns, frostbites, bedsores, penetrating lesions produced by nails, and human and animal bites, offer a suitable haven for proliferation of the organisms. Cases have resulted from the use of unsterile surgical supplies and biologic materials such as catgut. Infections of the post-partum uterus and the umbilical stump are now rare where modern obstetric techniques are used, but are common where these are not available. The disease also follows piercing of earlobes and circumcision performed under unhygienic conditions.

Clostridium tetani is a strict anaerobe and proliferates only in the presence of an oxidation-reduction potential far lower than that existing in normal living tissue. A fall in potential may occur in the presence of necrotic tissue, of soil or other foreign materials, or of tetanus toxin itself. Once the organism begins to grow, it produces toxin and thereafter can maintain the conditions necessary for continued multiplication. If conditions for growth are not optimal, tetanus spores may persist in the body for many months or years, in a dormant but viable state. If tissues are traumatized later, as in a surgical procedure, tetanus may then develop.

Tetanus bacilli grow locally in a wound, show little capacity to invade, and are in themselves harmless. They cause disease only by virtue of exotoxin elaborated during growth. Two toxins are produced, tetanolysin and tetanospasmin. Tetanolysin lyses red corpuscles in vitro and may also damage leukocytes. Its clinical significance is unknown, but it may contribute to tetanus infection by causing local tissue necrosis and by antiphagocytic action. Tetanospasmin is a protein with a molecular weight of 67,000. It is a potent neurotoxin, and it is estimated that a dose of 0.13 mg is lethal for man.

The toxin acts on the internuncial cells in the vicinity of the anterior horn cells of the spinal cord, causing a reduction of the central inhibitory balancing influences on motor neurone activity. This results in intensified reflex response to afferent stimuli, leading to exaggerated motor activity, spasticity of skeletal muscles, and paroxysmal seizures. The toxin also acts on the medullary centers. Tetanospasmin has a strong affinity for certain nerve tissues, and once combined with receptor cells, it cannot be neutralized by antitoxin. Nevertheless, the toxin is inactivated eventually by some unknown mechanism because patients who recover from tetanus show no residual neurologic defects.

The route by which toxin travels from the local lesion

to the central nervous system is a matter of controversy. There is good experimental evidence to support the theory that toxin can enter the neuromuscular end organs, pass centripetally up the axones of motor nerves to the cord, and then spread throughout the central nervous system. This pathway may account for the rare case of local tetanus. Ordinarily, most of the toxin is carried from the local lesion to the nervous system via the bloodstream, and this sequence of events probably obtains in generalized tetanus.

MANIFESTATIONS. The incubation period varies from 2 days to several months, but in two-thirds of cases it falls within the range of 6 to 15 days. Some patients have prodromal symptoms of restlessness and headache. In others, the first symptoms are caused by the developing muscular rigidity, with vague discomfort in the jaws, neck, or lumbar region. Among the first muscles to show involvement are those innervated by the fifth, seventh, ninth, tenth, eleventh, and twelfth cranial nerves. Spasm of the muscles of mastication causes trismus. This highly characteristic phenomenon gives the disease its common name of *lockjaw*. Sustained contraction of the facial muscles produces a distorted grin called *risus sardonicus*. Spasm of the pharyngeal muscles makes swallowing difficult. Stiff neck and opisthotonos are also among the early signs. Progressively, other muscle groups become involved, with tightness of the chest and rigidity of the abdominal wall, back, and limbs. The distribution of muscular rigidity may vary, as may the sequence of appearance of spasm. The *period of onset* of tetanus is considered to be the elapsed time from the first symptom until the appearance of reflex convulsive spasms. If this interval is less than 24 hr, the disease is most severe, and the fatality rate high.

The patient is conscious and mentally clear, restless, and apprehensive, and has much pain from muscular spasms. Coughing and swallowing become difficult, and breathing laborious. There is profuse perspiration. Fever is usually low-grade unless complications are present. The wound through which C. *tetani* was introduced is usually evident, although in 10 to 20 percent of patients it cannot be found. The tendon reflexes are hyperactive, often with sustained clonus, but there are no sensory changes. The symptoms and signs increase in severity for several days. Generalized tonic convulsions appear in all but the milder cases and are accompanied by spasm of the larynx and the respiratory muscles. Convulsions are precipitated by various stimuli such as a sudden noise, a hypodermic injection, or a jostling of the bed. The hypertonia sometimes disappears prior to death. If the patient survives, the intensity of muscle spasm begins to diminish slowly after 2 to 3 weeks, and complete recovery may take several months. Occasionally, in mild cases, there is only muscle rigidity without seizures. Sometimes the administration of tetanus antitoxin forestalls the development of generalized tetanus but not of local tetanus involving the muscles around the site of injury.

Complications. Complications are frequent. *Atelectasis* is common and may be followed by pneumonia, which

seriously lessens the chances of recovery. *Venous thrombosis* may occur and may be followed by pulmonary embolization. Acute *gastric ulcers* with hemorrhage or perforation occur. Constipation and fecal impaction, and urinary retention, are common. Urinary tract infections often develop in patients requiring catheterization. Traumatic *glossitis* is frequent and is an important cause of airway obstruction. *Compression fractures* of vertebras sometimes result from the convulsive seizures. *Decubitus ulcers* are likely to occur in patients under heavy sedation. *Serum sickness* may appear from 3 to 12 days after administration of equine antitoxin. Footdrop and muscle contractures sometimes follow prolonged unconsciousness with the limbs in poor position.

Death can result from several causes. Tetanus toxin itself can be lethal as a result of damage to the medullary centers, especially the respiratory center. Asphyxia from respiratory muscle or laryngeal spasm or from aspiration of secretions, vomitus, or food may be the immediate cause of death. Other causes include pneumonia, pulmonary embolism, and the complications of drugs used to control muscle hyperactivity, which may lead to oversedation and respiratory paralysis. Exhaustion, inanition, and electrolyte imbalance are contributory factors.

LABORATORY FINDINGS. The diagnosis of tetanus must be based on the clinical picture, and laboratory examinations are of little assistance. It is difficult to isolate the organism from the local lesion, and it is a laborious task to identify it precisely. Furthermore, the presence of C. *tetani* in a wound does not necessarily indicate that the patient has tetanus. The intoxication itself produces no change in the leukocyte count, but leukocytosis may accompany secondary infection. The cerebrospinal fluid is often under increased pressure but is otherwise not remarkable. The urine is normal in uncomplicated tetanus.

DIFFERENTIAL DIAGNOSIS. Fully developed tetanus is unlikely to be confused with other diseases. A frequent diagnostic problem is differentiation of serum sickness from early tetanus. Many injured patients are given equine tetanus antitoxin, and some subsequently develop serum sickness with temporomandibular arthralgia and trismus. Usually arthralgia of other joints is also present, together with urticaria and generalized adenitis. Other conditions in which trismus occurs include peritonsillar abscess and local infections of the mouth and cervical region. The phenothiazine group of tranquilizers may cause extrapyramidal tract symptoms with dystonic involvement of facial and pharyngeal muscles. Normal spinal fluid in tetanus eliminates confusion with meningitis. The clinical picture of strychnine poisoning, with hyperexcitability of the muscles, opisthotonos, risus sardonicus, and tonic convulsions, may mimic tetanus closely, except that the muscles are relaxed between seizures in strychnine intoxication, while spasm tends to persist in tetanus. In rabies, inability to swallow is often an early symptom, with drooling of saliva and spasms of the muscles of deglutition, followed by fever, anxiety, excitement, delirium, hyperesthesia, and convulsions.

TREATMENT. This is a grave disease for which there is no specific treatment. Nevertheless, careful and constant attention to certain supportive measures often will change the outcome from death to recovery.

Nursing Care. There is no disease in which meticulous, gentle nursing care is of greater importance, and it is essential that a trained attendant be at the bedside at all times. The patient should be in a quiet darkened room, where external stimuli are kept to a minimum. Secretions which accumulate in the pharynx must be removed by suction and postural drainage. A padded tongue depressor should be placed between the teeth to prevent tongue biting during convulsions. Bedsores can be avoided by use of a foam rubber or an alternating pressure-pad mattress, by changing the patient's position, and by special attention to skin care. Catheterization should be avoided if possible, because it precipitates convulsive seizures and inevitably leads to infection. Enemas are given as needed. Foot drop and wrist drop can be prevented by suitable positioning.

Sedatives and Muscle Relaxants. A most important feature in therapy is the use of medications to prevent acute tetanic seizures and to induce relaxation of muscle spasm. An ideal drug should also depress consciousness without rendering the patient comatose or depressing respiration. No single drug fulfills these criteria. Sedatives act by reducing sensory stimuli to the central nervous system, and several, including barbiturates, chloral hydrate, paraldehyde, and tribromoethanol, have been useful. Some of the centrally acting muscle relaxants and spinal depressants are effective because they diminish reflex activity and motor output. These include diazepam, chlorpromazine, mephenesin, meprobamate, and methocarbamol. It is recommended that at least two agents be employed, one from each group. This will permit a smaller dosage of each and will minimize toxic effects and the likelihood of tachyphylaxis. One of the drugs should be used in a relatively fixed dose as a basal medication; the dose of the second is varied to suit the immediate clinical requirements. An excellent combination is diazepam (up to 2 mg per kg in 24 hr) and thiopental sodium, given intravenously as a slow drip in a dilution of 0.5 to 1 Gm per liter of saline. The rate of flow must be titrated carefully to produce sleep without coma, but may be speeded up to control a seizure. Narcotics are contraindicated.

Another approach to control of convulsions is to use neuromuscular blocking agents of the curare group. This technique has been popular in Europe, but has found few advocates in the United States. These medications must be given in subparalyzing doses, aimed at controlling convulsions without interfering with respiration. Alternatively, the patient can be paralyzed deliberately and maintained with constant artificial respiration. These methods are obviously complex and dangerous and should be undertaken only by an experienced and skillful therapeutic team.

Antiserum. Antiserum has no curative action in tetanus, because it does not affect the toxin which has combined with nerve tissue. Its only action is to neutralize newly formed toxin as it is produced in the lesion and before it has reached susceptible nerve cells. There is actually little statistical proof that administration of antiserum materially alters the course of clinically developed tetanus; nevertheless, it should be used. Horse serum antitoxin was introduced in World War I and was the standard preparation for many years. Technical advances ultimately permitted the development of human tetanus immune globulin (TIG), which is now generally available in the United States. TIG is so far superior to equine antiserum that horse serum should be used only if TIG is unobtainable. The additional cost of TIG is more than offset by the elimination of morbidity and expense associated with the hypersensitivity reactions which were so frequent after administration of horse serum.

1. Homologous antitoxin (TIG). Allergic reactions are practically unknown, making sensitivity testing unnecessary. This material must be given intramuscularly. Being a human gamma-globulin, its predictable half-life is 25 days or more. Little experience has accumulated on the use of TIG in treatment of human tetanus, and consequently no consensus has been established regarding dosage. From 3,000 to 6,000 units appear to be more than ample, and the drop in titer is so slow that adequate protective levels are assured throughout the recovery period.

2. Heterologous antitoxin. Careful tests for horse serum sensitivity must be performed. If these are negative, 50,000 International Units of serum are given slowly intravenously in 250 ml normal saline solution, containing 1.0 ml of 1:1,000 aqueous epinephrine. The intravenous route is preferable because maximal plasma levels of antibody are achieved immediately, while following intramuscular injection, the plasma titer rises only gradually over a 2-day period. Ten thousand units of antitoxin are infiltrated around the local lesion because a considerable reservoir of toxin is present in this region. Horse serum should never be given intraspinally. Repeated doses are not necessary except in unusual cases involving extensive, slow-healing wounds. In such instances readministration may have to be considered after several weeks, but this involves a serious hazard of an allergic reaction and in this situation every effort to obtain TIG should be made. An alternative measure is to administer a unit of plasma obtained from a donor who has previously been actively immunized and has recently received a booster dose of tetanus toxoid.

Initiation of Active Immunization. There are sound reasons to advise that active immunization with toxoid should be commenced at the onset of therapy of tetanus. Even though it will be somewhat diminished by the simultaneous administration of a large excess of antiserum, an antigenic stimulus will be instituted. Consequently, toxoid should be given every 3 days over a period of 2 weeks. These injections should be considered *in toto* as the first dose of a primary immunization series. Another dose administered 3 weeks later will then stimulate production of the patient's own antibodies to replace the waning antibody introduced passively. Administration of toxoid provides protection in situations where the organism is not eradicated and where there may be late production of toxin.

Treatment of Local Lesion. The patient should receive sedatives and antiserum before the wound is manipulated. The lesion is then treated according to the same surgical principles that would be applicable if tetanus were not present. Specifically, a limb should not be amputated simply because the patient has tetanus. Meticulous debridement is essential.

Feeding. Oral feeding is usually hazardous or impossible because of trismus and dysphagia. Intravenous feeding is necessary during the first days of illness, and particularly in heavily sedated or unconscious patients. Nasogastric tube feeding should be avoided as long as danger of aspiration persists. Electrolyte balance requires careful regulation.

Management of Respiratory Tract. It is essential that respiratory tract obstruction be prevented or corrected, because this complication leads to anoxia, atelectasis, and pneumonia. Tracheostomy has proved to be a valuable therapeutic adjunct and should be used in most moderately or severely ill patients. Following this procedure convulsive spasms often diminish and less sedation is required.

Other Therapeutic Measures. The tetanal infection itself requires the use of an antibiotic, because antitoxin does not have antimicrobial properties. Conversely, antibiotics do not possess antitoxic properties. Penicillin G in dosage of 2.4 million units a day and tetracycline in dosage of 2.0 Gm per day are both useful, and one of them should be given. Corticosteroids have not been found to improve the clinical course. Several reports have indicated that hyperbaric oxygen may be of benefit, but the data are too meager to permit evaluation.

PREVENTION. Active Immunization. Tetanus toxoid is the most effective nonliving immunizing agent known. Active immunization can be achieved safely and almost infallibly, the rare exceptions being individuals who have diseases associated with deficient antibody production. The immunity is antitoxic rather than antibacterial in nature. Two types of toxoids are in general use, an alum-precipitated, or adsorbed type and a fluid type. The alum-precipitated type is the more effective immunizing agent and should be used for all primary immunization.

Primary immunization is achieved by giving two doses, interrupted by an interval of at least 3 weeks, and preferably one of 4 to 12 weeks. Permanent immunity requires a third reinforcing dose after 6 to 12 months. In experimental animals it has been shown that some resistance to infection has developed within 10 days after the initial dose of toxoid, and circulating antibody can be found in small quantity in man within 4 weeks after the first dose. The titer rises sharply within a few days after the second dose has been given, and the individual may be considered temporarily immune after 10 days. The reinforcing third dose is followed by a very high antibody titer and is necessary to induce lasting immunity. There will be an antibody response of some

degree even if the interval between the first and second doses of toxoid is as long as 12 years. Once basic immunization is accomplished, the normal person has an extraordinary capacity to respond with an effective antibody titer after a booster dose. Animal studies show a protective response within 24 hr, and a measurable rise in titer appears within 4 to 7 days, even when the recall dose is given as long as 22 years after primary immunization. Some authorities speculate that immunity persists for life; nevertheless, it seems prudent to give boosters at 10-year intervals.

Active immunization is the only really effective way of contending with the problem of tetanus, and should be a universal practice. Half the cases of tetanus in the United States involve wounds so trivial that they are disregarded by the patient or are considered by the physician to be too insignificant to warrant antitoxin prophylaxis. It is especially important to emphasize immunization in certain tetanus-prone groups. Tetanus neonatorum accounts for 10 to 30 percent of all cases in many parts of the world, and these could be prevented readily by immunizing the pregnant mothers. Many people are highly exposed to injury in their occupations and urgently require protection. The potential hypersensitivity to horse serum was formerly a major problem in all patients with an allergic diathesis and in those who had previously received equine antitoxin. This danger has diminished as human gamma-globulin has come into wider use.

A good time to initiate basic immunization is at the time of treatment of an acute injury. Tetanus toxoid is given in one limb, and if TIG is necessary, it is administered in another part of the body. In this manner, they do not significantly neutralize each other, and as passive protection slowly wanes, the patient begins to produce his own antibody.

Hypersensitivity reactions to tetanus toxoid are becoming more common, probably because of repeated injections. They are rarely seen before the age of twenty and become more frequent with advancing age. Usually they are of the delayed tuberculin type and are unpleasant but not serious. More severe local reactions of the Arthus type are seen occasionally. There have been rare reports of accelerated serum sickness or anaphylactic types of response. These reactions are associated with high antibody titers in the reacting individuals. Therefore, boosters should not be given with unnecessary frequency. Routine boosters every 10 years are sufficient, and in the event of an injury, one is needed only if more than a year has elapsed since the previous booster. If a local reaction is encountered, then future injections can be administered successfully by giving an initial dose of 0.05 ml of toxoid, followed by one or more fractional doses at intervals of several days.

Passive Immunization. Tetanus-immune human gamma-globulin is much to be preferred over horse antiserum. The prophylactic dose for an adult is 250 units given intramuscularly, and for a child it is 4 units per kg body weight. The dose may be doubled in those with highly contaminated lesions. TIG will give adequate protection for at least 1 month, and can be repeated without fear of an allergic reaction. If TIG is not available, then equine antiserum must be given subcutaneously in a dose of 1,500 to 5,000 units, depending on the severity of the wound and the degree of delay in administration. Hypersensitivity reactions are reported in 2.5 to 9 percent of patients who have not had previous serum injections and in up to 24 percent of those who have. Tests for serum sensitivity are likely to identify patients who are candidates for immediate anaphylactic reactions, but will not point out those who will develop serum sickness. Plasma antibody titers may persist for only a few days in persons who have had previous experience with horse serum. Attempts to desensitize are dangerous and probably fruitless and are not recommended.

Procedure after Injury. Of first importance is thorough and prompt cleansing and debridement. Certain types of injuries are more likely to be complicated by tetanus infections, including burns, compound fractures, deep or puncture wounds, those contaminated by soil, those over 3 hr old, wounds already otherwise infected, and those containing devitalized or avascular tissue. In addition to thorough debridement, penicillin or tetracycline should be given to prevent an incipient tetanal infection.

If the patient is known to have had basic tetanus immunization, and the last booster was given more than 1 year previously, then he should receive a toxoid booster. This will suffice except under unusual circumstances, when fortifying active immunity by giving antitoxin should be considered in addition. These circumstances are last toxoid booster more than 10 years previously; treatment delayed more than 24 hr after the injury; an extensive, mutilating, tetanus-prone injury; a patient who has a disease associated with poor production of gamma-globulin.

A decision must be made concerning the administration of TIG in the patient who has not had or has not completed a primary immunization series. Frequently, the history concerning this point is uncertain and when doubt exists it should be assumed that the patient has not been immunized. TIG is not needed if the wound is clean and minor, is treated soon after the injury, and can be debrided thoroughly. Those with more serious wounds are given TIG. Active immunization is initiated in all patients immediately, whether or not TIG is given.

PROGNOSIS. Case fatality rates average 30 to 50 percent but vary markedly. The rate is much higher in the very young, in the aged, in drug addicts, and in those who develop pneumonia or other secondary infections. It is higher if the incubation period is less than 7 days or if the period of onset is less than 24 hr. Most deaths occur within the first 10 days of illness. Survivors make a complete recovery from tetanus, although there may be residual effects from the various therapeutic measures used or from complications such as compression fractures. Those who recover are not immune to reinfection.

REFERENCES

Eckmann, L.: "Tetanus Prophylaxis and Therapy," New York, Grune & Stratton, Inc., 1963.

Edsall, G.: Current Status of Tetanus Immunization, Arch. Environ. Health, 8:731, 1964.

Laurence, D. R., and R. A. Webster: Pathologic Physiology, Pharmacology, and Therapeutics of Tetanus, Clin. Pharmacol. Therap., 4:36, 1963.

Smith, L. DeS.: *Clostridium Tetani,* pp. 88–107 in "Introduction to the Pathogenic Anaerobes," Chicago, University of Chicago Press, 1955.

Wright, G. P.: The Neurotoxins of *Clostridium Botulinium* and *Clostridium Tetani,* Pharmacol. Rev., 7:413, 1955.

171 BOTULISM
M. Glenn Koenig and David E. Rogers

DEFINITION. Botulism is a specific form of poisoning which results from absorption of toxin produced by *Clostridium botulinum.* The clinical picture is characterized by dilated fixed pupils, dry mucous membranes, progressive muscular paralysis, and high fatality rate.

HISTORY. The disease was first recognized over 200 years ago by South German physicians who adopted the term *botulismus* for the often fatal syndrome which sometimes followed the consumption of spoiled sausage (*botulus* is Latin for sausage). Studies by Van Ermengem in 1895 identified a gram-positive, spore-forming anaerobic bacillus as the etiologic agent and showed that a toxin produced by these bacilli was responsible for the disease.

Botulism was rare in the United States prior to World War I. The growth of commercial and home canning at this time led to a great increase in cases. A series of studies by Dr. K. F. Meyer and his associates in the early 1920s defined the habitat of *C. botulinum,* the foods often incriminated, and the conditions necessary for the destruction of *C. botulinum* spores. This knowledge led to the virtual elimination of botulism from the commercial canning industry. Since then clinical botulism has been infrequent in the United States and has usually followed consumption of improperly canned, home-preserved foods. In 1963 several outbreaks of type E disease followed consumption of certain commercially processed fish products. The introduction of new methods of packaging may have contributed to this problem.

ETIOLOGY. Six immunologically distinct strains of *C. botulinum,* designated as types A, B, C, D, E, and F, have been described. Each type elaborates an antigenically specific toxin which is liberated during growth and autolysis. Type A, B, and E toxins have been implicated most frequently in human disease in the United States. Only two outbreaks of type F botulism have been reported. The first occurred on the Danish island of Langeland following the ingestion of homemade liver paste. The second, which has been presumptively identified as type F, involved an outbreak in California traced to home-processed venison jerky. Types C and D produce disease almost exclusively in animals including wild water fowl, cattle, horses, and mink.

Type A and B spores are widely distributed in soil throughout the world. Type A spores are most common in the United States, especially along the Pacific Coast and the Rocky Mountain states. Type B spores have been found more frequently in the Eastern states and in Europe. Type E spores have been demonstrated in lakeshore mud, coastal sand, and sea bottom silt in northern latitudes. Fish apparently contaminate their intestinal tracts with type E spores, accounting for the high incidence of type E strains in fish-borne botulism. Type F spores have been found in marine sediments collected off the coast of California and Oregon and in salmon taken from the Columbia River.

Botulinum toxins are the most potent poisons known. Types A through E have been highly purified and identified as simple proteins. Original estimations of molecular weights have ranged from 900,000 for type A toxin to 18,600 for type E. Recent studies suggest that some botulinus toxins may depolymerize into units of lower molecular weight while maintaining or even increasing in toxicity. While antigenically distinct, all the toxins appear to produce identical symptoms in man and experimental animals, although there are marked differences in specific host susceptibility to the different toxins.

Spores of *C. botulinum* can withstand 100°C for several hours. Moist heat at 120°C for 30 min will destroy spores of all types, but the toxins are considerably more heat-labile. All varieties of toxin are destroyed by boiling for 10 min, or by temperatures of 80°C for 30 min.

PATHOGENESIS. Most human botulism follows the ingestion of food stuffs contaminated with preformed botulinus toxin. Rarely, wounds secondarily infected with *C. botulinum* have been the portal of entry. There is no convincing evidence that the botulinus bacillus produces toxin in the human gastrointestinal tract. Clinical botulism can occur only when the following conditions are met: (1) a food product is contaminated with viable *C. botulinum* bacilli or spores, (2) proper conditions for germination of the spores exist, (3) time and conditions allow production of toxin prior to eating, (4) the produce is not heated or is heated insufficiently to destroy botulinus toxin, (5) the toxin-containing food is ingested by a susceptible host (Table 171-1). While a relatively anaerobic

Table *171-1*. IMPORTANT FACTORS IN THE PATHOGENESIS OF BOTULISM

Spores	Toxin production	Toxin
1. Survive at 6°C (42.8°F) for several months 2. Can withstand boiling for several hours 3. Destroyed at 120°C (248°F) after 30 min	1. Strict anaerobic conditions not always required 2. Can occur at 6°C (42.8°F) 3. Optimal temperature 30°C (86°F) 4. Reduced at low pH's	1. Destroyed at 80°C (176°F) after 30 min or 100°C for 10 min 2. Unstable at high pH's 3. Type E toxin activated by trypsin

environment and temperatures above 80°F are optimal for toxin production, strict anaerobic conditions are not necessary and toxin production by some type E strains has been observed at temperatures as low as 6°C (42.8°F).

Home-canned string beans, corn, beets, spinach, asparagus, chili peppers, dill pickles, olives, tomatoes, figs, apricots, okra, mushrooms, peaches, home-processed venison jerky, gefilte fish, and albacore salad have been sources of botulism in the United States. Between 1941 and 1967, commercially processed foods have been implicated in only eight outbreaks (canned liver paste, type A; cheese, type unknown; smoked ciscoes, smoked whitefish, smoked whitefish chubs, and canned tuna fish, all type E; and possibly luncheon meat, type unknown).

Many type A and B strains of *C. botulinum* are proteolytic, and food frequently undergoes obvious putrefaction during their growth. Type E strains do not elaborate proteolytic enzymes, and foodstuffs containing type E toxin may not undergo spoilage and may look and taste perfectly normal.

Botulinus toxin is primarily absorbed in the stomach and upper small bowel. Despite its protein nature, it appears relatively resistant to inactivation by proteolytic enzymes. Indeed, the toxicity of type E toxin may be enhanced by tryptic digestion during passage through the upper gastrointestinal tract. Toxin which reaches the lower small bowel and colon may be slowly absorbed from these sites and may account for the delayed onset and the prolonged symptomatology observed in many patients.

Botulinus toxins exert a highly specific pharmacologic action, blocking transmission in cholinergic nerve fibers while sparing adrenergic fibers. Experimental studies have demonstrated that small amounts of toxin interrupt neural impulses close to the point of final branching of terminal nerve fibrils, but short of the motor end plate, and prevent release of acetylcholine. Nevertheless, muscle reactivity to acetylcholine applied directly to the motor end plate remains unimpaired. This contrasts with the action of curare, which prevents muscular response to acetylcholine. Some studies have suggested that botulinus toxins may exert some central inhibitory effects on cholinergic internuncial neurones in the spinal cord, but the clinical importance of this central action is uncertain.

CLINICAL MANIFESTATIONS. Botulism may vary from a mild illness for which patients seek no medical advice to a fulminant disease which ends in death within 24 hr. Symptoms usually begin 12 to 36 hr after ingestion of toxin, although extremes of 3 hr to 14 days are recorded. In general, the earlier the symptoms appear, the more serious the disease. Nausea and vomiting occur in approximately one-third of patients with type A or B disease and are very severe with type E intoxication. Weakness, lassitude, dizziness, and vertigo are early complaints. Severe dryness of the mouth and throat, sometimes associated with pharyngeal pain, is also noted. Neurologic symptoms may occur simultaneously or may be delayed for 12 to 72 hr. Blurred vision, diplopia, dysphonia, dysphagia, and weakness are followed by involvement of the muscles of respiration.

On examination, patients are usually alert, oriented,

and afebrile even with severe disease. Rarely, marked somnolence is noted. Difficulties in speech and deglutition may be obvious. The pupils are dilated and fixed. Extraocular palsies may be present but are less common than pupillary signs. The mucous membranes of the mouth and tongue are dry and crusted. Weakness of striated muscle groups, particularly the neck, proximal extremities, and muscles of respiration, appears as the disease progresses, but superficial and deep tendon reflexes remain *intact*. Abdominal distension with absent bowel sounds may be marked. Urinary retention may be present.

Respiratory paralysis may occur with startling swiftness. Failure of respiration, airway obstruction, and secondary pulmonary infection are the major causes of death. Sudden cardiac arrest has occurred in some patients with severe respiratory involvement, but whether this is secondary to anoxia or a primary action of botulinus toxin is unknown.

In patients recovering from botulism, return of function of the muscles of respiration, deglutition, and speech may be rapid, and improvement is often apparent within a week. General weakness, constipation, and ocular abnormalities may persist for weeks and sometimes several months.

LABORATORY FINDINGS. Routine laboratory studies do not aid in diagnosing clinical botulism. The cerebrospinal fluid is normal. Electrocardiographic abnormalities including minor disturbances in conduction, nonspecific T-wave and S-T segment changes, and various disorders of rhythm have been described. *The diagnosis of botulism rests on clinical grounds* and can be established only by the identification of botulinus toxin in the suspected food or in the patient. If available, portions of the suspected food should be suspended in saline and injected into mice intraperitoneally. If toxin is present, the animals will develop typical botulism and usually will die within 24 hr. Mice protected with specific antiserums survive. Fresh serum from patients suspected of having botulism should also be injected intraperitoneally in 1-ml amounts into mice with and without added type A, B, E, and F antiserums. Detection of circulating toxin in this manner has been useful in diagnosing type B and E intoxications and at least one outbreak of type A disease.

DIFFERENTIAL DIAGNOSIS. When the full clinical syndrome is evident, the symptoms and signs of botulism are sufficiently characteristic to lead to prompt diagnosis. In many instances the sequential appearance of findings can be confusing, particularly when no clear-cut history of ingestion of home-canned foods has been elicited.

The cranial nerve palsies, muscle weakness, and respiratory paralysis can lead to confusion with myasthenia gravis, Guillain-Barré syndrome, acute poliomyelitis, or stroke. A negative Tensilon test, normal cerebrospinal fluid, lack of sensory abnormalities, preservation of deep tendon reflexes, mental clarity, and absence of corticospinal tract signs in patients with botulism help to exclude these other possibilities.

Certain nonneurologic phenomena also have led to misdiagnosis. The pharyngeal pain, erythema, and dysphagia seen in some patients can suggest streptococcal or viral pharyngitis. The widely dilated pupils plus a dry mouth and mucous membranes resemble signs found in atropine, belladonna, or Jimson weed poisoning. The lack of nervous system excitement and hallucinations and the delay in onset of symptoms observed in botulism should exclude these possibilities. Nausea, vomiting, abdominal distension, constipation, and ileus may lead to consideration of intestinal obstruction. The dilated pupils and general paralytic phenomena should aid in differentiation.

Unexplained postural hypotension; dilated, unreactive pupils; extremely dry mucous membranes; and progressive muscle paresis occurring in a previously healthy afebrile patient should suggest botulism.

TREATMENT. Patients with botulism die of respiratory failure. *Early* tracheostomy and prompt use of the tank or other mechanical respirator can be life-saving. Cleansing enemas should be administered to remove any unabsorbed toxin from the colon. As soon as the clinical diagnosis of botulism has been made, appropriate skin testing for serum sensitivity should be carried out; if this is negative, 100,000 units of type A and type B antitoxin and 10,000 units of type E antitoxin should be administered intravenously. Patients sensitive to horse serum must be desensitized before antitoxin is given. Because each toxin is antigenically specific, there is no cross protection between antitoxins. Only a bivalent type A, B antitoxin is made commercially in the United States, but type E antitoxin can be obtained from the National Communicable Disease Center, Atlanta, Georgia. Because botulism antitoxin remains in the circulation for over 30 days, it is recommended that the total therapeutic dose be given immediately, rather than administering it in multiple small doses over a longer period. Antitoxin in one-third to one-half the therapeutic dose should be given prophylactically to individuals who are known to have eaten contaminated food but have not yet developed symptoms.

While older reports and certain animal experiments suggest that antitoxin does not alter the course of type A botulism once symptoms have appeared, the use of type-specific antitoxin has reduced mortality significantly in several outbreaks of type E disease. These reports suggest that antitoxin therapy should be vigorous and that the antitoxin treatment of type A and B botulism should be reassessed.

Because there is no evidence to suggest that *C. botulinum* can multiply in the gastrointestinal tract in man, antibiotics should be reserved for specific infectious complications.

PROGNOSIS. Type A strains have been the most frequent cause of botulism in the United States. Mortality rates of 60 to 70 percent have been reported in most outbreaks. Type B disease, which has been more common in Europe, has had consistently lower fatality rates of 10 to 30 percent. Type E botulism has produced outbreaks in northern latitudes among people eating raw fish (Japanese, Canadian Eskimos) with mortality rates ranging from 30 to 50 percent in large series. With more rapid diagnosis, aggressive management of respiratory paralysis, and use of polyvalent antitoxin, it seems likely these figures will be improved. Once the patient has survived the paralytic illness, the outlook for complete recovery is excellent.

REFERENCES

Dack, G. M.: "Food Poisoning," 3d ed., pp. 59–108, Chicago, University of Chicago Press, 1956.

Koenig, M. G., D. J. Drutz, A. I. Mushlin, W. Schaffner, and D. E. Rogers: Type B Botulism in Man. Am. J. Med., 42:208, 1967.

——, A. Spickard, M. A. Cardella, and D. E. Rogers: Clinical and Laboratory Observations on Type E Botulism in Man, Medicine, 43:517, 1964.

Rogers, D. E.: Botulism: Vintage 1963, Editorial, Ann. Intern. Med., 61:581, 1964.

172 OTHER CLOSTRIDIAL INFECTIONS
Edward W. Hook

INTRODUCTION AND HISTORY. Bacteria of the genus *Clostridium* are normal inhabitants of soil and the gastrointestinal tracts of man and animals. Most of the 93 species that have been described are saprophytic, but some are infectious for man and animals, usually under conditions of lowered host and tissue resistance. Infections with these organisms are often associated with profound systemic manifestations, and all pathogenic clostridia, except *Clostridium tetani* and *C. botulinum*, are capable of causing extensive tissue destruction. Diseases caused by these other clostridia are gas gangrene, cellulitis, postabortal and puerperal sepsis, and on occasion pneumonia, pleurisy, peritonitis, meningitis, endocarditis, cystitis, or bursitis. In addition, ingestion of food contaminated with certain clostridia may cause enterocolitis.

Hippocrates and Celsus were aware of the relationship between penetrating wounds and gas gangrene, but the nature of this disorder was not appreciated until the discovery of pathogenic clostridia by Pasteur, Novy, and Welch. The incidence of gas gangrene diminished markedly with the advent of antiseptic surgery in the latter half of the nineteenth century, but increased again to epidemic proportions during the trench warfare of the First World War. The rarity of serious clostridial infections in United Nations troops in Korea and in United States troops in more recent military actions attests to the advances in surgical management of war wounds. Gas gangrene and clostridial cellulitis are still encountered in neglected civilian injuries, and clostridial infections of the uterus account for a large proportion of deaths from criminal abortions.

ETIOLOGY. Wounds complicated by gas gangrene usually contain a mixture of pathogenic and saprophytic clostridia, often including *C. tetani*, as well as a variety of other bacteria. *Clostridium perfringens* (*welchii*), *C. novyi* (*oedematiens*), or *C. septicum* (*Vibrion septique*) can be cultured from most cases of gas gangrene and clostridial cellulitis, and *C. perfringens* causes virtually all clostridial infections of the uterus. *Clostridium bi-*

fermentans, C. histolyticum, and *C. fallax* are less virulent organisms that occasionally cause gas gangrene but are more commonly associated with localized cellulitis. Proliferation of *C. botulinum* in wounds occasionally leads to clinical manifestations of botulism.

The clostridia of gas gangrene and related infections are anaerobic or microaerophilic gram-positive bacilli that produce abundant gas in artificial media and form subterminal endospores. *Clostridium perfringens* is encapsulated and nonmotile, rarely sporulates in artificial media, and produces spores that can usually be destroyed by boiling.

EPIDEMIOLOGY AND PATHOGENESIS. Clostridia do not penetrate intact skin or mucous membranes, but frequently gain access to tissues through wounds or perforated abdominal viscera. Although these organisms can be cultured from one-third to two-thirds of severe traumatic wounds, gas gangrene develops in only an occasional case. The most important prerequisite for the conversion of clostridial contamination of a wound to a progressive infection is an environment with low oxidation-reduction potential, which permits spore germination and anaerobic growth. Local oxidation-reduction potential can be reduced by failure of the blood supply to a contaminated area, by the presence of foreign bodies such as clothing, dirt, or fragments of metal or wood, or by the multiplication of other bacteria in the wound. Once multiplication and toxin production are established, rapid invasion and destruction of healthy tissue follow.

The pathogenicity of clostridia is related to the capacity of these organisms to form exotoxins which destroy tissue cells. The nature and amount of toxins vary considerably for different species and strains. For example, at least 12 different extracellular "toxins" are produced by *C. perfringens*. Alpha toxin, a lecithinase, is clearly the most important and is the principal tissue-destroying, hemolytic, and lethal toxin. Other *C. perfringens* products include collagenase, hyaluronidase, hemolytic theta toxin, leukocidin, deoxyribonuclease, and fibrinolysin.

Gas gangrene is characterized by marked systemic symptoms and a local reaction with extensive necrotizing myositis, edema, thrombosis of small vessels, interstitial gas bubbles, and minimal infiltration of leukocytes. The local reaction in infected tissue can be explained by the action of clostridial toxins, especially alpha toxin, but the factors responsible for the general reaction are unknown. Alpha toxin, or other clostridial toxins, have not been demonstrated in circulating blood during the course of severe clostridial myonecrosis.

CLINICAL MANIFESTATIONS. Clostridial Myonecrosis (Gas Gangrene, Clostridial Myositis). Gas gangrene develops in anoxic devitalized tissues in which the arterial circulation has been compromised by trauma, constricting tourniquets or casts, or obliterative arterial disease. Infection is most frequent after extensive injury to skeletal muscle, particularly of the thigh and buttock, and is more common in wounds complicated by compound fractures of lodgment of foreign bodies. Once infection is established, it spreads to involve healthy muscle undamaged by previous trauma or ischemia.

The incubation period is usually 1 to 4 days but may vary from 3 hr to 6 weeks or longer. The earliest symptom is sudden, severe pain in the injured part. The distal portion of an involved limb becomes cold and edematous within a few hours, and eventually pulseless and gangrenous. The wound drains a watery, brown, or hemorrhagic material which may have a peculiar sweet odor. The appearance of the wound is usually not that of a pyogenic inflammatory lesion. Depending on the duration of the process, the surrounding skin may be normal, white, and tense, or dusky brown and reddish. Vesicles or hemorrhagic bullae may develop, particularly in *C. septicum* infections. Gas is usually not detectable in the tissues by palpation except in advanced lesions; although it is visible easily by x-ray. Occasionally, tiny bubbles may be seen in the discharge from the wound, and rarely, crepitation can be detected at an early stage by auscultation with the stethoscope. The involved muscle appears dark red or black and may herniate through the wound.

Systemic manifestations developing shortly after onset of severe pain and swelling of an injured extremity strongly suggest gas gangrene. The patient is prostrated, pale, and motionless but is usually well oriented, alert, and extremely apprehensive. The temperature usually does not exceed 101°F and may be normal. As the illness progresses, there may be anorexia, vomiting, profuse watery or bloody diarrhea, and eventually circulatory collapse. The pulse rate usually exceeds 120 beats per minute and is elevated out of proportion to the temperature. Massive intravascular hemolysis is rare in patients with clostridial myositis. Pericardial effusion is sometimes noted. Delirium and coma may precede death, but more commonly the patient dies suddenly several days after onset of illness, often during surgery or anesthesia. Acute renal failure is occasionally a late complication.

Gas gangrene has been described after hypodermic injection, especially injection of epinephrine. Minor trauma also occasionally activates clostridial spores dormant in scar tissue and leads to development of myonecrosis years after original injury.

Gas gangrene must be differentiated from nonclostridial infections of gangrenous limbs caused by anaerobic streptococci or aerobic gas-forming coliform bacilli.

Clostridial Cellulitis. This is a relatively benign infection of skin and subcutaneous tissues that occurs in a small proportion of wounds contaminated with pathogenic clostridia. The disease is characterized by spreading necrosis of superficial tissues and a profuse, foul-smelling, brown seripurulent exudate. Gas, which crepitates on palpation, invariably forms in the subcutaneous tissues and may involve an entire limb or form a localized gas pocket. In clostridial cellulitis, the underlying skeletal muscle is not involved, pain is not severe, and the only systemic manifestations are slight fever and moderate tachycardia. It can usually be differentiated from group A streptococcal cellulitis by the presence of subcutaneous gas and the absence of erythema.

Postabortal and Puerperal Sepsis. Uterine infections with *C. perfringens* usually occur after incomplete abortions induced under unsterile conditions and occasionally after spontaneous abortions, prolonged labor at term, ruptured membranes, or operative interference with pregnancy. The organisms presumably invade the damaged endometrium through the retained products of conception. The earliest symptoms may be related to instrumentation and consist of metrorrhagia, suprapubic and back pain, chills, and fever. Fever of 100 to 103°F, often with chills, usually recurs several days after abortion, but the incubation period can be as short as 6 hr. Vaginal bleeding is almost invariably present, and there is often a brown, foul-smelling vaginal discharge containing necrotic tissue. The cervix is soft and patulous, and the uterus and adnexae are usually very tender. The lower abdominal wall is often tense, or signs of generalized peritonitis may be present, secondary to perforation of the uterus or parametrial extension of infection. Nausea, vomiting, and profuse diarrhea are often prominent.

Systemic manifestations usually appear with dramatic suddenness. Massive intravascular hemolysis, accompanied by hemoglobinemia, hemoglobinuria, and jaundice, is often the most striking feature of the disease. Icterus may appear within hours after onset of illness. As in gas gangrene, the clinical picture may be dominated by circulatory collapse with hypotension, extreme tachycardia, cyanosis, hyperpnea, and pulmonary edema. Despite severe prostration, the patient is frequently well oriented, alert, and apprehensive. The mortality rate in postabortal or puerperal sepsis caused by *C. perfringens* is 40 to 70 percent. Death may occur a few hours after onset or be delayed for several days. Acute renal failure secondary to shock, dehydration, or hemolysis occurs frequently.

Unusual local complications of the uterine infection are gas gangrene of the vagina and rectum and clostridial cellulitis of the anterior abdominal wall following cesarean section or hysterectomy. At times, the infectious process is confined to the endometrium and myometrium with intrauterine gas formation (physometra).

Diseases to be considered in the *differential diagnosis* include perforated uterus, ruptured ectopic pregnancy, ingestion of toxic abortifacients, streptococcal or staphylococcal puerperal sepsis, pelvic thrombophlebitis with septic pulmonary emboli, acute hepatic necrosis of pregnancy, and sickle-cell crisis.

Clostridium Perfringens Food Poisoning. Meat and meat products contaminated with *C. perfringens* are frequently responsible for outbreaks of acute gastroenteritis. The strains of *C. perfringens* that cause food poisoning differ from those causing gas gangrene by forming spores that resist boiling for 1 to 4 hr. These strains are widespread in nature, and have been isolated from a high proportion of raw meat samples, from animal feces, and from stools of 2 to 5 percent of normal human beings.

Typical symptoms of diarrhea with abdominal pain develop 8 to 24 hr after ingestion of meat, stew, or soup which has been stored at a warm temperature for several hours after cooking. Nausea is common but vomiting is rare. Systemic manifestations are usually absent, and recovery is uneventful after 12 to 24 hr.

Clostridium perfringens food poisoning can be reproduced experimentally in man by feeding the actively growing organisms. However, gastroenteritis does not occur after ingestion of bacteria-free filtrates of cultures of food-poisoning strains.

A severe form of clostridial infection termed "enteritis necrotans" was observed in Germany after World War II. This disease was characterized by hemorrhagic necrosis of the small intestine, bloody diarrhea, severe dehydration, shock, and death. A similar infection termed "necrotizing jejunitis" has been described in natives of New Guinea who had eaten inadequately cooked pork.

Miscellaneous Clostridial Infections. Clostridia can be isolated not infrequently from bile obtained at elective cholecystectomy in patients without symptoms of clostridial infection. Clostridial cellulitis or myonecrosis may occasionally follow surgical procedures, particularly surgery on the gastrointestinal tract or gallbladder. Pathogenic clostridia are occasionally introduced into the abdomen, thoracic cavity, or cranium through penetrating wounds. Primary pneumonia in the absence of a penetrating wound or distant focus has been described. Clostridial pleurisy may involve the underlying lung but is usually an indolent localized infection with minimal systemic manifestations. Meningitis is usually secondary to a puncture wound of the skull and is often associated with a necrotizing cerebritis. Clostridial peritonitis may follow perforation of the gallbladder, appendix, or other viscus and is usually rapidly fatal. Clostridial septicemia occurs occasionally in patients with leukemia or other neoplastic processes who are treated with antimetabolites and anti-inflammatory glucocorticoids. The primary infection is in the gastrointestinal tract, which is usually the site of extensive neoplastic disease. Cystitis with pneumaturia, gaseous cholecystitis, endocarditis, and bursitis after needle aspiration are other examples of rare clostridial infections.

LABORATORY FINDINGS. The diagnosis of gas gangrene, clostridial cellulitis, postabortal sepsis, or other clostridial infections is based primarily on clinical criteria. Smears of wound exudate, uterine scrapings, or cervical discharge may show abundant large gram-positive rods, as well as other organisms. Spores are rarely observed in smears of exudates. Thioglycollate broth, deep meat broth, and blood-agar plates incubated in an anaerobic jar should be inoculated for definitive identification of specific clostridia. However, interpretation of positive wound cultures is difficult because clostridia are frequent contaminants. *Clostridium perfringens* bacteremia is common in postabortal infections but rare in gas gangrene.

Polymorphonuclear leukocytosis occurs frequently in gas gangrene and invariably in postabortal sepsis; total blood leukocyte counts range from 15,000 to 40,000 cells per mm and occasionally exceed 60,000 cells per mm. Marked thrombocytopenia develops in about 50 percent of patients with clostridial sepsis. The urine frequently contains protein and casts. Renal insufficiency may lead to severe uremia.

X-ray examination sometimes provides the first clue leading to the correct diagnosis by revealing the presence of gas in muscle, subcutaneous tissue, or uterus; however, demonstration of gas in tissues is not diagnostic

of clostridial infection. Other bacteria, especially *Aerobacter* or *Escherichia*, may be responsible for gas production, and occasionally air is sucked into a wound at the time of penetrating injury.

Profound alterations of circulating erythrocytes are common in postabortal sepsis but are much less frequent in other clostridial infection. Hemolytic anemia may develop with almost unbelievable rapidity; the red blood cell count occasionally decreases by 2 million cells per cu mm in less than 24 hr and is associated with hemoglobinemia, hemoglobinuria, and elevated levels of serum bilirubin. Spherocytosis, increased osmotic and mechanical fragility of the red blood cells, erythrophagocytosis, and methemoglobinemia have also been described.

TREATMENT. The traditional therapeutic approach to serious clostridial infection, such as diffuse, spreading myositis, is immediate surgical intervention with wide radical debridement followed by open drainage without closure. Early surgery not only aids diagnosis, but permits decompression of fascial compartments and excision of devitalized muscle and may obviate amputation. A number of authorities feel that hyperbaric oxygen therapy has modified this traditional approach to gas gangrene by assuming priority over radical surgical debridement. Hyperbaric oxygenation produces impressive, almost immediate improvement in patients with gas gangrene with rapid disappearance of systemic toxicity and prompt arrest of local spread of the gangrenous infection. Opinion differs about whether conservative debridement should be carried out before or after hyperbaric oxygen therapy. There is uniform agreement in recommending that patients with serious clostridial infections be transported immediately to a facility equipped to administer hyperbaric oxygen therapy. Oxygen toxicity consequent to hyperbaric oxygenation may lead to convulsions in some patients.

Curettage of the uterus should be performed for diagnosis and treatment of postabortal clostridial infections. Hysterectomy should be considered if metritis is present and if the condition of the patient is deteriorating. Perforation of the uterus may be present in some cases despite the lack of typical clinical findings.

Simple excision and adequate drainage usually suffice for treating clostridial cellulitis.

Penicillin is the antibiotic of choice for all clostridial infections and should be administered in doses of 20 million units a day. Tetracycline is also active against most strains of *Clostridium* and has been recommended as an adjunct to penicillin therapy.

The efficacy of polyvalent gas gangrene antitoxin is controversial. Many centers have discontinued the use of antitoxin in the management of patients with suspected gas gangrene or clostridial postabortal sepsis.

Intravenous infusions of blood, plasma-volume expanders, fluids, and electrolytes are required to combat shock, anemia, and dehydration. Renal insufficiency should be treated in the same manner as acute tubular necrosis from other causes.

The most reliable protection against gas gangrene is early and adequate wound debridement. Antitoxin is ineffective as a prophylactic agent. The use of clostridial toxoids for prophylactic immunization of individuals in hazardous occupations awaits evaluation.

REFERENCES

Boggs, D. R., E. Frei, and L. B. Thomas: Clostridial Gas Gangrene and Septicemia in Four Patients with Leukemia, New Engl. J. Med., 259:1255, 1958.

Clostridium Welchii Food-Poisoning, Editorial, Brit. Med. J., 2:1604, 1963.

Hitchcock, C. R., J. J. Haglin, and O. Arner: Treatment of Clostridial Infections with Hyperbaric Oxygen, Surgery, 63:759, 1967.

MacLennan, J. D.: The Histotoxic Clostridial Infections of Man, Bact. Rev., 26:177, 1962.

Mahn, E., and L. M. Dantuono: Postabortal Septicotoxemia Due to *Clostridium Welchii*. Seventy-five Cases from the Maternity Hospital, Santiago, Chile, 1948–1952, Am. J. Obstet. Gynecol., 70:604, 1955.

Murrell, T. G. C., L. Roth, J. Egerton, J. Samels, and P. D. Walker: Pig-Bel: Enteritis Necroticans: A Study in Diagnosis and Management, Lancet, 1:217, 1966.

Trippel, O. H., A. N. Ruggie, C. J. Staley, and J. VanElk: Hyperbaric Oxygenation in the Management of Gas Gangrene, Surg. Clin. N. A., 47:17, 1967.

173 CHOLERA
Charles C. J. Carpenter

DEFINITION. Cholera is an acute illness which results from colonization of the small bowel by *Vibrio cholerae*. The disease is characterized by its epidemic occurrence and the production of massive diarrhea with rapid depletion of extracellular fluid and electrolyte.

ETIOLOGY AND EPIDEMIOLOGY. *Vibrio cholerae* is a curved, aerobic, gram-negative bacillus with a single polar flagellum. It is rapidly motile and possesses both O and H antigens. Serologic identification is based on differences in the polysaccharide O antigens.

Cholera has been endemic in the Gangetic Delta of West Bengal and East Pakistan, and is often epidemic throughout South and Southeast Asia. The most recent pandemic spread of this disease, from 1961 to 1966, extended from the Celebes northward to Korea and eastward to Iraq and Southern Russia. The last major epidemic of cholera in the Western Hemisphere occurred during 1866–1867.

Several well-studied epidemics have clearly been waterborne, but direct contamination of food by infected feces probably contributes to spread during major outbreaks. Poor sanitation appears to be primarily responsible for the continuing presence of cholera, but as yet undefined host factors may also play an important role.

A chronic gallbladder carrier state has been observed in 4 to 5 percent of convalescent cholera patients. These chronic vibrio carriers may explain the persistence of the disease in endemic areas and also may provide a vehicle for spread outside of these areas. The basis for the annual cholera epidemics throughout the Gangetic Delta and for the periodic outbreaks throughout the remainder of South and Southeast Asia has, however, not been clearly delineated.

PATHOGENESIS. *Vibrio cholerae* produces an exotoxin which appears to be responsible for all known pathophysiologic aberration in cholera. This exotoxin causes secretion of isotonic fluid by all segments of the small bowel, but has no major effect on electrolyte absorption from the gut. The exotoxin-induced electrolyte secretion occurs in the absence of any demonstrable histologic damage to gut epithelial cells or to the capillary endothelial cells of the lamina propria. The former erroneous belief that extensive gut mucosal sloughing was a primary lesion in cholera was based upon autopsy studies. It is now clear that the observed intestinal denudation was secondary either to postmortem autolysis or to hypovolemic shock and played no etiologic role in fluid loss from the gut. Precise studies have demonstrated that the adult cholera stool is nearly isotonic, with sodium and chloride concentrations slightly less than those of plasma, a bicarbonate concentration approximately twice that of plasma, and a potassium concentration three to five times that of plasma. Disease caused by all known strains of *V. cholerae* results in the same stool electrolyte pattern. The basic pathophysiologic defect in cholera is extracellular fluid depletion with resultant hypovolemic shock, basedeficit acidosis, and progressive potassium depletion. There is no convincing evidence that the cholera vibrio invades any tissue, nor has the exotoxin been shown, in human disease, to affect any organ other than the small intestine.

MANIFESTATIONS. The extent of incubation period has not been defined, but generally is from 6 to 48 hr. This is followed by the abrupt onset of watery, generally painless diarrhea. In the more severe cases, the initial diarrheal stool may be in excess of 1,000 ml, and several liters of isotonic fluid may be lost within hours, leading rapidly to profound shock. Vomiting generally follows, but occasionally precedes the onset of diarrhea; the vomiting is characteristically effortless and not preceded by nausea. As saline depletion progresses, severe muscle cramps, commonly involving the calves, occur.

When first seen, the typical cholera patient is cyanotic, with pinched facies, scaphoid abdomen, poor skin turgor, and thready or absent peripheral pulses. The voice is faint, high-pitched, and often inaudible, and there are tachycardia, hypotension, and varying degrees of tachypnea. In all epidemics there are mild cases in which gastrointestinal fluid loss is not severe enough to require hospitalization.

The disease runs its course in 2 to 7 days, and subsequent manifestations depend on the adequacy of electrolyte repletion therapy. With prompt fluid and electrolyte repletion, recovery is remarkably rapid, and mortality exceptionally rare. However, if therapy is inadequate, the mortality is quite high. The important causes of death are hypovolemic shock, uncompensated metabolic acidosis, and uremia, which may follow acute tubular necrosis.

LABORATORY FINDINGS. In epidemics or in endemic

areas, the clinical picture should arouse strong suspicion immediately. The most reliable technique for identification of *V. cholerae* consists of direct plating of a sample of cholera stool on bile salt, gelatin-tellurite-taurocholate (GTT), or thiosulfate-citrate-bile salt-sucrose (TCBS) agar. On bile salt or GTT agar the organisms appear as typical translucent colonies within 24 hr. On TCBS agar, *V. cholorae* appears as distinct large yellow colonies at 24 hr. Further classification requires agglutination with type-specific antiserums. In mild or convalescent cases recovery of vibrios may be important to initial enrichment for 6 hr in alkaline peptone water followed by subculture on bile salt, GTT, or TCBS agar. Rapid diagnosis is possible either by directly observing immobilization of vibrios by type-specific antiserums with dark-field or phase microscopy or by identifying the organisms by immunofluorescent methods.

THERAPY. Successful therapy requires only prompt and adequate replacement of gastrointestinal losses of saline and alkali. Isotonic saline solution and isotonic sodium lactate (or bicarbonate), administered in a 2:1 ratio, should be rapidly infused, at 50 to 100 ml per min, until a strong pulse has been restored. The same fluids should subsequently be infused in quantities equal to the gastrointestinal losses. If losses cannot be measured accurately, intravenous fluids should be given at a rate sufficient to maintain a normal radial pulse and normal skin turgor. Overhydration can be avoided by careful observation of neck venous filling and auscultation of the lungs. Close observation is mandatory during the acute phase of the illness, because the cholera patient can lose as much as 1 liter of isotonic fluid per hr during the first 24 hr of the disease. Inadequate or delayed restoration of fecal fluid losses may result in a very high incidence of acute renal failure. Serious hypokalemic symptoms are rare in adults, and potassium repletion can usually be carried out orally; the dose is approximately 15 mEq potassium for each liter of stool produced. Hypokalemia contributes significantly, however, to the morbidity and mortality in inadequately treated pediatric cholera, and potassium, 8 to 12 mEq per liter, should be included in the intravenous fluids administered to pediatric patients.

Although adequate intravenous saline and alkali repletion alone results in rapid recovery of virtually all adult cholera patients, a dramatic reduction in the duration and volume of the diarrhea, and early eradication of vibrios from the stool, may be effected by antibiotic therapy. Oral tetracycline, 500 mg every 6 hr for the first 48 hr of treatment, has been most successful. Other antibiotics, including chloramphenicol and furazolidone, are also of value, but both appear to be slightly less effective than tetracycline.

PROGNOSIS. Under ideal conditions and with prompt and adequate fluid replacement, mortality approaches zero and significant sequelae are rare. Unfortunately, death rates as high as 60 percent still occur, especially during the initial phases of certain outbreaks. This high mortality reflects lack of pyrogen-free intravenous fluids in remote areas, the difficulties of initiating treatment promptly when large numbers of cases are occurring in poverty-striken populations, and the compromises which may have to be made under emergency conditions.

PREVENTION. Immunization by standard commercial vaccine, containing 10 billion killed organisms per ml, provides significant protection for a limited (4- to 6-month) period. Immunization with toxoid provides significant protection in experimental animals, but toxoid has not yet been tested in man. Careful hygiene provides the only sure protection against cholera.

REFERENCES

Carpenter, C. C. J., P. P. Mitra, and R. B. Sack: Clinical Studies in Asiatic Cholera I–VI, Bull. Johns Hopkins Hosp., 118:165, 1966.

Gangarosa, E. F., W. R. Beisel, C. Benyajati, H. Sprinz, and P. Piyaratn: The Nature of the Gastrointestinal Lesion in Asiatic Cholera and Its Relation to Pathogenesis: A Biopsy Study, Am. J. Trop. Med., 9:125, 1960.

Greenough, W. B. III, R. S. Gordon, Jr., I. S. Rosenberg, and B. I. Davies: Tetracycline in the Treatment of Cholera, Lancet, 1:335, 1964.

Wallace, C. K., P. N. Anderson, T. C. Brown, S. R. Khanra, G. W. Lewis, N. F. Pierce, S. N. Sanyal, C. V. Segre, and R. H. Waldman: Optimal Antibiotic Therapy in Cholera, Bull. World Health Organ., 39:239, 1968.

Watten, R. H., F. M. Morgan, Y. N. Songkhla, B. Vanikiati, and R. A. Phillips: Water and Electrolyte Studies in Cholera, J. Clin. Invest., 38:1879, 1959.

Section 9

Mycobacterial Diseases

174 TUBERCULOSIS
William W. Stead

DEFINITION. Tuberculosis is a necrotizing bacterial infection with protean manifestations and wide distribution.

In man, the lungs are most commonly affected, but lesions may occur also in the kidneys, bones, lymph nodes, and meninges or be disseminated throughout the body. Two stages of the infection are recognized: (1) primary tuberculosis, in which tubercle bacilli invade a host which has no specific immunity and which undergoes at least partial spontaneous healing as specific immunity develops; (2) postprimary or adult tuberculosis (often erroneously called "reinfection tuberculosis"), which is the result of progression of the infection in spite of specific immunity. Progression may occur shortly after primary infection or after a delay of years or even decades. In the Western world, where bovine tuberculosis has been controlled, the portal of entry in man is almost exclusively the lung.

HISTORY. Some human races (Caucasian, Mongolian) have lived with tubercle bacilli throughout much of their evolution. Lesions of bone typical of tuberculosis were noted in Neolithic man and Egyptian mummies. This is indicative of a cardinal feature of the infection: a tendency toward healing in its primary stage and chronic tissue destruction in its later stage. African, American Indian, and Eskimo peoples have had contact with the disease over a much shorter period. In them, it behaves much more like an acute infection and has a higher mortality in the primary and early postprimary phases and less tendency to develop an equilibrium between the host and parasite.

Tuberculosis was named because it tends to form nodules, or "tubercles," on serous surfaces and in tissues. For many years the chronic form (then often called phthisis or consumption) was thought to be a degenerative or hereditary disease unrelated to primary tuberculosis, which was obviously an infection. Laennec was the first to consider the chronic form as merely a later development in the same infection, but even Villemin's demonstration (1865) that material from both types of disease produced tuberculosis in animals and Koch's identification of the organism (1882) failed to convince their contemporaries. The validity of Laennec's clinical observations has been born out, and the "unitary concept" of tuberculosis is now accepted.

There has been a great drop in the prevalence of tuberculosis in the economically developed countries. The death rate from tuberculosis had already begun to fall by 1900 coincident with improvement in nutrition and standard of living. For the individual with active tuberculosis, however, the most important development occurred in 1944 with the discovery of streptomycin by Waksman and his associates. Hinshaw and Feldman showed the effectiveness of streptomycin against tuberculosis in animals and man. Lehmann discovered para-aminosalicylic acid (PAS), which was shown later to have an effect upon the disease when used with other agents. Isoniazid (INH) was discovered independently in 1951 by three groups of chemists and subsequently has been the most effective tuberculostatic agent discovered. Ethambutol (EMB) appears to have great potential in the treatment of cases in whom the bacilli have developed resistance to the other drugs.

ETIOLOGY. *Mycobacterium tuberculosis* is a rod of 2.0 to 4.0 μ in length and 0.3 μ in thickness. Its distinguishing staining property, i.e., resistance to decolorization by acid alcohol when stained with basic fuchsin, is related to the waxy component of the cell wall, probably specifically to its content of mycolic acid. "Acid-fastness" is dependent upon the structural integrity of the bacillus because it is lost when the organisms are damaged by grinding but is not affected by prolonged extraction with fat solvents.

Tubercle bacilli are strict aerobes and thrive best when there is a PO_2 of 100 mm Hg or more and a PCO_2 of about 40 mm Hg, and the organs most commonly affected by tuberculosis are those with relatively high oxygen tension. Metastatic foci are most common in the apexes of the lungs, where the PO_2 is in the range of 120 to 130 mm Hg in the upright position, followed by the kidney and the growing end of bones, where the PO_2 approximates 100 mm Hg. The liver and spleen, where the PO_2 is quite low, are rarely affected except in overwhelming disseminated infection.

Three strains of tubercle bacilli infect man: human, bovine, and avian. By far the greatest number of cases in the United States are caused by the human strain. Programs for eradication of bovine tuberculosis have been carried out with such vigor over the past 60 years that the disease now appears only sporadically in this country. Avian bacilli have little invasiveness for man.

Within the last 15 years several varieties of mycobacteria which resemble *M. tuberculosis* have been associated with chronic pulmonary infection (Chap. 176). The most common are *M. battey* and *M. kansasii*. In addition, certain pigmented mycobacteria (scotochromes) produce cervical adenitis in children (scrofula) and occasionally also chronic pulmonary lesions. These mycobacteria can be recognized in the laboratory by biochemical tests (nicotinic acid negative, catalase positive) and by lack of virulence for the guinea pig. The pathology in man produced by these related mycobacteria is indistinguishable from that of tuberculosis. However, they differ from *M. tuberculosis* in two important ways: transmission appears not to be airborne and they show little response to antituberculosis drugs.

TRANSMISSION. Most cases of tuberculosis among adults develop because of late recrudescence of dormant infection and are quite independent of recent exposure. The liquid caseum from a cavity in such a case abounds with tubercle bacilli, which are excreted in aerosolized droplets during coughing, sneezing, and talking. Droplets larger than 10 μ are usually caught on the mucociliary blanket and cleared from the lung without harm, but droplets of smaller size may reach the respiratory bronchiole and deposit the bacilli beyond the protective mucous blanket. There the organisms may invade tissues and establish an infection in the susceptible host. Persons who have been infected previously are sufficiently immune that naturally acquired inocula can be handled effectively by immune macrophages which lyse the invading organisms.

Transmission is usually due to close indoor contact of a susceptible (tuberculin-negative) host with a patient who is excreting tubercle bacili in large numbers (positive sputum smear). *Persons with primary tuberculosis excrete very few organisms and need not be considered contagious.* Bacilli often can be cultured from the dust in the room of a person with cavitary tuberculosis, but house dust is a very poor vehicle because of its large and irregular particles and their electrostatic charge. There is no evidence that tuberculosis is spread by hands, eating utensils, or fomites.

Tubercle bacilli are killed readily by boiling and by pasteurization at 60°C for 20 min. In countries where bovine tuberculosis has not been eradicated, pasteurization is especially important. Milk from a tuberculous cow often contains millions of bacilli per milliliter. In all likelihood the small number of organisms sprayed on food by a tuberculous food handler is no more dangerous than those from any other person excreting tubercle bacilli into the environment.

PREVALENCE AND INCIDENCE. There has been a great fall in prevalence of tuberculosis in the United States during the last 60 years. Early in this century surveys using the tuberculin skin test and autopsies indicated that over 80 percent of the population was infected *before* the age of twenty. In an autopsy study in 1946, Medlar found evidence of tuberculosis in 80 percent of the persons over the age of fifty living in New York City. In 1968 only 5 to 10 percent of young adults reacted to tuberculin (except in some urban areas), whereas about 50 percent of the persons over the age of fifty react. The declining incidence of the infection is most apparent among children and young adults and is due to a reduction in the number of open infectious cases, which, in turn, is attributable to an improved standard of living, reduced risk of late progression of infection, and prompter recognition and treatment of contagious cases.

LATENT INFECTION. The majority of persons who harbor tubercle bacilli have latent or dormant ("healed") tuberculosis. The terms *latent* or *dormant* are preferable to "healed," because in most instances the "scars" retain the potential for reactivation. Scars within the lung may remain dormant for many years and show no changes for years on roentgenogram only to reactivate and produce active infection. Figure 174-1 illustrates the most common sites in which dormant metastatic lesions may persist after the primary infection and undergo late progression to produce chronic postprimary tuberculosis.

MORBIDITY AND MORTALITY. The incidence of clinical disease must be distinguished from prevalence as shown by the tuberculin reaction. Of the 25 million persons in the United States who react to tuberculin, only 90,000 are known to have active tuberculosis and 230,000 have recovered from clinically apparent tuberculosis and are classified as "inactive" cases. Many of the remainder harbor dormant viable bacilli in latent foci but have not developed active disease. The morbidity rate in the United States was 24 per 100,000 in 1966, a reduction from 29 in 1961 and 53 in 1953.

Figures 174-2 and 174-3 illustrate some important facts concerning the natural history of tuberculosis in man. In the analysis of mortality from tuberculosis by 10-year cohorts (Fig. 174-2), it can be seen that the only significant mortality occurs among the older persons in the community, those who were most commonly infected early in life. Furthermore, the mortality experienced by

Fig. 174-1. Sites most commonly affected by tuberculosis:

1. Healed, calcified primary infection in right lung and hilar node (Ghon complex).

2. "Apical cap" and nodular scars (Simon foci) in right upper lobe due to hematogenous seeding during primary infection.

3. Recrudescence and coalescence of Simon foci, producing chronic inflammation and caseation necrosis (cavitation).

4. Dormant focus of tuberculosis in cervical lymph nodes, seeded by lymphatic drainage during primary infection.

5. Active tuberculosis in cervical lymph nodes, producing chronic inflammation and caseation necrosis.

6. Dormant focus of tuberculosis in kidney, seeded during primary infection.

7. Recrudescence of dormant renal focus producing inflammation and caseation necrosis. The male genital tract may become infected by organisms shed by a renal cavity.

8. Dormant focus of tuberculosis in vertebra.

9. Recrudescence of focus in vertebra, producing inflammation and caseation necrosis, with destruction of intervertebral disc.

(W. W. Stead: "Understanding Tuberculosis Today: A Handbook for Patients," Milwaukee, Marquette University Press, 1968.)

the cohorts to which these older persons belong was even greater in earlier years, particularly in their young adult life (Fig. 174-3).

Figure 174-2A shows the morbidity (active cases) from tuberculosis in Wisconsin in 1963, and morbidity was greatest in the older members of the population. However, when the age-specific morbidity is plotted against the age-specific prevalence (tuberculin reactors), there is a sharp peak in young adult life. The reduction in the number of tuberculin reactors among young adults accounts for the elimination of the peak of morbidity for that period in the general population. These data suggest that late reactivation of the original tuberculous infection is important in the pathogenesis of chronic tuberculosis.

Mortality has fallen steadily over the past 65 years. Tuberculosis has dropped from the leading cause of death with over 200 deaths per 100,000 in 1906 to 3.8 per 100,000 in 1966. Tuberculosis contributes to more deaths than the figures indicate because pulmonary scarring is important in the pathogenesis of cor pulmonale.

IMMUNITY

NATURAL RESISTANCE. The Caucasian and Mongolian races have a distinct natural resistance to tuberculosis consisting of the ability to develop an immune response to the infection, which enables them to recover from the primary infection. In them, primary infection usually subsides spontaneously; and reactivation generally produces a chronic disease which is characterized by cavitation and scarring.

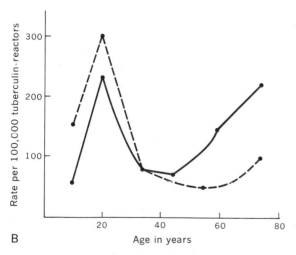

Fig. 174-2. *A.* Tuberculosis case rate per 100,000 population for each age group in Wisconsin, 1963. There is no peak in the young adult period because of the paucity of reactors to tuberculin of this age in Wisconsin today. (*Wisconsin Board of Health, Madison.*)

B. Tuberculosis case rate per 100,000 *tuberculin reactors* in each age group for Ontario, 1960. The predilection for reactors to develop active tuberculosis in young adult life and in old age can readily be seen. (*Grzybowski and Allen: Amer. Rev. Resp. Dis., 90:707, 1964; reproduced with permission of author and publisher.*)

Africans, American Indians, and Eskimos were spared tuberculous infection until extensive contact began with members of the white race in whom chronic tuberculosis was common. These people have less ability to develop an effective immune response to primary infection, and in them the infection tends to be more rapidly progressive.

SPECIFIC (ACQUIRED) IMMUNITY. Despite the immunity that infected animals have against reinfection, specific antibodies to tubercle bacilli have been difficult to demonstrate, and one of the unsolved problems in tuberculosis is why immune individuals develop progressive infection years or even decades after recovery from primary infection. Various metabolic and nutritional factors appear to impair immunity and release long-dormant bacilli.

TUBERCULIN HYPERSENSITIVITY. The most readily obtained evidence of a past or present infection with tubercle bacilli is the finding of hypersensitivity to tuberculin (protein derivative of the broth in which tubercle bacilli have been grown). Epidemiologic evidence strongly suggests that tuberculin hypersensitivity indicates that living tubercle bacilli are present. Whether the lesion in which they lie is active or inactive is often difficult to determine with certainty.

PATHOGENESIS AND PATHOLOGIC ANATOMY

PRIMARY TUBERCULOSIS. In the nonimmune subject tubercle bacilli can gain entrance to the body by several routes: lung, gastrointestinal tract, and direct cutaneous or percutaneous inoculation (as with an accident at the autopsy table). For practical purposes the only route that is of importance in the United States is the lung. The majority of primary lesions are in the lower two-thirds of the lungs, where ventilation is best and exposure to contamination of inspired air the greatest. Because they produce no toxins and no tissue reaction, tubercle bacilli initially are free to multiply without deterrence. They reach regional (hilar) nodes and even the bloodstream before their progress is inhibited by the gradual development of specific immunity over a period of several weeks. At this time the characteristic tissue reaction develops with epithelioid cell granulomata and caseation necrosis in the primary lesion, regional lymph nodes, and any site to which the bacilli have spread. The number of bacilli drops drastically with the appearance of caseation necrosis, suggesting that the process of caseation is important in the defense of the host. Thereafter the usual course of the primary infection is healing by a combination of resolution, fibrosis, and calcification.

SECONDARY STAGE. In the course of primary infection tubercle bacilli reach the general circulation in varying numbers. This event is marked only by fever and mild symptoms and is recognized as tuberculosis only when a patient is being observed closely because of a known recent exposure to tuberculosis. This stage is important in the pathogenesis of tuberculosis because it is the time when bacilli reach distant sites to establish metastatic foci of infection, which are the seeds from which post-primary chronic tuberculosis appears.

While bacilli presumably reach all organs in the secondary stage, they establish lesions with frequency in only a limited number of sites, which have one feature in common: a high tissue oxygen tension. The apex of the lung has the highest oxygen tension in the body and is the most frequent site for development of significant metastatic foci. It seems paradoxical that such a high PO_2 should exist in the poorly ventilated apexes, but this is due to a paucity of pulmonary circulation to that region when the body is in the upright position resulting in a high ventilation-perfusion ratio. Occasionally such metastatic foci progress and produce destructive tuberculosis in a short time, but more commonly the appearance of specific immunity causes the lesions to regress, scar, and become dormant. Such localized apical scars are often referred to as *Simon foci.*

Other sites at which distant metastatic lesions may develop with some frequency are the kidney, brain, and spine and long bones if infection occurs before closure of the epiphyses. Lesions in lymph nodes are probably the result of heavy seeding due to local drainage of the site of primary infection.

LATENT (DORMANT) INFECTION. Whenever a tuberculous lesion regresses and heals, the infection enters a latent phase in which infection persists without producing illness. Latent infection may remain dormant for life but may develop into active disease at any time.

TERTIARY STAGE (POSTPRIMARY TUBERCULOSIS). Chronic fibrocaseous tuberculosis may develop whenever a dormant lesion persists (Fig. 174-1). The most common site is the apical portion of the lung. At this stage bloodstream invasion is uncommon; the disease is characterized by localized areas of inflammation, necrosis abounding in bacilli, and proliferation of fibrous tissue.

OUTLOOK FOR PERSONS INFECTED WITH TUBERCULOSIS

Of new tuberculous infections, revealed by conversion of tuberculin reaction from negative to positive, 5 to 15 percent progress to serious disease within 5 years if left untreated. The risk of direct progression varies with age: it is greatest when infection begins in the first year of life or in young adults and adolescents. Among those remaining well for 5 years, a further 3 to 5 percent may be expected to develop late recrudescence at some time during life. The total morbidity in persons infected with *M. tuberculosis* is 8 to 20 percent. Both the early and the late appearance of chronic tuberculosis can be prevented if prompt treatment with INH is given when tuberculin "conversion" is discovered.

MANIFESTATIONS

I. Primary Infection

Uncomplicated primary tuberculosis often produces no significant clinical illness. It is usually diagnosed only

Fig. 174-3. Age-specific mortality from tuberculosis by 10-year cohorts, beginning with that of 1890–1900 (persons who were age 70–80 in 1966). Among earlier cohorts when the majority were infected in childhood, the peak death rate occurred during early adult life and declined steadily thereafter. In the later cohorts when few were infected during childhood, not many died as young adults. As shown also in Fig. 174-2A, the highest mortality rate was among the oldest persons in 1966. Tuberculosis should disappear as a health hazard in economically developed countries with the death of the oldest cohorts, who serve as the major reservoir of infection. The paucity of infection in later cohorts will furnish fewer cases of active tuberculosis. (*Adapted from S. Grzybowski, and J. Marr: Can. Med. Assoc., 89:737, 1963; published with permission.*)

when contacts of an open case are examined or when it progresses to a serious form of disease. The incubation period is 4 to 6 weeks from the time of inoculation to appearance of mild fever and malaise and tuberculin hypersensitivity. Symptoms usually subside without specific therapy because of the appearance of adequate specific immunity. Occasionally, however, the infection progresses either in the lung or by dissemination through the bloodstream. This turn of events is extremely serious unless detected and treated without delay.

Massive hematogenous dissemination is most common in very young children. For this reason any child under the age of three years who reacts to tuberculin should be given appropriate long-term antituberculosis chemotherapy. In older children primary infection only rarely progresses to a fatal form and usually passes totally unnoticed. The principal danger arises later during adolescence or early adulthood when the infection may undergo late progression.

Primary tuberculosis may produce pleurisy with effusion, cervical lymphadenitis, miliary tuberculosis, and meningitis. In addition, allergic manifestations, erythema nodosum and phlyctenular conjunctivitis, occasionally develop.

PRIMARY TUBERCULOSIS IN THE ADOLESCENT AND ADULT. In the United States 85 to 95 percent of young adults have never been infected with tuberculosis. Recently there have been several "epidemics" of tuberculosis among young men aboard ships of the U.S. Navy; in one case tuberculin-negative sailors were infected when late progression of infection occurred in a shipmate who had been infected years before. Persons working in the Peace Corps, Armed Forces, State Department, etc., who are assigned to countries where the prevalence of tuberculosis is high, are often heavily exposed to open cases of tuberculosis. If never previously infected or vaccinated with BCG, they may become infected as adults. As in children, clinical primary tuberculous infection in the adult usually produces only mild and nonspecific symptoms, but has a greater tendency to progress into a chronic phase. There may be an area of pneumonitis in any portion of the lung, but hilar adenopathy is not as prominent as in children. Whenever a young adult with the clinical picture of "flu" has a parenchymal infiltrate, a tuberculin test should be performed, particularly if there is any delay in clearing of the infiltrate. If the skin test is positive, the possibility of primary tuberculosis should be considered strongly because of the low incidence of positive reactions among young persons. The source of infection is usually an adult associate with cavitary tuberculosis.

II. Postprimary Tuberculosis

A. OF THE LUNGS. Chronic pulmonary tuberculosis may follow the primary infection directly or after a short, long, or very long period of dormancy (see Tertiary Stage in section on Pathogenesis and Pathologic Anatomy). Progressive disease has been observed to develop after 60 years of clinical dormancy. The most striking features of postprimary tuberculosis are (1) absence of recent exposure to an open case of tuberculosis (except in cases of direct progression from primary infection in adolescents and adults), (2) tendency to chronicity with liquefaction necrosis, and (3) production of fibrous tissue of repair. The last two phenomena are characteristic of the tissue responses in persons sensitized to tubercle bacilli. While the caseation necrosis of the primary stage is solid and paucibacillary, caseation produces liquefaction when it occurs in tissues previously sensitized. This liquid material contains abundant bacilli and may spread infection to other portions of the lungs and be aerosolized to contaminate the environment.

Symptoms. In most instances the onset of chronic pulmonary tuberculosis is insidious and the patient may be entirely asymptomatic. Many cases are discovered because a routine roentgenogram is taken as a part of a periodic health examination or upon admission to a hospital for some other illness.

The earliest symptoms are constitutional and probably result chiefly from the absorption of tuberculoprotein from the active lesion by the hypersensitive host. Abdominal symptoms may dominate the clinical picture. Fever is often present in the late afternoon or evening, but it is common for the patient to be unaware of it. A history of night sweats is merely a clue to the presence of an afternoon fever. It is common for the patient to be unaware of a fever as high as 102 to 103°F.

While fatigue and malaise may be noted by the patient, irritability, depression, or a need to rest at the end of the day, ascribed to excessive work, may be the only complaints.

Weight loss may precede symptoms, but is often passed off as being due to overwork or to voluntary caloric restriction. Often weight is well maintained until late in the course of the illness. When abdominal symptoms are present, anorexia may give rise to a rapid weight loss.

Headache may be noted occasionally, especially in the evening. Palpitation may occur during mild exertion. Menstruation is usually not disturbed until the disease is fairly far advanced when amenorrhea may develop.

Cough is frequent but not invariable and is often passed off as a "cigarette cough." When sputum is produced, it is usually odorless and green or yellow in color and is raised principally upon arising in the morning. Hemoptysis may accompany the cough and usually consists of streaked sputum with small amounts of blood.

In some patients the onset of pulmonary tuberculosis is relatively sudden, because of a rapid progression from a primary infection or from a massive spread from an area of liquefaction necrosis. A characteristic story is that the patient experiences a "bad cold" or "influenza" without awareness of any prior lung disease. The productive cough then persists while the constitutional symptoms partially abate, so that the patient feels that he is recovering. This situation may persist for several months before the patient notices enough constitutional symptoms to cause him to seek medical aid. When he does so, he may place more stress upon loss of weight or abdominal symptoms than upon the cough which he may attribute to smoking. Green or yellow sputum is often a clue that the cough is due to infection and not simply to smoking.

Physical and Roentgen Examinations. Early asymptomatic infiltrations due to tuberculosis are usually undetectable by physical examination, but may be extensive by x-ray. Crepitant inspiratory rales may be detected, especially when inspiration is preceded by full expiration and a small cough (posttussive rales). When larger lesions are present, especially with chronic cavitation, dullness to percussion and amphoric bronchial breath sounds may be elicited, but areas of recent excavation do not produce these signs. In tuberculous pneumonia the classical signs of pneumonia are present and even the white blood cell count may be elevated.

Long-standing tuberculosis with extensive fibrosis causes contraction and distortion of pulmonary tissue and of bronchi. In such instances, a wide variety of physical signs, such as bronchial breath sounds, coarse rales, deviation of the trachea, spasm and atrophy of various chest and neck muscles, and diminished movements of one hemithorax, may be noted. There is likely to be dullness over the apex of the involved lung.

However, because examination of the lungs in the early stages is so frequently unremarkable and the blood count and sedimentation rate are normal, *the importance of the chest roentgenogram in diagnosis of tuberculosis cannot be overemphasized.* In chronic tuberculosis the early infiltrate is usually in the apical and subapical areas. Cavitation is common but may require the use of planigraphy to demonstrate it. Because the chronic form of the disease is often a late manifestation of disseminated primary infection, nodular lesions are often present in the contralateral lung as well.

Of particular importance in the roentgen diagnosis is the comparison of the film with one or more examinations made months or years earlier, so that subtle changes can be detected in clinically dormant lesions. Because fibrous tissue does not change appreciably with time, any change in the lesions on serial films must be taken to indicate activity of the disease. Among 90 patients over the age of fifty with newly active chronic pulmonary tuberculosis, over 70 percent showed evidence of preexisting tuberculous scars. Comparison of films with previous examinations should become routine practice because it would permit detection and prophylactic treatment of slightly active lesions before liquefaction and spread of bacilli to other portions of the lungs and into the environment occur.

Other radiographic techniques which are of value in the proper evaluation of the lungs include *pulmonary oblique* views (taken at 20 to 25° rotation instead of 45 to 60°, as used for cardiac evaluation), sectional radiography (tomograms or planigrams), and the *apical lordotic* view, which shows the posterior segment of the upper lobe more clearly than the standard roentgenogram. The tomogram is of particular value in revealing the nodular and cavitary nature of indistinct pulmonary infiltrates.

Complications of Pulmonary Tuberculosis. Cavitation. When nodular lesions of tuberculosis become active and coalesce, areas of liquid necrosis develop. When necrosis includes a small bronchus, liquid material escapes into the bronchial tree and is expectorated, leaving a cavity within the lung parenchyma. At this stage, the sputum usually contains numerous tubercle bacilli.

Hemoptysis. In the majority of instances of bleeding from the lungs in tuberculosis, the blood arises from an ulceration of the bronchial mucosa and usually presents as streaks of bright red blood on the sputum. Bleeding usually subsides spontaneously if the patient lies quietly. Codeine in a dose of 15 mg or morphine, 8 mg, may be used to control cough. Many remedies have been advocated, but because bleeding usually stops spontaneously, it is difficult to demonstrate real effectiveness of any particular measure.

There is one type of hemoptysis which has a very different prognosis. When the blood is copious and dark (bluish red), its source is more likely a branch of the pulmonary artery, usually within the wall of a cavity. In the majority of instances the branches of the pulmonary artery in the vicinity of tuberculous cavities are thrombosed, but occasionally one remains open in the wall of a cavity, is eroded by the infection (Rasmussen's aneurysm), and may rupture. The majority of patients in whom this occurs exsanguinate before treatment can be administered, but if copious dark blood is expectorated and the patient survives, immediate resection of the cavitary area is indicated to prevent exsanguination.

Pleurisy with Effusion. The pleura overlying a tuberculous focus may become involved, resulting in pain on inspiration ("catch" in the side). Fibrous adhesions between the visceral and parietal pleural surfaces are usually the only residuals of such "dry pleurisy." A small caseous focus may erode through the visceral pleura and, in a hypersensitive host, produce pleurisy with effusion.

Tuberculous pleural effusion is most common in young adults between the ages of fifteen and twenty-five and occurs most commonly within the first 9 months after implantation of the primary infection. It frequently clears spontaneously, but this should not give a false sense of security because such a course is consistent with a tuberculous effusion. Pleural effusion may also develop in the course of chronic pulmonary tuberculosis (late recrudescence). The fluid is usually clear and light yellow in color. It is an exudate, which is characterized by lymphocytosis and high protein content (> 3 GM per 100 ml). The diagnosis is made best by needle biopsy of the parietal pleura. The management of unilateral tuberculous pleural effusion consists of the administration of effective antituberculous chemotherapy. When tuberculous effusion is bilateral, it is usually the result of disseminated tuberculosis and calls for prompt and vigorous chemotherapy with three effective agents.

The diagnosis of tuberculous pleural effusion is difficult because only about 20 to 25 percent of effusions yield tubercle bacilli upon culture and about an equal number of positive cultures result from gastric washings or sputum induced by inhalation of heated aerosol. Thus, in over 50 percent of the patients with tuberculous pleural effusion, bacteriologic proof of diagnosis is lacking at the time when therapy is most effective in preventing later development of overt tuberculosis. The percutaneous pleural biopsy has made a great contribution to the recognition of tuberculosis in the etiology of otherwise undiagnosed pleural effusion.

Tuberculous Pneumonia. The onset of tuberculosis occasionally is quite acute, resembling that of bacterial pneumonia. This form of tuberculosis is seen most often in Negroes, persons with diabetes, children with overwhelming primary infection, and elderly individuals in whom the lungs are flooded with bacilli discharged from an area of liquid necrosis. Chills, fever, productive cough, and pleuritic chest pain occur. Smear of the sputum usually reveals numerous tubercle bacilli.

Bronchopleural Fistula and Empyema. When a large caseous lesion erodes into the pleural space, the gross contamination often produces tuberculous empyema. The mechanism is the same as the production of exudative pleural effusion, but the extent of contamination is much greater. The caseous lesion may also erode a bronchus, giving rise to a *bronchopleural fistula* in addition to the empyema. Management is largely surgical and consists of establishing adequate drainage, in combination with the administration of three effective antituberculosis drugs.

Tuberculosis of Large Bronchi, Trachea, and Larynx. These organs are protected from implantation of *M. tuberculosis* by a covering of mucous secretion and become involved in advanced cavitary pulmonary tuberculosis with excretion of numerous tubercle bacilli. Ulceration of the bronchus may result in hemoptysis and a localized wheeze during respiration. The bronchial lumen also may be compromised without ulceration due to pressure of enlarged hilar lymph nodes associated with primary infection.

Prolonged hoarseness and pain in the throat accentuated by swallowing suggest tuberculous laryngitis. The abnormality is relatively easily detected by inspection of the vocal cords by indirect laryngoscopy. However, the lesion is fairly easily mistaken for a carcinoma of the larynx, even upon histologic examination. For this reason, a roentgenogram of the chest should be routine practice before performing a laryngectomy for carcinoma. Chemotherapy is highly effective for tuberculosis of mucous membranes.

Bronchiectasis. The smaller branches of the bronchial tree may be affected by tuberculosis either in the primary phase or in the chronic pulmonary phase. Localized dilatation of the bronchi may develop as a result of weakening of the bronchial wall and fibrous contraction of the parenchyma, just as happens with postviral suppurative pneumonia in childhood. Local obstruction by hilar nodes may also be present but is not a requisite for the development of bronchiectasis. When bronchiectasis occurs in an upper lobe, where drainage is good, it usually produces no symptoms. However, primary tuberculosis may damage bronchi in the lower portion of the lung, where poor drainage may permit pyogenic infection to occur years after the primary process has healed, resulting in a chronic cough productive of purulent sputum, often marked by periodic hemoptysis.

Gastrointestinal Tuberculosis. The gastrointestinal tract is relatively resistant to tuberculosis, but in advanced cavitary pulmonary disease associated with the excretion of numerous bacilli in the sputum, the gastrointestinal tract becomes infected usually in the ileocecal region. Symptoms consist chiefly of intermittent abdominal pain, cramping, and diarrhea. Occasionally the infection spreads through the wall of the intestine to give rise to tuberculous peritonitis, which is considered below.

Differential Diagnosis. The clinical picture presented by pulmonary tuberculosis varies widely and may simulate a great number of other diseases.

Carcinoma of the Lung. Tuberculosis is most commonly confused with carcinoma of the lung because the highest incidence of both diseases is in the upper lobe and in older men. Both cause loss of weight, chronic cough, blood-streaked sputum, and mild fever. In addition to bacteriologic studies for tubercle bacilli, sputum cytology and bronchoscopy should be employed to aid in the dif-

ferentiation. Comparison of prior roentgenograms may be of considerable help, but in some instances nothing short of a diagnostic thoracotomy will serve to make the distinction. When tuberculosis is considered among the diagnostic possibilities, antituberculosis chemotherapy should be instituted a few days before thoracotomy in order to avoid infectious complications in the event the lesion is tuberculous.

Mycotic Infections. Whenever tubercle bacilli cannot be isolated from a patient suspected of having tuberculosis, appropriate tests should be made for the various fungous infections, any of which may present a clinical picture indistinguishable from pulmonary tuberculosis. Reliable skin and serologic tests are available for coccidioidomycosis and histoplasmosis. Blastomycosis, actinomycosis, aspergillosis, nocardiosis, cryptococcosis, and sporotrichosis can be diagnosed only by demonstrating the organisms in a biopsy specimen or on culture.

Sarcoidosis. The typical patient with sarcoidosis is afebrile and has a negative tuberculin test and a roentgen picture of diffuse pulmonary infiltrations and hilar adenopathy, but the disease is very protean in its manifestations and may mimic tuberculosis. Scalene node and liver biopsies, as well as determination of serum protein and serum calcium, are of value in establishing this diagnosis. The Kveim test is of some value, but the antigen is not yet available commercially.

Aspiration Pneumonia, Lung Abscess. Pulmonary infection which is introduced by the drainage of contaminated saliva from a focus of pyorrhea during sleep occurs predominantly in the upper and midposterior segments of the lung and can mimic tuberculosis closely. The distinction can usually be made eventually, but much valuable time may be lost while the patient is erroneously treated for the wrong disease. The presence of foul sputum, hemoptysis, fever, and leukocytosis in a patient who has pyorrhea and has recently undergone surgery or who drinks to excess suggests a pyogenic lung abscess. While lung abscess is usually relatively acute, it may mimic tuberculosis in chronicity. If the differentiation cannot be made readily, it may be advisable to treat the patient with high dosages of intravenous penicillin for 1 to 2 weeks *before* initiating antituberculous chemotherapy. If the response is adequate and prompt, and there is some clearing by x-ray, a tentative diagnosis of lung abscess can be made. If not, antituberculous therapy can be instituted while the search continues for the etiologic agent.

Other Forms of Pneumonia. Several organisms (mycoplasma—(Chap. 207); adenovirus—(Chap. 206) can present clinical and roentgenologic appearances which at first are indistinguishable from pulmonary tuberculosis. Cold agglutinins and precipitin and complement fixation tests often establish the correct diagnosis. Cavitation is rare, and sputum examination does not yield tubercle bacilli. Primary tuberculosis may present with a localized infiltrate in the lung and slowly subside spontaneously coincident with tetracycline therapy, suggesting the diagnosis of mycoplasma pneumonia. However, tuberculous lesions usually fail to clear completely. A tuberculin skin test should be performed in all cases of "viral pneumonia," particularly if a pleural effusion, which is extremely rare in viral pneumonia, is present. A positive skin test in an adolescent or young adult with pneumonitis should be viewed seriously, in light of the infrequency of reactors at this age.

Pneumoconiosis. Pulmonary infiltrations associated with exposure to silicon dioxide (silicosis), beryllium, and cosmetic hair spray may present a roentgenographic appearance suggestive of tuberculosis. Silicosis can present great difficulty in diagnosis because it may produce conglomerate nodules and even cavitation that mimics tuberculosis. However, when the tuberculin skin test is positive in a patient with silicosis, smoldering tuberculosis is so likely to be present that prophylaxis with isoniazid is justified even in the absence of bacteriologic or clinical evidence of the infection.

Bronchiectasis. A productive cough due to infection in chronically dilated bronchi occurs much less frequently than formerly because of more effective antibiotic therapy for necrotizing pneumonias of childhood and the reduction in the number of children whose bronchi are damaged by primary tuberculosis. The lower and middle lobes (or lingula on the left) are most often involved, and a bronchogram effectively demonstrates the pathology. Tuberculosis should be considered as one possible cause of bronchiectasis. If the tuberculin test is positive, isoniazid should be administered prophylactically to prevent late progression of tuberculosis from coexistent Simon foci in the apexes whether or not these are visible radiographically.

Confusion Caused by Systemic Effects of Tuberculous Infection. Because of the insidious nature of tuberculosis, the clinical picture may be mistaken for that produced by several other disorders. Malaise, easy fatigability, inability to concentrate, anorexia, and weight loss may be mistaken for psychoneurosis. The tuberculin skin test and roentgenogram of the chest are usually of great aid in making this distinction. The symptoms may suggest *hyperthyroidism* or *diabetes mellitus*, but with a little care the distinction can be made. Tuberculosis should always be considered in the differential diagnosis of fever of unknown origin (Chap. 16). If the roentgenogram reveals a pulmonary infiltrate, the possibility of tuberculosis is increased, but in cases of disseminated or extrapulmonary tuberculosis, the chest roentgenogram may be normal. In these cases biopsy of an enlarged lymph node, bone marrow, or liver may be of help. Disseminated tuberculosis may present as *aplastic anemia*, particularly if associated with an obscure fever. Formerly, tuberculosis was overdiagnosed in patients presenting with general systemic symptoms. Today, however, because of a lessening awareness of tuberculosis, the principal danger is that tuberculosis will be overlooked. Furthermore, *tuberculosis may appear without reexposure in anyone who has ever been infected with it.*

B. CHRONIC TUBERCULOSIS OF OTHER ORGANS. Localized tuberculous infection may occur in a number of other organs, notably the lymph nodes, kidney, long bones, genital tract, brain, and meninges. Organisms reach these sites from the primary lesion either by lymphatic spread or by way of the bloodstream.

Tuberculosis of Lymph Nodes. The most common involvement of lymph nodes occurs in the hilus draining the lung involved with a primary infection. The enlargement is usually modest, but may be massive and give rise to obstruction and even ulceration of a major bronchus. The prognosis is good with proper chemotherapy, but the nodes may be slow in returning to normal. Surgical excision is indicated occasionally.

Cervical Adenitis. Cervical adenitis, or scrofula, has become relatively uncommon in the United States as a result of the elimination of tuberculous cattle and pasteurization of milk. Scrofula may present as a manifestation of the primary infection with human tubercle bacilli also. In Negroes, tuberculous cervical lymphadenitis occasionally appears as a late manifestation. The nodes may be quite large (several centimeters in diameter) and matted together in a mass with an area of soft fluctuation. The skin over the area is not usually red, hot, or tender. Swelling begins insidiously and usually is not accompanied by systemic symptoms. The skin may perforate with drainage of caseous material. Therapy consists of multiple-drug chemotherapy (see below). In some cases the offending organisms are unclassified mycobacteria, and for this reason cultures should be made of any pus.

Tuberculosis of the Kidney. Second to the upper lobes of the lungs, the kidney is the most common site for the late appearance of localized tuberculous infection. The mechanism of implantation is the same as that of the pulmonary apexes, namely, by hematogenous spread at the time of the primary infection. The oxygen tension in the cortical portion of the kidney approaches that in arterial blood, which enhances the growth and survival of tubercle bacilli for long periods of time. As in the lungs, foci of tuberculosis may remain dormant for many years and produce clinical disease late in life. The pathology is the same as is found in the lung: inflammation occurs, followed by caseation, liquefaction, and discharge of contaminated material into the collecting system and down the ureter to the bladder and in the male, to the genital tract.

Symptoms of renal infection are usually insidious and are often overlooked completely until the appearance of cystitis or epididymitis. Microscopic hematuria and pyuria with a "sterile" urine on culture for routine organisms should always call to mind tuberculosis and should lead to performance of a tuberculin test. If this is positive, the urine should be examined for tubercle bacilli by smear and culture of several early morning specimens. Painless gross hematuria from a chronic cavity in the kidney may occur on several occasions before the proper diagnosis is suspected and established. Intravenous pyelography may reveal a tuberculous cavity of the kidney connecting with the collecting system. Therapy consists of a multiple-drug regimen, including daily streptomycin and isoniazid. Therapy should be continued for 18 to 24 months to allow time for as complete healing as possible. The symptoms usually subside promptly with chemotherapy, and the patient may return to gainful employment when he feels clinically well. Resection of residual areas of destruction is only rarely necessary.

Genital Tuberculosis, Male. Infection of the genital tract in the male is probably always secondary to renal tuberculosis. Bacilli which are discharged from a cavitary lesion in the kidney may reach the seminal vesicles, prostate gland, and epididymis through their connections with the excretory tract. Symptoms begin insidiously, most commonly with pain in the scrotum due to inflammation of the epididymis and vas deferens or pain with ejaculation. On examination, the epididymis is found to contain one or more tender nodules. The prostate and/or seminal vesicles may be tender also. Therapy is the same as for tuberculosis of the kidney.

Genital Tuberculosis, Female. Tuberculosis of the female genital tract usually begins in the fallopian tube and is most common when the primary infection occurs during the childbearing period of life. It is uncommon in women whose primary infection occurred before puberty. Infection spreads from the tube into the uterus and may give rise to metromenorrhagia. Symptoms are usually mild and insidious and consist of abdominal pain, white vaginal discharge, and dyspareunia. Systemic symptoms and signs are uncommon, probably because the infection is indolent and localized. The most common manifestation is sterility, but ectopic pregnancy may also occur. Tuberculosis of the fallopian tube may contaminate the peritoneum and result in a tuberculous pelvic abscess or generalized peritonitis. Therapy consists of long-term multiple-drug chemotherapy.

Skeletal Tuberculosis. When primary tuberculosis occurs during childhood at the time of great metabolic activity and high oxygen tension at the epiphyseal lines, the chances for hematogenous lesions in the bones are increased. The greatest incidence of tuberculous osteomyelitis and arthritis is within 3 years after a primary infection in childhood, but late recrudescence may occur. The joints most commonly involved are the hip, knee, elbow, and wrist. Tuberculous tenosynovitis is most common about the wrist. Trauma may precipitate late activation of a dormant infection.

Tuberculous Spondylitis (Pott's disease). Implantation of bacilli in the vertebras may take place by the hematogenous route (if infection occurs before epiphyses close) or by spread of infection from a paraspinal lymph node draining tuberculous pleurisy or empyema. As with other forms of tuberculosis, lesions may not become manifest until late in life. The intervertebral disk is destroyed early, and narrowing of one such space on lateral x-ray of the spine may be the only detectable abnormality. A paravertebral abscess may be seen as a fusiform density extending the length of several vertebras. Chemotherapy with at least three drugs is usually quite effective, but the patient must be kept flat on an orthopedic bed to prevent damage to the spinal cord. Surgical drainage of the abscess and bony fusion of the involved vertebral bodies may be necessary to stabilize the spine and control the infection.

Tuberculous Peritonitis. The peritoneum may be implanted with tubercle bacilli by at least four mechanisms: (1) Spread through the wall of the infected intestine; (2) from a mesenteric lymph node; (3) from an infected fallopian tube; (4) from hematogenous seeding in the course of disseminated tuberculosis. Symptoms are insidious, but ultimately the patient has fever, night sweats, weakness, gastrointestinal symptoms, and abdominal pain. The disease occurs with increased frequency in alcoholics with cirrhosis in whom a clear tuberculous peritoneal exudate may be mistaken for ascites. Whenever ascitic fluid shows a lymphocytosis and a protein in excess of 3 Gm per 100 ml, tuberculous peritonitis should be considered. The diagnosis is most easily made by biopsy. Chemotherapy is highly effective but must be prolonged.

Tuberculous Pericarditis. Tuberculous infection may spread from the mediastinal lymph nodes or contiguous segments of lung to the pericardium in the same manner as to the pleura. The pathology is the same as with tuberculous pleurisy, with outpouring of a clear exudate from the serous surface, formation of granulomata, and subsequent fibrosis. The clinical picture is that of chronic pericardial tamponade, with hepatomegaly, edema, friction rub, cardiac enlargement during the active phase, and constriction during the phase of fibrosis. When such an illness is accompanied by afternoon fever or night sweats and a positive tuberculin reaction, tuberculosis should be strongly considered. The diagnosis is usually made by study of aspirated fluid or by open pericardial biopsy. Tuberculous effusion contains more than 3 Gm per 100 ml of protein and an increased number of white blood cells, predominantly lymphocytes. Therapy consists of a multiple-drug regimen as outlined below. Occasionally pericardiectomy is required if the process has become chronic and the pericardium fibrotic and unexpandable. However, adequate therapy early in the course of the disease usually obviates the need for pericardiectomy.

If tuberculous pericarditis has undergone spontaneous healing, the patient may present years later with the picture of chronic constrictive pericarditis (Chap. 272). Pericardiectomy is usually necessary at this stage to improve cardiac function but may be technically difficult due to extensive calcification extending into the myocardium.

Tuberculosis of the Adrenals. Occasionally hematogenous tuberculosis localizes in the adrenal glands and results in total destruction of the organs, giving rise to adrenal cortical insufficiency (Addison's disease). The condition must be differentiated from adrenal cortical atrophy, which is more common, and from other causes of adrenal destruction such as histoplasmosis. Therapy consists of the use of three antituberculosis agents plus adrenal hormone replacement therapy (Chap. 92).

Tuberculous Meningitis. Tuberculosis may involve the meninges either as a part of miliary tuberculosis or through reactivation and extension of infection from an old focus within the brain. In areas with a high incidence of tuberculosis, tuberculous meningitis is seen most commonly in young children in the first year of infection. In areas of low incidence, such as the United States today, meningitis is more common among adults as a result of late reactivation of dormant infection. Pathologically, the meninges contain small tubercles and a fibrinous exudate over the base of the brain.

Symptoms consist of headache, restlessness, and irritability usually accompanied by fever, malaise, night sweats, and loss of weight. Nausea and vomiting may be prominent. Stiffness of the neck and Brudzinski's sign are usually present. Spinal puncture usually reveals increased pressure, clear fluid containing an increased protein, reduced glucose (less than half the blood glucose), and 100 to 1,000 white blood cells, 80 to 95 percent of which are lymphocytes. Upon standing in a tube overnight a fine web of protein (pellicle) may form. A smear of this pellicle may reveal acid-fast bacilli, but culture of the fluid is often necessary to recover the organisms.

The differential diagnosis includes partially treated bacterial meningitis, fungal meningitides, and carcinomatosis of the meninges. There is considerable urgency in establishing the correct diagnosis because specific therapy is highly effective only if given early in the course of the illness. Irreversible brain damage can result from waiting 6 to 8 weeks for cultural proof of the diagnosis. When the diagnosis cannot be established readily, specific antituberculous chemotherapy should be instituted if the tuberculin is positive and the CSF findings are consistent with tuberculous meningitis. Therapy consists of at least two drugs including isoniazid, and steroids may be helpful in mitigating the inflammatory process. Intrathecal therapy is not indicated.

Low Sodium Syndrome. Older persons with tuberculous meningitis or overwhelming pulmonary tuberculosis occasionally manifest somnolence or coma associated with a very low serum sodium concentration (110 to 125 mEq per liter). This is probably due to inappropriate secretion of antidiuretic hormone, but this is not always demonstrable. It must be distinguished from adrenal insufficiency, which depresses the serum sodium concentration in concert with an elevated serum potassium. In addition to three antituberculosis agents, adequate sodium chloride should be administered, and water should be restricted.

III. Disseminated Tuberculosis

SILENT DISSEMINATION. Hematogenous dissemination of small numbers of tubercle bacilli is common during the primary infection, but usually produces little clinical illness. The principal importance of this event is the seeding of bacilli to sites far removed from the primary infection.

MASSIVE DISSEMINATION (MILIARY TUBERCULOSIS). When a liquid caseous focus empties its contents into a vein, there is a massive dissemination of tubercle bacilli throughout the body. The defense mechanisms are overwhelmed, and tubercles become established in all organs of the body. Without specific therapy death is almost certain.

Miliary tuberculosis is the most dreaded manifestation of tuberculosis. It may arise shortly after primary infection (progressive primary tuberculosis) or by reactivation of a dormant focus years or decades later. Because the resistance of the body is overwhelmed, lesions are not limited to those organs with an elevated PO_2 but are found in the liver, spleen, bone marrow, and meninges. One of the best diagnostic tests for miliary tuberculosis is biopsy of the liver, lymph node, or bone marrow in search of caseating granulomata.

Symptoms are usually nonspecific and consist of weight loss, weakness, gastrointestinal disturbances, fever, and sweats. The patient has usually had a course of penicillin or broad-spectrum antibiotics without control of the fever before the diagnosis comes to mind. Cough is not a prominent feature, but dyspnea may be. The correct diagnosis is often not suspected until the typical "miliary" pattern appears on the roentgenogram of the lungs. The white blood count may be normal or low, or may show a leukemoid pattern. One useful feature of the blood count is the finding of a decreased ratio of lymphocytes to monocytes (normal, 3:1). Proper therapy is dependent upon early and accurate diagnosis. Because histoplasmosis, coccidioidomycosis, blastomycosis, cryptococcosis, and other chronic infections may present similarly, it is imperative to obtain any material possible by biopsy or aspiration and perform appropriate stains and cultures.

SUBACUTE AND CHRONIC HEMATOGENOUS TUBERCULOSIS. Instead of a single massive invasion of the bloodstream, smaller numbers of tubercle bacilli may escape intermittently into the circulation and give rise to a variety of clinical manifestations including aplastic anemia, low-grade fever, lymphadenopathy, effusion into pleural and peritoneal cavities, and splenomegaly. There may be destructive lesions of bones, kidneys, subcutaneous tissue, or skin. This clinical picture is most common among Negroes of any age and in Caucasians of advanced years, and the process represents an overwhelming of immunity during reactivation of tuberculosis after years of dormancy.

The protean manifestations and bizarre clinical pictures caused by subacute and chronic forms of hematogenous tuberculosis provide a tremendous diagnostic challenge. To add to the confusion, the tuberculin reaction is often suppressed in persons with overwhelming infection. The solution to the clinical problem most commonly comes when the possibility of tuberculosis is considered. Confirmation must be sought from appropriate histologic and bacteriologic studies. Prognosis is uniformly bad without specific therapy, but improves with a multiple-drug regimen including INH.

DIAGNOSIS

TUBERCULIN SKIN TEST

Tuberculin (or its purified protein derivative—PPD) is derived from broth in which *M. tuberculosis* has been cultivated. It contains enough specific antigen to elicit a skin reaction in persons who are hypersensitive to tubercle bacilli whether from vaccination or from harboring the infection.

TECHNIQUE. The most reliable method of performing this test is to inject 0.1 ml of suitably diluted tuberculin intradermally, usually on the volar aspect of the forearm. An area of induration of 8-mm diameter at the site after 48 to 72 hr represents a positive result. The area is often erythematous, but only the diameter of the induration is considered significant. The usual *initial* dose is 5 tuberculin units (TU), or 0.0001 mg PPD (intermediate strength PPD), and should not exceed 10 TU in order to avoid large reactions accompanied by lymphangitis and systemic symptoms. This dose is the equivalent of a 1:1,000 dilution of "old tuberculin" (OT). If there is no reaction (or less than 8-mm induration), the test is read as negative and a stronger dose applied in the same manner, using second strength PPD or 1:100 OT, which gives a dose of 100 TU. If this test is also negative, the diagnosis of tuberculosis can be excluded with an accuracy of about 99 percent except in debilitated persons with overwhelming infection.

A positive reaction, particularly when elicited only by the stronger dose, does not necessarily indicate an infection with *M. tuberculosis,* but may be caused by an infection with one of the "unclassified" mycobacteria, i.e., *M. battey, M. kansasii,* or a scotochromogenic mycobacterium. However, a strong reaction to 5 TU of PPD usually indicates that the subject harbors an infection with *M. tuberculosis* which may be either dormant or active.

A positive tuberculin reaction can be suppressed temporarily by various factors: pneumonia, fracture of a hip, steroid therapy, or a severe toxic reaction from any disease, including overwhelming tuberculosis. Various studies have shown that as many as 15 to 30 percent of persons with bacteriologically active tuberculosis show no reaction to 5 TU of PPD. Furthermore, if there is reason to suspect an active tuberculosis or if the tuberculin is known to have been positive in the past, even a negative second strength PPD does not exclude tuberculosis. The diagnosis may be revealed by bacteriologic study.

BACTERIOLOGIC DIAGNOSIS

The only absolute proof of active tuberculosis is the cultural identification of *M. tuberculosis* from tissue or appropriate secretion: sputum, gastric washing, urine, CSF, serous effusion, or pus from an abscess or sinus. A useful preliminary examination, however, is to make a smear of the material and stain it for microscopic examination. Kenyon or Ziehl-Neelsen stain is used for standard microscopy and auromine-rhodamine stain for the more sensitive fluorescence microscopy. The smear is not a very sensitive method at best, but it has the virtue of giving immediate results and of identifying the contagious case who is excreting great numbers of organisms into the environment. For positive identification, cultures must be made on either solid egg medium (Löwenstein-Jensen) or Middlebrook 7H-10 medium using CO_2 (20 to 40 mm Hg) in the atmosphere to speed growth.

The most commonly examined material is sputum. When it can be produced spontaneously (usually in the early morning), it makes the most satisfactory material for both smear and culture. If none can be produced spontaneously, the patient may be asked to inhale a heated aerosol containing 10 percent each of glycerin and sodium chloride, which stimulates production of bronchial secretion. Sputum should never be collected over a 24-hr period because of the increased contamination associated with such prolonged collections. Guinea pig inoculation is no longer widely used for identification of *M. tuberculosis* because of the economic and technical advantages of culture methods.

When no sputum can be collected, as in young children or senile or psychotic persons, morning gastric contents may be aspirated and cultured. Diagnosis by smear of this material is less reliable than of sputum because of the occasional presence of saprophytic acid-fast bacteria in the stomach.

Multiple specimens may be needed before the organisms are recovered. This is particularly true in cases of primary tuberculosis, tuberculous pleurisy with effusion, and chronic tuberculosis of minimal extent. Also, old chronic tuberculous lesions may shed organisms only intermittently.

OTHER LABORATORY FINDINGS

HEMATOLOGY. The white blood cell count is usually not significantly elevated, except in tuberculous pneumonia, where it may suggest a pyogenic infection, and in miliary tuberculosis, where it may suggest leukemia (leukemoid reaction). Hemoglobin and hematocrit are usually normal unless a prolonged period of active disease has produced anemia of infection. The presence of 10 to 20 percent monocytes (equal to or greater than the number of lymphocytes) suggests severe and overwhelming tuberculosis. An elevated erythrocyte sedimentation rate indicates probable active infection, but a normal one is of little help in excluding activity. The ESR is usually elevated in advanced active tuberculosis, but is often normal with active lesions of lesser extent.

URINALYSIS. There are no specific changes except when a urinary lesion is present. Renal tuberculosis is not rare, and most often appears as "sterile" pyuria and hematuria. Cultures may have to be repeated several times before revealing *M. tuberculosis.*

MISCELLANEOUS. There is no satisfactory serologic test for diagnosing active tuberculosis such as exists for histoplasmosis and coccidioidomycosis. Biopsy of the liver, bone marrow, or lymph node can be of great aid in reaching a presumptive diagnosis of disseminated tuberculosis by revealing caseating granulomata. This finding may enable initiation of specific therapy in time to save a life; awaiting the results of culture may allow the situation to pass beyond the point of no return before the diagnosis is made and therapy is initiated.

TREATMENT

The availability of several effective chemotherapeutic agents during the past 20 years has completely changed the treatment of all forms of tuberculosis. While the healing of the lesions still must be accomplished by the processes of repair inherent in the host, inhibition of the organisms by properly selected drugs virtually assures a successful outcome providing that the offending organisms are susceptible to the drugs employed and the patient is not completely overwhelmed by infection.

Because healing depends upon host defenses aided by specific drug therapy, the total period of therapy must be quite long, that is, 18 to 24 months. However, only a small portion of this time need be spent in the hospital. For the remainder of the time the patient may live a rather normal life at home and may even return to work.

CHEMOTHERAPY

Ehrlich defined chemotherapy as the use of a chemical which would kill microorganisms without harm to the host. None of the agents used against tuberculosis would meet this criterion, because they merely inhibit growth or reproduction of the organisms. When streptomycin was first used in 1946–1947, it was frequently followed by relapse and the appearance of resistant bacilli because its action was bacteriostatic and served only as an aid to host defense mechanisms in overcoming the infection. From this observation stemmed the rational approach of using several drugs simultaneously in order to mitigate development of resistance and to achieve long-term inhibition of organisms while the body's rather slow defense mechanisms controlled the infection, permitting resolution of exudate and repair of tissue damage.

CHEMOTHERAPEUTIC AGENTS. The most widely used and valuable agents are streptomycin (SM), isoniazid (INH), para aminosalicylic acid (PAS), and ethambutol (EMB), a new synthetic agent released late in 1967.

It may seem a little surprising that the tubercle bacilli from the majority of "new" cases of tuberculosis in this country still show complete susceptibility to all these agents although SM and PAS have been in general use for 22 years and INH for 18. The reason for this is that the majority of cases of active tuberculosis among adults represent reactivation of foci of infection implanted years before the advent of chemotherapy. Furthermore, most new primary infections arise from implantation of organisms from such recently reactivated cases and not from patients who have received chemotherapy. The incidence of primary antibiotic resistance can be expected to rise in the United States as the few new infections caused by resistant organisms emerge from dormancy and reactivate.

Isoniazid. INH is the keystone of antituberculosis therapy, because it is very effective, is nontoxic, and is administered orally. In adults, it is most often given in a dose of 300 mg once a day (about 5 mg per kg). In children, larger doses are advisable (10 to 20 mg/kg/day). A few years ago, a controversy raged concerning the need for larger doses in certain adults who inactivate the drug rapidly, but clinical advantage of such large doses has not been demonstrated.

Streptomycin. Streptomycin was the first effective agent discovered for the treatment of tuberculosis and remains one of the most effective. It should only be used in conjunction with another agent, because organisms readily become resistant to it when it is used alone. The dosage is 1 Gm per day for most adults (0.5 Gm per day over the age of sixty) and 20 mg/kg/day in children. At the start of therapy it should always be given daily. After about 2 months, the frequency of administration may be changed to two or three injections each week in order to prolong the total period over which the drug can be administered without encountering serious vestibular toxicity. Several years ago it was the practice to administer streptomycin at these less frequent intervals from the start, but there are now adequate data to show that this practice results in a higher proportion of treatment failures and an increased number of cases with resistant organisms. Dihydrostreptomycin is no longer used because of its effects upon the auditory nerve producing deafness.

Para-aminosalicylic Acid. Para-aminosalicylic acid is of considerable value, but only as a companion agent for one or both of the drugs mentioned above. It may be given as the uncombined acid or as a sodium, potassium, or calcium salt. The dosage for adults is 12 Gm of the acid per day in divided doses (the salts must be administered in sufficient dosage to provide 12 Gm of the acid radical). All forms of PAS may be irritating to the gastrointestinal tract, and cause anorexia, nausea, cramping, and diarrhea. The sodium salt is contraindicated in patients with heart disease and hypertension in whom sodium needs to be restricted. The potassium salt is contraindicated in renal disease in which potassium may be retained. A more pure form of the acid (crystalized in the presence of ascorbic acid) is now available for which the daily dose is 6 Gm. This form produces considerably less gastric irritation, is better tolerated by patients, and is marketed as "PAS-C."

Ethambutol. Ethambutol is the most recent antituberculosis agent to receive FDA approval. Early results are very encouraging, particularly in the retreatment of tuberculosis in which the organisms are resistant to the more commonly used drugs. Optic toxicity presently limits its wide adoption for initial treatment regimens.

INDICATIONS FOR CHEMOTHERAPY

Because of the availability of several drugs, each with advantages and disadvantages, skill and experience are required to tailor therapy to each situation. The following is intended as a guide to choice of therapy.

ISONIAZID. INH may be given alone in several situations where the bacillary population is not great, no cavity is demonstrable by planigraphic radiograms, and in which the risk of producing strains of bacilli resistant to it is minimal:

1. Recent "converters" from negative to positive tuberculin skin test in whom there is no clinical or radiographic evidence of the infection

2. Young children who react to tuberculin and must be presumed to have been infected recently

3. Household contacts of an open case of tuberculosis

4. In postprimary tuberculosis of very minimal extent and questionable activity

5. As prophylaxis against the development of dormant infection into active disease when the tuberculin test is positive and the chest radiogram reveals Simon foci or other evidence of scarring from a previous infection

Chemoprophylaxis with INH is indicated when any of the following is also present because of their importance in late recrudescence of dormant infection: alcoholism, diabetes, debility due to age or any chronic disease, history of gastrectomy, silicosis, or prolonged steroid therapy for arthritis, asthma, sarcoidosis, etc.

ISONIAZID PLUS ANOTHER DRUG. When the tuberculous process is of somewhat greater extent and appears active, INH should be used in combination with at least one other effective agent in order to reduce the chance of emergence of strains resistant to INH. The most common regimen in use today is INH-PAS because of its demonstrated efficacy and the ease with which it can be given orally. Some prefer INH-SM despite the necessity of giving SM parenterally. It is likely that INH-EMB will gain in popularity because it is quite effective and not unpleasant to take. Two drugs should be continued for several months until resolution of the disease is well under way and the cultures of secretions are negative. Then INH should be continued alone for a total of 18 to 24 months, in order to permit solid healing.

ISONIAZID PLUS TWO DRUGS. Simultaneous use of three effective agents is indicated in far advanced or cavitary pulmonary tuberculosis, miliary tuberculosis, and in tuberculosis of the kidney, bone, spine, or meninges. These are all situations in which it is imperative to gain as rapid control of the infection as possible in order to prevent emergence of drug-resistant bacilli which may lead to relapse. Drugs may be used in combinations such as INH-SM-PAS, INH-SM-ENB, or INH-EMB-PAS. Because of its potency, INH should always be included in the regimen.

RETREATMENT OF "RESISTANT CASES." When the initial course of treatment has failed to eliminate organisms, several other agents are available which may be used in various combinations either alone or in combination with resectional surgery. Drugs should *never* be added one at a time to combat failure of therapy but in pairs to avoid emergence of resistant bacilli. "Secondary drugs" should be used only under experienced supervision in order to take full advantage of them along with resection or thoracoplasty, which must be timed properly to be effective. The drugs used in retreatment of "resistant cases" include ethambutol, viomycin, pyrazinamide, cycloserine, and ethionamide.

STEROID THERAPY. Therapy of arthritis, etc., with cortisone and its derivatives has been shown to increase the chance of reactivation of dormant tuberculosis. Yet, in patients who are very seriously ill with active tuberculosis, these agents may themselves be lifesaving. They should be used only when there is an immediate threat to life as shown by hypotension, debilitating fever, dyspnea, or an impending subarachnoid block in tuberculous meningitis. Prednisone should be used in dosage of 40 mg per day for 1 to 2 weeks and then 20 mg for another 8 weeks before gradual withdrawal. The effect upon temperature and general well-being may be dramatic, but there is little long-term benefit because patients who recover without steroids show no advantage. The frequency of side effects contraindicates the routine use of steroids in conjunction with chemotherapy. These agents should be reserved for patients in whom the infection poses an immediate threat to life and in whom the organism can be treated with effective agents simultaneously. There may be an exacerbation of signs and symptoms when steroid therapy is withdrawn, the "steroid rebound phenomenon."

TOXICITY. Reactions to INH are rare, but it occasionally produces peripheral neuropathy, especially in the feet, hepatitis, shoulder pain, skin rash, fever, anemia, and psychologic abnormalities. Pyridoxine in dosage of 50 to 100 mg per day may be used to counteract the neuropathy.

Streptomycin may produce vestibular damage with vertigo, which is noted first for a short time after each dose and later continuously. Impairment of hearing also occurs occasionally following prolonged usage. These symptoms require discontinuance of streptomycin. Circumoral paresthesia is common after each injection of the agent but is a side effect and not a toxic reaction. Streptomycin also has a mild toxic effect upon the renal tubules and should be used in reduced dosage in older persons and in those with borderline renal function. Blood urea nitrogen and vestibular function should be monitored in such cases.

The most serious toxic reactions occur with PAS. The gastrointestinal symptoms are more accurately termed side effects, but true toxicity is also common and may be serious. PAS becomes quite toxic if it is allowed to turn brown with age. For this reason, only fresh white (and dated) preparations should be used. Hypersensitivity reactions occur after about 15 to 30 days of administration and consist of gradually rising fever, malaise, generalized pruritic rash, and rising SGOT. Continuation of the drug in the face of such a reaction may give rise to serious hepatic toxicity or exfoliative dermatitis. The best course of action when fever develops in the course of chemotherapy is to stop all drugs until the reaction has completely subsided. Therapy then can be reinstituted one drug at a time, beginning with INH, then giving SM, and holding PAS until last. Desensitization to PAS can sometimes be accomplished, but it is usually advisable to substitute another agent such as ENB for it.

SURGICAL TREATMENT. Surgical resection of localized areas of diseased lung is of great importance in the management of selected cases of tuberculosis. The principal indications for resection are (1) persistence of cavity and excretion of bacilli, (2) persistence of bacilli in the sputum of a patient with a localized lesion, even in the absence of a demonstrable cavity, (3) drug-resistant bacilli if the infection is sufficiently localized, (4) need for a positive diagnosis where other methods have failed, and (5) bleeding or persistently positive sputum associated with tuberculous bronchiectasis.

These indications are gradually being modified. For

example, many patients with large "open negative cavities" are being discharged on medication if the sputum is repeatedly free of tubercle bacilli. The number of persons with an open negative status is increasing steadily, especially when resectional surgery carries an increased risk. Prolonged chemotherapy is particularly important in these patients to prevent reactivation.

Following a period of several months of chemotherapy, the inflammatory reaction is usually controlled and necessary resection of a localized area of disease can be accomplished with little risk. The dangers which attend resection of untreated tuberculosis, i.e., empyema, bronchopleural fistula, or spread of infection to another area of lung, are minimized by adequate preoperative chemotherapy.

Cavitary lesions which are removed following prolonged chemotherapy are usually positive for tubercle bacilli on both smear and culture. Residual closed necrotic foci, on the other hand, are often positive on smear and negative on culture and guinea pig inoculation. Failure of the organisms to grow does not indicate that they are dead but suggests that they are merely damaged by the combined effects of prolonged chemotherapy and the physicochemical properties of caseous material.

OUTMODED FORMS OF THERAPY. Therapeutic measures which are now largely of no more than historical interest are bed rest, removal to a salubrious climate, a diet rich in dairy products, collapse of the involved portions of lung by induction of pneumothorax, resection of ribs to permit collapse of underlying lung (thoracoplasty), pneumoperitoneum, surgical interruption of the phrenic nerve to allow the diaphragm on the involved side to rise, and introduction of masses of foreign materials (i.e., paraffin, lucite balls, or plastic sponge) into the extrapleural fascial plane adjacent to a cavitary lesion in the lung. A limited thoracoplasty is still used occasionally in the therapy of persistent tuberculous empyema and to lessen the risk of empyema developing in a large unfilled space after resection of a large amount of lung.

OVERALL PLAN OF MANAGEMENT AND PROGNOSIS. Because experience with the therapy of tuberculosis often is limited to tuberculosis hospitals or clinics, brief description of an overall therapeutic program seems appropriate. Usually it is desirable for patients with minimal noncavitary disease to be admitted to hospital or sanatorium for the initial laboratory and radiographic studies and initiation of therapy while they can be observed closely for signs of adverse reactions. The patient with minimal disease and negative sputum smears often can be discharged after this short initial period to continue chemotherapy at home.

In the case of moderately and far advanced cavitary tuberculosis in which bacilli are seen in the smear of the sputum, three drugs are often employed at first and the period of isolation must be longer. These patients, if cooperative, are usually ready for discharge home on therapy (usually on INH and PAS) after a few months. PAS is stopped after several more months and INH continued for about 2 years. In some instances the time required to achieve negative sputum may be prolonged, and resection of a cavity is necessary in about 5 percent of cases to stop excretion of tubercle bacilli. When all goes well, the majority of patients can return to their occupation shortly after discharge. When persistence of positive bacteriology or cavitation necessitates resectional surgery, the course is prolonged.

A favorable prognosis is dependent upon several factors: (1) Absence of other serious disease which may have been the trigger mechanism for development of dormant infection into active tuberculosis, (2) administration of adequate initial chemotherapy to control the active infection, and (3) cooperation of the patient in the prolonged chemotherapy necessary to permit healing. Alcoholism not only sets off late reactivation of dormant lesions but also serves as a serious handicap to patient cooperation in both the early intensive and the prolonged phases of therapy. The aid of social workers in the hospital and various social agencies is of great importance in the overall plan of treatment and rehabilitation.

PREVENTION AND ERADICATION OF TUBERCULOSIS

The decline in mortality from tuberculosis, which began with the improvement in living conditions which accompanied the industrial revolution, led several physicians early in this century to predict the eradication of tuberculosis by 1945. This prediction was based on the theory that the widespread infection with tuberculosis was harmless and that the danger lay in reinfections. Therefore, if reinfections could be prevented by isolation and treatment of contagious cases, the disease would rapidly disappear. It is clear, however, that active tuberculosis develops among adults largely from reactivation of old dormant foci acquired in earlier years rather than from reinfection, and eradication must await the natural disappearance of the organisms from the population through death of those who now harbor them, as well as prevention of contagious late recrudescence. This can best be accomplished by careful surveillance and prophylactic therapy with INH for those who harbor this infection. From study of Fig. 174-2, it can be seen that the disease is steadily disappearing in Western countries as the older, heavily infected segments of the population die off.

The major deterrent to the rapid disappearance of tuberculosis in the United States is the fact that such a high proportion of older persons harbor the infection in a dormant form. Such lesions may reactivate, cavitate, and disseminate as general health is impaired by old age, debility, alcoholism, steroid therapy, diabetes, gastrectomy, silicosis, or malignancy. These individuals may infect several grandchildren before active tuberculosis is detected. It is for this reason that many hospitals require routine chest roentgenograms on all hospital admissions. The most tuberculosis is no longer found among young women but in older men with chronic cough but little illness. Roentgenograms should be saved so that comparisons with subsequent films can be made in order to detect evidence of activity, before the sputum is positive for tubercle bacilli.

BIOLOGIC PROPHYLAXIS

BCG vaccine (Bacillus Calmette-Guérin), a live, attenuated strain of bovine tubercle bacilli, has been widely used in many countries to induce specific immunity against tuberculosis. In addition to reducing susceptibility to initial infection, BCG also prevents the serious effects of infections which do occur. There have been and still are conflicting opinions on the efficacy of BCG. Some authorities found no benefit from it, but most have shown the protection to be in the range of 80 percent. Its use is certainly warranted in countries where the prevalence of tuberculosis is high. In the United States today the prevalence is so low that vaccination is advisable only for tuberculin-negative persons in whom exposure is unavoidable: Peace Corps, State Department, and Armed Forces personnel assigned to countries of high prevalence and nursing and medical personnel in large city hospitals where tuberculosis continues to be common among older persons.

The question whether it is preferable to be tuberculin-negative or -positive often is raised. In the United States today, the chances for the reactor to develop a late recrudescence of dormant infection is greater than that of the nonreactor to contract an infection. On the other hand, if exposed to tuberculosis in a country of high prevalence, the nonreactor would have a greater risk of contracting a new active infection than the healthy reactor would have of developing a late recrudescence.

REFERENCES

Barry, V. C.: "Chemotherapy of Tuberculosis," Washington, Butterworth Scientific Publications, 1964.

Bentley, F. J., S. Grzybowski, and B. Benjamin: "Tuberculosis in Childhood and Adolescence," London, NAPT, 1954.

Canetti, G.: "The Tubercle Bacillus in the Pulmonary Lesion of Man," New York, Springer Publishing Co., Inc., 1955.

Dubos, R.: Acquired Immunity to Tuberculosis, Am. Rev. Resp. Dis., 90:505, 1954.

Gedde-Dahl, T.: Tuberculous Infection in the Light of Tuberculin Matriculation, Am. J. Hyg., 56:139, 1952.

Groth-Petersen, E., J. Knudsen, and E. Wilbek: Epidemiologic Basis of Tuberculosis Eradication in an Advanced Country, Bull. World Health Organ., 21:5, 1959.

Grzybowski, S., and E. A. Allen: The Challenge of Tuberculosis in Decline: A Study Based on the Epidemiology of Tuberculosis in Ontario, Canada, Am. Rev. Resp. Dis., 90:707, 1964.

——, and W. B. Marr: The Unchanging Pattern of Pulmonary Tuberculosis, J. Can. Med. Assoc., 89:737, 1963.

Pagel, W., F. A. H. Simmonds, N. MacDonald, and E. Nassau: "Pulmonary Tuberculosis," London, Oxford University Press, 1964.

Poulsen, A.: Some Clinical Features of Tuberculosis (No. 1), Acta Tuberc. Scand., 24-311, 1950; (No. 2) Acta Tuberc. Scand., 33:37, 1957.

Rasmussen, K. N.: The Apical Localization of Pulmonary Tuberculosis, Acta Tuberc. Scand., 34:245, 1957.

Smith, D. T.: Diagnostic and Prognostic Significance of the Quantitative Tuberculin Tests, Ann. Intern. Med., 67:919, 1967.

Stead, W. W.: Pathogenesis of a First Episode of Chronic Pulmonary Tuberculosis in Man: Recrudescence of Residuals of the Primary Infection or Exogenous Reinfection? Am. Rev. Resp. Dis., 95:729, 1967.

——: Pathogenesis of the Sporadic Case of Tuberculosis, New Engl. J. Med., 277:1008, 1967.

——, G. R. Kerby, D. P. Schlueter, and C. W. Jordahl: The Clinical Spectrum of Primary Tuberculosis in Adults: Confusion with Reinfection in the Pathogenesis of Chronic Tuberculosis, Ann. Intern. Med., 68:731, 1968.

175 LEPROSY (Hansen's Disease)
Charles C. Shepard

DEFINITION. Leprosy is a chronic granulomatous infection of man, which, in its various clinical forms, attacks superficial tissues, especially the skin, peripheral nerves, and nasal mucosa. The two major clinical types are *lepromatous* and *tuberculoid;* when the disease has features of both of these types it is called *borderline*. In addition an early *indeterminate* form is seen, which can later develop into one of the three types mentioned.

The earliest references to authentic leprosy are probably those in Indian and Chinese literature from about 1000 B.C. Møller-Christensen's archeo-osteological investigations indicate that leprosy was not present in the eastern Mediterranean area until 500 to 600 A.D. and that the disease then spread to western Europe in the following centuries. It remained a frequent disease in Norway less than a century ago.

At present there are probably 10 to 20 million patients with leprosy in the world. The disease is more common in tropical countries, in many of which 1 to 2 percent or more of the population is affected. It is also common in certain regions with cooler climates, such as Korea, China, and central Mexico. In the United States the chief leprosy areas are Texas, California, Hawaii, Louisiana, Florida, and New York. Part of the cases are acquired domestically, and part are acquired abroad, reflecting the increasing movement of people between the United States and the tropics.

ETIOLOGY. *Mycobacterium leprae,* or Hansen's bacillus, is the causal agent of leprosy. It is an acid-fast rod, found in enormous numbers in lepromatous lesions. Although it has not been cultivated in artificial medium, nor convincingly in tissue culture, it can be propagated in cooler tissues of small rodents, most consistently in the foot pads of mice. This development has made possible much recent experimentation, especially on drugs and vaccines. Because the organism grows slowly in mice, experiments usually require 6 to 12 months. A convenient and rapid method for estimating viability is the determination of the "solid ratio" or "morphologic index." Rationale for this measurement comes from the observation that only completely and solidly stained bacilli are infectious for mice.

Lepromin is a suspension of killed *M. leprae* prepared from the tissues of lepromatous patients. Intradermal injection elicits, somewhat irregularly, a tuberculinlike reaction at 48 hr (Fernàndez reaction) and, more consistently, a papular reaction at 4 weeks (Mitsuda reaction). The Mitsuda reaction is usually positive in tuberculoid patients and negative in lepromatous patients and is therefore an aid in clinical classification. However, because it is also positive in nearly all normal adults, it has no diagnostic value.

EPIDEMIOLOGY. Leprosy is frequently a family infection. Many patients give a history of prolonged exposure, and in close family contact (spouse-spouse) of untreated lepromatous patients the attack rate is 5 to 10 percent. Among young children of untreated lepromatous parents, 30 to 50 percent develop a mild, single-lesion type of leprosy which heals spontaneously. After the index case is under treatment, spread within the family apparently does not occur. Transmission from patients with tuberculoid leprosy is uncommon. The portal of entry is a matter of conjecture, but is probably either the skin or the nasal mucosa. The chief portal of exit is thought by some to be the ulcerated nasal mucosa of lepromatous patients.

The *incubation period* is frequently 3 to 5 years, but it has been reported to range from 6 months to several decades.

CLINICOPATHOLOGIC CLASSIFICATION. As is true of other chronic infections, such as syphilis and tuberculosis, the manifestations of leprosy are many and variable. The classification now in general use is based on clinical findings, histopathologic changes, and the lepromin test.

Lepromatous leprosy is one of the polar forms. The involvement is extensive, diffuse, and bilaterally symmetrical. Histologically there is a diffuse granulomatous reaction with the presence of large foam (Virchow) cells and many intracellular bacilli, frequently in spheroidal masses ("globi"). The lepromin reaction is usually negative.

Tuberculoid leprosy is the other polar type. Skin lesions are usually much fewer, and they are sharply demarcated. Neurologic involvement is relatively pronounced and may be severe. The histologic response contains epithelioid cells, and bacilli are few and sometimes difficult to demonstrate. The lepromin reaction is usually positive.

Borderline or *dimorphous* leprosy is a form in which the clinical features and histologic changes are a combination of the two polar types. The disease may change to the lepromatous or to the tuberculoid form (change from one polar type to the other is exceedingly rare, however).

In all types of leprosy peripheral nerve involvement is a constant feature. In any histologic section involvement of nerves will tend to be more severe than other tissues, and in some sections the nerves may be the only tissues involved.

PATHOGENESIS. *Mycobacterium leprae* probably enters the body through skin or upper respiratory mucosa. The early stages of infection have not been described accurately. There is evidence that the infection spreads through branches of the peripheral nerves. In lepromatous leprosy bacillemia is frequent and often so profuse that the organisms can be stained in smears of peripheral blood. Even in the most advanced lepromatous cases, destructive lesions are limited to the skin, peripheral nerves, anterior portion of the eye, upper respiratory passages above the larynx, testes, and structures of the hands and feet. The probable reason for the predilection of all these tissues is that they are all usually several degrees cooler than 37°C. Two sites of preferential involvement are the ulnar nerves near the elbow and the peroneal nerves where they pass around the head of the fibula; above and below these levels where these nerves take deeper courses, they are much less severely involved. In mice that have been experimentally infected in the foot pads, bacillary multiplication is maximal when the mice are kept at air temperatures at which the foot pad tissues are about 30°C; this is also the usual temperature of the most severely involved tissues of humans. In patients with lepromatous leprosy, collections of bacilli are also found in the liver and spleen, but these are probably scavenged from the blood.

Lepromatous leprosy is commonly held to be the result of a poor immune response and tuberculoid leprosy the result of strong immune response, but whether these different immune states precede the infection is not clear. Lepromatous patients have been shown to be deficient in the ability to develop delayed hypersensitivity, and their lymphocyte transformation in response to general stimulants is weak. Also mice that have been rendered immunologically deficient by thymectomy and irradiation respond to inoculation of *M. leprae* by developing a heavily bacilliferous infection which is histologically identical to lepromatous leprosy in man (and which spreads to the ears, nose, and uninoculated feet, i.e., the cooler tissues).

CLINICAL MANIFESTATIONS. Early Leprosy. The first signs of leprosy are usually cutaneous. One or more hypopigmented or hyperpigmented macules or plaques may be seen. There is little to distinguish them from other conditions, but they are frequently anesthetic. Often an anesthetic or paresthetic patch is the first symptom noted by the patient on careful examination, and skin involvement can also be found. When contacts are being examined, a single skin lesion is often noted, especially in children; usually a hypesthetic macule, the lesion is reported to clear in a year or two without treatment, but specific treatment is usually recommended. The earliest loss of sensation is that of temperature, followed by light touch (wisp of cotton) and then by pain (sharp or dull end of pin).

Tuberculoid Leprosy. Early tuberculoid leprosy is frequently seen as a hypopigmented macule, sharply demarcated and hypesthetic. Later the lesions are larger, and the margins are elevated and circinate or gyrate. There is peripheral spread and central healing. The lesions are usually few and not symmetrical. Nerve involvement occurs early, and the nerves leading from the lesions may be enlarged. The larger peripheral nerves may be palpably and visibly enlarged, especially the ulnar, peroneal, and greater auricular nerves. There may be severe neuritic pain. Muscle atrophy is frequent and especially involves the small muscles of the hand. Contractures of the hand are frequent, as is foot drop. Trauma, especially from burns and splinters and from excessive pressure, leads to secondary infection of the hands and to plantar ulcers. Later resorption and loss of phalanges is frequent. When the facial nerves are involved, there may be lagophthalmos, exposure keratitis, and corneal ulceration leading to blindness.

Lepromatous Leprosy. The skin lesions are macules, nodules, or papules. The macules are more often hypopigmented. The borders of the lesions are not sharp, and the raised lesions are convex (rather than concave as in tuberculoid disease). There is also diffuse infiltration between the lesions. The sites of predilection are the face (cheeks, nose, brows), ears, wrists, elbows, buttocks, and knees, and the involvement is often bilaterally symmetrical. In one form diffuse involvement with little or no nodulation progresses so subtly that the disease goes unnoticed. Loss of the eyebrows, especially the lateral portions, is common. Much later the skin of the face and forehead becomes thickened and corrugated ("leonine facies"), and the earlobes become pendulous.

Nasal symptoms (nasal "stuffiness," epistaxis, and obstructed breathing) are common and are sometimes presenting symptoms. Complete nasal obstruction, then laryngitis and hoarseness are frequent. Septal perforation and nasal collapse lead to saddle nose.

In adult males infiltration and scarring of the testes lead to sterility. Gynecomastia is common. Invasion of the anterior portion of the eye leads to keratitis and iridocyclitis. Painless inguinal and axillary lymphadenopathy occurs.

Neurologic involvement, of the same type as that seen in tuberculoid disease, tends to be less frequent in the lepromatous form. A "glove and stocking" type of hypesthesia is common in advanced lepromatous disease.

Reactional States. The general course of established leprosy is leisurely, but it is typically interrupted by episodes of rapid worsening. Several types are differentiated.

Erythema nodosum leprosum occurs only in lepromatous patients. It is particularly frequent during chemotherapy, especially toward the end of the first year of treatment. Painful, inflamed subcutaneous nodules develop, usually in crops. Each nodule subsides in a week or two, but more develop. Often there are fever, lymphadenopathy, and arthralgia. The reaction may last only a few weeks or may continue for long periods.

The bacilli of patients undergoing the reaction have greatly reduced viability as indicated by lack of infectivity for mice and by low "solid ratios."

Lepra reaction is an exacerbation of existing lepromatous lesions and fever. Probably most of the lepra reac-

tions in the older literature were in fact erythema nodosum leprosum.

The *Lucio phenomenon* is limited to patients with a diffuse nonnodular lepromatous disease; it is seen more often in Mexico, especially in Sinaloa, but has been observed in patients infected in the United States. In the reactions an arteritis leads to ulceration of the skin in a characteristic angular shape and subsequently to angular thin scars.

The reactional state in tuberculoid leprosy consists of exacerbation of skin lesions and worsening of neurologic disease, often with severe neuritic pain. Bacilli are said to become more numerous during these periods.

Complications. The crippling that follows involvement of the peripheral nerves has been mentioned. Leprosy is probably the most frequent cause of crippling of the hand in the world. Blindness also is common.

Amyloidosis is a frequent complication of lepromatous disease in the United States, but is less common elsewhere.

Patients with leprosy are said to be prone to develop other chronic infections. Tuberculosis is the chief cause of death in many leprosaria.

LABORATORY FINDINGS. There are no diagnostic blood changes. Lepromatous patients frequently have mild anemia, elevated erythrocyte sedimentation rate, and hyperglobulinemia. From 10 to 40 percent of lepromatous patients have false positive serologic tests for syphilis.

The differential diagnosis includes conditions such as lupus erythematosus, lupus vulgaris, sarcoidosis, yaws, dermal leishmaniasis, and the host of banal skin diseases. The skin lesions of leprosy, especially of tuberculoid disease, are characterized by hypesthesia, however, and peripheral nerve involvement can always be demonstrated. Peripheral neuropathy from other causes and syringomyelia are often confused with leprosy.

The combination of a chronic skin disease and peripheral nerve involvement should always lead to the consideration of leprosy.

The demonstration of acid-fast bacilli in the skin smears made by the scraped-incision method is required for diagnosis in many clinics. However, in tuberculoid disease, bacilli may be too few for demonstration. Wherever possible, a skin biopsy specimen, confined to the affected area, should be sent to a pathologist or dermatopathologist knowledgeable in leprosy.

The *lepromin* reaction has no diagnostic value.

TREATMENT. The discovery in 1943 that Promin, a sulfone, is effective against *M. leprae* ushered in a new era in the management of leprosy. Leprologists all over the world are able to use specific chemotherapy in the form of sulfones to cure or arrest the progress of the disease, to render the patients noninfectious, and to eliminate the need for segregation of leprosy patients from the general population. Just as chemotherapy alone has not eradicated tuberculosis, syphilis, or malaria, however, the sulfones have not ended leprosy as a world health problem. Even in parts of the world where chemotherapy is readily available, rehabilitation of patients with arrested leprosy for return to useful productive life has become a major concern. Physiotherapy and reconstructive surgery have assumed great importance in the management of leprosy.

Specific Chemotherapy. Promin, a conjugate of dapsone, was given intravenously, but it has been almost entirely replaced by the parent sulfone dapsone. The treatment of leprosy is largely in the hands of specialists, and hospitalization is advantageous for the first few months while the treatment is being established.

Dapsone (4,4'-diaminodiphenylsulfone, DDS, diaphenylsulfone) is effective and cheap. Oral treatment is begun with small doses and raised during the first few weeks to a maintenance dose of about 50 mg a day in adults. In a few months the bacilli lose infectivity for mice. The response of patient's bacilli to drugs can be observed by determinations of the solid ratio ("morphologic index"). When carefully done, this measurement is an accurate reflection of the viability of the bacilli. However, in lepromatous disease nonviable bacilli in large numbers (and probably a few viable bacilli) persist for many years, and treatment should be continued a year or two after the bacilli are no longer demonstrable in skin smears. Often this amounts to 6 years or more. In tuberculoid disease, especially in the milder cases, treatment is often discontinued after 2 years if the disease is clinically quiescent. Regularly scheduled follow-up is needed to detect possible relapses.

Other sulfones, such as Diasone or Sulphetrone, are used at times.

Sulfone resistance has been demonstrated by tests in mice on isolates from patients who had been treated many years with sulfone unsuccessfully. Apparently in these patients the initial response was favorable, but treatment was interrupted or irregular, and after 10 to 15 years there is no longer any response to therapy. Fortunately sulfone resistance is rare in patients treated initially with dapsone. Patients with sulfone-resistant bacilli are best treated with B663, a rimino-phenazine compound.

If given in the dosage mentioned, dapsone toxicity is rare. Dermatitis and hepatitis occur. With higher doses, anemia and methemoglobinemia are seen regularly.

The clinical response to adequate therapy is gradual, and the picture may be confused by reactional conditions (see below). However, progression of the disease stops and there is gradual improvement of skin lesions. Recovery from neurologic impairment is usually limited.

Some other drugs that have been recommended in leprosy are thiambutosine (a thiourea called SU 1906), Etisul (a mercaptan compound), isoniazid, streptomycin, and cycloserine. The precise value of these drugs is difficult to determine because of the complexities involved in clinical trials. These and other drugs are being investigated actively in experiments in mice.

Treatment of Reactional States. Moderate *erythema nodosum* (ENL) is managed by antipyretics and analgesics. If severe, it can be treated with corticosteroids and ACTH; the dosage is adjusted to alleviate severe distress but not to eliminate all signs of reaction. Sulfone therapy should be continued, if necessary in reduced dosage. In the past some leprologists have discontinued sulfone therapy at the first signs of ENL, but many now feel that such action is not warranted because it allows the emergence of viable bacilli. Corticosteroid therapy promotes the viability of *M. leprae* in mice not given antileprosy drugs.

Corticosteroids are helpful in severe reactional tuberculoid states also, but analgesics and antipyretics may be sufficient.

Several reports in the literature attest to the usefulness of thalidomide in reactional states. Because of its teratogenicity, however, the drug will not be released in the United States for many years. In countries where it is not banned, its use may be difficult to control, and for this reason its potential hazards outweigh its benefits.

Other Measures. Many of the deformities and disabilities of leprosy are preventable through proper attention from the beginning of treatment. Plantar ulcers, which are very common, may be prevented by rigid-soled footwear or walking plaster casts, and contractures of the hand may be prevented by physical therapy and application of casts. Reconstructive surgery is frequently necessary. Nerve and tendon transplants and release of contractures can give patients much more functional ability. Vocational retraining is often necessary for those with permanent disability. Plastic repair of facial deformities assist patients' acceptance in society. The psychologic trauma, which resulted from the prolonged segregation formerly practiced, is now minimized by permitting patients to continue therapy at home as soon as possible.

CONTROL. Early detection and treatment of the disease, which prevents the further development of deformities and which simplifies sulfone therapy, can be aided by education of physicians and laity in endemic areas. Because the disease is best treated by specialists, the establishment of clinics is helpful. Regular and complete skin examination of family contacts is essential. Field trials of BCG vaccination in endemic areas are showing favorable results, and BCG vaccination of family contacts even in nonendemic areas seems indicated. Chemoprophylaxis with low dosages of DDS may also be considered for family contacts. Removal of patients from the family and surroundings is probably not necessary, except perhaps in the first few months when therapy is being established, unless the patient does not follow regular treatment.

REFERENCES

Cochrane, R. G., and T. F. Davey (Eds.): "Leprosy in Theory and Practice," Baltimore, The Williams & Wilkins Company, 2d ed., 1964.

Fasal, P.: "Leprosy Occurs Everywhere," GP, 32:95, 1965.

Panel Reports from VIIIth International Congress on Leprology, Internat. J. Leprosy, 31:473, 1963.

Proceedings of Symposium on Sulfones by the U.S.-Japan Cooperative Medical Science Program, Internat. J. Leprosy, 35(4, pt. 2):563, 1967.

Wolstenholme, G. E. W., and M. O'Connor (Eds.): "Pathogenesis of Leprosy," Boston, Little, Brown and Company, 1963.

176 OTHER MYCOBACTERIAL INFECTIONS

Charles C. Shepard

Species of acid-fast bacteria morphologically similar to tubercle bacilli are widely distributed in nature as saprophytes or as pathogens of lower animals. Many examples are known of parasitism of amphibians and fishes by mycobacteria that cannot multiply at mammalian body temperatures. Among mammalian diseases that have been studied extensively are a chronic enteritis in cattle and sheep caused by *Mycobacterium paratuberculosis* (Johne's bacillus), a leprosylike disease of water buffalo and oxen called *lepra bubalorum* or *lepra bovinum,* and murine leprosy (of wild rats). The long-standing view that all other acid-fast bacilli were of importance in clinical medicine only because they might be confused with *M. tuberculosis* or *M. leprae* in smears or cultures has gradually given way to the realization that many other mycobacterial species are pathogenic for man, producing chronic *cutaneous disease, pulmonary disease,* or *lymphadenitis.*

Mycobacterium marinum (Balnei) (**"SWIMMING-POOL BACILLUS"**). This acid-fast organism inhabits swimming pools and gains entry to the human body through cutaneous abrasions on rough concrete. A few weeks later papules or nodules develop at the site and frequently ulcerate and enlarge to form superficial granulation tissue. The involved area usually is not extensive. Originally confused with skin tuberculosis, "swimming-pool granuloma" has now been described in many parts of the world including the United States. In Hawaii a much more chronic form lasting many years has been reported; exposure to swimming pools had usually not occurred. *Mycobacterium marinum* grows optimally at 25 to 35°C and poorly if at all at 37°C. This temperature range probably accounts for the lack of systemic spread; indeed regional lymph nodes remain uninvolved unless secondary pyogenic infection occurs.

The diagnosis is made by culturing the organism, usually from biopsy material on mycobacterial media at appropriate temperatures. Although it grows slowly on primary isolation, on transfer the organism is seen to be a rapid grower and photochromogenic (develops pigment only after exposure to light). Histologically the lesion is a nonspecific granuloma in which acid-fast bacilli can often be detected. Many, but not all, patients convert to tuberculin positivity during infection.

Treatment with antituberculous drugs, especially streptomycin, often appears to speed healing. Tests of antibiotic sensitivity are helpful in selecting drugs.

Prevention of the swimming pool outbreaks requires disinfection of the pool; reconstruction of the pool and elimination of rough surfaces may be necessary.

Mycobacterium ulcerans. This acid-fast organism produces extensive granulomatous ulceration which destroys subcutaneous tissue down to the muscle or fascia and extends peripherally under a characteristic undermined edge. Extensor surfaces of arms and legs are most often affected, but the trunk may also be involved. Histologically necrosis is prominent, and epithelialization of the ulcer floor extends under the overhanging margins. Systemic dissemination does not occur, although new lesions may develop at distant sites. In its natural course the disease may heal spontaneously in a year or two or may persist for many years with extensive ulcerations and contractures. Originally observed in southern Australia, the disease has since been described in central Africa and southeast Asia. Isolated cases and localized outbreaks, especially near rivers, have been described, but little is known of the distribution of the organism in nature.

Mycobacterium ulcerans grows optimally at 30 to 33°C and poorly if at all at 37°C. The organism grows very slowly, and colonies require 7 weeks to develop at optimal temperatures. Inoculation of mice foot pads is helpful in the isolation and identification of the organism. *Mycobacterium marinum* is easily differentiated on bacteriologic media because it is photochromogenic, grows rapidly and produces disease when inoculated into foot pads of mice much more rapidly than does *M. ulcerans.*

Treatment has been carried out with such antituberculosis drugs as streptomycin and isoniazid and the antileprosy drug dapsone. However, the rimino-phenazine compound B663 is the drug of choice. Surgical extirpation of the necrotic tissue and overlapping margins of the ulcer, followed by skin grafting, may be required.

PULMONARY DISEASE PRODUCED BY "ATYPICAL" ("Anonymous," "Unclassified") MYCOBACTERIA

DEFINITION. Mycobacterial species other than *M. tuberculosis* are known to be capable of causing chronic progressive pulmonary disease with fibrosis and cavitation closely resembling that of pulmonary tuberculosis.

ETIOLOGY. For a time the isolation from chronic pulmonary infections of mycobacteria other than *M. tuberculosis* or *M. bovis* caused widespread confusion. Fortunately recent taxonomic studies have brought order into the chaos. The nontuberculosis mycobacteria isolated from clinical sputum specimens were divided by Runyon into four groups. Of these group I (photochromogenic) is now given the species name of *M. kansasii.* Group III (nonphotochromogenic) includes several kinds of mycobacteria, but that responsible for human pulmonary disease is known as "*M. battey.*" Although closely related to *M. avium,* differences are usually distinct, and the species name *M. intracellularis* has been proposed for it. Of the nontuberculous mycobacteria isolated under circumstances that indicate their etiologic role in chronic pulmonary disease, about 90 percent are either *M. kansasii* or Battey mycobacteria. Group II (*scotochromogens,* produce pigment when grown in the dark) and group IV (rapid growers) are isolated from clinical disease less frequently. Isolation of nontuberculosis mycobacteria from clinical specimens does not have the same etiologic significance as the isolation of *M. tuberculosis,* because similar organisms can be isolated from sputum, saliva, etc., of healthy persons. Therefore it is necessary that before a nontuberculosis mycobacterium is accepted as the cause of the illness, it be isolated from several specimens and in significant numbers (more than 10 colonies per culture). However, when *M. kansasii* and Battey cultures are identified by appropriate additional tests, single isolations often have etiologic significance.

EPIDEMIOLOGY. The mode of transmission is unsettled. There is cross-sensitization between antigens of tubercle bacilli and other mycobacteria, but sensitization to the etiologic organism is usually greater. Comparative skin tests utilizing antigens from Battey bacilli and tuberculin indicate that many healthy individuals in the southeastern United States have been infected by organisms related to Battey bacilli, and in these areas chronic pulmonary disease that is not caused by *M. tuberculosis* is usually caused by Battey bacilli. In Texas and in Chicago *M. kansasii* is a more frequent causative agent than Battey bacilli. The proportion of new cases of chronic pulmonary disease caused by mycobacteria other than *M. tuberculosis* is not more than a few percent, but may be expected to increase as the number of infections due to *M. tuberculosis* decreases. In contrast to the experience with *M. tuberculosis* infections, multiple cases in the same family are very rare, and consequently enforced isolation is not indicated.

PATHOLOGY. Comparative studies of pulmonary tissue have failed to reveal consistent and reliable distinguishing features from infections due to *M. tuberculosis*. However, in *M. kansasii* infections the demarcation between diseased and normal lung is less distinct, and submucosal endobronchitis is more common. Extrapulmonary lesions are rare. Cervical adenitis due to *M. kansasii* or the scrofula type of group II is seen in children.

MANIFESTATIONS AND DIAGNOSIS. The symptoms and signs are those of pulmonary tuberculosis (Chap. 174), although there is some tendency for the disease to be more indolent. The diagnosis should be considered in single cases (without associated cases in the family). However, the diagnosis is established by isolations of the mycobacteria from the sputum. The laboratory should carry out tests for the production of nicotinic acid, at least on all isolates from new patients, because only *M. tuberculosis* consistently produces nicotinic acid. Differentiating tests can then be carried out in nicotinic acid–negative cultures.

TREATMENT. *Mycobacterium kansasii* infections usually respond to intensive antituberculous chemotherapy with isoniazid, streptomycin, and *para*-aminosalicylic acid. The cultures should be studied for drug susceptibility because many organisms are also susceptible to viomycin and ethionamide so that treatment can be adjusted in patients who respond poorly. Pulmonary resection has been found to be a valuable aid to chemotherapy, *after* the sputum cultures have become negative for *M. kansasii*.

Battey bacillus infections usually do not respond to antituberculosis chemotherapy. Fortunately, however, even though sputum cultures remain positive, pulmonary resections can be carried out with minimal risk of complication if the character and distribution of disease is suitable.

REFERENCES

Clancey, J. K., O. G. Dodge, H. F. Lunn, and M. L. Oduori: Mycobacterial Skin Ulcers in Uganda, Lancet, 2:951, 1961.

Clark, H. F., and C. C. Shepard: Effect of Environmental Temperatures on Infection with *Mycobacterium Marinum* (Balnei) of Mice and a Number of Poikilothermic Species, J. Bacteriol., 86:1057, 1963.

Kestle, D. G., V. D. Abbot, and G. P. Kubica: Differential Identification of Mycobacteria. II. Subgroups of Groups II and III (Runyon) with Different Clinical Significance, Am. Rev. Resp. Dis., 95:1041, 1967.

Lester, W.: Unclassified Mycobacterial Diseases, Ann. Rev. Med., 17:351, 1966.

Linell, F., and A. Norden: *Mycobacterium Balnei*: A New Acid-fast Bacillus Occurring in Swimming Pools and Capable of Producing Skin Lesions in Humans, Acta Tuberc. Scand., Suppl. No. 33, 1954.

Mollohan, C. S., and M. S. Romer: Public Health Significance of Swimming Pool Granuloma, Am. J. Public Health, 51:883, 1961.

Section 10

Spirochetal Diseases

177 SYPHILIS
Albert Heyman

DEFINITION. Syphilis is a chronic, infectious disease caused by *Treponema pallidum* and usually transmitted by sexual contact. It is capable of producing tissue destruction and chronic inflammation in almost any organ in the body and can produce a great diversity of clinical manifestations.

HISTORY. Considerable knowledge of the pathology and clinical aspects of syphilis was accumulated in the sixteenth to nineteenth centuries, but it was not until early in the present century that most of the fundamental information about the disease was uncovered. The etiologic agent, *T. pallidum*, was discovered by Schaudinn and Hoffmann in 1905. Soon afterward, Wassermann and his associates introduced serologic methods of diagnosis. In 1949, Nelson and Mayer introduced the *T. pallidum* immobilization test, following which other tests for demonstrating humoral antibodies were subsequently developed.

In 1910 Ehrlich announced the discovery of arsphenamine, and in 1917 Wagner von Jauregg demonstrated the value of malarial therapy for paresis. These were the two most important advances in the treatment of syphilis until 1943, when penicillin was found by Mahoney and his associates to be effective in the early stages of the disease. This drug has replaced the other forms of chemotherapy in syphilis.

ETIOLOGY. The *T. pallidum* is a slender spirochete with regular, evenly spaced spirals. It varies in length from 5 to 20 μ. When viewed under the dark-field microscope, *T. pallidum* shows characteristic motility, rotating on its long axis and moving slowly backward and forward. The spirals usually keep their uniform shape and size, although the body of the organism may bend at the middle. It does not have the quick, whipping movements of other spirochetes which are found in ulcerative lesions. The organism does not stain well with ordinary dyes and is best seen by silver impregnation methods in fixed tissues. For clinical purposes it can be demonstrated by dark-field microscopy.

Treponema pallidum is readily killed by soap, ordinary antiseptics, drying, and heat. It resists cold, however, and can be frozen and stored for long periods without loss of virulence. The organism does not remain viable, however, in whole blood or plasma which has been stored at refrigerator temperature for more than 96 hr.

Pathogenic forms of *T. pallidum* have not been cultivated and passed serially on artificial media. Strains of the organism which have been cultured are not virulent in animals and differ morphologically from pathogenic *T. pallidum*. Rabbits and monkeys can be experimentally infected with syphilis.

FREQUENCY. Although cases of primary and secondary syphilis in the United States are reportable by law, it is estimated that only a third of such patients treated by private physicians are reported to the local departments of health. For this reason exact information is not available as to the number of persons infected with syphilis in the United States (i.e., *prevalence*) or the number of new infections occurring each year (i.e., *incidence*). Both the incidence and prevalence of the disease have decreased considerably since World War II. In 1947, approximately 108,000 cases of primary and secondary syphilis were reported in this country to the Public Health Service, whereas in 1957 only 6,250 cases were reported. In the following 7 years, however, a disturbing rise in the incidence of new cases of syphilis appeared, and in 1966, more than 22,000 cases of primary and secondary syphilis were reported. The dramatic postwar decline in the incidence of syphilis was largely the result of the development of rapid-treatment methods, mass blood testing, and large-scale epidemiologic measures. Another factor responsible for the decline was the widespread use of penicillin for other diseases. As a result of this decrease in syphilis case rates, many of the states abandoned their public health control measures. The rise in the incidence of new cases leaves no doubt about the need for continuing intensive control programs. The incidence of new cases of syphilis has risen in the teen-age population, particularly in certain racial groups and in the lower socioeconomic classes.

PATHOGENESIS. Syphilis is usually transmitted by direct and intimate contact with moist infectious lesions in the skin and mucous membranes. Sexual contact is by far the commonest means of infection, but transfer of the disease by kissing or biting occasionally occurs. Indirect tranmission—i.e., by contaminated objects—is exceptional, because the organisms quickly die if allowed to dry. The disease can be spread by inoculation with infected blood, as in transfusion syphilis. Infection is transmitted to the fetus through the placenta. *Treponema pallidum* is apparently capable of penetrating the intact mucous membrane, but a small abrasion is probably required for inoculation to occur through the skin.

The natural resistance of man to virulent *T. pallidum* has been determined in volunteer subjects, in whom it was found that the ID_{50} for intracutaneous inoculation was approximately 57 organisms. Larger inocula produced larger ulcerative lesions and shorter incubation periods. Once the spirochete has penetrated the epithelium, it enters the lymphatics and can be demonstrated in the regional lymph nodes a few hours after experimental inoculation. From the lymph nodes the organism spreads rapidly throughout the body by way of the bloodstream. This spirochetemia may occur several weeks before appearance of the primary lesion at the site of inoculation. The early seeding of *T. pallidum* in various tissues is the basis for many of the later manifestations of the disease.

About 3 to 6 weeks after the organism has entered the body, a primary lesion, the *chancre*, develops at the site of inoculation. The chancre is usually a single ulceration of the skin or mucous membrane; it heals spontaneously. About 6 weeks after its appearance a generalized skin eruption, known as *secondary syphilis*, develops. In this stage, systemic manifestations are common. The signs of secondary syphilis also disappear spontaneously.

This sequence of events in early syphilis is variable. Infection without noticeable lesions probably occurs in a high percentage of cases, and many individuals with late syphilis are unable to recall either primary or secondary manifestations.

Following healing of the primary and secondary manifestations, the patient may show no outward signs of the infection (*latent syphilis*). Nevertheless, chronic, progressive, inflammatory changes may be taking place in the visceral organs or in the cardiovascular or central nervous system. Clinical evidence of cardiovascular syphilis or neurosyphilis may not develop for 10 to 20 years or more after the onset of the disease. Occasionally, the tissues of the host seem to become sensitized to the spirochetes, and large destructive lesions, called *gummas,* result. These lesions, which contain very few spirochetes, can occur in almost every organ of the body but are most frequent in the skin or bones.

Many patients with latent syphilis do not develop late manifestations and show no evidence of syphilis at autopsy. A study of patients with untreated early syphilis followed for a number of years showed that approximately one-third of them achieved spontaneous cures with the development of negative serologic tests. An equal number died of causes other than syphilis or developed latent syphilis with no clinical evidence of the disease other than a positive serologic test. The remaining third developed serious lesions of the cardiovascular or central nervous system or benign gummatous lesions of the skin or bones.

HISTOPATHOLOGY. The early lesions of syphilis are characterized by infiltration of the blood vessel walls and perivascular spaces with plasma cells, large mononuclear cells, and lymphocytes. Spirochetes can be demonstrated by silver impregnation stains. In the late lesions of syphilis there may be necrosis with granuloma or gumma formation. The necrosis is thought to be the result of an exaggerated or hypersensitivity response to a small number of organisms. Spirochetes are rarely found. These lesions heal slowly and often produce large scars.

IMMUNITY AND RESISTANCE. The development of immunity in a syphilitic patient may be considered from two standpoints: the resistance the patient develops to his own infection and the immunity he develops to reinfection.

Practically every patient with syphilis develops some resistance to his own infection. The degree of immunity determines whether the patient will achieve a spontaneous cure, the disease will remain latent, or late complications will develop. The factors responsible for the development of this type of immunity and the destruction of spirochetes are largely unknown. The serum of experimentally infected animals and patients with syphilis contains antibodies which immobilize and render noninfectious virulent strains of *T. pallidum.* These antibodies can be demonstrated in vitro by means of the *T. pallidum* immobilization (TPI) test. In human beings this immobilizing antibody appears during the early stages of syphilis and will usually persist indefinitely unless early adequate treatment for syphilis is instituted. The antibody is not present in the serum of normal persons nor in those with nonspirochetal diseases, but it occurs in the serum of patients with various treponematoses, such as bejel, yaws, and pinta. Although some workers have found a correlation in rabbits between the level of immobilizing antibody and the degree of immunity, other investigators have not confirmed their findings. The exact relationship between this antibody and the development of immunity, therefore, has not been established.

Humoral antibodies in syphilis have also been demonstrated by newer techniques such as the fluorescent antibody test and the Reiter protein complement fixation test. These procedures for detecting syphilitic antibodies are being used as diagnostic tests, particularly in cases in which there is doubt about the validity of the routine serologic methods.

Apparently the outcome of the syphilitic infection is influenced to some extent by the sex and race of the individual. Neurosyphilis, for example, occurs more frequently in men than in women, and in a higher proportion of whites than Negroes. Bone and cardiovascular syphilis are more common in Negroes.

Immunity to reinfection develops soon after the onset of the disease. In animals, immunity has been found to appear within 3 weeks after the initial infection and to increase progressively during a period of 6 months. In man, reinoculation usually results in a chancre if carried out within 15 days after the appearance of the primary lesion of the initial infection. Later than this a chancre seldom develops, but this resistance is relative. In rabbits with experimental syphilitic infection, resistance to reinfection increases with time during a 24-week period, as indicated by the need for an increasing number of virulent *T. pallidum* to produce infection.

Adequate treatment of patients with early syphilis may abort the development of immunity, and reinfections can occur. If treatment is delayed until after this period, immunity to reinfection becomes established and may remain throughout the lifetime of the individual. The question arises whether such immunity is caused by the persistence of treponemes or treponemal antigens in antibody-forming tissues. Recently, spirochetes having the characteristic motility and morphology of *T. pallidum* have been found in the anterior chamber of the eye in elderly patients with interstitial keratitis due to congenital syphilis and in other tissues in late syphilis. These organisms are also said to react to fluorescent antibody stains. Further investigations are necessary to establish whether such organisms are indeed *T. pallidum.*

If inadequate treatment is given during early syphilis and the patient's spirochetes are not completely destroyed, redissemination of the organisms may occur and produce infectious skin and mucosal lesions. This is the basis for the statement that poor treatment is worse than none at all. Once the patient has developed immunity to his own infection (usually within 4 years after the onset of the disease), inadequate treatment does not result in redissemination of organisms.

CLINICAL MANIFESTATIONS OF EARLY ACQUIRED SYPHILIS

PRIMARY STAGE. The period of incubation may vary from 10 to 90 days. The typical chancre is a solitary, indurated, nonpainful ulcer, which heals slowly with scar formation. It is often accompanied by painless enlargement of the regional lymph nodes, the *satellite bubo.* Primary syphilis is often atypical and may be manifested by small, multiple, or painful lesions which resemble many other conditions. Because of the frequent atypical appearance of the chancre, the clinical diagnosis or exclusion of primary syphilis can never be relied upon, and every genital lesion should have a dark-field examination.

Approximately 95 percent of primary lesions are found on or near the genitalia. In the male, the chancre frequently appears on the coronal sulcus or on the prepuce. Any part of the genitalia may be involved, however. Chancres of the external genitalia must be differentiated from chancroid, granuloma inguinale, lymphogranuloma venereum, carcinoma, and many other lesions which appear in this area. In the female, the primary lesion often appears on the labia and in the fourchette, but the perineum, pubis, clitoris, or urethra may be involved. Chancres of the cervix are frequent and are often mistaken for nonspecific erosions. About 5 percent of primary lesions occur on the lips, female breasts, or in the mouth.

In the diagnosis of primary syphilis, serologic tests cannot be relied upon entirely, because they are often negative in this stage of the disease. Moreover, a positive serologic reaction in a patient with a genital lesion may represent either latent infection associated with a nonsyphilitic lesion or else a biologic false positive reaction caused by another disease (i.e., lymphogranuloma venereum or chancroid). For this reason, a dark-field examination is of greatest importance in the diagnosis of this stage of the disease and should be done on the first visit of every patient suspected of having primary syphilis. If the initial dark-field examination is negative, material from the regional lymph nodes should be aspirated and examined. All local medication as well as antibiotics with treponemicidal activity should be withheld, but oral sulfonamides may be administered during this period of time. If the dark-field examinations and serologic tests for syphilis are negative, the serologic test should be repeated several times during the first 2 or 3 weeks and every few weeks thereafter for 3 months after the appearance of the lesion. If the patient develops a positive serologic reaction in a high or rising titer (with or without evidence of secondary manifestations), then antisyphilitic therapy should be begun. A single serologic test of low titer is not sufficient evidence for beginning antisyphilitic treatment if dark-field examinations are negative. Such tests should be confirmed several times for at least 2 weeks before treatment for syphilis is justified.

Penicillin or other spirocheticidal drugs should not be given as a therapeutic test to patients suspected of having primary syphilis. Healing of the genital lesion following such tests does not necessarily indicate the presence of syphilis, because nonsyphilitic lesions sometimes heal spontaneously. Biopsy of the genital lesions is often of value in the diagnosis of these patients.

SECONDARY STAGE. The secondary stage of syphilis usually develops about 6 weeks after appearance of the chancre and is manifested by a generalized skin eruption and systemic symptoms. Some patients have secondary lesions without ever being aware of a primary; others never develop secondary manifestations and enter the latent stage directly following the healing of the chancre.

The appearance of the *cutaneous lesions* of secondary syphilis varies considerably, so that they may be confused with many other skin eruptions. The lesions most often found are papules, maculopapules, or follicular papules. Occasionally, annular, pustular, or rupial lesions occur. Indeed, almost any type of skin eruption may appear except a vesicular one. The rash is usually widespread and frequently involves the palms, soles, and face, in addition to the trunk and extremities. The lesions are sometimes pruritic.

The *mucous membranes* of the mouth and genitalia are often involved in secondary syphilis. Syphilitic lesions of the mouth appear as painless, superficial erosions on the buccal surfaces, on the tongue, or inside the lip. When these lesions are covered with a thin, grayish exudate, they are known as *mucous patches*. They contain a large number of spirochetes but may be very inconspicuous, and the patient may not be aware of them. Lesions of the palate and tonsillar area can cause a persistent *sore throat*. So-called *split papules* are occasionally seen in secondary syphilis and may be mistaken for herpes, benign fissures, or the lesions of riboflavin deficiency.

Syphilitic mucosal lesions of the genitalia or perianal regions often become hypertrophic and are called *condylomata lata*. These lesions are broad, flat, wart-like excrescences which are found on the labia majora, perineum, and anal region. They are highly infectious and should be differentiated from condylomata acuminata, which are nonvenereal, pedunculated lesions (Chap. 227).

Although the clinical findings of secondary syphilis are often confined to the skin and mucous membranes, many patients will present evidence of *constitutional symptoms* and widespread spirochetal dissemination. Malaise, lassitude, headaches, fever, and myalgia are often noted. There may be a *generalized lymphadenopathy*. Localized areas of *alopecia* also occur, causing a "moth-eaten" appearance of the scalp.

Approximately 4 percent of patients with secondary syphilis have involvement of the eye, usually *iritis* or *neuroretinitis*.

Skeletal lesions occasionally occur in secondary syphilis and are manifested by localized areas of swelling and tenderness. *Arthralgia* and *hydrarthrosis* also occur, but changes in the joints cannot be detected by x-ray examination. An acute *nephrosis* with marked proteinuria, edema, and hypercholesterolemia is sometimes seen in secondary syphilis. Evidence of *central-nervous-system involvement*, such as paralysis of the cranial nerves or meningitis, may also appear in this stage of the disease.

It is apparent from the above description that secondary syphilis may be manifested by a great variety of apparently unrelated clinical symptoms. Although isolated lesions, such as iritis or periostitis, may not in themselves suggest the diagnosis, the recognition of other symptoms, such as sore throat, lymphadenopathy, or skin lesions will often make the diagnosis of secondary syphilis obvious. Whenever secondary syphilis is suspected, blood should be taken for a serologic test. This will be positive in practically 100 percent of the cases.

Conversely, if the serologic test is negative (and the possibility of technical errors has been excluded), secondary syphilis can be ruled out.

INFECTIOUSNESS AND EPIDEMIOLOGY

Syphilis is most infectious during the primary and secondary stages, when there are moist skin or mucosal lesions. The genital condylomas and the oral mucosal lesions contain large numbers of spirochetes and are more infectious than the dry skin lesions. The transmission of the disease by individuals or marital partners who deny having had open lesions is probably by way of small mucosal lesions which appear during the recurrent episodes of spirochetemia. Some secretions, such as saliva and semen, are frequently in contact with infectious mucosal lesions and may contain *T. pallidum*. The blood of patients with early syphilis has been shown to contain spirochetes and should not be used for transfusion. The serologic test is not always an indication of the infectiousness of the blood, because syphilis can be transmitted by transfusion from patients in the incubation period or in the sero-negative primary stage of the disease. The danger of transmitting syphilis either by transfusion or by direct contact is greatest in the first 4 years of the disease and is negligible after this period. In pregnancy, however, the disease can apparently be transmitted to the fetus for as long as 10 years or more after the onset of the disease, although the vast majority of congenital infections are acquired during the first 4 years of maternal infection.

It is important to determine the source of infection of patients with syphilis, particularly those with primary and secondary manifestations. It is equally important that the individuals to whom the patient may have transmitted the infection be located.

LATENT SYPHILIS

Latent syphilis is that stage of the disease in which there are no clinical signs or symptoms of the infection. Patients without signs or symptoms but with abnormal spinal fluid findings have a much more serious prognosis and are not regarded as having latent syphilis but are classified instead as having asymptomatic neurosyphilis.

Latent syphilis is by far the most frequent type of syphilis. Routine serologic testing is the only way in which the majority of patients with latent syphilis can be recognized.

Although the syphilitic infection is not clinically evident during the latent period, it may be producing serious changes in the viscera. Often the spirochete exists within the body throughout the entire lifetime of the host without producing any apparent effects upon health and longevity. Most patients with late latent syphilis develop sufficient resistance to their infection to prevent late clinical manifestations.

The diagnosis of latent syphilis is one of exclusion, and a careful history and physical examination should be made for clinical evidence of this disease. Because the diagnosis of latent syphilis is dependent upon the serologic test, false positive reactions must be ruled out. *Treponema pallidum* immobilization (TPI) tests or the newer treponemal antigen tests should be carried out routinely in patients with positive serologic tests in whom there is no history or clinical evidence of syphilis and in whom the diagnosis seems unlikely.

CLINICAL MANIFESTATIONS OF LATE ACQUIRED SYPHILIS

SKIN AND MUCOUS MEMBRANES. Late syphilis of the skin may appear as either small nodules or ulcerating gummas. The gumma begins as a painless, subcutaneous tumor which gradually softens and ruptures, exuding a viscous, gummy material. Spirochetes are seldom found in these lesions. The nodular form of late syphilis consists of slightly raised, reddish-brown lesions on the skin, which often coalesce to form arciform or serpiginous configurations.

Gummas also occur in the mucous membranes of the nose and throat, and may produce painful destructive lesions in the palate and nasal septum.

SKELETAL SYSTEM. Late osseous syphilis often presents a difficult diagnostic problem. The chief symptoms are pain, tenderness, and local warmth. The bones usually involved are the skull and tibia, although the clavicle, humerus, ribs, and nasopalatine structures are sometimes affected.

Syphilis of the skeletal system is often confused with other types of subacute or chronic osteomyelitis, primary or secondary neoplasms, or Paget's disease. The diagnosis can usually be made by close correlation of the serologic, clinical, and roentgenographic findings. In some instances, biopsy may be necessary.

The most common joint manifestation occurring in late syphilis is the *Charcot joint*, which is not caused directly by *T. pallidum* but develops as a consequence of destruction of the proprioceptive nerves in tabes dorsalis. It also occurs in other neurologic disorders, such as syringomyelia. The Charcot joint is usually confined to a single weight-bearing joint, such as the knee, ankle, or hip, and occasionally the spine. It begins as a painless swelling of the joint and is later manifested by hypermobility and loss of contour. The joint surface disintegrates, so that fragments of bone and cartilage can be felt within the joint capsule. Charcot joints often appear in arrested or "burnt-out" cases of tabes dorsalis—i.e., patients with normal blood and spinal fluid findings. Antisyphilitic drugs are of little value in treatment, and orthopedic measures are usually necessary.

LIVER. In patients with late syphilis the liver may contain multiple, minute, gummatous lesions or several very large ones. On healing, these lesions produce scarring and contraction of the surface, giving the liver the appearance of having several additional lobes—hence the name *hepar lobatum*. The most common finding on physical examination is a large, coarsely nodular, irregular liver. Ascites, jaundice, and splenomegaly are occasionally present. The serologic test for syphilis is almost always positive. Response to treatment is often dramatic, with rapid reduction in liver size and relief of symptoms.

STOMACH. Late syphilis of the stomach consists of a diffuse granulomatous infiltration of the stomach wall or a localized annular constriction about the pyloric area. Secondary ulceration and obstruction may occur, so that differentiation from carcinoma by roentgenographic examination is often impossible. Syphilis of the stomach may be suspected in young individuals on the basis of the roentgenographic appearance of the lesion and a positive serologic test, but exploratory laparotomy is usually indicated to confirm the diagnosis.

LARYNX. Syphilis of the larynx produces hoarseness without pain. Laryngoscopic examination may reveal gummatous infiltration of the vocal cords with secondary ulceration. The lesions may simulate carcinoma or tuberculosis, and biopsy is necessary for differential diagnosis. Treatment of this condition should be cautious, because intensive therapy has been known to produce edema, stridor, and suffocation. Patients with late syphilis may also develop hoarseness without pain as a result or recurrent nerve paralysis caused by aneurysm of the aorta.

KIDNEY AND GENITOURINARY TRACT. An acute nephrotic syndrome occasionally appears in early syphilis. In late syphilis, a specific type of interstitial nephritis may be present on postmortem examination without having produced a characteristic clinical picture. Gumma of the kidney is rare, but late syphilis of the bladder, testes, and penis is occasionally reported. Paroxysmal hemoglobinuria is sometimes caused by syphilis (Chap. 338).

In the female, late syphilis rarely involves the internal genital organs, but gummatous lesions sometimes appear in the breast.

Involvement of the endocrine glands, such as the adrenals, thyroid, and pituitary gland, is also infrequent.

CARDIOVASCULAR SYPHILIS. Cardiovascular syphilis is discussed fully elsewhere (Chaps. 270 and 277) and will be mentioned only briefly at this point. Cardiovascular syphilis is one of the most important of the late lesions of syphilis and probably accounts for the majority of deaths resulting from this disease. It is much more common in men than in women and seems to be more frequent in Negroes than in whites. It usually appears in the second to third decade after infection and may be associated with neurosyphilis and other late manifestations.

The fundamental lesion of cardiovascular syphilis is *aortitis. Treponema pallidum* causes destruction of the media, fragmentation of the elastic material, and eventual dilatation of the vessel. The base of the aorta is often involved, with dilatation of the valve ring and *aortic regurgitation.* If the weakening is localized, a saccular *aneurysm* may develop. The intima of the aorta becomes thickened, and occlusion of the orifices of the coronary arteries may occur. A few cases of multiple gummas of the myocardium have been reported, but the existence of a diffuse syphilitic myocarditis is a matter of controversy.

CENTRAL NERVOUS SYSTEM. Neurosyphilis, together with cardiovascular syphilis, accounts for about 90 percent of deaths caused by syphilis. Although all the tissues of the central nervous system are invaded by the spirochetes, the clinical symptoms may be arbitrarily divided into meningeal, vascular, and parenchymatous. Meningeal and vascular symptoms usually develop early in the course of the disease, whereas parenchymatous involvement, as manifested by tabes dorsalis and paresis, usually does not appear until 10 to 20 years after primary infection. Meningeal lesions are inflammatory and often reversible. Parenchymatous lesions, however, are likely to be degenerative with irreversible damage. The type of lesion which predominates, the structures involved, and the exact location of the lesion within the central nervous system are the three important factors which influence prognosis and response to treatment.

Gummas of the brain and spinal cord are occasionally observed. They produce symptoms similar to those caused by tumors of the central nervous system, and differentiation is difficult.

Asymptomatic Neurosyphilis. Asymptomatic neurosyphilis is that stage of the disease in which an abnormal spinal fluid exists without clinical signs or symptoms to indicate that the function of the central nervous system has been affected.

The outcome of asymptomatic neurosyphilis and the extent of the spinal fluid abnormalities appear to be definitely related, because patients with marked changes are more likely to develop signs and symptoms. The activity of the neurosyphilitic process is often related to the spinal fluid cell count and protein level. The presence of a positive spinal fluid Wassermann reaction indicates that infection of the central nervous system has occurred; the cells and protein indicate the activity of the condition. This concept maintains that if the spinal fluid is inactive —i.e., if the cell count and protein are normal—the syphilitic infection in the central nervous system has been arrested and no further therapy is needed. Although this concept is not completely accepted, it seems to hold true in the majority of patients.

The serologic reaction of the blood does not always parallel the spinal fluid findings. Patients with previous treatment may have a negative blood test and a strongly positive spinal fluid. This combination seldom occurs in untreated cases.

If the spinal fluid is completely negative 5 years after the onset of the disease, it rarely if ever becomes positive again.

Meningitis. In a small number of patients, involvement of the central nervous system may be manifested by an acute meningitis. This condition usually appears within the first 2 years after the onset of syphilis. It nearly always occurs in patients who have previously had inadequate therapy and may be associated with an infectious or mucocutaneous relapse.

The symptoms usually consist of headache, cranial nerve lesions, delirium, convulsions, or signs of increased intracranial pressure. *Papilledema* is frequently found in patients with syphilitic meningitis, and these cases are often diagnosed erroneously as brain tumors.

The serologic test for syphilis and the spinal fluid Wassermann are usually strongly positive. The spinal fluid may show a marked lymphocytosis, counts as high as 2,000 cells per cu mm having been observed. This condition is often confused with other forms of lymphocytic meningitis, such as tuberculous or virus meningitis. The immediate prognosis is good, but the ultimate prognosis is much more serious. If the patient does not receive adequate treatment, late manifestations of neurosyphilis or paresis are likely to develop.

Meningovascular Syphilis. Meningovascular syphilis is usually manifested by signs of thrombosis of one or more of the branches of the cerebral or spinal arteries. Because there is almost always some evidence of leptomeningitis, the term meningovascular syphilis is used to describe these cases.

The symptoms of this condition depend upon the location and size of the vessels involved. Monoplegia or hemiplegia, hemianesthesia, aphasia, or hemianopsia may occur. Cranial nerve palsies are frequent, and convulsions are often observed. Syphilitic endarteritis may also involve the cerebellar vessels. Patients with meningovascular syphilis sometimes develop psychotic behavior, and differentiation from paresis is often difficult.

In older patients it is often impossible to differentiate clinically between syphilitic vascular disease and a cerebral thrombosis of other etiology. In these cases the blood and spinal fluid findings provide the only means of differentiation. The blood serologic test is positive in the majority of patients with vascular neurosyphilis, and the spinal fluid usually shows a moderate increase of cells and protein with a positive serologic reaction. A diagnosis of meningovascular syphilis should not be made if the spinal fluid is normal.

The vessels and meninges of the spinal cord undergo changes identical with those in the brain. With thrombosis of the anterior spinal artery, the patient may suddenly develop signs of an acute *transverse myelitis* with paraplegia, loss of sensation, and fecal or urinary incontinence. Usually, however, meningovascular lesions of the spinal cord are insidious and produce chronic progressive paralyses and sensory disturbances. A number of neurologic syndromes result from more or less localized spinal cord lesions: syphilitic involvement of the pyramidal tract produces the so-called *Erb's spastic spinal paraplegia;* anterior horn cell degeneration causes a picture similar to *progressive muscular atrophy;* while a single localized *gumma* may simulate cord tumor.

The term *meningovascular syphilis* is also employed for a large group of patients with diverse signs and symptoms, such as *epilepsy, eighth nerve deafness,* other cranial nerve lesions, or chronic headaches. Pupillary abnormalities are frequently present and may consist of a variety of changes, such as miosis, dilatation, anisocoria, fixed pupils, or typical Argyll Robertson phenomenon.

Tabes Dorsalis (Locomotor Ataxia). Tabes dorsalis is a form of neurosyphilis in which there is selective degeneration in the posterior roots of the spinal nerves and the posterior columns of the spinal cord. Microscopically the dorsal roots may appear completely demyelinated, and there is marked loss of nerve fibers. The posterior columns of the spinal cord also show a loss of myelin and degeneration of the axones. Spirochetes are rarely found in these lesions. In the majority of cases tabes appears 20 to 30 years after the initial infection. It is found more commonly in men than in women.

Patients with tabes frequently develop severe, agonizing *shooting* or *"lightning"* pains in the legs. Girdle pains also occur in tabetics, along with paresthesias, numbness, and tingling of the trunk, hands, or feet. Another type of severe pain occurs in attacks of *gastric crisis.* About 10 percent of tabetic patients develop severe episodes of abdominal pain associated with nausea and vomiting. These attacks may last for days, resulting in dehydration and exhaustion. Patients with gastric crises are sometimes diagnosed as having acute surgical conditions, and unnecessary operations have been performed on them.

Ataxia is a major symptom in tabes and may be so severe that the patient is unable to walk or stand. Some patients develop a typical tabetic gait, which consists of slapping of the feet and walking on a broad base. The ataxia is worse in the dark, and the patient may sway or fall when standing with his eyes closed (Romberg's sign). The damage to the nerve fibers in the posterior columns not only results in ataxia but also produces loss of position sense, and the patient does not know without visual assistance the exact position of his toes or feet. Vibratory sensation in the legs is diminished or absent. There may be diminution of deep pain sensation to pressure on the testes or Achilles tendon, and areas of hypesthesia may be present on the trunk or in the hands and feet. The patella and Achilles tendon reflexes are sluggish or absent. Patients with tabes often show evidence of hypotonia and hyperextensibility of the joints. Degenerative lesions, such as chronic, nonhealing lesions of the skin and *Charcot joints,* are also found.

Involvement of the autonomic nervous system may occur in patients with tabes, and *postural hypotension* is occasionally present. Severe *paroxysmal hypertension,* associated with gastric crises, has also been observed and may simulate paroxysmal hypertension caused by pheochromocytoma.

Urinary difficulties occur in approximately 50 to 60 percent of patients with tabes. These often appear early in the disease and consist of hesitancy or difficulty in starting micturition. Later the patient develops complete loss of bladder sensation. Patients with tabetic bladder often give no history of urinary symptoms, and catheterization for residual urine should be done in all who have evidence of tabes. *Impotence* and loss of sexual desire are frequently noted.

Paralysis of the oculomotor nerves is common in tabes, resulting in diplopia, ptosis of the lids, or ophthalmoplegia. Pupillary abnormalities are also extremely common and may be manifested by the classic *Argyll Robertson phenomena,* i.e., miosis, reaction to accommodation but no reaction to light, poor response to atropine, and absence of ciliospinal reflex. This condition must be differentiated from *Adie's pupil,* which is usually unilateral, is larger than the normal pupil, and reacts slowly to both light and accommodation. Patients with Adie's pupils may also have absent or diminished tendon reflexes.

Atrophy of the optic nerve occurs in about 10 to 15 percent of patients with tabes. Seventy percent of patients with untreated optic atrophy become blind in 3 years and 90 percent in 5 years. On ophthalmoscopic examination the optic disk appears white and sharply defined. The physiologic cup is prominent, and the lamina cribrosa is abnormally conspicuous. Visual field defects and diminution of vision may be present with only slight changes in the color of the disks. To detect such cases of optic atrophy early, careful perimetry and visual acuity examinations should be made in all cases of neurosyphilis. Although improvement in vision is not to be expected in patients with optic atrophy, arrest of the atrophic process can usually be obtained by penicillin therapy in patients with early involvement.

In early cases of tabes the serologic test for syphilis is often strongly positive, and the spinal fluid may show definite abnormalities, such as increased cells and protein and a positive Wassermann reaction. In patients with long-standing tabes, however, the blood and spinal fluid findings may be misleading. Approximately one-fourth of such patients have negative blood serologic tests, while as many as 20 percent have normal spinal fluids. Tabes dorsalis must be differentiated from numerous other diseases of the spinal column, such as cord tumor, combined system disease, and syringomyelia, as well as various types of peripheral neuritis (particularly diabetic neuropathy). The response of tabes to treatment is often poor, and symptoms may progress despite all forms of therapy.

Paretic Neurosyphilis (Dementia Paralytica, Paresis, General Paralysis of the Insane). General paresis is a psychosis caused by extensive spirochetal invasion of the brain. On histologic examination the most prominent feature is degeneration of the nerve cells. Perivascular infiltration and endothelial proliferation of the small vessels are seen. *Treponema pallidum* can be demonstrated in the cerebral cortex and other portions of the brain.

Paretic neurosyphilis is more common in men than in women and usually develops between the ages of thirty-five and fifty. The onset is most often insidious; prodromal symptoms consist of headache, insomnia, difficulty in concentration, and easy fatigability. As the disease progresses, a gradual change in personality takes place, with increased irritability, memory loss, poor judgment, lack of personal care, and deviations in character. These alterations may occur over a period of several months. Many of them are noted by the patient's family only in retrospect and elicited only by close questioning. The onset of paresis is sometimes sudden and may be ushered in by convulsions, syncope, or a cerebral vascular accident.

The simple, demented type of psychosis is the most common. These patients show confusion, apathy, impaired memory, and defects in judgment. Memory is particularly poor for recent events. They are often unable to concentrate on simple calculations and show

little insight or concern about their illness. The grandiose form of paresis is manifested by euphoria, overactivity, ideas of grandeur, and megalomania. Auditory and visual hallucinations are not common in these patients, but delusions of wealth and prowess are frequent. The type of psychosis that prevails in a given case depends to a great extent upon the preparetic personality of the individual. As the disease progresses, however, the symptoms of euphoria, paranoia, or mania recede, and simple deterioration and dementia become the outstanding features.

Eventually the patients become completely bedridden and are unable to move and feed themselves.

On neurologic examination these patients may present various motor disturbances, such as *tremors* of the facial muscles, tongue, and outstretched hands. The patient's handwriting is altered because of the tremors and incoordination. The speech becomes slurred, and test phrases are mispronounced. Pupillary abnormalities are common, and deep reflexes are usually exaggerated. Some patients with paresis also have signs and symptoms of tabes—i.e., *taboparesis.*

The demented form of paresis must be differentiated from senile dementia and Alzheimer's disease. The manic and paranoic types must be distinguished from manic-depressive psychoses and schizophrenia. In the early stages of paresis, differentiation from neurasthenia is sometimes difficult, and spinal fluid examination may be the only means of diagnosis.

The spinal fluid in general paresis shows marked changes, with increased cells and protein, positive serologic test, and first-zone colloidal reaction. The diagnosis of paresis should never be made in the presence of a normal spinal fluid; a positive spinal fluid is present in 100 percent of untreated cases.

The course of untreated paresis is progressive, and death usually occurs within a few years after the onset of symptoms. The prognosis improves considerably with therapy, but the chances for complete recovery are at best about 50 to 60 percent.

SYPHILIS IN PREGNANCY

Syphilis in pregnancy is a special problem, because the fetus becomes infected after the fifth month of pregnancy by passage of *T. pallidum* through the placenta. This usually occurs in women with early untreated syphilis, but is sometimes observed in late syphilis. Pregnancy complicated by syphilis may terminate in a spontaneous abortion, a stillborn infant, or a premature or full-term infected child. The maternal infection, however, becomes attenuated as the duration of the disease increases, and the chances of the fetus being infected are less with each succeeding pregnancy.

Pregnancy is believed to have a beneficial influence upon the course of the syphilitic infection, and late manifestations of the disease seem to occur less frequently in multiparous women than in others. A serologic test for syphilis should be taken routinely at the first prenatal visit of every pregnant woman. The early recognition of syphilis in pregnancy followed by adequate treatment will prevent congenital syphilis in almost every instance.

CONGENITAL SYPHILIS

Infantile congenital syphilis is often an overwhelming infection; such infants are severely ill, malnourished, and dehydrated. The most common manifestations of the disease in infants are skin lesions, fissures, condylomas, persistent rhinitis, tenderness over the long bones, and pseudoparalysis.

The diagnosis of syphilis in the infant is best established by dark-field demonstration of *T. pallidum* from the cutaneous or mucosal lesions. A positive serologic test in the first 2 months of life does not always indicate syphilis in the infant, because reacting substances may have been transferred from the maternal circulation. A very high titer of the serologic reaction or a steady rise in titer, however, is indicative of congenital syphilis. Roentgenographic examination of the long bones may show characteristic areas of bone destruction and *osteochondritis.*

Late congenital syphilis frequently manifests itself in the second decade with signs of central-nervous-system involvement, such as eighth nerve deafness, optic atrophy, and *juvenile paresis.* The prognosis of congenital neurosyphilis is serious; these patients commonly show little response to treatment. Cardiovascular syphilis is rare in the congenital infection.

Patients with late congenital syphilis often exhibit typical stigmas, such as hypoplasia, wide spacing and notching of the central incisors (*Hutchinson's teeth*), frontal bossing, a highly arched palate, and *saber shins.* The first permanent molar is also frequently affected in congenital syphilis and shows a characteristic appearance, with several small atrophic cusps on the occlusal surface. This is known as a "mulberry molar." *Interstitial keratitis,* a frequent complication, usually appears in the second decade. It is characterized by pain, lacrimation, circumcorneal injection, and corneal opacity. The response to therapy is poor, and serious impairment of vision often results. Occasionally, hydrarthrosis of the knee joint (*Clutton's synovitis*) is associated with interstitial keratitis.

LABORATORY DIAGNOSIS

Dark-field demonstration of *T. pallidum* is most useful in the early stages of syphilis. It should be employed routinely on every genital lesion and on all cutaneous and mucosal lesions suspected of being syphilitic. In the hands of a competent microscopist, dark-field examination is reliable and establishes without doubt the diagnosis and stage of the infection.

SEROLOGIC TESTS. Serologic tests for syphilis (STS) are the most commonly used diagnostic procedures. In latent syphilis they are the only means by which the diagnosis can be made. The serologic tests are based upon the presence of an antibody-like substance (sometimes called *reagin*), which appears in the patient's serum soon after the onset of the disease. Syphilitic serum reacts with a lipoidal antigen made from an alcoholic extract of beef heart. Various modifications of flocculation tests for syphilis have been named after their originators (Kahn, Kline, and Hinton). The complement fixation technique or Wassermann test employs the same type of antigen, the Kolmer modification being the most commonly used in this country. The VDRL (Venereal Disease Research Laboratory) test is a rapid slide technique employing cardiolipin antigen. It has a high degree of sensitivity and specificity and has become the flocculation test of choice in most state laboratories and hospitals.

In addition to these serologic tests for syphilis using lipoidal or cardiolipin antigens, a number of other techniques have been developed which employ antigens made from whole-body virulent *T. pallidum* or from chemical fractions of this organism.

The most useful of the various tests to detect treponemal antibodies has been the *T. pallidum* immobilization test (TPI), which uses a live virulent strain of the organism as an antigen. It demonstrates a circulating treponemal antibody which persists for many years after the onset of the original infection and is little influenced by treatment unless this was carried out early in the course of the disease. Although the test is difficult to perform, it has been of value in distinguishing late syphilis from conditions causing biologic false positive reactions and in the diagnosis of patients who have clinical signs of late syphilis and in whom the tests for reagin are negative or inconclusive. Various other tests using treponemal antigens that were developed later include the *T. pallidum* agglutination (TPA), complement fixation (TPCF), and immunoadherence tests (TPIA). A standardized antigen of Reiter's strain of the cultivated spirochete is also commercially available and is being used in agglutination as well as complement fixation tests.

Perhaps the most practical of these methods has been the fluorescent treponemal antibody test (FTA). Investigations with this test have shown that syphilitic serum contains antibodies specific for *T. pallidum* as well as a low-titered nonspecific treponemal antibody which is also found in normal serums. False positive reactions to normal serums could, however, be avoided by testing the serum at a dilution of 1:200 (FTA 200 test). The FTA test has been refined further by removing the nonspecific group antibody from the serum by absorption with material derived from Reiter's strain of the cultivated spirochete. This improved technique, designated as the fluorescent treponemal antibody absorption test (FTA-ABS), has become a valuable addition to the current serologic methods for the diagnosis of syphilis. The FTA-ABS test has been shown to be more sensitive and more specific than the TPI in all phases of syphilis and promises to become the treponemal test of choice for differentiation of chronic biologic false positive reactions. It also appears to be of considerable value in the diagnosis of treated and untreated cases of late syphilis, even when the serologic tests using lipoidal or cardiolipin antigens are nonreactive. The fact that patients with such conditions maintain treponemal antibodies many years after supposedly adequate therapy has been related to the recent demonstration by fluorescent antibody stains that treponemes may be present in various body fluids and tissues such as aqueous humor and cerebrospinal fluid.

Although these and other new serologic procedures are now available, it is recommended that the standard reagin tests continue to be used for the routine serologic diagnosis of syphilis, because they are highly standardized, adequately sensitive, and inexpensive. Moreover, they are widely used and the results are readily understood and interpreted. Although treponemal tests such as the FTA-ABS may eventually supplant the standard reagin test as a primary screening device if the techniques can be simplified, in general they should be used primarily as confirmatory tests for the diagnosis of biologic false positive reactions. When the results of the various standard serologic tests are inconclusive and a biologic false positive reaction is considered, the patient's serum should be tested by one of the treponemal procedures. A close correlation has been shown between the results of the FTA-ABS and TPI tests. The FTA-ABS test is technically much simpler to perform, however.

It has been recommended that the results of serologic tests be reported as "reactive," "weakly reactive," and "nonreactive" in place of the previous terms "positive," "doubtful," or "negative." A nonreactive or negative standard reagin test does not always exclude syphilis, nor is a reactive or positive test always proof of the existence of the disease. The reagin serologic tests are nonreactive in the incubation period of syphilis, during the early weeks of the primary stage, and in many of the late manifestations such as cardiovascular disturbance and neurosyphilis (tabes dorsalis in particular). In approximately one-fourth of the patients with "adequately" treated late syphilis, the serologic tests using cardiolipin antigens may be nonreactive, whereas the TPI and FTA-ABS continue to be reactive. Reversal of the standard reagin tests from reactive to nonreactive may be indicative of the disappearance of nonspecific antibodies only, whereas the more specific treponemal antibody seems to persist despite presumably adequate therapy.

The height of the titer in serial serologic tests is of value in the diagnosis and management of the various stages of the disease. A sharply rising titer is usually found in recently acquired syphilis, while a stationary titer indicates an infection of some duration. A rapidly falling titer in the absence of therapy is evidence against the diagnosis of syphilis and may indicate a false positive reaction. The height of the titer has no bearing on the prognosis or outcome of the disease. Carefully titered tests are also important in determining the results of therapy; a continuing falling titer indicates a satisfactory response.

BIOLOGIC FALSE POSITIVE SEROLOGIC TESTS FOR SYPHILIS. Serologic tests for syphilis using lipoidal or cardiolipid antigens may be reactive in a great variety of non-spirochetal illnesses. These biologic false positive reactions are due presumably to the appearance in the patient's serum of substances which act like reagin and give positive flocculation and complement fixation reactions for syphilis. These reactions are usually transient, but in some instances may be positive for months or years.

Biologic false positive reactions are frequently observed in patients with vaccinia, infectious mononucleosis, malaria, leprosy, and upper respiratory diseases, as well as in spirochetal infections, such as yaws, pinta, and relapsing fever. Other infections which are occasionally associated with false positive reactions are lymphogranuloma venereum, chancroid, measles, chickenpox, atypical pneumonia, infectious hepatitis, rat-bite fever, and disseminated lupus erythematosus. In fact, any febrile disease or immunization is a potential cause of false positive tests. There is evidence that individuals with biologic false positive reactions of long duration may have autoimmune diseases or dysproteinemia. The biologic false positive STS has been shown to be associated with systemic lupus erythematosus and Hashimoto's thyroiditis. A false positive STS may serve as a forerunner to the eventual development of one of these autoimmune disorders.

The TPI test and other treponemal tests such as the FTA-ABS are often of considerable aid in the diagnosis of false positive reactions. These tests are almost always positive in late syphilis. A negative treponemal test is, therefore, of value in excluding the diagnosis of syphilis. A positive test, on the other hand, indicates the existence of a syphilitic infection even if the standard serologic tests are negative. In most cases, the false positive reaction will become negative within 6 months. If the patient continues to show a positive serologic test and if appropriate diagnostic procedures do not indicate a false positive reaction, antisyphilitic therapy should be instituted. If the patient becomes pregnant or is to be married, immediate treatment is indicated.

SERORESISTANCE. In many patients with syphilis the serologic test remains positive despite prolonged, intensive therapy. These patients are called seroresistant, or Wassermann-fast. One of the aims of therapy in early syphilis (particularly during the first 2 years of the disease) is to procure and maintain a negative serologic reaction. In late syphilis, however, seroresistance is of little clinical importance and has no relationship to the outcome of the disease.

In most patients with early syphilis the serologic test becomes negative within 6 months after therapy is begun. Occasionally the titer of the serologic reaction falls very slowly and the tests remain positive in low titer (i.e., less than 1:4 dilution) for as long as 1 to 2 years. In some patients with early syphilis there is very little serologic response to treatment, and the titer remains high for 6 to 9 months or more. This type of seroresistance is usually followed by clinical relapse, and these patients should be re-treated.

Neurosyphilis is frequently associated with seroresistance in both early and late cases, and the spinal fluid should be examined in every patient with a persistently positive serologic reaction.

The seroresistant patient is often discouraged over the failure to reverse the serologic test and becomes deeply concerned for fear that the infection is not arrested. In addition, he may be embarrassed in applying for a marriage license or employment when blood tests are a part of the premarital or preemployment examination. These patients should be reassured that the outcome of the disease is not related to the persistence of a positive serologic test. Seroresistance should not be an obstacle to marriage.

SPINAL FLUID TESTS. The spinal fluid must be examined in every patient with syphilis. This is the only method of detecting involvement of the central nervous system in the asymptomatic stage, of determining the efficacy of treatment, and of confirming the diagnosis of symptomatic neurosyphilis.

The spinal fluid cell count should be done within an hour after the fluid is withdrawn. A count of more than 8 lymphocytes per cu mm is considered abnormal. Even a small amount of blood in the spinal fluid will affect the accuracy of the various examinations. A quantitative determination of the spinal fluid protein should be done in every case.

Complement fixation tests for syphilis are generally regarded as being more sensitive than flocculation tests for examination of spinal fluid. The spinal fluid of patients with neurosyphilis has been found to contain immobilizing antibodies for *T. pallidum.*

The spinal fluid may also show biologic false positive complement fixation or flocculation reactions. This may be caused by a bloody tap or any condition which produces an increased protein in the spinal fluid. Brain tumor, bacterial or virus meningitis, encephalitis, or subarachnoid hemorrhage can produce a false positive test for syphilis in either syphilitic or nonsyphilitic patients.

The value of colloidal precipitation tests (gold and mastic reactions) has been overemphasized in the diagnosis of neurosyphilis. The zone of precipitation or the shape of the colloidal curve has little diagnostic significance.

BIOPSY. Biopsy is a valuable diagnostic procedure, especially for cutaneous lesions. In late syphilis involving the lymph nodes, testes, or larynx, it is indispensable.

TREATMENT

In patients with early syphilis adequate treatment can produce an absolute, or biologic, cure, with complete healing of lesions and reversal of serologic tests and spinal fluid findings. These patients become entirely well, are not infectious, and do not develop any of the late manifestations of the disease.

Treatment of late syphilis may not achieve these goals. Despite long and vigorous therapy the serologic tests in late syphilis often remain positive. Late syphilitic lesions are often associated with permanent damage, and treatment may produce little or no return of function.

EARLY SYPHILIS. In 1943 penicillin was found to be effective in the treatment of syphilis. The use of arsenicals, bismuth, or mercurials is rarely, if ever, indicated. Other antibiotics, such as chloramphenicol and the various tetracyclines have treponemicidal activity and produce healing of both early and late syphilitic lesions. The ultimate place of these drugs in the treatment of syphilis has not been established. They are probably not as effective as penicillin. Erythromycin and the tetracyclines have also been shown to have treponemicidal action, and doses of 20 to 30 Gm are recommended over a period of 10 to 15 days in patients in whom penicillin is contraindicated.

Procaine penicillin and benzathine penicillin G have generally replaced crystalline, aqueous penicillin, except perhaps in the very serious or far-advanced stages of infection. The minimal effective total dosage of penicillin is approximately 2.4 million units. Increasing the total amount of penicillin from 2.4 to 9.6 million units does not decrease the failure rate in early syphilis.

The total dosage of depot (procaine) penicillin usually prescribed is approximately 4.8 to 6 million units given in injections of 1.2 million units at 2- or 3-day intervals for a period of 8 to 12 days. This schedule will produce satisfactory results in about 90 percent of patients. The remaining 10 percent will show clinical or laboratory changes of either relapse or reinfection. Benzathine penicillin G is also effective in early syphilis when given in a single dose of 2.4 million units (1.2 million units in each buttock) or in 2 or 3 weekly injections of 1.2 million units each. It has the advantage from the public health standpoint of completing treatment in a minimum period of time but is not recommended as a routine method. Oral penicillin is not recommended for the treatment of syphilis. The other antibiotics with treponemicidal activity should be used only in patients in whom penicillin is contraindicated.

Jarisch-Herxheimer Reaction. Within a few hours after the first injection of either an arsenical or penicillin, about 50 percent of patients with early syphilis experience fever, malaise, headache, myalgia, and a flare-up of cutaneous lesions. This is presumed to be caused by release of breakdown products of spirochetes following the injection of treponemicidal agents. In early syphilis these symptoms disappear within several hours and leave no permanent tissue damage. In late syphilis such reactions can be disastrous if the lesions are located in such areas as the ostiums of the coronary arteries, the wall of an aneurysm, or the central nervous system.

Posttreatment Observation. After completing treatment, patients should return every month during the first year for quantitative serologic tests and examination for relapsing lesions. If the patient develops a recurrence of syphilitic lesions or evidence of neurosyphilis, or if there is a birth of a syphilitic child, retreatment is necessary. If the serologic test in patients with early syphilis shows no appreciable decrease within 6 months or if the titer is elevated (arbitrarily a dilution of 1:4 or higher) 1 year after completion of therapy, further treatment is indicated. A positive reaction in any dilution 18 months or more after completion of treatment of primary or secondary syphilis should be considered as evidence of treatment failure, and another course of penicillin is indicated.

Serologic tests should be taken at 3-month intervals during the second year after treatment and at 6-month intervals during the third, fourth, and fifth years. If at the end of 5 years the patient has no clinical evidence of syphilis and has a normal blood and spinal fluid, he may be considered completely cured.

A spinal fluid examination should be performed 6 months after the completion of treatment for early syphilis. If the spinal fluid is normal at this time and if the patient continues to show no evidence of clinical or serologic relapse, the examination need not be repeated until approximately 2 years following treatment. Patients having positive spinal fluid tests for syphilis 6 months or more after treatment for early syphilis should be re-treated.

Relapse and Reinfection. Evidence of relapse in early syphilis may occur as early as 4 weeks or as late as 2 years after treatment.

The prognosis of relapsing syphilis is more serious than the initial infection, and these patients should be re-treated with twice the original dose of penicillin, given over a longer period of time. Many patients with recurrent syphilis actually have a new infection rather than a relapse of their original infection. Although various criteria have been set up to distinguish relapse from reinfection, differentiation is often impossible.

SYPHILIS IN PREGNANCY. Congenital syphilis can be prevented by proper treatment of syphilis in pregnancy. Although women with syphilis of many years' duration are not likely to bear syphilitic children, further treatment of such patients during pregnancy is recommended. Although treatment with penicillin is of considerable value when given during the last months of pregnancy, it is best given before the fetus becomes grossly infected, i.e., before the last trimester.

All patients treated for syphilis in pregnancy should be observed very closely, and quantitative serologic tests for syphilis taken at least every month. Re-treatment during pregnancy is indicated if there is a rise in serologic titer following therapy, if a definite decrease in titer fails to occur in patients with early syphilis, or if the patient develops recurrent syphilitic lesions. A positive serologic test at the time of delivery does not necessarily indicate that treatment has been inadequate. The child born of a mother treated for syphilis should have a serologic test every 2 to 4 weeks until it is at least six months of age. Once the woman has received adequate amounts of penicillin for syphilis, it is not necessary to re-treat her during succeeding pregnancies if the titer of the serologic test is negative or remains low (less than 1:4).

CONGENITAL SYPHILIS. Infants with congenital syphilis should receive careful supportive care and adequate nutrition, in addition to antisyphilitic treatment. Penicillin is very effective; a total dosage of 200,000 units per kg body weight given in equally divided amounts every 3 hr to 7 to 10 days is adequate. Although the use of

procaine penicillin in a large series of these cases has not been reported, this type of penicillin should also give satisfactory results. Doses of 150,000 units of procaine penicillin in aqueous solution given every day for eight injections are recommended. Follow-up blood tests and the indications for re-treatment in early congenital syphilis are the same as in early acquired syphilis.

Treatment of interstitial keratitis is not altogether satisfactory. Penicillin therapy is recommended, but it does not always result in reduction of the inflammation or clearing of the corneal opacities. Occasionally, interstitial keratitis appears for the first time during, or immediately after, what appear to be adequate dosages of penicillin. It seems probable that this ocular manifestation represents a type of hypersensitivity phenomenon. Cortisone in aqueous suspension (5 mg per ml) or in ointment form should be applied to the involved eye every few hours day and night for several weeks. The inflammatory reaction often recurs, however, after the drug is discontinued, and repeated courses may be necessary until spontaneous regression appears. Hydrarthrosis (Clutton's synovitis) responds slowly to penicillin therapy.

LATE SYPHILIS. Latent Stage. The chief purpose in treating late latent syphilis is to prevent the development of gummatous lesions and cardiovascular syphilis. Patients with late latent syphilis have negative spinal fluids and rarely, if ever, develop neurosyphilis.

The value of penicillin has not been fully assessed in late latent syphilis. Because the prognosis of this stage of the disease is so good and the drug is known to be effective in both early and late symptomatic syphilis, it is presumed to be of value in patients with latent infection. The treatment schedules suggested for early syphilis, employing 4 to 6 million units of penicillin, are recommended. Failure of the serologic test to revert to negative after adequate treatment—i.e., *seroresistance*—is not necessarily a forerunner of late complications. Once the patient with late syphilis has had adequate treatment, additional penicillin therapy will not contribute significantly toward reversal of the blood test.

Skin, Bones, and Viscera. Gummatous lesions of the skin, mucous membranes, bones, and viscera usually respond promptly to penicillin therapy. The recommended total dosage of penicillin is greater than that employed in early syphilis and should be approximately 10 million units. This can be administered as 900,000 units of procaine penicillin given every 48 hr for 12 injections. The posttreatment observations and indications for re-treatment of these patients are the same as those recommended above. A high percentage of patients with late syphilitic lesions have abnormal spinal fluid findings, and a lumbar puncture is indicated in every patient before treatment is instituted.

Cardiovascular Syphilis. The value of antisyphilitic therapy in late cardiovascular syphilis is difficult to determine. Many syphilologists believe that treatment does not delay the ultimate development of myocardial failure or aneurysmal rupture. Treatment appears to be of some value, however, in early aortic regurgitation, uncomplicated aortitis, or small asymptomatic aneurysms. The risk of a serious Herxheimer reaction following initiation of penicillin treatment has been minimal. Preparatory bismuth therapy is probably of little value in preventing this type of reaction, and most workers begin treatment with penicillin. The total dosage is 10 to 15 million units of penicillin, given in schedules similar to those recommended for gummatous lesions. As in other types of late syphilis, the serologic test often remains positive after therapy. Proper management of congestive failure and restriction of physical activity of these patients are of paramount importance.

Neurosyphilis. The results of treatment of neurosyphilis depend largely upon the type and duration of the neuropathologic process. If the predominant lesion of the central nervous system is degenerative, as in tabes and optic atrophy, little response to any form of treatment can be expected. If the tissue reaction is chiefly inflammatory, as in syphilitic meningitis, rapid and almost complete return of function will occur.

Penicillin treatment of neurosyphilis is often followed by dramatic clinical response with prompt and favorable changes in the spinal fluid. Shortly after penicillin therapy, there is a rapid reduction in the spinal fluid cell count and protein. The spinal fluid serologic reaction, however, may not become negative for 5 years or more. Penicillin produced normal spinal fluid cell counts in 85 to 90 percent of patients treated for various types of neurosyphilis. The remaining 10 to 15 percent showed abnormal spinal fluid cell counts 6 to 12 months following treatment and were considered treatment failures.

It is generally agreed that the improvement in the clinical manifestations of neurosyphilis and in the spinal fluid abnormalities following penicillin is as good as that obtained with fever therapy. Penicillin alone is the treatment of choice in patients with asymptomatic neurosyphilis, syphilitic meningitis, meningovascular syphilis, and tabes. The optimum dosage schedule has not been definitely established, but doses of 10 to 15 million units are usually recommended either as the aqueous solution, 100,000 units every 3 hr, or as repository penicillin 900,000 units a day.

Treatment of the tabetic bladder may be very discouraging. Drugs, such as Mecholyl chloride and ergotamine, have been employed to increase bladder tone and contraction, but the results are variable. In early cases the patient can be trained to micturate at regular intervals and empty the bladder by pressure on the lower part of the abdomen. In late cases, surgical procedures (transurethral resection of the vesical neck, suprapubic cystotomy) may be necessary. Urinary tract infection should be prevented and instrumentation avoided as much as possible. Charcot joints are rarely improved by antisyphilitic therapy, and special orthopedic treatment is necessary. The management of patients with gastric crisis is sometimes very difficult. In the acute attack the patient should be heavily sedated. Morphine should be avoided. Large doses of atropine are said to be of value in relieving the symptoms of gastric crisis.

In most cases of advanced optic atrophy the use of penicillin or fever, alone or in combination, does not prevent the development of blindness. Patients with optic atrophy should be admitted to the hospital and given penicillin in aqueous solution, 200,000 units every 4 hr for 13 to 17 days, for a total dosage of 15 to 20 million units.

In paresis, penicillin alone often results in marked improvement in tremor, mental state, and speech and writing defects. It has been reported to produce entirely satisfactory results in about 20 percent and significant improvement in an additional 35 percent of a large series of patients with paresis treated in general hospitals. Early penicillin treatment of incipient paresis has resulted in clinical remission and ability to return to work in more than 80 percent of patients. Large amounts of penicillin —15 to 20 million units—are generally recommended, but doses as low as 6 million units have been found to be of value. Although the repository type of penicillin is said to be as effective as aqueous penicillin in paresis or optic atrophy, the aqueous preparation is preferred in moderately or severely affected patients. It should be given in schedules similar to those recommended for optic atrophy.

Fever therapy should not be used initially in either optic atrophy or paresis because its possible additive effects are not sufficient to justify the hazards associated with it. In selected patients in whom the neurosyphilitic process progresses despite adequate initial penicillin therapy, re-treatment with fever therapy and penicillin should be considered. Retreatment with penicillin alone, however, is indicated in progressive paresis if the initial course of treatment consisted of less than 6 million units. Penicillin alone should also be used to re-treat patients who show elevated spinal fluid cell counts a year or more after the initial therapy or in whom there was temporary clinical improvement after treatment but subsequent progression of the disease.

Careful neuropsychiatric and spinal fluid observations should be made following treatment of all patients with neurosyphilis. These should be done every 4 months during the first year, twice during the second year, and once a year thereafter, or until the spinal fluid is completely negative and permanent regression of symptoms seems apparent. In late neurosyphilis the spinal fluid serologic reaction often remains positive for many years, despite repeated courses of chemotherapy or fever; this does not in itself indicate progression or relapse of the neurosyphilitic process.

Herxheimer Reactions in Late Syphilis. Exacerbations of late syphilitic lesions are not infrequently observed following the initial administration of arsenicals or penicillin. Approximately one-half the patients treated for paresis become temporarily worse and show increased agitation and mental confusion during the first 24 hr of penicillin treatment. Other manifestations of Herxheimer's reaction, such as myelitis, convulsions, and exacerbation of lightning pains, have been reported.

There have been very few cases in which penicillin

therapy has produced an acute exacerbation of clinical manifestations of cardiovascular syphilis. Neither the use of small initial doses of penicillin nor preparatory treatment with bismuth seems indicated in an attempt to prevent Herxheimer's effects.

EFFECT OF PENICILLIN AND OTHER ANTIBIOTICS WHEN USED FOR OTHER DISEASES. The widespread use of penicillin and antibiotics with treponemicidal properties in the treatment of various other infections has created confusion in the diagnosis and management of syphilis. This is particularly true when gonorrhea is treated. Patients with gonorrhea may have acquired syphilis simultaneously. Although there is reason to believe that the use of penicillin and perhaps of the other antibiotics frequently aborts the syphilitic infection completely, they may at times only delay the appearance of the lesions or prevent their development. For these reasons it is recommended that all persons with gonorrhea treated with penicillin or the other spirocheticidal antibiotics should have serologic tests for syphilis at monthly intervals for at least 4 months. The appearance of fever several hours after the administration of penicillin for gonorrhea is suggestive of Herxheimer's reaction and of syphilis.

The management of patients with positive serologic tests who have had previous penicillin therapy for other nonrelated infections is sometimes difficult. If syphilitic infection is thought to be present, the decision as to further therapy should be based upon the amount of penicillin already administered, the type and duration of syphilitic infection, the result of the spinal fluid examination, and the titer of the serologic test.

PROPHYLAXIS

Syphilis and the other venereal diseases can be prevented in most instances by the proper prophylactic measures during and following sexual intercourse. Protection from contact with infectious genital lesions can be obtained to some degree by the use of a condom. The danger of infection can also be reduced if the genitalia are washed thoroughly with soap and water immediately after exposure. Although ointments containing various treponemicidal substances have been employed for many years as local prophylactic agents, the use of these compounds is no longer recommended. In small series of cases, penicillin has been shown to prevent infection in individuals who are known to have been sexually exposed to patients with primary or secondary syphilis. The use of penicillin in these cases is justified not only as an attempt to abort the infection in the exposed individual, but also to prevent reinfection of the original patient who often maintains sexual relations with the contact despite instructions to the contrary.

Procaine penicillin or benzathine penicillin G in doses of 2.4 million units should be given soon after exposure to persons who have had sexual contact with known or suspected cases of infectious syphilis. The administration of penicillin as a routine prophylactic measure following every extramarital sexual exposure is neither practical nor advisable. Persons receiving prophylactic treatment should be kept under observation and should have repeated serologic tests for at least 6 months.

The prophylactic treatment of nurses, physicians, or laboratory workers accidentally exposed to, or inoculated with, infectious material will depend largely upon the risk of infection in the individual case. Another indication for prophylactic treatment is in pregnant women who are sexually exposed to infectious patients. A full course of penicillin treatment in these cases is indicated in an effort to prevent fetal infection.

PSYCHOTHERAPY

There are still considerable stigma and psychologic trauma attached to the diagnosis of syphillis, and proper treatment requires more than the mere administration of chemotherapeutic agents. The sociologic and psychologic aspects of this disease are considerable. Patients often have a sense of shame and guilt, and some postpone or discontinue medical care. Others develop serious anxiety states and return repeatedly for reassurance that the disease has been arrested. Some individuals develop syphilophobia as a result of having heard or read of the serious effects of the disease. Every effort to relieve these patients of their anxiety by correcting mistaken ideas regarding the infection and by emphasizing the good prognosis should be made.

Upon learning the diagnosis, many patients either condemn their marital partners and threaten divorce or separation or else refuse to impart the information to their spouse. It is essential, however, that the marital partners of patients with infectious syphilis be examined at regular intervals for evidence of the disease.

REFERENCES

Atwood, W. G., J. L. Miller, G. W. Stout, and L. C. Norins: The TPI and FTA-ABS Tests in Treated Late Syphilis, J.A.M.A., 203:549, 1968.

Cannefax, G. R., L. C. Norins, and E. J. Gillespie: Immunology of Syphilis, Ann. Rev. Med., 18:471, 1967.

Harvey, A. M., and L. E. Shulman: Connective Tissue Disease and the Chronic Biologic False-positive Test for Syphilis (BFP Reaction), Med. Clinics N. Am., 50:1271, 1966.

Magnuson, H. J., E. W. Thomas, S. Olansky, B. I. Kaplin, L. deMello, and J. C. Cutler: Inoculation Syphilis in Human Volunteers, Medicine, 35:33, 1956.

Nicholas, L., and H. Beerman: Late Syphilis: A Review of Some of the Recent Literature, Am. J. Med. Sci., 254:549, 1967.

Tuffanelli, D. L., K. D. Wuepper, L. L. Bradford, and R. M. Wood: Fluorescent Treponemal-antibody Absorption Tests, New Engl. J. Med., 276:258, 1967.

178 YAWS
Albert Heyman

DEFINITION. Yaws is an infectious tropical disease caused by the *Treponema pertenue*. It is characterized by a primary cutaneous lesion, which is followed by a granulomatous skin eruption and, in some instances, by late destructive lesions of the skin and bones. The disease is also known as *frambesia, pain, bouba,* and *parangi.*

ETIOLOGY. The etiologic agent of yaws, the *T. pertenue,* is morphologically indistinguishable from *Treponema pallidum.* It further resembles the spirochete of syphilis, in that it produces a positive reaction with the Wassermann and flocculation tests for syphilis and is also susceptible to arsenicals, bismuth, and penicillin. Cross immunity between the two diseases has been observed in both man and experimental animals. There has been considerable controversy as to whether the two diseases were at one time identical and have been modified over the years by climate, race, and other factors.

EPIDEMIOLOGY. Yaws is confined entirely to the Tropics and is prevalent in the West Indies, South Pacific islands, equatorial Africa, and South America. The disease is usually acquired before puberty and is spread by direct contact with open lesions containing the spirochete. Transmission of the disease occurs rarely by sexual contact. Certain species of flies are also thought to be vectors of this infection. The disease is more common in natives with poor personal hygiene.

MANIFESTATIONS. Following an average incubation period of 3 to 4 weeks, a primary lesion, the *mother yaw,* appears at the site of inoculation. This is almost invariably extragenital and usually occurs on the legs. This lesion is a granuloma, which later ulcerates and heals with scar formation. About 6 to 12 weeks after the appearance of the lesion, a generalized eruption develops, consisting of large papules or granulomas on the face, neck, extremities, and buttocks. These lesions often occur about the mucocutaneous junctions, such as the mouth, nose, and rectum, and resemble condylomas of secondary syphilis. They heal slowly, but relapses may occur months or years after the onset of the initial yaw. The lesions of yaws often appear on the soles of the feet and produce painful ulcerations, so-called "crab yaws."

After several years, late destructive lesions may appear in the skin and bones. Periostitis and osteitis are found in the bones of the hands, arms, and legs, producing characteristic dactylitis and "saber shins." Destructive lesions appear about the nose and result in severe ulcerative areas (*gangosa*). Proliferative exostoses develop in the nasal portion of the maxillary bones; this is known as *goundou.* Juxtaarticular nodules are also seen in the late stage of the disease. Involvement of the aorta and the central nervous system has been reported, but these complications are rare.

DIAGNOSIS. The diagnosis of yaws can often be made on the appearance of the generalized skin eruption alone, but *T. pertenue* is easily demonstrated in the lesions. The Wassermann and flocculation tests for syphilis are usually positive. The lesions of yaws may be confused with those of leishmaniasis, leprosy, and tuberculosis. It is often impossible to differentiate between late lesions of yaws and late gummatous syphilis.

TREATMENT. Penicillin, the drug of choice in the treatment of yaws, produces prompt disappearance of the treponemes on dark-field examination and rapid healing of the lesions. The recommended dosage is a single injection of 1.2 million units of procaine penicillin in adults with early active lesions and proportionally less in children and in those with latent cases. The tetracyclines are thought to be less effective in the management of this condition. The World Health Organization has conducted large-scale campaigns to eradicate the disease in endemic areas, and some 40 million persons have been treated under its auspices. In high-prevalence areas, treatment has been given to the total population, with dramatic reduction in the incidence of new cases. As a result of these control measures and improvement in living standards of the native populations, yaws is rapidly receding in the equatorial portions of the world. The extensive and rapid travel now prevalent throughout the world and the large migration of West Indian and Middle Eastern natives to the English-speaking countries has led to the appearance of sporadic cases of infectious yaws and other types of treponematosis in several large cities in the United Kingdom.

REFERENCES

Hackett, C. J.: "An International Nomenclature of Yaws Lesions," World Health Organization Monograph Series, no. 36, 1957. (An atlas containing numerous photographs illustrating recommended terminology.)

——, and T. Guthe: Some Important Aspects of Yaws Eradication, Bull. World Health Organ., 15:869, 1956. (This reference is part of a symposium on treponematoses as a worldwide problem.)

Lanigan-O'Keefe, F. M., J. G. Holmes, and D. Hill: Infectious and Active Yaws in a Midland City, Brit. J. Dermatol., 79:325, 1967.

Turner, T. B., and D. H. Hollander: "Biology of the Treponematoses," World Health Organization Monograph Series, no. 35, 1957.

179 PINTA
Albert Heyman

DEFINITION. Pinta is an infectious disease of the skin caused by *Treponema carateum.* It is characterized by an initial papular lesion of the skin, followed by depigmented areas on the extremities and hyperkeratosis on the soles and palms. The disease is also known as *mal del pinto, azul,* and *carate.* Pinta is found almost entirely in the Western Hemisphere and is especially prevalent in Mexico and Colombia.

ETIOLOGY. *Treponema carateum,* the etiologic agent of pinta, is morphologically indistinguishable from *Treponema pallidum.* The exact relationship of this disease to other treponematoses (syphilis, yaws, and bejel) has not been definitely determined, and there are many similarities in the clinical manifestations of these infections. Pinta is usually transmitted from person to person by direct contact. It may also be spread by an insect vector.

MANIFESTATIONS. The primary lesion of pinta appears after an incubation period of 7 to 20 days as a non-ulcerative papule at the site of infection. This is followed 5 to 18 months later by a secondary eruption character-ized by flat erythematous and hyperpigmented lesions, called *pintids*. Late lesions develop after several years and appear as vitiligoid, slate blue, or variously colored patches of the skin. The hands, wrists, knees, and ankles are commonly involved, and hyperkeratoses of the palms and soles are also seen. Aortitis and spinal fluid abnor-malities similar to those found in neurosyphilis have been observed in some pinta patients. The Wassermann reac-tion of the blood and flocculation tests for syphilis are usually positive in the late stages of the disease.

TREATMENT. A single injection of 1.2 million units of procaine penicillin or benzathine penicillin G pro-duces rapid disappearance of the *T. caratum* from the lesions of pinta and a decline in serologic titer. It is the treatment of choice in this disease and is more effective than chloramphenicol or the tetracyclines.

REFERENCES

Beerman, H.: Pinta: A Review of Recent Etiologic and Clinical Studies, Am. J. Med. Sci., 205:611, 1943.
Hume, J. C.: Worldwide Problems in the Diagnosis of Syphilis and Other Treponematoses, Med. Clinics N. Am., 48:721, 1964.
Marquez, F., C. R. Rein, and O. Arias: Mal del Pinto in Mex-ico, Bull. World Health Organiz., 13:299, 1955.

180 BEJEL
Albert Heyman

DEFINITION AND ETIOLOGY. Bejel is a chronic infec-tious disease caused by a spirochete indistinguishable from *Treponema pallidum*. It is found chiefly among the children of Arab tribes in the Eastern Mediter-ranean area, being particularly prevalent in some sec-tions of Iraq, Syria, and Jordan. The illness is first manifested by ulcerations of the mucous membranes in the mouth and is thought to be spread by the use of common drinking utensils. It is rarely transmitted by sexual contact and is usually acquired by adults through close contact with an infected child as by kissing and fondling.

Treponemes are readily found on dark-field exami-nation of the lesions of the skin and mucous membranes. The disease is thought by Hudson to be an example of nonvenereal syphilis, the causative organism and the clinical manifestations having been modified for many generations by special epidemiologic and climatic factors.

Bejel resembles in many respects the cases of endemic syphilis which appeared for many years in certain areas of South Africa and Yugoslavia.

MANIFESTATIONS. The illness begins with ulcerations in the mouth and lips, but there may also be a diffuse papular eruption with moist lesions on the mucocu-taneous surfaces and skin folds. The late lesions re-semble gummatous syphilis and are manifested as ulcera-tions in the skin and mucous membranes. Osteitis and periostitis of the long bones and skull may develop. The nasal bones, palate and pharynx, particularly, may be involved in a destructive process. The heart and nervous system are rarely, if ever, affected. The illness also differs from venereal syphilis in that it is apparently not spread to the child in utero from an infected mother. The diag-nosis can be made by dark-field examination of the lesions or by the usual serologic tests for syphilis.

TREATMENT. A single injection of 1.2 million units of procaine penicillin seems to be effective. In patients with late osseous or ulcerative lesions, additional peni-cillin may be required.

REFERENCES

Hudson, E. H.: "Non-venereal Syphilis," Edinburgh, E. S. Livingston, Ltd., 1958.
Hume, J. C.: Worldwide Problems in the Diagnosis of Syphilis and Other Treponematoses, Med. Clinics N. Am., 48:721, 1964.
Wray, P. M.: Bejel in Sheffield, Brit. J. Venereal Dis., 42:25, 1966.

181 LEPTOSPIROSIS
Fred R. McCrumb, Jr., and T. E. Woodward

ETIOLOGY. The genus *Leptospira* comprises a large group of microorganisms possessing a high degree of antigenic specificity which forms the basis of their clas-sification. Leptospiral serotypes pathogenic for man are indistinguishable morphologically and, in general, have similar biochemical activities and cultural requirements. The organisms show a delicate spiral configuration about an axial filament which is readily demonstrated by elec-tron microscopy. Examination of the organisms in a fluid medium by dark-ground illumination reveals active motility with characteristic hooklike bending at one end or both ends. Within the genus there are at least 18 serogroups composed of a total of 124 serotypes. Among the 22 serotypes known to occur in the United States, 13 have been associated with human infection.

EPIDEMIOLOGY. The natural reservoir of leptospirosis is found among a broad spectrum of lower animal spe-cies; wild and commensal rodents are the major sources of infection in the classical endemic areas of the world. Leptospirosis is worldwide in distribution; however, the widest variety of serotypes is found in tropical or sub-tropical regions with an abundance of rainfall and a rich rodent fauna. Wherever agricultural practices have resulted in the emergence of a few rodent species, the spectrum of leptospiral serotypes becomes restricted. Natural infection of rats, mice, voles, opossums, cattle, swine, and dogs leads frequently to the development of a renal carrier state and the shedding of leptospiras in the urine of these hosts. Man may become infected whenever his activities bring him into an area frequented by animal carriers. Infected rodents rarely show any evidence of disease, and adult domestic swine may experience only an increased incidence of abortion. In contrast, well-defined clinical illness occurs in dogs and cattle, which may die from the infection.

Leptospiras are transmitted to man most frequently through water contaminated by the urine of carrier animal hosts, although direct contact with infected tissues is important among veterinarians, abbatoir workers, and farmers. The occupational hazard of leptospirosis is greatest among rice-field workers, cane cutters, miners, sewer workers, operational military personnel, farmers, veterinarians, and employees of animal processing plants. The age and sex distribution of leptospirosis is determined largely by occupational or avocational risk rather than by age or sex influences on susceptibility to infection. A notable exception to the general preponderance of leptospirosis among adult males is the high attack rate in female rice-field workers in Italy.

Recognition of leptospirosis as a human health problem in the United States is a recent medical achievement. By 1956, fewer than 500 cases of this disease in man had been reported in this country. The total number of cases reported by 1961 still numbered under 1,000; however, additional serotypes had been associated with human infections. Among the 22 serotypes associated with infections in lower animals, *L. icterohaemorrhagiae, L. canicola, L. pomona, L. grippotyphosa, L. autumnalis, L. australis, L. bataviae, L. hebdomadis, L. ballum,* and *L. pyrogenes* have been identified as causes of human infection in this country. The first three of these serotypes are most frequently associated with infection in man.

PATHOGENESIS. Leptospiras gain access to the body by way of the skin and mucous membranes. Cutaneous transmission of leptospiras must occur commonly because skin is exposed frequently to the media through which this disease is acquired, particularly in workers whose occupation results in trauma to skin of the hands and lower extremities. Accidental contamination of the buccal mucous membranes or conjunctivas has been followed by leptospiral infections in laboratory workers, and outbreaks of this disease have been related to the consumption of contaminated food or water. Transmission from man to man is rare, probably because leptospiras are unable to survive in acid urine.

Infection in man is regularly associated with entry of leptospiras into the blood and dissemination to various organs. Adequate histopathologic studies have been limited to fatal cases wherein tissue changes were extreme. Renal changes consist of cloudy swelling of tubular epithelium and focal areas of interstitial nephritis characterized by infiltration with lymphocytes and plasma cells. Dissociation of hepatic cords and cloudy swelling of parenchymal and Kupffer cells are frequent in patients dying of leptospirosis. Obstruction of bile capillaries may be observed but is not a consistent finding. Hepatic dysfunction may be much more severe than the histopathologic abnormalities would suggest. The mechanism of hemorrhagic manifestations in leptospirosis is not clearly understood. Inflammatory lesions are observed in skeletal muscle as well as in myocardium. Perivascular inflammation is present in the brain and meninges of patients with signs of central-nervous-system involvement. Leptospiras are demonstrated irregularly in renal and hepatic tissues by silver impregnation staining, but this procedure is not a suitable substitute for cultural methods.

CLINICAL MANIFESTATIONS. Leptospirosis was first recognized and described as a distinct clinical entity in 1883 by Landouzy. Three years later, Weil observed several patients with fever, jaundice, and hemorrhages associated with hepatic and renal failure. This form of leptospirosis, since known as *Weil's disease,* is characterized by unusual severity and a high mortality rate. In contrast to the leptospiras producing Weil's disease, most serotypes produce self-limiting disease of varying severity, rarely lasting more than 7 days. The vast majority of infections are benign and do not conform to Weil's description of severe leptospirosis.

Leptospiral infections in man are characterized by the abrupt onset of high fever, prostration, headache, nausea and vomiting, conjunctival injection, and myalgia after an incubation period of 3 to 19 days, usually 7 to 13 days. The febrile phase of the illness usually ends after 1 week, and in milder infections, other evidence of disease subsides with defervescence. Mild relapses lasting 2 to 3 days are not uncommon. Although the term Weil's disease is used to describe severe leptospiral illnesses caused by *L. icterohaemorrhagiae,* milder infections with this organism are not rare, and other leptospiral serotypes can produce severe and even fatal forms of the disease. The frequency with which icterus and renal failure occur varies with the geographic area, because certain serotypes commonly associated with severe infections are more prevalent in some countries than in others.

Headache is present in nearly all patients with leptospirosis, and about 50 percent of patients complain of severe retrobulbar pain. *Conjunctival injection* is noted in 85 percent of patients, and is marked in the severely ill. *Rash* appears between the fourth and eighth days of disease in about 25 percent of patients, and there is a tendency for it to become hemorrhagic in those with a serious infection. The eruption usually consists of small macules or maculopapules distributed over the trunk and extremities. *Gastrointestinal disturbances* consisting of anorexia, nausea, vomiting, and abdominal pain occur in nearly all patients with leptospirosis, and protracted vomiting and headache frequently constitute the most distressing features of the illness. *Cough* is a common complaint and is productive of blood-streaked sputum in about 25 percent of those with this symptom. Roentgen examination of the chest may reveal pneumonitis, a feature which has not received much attention.

Severe *hemorrhagic manifestations* of leptospirosis are

uncommon except in profoundly ill patients; however, some evidence of bleeding is observed in 30 to 50 percent of all patients. Hematemesis and hemoptysis are the most common hemorrhagic manifestations, followed in frequency by conjunctival hemorrhage, epistaxis, petechiae, and melena. There may be moderate lymphadenopathy, but splenomegaly is rare.

Nuchal rigidity occurs in 30 to 40 percent of patients. In some instances, the clinical picture is that of aseptic meningitis and may be indistinguishable from the same syndrome caused by mumps, lymphocytic choriomeningitis, and certain enterovirus infections. When other evidence of leptospirosis is inconspicuous or absent in patients with aseptic meningitis, some time may elapse before the true cause is suspected. Iridocyclitis manifested by photophobia and circumcorneal injection occurs in fewer than 5 percent of patients with leptospirosis.

The incidence of clinically overt jaundice varies considerably, depending on the infecting serotypes encountered. Icterus is found in 75 percent of patients infected with *L. icterohaemorrhagiae* but only in 5 to 10 percent of persons infected with serotypes such as *L. grippotyphosa*, *L. canicola*, and *L. pomona*. Jaundice usually appears toward the end of the first week of illness as the fever is subsiding. Those with marked liver involvement show evidence of progressive hepatic dysfunction, and recovery may not occur for 2 or 3 weeks. Hepatomegaly and liver tenderness are common findings in patients with jaundice.

Severe leptospiral infections are also characterized by renal failure manifested by oliguria, proteinuria, and azotemia. Fatal leptospirosis is almost always ascribable to renal failure, although hepatic insufficiency complicates the illness, and massive hemorrhage may cause death. Mortality rates range from less than 1 percent to as high as 10 percent in different regions, depending on the incidence of severe forms of the disease.

LABORATORY FINDINGS. Although normal peripheral blood leukocyte counts are the rule in uncomplicated leptospirosis, neutrophilic leukocytosis of 12,000 to 15,000 cells per cu mm may be observed in severely ill patients, and counts of 25,000 to 40,000 cells per cu mm occur in Weil's disease. Urinary abnormalities are noted in about 80 percent of patients with leptospirosis; proteinuria, cylindruria, pyuria, and hematuria are frequent and constitute important diagnostic clues. Return to normal renal function usually is rapid, and there is no evidence that permanent renal damage results from leptospiral infections.

Hyperbilirubinemia, abnormal flocculation tests, hypoalbuminemia and hyperglobulinemia, and abnormalities in alkaline phosphatase, SGOT (serum glutamic oxalic transaminase), SGPT (serum glutamic pyruvic transaminase), and LDH (lactic dehydrogenase) can be demonstrated in over 50 percent of patients without clinical evidence of liver disease. Recovery of normal liver function is rapid as the clinical manifestations of the illness subside.

Leptospirosis has been shown to be the cause of approximately 4 percent of all cases of aseptic meningitis in several well-studied series (Chap. 361). However, the frequency with which the central nervous system is involved in leptospirosis is not known. Mild pleocytosis (40 to 500 cells) with mononuclear cells characterizes leptospiral aseptic meningitis. Modest elevation of cerebrospinal fluid protein is usual, but glucose and chloride concentrations remain normal. The cerebrospinal fluid quickly reverts to normal during early convalescence.

LABORATORY DIAGNOSIS. Leptospiras can be isolated from the blood of most patients during the acute phase of the illness. Many leptospiral serotypes do not produce overt disease in guinea pigs and hamsters, and isolation of these organisms ultimately requires the use of cultural techniques. For this reason, the use of laboratory animals to diagnose leptospirosis should be limited to situations in which the only material available for isolation of the causative organism is contaminated. The simplest artificial medium for culturing of leptospiras is prepared by mixing a small amount of peptone with distilled water and adding sterile inactivated rabbit serum in a final concentration of 7 to 10 percent. This medium is dispensed in 10-ml amounts into screw-capped tubes or rubber-stoppered bottles and may be stored in a refrigerator for several months. It is imperative to use small inoculums when attempting to recover leptospiras to avoid inhibition of these organisms by excessive quantities of blood. When single drops of whole venous blood are inoculated into each of five tubes at the bedside, positive results may be expected in 75 to 90 percent of cultural attempts made during the first 3 days of illness. As the disease progresses, the intensity and regularity of leptospiremia decrease. Because of the intermittent nature of leptospiruria and the adverse effect of low pH and bacterial contamination, culture of urine is not recommended. Leptospiras also have been recovered from cerebrospinal fluid.

Incubation of cultures is carried out at 32°C, and in order to avoid the risk of contamination of the medium, dark-field examination of the cultures is performed at weekly intervals, beginning 10 days after inoculation.

Several serologic tests may be employed in the diagnosis of leptospirosis. The classical microscopic agglutination-lysis test is cumbersome because of its type specificity and the need to maintain a large number of stock cultures. In addition the use of viable antigens creates a risk of laboratory infection. For these reasons this procedure should be confined to reference centers and research laboratories where serotyping of leptospiral isolates is a major activity.

Tests employing antigen pools or broadly reactive antigens with generic specificity, permitting the recognition of antibody against most leptospiral serotypes, should be employed by diagnostic laboratories. The slide agglutination test developed by Galton employs formolized antigens in four pools representing 12 serotypes. In recent years this procedure has been widely used and is probably the best diagnostic test. Two other serologic tests with broad reactivity have been employed successfully in the diagnosis of human infection. Complement-fixing antibodies can be detected in the serum of patients convalescing from leptospirosis using sonicated antigen derived from *L. icterochaemorrhagiae, L. grippotyphosa,* and *L. tarassovi.* Antigen with similar group reactivity prepared from *L. biflexa* permits detection of antibody resulting from infection with a wide variety of serotypes. In this procedure, antigen adsorbed onto sheep erythrocytes will cause hemolysis of these cells in the presence of complement and leptospiral antibody. The hemolytic test has the attributes of broad reactivity and a high degree of sensitivity in the detection of antibody in man but is relatively insensitive when employed with bovine or porcine serum. Measurement of antibody using an indirect immunofluorescent technique has been reported. However, its utility as a routine diagnostic procedure is not established.

DIFFERENTIAL DIAGNOSIS. Leptospirosis should be considered a possible cause of any febrile disease characterized by headache, gastrointestinal symptoms, conjunctival injection, and myalgia. The presence of urinary abnormalities and a history of contact with water frequented by rodents or domestic animals should arouse further suspicion. The diagnosis should not be reserved for patients with jaundice, because a majority of leptospiral infections is not associated with clinically overt icterus. Leptospirosis should be considered in the differential diagnosis of all cases of aseptic meningitis. Other acute febrile illnesses with which leptospirosis may be confused include influenza, the rickettsioses, enteric fevers, brucellosis, and dengue. Late manifestations of leptospirosis may resemble infectious hepatitis, hemolytic and obstructive jaundice, and acute glomerulonephritis.

TREATMENT. Evaluation of antibiotics in human leptospirosis is complicated by the relatively short course of the acute infection and the lack of suitably controlled studies. Penicillin, streptomycin, and the tetracyclines inhibit the growth of leptospiras in vitro and will control experimental infections in hamsters and guinea pigs. Streptomycin and tetracyclines eliminate leptospiras from the kidneys of canine carriers of *L. canicola.*

Opinions differ regarding the usefulness of penicillin and tetracyclines in the treatment of human leptospirosis. It is agreed that chloramphenicol does not favorably alter the course of this disease. The use of tetracyclines, penicillin, streptomycin, and chloramphenicol in one controlled study failed to reveal a shortening of the febrile course or a reduction in the incidence of complications as a result of antibiotic therapy. Other evidence supports the concept that penicillin results in a shorter febrile course and in a lower incidence of complications. On the basis of most studies, the use of 4 to 6 million units of penicillin G daily in divided dosage during the febrile phase of the illness is probably indicated.

Most leptospiral infections are not severe and subside without complications even in untreated patients. Because acute renal failure in leptospirosis is reversible, its management should make use of all available therapeutic aids, including hemodialysis. Rarely, hemorrhage may result in enough blood loss to warrant replacement.

REFERENCES

Alston, J. M., and J. C. Broom: "Leptospirosis in Man and Animals," London, E. & S. Livingstone, Ltd., 1958.

Doherty, R. L.: A Clinical Study of Leptospirosis in North Queensland, Australasian Ann. Med., 4:53, 1955.

Edwards, G. A., and B. M. Domm: Human Leptospirosis, Medicine, 39:117, 1960.

Fairburn, A. C., and S. J. G. Semple: Chloramphenicol and Penicillin in the Treatment of Leptospirosis among British Troops in Malaya, Lancet, 1:13, 1956.

Hall, H. E., J. A. Hightower, R. Diaz-Rivera, R. J. Byrne, J. E. Smadel, and T. E. Woodward: Evaluation of Antibiotic Therapy in Human Leptospirosis, Ann. Intern. Med., 35:981, 1951.

Heath, C. W., A. D. Alexander, and M. M. Galton: Leptospirosis in the United States, Analysis of 483 Cases in Man, 1949–1961, New Engl. J. Med., 273:857, 1965.

McCrumb, F. R., Jr., J. L. Stockard, C. R. Robinson, L. H. Turner, D. G. Lewis, C. W. Maisey, M. F. Kelleher, C. A. Gleiser, and J. E. Smadel: Leptospirosis in Malaya: I. Sporadic Cases among Military and Civilian Personnel, Am. J. Trop. Med. Hyg., 6:238, 1957.

World Health Organization Tech. Rep. Ser., no. 380, 1967.

182 RELAPSING FEVER
E. H. O. Parry and Robert G. Petersdorf

DEFINITION. Relapsing fever, an acute infectious disease caused by spirochetes of the genus *Borrelia,* has two varieties which depend on the vector—the louse-borne disease and the tick-borne.

ETIOLOGY. Spirochetes of the genus *Borrelia* are 10 to 20 μ long and slender, and move in a corkscrew fashion. *Borrelia recurrentis* is the causative organism of louse-borne relapsing fever. Many strains of *Borrelia* have been found in the tick-borne disease, and they are known by their vector. Culture of the organisms is difficult.

EPIDEMIOLOGY AND PATHOGENESIS. The louse-borne disease is disappearing rapidly but is still endemic in Ethiopia, and may occur in East Asia also. Major epidemics followed World War I, when millions of cases were seen in Eastern Europe. Soldiers returning home introduced the disease to the Sudan belt of Africa; from there it moved slowly eastwards, with the mortality rate reaching 30 percent in some areas. A similar but less-virulent epidemic crossed Africa after World War II. In a small epidemic in Kenya in 1945 the mortality rate was 40 percent in untreated cases.

The tick-borne disease appears sporadically in many parts of the world, probably as a manifestation of an endemic focus in each place. It is the form which is sometimes seen in the United States.

Infection of man occurs if an infected louse is crushed against an abrasion or wound, or if a person is bitten by an infected tick. In both types, the organism enters the bloodstream and is able to spread via the hematogenous route.

MANIFESTATIONS. In general, patients with louse-borne disease are more seriously ill than those with the tick-borne disease. The incubation period varies between 4 and 12 days. Symptoms are not specific: fever, sweating, headache, and upper abdominal discomfort are the commonest. Cough, painful limbs, and bleeding—particularly epistaxis—also occur. Pregnant women often abort. The clinical picture varies from mild fever only, to one of severe toxicity characterized by confusion, jaundice, and purpura. The liver and spleen are enlarged and tender in about 20 to 80 percent of cases; jaundice, often accompanied by purpura, is seen in 10 to 70 percent. A gallop rhythm, low arterial pressure, and tachycardia are found; tachypnea, sometimes as high as 70 breaths per min, is characteristic of most cases. Tender skeletal muscles and, more rarely, neck stiffness, confusion, and even transient focal neurologic signs may be seen. The temperature may be as high as 105°F when the patient is first seen. Very rarely the picture of hypovolemic "endotoxin shock" occurs.

The term *relapsing fever* was introduced to describe the cycles of fever, i.e., periods of fever lasting for 7 to 10 days and separated by fever-free intervals of from 4 to 7 days. Relapses are rarely seen now that antibiotics are used.

PATHOLOGIC PHYSIOLOGY. In the louse-borne disease, cardiorespiratory changes, which may be very severe, occur in most cases. The electrocardiogram reveals evidence of myocardial damage in 30 percent of patients; a prolonged QTc interval, ventricular ectopic beats, and nonspecific S-T segment and T-wave changes are seen. After spirochetes disappear and the peak of the reaction is over, electrocardiographic evidence of acute right-sided heart strain may be found, and the pulmonary arterial pressure may rise transiently. The central venous pressure, which may also rise about 4 hr after spirochetes disappear, can be lowered by rapidly acting intravenous digitalis preparations. Overt pulmonary edema is rare.

At the peak of the reaction, marked overbreathing causes respiratory alkalosis. Arterial oxygen saturation decreases because of maldistribution of pulmonary blood flow. The increase in venous admixture coincides with a sudden fall in pulmonary vascular resistance. Cardiac output and systemic arterial pressure are greatly increased at this time. These changes are not related simply to the rise in body temperature, and there is no cerebrospinal fluid acidosis to explain the respiratory stimulation. Hydrocortisone suppresses the fever before the onset of rigors but does not prevent or modify the systemic reaction after tetracycline.

After the peak there is a progressive fall in arterial pressure to very low levels. The hypotensive phase lasts many hours and is the result of a decrease in cardiac output and of persistent peripheral vasodilatation. Ventilation gradually decreases and metabolic acidosis develops, while arterial glucose, lactate, and pyruvate concentrations increase. Continuous "100 percent" oxygen therapy is clinically beneficial and prevents these metabolic abnormalities.

The fully established syndrome of disseminated intra-vascular coagulation has been reported but is rare. However, thrombocytopenia is seen in most cases.

LABORATORY FINDINGS. The hemogram varies. Moderate anemia is common; its mechanism is uncertain. The leukocyte count is not normally raised before treatment: an "overshoot" leukocytosis, with many immature forms, occurs after the leukopenia which accompanies treatment. The sedimentation rate is elevated. The thrombocytopenia is associated with normal megakaryocytes in the bone marrow. The prothrombin time is often prolonged. Hepatic function tests reveal abnormal hepatocellular function. In severe cases, the total serum bilirubin level may reach 16 mg per 100 ml. Azotemia, apparently unrelated to extracellular fluid depletion, is common among jaundiced patients. The first investigation, and the only one essential to the diagnosis, is examination of thick and thin blood films, stained with Fields', Giemsa, and Leishman's stains. In the louse-borne disease, spirochetes are easily visible; in tick-borne disease their identification may be more difficult. Spirochetes may also be seen by phase-contrast microscopy with dark-field illumination.

DIFFERENTIAL DIAGNOSIS. Many infections in which the first symptom is fever of unknown origin, including malaria, salmonellosis (including typhoid), typhus, dengue, rat-bite fever, and Weil's disease, must be considered. Practically, the issue should not remain long in doubt if blood films are repeatedly searched for spirochetes, an essential practice in patients with fever of unknown origin in areas where the louse- and tick-borne diseases occur.

TREATMENT. The peripheral blood is quickly cleared of spirochetes by penicillin, tetracycline, and chloramphenicol. The best initial dose and the duration of treatment are not yet known.

Repeated small doses, e.g., 80,000 to 100,000 units, of penicillin clear the blood slowly and with a less-severe systemic reaction than the more usual 500,000 units, but spirochetes may persist in the brain after penicillin therapy. Tetracycline, probably the best drug, should be given in dosage of 250 mg on the first day and continued for 4 days in a daily dose of 1 Gm; however, this long a course may be unnecessary.

During epidemics, when economic factors may be important and follow-up may be impossible, a single dose of 1.2 million units of crystalline-procaine penicillin, or 1.5 Gm chloramphenicol on the first 2 days only, probably will be curative in the vast majority of patients.

The more ill patients should be hospitalized and, ideally, should receive intensive care during and after the reaction to treatment. At this time continuous oxygen therapy to prevent lactic acidosis and a digitalis preparation to support the myocardium are desirable. The patient should be nursed lying flat; hypotension can be corrected by raising the foot of the bed, but vasopressor drugs may be needed. In the face of possible myocardial damage, rapid infusion of plasma expanders may be dangerous, but it is important to maintain extracellular volume and to replace fluid lost through sweating and overventilating.

Vitamin K should be given parenterally to all patients.

Heparin is indicated if intravascular coagulation is found.

Any patient with a prolonged QTc interval on the electrocardiogram should be kept at bed rest until the QTc interval is normal.

EFFECTS OF TREATMENT. Spirochetes disappear from the peripheral blood about 1 hr after an adequate dose of penicillin or tetracycline. The arterial pressure, heart rate, respiratory rate, and temperature rise abruptly and transiently at this time, and there is a profound leukopenia. About 4 hr later, the arterial pressure has fallen substantially and the leukocyte count has returned to, or above, normal again.

This Jarisch-Herxheimer reaction is alarming; the patient shivers and groans and may vomit; transient neurologic signs may occur also. The calm which follows it may be deceptive because the marked pathophysiologic alterations, as described above, may be masked.

PROGNOSIS. When epidemics strike a nonimmune population, the high mortality rate due to the louse-borne disease shows the potential menace of this disease. Most patients, however, recover quickly and completely; relapses do not occur if antibiotic therapy is adequate. Adverse signs are deep jaundice, uncontrolled bleeding, and a grossly prolonged QTc interval.

Typhus and enteric fever may occur simultaneously with louse-borne relapsing fever, and they probably contribute to the mortality rate, particularly during epidemics.

REFERENCES

Bryceson, A. D. M., E. H. O. Parry, C. S. Leithead, P. L. Perine, D. Vukotich, and D. A. Warrell: Louse-borne Relapsing Fever in Ethiopia, Quart. J. Med. (in press).

Felsenfeld, O.: Borreliae, Human Relapsing Fever, and Parasite-Vector-Host Relationships, Bacteriol. Rev., 29: 46, 1965.

Heisch, R. B.: Studies in East African Relapsing Fever, E. African Med. J., 27:1, 1950.

183 RAT-BITE FEVER
(Spirillum minus Infection)

Ivan L. Bennett, Jr., and
Robert G. Petersdorf

DEFINITION. Rat-bite fever (sodoku) is an acute infectious disease caused by *Spirillum minus* and characterized by relapsing fever and a skin eruption.

ETIOLOGY. The causative organism is a spirillum 2 to 5μ in length; it has two to five broad spirals and is propelled by flagella. The organism is easily identified in dark-field preparations by its quick, darting motility. It is found occasionally in the blood of apparently healthy rats, mice, guinea pigs, and monkeys.

EPIDEMIOLOGY. In man, infection by S. *minus* is almost always acquired through the bite of a rat. It is commonest in infants and young children but may also occur in adults, particularly in laboratory workers. Rats may attack sleeping persons and will bite anyone attempting to catch or handle them. Documented examples of infection from the bite of a mouse are known.

MANIFESTATIONS. Because of the long incubation period (1 to 6 weeks), the initial lesion may have healed before the onset of systemic symptoms. Often, however, one finds swelling and redness at the site of the eschar and swelling of regional lymph nodes. A chill may occur at the onset of a febrile period. Bouts of fever last 2 to 4 days and are separated by afebrile periods, also lasting 2 to 4 days. During febrile episodes there are malaise, headache, sweating, photophobia, nausea, and vomiting. In 75 percent of cases a *skin eruption* occurs, usually on the extremities. The rash is frequently asymmetric in its distribution and most commonly consists of reddish or purplish macules, which may become large and confluent. Arthritis is rare; if present it usually involves the large joints. The disease tends to run a prolonged course, usually 4 to 8 weeks, but cases have been reported in which clinical manifestations continued for more than a year. Subacute bacterial endocarditis due to this organism has been observed.

LABORATORY FINDINGS. The total leukocyte count may be normal, or there may be a leukocytosis up to 20,000. Biologic false positive serologic tests for syphilis occur in 50 percent of patients. The S. *minus* seldom can be found in the blood or tissues of patients by direct dark-field examination and cannot be cultured. Mice or guinea pigs should be inoculated intraperitoneally with the patient's blood. *Spirillum minus* can usually be found in the blood or peritoneal fluid of the animal by dark-field examination 5 to 15 days later. Laboratory animals may be naturally infected with S. *minus,* and precautions must be taken to ensure that the animals are free of infection before inoculation.

DIFFERENTIAL DIAGNOSIS. It is important to inquire about rat bite in all patients with a relapsing type of fever. In patients with a history of rate bite, the principal problem is in differentiating between infection with S. *minus* and that with *Streptobacillus moniliformis*. This cannot be done with certainty on clinical grounds, but a prolonged incubation period, relapsing instead of sustained fever, and few or no manifestations of arthritis suggest a diagnosis of S. *minus* infection. Laboratory tests should be made for both organisms. The significance of a previous rat bite may not be appreciated in cases with a long incubation period, and the disease may be confused with other infections characterized by relapsing fever, such as malaria, meningococcemia, and *Borrelia recurrentis* infection.

TREATMENT. Penicillin, in dosage of 300,000 to 600,000 units twice a day intramuscularly, is the drug of choice. In patients allergic to penicillin, a tetracycline in dosage of 2 Gm a day for 7 days may be used.

PROGNOSIS. Patients treated with penicillin become afebrile within 24 to 72 hr, and complete recovery is the rule.

REFERENCES

Roughgarden, J. W.: Antimicrobial Therapy of Rat-bite Fever, Arch. Intern. Med., 116:39, 1965.

Section 11

Diseases Caused by Fungi

INTRODUCTION

Abraham I. Braude

Except for their etiology, fungous infections differ little from bacterial infections. The close relationship between bacteria and fungi is apparent from transitional forms connecting the two classes, and from the similarity of the pathologic changes and clinical manifestations induced by them.

The intermediate, or transitional, forms are represented by the *Actinomycetes.* These possess the characteristic branched mycelium of fungi but divide by segmentation into gram-positive bacillary or coccoid forms. The acid-fast property of one species, *Nocardia asteroides,* indicates a relationship to the tubercle bacillus. The *Actinomycetes* also differ from fungi in their susceptibility to phages, their unorganized nuclei, and their sensitivity to antibiotics, which attack bacteria, but not to the antifungal polyene antibiotic amphotericin B. The *Actinomycetes* do not possess the sterols which complex with polyene antibiotics and injure the cell membranes of fungi. Finally, actinomyces, like bacteria but unlike fungi, contain neither chitin nor cellulose in their cell walls. Although actinomycosis and nocardiosis are placed among the fungous diseases in this book, the causative agents are unequivocally classed with the bacteria.

An important characteristic of pathogenic fungi is dimorphism, growth in two distinct forms under different environmental conditions. The fungi responsible for blastomycosis, sporotrichosis, and histoplasmosis assume unicellular "yeast" forms in infected tissues but grow as mycelia and produce asexual spores on Sabouraud's agar. The reverse is true for the fungus causing moniliasis. Another type of dimorphism is found in coccidioidomycosis. The organism responsible for this infection is multicellular in vivo and in vitro, but its form differs under the two conditions. In tissues it is a sac filled with spores, but on agar it grows as a segmented mycelium. *Cryptococcus neoformans* is the only pathogenic fungus that fails to change form when environmental conditions vary.

Mycotic diseases are not transmitted from one person to another. Many fungous infections are acquired by inhalation of spores growing freely in nature. These spores may be rectangular unicellular mycelial fragments known as *chlamydospores,* or spherical bodies borne on thin mycelial stalks and called *conidia.* Some infections, such as sporotrichosis, result from inoculation of spores directly into the skin.

A few fungous diseases are endogenous in origin. *Actinomyces israeli* and *Candida albicans* are normal residents of the bowel and mouth. When resistance is lowered, endogenous infection with either agent can develop. Actinomycosis is often preceded by tooth extraction, and overgrowth of normal saprophytic bacteria by *C. albicans* in the course of antibiotic therapy can lead to moniliasis.

The mechanisms whereby fungi produce disease are obscure. *Cryptococcus neoformans* has a polysaccharide capsule similar to that of the pneumococcus which seems to protect the yeast from phagocytosis. This capsular material also produces mechanical injury in the nervous system. It is possible that the thick walls of other fungi such as *Blastomyces dermatitidis* and *Coccidioides immitis* also protect against leukocytes. Some fungi are ingested by phagocytes but seem to flourish within them. In histoplasmosis, for example, the parasites are found in enormous numbers within reticuloendothelial cells. The endothelium of small vessels can become so packed with histoplasma organisms that blood flow is compromised.

Another possible factor in the pathogenesis of these infections is hypersensitivity. In most fungous diseases the patient exhibits marked local or even systemic reactivity to intradermal injection of the causative organism. In coccidioidomycosis this type of reaction is closely associated with the development of erythema nodosum and pleural effusions. The occurrence of necrosis at the site of injection of fungous antigens suggests that hypersensitivity may be responsible for necrosis of infected tissues. In other patients, however, widespread destruction of tissue may occur despite absence of dermal sensitivity.

Despite the differences in morphology and life cycle of fungi and bacteria, both elicit similar pathologic changes and clinical manifestations. For this reason, specific diagnosis can seldom be made without demonstration of the causative organism. Fortunately, most pathogenic fungi are easily seen in infected tissues or exudates. In a few circumstances, however, it is necessary to rely upon epidemiologic and immunologic methods for diagnosis.

The following chapters deal only with those infections in which fungi penetrate beneath the skin and mucous membranes to involve the underlying tissues and viscera.

184 ACTINOMYCOSIS
Abraham I. Braude

DEFINITION. Actinomycosis is a noncontagious suppurative infection produced by an anaerobic organism normally resident in the mouth. The disease is characterized by chronic inflammatory induration and sinus formation.

ETIOLOGY. The causative agent is a branching gram-positive filamentous organism. Two separate anaerobic species of the genus *Actinomyces* have been recognized: *Actinomyces bovis* is responsible for actinomycosis in cattle, and *A. israeli,* for human actinomycosis.

Actinomyces israeli and *A. bovis* differ from other actinomyces in their intolerance of free oxygen and failure to grow on Sabouraud's medium. On blood agar, colonies require 4 to 6 days of anaerobic incubation at 37°C to reach a size of 1 to 2 mm. Although most strains require anaerobic conditions for isolation, some can be subcultured aerobically in 10 to 20 percent carbon dioxide. *Actinomyces israeli* has never been found outside man or animal, and case-to-case transmission is unknown.

PATHOGENESIS. The oxidation-reduction potential of normal tissues is probably too high for multiplication of *A. israeli,* but devitalized tissues allow it to reproduce, gain a foothold, and spread. The frequency of actinomycotic lesions of the face and neck may be explained by the greater population of *A. israeli* on surfaces of teeth, in carious teeth, and in tonsillar crypts and by the frequent trauma to which these tissues are subjected by eating, by dental procedures, or by infection with oral bacteria. Anaerobic conditions also prevail in atelectatic areas of the lung after aspiration of *A. israeli* so that pulmonary actinomycosis can develop. It is also possible that pulmonary actinomycosis may arise hematogenously from an infected focus in the mouth. The mediastinal form of thoracic actinomycosis probably spreads from the esophagus into the superior or posterior mediastinum, quickly involving the pleura to produce early pleural effusion or empyema, and then tends to attack the adjacent ribs and vertebral bodies. Eventually mediastinal actinomycosis produces abscesses which point in the paravertebral region. The exact mode of development of abdominal actinomycosis is unknown, but the frequency with which the cecal region is involved suggests that the conditions here favor devitalizing injury. Occasionally, perforation by a foreign body precedes infection.

From foci in the jaw, lung, or bowel, actinomycosis may spread by contiguity or through the bloodstream to the liver, spine, brain, kidneys, genitalia, spleen, and subcutaneous tissues. Lymphatic spread is rare.

The inflammatory reaction to *A. israeli* is characterized by three features: (1) chronic suppuration, (2) extensive necrosis, and (3) intense fibrosis. The so-called "sulfur granules" which are prominent in the inflammatory lesion of actinomycosis are composed of intertwined mycelial filaments.

CLINICAL MANIFESTATIONS. The essential feature of actinomycosis is a painful, indurated swelling. This lesion may appear over the jaw a week or more after such trauma as tooth extraction or compound fracture of the mandible. As it increases in size, points of suppuration, the openings of fistulas, appear on the bluish-red surface of the edematous skin. Cervical lymphadenopathy is rare.

The lower lobes of the lung are frequently affected; then the disease suddenly becomes evident when the pleura and chest wall are involved by direct extension from the lung. Until then the patient may notice only fever, cough, and expectoration. Physical examination at this time reveals a diffuse, tender, indurated thoracic swelling with pulmonary consolidation and empyema.

Abdominal actinomycosis is often mistaken for appendicitis, carcinoma of the cecum, tuberculosis, or amebiasis. Patients with abdominal actinomycosis are subjected to surgery for drainage of a supposed appendiceal abscess, and the true nature of the disease is recognized only when an indurated draining sinus remains and stubbornly refuses to heal. Actinomycosis may also be mistaken for tumor of the reproductive organs in women or for tuberculous psoas abscess. Peritonitis is rare.

In the rare case of hematogenous disseminated actinomycosis, lesions appear in all parts of the body. Painful indurated nodules under the skin of the legs, arms, back, and scalp are prominent and nonsuppurative effusions of the pleura or pericardium develop.

DIAGNOSIS. The disease is easily recognized by detecting *A. israeli* in pus obtained from sinuses, empyema fluid, or abscess cavities. Interpretating actinomyces in sputum is difficult because the organisms are normal inhabitants of the mouth. Sulfur granules vary in size from several microns to 3 mm in diameter. Large granules are nearly always found if a thorough search is made by diluting the pus with saline solution and filtering through gauze. They are white, yellow, or brown and stand out sharply against the background of blood-tinged pus. The conclusive finding is the demonstration of gram-positive filaments or bacilli which fail to grow aerobically. Granules of other organisms (staphylococci, nocardias, monosporia), fragments of caseous material, and clumps of pus cells or fibrin may be confused with actinomycotic granules. The technique for recovery of *A. israeli* from the infected material differs from that of other pathogenic fungi in two important respects: (1) animal inoculation is of no value, and (2) Sabouraud's medium will not support its growth. Cultural isolation of *A. israeli* is not difficult if anaerobic methods are used. A small microaerophilic gram-negative bacillus, *Actinobacillus actinomycetemcomitans,* is often associated with *A. israeli* in actinomycosis. Anaerobic streptococci, *Bacteroides,* and other anaerobes are also present frequently. Hence actinomycosis is characteristically a mixed anaerobic infection.

Biopsy may establish the diagnosis if the actinomycotic colony ("ray fungus") is observed microscopically. Demonstration of the organism may be difficult, requiring careful search of many sections.

Intradermal or serologic tests with *A. israeli* or its fractions are of no diagnostic aid. Radiologic examination may suggest actinomycosis if consolidation of the lungs and periosteal proliferation of the ribs are found because this combination rarely occurs in other conditions. The appearance of the spine in lateral views may be almost pathognomonic because the areas of absorption and newly formed bone give a picture of a coarse sieve not seen in any other vertebral disease.

TREATMENT. Penicillin and the tetracycline antibiotics are so effective that the disease is disappearing through the wide use of these drugs in conditions that would otherwise evolve into actinomycosis. When either is administered in large doses over long periods of time, remarkable improvement may be expected even when the purulent foci are inaccessible to surgical drainage. Many reports indicate that the tetracycline drugs (chlortetracycline, oxytetracycline, tetracycline) are superior to penicillin. When the tetracyclines are given in doses of 500 mg every 6 hr, there is a reduction in pain and swelling within a few days as well as gain in strength, increase in weight, and prompt defervescence. Treatment should be continued for several weeks after the patient appears cured. Because penicillin is no more effective than the tetracyclines and because it requires repeated intramuscular or intravenous injection of large doses for long periods of time, it should be reserved for patients who cannot tolerate tetracycline drugs. The optimum dose of penicillin is not known, but at least 4 million units daily should be given intramuscularly.

Surgical drainage or excision of accessible actinomycotic lesions is a valuable adjunct to chemotherapy, although surgery alone is of little value. Older treatments such as iodides, irradiation, or the sulfonamides have no place in the treatment of actinomycosis, and amphotericin B is of no value.

REFERENCES

Cope, V. Z.: "Actinomycosis," London, Oxford University Press, 1938.

Drake, C. H., M. T. Sudler, and R. I. Canuteson: A Case of Staphylococcic Actinophytosis (Botryomycosis) in Man, J.A.M.A., 123:339, 1943.

Garrod, L. P.: Actinomycosis of the Lung: Etiology, Diagnosis, and Chemotherapy, Tubercle, 33:258, 1952.

Lane, S. L., A. Kutscher, and R. Chaves: Oxytetracycline in the Treatment of Orocervical-Facial Actinomycosis: Report of Seven Cases, J.A.M.A., 151:986, 1953.

McVay, L. V., Jr., and D. H. Sprunt: A Long-term Evaluation of Aureomycin in the Treatment of Actinomycosis, Ann. Intern. Med., 38:995, 1953.

Nichols, D. R., and W. E. Herrell: Penicillin in the Treatment of Actinomycosis, J. Lab. Clin. Med., 33:521, 1948.

Rosebury, T.: The Parasitic Actinomycetes and Other Filamentous Microorganisms of the Mouth: A Review of Their Characteristics and Relationships of the Bacteriology of Actinomycosis and of Salivary Calculus in Man, Bacteriol. Rev., 8:189, 1944.

185 CRYPTOCOCCOSIS
Abraham I. Braude

DEFINITION. Cryptococcosis is a highly fatal infection caused by *Cryptococcus neoformans*, an encapsulated yeast with a special predilection for the central nervous system. Cryptococcosis may also involve the lungs, bones, and skin and occurs with increased frequency in patients with leukemia or lymphoma.

ETIOLOGY. Members of the genus *Cryptococcus*, to which *C. neoformans* belongs, form neither mycelia nor spores and reproduce entirely by budding. The cells of *C. neoformans* are spherical, measure 5 to 15 μ in diameter, retain the Gram stain, and are surrounded by a capsule which may have a diameter three times that of the cell. The capsular material contains a polysaccharide which is responsible for the slimy appearance of the yeast in culture and for the myxomatous character of cryptococcal lesions.

The organisms grow readily on various media at room temperature and at 37°C. On Sabouraud's glucose agar, visible growth appears within a few days at 37°C and gradually becomes brownish and slimy. Unlike other pathogenic yeastlike fungi, cryptococci never form mycelia. Most cells of *C. neoformans* are killed in 24 hr at temperatures of 40.6°C or higher.

PATHOGENESIS AND PATHOLOGY. Cryptococci resembling *C. neoformans* have been isolated from soil, pigeon droppings, the surface of fruit, and from the skin and intestinal tract of normal man. Hence it is possible for infections to be of either endogenous or exogenous origin. The organism reaches the nervous system in most cases. Although neurologic disturbances overshadow others, there is good evidence that infection is usually established in the lung and other viscera before dissemination to the brain and the meninges occurs. Often the pulmonary foci give rise to no clinical findings, although they can be detected if a careful search is made at postmortem examination.

The cryptococcus does not evoke the active inflammatory response observed with other fungi or bacteria. The cellular reaction is very slow to develop and is seldom intense. The cryptococcus seems to meet little resistance and frequently proliferates so freely that macroscopic masses of gelatinous yeasts fill the lesions. Older lesions occasionally show granulomatous reactions. The small number of cryptococci observed within granulomas suggests that mononuclear cells can destroy the organism. This may account in part for the fact that lymphomatous diseases involving the mononuclear cells lower resistance to cryptococcal infection. At other times, however, many cryptococci are present within mononuclear and giant cells. It is unusual to see necrosis in cryptococcosis.

Granulomas or gelatinous cryptococcal masses may appear in the nervous system, lungs, bones, or skin. In the nervous system, lesions usually develop in the meninges at the base of the brain, with resulting involvement of the brain stem, cranial nerves, and cerebellum. Large masses of yeast may accumulate in the subarachnoid space and extend diffusely along perivascular spaces into the brain substance to produce cystic nodules. Because the fungal masses shrink after fixation of the brain in formalin, cyst-like spaces remain. In the lung, scattered miliary nodules, diffuse pneumonic infiltrations, or solitary masses easily mistaken for pulmonary neoplasms may occur. Calcification or hilar lymphadenopathy is extremely rare. These characteristics of the cryptococcal pulmonary lesions are helpful in distinguishing the disease from tuberculosis, sarcoidosis, and other mycoses. In contrast to cryptococcal meningoencephalitis, serious predisposing diseases accompany pulmonary cryptococcosis in only 10 percent of patients.

CLINICAL MANIFESTATIONS. Most patients with cryptococcal infection present only after the onset of neurologic manifestations. Complaints of severe headache, diplopia, dizziness, ataxia, vomiting, tinnitus, memory disturbances, or Jacksonian convulsions are common. Fever is usually low-grade or may be absent. Many patients die within a few months, but some have lived for many years as the disease undergoes remissions and relapses.

When pulmonary infection is present in the absence of meningoencephalitis, the patient is generally free of constitutional symptoms. The disease is detected when roentgenographic examination of the chest shows a dense, usually solitary infiltration of the lower portions of the lung. Cough may be a prominent feature of diffuse cryptococcal pneumonia. Cavities are not rare.

Involvement of bones in the absence of disseminated disease is rare, and cryptococcosis of joints is almost always secondary to adjacent osseous lesions.

Disseminated infection may also produce multiple nodules or papules in the skin. These range from a few millimeters in diameter to masses resembling strawberries in size and color.

The possibility of underlying Hodgkin's disease, lymphosarcoma, leukemia, or diabetes should be considered in every patient with cryptococcosis.

DIAGNOSIS. Cryptococcal meningitis must be distinguished from other diseases which present as aseptic meningitis, including brain abscess, tuberculous meningitis, coccidioidal meningitis, and carcinomatous meningitis. In each of these, the spinal fluid is sterile by ordinary cultural methods and may contain from a few to several hundred mononuclear cells, an increased amount of protein, and a reduced concentration of glucose. Because *C. neoformans* is recovered with much greater ease than the etiologic agents of the other diseases, culture of the spinal fluid is the decisive procedure in differential diagnosis. The cryptococcus is isolated on Sabouraud's agar at room temperature and usually grows after 1 to 2 weeks. In tuberculous and coccidioidal meningitis positive cultures are much less common, and in uncomplicated brain abscess the spinal fluid is sterile. Cryptococcal cells may also be found by direct microscopic examination of sediment from centrifuged spinal fluid. Mixing a drop of sediment with India ink facilitates the recognition of the mucinous capsule. The organism can be cultured from the blood and urine in 25 to 35 percent of patients with cryptococcal meningitis. Lung biopsy is essential for diagnosis in most cases of pulmonary infection. In tissue removed by biopsy, intracellular forms with small capsules may resemble *Histoplasma capsulatum* but can be differentiated by mucicarmine, which stains the capsular mucopolysaccharide peculiar to *C. neoformans*. Biopsied material should also be inoculated onto Sabouraud's glucose agar and intraperitoneally in white mice. *Cryptococcus neoformans* is highly pathogenic for these animals and is readily demonstrated microscopically in sections or smears of their brains. In many cases, the patients' serums give positive complement fixation tests for either cryptococcal antigen or antibody. Circulating antigens appear to indicate continuing disease, while antibodies are found only after treatment, when the cryptococcus and its antigens are disappearing from the body fluids.

TREATMENT. All forms of cryptococcosis usually improve after intravenous infusions of 75 to 100 mg amphotericin B daily. These maximum daily doses are reached only after gradual increments of the initial dose of 1 mg. When maintenance levels are reached, the drug should be given every other day. Patients without meningoencephalitis can be cured with total doses of less than 1.5 Gm, but 3.0 Gm is probably required for infections of the nervous system. If relapse occurs after intravenous treatment, amphotericin B may be dissolved in the spinal fluid and 0.5 mg injected intrathecally on alternate days in conjunction with intravenous administration. Strict precautions must be taken during intrathecal injection to avoid bacterial contamination and drug overdosage. One milligram amphotericin B intrathecally may cause fever, temporary paralysis of the bladder and legs, and arachnoiditis. The chief dangers of intravenous amphotericin B are anemia, hypokalemia, and renal damage. The anemia frequently occurs after prolonged treatment and is normocytic, normochromic, and reversible. The hypokalemia develops with or without impaired renal function and requires prophylactic potassium supplements. Disturbances in renal function should be expected. Azotemia, impaired urine concentration, and microscopic hematuria with granular casts are the main findings but are reversible if caught in time. Treatment should be discontinued if the blood urea nitrogen exceeds 40 mg per 100 ml and resumed when it approaches normal levels. Serious and permanent renal damage with nephrocalcinosis has occurred in patients given a total dosage greater than 5.0 Gm.

REFERENCES

Butler, W. T., D. W. Alling, A. Spickard, and J. Utz: Diagnostic and Prognostic Value of Clinical and Laboratory Findings in Cryptococcal Meningitis, New Engl. J. Med., 270:59, 1964.

Campbell, G. D.: Primary Pulmonary Cryptococcosis, Am. Rev. Resp. Dis., 94:236, 1966.

Littman, M. L., and L. E. Zimmerman: "Cryptococcosis," New York, Grune & Stratton, Inc., 1956.

Walter, J. E., and R. D. Jones: Serodiagnosis of Clinical Cryptococcosis, Am. Rev. Resp. Dis., 97:275, 1968.

186 BLASTOMYCOSIS
Abraham I. Braude

DEFINITION. Blastomycosis is a fungous infection of the skin and viscera, caused by *Blastomyces dermatitidis* in North America and by *Paracoccidioides brasiliensis* in South America. South American blastomycosis (paracoccidioidal granuloma) produces massive lymphadenopathy and destructive lesions of the nasopharynx and bowel not found in its North American counterpart.

ETIOLOGY. In infected tissues *B. dermatitidis* has the appearance of a yeast, forming single buds from 3 to 24 μ in diameter. Two features aid in recognition: (1) its thick wall, spoken of as "double-contoured," because the inner and outer margins can be seen, and (2) the wide opening between parent cell and bud at the base of attachment.

In culture, *B. dermatitidis* is dimorphic and appears as the wrinkled, waxy yeast form on blood agar incubated at 37°C, or as a mold with branching hyphae on Sabouraud's agar at room temperature. On microscopic examination the cultured yeast may be identical with that in the infected lesions or may have abortive mycelia. The mycelia give rise to oval or pear-shaped exogenous spores.

Multiple buds on the yeastlike cell of *P. brasiliensis* distinguish it morphologically from *B. dermatitidis*. The tiny multiple buds have the appearance of a crown of small beads attached to the cell wall. The fungus reproduces by budding both in tissues and when cultured at 37°C. At room temperature it produces mycelia but not true spores.

PATHOGENESIS AND PATHOLOGY. The skin has been proposed as a portal of entry in North American blastomycosis because cutaneous lesions are prominent and because infections may follow injury to the skin. The lung is also a likely portal, but the fungus has never been cultured from the soil.

In most cases of South American blastomycosis the portal of entry is the nasopharynx. Here the fungus produces a destructive lesion with gross swelling and ulceration and eventual extension to the cervical lymph nodes. Occasionally, the primary lesion is inconspicuous and massive enlargement and suppurative necrosis of the regional lymph nodes predominate. In addition to the nasopharynx, primary lesions may occur in the lymphoid tissue of the cecal and appendiceal regions.

Characteristic pathologic features are found in the lung and skin in both North and South American forms. Pulmonary lesions vary in size from miliary granulomatous nodules to confluent areas of diffuse pneumonia involving an entire lobe. The granulomas may undergo caseation and fibrosis. Differentiation from tuberculosis is facilitated by finding the yeast in giant cells or other phagocytes.

In the skin, microabscesses lie just beneath the epidermis and are surrounded by a granulomatous reaction. The epidermis itself often becomes so hyperplastic that it resembles an epithelioma.

In both North and South American varieties, the infection may spread to the lymph nodes, brain, bones, urogenital tract, liver, spleen, and adrenals.

CLINICAL MANIFESTATIONS. In the typical case of systemic North American blastomycosis the onset is insidious. The patient may seek medical attention because of a persistent "chest cold," low-grade fever, weight loss, or progressive disability. Physical examination and roentgenogram of the chest disclose evidence of pneumonia, which may involve any segment or lobe of the lung. Cavitation is frequent, and mediastinal lymph nodes may

be prominent. Hemoptysis, purulent sputum, chest pain, and dyspnea appear as the disease progresses. Although the pulmonary infection may subside spontaneously, extrapulmonary lesions of the skin, bones, joints, and viscera eventually call attention to dissemination. These metastatic suppurative lesions are accompanied by an increase in fever, sweats, chills, and weakness. Death in the untreated infection sometimes occurs in less than 6 months, but most patients live for a year or two. The overall mortality in systemic blastomycosis is said to be 92 percent in patients who have been followed for 2 years or longer without specific therapy.

Primary infection of the skin by *B. dermatitidis* (Gilchrist's disease) first appears on unclothed areas such as the hands, face, or forearm but not the scalp, palms, or soles. The infection begins as a firm nodule surrounded by similar lesions which tend to coalesce. Suppuration in the center of the nodule is followed by partial healing and fibrosis as extension occurs peripherally. The hyperplastic epithelium gives these lesions a hard, raised, wartlike margin. When fully developed, blastomycosis of the skin presents the appearance of one or more ragged ulcers with partially healed centers and thick raised margins. The primary cutaneous infection may be confined to the skin for months or years.

The first symptoms in South American blastomycosis usually result from painful ulcers of the mouth or nose, although loss of appetite, abdominal pain, vomiting, and diarrhea may be the first complaints. In other cases, massive lymphadenopathy is the first manifestation. In the usual infection, however, there is a progressive extension of lesions from the mouth and neighboring skin. The lymph nodes undergo suppurative necrosis, and sinuses rupture through the overlying skin. The patient has severe pain, fever, inability to eat, and cachexia. Depending on the rapidity of spread to the viscera, bones, and central nervous system, the untreated disease is fatal after a few months or several years.

DIAGNOSIS. Pulmonary blastomycosis closely resembles tuberculosis, carcinoma of the lung, aspiration pneumonitis, and other fungous infections, including coccidioidomycosis, actinomycosis, nocardiosis, and histoplasmosis. Differentiation must be based on the recovery of the etiologic agent, because neither clinical nor epidemiologic features are specific. Most cases of North American blastomycosis are found in the Southeastern United States and in the Mississippi River Valley, but the disease occurs throughout the United States and Canada. Occupational history, sex, race, and age are of no diagnostic aid.

It is usually possible to find either *B. dermatitidis* or *P. brasiliensis* by microscopic examination of biopsied material, sputum, or pus. The yeastlike forms can be observed if a drop of purulent material is first mixed on a slide with a drop of 10 percent potassium hydroxide and kept at room temperature for 30 min. The multiple buds covering the entire surface of *P. brasiliensis* are connected by a narrow neck to the parent cell, while buds of *B. dermatitidis* are connected by a wide communication. *Blastomyces dermatitidis* is isolated by culturing pus on Sabouraud's agar at room temperature and on blood agar at 37°C. *Paracoccidioides brasiliensis* can also be isolated on blood agar at 37°C but grows so slowly that more than a month may elapse before colonies appear. Inoculation of mice or other animals is usually not successful in recovering either fungus.

The diagnostic value of the skin test for blastomycosis is limited. The complement fixation test in both North and South American blastomycosis is positive in high titer with serums of patients who have systemic infections. The results of intradermal and serologic tests may be of prognostic value. Patients with marked dermal hypersensitivity and low serum titers of complement-fixing antibody are said to have a better prognosis in North American blastomycosis than those with negative skin tests and high complement fixation titers.

TREATMENT. Amphotericin B is curative in both North and South American blastomycosis. North American blastomycosis also responds, but less favorably, to 2-hydroxystilbamidine, while South American blastomycosis is resistant to it. Either drug is given daily or every other day by slow intravenous drip in increasing doses. The maximum daily dose of amphotericin B is 75 to 100 mg, and that of 2-hydroxystilbamidine is 250 mg. Complete arrest of North American blastomycosis has been observed after a total of 1.0 Gm amphotericin B; 4 to 10 Gm of 2-hydroxystilbamidine may be required. Anesthesia over the distribution of the trigeminal nerve is the main untoward reaction from 2-hydroxystilbamidine; it persists after treatment. Surgical excision of pulmonary cavities or destroyed tissues is sometimes necessary in addition to chemotherapy.

In South American blastomycosis the sulfonamide drugs produce dramatic clinical remissions of most forms of the disease, but relapses invariably occur unless the patient is maintained on continuous therapy. Sulfadiazine in doses of 4 to 6 Gm daily has been successful in arresting the disease.

REFERENCES

Harrell, E. R., and A. C. Curtis: North American Blastomycosis, Am. J. Med., 27:750, 1959.

Lacaz, C. S.: South American Blastomycosis, Anales Fac. Med. Univ. São Paulo, 29:1, 1955–1956.

Martin, D. S., and D. T. Smith: Blastomycosis (American Blastomycosis, Gilchrist's Disease): Review of the Literature, Am. Rev. Tuberc., 39:257, 1939.

Smith, J. G., J. S. Harris, N. F. Conant, and D. T. Smith: An Epidemic of North American Blastomycosis, J.A.M.A., 158:641, 1955.

187   COCCIDIOIDOMYCOSIS

Abraham I. Braude

DEFINITION. Coccidioidomycosis is an infection acquired by inhalation of *Coccidioides immitis,* a fungus existing only in the mycelial phase in nature and converted to a spherule in tissues. Although most infections are mild or unapparent, *C. immitis* may produce a fatal disseminated disease with destructive lesions in the lungs, lymph nodes, spleen, liver, bones, kidneys, and brain.

ETIOLOGY. *Coccidioides immitis* grows readily at room temperature or at 35°C and produces white, cottony mycelia. As the culture ages, the segmented mycelium breaks up into thick-coated rectangular *arthrospores,* $2 \times 4 \mu$ in size. These arthrospores can survive in stored cultures and are highly infectious for laboratory personnel. The mycelium and its spores are pathogenic for various laboratory animals. The mycelial form is converted to a thick-walled spherule filled with endospores in animal tissues and under special cultural conditions.

PATHOGENESIS AND PATHOLOGY. Coccidioidomycosis is acquired by inhalation of *chlamydospores* in endemic areas in the semiarid regions of the Southwestern United States and the Chaco district of Argentina. The majority of infections occur during the dry seasons, particularly after exposure to dust storms. The fungus grows in the soil in rainy weather and becomes disseminated in dust during dry weather. *Coccidioides immitis* is isolated from soil and from desert rodents.

The inhaled spores are carried to the terminal bronchioles and alveoli, where the first reaction is an outpouring of polymorphonuclear leukocytes, fluid, and a few mononuclear cells. In most cases, the organism is probably killed, or at least arrested, at a stage when the lesion is too small to be detected by clinical means. In others, the organisms proliferate and elicit an inflammatory response which appears to depend on the rate of multiplication of the fungus. The phase of rapid multiplication is manifested by frequent discharge of endospores from the ripened spherules and elicits suppuration and an exudate rich in polymorphonuclear leukocytes. The phase of slow multiplication, with infrequent rupture of spherules, produces a granulomatous reaction in which epithelioid cells and giant cells predominate. Although polymorphonuclear leukocytes congregate about the point of rupture of a spherule and actually invade the broken capsule, attempts at phagocytosis by these cells are unsuccessful. As the released endospores develop into spherules, the neutrophilic reaction gives way to proliferating mononuclear cells which often are able to ingest the fungus.

Either phase of this inflammatory cycle may predominate, or a mixture of the two may be found. Rapidly progressive infections produce large areas of confluent suppurative pneumonia and necrosis. In contrast, granulomatous lesions contain exudates composed almost exclusively of mononuclear cells and giant cells which fill alveoli but leave their walls intact. Both reactions are accompanied by involvement of the overlying pleura and of the hilar and mediastinal lymph nodes. Ultimately the bronchopneumonia in most patients resolves or heals by fibrosis; in others, the lesions are permanently arrested but persist as cavities or solid nodules.

Recovery is accompanied by the development of hypersensitivity to the fungus. This hypersensitivity is apparently responsible for at least two special manifestations: (1) *erythema nodosum,* a sterile, focal, nodular granulomatous reaction usually limited to the skin of the lower extremities and characterized by extravasation of red cells into the lesion; (2) *pleural effusion*. It is believed that rupture of a pleural granuloma discharges antigenic material onto the sensitized pleural membranes.

In patients who do not develop dermal hypersensitivity, the infection spreads systemically to involve lymph nodes, spleen, bones, liver, kidney, meninges, skin, adrenals, and pericardium. In the meninges, the reaction may take two forms: (1) the granulomatous reaction is commoner and produces a firm plastic lesion which encloses the brainstem and other structures in a rigid mass of tissue; (2) the suppurative reaction results in outpouring of polymorphonuclear leukocytes with little granulomatous change. In either type, but especially in the granulomatous, involvement of the brainstem may lead to severe hydrocephalus.

CLINICAL MANIFESTATIONS. The infection may be either benign or disseminated. The benign infection, so-called "desert fever," is self-limited, and as many as 50 percent of benign infections are asymptomatic. The remainder are accompanied by influenza-like symptoms. After an incubation period of 1 to 3 weeks, the patient experiences fever, chills, fatigue, headache, severe arthralgia, and symptoms of respiratory infection. The most frequent complaint is poorly localized chest pain, aggravated by breathing or coughing. A nonproductive cough is common, but hemoptysis is infrequent. Physical findings are scant except in patients who develop erythema nodosum or pleural effusion. Although hydrothorax may be massive and require repeated thoracenteses, it eventually resorbs without further difficulty.

Despite the paucity of signs in the chest, prominent abnormalities are found in roentgenograms. These include focal areas of infiltration, hilar and mediastinal lymphadenopathy, nodules or cavities, and pleural effusion. The commonest are single or multiple infiltrates which may appear in any segment and can simulate tuberculosis if the upper lobe is involved. They usually resolve after several weeks.

In about 2 percent of benign infections a solid or cavitary pulmonary lesion remains. The typical cavity of coccidioidomycosis is peripheral, has a thin wall, and gives a cystlike appearance in roentgenograms. Bronchoscopic examination may disclose stenosis and ulceration of the bronchus. Residual solid lesions may be as large as 3 cm in diameter. Both solid and cavitary lesions are commoner in the upper lobes. Calcification is rare.

In a few individuals (0.05 to 0.2 percent), the primary infection progresses to the disseminated form of the disease. Dissemination usually occurs within a few months of infection. Dark-skinned persons and pregnant women are more vulnerable. Among Negroes and Filipinos, 85 to 90 percent with dissemination die, as compared to 50 percent of whites. Patients who develop progressive coccidioidomycosis do not give a history of erythema nodosum.

The course of disseminated infection is marked by fungating or ulcerating skin lesions, multiple pulmonary nodules or cavities, widespread destructive lymphadenopathy, osteomyelitis, and meningitis. Weight loss, fever, and weakness are the outstanding systemic manifestations, and the course is often rapid, with death occurring in less than a year. If vital organs are spared, however, patients with disseminated coccidioidomycosis may feel surprisingly well, continue to work, and even gain weight despite the presence of large numbers of *C. immitis* in the sputum or subcutaneous abscesses. The meningeal form is invariably fatal, but even it is compatible with survival for several years. In the presence of meningitis with progressive hydrocephalus, patients experience severe headaches, cranial nerve palsies, memory disturbances, and disorientation. The spinal fluid shows 100 to 200 cells, mostly mononuclear, elevated protein levels, and frequently a reduction in glucose concentration.

DIAGNOSIS. Except in meningitis, *C. immitis* is easily recovered from the lesions of disseminated coccidioidomycosis by direct examination and cultures of exudates or biopsied tissues. The characteristic spherule with endospores is seen best in purulent material treated with 20 percent potassium hydroxide. Occasionally, in biopsied tissue, spherules may all be immature and contain no endospores, making them indistinguishable from *B. dermatitidis*. Cultural identification becomes essential for diagnosis. On Sabouraud's agar, mycelial growth appears in 4 to 8 days, and inoculation of mice produces multiple necrotic lesions containing spherules. In meningitis, only a few spherules appear in the spinal fluid, despite the presence of large numbers in the granulomatous exudate around the brain stem. Occasionally, the culture of 20 to 30 ml of spinal fluid yields positive results, but sometimes the diagnosis can be based only on serologic tests.

Serologic tests are performed with coccidioidin, a filtrate from cultures of *C. immitis*. By the third week of primary infection, precipitins are found in the serum of 91 percent of patients with symptomatic infection but in only 7 percent of asymptomatic individuals. Complement-fixing antibodies appear later and persist longer than precipitins in nondisseminated coccidioidomycosis; they are almost always present in the disseminated disease. Intradermal tests with coccidioidin are of value in the recognition of primary benign infections because they become positive before precipitins appear, but in disseminated infection the skin test is frequently negative.

The roentgenographic appearance of pulmonary lesions is suggestive of primary coccidioidomycosis if hilar lymphadenopathy progresses while the parenchymal infiltrate is subsiding or if the adenopathy is associated with multiple areas of pneumonitis. A residual smooth, thin-walled cavity without surrounding parenchymal infiltration is also characteristic of the primary form of the disease. Other residual lesions include calcified or noncalcified nodular foci and localized bronchiectasis. In disseminated pulmonary infection the commonest picture is that of multiple infiltrates accompanied by pleural involvement and prominent hilar or mediastinal lymphadenopathy.

The only remarkable hematologic finding is eosinophilia, which may reach 35 percent of the total leukocyte count in the primary disease, especially if erythema nodosum is present.

TREATMENT. Intensive intravenous treatment with amphotericin B in daily doses of 1.0 mg per kg body weight appears to be effective in some cases of extrameningeal coccidioidomycosis. Coccidioidal meningitis is extremely resistant to amphotericin B therapy and should be treated with repeated intrathecal injections of 0.5 mg of this drug. The total dose necessary varies from less than 1.0 Gm to more than 10.0 Gm intravenously and as much as 45 mg intrathecally. Severe nausea, venous thrombosis, and reversible impairment of renal and hepatic function often interrupt the treatment schedule, but persistent administration of amphotericin B in the face of troublesome side effects has occasionally produced improvement. A fall in titer of complement-fixing antibodies and a return of coccidioidin skin sensitivity are evidence of effective treatment. Drug therapy may have to be supplemented by surgical removal of peripheral granulomas.

Primary surgical excision of residual pulmonary foci is indicated if these lesions become troublesome because of secondary infection or hemoptysis. Dissemination of the disease from these foci almost never occurs.

REFERENCES

Baker, O. B., and A. I. Braude: A Study of Stimuli Leading to the Production of Spherules of Coccidioidomycosis, J. Lab. Clin. Med., 47:169, 1956.

Emmons, C. S.: Isolation of *Coccidioides* from Soil and Rodents, Public Health Rept. U.S., 57:109, 1942.

Fiese, M. J.: "Coccidioidomycosis," Springfield, Ill., Charles C Thomas, Publisher, 1958.

Forbus, W. D., and A. M. Bestebreurtje: Coccidioidomycosis: A Study of 95 Cases of the Disseminated Type with Special Reference to the Pathogenesis of the Disease, Mil. Surg., 99:654, 1946.

Harris, R. E.: Coccidioidomycosis Complicating Pregnancy, Obstet. Gynecol., 28:401, 1966.

Peck, W. A., and S. S. Romendick: Coccidioidomycosis: A Roentgen Study, Texas State J. Med., 52:86, 1956.

Smith, C. E., M. T. Saito, and S. A. Simons: Pattern of 39,500 Serologic Tests in Coccidioidomycosis, J.A.M.A., 160:546, 1956.

Taylor, A. B., and A. K. Briney: Observations on Primary Coccidioidomycosis, Ann. Intern. Med., 30:1224, 1949.

188 HISTOPLASMOSIS
Abraham I. Braude

DEFINITION. Histoplasmosis is a protean infection caused by the dimorphic fungus *Histoplasma capsulatum,* an organism found as a tiny body within reticuloendothelial cells. The disease varies from mild or unnoticed respiratory infection to widely disseminated lethal disease characterized by fever, anemia, hepatomegaly, splenomegaly, leukopenia, pulmonary lesions, ulcerations of the gastrointestinal tract, and adrenal necrosis.

ETIOLOGY. Although *H. capsulatum* grows on Sabou-raud's agar at room temperature as a spore-bearing mold, it is transformed after animal inoculation into nonencapsulated oval yeastlike cells measuring $2 \times 4 \mu$. In histologic section the protoplasm is shrunken so that the unstained space beneath the cell wall has the appearance of a capsule. The name *capsulatum* is based on a misinterpretation of the nature of this unstained space. The fungus also grows in the yeastlike phase if incubated at 37°C in sealed tubes of blood agar. The most distinctive cultural feature, however, is the tuberculate *chlamydospore* found only on mycelia; it is round, $10 \times 20 \mu$ in diameter, and covered with warty projections. Another smaller spore, not distinguishable from that of *Blastomyces dermatitidis,* is also present on the mycelium. A newly recognized species, *Histoplasma duboisii,* resembles *B. dermatitidis* and is responsible for an infection in Africa that involves the skin and bones but not the lung.

PATHOLOGY AND PATHOGENESIS. The source of human infection is probably soil containing spores of *Histoplasma.* Several studies have emphasized the isolation of the fungus from soil in areas inhabited by chickens, birds, and bats. City dwellers are often exposed to histoplasma growing in soil under trees which shelter starlings. In most cases the portal of entry is the lung, where a primary complex may be formed by extension of infection from the pulmonary focus to the regional lymph nodes. Infection through the gastrointestinal tract probably occurs in patients whose initial lesions are in the mouth and pharynx.

The basic pathologic process is multiplication of *H. capsulatum* in cells of the reticuloendothelial system. The yeast form multiplies extensively and greatly distends the cells. As proliferating histiocytes encroach on parenchymal cells, the infected organ becomes enlarged. The liver, lymph nodes, lung, spleen, adrenal glands, bowel, and marrow may be affected in disseminated histoplasmosis.

In addition to the diffuse lesions of the reticuloendothelial system, the tissues contain nodular accumulations of epithelioid cells and giant cells of the Langhans type. The noncaseous granuloma probably represents an effective defensive action, and histoplasma organisms are difficult to demonstrate in the epithelioid cells of such a lesion.

Caseous necrosis may accompany both types of lesion. The adrenals, which are involved in nearly all disseminated infections, are often massively enlarged. Caseous necrosis is usually present in the center of the pulmonary granulomas, which resemble those of cavitary pulmonary tuberculosis. Necrotizing histoplasmosis may also take the form of renal papillitis. Extracellular forms of histoplasma are readily found in the necrotic areas of all organs by special stains (periodic acid–Schiff, Gridley). These extracellular organisms may be much larger than the intracellular ones, appear distorted, and occasionally assume the mycelial form.

CLINICAL MANIFESTATIONS. The signs and symptoms of histoplasmosis range from those of a slight self-limited infection to fatal disseminated disease. The high incidence of positive intradermal reactions to histoplasmosis in healthy persons in many parts of the world indicates that most infections by *H. capsulatum* are inapparent or very mild. This variability in severity is observed among different persons involved in the same outbreak. Severe infections are characterized by prolonged fever, dyspnea, chest pain, weight loss, prostration, widespread pulmonary infiltrates, hepatomegaly, and splenomegaly. Other infected persons may have only a benign acute pneumonitis lasting a week or less, while still others are entirely free of symptoms. Widespread ill-defined noncalcified pulmonary infiltrates of miliary size or larger are found in symptomatic infections and may also be present, although less extensively, in the asymptomatic ones. Eventually, pulmonary lesions either disappear or calcify. In the east central part of the United States there is a high incidence of pulmonary calcification in persons who have negative tuberculin and positive histoplasmin skin tests. In some epidemics of acute histoplasmosis, erythema nodosum and erythema multiforme have been prominent in middle-aged women.

Least resistance to histoplasmosis is encountered in young infants and in adults after the fifth decade. Most cases of disseminated infection have occurred at these extremes of life, but with somewhat different clinical manifestations in the two groups. In the infant there are fever, emaciation, anemia, and leukopenia, and evidence of widespread involvement of many viscera including the liver, spleen, lung, bowel, lymph nodes, adrenals, skin, kidney, brain, eye, or endocardium. Although the same degree of dissemination may occasionally occur in the adult, usually visceral involvement is less widespread. Unlike the disease in infancy, adult histoplasmosis shows a marked predilection for men. Histoplasmosis of the lips, mouth, nose, and larynx occurs almost exclusively in adults and is the initial manifestation in about one-third of the fatal cases. Among the various syndromes encountered are subacute vegetative endocarditis, massive lymphadenopathy resembling tuberculosis or lymphoma, various forms of pneumonia, cerebral histoplasmoma, and meningitis. The last is characterized by signs of basilar localization with spinal fluid findings and a clinical course identical with those of tuberculous meningitis.

In addition to the acute benign and disseminated infections, chronic localized histoplasmosis occurs in adults. Although frequently accompanied by necrosis or ulceration, this form is basically a granuloma, with a tendency to remain localized.

Two main clinical types of chronic localized histoplasmosis are encountered: (1) *Pulmonary.* This may resemble pulmonary tuberculosis in all respects. The patient may be asymptomatic or may complain of a chronic and occasionally productive cough. Roentgenograms will show lesions identical with those of reinfection tuberculosis, sometimes with cavitation, and accompanied by consistently positive cultures of sputum for *H. capsulatum.* (2) *Mucocutaneous.* Ulcers of the mouth, tongue, pharynx, gums, larynx, penis, or bladder are rare lesions found only in adults. Regional lymphadenopathy is common in these types.

In African histoplasmosis, the predominant lesions are in the skin. These may rupture through the epidermis or encroach on underlying bone. In the disseminated form, multiple lesions involve the lymph nodes, bone, skin, liver, and spleen, but, in contrast to *H. capsulatum* infections, the lungs are spared.

DIAGNOSIS. Isolation of *H. capsulatum* is not difficult in disseminated or chronic localized infections if cultures are made of bone marrow, blood, biopsied lesions, sputum, or exudate from an ulcer. After incubation of infected material on Sabouraud's agar at room temperature there appears a white cottony colony which later turns brown and produces the diagnostic tuberculate chlamydospores. Material may also be cultured at 37°C on Francis' medium or blood agar, but the growth is yeastlike, and the diagnostic spores are not found. Isolation from sputum is best accomplished in mice, because contaminants are suppressed and the mouse is extremely susceptible to infection by histoplasmas. The animal does not die, but subculture of the spleen 1 month later on Sabouraud's agar yields the organism. Histoplasmas may also be seen in bone marrow, material from open or biopsied lesions, and occasionally in blood smears of terminally ill patients. Special fungous stains (periodic acid–Schiff, Gridley) should be used. Certain intracellular forms of *Cryptococcus neoformans* may be indistinguishable from histoplasma in histologic sections, unless strains for the cryptococcal mucinous capsule are employed.

In cases from which *H. capsulatum* cannot be isolated, indirect clues to identification are (1) history of exposure to soil or dust in an endemic area, (2) positive complement fixation tests, (3) positive histoplasmin skin tests, and (4) development of miliary calcifications in the lung. Although these criteria are not dependable individually, they appear to be reliable when used together. The serologic and skin tests are frequently negative in culturally proved cases of histoplasmosis, and their specificity is not fully established. Histoplasmin skin tests may confuse the serologic picture by producing complement-fixing antibodies to mycelial antigens, but not to yeast-phase antigens.

Histoplasmosis must be differentiated from tuberculosis, sarcoid, leukemia, infectious mononucleosis, Hodgkin's disease, brucellosis, and kala-azar. Because cortisone is frequently of value in sarcoid but can cause dissemination in histoplasmosis, differential diagnosis between these two diseases is critical. Biopsied tissue in both diseases contains morphologically identical granulomas. For this reason the diagnosis of sarcoid should be withheld until tissues have been examined with special fungous stains. In kala-azar the intracellular Leishman-Donovan body bears a close resemblance to *H. capsulatum,* and cultural isolation of the fungus may be important in distinguishing between the two.

TREATMENT. Amphotericin B, in intravenous doses of 50 to 100 mg daily, is effective in all forms of histoplasmosis. Treatment given daily, or on alternate days, must be continued for periods varying from 1 to many months. Sulfadiazine has also been effective in adults in oral doses of 6 Gm daily and may be given in conjunction with intravenous amphotericin B.

REFERENCES

Binford, C. H.: Histoplasmosis: Tissue Reaction, and Morphologic Variations in the Fungus, Am. J. Clin. Pathol., 25:25, 1955.

Loosli, C., J. T. Grayston, E. R. Alexander, and F. Tanzi: Epidemiological Studies of Pulmonary Histoplasmosis in a Farm Family, Am. J. Hyg., 55:392, 1952.

Parsons, R. J., and C. J. D. Zarafonetis: Histoplasmosis in Man: Report of Seven Cases and Review of Seventy-one Cases, Arch. Intern. Med., 75:1, 1945.

Sellers, T. E., Jr., W. N. Price, Jr., and W. M. Newberry, Jr.: Epidemic of Erythema Multiforme and Erythema Nodosum Caused by Histoplasmosis, Ann. Intern. Med., 62:1214, 1965.

Shapiro, J. L., J. J. Lux, and B. E. Sprofkin: Histoplasmosis of the Central Nervous System, Am. J. Pathol., 31:319, 1955.

Sweany, Henry C.: "Histoplasmosis," Springfield, Ill., Charles C Thomas, Publisher, 1960.

189 SPOROTRICHOSIS
Abraham I. Braude

DEFINITION. Sporotrichosis is a chronic infection due to *Sporotrichum schencki*. It is characterized by the formation of suppurating nodules along the lymphatics of the skin and subcutaneous tissues. Hematogenous dissemination is rare.

ETIOLOGY. The fungus *S. schencki* is dimorphic. On Sabouraud's agar at room temperature its growth is mycelial, but in the tissue it takes the form of tiny, cigar-shaped yeast cells. The yeast phase also develops in vitro by incubation at 37°C on blood agar containing cystine.

PATHOGENESIS AND PATHOLOGY. The fungus lives as a saprophyte on vegetation and penetrates the hands when the skin is broken. Many cases have followed injury by thorns, and an outbreak of sporotrichosis occurred among South African natives exposed to *S. schencki* growing on timbers supporting a gold mine. In this country, it is primarily an occupational disease in people working with plants. Sphagnum moss is an important source of infection, and its increased use as mulch may lead to a greater occurrence of sporotrichosis.

After penetrating the skin, the fungus spreads up the extremities and evokes nodular lesions along the thickened lymphatics. Microscopically the nodules are granulomas with central necrosis. In exceedingly rare infections the organism may become disseminated throughout the subcutaneous tissues, the liver, testicles, bone, and kidney. Disseminated disease is not usually accompanied by primary infections of the extremities, and its portal of entry is believed to be the gastrointestinal tract.

CLINICAL MANIFESTATIONS. There is a marked disproportion between symptoms and findings. A chain of hard, reddened discrete lumps extends up the arm or leg to the axilla or groin, and the intervening lymphatics are red and thickened, but there is no pain, fever, or other constitutional symptom. Older nodules may rupture to produce fistulas or ulcers. In the rare patient with disseminated sporotrichosis, constitutional symptoms may be marked and the disease is rapidly fatal. Unlike other disseminated mycoses, sporotrichosis almost never involves the lungs or central nervous system. Instead, it has a predilection for bone, joints, periosteum, and muscle.

Without treatment, sporotrichosis does not heal, and the lesions often become secondarily infected with bacteria.

DIAGNOSIS. The fungus cannot be seen upon microscopic examination of biopsied material or pus in most cases. Cultural isolation is invariably successful, however, if pus is aspirated from an unbroken nodule and inoculated onto Sabouraud's agar. The growth at first has the soft creamy character of bacterial colonies and later develops a wrinkled dark-brown appearance without the cottonlike filament of most molds. Microscopically, typical clusters of pear-shaped spores are found at the tips of conidiophores arising from the tangled mass of delicate branched mycelia. If the mold or the pus is inoculated intraperitoneally into mice or rats, numerous yeast forms will be seen in lesions of the peritoneal cavity or testicle, where they take the form of gram-positive cigar-shaped rods within polymorphonuclear leukocytes.

Recovery of the organism by these techniques permits ready differentiation of sporotrichosis from other chronic infections of the subcutaneous tissues such as syphilis, tularemia, blastomycosis, coccidioidomycosis, and tuberculosis. The hard sporotrichotic lesions are sometimes mistaken for syphilitic gummas, and their response to iodides is interpreted as therapeutic proof of the diagnosis.

TREATMENT. The common lymphangitic form of sporotrichosis is almost invariably dramatically cured by saturated potassium iodide. This should be given orally in starting doses of 10 drops t.i.d. after meals and gradually increased to the point of maximum tolerance. Treatment should be continued for a month after lesions disappear. Additional local therapy may be required for cutaneous ulcers, which should be painted with tincture of iodine. It may also be necessary to excise the epidermal lesions, because these may not subside with oral iodides. Systemic sporotrichosis is also resistant to iodides, but it responds well to intravenous treatment with amphotericin B, given in a total dose of 1.5 to 2.0 Gm over a period of 6 to 8 weeks.

REFERENCES

Kedes, L. H., J. Siemienski, and A. I. Braude: The Syndrome of the Alcoholic Rose Gardener: Sporotrichosis of the Radial Tendon Sheath, Ann. Intern. Med., 61:1139, 1964.

Wilson, D. E., J. J. Mann, J. E. Bennett, and J. P. Utz: Clinical Features of Extracutaneous Sporotrichosis, Medicine, 46:265, 1967.

190 MONILIASIS (Candidiasis)
Abraham I. Braude

DEFINITION. Moniliasis is a common mild mucocutaneous infection due to *Candida albicans*. This fungus is also an unusual cause of widespread visceral infection.

ETIOLOGY. Among the many species of *Candida*, only *C. albicans* is a common pathogen for man. On the usual nutrient laboratory media *C. albicans* grows as a budding yeast in creamy white colonies, but it produces both mycelia and yeastlike cells in infected tissues. *Candida parapsilosis* is only important as a cause of endocarditis. *Candida guilliermondii* and *Candida tropicalis* have also been isolated rarely in endocarditis.

PATHOGENESIS. *Candida albicans* resides normally on the mucous membranes and is frequently cultured from the mouth and feces of persons in good health. The rate of cultural isolation from feces in numerous surveys has ranged from 14 to 19 percent. In debilitated infants, and sometimes in adults, the fungus may produce white patches on the buccal mucosa and initiate mild inflammatory reaction in the underlying tissues. At times chronic moniliasis of the oral mucosa induces chronic hyperplastic changes that resemble leukoplakia. In pregnancy and diabetes, *C. albicans* frequently causes a mild superficial infection of the vagina. Presumably, the high glycogen content of the vaginal mucosa in pregnancy and the glycosuria of diabetes favor its growth. Candida multiplies excessively in the bowel or mouth if the normal bacterial flora is suppressed by chemotherapy. Although true infection seldom accompanies this overgrowth of candida, the large inoculum provides a threat in debilitated persons, who may develop aspiration pneumonia or even candidemia. The kidney and brain bear the brunt of hematogenous infection, but lesions also occur in the thyroid, myocardium, endocardium, pancreas, adrenals, and liver. The visceral lesions are granulomatous nodules or abscesses containing both mycelia and yeastlike cells.

A striking susceptibility to moniliasis of the skin and nails is seen in children with congenital hypoparathyroidism. Extensive cutaneous moniliasis occurs in infants with the Swiss type of agammaglobulinemia (alymphocytosis), but not in those with the Bruton form (Chap. 69).

CLINICAL MANIFESTATIONS. No systemic disturbances accompany the local signs of mucocutaneous infection. Infection of the mucous membranes, known as *thrush*, gives rise only to soft white patches on the tonsils, cheeks, gums, and tongue. These patches are easily removed and leave a reddened surface. Although usually self-limited, the disease may become chronic and spread to other mucosal surfaces or intertriginous areas in the groins, the antecubital fossae, the interdigital folds, the inframammary areas, the umbilicus, and the axillas. Eczematoid lesions and vesicles are also found in vulvovaginal moniliasis of pregnancy or diabetes.

Aspiration pneumonia is probably the chief form of visceral moniliasis. It is seen in debilitated persons, often in the course of intensive therapy with tetracycline or other antibiotics, and may be accompanied by mixed infection with bacteria. Cough, chest pain, and high fever are prominent.

Bloodstream infections are seen in the late stages of severe debilitating disease and seem to occur most commonly in children receiving intensive antibiotic therapy. Acute disseminated moniliasis may be suspected in debilitated adults who suddenly develop fever, shock, azo-temia, depressed sensorium, and gastrointestinal bleeding after receiving continuous antibiotic treatment. Monilia also may cause vegetative endocarditis, a disease that has been described mainly in narcotic addicts. Meningitis is another rare form of moniliasis; it produces a clinical syndrome similar to tuberculous meningitis.

DIAGNOSIS. In thrush, the organisms are seen upon microscopic examination of the white patches as a tangled mass of mycelia and yeastlike cells. They grow readily on Sabouraud's agar. In fungemias the fungus can be isolated repeatedly from the blood. Pulmonary moniliasis may be difficult to recognize, because *C. albicans* is a normal resident of the oropharynx and may appear in the sputum in the absence of respiratory infection. For this reason, it is often impossible to be certain of the diagnosis of pulmonary moniliasis unless the organism is demonstrated in pulmonary lesions at autopsy or surgery.

TREATMENT. Oral and vaginal thrush are best treated topically. Nystatin oral suspension is used in the mouth and nystatin or candicidin tablets in the vagina. Topical therapy with nystatin ointments, amphotericin B lotion, or alcoholic solutions of gentian violet is effective in cutaneous moniliasis. Nystatin oral tablets may also be of some benefit in preventing candidal pneumonia or septicemia in debilitated persons whose mouth and intestines have become overgrown with candida during treatment with antibiotics. Intravenous amphotericin B in doses of 1.0 mg per kg body weight daily is effective in treating systemic moniliasis.

REFERENCES

Benham, R. W., and A. M. Hopkins: Yeast-like Fungi Found on the Skin and in the Intestines of Normal Subjects, Arch. Dermatol. Syphilol., 28:532, 1933.

Braude, A. I., and J. Rock: The Syndrome of Acute Disseminated Moniliasis in Adults, A.M.A. Arch. Intern. Med., 104:91, 1959.

Merchant, R. K., D. B. Luria, P. H. Geisler, J. H. Edgcomb, and J. P. Utz: Fungal Endocarditis: Review of the Literature and Report of Three Cases, Ann. Intern. Med., 48:242, 1958.

Winner, H., and R. Hurley: "Candida Albicans," Boston, Little, Brown and Company, 1964.

191 MUCORMYCOSIS
Abraham I. Braude

DEFINITION. Mucormycosis (phycomycosis) is a rare but malignant infection of cranial, pulmonary, and abdominal blood vessels due to fungi of the order Mucorales. The most frequent manifestations are ophthalmoplegia and meningoencephalitis.

ETIOLOGY. The etiologic agent has rarely, if ever, been cultured from the brain or spinal fluid even when expert mycologic techniques were used with fresh cerebral tissues known to harbor the characteristic mycelium. The mycelium is broad, branching, and aseptate, with a diameter of 6 to 15 μ. The fungus *Rhizopus oryzae,* a species of the order Mucorales, has been recovered from the paranasal sinuses of patients with fatal mucormycosis, and the mycelia in culture were identical in appearance with those in the brain. Because known members of the order Mucorales grow readily on ordinary media, the failure of cultural isolation from the brain remains a puzzle. In addition to *R. oryzae,* it has been possible to isolate *Absidia corymbifera, Rhizopus arrhizus,* and *Mucor pusillus* from infected foci outside the nervous system. A benign form of tropical subcutaneous phycomycosis is caused by *Basidiobolus ranarum.*

PATHOGENESIS. These fungi abound in soil, manure, and starchy foodstuffs, but become pathogenic for man only in rare cases of diabetic acidosis and even less commonly in patients debilitated by uremic acidosis, leukemia, irradiation, or radiomimetic drugs. The usual portal of entry appears to be the nasal turbinates or paranasal sinuses; from there the organism is thought to extend along the invaded vessels to the retroorbital tissues and cerebrum. Thrombosis of arteries and veins leads to multiple infarcts throughout the brain, but only a minimal inflammatory response is found. Cerebral mucormycosis may be associated with hematogenous spread to pulmonary and intestinal vessels. Pulmonary and intestinal infarction may also develop as a primary infection apparently after inhalation or ingestion of the fungus. Organisms probably penetrate the walls of bronchi or intestine and infect the adjacent hilar or mesenteric vessels. Intestinal mucormycosis takes the form of hemorrhagic segmental infarction of the ileum or colon. Invasion of coronary arteries may produce myocardial infarction.

CLINICAL MANIFESTATIONS. Cerebral mucormycosis is characterized by three features: (1) uncontrolled diabetes with acidosis, (2) ophthalmoplegia, and (3) signs of acute diffuse cerebrovascular disease. If the portal of entry is the nose, a fourth feature is a black nasal turbinate and malar anesthesia. When the patient is first seen, drowsiness and semistupor are usually attributed to the metabolic disturbance, but the cerebral manifestations persist and progress after the acidosis is corrected. Headache and fever are prominent, and paranasal sinusitis is frequently present.

In addition to complete internal and external ophthalmoplegia, there may be edema of the eyelids and retina, proptosis, and signs of retinal vascular occlusion. Nuchal rigidity and mild mononuclear pleocytosis in the spinal fluid have also been described. Pulmonary mucormycosis may start gradually or suddenly with chest pain, fever, hemoptysis, and a friction rub. A few cases have been described in which the orbit or sinuses were infected without extension to the brain. In tropical Africa, subcutaneous phycomycosis is relatively common. This benign disease is caused by fungi belonging to the genus *Basidiobolus* and produces a woody-hard, freely movable lump in the thighs, buttocks, and forearms, with no constitutional disturbances. Most patients are children. The Sassoon Hospital syndrome, a remarkable disorder attributed to the toxin of *Rhizopus nigricans,* is characterized by epidemic polyuria and polydipsia.

DIAGNOSIS. The syndrome of cerebral mucormycosis is so characteristic that it can be recognized by its clinical features alone. The fungus can be found in sections and cultures of the infarcted nasal turbinate or paranasal sinus.

PROGNOSIS. Untreated cerebral mucormycosis is almost invariably fatal. Rare cases of recovery have followed control of diabetic acidosis.

TREATMENT. A few patients with cerebral mucormycosis have recovered after treatment with amphotericin B in doses of 50 to 70 mg intravenously daily. The total doses were approximately 2.2 Gm. Treatment should also be directed toward rapid correction of the hyperglycemia and acidosis as well as local excision of infected tissue in the nose, paranasal sinuses, or orbit. Surgical removal of infected lung has been successful. Subcutaneous African phycomycosis has improved during treatment with oral potassium iodide.

REFERENCES

Baker, R. D.: Mucormycosis—a New Disease? J.A.M.A., 163:805, 1957.

Bauer, H., L. Ajello, E. Adams, and D. Hernandez: Cerebral Mucormycosis: Pathogenesis of the Disease: Description of the Fungus *Rhizopus oryzae* Isolated from a Fatal Case, Am. J. Med., 18:822, 1955.

Burkitt, D. P., A. M. M. Wilson, and D. B. Jelliffe: Subcutaneous Phycomycosis: A Review of 31 Cases Seen in Uganda, Brit. Med. J., 1:1669, 1964.

Burrow, G. N., R. B. Salmon, and J. P. Nolan: Successful Treatment of Cerebral Mucormycosis with Amphotericin B, J.A.M.A., 183:370, 1963.

192 NOCARDIOSIS
Abraham I. Braude

DEFINITION. Nocardiosis, an infection caused by an aerobic actinomycete, may produce lung abscesses and spread to the brain and elsewhere; or it may appear as a chronic deforming granulomatous infection limited to the foot (maduromycosis).

ETIOLOGY. Pulmonary and disseminated nocardiosis usually result from infection with *Nocardia asteroides.* This organism is relatively acid-fast, and its bacillary form resembles the tubercle bacillus. The following properties of *N. asteroides* permit easy differentiation from the tubercle bacillus: (1) rapid growth on Sabouraud's medium or on 10 percent blood agar with colonies appearing in 3 to 14 days at room temperature; (2) the presence in exudates of long-branched mycelial forms in addition to the bacillary forms; (3) rapid killing of guinea pigs and rabbits inoculated intraperitoneally and the recovery of *N. asteroides* from miliary nodules in the abdominal viscera; death of guinea pigs occurs in less than a week from pathogenic strains; (4) intense gram-positive staining reaction.

PATHOGENESIS. *Nocardia asteroides* can be recovered readily from soil. Nocardiosis appears, therefore, to be an exogenous infection usually having its portal of entry in the lungs. In almost every patient with nocardiosis (other than maduromycosis) the earliest and most extensive lesions are pulmonary acute suppurative foci containing acid-fast, branching nocardial filaments. A well-defined wall is absent, a fact which probably accounts for the marked tendency of nocardial abscesses to spread to the brain and to a lesser extent to the spleen, skin, peritoneum, and kidney. Occasionally noncaseating granulomas are found. Susceptibility to nocardiosis is increased in Cushing's syndrome, in pulmonary alveolar proteinosis, and in some patients with lymphomas or leukemia after antitumor chemotherapy.

CLINICAL MANIFESTATIONS. The chief symptom is cough, usually productive of a thick, sometimes bloody, sputum. Chest pain and dyspnea are common. These symptoms are usually accompanied by fever, sweats, chills, leukocytosis, weakness, anorexia, and weight loss. The illness may be prolonged and present the picture of a chronic pulmonary infection resembling tuberculosis, lung abscess, or unresolved suppurative pneumonia. In nearly one-third of the patients this syndrome is interrupted suddenly by the acute neurologic changes of metastatic brain abscess. At this time the patient may have severe headache and focal sensory or motor disturbances. The protein, cells, and pressure of the spinal fluid are increased, but the concentration of glucose is not reduced unless the meninges are also infected. Occasionally, symptoms of brain abscess are the first clinical manifestations of nocardiosis, especially in patients with Cushing's syndrome secondary to adrenal steroid therapy. Infection of the skin is frequent and produces numerous scattered abscesses or single draining sinuses of the hand, chest wall, or buttocks.

The disease is usually fatal, but the duration varies from months to years.

DIAGNOSIS. Because patients with nocardiosis are usually suspected of having tuberculosis, their sputums are likely to be examined for tubercle bacilli. The usual methods for concentrating tubercle bacilli often inactivate *N. asteroides*, however, and the fungus may not be recovered after such treatment despite the readiness with which it otherwise grows on a variety of media. *Nocardia asteroides* may also be overlooked in smears stained by the Ziehl-Neelsen method, because it is less resistant than the tubercle bacillus to the decolorizing action of acid alcohol. If nocardiosis is suspected on clinical grounds, precautions must be taken, therefore, against killing the organism by sputum concentration methods and against overdecolorizing it. The first can be avoided by concentrating with trisodium phosphate; the second by using a weak solution of acid alcohol.

Although sulfur granules are not found in pulmonary or disseminated nocardiosis, the gram-positive filamentous organisms in nocardial exudates often resemble *Actinomyces israeli*. The two pathogens can be distinguished, however, by the ease with which *N. asteroides* is cultivated on Sabouraud's medium or blood agar aerobically, by its acid-fast staining characteristics, and by its pathogenicity for guinea pigs and rabbits. If biopsy material is available, the nongranulomatous and minimally fibrotic character of the nocardial suppurative reaction also helps to distinguish it from that seen in infections due to *A. israeli*. The absence of tubercles, of course, is valuable in differential diagnosis from tuberculosis.

TREATMENT. Sulfadiazine is sometimes successful in the treatment of nocardiosis. Penicillin and the tetracycline derivatives appear ineffective, and resistance of nocardiosis to these drugs may be used in distinguishing it from actinomycosis due to *A. israeli* and from other pulmonary infections which respond to these antibiotics. Patients with nocardiosis should receive 8 to 12 Gm sulfadiazine daily. Despite the poor clinical results with penicillin and tetracycline, in vitro tests are warranted to determine the sensitivity of each new strain of *N. asteroides* to various antibiotics. An antibiotic selected on this basis can be used to supplement the sulfonamides.

REFERENCES

Andriole, V. T., M. Ballas, and G. L. Wilson: The Association of Nocardiosis and Pulmonary Alveolar Proteinosis, Ann. Intern. Med., 60:266, 1964.

Danowski, T. S., W. M. Cooper, and A. I. Braude: Cushing's Syndrome in Conjunction with *Nocardia Asteroides* Infection, Metabolism, 11:2, 1962.

Henrici, A. T., and E. L. Gardner: The Acid-fast Actinomycetes: With a Report of a Case from Which a New Species Was Isolated, J. Infect. Dis. 28:232, 1921.

Weed, L. A., H. A. Andersen, C. A. Good, and A. H. Baggentos: Nocardiosis: Clinical, Bacteriologic and Pathologic Aspects, New Engl. J. Med., 253:1138, 1955.

193 OTHER DEEP MYCOSES
Abraham I. Braude

ASPERGILLOSIS

DEFINITION. Aspergillosis is an infection produced by *Aspergillus fumigatus* and other species of *Aspergillus*, a group of fungi of low pathogenicity for man unless resistance is overcome by an overwhelming inoculum or debilitating illness. The disease may become disseminated or remain localized to the lung, ear, orbit, or paranasal sinuses.

ETIOLOGY. Asperigilli assume the mycelial form both in culture and in infected tissues. They are hardy, widely prevalent organisms and grow rapidly on all culture media at room temperature or 35°C as colored woolly colonies peppered with dark dots. They are composed of segmented mycelia that bear masses of small round spores on a knoblike swelling at the end of specialized mycelial stalks known as conidiophores.

PATHOGENESIS AND PATHOLOGY. Primary infection of the lung sometimes develops after inhalation of massive numbers of spores from mycelia growing on grain. Pulmonary aspergillosis was an occupational disease in persons who fattened squabs by forcing masticated grain from their mouths into the esophagus of the birds. Secondary pulmonary infection may be superimposed on tuberculous cavities, bronchiectasis, and bronchogenic carcinoma or may become established after resistance is lowered by leukopenia, Hodgkin's disease, irradiation, and other debilitating processes. Excessive use of adrenal steroids or antibiotics is also thought to favor secondary invasion by aspergillus. The most distinctive pulmonary lesion is the aspergilloma, a mycelial mass in a fibrous cavity lined with bronchial epithelium. Chronic granulomatous lung lesions resembling tuberculosis have also been described. More destructive infections take the form of bronchopneumonia and lung abscesses. Thrombosis of pulmonary vessels by invading mycelia leads to local necrosis with hemorrhage and to hematogenous abscesses in the brain, lung, kidney, spleen, heart, and thyroid. Primary infections of the ear, orbit, and nasal sinuses may also be invasive and extend locally into the middle ear and brain. In all lesions, mycelia are prominently observed in tissues stained with Schiff's periodic acid or hematoxylin and eosin.

CLINICAL MANIFESTATIONS. In pulmonary aspergillomas the chief symptom is hemoptysis. Aspergillus lung abscesses and granulomas are associated with cough and fever. In fulminating disseminated infections, pulmonary manifestations are often overshadowed by coma and other signs of cerebral infection. Fever, joint pains, and skin eruptions lasting for a few weeks or months may also accompany disseminated aspergillosis. A syndrome of allergic aspergillosis occurs in asthmatics who develop hypersensitivity to aspergillus antigens. These patients are subject to recurrent episodes of localized pulmonary infiltrations with blood eosinophilia, increased wheezing, cough, fever, and pleuritic pain. Allergic aspergillosis is said to be the most frequent cause in Great Britain of transient lung infiltrates with eosinophilia. A form of allergic aspergillosis, known as hemp disease, produces asthma in people working in rope factories.

DIAGNOSIS. Cultures of aspergilli have no diagnostic value unless they are obtained directly from infected tissues. They may be present in the mouth and in sputum cultures in the absence of aspergillus infection, and they may contaminate uninfected biopsy specimens unless strict sterile precautions are observed. Cultural findings should be confirmed by demonstration of the characteristic septate mycelia in biopsy material. Diagnosis should not be based alone on the morphology of the fungus in tissue section without simultaneous culture, because its mycelia may be confused with those found in the tissues in candidiasis and mucormycosis. In chronic aspergillomas the sputum cultures may sometimes become negative after the fungus loses its ability to sporulate.

Aspergillomas of the lung can usually be recognized by the unique appearance in roentgenograms of a crescentic radiolucency surrounding a circular mass. In other forms of pulmonary aspergillosis the roentgenogram is not diagnostic and may resemble that of bronchogenic carcinoma, bacterial lung abscess, and tuberculosis. In allergic aspergillosis, the sputum may contain small plugs composed of eosinophilic and mycelial fragments, and serum precipitins against aspergillus antigens are found by double diffusion in agar gel. Such precipitins are also present constantly in pulmonary aspergillomas.

TREATMENT. Localized lesions have been successfully excised from both the lung and the brain. The value of chemotherapy has not been established in systemic infections, but intravenous amphotericin B shows enough promise to warrant its use.

GEOTRICHOSIS

DEFINITION. Geotrichosis is the name given to certain disorders of the mouth, bronchi, and intestinal tract from which *Geotrichium candidum* has been isolated. This fungus has not been established as a human pathogen, and the validity of geotrichosis as a disease entity remains questionable.

ETIOLOGY. The fungus *G. candidum* may resemble *Coccidioides immitis* in culture because its septate mycelium fragments into large square-ended arthrospores. *Geotrichium candidum* does not form sporangia in vivo, however, and its soft creamy colonies on solid medium are easily distinguished from those of *C. immitis*.

PATHOGENESIS. Geotrichium is a normal inhabitant of the pharynx and bowel and may proliferate locally to produce visible white colonies on the mucous membranes. It may also appear in devitalized tissues and secretions of the nasopharynx, bronchopulmonary tree, and colon but probably not as a primary pathogen.

CLINICAL MANIFESTATIONS. Geotrichosis is reported to cause pulmonary cavities and colitis. In bronchopulmonary geotrichosis, the patient coughs up gelatinous sputum tinged with blood, and in rare cases thin-walled cavities like those of coccidioidomycosis have been described.

DIAGNOSIS. In secretions and exudates, *G. candidum* has the appearance of oval or barrel-shaped spores measuring up to 8 to 10 mm in diameter. They are easily recovered on Sabouraud's agar at room temperature.

TREATMENT. Lesions resembling thrush respond to local application of 1:10,000 solution of gentian violet. Bronchopulmonary geotrichosis is said to respond to oral treatment with potassium iodide, and intestinal geotrichosis is treated by oral administration three times daily of capsules containing 0.32 mg gentian violet.

MYCETOMA

DEFINITION. Mycetoma is a chronic destructive infection of the skin, subcutaneous tissues, fascia, and bone. The infection produces a localized swelling containing multiple fistulas which extrude mycotic granules.

ETIOLOGY. The most frequent cause of mycetoma in the United States is a higher fungus known as *Monosporium apiospermum*, the "imperfect" form of the ascomycete *Allescheria boydii*. It grows rapidly on Sabouraud's agar as a cottony mycelium bearing asexual spores either singly or in small groups at the tips or sides of conidiophores. Other higher fungi isolated in mycetoma include members of such diverse genera as *Aspergillus*, *Penicillium*, *Madurella*, *Cephalosporium*, and *Phialophora*.

Members of the genus *Nocardia* are important causes of mycetoma outside the United States. *Nocardia madurae* is found in southeastern Asia and *N. brasiliensis* in South America and Mexico.

PATHOGENESIS AND PATHOLOGY. The fungi found in mycetoma are inhabitants of the soil and enter the tissues of the bare foot and leg, presumably after trauma. The chest wall is infected by sacks, contaminated with soil, and carried over the shoulder. The buttocks, abdomen, and arm are also infected.

The infection begins in the outer tissues and burrows through to destroy bone, muscle, and connective tissue indiscriminately. The areas of destruction show chronic suppuration with fibrosis and are connected by multiple fistulas which rupture to the outside. Mycotic granules are seen in the suppurative foci. The prolonged proliferation of granulation and scar tissue leads to enlargement of the affected part.

CLINICAL MANIFESTATIONS. The earliest sign is usually a small swelling on the sole or dorsum of the foot which undergoes a recurring cycle of swelling, suppuration, and healing. Later, similar lesions appear on other parts of the foot, and over a period of months destruction of deeper tissues is manifested by slight or moderate pain, generalized swelling, and redness. The course is intermittently progressive, and there may be periods of remission. Ultimately the foot becomes a swollen, deformed mass of destroyed tissue with many fistulous openings through which mycotic granules are discharged. The infection does not spread hematogenously to other parts, but in rare instances there is direct extension along lymphatics. Death may occur from secondary bacterial infection.

DIAGNOSIS. The characteristic granules are 0.5 to 2 mm in diameter and may be white, yellow, black, or red. Nocardial granules are easily distinguished from those of *Aspergillus boydii* and other higher fungi by direct microscopic examination. They are masses of radiating gram-positive filaments; those of higher fungi contain large segmented hyphae and numerous chlamydospores. Either type of granule grows rapidly on Sabouraud's agar.

Roentgenograms disclose destruction of bone which is more extensive than the external appearance and pain might indicate.

TREATMENT. Nocardial mycetomas should be treated with oral sulfonamides, and those due to higher fungi with intravenous and local amphotericin B. Antibacterial chemotherapy is valuable in arresting secondary infection. There is no dependable cure, however, and many cases eventually require amputation.

CHROMOBLASTOMYCOSIS

DEFINITION. Chromoblastomycosis is an infection of the skin produced by several species of the genus *Phialophora* and characterized by slowly progressive cauliflower-like lesions of the skin of agricultural workers in tropical or subtropical regions.

ETIOLOGY. The three species *P. pedrosi*, *P. compactum*, and *P. verrucosa* cannot be distinguished upon microscopic examination of infected tissue, in which all appear as small clusters of spores with thick, dark-brown walls. On culture, however, the three differ in their methods of sporulation. The species most commonly found, *P. pedrosi*, exhibits three types of spore formation: (1) branching chains of spores borne at the tips of long conidiophores, (2) clusters of spores forming sleeves about the hyphae, and (3) balls of spores arising in the cuplike ends of very short flask-shaped conidiophores. *Phialophora verrucosa* forms only the third type of spore, and *P. compactum* is recognized by chains of spores arranged in compact masses. On Sabouraud's agar all three grow very slowly and will produce deeply pigmented olive or black colonies.

PATHOGENESIS AND PATHOLOGY. The fungi undoubtedly live in the soil or vegetation and enter the skin of agricultural workers. The disease occurs mostly on the lower extremity of barefoot workmen, but sometimes on the upper extremity or buttocks.

Three pathologic processes are found: (1) microabscesses in the dermis containing numerous fungi, (2) extensive fibrosis, and (3) epidermal hyperplasia and hyperkeratosis. The lesions progress along the lymphatics but only rarely beyond them, and they do not penetrate deeply to involve bone. A few cases of brain abscesses have occurred.

CLINICAL MANIFESTATIONS. The earliest lesion is a papule, which develops into a well-circumscribed bluish lesion with a warty, raised margin. Although it resembles the cutaneous form of North American blastomycosis at this early stage, it does not spread peripherally. Instead, adjacent new lesions appear over a period of years and, as the epithelial hyperplasia and hyperkeratosis increase, the entire area assumes a cauliflower-like appearance. Eventually the whole extremity is covered. Pain and constitutional symptoms are absent unless secondary bacterial infection occurs or elephantiasis develops as a result of lymphatic scarring.

DIAGNOSIS. The typical dark-brown septate bodies are seen in large numbers in biopsied tissue or pus, and brown hyphae can be found in crusts treated with 10 percent potassium hydroxide. For specific identification, however, it is necessary to culture the slowly growing fungus on Sabouraud's agar.

TREATMENT. Early in the disease, the lesions may be destroyed by electrocoagulation or removed by surgical excision. Later in the course, excision of the larger nodules leaves indolent ulcers which heal very slowly.

Saturated solution of potassium iodide, given to tolerance orally, as in sporotrichosis, is said to be effective when combined with weekly injections of calcipherol. Local injection into the lesions of 0.035 mg amphotericin B in 7 ml of 2 percent procaine solution at weekly intervals has been used because the organisms are resistant to the levels achieved after intravenous injection. This local treatment produced complete resolution of lesions in a limited trial and should be tried. In general, the treatment of chromoblastomycosis has been disappointing. The disease is never fatal, however, and the usefulness of the limb is retained despite its unsightly appearance.

RHINOSPORIDIOSIS

DEFINITION. Rhinosporidiosis produces small tumorlike masses usually confined to the nose and nasopharynx. An endosporulating fungus seen in the tissues cannot be cultured on laboratory media.

ETIOLOGY. The fungus *Rhinosporidium seeberi* is placed in the class Phycomycetes and family Coccidioidaceae because characteristic giant sporangia develop in the tissues. These thick-walled endospore-filled sporangia may reach 500 μ in diameter but otherwise resemble the smaller spherules of *Coccidiodes immitis*.

PATHOGENESIS AND PATHOLOGY. The disease is probably acquired by bathing or diving into infected water. In India, where rhinosporidiosis reaches endemic proportions, its rarity in women is attributed to social taboos that prohibit their bathing in open places. The characteristic lesion is a vascularized papillomatous proliferation of the nasal or pharyngeal mucous membrane containing sporangia in various stages of maturity. Red cells, inflammatory cells, and extruded endospores fill the interstitial tissue. As sporangia enlarge they compress the columnar epithelium of the nose or the squamous epithelium of the pharynx and allow endospores to escape and reinoculate the adjacent tissue.

CLINICAL MANIFESTATIONS. Single or multiple pedunculated fleshy red masses appear in the nares or pharynx and produce symptoms of rhinitis, epistaxis, and nasal obstruction. In exceptional cases hoarseness may develop from laryngeal infection. The conjunctivas and lacrimal sac may also be involved.

DIAGNOSIS. The characteristic sporangia are easily identified in biopsied tissue section. Because the only endemic foci are in India, most patients are Asiatic.

TREATMENT. The lesions can be completely removed surgically or by electrocautery. Electrocautery is preferred because surgery leaves open incisions in which spores can be implanted.

REFERENCES

Aspergillosis

Finegold, S. M., D. Well, and J. F. Murray: Aspergillosis: A Review and Report of Twelve Cases, Am. J. Med., 27:463, 1959.

Grcevic, N., and W. F. Mathews: Pathologic Changes in Acute Disseminated Aspergillosis, Am. J. Clin. Pathol., 35:536, 1959.

Naji, A. F.: Bronchopulmonary Aspergillosis, A.M.A. Arch. Pathol., 68:282, 1959.

Pepys, J., R. W. Reddell, K. M. Citron, Y. M. Clayton, and E. I. Short: Clinical and Immunological Significance of *Aspergillus Fumigatus* in the Sputum, Am. Rev. Resp. Dis., 80:167, 1959.

Chromoblastomycosis

Barwasser, N. C.: Chromoblastomycosis: Thirteenth Reported Case in the United States, J.A.M.A., 153:556, 1953.

Binford, C. H., G. Hess, and C. W. Emmons: Chromoblastomycosis, Arch. Dermatol. Syphilol., 49:398, 1944.

Conway, H., and W. Berkeley: Chromoblastomycosis (Mycetoma Form) Treated by Surgical Excision, A.M.A. Arch. Dermatol. Syphilol., 66:695, 1952.

Geotrichosis

Kunstadter, R. H., A. Milzer, and F. Whitcomb: Bronchopulmonary Geotrichosis in Children, Am. J. Dis. Child., 79:82, 1950.

Smith, D. T.: Geotrichosis, J. Chronic Dis., 5:532, 1957.

Mycetoma

Ajello, L.: Soil as Natural Reservoir for Human Pathogenic Fungi, Science, 123:876, 1956.

Rhinosporidiosis

Purandare, N. M., and S. M., Deoras: Rhinosporidiosis in Bombay, Indian J. Med. Sci., 7:603, 1953.

Section 12

The Rickettsioses

194 GENERAL CONSIDERATIONS AND PATHOLOGY

Theodore E. Woodward and
Elizabeth B. Jackson

The rickettsial diseases of man consist of a variety of clinical entities caused by microorganisms of the family *Rickettsiaceae*. The rickettsias are obligate intracellular parasites about the size of bacteria and are usually seen microscopically as pleomorphic coccobacilli. Each of the rickettsias pathogenic for man is capable of multiplying in one or more species of arthropod as well as in animals and man. Indeed, the majority of the rickettsias are maintained in nature by a cycle which involves an insect vector and an animal reservoir, and infection

Table 194-1. RICKETTSIAL DISEASES

Group	Disease		Geographic distribution	Natural cycle		Transmission to man	Serologic diagnosis	
	Type	Agent		Arthropod	Mammal		Weil-Felix reaction	Complement fixation
Spotted fever	Rocky Mountain spotted fever	*R. rickettsii*	Western hemisphere	Ticks	Wild rodents; dogs	Tick bite	Positive OX-19 OX-2	Positive group- and type-specific
	Boutonneuse fever	*R. conorii*	Africa, Europe, Middle East, India					
	Queensland tick typhus	*R. australis*	Australia		Marsupials, wild rodents			
	North Asian tick-borne rickettsiosis	*R. sibirica*	Siberia, Mongolia		Wild rodents			
	Rickettsial-pox	*R. akari*	United States, Russia, Africa(?)	Blood-sucking mite	House mouse, other rodents	Mite bite	Negative	
Typhus	Endemic (murine)	*R. mooseri*	Worldwide	Flea	Small rodents	Infected flea feces into broken skin	Positive OX-19	Positive group- and type-specific
	Epidemic	*R. prowazeki*	Worldwide	Body louse	Man	Infected louse feces into broken skin	Positive OX-19	
	Brill-Zinsser disease	*R. prowazeki*	Worldwide	Recurrence years after original attack of epidemic typhus			Usually negative	
	Scrub	*R. tsutsuga-mushi*	Asia, Australia, Pacific islands	Trombiculid mites	Wild rodents	Mite bite	Positive OX-K	Positive in about 50% of patients
Q fever		*R. burnetii*	Worldwide	Ticks	Small mammals, cattle, sheep, goats	Inhalation of dried infected material	Negative	Positive
Trench fever		*R. quintana*	Europe, Africa, North America	Body louse	Man	Infected louse feces into broken skin	Negative	None available

of man is unimportant in the cycle. Epidemic typhus presents a number of points of dissimilarity to most of the other rickettsioses, because the natural cycle of infection involves only man and the louse. Moreover, the agent of epidemic typhus has not established a well-organized parasitic relationship which ensures its perpetuation either in its mammalian host and reservoir (man) or in its arthropod host (louse). Man frequently dies from epidemic typhus; only rarely do recovered patients serve as a reservoir and infect their body lice.

Furthermore, the louse is relatively poorly adapted to perpetuation of the rickettsias, which induce a fatal disease in this arthropod. In contrast, most rickettsias cause only a mild disease in their mammalian hosts and do not affect their vector adversely; indeed, a number are transmitted transovarially in arthropods from one generation to the next.

A compendium of information on the rickettsial diseases is presented in Table 194-1. Because each of the rickettsioses responds therapeutically to tetracyclines or chloramphenicol, the table mentions no therapy. Procedures for diagnostic isolation of the rickettsias are omitted because they generally are less useful than serologic methods, and the techniques which they require are highly specialized and hazardous. Information on isolation may be found in textbooks devoted to viral and rickettsial diseases.

HISTORY OF THE RICKETTSIAL DISEASES. Of all the afflictions of mankind the rickettsial diseases, particularly epidemic typhus, rank among the foremost as a cause of human suffering and death. Classical typhus fever undoubtedly existed during ancient times, although Zinsser cites an outbreak of illness in 1083 in a monastery near Salerno, Italy, as the first probable recorded incidence of this disease. Typhus fever, through its able transmitter, the body louse, has always identified itself intimately with wars, famines, and human catastrophes of all kinds. Alone it has cast a decisive vote in the outcome of many military campaigns.

The record of deaths from epidemic typhus in this century in the Balkan countries and in Poland and Russia reaches astounding figures. Serbia in 1915 suffered an epidemic of major proportions, with 150,000 dead and a mortality rate ranging from 20 to 60 percent. Typhus ravaged Russia and eastern Poland from 1915 to 1922, infecting 30 million of the inhabitants and causing an estimated 3 million deaths.

The past two decades have seen the development of excellent methods for the prevention and treatment of the rickettsioses of man. In fact, these measures have been so successful that the rickettsioses have become of minor importance in the United States and in many other countries. Although conquered, the rickettsioses have not been eliminated, and they could again become rampant if the will to control them, the present high standards of sanitation, and the necessary industrial capacities for production of effective insecticides and therapeutic agents should be decreased through war or disaster. It is worthwhile to review the classical milestones representing the clinical and scientific contributions which have resulted in the understanding and conquest of the rickettsial infections.

Gerhard in 1836 differentiated typhoid fever from louse-borne typhus fever. In 1899, Maxcy described the clinical manifestations of Rocky Mountain spotted fever. In a series of studies from 1906 to 1909, Ricketts, for whom the rickettsial microorganisms are named, successfully transmitted this disease to guinea pigs, incriminated the wood tick as a vector, and observed rickettsias in smears prepared from tick tissues.

Nicolle in 1909 reproduced typhus fever in monkeys and demonstrated transmission by the body louse. Von Prowazek in 1914 and Da Rocha-Lima in 1916 demonstrated small microorganisms in the tissues of lice taken from typhus patients.

Brill in 1910 recognized a febrile disease in patients in New York City as an example of mild epidemic typhus unassociated with lousiness. Zinsser in 1934 postulated that this disease was a recurrent form of typhus occurring in patients during periods of stress or waning immunity. Subsequent studies have confirmed Zinsser's hypothesis. This entity is now called Brill-Zinsser disease.

Weil and Felix, working with typhus patients in Poland in 1915, recognized that agglutinins for certain proteus organisms appeared in the serum of convalescent patients. The Weil-Felix reaction, although nonspecific, affords a simple and valuable screening method for several rickettsioses.

In 1926 Maxcy, on purely epidemiologic evidence, surmised that typhus in the United States had its reservoir in rodents and was transmitted to man by ticks or fleas. Confirmation of Maxcy's hypothesis was obtained in Baltimore in 1930 by Dyer and others when they isolated rickettsias from the brains of rats and shortly thereafter incriminated the flea as a vector. This disease, caused by *Rickettsia moorseri* and now designated endemic or murine typhus, is distinct from epidemic typhus and Brill-Zinsser disease.

The development of suitable vaccines and specific diagnostic antigens was impeded until it was possible to prepare appreciable quantities of highly infectious rickettsial material in the laboratory. The most important steps were (1) the Weigl vaccine (1930), a phenolized suspension of gut tissue obtained from body lice which had been injected intrarectally with the rickettsias of epidemic typhus; (2) the killed murine typhus vaccine prepared by Casteneda (1939) from lung tissues of rats injected intranasally; and (3) the inactivated Rocky Mountain spotted fever vaccine obtained by Cox (1941) from infected yolk sacs of embryonated hen eggs. Each of the developments was applied in principle to other rickettsial agents, but the low cost and relative simplicity of the egg techniques have led to their general use for preparation of vaccines and diagnostic antigens. The specific diagnostic complement fixation tests for the rickettsial diseases now used in the United States stem directly from the pioneering work of Bengston on Q fever and of Plotz on the spotted and typhus fevers during the early 1940s.

The years of World War II saw many strides in the conquest of the rickettsioses; perhaps greatest among these were the highly successful attacks on the arthropod vectors. The lousicide DDT proved to be ideal for control when dusted on the clothes of infested persons. The epidemic at Naples during the winter of 1943 to 1944 established a milestone, because it was the first to be suppressed by the use of insecticides. On the other side of the world, scrub typhus (mite-borne typhus) was creating a major problem in military medicine in the Pacific area. Here, too, the major contributions to successful control were concerned with application of miticidal chemicals to the person and his clothes.

Hyperimmune rabbit serum (Topping, 1939) ameliorated the course of Rocky Mountain spotted fever if given during the early stages, and para-aminobenzoic acid (Yeomans, 1944) was found to be effective in typhus fever, but the advent of broad-spectrum antibiotics, first chloramphenicol, then chlortetracycline in 1948, and later oxytetracycline, provided dramatic therapeutic results in each of the rickettsioses.

Table 194-1 includes several rickettsial diseases which have not been mentioned in this historical review. Although important in themselves, none except Q fever has been the subject of work which contributed broad principles applicable to the group.

PATHOGENESIS. Rickettsial diseases of man develop following infection through the skin or the respiratory tract. Agents of the typhus and spotted fever group are introduced through the bite of the infected arthropod vector. Ticks and mites, which transmit the spotted fevers and scrub typhus, inoculate the rickettsias directly into the dermis during feeding. The louse and flea, which transmit epidemic and murine typhus, respectively, deposit infected feces on the skin; infection occurs when organisms are rubbed into the puncture wound made by the arthropod. The rickettsia of Q fever gain entry through the respiratory tract by inhalation of infected dust; moreover, the respiratory route is occasionally implicated in epidemic typhus when infection results from inhalation of dried infected louse feces.

Although organisms probably multiply at the original site of entry in all instances, local lesions appear with regularity only in certain diseases, namely, the initial cutaneous lesions of scrub typhus, rickettsialpox, and boutonneuse fever and the pneumonitis which develops in about half the persons infected with Q fever.

Volunteers infected with either scrub typhus or Q fever develop rickettsemia late in the incubation period, often some hours before the onset of fever. Similar events probably occur in all the rickettsial diseases; certainly circulating rickettsias can be detected during the early febrile period in practically all patients. Little is known about the pathogenesis of infection during the midportion of the incubation period. However, it is reasonable to assume that, during this time in patients with typhus or spotted fever, a transient low-grade rickettsemia results from release of organisms multiplying at the initial site of infection and that this seeds infection in the endothelial cells of the vascular tree. Vascular lesions developing at such sites could account for the pathologic changes, including the rash.

Rickettsia apparently invade and proliferate in the endothelial cells of small blood vessels. Endothelial cell destruction occurs from the proliferation of organisms and eventual disruption. Rickettsia may exert a cytotoxic effect on endothelial cells; in mice the rickettsial toxin causes remarkable increase in capillary permeability, independent of proliferation. Whether later manifestations in rickettsial diseases result from immunopathologic mechanisms is unknown.

The underlying cause of the toxic-febrile state which characterizes the rickettsial diseases remains unknown. Several rickettsial species contain type-specific toxins which are lethal for mice; these may play a role.

PATHOLOGY. The basic lesions in the spotted and typhus fever groups are in the small vessels. The most diverse and extensive of these are found in Rocky Mountain spotted fever. Here swelling, proliferation, and degeneration of the endothelial cells occur, frequently with thrombus formation which partially or completely obliterates the lumen. The muscle cells of the arteriole undergo swelling and fibrinoid changes. The adventitial tissues are infiltrated with mononuclear leukocytes, lymphocytes, and plasma cells. The vascular damage is scattered along the arteries, veins, and capillaries, with normal architecture prevailing throughout most of the vascular bed. The changes in murine, epidemic, and scrub typhus fevers resemble those in Rocky Mountain spotted fever, but thrombosis is uncommon and involvement of the musculature is rare.

The vascular changes, with resultant lesions in adjacent parenchymatous tissues, occur throughout the body but are most conspicuous in the heart, lung, and brain. Interstitial myocarditis occurs in each of these diseases but is usually most extensive in Rocky Mountain spotted fever and in scrub typhus. In the brain, the glial nodule is found in all members of the group; but microinfarcts in the brain tissue or in the myocardium are most often observed in spotted fever.

A rickettsial pneumonitis occurs, at least to some extent, in many patients with spotted or typhus fever and is the characteristic pathologic change in patients with Q fever. The process is patchy and consists macroscopically of areas of congestion and edema with gray granular consolidation. Microscopically, in the consolidated areas the alveoli are filled with compact fibrinocellular exudate containing lymphocytes, plasma cells, large mononuclear cells, and erythrocytes, but few if any polymorphonuclear leukocytes.

Rickettsias can occasionally be observed microscopically in sections of tissue. However failure to demonstrate rickettsias in histologic section is of no diagnostic significance.

LABORATORY DIAGNOSIS. Diagnostic procedures which depend on isolation of the etiologic agent from blood or other clinical material are expensive, time-consuming, and hazardous to laboratory personnel. Except in unusual circumstances the currently available serologic tests are adequate for laboratory confirmation of the clinical diagnosis in each of the rickettsial diseases.

As in most serologic diagnostic procedures the demonstration of a rise in titer of specific antibody during convalescence is of prime importance in establishing the laboratory confirmation. Table 194-2 summarizes the serologic results usually encountered in persons who suffer from rickettsial diseases in the United States. The Weil-Felix test employing Proteus strains OX-19 and OX-2 gives positive results in patients with spotted fever and murine typhus and negative results in those with rickettsialpox and Q fever. It is useful as a screening proce-

Table 194-2. SEROLOGIC DIAGNOSIS OF RICKETTSIAL DISEASES OF THE UNITED STATES

Group	Disease	Weil-Felix reaction				Complement fixation tests with type-specific antigen				
		Proteus	Illustrative titer		Cases with diagnostic titer	Rickettsial antigen	Illustrative titer			Cases with diagnostic titer
			10th day	20th day			10th day	20th day	30th day	
Spotted fever	Rocky Mountain spotted fever	OX-19	40	320	Most	R. rickettsii	20	160	80	Most
		OX-2	20	160						
	Rickettsialpox	OX-19	0	0	None	R. akari	0	64	128	Most
		OX-2	0	0						
Typhus.....	Murine typhus	OX-19	160	640	Most	R. mooseri	0	160	160	Most
		OX-2	10	40						
	Brill-Zinsser disease	OX-19	160	20	Infrequent	R. prowazeki	1,280	640	320	Most
		OX-2	0	0						
	Q fever	OX 19	0	0	None	R. burnetii	10	80	160	Most
		OX-2	0	0						

dure but cannot be relied upon to differentiate spotted fever from murine typhus. In patients with Brill-Zinsser disease the *Proteus* OX-19 reaction is usually negative or low in titer.

Complement fixation tests employing group-specific rickettsial antigens provide data which clearly differentiate the most common infections, i.e., murine typhus, Rocky Mountain spotted fever, and Q fever. Moreover, if type-specific rickettsial antigens are employed, it is generally possible to distinguish rickettsialpox from spotted fever and Brill-Zinsser disease from murine typhus.

Antibodies during response to a primary infection of epidemic typhus or Rocky Mountain spotted fever are usually 19S globulins. In patients with Brill-Zinsser disease, which is a recrudescence, antibodies occur more quickly—within several days after onset of illness—rise to a higher titer, and are 7S globulins.

Specific antibiotic therapy has little effect on the time of appearance of antibodies or on their ultimate titer, provided treatment is instituted some days after onset of the illness. However, if the illness is cut short by early and vigorous treatment, antibody production may be delayed for a week or so, and also the maximal titers attained may be below those illustrated in Table 194-2. Under these circumstances a sample of blood taken 4 to 6 weeks after onset of illness should also be tested.

An additional serologic test is based on the agglutination of sheep or human O erythrocytes after sensitization with a serologically active fraction of rickettsias designated ESS (erythrocyte-sensitizing substances). Erythrocytes exposed to the typhus ESS are specifically agglutinated by serums of patients as early as the eighth febrile day. The ESS test is simple and inexpensive.

The immunofluorescent antibody test is a very useful procedure for detecting rickettsia in the tissues of pa-tients with the typhus group of rickettsioses, the spotted fevers, and Q fever. The technique also visualizes rickettsia in ticks and the tissues of animals.

Except for normochromic anemia, which occurs in patients severely ill with rickettsial diseases, there are no other distinctive alterations in the hematologic picture. The white blood cell count in Rocky Mountain spotted fever, rickettsialpox, murine and epidemic typhus, Brill-Zinsser disease, Q fever, and others is usually within the normal range: 6,000 to 10,000 cells per cu mm. Leukopenia is occasionally observed, and in the presence of complications, such as superimposed infections and extensive vascular lesions, moderate leukocytosis occurs. The differential blood count is usually normal.

195 ROCKY MOUNTAIN SPOTTED FEVER

Theodore E. Woodward and Elizabeth B. Jackson

DEFINITION. Rocky Mountain spotted fever is an acute febrile illness caused by *Rickettsia rickettsii*, transmitted to man by ticks. The disease is characterized by sudden onset with headache and chills and by fever which persists for 2 to 3 weeks. A characteristic exanthem appears on the extremities and trunk about the fourth day of illness. Delirium, shock, and renal failure occur in the severely ill.

ETIOLOGY AND EPIDEMIOLOGY. The causative microbe *R. rickettsii* is the prototype for the rickettsial group of agents. The minute organisms are purple when stained by Giemsa's method or red by Macchiavello's technique; most are gram-negative. They are surrounded by a halo as if encapsulated. These organisms often occur in pairs and possess a cell wall similar in structure and chemical composition to that of gram-negative bacteria; there is a cell membrane, cytoplasmic granules corresponding to ribosomes, and procariotic organization of nuclear material. The cell membrane is selectively permeable; the cell wall is the focus of important antigens and an endotoxin-like substance.

The rickettsias grow in the nucleus and the cytoplasm of infected cells of ticks, mammals, and embryonated eggs; the intranuclear situation of the organisms is shared by the other members of the spotted fever group, but not by rickettsias of the typhus group. *Rickettsia rickettsii* is readily disinguishable from the agents of the typhus fevers by cross-immunity tests in guinea pigs and by complement fixation tests employing antigens prepared from infected yolk sac tissues. The differentiation of *R. rickettsii* from closely related members of the spotted fever group frequently requires elaborate procedures. Strains of the agent of Rocky Mountain spotted fever vary considerably in their virulence for man and animals.

The first reports of spotted fever in Idaho and Montana during the final decade of the last century led to the name Rocky Mountain spotted fever. However, the disease has been reported in all states except Maine and Vermont, as well as in Canada, Mexico, Colombia, and Brazil. Although related diseases are found on other continents, this particular infection is limited to the Western Hemisphere. Formerly about 500 but currently about 200 cases of spotted fever occur annually in the United States. The mortality in the days before specific therapy was about 20 percent but has decreased to about 5 percent. Although the attack rate per unit of population is highest in Wyoming, almost half the cases occur in the South Atlantic states, with the greatest number of these in Virginia, North Carolina, Georgia, and Maryland.

A number of species of ticks are found infected with *R. rickettsii* in nature, but only two are important in transmitting spotted fever to man. These are *Dermacentor andersoni*, the wood tick, which is the principal vector in the West, and *D. variabilis*, the dog tick, which assumes this role in the East. Infected female ticks transmit the agent transovarially to at least some of their offspring. Ticks which become infected, either through the egg or at one of the stages during their development cycle by feeding on an infected mammal, harbor the rickettsias throughout their lifetime, which may be several years. Thus, the tick serves as a reservoir in addition to being a vector. Small wild mammals are suspected of playing an important role in spreading the rickettsias in nature by infecting ticks which feed on them during rickettsemia.

Disease in man is generally acquired from the bite of an infected tick. Transmission is unlikely unless the tick remains attached for a number of hours. Infection may also be acquired through abrasions in the skin which become contaminated with infected tick feces or tissue juices; hence, the hazard associated with crushing ticks between the fingers when removing them from persons or animals.

There are seasonal variations in the incidence of cases of spotted fever, as well as differences in age and sex distribution of cases. In each instance these differences are related to exposure to ticks. Most cases are seen during the period of maximal tick activity, i.e., late spring and early summer. About half the cases in the Western states occur in men over forty, whereas half those in the Eastern states were in children under fifteen. This age distribution is undoubtedly influenced by propinquity to the wood and dog ticks, respectively. Mortality increases with age of the patient.

CLINICAL MANIFESTATIONS. Incubation Period and Prodromata. A history of tick bite is elicited in approximately 80 percent of patients. The incubation period varies between 3 and 12 days with a mean of 7. A short incubation period usually indicates a more serious infection.

Onset. In nonvaccinated persons, the onset is usually abrupt, with severe headache, a sudden shaking rigor, prostration, generalized myalgia, especially in the back and leg muscles, nausea with occasional vomiting, and fever which reaches 103 to 104°F within the first 2 days. Pain in the abdominal muscles may be severe, and arthralgia is not uncommon. Deep muscle palpation often elicits tenderness. Occasionally the debut of illness in children and adults is mild, accompanied by lethargy, anorexia, cephalgia, and low-grade fever. These symptoms are similar to those of many acute infectious diseases, making specific diagnosis difficult during the first few days.

Pyrexia. Fever continues for approximately 15 to 20 days in untreated cases. The febrile course in children may be shorter. Hyperthermia of 105°F or greater is of unfavorable prognostic significance, although fatalities may occur when the patient is hypothermic, with concurrent vasomotor collapse. Fever generally terminates by lysis over a period of several days, but rarely does so by crisis. Recurrent fever is uncommon except in the presence of secondary pyogenic complications.

The *headache* is generalized and excruciating, and frequently more intense over the frontal area. It persists throughout the first and second week of illness in untreated cases. Malaise continues for the first week; irritability is notable, and the patient shuns distractions such as questioning and examination.

Cutaneous Manifestations. The rash which is present in practically all cases is the most characteristic and helpful diagnostic sign. It usually appears on the fourth febrile day; the range is 2 to 6 days. The initial lesions are on the wrists, ankles, palms, soles, and forearms. The first lesions are macular, nonfixed, pink, irregularly defined, and measure 2 to 6 mm. A warm compress applied to the extremity accentuates the rash in the early stages. The exanthem is most prominent when the temperature is elevated. After 6 to 12 hr, the rash extends centripetally to the axilla, buttocks, trunk, neck, and face. (This is in contrast to the eruption of typhus fever, which begins on the trunk and spreads centrifugally, rarely involving the face, palms, or soles.) The rash becomes maculopapular after 2 to 3 days (it may be felt by light palpation) and assumes a deeper red hue. By about the fourth day it is petechial and fails to fade on pressure. Not uncommonly, the hemorrhagic lesions coalesce to form large ecchymotic blemishes; these lesions tend to form over bony prominences and may ultimately slough to form indolent, slow-healing ulcers. Patients who have had the typical rash show brownish discolorations at the site for several weeks during convalescence. In milder cases, the rash does not become purpuric and may disappear within a few days. Antibiotic therapy may abort the early exanthem; the later fixed lesion fades less rapidly with specific therapy.

The application of tourniquets for several minutes, or the occasional taking of the blood pressure, may provoke additional petechiae (Rumpel-Leede phenomenon), further evidence of capillary abnormalities.

Cardiovascular and Respiratory Features. During the early stages, the pulse is full and regular but accelerated in proportion to the height of the temperature, and the blood pressure is well sustained. During the peak of illness in seriously ill patients, the pulse is rapid and feeble, and hypotension of 90 mm Hg is common. If circulatory failure is sustained, the resultant hypoxia and shock lead to agitation and delirium and contribute to the formation of ecchymoses and gangrene of fingers, toes, genitalia, buttocks, earlobes, and nose. Cyanosis of the peripheral parts of the body is common. Venous pressure determinations show no elevation. A reduction of the total blood volume is occasionally found, as are evidences of myocardial impairment as shown by low voltage of ventricular complexes, minor S-T segment deflections, and occasionally delay in atrioventricular conduction on the electrocardiogram. These changes are transient and nonspecific. Severely ill patients have a puffy appearance of the face, hands, ankles, feet, and lower sacrum.

Respirations are either normal or slightly accelerated. Cough may be harassing and nonproductive, and localized pneumonitis may occur, but pulmonary consolidation is extremely rare. Pulmonary edema may develop after injudicious use of intravenous fluids.

Hepatic and Renal Manifestations. In the majority of patients, there is little alteration in renal or hepatic function. The liver may be enlarged, but jaundice is unusual. Oliguria commonly occurs in the seriously ill, and anuria may mark the critically ill patient. Azotemia is common and when marked, is a very unfavorable sign. Abnormalities in liver function are probably responsible for the hypoproteinemia, with reduction in the albumin fraction.

Neurologic Manifestations. The principal neurologic manifestations are headache, restlessness, and varying degrees of insomnia. Stiffness of the back is common. The cerebrospinal fluid is clear, with normal dynamics and normal chemical constituents. Coma and muscular rigidity may occur. Athetoid movements, convulsive seizures, and hemiplegia are grave manifestations. Deafness during the active stages of the disease is not uncommon. As a rule, all neurologic signs abate without residua. Findings based upon follow-up examinations and electroencephalograms may be interpreted as indicative of minor residual brain damage for a year or more following

recovery of certain patients from Rocky Mountain spotted fever.

Other Physical Manifestations. Patients become dehydrated, with extreme dryness of lips, gums, tongue, and pharynx. The skin is hot and dry, the conjunctivas are frequently injected, and the eyes suffused. Photophobia is common in the early stages of illness. Petechial hemorrhages may be noted in the conjunctivas or in the retina. The spleen is enlarged in approximately one-half the cases and is firm and nontender. Abdominal distension is frequent, and occasionally some degree of intestinal ileus is observed. Constipation is usual.

COURSE OF DISEASE. In mild and moderately severe cases given no specific antibiotic therapy, the disease abates within 2 weeks, and convalescence is rapid. In fatal cases death usually occurs during the latter part of the second week as a result of toxemia, vasomotor weakness, and shock or renal failure.

In vaccinated individuals who contract the disease, the illness is mild, with a short febrile course and an atypical rash.

COMPLICATIONS AND PROGNOSIS. If the serious manifestations of spotted fever mentioned above are regarded as intrinsic parts of the disease, then complications are uncommon and consist mainly of secondary bacterial infections, namely, bronchopneumonia, otitis media, and parotitis. Thrombosis of major blood vessels may result in gangrene of a portion of an extremity. Hemiplegia and peripheral neuritis are rare sequelae.

The overall mortality rate for spotted fever was formerly about 20 percent. Death occurred in more than half of persons over forty years of age but mortality was much lower in children and young adults. Since the introduction of the broad-spectrum antibiotics and the development of more precise knowledge regarding correction of the physiologic abnormalities which develop during the disease, fewer deaths occur from this infection. Some of the fatalities can be attributed to failure to consider spotted fever in the differential diagnosis.

DIFFERENTIAL DIAGNOSIS. During the early stages of infection before the rash has appeared, differentiation from other acute infections is difficult. History of tick bite while living or traveling in a highly endemic area is helpful. The rash of meningococcemia (Chap. 142) resembles Rocky Mountain spotted fever in certain aspects, because it is macular, maculopapular, or petechial in the chronic form, and petechial, confluent, or ecchymotic in the fulminant type. The meningococcic skin lesion is tender and develops with extreme rapidity in the fulminant form, whereas the rickettsial rash occurs on about the fourth day of disease and gradually becomes petechial. The exanthem of rubeola rapidly becomes confluent, while that of rubella almost never becomes petechial.

Murine typhus is a milder disease than Rocky Mountain spotted fever; the rash is less extensive, nonpurpuric, nonconfluent; and renal and vascular complications are uncommon. Not infrequently differentiation of these two rickettsial infections must await the results of specific serologic tests. Epidemic typhus fever is capable of causing all the pronounced clinical, physiologic, and anatomic alterations seen in patients with Rocky Mountain spotted fever, i.e., hypotension, peripheral vascular collapse, cyanosis, skin necrosis and gangrene of digits, renal failure with azotemia, and neurologic manifestations. However, the rash of classical typhus is noted initially in the axillary folds and on the trunk and later extends peripherally, rarely involving the palms, soles, or face. The serologic patterns in these two diseases are distinctive when specific rickettsial antigens are employed in tests. Moreover, louse-borne typhus is not recognized in the United States except in the form of Brill-Zinsser disease (recurrent typhus fever). Rickettsialpox, although caused by a member of the spotted fever group of organisms, is usually readily differentiated from Rocky Mountain spotted fever by the initial lesion, the relative mildness of the illness, and the early vesiculation of the maculopapular rash. The Weil-Felix reaction is positive in Rocky Mountain spotted fever and in murine and epidemic typhus, but is negative in rickettsialpox. Agglutinins against *Proteus* OX-19 and OX-2 appear in the serum of patients with spotted fever, but only those against OX-19 are generally found in murine and epidemic typhus.

THERAPY. General. Certain physiochemical changes occurring in the patient seriously ill with one of the diseases of the typhus–spotted fever group should be understood before outlining a therapeutic regime. These changes are circulatory collapse, coma, oliguria and anuria, azotemia, anemia, hypoproteinemia, hypochloremia, and edema of the underlying tissues. These alterations are often absent in the mildly ill, and in them management is much less complicated. The therapeutic principles necessary for the treatment of all rickettsioses are (1) specific chemotherapy and (2) supportive care. Attention to both is mandatory for the seriously ill patient first recognized late in the disease. During the first week in the moderately ill patient, supportive therapy may be less energetic, because specific chemotherapy usually suffices. The early mild case may be successfully treated at home, while the later case should receive hospital care.

Therapeutic measures advisable for the management of Rocky Mountain spotted fever will be described in detail. Variations of this regimen which apply to the other rickettsioses are described in subsections relegated to other diseases of the typhus–spotted fever group and Q fever.

Specific Therapy. Specific therapy is most effective when initiated during the early stages of disease coincident with the appearance of the rash. When therapy is delayed until the rash has become hemorrhagic and widespread, the response is less dramatic. The antibiotics of choice are chloramphenicol and the tetracyclines, which are effective because of their rickettsiostatic properties. They are not rickettsiocidal.

The following antibiotic regimen is considered optimal: For chloramphenicol, an initial dose of 50 mg per kg body weight, and for tetracycline, 25 mg per kg body weight. Subsequent daily doses are the same as the initial loading dose, with the requirement divided equally and

given it at 6- to 8-hr intervals. Antibiotic treatment is continued until the patient is improved and has been afebrile approximately 24 hr. In patients too ill to take oral medication, an intravenous preparation of one of the antimicrobials may be employed for the loading dose.

Adrenal cortical hormones may need to be utilized for their antitoxemic effects, in patients first observed late in the course of severe illness. Large doses for brief periods (5 to 7 days) are recommended.

Table 195-1 summarizes information on the duration of disease and the mortality in the major rickettsioses prior to and since the introduction of specific antibiotic therapy.

Table 195-1. EFFECT OF SPECIFIC ANTIBIOTICS ON THE COURSE OF THE MAJOR RICKETTSIOSES

Disease	Untreated		Treated	
	Average duration of fever, days	Mortality, %	Average duration of fever after start of treatment, days	Mortality, %
Rocky Mountain spotted fever......	16	21	3	0
Epidemic typhus.....	14	30	2	0
Murine typhus	12	2	2	0
Scrub typhus .	14	15	1	0

Duration of Therapy and Therapeutic Response. Therapy with antibiotics is continued until the toxemia has abated, the general condition has markedly improved, and the temperature has remained at normal levels for 24 hr. In uncomplicated cases of spotted fever, there is symptomatic improvement within 24 hr and temperature becomes normal in 60 to 72 hr.

SUPPORTIVE CARE. Nursing Care. Frequent turning of the patient relieves pressure from prominent bony parts and also militates against the development of aspiration pneumonia. Proper mouth care with frequent swabbing of the oral cavity may avert the development of parotitis and gingivitis. Sucking of the juice of a lemon or the oral use of glycerin or mineral oil is helpful.

Protein Balance. A generous intake of protein should be provided by frequent feedings as soon as the disease is suspected, in order to avoid subsequent protein deficiency. Usually food is well tolerated by patients with rickettsial disease, and the daily diet should provide 3 to 5 Gm protein per kg normal body weight, with adequate carbohydrate and fat to make it palatable. When the patient is uncooperative, the diet may be supplemented by hourly liquid protein feedings via stomach tube, provided that there is no abdominal distension.

At the critical stage, when hypoproteinemia is present and changes in capillary permeability lead to edema and vascular embarrassment, careful attention is given to the parenteral administration of protein supplements. When indicated by hematologic studies, whole-blood transfusions given slowly are helpful, or if the total red cell mass is adequate, one of the preformed protein supplements is beneficial. Intravenous albumin may be particularly useful, because it also aids in the reduction of tissue edema. The judicious administration of one of the plasma expanders at this stage may have a definite favorable effect upon impending circulatory collapse. If the patient is anuric and azotemia is pronounced, overloading the circulation with protein supplements and fluids should be avoided. The type and amount of parenteral therapy should be governed by clinical judgment and very careful laboratory studies. Frequent determinations of hemoglobin, hematocrit, electrolytes, and protein, sometimes at intervals of a few hours during crucial periods, are necessary in order to ascertain abnormalities and to permit institution of corrective measures.

COMPLICATIONS. *Pyogenic complications,* including otitis media and parotitis, are encountered in patients severely ill with Rocky Mountain spotted fever and other rickettsioses. These localized infections respond to therapy with appropriate antibiotics combined with ordinary supplemental surgical measures.

Pneumonitis usually develops as a result of specific rickettsial action. The sputum is scant but should be examined to determine whether superimposed infection is present. Specific therapy is guided by the results of these laboratory studies. The pneumonitis generally responds to the antibiotic therapy the patient is receiving, but if staphylococcal pneumonia is suspected, a penicillinase-resistant penicillin should be added to the broad-spectrum drug.

Circulatory failure of peripheral or central origin is combated by careful administration of electrolytic and protein supplements. Heart failure may develop rarely from the disease or as a result of overzealous intravenous alimentation and is recognized by the common signs of rapid pulse, gallop rhythm, increase in venous pressure, and muffled cardiac sounds. When the clinical signs reveal unmistakable evidence of cardiac failure, digitalis may be employed in the usual manner. Oxygen therapy by nasal tube, mask, or tent improves the cardiac and circulatory status and is helpful in hypoxic patients with involvement of the central nervous system.

PREVENTION. Prevention is attained primarily by avoidance of tick-infested areas. When this is impractical, prophylactic measures include (1) spraying the ground with dieldrin or Chlordane for area control of ticks, (2) application of repellents such as diethyltoluamide or dimethylphthalate to clothing and exposed parts of the body, or in very heavily infested areas the wearing of clothing which interferes with attachment of ticks, i.e., boots and a one-piece outer garment, preferably impregnated with repellent, and (3) daily inspection of the entire body, including the hairy parts, to detect and remove attached ticks. In removing attached ticks great care should be taken to avoid crushing the arthropod, with resultant contamination of the bite wound; touching

the tick with gasoline or whisky encourages detachment but gentle traction with tweezers applied close to the mouth parts may be necessary; the skin area should be disinfected with soap and water or other antiseptics. Similarly, precautions should be employed in removing engorged ticks from dogs and other animals, because infection through minor abrasions on the hands is possible. Vaccines containing *R. rickettsii* are available commercially and should be used for those exposed to great risk, namely, persons frequenting highly endemic areas and laboratory workers exposed to the agent. Because the broad-spectrum antibiotics are such excellent therapeutic agents in spotted fever, there has been less impetus for vaccination of persons who run only a minor risk of infection.

196 OTHER TICK-BORNE RICKETTSIAL DISEASES

Theodore E. Woodward and Elizabeth B. Jackson

DEFINITION. Boutonneuse fever, North Asian tick-borne rickettsiosis, and Queensland tick typhus, three diseases occurring in the Eastern Hemisphere, are caused by rickettsias closely related to one another and to the agent of Rocky Mountain spotted fever. Each is transmitted by the bite of an ixodid tick. These mild to moderately severe illnesses are characterized by an initial lesion (called *tache noire* in boutonneuse fever), a fever of several days to 2 weeks, and a generalized maculopapular erythematous rash which appear on about the fifth day and usually involves the palms and soles. Specific complement-fixing antibodies appear in the patients' serums during convalescence, but agglutinins to *Proteus* OX-19 (Weil-Felix reaction) are frequently found only in low titer.

ETIOLOGY AND EPIDEMIOLOGY. The etiologic agents of these three diseases are all members of the spotted fever group of rickettsias. Together with *Rickettsia rickettsii* and *R. akari* they possess common group antigens which are readily demonstrated by agglutination and complement fixation.

Boutonneuse fever, which may be regarded as the prototype of the three, is caused by *R. conorii.* Modern serologic methods employing specific rickettsial antigens have shown this rickettsia to be the causative agent for a single widely disseminated disease known by various local names. Information on the distribution and etiology of the various tick-borne rickettsial diseases is contained in Table 194-1.

In general, the epidemiology of these tick-borne rickettsioses resembles that of spotted fever in the Western Hemisphere. Ixodid ticks and small wild animals maintain the rickettsias in nature; man, if he intrudes accidentally into the cycle, is a dead end in the transmission chain. In certain areas, the cycle of boutonneuse fever involves domiciliary environments, with the brown dog tick *Rhipicephalus sanguineus* as the dominant vector.

CLINICAL MANIFESTATIONS. These three tick-borne rickettsioses, which occur in different parts of the Eastern Hemisphere, resemble one another closely. The clinical course is usually milder than that of spotted fever, with a shorter febrile period and fewer severe complications; fatalities are rare and generally limited to the aged and debilitated. The initial lesion, which is present in most cases at the onset of fever, heals slowly; the regional lymph nodes are enlarged. The rash usually remains papular and only in severe cases becomes hemorrhagic.

The clinical picture, including the primary lesion, the geographic location, and epidemiologic considerations are helpful in establishing the diagnosis. The typhus fevers, meningococcal infections, and measles must be considered in the differential diagnosis; the serologic reactions, i.e., Weil-Felix and complement fixation tests, are of value here.

TREATMENT AND PREVENTION. Chloramphenicol and the tetracyclines are effective therapeutic agents for boutonneuse fever. Patients generally become afebrile after 2 to 3 days of treatment, and recovery is rapid. The therapeutic procedures are comparable to those used in spotted fever (Chap. 195). Presumably these measures are also applicable to North Asian tick-borne rickettsiosis and Queensland tick typhus.

The major effective methods of control are concerned with avoidance of tick bites; these include application of newer repellents and prompt removal of attached ticks. Effective vaccines are not available commercially.

197 RICKETTSIALPOX

*Theodore E. Woodward and
Elizabeth B. Jackson*

DEFINITION. Rickettsialpox is a mild, nonfatal, self-limited, febrile illness caused by *Rickettsia akari*, which is transmitted from mouse to man by mites. It is characterized by an initial skin lesion at the site of the mite bite, a week's febrile course, and a papulovesicular rash.

ETIOLOGY AND EPIDEMIOLOGY. Rickettsialpox was first recognized in New York City in 1946, and about 180 cases were reported annually for several years thereafter. It has been diagnosed in several other areas of the United States, and outbreaks have been reported in European Russia. The vector is a small, colorless mite, *Allodermanyssus sanguineus* (Hirst), which infests small mice and rodents. House mice serve as the reservoir of infection.

Rickettsia akari is morphologically and biologically similar to other rickettsias and is antigenically related to, but distinct from, *R. rickettsii*, the cause of Rocky Mountain spotted fever. Mice, guinea pigs, and fertile hen eggs are susceptible to experimental infection. Diagnostic antigens prepared from infected yolk sacs are used in complement fixation tests.

CLINICAL MANIFESTATIONS. The initial skin lesion appears about 7 to 10 days after the mite bite as a firm red papule 1 to 1.5 cm in diameter. In a few days, the center vesiculates, and the papule is sourrounded by an area of erythema. The regional lymph glands are moderately enlarged. The primary lesion, which is never painful, becomes covered with a black scab; it heals slowly, and a small scar is visible on separation of the crust.

The febrile phase begins 3 to 7 days following the initial lesion, and exanthem may accompany the fever or begin several days later. The onset of fever is sudden, with chilly sensations or frank chills, headache, sweats, myalgia, anorexia, and photophobia. The pyrexia ranges from 103 to 104°F and continues for about a week, occasionally with morning remissions.

The exanthem is maculopapular-vesicular, generalized in distribution, and may be abundant or scant. The lesions may involve the oral cavity but not the palms or soles. In a week, the vesicles dry and form scabs which eventually scale but leave no scar.

The constitutional symptoms are generally mild, and the course of illness is uncomplicated. No fatal cases have been reported.

The disease may be confused with varicella (chickenpox—Chap. 224), which is different because it occurs usually in childhood and has no initial lesion and the papular cutaneous lesion is entirely transformed into a vesicle. Variola (smallpox—Chap. 223) is accompanied by a more severe constitutional reaction, and the vesicles become pustules. The skin lesions of the other rickettsioses differ in their lack of vesiculation. The Weil-Felix reaction is usually negative in this rickettsial disease, but the specific complement fixation test is a useful laboratory diagnostic aid even though there is considerable crossing with materials from Rocky Mountain spotted fever.

TREATMENT AND PREVENTION. Chloramphenicol and the tetracycline antibiotics are all effective for treating patients with rickettsialpox. The temperature reaches normal levels in about 2 days, and recovery is rapid.

Control measures should be directed toward elimination of house mice and the vector mites responsible for transmitting the disease.

198 MURINE (Endemic) TYPHUS FEVER

*Theodore E. Woodward and
Elizabeth B. Jackson*

DEFINITION. Murine typhus fever is an acute febrile disease caused by *Rickettsia mooseri* and transmitted to man by fleas. The clinical illness is characterized by fever of 9 to 14 days, headache, a maculopapular rash appearing on the third to fifth day, and myalgia.

ETIOLOGY AND EPIDEMIOLOGY. *Rickettsia mooseri* resembles other rickettsias in morphologic properties, staining characteristics, and intracellular parasitism. Under the electron microscope *R. mooseri* contains dense masses of nuclear material in a less dense homogeneous protoplasmic substance, the whole of which is surrounded by a limiting membrane. It differs from *R. rickettsii* in that it always multiplies within the cytoplasm of cells, in contrast to the intranuclear and cytoplasmic positions of spotted fever rickettsias.

Invasion of the body by *R. mooseri* provokes specific and nonspecific immunologic responses. Utilizing highly purified antigens, specific antibodies may be demonstrated readily by complement fixation and agglutination reactions. The positive Weil-Felix reaction which occurs in this disease is nonspecific, because it is attributable to the presence of a common carbohydrate antigen in *Proteus* OX-19 and *R. mooseri* and because the reaction is also positive in epidemic typhus and spotted fever. A number of investigators have demonstrated group-specific rickettsial antigens common to both *R. mooseri* and *R. prowazeki*, namely, a heat-stable complement-fixing substance. Furthermore, both murine and epidemic rickettsias possess toxic factors which are lethal to mice and rats and can be neutralized by convalescent serum from man or lower animals.

The common vector of *R. mooseri* for rats and man is the rat flea (*Xenopsylla cheopis*). In nature, the rat louse (*Polypax spinulosis*) may transmit the agent among rodents. Customarily, rat fleas become infected on ingestion of blood from diseased rats; the rickettsias multiply within the intestinal cells of the arthropod and are excreted in the feces. Infection in man occurs following the flea bite and contamination of the broken skin by rickettsia-laden feces. Dried flea feces may also infect via the conjunctivas or the upper part of the respiratory tract.

Rats and mice are naturally infected with murine typhus, and although the rodent disease is nonfatal, viable rickettsias persist in the brain for variable periods.

Murine typhus is one of the most benign and widespread of the rickettsioses in the United States. Prevalent in the Southeastern and Gulf Coast states, it has been identified in most of the other states and in harbor centers throughout the world wherever rats and fleas abound. Through control of rats and their fleas a sharp decline in incidence has occurred since 1951, particularly in the Southern United States; about half the cases reported annually now occur in Texas. In urban areas the disease is more prevalent during the summer and fall months and occurs predominantly among persons working in proximity to granaries or food depots. Recently there has been an extension to certain rural areas because changing agricultural practices have provided rats with ready access to adequate food supplies.

CLINICAL MANIFESTATIONS. Incubation Period and Prodromata. According to experimental observations, the incubation period ranges from 8 to 16 days, with a mean of 10. Common prodromata are headache, backache, arthralgia, and chilly sensations. Nausea, malaise, and transient temperature rises may precede the true onset of disease.

Onset and General Symptoms. A frank shaking chill and often repeated rigors are present at the onset, associated with a severe frontal headache and fever. This triad of headache, chill, and pyrexia is usually followed within a few hours by nausea and vomiting. Prostration, malaise, and weakness are sufficient to enforce cessation of activity in adults, in contrast to the course in children, whose illness is less severe. Occasionally, mild symptoms make it difficult to define the actual onset.

Pyrexia. The usual febrile course in murine typhus lasts for about 12 days in adults, and the temperature ranges from 102 to 104°F but may reach 105 to 106°F in children. The temperature may reach high levels abruptly after onset or ascend in a stepwise manner during the first few days. With the appearance of the rash, fever is usually sustained, with partial daily remissions which occasionally reach normal levels in the morning. Defervescence is generally by lysis over several days but sometimes occurs by abrupt crisis. Transient mild fever of 100°F is not uncommon during early convalescence. A few patients experience only low-grade fever throughout, but this does not necessarily connote a mild illness.

Cutaneous Manifestations. The early lesions, which are sparse and discrete, are hidden in the axillas and inner surface of the arm. Most patients then develop with surprising suddenness a generalized, dull red macular rash of the upper part of the abdomen, shoulders, chest, arms, and thighs. The individual lesions are discrete and pea-size, with an ill-defined border, and fade on pressure during the first 24 hr. They later become maculopapular, in contrast to the exanthem of epidemic typhus, which is persistently macular. The distribution over the trunk with sparse involvement of the extremities, palms, soles, and face differs from the peripheral distribution and facial involvement of Rocky Mountain spotted fever. The murine rash generally appears initially on the fifth febrile day, but rarely it is seen concurrently with the onset of fever or developing as late as the seventh day.

Eighty percent of patients develop a rash which persists for 4 to 8 days and fades before defervescence. The cutaneous manifestations vary greatly in intensity and duration and may be fleeting. They are readily overlooked in dark-skinned patients, in whom they should be searched for by light palpation and indirect lighting.

Cardiovascular and Respiratory Features. An irritating, nonproductive cough is frequent and is occasionally associated with moderate hemoptysis. Early in the second week, rales may be detected in the basilar lung areas. These changes are generally rickettsial rather than bacterial in origin and respond to the broad-spectrum antibiotics but not to penicillin or sulfonamide therapy. Pulmonary congestion occurs in extremely ill and elderly patients.

Accelerated pulse, hypotension, and general circulatory weakness occur in this disease, although less frequently than in patients with epidemic typhus or Rocky Mountain spotted fever (Chap. 195).

Neurologic Manifestations. Headache is the most common neurologic manifestation of murine typhus and may dominate the clinical picture. It is frontally localized and continues into the second week of illness. In the early stages the facial expression is strained, and the patient resents distraction. Stupor and prostration may occur in the second week, and in severe cases, there may be muttering delirium, extreme agitation, or coma. Coma in elderly patients after 2 weeks of illness presages death. Nuchal rigidity and general spasticity often suggest meningitis, although the spinal fluid is normal except for slight increases in pressure and lymphocytes (5 to 30 per cu mm). Transient partial deafness occurs occasionally in murine typhus patients, but rarely is there localized neuritis or hemiplegia. Neurologic sequelae are unusual. Children experience minimal neurologic changes.

Other Physical Manifestations. During the first 2 days of illness the patient may be nauseated and vomit, but vomiting later in the illness should arouse suspicion of an intercurrent complication. Abdominal pain, particularly in dehydrated patients, is bothersome; when associated with diarrhea it responds to intravenous alimentation. A sluggish, constipated bowel is occasionally observed. Hepatomegaly and jaundice are unusual. There is splenomegaly in approximately 25 percent of patients.

Photophobia, retroocular pain, suffusion of the eyes, and congestion of the conjunctivas are common manifestations but are less severe than in the other typhus and spotted fevers.

Renal function is usually unaltered except in elderly patients with prolonged hypotension. Under these circumstances, in seriously ill patients, azotemia may develop to the degree observed in epidemic typhus. The blood chloride level is low in severe murine typhus, as in the epidemic type; hypochloremia of 80 mEq per liter may be observed. Hypoalbuminemia is also encountered.

COURSE OF DISEASE AND COMPLICATIONS. After defervescence, murine typhus patients recover rapidly. Fatalities occur between the ninth and twelfth days in elderly or debilitated patients, usually as a result of circulatory and renal failure or intercurrent bacterial infection.

PROGNOSIS. The mortality in murine typhus was low even before the introduction of modern specific therapy. Only one death occurred in 114 cases studied by Maxcy and none in the 180 reported by Stuart and Pullen.

DIFFERENTIAL DIAGNOSIS. Because murine typhus and Rocky Mountain spotted fever occur in many of the same states, the problem of differential diagnosis often arises. Flea-borne murine typhus, which is predominantly an urban disease, is more likely to occur in late summer and autumn. In contrast, spotted fever is a rural and suburban disease in which exposure to ticks is important. Most cases occur in the spring and summer.

TREATMENT AND PREVENTION. The therapeutic procedures are comparable to those used in spotted fever. Both chloramphenicol and the tetracycline antibiotics have controlled the disease.

Prevention of murine typhus in man is attained by reducing the natural reservoir and vector by applying measures for eliminating rodents and employing DDT in rat-infested areas to control fleas.

199 EPIDEMIC (Louse-borne) TYPHUS FEVER AND BRILL–ZINSSER DISEASE (Recrudescent Typhus)

Theodore E. Woodward and Elizabeth B. Jackson

EPIDEMIC (Louse-borne) TYPHUS FEVER

DEFINITION. The classical epidemic form of typhus is a severe, febrile disease caused by *Rickettsia prowazeki* and transmitted to man by the body louse. Intense headache, continuous pyrexia of about 2 weeks, a macular skin eruption appearing on about the fifth febrile day, malaise, and vascular and neurologic disturbances represent the principal clinical features. Confirmation of the diagnosis is made by demonstration of *Proteus* OX-19 agglutinins and of specific complement-fixing antibodies in convalescence. The broad-spectrum antibiotics are specific therapeutic agents.

ETIOLOGY AND EPIDEMIOLOGY. The causative microbe, *R. prowazeki*, is closely related to *R. mooseri*, which causes murine typhus; indeed, the two have a number of common antigens. *Rickettsia prowazeki* was the first of the rickettsias shown to have its own enzyme system, which permits it to respire independently of the host cell.

Man generally is infected when rickettsia-laden louse feces are rubbed into the broken skin; scratching the louse bite facilitates this process. *Pediculus humanus corporis*, which is peculiarly adapted to man, is the only important vector of epidemic typhus. It dies of its infection and fails to transmit rickettsias to its offspring. There is no known animal habitat of *R. prowazeki*; it is maintained by a cycle involving man-louse-man. New epidemics apparently originate from patients with Brill-Zinsser disease (recurrent epidemic typhus). Inhalation of dust containing dried louse feces may rarely cause infection.

Epidemic typhus, if uncontrolled, behaves as a cyclic disease in a susceptible population, extending over a 3-year period. During the first year there is a gradual seeding of cases throughout the group; during the second there is epidemic spread; and during the third the epidemic tapers off, because the majority of persons have become immune. Outbreaks of epidemic typhus last occurred in the United States in the nineteenth century, and its presence is now recognized only in the form of Brill-Zinsser disease.

CLINICAL MANIFESTATIONS. A classic clinical description of Old World typhus is provided in the 1922 monograph of Wolbach, Todd, and Palfrey. Epidemic typhus resembles murine typhus but is more severe. After an incubation period of about 7 days an abrupt onset of headache, chill, and rapidly mounting fever ushers in the illness. Cephalgia, malaise, and prostration continue unabated until the rash appears on the fifth febrile day. It is initially macular in the axillary folds but ultimately invades the trunk and extremities as a pink, irregular macular lesion which becomes fixed, petechial, and confluent in the later stages.

Neurologic features range from headache and general spasticity to extreme agitation, stupor, and coma. Circulatory disturbances consisting of tachycardia, hypotension, and cyanosis are more profound than those observed in murine typhus and are almost as severe as in Rocky Mountain spotted fever. Ultimately, in untreated cases azotemia often reaches high levels as a result of vascular and renal failure, and death occurs late in the second week of illness. Furthermore, thrombosis of major blood vessels and cutaneous gangrene develop in a manner similar to that seen in the virulent form of Rocky Mountain spotted fever.

The complications and sequelae of epidemic typhus are more severe than those in murine typhus, but not as severe as those in Rocky Mountain spotted fever. However, during certain outbreaks, epidemic typhus was fatal in 60 percent of those infected, and convalescence in survivors was prolonged. Broad-spectrum antibiotics have eradicated mortality in this dread disease, provided therapy is instituted before irreversible changes have been established in the tissues.

DIFFERENTIAL DIAGNOSIS. Differentiation of epidemic typhus from the various rickettsioses and other diseases with which it may be confused is described in Chap. 195. The disease in epidemic form never occurs in the absence of lousiness in the general population. Under the conditions in which typhus epidemics are likely to occur, other diseases which may cause confusion include malaria, relapsing fever, pneumonia, and tuberculosis. Classic typhus contracted by a previously vaccinated person is usually mild and may be clinically indistinguishable from murine typhus except by serologic methods.

TREATMENT AND PREVENTION. Both chloramphenicol and the tetracycline antibiotics have been found to be highly efficient therapeutic agents in epidemic typhus. Usually the patient becomes afebrile after 2 days of treatment. The therapeutic procedures are comparable to those used in spotted fever.

The most effective measures for controlling epidemic typhus are those which eliminate lousiness. DDT or lindane powder when dusted into clothing is suitable for this purpose. If resistant lice are found, malathion may prove effective.

A commercially available vaccine prepared from formalin-treated suspensions of infected yolk sac tissue is an effective immunizing agent.

BRILL-ZINSSER DISEASE

(Recrudescent Typhus)

DEFINITION. Brill-Zinsser disease is a recrudescent episode of epidemic typhus fever which occurs years after the initial attack. Nathan Brill in 1898 observed a sporadic disease which resembled typhus fever among nonlousy inhabitants of New York City. Zinsser, in 1934, suggested on the basis of epidemiologic and immunologic considerations that this was a recurrent form of typhus encountered in persons who had recovered from the epidemic disease while residing in countries where it was prevalent. Additional information has gradually accumulated in support of this hypothesis.

Murray and Snyder were successful in regularly isolating rickettsias indistinguishable from *R. prowazeki* from lice fed on patients during the active stages of illness.

CLINICAL MANIFESTATIONS. The clinical entity, not always mild, resembles epidemic typhus in the character of the rash, circulatory disturbances, and hepatic, renal, and nervous system changes. Recovery is the rule. The Weil-Felix reaction with the various *Proteus* antigens is usually negative, or positive in very low titer. The specific complement fixation reaction is valuable in establishing the diagnosis. In Brill-Zinsser disease the specific complement-fixing antibodies appear as early as the fourth day after the onset of illness; the peak response is attained by the eighth to tenth days. Specific antibody titers in the primary attack of epidemic typhus begin later, about the eighth to twelfth day, with maximum titers on about the sixteenth day after onset. Antibodies in Brill-Zinsser disease and the primary attack are associated with 7S and 19S globulins, respectively.

The therapeutic procedures are comparable to those used in spotted fever.

200   SCRUB TYPHUS

Theodore E. Woodward and
Elizabeth B. Jackson

DEFINITION. Scrub typhus is limited to eastern and southeastern Asia, India, northern Australia, and the adjacent islands. It is caused by *Rickettsia tsutsugamushi* and characterized by a primary lesion at the site of the bite of an infected mite, a fever of about 2 weeks' duration, a cutaneous rash which develops about the fifth day, and the appearance late in the second week of agglutinins against the OX-K strain of *Proteus* bacillus. The broad-spectrum antibiotics are specific therapeutic agents.

ETIOLOGY. The agent of scrub typhus resembles other rickettsias in its physical properties but differs from them in antigenic structure, vector, and reservoir. The disease is transmitted by larvae of several species of mites, especially *Trombicula akamushi* and *T. deliensis*. These tiny chiggers attach themselves to the skin and during the process of obtaining a meal of tissue juice may acquire infection from the host or transmit rickettsias to the vertebrate. The infection is maintained in nature by a cycle involving mites and small rodents and by transovarial transmission in mites; human infection represents an accident attributable to propinquity.

CLINICAL MANIFESTATIONS. About 10 to 12 days after infection, illness begins abruptly with chilliness, severe headache, fever, conjunctival injection, and moderate generalized lymphadenopathy which is most prominent in the nodes draining the area of the primary lesion. The initial lesion at the beginning of fever is evidenced by an erythematous indurated area 1 cm in diameter, surmounted by a multiloculated vesicle; within a few days the vesicle ulcerates and becomes covered with a black crust.

Fever increases progressively during the first week, generally reaching 104 to 105°F, but the pulse remains relatively slow, 70 to 100 per min. The red macular rash, which begins on the trunk about the fifth day and spreads to the extremities, sometimes becomes maculopapular but usually fades in a few days. The course of the disease and the complications resemble those of endemic and epidemic typhus; however, interstitial myocarditis is more prominent than in the other typhus fevers.

PROGNOSIS. Prior to the introduction of the broad-spectrum antibiotics the mortality varied from 1 to 60 percent, depending on the geographic area and the virulence of the local strains of *R. tsutsugamushi*, and convalescence was prolonged. With modern therapeutic methods, deaths are extremely rare and convalescence is short.

DIFFERENTIAL DIAGNOSIS. Scrub typhus is to be differentiated from the other members of the typhus and the spotted fever group of diseases as well as from measles, typhoid fever, and meningococcal infections. The geographic localization of scrub typhus, the primary lesion, and the occurrence of OX-K agglutinins are especially useful in establishing the diagnosis.

TREATMENT AND PREVENTION. Chloramphenicol and the tetracycline antibiotics are valuable specific therapeutic agents in scrub typhus. The therapeutic procedures are comparable to those used in spotted fever. In fact, scrub typhus is more amenable to drugs than are the other rickettsial infections, and patients with this disease regularly become afebrile and are decidedly improved within 24 to 36 hr after beginning treatment, irrespective of the stage of disease.

Prevention of disease in the individual is accomplished by the application of miticidal chemicals (dibutyl phthalate, benzyl benzoate, diethyltoluamide, and others) to clothing and the skin. There is no satisfactory vaccine.

201 Q FEVER

Theodore E. Woodward and
Elizabeth B. Jackson

DEFINITION. Q fever is an acute infectious disease caused by *Coxiella burnetii* and characterized by a sudden onset of fever, malaise, headache, weakness, anorexia, and interstitial pneumonitis. Rickettsemia occurs during the febrile period, and specific complement-fixing antibodies are present during convalescence. In contrast to the other rickettsioses, the disease is not associated with a cutaneous exanthem or agglutinins for the *Proteus* bacteria (Weil-Felix reaction).

ETIOLOGY AND EPIDEMIOLOGY. *Coxiella burnetii* possesses the general properties of other rickettsias but is somewhat more resistant to inactivation in unfavorable

environments and more pleomorphic than the others. Its infectivity after drying under natural conditions is of importance in the spread of infection to man. Its pleomorphism, which ranges from diplobacillary structures measuring 1.5 μ in length to tiny spheres about 0.2 μ in diameter, contributes to its filtrability through Berkefeld N candles. This filtrability led Cox (1939) to suggest the name *Rickettsia diaporica* for the first American isolate, but the name was subsequently abandoned when this agent was found to be identical with that causing Q fever in Australia. *Coxiella burnetii* has a wide host range in nature, but guinea pigs and embryonated eggs are the common laboratory hosts employed for its propagation.

Strains of *C. burnetii* differ in their ability to fix complement in the presence of serums from convalescent patients. This phenomenon is explained by "phase variation" of *C. burnetii*, and organisms may convert from one phase to another. Newly isolated strains from animals and ticks are characteristically in phase I. After passage in embryonated chicken eggs, phase I strains are converted to phase II strains. Any phase II strain of *C. burnetii* can be converted to phase I by passage in a susceptible animal. Knowledge of phase variation is pertinent to the interpretation of serologic reactions. Also phase I rickettsias are used for prophylactic vaccines.

Human cases of Q fever are contracted by inhalation of infected dusts, by handling infected materials, and possibly by drinking milk contaminated with *C. burnetii*. The disease in Australia is enzootic in animals, especially bandicoots, and is transmitted in nature by ticks. Rickettsia-laden tick feces may contaminate cattle hides, and inhalation of this material has caused infection in man. In the United States, a number of species of ticks are naturally infected, among them *Dermacentor andersoni* and *Amblyomma americanum*, and in North Africa transovarial transmission of the agent in indigenous ticks has been demonstrated. Sheep, goats, and cows have been found to be naturally infected in North America and in Europe, and *C. burnetii* has been recovered from the milk of such animals. Milk, as well as infected excretions from livestock, probably accounts for certain outbreaks of human disease following inhalation by cows of infected dust from barns and pens. The method of spread of Q fever was not clearly established among stockyard workers in Texas and Illinois, wool processors in Pennsylvania, employees in a rendering plant in New York, and laundry workers in Montana, who hauled dirty linen from a laboratory engaged in studies in Q fever; however, the air-borne route of dried contaminated material seems the most likely. A number of epidemics have occurred among laboratory workers engaged in studies on *C. burnetii*. The disease is not transmitted from man to man.

CLINICAL MANIFESTATIONS. After incubation of approximately 19 days (the range is 14 to 26), the disease begins with headache, chilly sensations, fever, malaise, myalgia, and anorexia. For several days, the temperature ranges from 101 to 104°F; the entire course rarely exceeds 2 weeks and usually ranges from 3 to 6 days. There may be wide fluctuations in the fever. Respiratory and gastrointestinal symptoms are not conspicuous in the early stages. Headache and fever predominate. A dry cough and chest pain occur after about 5 days, when rales are usually audible. Roentgenographic findings indistinguishable from those of primary atypical pneumonia are present usually by the third to fourth day of disease, first as patchy areas of consolidation involving a portion of one lobe, giving a homogeneous ground-glass appearance. These manifestations persist beyond the febrile period and may appear in patients who are unaware of pulmonary involvement. Complications are rare, and coincident with defervescence the appetite begins to return. Convalescence progresses slowly for several weeks, during which time the principal disability is weakness. It is not uncommon for patients to lose 15 to 20 lb during the active stages of disease. Several investigators have emphasized that the disease may be protracted in approximately 20 percent of cases, with fever persisting for longer than 4 weeks, particularly in elderly patients. Occasionally relapse occurs, especially in patients treated with antibiotics during the first several days of disease.

Hepatitis, with the development of clinically detectable icterus, occurs in approximately one-third of patients with the protracted form. This form of Q fever is characterized by fever, malaise, absence of headache or respiratory signs, and hepatomegaly with right upper quadrant pain. Liver biopsy specimens show diffuse granulomatous changes with multinucleated giant cells (see Fig. 201-1) and scattered infiltrations of polymorphonuclear leukocytes, lymphocytes, and macrophages. *Coxiella burnetii* may be demonstrated in such specimens with the fluorescent antibody technique. Therefore, Q fever must be included in the differential diagnosis of liver granulomatas such as tuberculosis, sarcoidosis, histoplasmosis, brucellosis, tularemia, syphilis, and others.

Endocarditis also has been reported, and *C. burnetii* has been identified by smear and isolation in vegetations on the heart valves obtained at operation or autopsy. The aortic valve is most commonly involved. It is important, therefore, to suspect the possibility of Q fever in cases of apparent subacute bacterial endocarditis with persistently negative blood cultures. Operative intervention with replacement of damaged valves is necessary for recovery because the available antibiotics are not rickettsicidal. A high complement-fixing antibody titer is present in both endocarditis and granulomatous hepatitis.

PROGNOSIS. Few fatalities have been recorded and, except for the patient with protracted illness and hepatic involvement or endocarditis, the course of disease is generally uncomplicated and benign.

TREATMENT AND CONTROL. The tetracycline antibiotics and chloramphenicol are effective in the treatment of patients with Q fever. Most patients, when treated early in the course of disease, respond promptly and recover without relapses. The therapeutic procedures are comparable to those used in spotted fever.

Fig. 201-1. Q fever hepatitis showing granulomatous changes in an adult male with fever, myalgia, and right upper quadrant pain. Note multinucleated giant cell. *Coxiella burnetii* was demonstrated by fluorescent antibody test, and complement fixation reaction was positive.

Chloramphenicol has been uniformly effective in treatment of patients with granulomatous hepatitis.

Control of Q fever depends primarily on immunization of susceptible persons with specific vaccines. Vaccines made from phase I rickettsias are potent and afford considerable protection to slaughterhouse and dairy workers, herders, rendering-plant workers, woolsorters, tanners, laboratory workers, and others at risk. Measures should be taken to avoid exposure to infected aerosols; milk from infected domestic livestock must be pasteurized or boiled.

202 TRENCH FEVER
Theodore E. Woodward and
Elizabeth B. Jackson

DEFINITION. Trench fever is a febrile disease transmitted from man to man by the body louse, *Pediculus* *humanus corporis.* It is characterized by a sudden onset with headache and severe pain in the muscles, bones, and joints. In most cases the fever and other symptoms assume a relapsing character. Fatalities are rare. The disease is also known as Shin bone fever, Wolhynian fever, His-Werner disease, and Quintan fever.

HISTORY. Trench fever, first described as a distinct clinical entity in 1915, was widespread on the Eastern and Western fronts during World War I, constituting one of the major medical problems. Intensive investigation by British and American commissions as well as by German workers provided much basic information. In the years between the two world wars the disease ceased to be recognized, but it reappeared in epidemic form during World War II among German troops on the Eastern front.

ETIOLOGY AND EPIDEMIOLOGY. *Rickettsia quintana,* the etiologic agent, grows extracellularly in the louse gut, in contrast to other pathogenic rickettsias which can only multiply within cells. Although a subclinical infection can be produced in several species of monkeys by inoculation of *R. quintana,* until 1961 this agent had not been cultivated in the laboratory. Hence, the classic method of identification of trench fever has been by xenodiagnosis. In this test, "clean" laboratory-bred lice which ingest blood from a trench fever patient develop a characteristic histologic picture of extracellular rickettsias in the lumen of their gut.

In 1961 Vinson and Fuller reported the cultivation of a European strain of *R. quintana* on blood agar inoculated with blood from a volunteer patient with trench fever. Later, Vinson induced typical trench fever in volunteers with a Mexican strain isolated and propagated on blood agar. *Rickettsia quintana* grown in vivo in the louse gut and in vitro on blood agar are identical morphologically and tinctorially.

Man is the only known reservoir of infection. The louse does not transmit the organism transovarially but acquires its infection by ingesting the blood of a person with rickettsemia. The organisms multiply extracellularly in the louse gut, without injury to this host, and are excreted in large numbers with the feces. Man becomes infected by the inoculation of the contaminated feces into his abraded skin or conjunctivas. *Rickettsia quintana* may be recovered periodically from human blood for several years after convalescence from an acute attack. Trench fever is known to exist in Mexico, Tunisia, Eritrea, Poland, the U.S.S.R., and possibly China.

PATHOLOGY. Since there have been no recorded fatalities, histologic examination has been confined to excised macules of the skin, which have shown nonspecific perivascular infiltrates without the involvement of the vessel walls that is seen in typhus fever.

CLINICAL MANIFESTATIONS. A variety of clinical manifestations is displayed in trench fever, ranging from a mild afebrile disease to a debilitating illness with a protracted clinical course involving numerous relapses. Following an incubation period of 10 to 30 days the onset may be insidious or dramatically abrupt. The acute disease is characterized by malaise, headache, fever, and bone and body pain, especially severe in the shins. In some cases only one fever peak occurs; in others the fever continues for from 5 to 7 days; and in others there is an initial febrile episode lasting 1 to 3 days followed by relapses which characteristically occur at 4- to 5-day intervals. In some cases the fever and symptoms are continuous for 2 or 3 weeks. Enlargement of the spleen and a red macular rash occur in 70 to 80 percent of the cases. Pain and soreness in the muscles usually recur with each febrile relapse.

The disease is marked by a persistent rickettsemia, which is present during the initial attack and which continues during the relapses, throughout the asymptomatic periods between relapses, and for months or even years after cessation of physical symptoms. A relapse has been reported 10 years after the original attack.

PROGNOSIS. The disease has no known mortality, but its duration is quite variable. About 85 percent of patients are able to return to work within 2 months of onset, but about 5 percent of all cases become chronic. Recovery is even more delayed in the aged and debilitated.

DIFFERENTIAL DIAGNOSIS. During epidemics, typical cases are easily diagnosed on the basis of symptoms. The disease may be differentiated from influenza, typhoid, typhus, dengue, and relapsing fever by the specific laboratory tests available for the diagnosis of each of these diseases.

TREATMENT AND PREVENTION. *Rickettsia quintana* is highly sensitive in vitro to the broad-spectrum antibiotics, but no reliable information has been obtained about the value of these drugs in treating trench fever. The treatment is symptomatic. Aspirin is used to control pain and discomfort, but codeine may be necessary. The patient should remain in bed for a week or more after complete cessation of subjective and objective evidence of infection. He should be kept under observation for several months and returned to bed at the first sign of relapse.

The methods employed to control epidemic typhus should be equally efficacious in controlling trench fever. These are based on the elimination of lousiness and the improvement of living conditions with provision for frequent bathing and washing of clothing. DDT or lindane powder should be applied by a hand or power duster at appropriate intervals to clothes and persons of populations living under conditions favoring lousiness. If resistant lice are found, malathion or other effective lousicides may be substituted as a dusting powder.

REFERENCES

Allen, A. C., and S. Spitz: A Comparative Study of the Pathology of Scrub Typhus (Tsutsugamushi Disease) and Other Rickettsial Diseases, Am. J. Pathol., 21:603, 1945.

Andrew, R., J. M. Bonin, and S. Williams: Tick Typhus in North Queensland, Med. J. Australia, 2:253, 1946.

Audy, J. R., and J. L. Harrison: A Review of Investigations

on Mite Typhus in Burma and Malaya, 1945–1950, Trans. Roy. Soc. Trop. Med. Hyg., 44:371, 1951.

Blake, F. G., K. F. Maxcy, J. F. Sadusk, Jr., G. M. Kohls, and E. J. Bell: Studies on Tsutsugamushi Disease (Scrub Typhus, Mite-borne Typhus) in New Guinea and Adjacent Islands: Epidemiology, Clinical Observations and Etiology in the Dobadura Area, Am. J. Hyg., 41:243, 1945.

Derrick, E. H.: The Epidemiology of Q Fever: A Review, Med. J. Australia, 1:245, 1953.

Ferguson, I. C., J. E. Craik, and N. R. Grist: Clinical, Virological and Pathological Findings in a Fatal Case of Q Fever Endocarditis, Brit. J. Clin. Pathol., 15:235, 1962.

Freyche, M. J., and Z. Deutschman: Human Rickettsioses in Africa, Epidemiol. Vital Statistics Rept. (WHO), 3:160, 1950.

Gear, J.: The Rickettsial Diseases of Southern Africa: A Review of Recent Studies, South African J. Clin. Sci., 5:158, 1954.

Greenberg, M.: Rickettsialpox in New York City, Am. J. Med., 4:866, 1948.

Harrell, G. T.: Rocky Mountain Spotted Fever, Medicine, 28:333, 1949.

——: Rickettsial Involvement of the Nervous System, Med. Clin. N. Am., 37:395, 1953.

Harris, B. P.: Aureomycin in Tick Typhus, East African Med. J., 29:403, 1952.

Huebner, R. J., W. L. Jellison, and C. Pomerantz: Rickettsialpox, a Newly Recognized Rickettsial Disease: IV. Isolation of a Rickettsia Apparently Identical with the Causative Agent of Rickettsialpox from *Allodermanyssus Sanguineus*, a Rodent Mite, Public Health Rept. U.S., 61:1677, 1946.

Lennette, E. H.: Epidemiology of Q Fever, Arch. Inst. Pasteur (Tunis), 36:521, 1959.

Ley, H. L., Jr., and J. E. Smadel: Antibiotic Therapy of Rickettsial Diseases, Antibiot. Chemotherapy, 4:792, 1954.

Lillie, R. D., T. L. Perrin, and C. Armstrong: An Institutional Outbreak of Pneumonitis: III. Histopathology in Man and Rhesus Monkeys in the Pneumonitis Due to the Virus of "Q" Fever, Public Health Rept. U.S., 56:149, 1941.

Marmion, B. P., and M. G. P. Stoker: The Epidemiology of Q Fever in Great Britain: An Analysis of the Findings and Some Conclusions, Brit. Med. J., 2:809, 1958.

Maxcy, K. F.: Typhus Fever in the United States, Public Health Rept. U.S., 44:1735, 1929.

Mohr, C. O., and W. W. Smith: Eradication of Murine Typhus Fever in a Rural Area, Bull. World Health Organ., 16:255, 1957.

Moulton, F. R. (Ed.): "The Rickettsial Diseases of Man," Washington, American Association for the Advancement of Science, 1948.

Murray, E. S., G. Baehr, G. Shwartzman, R. A. Mandelbaum, N. Rosenthal, J. C. Doane, L. B. Weiss, S. Cohen, and J. C. Snyder: Brill's Disease: I. Clinical and Laboratory Diagnosis, J.A.M.A., 142:1059, 1950.

—— and J. C. Snyder: Brill's Disease: II. Etiology, Am. J. Hyg., 53:22, 1951.

Ormsbee, R. A., E. J. Bell, D. B. Lackman, and G. Tallent: The Influence of Phase on the Protective Potency of Q Fever Vaccine, J. Immunol., 92:404, 1964.

Parker, R. R.: Rocky Mountain Spotted Fever, J.A.M.A., 110:1185, 1938.

Plotz, H., B. L. Bennett, K. Wertman, M. J. Snyder, and R. Gauld: Serological Pattern in Typhus Fever: I. Epidemic, Am. J. Hyg., 47:150, 1948.

Pratt, H. D.: The Changing Picture of Murine Typhus in the United States, Ann. N.Y. Acad. Sci., 70:516, 1958.

Price, E. G.: "Fighting Spotted Fever in the Rockies," Helena, Mont., Naegele Printing Co., 1948.

Ricketts, H. T.: "Contributions to Medical Science by Howard Taylor Ricketts 1870–1910," Chicago, University of Chicago Press, 1911

Rose, H. M.: The Clinical Manifestations and Laboratory Diagnosis of Rickettsialpox, Ann. Intern. Med., 31:871, 1949.

Smadel, J. E.: Influence of Antibiotics on Immunologic Responses in Scrub Typhus, Am. J. Med., 17:246, 1954.

——: Status of the Rickettsioses in the United States, Ann. Intern. Med., 51:421, 1959.

—— (Ed.): "Symposium on Q Fever," Med. Sci. Publ. 6, Walter Reed Army Institute of Research, Washington, U.S. Government Printing Office, 1959.

—— and E. B. Jackson: Rickettsial Infections, pp. 743–772 in "Diagnostic Procedures for Viral and Rickettsial Diseases," 3d ed., New York, American Public Health Association, 1964.

Snyder, J. C.: Typhus Fever Rickettsiae, pp. 1059–1094 in "Viral and Rickettsial Infections of Man," 4th ed., F. L. Horsfall, Jr., and I. Tamm (Eds.), Philadelphia, J. B. Lippincott Company, 1965.

Stoker, M. G. P., and P. Fiset: Phase Variation of the Nine Mile and Other Strains of *Rickettsia Burnetii*, Can. J. Microbiol., 2:310, 1956.

—— and B. P. Marmion: The Spread of Q Fever from Animals to Man: The Natural History of a Rickettsial Infection, Bull. World Health Organ., 13:781, 1955.

Strong, R. P.: Trench Fever, pp. 984–996B in "Stitt's Diagnosis, Prevention and Treatment of Tropical Diseases," 7th ed., New York, McGraw-Hill Book Company, 1944.

Stuart, B. M., and R. L. Pullen: Endemic (Murine) Typhus Fever: Clinical Observations of One Hundred and Eighty Cases, Ann. Intern. Med., 23:520, 1945.

Vinson, J. W.: Etiology of Trench Fever in Mexico, pp. 109–114 in "Industry and Tropical Health: V," Boston, Harvard School of Public Health, 1964.

Section 13

Introduction to Viral Diseases

203 PROPERTIES AND CLASSIFICATION OF VIRUSES

Robert R. Wagner

VIRUS STRUCTURE AND FUNCTION. The viruses occupy a special taxonomic position as the simplest and most distinctive forms in the biologic universe. Separate classes of viruses infect bacteria (the bacteriophages), plants, or animals. Unlike true organisms, such as bacteria or fungi, viruses are obligate intracellular parasites which derive energy exclusively from metabolism of the cells that they infect. Two stages occur in the life cycle of all viruses: the replicative (intracellular) and the infectious (extracellular). Extracellular virus particles, *virions,* are metabolically inert, consisting of an internal core of nucleic acid surrounded by a protein coat or *capsid.* The capsid is made up of symmetrically arranged subunits known as *capsomeres.* The size, shape, number, and spacing of capsomeres can be determined by electron microscopy and x-ray diffraction. Two major groups have been recognized on the basis of capsid morphology: (1) The *helical viruses* appear as hollow rods in which the capsomeres are radially distributed around a single coil, or helix, of nucleic acid; (2) the *polygonal viruses* assume a perfect geometric shape, usually an icosahedron (a symmetric 20-sided structure), in which the capsomeres are arranged in a shell around a molecule of nucleic acid. The capsids of larger and more complex animal viruses, both helical and polygonal, may be surrounded by a lipid-containing envelope derived from the host cell. The known functions of capsids are to protect the nucleic acid from nucleases and to initiate infection by providing specific receptors for virion attachment to corresponding sites on the surface of cells. In contrast to animal and plant viruses, many bacteriophages are equipped with a tail which injects viral nucleic acid through the rigid bacterial cell wall.

The true infectious moiety of any virus is a giant molecule of deoxyribonucleic acid (DNA) or ribonucleic acid (RNA), never both. Nucleic acid alone, stripped of its protein capsid, can infect cells, although less efficiently than intact virions. Viruses vary considerably in their complexity and content of nucleic acid. The RNA of the tiny f_2 bacteriophage contains approximately 1,600 nucleotides and provides genetic information for synthesis of only three or four proteins. In contrast, the DNA of the large vaccinia virus is composed of almost 500,000 nucleotides, considerably greater than the nucleotide content of organisms of the genus *Mycoplasma.*

Viral nucleic acid has three major functions: (1) It is a template on which nucleic acid is replicated. (2) It contains the genetic information for manufacture of enzymes required for the synthesis of viral nucleic acid and protein. Protein synthesis by double-stranded DNA viruses is mediated by transcription of messenger RNA that is complementary in base sequences to viral DNA. Protein synthesis by viral RNA is preceded by formation of a complementary RNA species (minus strand) to form a double-stranded RNA "replicative form" and a "replicative intermediate" composed of double-stranded and single-stranded regions. (3) Viral nucleic acid can mutate and can also mate with nucleic acid of a homologous virus by recombination, giving rise to progeny that differ from the parents. In addition, the DNA of certain bacteriophages can become integrated with the DNA of bacterial cells, a process known as lysogeny, during the course of which new information may be imparted to the cell by genetic transduction. Malignant transformation of animal cells by DNA tumor viruses may involve a similar process.

INFECTION AT THE CELLULAR LEVEL. Viral infection is initiated after random collision between one or more virions and a susceptible cell. The concept of virus *tropism,* implying attraction of virus to a particular cell, is no longer tenable and should be discarded. The initial stage of infection is *adsorption* (physical attachment) of virion capsid to cell membrane at specific receptor sites. The nature of the chemical bonds between the capsid and cell membrane is unknown, but the receptor for myxoviruses has been identified as neuraminic acid. The absence of cellular receptors precludes infection, which explains, for example, the complete resistance of most nonprimate cells to intact polio virions. Following adsorption, *penetration* of animal viruses takes place by dissolution of the outer envelope of the virus fused at the cell surface or by phagocytosis of the entire virion. Large animal viruses can be seen by electron microscopy to be transported across the cytoplasmic membrane engulfed in a cytoplasmic vacuole. At this stage, the outer envelope is stripped off (presumably by lysosomal enzymes), freeing the viral nucleocapsid. During penetration by poxviruses, a new "uncoating enzyme" is synthesized by the viral genome, which digests the capsid and frees the viral DNA.

After penetration and decapsidation, there is always an *eclipse* period, of variable duration for each virus-cell system, during which time no infectious virus can be detected in the cell. *Biosynthesis* of viral proteins and nucleic acid begins during this stage of infection and continues in an orderly sequence. The first products synthesized under genetic control of viral DNA or RNA are nucleotide kinases, synthetases, polymerases, and other enzymes required for synthesis of viral nucleic acid. Synthesis of viral nucleic acid then begins, accompanied by, or followed by, onset of synthesis of viral structural protein. Ribosomes, amino acids, nucleotides, transfer RNA, activating enzymes, and energy all are supplied by the infected cell. Viral nucleic acid condenses with structural protein in a poorly understood and inefficient process called *maturation*. Among every population of animal viruses are many "incomplete" or noninfectious forms which result from inefficient incorporation of viral nucleic acid within the capsid. Bacteriophage can also incorporate cellular genes, which can then be transferred to other bacterial cells, a process known as *transduction*. The final step in the infectious process is *release* of virions by leakage from the living cell or by lysis of the cell. The released virus can then infect other cells, and the cycle is repeated.

Different viruses multiply and mature in different parts of the cell. Herpes simplex virus and adenoviruses, for example, form within the nucleus as a crystalline array. These crystals are the intranuclear inclusion bodies seen in stained infected cells. Intranuclear viruses are released from cells slowly and poorly. In contrast, influenza and other myxoviruses mature at the periphery of the cell just under the cytoplasmic membrane. Mature myxovirus particles protrude from the cell surface as fingerlike projections enveloped by cytoplasmic membrane, which then pinch off to become free virions almost as soon as they are formed.

Certain other cytopathologic changes appear to be common to many viral infections. Dissolution of nucleoli and clumping and margination of nuclear chromatin are frequently seen. RNA granules often appear in the cytoplasm and are extruded into the surrounding medium. Eventually, the cytoplasm may disappear, leaving a pyknotic nucleus. However, not all viral infections result in cell death. There is considerable variation in the degree to which viruses compromise the normal metabolism of infected cells. The RNA of poliovirus, for example, can code for proteins that cut off cellular RNA and protein synthesis. The tumor viruses, on the other hand, can induce malignant transformation that results in enhanced cellular proliferation and DNA synthesis. These "transformed" cells also acquire new virus-specific nuclear and cytoplasmic membrane antigens and, in some cases, can be transplanted to animals where the cells grow as malignant tumors. Measles and herpes simplex viruses alter cytoplasmic membranes,

causing them to fuse with adjacent uninfected cells, with formation of giant cells (syncytia, polykaryocytes) that are characteristic of infection with these viruses.

CHEMOTHERAPY. An important characteristic of all true viruses is their complete insusceptibility to antibiotics commonly used for treatment of bacterial infections. Contrary to popular belief, however, many antibiotics and other chemical compounds are known to inhibit viral multiplication. The main difficulty is that most of these agents also compromise the integrity of the cell to varying degrees. Nevertheless, specific inhibitors of nucleic acid or protein biosynthesis have been valuable tools in studying viral multiplication and hold out promise for eventual chemotherapy of human viral infections. Several compounds inhibit multiplication of DNA viruses without affecting most RNA viruses:

1. Mitomycin C is an antibiotic that causes depolymerization of viral and cellular DNA in a manner reminiscent of ionizing radiation.

2. Actinomycin D specifically binds to viral or cellular DNA and blocks transcription of messenger RNA. Most RNA viruses synthesize RNA by a pathway independent of DNA and, therefore, are not influenced by actinomycin D. Exceptions to this rule are the reoviruses, which contain double-stranded RNA, and influenza virus and Rous sarcoma virus, which appear to require the transcriptive function of cellular DNA for replication.

3. Halogenated pyrimidines, the best known of which is 5-iodouracildeoxyriboside (IUdR), act primarily as competitive antagonists of thymidine incorporation into DNA. IUdR may be partially effective in treatment of herpes simplex keratitis, although the results of clinical trails are equivocal and resistant mutants are common.

Competitive antagonists of viral (and cellular) protein synthesis also inhibit viral multiplication. Puromycin, a structural analogue of aminoacyl–soluble RNA, reversibly blocks incorporation of amino acids into the growing peptide chain on mammalian or bacterial ribosomes. The antiviral action of puromycin is similar, in some respects, to that of chloramphenicol on bacterial growth. Substituted amino acids, such as p-fluorophenylalanine, are incorporated into peptide chains, resulting in formation of "fraudulent" proteins. Isatin β-thiosemicarbazone inhibits transcription of late messenger RNA of poxviruses and is partially effective in chemoprophylaxis of smallpox.

Little success has been achieved in the search for compounds that selectively inhibit viruses without altering nucleic acid or protein metabolism of cells. Two that have been studied in the laboratory are guanidine hydrochloride and α-hydroxybenzylbenzimidazole, both of which inhibit multiplication of polioviruses, a few other enteroviruses, and some rhinoviruses. These compounds are thought to block synthesis of poliovirus RNA by interfering with the specific viral RNA polymerase. Unfortunately, resistant mutants soon outgrow the susceptible viruses.

Table 203-1. A CLASSIFICATION OF VIRUSES AND PSEUDOVIRUSES* THAT INFECT MAN

Generic name and properties†	Prototype viruses (common name)	Major antigenic types	Best available methods of virus isolation	Principle modes of transmission	Usual clinical manifestations
Mycoplasma (PPLO)* DNA + RNA 125 × 250 mμ Protoplast-like	*M. pneumoniae* (Eaton agent) *M. hominis* *M. salivarium*	1 2 1	Enriched cell-free medium, chick embryos	Respiratory Genitourinary Oral	Pneumonia, URI, myringitis Urethritis Saprophyte
Psittacosis* (*Chlamydozoaceae*) DNA + RNA 250 × 400 mμ Complex, cell wall	Psittacosis Lymphogranuloma Trachoma Inclusion conjunctivitis	1 1	Yolk sac of chick embryo, mouse Yolk sac of chick embryo	Respiratory Venereal Eye Eye, venereal	Pneumonia Bubo, proctitis Keratitis Conjunctivitis
Poxvirus DNA 200–300 mμ Complex structure Enveloped	Smallpox Vaccinia-cowpox Molluscum contagiosum Myxoma (rabbits) Orf-Milker's nodules	1 ? 1 2	Chick embryo, mouse, rabbit, cell cultures Human volunteers Rabbit (European) Cell cultures	Respiratory Skin Skin Skin Skin	Pustular exanthem Local papule, pustule Papules Hemorrhages, tumors Papules, pustules
Herpesvirus DNA 100–200 mμ Polygonal Enveloped	Herpes simplex Monkey B Chickenpox-herpes zoster Cytomegalovirus Epstein-Barr (EB) virus	1 1 1 1 ?	Cell cultures Monkey cell cultures Human cell cultures Human cell cultures Leukocyte cultures	Mucous membranes Skin (monkey bite) Respiratory latent Transplacental, respiratory(?) Not known	"Cold sores," stomatitis Encephalitis Vesicles, pneumonia Radiculitis, vesicles Hepatitis, pneumonia encephalitis Burkitt lymphoma Infectious mononucleosis
Myxovirus and *Paramyxovirus* RNA 100–200 mμ Helical Enveloped	Influenza A, B, C Parainfluenza Mumps Measles German measles (rubella) Respiratory syncytial (RS virus)	3 4 1 1 1 1	Chick embryo Human cell cultures Chick embryo, cultures Human cell cultures Monkey cell culture interference Human cell cultures	Respiratory Respiratory Respiratory Respiratory Respiratory Respiratory	Influenza, pneumonia URI, croup, pneumonia Parotitis, orchitis, meningitis Macular rash, pneumonia Macular rash, congenital malformations Bronchiolitis, croup, pneumonia
Reovirus RNA, 75 mμ, polygonal	Reoviruses	3	Various cell cultures	Respiratory, enteric	URI, fever, hepatitis, encephalitis
Rhabdovirus‡ RNA 65 × 180 mμ Helical Enveloped	Vesicular stomatitis Rabies	2 1	Cell cultures Mouse	Skin and mucosa Animal bites	Vesicles Encephalitis
Adenovirus DNA, 70 mμ cubic	Adenoviruses	44+	Human cell cultures	Respiratory, eye, enteric(?)	Pharyngitis, pneumonia, conjunctivitis
Arborvirus (Arbor, arthropod-borne viruses) RNA 50–100 mμ Polygonal Enveloped(?)	Equine encephalitis Semliki Forest Japanese B Russian tick-borne Yellow fever Dengue Morituba, Oriboca Rift Valley Colorado tick fever Sandfly fever	1 Group A 1 or more Group B Group C Many ungrouped	Cerebral injection of newborn mice, some in tissue culture	Mosquito bite Mosquito bite Tick bite, oral Mosquito bite Mosquito bite Mosquito bite Mosquito bite Tick bite Sandfly bite	Encephalitis, dengue-like fever, mild fever, hemorrhagic fever, hepatitis or asymptomatic
Papovavirus DNA 25–45 mμ Polygonal	"Warts" (human) Papilloma (rabbit) Polyoma (mouse) Simian virus 40	1 1 1 1	Human volunteers Rabbit skin Mice, hamsters Monkey cell culture	Skin Skin Unknown, enteric(?) Unknown	Warts (verrucae) Papilloma of skin Sarcomas Sarcomas (hamsters)
Picornavirus RNA, 15–30 mμ, polygonal *Enterovirus* *Rhinovirus* Others	Poliovirus Coxsackie A Coxsackie B ECHO Common cold Encephalomyocarditis Foot-and-mouth disease	3 24+ 6 30+ Many 1 7	Primate cell culture Infant mouse Cell culture, mice Human cell culture Primate cell cultures Mouse, cell cultures Cell cultures	Enteric Enteric Enteric Enteric, respiratory Respiratory Unknown Skin and mucosa	Paralysis, encephalitis Herpangina, fever Pleurodynia, meningitis Meningitis, macular rash Afebrile URI Fever, encephalitis Vesicles, fever
Unclassified viruses	Lymphocytic chorio-meningitis Human hepatitis	1 2(?)	Adult mouse Human volunteers	Respiratory Enteric, injection	Meningitis Hepatitis

* *Mycoplasma* and psittacosis groups are bacteria rather than viruses but cause viruslike illnesses.
† Classification of true viruses is based on content of either DNA or RNA, diameter in millimicrons, polygonal or helical symmetry of capsomeres, presence or absence of outer envelope. These properties have not been thoroughly investigated for those viruses listed in "unclassified" group.
‡ Tentative terminology.

940

CLASSIFICATION. The primary bases for virus classification are chemical composition, morphology, size, physical properties and antigenicity. Biologic properties of viruses are neither distinctive nor stable enough to serve as criteria. All viruses can be divided into two major categories, depending on whether their genetic information is in the form of DNA or RNA. Each of these two categories can be further subdivided into those with polygonal or helical arrangement of protein capsomeres. The presence or absence of an outer envelope derived from the host cells is also useful but not always definitive. The number of capsomeres has also been proposed as a basis for classification. The size of viruses must also be considered, but this criterion is also of limited value because of wide variation among certain groups of viruses. The typing of viruses within major groups or subgroups is largely based on antigenicity.

The viruses infectious for man are classified in Table 203-1 under the generic names that are widely accepted. Eight major groups are listed, along with their distinguishing characteristics, as well as several viruses not yet classified because of insufficient information. Also included under the heading *pseudoviruses*, because of prevailing clinical custom, are the true microorganisms of the *Mycoplasma* group and the agents that cause psittacosis, lymphogranuloma venereum, and trachoma, which belong more properly with the rickettsias and bacteria.

Viruses continually undergo mutations to forms which lose the capacity to infect certain types of cells or to cause disease but which in other respects remain indistinguishable from the original strains. However, it is feasible and convenient to categorize viruses that infect man by their portal of entry and initial site of multiplication. Such a system has the advantage of characterizing viruses by their usual mode of transmission and epidemiology. Table 203-1 summarizes the salient epidemiologic, cultural, and clinical features of viruses of real or potential medical significance. These characteristics conform reasonably well to the group classifications based on physicochemical properties.

REFERENCES

Andrewes, C. H., and H. G. Peirera: "Viruses of Vertebrates," 2d ed., Baltimore, The Williams & Wilkins Company, 1967.

Davis, B. D., R. Dulbecco, H. N. Eisen, H. S. Ginsberg, and W. B. Wood, Jr.: "Microbiology," New York, Harper and Row Publishers, Incorporated, 1967.

Fenner, F.: "The Biology of Animal Viruses," vol. I., "Molecular and Cellular Biology," New York, Academic Press, Inc., 1968.

Morgan, C., and H. M. Rose: Structure and Development of Viruses as Observed in the Electron Microscope. VIII. Entry of Influenza Virus, J. Virol., 2:925, 1968.

Stent, G. S.: "Molecular Biology of Bacterial Viruses," San Francisco, W. H. Freeman and Company, 1963.

Tamm, I., and H. J. Eggers: Specific Inhibition of Replication of Animal Viruses, Science, 142:24, 1963.

Wagner, R. R.: Chemical and Biologic Approaches to the Therapy of Viral Diseases, Am. Rev. Resp. Dis., 88:404, 1963.

204 PATHOGENESIS OF VIRAL DISEASES

Robert R. Wagner

The events that occur during the course of viral infection in a single cell (Chap. 203) differ in no important respect from the sequence that leads to infection of multicellular organisms, including man. To initiate infection, a virus must make contact with a susceptible cell in the respiratory tract, intestine, skin, or eye. Newly formed virus is released and transmitted to adjacent cells at the primary focus. Certain viruses remain localized to the original site of infection and draining lymph nodes. Others invade the blood directly from infected capillary endothelium or by way of lymphatic vessels, and are disseminated to distant organs. Viremia is detectable when the rate of invasion exceeds the rate of clearance by reticuloendothelial cells. Most viruses are carried in plasma, but certain myxoviruses and arborviruses are attached to erythrocytes; the poxviruses and measles virus are transported in or on circulating monocytes, lymphocytes, and platelets. Plasma-borne viruses are rapidly cleared; viruses associated with formed elements persist in the circulation for a longer time.

Whether infection remains localized or becomes generalized and whether localized or systemic infection results in disease are largely determined by the genetic constitution of the virus and of the host. Most viral infections of man do not cause recognizable disease. *Virulence* is the disease-producing capacity of a particular virus in a particular host. It usually reflects the degree of tissue damage, which, in turn, is a function of the degree to which the virus multiplies. A strain of poliovirus, for example, is said to be virulent for man if infection of the intestine leads sequentially to viremia, dissemination to the central nervous system, multiplication of virus in anterior horn cells, cell death, and paralysis in a high proportion of cases. Immunologic responsiveness, other host factors, the infecting dose, and environmental conditions also determine the outcome of infection.

TISSUE REACTIONS TO VIRAL INFECTIONS. These vary from rapid cell destruction to indetectable changes. Cellular necrosis may be the result of virus-induced rupture of lysomes and intracellular discharge of autolytic enzymes. Inflammation is usually characterized by the presence of macrophages, but polymorphonuclear leukocytes may predominate if infection causes extensive tissue necrosis or hemorrhage. Although the extent of damage, and hence the severity of the disease, varies considerably, the types of responses to different viruses are often quite similar. For example, many viruses can infect the meninges and produce the syndrome of aseptic meningitis (Chap. 215). Conversely, a virus such as Coxsackie B can cause a variety of illnesses, including fatal myocarditis, pleurodynia, meningitis, and encephalitis.

Certain viruses stimulate cellular proliferation. Vaccinia virus sometimes induces hyperplasia, and influenza virus regularly causes squamous metaplasia of bronchial epithelium. Hundreds of viruses, among them certain strains of human adenoviruses, have now been found to be capable of causing neoplasms in animals. The Stewart-Eddy polyoma virus has been particularly well studied and has been shown to be responsible for widespread epizootics of malignant tumors in mice. Polyoma virus also infects other rodents, including newborn hamsters. Neoplastic viruses with widely varying biologic properties have been isolated from vertebrate species ranging from fish to primates. Thus far, only warts have been proved to be virus-induced tumors of man. However, a herpesvirus-like agent, the Epstein-Barr (EB) virus, present in cultured leukocytes may be the cause of Burkitt lymphoma and infectious mononucleosis. It will not be surprising if more human neoplasms are found to be caused by viruses.

Certain chronic neurologic diseases in domestic animals have been attributed to an ill-defined group of agents known as "slow viruses" (Chap. 219). A filtrable, transmissible agent with unusual physical properties has been isolated from sheep dying with scrapie, a demyelinating encephalopathy. Similar pathologic lesions are seen in sheep infected with a myxovirus-like agent known as the Visna virus. Both of these diseases bear certain resemblances to multiple sclerosis. These observations coupled with indirect evidence that measles virus can cause allergic encephalitis have stimulated a search for viruses as potential causative agents of multiple sclerosis and similar neurologic diseases of man.

IMMUNITY TO VIRAL DISEASES. Acquired resistance to viral infections takes several forms. Probably the most important is specific immunity induced by natural exposure to a virus or by vaccination. Injection of a sufficient antigenic mass of virus induces the formation of rapidly sedimenting (19S or γM) antibody within several days, followed by the appearance of smaller, more slowly sedimenting (7S or γG) antibody. Although identical in specificity, 7S antibody is more efficient than 19S antibody in neutralizing the same virus. The predominant antiviral antibody present on mucosal surfaces is γA globulin. Antibody in the circulation and extracellular fluid is a barrier to cross infection of cells. If reinfection with the same or an antigenically related virus occurs even after a long interval, a prompt anamnestic response often prevents spread of infection from the primary focus and the host's reaction to infection is mild or asymptomatic. The content of antibody (γA) in nasal secretions is thought to be one factor in immunity to rhinoviruses and other respiratory viruses. Similarly, viruses that persist in the tissues for many years after a primary infection are prevented from causing widespread disease by continual formation of antibody.

Secondary herpes simplex, for example, usually remains localized to the lips rather than becoming disseminated, as may occur in primary infection (Chap. 226).

Factors other than antibody production also influence the outcome of infection on first exposure to a virus. It is common for the acute manifestations of a viral disease to abate before neutralizing antibody can be detected in the circulation. Children with hypogammaglobulinemia have been noted to recover from measles, mumps, chickenpox, poliomyelitis, and viral respiratory infections in a normal manner. Furthermore, these children rarely show evidence of reinfection with a virus, in contrast to their tendency to undergo repeated infections by the same bacteria. However, vaccinia gangrenosa (Chap. 223) and severe viral hepatitis are unusually frequent in children with hypogammaglobulinemia.

A form of immunologic tolerance may play a significant role in resistance to congenital viral infections. Mice infected in utero, or a few hours after birth, with lymphocytic choriomeningitis virus resist reinfection with the same virus for many months. These resistant animals form little or no circulating antibody to the virus, but viral antibody and antigen-antibody complexes are found sequestered in the kidney, sometimes associated with glomerulonephritis. An analogous situation may obtain in congenital infections of man with salivary gland virus (Chap. 232). This virus often lies dormant in the tissues for many years without causing cytomegalic inclusion disease or other manifestations of infection.

Infection with one virus may also confer resistance to infection with an antigenically related or unrelated virus, a phenomenon known as *viral interference*. This observation is of practical significance in scheduling the sequence of oral vaccination with the Sabin strains of attenuated polioviruses. If all three poliovirus types are administered together, type 2 may inhibit enteric multiplication of the other two types, with consequent depression of antibody response to them. Latent enteric infection with ECHO or other enteroviruses has also been noted to prevent infection with virulent polioviruses. Experimental studies indicate that one type of viral interference is caused by a nonviral protein, called *interferon,* which is produced by infected cells. The suggestion has been made that recovery from certain viral infections may be attributable to endogenous production of interferon.

VACCINATION. Purified concentrated virus inactivated by formalin or attenuated infectious virus can be used as vaccines. Their success depends, in large measure, on the antigenic mass originally injected or on the multiplication of attenuated virus to equivalent titers. Repeated administration is often required and, even then, immunity is likely to be less pronounced and of shorter duration than that following recovery from natural infection.

The efficacy of a vaccine is judged from several standpoints. The first consideration is its safety for those receiving it and for their contacts. Secondly, a vaccine must induce a significant antibody response and, in so doing, reduce morbidity and mortality after natural exposure to the virus. Rarely is prevention of infection per se considered to be an important goal of vaccination. In fact, asymptomatic infection after vaccination can serve to enhance and prolong the immune response.

PERSISTENCE AND LATENCY. Many viruses persist in host tissues for months or years without causing overt disease. A flare-up of these latent infections may be induced by trauma, intercurrent disease, decline in antibody titers, or unknown stimuli. Experiments with tissue cultures and laboratory animals reveal that persistence of virus in tissue results from an interplay of various factors peculiar to each virus and its host. Latency is promoted by the presence of antibody or other viral inhibitors that prevent extensive cell-to-cell spread of virus. If antibody is withdrawn, viral multiplication often resumes, with concomitant cellular necrosis. Congenital viral infections tend to be latent for long periods of time, possibly through the mechanism of immunologic tolerance. One of the most important causes of virus persistence is thought to result from endogenous production of interferon by chronically infected cells. An equilibrium can be established in tissue culture when a small proportion of the cells in a population produces infectious virus and the same or different cells produce interferon.

DIAGNOSIS. Although similar in principle to diagnostic bacteriology, laboratory diagnosis of viral diseases often entails procedures that are far more time-consuming and costly. Therefore, the decision to undertake virus diagnostic studies must be based on sound clinical judgment and a carefully reasoned evaluation of the public health implications of the disease in question. Specimens sent to the virus laboratory as part of a "complete" diagnostic work-up are usually valueless. The laboratory procedures to be followed vary considerably for different viral diseases and frequently depend on the duration of illness and whether the infection has occurred sporadically or during an epidemic. The virologist relies heavily on knowledge of diseases endemic in a community, their seasonal incidence, the geographic distribution of certain viruses, and the potential animal reservoirs and insect vectors of an area. The presence of characteristic histopathologic lesions may contribute more to a retrospective diagnosis of diseases such as rabies, yellow fever, measles, cytomegalic inclusion disease, and poliomyelitis than will be gained by virus isolation and serologic studies. The diagnosis of infectious hepatitis is based entirely on clinical or pathologic findings.

The advent of tissue culture and cell culture methods has greatly facilitated isolation of certain viruses (see Table 203-1), but because of variation in cellular susceptibility to viral infection, it is often essential to choose the type of tissue culture on the basis of the virus anticipated to be present. Despite continuing advances in technique, viruses are generally difficult to isolate and even more difficult to identify. Some cause characteristic cytopathologic changes in culture, but

cellular reactions to others often lack specificity. The histochemical technique of immunofluorescence is another reliable means for rapid identification of viral antigen within cells.

A serious problem in diagnostic virology is the frequency with which uninoculated tissue cultures are contaminated with latent viruses that may induce cytopathic effects indistinguishable from those caused by the virus one is attempting to isolate. For example, cultures of renal epithelium from presumably healthy monkeys often contain measles or other viruses. Another major difficulty stems from the observation that feces and nasopharyngeal secretions may contain viruses other than, or in addition to, those originally suspected of causing a patient's illness. To cite but two examples, the ECHO viruses were discovered during studies of poliomyelitis, and some of the parainfluenza viruses were originally isolated during an influenza epidemic. In several instances, identification of new viruses has led to recognition of new disease entities, the existence of which had not been suspected on clinical grounds alone.

Final identification of viruses and the diagnosis of viral diseases almost invariably depend on immunologic tests. Each diagnostic laboratory maintains a supply of viral antigens and standard reference antiserums. When a virus is isolated, it is identified in terms of its immunologic reactivity compared with known viruses. The most useful serologic procedures in virology are complement-fixation and neutralization of infectivity. Virus neutralization is the most sensitive immunologic test yet devised. Precipitin reactions in fluid medium or by agar gel diffusion can be performed only with highly concentrated preparations of virus and specific antibody. For those viruses which readily agglutinate erythrocytes, such as the myxoviruses, antibody can be assayed by hemagglutination inhibition or by hemadsorption inhibition. It is important to keep in mind that different serologic tests may measure different antigenic components of the same virus. All members of the adenovirus group, for example, share a common complement-fixing antigen, but each can be typed by specific neutralizing antibody.

In the final analysis, only an antibody response in the host constitutes definitive evidence of infection with a specific virus. Therefore, it is essential to obtain serum specimens at properly spaced intervals. The result of a single serologic test is often misleading because it may be impossible to determine whether the antibody represents a response to infection in the recent or distant past.

REFERENCES

Burdette, W. J. (Ed.): "Viruses Inducing Cancer," Salt Lake City, University of Utah Press, 1966.

Fenner, F.: "The Biology of Animal Viruses," vol. II, "The Pathogenesis and Ecology of Viral Infections," New York, Academic Press, Inc., 1968.

Finter, N. B. (Ed.): "Interferons," Amsterdam, North-Holland Publishing Company, 1966.

Mims, C. A.: Aspects of the Pathogenesis of Virus Diseases, Bacteriol. Rev., 28:30, 1964.

Svehag, S. E., and B. Mandel: The Formation and Properties

of Poliovirus-neutralizing Antibody, J. Exp. Med., 119:1, 21, 225, 1964.

Section 14

Viral Diseases of the Respiratory Tract

205   GENERAL CONSIDERATIONS OF RESPIRATORY VIRAL DISEASE

Vernon Knight

The viral respiratory diseases as a group are responsible for one-half or more of all acute illnesses, and although influenza virus is the only agent among them which causes significant mortality in adults, several different viruses make a large contribution to the 20 percent of childhood mortality due to respiratory disease. Respiratory disease morbidity, due primarily to virus infections, causes 30 to 50 percent of time lost from work in adults, and from 60 to 80 percent of time lost by children from school. These diseases are worldwide, and although studies in many areas are scanty, reports from Great Britain, Western Europe, U.S.S.R., Czechoslovakia, Latin America, and the Orient indicate many common denominators in the problems of etiology, prevalence, and severity.

Viral respiratory diseases are associated with a spectrum of host responses ranging from asymptomatic carriers to severe and sometimes fatal pneumonias. There is a recurring pattern of severe illness in infants and young children and milder disease with increasing age. There are a few clinical and epidemiologic entities which can be recognized without laboratory aids, such as acute respiratory disease (ARD) in military recruits, caused by adenovirus type 4, and rhinovirus coryza in adults. The causative agent in a large proportion of cases, however, cannot be identified without virologic study. Although it is presently impractical and unnecessary to diagnose the etiology of most respiratory viral illnesses in individual patients, an understanding of this group of diseases is best when based on etiologic relationships.

EPIDEMIOLOGY IN THE UNITED STATES

There are at present at least 153 serotypes, representing 12 groups of viruses, which have been or may be associated with acute respiratory illness in man. With the capacity to isolate this large group of agents and with the recognition of the importance of the pleuropneumonia-like organism (PPLO), *Mycoplasma pneu-*

moniae (Chap. 207) in respiratory illness, it has been possible in some studies to define the cause of many respiratory illnesses. In all studies, a majority of illnesses was caused by viruses. It seems probable that the inability to identify etiologic agents is greater than can be accounted for by lack of efficient application of known diagnostic methods and that additional viral and possibly other causes of respiratory illness remain to be discovered. For example, agents with morphologic characteristics similar to the infectious bronchitis virus of chickens (IBV) have been isolated from man, and were associated with mild respiratory illness. They may represent an additional etiologic category of human respiratory disease.

NATIONAL HEALTH SURVEY. There has been considerable progress in determining the cause of respiratory disease chiefly resulting from the National Health Survey, which, since 1957, has made annual estimates from selected population samples of the incidence of acute respiratory illness in the United States. These studies were designed to show the socioeconomic impact of illness, and cases were reported only if they caused restriction of daily activity or required medical care. There were 259 million cases of acute respiratory illness in the United States between July 1, 1961, and June 30, 1962, an average of 1.4 illnesses per person per year. A similar incidence has been noted in every year of the survey. The percentage distribution of these illnesses according to clinical diagnosis (International Classification of Diseases, 1955 revision) is shown in Table 205-1.

Except for streptococcal sore throat, some cases of bacterial pneumonia, sinusitis, etc., the remaining cases were undoubtedly largely of viral origin. It seems that some illnesses were incorrectly reported as influenza, but in other respects, the diagnostic categorization correlates well with smaller studies in which the specific cause of respiratory disease has been determined.

ETIOLOGY. An example for comparison of the specific causes with the descriptive diagnoses above is a study of acute respiratory illness in university students and military personnel in Louisiana and Mississippi. Cases were admitted to the study on the basis of a request for medical care at a dispensary. Diagnostic categories consisted of mild or acute febrile upper respiratory illness, with or without pharyngitis. These would include

Table 205-1. PERCENTAGE DISTRIBUTION BY DIAGNOSIS
OF 259 MILLION ACUTE RESPIRATORY CONDITIONS:
UNITED STATES, JULY, 1961, TO JUNE 1962

Condition	Percentage of total
Common cold	43.1
Influenza	28.6
The "virus"	9.6
Sinusitis, pharyngitis, tonsillitis, laryngitis, etc.	11.3
Pneumonia Bronchitis Influenza with digestive manifestations Other	6.1
Streptococcus sore throat	1.3
Total	100.0

SOURCE: Condensed from National Health Survey.

a large majority of the illnesses described in Table 205-1. No cases of pneumonia were included. The etiologic

Table 205-2. ETIOLOGY OF ACUTE RESPIRATORY ILLNESS
IN MILITARY RECRUITS AND UNIVERSITY STUDENTS,
NEW ORLEANS, 1958–1960

Agent	Students, %	Recruits, %
Rhinovirus	45.0	38.7
Parainfluenza type 1, 2, 3	9.4	6.8
Influenza (A_2, B)	9.2	5.8
Respiratory syncytial virus	5.3	7.9
Herpes simplex	4.1	2.9
Adenovirus	1.3	11.4
	74.3	73.5
Beta-hemolytic streptococci	3.0	5.7
Mycoplasma pneumoniae	5.5	7.0
	9.1	12.7
Unknown	16.6	13.8
Total	100.0	100.0

diagnosis was made in about 85 percent of cases (Table 205-2). Rhinovirus illness was most frequent (45.0 percent of students and 38.7 percent of recruits). Adenovirus illness was uncommon in students (1.3 percent) in contrast to 11.4 percent in recruits. Respiratory syncytial, parainfluenza, and influenza viruses made up the remainder of the illnesses, except for the small percentage of beta-hemolytic streptococcal and M. pneumoniae infections. The small percentage of herpes simplex infections represented cases in which illness was associated with a fourfold or greater rise in titer of antibody to this agent. Whether these rises represented primary or secondary infection is uncertain. The frequency of herpes labialis complicating febrile illness, the regular isolation of herpes simplex from asymptomatic persons, and the uniform presence of serum antibody to this agent in the adult population make it difficult to interpret the role of this virus in respiratory infection in the adult. Acute respiratory illness probably occurs as a consequence of primary herpes simplex infection in children.

The distribution of the virus-caused illnesses in this study is not representative of all population groups. Nevertheless, in other studies with differences in age, sex, locale, and severity of cases, these six groups of viruses have been responsible for a great majority of the diagnosed illness. They represent at least 90 different serotypes, but a much smaller number of serotypes is responsible for most of the cases in any one area at any one time.

A classification and summary of characteristic properties of these agents appear in Table 205-3 (see also Table 203-1). It is remarkable that agents of such widely varying properties can produce respiratory illnesses in man which are so clinically similar.

FREQUENCY AND SEVERITY. The National Health Survey and the above study included only cases in which there was an appreciable severity of illness. For example in the National Health Survey in the period of July 1961 to June 1962, loss of time from work or school

Table 205-3. CLASSIFICATION AND CHARACTERISTIC PROPERTIES OF HUMAN RESPIRATORY VIRUSES

Nucleic acid core	Capsidal symmetry	Enveloped	Ether and/or chloroform sensitivity	pH 3.0 liability	Virus particle size, mμ	Virus group
DNA (deoxyviruses)	Cubic	Naked	Resistant	Stable	60–85	Adenoviruses
		Enveloped	Sensitive	Labile	180–250	Herpesviruses
RNA (riboviruses)						Picornaviruses:
	Cubic	Naked	Resistant	Stable	28	Enteroviruses (Coxsackie virus, ECHO virus, and poliovirus)
				Labile	17–18	Rhinoviruses
						Myxoviruses:
	Helical	Enveloped	Sensitive	Labile	80–120	Influenza
					150–250	Parainfluenza
					90–120	Respiratory syncytial

SOURCE: Condensed from B. I. Wilner, "A Classification of the Major Groups of Human and Lower Animal Viruses," 2d ed., Berkeley, Calif., Cutter Laboratories, 1964.

Fig. 205-1. Incidence of acute upper and other respiratory conditions per 100 persons per quarter. (*National Health Survey, U.S. Public Health Service, Publ. 1000, 1963.*)

averaged 4.2 days for the 80 percent (207 million) of cases in which some restriction of activity was reported. About 50 percent, or 130 million, of persons sought medical attention although at least 52 million reported no restriction of activity.

In other studies, milder illness has been included, with a corresponding rise in annual frequency of reported cases. The Cleveland Family Study found an annual rate of illness of 6.2 per person per year, amounting to an estimated more than 1 billion cases annually in the United States. The greatest proportion of these illnesses were so mild that they constituted no hazard to health, but they are of significance in the spread of infection. In addition, it is known that wholly asymptomatic virus infections occur.

AGE, SEX, AND SEASONAL VARIATION. All studies have been in agreement that infants and young children have the greatest number of viral respiratory infections and children under six may have twice as many illnesses per year as the average of the population. Females have more illness than males; the excess is most marked during adult years and amounts to about 25 percent. There are prominent seasonal differences in the frequency of acute respiratory illness; these are shown in Fig. 205-1 from the National Health Survey. In the January-March quarter, the rates are highest (solid line), with values approximating 30 cases per 100 persons. Illness is least frequent during the summer, about

one-third of the maximum at 10 per 100 persons. The characteristic 2- to 3-year epidemic pattern of influenza is also shown.

In the following chapter (Chap. 206) consideration is given to four of the six groups of viruses chiefly responsible for respiratory disease, i.e., rhinoviruses, adenoviruses, respiratory syncytial viruses, and parainfluenza viruses. Included also is a description of the small contribution to respiratory illness of the enteroviruses, Coxsackie virus A and B, ECHO virus, and poliovirus (these viruses are discussed in detail in Chaps. 210 to 212). Influenza is described separately in Chap. 208. Pneumonia due to *M. pneumoniae* (Eaton agent) will be considered in this section (Chap. 207) for clinical reasons, although the causative agent is a pleuropneumonia organism, not a virus. Psittacosis has been included in this section in Chap. 209 for clinical reasons, although the causative agent is not a virus.

REFERENCES

Acute Conditions, Incidence and Associated Disability, United States, July 1961–June 1962, National Health Survey, U.S. Public Health Service Publ. 1000, Series 10, No. 1, 1963.

Dingle, J. H., G. F. Badger, A. E. Feller, R. G. Hodges, W. S. Jordan, and C. H. Rammelkamp: A Study of Illness in a Group of Cleveland Families: I. Plan of Study and

Certain General Observations, Am. J. Hyg., 58:16, 174, 1953.

Loosli, C. G. (Ed.): Conference on Newer Respiratory Disease Viruses, Am. Rev. Resp. Dis., 88(Suppl):1–419, 1963.

Mogabgab, W. J.: Viruses Associated with Upper Respiratory Illnesses in Adults, Ann. Intern. Med., 59:306, 1963.

206 COMMON VIRAL RESPIRATORY ILLNESSES
(Rhinoviruses; Adenoviruses; Respiratory Syncytial Virus; Parainfluenza Virus; Coxsackie Virus, ECHO Virus, and Polioviruses)

Vernon Knight

RHINOVIRUS INFECTIONS

ETIOLOGY. Pelon and Mogabgab and associates in 1956 described a new agent isolated from recruits with respiratory illness which was subsequently designated *ECHO virus, type 28.* In 1960, Hitchcock and Tyrrell isolated new agents from cases of common cold which they named *rhinoviruses.* Subsequently a large number of agents with properties similar to ECHO virus, type 28, and rhinoviruses have been isolated. At present, 55 types are known, and others are certain to be found. Some of the properties of rhinoviruses are shown in Table 205-3. Some rhinoviruses produce cytopathic effects in monkey kidney cell culture (M strains); others are not cytopathic for monkey cells but will grow in cells of human origin (H strains).

EPIDEMIOLOGY. As much as 40 percent of acute respiratory illness in adults may be caused by rhinoviruses. On the basis of the large number of serotypes, it can be presumed that the recognized contribution of these agents to acute respiratory illness will increase. Infections occur throughout the year but are most frequent in the late winter and early spring. In a limited study of the distribution of serotypes over a continuing period of observation in children, university students, and industrial employees, multiple serotypes were found to circulate simultaneously. Individual types usually persist for only a few months, however, and do not recur during succeeding seasons. Adults commonly exhibit antibody against several serotypes, whereas young children (except for the very young with maternal antibody) are relatively free of antibody. In studies in children and adults a small percentage of non-ill controls have yielded positive cultures for rhinoviruses, but in the main, the presence of rhinoviruses in the respiratory tract is associated with illness.

Most patients develop appreciable titers of type-specific antibody, and measurable levels persist for 2 to 4 years. In screening of prisoner volunteers for participation in experiments with rhinoviruses, it was found that only one-third of men are entirely free of antibody to four rhinovirus serotypes. However, illness and virus shedding can be readily induced in volunteers unless very high titers of antibody are present. Clearly, then, a high proportion of children and adults are susceptible to infection and illness with rhinoviruses. However, with some homologous and heterologous types of rhinovirus there is almost complete resistance to reinfection for several weeks following infection which is not dependent on serum antibody.

CLINICAL MANIFESTATIONS. The incubation period for rhinovirus infections in volunteers is 1 to 2 days. The common cold syndrome induced in volunteers resembles naturally occurring cases in adults. Within 24 hr of inoculation there are scratchy throat, nasal congestion and discharge, malaise, and mild headache. There is no fever, as is usual in the disease. Nasal secretions measured in grams increase sharply between day 1 and 2 and then as promptly return to preillness values. Recovery is rapid and complete. Virus shedding begins a few hours after inoculation and continues for almost 2 weeks. Type-specific neutralizing antibody rises to 1:128 at 21 days.

Table 206-1. ILLNESS ASSOCIATION WITH RHINOVIRUS INFECTIONS

Diagnosis	Adults (61)	Children (32)	Adult volunteers with nasopharyngeal inoculation (31)
	%	%	%
Common cold........	58 (92)	14 (44)	26 (84)
Croup..............	......	1 (3)	
Bronchitis..........	1 (2)	7 (23)	2 (6)
Bronchiolitis........	......	3 (9)	
Bronchopneumonia....	......	3 (9)	
No disease..........	2 (3)	4 (12)	3 (10)

SOURCE: Hamparian et al., Proc. Soc. Exp. Biol. Med., 117:469, 1964; and Cate et al., J. Clin. Invest., 43:56, 1964.

Table 206 summarizes clinical experience with naturally occurring rhinovirus infections in adults and children and artificial infection in volunteers. The great majority of adults have only a common cold syndrome, with a rare case of bronchitis as the only other form of illness. In contrast, more than one-half of children develop bronchitis, bronchiolitis, or bronchopneumonia. Although these findings resemble those of respiratory syncytial (RS) virus infection, rhinovirus disease is generally milder than that due to RS virus.

LABORATORY FINDINGS. In illness with rhinovirus there is usually a slight neutrophilia, which is the only significant alteration in leukocyte count which has been observed in this infection. Similar leukocyte responses are found in illness with rhinovirus, influenza virus, Coxsackie virus A, type 21, and adenovirus type 4. About one-third of volunteers develop elevations in sedimentation rates ranging from 27 to 50 mm per hr.

COMPLICATIONS. No serious complications have been reported with rhinovirus infections.

DIFFERENTIAL DIAGNOSIS. Among the respiratory viruses, rhinovirus infection most consistently results in coryzal illness. In any one case, however, the illness cannot be distinguished from coryza due to other agents. Except for rare confusion with an atypical case of streptococcal sore throat, only respiratory viral diseases need be considered in differential diagnosis.

TREATMENT AND PREVENTION. There is no specific treatment, and no vaccines are currently available for rhinovirus infections. Rest, analgesics, antihistamines, and nose drops are advised, depending on symptomatic needs.

ADENOVIRUS INFECTIONS

ETIOLOGY. The adenovirus group contains 31 human and 17 animal serotypes. Strains of types 3, 7, 11, 12, 14, 16, 18, 21, and 31 have been shown to cause sarcomas when injected into newborn hamsters.

Adenoviruses share a common antigen which is associated with a structural subunit of the protein coat of the

virus called a hexon. An antigenic determinant on this protein is the basis for a diagnostic complement fixation test. Type specificity in neutralizing antibody tests depends on antigenic determinants present on hexons and on another protein subunit designated the fiber, which is part of another structure in the virus coat called a penton. Except for types 12 and 18, hemagglutination inhibition (HI) tests also permit type-specific identification. Adenovirus hemagglutinins, the bases for the HI test, are variably associated with fiber subunit, with the complete penton subunit, and with the intact virion. Human adenoviruses grow well in continuous cell lines of epithelial origin.

EPIDEMIOLOGY. Adenoviruses were first isolated in 1953 by Rowe and his associates from human adenoids after elective surgery. Association with respiratory illness in military personnel was described a short time later by Hillenman and Werner. Even though serologic surveys suggest an appreciable prevalence of infection with many serotypes, definite virus-associated illness is now limited to about 10 serotypes. These serotypes produce five major patterns of illness, all of which occur in epidemics. A summary of these is presented in Table 206-2.

Acute respiratory disease (ARD), a respiratory illness of military recruits, was described by the U.S. Army Commission on Respiratory Disease before adenoviruses

Table 206-2. ILLNESS ASSOCIATED WITH ADENOVIRUS INFECTION

Disease	Occurrence	Order of association (serotypes)		Respiratory tract involvement				Fever and constitutional reaction	Other
		Common	Less common	Common cold	Pharyngitis	Bronchitis	Pneumonia		
Acute respiratory disease (ARD)	Epidemic in winter and spring in military recruits	4, 7	3, 14, 21	Often present	*Most frequent,* usually with fever, often with laryngitis	Frequent, usually with fever and laryngitis	Infrequent complication of ARD, but adenovirus pneumonia is an important type of pneumonia in recruits	Headache, malaise, often high fever for several days	Usually no other involvement
Pharyngoconjunctival fever	Summer epidemics in civilians, often in school-age children related to swimming pools. Sporadic cases of conjunctivitis may occur without pharyngitis.	3, 7	4, 14	Often present	*Most frequent,* usually with fever and cervical lymphadenopathy, hoarseness	Uncommon	Rare	Headache, malaise, high fever for several days	Acute follicular conjunctivitis, usually unilateral, occurs with varying frequency. Preauricular lymphadenopathy common with conjunctivitis
Febrile pharyngitis	Sporadic or epidemic, resembles ARD, often in children	3, 7	1, 2, 5	Often present	*Most frequent,* usually with fever	Frequent, especially in older children	Infrequent but severe complications	High fever, malaise, headache	Nausea, vomiting, and diarrhea may occur, especially in infants
Pneumonia in children	Highly fatal illness in infants, sporadic or epidemic	3, 7		Occurs	Very frequent	Very frequent	Primary, with acidophilic necrosis of tracheal and bronchial mucosa resembling tissue culture CPE	High fever, prostration	Conjunctivitis, skin rash, diarrhea, intussusception, and CNS invasion in some cases
Keratoconjunctivitis (EKC)	Epidemic disease in shipyard workers; also spread from infected eye solutions	8	11	Unusual	Uncommon	Not reported	Not reported	Usually afebrile	Usually unilateral severe, acute conjunctivitis followed by corneal subepithelial keratosis; preauricular lymphadenopathy common

were discovered. Later testing of serum from some of these patients revealed that these infections were caused by adenoviruses. Other studies have shown regular winter and spring outbreaks of ARD in military recruits in the United States caused by adenovirus types 4 and 7, and with lesser frequency by type 3. Types 14 and 21 have caused similar outbreaks in military personnel in the Netherlands and elsewhere. In military groups, 15 to 50 percent of acute respiratory illness is caused by adenoviruses, but in civilian adults, only about 2 percent of respiratory illnesses are due to adenoviruses, and in children only about 6 percent.

Febrile pharyngitis due to adenoviruses is usually a disease of civilians, often occurring sporadically or in small outbreaks in children. Its manifestations are summarized in Table 206-2. *Pharyngoconjunctival fever* is febrile pharyngitis associated with acute follicular conjunctivitis. This disease occurs as summer epidemics, frequently among children in relation to exposure in swimming pools. Although it is not limited to swimming pool exposure, it is believed that eye irritation from water, sun, or chlorine may be a factor in its initiation. Conjunctivitis may occur without pharyngitis.

Pneumonia due to adenovirus infection is rare in civilian adults, but it now seems certain that an atypical pneumonia due to adenovirus infection occurs in military recruits, usually as an extension of ARD. In infants and children, sporadic and epidemic occurrence of highly fatal adenoviral pneumonia has been described in several parts of the world. These have been principally caused by types 3 and 7. The severity of disease in this young age group may reflect the lack of prior experience with these agents, but other factors such as size and route of inoculation, general health, or greater susceptibility due to immaturity may be important.

Epidemic keratoconjunctivitis due to type 8 and less often to type 11 or other serotypes is described in Chap. 228.

Incubation Period. The period of incubation for pharyngoconjunctival fever and ARD is 5 to 10 days. A similar incubation period has been noted for induced disease in volunteers. Incubation periods for the other naturally occurring syndromes have not been established but are probably similar.

PATHOGENESIS. Illness in volunteers is produced when the conjunctival sac is swabbed with suspensions of adenovirus. In these cases, conjunctivitis occurs and there is sometimes respiratory involvement. The initiation of illness appears to require a significant degree of conjunctival irritation. A second method of producing illness is administration of virus aerosol by inhalation. Volunteers inoculated in this way have developed ARD and primary atypical pneumonia.

These observations suggest the existence of at least two routes of inoculation for naturally occurring respiratory illness with adenoviruses: (1) ocular inoculation associated with eye irritation such as may occur in outbreaks around swimming pools, with the development of *pharyngoconjunctival fever;* (2) inoculation through inhalation of infectious aerosol generated by sneezing and

coughing of ill recruits under the crowded circumstances incidental to recruit training. This exposure results in *ARD or primary atypical pneumonia.* The route of inoculation of infants is less likely to be limited to aerosolized virus, and the occurrence of pneumonia may represent primarily a lack of resistance in this young age group.

The regular production of virus infection without illness by nasopharyngeal inoculation in volunteers suggests that a similar circumstance may occur naturally as an explanation for the high frequency of antibody to many serotypes in the population. This antibody may also result from intragroup cross reactions among serotypes in the three broad immunologic groups of adenovirus.

CLINICAL MANIFESTATIONS. *Acute respiratory disease* is an acute febrile illness lasting about 1 week and characterized by fever, cough, hoarseness, and sore throat. Fever has gradual onset and reaches a maximum of 103 to 104°F on the second or third day. There are associated malaise and often headache. Pharyngitis is the most prominent localized manifestation of the disease, and reaches maximum severity after about 3 days. There may also be regional lymphadenopathy, pharyngeal injection, some edema, frequent lymphoid follicular hyperplasia, but little or no faucial exudate. Nasal obstruction and discharge occur in almost one-half of cases, but these abnormalities are not usually conspicuous. Cough is almost always present, and hoarseness is also frequent.

Many clinical and laboratory features of ARD are represented in Fig. 206-1, a case caused by inhalation of aerosol containing adenovirus type 4. This volunteer had no measurable antibody to the agent before inoculation. Five days after inoculation he developed a febrile pharyngitis which increased in severity for 2 or 3 days and then gradually improved. There were also cough, hoarseness, malaise, and headache. Shedding of virus from nose, throat, and rectum continued for at least 4 weeks, long after recovery from illness. The white cell count remained at preinoculation levels for the first few days of illness but declined to low values 1 week after onset of symptoms. This late leukopenia is in accord with observations in other volunteers and with limited observations on naturally occurring disease. There was also a significant rise in blood sedimentation rate.

Pharyngoconjunctival fever is usually a milder respiratory illness than ARD, although fever may be high for 5 or 6 days. Nontender submandibular lymphadenopathy is common even in the absence of sore throat. Lower respiratory tract involvement has not been described. Conjunctivitis is mild to moderate but may last longer than respiratory symptoms. It is an acute, nonpurulent, follicular conjunctivitis. In most cases, it is unilateral, and pre-auricular lymphadenopathy is rare. There is usually no involvement of the cornea or uveal tract.

Febrile pharyngitis without conjunctivitis resembles the foregoing illness, except for the absence of conjunctivitis.

Adenoviral pneumonia in children occurs as a primary illness and is associated with as much as 15 percent mortality. Pediatric texts should be consulted for further details.

Fig. 206-1. Acute respiratory disease (ARD) produced in a volunteer by aerosol inoculation. (*Case of Dr. Robert B. Couch, National Institutes of Health.*)

DIFFERENTIAL DIAGNOSIS. The differential diagnosis of ARD should include the respiratory viral diseases described in the present chapter and influenza (Chap. 208), nonpneumonic forms of *Mycoplasma pneumoniae* infection (Chap. 207), streptococcal sore throat, and purulent sinusitis. Pharyngitis and upper respiratory illness may also accompany the onset of infectious hepatitis and infectious mononucleosis.

Differential diagnosis of *pharyngoconjunctival fever,* when conjunctivitis is prominent, includes leptospirosis, influenza, measles, herpangina, and the nonpurulent conjunctivitides, such as inclusion conjunctivitis and physical or chemical trauma to the eye.

TREATMENT. There is no specific treatment for adenovirus infection. In one study, adenovirus conjunctivitis in volunteers did not respond to 5-iodo-2′ deoxyuridine by local application. In vitro this compound prevented DNA synthesis by adenoviruses, and failure of the therapeutic trial may have resulted from inadequate contact of the drug with infected tissues. The considerable toxicity of the drug when given systemically has prevented its further study.

Treatment is limited to alleviation of general discomfort, headache, and coughing with analgesics, cough syrup containing terpin hydrate, codeine, antihistamines, or other antitussives.

PREVENTION. Communicability of adenovirus infection probably extends from a day or so before onset of illness to recovery, and conventional precautions against respiratory spread should be employed during acute illness for patients in the hospital and to the extent reasonably possible in care of patients at home.

Avoidance of swimming pools during outbreaks of pharyngoconjunctival fever is recommended. Patients

with epidemic keratoconjunctivitis should be kept from work, and care should be exercised to prevent spread of discharges from infected eyes.

Early studies on volunteers revealed that type-specific antibody provided substantial protection against live virus challenge. Formalin-treated vaccines against types 3, 4, and 7 offer significant protection against infection, but their use has largely been limited to military recruits. A vaccine for type 4 adenovirus infection consisting of live virus incorporated into an enteric-coated capsule may soon become available.

RESPIRATORY SYNCYTIAL VIRUS INFECTION

ETIOLOGY. Respiratory syncytial virus (RS) is classified as a subgroup of the myxoviruses. It is of medium size (90 to 120 mμ), RNA in type, of helical symmetry, and is destroyed by ethyl ether. In tissue culture, it causes formation of giant cells, or syncytia, from which its name was derived. It grows well in several human primary and continuous cell lines and in primary rhesus monkey kidney culture. There is a soluble complement-fixing antigen which, with the neutralization test, permits virus identification and serologic studies. RS virus contrasts with other myxoviruses because it does not grow or cause detectable changes in mice, guinea pigs, rabbits, or chick embryos and does not cause hemagglutination or hemadsorption.

EPIDEMIOLOGY. Since the first recovery of RS virus from a chimpanzee with a coryzal illness by Morris and his associates in 1956, epidemiologic studies have delineated a very substantial role of this agent in acute respiratory disease in children. Illness in young children occurs most commonly in epidemics in the late winter and early spring. Attack rates are nearly 100 percent among susceptibles, who are mostly children under four years of age. In older children and adults, the disease appears in nonepidemic patterns. The limitation of epidemic disease to the younger age group is also evidence for unchanging antigenicity of the agent, in contrast to the situation with influenza virus, in which antigenic shifts are associated with recurrent epidemics in persons of all ages.

In serologic surveys of several hundred Federal prisoners for selection as volunteers, all were found to possess a measurable titer of neutralizing antibody to RS virus. Mild upper respiratory illness appears to be the only clinical manifestation of RS virus infection in adults.

It is probable that RS virus is transmitted by means of infected respiratory secretions but, as with other respiratory viral diseases, the mechanism has not been more precisely defined. The incubation period of naturally occurring disease in children is about 4 days, and in adult volunteers who developed common cold syndromes, the average incubation period was approximately 5 days. Virus was generally recovered from volunteers a day or so before the onset of illness, and throat swabs yielded a higher proportion of positive cultures than nasal swabs. Virus shedding continues for 3 to 4 days after onset of illness.

CLINICAL MANIFESTATIONS. Table 206-3 gives data on

Table 206-3. ILLNESS WITH RESPIRATORY SYNCYTIAL VIRUS IN CHILDREN AND ADULTS

Subjects	Upper respiratory illness (rhinitis, pharyngitis, cough, malaise), %	Bronchitis, %	Bronchiolitis, %	Bronchopneumonia, %
Children,* 108 cases, 8 years old and younger........	46	16	9	21
Adults,† 20 volunteers...........	100	None	None	None

* 91% with fever, average 102°F.
† No fever.
SOURCE: McClelland et al., New Engl. J. Med., 264:1169, 1961; Reilly et al., New Engl. J. Med., 264:1176, 1961; and Kravetz et al., J.A.M.A., 176:657, 1961.

the clinical syndromes associated with RS virus infection. Somewhat less than one-half of children had symptoms defined as a common cold; the remainder had bronchiolitis or bronchopneumonia. Fever was present in 91 percent of all children, with an average elevation of 102°F. Cough was almost invariably present, and severe malaise was frequent. Pharyngitis was not usually severe. Fatalities have been reported in infants.

In contrast, naturally occurring illness or induced disease in adult volunteers is a mild syndrome characterized by rhinitis and pharyngitis. Intranasal inoculation of virus into a normal volunteer was followed in 4 days by an afebrile illness consisting of nasal obstruction, clear, profuse nasal discharge, headache, malaise, and slight cough. On the second day of illness, nasal secretion amounted to more than 30 Gm. Improvement was rapid, and recovery was nearly complete 8 days after inoculation. Virus shedding preceded symptoms by 2 days and continued during the first 4 days of illness.

LABORATORY FINDINGS. In children, leukocytosis occurs with some frequency, but no significant hematologic changes were observed in adult volunteers. Bacterial flora of the nasopharynx and other laboratory indices show no significant alterations in either age group.

COMPLICATIONS. Except for progression to overwhelming lower respiratory tract disease in a few young children, no special complications are known. There is no evidence of secondary bacterial infection or systemic invasion by the virus in children. In adults, bacterial sinusitis is occasionally encountered.

DIFFERENTIAL DIAGNOSIS. The resemblance of this disease in children to influenza has been suggested. In addition, illness with other respiratory viruses, especially adenovirus and parainfluenza, may be difficult to distinguish. Finally, M. pneumoniae infections or bacterial pneumonias may cause difficulty in diagnosis. In adults, the differential diagnosis should include rhinovirus and parainfluenza infection and, less often, other respiratory viral diseases and M. pneumoniae infection.

TREATMENT. As with the other respiratory viral diseases, treatment should include rest and palliative medications such as aspirin, nose drops, and medication for sleep when restlessness occurs. The possibility of bacterial sinusitis in adults should be kept in mind and antimicrobial treatment, drainage procedures, or other therapy instituted when necessary.

PREVENTION. No vaccine is available. The infection spreads rapidly among children in institutions and poses a threat to debilitated or very young children. Rigid isolation procedures should be enforced in such circumstances, but their effectiveness cannot be assured. Suspected cases should avoid contact with children.

PARAINFLUENZA VIRUS INFECTIONS

ETIOLOGY. The first agent of this group of myxoviruses to be isolated was the Sendai virus (parainfluenza type 1). It was obtained in mice following intranasal inoculation with material from the lung of a child with a fatal case of pneumonia. In view of later isolations of parainfluenza type 1 from mice, the human origins of this first isolate has been questioned. Subsequently, human strains were isolated in tissue culture in the period 1956 to 1960. On the basis of antigenic differences, they are divided into four types. They agglutinate avian and mammalian erythrocytes and grow slowly in tissue culture, and only type 2 produces readily visible cytopathic effects. Growth of these agents in tissue culture is detected by addition of guinea pig erythrocytes, which absorb on the surface of infected cells to form rosettes, a process known as hemadsorption. Parainfluenza viruses have antigens common to Newcastle disease and mumps viruses, but influenza virus does not share these. Parainfluenza serotypes are distinguished by complement fixation, hemagglutination-inhibition, or tissue culture neutralization tests.

Primary monkey or primary human embryonic kidney cell cultures are suitable for isolation. Other human primary and continuous lines support growth of these agents less well. They grow slowly or not at all in embryonated chicken eggs.

Animal counterparts to the first three types have been identified; type 1 (Sendai virus) has been isolated from mice and pigs, type 2 (simian viruses 5 and 41) has been isolated from monkeys, and type 3 (shipping fever virus) has been recovered from cattle.

EPIDEMIOLOGY. The first three types of parainfluenza viruses have been found in many parts of the world; type 4 has so far been isolated only in the United States. Infection with parainfluenza viruses occurs early in life. By the age of eight years, a majority of children show antibody to types 1 to 3, and, although studies are limited, it appears that most adults have antibody to all four types.

In children, illness with parainfluenza viruses occurs throughout the year, with seasonal increases in the winter and spring. Studies of institutional outbreaks suggest that type 3 virus spreads more rapidly than types 1 and 2. Heterotypic rises are frequent, with antibody to type 3 developing in half the cases with type 1 infection. In both children and adults, reinfection is frequent. In one outbreak, 96 percent of children without antibody, 67 percent with low levels, and 33 percent with high levels of antibody became infected. In adults, the disease is almost invariably a reinfection and, presumably for this reason, is much milder than in children.

The total contribution of parainfluenza infections to respiratory illness is quite variable, its frequency increasing in institutions in which general health status is lower than average and levels of sanitation and personal hygiene are less than optimum. In the United States, the percentage contribution of parainfluenza infections in several studies of children has varied from 4.3 to 17. The milder illness which occurs in adults has usually constituted less than 5 percent of respiratory illnesses.

CLINICAL MANIFESTATIONS. In all age groups, the incubation period appears to be 5 to 6 days. The disease is most serious in infants and children, the characteristic syndrome being laryngotracheobronchitis, or croup. In a study of croup in a large children's hospital, a third of the cases were due to parainfluenza infections. Much of the bronchiolitis, bronchitis, and bronchopneumonia in children was also caused by these agents. The average age of the children with croup was two years.

In older children the disease is less serious, usually without evidence of pulmonary involvment, and in adults, the virus produces a common cold syndrome with hoarseness and cough.

Fever is a constant feature of illness in children but is less frequent in adults. A description of selected febrile cases observed in a community outbreak appears in Table 206-4. Nasal discharge was a common occurrence at all ages, although this is not reflected in the small number of cases in the five- to fourteen-year age group described in the table. Cough and hoarseness were common, and stridor, indicative of croup, was present in many of the infants and children.

Table 206-4. CLINICAL FEATURES OF ILLNESS WITH PARAINFLUENZA VIRUSES

Clinical features	0–4 years, 14 cases, %	5–14 years, 7 cases, %	Adults, 11 cases, %
Fever	100	100	100
Cough	100	100	90
Hoarseness	92	86	72
Stridor	43	29	
Sore throat	36	71	72
Nasal discharge	64	28	56
Headache	7	43	72
Depression	...	...	45

SOURCE: Condensed from Banatvala et al., Brit. Med. J., 1:537, 1964.

Physical findings are not distinctive. The throat is reddened, with little or no exudate. There may be tender submandibular lymphadenopathy.

LABORATORY FINDINGS. In adult volunteers given type 2 virus, leukocyte counts were not abnormal. In children there is a considerable variation in leukocyte counts early in illness, making it difficult to distinguish this disease from pneumococcal and other bacterial infections. After a few days, however, leukocyte counts tend to become normal or low. Detailed studies of blood counts in proved cases have not been reported. No characteristic alterations have been reported in other laboratory indices such as liver or renal function tests, electrocardiograms, and urinalyses.

COURSE AND COMPLICATIONS. In children, *otitis media* has occurred as a complication more often with parainfluenza than with the other infections. It may be caused by pneumococci, streptococci, or *H. influenza.* The illness is characterized by slow resolution of pulmonary involvement and long persistence of cough and other symptoms. In very young or debilitated children, the outcome can be fatal. In adults, bacterial sinusitis may occur, and in persons with chronic bronchitis, emphysema, or bronchiectasis, the possibility of pulmonary bacterial superinfections should be considered.

TREATMENT. There is no specific treatment. Therapy is limited to symptomatic measures and efforts aimed at early detection and treatment of bacterial complications such as otitis media or pneumonia. Nursing care is important in pediatric cases, especially children with croup, and reference should be made to appropriate pediatric sources for procedures to be followed.

Table 206-5. RESPIRATORY ILLNESS ASSOCIATED WITH COXSACKIE VIRUS A AND B, ECHO VIRUS, AND POLIOVIRUS

Diagnosis	Description	Associated viruses
Herpangina..................	Febrile pharyngitis, anorexia, and discrete vesicular eruption on anterior faucial pillars. Occurs chiefly in children in summer and early fall outbreaks. Similar illnesses without eruption caused by the same viruses probably occur. An illness with nonulcerating nodules on anterior pillars caused by Coxsackie A 10 has also been described.	Coxsackie virus A 1 through 6, 8, 10, and 12
Febrile respiratory illness ("summer grippe")	Undifferentiated febrile illness marked by headache, sore throat, and anorexia occurring in summer or early fall. Includes epidemics in recruits of similar disease with Coxsackie A 21, in which illness patterns have been confirmed by experimental inoculation of volunteers.	Coxsackie virus A 21, 24, Coxsackie virus B 2, 3, 5 (?), ECHO virus 1, 3, 6, 19, 20, and polioviruses
Upper respiratory illness associated with gastroenteritis	Cases occurring largely in infants and exposed mothers.	ECHO virus 1, 11, 19, 20
Acute laryngotracheobronchitis (croup)	Winter outbreaks in nurseries and institutions. Association less definite than with other syndromes.	Coxsackie virus A 9, B 5, and ECHO virus 11
Pneumonitis and pleuritis......	Largely confined to young infants and children; of uncommon occurrence	Coxsackie virus A 9, B 4, 5, ECHO virus 9, 19, 20

In adults, analgesics, antihistamines, and small doses of codeine for cough are generally sufficient.

PREVENTION. Vaccines against parainfluenza virus infections are not available. In hospitals, respiratory precautions should be carried out. At home, bed rest or room isolation during acute illness is advised, with special effort to avoid contact with very young children or aged persons.

COXSACKIE, ECHO, AND POLIOVIRUS INFECTIONS

Diseases produced by these agents are described in Chaps. 210 through 212 and 216. Table 206-5, however, summarizes the respiratory illnesses sometimes seen in infections by these viruses.

REFERENCES

General

Loosli, C. G. (Ed.): Conference on Newer Respiratory Disease Viruses, Am. Rev. Resp. Dis., 88(Suppl.):1–419, 1963

Adenoviruses

Bell, J. A., W. P. Rowe, J. I. Engler, R. H. Parrott, and R. J. Huebner: Pharyngoconjunctival Fever: Epidemiological Studies of a Recently Recognized Disease Entity, J.A.M.A., 157:1083, 1955.

Commission on Respiratory Diseases: Clinical Patterns of Undifferentiated and Other Acute Respiratory Diseases in Army Recruits, Medicine, 26:441, 1947.

Girardi, A. J., M. R. Hilleman, and R. E. Zwickey: Tests in Hamsters for Oncogenic Quality of Ordinary Viruses Including Adenovirus Type 7, Proc. Soc. Exp. Biol. Med., 115:1141, 1964.

Kasel, J. A., P. A. Banks, R. Wigand, V. Knight, and D. W. Alling: An Immunologic Classification of Heterotypic

Antibody Responses to Adenoviruses in Man, Proc. Soc. Exp. Biol. Med., 119:1162, 1965.

Ward, T. G., R. J. Huebner, W. P. Rowe, R. W. Ryan, and J. A. Bell: Production of Pharyngoconjunctival Fever in Human Volunteers Inoculated with APC Viruses, Science, 122:1086, 1955.

Coxsackie, Echo, and Polioviruses

Kibrick, S.: Current Status of Coxsackie and ECHO Viruses in Human Disease, pp. 27–70 in "Progress in Medical Virology, 6," J. L. Melnick (Ed.), Basel and New York, S. Karger AG, 1964.

Spickard, A., H. Evans, V. Knight, and K. Johnson: Acute Respiratory Disease in Normal Volunteers Associated with Coxsackie A-21 Viral Infection: III. Response to Nasopharyngeal and Enteric Inoculation, J. Clin. Invest., 42:840, 1963.

Parainfluenza Virus

Banatvala, J. E., T. B. Anderson, and B. B. Reiss: Parainfluenza Infections in the Community, Brit. Med. J., 1:537, 1964.

Chanock, R. M., R. H. Parrott, M. K. Cook, B. E. Andrews, J. A. Bell, T. Reichelderfer, A. Z. Kapikian, F. M. Mastrata, and R. J. Huebner: Newly Recognized Myxoviruses from Children with Respiratory Disease, New Engl. J. Med., 258:207, 1958.

Johnson, K. M., R. M. Chanock, M. K. Cook, and R. J. Huebner: Studies of a New Human Hemadsorption Virus: I. Isolation, Properties, and Characterization, Am. J. Hyg., 71:81, 1960.

Respiratory Syncytial Virus

Kravetz, H. M., V. Knight, R. M. Chanock, J. A. Morris, K. M. Johnson, D. Rifkind, and J. P. Utz: Respiratory Syncytial Virus: III. Production of Illness and Clinical Observations in Adult Volunteers, J.A.M.A., 176:657, 1961.

McClelland, L., M. R. Hilleman, V. V. Hamparian, A. Keller, C. M. Reilly, D. Cornfeld, and J. Stokes, Jr.: Studies of

Acute Respiratory Illness Caused by Respiratory Syncytial Virus: 2. Epidemiology and Assessment of Importance, New Engl. J. Med., 264:1169, 1961.

Reilly, C. M., J. Stokes, Jr., L. McClelland, D. Cornfeld, V. V. Hamparian, A. Ketler, and M. Hilleman: Studies of Acute Respiratory Illness Caused by Respiratory Syncytial Virus: 3. Clinical and Laboratory Findings, New Engl. J. Med., 264:1176, 1961.

Rhinoviruses

Cate, T. R., R. B. Couch, and K. M. Johnson: Studies with Rhinoviruses in Volunteers: Production of Illness, Effect of Naturally Acquired Antibody, and Demonstration of a Protective Effect Not Associated with Serum Antibody, J. Clin. Invest., 43:56, 1964.

Hamparian, V. V., M. B. Leagus, M. R. Hilleman, and J. Stokes, Jr.: Epidemiologic Investigations of Rhinovirus Infections, Proc. Soc. Exp. Biol. Med., 117:469, 1964.

207 PNEUMONIA CAUSED BY MYCOPLASMA PNEUMONIAE

Vernon Knight

SYNONYMS. Primary atypical pneumonia, Eaton's agent pneumonia, cold agglutinin-positive pneumonia, "virus" pneumonia.

DEFINITION. Pneumonia caused by *Mycoplasma pneumoniae* is characterized by fever, pharyngitis, cough, and

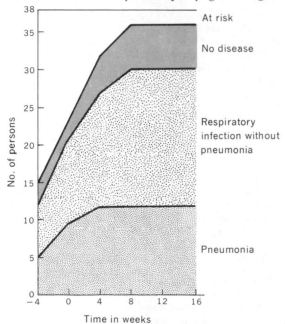

Fig. 207-1. Cumulative incidence of *M. pneumoniae* infection and clinical response in 38 exposed family members. The final case of pneumonia appeared 8 weeks after the first case. Respiratory infection without pneumonia continued to occur for 12 weeks after onset of the first case. This slow course of family spread is typical of such outbreaks. (*Balassanian and Robbins; N. Eng. J. Med., 277:719, 1967; with permission.*)

pulmonary infiltration, often multilobular, in which roentgenographic signs are more extensive than indicated by physical examination. This organism is also the cause of upper respiratory illness without pneumonia and of asymptomatic infection.

ETIOLOGY. *Mycoplasma pneumoniae*, one of several species of human and animal pleuropneumonia-like organisms (PPLO), is one of the smallest organisms (150 to 250 mμ) capable of replication in cell-free media. It lacks a cell wall, requires cholesterol for development of its limiting membrane (not a requirement for saprophyte types), and has exacting nutritional requirements. It grows on or beneath the surface of agar slants in a small, round, granular colony without the "fried egg" peripheral zone characteristic of many other PPLO. It is inhibited in vitro by tetracycline derivatives, streptomycin, kanamycin, erythromycin, oleandomycin, chloramphenicol, and gold salts. It is not inhibited by penicillin, sulfonamides, or thallium acetate. It is distinguished from other human mycoplasmas by rapid hemolysis of guinea pig erythrocytes and utilization of glucose and other sugars. It also hemolyzes human and rat erythrocytes. It may also be distinguished from other mycoplasmas by fluorescent antibody, complement fixation, growth inhibition, and indirect hemagglutination tests all of which are useful for serologic diagnosis of human infection. In addition to growth on agar, the organism grows on the surface of cells of embryonated eggs and monkey kidney cell culture with little evidence of cytopathic effect. In human cell cultures, however, there is intracellular growth with cytopathic effects.

EPIDEMIOLOGY. In the general population *M. Pneumoniae* infection is characterized by intrafamily spread. In most cases the infection is introduced into the family by a schoolchild. Once introduced, most family members become infected. The time course of the infection and associated illnesses in six involved families is described in Fig. 207-1. Spread through these families required about 8 weeks; pneumonia occurred in one-third of the infected family members. In family outbreaks, pneumonia occurs with greatest frequency among school-age children with a predominance in males. The disease is rare above age forty. *Mycoplasma pneumoniae* pneumonia occurs throughout the year, although prolonged wintertime outbreaks may occur in college groups or communities. The total incidence of *M. pneumoniae* pneumonia in a study in Seattle was 1.3/1,000/year, which constituted about 10 percent of pneumonia from all causes.

In the military, *M. pneumoniae* infections account for a small proportion of upper respiratory illness in recruits, in one study 6.3 percent. However, it accounted for almost one-half of cases of pneumonia in the same military population. The disease appears to be endemic at military bases, and onset of cases is greatest during the second to fifth months of training.

Mycoplasma pneumoniae is probably spread by means of infected respiratory secretions. The organisms can be cultured from sputum of naturally occurring cases and from volunteers inoculated artificially. Primary atypical pneumonia has been induced in volunteers both by nasopharyngeal inoculation and by inhalation of a small-particle aerosol containing the agent. Studies in volunteers reveal that naturally acquired antibody is associated with a high degree of resistance to infection.

CLINICAL MANIFESTATIONS. From studies in military recruits and normal volunteers, the incubation period appears to vary from 9 to 12 days. Illness due to *M. pneumoniae* usually begins with symptoms of upper respiratory illness, which, in a small percentage of cases, progresses to bronchitis and pneumonia. Cough is almost universal in pneumonia and is frequent in cases without pulmonary involvement. Blood-flecked sputum may occur in the more severe cases, but gross hemoptysis is rare. A variety of other respiratory and systemic complaints may occur. Fever, nasal congestion, and sore throat are common. Cervical adenopathy is not frequent. In pneumonia, harsh or diminished sounds are frequent but bronchial breathing is uncommon. Fine inspiratory rales are found in most patients but are not impressive. Pleural rubs and pleural effusion are infrequent. Studies on the distribution of pneumonia show frequent bilateral involvement in the lower lobes. Involvement of a single lower lobe is less common, and upper lobe involvement is rare. Pulmonary infiltrates may occur as an isolated area in the lung periphery but more often spread from the hilum.

The disease is variable in severity, but high fever may persist for 1 to 2 weeks in untreated cases. X-ray changes last for as long as 3 weeks in untreated cases, but for 7 to 10 days in treated cases. Even in untreated cases, complications are rare and consist of occasional purulent sinusitis, persistent cough, and, rarely, pleurisy. Prolonged weakness and malaise follow the untreated illness in adults.

Many features of naturally occurring illness are presented in a case of disease induced in a volunteer (Fig. 207-2). On day 10 after inoculation, temperature elevation was first noted; by day 12 the temperature was almost 40°C (104°F). Right lower lobar infiltration was detected on day 12. On day 13 a small area of infiltration was observed near the left cardiac border in the left lower lobe. Neither infiltrate was especially dense. Rapid recovery ensued with treatment with demethylchlortetracycline. There was no leukocytosis, but the sedimentation rate was increased on day 15 to 65 mm per hr. *Mycoplasma pneumoniae* was isolated from sputum specimens in tissue culture on four occasions. Fluorescent antibody increased from a nonmeasurable value to a serum dilution of 1:160 by day 24. Cold agglutinin titers increased from

S.m. 33YOW♂

Fig. 207-2. Case of primary atypical pneumonia in a volunteer produced by inoculation with *Mycoplasma pneumoniae*. After an incubation period of about 10 days bilateral mild atypical pneumonia developed. Although the apparent response to treatment with demethylchlortetracycline in this case is not proof of drug effect, it is indicative of the favorable response seen in a large controlled study with this drug. (*Rifkind et al.: Rev. Resp. Dis., 85:479, 1962.*)

1:8 to 1:256. *Streptococcus MG* agglutinins did not appear. This patient also developed a hemorrhagic myringitis bilaterally, which healed promptly with recovery from pneumonia.

Ear involvement consisting of congestion of the tympanic membrane, bullous, and, rarely, hemorrhagic myringitis may occur in as many as 10 percent of cases, most often in children.

Studies with volunteers have revealed, in addition to pneumonia, the occurrence of febrile and afebrile upper respiratory illness characterized by nonexudative pharyngitis and tracheobronchitis, often associated with cough, headache, and nasal congestion. This disease persists for 1 to 2 weeks and is followed by uncomplicated recovery. This is a common manifestation of *M. pneumoniae* infection in the general population at all ages.

LABORATORY FINDINGS. During acute illness leukocytosis in the range of 10,000 to 15,000 per cu mm occurs in about 25 percent of cases. Increase in sedimentation rate above 40 mm per hr occurs in at least two-thirds of cases. Urinalysis, electrocardiograms, and fluid and electrolyte and liver function studies show no characteristic changes. The complement fixation, fluorescent antibody, indirect hemagglutination, and growth inhibition tests all yield highly specific diagnostic information. The simplicity of the complement fixation test recommends it for general use. Fourfold rises in titer often occur within 2 weeks, and maximum rise is achieved in 4 weeks. In atypical pneumonia, agglutinins to *Streptococcus MG* have been reported to develop in varying frequency. Higher titers are correlated with more severe illness. Of probably greater diagnostic value than *Streptococcus MG* agglutination is the appearance late in illness of cold agglutinins for human, type O red cells. The test may be positive in as high as 90 percent of severely ill patients but is less often positive in nonpneumonic cases.

DIFFERENTIAL DIAGNOSIS. Pneumonia due to *M. pneumoniae* is to be distinguished from pneumonia of all other types. It is usually less severe and is associated with less dense pulmonary infiltration than pneumococcal and other bacterial pneumonias. The discovery of pulmonary infiltrate in the absence of symptoms or physical signs may initially suggest acute pulmonary tuberculosis. In military populations adenovirus pneumonia must be excluded. Pneumonic involvement as a direct result of influenza viral infection or its complication by pneumococcal, streptococcal, staphylococcal, or *H. influenza* infection may cause difficulty in diagnosis. Q fever, psittacosis, and tularemia are less frequent causes of pneumonia which may be difficult to distinguish from *M. pneumoniae* infection. In children, especially young infants, pneumonia due to respiratory syncytial, parainfluenza, adenovirus, and influenza viruses may resemble *M. pneumoniae* infection. Cases of undiagnosed pneumonia, despite careful workup, are a regular finding in both military and civilian populations, suggesting that other causes of pneumonia remain to be discovered.

TREATMENT. Demethylchlortetracycline and other tetracycline derivatives, erythromycin, and triacetyloleandomycin are effective in treatment of pneumonia due to *M. pneumoniae*. Demethylchlortetracycline may be given to adults in daily doses of 0.9 Gm; tetracycline, 1.5 Gm; erthromycin stearate or ethyl succinate, 1.5 and 1.2 Gm per day, respectively. Response to treatment is characterized by prompt defervescence, rapid clearing of x-ray signs of pneumonia, and disappearance of malaise and weakness. Persistent cough, despite treatment, is a relatively common finding, especially in women.

Treatment temporarily reduces the frequency of positive cultures from the respiratory tract, but shedding may continue for several weeks after treatment, a finding similar to that in psittacosis pneumonia. Relapse of *M. pneumoniae* pneumonia occurs occasionally following treatment, but such cases respond to retreatment.

PREVENTION. Although antibody is apparently highly protective, effective vaccines are not yet available. For patients in the hospital respiratory precautions are advisable during the first day or so of treatment. Acutely ill patients at home should be isolated from very young children and persons in whom a complicating respiratory illness would constitute a special hazard.

REFERENCES

Foy, H. M., J. T. Grayston, G. E. Kenny, E. R. Alexander, and Ruth McMahan: Epidemiology of *Mycoplasma Pneumoniae* Infection in Families, J.A.M.A., 197:137, 1966.

Kingston, J. R., R. M. Chanock, M. A. Mufson, L. P. Hellman, W. D. James, H. H. Fox, M. A. Manko, and J. Boyers: Eaton Agent Pneumonia, J.A.M.A., 176:118, 1961.

Mogabgab, W. J.: *Mycoplasma Pneumoniae*, and Adenovirus Respiratory Illnesses in Military and University Personnel, 1959–1966, Am. Rev. Resp. Dis., 97:345, 1968.

Rifkind, D., R. Chanock, H. Kravetz, K. Johnson, and V. Knight: Ear Involvement (Myringitis) and Primary Atypical Pneumonia Following Inoculation of Volunteers with Eaton Agent, Am. Rev. Resp. Dis., 85:479, 1962.

208 INFLUENZA
Robert R. Wagner

DEFINITION. Influenza is an acute respiratory infection of specific viral etiology characterized by sudden onset of headache, myalgia, fever, and prostration. The terms *influenza* and "flu" should be restricted to those cases with clear-cut epidemiologic or laboratory evidence of infection with influenza viruses.

HISTORY. Influenza is an Italian word meaning "influence" (originally referring to the influence of the stars or the cold), which first came into common English usage during the European epidemic of 1743. In most non-English-speaking countries, the disease is referred to by the French word "grippe," or its equivalent. According to the best available records, influenza was uncommon in Europe during the nineteenth century until the pandemic of 1889. Subsequently, the frequency and severity of epidemics increased, culminating in the disastrous pandemic of 1918, which caused an estimated 20 to 40 million deaths. The isolation of the causative virus in 1933 by Smith, Andrewes, and Laidlaw led to the development of simple diagnostic tests, which have greatly advanced knowledge of the disease. The pandemic of 1957 was, perhaps, the most thoroughly studied and documented major epidemic in the annals of medicine.

ETIOLOGY. There are three distinct antigenic types of influenza virus, designated A, B, and C, in the order in which they were discovered. Infection with one type confers no immunity to infection with the other two. They are all approximately 100 $m\mu$ in diameter, visible as spheres or filaments by electron microscopy, and are biologically related by their infectivity for chick embryos, capacity to agglutinate erythrocytes, and affinity for the respiratory epithelium of various mammals. Influenza viruses are the prototypes of the myxovirus group and are related to the larger paramyxoviruses, which include mumps, Newcastle disease, measles, and the parainfluenza viruses. These viruses are composed of a helical ribonucleoprotein core wound up in a lipid-containing envelope from which protrude protein spikes that serve as attachment organs and principal antigenic sites.

EPIDEMIOLOGY. Influenza B and C usually occur sporadically or in localized outbreaks, particularly in schools and military camps. Influenza A viruses are the cause of major epidemics which tend to recur at intervals of 2 to 4 years in the winter months. The factors responsible for this periodicity are the decline in effective immunity of a population in interepidemic periods and the emergence every few years of new strains of virus. A marked change in the antigenicity of type A viruses occurred in 1946–1947, when viruses extant between 1933 and 1945 completely disappeared and were replaced by strains designated as influenza A' or A_1.

A further alteration in the serotype of influenza A viruses was detected in China early in 1957. These A_2 or "Asian" influenza viruses were widely disseminated in the Orient in the following spring, giving rise to the pandemic of 1957. On the basis of laboratory studies and international epidemic intelligence, accurate predictions were made within a month of the first outbreaks in East Asia that influenza would spread throughout the world. A second pandemic wave occurred early in 1958, and major epidemics of the same type recurred in the winter of 1959–1960. Since the pandemic of 1957, virtually everyone in urban populations has acquired antibody to A_2 influenza virus. A new antigenic variant of influenza virus appeared in Asia in 1968 and has tentatively been designated A_3.

Influenza A epidemics start abruptly, reach a peak in 2 to 3 months, and subside almost as rapidly. The attack rate is variable but was noted in 1957 to exceed 50 percent of urban populations. An additional 25 percent of individuals may show serologic evidence of infection without clinical manifestations. Experiences in 1957 proved conclusively that crowding, even in summer months or in tropical countries, is the major factor predisposing to epidemics. Schoolchildren, in particular, are the primary focus and disseminators of infection in the United States. The end of summer recess in September brings a highly susceptible population into close proximity and facilitates rapid spread. If the general immunity of a population is at low levels, community-wide epidemics may occur within a few weeks of the opening of schools. If, on the other hand, immune individuals predominate, the case rate will rise slowly and may not reach epidemic proportions, or may do so later in the winter.

PATHOGENESIS. Influenza is primarily an infection of the respiratory epithelium that is transmitted from man to man by inhalation of infective droplet nuclei. Influenza A viruses have been recovered in nature from swine and horses, but these animals probably do not transmit the infection to man. Detailed experimental studies of the pathogenesis of the disease have been made in ferrets and mice. After intranasal inoculation, the virus multiplies to maximum titers in 24 to 48 hr and rapidly involves the entire tracheobronchial tree. At first, the mucosa becomes boggy and hyperemic and loses its normal ciliary activity. This may shortly be followed by necrosis of respiratory epithelium, invasion by leukocytes, pulmonary consolidation, and abnormal regeneration of metaplastic squamous epithelium in the bronchi and bronchioles. The infection is largely confined to the respiratory tract and hilar lymph nodes of adult animals; viremia is a transient and inconstant feature. However, virus has been isolated from heart, kidney, and other extrapulmonary tissues in fatal human infections, suggesting that virus products can enter the circulation and may account for systemic manifestations of the disease.

The findings at autopsy are pulmonary hemorrhages, necrosis of bronchial epithelium, bronchiolitis, squamous metaplasia of respiratory epithelium, and marked edema of alveolar septums and spaces. Fatal human infections can be caused by the influenza virus itself or by combined viral and bacterial infections.

MANIFESTATIONS. The disease assumes its typical form during major epidemics of influenza A, but clinical differentiation between influenza A and B is not possible in localized outbreaks. Sporadic infections with either influenza A or B are likely to result in relatively minor illnesses, with predominantly respiratory symptoms, similar to those of common respiratory disease (Chap. 206). Influenza C is particularly difficult to recognize because of its mildness. Although the manifestations and severity of influenza A vary from year to year, cases in a single epidemic often follow a remarkably similar pattern. The clinical description that follows is a composite picture of epidemic influenza A of the past three decades.

The *incubation period* is usually 18 to 36 hr but may be as long as 3 days. Mild prodomal symptoms of cough, malaise, and chilliness are sometimes present, but extremely sudden onset is often such a characteristic feature that many patients can recall its exact time. The most common initial symptom is severe generalized or frontal *headache*, frequently accompanied by stabbing retro-orbital pain that is accentuated by lateral or upward gaze. Diffuse *myalgia*, particularly marked in the legs and over the lumbosacral area, occurs in more than half the cases.

Pain and spasm of the abdominal muscles may simulate acute peritonitis, and incapacitating periarticular pains are sometimes confused with acute arthritis. *Feverishness* and *chilliness*, or occasionally true rigors, may be the first manifestations, but more often they are preceded by headache and myalgia. The temperature rises abruptly to a maximum of 100 to 103°F several hours after onset; rarely it may reach 106°F. Thereafter, the fever and pain usually subside over a 2- to 3-day period but may persist for as long as a week. A common variant in the temperature course is rapid defervescence after the initial peak, with a secondary rise to the original level on the following day. In general, severity of illness parallels the height and duration of the fever. The pulse rate is usually slow in relation to the fever, but marked tachycardia may occur in severely ill patients.

Prostration of some degree is almost invariable and is often the most prominent and alarming manifestation. The face is flushed, and the skin is hot and dry; however, profuse sweating and cold, mottled extremities are sometimes noted. Anorexia, nausea, and constipation are frequent secondary symptoms, but vomiting and diarrhea are rare. There is no evidence that influenza viruses infect the gastrointestinal tract, and the term *intestinal flu* is a misnomer. Meningoencephalitis, polyneuritis, cranial nerve palsies, transient nerve deafness, aphasia, hemiplegia, psychoses, and other neurologic disorders have been described in association with influenza but are very unusual. Hypotension, heart block, peripheral vasoconstriction, and fatal myocarditis have also been reported in a few cases. The exact relationship of these neurologic and cardiovascular disorders to influenza viral infection has not been determined. The incidence of abortion appears to be increased when influenza occurs during the first trimester of pregnancy.

Respiratory symptoms may be present at the onset but become most prominent when the systemic manifestations and fever begin to subside. They are frequently less pronounced than in common respiratory disease and may be entirely absent. Sneezing, watery nasal discharge, or stuffy nose occurs in most cases; hoarseness and epistaxis are less frequent. Conjunctival suffusion and burning, and itching, watery eyes are often noted. The throat may feel dry, and the pharynx often appears slightly injected. *Cough* develops during the course of the illness in more than three-fourths of the cases, and in about a third of these it is productive of small amounts of tenacious, mucoid sputum. *Chest pain,* usually substernal in location and accentuated by coughing but not by breathing, is present in almost half the patients. Pleurisy and pleural effusion are uncommon. Slight hyperpnea is often noted, but the most ominous, although infrequent, signs are dyspnea and cyanosis, which signal bronchiolar or pneumonic involvement. Physical examination of the lungs is often negative in uncomplicated influenza, but scattered rhonchi, wheezes, and showers of moist rales have been reported in 5 to 40 percent of cases in different epidemics. Influenzal bronchiolitis should be suspected if rales persist in the absence of x-ray evidence of pneumonitis and if the patient raises mucopurulent or blood-tinged sputum.

The chief *complications* of influenza are secondary bacterial infections of the paranasal sinuses, middle ear, bronchi, and lungs. The incidence of bacterial pneumonia is greatly increased during influenza epidemics; even mild or asymptomatic infections with influenza viruses predispose to pneumococcal and other types of pneumonia. The most serious complication is staphylococcal pneumonia, which tends to run a fulminant, often fatal, course.

During the 1958 epidemic a fulminating pneumonia characterized by severe dyspnea and cyanosis, scanty sputum containing gross blood, leukopenia, scanty physical findings in the lung in the face of large perihilar infiltrates, and a rapidly fatal course was described. Although staphylococci were isolated from the sputum, these patients failed to respond to appropriate antimicrobials. Furthermore, influenza virus was cultured from the lungs of some patients, suggesting that influenza virus rather than secondary bacterial infection played the major role in producing lung damage. In subsequent epidemics, this type of "influenza pneumonia" has been rare. Superinfection with *Hemophilus influenzae,* so common in the pandemic of 1918, is rarely encountered now.

Recovery from uncomplicated influenza is often complete in 2 to 3 days or, occasionally, in a week, but convalescence may be prolonged by "postinfectious asthenia" and depression, particularly in elderly persons. Minor relapses with fever can occur but are uncommon.

The *mortality* rate from all causes always increases markedly during epidemics of influenza. In the fall and winter of 1957–1958 it was estimated that 40 million persons in the United States became ill with influenza and the total numbers of influenza-associated deaths was reported to be in excess of 8,000. In addition, approximately 60,000 more deaths from various causes occurred during this period than would be expected under normal conditions. The greatest incidence of excess mortality occurred among infants under one year of age and adults over sixty years of age. Data from small series of cases clearly indicate that influenza is frequently fatal in individuals with preexisting pulmonary or cardiac disease, regardless of age. Chronic rheumatic heart disease with mitral stenosis, in particular, appears to predispose to fatal influenzal pneumonia.

LABORATORY FINDINGS. Virus is isolated most readily during the acute phase of the disease by inoculation of broth garglings into the amniotic cavity of chick embryos or into tissue cultures of monkey kidney or human cells. Serologic diagnosis can be made most reliably by hemagglutination-inhibition or complement fixation tests, using paired serum samples obtained in both the acute and convalescent phases. However, type-specific antibody against soluble complement-fixing antigens of influenza A virus often appears in the circulation of patients during the acute illness.

X-ray of the lungs in uncomplicated influenza is usually normal but occasionally reveals increased vascular markings, basilar streaking, small areas of patchy infiltration, atelectasis, nodular densities, or pleural effusion. The blood leukocyte count may be low 2 to 4 days after onset of illness, but is often normal or slightly elevated.

Leukocytosis with counts above 15,000 cells per cu mm indicates secondary bacterial infection, but leukopenia can occur in severe staphylococcal pneumonia. Slight proteinuria is common during the height of the febrile illness.

DIFFERENTIAL DIAGNOSIS. Many bacterial and viral infections simulate influenza at their onset, but few febrile diseases have such a self-limited course. The pattern of clinical manifestations becomes readily apparent during an epidemic, but many influenza outbreaks are associated with an increased incidence of other respiratory infection of viral and bacterial etiology. Noninfluenzal respiratory diseases (Chap. 206) are generally characterized by more gradual onset, milder systemic manifestations, and predominant symptoms of coryza, rhinorrhea, pharyngitis, and conjunctivitis.

TREATMENT. Antibiotics do not affect the course of uncomplicated influenza, nor is there any evidence that they prevent complications. Specific chemotherapy should be reserved for secondary bacterial infections. Clinical trials have shown some effectiveness of adamantanamine hydrochloride, a symmetrical amine which inhibits cellular penetration of influenza virus, as a chemoprophylactic agent, but the results are not impressive. Codeine affords relief from incapacitating cough and is more effective than salicylates for symptomatic treatment of headache and myalgia; salicylates often increase discomfort by causing drenching sweats and chills. Bed rest and gradual return to full activity are advisable.

PROPHYLAXIS. Formalinized egg vaccines containing a mixture of influenza A, A$_1$, A$_2$, and B viruses are the standard preparations available commercially in the United States. The British favor the use of a monovalent vaccine presently prepared from a more concentrated suspension of influenza A$_2$ virus. Infectious attenuated virus administered intranasally has been widely used for influenza immunization in the Soviet Union, but its safety and efficacy have not been proved. The most promising results have been obtained in the American Armed Forces by preliminary trials of adjuvant influenza vaccines emulsified with mineral oil and Arlacel A. Although they stimulate the production of serum antibodies, the prophylactic value of influenza vaccines is limited by the following factors: (1) infection can occur in spite of high levels of serum antibody; (2) antibody concentration is low at the site of infection in the respiratory tract; (3) vaccines sometimes do not contain antigens prepared from the most recent strains of virus; and (4) even under optimal conditions, their protective effect often lasts for only a few months.

The U.S. Public Health Service strongly recommends routine yearly immunization with polyvalent influenza vaccine for high-risk groups, including persons of all ages who suffer from chronic rheumatic heart disease, other cardiovascular diseases, chronic bronchopulmonary diseases, diabetes mellitus, or Addison's disease; also pregnant women and persons sixty-five years of age, or older, regardless of their previous state of health. For initial immunization it is advisable to administer the vaccine subcutaneously in two divided doses of 1 ml each, the first injection in September and the second several weeks or months later. A single subcutaneous dose of 1 ml given each autumn is satisfactory as a yearly booster. Intradermal injection of vaccine is far less satisfactory because a sufficient antigenic mass cannot be administered by this route.

Influenza vaccination is generally safe but not completely innocuous. Fatal anaphylactic reactions and purpura have been reported in individuals sensitive to egg proteins, and inactivated virus itself is pyrogenic and can sometimes produce an illness similar to active influenza. Influenza vaccine should be administered only advisedly and in much smaller doses to infants and young children, in whom severe febrile reactions may result in convulsions and death. Most influenza vaccines are contaminated with bacterial pyrogens. Large-scale purification of virus by zonal centrifugation shows considerable promise for production of vaccines from pure viral antigens.

REFERENCES

Davenport, F. M.: Factors of Importance in the Control of Influenza, Med. Clin. N. Am., 47:1185, 1963.

Loosli, C. G. (Ed.): Proceedings of the International Conference on Asian Influenza, Bethesda, Maryland, February, 1960, Am. Rev. Resp. Dis., 93:2, February, 1961.

Louria, D. B., H. L. Blumenfeld, J. T. Ellis, E. D. Kilbourne, and D. E. Rogers: Studies on Influenza in the Pandemic of 1957-1958: II. Pulmonary Complications of Influenza, J. Clin. Invest., 38:213, 1959.

Petersdorf, R. G., J. J. Fusco, D. R. Harter, and W. S. Albrink: Pulmonary Infections Complicating Asian Influenza, Arch. Intern. Med., 103:262, 1959.

Reimer, C. B., R. S. Baker, R. M. van Frank, T. E. Newlin, G. B. Cline, and N. G. Anderson: Purification of Large Quantities of Influenza Virus by Density Gradient Centrifugation, J Virol., 1:1207, 1967.

Zhdanov, V. M., V. D. Solov'ev, and F. G. Epshtein: "The Study of Influenza; A Translation from the Russian *Ucheniye o Grippe*," Public Health Service Publ. 792, Bethesda, Md., U.S. Department of Health, Education, and Welfare, 1960.

209 PSITTACOSIS
Vernon Knight

DEFINITION. Psittacosis is an infectious disease of birds caused by an organism that has a number of properties in common with gram-negative bacteria. Transmission of infection from birds to man results in a febrile illness characterized by pneumonitis and systemic manifestations. Inapparent infections or mild influenza-like illnesses may also occur. The term *ornithosis* is sometimes applied to infections contracted from birds other than parrots or parakeets, but *psittacosis* is the preferred generic term for all forms of the disease.

ETIOLOGY. The causative agent *Chlamydia psittaci* is a gram-negative obligate intracellular parasite, formerly classified as a virus. Now, along with the rickettsias, it may be considered specialized bacteria. The chlamydias, like rickettsias, synthesize RNA and DNA, reproduce by binary fission, and are susceptible to antimicrobial drugs. In contrast to rickettsias, the chlamydias are dependent on their hosts for metabolic energy. During intracellular growth, the chlamydias exhibit a large (1 μ) replicating form without a rigid cell wall, from which small (0.3 to 0.4 μ) infectious forms with a rigid cell wall are derived. The cell walls are thinner than those of bacteria, contain murein, and have a high lipid content characteristic of gram-negative bacteria. Recently, slight but definite homology of the DNA of members of the *Chlamydia* genus with the DNA of *Neisseria meningitidis* was shown. The psittacosis agent is the prototype of a biologically and antigenically homogenous class of microorganisms that includes the causative agents of lymphogranuloma venereum, trachoma, and 30 or more mammalian parasites which rarely produce human disease.

EPIDEMIOLOGY. Psittacosis is widely distributed throughout the world, and almost any avian species can harbor the agent. Psittacine birds are most commonly infected, but human cases have been traced to contact with pigeons, ducks, turkeys, chickens, and many other birds. Psittacosis may be considered an occupational disease of pet-shop owners, poultry raisers, pigeon fanciers, taxidermists, and zoo attendants. The incidence of human infection in the United States rose steadily from 1930, owing in large measure to the increasing popularity of parrots and parakeets as pets and, as subsequently recognized, transmission of infection by barnyard fowl and pigeons. The number of reported cases reached a peak in 1956 and gradually declined thereafter. By 1963 the disease had again become relatively uncommon coincident with acceptance of control measures such as incorporation of tetracyclines in poultry feed.

The agent is present in nasal secretions, excreta, tissues, and feathers of infected birds. Although the disease can be fatal, infected birds frequently show only minor evidences of illness such as ruffled feathers, lethargy, and anorexia. Asymptomatic avian carriers are common, and complete recovery may be followed by continued shedding of the organism for many months.

Psittacosis is almost always transmitted to man by the respiratory route. On rare occasions the disease may be acquired from the bite of a pet bird. Intimate and prolonged contact is not essential for transmission of the disease; a few minutes spent in an environment previously occupied by an infected bird has resulted in human infection. The severity of the disease in man bears no apparent relationship to closeness or duration of contact. Human-to-human transmission of a psittacosis-like agent has occurred particularly among hospital personnel, with severe and sometimes fatal infections. There is evidence that these "human" strains are more virulent than native avian organisms. There is no record of infection acquired by eating poultry products.

PATHOGENESIS. The psittacosis agent gains entrance to the body through the upper part of the respiratory tract and eventually localizes in the pulmonary alveoli and the reticuloendothelial cells of the spleen and liver. Invasion of the lung parenchyma probably takes place by way of the bloodstream rather than by direct extension from the upper air passages. A lymphocytic inflammatory response occurs on both the interstitial and respiratory surfaces of the alveoli as well as in the perivascular spaces. The alveoli walls and interstitial tissues of the lung are thickened, edematous, necrotic, and occasionally hemorrhagic. Histologically, the affected areas show alveolar spaces filled with fluid, erythrocytes, and lymphocytes. The picture is not pathognomonic of psittacosis unless macrophages containing characteristic cytoplasmic inclusion bodies (LCL bodies) can be identified. The respiratory epithelium of the bronchi and bronchioles usually remains intact.

MANIFESTATIONS. The clinical manifestations and course of psittacosis are extremely variable. After an *incubation period* of 7 to 14 days, or longer, the disease may start abruptly with shaking chills and high fever, but the onset is often gradual with increasing fever and malaise over a 3- to 4-day period. Headache is almost always a prominent symptom; it is usually diffuse and excruciating and often the patient's chief complaint. Generalized myalgia is also common. Spasm and stiffness of the muscles of the back and neck may lead to an erroneous diagnosis of meningitis. A faint, macular rash (Horder's spots) simulating the rose spots of typhoid fever has been described. Lethargy, mental depression, agitation, insomnia, and disorientation have been prominent features of the illness in some epidemics, but not in others; delirium and stupor occur near the end of the first week in severe cases. Occasional patients are comatose when first seen, and the diagnosis of psittacosis may be missed in this circumstance. Gastrointestinal complaints such as abdominal pain, nausea, vomiting, or diarrhea are present in some cases; constipation and abdominal distension sometimes occur as late complications. Icterus, the result of severe hepatic involvement, is a rare and ominous finding. Symptoms of infection of the upper part of the respiratory tract are not prominent, although mild sore throat, pharyngeal injection, and cervical adenopathy are often present; and on occasion may be the only manifestation of illness. Epistaxis is encountered early in the course of nearly one-fourth of the cases. Photophobia is also a common complaint.

A dry, hacking cough is characteristic of psittacosis; it is usually nonproductive, but small amounts of mucoid or bloody sputum may be raised as the disease progresses. Cough may appear early in the course of the disease or as late as 5 days after the onset of fever. Chest pain, pleurisy with effusion, or a friction rub may all occur but are not usual. Pericarditis and myocarditis have been reported. Most patients have a normal or slightly increased respiratory rate; marked dyspnea with cyanosis occurs only in severe psittacosis with extensive pulmonary involvement. In psittacosis, as in most nonbacterial pneumonias, the physical signs of pneumonitis tend to be less prominent than symptoms and x-ray findings would suggest. The initial examination may reveal fine, sibilant rales, or clinical evidence of pneumonia may be completely lacking. Rales usually become audible and more numerous as the illness progresses. Signs of frank pulmonary consolidation are usually absent.

Patients without cough or other clinical evidence of respiratory involvement present the problem of a fever of unknown origin. The pulse rate in psittacosis is slow in relation to the fever. When splenomegaly is present in a patient with acute pneumonitis, psittacosis should be considered. Inability to feel the spleen is of no diagnostic significance, however; the reported incidence of splenomegaly has ranged from 10 to 70 percent in different series of proved cases. Nontender hepatic enlargement also occurs, but jaundice is rare. Thrombophlebitis is not unusual during convalescence; indeed, pulmonary infarction is sometimes a late complication and may be fatal.

In untreated cases of psittacosis, sustained or mildly remittent fever persists for 10 days to 3 weeks, or occasionally as long as 3 months. Defervescence is by lysis, rarely by crisis, and is accompanied by abatement of respiratory manifestations. Psittacosis contracted from parrots or parakeets is more likely to be a severe, prolonged illness than infections acquired from pigeons or barnyard fowl. Relapses occur but are rare. Secondary bacterial infections are uncommon. Immunity to reinfection is probably permanent.

LABORATORY FINDINGS. The x-ray of the lungs in psittacosis mimics a great variety of pulmonary diseases. The pneumonic lesions are usually patchy in appearance but can be hazy, diffuse, homogeneous, lobar, atelectatic, wedge shaped, nodular, or miliary. The white blood cell count is normal or moderately decreased in the acute phase of the disease but may rise in convalescence. The erythrocyte sedimentation rate is frequently not elevated. Transient proteinuria is common. The cerebrospinal fluid sometimes contains a few mononuclear cells but is otherwise normal. Cold agglutinins are rarely present in the serum of patients with psittacosis.

The diagnosis of psittacosis can be confirmed only by isolation of the causative microorganism or serologic studies. The agent is present in the blood during the acute phase of the disease and in the bronchial secretions for weeks or sometimes years after infection, but it is often difficult to isolate. Psittacosis is most readily diagnosed by the demonstration of a rising titer of complement-fixing antibody in the patient's blood. An acute and convalescent specimen should always be tested. Even a low titer of antibody during the acute febrile phase constitutes presumptive evidence of psittacosis. The prompt initiation of treatment with tetracycline has been shown to delay antibody rise in convalescence for several weeks or months. Interpretation of a single complement fixation test may sometimes be difficult because of the antigenic cross reaction between the agents of psittacosis and lymphogranuloma venereum.

DIFFERENTIAL DIAGNOSIS. A history of exposure to birds may be the only clinical basis for differentiating psittacosis from a great variety of infectious and noninfectious febrile disorders. A partial list of pneumonic diseases that may be confused with psittacosis includes primary atypical pneumonia, Q fever, coccidioidomycosis, tuberculosis, carcinoma of the lung with bronchial obstruction, and bacterial pneumonias. In the early stages, before pneumonitis appears, psittacosis may be mistaken for influenza, typhoid fever, miliary tuberculosis, infectious mononucleosis and, less commonly, rheumatic fever or bacterial endocarditis.

TREATMENT. The tetracyclines are consistently effective in the treatment of psittacosis. Defervescence and alleviation of symptoms usually occur in 24 to 48 hr after instituting therapy with 2 Gm daily. To avoid relapse, treatment should probably be continued for at least 7 days after defervescence. The disease will usually respond to penicillin if a daily dose of at least 2 million units is used. In severe cases, oxygen and other supportive measures are indicated.

REFERENCES

Meyer, K. F.: The Ecology of Psittacosis and Ornithosis, Medicine, 21:175, 1942.

——: Psittacosis-Lymphogranuloma Venereum Agents, pp. 1006–1041 in "Viral and Rickettsial Infections of Man," 4th ed., F. L. Horsfall, Jr., and I. Tamm (Eds.), Philadelphia, J. B. Lippincott Company, 1965.

Moulder, J. W.: "The Life and Death of the Psittacosis Virus," Hosp. Practice, June, 1968.

Seibert, R. H., W. S. Jordan, Jr., and J. H. Dingle: Clinical Variations in the Diagnosis of Psittacosis, New Engl. J. Med., 254:925, 1956.

—— et al.: Epidemiological Studies of Psittacosis in Cleveland, Am. J. Hyg., 63:28, 1956.

Section 15

Enteric Viruses

INTRODUCTION

A. Martin Lerner

It has been more than two decades since Dalldorf and Sickles isolated the first Coxsackie viruses by inoculating suspensions of feces from two children with paralytic poliomyelitis into suckling mice. Subsequently some 67 enteroviruses, including polio-, Coxsackie, and ECHO viruses, have been shown to multiply in the human gastrointestinal tract (see Table). Enteroviruses have been recovered where attempts have been made; their distribution appears global. With notable exceptions such as Coxsackie virus A, type 21, and ECHO virus, type 28 (which are predominantly respiratory pathogens and are only incidentally isolated from feces), enteroviruses, like salmonellas, periodically multiply within the human alimentary canal and sometimes concomitantly produce disease. Available information suggests there is no "normal" enteric virus flora. In addition to enteroviruses, adenoviruses (Chap. 206) and reoviruses (Chap. 214) are

CLASSIFICATION OF ENTEROVIRUSES

I. Picornaviruses of human origin
  A. Enteroviruses
    1. Polioviruses (3 types)*
    2. Coxsackie virus A (24 types)
    3. Coxsackie virus B (6 types)
    4. ECHO viruses (34 types)†
  B. Rhinoviruses (see Chap. 206)
  C. Unclassified
II. Picornaviruses of lower animals

* Typing is by neutralization of infectivity with immune serums in either suitable tissue cultures or suckling mice.

† ECHO virus, type 10, has been reclassified as belonging to another taxonomic group, now known as reoviruses.

commonly recovered from stools.

Coxsackie viruses are named for the village of Coxsackie on the banks of the Hudson River in the State of New York, where the first isolations were made. ECHO viruses are descriptively named: E, for their *enteric* residence; C, the filterable agents produced *cytopathic* effects in tissue cultures of rhesus kidney; H, *human*; O, *orphan*, indicating that their relationship to disease remained to be established. They were viruses "in search of a disease." It is increasingly evident that a wide variety of illnesses may result from enterovirus infections. As observations accumulate, the list of these illnesses is continually being refined (see table on page 963). Etiologic associations are difficult to establish because they require virologic, serologic, epidemiologic, and volunteer studies. Moreover, these are viruses often isolated from the pharynx or anus, where they multiply without causing significant injury to tissues. More meaningful are isolations from blood, vesicular fluids of patients with rashes, urine, cerebrospinal fluid, or tissues taken by biopsy or at autopsy. Coxsackie or ECHO viruses have been recovered from lung, heart, pericardial fluid, liver, spleen, testicle, kidney, muscle, and brain.

CHARACTERISTICS OF THE VIRUSES. Enteroviruses consist of a ribonucleic acid core surrounded by a capsid of protein. The outer coat determines species, tissue, and age specificities as well as antigenic quality. The RNA of the virus within infected cells transcribes and translates its own genetic information independent of the host DNA. Particle diameters are 15 to 30 mμ. Enteroviruses are quite stable in acid and in lipid solvents. They can be protected from thermal inactivation by certain cations.

When inoculated into suckling mice, group A Cox-

sackie viruses induce primarily an inflammatory myositis, whereas group B viruses cause lesions of the central nervous system and other viscera. Coxsackie virus B and ECHO viruses are cytopathogenic for cultures of monkey kidney cells, but this is not the case for Coxsackie viruses of group A. These distinctions are not invariable. Type 6 and type 9 ECHO viruses have been adapted to produce lesions in baby mice. Some strains agglutinate human erythrocytes obtained from adult or umbilical cord blood. None of the Coxsackie or ECHO viruses have been adapted to grow in embryonated eggs.

EPIDEMIOLOGY. Fecal-oral contact is the usual method of contagion and toddlers often bring enteroviruses into a household. Personal hygiene inhibits the infectious cycle. Insects may act as passive vectors. ECHO virus, type 6, can multiply in the gastrointestinal tracts of dogs. This has not been noted with other Coxsackie or ECHO viruses, and with ECHO virus 6 canine to human transmission has not been demonstrated. Respiratory transmission by droplets or their nuclei also occurs.

The incubation period is 2 to 5 days. Multiple concurrent infections within a family are not unusual. Clinical manifestations of infection vary within the family and community. For example, a two- or three-year-old child may have a mild fever with rash, while an older sibling may suffer from pleurodynia, myocarditis, or one of a number of syndromes heralding involvement of the central nervous system (see table on page 963). The mechanism of the variation in expression of enterovirus disease is not well understood, but may relate to developmental changes in the numbers or availability of specific receptors at the surfaces of susceptible cells.

Enterovirus infections are most common during summer months. Prevalence is mirrored by virus isolations from samples of sewage. Serotypes present in a community vary from year to year. The level of immunity of a populace as reflected by the prevalence of type-specific neutralizing antibodies in serums apparently determines the likelihood of infection by a particular enterovirus.

VIRUS ISOLATION. Primary multiplication occurs in epithelial and paraepithelial lymphatic cells of the pharynx. During this early period of infection the patient may be asymptomatic or have mild malaise, sore throat, or low-grade fever. Similarly virus later multiplies in the intestines. If a critical virus concentration within the pharynx results, viremia follows. During the viremic phase the patient is asymptomatic. Secondary foci of virus multiplication may occur in various tissues (skin, muscle, heart, nervous system, etc.). Major illness of moderate to serious severity sometimes results (see table on page 963). Occasionally (especially during infancy) aspirations of pharyngeal virus lead to lower respiratory infection.

Virus may be isolated from the throat during the minor illness and for as long as a week thereafter. Virus shedding persists in feces for a longer interval, but permanent fecal damage does not occur. Viremia can be documented during the incubation period until type-specific neutralizing antibodies appear.

ILLNESSES (OR SYNDROMES) ASSOCIATED WITH COXSACKIE OR ECHO VIRUS INFECTIONS

Classification	Viruses (not inclusive)		
	Coxsackie virus, group		ECHO virus, types
	A, types	B, types	
I. No Illness (probably 75% of infections).......................	1–24	1–6	1–8,* 11–34
II. Mild or moderate illness			
A. Undifferentiated mild febrile illness (nonspecific).............	1–24	1–6	1–8, 11–34
B. Upper respiratory syndromes (rhinitis pharyngitis, including herpangina and lymphonodular pharyngitis, and conjunctivitis)	1–10, 16, 21,† 22, 24	1–5	1, 3, 6, 9, 16, 19, 20, 28
C. Laryngotracheitis..	9	5	11
D. Exanthems (various)......................................	5, 9, 16	3, 5	2, 4, 9, 11, 16
E. Lymphadenitis, with or without splenomegaly................	5, 6, 9	5	4, 9, 16, 20
F. Pleurodynia (sometimes with pleural effusion)................	4, 6, 10	1–5	1, 6, 9
G. Orchitis..	....	1–5	9
H. Gastroenteritis....	... .	3, 4	2, 3, 6–9, 11–14, 18, 19, 22–24
III. Severe or life-threatening illness			
A. Hepatitis...	4, 9	5	4, 9
B. Hemolytic-uremic syndrome..............................	4		
C. Pneumonia...	9	1, 4	3, 8, 9, 19, 20
D. Cardiac			
1. Myocarditis/pericarditis.............................	1, 4, 9, 16	1–5	3, 6–9, 22
2. Chronic myocardopathy‡			
3. Subendocardial fibroelastosis‡........................	....	3	
4. Endocardial deformities‡			
5. Congenital malformations†	3, 4		
E. Neurologic			
1. Aseptic meningitis/encephalitis including variants (b-f).....	7, 9, 16	1–5	1–9, 11–23, 25, 30–32
2. Acute cerebellar ataxia.......	3, 4		
3. Benign intracranial hypertension			
4. Transverse myelitis			
5. Postencephalitic Parkinsonism			

* Asymptomatic infection is less common with ECHO virus, type 9. Variation in attack rates among types (and strains of a single type) occurs.

† Coxsackie virus A, type 21, is also known as Coe virus.

‡ Suggested (and probable), but cause not established.

PROTECTIVE RESPONSES AND SEROLOGIC DIAGNOSIS. Intracellular virus multiplication stimulates the production within the infected cell of interferon, a small protein with a molecular weight of about 20,000 that inhibits virus maturation. Virulent infections lead to rapid cellular lysis and the release of lesser quantities of interferon. About 3 days after the onset of infection specific antibodies appear in saliva and serum. These immunoglobulins combine with extracellular virus to limit spread of virus; virus-antibody complexes are eliminated by phagocytosis.

Secretory immunoglobulins in saliva and succus entericus are IgA while the earliest antibodies to appear in serum are IgM (Chap. 68). Both species of macromolecules have complement-fixing and neutralizing qualities. Within 3 to 4 weeks complement-fixing antibodies reach their peak and decline. Neutralizing antibodies of higher avidity (IgG) replace the IgM molecule

about 2 weeks after the onset of infection and persist, providing permanent type-specific immunity.

This information is important in practical diagnosis because IgM molecules are susceptible to reduction and resultant biologic inactivation with sulfhydryl active compounds such as 2-mercaptoethanol (2-ME). IgG immunoglobulins are resistant to 2-ME. IgG antibodies to Coxsackie and ECHO viruses traverse the placenta freely, but IgM immunoglobulins do not. IgA antibodies in colostrum and milk are not absorbed, but apparently provide some local protection in the intestines of nursing babies. Passively acquired antibodies in serum protect the newborn from viremia for 3 to 6 months, because they inhibit active synthesis of virus, but these antibodies in serum may not protect the respiratory tract where active synthesis of secretory antibody in saliva and nasal secretions is required.

A fourfold rise in neutralizing antibodies or a titer

which is diminished by 2-ME indicates recent infection. When applicable, hemagglutination inhibition tests are simple and practical. Results parallel those obtained in neutralization tests. Complement-fixing antibodies to enteroviruses are not type-specific and are less useful in diagnosis.

OTHER LABORATORY FINDINGS. Enterovirus infections are acute; persistent or chronic infections do not occur. Marked changes in concentrations of hemoglobin or plasma proteins are unusual. Occasionally hemolysis occurs (Chap. 210). White blood cell counts and the erythrocyte sedimentation rates are only mildly elevated. If there is necrosis of the liver or lung, neutrophilic leukemoid reactions may be noted. Hyperbilirubinemia, elevated transaminase and alkaline phosphatase levels, and delayed excretion of Bromsulphalein may be seen in hepatitis. Albuminuria often occurs transiently, but hematuria is rare.

TREATMENT. Antiviral chemotherapy is not available, and the 64 antigenic varieties of Coxsackie and ECHO viruses make vaccine prophylaxis impractical. Pooled human gamma globulin contains enterovirus antibodies, but during serious infections its administration has no therapeutic effect. Most human enterovirus infections are mild, and gamma globulin prophylaxis is rarely warranted. As with poliomyelitis, tonsillectomies and other inoculations probably are best delayed during an outbreak of enterovirus disease. In a murine model of Coxsackie virus A 9 myocarditis, virus was isolated in high titer from hearts of a significantly greater proportion of mice vigorously exercised daily by swimming, and rest is probably the best symptomatic therapy. It has also been shown repeatedly in the laboratory that during the acute phase of infection administration of steroids appreciably increases quantities of virus in tissues and the degree of ensuing injury. Therefore, at least during the acute phase of enterovirus infections, steroids are contraindicated.

REFERENCES

Gelfand, H. M.: Occurrence in Nature of Coxsackie and ECHO Viruses, Progr. Med. Virol., 3:193, 1961.

Horstmann, D. M.: Clinical Virology, Am. J. Med., 38:738, 1965.

Huebner, R. J.: The Virologist's Dilemma, Ann. N.Y. Acad. Sci., 67:430, 1957.

Kibrick, S.: Current Status of Coxsackie and ECHO Viruses in Human Disease, Progr. Med. Virol., 6:27, 1964.

210 COXSACKIE VIRUSES, GROUP A

A. Martin Lerner

Group A Coxsackie viruses cause herpangina, lymphonodular pharyngitis, upper and lower respiratory disease, cutaneous eruptions, hepatitis, aseptic meningitis, paralytic disease, and some sudden deaths in infancy. Pharyngeal multiplication can produce diffuse moderate reddening, but purulent exudate is absent. More characteristic is herpangina (Chap. 227), a common febrile illness characterized by small papular vesicular or ulcerative lesions on the anterior pillars, soft palate, tonsils, pharyngeal mucous membrane, and posterior part of the buccal mucosa. Zahorsky in 1920 and again in 1924 described the entity, and its viral etiology was established by Huebner in 1951. Herpangina has been seen during infections with Coxsackie viruses group A, types 1 to 10, 16, and 22. Vesicular lesions of herpangina have also been described in patients with illnesses due to Coxsackie viruses group B, types 1 to 5, and ECHO viruses, types 9 and 17. Coxsackie virus A 10 may induce *acute lymphonodular pharyngitis*. Lesions here are raised, discrete, white to yellow 3 to 6-mm papules surrounded by a zone of erythema. All of the papules appear at the same time, do not ulcerate, and occur on the uvula, anterior pillars, and posterior pharynx.

Coxsackie virus A 21 (Coe virus) is predominantly a respiratory pathogen and is isolated regularly from the throat and occasionally from feces. It has been associated with several outbreaks in military recruits of a common coldlike illness.

The first enterovirus etiologically implicated in causation of pneumonias was Coxsackie virus A 9. Subsequently, a number of other enteroviruses have been implicated (see table on page 963). Fatal cases occurred in infants or young children. Hyperpnea, cyanosis hyperpyrexia, leukocytosis (or leukemoid reactions), and subsequently coma have been characteristic. Alveolar capillary block syndromes and diffuse bronchopneumonia with alternate areas of atelectasis and emphysema have been found. Histopathologic examination show mixed alveolar septal infiltration without necrosis or giant cells.

A striking cutaneous vesicular eruption, *hand, foot-and-mouth disease* (Chap. 227), has repeatedly been associated with infections due to Coxsackie virus group A, type 16, infants and children with Coxsackie virus group A, type 4, infections have been described with respiratory or gastrointestinal symptoms, acute renal disease, thrombocytopenia, and hemolytic anemia. Reticulocytosis, albuminuria, and hematuria accompany this constellation of findings, which has been described as the *hemolytic-uremic syndrome*. Aseptic meningitis with occasional paralytic disease (especially due to A 7) also occurs.

REFERENCES

Dalldorf, G., and G. M. Sickles: An Unidentified, Filterable Agent Isolated from the Feces of Children with Paralysis, Science, 108:61, 1948.

Huebner, R. J., R. M. Cole, E. A. Beeman, J. A. Bell, and J. H. Peers: Herpangina: Etiological Studies of a Specific Infectious Disease, J.A.M.A., 145:628, 1951.

Lerner, A. M., J. O. Klein, H. S. Levin, and M. Finland: Infections Due to Coxsackievirus Group A, Type 9, in Boston, 1959, with Special Reference to Exanthems and Pneumonia, New Engl. J. Med., 263:1265, 1960.

211 COXSACKIE VIRUSES, GROUP B

A. Martin Lerner

Infections with group B Coxsackie viruses cause a number of upper respiratory syndromes, exanthems, diarrheas, pleurodynia, orchitis, pneumonia, and cardiac and central nervous system disease. Pleurodynia and cardiac disease due to enteroviruses are predominantly associated with this group of enteroviruses (see table on page 963).

PLEURODYNIA (Epidemic Myalgia, Bornholm Disease, Devil's Grip). Prodromal symptoms of malaise, sore throat, and anorexia are interrupted by increasing debility, fever, and sudden onset of muscle, pleuritic, and abdominal pain. Pain is sharp, severe, and paroxysmal over the lower ribs or substernal area. It is accentuated by moving, breathing, coughing, sneezing, and hiccuping and may be referred to the shoulders, neck, or scapulas. Pain and spasm of anterior abdominal muscles occur in about half the cases, often in combination with chest pain. Muscle tenderness is usually not prominent but some patients complain of intense cutaneous hyperesthesia and paresthesia over the affected area. The illness usually lasts 3 to 7 days, but relapses may occur. Among differential diagnoses are myocardial infarction and acute surgical disease of the abdomen. Coxsackie viruses B have been isolated from striated muscle of patients with pleurodynia during epidemics. Occasionally pleuritis is accompanied by effusion, and virus has been isolated from pleural fluid. Bornholm disease may occur at any age, but is commonest in children and young adults.

Early in the course of illness, meningitis, myocarditis, or hepatitis may ensue. In patients with jaundice, liver biopsy shows subacute portal triaditis and intense cloudy swelling of central-zone hepatocytes. Orchitis is a late complication in 3 to 5 percent of cases of pleurodynia.

CARDIAC DISEASE. Acute "idiopathic" myocarditis is predominantly a disease caused by group B Coxsackie viruses. When congenital or neonatal infection occurs, the course is often rapidly fatal with concomitant myocarditis, encephalitis, hepatitis, and sometimes adrenal necrosis. Later in childhood or in adult life, the heart and pericardium usually are involved as the single site of disease. Cardiac inflammation and necrosis vary in intensity. Pericarditis may dominate the clinical picture with fever, precordial pain, friction rub, and even cardiac tamponade. There may be prominent signs of myocarditis with myocardial failure or arrhythmias. Illnesses are usually self-limited and recovery complete. Strict bed rest until all electrocardiographic changes have reverted to normal or are stationary is indicated. This may require 4 to 6 weeks. Because steroids increase virulence of Coxsackie B myocarditis in mice, they are contraindicated. Some infections heal with significant myocardial scarring. Seventeen of forty hearts from autopsies of patients dying when less than thirty years of age were positive by fluorescent antibody staining for Coxsackie virus antigen in the myocardium. Chronic focal interstitial myocarditis was present in each of the positive cases. Viral antigens were found in both the myocardium and the mitral valve in three cases. There is epidemiologic evidence implicating Coxsackie virus B, types 3 and 4, in congenital heart disease. Most infections in pregnant mothers were subclinical and occurred in the first trimester. There are other data implicating group B Coxsackie viruses in congenital subendocardial fibroelastosis. All these findings need further study for confirmation.

REFERENCES

Bain, H. W., D. W. McLean, and S. J. Walker: Epidemic Pleurodynia (Bornholm's Disease) Due to Coxsackie B5 Virus: The Interrelationship of Pleurodynia, Benign Pericarditis and Aseptic Meningitis, Pediatrics, 27:889, 1961.

Brown, G. C., and T. N. Evans: Serologic Evidence of Coxsackievirus Etiology of Congenital Heart Disease, J.A.M.A., 199:151, 1967.

Burch, G. E., S. C. Sun, H. L. Colcolough, R. S. Sohal, and N. P. DePasquale: Coxsackie B Viral Myocarditis and Valvulitis Identified in Routine Autopsy Specimens by Immunofluorescent Technique, Am. Heart J., 74:13, 1967.

Johnson, R. T., B. Portnoy, N. G. Rogers, and E. L. Buescher: Acute Benign Pericarditis: Virologic Study of 34 Patients, Arch. Intern. Med., 108:823, 1961.

Kibrick, S.: Viral Infections of the Fetus and Newborn, Perspectives Virol. Symp. New York, 2:140, 1961.

Sutton, G. C., H. B. Harding, R. P. Trueheart, and H. P. Clark: Coxsackie B4 Myocarditis in an Adult: Successful Isolation of Virus from Ventricular Myocardium, Clin. Aviat. Aerospace Med., 38:66, 1967.

Sylvest, E.: "Epidemic Myalgia: Bornholm Disease," London, Oxford University Press, 1934.

Tilles, J. G., S. H. Elson, J. A. Shaka, W. H. Abelmann, A. M. Lerner, and M. Finland: Effects of Exercise on Coxsackie A9 Myocarditis in Adult Mice, Proc. Soc. Exp. Biol. Med., 117:777, 1964.

212 ECHO VIRUSES

A. Martin Lerner

ECHO virus infections may be asymptomatic or may cause mild, moderate, or life-threatening illness (see table on page 963). Mild to moderate are undifferentiated fevers, upper respiratory infections, various rashes (Chap. 222), pleurodynia, and diarrheas (Chap. 213). Pneumonias, myocarditis, and neurologic involvement can be serious. Illnesses due to ECHO viruses do not differ from those caused by Coxsackie viruses.

NEUROLOGIC MANIFESTATIONS. There may be a mild prodromal malaise, but major illness usually begins with increased fever, headache, and stiff neck. Papilledema, Kernig, Brudzinski, and Babinski signs may be present. Localizing sensory or motor deficits are unusual. Confusion and delirium reflect an accompanying diffuse inflammatory reaction in the substance of the brain. These acute findings may persist for 4 to 7 days. Cerebrospinal fluid pleocytosis is usually less than 500 cells per cu mm. Early there may be as many as 90 percent polymorphonuclear leukocytes, but within 48 hr the cellular response becomes completely mononuclear. Persistence of polymorphonuclear leukocytes suggests a pyogenic focus (intracerebral, subdural, or epidural) (Chap. 360). Gram stain and appropriate spinal fluid cultures must be done to exclude bacterial meningitis, tuberculosis, or mycotic meningitis. Protein concentration in the cerebrospinal fluid is moderately elevated, but glucose is normal. Early in the illness, ECHO viruses may be isolated from spinal fluid. Hospitalization for several weeks may be required, and the CSF should be checked prior to discharge. At that time, it should contain only a few lymphocytes per cubic millimeter.

Throat and rectal swabs, serum, and cerebrospinal fluid should be collected as early as possible for attempts at virus isolation. Acute and convalescent serums should be studied for type-specific neutralizing antibodies.

It is not possible clinically to distinguish aseptic meningitis due to various enteroviruses from that caused by mumps. Localizing findings, hemiplegias, prolonged fevers, oculogyric crises, coma, and bloody spinal fluid are differential features of herpes simplex encephalitis (Chaps. 218 and 361). Although ECHO virus aseptic meningitis most often is self-limited and recovery complete, about 10 percent of patients have serious involvement of the central nervous system. Minor muscle weakness with reflex changes may persist for weeks to months, but over 95 percent of patients recover completely within a year. Occasionally choreiform movements, ataxia, nystagmus, transverse myelitis, coma, bulbar involvement, and death result.

REFERENCES

Horstmann, D. M., and N. Yamada: Enterovirus Infections of the Central Nervous System, Assoc. for Res. in Nervous & Mental Dis. Res. Pub., 44:236, 1968.

Karzon, D. T., N. S. Hayner, W. Winkelstein, Jr., and A. L. Barron: Epidemic of Aseptic Meningitis Syndrome Due to ECHO Virus Type 6. II. Clinical Study of ECHO 6 Infection, Pediatrics, 29:418, 1962.

Lepow, M. L., D. H. Carver, H. T. Wright, Jr., W. A. Woods, and F. C. Robbins: A Clinical, Epidemiologic and Laboratory Investigation of Aseptic Meningitis during the Four Year Period, 1955–1958. I. Observations Concerning Etiology and Epidemiology, New Engl. J. Med., 266:1181, 1962.

Sabin, A. B., E. R. Krumbiegel, and R. Wigand: ECHO Type 9 Virus Disease: Virologically Controlled Clinical and Epidemiologic Observations during 1957 Epidemic in Milwaukee with Notes on Concurrent Similar Diseases Associated with Coxsackie and Other ECHO Viruses, J. Dis. Child., 96:197, 1958.

213 VIRAL GASTROENTERITIS
A. Martin Lerner

Sporadic endemic cases of nonbacterial diarrheas as well as acute outbreaks occur in summer or winter and have been termed "winter vomiting diseases" or "intestinal flu." There is no association of gastrointestinal symptoms with influenza virus. Diarrhea may occur as a minor manifestation of enterovirus disease during a summer outbreak, but this is not a usual occurrence. In individuals and in epidemiologically controlled series, Coxsackie viruses, types B 3 and 4, as well as ECHO viruses, types 2, 3, 6 to 9, 11 to 14, 18, 19, and 22 to 24 have been implicated etiologically. Administration of oral attenuated poliovirus vaccines also has induced gastroenteritis.

Outbreaks of vomiting and diarrhea due to ECHO viruses occurring in winter are brief but debilitating illnesses. Malaise and several watery stools may herald the onset. Fever occurs but is not always present. Within 24 hr, repeated vomiting, retching, and chilliness ensue and there may be abdominal cramps and myalgia. The disease is highly contagious, and multiple cases occur within the family at one time or following closely one upon another. Recovery from the acute episode within 48 hr is usual, but mild diarrhea may persist for several weeks. During initial chilliness and cramping, ECHO viruses have been isolated from the blood, posterior pharyngeal wall, and rectal swabs. Shedding of virus is brief, and virus isolation is often unsuccessful within 36 hr after onset.

Reoviruses and adenoviruses have been implicated in similar gastroenteritides. Nevertheless, even during epidemiologic surveillances, most episodes of nonbacterial gastroenteritis remain undiagnosed. Differential diagnosis includes staphylococcal enterotoxin diarrhea (Chap. 137), salmonellosis (Chap. 150), and shigellosis (Chap. 151). Cases of dual bacterial-viral infection have occurred, but no obvious increase in virulence has been evident.

REFERENCES

Behbehani, A. M., and H. A. Wenner: Infantile Diarrhea (A Study of the Etiologic Role of Viruses), Am. J. Dis. Child., 111:623, 1966.

Goodwin, M. H., Jr., G. J. Love, D. C. Mackel, K. R. Berquist, and R. S. Gandin: Observations on the Association of Enteric Viruses and Bacteria with Diarrhea, Am. J. Trop. Med. Hyg., 16:178, 1967.

Klein, J. O., A. M. Lerner, and M. Finland: Acute Gastroenteritis Associated with ECHO Virus, Type 11, Am. J. Med. Sci., 240:749, 1960.

Ramos-Alvarez, M., and J. Olarte: Diarrheal Diseases of Children: The Occurrence of Enteropathogenic Viruses and Bacteria, J. Dis. Child., 107:218, 1964.

214 REOVIRUSES
A. Martin Lerner

Reoviruses were discovered inadvertently in studies of the intestinal viral flora of healthy children and adults. They were initially classified as ECHO virus, type 10, but were later reclassified. They were named to emphasize their (1) *respiratory* or (2) *enteric* human origins and their (3) *orphan* status.

Reoviruses are quite different from picornaviruses. They are about 2½ times larger (70 mμ in diameter) and show icosohedral symmetry. Their RNA is unique because it is a double-stranded helix like DNA and is also resistant to ribonuclease. Reoviruses are the only animal viruses with this type of RNA. The capsid is protein and consists of 92 hollow capsomeres. Unlike that of enteroviruses, the cytopathic effects of reovirus are nonlytic. Reoviruses multiply in primate and nonprimate tissue cultures, and the particles hemagglutinate human or avian erythrocytes. On the basis of hemagglutination inhibition tests with type-specific serums, there are 3 serotypes.

Human infections with reoviruses are common, and their distribution is worldwide. Like Coxsackie and ECHO viruses, reoviruses spread by enteric and respiratory routes. By adult life, 50 to 80 percent of several widely scattered populations in this hemisphere have had reovirus infections as measured by the presence of persistent neutralizing or hemagglutinating antibodies. Infections are more frequent in winter but can occur in any season. Reoviruses have been isolated from human nasal secretions, posterior pharyngeal and rectal swabs, spinal fluid, brain, and lung. They have been recovered from tissues of Burkitt's lymphoma. In addition, reovirus isolations or serologic data indicate that natural infections occur in cattle, dogs, mice, horses, swine, and monkeys. Although animal to human contagion has not been demonstrated, its possibility is likely.

Widespread evidence of infection and few associations with disease indicate that most infections with reoviruses are probably asymptomatic. Isolations of virus and fourfold rises in HIA (hemagglutination inhibition antibodies) in individual patients with common colds, nonspecific febrile illness, exanthem, and diarrhea suggest that these viruses may be causative in these common syndromes, but adequate epidemiologic controls are not available, and these observations need to be confirmed. More provocative are data from three thoroughly studied fatal cases with encephalitis, myocarditis, hepatitis, or interstitial pneumonias. In these patients reoviruses and no other bacterial or viral pathogens were isolated.

REFERENCES

El-Rai, F. M., and A. S. Evans: Reovirus Infections in Children and Young Adults, Arch. Environ. Health, 7:700, 1963.

Gomatos, P. J. and I. Tamm: The Secondary Structure of Reovirus RNA, Proc. Nat. Acad. Sci., 49:707, 1963.

Rosen, L.: Serologic Grouping of Reoviruses by Hemagglutination-Inhibition, Am. J. Hyg., 71:242, 1961.

———, H. E. Evans, and A. Spickard: Reovirus Infections in Human Volunteers, Am. J. Hyg., 77:29, 1963.

Sabin, A. B.: Reoviruses: New Group of Respiratory and Enteric Viruses Formerly Classified as ECHO, Type 10 Is Described, Science, 130:1387, 1959.

Tillotson, J. R., and A. M. Lerner: Reovirus, Type 3 Associated with Fatal Pneumonia, New Engl. J. Med., 276:1060, 1967.

Section 16

Viral Diseases of the Central Nervous System

215   LYMPHOCYTIC CHORIOMENINGITIS

*Harry N. Beaty and
Robert G. Petersdorf*

DEFINITION. Lymphocytic choriomeningitis (LCM) is an acute systemic viral infection which is frequently accompanied by the clinical syndrome of "aseptic meningitis" (Chap. 361) in man.

ETIOLOGY. The agent responsible for LCM has not been identified definitively. It is probably a small RNA virus which is heat labile and readily inactivated by formalin or ultraviolet light. Many different strains of the virus have been identified on the basis of tissue tropism and pathogenicity, but none is antigenically distinct. The agent can be propagated readily in chick embryo and cell cultures from chick or mouse embryo, mouse or monkey kidney, and certain established diploid cell lines.

EPIDEMIOLOGY. The virus of LCM is probably worldwide in distribution, but the disease is uncommon in man. Although natural infection occurs in a variety of animals, mice are the major reservoir for the virus and represent the only species in which latent, asymptomatic infection occurs. The latency of mouse infection depends upon immunological tolerance, and animals infected *in utero* or shortly after birth excrete the virus for life without overt disease. In man, LCM has followed direct contact with wild mice or infected rodents in experimental laboratories, and it is assumed that contact with contaminated mice or their excreta is the major mechanism for spread of this infection. Lymphocytic choriomeningitis occurs throughout the year, but is somewhat more frequently encountered in the colder months when human contact with wild rodents is greatest. Transmission of the virus by arthropod vectors has been accomplished experimentally but has not been demonstrated to occur naturally. Man-to-man transmission probably does not occur.

PATHOGENESIS. In natural infection, the portal of entry is probably through the respiratory tract. Virus multiplication occurs initially in the respiratory epithelium, and in some patients symptoms of an upper-respiratory-tract infection or influenza-like illness develop. Dissemination of virus to secondary extraneural sites of growth, possibly in reticuloendothelial cells, may be an important step in the pathogenesis of central-nervous-system disease. The virus multiplies in these sites, and when sustained viremia develops it crosses the "blood-brain barrier" and infects meningeal cells. In mice, the resulting meningitis, which is characterized by lymphocytic infiltration, is attributed to immunologic reactivity. It is postulated that this immune response is mediated by lymphocytes which were sensitized while the virus multiplied in the reticuloendothelial system and is directed against viral antigen in infected host cells. Support for this hypotesis is derived from the observation that disease can be prevented by neonatal thymectomy, irradiation, or immunodepressant drugs. There is only limited circumstantial evidence that a similar pathogenetic mechanism operates in man, but the concept that LCM is a virus-induced autoimmune disease is intriguing and deserves further study.

MANIFESTATIONS. Infection of man by the LCM virus produces a variety of clinical manifestations. Serologic surveys indicate that inapparent or unrecognized infection is common. It is also clear that symptomatic infection in man ordinarily consists of a clinically nonspecific, grippelike illness which resembles influenza. Neurologic manifestations appear only infrequently and take the form of aseptic meningitis or encephalitis.

The exact incubation period is not known, but it is probably only a few days. Initially, symptoms consist of remittent fever, anorexia, malaise, generalized aching, headache, and respiratory manifestations ranging from pharyngitis, cough, and bronchitis, to frank pneumonia. Fever and discomfort often vary in their intensity, abating somewhat and then recurring over a period of 1 to 3 weeks. Many patients then recover completely. In others, however, apparent convalescence is interrupted by a recurrence of fever and the abrupt onset of headache, photophobia, and signs of meningeal irritation. This second stage of the disease ordinarily lasts 7 to 10 days, and prompt recovery is the rule. However, relapses or recurrences of meningeal symptoms are seen occasionally. A few patients have transient erythematous or papular rashes during the meningeal phase.

Patients with aseptic meningitis almost always recover without sequelae. Fatality is also uncommon with encephalitis, but 25 to 30 percent of patients develop paralysis, and convalescence may be prolonged. Arthralgia and frank arthritis may be seen during recovery from the acute systemic illness, and in a few well-documented cases of infection with the LCM virus, orchitis has been observed.

LABORATORY FINDINGS. Leukopenia with granulocytopenia and relative lymphocytosis is commonly seen in association with the acute systemic illness. If meningitis develops, the leukocyte count is often normal, but may be elevated with a predominance of polymorphonuclear leukocytes. The cerebrospinal fluid pressure may be increased, and protein concentrations usually range from 5 to 200 mg per 100 ml. The glucose concentration in the spinal fluid is usually normal, but levels of 35 to 40 mg per 100 ml have been observed. The cell count usually ranges from 100 to 3,000 cells per cu mm with 90 percent lymphocytes.

The diagnosis of LCM often can be established with certainty by recovery of the virus from blood or spinal fluid. In most patients, however, the diagnosis is established only by serologic studies. Complement-fixing antibodies are usually detectable 1 to 2 weeks after the onset of infection, and neutralizing antibody appears after 6 to 8 weeks. Immunofluorescent studies have detected antibody to the LCM virus early in the course of the illness, and its appearance seems to parallel the development of the neurologic phase.

DIAGNOSIS. Lymphocytic choriomeningitis must be differentiated from the many other causes of the clinical syndrome of aseptic meningitis. A detailed discussion of this syndrome appears in Chapter 361.

TREATMENT. The management of infections with the LCM virus is purely supportive and symptomatic.

REFERENCES

Baum, S. G., A. M. Lewis, Jr., W. P. Rowe, and R. J. Huebner: Epidemic Nonmeningitic Lymphocytic Choriomeningitis Virus Infection, New Engl. J. Med., 274:934, 1966.

Farmer, T. W., and C. A. Janeway: Infections with the Virus of Lymphocytic Choriomeningitis, Medicine, 21:1, 1942.

Hotchin, J.: The Biology of Lymphocytic Choriomeningitis Infection: Virus-induced Immune Disease, Cold Spring Harbor Symp. Quant. Biol., 27:479, 1962.

Johnson, R. T., and C. A. Mims: Pathogenesis of Viral Infections of the Nervous System, New Engl. J. Med., 278:23, 1968.

Meyer, H. M., Jr., R. T. Johnson, I. P. Crawford, H. E. Dascomb, and N. G. Rogers: Central Nervous System Syndromes of Viral Etiology, Am. J. Med., 29:334, 1960.

216 POLIOMYELITIS
Louis Weinstein

DEFINITION. Poliomyelitis is a common acute viral infection which occurs naturally only in man and produces a wide variety of clinical manifestations. In its most severe form, it involves parts of the central nervous system. In most instances, the nervous system is not invaded; infection may take place without apparent illness, or may result in the production of nonspecific syndromes.

ETIOLOGY. The causative agent of poliomyelitis is an RNA virus of the Picorna group, 8 to 30 mu in diameter, pathogenic for man and primates. Three antigenically distinct types have been defined: type I (Brunhilde), type II (Lansing), and type III (Leon). Cross neutralization is demonstrable in highly immunized experimental animals, but infection in man with one type does not protect against invasion by another. Poliomyelitis virus grows well in tissue culture.

Under proper conditions, the virus may remain viable in water or sewage for as long as 4 months. It is not killed by ether, Merthiolate, tincture of Zephiran, ethyl alcohol, or low concentrations of mercury, oxidizing agents, 2% tincture of iodine, ultraviolet light, and 10-min exposure to a chlorine concentration of 0.05 ppm.

EPIDEMIOLOGY. Poliomyelitis is worldwide, but epidemics have been limited to a relatively small number of areas. That infection is much more prevalent than is suggested by the number of clinically recognized cases is proved by the widespread distribution of neutralizing antibody in populations all over the world. Poliomyelitis occurs with the highest frequency from July through September in the North Temperate Zone, although it may appear as early as April or as late as December. In tropical or subtropical regions, the season may be prolonged.

In areas of poor sanitation, most individuals develop neutralizing antibodies in early childhood, while in other localities, the peak of population immunity is not reached until fifteen years of age or older. Urban dwellers become immune earlier than those who live in rural areas. In lower-income groups, evidence of contact with poliomyelitis virus appears at a younger age than in individuals whose financial status is good.

Poliomyelitis was most common in the preschool child until World War II but has been increasing in older age groups. In some epidemics since the war, 25 to 30 percent of patients have been older than fifteen years of age. Paralytic disease has been described in the neonatal period and as late as the sixth decade but is very uncommon at these age extremes.

PATHOGENESIS. Man is the sole reservoir of poliomyelitis virus. Carriers, especially those with unapparent infection, are most important in transmission of the virus. A history of contact with recognized cases is uncommon. Milk was incriminated as the source of infection in one epidemic.

Virus is recoverable from pharyngeal secretions for only a few days but is demonstrable in the feces for several weeks. The intestinal tract is the main source from which virus is disseminated. The mode of infection, therefore, is fecal-oral, the same as in salmonellosis, shigellosis, and other enteric infections. Large quantities of virus are present in sewage drained from areas in which the infection is present. Flies trapped in areas close to patients with poliomyelitis may carry the virus. Attempts to reduce the spread of disease in epidemics by eradication of the fly population, however, have not been successful. Poliomyelitis is as highly communicable as measles or varicella; in individuals under fifteen years of age, infection, with or without clinical manifestations, occurs in 100 percent of household and 87 percent of daily contacts.

The following sequence of events has been postulated as the basis for infection: (1) The virus enters the body by way of the mouth, begins to multiply in the oropharynx and lower part of the intestinal tract, and can be transmitted from either area. The site of viral growth is probably extraneural. Virus is present in pharyngeal secretions and stool during the incubation period; it has been demonstrated in the feces as long as 19 days prior to onset of the disease. (2) The phase of "minor illness" (described below) develops in association with the presence of the virus in the blood, throat, and feces; the viremia persists for only a few days until antibodies make their appearance. The virus in the intestinal tract penetrates the lymphatic channels and enters the bloodstream, from which it is disseminated. (3) The final stage in the pathogenesis of poliomyelitis is invasion of the nervous system. It has been suggested that the virus enters the nervous system from the blood in the area postrema of the medulla oblongata because this is more permeable than other parts of the brain to dyes injected intravascularly; it has also been postulated, however, that viral invasion of the nervous system occurs at many points by direct passage of virus from capillaries to neurones. Once the virus has reached the nervous system, it spreads along nerve fibers.

Strains of poliomyelitis virus vary greatly in their ability to invade nervous tissue and to destroy neurones. Repeated passage in animals or tissue cultures induces changes in invasive capacity without affecting the basic antigenic character of the agent. The early presence of detectable antibody results from multiplication of virus in nonnervous tissue, and accounts for the short persistence of virus in the pharynx and blood, sites in which antibody is demonstrable. The persistence of virus in the nervous system and intestine is probably due to the difficulty which antibody has in reaching these areas.

The most important determinant of human susceptibility to poliomyelitis is serum antibody. Previous inapparent infection and illness without invasion of the nervous system are common. Many children and most adults possess neutralizing antibody for all three types of virus; this probably accounts for the relative infrequency of the disease in older age groups. Infants under six months old rarely get poliomyelitis because immunity is passively transferred from the mother. Babies born to women in the acute phase of poliomyelitis can develop the disease shortly after birth. Sex plays a role in determining susceptibility. Among children, males are affected more often than females; the opposite is true in adults. Pregnancy increases the risk of clinically apparent poliomyelitis, and multiparous females are more susceptible than primiparas. The disease is somewhat more frequent in the second than in the first or third trimesters. Menstruation or ovulation appears to heighten susceptibility. Absence of the tonsils and adenoids, regardless of the time of their removal, is associated with a marked increase in incidence of bulbar poliomyelitis. Chilling or physical exertion after invasion by the virus leads to more frequent development of paralytic poliomyelitis, especially in adults.

CLINICAL MANIFESTATIONS. The incubation period of poliomyelitis varies from 3 to 35 days; about 80 percent of cases occur 6 to 20 days after contact with the virus.

The infection may assume one of four forms: (1) inapparent infection, (2) "minor illness," (3) nonparalytic poliomyelitis, (4) paralytic poliomyelitis.

Inapparent Infection. As much as 95 percent of infection with the poliomyelitis virus occurs in this form. There are no symptoms, but the virus is present in the pharynx, intestine, and probably the blood. Type-specific neutralizing antibody usually develops.

"Minor Illness." The entire course of poliomyelitis may consist of a nonspecific illness without clinical or laboratory evidence of central-nervous-system invasion; this is "abortive" poliomyelitis. Three syndromes have been observed: (1) upper respiratory manifestations, consisting of fever of varying degree, pharyngeal discomfort, with or without coryza, and reddening and swelling of the lymphoid tissues of the throat; (2) gastrointestinal disturbances, with nausea, vomiting, diarrhea or constipation, and abdominal discomfort, accompanied by moderate fever; (3) grippelike disease with fever and generalized aching of muscles, bones, and joints, resembling influenza. Virus can be demonstrated in the pharynx, feces, and blood in the early stages of these "minor" illnesses. Type-specific neutralizing and complement-fixing antibodies develop during convalescence.

Nonparalytic Poliomyelitis. Nonparalytic poliomyelitis consists of prodromal manifestations, signs of meningeal irritation, and abnormalities of the spinal fluid. The prodrome is similar to that of the "minor" illnesses and is usually present for several days before the onset of other signs. Stiffness of the neck and back (Kernig's sign), and, with severe meningeal irritation, leg and neck (Brudzinski's sign) are present. The tripod (patient extends arms behind back with hands on bed for support when sitting up) and Hoyne's signs (head falls back when, with patient in supine position, shoulders are elevated) can be elicited in paralytic or nonparalytic poliomyelitis but are not pathognomonic.

Spinal Fluid. The spinal fluid usually contains between 25 and 500 cells, and rarely as many as 1,000 to 2,000. Very early in the disease, there is often a preponderance of neutrophils (up to 80 percent); within a few days, however, mononuclear cells predominate. The protein is normal or slightly elevated at the beginning of the illness but may increase to between 50 and 100 mg per 100 ml. The sugar content is normal. These spinal fluid findings are typical of *aseptic meningitis* (Chap. 361) and indicate an inflammatory reaction of the meninges but are not diagnostic of poliomyelitis. They are also present in healing bacterial meningitis, tuberculous meningitis, scarlet fever, pertussis encephalopathy, leptospiral meningitis, syphilis, mumps meningitis, Coxsackie virus infections, herpes simplex meningitis, infectious mononucleosis, trichinella meningitis, brain abscess, multiple sclerosis, tumors of the brain or spinal cord, allergic reactions involving the nervous system, postinfectious encephalitides, "infectious" polyneuritis, and lymphocytic choriomeningitis.

The diagnosis of nonparalytic poliomyelitis on clinical grounds alone is impossible, because the signs, symptoms, and laboratory findings are completely nonspecific. Viral and immunologic studies suggest that fewer than 40 percent of cases of "nonparalytic poliomyelitis" are actually this disease; mumps meningitis without salivary gland involvement (Chap. 231) and Coxsackie virus disease (Chaps. 210 and 211) are the two most common differential diagnoses.

The course of nonparalytic poliomyelitis is benign. Defervescence occurs in 3 to 5 days, but meningeal irritation may persist for 2 weeks. No changes in muscle and nerve function are detectable. The white blood cell count may be as high as 15,000 in the early stage of the disease but is usually normal within a week.

Paralytic Poliomyelitis. The syndrome of paralytic poliomyelitis consists of prodromal manifestations ("minor" illness), signs of meningeal irritation, abnormal spinal fluid, and signs of involvement of motor nerve cells in the spinal cord, brain, or cranial nerve nuclei, resulting in paresis or paralysis of various muscles. Lesions may also be present in parts of the nervous system other than anterior horn cells; the precentral gyrus, the reticular formation in the medulla, the roof nuclei and vermis of the cerebellum, Auerbach's and Meissner's plexuses, and sympathetic ganglions are usually involved in fatal cases. Seldom, however, are there clinical signs pointing to disease of these parts. "Skip" areas are common in spinal paralytic disease; involvement of the cervical and lumbar cord is often present with no dysfunction of the thoracic portion.

Paralytic poliomyelitis may be subdivided into the following types:

  I. Spinal
    A. Cervical
    B. Thoracic
    C. Lumbar
    D. Any combination of A, B, and C
 II. Bulbar
    A. Upper cranial nerve involvement—III, IV, V, VI, VII, VIII
    B. Lower cranial nerve involvement—IX, X, XI, XII
    C. Involvement of cardiorespiratory centers
III. Bulbospinal
 IV. Polioencephalitis—paralytic or nonparalytic
    A. Diffuse encephalitis
    B. Focal encephalitis
    C. Cerebellar involvement (?)
    D. Bulboencephalitic disease
    E. Spinal-encephalitic disease

Prodromal manifestations are often absent in paralytic poliomyelitis. In some cases, the illness is biphasic in character. The disease starts with fever and manifestations of one of the "minor" illnesses. After several days, all symptoms disappear; in 5 or 10 days, there are recrudescence of fever, the development of signs of meningeal irritation, and the appearance of paralysis. The commonest prodromal symptoms in adults are generalized muscle and bone discomfort. In children, upper-respiratory-tract syndromes are most frequent. The spinal fluid findings in paralytic poliomyelitis are the same as those in the nonparalytic disease. Paralytic poliomyelitis may be accompanied by a completely normal spinal fluid throughout its entire course, but this occurs in no more than 0.5 percent of cases. In some patients, decrease in number of cells in the spinal fluid is accompanied by a progressive rise in protein, which may reach levels high enough to cause confusion with the cytoalbuminologic dissociation observed in "infectious" polyneuritis.

Spinal Paralytic Poliomyelitis. In the early stages of spinal paralytic poliomyelitis, cramping pain in the muscles innervated by the affected neurones and hyperesthesia of the overlying skin are present. The discomfort may be very severe; muscle "spasm," the exact mechanism of which is not clear, is usually detectable. In some instances, increase in muscle weakness is very slow; in others, it becomes widespread within 48 hr Rarely, a rapidly ascending paralysis of the Landry type is observed. Age is one factor in determining the extent of involvement. In children less than five years old, paresis of one leg is most common. In patients between five and fifteen years of age, weakness of one arm, or paraplegia, is most frequent, while in adults (sixteen to sixty-five years old), quadriplegia is observed most often. Dysfunction of the urinary bladder is at least ten times more frequent in adults than in children. Paralysis of the muscles of respiration is most common in those older than sixteen years of age. Infants younger than one year are subject to very extensive involvement. Among adults, men develop quadriplegia, respiratory paralysis, and loss of bladder function more frequently than do women. Pregnancy does not increase the severity of the disease unless parturition takes place during the acute phase. There is a definite association of inoculation of antigenic materials ("triple vaccine," for example) with involvement of the muscles around the site of injection.

When the *cervical cord* is involved, there is paresis or paralysis of the muscles of the shoulders, arms, neck, and diaphragm. Very early in the disease, the reflexes in the arms remain intact; they diminish rapidly, however, and are usually absent by the time paralysis has become established. Coarse twitching of the affected muscles is common. With cervical cord disease, there is always danger of respiratory paralysis due to spread of the infection to the motor nuclei of the phrenic nerves and medulla.

Weakness of the muscles of the chest, upper portion of the abdomen, and spine follows involvement of the *thoracic portion* of the spinal cord. Difficulty in breathing results from dysfunction of the intercostal and other thoracic muscles. The chest wall may be in "spasm" and may appear rigid despite the presence of only a minor degree of paresis.

Disease of the *lumbar portion of the spinal cord* produces weakness of the legs and inferior portions of the abdomen and back. Again, pain, tenderness, "spasm," and twitching herald the oncoming paralysis, and the reflexes are abolished with the development of flaccid paralysis. In adults, complete paraplegia is not infrequent. Paralysis of the urinary bladder, usually temporary, occurs in about one-third of patients over sixteen years of age and is rarely observed in the absence of weakness of the legs.

The abdominal and cremasteric reflexes usually disappear before muscle weakness is marked in paralytic poliomyelitis and may be absent during the entire course of the disease. An extensor plantar response (positive Babinski's sign) is rare; its persistence is incompatible with poliomyelitis. Hyperesthesia of the skin is frequent, but sensory loss does not occur. Constipation, abdominal cramps, and metiorism are common and are due to ileus resulting from involvement of the autonomic nervous system and weakness of the abdominal muscles. When the disease is severe, sympathetic nervous system disturbances, with tachycardia, hypertension, abnormal sweating, and cyanosis and coldness of the involved extremities, are present.

Fever in spinal paralytic poliomyelitis is usually present for the first few days of the disease and disappears by lysis. In about 90 percent of cases, there is little or no extension of paralysis 48 hr after defervescence has occurred. In about 10 percent, however, considerable progression of weakness may continue for as long as a week or more.

Bulbar Poliomyelitis. The incidence of bulbar poliomyelitis differs from one epidemic to another and varies between 6 and 25 percent. In patients subjected to tonsilloadenoidectomy within 30 days of onset of the disease and in those in whom the operation was carried out years before, the bulbar form of infection is present in about 85 percent of cases. Pure bulbar involvement (without any signs of spinal cord involvement) is commonest in children; adults with bulbar disturbances usually have associated spinal paralyses. The syndromes which develop depend on the area of the brainstem involved, and result from damage to the medulla, pons, and midbrain. Signs and symptoms are produced by (1) dysfunction of the upper cranial nerve nuclei, (2) damage to the lower cranial nerve nuclei, and (3) disturbances of the respiratory and vasomotor regulating centers in the medulla. Combined bulbar and diffuse or focal encephalitis or spinal involvement may occur.

1. *Upper Cranial Nerve Nuclei—III, IV, V, VI, VII, VIII.* Isolated ocular nerve palsies, total external ophthalmoplegia, pupillary disorders, and Horner's syndrome occur. There may be unilateral or bilateral involvement of the fifth nerve, with difficulty in chewing and closing the mouth, as well as deviation of the jaws. Paralysis of the seventh cranial nerve is common and usually unilateral; the entire face or only the upper or lower parts may be affected. Disturbances of vestibular function and deafness resulting from damage to the nucleus of the eighth nerve occur infrequently.

2. *Lower Cranial Nerve Nuclei—IX, X, XI, XII.* Life may be endangered when the muscles of deglutition are paralyzed because of involvement of the nucleus ambiguus in the medulla. Hoarseness and laryngeal stridor follow weakness or paralysis of the vocal cords. Unilateral or bilateral weakness of the tongue, sternocleidomastoid, and trapezius muscles may be present. Inability to swallow results in pooling of saliva and food in the pharynx,

with obstruction to the airway. Aspiration into the larynx, reflex spasm of the glottis, and abductor paralysis of the vocal cords constitute very serious threats to life. Minor or major pareses of the soft palate and pharyngeal muscles are detectable by a nasal quality of the voice.

3. *Disease of the medullary respiratory center* produces irregularity of the rhythm, depth, and rate of breathing. Respirations are shallow, and as the disease progresses, there are progressively longer periods of apnea until breathing stops completely. The thoracic muscles and diaphragm are not weak, unless spinal involvement is present. Hiccuping is frequent in the early phase of respiratory center dysfunction. Hypoxia, without visible cyanosis, is common and contributes to the intensity of the manifestations. In the late stages, cyanosis, unresponsive to oxygen administration, is common, and temperature, pulse rate, and blood pressure are elevated. The final event is usually irreversible shock.

Involvement of the circulatory regulating center includes a cherry-red color of the lips, flushed skin, rapid, irregular pulse, small pulse pressure when the blood pressure is normal, and moderate to severe hypotension. Hyperthermia, cold, mottled, clammy skin, shallow respiration, and anxiety, restlessness, and confusion appear as the circulation becomes impaired and irreversible shock develops.

Polioencephalitis. Encephalitic symptoms occur as isolated syndromes, or together with bulbar or spinal poliomyelitis. The incidence of polioencephalitis is variable; one small epidemic in which most of the patients had this type of disease has been described. The diffuse form is characterized by confusion, agitation, anxiety with a feeling of impending doom, or somnolence. Quivering and jerking of the facial muscles and extremities, flushing of the face, tremor of the hands, and restless movements occur. Insomnia may be severe. In fatal cases, confusion is marked and progresses to lethargy and death.

In focal polioencephalitis, there may be clinical evidence of brain damage, or the lesions may be silent and demonstrable only at necropsy. Visual-verbal agnosia, myoclonic jerks, grand mal convulsions, which occasionally persist for a long time after recovery, spastic hemiparesis, ataxia of one arm or leg, and hydrocephalus have been described.

DIAGNOSIS. The diagnosis of paralytic poliomyelitis can usually be made on clinical grounds. The outstanding manifestations are a lower motor neurone lesion which develops rapidly and is characterized by flaccid weakness and hypo- or areflexia. Signs of upper motor neurone disease or decreased sensation are not compatible with poliomyelitis. Among the diseases which may cause confusion, especially in their early stages, are toxic, "infectious," or idiopathic polyneuritis, the postinfectious encephalitides, viral encephalitides, trichinosis, acute rheumatic fever, cerebrovascular accidents with paralysis, acute syphilitic meningitis (frequent cranial nerve palsies), meningomyeloencephalitis resulting from sensitization to foreign protein (horse serum, rabies vaccine,

pertussis vaccine), osteomyelitis, scurvy, acute multiple sclerosis, pseudobulbar palsy, myalgic meningoencephalitis (Iceland, Tallahassee, or Coventry disease), spinal epidural abscess or tumor, neoplasms of the brain and spinal cord, Coxsackie virus infection, the encephalitis of the preicteric phase of infectious hepatitis, infectious mononucleosis with neurologic involvement, infections due to the enteric cytopathogenic human "orphan" (ECHO) viruses, focal embolic encephalitis associated with subacute bacterial endocarditis, tuberculous meningitis with hemiplegia or cranial nerve (especially the sixth) palsies, and brain abscess. Study of these diseases over a period of a few days to a week after onset clarifies the situation in most instances. The only positive method of establishing the diagnosis of paralytic poliomyelitis is the isolation of the virus from the stool or pharyngeal secretions (spinal cord or brain at necropsy) and the demonstration of a rise in the level of neutralizing antibody to the isolated strain in acute- and convalescent-phase serums. If virus cannot be isolated, the three type strains maintained in tissue culture may be used; a significant rise in titer of neutralizing antibody against a specific serotype is diagnostic.

COMPLICATIONS. Complications occur most frequently when the respiratory muscles are involved because of involvement of spinal or bulbar motor neurones; they are, at times, the direct cause of death. Disturbances in water and electrolyte balance are common in patients receiving continuous artificial respiration. Fever and the sweating which follow enclosure in a tank respirator during the summer months, together with vomiting, diarrhea, inability to take food, and disturbances in carbon dioxide related to improperly regulated ventilation, produce a complicated series of chemical disturbances. Edema and low electrolyte levels often follow overenthusiastic hydration and have been misinterpreted as evidence of a salt-wasting syndrome. Myocarditis is not uncommon in poliomyelitis; it is probably due to direct viral invasion. ECG changes, mainly T and ST-T and P-R abnormalities, are present in from 10 to 20 percent of cases. Interstitial infiltration of the myocardium with round cells and mild muscle changes are not infrequent. Severe myocardopathy has been thought to be responsible for death in some cases. Hypertension may develop by two mechanisms: (1) transient elevation of blood pressure due to hypoxia, and (2) persistent hypertension secondary to hypothalamic involvement, which may become "malignant" and lead to severe retinopathy, convulsions, and mental deterioration.

Pulmonary edema and shock, the exact pathogenesis of which is not known, are usually the terminal events in fatal cases of poliomyelitis. Phlebothrombosis of the legs, with or without pulmonary embolism, is not uncommon, even in young adults. All methods of artificial respiration produce hemodynamic disturbances, which are countered by reflex mechanisms acting to maintain normal blood pressure and cardiac output. When patients are placed in respirators under negative tank pressure (positive intratracheal pressure) after hypotension and impending shock are already present, the peripheral vascular collapse often is made worse. Acute and marked dilatation of the stomach and large bowel, perforation of the cecum, acute ulceration of the duodenum, stomach, and esophagus, the formation of multiple erosions of the entire gastrointestinal tract with considerable bleeding and paralytic ileus have been observed. Marked depression of prothrombin, with massive spontaneous hemorrhage, occurs in individuals with severe poliomyelitis, especially if they are receiving large doses of broad-spectrum antibiotics orally. Severe bulbar (ninth and tenth cranial nerves) or bulbospinal disease with paralysis of the respiratory muscles is accompanied by the risk of major atelectasis.

Bacterial infection is one of the most dangerous complications of paralytic poliomyelitis. Pneumonia is quite common in patients with paralysis of the muscles of respiration or deglutition. The incidence of pulmonary infection is greatly increased by tracheostomy and is highest in the respirator patient subjected to this operation. The organisms involved most often are *Staphylococcus aureus* and gram-negative bacilli, many strains of which are not sensitive to the commonly used antimicrobial agents. Chemoprophylaxis is of no value in preventing secondary bronchopulmonary bacterial invasion.

The other common site of infection in poliomyelitis is the urinary tract because of the necessity for chronic catheterization in patients with paralysis of the bladder; chemoprophylaxis is usually ineffective, although closed catheter drainage may be effective in keeping the urine sterile for as long as a week. The responsible organisms are those usually found in urinary tract infections and are often insusceptible to antibiotics and sulfonamides. Renal stone formation is frequent and may be responsible for renal colic, obstruction of the pelvis, and pyonephrosis, pyelonephritis, renal decompensation, hypertension, and vascular disease. The factors which contribute to renal lithiasis are immobility with hypercalcuria, infection, stasis, dehydration, and excessive calcium intake. Attempts to control this problem consist of the liberal administration of fluids, decrease of calcium intake, acidification of the urine, administration of salicylate, and early mobilization.

A syndrome resembling rheumatoid arthritis, with redness, swelling, pain, and tenderness of the larger joints, is observed rarely in the convalescent phase of paralytic poliomyelitis. A variety of skin rashes may occur, including miliaria, seborrhea, and purpuric, morbilliform, or exfoliative eruptions due to drug sensitization. Bedsores are common in respirator patients because of the difficulty in moving them about. Markedly paralyzed individuals, especially those whose life is threatened by respiratory difficulty, frequently experience very difficult emotional problems. Disorientation, acute panic states, Korsakoff-like syndromes, and acute psychoses have been noted. Chronic anxiety and depression are almost universal in adults with severe neurologic involvement and probably reflect the sudden impact of a crippling disease, rather than brain damage due to viral invasion.

IMMUNITY. One attack of poliomyelitis usually confers lifelong immunity against reinvasion by the same sero-type. Both neutralizing and complement-fixing antibodies appear early in the disease; complement-fixing antibodies persist for several years after infection, while neutralizing antibodies persist throughout life. Theoretically, an individual could have three episodes of the disease, because immunity is strictly type-specific. Most adults and many children have poliomyelitis, without nervous system invasion, two or three times, as shown by the presence of neutralizing antibody for more than one virus type. There are, however, well-documented instances of two episodes of paralytic infection separated by a number of years in the same individual.

TREATMENT. Cases of *abortive poliomyelitis* should receive no therapy except for symptomatic relief.

The management of *nonparalytic poliomyelitis* involves primarily the relief of the headache, pain in the back, and "spasm" of the legs. Rest in bed with the mattress supported by a board may be of value in preventing paralysis and is helpful in reducing back pain. The application of wet heat, in the form of "hot packs," to the affected muscles produces considerable relief. Analgesics such as meperidine and codeine are very useful and are preferable to morphine derivatives. Antimicrobial agents are useless because they have no effect on the primary disease and do not decrease the risk of secondary infection. Neuromuscular examination should not be carried out more often than every 3 to 4 days. Bed rest is terminated as soon as severe discomfort is absent in order to reduce the risk of phlebothrombosis and pulmonary embolism. Every patient thought to have nonparalytic poliomyelitis should have careful assessment of muscle function and an orthopedic follow-up study for 2 to 3 months after recovery. The purpose of these measures is to detect and correct minor degrees of weakness which may become apparent only when muscles which appear normal at rest are taxed by the exertion of normal physical activity.

The treatment of *paralytic poliomyelitis* involves (1) the use of all measures to spare the life of the patient threatened by involvement of vital areas, (2) relief of discomfort, (3) maintenance of weak muscles in as good a condition as possible, (4) immediate recognition and treatment of medical complications, (5) prophylaxis and therapy of emotional disorders, (6) surgical treatment of correctable defects, and (7) social, economic, occupational, and physical rehabilitation.

Patients with paralysis of swallowing, loss of function of the respiratory muscles, pulmonary edema, or shock are in great danger of death. Dysfunction of the ninth and tenth cranial nerves is most important because of the danger of fatal airway obstruction. For this reason, it has been suggested that tracheostomy be performed in all such cases. However, thorough study has indicated that this operation is followed by a much higher incidence of bronchopulmonary infections due to organisms difficult to eradicate with antibiotic agents than occurs when the procedure is not carried out. In some cases, however, tracheostomy becomes necessary, despite the risk. The indications for this operation are (1) abductor paralysis of the vocal cords; (2) pneumonia with inability to clear the lungs of exudate; (3) repeated bouts of major atelectasis requiring tracheal catheterization or bronchoscopy; (4) inability to keep the airway relatively free of secretions—this is often purely a matter of availability of a sufficient complement of experienced personnel.

Decreased movement of the diaphragm or intercostal muscles dictates frequent determination of vital capacity. When this is reduced to 50 percent of normal or less, artificial respiration must be given with a tank or cuirass type of chest respirator. Details of this type of treatment are discussed in Chap. 295. An electrophrenic respirator is indicated when the respiratory center is involved because tank respiration may actually increase the difficulties imposed by respiratory center dysfunction. Indirect stimulation of one phrenic nerve through the skin is usually sufficient.

Shock is easier to prevent than to treat. Assurance of adequate oxygen saturation, prevention of dehydration, and early treatment of superimposed bacterial infection are of prophylactic value. When marked hypotension develops, vasoconstricting agents such as norepinephrine are often helpful in restoring blood pressure to normal. As a rule, however, these drugs become ineffective as their use is prolonged. Plasma infusions may be of some help. Hypotension appearing during artificial respiration may respond to alternating positive and negative tank pressures of approximately the same degree.

The relief of discomfort is one of the most important problems in paralytic poliomyelitis. Hot wet packs, diathermy, warm baths, and dry heat reduce pain due to muscle "spasm." Analgesic drugs should be used whenever necessary, but morphine derivatives should be avoided. Changing the position of paralyzed limbs and moving the patient about in bed are effective in reducing pain.

Weak muscles must be maintained in as good condition as possible until neural function returns; the time, degree, and extent of resumption of function are unpredictable, but treatment should be continued for at least 2 years and is managed best by the physiotherapist who has had experience with poliomyelitis. Daily physiotherapy is usually started 3 to 4 days after complete defervescence and after there is no further extension of weakness. Exercise against resistance is thought to be most beneficial, but in many clinics, exercise in water to remove the effects of gravity is standard practice.

The prevention and treatment of the emotional disorders which accompany severe paralytic poliomyelitis best are carried out by the attending physicians and nurses. Although the help of the psychiatrist is necessary in difficult situations, the importance of physicians, nurses, and attendants who are in constant contact with the patient and are properly oriented toward these problems cannot be overemphasized.

Maximal return of muscle function usually is established at the end of 2 years following the onset of paralytic poliomyelitis. A review of the clinical problem by an orthopedic surgeon should be carried out if residual palsies remain, and a program of surgical rehabilitation should be set in motion.

The impact of paralytic poliomyelitis on the social and economic status of adults is often very severe. Every effort must be made to enlist the cooperation of social service agencies to minimize the disruptive effects of the disease. Many patients require occupational rehabilitation because of inability to perform the work in which they were engaged prior to being crippled. For others, the use of devices, such as movable splints and hooks, is very helpful in physical rehabilitation.

PROGNOSIS. The overall mortality rate for poliomyelitis is about 5 percent. Patients with abortive or nonparalytic disease recover completely. About 2 to 5 percent of children and 15 to 30 percent of adults (increasing with age) with paralytic infection die. When bulbospinal involvement, especially with medullary or phrenic and intercostal nerve dysfuntion, is present, the fatality rate varies between 25 and 75 percent and is greatly influenced by age and the presence of shock, pulmonary edema, superimposed infection, or other medical complications.

Many persons with paralytic poliomyelitis recover completely. In a considerable number, muscle function returns to some degree. Only a few remain totally paralyzed. The more life-threatening the disease in the acute stage, the more frequent is complete functional recovery, if the patient survives. For example, paralysis of the respiratory center usually disappears completely. Dysfunction of the ninth and tenth cranial nerves is followed by total recovery in most instances, although mild palatopharyngeal weakness occasionally may persist for life. Paralysis of the muscles of respiration often disappears completely. In some cases, the final vital capacity, although reduced, is adequate to maintain ventilation, even with moderate physical exertion. In very few instances is chronic respirator care necessary. Weak extremities regain about 60 percent of the total strength that they will ever recover in 3 months, and 80 percent, within 6 months. Improvement may continue for as long as 2 years. The final degree of functional return depends on the number of neurones destroyed.

PREVENTION. Because 90 to 95 percent of cases of poliomyelitis are inapparent, or "minor" infections, and are not diagnosed, the prevention of the disease by isolation is very difficult. The common practice of isolating clinically evident cases is of much greater individual than public health benefit. The usual period of isolation is about 2 weeks, although virus may be present in the feces for a much longer period. Contact with known cases should be avoided. Restriction of community activities such as swimming or gathering of people is not indicated except with large epidemics, when it is more effective in allaying panic than in reducing infection. Pregnant women should take special precaution because of the increased susceptibility to the disease during pregnancy. Tonsillectomy is contraindicated in areas where poliomyelitis is present. All individuals with "minor" illnesses during the poliomyelitis season should limit their physical activity and avoid chilling until all symptoms have disappeared.

Active immunization against paralytic poliomyelitis has been successful by means of parenteral administration of formalin-inactivated strains of the three viral serotypes grown in monkey kidney tissue culture. The vaccine is

60 to 70 percent effective against type 1 and 85 to 90 percent effective against types 2 and 3. A booster dose should be given within 2 years after initial injection series. The effectiveness of this vaccine is evidenced by the fact that, in the year (1955) in which it was introduced, there were 28,985 cases of poliomyelitis in the United States. Two years later, only 2,218 cases were reported. Formalin-inactivated vaccine does not decrease the incidence of nonparalytic poliomyelitis. It has no effect on the intestinal phase of the disease and fails, therefore, to interrupt the spread of virus from one vaccinated person to another. Another drawback is the necessity to give "booster" doses for the maintenance of a protective level of antibody. Although four doses are presently recommended, whether more injections are necessary has not been determined.

Oral administration of attenuated strains of poliovirus is highly effective in stimulating antibody production and preventing infection and is the method of choice for protecting a population. The virus preparations are easily handled and are stable. They may be stored in a conventional refrigerator up to 30 days. Once a vial has been used in part, the rest of its contents should be discarded after 7 days.

Vaccine virus multiplies in the intestinal tract and remains at this site. Viremia occurs rarely, and then only with some strains. Live vaccine virus spreads and infects contacts of vaccinated individuals. The incidence of spread is lowest in high-income groups (about 9 percent) following feeding of infants. This type of immunization in the presence of epidemic poliomyelitis may lead to replacement of the "wild" paralytogenic strain by the one in the vaccine, and may actually abort spread of the disease.

Significant levels of antibody develop in 90 to 100 percent of persons receiving live virus vaccine; they develop more rapidly and persist longer than those which follow the use of formalinized vaccines. Intestinal immunity is present after feeding of the "live" preparations so that minimal or no multiplication in the bowel occurs on exposure to "wild" strains of virus.

The highest levels of poliomyelitis-neutralizing antibody appear when monovalent oral vaccines are administered. The recommended order of administration is type 1, followed within no less than 8 weeks by type 3, which, in turn, should be followed in 6 or more weeks by type 2. If the polyvalent vaccine (all three types) is given to adults, two doses are fed 8 weeks apart. If newborns are given vaccine, the viruses should be refed at a later date because about 50 percent of neonates fail to develop significant levels of immunity if treated shortly after birth. Immunization of breast-fed infants should be delayed until they are taking regular diets. It has been suggested that a community-wide program of vaccine virus feeding followed by routine immunization of infants in the first year of life may result in eradication of poliomyelitis. The efficacy of this procedure is emphasized by the fact that there were only 66 cases of poliomyelitis recorded in the United States during the first 9 months of 1966. Immunization with live vaccine is best carried out during the cooler months of the year. The widespread prevalence of other enteroviruses in the intestinal tract, especially in children, may result in a low level of immunization because these may interfere with the implantation of the vaccine strains. Although the necessity for "booster" doses of this preparation in older children and adults has not been proved, many physicians are administering the triple vaccine 1 to 2 years after primary immunization; some are giving a second "booster" 1 to 2 years after the first.

The administration of live poliomyelitis virus vaccines to millions of persons in many areas of the world has demonstrated very convincingly the very high degree of protection (over 90 percent) against paralytic poliomyelitis conferred by this preparation and a tendency for epidemic strains to be replaced by those present in the vaccine. The vaccines are remarkably safe. Although instances of the disease are thought to have been associated with feeding of each of the three strains (0.4 cases per million doses for type 3, 0.16 per million doses for type 1, and 0.02 per million doses for type 2), it has been suggested that the greatest risk of developing active disease produced by the vaccine strain is related to the administration of the type 3 preparation to individuals in the age range of twenty to thirty-nine years. However, firm proof of the association of vaccine virus and the development of poliomyelitis is lacking, and the possibility has been raised that the "compatible" cases have been caused by wild strains of poliomyelitis virus or other enteroviruses present in the intestinal tract at the time the vaccine was administered. Type 1 vaccine strain has been incriminated in a case of paralytic poliomyelitis in a young child with marked hypogammaglobulinemia. Children known to have this defect should probably not receive this agent.

REFERENCES

Grulee, C. G.: Differential Diagnosis of Poliomyelitis, J.A.M.A., 152:1587, 1953.

Henderson, D. A., J. J. Witte, L. Morris, and A. D. Langmuir: Paralytic Disease Associated with Oral Polio Vaccines, J.A.M.A., 190:41, 1964.

Hodes, J. L.: Treatment of Respiratory Difficulty in Poliomyelitis, in "Poliomyelitis, Papers and Discussions Presented at the Third International Poliomyelitis Conference," Philadelphia, J. B. Lippincott Company, 1955.

Horstmann, D. M.: The Epidemiology and Pathogenesis of Poliomyelitis, Bull. N.Y. Acad. Med., 29:909, 1953.

———, M. D. McCollum, and A. D. Mascola: The Incidence of Infection among Contacts of Poliomyelitis Cases, J. Clin. Invest., 34:1573, 1955.

Report of Special Advisory Committee on Oral Poliomyelitis Vaccines to the Surgeon General of the Public Health Service: Oral Poliomyelitis Vaccines, J.A.M.A., 190:49–51, 1964.

Sabin, A. B.: Commentary on Report on Oral Poliomyelitis Vaccines, J.A.M.A., 190:52–55, 1964.

———: Poliomyelitis. Accomplishments of Live Virus Vaccine. First International Conference on Vaccines against Viral and Rickettsial Diseases, Bull. World Health Organ., p. 171, 1967.

Symposium on Poliomyelitis, Pediat. Clin. N. Am., 1:1, 1953.

Symposium on Poliomyelitis Vaccination, J.A.M.A., 158:1239, 1955.

Weinstein, L.: Diagnosis and Treatment of Poliomyelitis, Med. Clinics N. Am., p. 1377, September, 1948.

——: The Influence of Muscular Fatigue, Tonsilladenoidectomy and Antigen Injections on the Clinical Course of Poliomyelitis, Boston Med. Quart., 3:11, 1952.

——: Influence of Age and Sex on Susceptibility and Clinical Manifestations in Poliomyelitis, New Engl. J. Med., 257:47, 1957.

——: Cardiovascular Disturbances in Poliomyelitis, Circulation, 15:735, 1957.

217 RABIES
Robert R. Wagner

DEFINITION. Rabies (hydrophobia, lyssa) is a fatal viral infection of the nervous system transmitted in saliva of rabid animals.

HISTORY. Some of the earliest extant writings contain suggestive references to mad dogs. Aristotle (*c.* 335 B.C.) described the transmission of rabies from dogs to other animals, and Celsus (*c.* A.D. 100) recognized that hydrophobia in man was caused by the bite of a rabid dog. The prevalence of the disease in man increased markedly in the eighteenth century following a European epizootic of canine rabies. The first effective control measures were instituted in Scandinavia, resulting in elimination of the disease there by 1826. Galtier's report in 1879 of transmission of rabies to laboratory rabbits led to the classical studies by Pasteur and his associates of "fixed" virus for vaccine production. Histologic diagnosis of infection became possible after Negri in 1903 described the characteristic cellular inclusion bodies of the disease.

ETIOLOGY. Rabies is a complex, cylindrical, RNA-containing virus that has been tentatively assigned to the rhabdovirus group along with the virus of vesicular stomatitis. Rabies virus is infectious for nervous tissue of all warm-blooded animals and can also be grown in tissue culture and chick embryos. The term *street virus* is used to designate the agent of the naturally occurring disease. *Fixed viruses* are rapidly multiplying strains used in vaccine production which have lost their infectivity for salivary gland tissue after passage in laboratory animals. There is only one antigenic type of the virus.

EPIDEMIOLOGY. All mammals are potential vectors, but carnivores are responsible for most cases in man and animals. Virus is present in saliva for several days before symptoms develop and persists until the time of death. Rabies is usually contracted from bites, occasionally from scratches or abrasions contaminated with infected saliva, or rarely by penetration of mucous membranes. Although dogs were formerly the principal cause of human rabies in the United States, wild animals now constitute a more important source of infection. The usual form of the disease in dogs, called *furious rabies*, is characterized by progressive agitation, aimless wandering, difficulty in swallowing, frothing at the mouth, labored respirations,

feeble bark, ataxia, convulsions, and vicious, indiscriminate attacks on all creatures and inanimate objects. Paralysis and stupor usually develop 2 to 3 days before death and are the sole manifestations (*dumb rabies*) in about one-fifth of infected dogs.

Although quarantine, killing of stray animals, and vaccination are effective in controlling canine rabies, large reservoirs of infection exist in wild animals, such as the wolf in Eastern Europe and Western Asia, the jackal in India and North Africa, and the mongoose in South Africa. During 1964, an epizootic of rabies in foxes was prevalent in Tennessee and adjacent states, where enzootic foci still exist, and the disease is also found in skunks, raccoons, coyotes, squirrels, bobcats, mountain lions, and other animals throughout the world. Vigorous control measures have eliminated all foci of rabies in domestic and wild animals of Scandinavia and the British Isles and prevented importation of the disease into Hawaii and Australia.

The vampire bat transmits a paralytic form of the disease to cattle and horses and constitutes an important reservoir of rabies in South and Central America, Mexico, and the West Indies. Vampire bats are occasionally nocturnal predators of man, attacking silently to take their blood meal without the sleeping victim's knowledge. Human rabies acquired from bites of common bats was first recognized in the United States in 1951 to 1953, and subsequent surveys have revealed that the disease occurs in many insectivorous and herbivorous species.

Rabies is almost invariably a rapidly fatal infection in all mammals except vampire and insectivorous bats, which can continue to transmit the disease for many months. Abortive infection with subsequent immunity can be produced experimentally in mice.

PATHOGENESIS. Rabies virus spreads from the site of inoculation along sensory nerve pathways to the posterior columns of the spinal cord, if the bite is on the extremities or trunk, or by cranial nerves to the brain stem from face wounds. The salivary glands, intestine, pancreas, renal tubules, and adrenal medulla are involved by extension along the autonomic nerves. Viremia may occur. Focal inflammation, neuronophagia, demyelinization, hemorrhages, and perivascular infiltration by mononuclear cells occur throughout the nervous system, but these changes are most marked in the basal ganglia, subcortical areas, and spinal cord. Rabies can be distinguished from other viral encephalitides if the pathognomonic Negri bodies are found. These are eosinophilic inclusion bodies, 0.5 to 10 μ in diameter, demonstrable in the cytoplasm of nerve cells by special stains. In all animals, including man, they are found in greatest abundance in Ammon's horn of the hippocampus and to a lesser extent in pyramidal cells of the cerebral cortex, Purkinje cells of the cerebellum, and nuclei of the basal ganglions.

MANIFESTATIONS. The *incidence* of rabies in unvaccinated individuals bitten by rabid animals is about 15 percent, but varies from 5 to 70 percent, depending on the amount of virus in the saliva and the location and depth of the wounds. It may be difficult to obtain a history of animal exposure if the disease is acquired from minor bites or scratches. The *incubation period* is usually 30 to 70 days but can be as short as 10 days or, rarely, more than a year. Short incubation periods occur after face or arm bites, multiple wounds, or wolf bites. Prodromal symptoms of fever with temperatures of 100 to 102°F, headache, malaise, nausea, vomiting, sore throat, and persistent loose cough are often present for 1 to 4 days. The most significant early manifestations, in about 80 percent of cases, are tingling, paresthesias, and dull or stabbing pain at the site of the bite, often radiating to the hip, shoulder, or neck, and to distal parts of the involved extremity. The wound may be inflamed and excoriated by the patient's scratching. The first, or *excitement*, phase of the disease is characterized by increasing agitation, marked restlessness, excessive motor activity, aimless pacing, dysarthria, and occasionally, visual or auditory hallucinations. Episodes of unreasoning fear and rage alternate with profound depression. The patient may become destructive, wildly apprehensive, and combative if restrained but usually does not attack his attendants. Spasmodic gross muscle contractions and generalized clonic or tonic convulsions with opisthotonos develop shortly after the onset, often precipitated by loud noises, bright lights, touch, or even drafts. Respirations become shallow and irregular, the pulse becomes rapid and thready, and the temperature usually exceeds 103°F. There may be involvement of the autonomic nervous system manifested by dilated, irregular pupils, excessive lacrimation, sweating, and salivation. Many patients also exhibit vertigo, nystagmus, optic neuritis with central blindness, diplopia, strabismus, or facial palsy. Paralysis of the vocal cords results in hoarseness or aphonia. Hyperactive deep tendon reflexes, Babinski signs, and nuchal rigidity are often present.

The most characteristic feature of the disease is severe, painful *contractions of the pharyngeal muscles*, initially precipitated by attempts to swallow fluids. This usually develops 1 to 3 days after onset and progresses until the mere sight, sound, mention, or even thought of water causes reflex spasms of the muscles of deglutition and respiration, leading to bouts of apnea, cyanosis, and generalized convulsions. Most patients manifest a *fear of water (hydrophobia)* and to avoid swallowing allow frothy saliva to drool from the mouth. Death usually follows a generalized convulsion with prolonged apnea.

Patients who survive the excitement stage of the disease develop *generalized flaccid paralysis*, often evident at first in the bitten extremity. Muscle spasms and pharyngeal contractions cease, and agitation gives way to depression, apathy, hyporeflexia, and coma. The ability to swallow may return temporarily, and there is often transient slowing of the pulse and respirations. The bladder usually becomes atonic. Generalized paralysis, resembling the Guillain-Barré syndrome, is occasionally the only neurologic manifestation. Rabies acquired from vampire bats, which frequently bite the toes, usually takes the form of Landry's ascending paralysis without excitation or pharyngeal spasm. Death usually occurs 2 to 3 days after onset of paralytic rabies but may be delayed for several weeks.

LABORATORY FINDINGS. The blood leukocyte count may be elevated, occasionally to 30,000 cells per cu mm, with an increased number of polymorphonuclear and large mononuclear cells. Glycosuria, acetonuria, proteinuria, and oliguria are present in most cases. The cerebrospinal fluid is usually normal but may contain slightly increased amounts of protein and as many as 100 mononuclear cells per cu mm. Virus may be present in saliva or, rarely, in cerebrospinal fluid. Serum antibodies can be determined by neutralization or complement fixation tests, but serologic studies are of little value for retrospective diagnosis, because almost all surviving patients have received vaccine or immune serum. Definitive diagnosis is usually made at autopsy by demonstrating Negri bodies or by isolation of rabies virus from the brain. The histochemical technique of staining brain or parotid tissue with fluorescent antibody has proved to be an accurate and rapid method of diagnosis.

DIFFERENTIAL DIAGNOSIS. *Hysterical reactions* to dog bites and *allergic encephalomyelitis caused by rabies* vaccine are sometimes difficult at first to differentiate from rabies. Paralytic rabies may be confused with poliomyelitis or the *Guillain-Barré syndrome*, particularly when a history of animal bite cannot be obtained or the incubation period exceeds 3 months. Many of the manifestations of *tetanus*, except trismus, resemble those of rabies. *Delirium tremens* and *intoxication with belladonna alkaloids* occasionally simulate rabies.

TREATMENT. There are about 5,000 cases of rabies in animals reported annually in the United States. The incidence of recognized cases in man has declined from 56 in 1946 to a single case in 1963. However, approximately 50,000 persons each year are considered to be exposed to rabies and receive vaccine treatment. The basic principle in the treatment of individuals exposed to rabies is to furnish sufficient antibody to prevent the virus from involving the central nervous system. Semple's vaccine, prepared from fixed virus grown in rabbit brain and inactivated with phenol, was formerly used for this purpose in the United States.

A vaccine prepared in duck embryos, and free of brain tissue, is now recommended for human use in the United States. A course of 14 daily inoculations is usually given to an individual exposed to rabies. Prophylactic immunization is best accomplished in dogs and other domestic animals by injection of a single dose of live, attenuated virus of the Flury strain. Passive immunization with antirabies horse serum, used as an adjunct to vaccination, appears to afford enhanced resistance to infection, particularly in heavily exposed individuals. The local treatment of bites consists of thorough cleaning with strong soap or detergent solutions and infiltration of the area with immune serum. Cauterization or debridement of the wound is no longer recommended.

The chief hazards of Semple's vaccine are *hypersensitivity reactions* with severe local erythema, often accompanied by fever and arthralgia, in about 5 percent of cases and *peripheral neuritis* or *allergic encephalomyelitis* caused by the rabbit brain tissue in 1 of 600 to 10,000 vaccinated individuals. Encephalomyelitis usually occurs

1 to 3 weeks after the first injection of vaccine and is characterized by the sudden onset of chills, fever, headache, and vomiting, followed by disorientation, dysarthria, ataxia, paresthesias, cranial nerve palsies, visual disturbances, and, frequently, hemiparesis or paraplegia. Increased concentrations of protein in the cerebrospinal fluid and mononuclear pleocytosis are noted in the majority of cases. The mortality rate varies from 0 to 25 percent, and about one-third of patients who recover from allergic encephalomyelitis have residual neurologic disorders.

The decision to proceed with antirabies treatment must depend on the risk of exposure in individual cases. Sudden, unprovoked attacks by any animals are rare and should be considered presumptive evidence of exposure to rabies.

Vaccine should be administered promptly if a person is bitten by an animal that escapes, is clinically rabid, or shows histologic evidence of infection. However, Negri bodies are not demonstrable in 12 percent of animals with rabies proved by virus isolation. Healthy dogs or cats that inflict minor bites or scratches contaminated with saliva should be impounded and observed for 7 days. No treatment is required if the animal remains healthy. Immune serum should be administered within 24 hr to all individuals who incur severe or multiple bites, regardless of whether the animal shows signs of rabies at the time. Every bat bite should be considered to be an exposure to rabies.

Prophylactic vaccination is advisable for a small, but selected, "high-risk" segment of the population of the United States, including veterinarians, spelunkers, dog catchers, and postmen. After a primary course of duck embryo vaccine, a single booster injection induces a prompt antibody response. Semple rabbit-brain vaccine should not be used for repeated revaccination because of the increased risk of allergic encephalomyelitis in individuals sensitized to rabbit brain tissue.

No specific treatment is available if clinical manifestations develop. The patient should be kept in a quiet, darkened, draftless room and disturbed as little as possible. Large doses of barbiturates are more effective than opiates in lessening anxiety, delirium, and the frequency of pharyngeal spasms and convulsions. Parenteral administration of fluids is often required.

PROGNOSIS. Thus far, rabies has been an invariably fatal disease in man. However, every patient should receive all possible supportive treatment in the hope that the diagnosis is in error.

REFERENCES

Applebaum, E., M. Greenberg, and J. Nelson: Neurological Complications Following Antirabies Vaccination, J.A.M.A., 151:188, 1953.

Gibbs, F. A., et al.: Comparison of Rabies Vaccines Grown on Duck Embryo and on Nervous Tissue, New Engl. J. Med., 265:1002, 1961.

Hildreth, E. A.: Prevention of Rabies, or the Decline of Sirius, Ann. Intern. Med., 58:883, 1963.

Hummeler, K., H. Koprowski, and T. J. Wiktor: Structure and Development of Rabies Virus in Tissue Culture, J. Virol., 1:152, 1967.

Johnson, H. N.: Rabies Virus, pp. 814–840 in "Viral and Rickettsial Infections of Man," 4th ed., F. L. Horsfall and I. Tamm (Eds.), Philadelphia, J. B. Lippincott Company, 1965.

Koprowski, H.: Rabies. Pediat. Clin. N. Am., 2:55, 1955.

Roueché, B.: The Incurable Wound, pp. 36–67 in "The Incurable Wound and Further Narratives of Medical Detection," Boston, Little, Brown and Company, 1958.

Sulkin, S. E.: The Bat as a Reservoir of Viruses in Nature. Progr. Med. Virol., 4:157, 1962.

218 VIRAL ENCEPHALITIS
Jay P. Sanford

DEFINITION. The clinical picture of encephalitis (fever, neurologic signs indicating cerebral involvement, i.e., alterations in cerebration, seizures, cranial nerve weakness, meningeal irritation, and pleocytosis in the cerebrospinal fluid) can result from cerebral damage due to a large number of infections as well as noninfectious causes. Of the more than 3,000 patients reported with encephalitis during 1966, 34 percent were classified as postinfectious. This is a broad category which includes mumps, measles, varicella, herpes, influenza, and rubella. An enteroviral etiology (poliovirus, Coxsackie virus, and ECHO virus) was considered in approximately 4 percent, while 14 percent were due to arboviruses. In the remaining 48 percent, the etiology was not determined. Four arboviruses are presently recognized as numerically important causes of encephalitis in the United States: St. Louis encephalitis virus, Eastern equine encephalitis virus, Western equine encephalitis virus, and the California encephalitis group of viruses. With few exceptions, for the last 12 years in the United States, St. Louis encephalitis virus has been the most common cause of arboviral encephalitis in humans.

Encephalitis lethargica, or Von Economo's disease, and subacute inclusion encephalitis, diseases of presumed but not unequivocally proved viral etiology, are described in Chap. 361.

ETIOLOGY. Despite the diversity of specific viral etiologies (Table 218-1), in individual patients, the clinical manifestations of encephalitis are very similar, and preclude an etiologic diagnosis without ancillary information regarding epidemiologic and serologic features. The clinical picture for the broad entity of arbovirus encephalitis will be discussed, then the specific epidemiologic and prognostic features which characterize the major types will be presented.

CLINICAL MANIFESTATIONS. The clinical features of arbovirus encephalitis differ among age groups. In infants under one year of age, the only consistently noted symptoms are sudden onset of fever which is often accompanied by convulsions. Convulsions may be either generalized or focal. Typically the fever ranges between

Table 218-1. SUMMARY OF VIROLOGIC AND EPIDEMIOLOGIC FEATURES OF ARBOVIRUSES ASSOCIATED WITH CENTRAL NERVOUS SYSTEM INVOLVEMENT IN MAN

Virus	Serologic group	Vector	Known geographic range of infection
Eastern equine encephalitis.........	A	Mosquito	Eastern Canada, United States, Mexico, Dominican Republic, Jamaica, Panama, Trinidad, Brazil, Colombia, Argentina
Western equine encephalitis.........	A	Mosquito	Canada, United States, Mexico, Brazil, Argentina
Venezuelan equine encephalitis......	A	Mosquito	Florida, Mexico, Panama, Colombia, Venezuela, Trinidad, Brazil, Ecuador
Central European encephalitis.......	B	Tick	Central and Eastern Europe
Diphasic meningoencephalitis.......	B	Tick	Central and Eastern Europe
Ilheus....................	B	Mosquito	Northern South America, Trinidad, Central America, Florida
Japanese encephalitis..............	B	Mosquito	Japan, China, Malaya, Taiwan, Thailand, Vietnam, Burma, Guam, Philippines, Korea, Australia, New Zealand
Kyasanur Forest disease............	B	Tick	India
Louping ill.......................	B	Tick	Great Britain, Eire
Medoc.........................	B		United States
Murray Valley encephalitis..........	B	Mosquito	Australia, New Guinea
Negishi.........................	B	?	Japan
Powassan.......................	B	Tick	Canada
Russian spring-summer encephalitis..	B	Tick	U.S.S.R.
St. Louis encephalitis..............	B	Mosquito	United States, Caribbean Islands, Panama, Brazil, Argentina
West Nile.......................	B	Mosquito	South and West Africa, Rhone Delta, Near East, Israel, India, Malaysia, Borneo
California encephalitis.............	California complex	Mosquito	United States
Phlebotomus, Naples..............	Phlebotomus	Sandfly	Italy, Egypt, Iran, West Pakistan

SOURCE: Adapted from the World Health Organization Technical Report Series, 1961, p. 219.

102 and 104°F. Other physical findings may include tenderness of the fontanelle, rigidity of the extremities, and abnormalities in reflexes.

In children between five and fourteen years of age, subjective symptoms are more easily elicited. Headache, fever, and drowsiness of 2 to 3 days' duration before seeking medical attention are common. The symptoms may then subside or become more intense and may be associated with nausea, vomiting, muscular pain, photophobia, and less frequently, convulsions (less than 10 percent). On examination, the child is acutely ill, febrile, and lethargic. Nuchal rigidity and intention tremors are often present and on occasion, muscular weakness can be demonstrated.

In adults, the initial symptoms commonly include the fairly abrupt onset of fever, nausea with vomiting, and severe headache. The headache is most often frontal but may be occipital or diffuse in location. Mental aberrations, represented by confusion and disorientation, usually appear within the subsequent 24 hr. Other symptoms may include diffuse myalgia and photophobia. The abnormalities on physical examination predominantly relate to the neurologic examination, although conjunctival suffusion is frequently seen and skin rashes may occur. Disturbances in mentation are among the most outstanding clinical features. These range from coma through severe disorien-

tation to subtle abnormalities detected only by cerebral function tests such as the subtraction of serial sevens. A small proportion of patients show only lethargy, lying quietly, apparently asleep unless stimulated. Tremor is common and is observed more frequently in individuals over forty years of age. The tremors vary in location and may be continuous or intention in type. Cranial nerve abnormalities resulting in oculomotor muscle paresis and nystagmus, facial weakness, and difficulty in deglutition may occur, and are usually present within the initial several days. Objective sensory changes are unusual. Hemiparesis or monoparesis may occur. Reflex abnormalities are also common; these include exaggerated palmomental reflexes, and suck and snout reflexes. Superficial abdominal and cremasteric reflexes are usually absent. Changes in the tendon reflexes are variable and inconstant. The plantar response may be extensor and fluctuates almost hourly. Dysdiadochokinesia often exists.

The duration of the fever and neurologic symptoms and signs can vary from several days to a month but usually ranges from 4 to 14 days. Clinical improvement generally follows the subsidence of the fever within several days unless irreversible anatomic changes have occurred.

LABORATORY DATA. Erythrocyte values are usually normal. Total leukocyte counts often reveal both a slight to moderate leukocytosis (occasionally greater than 20,000 per cu mm) and neutrophilia. Examination of the cerebrospinal fluid usually reveals several hundred cells per cu mm, but on occasion cloudy cerebrospinal fluid with cells in excess of 1,000 per cu mm may be seen. Within the first several days of illness, polymorphonuclear neutrophiles may predominate. The initial cerebrospinal fluid protein is often slightly elevated but may exceed 100 mg per 100 ml on occasion. The level of spinal fluid sugar is normal; a significant decrease should raise serious consideration of an alternative diagnosis. As the illness progresses, mononuclear cells in the cerebrospinal fluid tend to increase so that they predominate and the protein concentration may increase. Other laboratory studies have been performed only sporadically, but abnormalities may include hyponatremia, often due to the inappropriate secretion of antidiuretic hormone, and elevations in serum creatine phosphokinase.

DIAGNOSIS. Specific diagnosis requires the isolation of the virus or detection of antibodies with a rising titer between the acute phase of disease and convalescence. Antibodies can be detected by hemagglutination inhibition, complement fixation, or virus neutralization techniques.

TREATMENT. Treatment is entirely supportive and requires meticulous attention in the comatose patient.

EASTERN EQUINE ENCEPHALITIS

Eastern equine encephalitis, a Group A arbovirus, was first isolated in 1933 from the brain tissue of horses during an outbreak of equine illness in New Jersey. The first recognized human outbreak occurred in Massachusetts in 1938.

EPIDEMIOLOGY. The virus is distributed along the eastern coast of the Americas from northeastern United States to Argentina. Viral isolations also have been reported in the Philippines, Thailand, Czechoslovakia, Poland, and the USSR, but the question of type specificity has not been resolved. In the northeastern United States, epidemics occur in the late summer and early fall. Epizootics in horses precede the occurrence of human cases by 1 to 2 weeks. The disease affects mainly infants, children, and adults over fifty-five years of age. There is no sex preponderance. Inapparent infection occurs in all age groups, suggesting that the decreased likelihood of developing overt infection in the fifteen to fifty-four-year age group is not the result of decreased exposure. The ratio of inapparent infection to overt encephalitis approximates 25 to 1.

The natural reservoir is unknown. Isolations have been made from numerous species of wild birds and also from amphibians, reptiles, and mammals. The natural vector is the mosquito, including *Aëdes sollicitans* and *Culiseta melanura*. *Aëdes sollicitans*, a salt-marsh mosquito which is an avid human feeder, has been postulated as the epidemic vector, while *Culiseta melanura* is important in bird-to-bird transmission. Equine animals and man are probably "dead ends" in the transmission cycle, and infection in them is accidental.

PATHOLOGY. An outstanding feature is the predominance of neutrophilic leukocytes in the infiltrates. Foci of

tissue damage represented by rarefaction necrosis are common. Neuronolysis also is very common. Large perivascular collections of neutrophiles and activated histiocytes are frequently detected in the white matter of the cortex. Other sites of predilection are the thalamus, putamen, substantia nigra, and pons.

CLINICAL MANIFESTATIONS. While human infections have been thought usually to result in serious, if not fatal, central-nervous-system involvement, the detection of inapparent infection as well as relatively mild disease establishes the occurrence of milder forms. In many patients, the cerebrospinal fluid is cloudy and contains in excess of 1,000 cells per cu mm.

DIAGNOSIS. The hemagglutination-inhibition or neutralization tests are the serologic methods of choice. The complement fixation test may be negative in patients with confirmed infections.

PROGNOSIS. The mortality in clinical infection exceeds 50 percent. In the most severe cases, death occurs between the third and fifth days. Children under ten years of age have a greater likelihood of surviving the acute illness, but also have a greater likelihood of developing severe disabling residuals: mental retardation, convulsions, emotional lability, blindness, deafness, speech disorders, and hemiplegia.

WESTERN EQUINE ENCEPHALITIS

The virus of this disease is a Group A arbovirus and was isolated in 1930 in California from horses with encephalitis. In 1938 it was recovered from a fatal human infection.

EPIDEMIOLOGY. Western equine encephalitis virus has been isolated in the United States, Canada, Brazil, British Guiana, and Argentina. Human disease has been diagnosed only in the United States, Canada, and Brazil. In the United States, the virus is found in virtually all geographic areas. The central valley of California represents an important endemic area. The disease occurs mainly in early and midsummer. Wild birds, which develop viremia of sufficiently high titer to infect mosquitoes on feeding, are the basic reservoir, although nonavian vertebrate hosts may be important. Both laboratory and field observations point to the importance of *Culex tarsalis* as the principal vector in the western United States. In areas east of the Appalachian Mountains, another vector must be operative. The virus has been repeatedly isolated from *Culiseta melanura;* however, the importance of this mosquito has been questioned, since it is not primarily a man-biting mosquito. The ratio of inapparent infection as evidenced by serologic survey studies and disease varies from 58 to 1 in children to 1,150 to 1 in adults. Approximately one-fourth of patients are less than one year of age. The highest attack rates occur in individuals fifty years or older.

PATHOLOGY. The outstanding feature is the presence of many foci of rarefaction necrosis, which are most numerous in the striatum, then the globus pallidus, cerebral cortex, thalamus, and pointine tegmentum. A number of foci contain neutrophiles and resemble "abscesses."

Perivascular collections of lymphocytes and ameboid cells are common. Occasional chronic cases have been characterized by severe cystic transformation in the basal ganglia, cerebral white matter, and cerebral cortex.

PROGNOSIS. The fatality rate approximates 2 to 3 percent in laboratory confirmed cases. The incidence and severity of sequelae are related to age. Sequelae among very young infants are frequent and severe (61 percent in a group of patients less than three months old) and consist of upper motor neurone impairment, involving the pyramidal tracts, extrapyramidal structures, and cerebellum and result in behavioral problems and convulsions. Both the incidence and severity of sequelae diminish rapidly after one year of age. Adults may complain of nervousness, irritability, easy fatigability, and tremulousness for 6 months or longer after the acute illness. Probably not more than 5 percent of adults have sequelae which are sufficiently severe to be of practical significance. Postencephalitic seizures are rare.

VENEZUELAN EQUINE ENCEPHALITIS

Venezuelan equine encephalitis virus was first reported in 1938 following studies of an epizootic disease in horses, donkeys, and mules in Venezuela known as "crazy plague."

EPIDEMIOLOGY. Disease has been confirmed in man by virus isolation in Venezuela, Colombia, and Panama. Serologic evidence of infection has also been found in persons in Trinidad, Ecuador, and Florida. The natural transmission cycle of the virus is unknown. The virus has been isolated from a variety of mosquito species, including *Aëdes taeniorhynchus* and *Aëdes escapularis,* and also from wild rodents. While several species of wild birds develop an asymptomatic viremia after experimental exposure, the role of wild birds as a reservoir is not clear. Studies on birds in Venezuela have failed to demonstrate either virus or antibodies, while in Colombia several species of wild birds have been shown to possess VEE antibodies, and the virus has been isolated from birds in Panama. During the initial 3 days of illness, viremia has been detected in approximately two-thirds of patients. The levels of viremia are sufficiently high so that man also could serve as a reservoir. VEE virus also can be isolated by pharyngeal swab in a few patients, suggesting the potential for person-to-person transmission. The available observations make it reasonable to consider that the natural vector is a mosquito, although natural infection can probably take place without an arthropod vector. Laboratory infections have occurred and are probably due to inhalation of aerosols.

PATHOLOGY. In the liver, there is focal necrosis of hepatic cells and prominence of the Kupffer's cells. The hepatic changes are similar to those in yellow fever and Bolivian hemorrhagic fever. Lymph nodes appear depleted and follicles are difficult to discern. The marked depletion of lymphoid tissues is compatible with experimental data. There may be slight turbidity of the leptomeninges with hyperemia and flattening of the cerebral convolutions. If death occurs within the first 2 days, there is swelling of vascular endothelium and transudation of fluid into Virchow-Robin spaces. Later findings include many foci of necrosis which are characterized by glitter cells and glial proliferation. The nuclei of the brainstem and surrounding tissue were most affected.

CLINICAL MANIFESTATIONS. In man, infection with Venezuelan equine encephalitis virus usually results in an acute febrile illness without neurologic complications. The illness is similar to dengue with fever of 1 to 4 days and delayed convalescence. In one case report, palatine petechiae were noted and the patient vomited "coffee grounds" material. Other hemorrhagic features were not described. In an epidemic in Venezuela in 1962, almost 16,000 cases of acute disease were evaluated; 38 percent were classified as encephalitis, but only 3 to 4 percent had severe neurologic abnormalities: convulsions, nystagmus, drowsiness, delirium, or meningitis. The mortality rate was estimated to be less than 0.5 percent, and nearly all deaths occurred in young children.

JAPANESE ENCEPHALITIS

The name Japanese B encephalitis was employed during an epidemic which occurred in 1924 to distinguish it from Von Economo's disease which was designated as type A encephalitis. The designation as Japanese B no longer seems useful, and the term Japanese encephalitis should be employed.

EPIDEMIOLOGY. Japanese encephalitis virus infection is known to occur in eastern Siberia, China, Korea, Taiwan, Japan, Malaya, Vietnam, Singapore, Guam, and India. In temperature climates, the disease shows a late summer, early fall seasonal incidence. In tropic climates there is no seasonal variation. The mosquito, *Culex tritaeniorhynchus,* is the major vector species. It is a rural mosquito which breeds in rice fields and preferentially bites large domestic animals, such as pigs, but also feeds on birds and man. Man is an accidental host in the transmission cycle. In several outbreaks, a higher incidence of cases has been reported in children than in adults.

PATHOLOGY. Japanese encephalitis is characterized by intense neuronophagia. Gliomesenchymal nodules are found in the cerebral cortex and the molecular and Purkinje cell layers of the cerebellum. In the thalamus and substantia nigra, foci of tissue breakdown are found. Perivascular infiltration adjacent to damaged nerve tissue occurs. Relatively severe involvement of the spinal cord also may occur.

CLINICAL MANIFESTATIONS. The occurrence of severe rigors at the onset has been noted in almost 90 percent of patients. Localized paresis is found more often than with other arboviral encephalitides, e.g., 31 percent, with predominantly upper extremity involvement. Weight loss has been very striking, averaging 26 lb in one report. The failure of the temperature to lyse, appearance of diaphoresis, tachypnea, and the accumulation of bronchial secretions are grave prognostic signs.

PROGNOSIS. The immediate mortality rate has varied from 7 percent to 33 percent or higher. The rate of occurrence of sequelae varies inversely with the fatality rate; in those series with high fatality rates (33 percent), sequelae occurred in 3 to 14 percent. In another series with a fatality rate of 7.4 percent, the sequelae rate was 32 percent. Sequelae consisted of neurologic or intellectual defects and psychiatric complaints.

ST. LOUIS ENCEPHALITIS

St. Louis encephalitis was first recognized as an entity during a major outbreak in St. Louis, Mo., and the surrounding area in 1933. St. Louis encephalitis is the most common type of arbovirus encephalitis in the United States.

EPIDEMIOLOGY. In the United States, epidemics of St. Louis encephalitis fall into two epidemiologic patterns. One pattern is found in the west, where mixed outbreaks of Western equine encephalitis and St. Louis encephalitis have occurred primarily in irrigated rural areas. The vector has been *Culex tarsalis*. The second pattern occurred in the original St. Louis outbreak and the numerous subsequent epidemics in the Midwest, New Jersey, and Florida. These outbreaks have been more urban in location and are characterized by a marked tendency for the development of encephalitis in older persons. In such urban-suburban epidemics, the epidemic vector has been mosquitoes of the *Culex pipiens-quinquefasciatus* complex with the exception of the Florida epidemic, in which *Culex nigripalpus* was incriminated. The presence of St. Louis virus outside of the United States has been proven by isolations in Trinidad, Panama, and Jamaica. However, except in Jamaica, no case of encephalitis due to this virus has been reported outside of the United States. The basic transmission cycle is that of wild bird-mosquito-wild bird. The mechanism by which the virus overwinters has not been defined. The disease in man usually appears in midsummer to early fall. There is no sex predominance. Man represents an accidental host and plays no role in the basic transmission cycle. Serologic studies following most urban epidemics indicate that infection rates are similar in all age groups, and the increasing age-specific attack rate for clinical encephalitis which is typical of urban St. Louis encephalitis is probably due to age differences in host susceptibility to overt disease rather than to a higher rate of infection.

PATHOLOGY. The basic lesions are small perivascular hemorrhages and cuffing by round cells. Nerve cell damage occurs in small clusters of cells in the gray matter. The lesions of St. Louis encephalitis predominate in the thalamus and substantia nigra, but the cerebral cortex may be slightly to moderately affected. There is usually little neuronophagia.

CLINICAL MANIFESTATIONS. Infection with St. Louis virus most commonly results in an inapparent infection. Of the patients with confirmed disease, approximately three-fourths have clinical encephalitis, while the remainder present with aseptic meningitis, febrile headaches, or nonspecific illness. Virtually all patients over forty years of age have encephalitic manifestations. Urinary frequency and dysuria have been symptoms in approximately 20 percent of patients despite sterile routine aerobic urine cultures. The basis for the urinary tract symptoms is not understood.

DIAGNOSIS. The occurrence of either encephalitis or aseptic meningitis as manifested by febrile illness with cerebrospinal fluid pleocytosis in the months of June through September in an adult, especially over thirty-five years of age, should raise the suspicion of St. Louis encephalitis. Because approximately 40 percent of patients with St. Louis encephalitis have antibodies detectable by hemagglutination inhibition at the onset of illness, acute serum for serologic studies should be submitted promptly to a competent laboratory.

PROGNOSIS. The case fatality ratio in the original St. Louis epidemic was 20 percent. In most subsequent outbreaks the mortality has varied from 2 to 12 percent. Subjective nervous complaints including nervousness, headaches, and easy fatigability and excitability appear to be the most common residuals. Late organic defects such as speech defects, difficulty in walking, and disturbances in vision were demonstrated in approximately 5 percent of patients 3 years following infection.

CALIFORNIA ENCEPHALITIS

A neurotropic virus which was named the California virus was isolated in 1943 and 1944 from three separate pools of mosquitoes in Kern County in the San Joaquin Valley of California. In 1945, serologic evidence of infection by this virus was demonstrated in three patients. Since 1963, a large number of isolations of what is now known to be the California group of viruses have been made. Cases of encephalitis and inapparent infection have been discovered, and the California group of viruses is now well established as a significant cause of encephalitis in the United States.

EPIDEMIOLOGY. The epidemiology has not been well elucidated. Infection has been demonstrated to occur in the Midwest, especially in Ohio, Indiana, and Wisconsin, as well as along the Eastern Seaboard. Birds do not appear to be an important host of the California viruses. Most of the potential host isolations have been from mammals. Virus has been isolated from *Aëdes triseriatus* mosquitoes. Some tick isolations also have been made. A basic transmission cycle involving small mammalian hosts and *Aëdes* species of mosquitoes has been suggested. Most of the illnesses have occurred in the late summer and early fall. One-half of the patients are children six years of age and younger. The home or recreational area of patients has been found to be in areas of high mosquito incidence.

DIAGNOSIS. Neutralizing and hemagglutination-inhibition antibodies are usually present a few days after the reported onset of disease. Complement fixing antibodies usually are detectable 10 to 12 days after the onset of illness.

PROGNOSIS. The case fatality ratio is low, and most patients recover. Follow-up studies have not been underway for sufficient time to evaluate sequelae; however, complaints of emotional lability, difficulty in learning in school, and personality problems have been frequent.

OTHER ARBOVIRUSES WITH CENTRAL-NERVOUS-SYSTEM INVOLVEMENT

There is a large group of additional arboviruses which have been associated with encephalitis or aseptic meningitis. Some of these agents are listed in the table. While the epidemiology of each of these agents differs, the general features are sufficiently similar to require laboratory support for their differentiation.

REFERENCES

Altman, R., M. Goldfield, and O. Sussman: The Impact of Vector-borne Viral Diseases in the Middle Atlantic States, Med. Clinics, No. Am., 51:661, 1967.

Briceno Rossi, A. L.: Rural Epidemic Encephalitis in Venezuela Caused by a Group A Arbovirus (VEE), Progr. Med. Virol., 9:176, 1967.

Casals, J., and D. H. Clarke: Arboviruses; Group A, p. 583 in "Viral and Rickettsial Infections of Man," 4th ed., F. L. Horsfall, Jr., and I. Tamm (Eds.), Philadelphia, J. B. Lippincott Co., 1965.

Cramblett, H. C., H. Stegmiller, and C. Spencer: California Encephalitis Virus Infections in Children. Clinical and Laboratory Studies, J.A.M.A., 198:108, 1966.

Dickerson, R. B., J. R. Newton, and J. E. Hansen: Diagnosis and Immediate Prognosis of Japanese B Encephalitis. Observations Based on More Than 200 Patients With Detailed Analysis of 65 Serologically Confirmed Cases, Am. J. Med., 12:277, 1952.

Feemster, R. F., and W. Haymaker: Eastern Equine Encephalitis, Neurology, 8:882, 1958.

Finley, K. H., W. A. Longshore, Jr., R. J. Palmer, R. E. Cook, and N. Riggs: Western Equine and St. Louis Encephalitis. Preliminary Report of a Clinical Follow-Up Study in California, Neurology, 5:223, 1955.

Johnson, K. M., A. Shelokov, P. H. Peralta, G. J. Dammin, and N. A. Young: Recovery of Venezuelan Equine Encephalomyelitis Virus in Panama, Am. J. Trop. Med. Hyg., 17:432, 1968.

Lennette, E. H., and H. Koprowski: Human Infection With Venezuelan Equine Encephalomyelitis Virus, J.A.M.A., 123:1088, 1943.

Luby, J. P., S. E. Sulkin, and J. P. Sanford: The Epidemiology of St. Louis Encephalitis (SLE): A Review, Ann. Rev. Med., 1969 (in press).

National Communicable Disease Center: Neurotropic Viral Diseases Surveillance, Encephalitis, Annual Encephalitis Summary, 1966, April 30, 1968.

Thompson, W. H., and S. L. Inhorn: Arthropod-borne California Group Viral Encephalitis in Wisconsin, Wis. Med. J., 66:250, 1967.

Weaver, O. M., S. Pieper, and R. Kurland: Japanese Encephalitis: Sequelae, Neurology, 8:887, 1958.

219 DISEASES CAUSED BY SLOW VIRUSES

Donald H. Harter

Slow virus diseases are characterized by a long asymptomatic period, often on the order of months or years, between the introduction of the infectious agent and the appearance of clinical illness.

The factors responsible for this protracted incubation period have not been defined. Viruses causing slow infections do not appear to have any unique or common features, and the slowness of the disease may be due in large measure to the manner in which the host reacts or accommodates to the virus.

Some slow viruses provoke a conventional inflammatory response during the time they are clinically silent; others are able to reside within cells for long periods without causing detectable cytopathic changes. The role of immunity in slow virus infection is largely unknown. One possibility is that the agent is kept in check by the host's immunologic defenses during the long incubation period and that disease occurs when these defenses fail.

In animals, slow viruses are known to produce a variety of pulmonary, hepatic, renal, and neurologic disorders. At present, there are only three definitely identified slow virus infections of man. These are three infrequently encountered neurologic diseases: kuru, progressive multifocal leukoencephalopathy, and subacute sclerosing panencephalitis. Of these three, only kuru has been shown to be caused by a slow virus; in the other two a "viruslike" particle or viral component have been identified, but it has not been transmitted to experimental animals.

KURU

Kuru, or "trembling with fear," is a progressive and fatal neurologic disorder which occurs exclusively among natives of the New Guinea Highland.

Difficulty in walking is usually the first sign of kuru. This usually progresses from a minor disturbance in gait rhythm to marked side to side lurching and staggering. Eventually ambulation becomes incoordinated and the patient is unable to use his limbs. As the disease progresses, cerebellar involvement (intention tremor, inability to perform rapid alternating movements, slurring of speech, hypotonia), abnormal involuntary movements resembling myoclonus, athetosis, or chorea, and convergent strabismus appear. Dementia develops in the later phases of the disease. The illness terminates fatally in 4 to 24 months, usually from decubitus ulcers or bronchopneumonia. Approximately 80 percent of adults afflicted with the disease are women.

Pathologic changes are limited to the central nervous system and include widespread neuronal loss, intense astrocytic and microglial proliferation, loss of myelinated fibers, and the presence of plaquelike bodies. Perivascular cuffing by lymphocytes and mononuclear cells has been observed occasionally.

It was the close similarity between the neuropathologic and clinical findings found in kuru and in *scrapie*, a slow infectious disease of sheep, that suggested the possibility that kuru was caused by a virus or other infectious agent. The infectious origin of kuru was confirmed subsequently by the appearance of a kurulike syndrome in chimpanzees 18 to 21 months after intracerebral inoculation of suspensions of brain from human cases. Furthermore, the kuru syndrome has been transmitted from chimpanzee to chimpanzee by intracerebral passage with shortening of the incubation period to 12 months. The chimpanzee has been the only animal found to be susceptible to experimental kuru. Although a number of known and novel viruses have been recovered from tissue explants prepared from chimpanzees with the kuru syndrome, the specific agent responsible for the disease has not yet been characterized.

Cannibalism has been considered as a possible mode to transmission of kuru. Native custom in the New Guinea dictates that marrow, viscera, and brain be cooked and eaten. The marked predilection of kuru for the adult female may be explained by the observation that cannibalism appears more prevalent among women and that males who practice cannibalism seldom eat the bodies of women. The recent influx of foreign settlers into the kuru area has led to increasing rejection of cannibalistic practices and this, in turn, may be responsible for the progressive decline in the number of cases of kuru since 1960.

PROGRESSIVE MULTIFOCAL LEUKOENCEPHALOPATHY

This rare neurologic condition first described in 1958 usually occurs in patients who have lymphomas, carcinomatosis, or sarcoidosis.

The disease affects adults of both sexes and its duration from onset of symptoms to death is 3 or 4 months. The neurologic signs and symptoms show diffuse, asymmetrical involvement of the cerebral hemispheres. Hemiplegia, hemianopsia, aphasia or dysarthria, and organic mental changes are frequent, and incomplete or complete transverse myelitis may develop. Headache and convulsive seizures are rare, but electroencephalographic abnormalities consisting of diffuse slow-wave activity are often present.

The pathologic changes consist of multiple areas of demyelination with little or no perivascular infiltration. The presence of distinctive intranuclear inclusions in oligodendrocytes first suggested that the disease was of a viral etiology. Electron microscopic observations show the intranuclear inclusion bodies to be composed of closely packed spheres which have the physical dimensions and properties of members of the polyoma, SV 40 and K virus subgroup of the papova viruses. The papova group consists of several tumor-producing virus, including the human wart virus.

The disease has not been transmitted to animals.

It has been postulated that the patient's initial underlying illness so alters immunologic responsiveness that the virus is able to enter and multiply within the central nervous system. The demyelination which occurs may be related to virus-induced damage of oligodendroglia, cells which appear to be required for the normal maintenance of myelin.

SUBACUTE SCLEROSING PANENCEPHALITIS (Inclusion Body Encephalitis)

This progressively fatal disease of children and adolescents has been suspected to be of viral origin since its initial description by Dawson in 1932. Although recent findings have given further support to a viral etiology, infective virus has not yet been recovered from the brains of patients with the disease.

Subacute sclerosing panencephalitis occurs between four and twenty years of age; 80 percent of patients are under eleven. Onset is usually insidious, and mental deterioration, often expressed by a decline in the patient's school work, is the presenting symptom. Incoordination, ataxia, and myoclonic jerks develop along with abnormalities of the pyramidal and extrapyramidal motor systems. The patient becomes bedridden within 6 to 9 months. Death occurs from superimposed pulmonary or urinary tract infections or from decubiti. Neither fever nor signs of meningeal irritation occur. The cerebrospinal fluid gamma-globulin, as determined by electrophoresis, quantitative immunochemical assay, or colloidal gold curve is elevated, but the fluid is otherwise normal. The electroencephalogram typically shows a "burst suppression" pattern characterized by synchronous and symmetrical spike and high voltage slow wave activity. Brain biopsy may be required to make a definitive antemortem diagnosis.

There is no effective treatment for the disease.

Pathologic findings include round cell infiltration about small cerebral arteries and veins, intranuclear and intracytoplasmic inclusions in neurones and glial cells, and varying degrees of demyelination.

There is considerable evidence pointing to measles virus as the etiologic agent. The electron microscope shows the intranuclear inclusions to be composed of hollow tubular filaments resembling the internal nucleic acid component of members of the subgroup II myxoviruses. Staining of brain tissue from patients with the disease with fluorescent antibody demonstrates measles virus antigen in the inclusions. Furthermore, a significant number of patients with the disease have elevated serum levels of measles antibody and increases in measles antibody titers have been observed as the disease progresses. As a group, patients with inclusion body encephalitis have higher levels of measles antibody than are found during convalescence from measles.

Attempts to transmit the disease to animals have met with variable results, and reported failures outnumber reported successes.

Subacute sclerosing panencephalitis appears many years after the patient's initial experience with rubeola and may represent an unusual response of the nervous system to viral infection. It is possible that a viral carrier state becomes established within the nervous system wherein cells may continue to elaborate intracellular viral antigen without producing detectable amounts of mature infective virus. The implications of this concept for other diseases of the central nervous system such as parkinsonism or multiple sclerosis remains in the realm of speculation.

REFERENCES

Abinanti, F. R.: The Possible Role of Microorganisms and Viruses in the Etiology of Chronic Degenerative Diseases of Man, Ann. Rev. Microbiol., 21:467, 1967.

Conference on Measles Virus and Subacute Sclerosing Panencephalitis, J. L. Sever and W. Zeman (Eds.), Neurology, vol. 18, Part 2, 1968.

Gajdusek, D. C.: Slow-virus Infections of the Nervous System, New Engl. J. Med., 276:392, 1967.

Richardson, E. P.: Progressive Multifocal Leukoencephalopathy, New Engl. J. Med., 265:815, 1961.

Section 17

Diseases with Lesions of Skin or Mucous Membranes

220 MEASLES (Rubeola)

John C. Ribble

DEFINITION. Measles (the term derives from an Anglo-Saxon word for spot) is an acute febrile eruption which for centuries has been one of the most common diseases of civilized man. With the development of effective prophylactic measures it promises to become a rarity.

HISTORY. Measles probably did not exist before the building of large cities, inasmuch as perpetuation of the disease in present day isolated communities of less than 500,000 persons does not occur. Rhazes wrote about the disease in the tenth century, but indicated that it had been described as early as the first century by a Hebrew physician. Sydenham in the seventeenth century wrote a full account of the disease as he encountered it in England and differentiated it from other exanthems. In 1905 measles was transmitted by the blood of infected persons to human volunteers and in 1911 to monkeys by both blood and nasopharyngeal secretions that had previously been passed through bacteria-retaining filters. Enders and Peebles in 1954 obtained from patients with measles an agent that produced cytopathic changes in cell cultures. This achievement has allowed the investigation of the characteristics of the measles virus and the pathogenesis of the disease and its complications and has established means for the development of diagnostic and prophylactic measures.

ETIOLOGY. The measles virion is composed of a central core of ribonucleic acid with a helically arranged protein coat encased in a lipoprotein envelope with small spike-like structures. The virion is 1,200 to 2,500 Å in diameter, and in structure and size resembles some of the myxoviruses.

The measles virus is isolated most easily from infected persons utilizing primary cultures of monkey or human kidney, although primary isolations have been accomplished using human amnion or chorion or dog kidney. After several passages, the virus can be propagated on a number of stable cell lines of human origin, human leukocytes, and primary cultures from other animals, including chick embryo cells upon which many of the vaccine strains are grown.

Measles virus infection of cells in culture results in the formation of multinucleated giant cells, many with eosinophilic intranuclear, and intracytoplasmic inclusions. The number of infectious particles of measles virus can be determined by visible plaque formation in suitably prepared cell layers or by using immunofluorescence techniques.

EPIDEMIOLOGY. Measles occurs naturally only in human beings, although infection with the virus can be demonstrated in laboratory colonies of monkeys exposed to infected individuals. Before active immunization became widespread, epidemics of measles occurred every 2 or 3 years, with the result that about 95 percent of town and city dwellers developed the disease before the age of fifteen years. The virus is transmitted by transfer of nasopharyngeal secretions, either directly or in airborne droplets to the respiratory mucous membranes or conjunctivae of susceptible individuals. Persons infected with the virus may transmit the disease during a period which extends from 4 days before, until 5 days after skin lesions have appeared. Measles is a disease of childhood in populous areas, but may occur at any age in remote isolated communities if the disease is introduced. Infants are uncommonly affected under the age of six to eight months because of the persistence for this period of time of antibody acquired by transplacental transmission from the mother.

PATHOGENESIS AND PATHOLOGY. It is probable that after infection, measles virus multiplies in the epithelium of the respiratory tract and is disseminated by way of the blood to distant sites. For a few days before, and for 1 or 2 days after the rash appears, the virus can be isolated from blood or washed white cells, conjunctiva, lymphoid tissue, and respiratory mucous membranes and secretions. The virus can be obtained from urine for as long as 4 days after the onset of the eruption.

The skin and mucous membrane lesions (Koplik's spots) consist of vesicle formation and epithelial necrosis and may be due either to direct infection of these areas or, as suggested by Enders, to the action of complexes of measles antigen and antibody. Large multinucleated cells (Warthin-Finkeldy cells) are characteristic of measles virus infection and can be found in hyperplastic lymphoid tissues, respiratory epithelium and secretions, and in urine. An unusually high number of white cells from patients with the disease contain broken chromosomes. The epithelium of the respiratory passages may become necrotic and slough, leading to secondary bacterial infection; in addition, interstitial pneumonia with giant-cell infiltration may be observed. Changes in the brain of patients with encephalitis resemble those seen in other postviral encephalitides and consist of focal hemorrhage, congestion, and demyelinization.

MANIFESTATIONS. The time from exposure to the development of the first symptoms of measles infection is usually 9 to 11 days, and from exposure to the appearance of rash is about 2 weeks. The initial manifestations of the disease are malaise, irritability, fever as high as 105°F, conjunctivitis with excessive lacrimation, edema of the eyelids and photophobia, moderately severe hacking cough, and nasal discharge. Koplik's spots, small red irregular lesions with blue-white centers, appear one or two days before the onset of the rash on the mucous membranes of the mouth and occasionally on the conjunctiva or intestinal mucosa. The findings of the prodromal illness subside or disappear within 1 or 2 days after the outbreak of skin lesions, although the cough may persist throughout the course of the disease.

The red maculopapular rash of measles breaks out first on the forehead, spreads downward over the face, neck, and trunk and appears on the feet on the third day. The density of lesions is greatest on the forehead, face, and shoulders, where coalescence of individual spots usually occurs. The lesions in each area persist for about 3 days and disappear in the same order in which they appeared, resulting in total duration of rash of about 6 days. As the maculopapules fade, a brown discoloration of the skin may be noticed, and finely granular skin may be desquamated. In adults the duration of fever may be longer, the rash more prominent, and the incidence of complications higher.

The course of measles can be altered by the administration of gamma-globulin soon after exposure. The incubation period may be prolonged for as long as 20 days. The prodromal period of the modified disease may be shorter, the fever, respiratory symptoms, and conjunctivitis milder, and the rash less marked; Koplik's spots may not be present. An atypical, severe form of measles is seen in some persons who have received inactivated measles vaccine several years before exposure. The prodromal period with prominent fever, headache, myalgias,

and abdominal symptoms lasts for 2 to 3 days and is followed by an eruption of maculopapules, vesicles, and petechiae. In contrast to natural measles, the rash begins on the feet and progresses toward the head and is especially prominent on the legs and in body creases. Peripheral edema and pneumonia have been prevalent in this form of atypical measles.

COMPLICATIONS. Measles, usually a benign self-limited disease, may be associated with a number of complicating illnesses. Viral involvement of the respiratory tract may lead to croup, bronchitis, bronchiolitis, or rarely to interstitial pneumonia, which is seen most often in children suffering from a severe systemic disease such as leukemia, and which is characterized by severe respiratory symptoms, pulmonary infiltrations, and the presence in the lungs of giant cells. It may occur in the absence of the typical measles exanthem. Conjunctivitis, which is seen regularly in the course of uncomplicated measles, may occasionally progress to permanent corneal ulceration, keratitis, and blindness. Myocarditis characterized by transient changes in the electrocardiogram occurs in about 20 percent of patients with measles, but clinical evidence of cardiac dysfunction is rare. Viral involvement of the mesenteric lymph nodes and appendix may result in abdominal pain and signs of peritoneal inflammation so severe that surgical exploration is considered. The situation is especially confusing if the evidence of appendiceal involvement become manifest during the preeruptive phase of the disease. Measles infection of pregnant women results in death of the fetus in about 20 percent of the cases; however, a teratogenic effect such as that observed in rubella has not been demonstrated.

Superimposed bacterial pneumonia caused by streptococci, pneumococci, staphylococci, or *H. influenza* is considerably more common than giant-cell pneumonia and may progress to formation of empyema or lung abscess. Bacterial otitis media is a frequent sequela of measles infection in children. In tropical areas stomatitis, probably of bacterial etiology, progressing to cancrum oris may be encountered during the course of measles.

In addition to conditions associated with consequences of viral infection and the complications resulting from superimposed bacterial infection, there are several situations which may arise after measles infection which are of uncertain pathogenesis. Clinically apparent *encephalomyelitis* occurs in every 1 of 1,000 patients with measles. It begins 4 or 5 days after the appearance of the eruption and is characterized by return of high fever, headache, drowsiness, and coma, and in some patients by focal brain or spinal cord involvement. Death occurs in about 10 percent of affected individuals, and persistent signs of central nervous system damage including mental changes, epilepsy, and paralysis are encountered. Electroencephalographic abnormalities without other signs of CNS dysfunction may be demonstrated in 50 percent of patients with otherwise uncomplicated measles. There is no evidence that encephalomyelitis is due to direct invasion of the nervous system by measles virus, and it is postulated that the disease has an allergic origin. An extremely rare condition, *subacute sclerosing panencephalitis*, is now thought to be a late complication of measles. *Thrombocytopenia* may occur 3 to 15 days after the onset of the rash and results in purpura as well as bleeding from mouth, intestine, and genitourinary tract. Measles is associated with disappearance of delayed hypersensitivity to tuberculin, exacerbation of existing tuberculosis, and an increased incidence of new tuberculous infections.

LABORATORY FINDINGS. Leukopenia is frequent in the prodromal phase of measles, and the appearance of leukocytosis suggests bacterial superinfection or another complication. During the prodrome and in the early eruptive phase, Warthin-Finkeldy cells can be identified in stained preparations of sputum, nasal secretions, or urine, and the measles virus can be isolated by inoculation of the same materials into appropriate cell cultures. Complement fixation, neutralization, and hemagglutination-inhibition tests are available for serologic confirmation of measles. Spinal fluid of patients with encephalomyelitis may contain increased protein and 500 to 1,000 lymphocytes. Bacterial infection can be identified by appropriate cultures.

DIFFERENTIAL DIAGNOSIS. Measles with its prodrome, Koplik's spots, and characteristic rash, is infrequently confused with other diseases. Rubella is a shorter, milder disease with more prominent lymphadenopathy. Infectious mononucleosis and toxoplasmosis can be identified by the presence of atypical lymphocytes and by a serologic test respectively. Drug reactions and secondary syphilis may display skin lesions similar to the measles rash. The atypical form of measles in patients previously immunized with inactivated vaccine may suggest Rocky Mountain spotted fever.

PROPHYLAXIS. Measles can be prevented by the administration of 0.25 mg per kg gamma-globulin within 5 days of exposure. Passive immunization should be considered for any susceptible person exposed to the disease, but is especially important for children under three years of age, for pregnant women, for patients with tuberculosis, and for those patients in whom immune mechanisms are impaired. A modified, less severe form of the disease which results in some degree of active immunity may be observed if 0.05 mg per kg of gamma-globulin is given within 5 days of exposure (see Manifestations). Administration of antibiotics does not decrease the frequency or severity of bacterial superinfections.

Active immunity can be induced by the use of live attenuated measles virus without spread to contacts of vaccinated individuals. The administration of Edmonston strain vaccines, prepared either in chick embryo or dog kidney cells, frequently results in a febrile illness beginning about 6 days after vaccination, a mild rash, and occasionally respiratory symptoms and Koplik's spots. To modify these manifestations of disease, gamma-globulin, 0.01 mg per kg in a separate syringe and at a different site may be given concomitantly. A further attenuated vaccine (Schwarz) is associated with fewer manifestations of disease and is administered without gamma-globulin. Vaccination with these preparations induces antibody formation in more than 95 percent of susceptible individuals. The magnitude of serologic response following use of the Edmonston strain approximates that seen after natural measles and is slightly greater than that induced by the Schwarz vaccine or Edmonston strain vaccine plus gamma-globulin. Vaccination results in protection for at least 2 or 3 years, but the total duration of immunity is not known. Live measles vaccine should not be given to pregnant women, to those sensitive to egg proteins or dog dander, to patients with tuberculosis, to patients with leukemia or lymphoma, or to those who are receiving therapy which depresses immune response.

There is no indication for the use of inactivated vaccine because of severe atypical measles which has been observed in persons immunized with it (see Manifestations).

TREATMENT. No therapy is indicated for uncomplicated measles. Gamma-globulin, although effective in prophylaxis, is of no value once symptoms are evident. Bacterial infections should be treated with appropriate antibiotics (Chaps. 135, 138, 139, 140, and 152).

REFERENCES

Enders, J. F., and T. Peebles: Propagation in Tissue Cultures of Cytopathogenic Agents from Patients with Measles, Proc. Soc. Exp. Biol. Med., 86:277, 1954.

Fulginiti, V. A., J. Eller, A. Downie, and C. Kempe: Altered Reactivity to Measles Virus, Atypical Measles in Children Previously Immunized with Inactivated Measles Virus Vaccines, J.A.M.A., 202:1075, 1967.

Katz, S. L.: Measles, Its Complications, Treatment, and Prophylaxis, Med. Clinics N. Am., 46:1163.

Krugman, S., and R. Ward: Infectious Disease of Children, 3d ed., St. Louis, The C. V. Mosby Company, 1964.

Report of the Committee on the Control of Infectious Diseases, 15th ed., American Academy of Pediatrics, 1966.

221 RUBELLA (German Measles)
John C. Ribble

DEFINITION. Rubella, a febrile disease with rash and lymphadenopathy, is usually a benign condition, but when it occurs in pregnant women it may lead to infection and serious disorders of the fetus.

ETIOLOGY. In the late 1930s and 1940s rubella was transmitted to humans and monkeys, and in 1962 a viral agent was recovered in cell cultures inoculated with nasopharyngeal secretions of infected persons. Human primary amnion cells infected with rubella virus display rounding, clumping of nuclear chromatin, and eosinophilic intranuclear inclusions. Rubella virus can be detected indirectly in monkey kidney cells by the interference or exclusion method. In this system, cells infected with rubella appear normal, but are resistant to viruses such as ECHO 11 or Coxsackie A9 that ordinarily produce cytopathic effects in monkey kidney cells. Complement-fixing antigen, and a hemagglutinin active at 4°C against red cells from young chickens have been identified.

PATHOGENESIS AND PATHOLOGY. Rubella can be induced in susceptible persons by the instillation of infected materials into the nasopharynx, and natural infection is probably induced in the same way. Virus is present in blood, throat washings, and stools for several days before the exanthem becomes apparent. It can be detected in blood for 1 or 2 days, and in throat washings and stools for as long as 2 weeks after appearance of rash. Lymph nodes show edema, hyperplasia, and loss of follicles.

Congenital rubella results from transplacental transmission of virus to the fetus from an infected mother, and may be associated with growth retardation, infiltration of liver and spleen by hematopoietic tissue, interstitial pneumonia, decreased number of megakaryocytes in the bone marrow, and various structural malformations of the cardiovascular and central nervous systems. The virus may persist in the fetus during intrauterine life and for many months after birth.

EPIDEMIOLOGY. Rubella is less contagious than measles, and large-scale epidemics are not common. In 1964, however, more than 1,800,000 cases of rubella were reported in the United States. Immunity to rubella is considered to be lifelong, but indirect epidemiologic evidence has raised the possibility that second subclinical attacks may occur.

MANIFESTATIONS. The time from exposure to the appearance of the rash of rubella is 14 to 21 days, usually about 18 days. In adults there may be a prodromal illness preceding the exanthem by 1 to 7 days and consisting of malaise, headache, fever, mild conjunctivitis, and lymphadenopathy. In children the rash may be the first manifestation of disease. It is apparent from serologic studies that rubella infection may be associated with no signs or symptoms, or may result in lymph node enlargement without skin lesions; however, rash without lymphadenopathy is uncommon. Respiratory symptoms are mild or absent. Small red lesions (Forcheimer spots) occasionally may be seen on the soft palate, but are not pathognomonic of the disease.

The rash begins on the forehead and face and spreads downward to the trunk and extremities. The small pink, maculopapular lesions, of lighter hue than those of measles, are usually discrete but may coalesce to form a diffuse erythema suggestive of scarlet fever. The rash may last from 1 to 5 days, but is most commonly present for 3 days. Enlarged, tender lymph nodes appear before the rash, are most impressive during the early eruptive phase, and may persist several days after the rash has disappeared. Splenomegaly or generalized lymphadenopathy may occur, but the postauricular and suboccipital nodes are most strikingly involved. Arthralgias and slight joint swellings may be a complication of rubella, especially in young women. The pain and swelling, usually in the small joints, are most marked during the period of rash and may persist for several days after other manifestations of rubella have disappeared. Purpura with or without thrombocytopenia may occur and be associated with hemorrhage. Encephalomyelitis following rubella resembles other postinfectious encephalitides and is much less common than encephalitis following measles.

The syndrome of *congenital rubella* has conventionally been thought to consist of heart malformations—patent ductus arteriosus, interventricular septal defect, or pulmonic stenosis; eye lesions—corneal clouding, cataracts,

chorioretinitis, and microphthalmia; microcephaly, mental retardation, and deafness. In the American epidemic of 1964 thrombocytopenic purpura, hepatosplenomegaly, intrauterine growth retardation, interstitial pneumonia, and metaphyseal bone lesions were encountered frequently in association with the previously recognized manifestations, leading to the term *expanded rubella syndrome.* Any combination of lesions may be seen in an individual infant.

Congenital rubella is usually the result of maternal infection during the first trimester of pregnancy, although well documented cases have resulted from infection several days prior to conception; deafness may occur as a result of infection in the fourth month. In the 1964 epidemic, about 10 percent of women with clinically recognized rubella during the first trimester gave birth to infants with the rubella syndrome. Serologically identified, asymptomatic maternal rubella can also result in fetal disease. If exposure of a pregnant woman occurs in the first trimester, rubella antibody levels should be obtained immediately and 2 or 3 weeks later. The combination of determinations may allow the detection of seroconversion occurring in subclinical infection, aid in the diagnosis of rubella if an exanthematous disease develops, or suggest remote past infection and immunity to the disease.

DIAGNOSIS. Rubella is frequently confused with other mild diseases such as those described in Chap. 222, infectious mononucleosis (Chap. 255), or acquired toxoplasmosis (Chap. 244). A certain diagnosis of rubella can be made by virus isolation and identification, or by changes in antibody titers. Rubella antibodies may be present by the second day of rash and increase in quantity over the next 2 or 3 weeks. There are no other laboratory findings helpful in the diagnosis of rubella, although lymphocytosis with atypical lymphocytes may occur. Congenital rubella should be differentiated by appropriate serologic tests from congenital syphilis, toxoplasmosis, and cytomegalic inclusion virus disease.

PREVENTION. In adults and children rubella is usually a mild disease with infrequent complications. However, the severity of congenital infection has prompted efforts to prevent the disease. Administration of gamma-globulin to exposed persons can abort the clinical disease, but seroconversion and transmission of the disease from mother to fetus may occur despite the administration of large amounts of gamma-globulin soon after exposure.

Active immunization, as indicated by antibody response, and prevention of disease in exposed vaccinated persons has been accomplished by the administration of live attenuated rubella virus grown in monkey kidney cells. The attenuated virus is excreted in the nasopharyngeal secretion of vaccinees and the possibility of transmission to susceptible persons has led to caution in the widespread use of the vaccine. Despite the fact that rubella vaccine remains experimental, it is likely that it will be adapted to general use.

REFERENCES

Cooper, L. Z., J. Giles, and S. Krugman: Clinical Trial of Live Attenuated Rubella Virus Vaccine, Am. J. Dis. Child., 115:655, 1968.

Green, R. H., et al.: Studies of the Natural History and Prevention of Rubella, Am. J. Dis. Child., 110:348, 1965.

McCarthy, K., C. Taylor-Tobinson: Rubella, Brit. Med. Bull., 23:185, 1967.

Sever, J. L., et al.: Rubella Antibody Determinations, Pediatrics, 40:789, 1967.

——, K. Nelson, and M. Gilkeson: Rubella Epidemic, 1964. Effect on 6,000 Pregnancies, Am. J. Dis. Child., 110:395, 1965.

222 OTHER VIRAL EXANTHEMATOUS DISEASES

John C. Ribble

In addition to the diseases such as measles, rubella, and chickenpox which historically have been associated with prominent skin lesions, there are other virus infections in which skin manifestations may occur. A transient maculopapular eruption may be seen during the course of infectious mononucleosis, cytomegalic inclusion disease, cat-scratch fever, psittacosis, and illnesses caused by arboviruses. Exanthem subitum and erythema infectiosum are mild exanthematous diseases which have been recognized by their distinctive clinical features and which are presumably of viral origin. The study of epidemics using techniques of virus isolation has identified exanthematous diseases associated occasionally with adenovirus and reovirus infection, and more frequently with illnesses caused by enteroviruses.

EXANTHEM SUBITUM (Roseola infantum)

Exanthem subitum is a benign disease of infants six to twenty-four-months of age that is characterized by a high fever and rash. The disease can be transmitted to humans and monkeys by the transfer of blood obtained from a patient during the first few days of illness. The infectious agent is probably a virus, although it has not been isolated. The first manifestation of disease, after an incubation period of 10 days, is the abrupt onset of fever which lasts for 3 to 5 days and may be as high as 105°F. There may be mild pharyngitis, slight lymph node enlargement, and convulsions may occur during the height of the fever. On the fourth or fifth day of illness, there is a sudden drop in temperature to normal or below normal. Several hours after defervescence the rash suddenly and surprisingly appears. It is characterized by faint maculopapules over the neck and trunk and may extend to the thighs and buttocks; it may last for only a few hours or may be present for a day or two. Leukopenia is frequent during the febrile period. The disease is benign and not associated with complications, although occasionally an infant may show sequelae as a result of febrile convulsions.

ERYTHEMA INFECTIOSUM (Fifth Disease)

Erythema infectiosum is a mild febrile exanthematous disease without a prodrome. The incubation period is probably 5 to 10 days, but it has not been ascertained precisely. The first manifestations are low-grade fever and a bilaterally symmetrical rash, most prominent on the face but also found on the arms, legs, and trunk but not on the palms or soles. The rash is most marked on the cheeks, giving a "slapped face" appearance. The lesions are maculopapular and tend to be confluent, forming slightly raised blotchy areas and reticular or lacy patterns. The rash usually lasts about a week, and during this time it may disappear, only to reappear in the same areas a few hours later. The waxing and waning eruption may occasionally persist for several weeks. Mild joint pain and swelling have been observed in a large proportion of adults with the disease. Erythema infectiosum affects all ages but is most common in children of school age and may occur in epidemic form. The mode of transmission of the disease is not known and an infectious agent has not been recovered.

ENTEROVIRAL EXANTHEMS

Many individual enteroviruses have been associated with rash—poliomyelitis virus only rarely, Coxsackie B5, A2, A4, and A9, and ECHO viruses 2, 3, 4, 5, 6, 11, 14, 18, 19, occasionally. Three enterovirus infections are frequently associated with rashes and have been studied extensively enough to warrant individual description.

HAND, FOOT, AND MOUTH DISEASE (COXASCKIE A16 INFECTION). (Chap. 227.)

BOSTON EXANTHEM (INFECTION WITH ECHO VIRUS 16). This is probably a common infectious disease of childhood. It was described first and most extensively during an epidemic in Boston in 1951, as a finding in many patients with ECHO virus type 16 infection. Children who were infected usually had a disease characterized by exanthem and low-grade fever, while adult family contacts developed high fever, prostration, and signs of aseptic meningitis with absent or fleeting rash. The first manifestation of the disease in children was fever of 101 to 102°F, lasting for a day or two, pharyngitis with ulcerated lesions resembling herpangina, and slight enlargement of the cervical and postauricular lymph nodes. The rash appeared during or after defervescence and consisted of small pink maculopapules on the face, upper chest, and occasionally on the whole body, including the palms and soles. The rash lasted for 1 to 5 days, and there were no important complications or sequelae. The disease resembled exanthem subitum but occurred in children of all ages and in adults.

INFECTION WITH ECHO VIRUS 9. Infection with this virus has occurred in epidemics among children and adults and has been characterized by a febrile disease with a high incidence of aspetic meningitis. The incubation period is 5 to 8 days. About 30 percent of patients have a rash which may occur with or without meningitis, is usually maculopapular, presents at the onset of the disease, appears first on the face and neck, spreads to the trunk and extremities, may involve the palms and soles, and persists for 3 to 5 days. Petechiae with or without maculopapules have been recognized, and when seen in association with meningitis, there may be confusion with meningococcal meningitis. A vesicular eruption with crusting lesions has been seen occasionally. An exanthem on the buccal mucosa and soft palate occurs in about 30 percent of patients and consists of small red areas with white centers which resemble Koplik's spots. The disease is usually benign, but rarely has been associated with permanent central-nervous-system damage.

REFERENCES

Ager, E. A., T. D. Y. Chin, and J. Poland: Epidemic Erythema Infectiosum, New Engl. J. Med., 275:1326, 1966.

Lerner, A. M., et al.: New Viral Exanthems, New Engl. J. Med., 269:678, 736, 1963.

Miller, G. D., and J. Tindall: Hand, Foot and Mouth Disease, J.A.M.A., 203:827, 1968.

Neva, F. A., R. Reemster, and I. Gorbach: Clinical Epidemiological Features of Unusual Epidemic Exanthem, J.A.M.A., 155:544, 1954.

Wenner, H. A., and T. Lou: Virus Diseases Associated with Cutaneous Eruptions, Progr. Med. Virol., 5:219, 1963.

223 SMALLPOX, VACCINIA, AND COWPOX

John C. Ribble

Poxviruses are a group of large (200 to 320 mμ), brick-shaped, DNA-containing viruses that possess a common antigen and have a predilection for skin. Many of the poxviruses, such as myxoma and fowlpox agents, cause disease mainly in lower animals. Smallpox (variola major), alastrim (variola minor), vaccinia, and cowpox agents are closely related members of the poxvirus group that cause human disease. All of these viruses grow and produce pox on the chorioallantoic membrane of chick embryos incubated at 37°C and can be cultivated in cells from various mammalian tissues with formation of intracytoplasmic inclusions, rounding, fusion, and heaping up of cells, and eventual degeneration of the infected area. The poxviruses responsible for human disease may be distinguished from each other by minor antigenic differences and by the type and severity of lesions they induce in experimental animals and man. Smallpox and alastrim viruses produce smaller pox on the chorioallantoic membrane than vaccinia. Pock production by vaccinia virus can be demonstrated at incubation temperatures of 39 to 40°C, whereas the smallpox and alastrim agents do not induce lesions at this temperature. The alastrim virus causes pock formation only below 38°C, but the variola major virus can induce lesions at temperatures above 38°C but below 39°C.

SMALLPOX (Variola)

DEFINITION. Smallpox is a severe contagious, febrile disease characterized by a vesicular and pustular eruption. Alastrim is a similar but milder illness.

PATHOGENESIS AND PATHOLOGY. The virus gains access to the body by the respiratory tract and multiples at unidentified sites, probably lymph nodes or liver. After several days, during which there are no evidences of infection, viremia ensues, with production of swelling of the endothelium of blood vessels in the corium and perivascular inflammation. Loculated vesicles are the result of cellular destruction and exudation of serum. The infected epithelial cells are swollen and contain intracytoplasmic inclusions surrounded by a halo (Guarnieri's bodies). The extent of skin involvement is greater in smallpox than in chickenpox and reaches into the corium. Pitting, most commonly seen on the face, is said to result from destruction of sebaceous glands which are abundant in this area. The liver, spleen, and lymph nodes may be enlarged and may show focal accumulations of large mononuclear cells.

EPIDEMIOLOGY. A patient with smallpox is infectious from a day before the rash appears until the lesions have healed and the scabs have fallen off. During the early phase of the illness, the virus is transmitted in nasopharyngeal secretions; when the eruption is fully formed, the lesions themselves are a major source of infectious material. Variola virus may contaminate clothing, bedding, dust, or other inanimate objects and remain infectious for months, necessitating disinfection of articles in the patient's environment. Although smallpox is usually disseminated by a patient with the disease, it is possible that the virus may be transmitted by an individual, especially a partially immune person, who has an inapparent or very mild infection. Long-term completely asymptomatic carriers have not been recognized, nor has aerial transmission over long distances been convincingly demonstrated. Smallpox is still a major world health problem and exists in endemic form in India, Indonesia, and parts of Africa; alastrim is prevalent in South America, especially in Brazil.

MANIFESTATIONS. Smallpox can be divided into a prodrome, an early eruptive phase, and a period of vesiculation and pustule formation. The prodrome is characterized by fever of 102 to 106°F, headache, myalgia especially in the back, abdominal pain, vomiting, and in some patients by a transient, blotchy, erythematous eruption. After 3 or 4 days the fever subsides, the symptoms decrease, and the patient seems to recover. It is at this time, when the patient is afebrile, that the focal eruption begins. Early manifestations are painful ulcers on the buccal mucosa, and macules which appear first on the face and forearm, and rapidly become firm, shotty papules. The papules increase in number and spread from the face and distal extremities to involve the trunk. The individual lesions may remain discrete and scattered or they may become confluent and involve most of the body. They are most concentrated on the face and distal extremities including the palms and soles and are relatively sparse in the axilla. On the third or fourth day after the appearance of the focal rash, the papules progress to vesicles containing clear fluid, which, over the next few days, becomes cloudy due to infiltration by pus cells and desquamated epithelial cells; hemorrhage into the vesicles and surrounding skin may also be seen. During the course of smallpox, the lesions at any one time, in one area, are all at the same stage of evolution. At the time the vesicles become pustular, there is recurrence of fever, which may persist until healing occurs. The pustules umbilicate and form crusts and scabs which usually fall off 3 weeks after the beginning of illness, leaving small scars or deep pits.

The above description applies to disease of moderate severity. A milder illness may occur in previously immunized persons or in some who have no history of vaccination. It is characterized by the usual incubation period and prodrome, but is followed either by focal eruption of fewer than 100 papules, or by a rash resembling chickenpox. Smallpox with prodrome, but no eruption of any kind, has been recognized (*variola sine eruptione*). The disease may also occur in a rapidly fulminating form ("sledgehammer smallpox"). After the usual incubation period, the patient develops an initial illness characterized by severe prostration, fever, bone-marrow depression, hemorrhagic skin lesions, bleeding from the mouth and intestine, shock, coma, and death. The disease progresses from inception to death within 3 or 4 days without evidence of the typical focal skin lesions.

Alastrim is similar to mild and moderate forms of variola major in that it has the same incubation period and prodromal illness, but the skin eruption is less extensive, and fatalities are extremely rare and are related to secondary infections.

COMPLICATIONS. Bacterial superinfections of the lesions, usually with *S. aureus,* may occur in the late pustular stage. Viral infections of the trachea, pharynx, and larynx, and superimposed bacterial pneumonia, may be seen in severe forms of smallpox. Mild conjunctivitis is quite common, and iritis and keratitis have been recognized. Encephalomyelitis may occur in the late stage of the disease and is similar to other postinfectious encephalitides. Osteomyelitis and joint effusions may complicate the disease.

LABORATORY FINDINGS. Leukopenia is present during the prodromal illness, and there is usually leukocytosis during the pustular stage. Rapid diagnosis of poxvirus infection can be made by finding of characteristic brick-shaped particles in preparations of vesicle fluid examined by electron microscopy. Specific precipitation in agar using antigen prepared from lesions and antivariola or antivaccinia immune serum may also allow detection of poxvirus within a few hours. These tests do not distinguish variola from vaccinia or other poxviruses but do allow rapid differentiation from herpes simplex and varicella-zoster viruses. For definitive identification the virus must be grown in cell culture or on the chorioallantoic membrane and examined for its biologic characteristics.

DIFFERENTIAL DIAGNOSIS. The major problem in differential diagnosis is in distinguishing smallpox from chickenpox. Smallpox is preceded by a longer prodrome than chickenpox and its eruption vesiculates over a period of days instead of hours. The smallpox lesions are all characteristically in the same stage of development, whereas those of chickenpox may, in one area, display all stages of evolution. Electron microscopy and agar pre-cipitation techniques (see above) are especially useful in distinguishing between smallpox and chickenpox.

PROPHYLAXIS. Smallpox may be prevented among the patient's contacts by vaccination. Because this procedure is most successful if carried out during the early part of the incubation period, all exposed persons, regardless of previous immunization, should be vaccinated immediately upon recognition of exposure. Large controlled clinical trials have demonstrated that oral administration of 1-methylisatin-3-thiosemicarbazone (methisazone), a drug which interferes with poxvirus multiplication, can prevent smallpox and alastrim in patients exposed to these diseases. The use of the drug together with prompt vaccination results in greater chance of protection than either measure alone. A drawback to the use of methisazone is its tendency to induce vomiting. The combined use of vaccination and parenteral administration of vaccinia immune globulin early in the incubation period is effective in the prevention of smallpox in exposed individuals.

TREATMENT. There is no specific therapy for smallpox. Thiosemicarbazone, although effective in prophylaxis, has not been shown to be of value in the treatment of established cases. Fluid deficits incurred by lack of intake and by loss from affected areas should be replaced by the administration of appropriate solutions. During the vesicular and pustular phases of the disease, an attempt should be made to prevent bacterial infection by the use of sterile sheets and sterile nursing procedures. Antihistamines may be helpful in decreasing pruritus. Bathing and application of lotions or ointments should be avoided. Later in the course of the illness, when desquamation has begun, showers or baths may be helpful in removing desquamating tissue.

Administration of parenteral penicillin, beginning on the fifth day of rash, has been reported to decrease the incidence of infection of skin lesions and the formation of boils and abscesses due to penicillin-sensitive bacteria. Inasmuch as penicillin-resistant staphylococci are frequently responsible for bacterial infections, the use of penicillinase-resistant penicillin may be of value, but its efficacy as a prophylactic agent in smallpox has not been evaluated. If bacterial infection is demonstrated, an antibiotic active against the infecting organism should be given by the parenteral route. Topical antibiotics should be avoided.

VACCINIA

Vaccinia is a virus disease of the skin which is induced by inoculation for the prevention of smallpox. The exact origin of the vaccinia virus is obscure. The material used by Jenner for vaccination was derived from cowpox lesions, and the infectious agent was propagated for many years by successive passage from person to person using exudate from fresh skin lesions. The original agent possibly became contaminated with variola virus during the period when transfer was being carried out without strict controls. It has been suggested that vaccinia virus is a hybrid of cowpox and variola agents, a contention supported by the finding that laboratory-induced hybrids of variola and cowpox viruses have many of the characteristics associated with vaccinia.

VACCINATION. Live, lyophilized vaccinia virus prepared from vesicle fluid of infected calves is commercially available and maintains potency for 18 months at 46°F. It is dissolved in a diluent solution just prior to use. The usual method for vaccination is to apply a small drop of vaccine to the skin over the deltoid muscle and to press a sterile needle through the vaccine several times in such a way that only the superficial layer of skin is entered. Vaccination should always induce some form of skin reaction; complete absence of any kind of lesion indicates that the vaccine was not viable or was not administered properly. The reaction which occurs in nonimmune individuals is characterized by a red papule at the site of inoculation 3 to 5 days after vaccination. The papule becomes vesicular on about the fifth or sixth day and pustular by the ninth or eleventh day after inoculation. The vesicle and pustule may be surrounded by a large area of erythema. About 2 weeks after vaccination, the pustule dries and develops a crust which falls off by the end of the third week, leaving a scar. Fever, malaise, and irritability are common in children during the vesicular and pustular phases, and axillary lymphadenopathy may develop and persist for several months. In the partially immune person, a modified reaction develops without fever or constitutional symptoms. A papule appears on the skin within 3 days, vesiculates in 5 to 7 days, and heals without much scarring. In an immune person a small papule forms in 3 days, but it does not vesiculate or result in scarring.

COMPLICATIONS. Healing of the primary vaccinal lesion may not occur, and there may be during a period of weeks or months progressive necrosis with destruction of large areas of skin, subcutaneous tissue, and underlying structures (*vaccinia gangrenosum*). In addition to the local destruction, there may be metastatic lesions on other parts of the skin surface and in bone and viscera. Vaccinia gangrenosum occurs most frequently in persons with disorders of immunity and if untreated, is nearly always fatal. *Eczema vaccinatum* (Plate 3) is a serious complication that is seen in persons with eczema or other type of chronic dermatosis. Widespread infection in the previously affected areas, as well as in normal skin, may result from direct vaccination of an eczematous patient or from exposure to a recently vaccinated individual. *Generalized vaccinia* in patients without preexisting skin disease is characterized by a few satellite lesions surrounding the inoculation site or by widely disseminated pox resembling the primary vaccination lesion. This condition may be mild, and recovery is to be expected. Vaccinia virus may be transferred from the primary inoculation site to the eye or other sites by scratching. *Postvaccinal encephalomyelitis* appears from 2 to 25 days after vaccination. The patient becomes severely ill quite suddenly, with nuchal rigidity, drowsiness, vomiting, convulsions, coma, and signs suggesting disease of the spinal cord. The period of coma lasts for a few days, and in those who recover there are usually no permanent sequelae. Death occurs in about half of the patients with encephalo-

myelitis. *Erythema multiforme bullosum* or diffuse blotchy erythema may occur in vaccinated patients 7 to 10 days after vaccination, and are thought to be allergic reactions to the virus or other components of the vaccine.

The incidence of complications has been compiled by the National Communicable Disease Center. The frequencies of the various adverse effects per million primarily vaccinated persons are vaccinia gangrenosum, 1.1; eczema vaccinatum, 8.7; generalized vaccinia, 20.8; vaccinal lesions resulting from accidental implantation of virus, 13.6; postvaccinal encephalitis, 1.9; other complications, 6.7. The survey indicated that complications are two or three times more frequent in infants under one year of age than in any other age group, and it is recommended that first vaccination be performed sometime between the first and second birthdays. As many as two-thirds of the complications could have been prevented if vaccination had been avoided in patients with eczema, family members of patients with eczema, persons with agammaglobulinemia, blood dyscrasias, or lymphoma, or patients being treated with adrenal steroids of immunosuppressive drugs. Because of the severity and frequency of adverse effects, the rarity of smallpox in this country, and the documented efficacy of thiosemicarbazone prophylaxis, some physicians have questioned the wisdom of routine vaccination in the United States. On the other hand, the possibility of rapid spread of smallpox in a completely nonimmunized population, the difficulty in making a prompt accurate diagnosis, and the avoidability of many complications of vaccination have convinced others that routine immunization should be continued. Attenuated strains of vaccinia virus that produce fewer adverse reactions have been developed and may be generally available soon.

TREATMENT. Patients with vaccinia gangrenosum, eczema vaccinatum, generalized vaccinia, and vaccinia of the eye should be treated promptly with vaccinia immune globulin, which is available through the American Red Cross. Some experience indicates that thiosemicarbonaze, together with vaccinia immune globulin, is more effective therapy for vaccinia gangrenosum than the use of globulin alone. No specific therapy is available for patients with postvaccinal encephalitis.

COWPOX

Cowpox is primarily a disease of the teets and udders of cows. Man is almost always infected by milking, but occasional spread to contacts may occur from an infected person. The human disease is characterized by low-grade fever and by small papules on the fingers and hand which go through vesicular and pustular stages resembling the course of vaccinia infection. The lesions may be ruptured by trauma and spread to immediately adjacent areas on the hand and continue to ulcerate for several weeks. Edema, lymphangitis, and axillary lymph node enlargement are common. Very rare cases of postcowpox encephalitis and serious infections of eczematous persons have been reported. In general, the disease is benign, heals without scarring, and is usually uncomplicated.

REFERENCES

Bedson, H. S., K. Dumbell: Smallpox and Vaccinia, Brit. Med. Bull., 23:119, 1967.

Dixon, C. W.: "Smallpox," London, J. & A. Churchill, 1962. Joklik, W. K.: The Poxviruses, Bacteriol. Rev., 30:33, 1966.

Neff, J. M., et al.: Complications of Smallpox Vaccination. National Survey in the United States, 1963. New Engl. J. Med., 276:125, 1967.

224   CHICKENPOX (Varicella)

John C. Ribble

DEFINITION. Chickenpox is a contagious disease characterized by fever and a disseminated vesicular eruption. Chickenpox and herpes zoster (Chap. 225) are different manifestations of infection with the same viral agent.

ETIOLOGY. In 1953 a virus was recovered from patients with chickenpox and herpes zoster that produced intranuclear, eosinophilic inclusions and multinucleated giant cells in lines of cells derived from various monkey and human tissues. The varicella-zoster virus in culture spreads from cell to adjacent cell by direct invasion, rather than by way of suspending medium, and can be passed to other tissue cultures only by transfer of infected cells. The structure of the varicella-zoster virion resembles that of herpes simplex; however, the difficulty in recovery of cell-free virus has hampered the investigation of its chemical composition. Complement-fixing antigens can be detected in vesicle fluid and in suitable preparations of infected cell cultures. No hemagglutinin has been identified.

PATHOGENESIS AND PATHOLOGY. Varicella is presumably transmitted by the respiratory route, although the virus has only rarely been isolated from nasopharyngeal secretions of infected persons. Virus multiplication occurs at some unidentified site and probably results in intermittent viremia, as suggested by the successive crops of widely spaced lesions. Focal viral infection of blood vessels in the corium, with intranuclear inclusions in endothelial cells, results in degeneration of epidermis and formation of vesicles containing serum, epithelial and inflammatory cells, and multinucleated giant cells. Virus can be isolated from vesicle fluid, but not from crusting lesions or scales, for 3 days after eruption. In patients with varicella pneumonia the tracheobronchial mucosa, the alveolar septa, and the interstitial areas of the lungs are edematous and contain monocytic inflammatory cells, cells with intranuclear inclusions and giant cells. The nodular areas of pneumonia may eventually become calcified. The changes in the central nervous system in patients with varicella encephalomyelitis resemble those seen in measles.

EPIDEMIOLOGY. Chickenpox is a highly contagious disease with attack rates of 70 percent or more among susceptible persons exposed to a patient with the disease. The infectious period extends from a day or two before the rash until as long as 6 days after the appearance of new skin lesions. Patients with herpes zoster may be the source of an outbreak of chickenpox among susceptible contacts. Children from five to eight years of age are most commonly affected, but younger children, including newborn infants, and adults may develop chickenpox; an estimated 2 to 20 percent of cases occur in persons over the age of fifteen years. In the United States the disease is endemic, with superimposed epidemics every 2 to 5 years, usually the winter or spring.

MANIFESTATIONS. The incubation period from the time of exposure to the appearance of rash is 10 to 21 days, most often 14 to 17 days. There may be a 1- or 2-day prodrome with fever and malaise, but these symptoms usually begin when the rash appears. The first skin manifestations are pruritic maculopapules that evolve in a few hours to thin-walled vesicles which contain clear fluid and are surounded by a red border. During the next day the erythmea diminishes and the vesicles collapse in the center, forming annular or umbilicated lesions which dry further and form scabs that fall off after several days without scarring. New maculopapules continue to erupt during the first 3 or 4 days of illness and go through a similar evolution. The findings at one time, in one area, of skin lesions in all stages of development—maculopapules, vesicles, umbilicated lesions, and scabs—is characteristic of chickenpox. The rash is most concentrated on the trunk, but pox are frequently seen on the face and scalp, occasionally on the mucosal surfaces of the mouth or conjunctiva, and rarely on the palms or soles.

Chickenpox in adults is often more severe than the disease in children, with more profuse rash, higher fever, and greater incidence of pneumonia.

COMPLICATIONS. Hemorrhage into vesicles and surrounding skin may be seen in adults with severe chickenpox or in children receiving adrenal steroids. Infection of the varicella lesions by bacteria, most commonly S. *aureus*, results in delayed healing and scarring of skin, and occasionally in bacteremia.

Of adults with chickenpox, 15 percent develop *primary varicella pneumonia*, and adult patients account for 90 percent of the patients who develop this complication. Pneumonia is invariably associated with skin lesions and appears 1 to 6 days after onset of rash. The degree of pulmonary involvement is to some extent correlated with the severity of the rash; patients may be virtually asymptomatic or may develop serious, life-threatening disease. Tachypnea, dyspnea, cough, and fever of 102°F or more are present in most patients with symptomatic pneumonia; cyanosis, pleuritic chest pain, and hemoptysis each occur in 20 to 40 percent of the recorded cases. The physical examination may disclose no abnormalities, or there may be intercostal retractions, a few rhonchi, wheezes, scattered râles, and rarely, evidence of pleural effusion. In contrast to paucity of physical signs, roentgenograms demonstrate widespread nodular infiltration of both lungs, most prominent at the hila and least evident at the apices. Vital capacity is decreased, arterial oxygen saturation is diminished, and the airways may be blocked by tenacious bronchopulmonary secretions. Most patients with varicella pneumonia show symptomatic improvement at the time the rash begins to wane; however, seriously ill patients can remain febrile and dyspneic for as long as 2 weeks. Roentgenographic evidence of disease diminishes at the time of clinical improvement, but may persist for several weeks. Abnormalities of pulmonary gas diffusion have been demonstrated several months after apparent recovery.

Encephalomyelitis is a less frequent complication of chickenpox than of measles and occurs predominantly in children. It begins 3 to 14 days after the onset of rash with drowsiness and irritability progressing to vomiting, convulsions, and coma which lasts for 4 or 5 days. As the patient regains consciousness, evidence of CNS abnormalities may be apparent. Varicella encephalomyelitis is frequently associated with cerebellar dysfunction either isolated or associated with other nervous disorders such as hemiparesis, athetosis, cranial nerve abnormalities, and various spinal syndromes.

Patients who *contract varicella while receiving steroids* may have recurrent crops of new skin lesions for as long as 3 weeks. They have a higher incidence of hemorrhagic and progressive gangrenous lesions and occasionally develop a fatal disseminated disease with viral infection in all the viscera. The fatal form of the disease has been encountered most frequently in children being treated with steroids for leukemia or other disease of the hematopoietic system, but it has also been seen in those receiving therapy for rheumatic fever and allergic disorders. Other complications of chickenpox such as myocarditis, corneal lesions, iritis, nephritis, orchitis, and appendicitis have been recognized but are rare. Congenital infection with varicella can occur, and infants born of mothers with chickenpox may display the typical skin lesions. Evidence of congenital malformations as a result of infection in early pregnancy is not convincing.

LABORATORY FINDINGS. Multinucleated giant cells and epithelial cells with eosinophilic intranuclear inclusions can be identified in material scraped from the base of a vesicular lesion or in sputum from patients with varicella pneumonia. For specific diagnosis, virus can be isolated from vesicular fluid and complement fixation tests can be performed. The white blood count in patients with uncomplicated chickenpox is normal. The spinal fluid in patients with encephalomyelitis contains increased protein and as many as 3,000 lymphocytes per cu mm.

DIFFERENTIAL DIAGNOSIS. Chickenpox can usually be diagnosed by the history of recent exposure and the character of the rash. In situations where smallpox is a possibility, differentiation from chickenpox can be attempted by noting the distribution and evolution of the rash and by examination of cells from vesicles, but definitive diagnosis can be made only by identification of the virus. Disseminated vaccinia lesions similar to chickenpox may occur in patients, especially those with disorders of immunity or eczema, who have recently been vaccinated or exposed to a vaccinated person. Herpes simplex infection in patients with chronic eczema or neurodermatitis may present as a varicelliform eruption confined to previously involved areas of skin; the diagnosis can be confirmed by virus isolation. Rickettsialpox can be differentiated from chickenpox by the presence of an eschar in the area of mite bite, prominent headache, and specific complement-fixing antibodies to *R. akari.*

PROPHYLAXIS. Chickenpox can be modified but not completely prevented by the administration of 0.2 to 0.3 ml per lb gamma-globulin. If exposure occurs, passive immunization should be attempted in pregnant women without a history of chickenpox, newborn infants, and nonimmune persons on steroid therapy.

TREATMENT. The patient with uncomplicated chickenpox should receive local applications for the relief of itching. Secondary bacterial infections should be treated with appropriate antibacterial agents. Patients with varicella pneumonia require skillful nursing care, removal of bronchial secretions, administration of oxygen, and on occasion ventilatory assistance, such as positive pressure breathing. Adrenal steroids have been considered by some to be beneficial in the treatment of varicella pneumonia, but convincing evidence of their efficacy in this condition is not available. Patients suspected of having varicella-zoster infection of the eye should be promptly treated by an ophthalmologist.

REFERENCES

Brunnell, P. A.: Varicella-zoster Infections in Pregnancy, J.A.M.A., 199:315, 1967.

Gordon, J. E.: Chickenpox: An Epidemiological Review, Am. J. Med. Sci., 244:362, 1962.

Ross, A.: Modification of Chickenpox in Family Contacts by Administration of Gamma Globulin, New Engl. J. Med., 267:369, 1962.

Triebwasser, J. H., R. Harris, R. Bryant, and E. Rhoades: Varicella Pneumonia in Adults: Report of Seven Cases and a Review of Literature, Medicine, 46:409, 1967.

Weller, T. H., H. Witton, and E. Bell: Etiologic Agents of Varicella and *Herpes zoster,* J. Exp. Med., 108:843, 1958.

225 HERPES ZOSTER
Lewis L. Coriell

DEFINITION. Herpes zoster, or shingles, is an acute infectious disease of man. It is caused by a virus and is characterized by unilateral, segmental inflammation of the posterior root ganglions or extramedullary ganglions of cranial nerves and by a painful vesicular eruption of the skin along the peripheral distribution of the involved nerve.

HISTORY. The disease was called zona ("girdle") by the Greeks because of the bandlike distribution of the eruption about the trunk. Bokay (1888) suggested a possible etiologic relationship between zoster and varicella, and Lipschutz (1921) defined the specific histopathology of the skin lesions. Serial cultivation of the virus in tissue culture of human fibroblasts (1953) enabled Weller to show that the viruses of varicella and herpes zoster were identical serologically.

ETIOLOGY. The virus of herpes zoster is relatively large (204 x 240 μ). It is strictly a parasite of man. Electron micrographs of a vesicle fluid have shown it to be similar in size and shape to the virus of varicella. The virus may be plentiful in early vesicles but is typically scanty after 24 hr. Zoster is now considered to be a reactivation of a latent varicella virus in a partially immune individual, although the mechanism of reactivation is not clear.

EPIDEMIOLOGY. Infection is rare in children but increases in frequency, severity, and duration with age. It occurs in all seasons and is slightly more frequent in males than in females. In the United States the majority of patients with herpes zoster gives a history of a previous attack of varicella. Epidemics have occurred in schools and barracks but are not common. Outbreaks of herpes zoster have occurred in contacts of a patient with varicella, and vice versa. The grouping of these secondary infections suggests that zoster is infectious only during the first 2 or 3 days after appearance of the eruption. Secondary zoster following trauma such as spinal puncture, administration of arsenic or bismuth, spinal cord tumor, tabes, and lymphatic leukemia suggests that the virus may remain dormant in the tissues for long periods. The disease appears to be more common in persons who are overworked or ill.

PATHOGENESIS. Whether the virus enters the skin and travels up the sensory nerve or extends peripherally has not been established. The virus has been demonstrated only in the skin lesions, although an inflammatory reaction is a constant finding in the segmental nerve, its sensory ganglion, and the posterior horn of the spinal column (posterior poliomyelitis). The regional lymph nodes show an acute inflammatory reaction.

The skin vesicle is confined to the epidermis, while the corium is congested and infiltrated with inflammatory cells. In the margin of the vesicle are epithelial cells undergoing balloon degeneration. Some of the cells contain eosinophilic intranuclear inclusion bodies which displace the basichromatin to the periphery of the enlarged nucleus. Multinucleated giant cells may be present, each nucleus containing an inclusion body. Within 2 or 3 days, inflammatory cells fill the vesicle, and healing progresses from below, frequently with slight scarring.

MANIFESTATIONS. The incubation period varies from 7 to 21 days. The preeruptive stage consists of fever and constitutional symptoms, with pain, paresthesias, or hyperesthesia over the distribution of the involved nerve for 2 to 4 days. Following this, an erythematous dermatitis appears, which quickly becomes papular and vesiculates, with large or small grouped vesicles on an erythematous base. The vesicles, at first clear, become cloudy within 2 to 3 days, then crust and dry after 5 to 10 days. The eruption may appear first near the spinal column, with successive crops over the distal distribution of the nerve. The pain and vesicular band, following radicular lines, run transversely around the trunk or vertically over the arm and leg. The lesions are almost always unilateral. Headache and meningismus are not uncommon. Pain is frequently slight or absent in young children but may be intense and not completely controlled by analgesic drugs in adults. It is variously described as aching, soreness, burning, gnawing, shooting, stabbing, or neuralgic.

The regional lymph nodes are enlarged and tender. Secondary bacterial infection of the ruptured vesicles is common. Over 75 percent of cases occur between the second dorsal and second lumbar vertebras; cases are rare below the elbow or knee. Involvement of the fifth cranial nerve is next in frequency, and in 50 percent the globe of the eye is affected. When the nasociliary branch of the semilunar ganglion is involved, the cornea, sclera, or ciliary body may be permanently damaged; the first branch of the fifth nerve is affected more frequently then the second or third. Disease of the geniculate ganglion may lead to zoster of the concha of the ear, the external auditory canal, or the soft palate, and to loss of taste (Hunt's syndrome); these manifestations are often accompanied by paralysis of the seventh nerve. Paralysis is not uncommon in cephalic and cervical zoster but is rare in zoster of the trunk. Second attacks of herpes zoster are exceedingly rare and should suggest the alternate diagnosis of localized herpes simplex. In some patients, a generalized vesicular eruption simulating varicella appears shortly after the appearance of the localized lesion (zoster generalisata).

The total course of the disease from onset to complete recovery is 10 days to 5 weeks. In the age group up to nineteen years, 90 percent of patients recovered within 14 days, while in the forty- to fifty-nine-year age group, only 45 percent of lesions cleared in this interval. If all the vesicles appear within 24 hr, the total illness is usually short; if crops of vesicles appear up to 7 days, the total duration was progressively longer.

A serious complication is the syndrome of postherpetic neuralgia, which is limited to aged patients with arteriosclerosis. It usually involves only the trunk or the ophthalmic division of the trigeminal nerve. Frequently there is an interval between the acute phase and full unfolding of severe pain, which is of such severity and intensity that the patients cannot rest or sleep, and which may persist for weeks or months.

LABORATORY FINDINGS. The fluid from unruptured vesicles is sterile bacteriologically, but a smear stained with Giemsa shows multinucleated giant cells and type A inclusion bodies. The cerebrospinal fluid is abnormal in 40 percent of cases; pressure may be increased, and a pleocytosis of up to 300 mononuclear cells has been observed.

DIFFERENTIAL DIAGNOSIS. In the preeruptive stage, the diagnosis is difficult, and the disease is usually confused with many other more common causes of pain, such as pleurisy, appendicitis, "lumbago," pleurodynia, or collapsed intervertebral disk. After the unilateral eruption appears, the clinical features are so characteristic that the diagnosis is simple. Occasionally, localized herpes simplex along the distribution of a segmental nerve may simulate zoster, including the localized pain and tenderness. The diagnosis of herpes simplex infection can be confirmed in the laboratory.

TREATMENT. Treatment is directed toward increasing the patient's comfort and preventing secondary infection.

The average case of herpes zoster is self-limited and presents no serious complications. The two unsolved problems are the syndrome of postherpetic neuralgia and ophthalmic zoster. In the acute phase, pain is usually controlled by aspirin and codeine, combined with mild sedation; local anesthetic ointments are not very effective. A petrolatum gauze pad bandage to prevent painful trauma by clothing may be helpful. The skin lesions are adequately managed with applications of calamine lotion in most cases. Adhesive tape strapping should not be applied for the preeruptive pain of herpes zoster because it will lead to extensive loss of epidermis upon removal of the tape. Antibiotics have no effect on the virus but may be indicated to control secondary infection, particularly in ophthalmic zoster or severe spinal involvement with secondary infection. In ophthalmic involvement the choice of antibiotic should be guided by bacterial cultures and sensitivity tests. Idoxuridine (IDU) is of no value. Treatment of lesions of the eye should be supervised by an ophthalmologist. Early relief of pain and inflammation follows the use of cortisone and corticotropin. Cycloplegic eyedrops are used for iridocyclitis.

Severe postherpetic pain may be resistant to all types of management. One theory advanced to explain this is the activation of self-contained pain circuits in and above the thalamus. The following procedures are based on the supposition that the defect is central: injection of dorsal root ganglion with alcohol or irradiation with x-ray, dorsal rhizotomy, cordotomy, and lobotomy. On the theory of peripheral nerve abnormality are based vitamin B therapy, procainization or excision of skin, surgical pituitrin, paravertebral block, intravenous tetraethylammonium chloride, and sympathetic ganglionectomy. Other empirical procedures which have been helpful in certain cases include autohemotherapy, sodium iodide, moccasin venom, and Protamide. The multiplicity of recommended procedures is eloquent evidence that none is entirely satisfactory.

PROGNOSIS. It is very unusual for serious complications to follow inflammation of the spinal ganglions. Partial paralysis of the third, fourth, sixth, and seventh cranial nerves, or hypesthesia, may persist for some time. Significant impairment of vision occurs in many cases of zoster ophthalmicus.

REFERENCES

Bailey, P.: Herpes Zoster, Postgrad. Med., 12:127, 1952.

Blank, H., L. L. Coriell, and T. F. McN. Scott: Human Skin Grafted upon the Chorioallantois of the Chick Embryo for Virus Cultivation, Proc. Soc. Exp. Biol. Med., 69:341, 1948.

Rake, G., H. Blank, L. L. Coriell, F. P. O. Nagler, and T. F. McN. Scott: The Relationships of Varicella and Herpes Zoster: Electron Microscope Studies, J. Bacteriol., 56:293, 1948.

Scheie, H. G., and M. C. Alper: Treatment of Herpes Zoster Ophthalmicus with Cortisone or Corticotropin, A.M.A. Arch. Ophthalmol., 53:38, 1955.

Weller, T. H.: Varicella-Herpes Zoster Virus in "Horsfall and Tamm Viral and Rickettsial Infections of Man," 4th ed., Philadelphia, J. B. Lippincott Company, 1967.

226 HERPES SIMPLEX
Lewis L. Coriell

DEFINITION. Herpes simplex is an infectious disease caused by a virus. Classically, it appears in recurrent attacks as clusters of vesicles on the face, lips, and mucocutaneous junctions. The initial infection in some individuals may be serious or even fatal. Infection of the central nervous system, the eye, the skin in eczematous patients, the viscera, or the mouth and throat in gingivostomatitis are the common forms of "primary" herpes simplex.

HISTORY. Gruter, in 1914, first transferred infection from the cornea of a patient to the cornea of a rabbit and, subsequently, back to the cornea of a blind man, reproducing a typical dendritic ulceration of the cornea. In 1938 Dodd, Buddingh, and Johnston isolated herpes simplex virus from the mouths of children suffering with febrile ulcerative stomatitis (acute herpetic gingivostomatitis).

ETIOLOGY. The virus of herpes simplex (*Herpesvirus hominis*, HVH) passes ordinary bacterial filters, measures 180 to 200 mμ in diameter, and is composed of a central core of double stranded DNA, an envelope with 162 capsomers arranged as an icosahedron, a surrounding granular zone, and an outer membrane with short projections. It is present in early vesicles. It may be propagated on the cornea or in the brain of several laboratory animals, on the chorioallantoic membrane of embryonated eggs, or in tissue culture. Two serologic types can be distinguished by microquantal neutralization tests. Type 2 isolates are usually associated with infection of the adult genital tract, and type 1 strains, with infection from all other sites.

EPIDEMIOLOGY. The serums of most adults (70 to 90 percent) contain neutralizing antibodies against herpes simplex; many of these individuals experience recurrent manifestations of disease. Fever, whether due to infectious diseases or artificially induced ("fever blister"), and the common cold ("cold sore") are probably the most frequent precipitants of recurrent herpes; emotional disturbance, physical fatigue, sunburn, menstruation, and food allergy are other incitants. The virus remains latent in the tissues between attacks but is sufficiently active to stimulate antibody production. Virus has frequently been found in the saliva when there was no clinical evidence of disease. Adults who have never been infected may contact a primary infection. Full-term newborn infants are usually immune by virtue of transplacental transfer of antibodies, which they gradually lose after the first few months of life. However, by the fifth year, the percentage of children with specific neutralizing antibodies approaches that observed in adults, indicating a high infection rate during infancy. The clinical syndromes recognized as primary infection in this age group account for only 15 percent of serologic infections. Herpes simplex has evolved an unusually successful host-parasite relationship with man. Most individuals harbor the virus from infancy to old age with little inconvenience to themselves, and even the primary contact in infancy is usually not accompanied by manifest clinical disease. The association of type 2 herpes virus with the genital tract or closely related sites suggests that it is commonly transmitted by venereal contact, whereas type 1 is spread by contact with oral secretions or from recurrent vesicles of the mucocutaneous junction about the face.

PATHOGENESIS. It is probable that during latent periods the virus lives within cells, because the extracellular fluid contains sufficient neutralizing antibody to inactivate the virus. The various precipitating factors which induce recurrent disease may have a common denominator in altered physiology of the host cell which permits the virus to multiply, but little specific information is available on this point. Skin biopsies taken during the early vesicular stage show congestion of the dermis, with swelling and ballooning degeneration of prickle cells of the epidermis. In some of these, the nuclear basichromatin is collected at the periphery and the entire central area of the enlarged nucleus is filled with a homogeneous mass which at first stains blue and later red with hematoxylin and eosin. This is the type A inclusion body, found wherever there is active herpes simplex infection. Multinucleated giant cells, with each nucleus containing an inclusion body, are frequently seen in biopsies of infected human skin.

The intraepidermal vesicle does not extend below the basement membrane and hence does not cause scarring, although depigmentation may persist for some time in dark-skinned persons. In the healing phase, the vesicle and corium are densely infiltrated with inflammatory cells.

MANIFESTATIONS. *Recurrent herpes simplex* is a circumscribed eruption, consisting of closely grouped, thin-walled vesicles on an erythematous base, which tends to recur repeatedly in the same area of the skin, particularly at mucocutaneous junctions. It begins as a mild itching or burning lesion which rapidly becomes papular and vesicular, and then passes successively through crusting, scab formation, and desiccation, the whole process taking 3 to 14 days. Typically, there is no fever, regional lymphadenopathy, or other signs of systemic illness. The disease is self-limited and is commonly identified with its anatomic location—herpes facialis, labialis, nasalis, progenitalis, or vulvovaginalis.

Herpetic keratoconjunctivitis (Chap. 228) is characterized usually by swelling and congestion of the conjunctiva, with superficial opacities in the cornea and a palpable preauricular lymph node. Bacterial cultures are sterile; hyperesthesia is a prominent sign. The presence of typical herpetic vesicles on the eyelids may aid in the diagnosis; however, the recurrent attacks are frequently confined to the cornea in the form of dendritic ulcers or, less often, as punctate, marginate, or discoform ulcers. The corneal ulcerations may persist for several weeks and respond poorly to local therapy; they are superficial, but repeated attacks pose a threat to vision.

Traumatic herpes designates those cases where the primary infection occurs at the site of a skin abrasion on the hand, elbow, finger, or other area not commonly associated with the disease. Recurrences have been observed at the same site over a period of many years.

Acute herpetic gingivostomatitis is the commonest form of primary infection and is seen most frequently in children one to four years of age, less often in adults. It is characterized by gradual or sudden onset, with fever, malaise, sore mouth and throat, and extreme irritability, sometimes alternating with lethargy. The temperature may reach 104°F, but is usually 101 to 103°F. Physical examination reveals multiple painful shallow aphthous ulcers on a red base on the buccal mucous membranes, tongue, or oropharynx. The gums are swollen, bleed easily, and are typically most inflamed at the gingival margin. The regional lymph nodes are large and tender. Fever and pain usually persist for 6 to 8 days, followed by gradual healing of the ulcers during the following week. The ulcers may be confined to, or appear first in, the pharynx (herpetic pharyngitis), and in such cases the diagnosis is commonly missed.

Eczema herpeticum (Kaposi's varicelliform eruption) is a rarer manifestation of primary infection which occurs in persons with eczema or neurodermatitis. Large areas of abnormal skin are involved, the grouped vesicles usually appearing in crops over a period of several days; hence the similarity to varicella. The temperature may reach 106°F, and marked prostration is not uncommon. The fever subsides during the second week, coincident with the crusting and healing of the skin lesions.

Meningoencephalitis was formerly thought to be a rare form of primary herpes in man, but complement fixation tests indicate that 5 to 7 percent of cases of aseptic meningitis may be due to this virus. It is accompanied by fever, headache, gastrointestinal symptoms, and signs of meningeal irritation and encephalitis. Patients with herpes encephalitis frequently manifest personality changes, bizarre behavior, hallucinations, and aphasia in the early stages of disease indicating localization in the temporal lobe.

In addition to the syndromes described above, herpes simplex has been known to occur in segmental nerve distribution simulating herpes zoster. The occurrence of repeated attacks in the same area is diagnostic.

Visceral herpes simplex, characterized by fulminating generalized infection with fever, viremia, and necrotic lesions in the liver and other viscera, and frequently terminating in death, is a clinical entity in newborn infants. Skin lesions are not always present. Most cases have been in premature infants or have occurred when the mother herself had a primary herpetic infection. In several cases the mother was known to have had repeated bouts of herpes vulvovaginitis.

LABORATORY FINDINGS. The total leukocyte count is usually normal or only slightly increased, with a normal differential. The diagnosis can be confirmed in the laboratory by (1) isolation and identification of the virus, (2) demonstration of typical eosinophilic intranuclear inclusions or fluorescence in tissue biopsy or vesicle fluid, or

(3) in primary infections, a rising titer of specific neutralizing antibodies. The acute phase serum should be collected before the fifth day of illness, because antibodies appear early. In central-nervous-system infection, the spinal fluid pressure and protein are slightly increased, and the sugar is normal. A pleocytosis up to 500 cells is observed; many polymorphonuclear leukocytes occur early, and change later to mononuclear cells; the virus may not be present in spinal fluid.

DIFFERENTIAL DIAGNOSIS. The history and clinical appearance of the recurrent skin and eye manifestations are usually sufficient to establish the diagnosis.

The laboratory tests enumerated above are confirmatory in doubtful cases and are essential for absolute diagnosis in the primary manifestations. Herpetic gingivostomatitis is often confused with Vincent's angina (Chap. 168), which responds dramatically to penicillin. Recurrent solitary aphthous ulcers in the mouth are not caused by herpes simplex.

In herpangina, caused by group A Coxsackie virus (Chap. 210), the vesicles are confined to the posterior part of the mouth, and the disease occurs in epidemics. Large bullae, recurrent attacks, and normal lymph nodes are seen in erythema multiforme (Chap. 400).

Eczema herpeticum may be easily confused with secondary bacterial infection of eczema. Extensive weeping and crusting may obscure the grouped vesicular nature of the lesion before the crusts are removed with wet dressings. Eczema vaccinatum (generalized vaccinia) (Chap. 223), usually presents with larger vesicles with a central indentation. Herpetic meningoencephalitis must be differentiated from bacterial and viral encephalitides, particularly enterovirus encephalitis, poliomyelitis, lymphocytic choriomeningitis, and postinfectious encephalitis. Early appearance of temporal lobe symptoms is suggestive.

TREATMENT. In early herpetic keratitis and dentritic ulcers, Idoxuridine (IDU) or other thymidine analogues are usually beneficial. Results are not so favorable if the stroma or iris is involved. Good results have also been reported with local application of interferon. Corticosteroids are usually contraindicated in herpes simplex eye infections, but may be helpful in stromal lesions and in herpes zoster lesions. Therapy of eye lesions should always be supervised by an ophthalmologist.

Parenteral thymidine analogues given early in encephalitis may be beneficial, but to achieve rapid confirmation of the diagnosis may require a brain biopsy and hence the frequency of temporal lobe symptoms is stressed.

Antibiotics may be helpful in controlling secondary bacterial infection. In acute gingivostomatitis, the maintenance of adequate hydration and nutrition is aided by the local application, before meals, of 1 percent Pontocaine. A detergent mouthwash helps to maintain oral hygiene and inhibits bacterial proliferation. In eczema herpeticum and visceral disease, supportive therapy, fluid replacement, blood transfusions, and appropriate antibacterial measures are indicated. Convalescent serum and γ-globulin have not been beneficial.

PROGNOSIS. Except for complications following infection of the cornea, recurrent herpes has few sequelae. The primary manifestations have a self-limited course except for meningoencephalitis and visceral disease, which are sometimes fatal, and eczema herpeticum, in which the mortality rate may be 20 percent.

REFERENCES

Dodd, K., J. Buddingh, and L. Johnston: Herpetic Stomatitis, Am. J. Dis. Child., 58:907, 1939.

Dohlman, C. H.: Annual Review—Cornea and Sclera, A.M.A. Arch. Ophthalmol., 71:249, 1964.

Dowdle, W. R., A. J. Nahmias, R. W. Harwell, and F. P. Pauls: Association of Antigenic Type of Herpesvirus Hominis with Site of Viral Recovery, J. Immunol., 99: 974, 1967.

Johnson, R. T., L. C. Olson, and E. L. Buescher: Problems in Laboratory Diagnosis of Herpes Simplex Infection of the Nervous System, Arch. Neurol., 18:260, 1968.

Lynch, F. W., C. A. Evans, V. S. Bolin, and R. J. Steves: Kaposi's Varicelliform Eruption: Extensive Herpes Simplex as a Complication of Eczema, Arch. Dermatol. Syphilol., 51:129, 1945.

Marshall, W. J. S.: Herpes Simplex Encephalitis Treated with Idoxuridine and External Decompression, Lancet, II:579, 1967.

Pauls, F. P., and W. R. Dowdle: A Serologic Study of Herpesvirus Hominis Strains by Microneutralization Tests, J. Immunol. 98:941, 1967.

Scott, T. F. McN.: Infection with the Virus of Herpes Simplex, New Engl. J. Med., 250:183, 1954.

Zuelzer, W., and C. Stuhlberg: Herpes Simplex Virus as the Cause of Fulminating Visceral Disease and Hepatitis in Infancy, A.M.A. J. Dis. Child., 83:421, 1952.

227 MINOR VIRAL DISEASES OF THE SKIN AND MUCOSAL SURFACES

Alvin E. Friedman-Kien

HERPANGINA

Herpangina is a specific, benign, infectious disease of childhood, although it is not uncommon in young adults. It is caused by Group A Coxsackie viruses types 2, 3, 4, 5, 6, 8, and 10. It occurs throughout the world in epidemic form, usually in the summer and early fall. Similar disorders have been attributed to ECHO and Coxsackie B viruses (Chap. 210).

The incubation period for herpangina is about 4 to 6 days. Children between the ages of one and seven are most commonly afflicted. Immunity persists for at least 1 year; reinfection with another strain of the virus can occur.

Herpangina is characterized by sudden onset of fever, temperatures often rising to 104°F, severe sore throat, nausea, and vomiting. Anorexia, dysphagia, excessive salivation, and severe malaise are common. The throat and posterior portions of the mouth are usually quite red and injected and are covered with numerous minute vesicles (1 to 2 mm in diameter), which quickly rupture, erode and enlarge to form 3 to 4 mm punched-out, shallow ulcers with grayish centers surrounded by deep red areolas. The number and size of the lesions increase for 2 to 3 days and heal within 4 or 5 days. The anterior faucial pillars of the pharynx, the tonsils, and the soft palate are usually involved. Occasionally, similar vesicles are found in the vaginal mucosa.

The systemic and local symptoms begin to regress within 4 to 5 days, and total recovery occurs within 7 days. Headache, coryza, and other respiratory tract symptoms are absent. Myalgia and arthralgia are rare. Mild cervical lymphadenopathy is sometimes noted. Parotitis and aseptic meningitis have been reported.

Recovery from the illness is always uneventful. Treatment is confined to topical symptomatic measures; frequent mouthwashes and gargles with topical anesthetics such as Benadryl elixir or butacaine are soothing. A fluid or soft diet is advisable. Demonstration of a Coxsackie virus from one of the vesicles, or isolation from pharyngeal washing and/or stool may be helpful, especially when combined with a demonstrable rise in antibody titer in the convalescent as compared to the acute serum.

Differential diagnosis should include a primary herpes simplex infection which may produce a severe oropharyngeal eruption. However, herpes does not usually occur in epidemics and the herpetic lesions are more typically confined to the anterior portions of the mouth, such as the lips and tongue. With herpes, the gingiva are typically red and edematous. Aphthous stomatitis, bacterial pharyngitis, and the oropharyngeal lesions of viral exanthems, such as chickenpox and measles, may be confused initially with herpangina. The natural course of the disease will help clarify the diagnosis.

FOOT-AND-MOUTH DISEASE

Foot-and-mouth disease is a fairly common epidemic viral disease of farm animals in Europe, Asia, and Africa. It is rarely known to affect man. The causative agent is the smallest virus known to infect animals. A few cases have been reported in children and adults who had been exposed by contact with an infected stock of animals, by ingestion of meat or dairy products, or from exposure to the hides or excretions of sick animals. The incubation period seems to range between 2 to 18 days. Multiloculated vesicles appear on the skin and mucous membranes. Intranuclear inclusion bodies have been observed in the epidermal cells at the base of the vesicles and in the surrounding tissue.

The onset of the infection is characterized by fever, headache, malaise, and dryness and burning sensation of the oral mucosa. Within 2 to 3 days loculated vesicles develop on the lips, tongue, and buccal mucosa. The palms and soles and interdigital skin may also show such lesions. Generalized pruritus may occur. The vesicles go on to develop into irregularly shaped, painful ulcers which may become edematous and bleed easily. At times either the mouth or the hands alone may be involved. Rarely,

other areas of the skin may be affected. The course of the disease is usually mild; the temperature falls rapidly, and the lesions begin to heal after 6 or 7 days. Total healing is complete by 2 to 3 weeks, leaving no scars.

Diagnostic confirmation depends upon a rise in specific complement-fixing antibody titers. The virus can be isolated in tissue cultures, guinea pigs, and chick embryos. In the United States, strict regulations of quarantine and meat inspection have limited the occurrence to a few outbreaks near the Mexican border. Treatment is symptomatic.

HAND, FOOT, AND MOUTH DISEASE

Hand, foot, and mouth disease represents a syndrome characterized by a vesicular eruption of the skin and the mouth. It has been reported to occur in epidemics in the United States, England, and Australia. Laboratory studies suggest that the disease is associated with Coxsackie A viruses, types 16, 5, and others. The infection occurs primarily in children. The disease is mild, running its course in 4 to 8 days. A transient, low-grade fever may be present at the onset. The most troublesome symptom is stomatitis. Initially vesicles appear in random distribution on the tongue, buccal mucosa, gingiva and palate, usually sparing the pharynx. These vesicles are few in number and are somewhat larger than those seen in herpangina. The vesicles quickly develop into shallow, whitish ulcerations with red areolas.

Lesions on the skin are not always present, but are typically vesicular, approximately 4 or 5 mm in size. They are characteristically few in number, ovoid or elongated in shape, grayish in color, surrounded by a fine, red margin. These vesicles appear on the dorsum of the fingers and especially about the periungual region and the heel margin. Occasionally vesicles may be found on the palms or soles. They usually start to disappear within a few days after onset. On rare occasions a more diffuse, vesicular eruption and exanthematous rash have been reported, with particular concentration of such lesions on the buttocks.

The differential diagnosis includes herpangina, aphthous stomatitis, and other Coxsackie and ECHO virus infections. The confirmation of the exact diagnosis depends upon viral and serologic studies.

VESICULAR STOMATITIS

Vesicular stomatitis is a viral illness of horses, cattle, and pigs, but it occasionally affects man. The disease occurs in the United States and South America. The mode of natural spread among livestock is unknown, but the disease is probably transmitted by direct and indirect contact. Epidemics do not occur in freezing weather, and it is therefore assumed that the virus is arthropod-borne in nature. The virus has been isolated from flies and mosquitoes. Two antigenically distinct viruses are known to cause the disease in the United States, the Indiana type and the New Jersey type. The incubation period is 2 to 6 days. In man the disease is mild and self-limited, the symptoms are similar to those of influenza. The virus has been studied and used extensively in experimental laboratories. Consequently, several cases have been reported in laboratory personnel as well as farm workers.

The sudden onset is characterized by fever up to 104°F, lasting 24 hr, chills, and profuse sweating. Myalgias, malaise, headache, and aching of the eyes are common. The symptoms are worse on the second day. One-third of the patients develop sore throats with cervical and submandibular adenopathy. The tongue and mucous membranes may become sore as well, and conjunctivitis may occur. In a few cases, small, subcorneal, intraepithelial vesicles appear on the fingers. Symptoms last only 3 to 4 days, but relapses can occur. Inapparent infections have been demonstrated by a rise of both complement-fixing and neutralizing serum antibodies in laboratory workers. Differential diagnosis must include hand, foot, and mouth disease, herpangina, and other mucocutaneous syndromes. Viral isolation from patients is rare, but the comparison of acute and convalescent sera in a suspected case will help to confirm the diagnosis.

WARTS (Verrucae)

Warts are an infectious disease of the skin and contiguous mucous membrane. The etiologic agent is a member of the Papova group of viruses that includes the animal papilloma viruses, the polyoma, simian vacuolating viruses, such as SV_{40} and SV_5. These viruses have been shown to induce tumors in experimental animals and to cause in vitro transformation of tissue cultures.

The human wart virus, which is a DNA virus measuring about 45 mμ in diameter, has been extracted from human lesions and has been used experimentally to induce the formation of warts at inoculated sites in the skin of human volunteers. The incubation period based on the experimental inoculations varies between 1 to 20 months, averaging about 4 months. The virus has been shown electronmicroscopically to parasitize the nuclei of epidermal cells. The successful isolation of the human wart virus in tissue culture has not been accomplished conclusively.

The skin lesions induced by the wart virus are due to an abnormal proliferation of epidermal cells. The lesions, which are skin-colored, may occur as single lesions or in multiples widely disseminated over the entire body. Although the same virus is thought to cause all varieties of human warts, the character of the lesion depends upon the local response of the affected skin to the virus host. Immunity may also play a role. For convenience, lesions are classified according to location and morphology.

Common warts (*verrucae vulgares*) are usually seen on the hands or under and about the fingernails. These lesions are rough surfaced, horny papules which can vary in size from 1 mm to 2 cm in diameter. Confluency of clustered lesions occurs frequently. The lesions are asymptomatic.

Plantar warts occur mostly beneath pressure points on the soles of the feet and are frequently quite painful. The surface lesions are flat, firm, stippled, and horny. They may occur individually or in a mosaiclike cluster. The mass of plantar warts is beneath the skin surface. These warts are generally larger than one might expect. They have conical shape, the pointed end projected inward. This configuration is probably due to the pressure imposed by walking. Plantar warts are most common in teenagers; females seem slightly more susceptible than males.

The differential diagnosis of plantar warts includes calluses and corns. The normal epidermal ridges are continuous across the surface of calluses and corns, whereas the surface of warts disrupts the normal pattern. Local foreign body reactions and congenital keratotic lesions of the palms and soles also have to be ruled out.

Flat warts (*verrucae planae*) are skin-colored, smooth, flat or slightly elevated, round or polygonal papules that vary between 1 and 5 mm in diameter. They almost always occur in multiples, up to several hundred. The common sites are the face, neck, chest, dorsum of the hands, flexor surface of the forearms, and shins. The mucous membranes are rarely involved. The surface of these lesions show a stippled appearance when examined under a magnifying glass. Flat warts are most frequently confused with the lesions of lichen planus. Multiple lesions on the dorsum of the hands may be mistaken for one of the inherited disorders known as acrokeratosis verruciformis, epidermodysplasia verruciformis, or Darier's disease.

Filiform warts are most frequently seen in adult males, and usually occur in the bearded area of the face. The lips and eyelids are often involved. The lesions are horny, fingerlike projections which may grow to considerable length if left unattended. They occur in multiples, but are seen occasionally as individual lesions. Differential diagnosis includes cutaneous horns.

Digitate warts are seen on the scalp of adults as clusters of fleshy fingerlike projections. They must be differentiated from epidermal nevi.

Condylomata acuminata (*moist warts*), also known as venereal or fig warts, are the lesions which occur at the mucocutaneous junctions of the skin in the genital and perianal areas. Rare cases have been seen about the areola of the nipple in females, the margins of the mouth, both the inguinal and axillary folds, and in the interdigital skin between the toes.

These warts are pink-to-red in color and moist and soft. They may be pedunculated or elongated. Clusters of these warts may resemble a cauliflower in appearance. They may occur in great numbers and can become macerated and malodorous because of their location. These warts are most often seen in young adults, but children as well as adults are affected. The eruption of moist warts is frequent and more severe in pregnancy. Although the lesions have been known to be transmitted between sexual partners, it is a misconception that these lesions are usually venereal in origin.

Condylomata acuminata, unlike other warts, are most effectively treated with the repeated topical application of a 25 percent podophyllum resin in tincture of benzoin. A single, persistent, fungating lesion on the penis, resistant to this treatment, should be biopsied to rule out a malignancy, such as squamous cell carcinoma or a rare, abnormal growth, known as the Buschke-Lowenstein tumor. The more sessile condylomata lesions of secondary syphilis may be confused with viral-induced and genital warts.

Warts often tend to recur, even after apparently adequate treatment. The variety of methods used for removal are primarily destructive, such as electrodesiccation and curettage, surgical excision, x-ray, or cryosurgery by applying liquid nitrogen or dry ice. Repeated paring of warts, followed by the application of caustic agents such as mono- or trichloracetic acid, salicylic acid, phenol, or silver nitrate is very helpful. It is important to avoid radical means of therapy, because all warts will eventually disappear spontaneously, leaving no scar, suggesting the development of an immune response. However, warts may persist and spread within the same host for several years.

ORF (Ecthyma Infectiosum)

Orf is an infectious disease which primarily affects the mouth and lips of sheep. It is caused by a specific virus which has been isolated in tissue culture. The disease is transmitted between animals and also from virus-contaminated, dried crusts of lesions found in grazing pastures. The virus may remain in an infective state for several months or years. The disease has a worldwide distribution. The mouths of young lambs are most often affected; infection confers lifelong immunity. Human infection occurs in shepherds, butchers, veterinarians, and children who play with sheep.

In man, the incubation period is about 5 to 6 days. The eruption may occur as single or multiple lesions on the hands and other exposed parts of the body. Initially, a small, reddish-blue papule appears and rapidly enlarges to form a 2 to 3 cm hemorrhagic bulla. Itching is intense and the bulla ruptures to form an umbilicated, erythematous ulcer which develops a gray-white crust. Systemic manifestations are rare, except for occasional low-grade fever and mild regional lymphangitis and lymphadenopathy. A transient macular and papular red rash may occur on the trunk during the second week of the disease. Spontaneous healing occurs within 3 to 6 weeks.

The disease should be suspected when the characteristic lesions develop in individuals exposed to sheep. The diagnosis can be confirmed by virus isolation in the laboratory as well as a comparative rise of antibody titers in acute and convalescent sera.

Differential diagnosis must include milkers' nodule, anthrax, tularemia, primary inoculation tuberculosis, and cowpox.

MILKERS' NODULE (Paravaccinia, Milkers' Warts)

Milkers' nodule is a benign, poxvirus disease contracted from infected cows. The disease has a worldwide distribution. Nodules and ulcers occur on the teats of infected dairy cattle. In man, lesions appear within 5 to 7 days after milking an infected cow. They usually occur on the hands, but other exposed parts of the body, such as the face, may be inoculated. The virus has been isolated in bovine kidney tissue culture and resembles the orf virus. The early, flat, dark red papules enlarge up to 1 to 2 cm in diameter within a week and develop into solid, elastic, shiny, brownish-purple, highly vascular nodules. No pus or fluid accumulates. The nodules may be slightly tender, and mild regional lymphadenopathy may occur. Mild temperature elevations have been reported. Gradually an opaque, gray, slightly depressed eschar develops over the surface of the nodules' red granulation tissue. The lesion is surrounded by an areola of erythema. Resolution occurs within 5 to 6 weeks without scarring. One infection provides permanent immunity. The virus can be isolated in tissue culture, but this is not a practical routine procedure. There is no cross immunity between milkers' nodule, cowpox, and vaccinia.

Differential diagnosis between milkers' nodule and warts may not be possible on clinical grounds. Pyogenic granuloma and cowpox should also be considered.

MOLLUSCUM CONTAGIOSUM

Molluscum contagiosum is an infectious disease of the skin and mucous membranes caused by one of the largest known viruses. It is limited to man and most frequently occurs in childhood. Although the virus has not been grown in the laboratory, it has been classified morphologically on the basis of electronmicroscopy with the pox group of viruses. No cross-antigenicity with other pox viruses has yet been demonstrated. The mode of transmission is unknown. The disease has a worldwide distribution and has occurred in epidemics within children's institutions, between wrestlers, and members of the same family. Infections have been transmitted between genitalia during sexual intercourse and from the mouth of a suckling baby to its mother's breast. Successful experimental inoculation of lesion extracts to the skin of human volunteers has been reported. The incubation period varies between 2 weeks and 2 months. Recent fluorescent-antibody and gel-diffusion immunologic studies have shown demonstrable antibody in the serum of infected individuals.

The lesions may vary in number and size, ranging from 1 mm up to "giant" lesions of 1 to 2 cm in diameter, and average about 4 mm. They are elevated, waxy, pearly white papules which show an umbilicated central pore. By squeezing such a papule, one can express from the pore a curdlike, cheesy material, which, upon electronmicroscopic examination, proves to be loaded with virus particles. Ordinary light microscopy smears of the curd show a specific diagnostic picture of clusters of cells containing eosinophilic, giant cytoplasmic inclusion bodies. The papules may appear alone or in groups. Autoinoculation is frequent; the lesions are usually present for 6 months to a year, but may persist and spread for 3 to 4 years. The face, especially the eyelids, the trunk, and anogenital areas are most commonly involved. The conjunctiva, lips, and buccal mucosa may rarely be involved.

Molluscum lesions are frequently traumatized and become secondarily infected, but injury seems to cause individual lesions to resolve. Spontaneous regression eventually occurs without scarring.

Treatment by sharp curettage clears up the lesions with little, if any, scarring.

Diagnosis of multiple lesions is fairly simple. A single lesion may be confused with a keratoacanthoma, basal cell epithelioma, or pyogenic granuloma. The diagnosis can be made histologically.

REFERENCES

Friedman-Kien, A. E., W. P. Rowe, W. G. Banfield: Milkers'

Nodule: Isolation of a Virus from a Human Case, Science, New York, 140:1335, 1963.

Friedman-Kien, A. E., and J. Vilcek: Induction of Interference and Interferon Synthesis by Non-replicating Molluscum Contagiosum Virus, J. Immunol., 99:1092, 1967.

Huebner, R. J., R. M. Cole, E. A. Beeman, J. A. Bell, and J. H. Peers: Herpangina: Etiological Studies of a Specific Infectious Disease, J.A.M.A., 145:628, 1951.

Kibrick, S.: Current Status of Coxsackie and ECHO Viruses in Human Disease, Progr. Med. Virol., 6:27, 1964.

Nagington, J., and C. H. Whittle: Human Orf: Isolation of the Virus by Tissue Culture, Brit. Med. J., 2:1324, 1961.

Patterson, W. C., L. O. Mott, and E. W. Jenney: A Study of Vesicular Stomatitis in Man, J. Am. Vet. Med. Ass., 133: 57, 1958.

Section 18

Viral Diseases of the Eye

228   VIRAL INFECTIONS OF THE EYE

J. T. Grayston

The eye and its adnexal tissues may be secondarily infected during the course of many cutaneous and systemic viral diseases. Sometimes, these infections lead only to minor disturbances, examples of which are transient loss of pupillary accommodation in dengue, and inflammatory lesions of the eyelid and conjunctiva in chickenpox and pharyngoconjunctival fever. However, serious and permanent visual disorders can result if the cornea is infected with viruses such as herpes simplex, herpes zoster, vaccinia, or smallpox. In addition, congenital rubella is an important cause of cataracts and microphthalmos, and cytomegalic inclusion disease may involve the retina and the other ocular tissues.

The diseases described in this chapter are caused by microorganisms that characteristically produce localized eye lesions without infecting other tissues. Although they are mainly of concern to ophthalmologists, they sometimes enter into the differential diagnosis of systemic disorders that involve the eye. Knowledge of the epidemiology of the diseases will aid in their recognition.

TRACHOMA AND INCLUSION CONJUNCTIVITIS (Inclusion Blennorrhea)

DEFINITION. Trachoma remains the world's most important cause of blindness and loss of sight. It has been estimated that there are 500 million cases of trachoma throughout the world. Inclusion conjunctivitis is a self-limited disease that is often not diagnosed. It occurs both in the developed western countries and in underdeveloped tropical areas.

ETIOLOGY. Although the agents that cause these diseases are obligate, intracellular microorganisms, they are not true viruses because they have cell walls with chemical and metabolic properties similar to bacteria and are affected by broad-spectrum antibiotics. They are closely related to the agents of psittacosis and lymphogranuloma venereum. The organisms causing *TR*achoma and *I*nclusion *C*onjunctivitis (now called *TRIC* agents) are virtually indistinguishable in the laboratory. They grow only in the epithelium of the eye and the genital tract. By formation of inclusion bodies they can be identified in Giemsa-stained smears of conjunctival cells obtained from scrapings. The organisms may be isolated and grown in the yolk sacs of embryonated chicken eggs. Only primates are susceptible to eye infections with these organisms. They do not grow in mice or other laboratory animals. High-titer yolk sac material produces death in mice following intravenous injection, and can be prevented by prior immunization. This forms the basis of a mouse toxicity prevention test that permits classification of the organisms into several serologic groups.

EPIDEMIOLOGY. Trachoma is now a rare eye disease in the United States. The only important endemic focus remains in the Indians of the Southwest. Acute relapse of old trachoma may be seen occasionally following treatment with cortisone eye ointment. The disease has been most prevalent and severe in North Africa, Egypt, the Middle East, and northern India. It is prevalent in China and southeast Asia in a milder form which is characterized by prolonged low-grade activity and a relatively high incidence of late sequelae. Transmission of the disease in endemic areas is probably through close personal contact. Although hot, dry, dusty, climate and abundant flies have been implicated in the epidemiology of the disease, their role may be primarily to promote seasonal bacterial conjunctivitis and to contribute to destruction of the eye once the normal physiologic function of the lid is upset by trachoma scar formation.

CLINICAL MANIFESTATIONS. Initially, trachoma is a follicular conjunctivitis that is not different from many other follicular conjunctivitises. Epithelial keratitis is present during active disease. As the disease progresses there is pannus formation, infiltration of leukocytes, and ingrowth of new blood vessels into the cornea. These findings along with the more mature neurotic follicles permit the clinical diagnosis of trachoma. Healing of the follicles leaves characteristic scars in the conjunctiva and if severe, leads to distortion of the lid and to contractures. The lid margins may be inverted (entropion) and some eyelashes turned inward (trichiasis). Abnormal dryness (xerosis) may result from loss of secretory cells. Ingrowth of vessels may continue until the cornea is completely covered (*pannus totalis*). Loss of sight or complete blindness may be due to trauma and bacterial infections resulting from the distorted lid and dry conjunctivas or from the pannus.

DIAGNOSIS. The diagnosis is usually established on clinical grounds alone. While not difficult, demonstration of typical inclusion bodies in smears requires some experience to avoid confusion with many artifacts. In chronic inactive disease, inclusions are rare. While isolation of the organism is feasible in the acute stage, it is often unsuccessful in chronic disease. There is no useful serologic test in diagnosis. There is a tendency to over-diagnose trachoma both in endemic countries and in Westerners. Follicular conjunctivitis in Americans exposed in endemic countries is very rarely trachoma.

TREATMENT. Broad-spectrum antibiotics and sulfonamides are effective both in vitro and in vivo. Prolonged therapy usually is required to effect a cure of chronic trachoma. Reinfection, and perhaps relapse, is common in endemic areas. Tetracycline eye ointments have been used most extensively. Administration two to four times a day for 6 weeks often will result in a cure. Intermittent therapy with topical applications two times a day for 1 week each month for 6 months has been proposed as a more effective regimen. Erythromycin has also been used successfully in eye ointments. Sulfonamides have been used both orally and topically. Except for their toxicity, long-acting sulfonamides would be ideal for treatment in endemic countries. Combined oral sulfonamides and tetracycline eye ointment have been effective in curing the acute disease following experimental or laboratory infections. Because of reinfection, inadequate length of treatment, or suboptimal dosage, most treatment campaigns in countries with endemic trachoma have failed to reduce the disease significantly. Surgical repair of entropion with or without trichiasis is a useful method of decreasing the risk of visual loss.

PREVENTION. Since the organism was first isolated in 1957, there have been efforts to develop an effective vaccine. Experimental vaccines have produced short-term prevention of infection, but vaccines effective for general use are not available. General hygienic measures associated with improved living standards are effective in the elimination of trachoma.

INCLUSION CONJUNCTIVITIS

While trachoma seems to be spread from eye to eye, genital transmission of inclusion conjunctivitis has been recognized. Inclusion blennorrhea of the newborn may be differentiated from neonatal gonococcal ophthalmia by its longer incubation period (5 to 14 days versus 1 to 3 days). It invariably has an acute onset with profuse mucopurulent exudate. There may be pseudomembrane formation. In older children and adults there is prominent follicular formation in the conjunctivas. These follicles do not develop the neurotic changes seen in trachoma. The illness lasts weeks in infants or a few months in adults and does not involve pannus formation or residual conjunctival scars. Topical tetracycline therapy for 2 weeks promptly controls the disease.

A clinical form of inclusion conjunctivitis intermediate between trachoma, with punctate keratitis and micropannus, has been described in adults.

Inclusion conjunctivitis often is associated with venereal infection. Clinical conjunctivitis seems to be relatively rare, while transmission of the organism by the venereal route is not uncommon. Genital-tract disease also may be caused by TRIC agents, but they can also be isolated from normal genital tracts. The importance of TRIC agents in the etiology of nongonococcal urethritis and of cervicitis is unknown.

EPIDEMIC KERATOCONJUNCTIVITIS (EKC)

EKC is an infectious conjunctivitis with characteristic subepithelial punctate keratitis that is endemic in the Near and Far East with yearly seasonal outbreaks. The disease was unknown in the continental United States until its introduction from Hawaii during the Second World War, at which time there were large outbreaks among shipyard workers. The disease has been recognized sporadically in sailors returning from the Orient. The etiologic agent of the epidemic disease is adenovirus type 8, which may produce more serious ocular disease than the adenoviruses that cause pharyngoconjunctival fever (Chap. 206). Several other adenovirus types cause EKC but have not been associated with epidemics. In the United States, EKC occurs mainly in localized outbreaks around ophthalmologists' offices and eye clinics. This is because solutions used for sterilization of instruments do not kill the hardy adenovirus. The incubation period varies from 5 to 10 days. The disease begins unilaterally with mild or severe follicular conjunctivitis which is often associated with pseudomembrane formation and sometimes with iritis and subconjunctival hemorrhages. Transient fever, headache, and malaise are the only systemic manifestations. The preauricular lymph node on the affected side is usually enlarged. Within a few days, the cornea becomes inflamed, with resultant pain, lacrimation, photophobia, and blurred vision. The contralateral eye is involved several days after the original in about 50 percent of cases. Subepithelial punctate corneal opacities in the central area without ulceration appear 1 to 3 weeks after onset and, rarely, may persist for years. They result in surprisingly little impairment of visual acuity. Milder infections have been recognized among family contacts of affected individuals, but the incidence of secondary cases is generally low. There is no specific therapy. The disease is self-limited. Epidemics can be controlled by adequate sterilization of ocular instruments, by boiling them for 10 minutes, and strict sanitation of common use facilities in factories.

NEWCASTLE DISEASE

Human infection with this avian virus, which is related to influenza, occurs mainly in poultry workers and virologists. In man, accidental introduction of contaminated material into the eye is followed in 24 to 72 hr by conjunctivitis, edema of the lids, and profuse lacrimation. The cornea is not involved, and photophobia is unusual.

Constitutional symptoms are absent or mild. Recovery is complete in 10 to 14 days. The diagnosis may be confirmed by virus isolation in embryonated eggs.

REFERENCES

Grayston, J. T., Y. F. Yang, P. B. Johnston, and L. S. Ko: Epidemic Keratoconjunctivitis on Taiwan, Am. J. Trop. Med. Hyg., 13:492, 1964.

Hanna, L. (Chairman, program committee): "Conference on Trachoma and Allied Diseases." Am. J. Ophthalmol., 63: 1027, 1967.

Jawetz, E.: The Story of Shipyard Eye, Brit. Med. J., 1:873, 1959.

———, and P. Thygeson: Trachoma and Inclusion Conjunctivitis Agents, p. 1042 in "Viral and Rickettsial Infections of Man," Horsfall and Tamm, 4th ed., Philadelphia, J. B. Lippincott Company, 1965.

Nelson, C. B., B. S. Pomeroy, K. Schroll, W. E. Park, and R. J. Lindeman: Outbreak of Conjunctivitis Due to Newcastle Disease Virus (NDV) Occurring in Poultry Workers, Am. J. Public Health, 42:672, 1952.

Section 19

Viral Diseases Affecting Lymphoid Tissue

229 LYMPHOGRANULOMA VENEREUM

Albert Heyman

DEFINITION. Lymphogranuloma venereum is an infectious disease usually transmitted by sexual contact and characterized by a small primary lesion, regional lymphadenitis, and constitutional symptoms. The disease is known by a variety of names, such as *lymphogranuloma inguinale, lymphopathia venereum,* and *climatic bubo,* but the name generally preferred is *lymphogranuloma venereum.* This disease should not be confused with granuloma inguinale, an ulcerative infection of the skin caused by the Donovan body (Chap. 164).

ETIOLOGY. The etiologic agent of lymphogranuloma venereum is closely related to that of psittacosis (Chap. 209). When stained by special methods, the organisms can be seen with the ordinary microscope as small spherical granules or elementary bodies. The agent is also distinctive in that it is susceptible to sulfonamide therapy. It produces meningoencephalitis in mice and monkeys and can be cultured in the yolk sac of the chick embryo. Infected yolk sac tissues are used as diagnostic antigens for intradermal (Frei) tests and complement fixation reactions. There are serologic cross reactions, however, with psittacosis and certain other agents (meningopneumonitis, feline pneumonitis).

INCIDENCE. Lymphogranuloma venereum exists in almost every part of the world but is especially prevalent in tropical and subtropical countries. It is frequently seen in the southeastern portion of the United States, particularly among Negroes. There is no accurate information regarding the incidence of the disease. Only 625 new cases were reported in the United States in 1966, but it is likely that the incidence is much higher. An increased incidence has been noted recently in American soldiers returning from Southeast Asia.

PATHOGENESIS. Lymphogranuloma venereum is nearly always transmitted by sexual contact. The incubation period varies from 2 to 30 days. A small evanescent lesion may appear at the site of inoculation, but more often the first sign of the infection is inflammation and suppuration of the inguinal lymph nodes. The virus is apparently disseminated throughout the body by way of the bloodstream; it has been isolated from the primary lesion, the regional lymph nodes, the blood, and the spinal fluid. Severe systemic manifestations, such as meningoencephalitis, keratitis, cutaneous lesions, and arthritis may occur. Specific evidence of immunity to the virus, including skin sensitivity of the tuberculin type, and complement-fixing humoral antibodies, can be demonstrated in almost every patient shortly after the onset of the disease. Positive skin and complement fixation reactions persist for several years. Patients with lymphogranuloma venereum frequently have an increase in serum globulin concentrations.

Following the initial infection, the patient may remain asymptomatic for a long period of time but may eventually develop late manifestations of the disease, such as rectal strictures or elephantiasis of the genitalia.

The early histologic lesion of lymphogranuloma venereum consists of a granuloma forming about a small blood vessel and composed of large mononuclear cells. The vessel is eventually compressed and obliterated, and necrosis occurs in the center of the granuloma. The "stellate" abscesses which are formed in this manner are characteristic of the fully developed acute lesions of this disease.

CLINICAL MANIFESTATIONS. The initial lesion of lymphogranuloma venereum is seldom noted because it is transitory and inconspicuous. Those which are observed consist of single, small, shallow ulcerations on the external genitalia. Shortly after the appearance of the initial lesion there are enlargement and suppuration of the regional lymph nodes. The usual site is the inguinal or femoral region, and this lymphadenitis is called the *bubo*. The typical lymphogranuloma bubo develops slowly, is bilateral, and forms an ill-defined, lobulated mass. Suppuration usually follows, producing multilocular areas of fluctuation which may rupture spontaneously, forming one or more draining fistulas.

The majority of patients with buboes show constitutional reactions: headache, malaise, fever, and anorexia. Occasionally the virus causes inflammation of distant areas, and "aseptic meningitis," pericarditis, and conjunctivitis have been observed. Generalized skin eruptions and arthritis have also been described; these apparently have been provoked occasionally by the performance of skin tests for the disease.

Many years after the onset of the infection, the patient may develop a proctitis associated with rectal bleeding and a purulent discharge. Eventually there is scar formation, and a complete fibrous ring may develop, producing a *rectal stricture*, which may necessitate colostomy. Rectal lesions are found predominantly in women and are the result of the lymphatic drainage from the posterior part of the vulva and the vagina into the perirectal and retroperitoneal lymph nodes. In the male the lymph vessels drain from the penis to the inguinal area and thence to the deep iliac nodes.

Another late complication of lymphogranuloma venereum is elephantiasis of the external genitalia. This is known as *esthiomene* and is caused by interference with lymphatic drainage. Ulceration is frequent, and secondary infection may cause marked destruction of the genitalia.

DIAGNOSIS. Isolation of the virus is the most accurate means of diagnosis, but it is too laborious for general use. The diagnosis is usually based upon the clinical findings, together with a positive intradermal test and complement fixation reaction. Commercial antigens are available for these. A positive skin (Frei) test is of limited value, as it merely indicates that the patient has been infected with the virus at some previous time. In a recently acquired infection, the complement fixation test will usually be positive in a high titer (1:80 to 1:640). Furthermore, a change in the titer of circulating antibodies may be found in successive tests. Biopsy of the primary lesion or of a lymph node should be done whenever feasible because the histologic picture is sufficiently characteristic to permit a diagnosis and to differentiate this disease from other venereal infections.

TREATMENT. Sulfonamide therapy has been the standard treatment of the early manifestations of lymphogranuloma venereum. Sulfadiazine, in doses of 4 Gm a day for 2 to 3 weeks, usually results in disappearance of symptoms and lesions. The tetracyclines (500 mg every 6 hr) have also been found to be of value in the treatment of buboes, draining sinuses, and early proctitis, and seem to be as effective as the sulfonamides. There is evidence to suggest that sulfonamide therapy may not destroy the virus completely and that it may persist in the body after the acute infection has subsided. The late manifestations of the disease, such as rectal stricture and elephantiasis, do not usually respond to any form of medication, and treatment is chiefly surgical. Buboes which have become fluctuant should be aspirated to prevent spontaneous rupture and subsequent sinus formation.

REFERENCES

Abrams, A. J.: Lymphogranuloma Venereum, J.A.M.A., 205: 199, 1968.

Favre, M., and S. Hellerstrom: The Epidemiology, Aetiology and Prophylaxis of Lymphogranuloma Inguinale, Acta Dermato-Venereol., 34-Suppl., 30:1, 1954.

Heyman, A.: The Clinical and Laboratory Differentiation between Chancroid and Lymphogranuloma Venereum, Am. J. Syph., Gonor., Vener. Dis., 30:279, 1946.

Koteen, H.: Lymphogranuloma Venereum, Medicine, 24:1, 1945.

Sigel, M. M.: "Lymphogranuloma Venereum," Coral Gables, Fla., University of Miami Press, 1962.

230 CAT-SCRATCH DISEASE
Ivan L. Bennett, Jr. and Robert G. Petersdorf

DEFINITION. Cat-scratch disease is an infection characterized by indolent, occasionally suppurative, regional lymphadenitis, secondary to a primary cutaneous lesion at the site of inoculation, usually a minor trauma. Because more than 90 percent of the reported cases have originated from cat scratches and a history of close contact with cats is often elicited, the name *cat-scratch disease* has become popular. However, a similar disorder has been acquired from splinters, thorns, beef-bone fragments, etc., and in a fair percentage of patients no inciting trauma is recalled. Other names such as *nonbacterial regional lymphadenitis* or *benign inoculation reticulosis* have been suggested but have not been widely used.

ETIOLOGY. A specific etiologic agent has not been identified. Bacterial cultures of involved nodes are uniformly negative. The disease has been transmitted by inoculation of pus from suppurating nodes into monkeys and man, but these studies have not been confirmed, and numerous attempts to isolate a virus have failed. Intranuclear and intracytoplasmic inclusions are occasionally seen in histologic preparations of infected nodes but are absent in most specimens. Complement-fixing antibodies for lymphogranuloma venereum antigen are demonstrated in serums of about 25 percent of patients with this disease, suggesting that a virus related to the lymphogranuloma-psittacosis group may be the causative agent. Photochromogenic acid-fast bacilli have been reported to cause suppurative lymphadenitis in children, and it may be that anonymous mycobacteria are responsible for some cases of cat-scratch disease (Chap. 176).

EPIDEMIOLOGY. Careful observation of cats thought to be responsible for the disease has revealed no evidence of illness; these animals do not react to intradermal injection of antigen. These facts, together with evidence that other forms of trauma transmit the disease, indicate that the infecting agent is simply transmitted passively by the cat's claws or, perhaps, its excreta. Cats may act as long-term carriers, a hypothesis supported by the familial occurrence of several infections interspersed by months or years.

PATHOLOGY. The histopathologic appearance of lymph nodes has three characteristics: (1) Early lesions show reticulum cells hyperplasia; (2) intermediate lesions show granuloma formation; and (3) late lesions show microabscesses. These reactions are not readily distinguished from those induced by the tubercle bacillus. However, acid-fast bacilli are invariably absent.

MANIFESTATIONS. The incubation period is from a few days to several weeks. Systemic symptoms are usually mild, consisting of headache, fever, and malaise, which subside within a few days. Shaking chills and fever as high as 104°F can occur but are unusual. A transient macular or vesicular rash which subsides within 48 hr is rarely present during the early stages. Erythema nodosum and multiforme have been reported.

In a typical case the *primary* lesion consists of a raised, slightly tender papule crowned by a small vesicle or eschar; it often resembles an indolent furuncle or insect bite. Multiple primary lesions have been described. Some patients do not exhibit a lesion.

Regional adenopathy becomes evident in a few days or as long as 6 weeks after infection. The axillary and epitrochlear, femoral, or (most commonly) the cervical nodes on one side become visibly swollen and tender, often with redness of the overlying skin. The nodes occasionally suppurate, soften, and drain spontaneously; fistulas heal completely with only slight scaring. Usually the tenderness subsides gradually, and nontender, firm, enlarged nodes remain palpable for some weeks or even months. There is no generalized glandular enlargement, and the spleen is not palpable.

It seems probable that clinical forms of this infectious disease other than that described above may be delineated. A few cases of *encephalitis* associated with localized adenopathy and a positive skin test have been reported. European authors have suggested that *nonspecific*

mesenteric lymphadenitis in children is an abdominal form of cat-scratch disease, and in at least one reported case a previously negative skin test became positive after an illness diagnosed at laparotomy as mesenteric adenitis. A number of cases of so-called "Parinaud's oculoglandular syndrome," characterized by conjunctivitis and regional lymphadenopathy and previously thought to be due to infection by *Leptothrix*, have been reported to show positive skin tests for cat-scratch disease. Evidence for a primary *pulmonary* form is scant but suggestive, and at least two cases of possible bone involvement in the form of osteolytic foci have been described. Thrombocytopenic purpura has also been reported as a complication of this disease.

DIAGNOSIS. The following criteria should be fulfilled before a diagnosis of cat-scratch disease is established: (1) regional lymphadenopathy, (2) history of contact with cats, (3) positive intradermal skin test, (4) biopsy of lymph node with demonstration of histopathologic changes consistent with cat-scratch disease (this may not be necessary if the skin test is positive), and (5) failure to demonstrate other possible causative agents.

Specific diagnosis is made by means of a skin test. Antigen for this is prepared from pus aspirated from infected lymph nodes; it is inactivated by heating at 60°C for 2 hr and for 1 hr on the succeeding day. A positive reaction is of the delayed, tuberculin type, appearing in 24 to 48 hr. Patients in this country have reacted to antigens prepared from European countries, and vice versa—evidence that the disease is widespread and that strain differences in skin-test antigens are not significant. Skin reactivity to the antigen persists for at least 4 years and is probably permanent.

The skin test has several limitations: (1) Each batch of antigen must be tested against patients known to have had the disease; (2) different batches of antigen differ in potency; (3) the antigen may deteriorate with time; (4) approximately 10 percent of normal individuals have false positive reactions; (5) there is a remote chance of carrying hepatitis virus in the antigen. An alternative diagnostic test which has some promise requires incubation of the patient's blood with standard skin-test antigen. A decrease in leukocytes (cytolysis) is evidence for a positive test.

Other laboratory abnormalities include mild leukocytosis (up to 15,000), mild eosinophilia, and elevated sedimentation rate. The Frei test is negative.

Cat-scratch disease is a benign illness, and the prognosis is uniformly good. Its main clinical importance lies in its possible confusion with other more serious diseases of the lymphatics. Diseases to be considered are tularemia, lymphatic tuberculosis, sporotrichosis, lymphogranuloma venereum, and bacterial adenitis. Because of the indolent character of the adenopathy, Hodgkin's disease or other lymphomas may be suspected. Appropriate serologic and cultural tests serve to rule out other infections; biopsy may be needed to exclude tumor, but a positive skin test with cat-scratch antigen effectively rules out the necessity for such procedures.

TREATMENT. In instances of node suppuration, aspiration of accumulated pus affords relief of pain (and incidentally, serves as a source of material for the preparation of skin-test antigen). Penicillin and streptomycin are ineffective. Tetracycline drugs sometimes shorten the course of the disease, but their effect is usually not dramatic.

REFERENCES

Boyd, G. L., and G. Craig: Etiology of Cat-scratch Fever, Pediatrics, 59:313, 1961.

Brooksaler, F. S., and S. E. Sulkin: Cat-scratch Disease, Postgrad Med., 36:366, 1964.

Daniels, W. B., and F. G. MacMurray: Cat-scratch Disease, Report of 160 Cases, J.A.M.A., 154:1247, 1954.

Margileth, A. M.: Cat-scratch Disease as a Cause of Oculoglandular Syndrome of Parinaud, Pediatrics, 20:1000, 1957.

Rice, J. E., and R. M. Hyde: Rapid Diagnostic Method For Cat-scratch Disease, J. Lab. Clin. Med., 71:166, 1968.

Stevens, H.: Cat-scratch Fever Encephalitis, A.M.A. J. Dis. Child., 84:218, 1952.

Section 20

Other Systemic Viral Diseases

231 MUMPS
Robert G. Petersdorf

DEFINITION. Mumps is an acute communicable disease of viral origin characterized by painful enlargement of the salivary glands, and, sometimes, particularly in adults, involvement of the gonads, meninges, and pancreas.

ETIOLOGY. The causative agent of mumps is a virus of intermediate size which has been classified among the myxoviruses; serologic cross reactions have been demonstrated between it and some other members of this group. The virus of mumps causes agglutination of erythrocytes of certain species, produces hemolysis, and has two components capable of fixing complement, the soluble, or S, and the viral, or V, antigens. It elicits a delayed allergic reaction when used as an antigen in persons who have had mumps. The virus can be cultivated in the chick embryo and propagated in tissue cultures of HeLa cells and monkey kidney cells. In general, tissue cultures are a more sensitive means of isolating mumps virus than are chick embryos.

EPIDEMIOLOGY. Man is the only natural host for mumps. The disease is worldwide and is endemic in urban communities. Epidemics are relatively infrequent and are confined to closely associated groups who live in orphanages, army camps, or schools. The disease is most frequent in spring, and occurrence is highest in April and May. Although mumps is generally considered less "contagious" than the common exanthems, measles and chickenpox, this difference may be more apparent than real because most mumps infections tend to be inapparent clinically, at least in children, and 80 percent of an adult population had serologic evidence of previous infection with mumps.

Infections are rare before the age of two and then increase rapidly in frequency, reaching a peak at age six to ten. Clinical mumps may be more common in males than in females. Adults are usually infected through direct contact. In North American cities, most infections are contracted from schoolmates and infected family members. The virus is transmitted in infected salivary secretions, although its isolation from urine suggests that the virus may spread via this route. Mumps virus is rarely cultured from stools. The saliva is infectious for approximately 6 days prior to the onset of parotitis, and virus has been cultured for as long as 2 weeks after onset of swelling. Viruria also persists for several weeks in some patients. Despite this prolonged secretion, epidemiologic evidence suggests that the peak of infectivity occurs a day or two before onset of parotitis and subsides rapidly after appearance of glandular enlargement.

One attack of clinical or subclinical mumps confers lasting immunity, and second attacks are most unusual. Unilateral parotitis affords protection just as effectively as does bilateral disease.

PATHOGENESIS. The virus enters via the oral route; during the incubation period of 18 to 21 days, it presumably multiplies in the salivary glands, from which it is disseminated via the bloodstream to other organs, including the meninges, gonads, pancreas, breasts, thyroid, heart, liver, kidneys, and cranial nerves. An alternative, but less likely, hypothesis is that salivary adenitis is secondary to viremia and that the primary locus of multiplication is elsewhere in the respiratory tract.

MANIFESTATIONS. Salivary adenitis. The onset of parotitis is usually sudden, although it may be preceded by a prodromal period of malaise, anorexia, chilly sensations, feverishness, sore throat, and tenderness at the angle of the jaw. In many cases, however, parotid swelling is the first indication of illness. The swollen gland extends from the ear to the lower portion of the mandibular ramus and to the inferior portion of the zygomatic arch. The skin over the gland may be red, hot, and taut, and there may be reddening and pouting of the orifice of Stensen's duct. There are often considerable pain and tenderness, although at times these are absent. The edema of mumps has been described as "gelatinous," and when the involved gland is tweaked, it rolls like jelly. Swelling may involve the submaxillary and sublingual glands, and may extend over the anterior chest, as "presternal edema." Swelling of the glottis occurs rarely but may require tracheostomy. Parotitis is bilateral in two-thirds of cases and remains confined to one side in the remainder. The second gland tends to swell as the first is subsiding, usually 4 to 5 days after onset. In general, parotitis is accompanied by fever of 100 to 103°F, malaise, headache, and anorexia, but systemic symptoms may be virtually absent, particularly in children. In most patients the chief complaints refer to difficulty in eating, swallowing, and talking.

Orchitis. Mumps is complicated by orchitis in 20 percent of postpubertal males. Testicular involvement usually appears 7 to 10 days after onset of parotitis, although it may precede it or appear simultaneously. Occasionally, orchitis occurs in the absence of parotitis. Gonadal involvement is unilateral in approximately 75 percent of patients. Orchitis is heralded by recrudescence of malaise and appearance of chilly sensations, headache, nausea, and vomiting. Shaking chills and high fevers with temperatures between 103 and 106°F are frequent. The testicle becomes greatly swollen and exquisitely painful. The epididymis is often palpable as a swollen tender cord. Occasionally there may be epidydimitis without orchitis. Swelling, pain, and tenderness persist for 3 to 7 days and gradually subside; lysis of fever usually parallels abatement of swelling. Occasionally, the temperature falls by crisis. Mumps orchitis is followed by progressive atrophy of the testicle in one-half the cases. Even after bilateral orchitis, sterility is unusual, provided no significant atrophy has taken place. However, if bilateral testicular atrophy occurs after mumps, sterility or subnormal sperm counts are quite common. Pulmonary infarction has been noted to follow mumps orchitis. This may be the result of thrombosis of the veins in the prostatic and pelvic plexuses in association with the testicular inflammation. Priapism is a rare but painful complication of mumps orchitis.

Pancreatitis. Pancreatic involvement is a potentially serious manifestation of mumps, which may rarely be complicated by shock or pseudocyst formation. It should be suspected in patients with abdominal pain and tenderness, and clinical or epidemiologic evidence of mumps. It is difficult to document, since hyperamylasemia, the hallmark of pancreatitis, is also often present in parotitis. Many times the symptoms resemble those of gastroenteritis, and it is conceivable that the high incidence of gastrointestinal symptoms seen in association with the mumps epidemic in Great Britain in 1961 was due to involvement of the pancreas. Although diabetes or pancreatic insufficiency rarely follows mumps pancreatitis, several children have developed "brittle," diabetes, i.e., difficult to manage, within a few weeks after mumps.

Central Nervous System Involvement. Nearly half the patients with mumps have an increased number of cells, usually lymphocytes, in the cerebrospinal fluid, although symptoms of meningitis, stiff neck, headache, and drowsi-

ness are less common. Mumps should be recognized as capable of presenting a picture of mild paralytic poliomyelitis; definition of the cause depends on isolation of virus from the cerebrospinal fluid or serologic confirmation of mumps in the absence of changing antibody titers to poliomyelitis viruses. Rarely mumps may cause a fulminating encephalitis, transverse myelitis, or the Guillain-Barré syndrome. Although meningitis may occur in association with parotitis, it is often the sole manifestation of mumps virus infection, and some 10 to 15 percent of cases of aseptic meningitis in the United States are caused by mumps virus. Mumps meningitis is benign, and the only significant residuum, nerve deafness, is rare, and tends to be unilateral.

OTHER MANIFESTATIONS. Mumps virus tends to involve glandular tissues; inflammation of the lacrimal glands, thymus, thyroid, breasts, and ovaries occurs occasionally. *Oöphoritis* may be recognized by persistence of pain in the lower part of the abdomen and fever. It does not result in sterility. Mumps virus has been implicated in the causation of subacute *thyroiditis;* 10 of 11 patients who acquired this illness at a time when the incidence of mumps was high gave serologic evidence of infection with mumps virus, and mumps virus was isolated from the thyroid gland in two cases. A case of myxedema following mumps thyroiditis has been reported. Ocular manifestations of mumps include dacryoadenitis, optic neuritis, keratitis, iritis, conjunctivitis, and episcleritis. Although these conditions interfere with vision transiently, complete resolution is the rule. Mumps *myocarditis* evidenced primarily by transient abnormalities in the electrocardiogram is relatively common, but does not produce symptomatic disease or impair cardiac function. Similarly, *hepatic* involvement may be manifested by mild abnormalities in liver function, but icterus and other clinical signs of hepatic damage are extremely rare. *Thrombocytopenic purpura* as a complication of mumps has been described, and an occasional patient has a leukemoid reaction involving predominantly lymphocytes.

A rare but interesting manifestation of mumps is *polyarthritis*. It is most common in males between the ages of twenty and thirty. Joint symptoms begin 1 to 2 weeks after subsidence of parotitis, and usually the large joints are involved. The illness lasts about 6 weeks, and complete recovery is the rule. It is not clear whether arthritis is due to viremia or whether it is a "hypersensitivity reaction."

Acute hemorrhagic glomerulonephritis in the absence of streptococcosis has been reported after mumps. The relationship of these two diseases is not clear.

LATE COMPLICATIONS. With the exception of the rare cases of encephalitis, myelitis, or polyneuritis which follow mumps, and the occasional patient who is sterile following bilateral testicular involvement or who develops nerve deafness, mumps leaves no sequelae. There is no firm evidence that stillbirths and offspring with congenital defects are more common among mothers who have mumps during pregnancy. However, the finding that infants with endocardial fibroelastosis have positive mumps skin tests (but no serologic or virologic evidence of mumps infection), raises the question of intrauterine infection, as well as the possible causal relationship of mumps virus to this lesion.

LABORATORY FINDINGS. In uncomplicated parotitis, the blood leukocyte count is normal, although there may be mild leukopenia with relative lymphocytosis. Patients with mumps orchitis, however, may have a marked leukocytosis with a shift to the left. In meningoencephalitis, the white blood cell count is usually within normal limits. The erythrocyte sedimentation rate is usually normal but may rise with testicular or pancreatic involvement. The serum amylase level is elevated both in pancreatitis and in salivary adenitis. It may also be elevated in some patients in whom the sole evidence of mumps is meningoencephalitis, and probably reflects subclinical involvement of the salivary glands. In contrast to the amylase, serum lipase level is elevated only in pancreatitis, in which hyperglycemia and glucosuria also occur. The cerebrospinal fluid contains 0 to 2,000 cells per cu mm, almost all mononuclears. The pleocytosis in mumps meningitis tends to be greater than in aseptic meningitides caused by the poliomyelitis, Coxsackie, and ECHO viruses. There is no relationship between the cell count and the severity of central nervous system involvement. Transient hematuria and mild reversible abnormalities in renal function including inability maximally to concentrate the urine, excrete PSP, and clear creatinine, occur in association with the viruria of mumps.

The definitive diagnosis of mumps depends on isolation of the virus from blood, saliva, cerebrospinal fluid, or urine. However, even with the simplification of viral isolation by means of tissue culture techniques, culture of the virus is rarely necessary. When an etiologic diagnosis is needed, as in aseptic meningitis, or atypical cases of parotitis, the complement fixation test is highly reliable, simple, and inexpensive. It becomes positive during the second week of the disease, and titers remain elevated for at least 6 weeks. Paired serums should be obtained, and a fourfold rise in titer is necessary to confirm recent infection. The hemagglutination inhibition reaction is demonstrable somewhat later and persists for several months.

The serum neutralization test is the most sensitive indicator of previous mumps infection and should replace the skin test (intradermal injection of killed mumps virus, which produces a delayed reaction of the tuberculin type). The skin test is of no value in the diagnosis of acute mumps.

DIAGNOSIS. The diagnosis of mumps during an epidemic is usually obvious. Sporadic cases, however, must be distinguished from other causes of parotid enlargement. *Bacterial parotitis* usually occurs in debilitated patients with severe underlying diseases such as uncontrolled diabetes mellitus, cerebrovascular accidents, or uremia. It may also follow surgical operations. The parotid glands are swollen and tender, and pus can be expressed from the orifices of Stensen's ducts. Marked polymorphonuclear leukocytosis is present. The disease is usually acquired in the hospital, and *Staphylococcus aureus* is the causative organism. Dehydration followed by inspissation of secretions in the salivary ducts is an important predisposing factor. *Calculus* in a salivary duct is usually detectable by palpation or by injection of radioopaque media into Stensen's duct. *Drug reactions* may produce tender swellings of the parotid and other salivary glands. "Iodine mumps" is the commonest type. It may follow such procedures as intravenous urography; mercurialism and the antihypertensive agent, guanethidine, may also cause parotid enlargement and tenderness. Careful history usually serves to clarify the cause of these reactions. Cervical adenitis caused by streptococci, "bull-neck" diphtheria, infectious mononucleosis, cat-scratch disease, sublingual cellulitis (Ludwig's angina), and cellulitis of the external auditory canal are usually easy to distinguish from mumps by careful examination. Parotid tumors, and chronic infections like actinomycosis, tend to follow a more indolent course, with slowly progressive swelling. The common "mixed tumor" of the parotid is well circumscribed, nontender, and very firm, almost cartilaginous on palpation. Parotid swelling and fever, often accompanied by lacrimal adenitis and uveitis (Mikulicz's syndrome), may occur in tuberculosis, leukemia, Hodgkin's disease, and lupus erythematosus. The onset may be sudden, but the process is usually painless and of long duration. "Uveoparotid fever" of similar type may be the first manifestation of sarcoidosis; in this disease parotid swelling is frequently accompanied by single or multiple palsies of cranial nerves —in particular, the facial—and is referred to as Heerfordt's syndrome. Presternal edema may also be a manifestation of malignant lymphoma involving retrosternal lymph nodes. Bilateral painless parotid swelling unassociated with fever is found in patients with Laennec's cirrhosis, chronic alcoholism and malnutrition. There is a chronic inflammation of the parotid and other salivary glands which is often associated with atrophy of the lacrimal glands and occurs most commonly in women past the menopause. With cessation of lacrimal and salivary function, there may be striking dryness of the conjunctiva and cornea (keratoconjunctivitis sicca) and of the mouth (xerostomia). These patients may also have a variety of systemic manifestations, including arthritis of the rheumatoid type, splenomegaly, leukopenia, and hemolytic anemia. When dryness of the mucosal surfaces is a prominent feature, the name *Sjögren's syndrome* is often applied, although some insist that *Mikulicz's disease* (as opposed to the syndrome accompanying other diseases) is the proper term (Chap. 390). The chronicity of the process and its occurrence in elderly women make confusion with mumps unlikely. Finally, benign hypertrophy of both masseter muscles, presumably due to habitual clenching and grinding of teeth, may be confused with painless parotid swelling. The causes of aseptic meningitis are listed in Chap. 361.

Orchitis occurring in the absence of parotitis is likely to remain undiagnosed. Serologic testing may later confirm the diagnosis of mumps. Orchitis may occur in association with acute bacterial prostatitis and seminal vesiculitis. It is a rare complication of gonorrhea. Occasionally testicular inflammation accompanies pleurodynia, leptospirosis, melioidosis, relapsing fever, chickenpox, brucellosis, and lymphocytic choriomeningitis.

TREATMENT. There is no specific treatment for infections with the mumps virus. Patients with parotitis should receive mouth care, analgesics, and a bland diet. Bed rest is advisable only as long as the patient is febrile; contrary to popular belief, physical activity has no influence on the development of orchitis or other complications. Patients with epididymoorchitis may be acutely ill and in great pain. Many advocated forms of treatment, including surgical decompression of the testicle, infiltration of the spermatic chord with local anesthetics, estrogens, convalescent serum, and broad-spectrum antibiotics, have not been regularly effective. Despite failure to document their effectiveness in controlled studies, adrenal steroids have been of considerable benefit in diminishing fever, as well as testicular pain and swelling, and in restoring the sense of well-being in a number of patients. It is important to give a single large dose, corresponding to 300 mg cortisone or 60 mg prednisone, initially. During the ensuing 24 hr the same quantity should be given in divided dosage. Subsequently, administration of the hormone can be tapered over 7 to 10 days. Adrenal steroids have not exerted an adverse effect on concomitant pancreatitis or meningitis, although they have not benefited patients with meningeal involvement, and their withdrawal has usually been accompanied by a sharp recrudescence of symptoms. Adrenal steroids have not prevented the appearance of parotid involvement on the contralateral side.

Mumps arthritis is usually mild and requires no treatment. Mumps thyroiditis may subside spontaneously, but excellent relief has been obtained with adrenal hormones.

PROPHYLAXIS. A live attenuated mumps virus vaccine (Jeryl Lynn strain) prepared in chick embryo cell culture has been highly effective in producing significant rises in mumps antibody in individuals who are seronegative prior to vaccination. The vaccine also has boosted antibody levels in seropositive vaccinees, and has afforded 95 percent protection to individuals exposed to mumps. The vaccine produces an inapparent, noncommunicable infection which is not associated with fever or mumpslike symptoms. It confers excellent protection for at least 2 years, but its long-term effectiveness is not yet known. Protection has been demonstrated in both children and adults.

Live mumps vaccine should be given to children approaching adolescence, adolescents, and adults, especially men who have not had mumps. Individuals living in groups or in institutions should be vaccinated, particularly because it has been shown that isolation of mumps patients does not prevent transmission of the infection. Mumps is a mild infection in young children and vaccination of all children is not recommended. The vaccine should be given in dosage of 0.5 ml subcutaneously. A single dose suffices, and simultaneous administration of gamma-globulin does not interfere with development of mumps antibody.

Vaccination is contraindicated in babies under the age of one because of the interfering effect of maternal antibody, in individuals with a history of hypersensitivity to egg proteins, and in patients with febrile illnesses, leukemia, lymphoma, generalized malignancies or those receiving steroids, alkylating drugs, antimetabolites and irradiation.

It is not known whether the vaccine will prevent infection when administered after exposure, but no contraindication to its use in this situation exists. Specific mumps-immune globulin has been effective in aborting orchitis when given 1 to 2 days after exposure, although it may not prevent parotitis. Ordinary gamma-globulin is not effective in preventing mumps.

REFERENCES

Candel, S.: Epididymitis in Mumps, Including Orchitis: Further Clinical Studies and Comments, Ann. Intern. Med., 34:20, 1951.

Caranasos, G. J., and J. R. Felker: Mumps Arthritis, Arch. Intern. Med., 119:394, 1967.

Eylan, E., R. Zuweky, and C. Shaba: Mumps Virus and Subacute Thyroiditis: Evidence of a Causal Association, Lancet, 1062, 1957.

Hilleman, M. R., R. E. Weibel, E. B. Buynak, J. R. Stokes, and J. E. Whitman, Jr.: Live Attenuated Mumps-Virus Vaccine, New Engl. J. Med., 276:252, 1967.

Kocen, R. S., and E. Critchley: Mumps Epididymo-orchitis and Its Treatment with Cortisone, Brit. Med. J. 2:20, 1961.

Meyer, M. B.: An Epidemiologic Study of Mumps; Its Spread in Schools and Families, Am. J. Hyg., 75:259, 1962.

Petersdorf, R. G., and I. L. Bennett, Jr.: Treatment of Mumps Orchitis with Adrenal Hormones: Report of 23 Cases with a Note on the Hepatic Involvement in Mumps, A.M.A. Arch. Intern. Med., 99:222, 1957.

St. Geme, J. W., Jr., G. R. Noren, and P. R. Adams: Proposed Embryopathic Relationship Between Mumps Virus and Primary Endocardial Fibroelastosis, New Engl. J. Med., 275:339, 1966.

Weibel, R. E., J. Stokes, Jr., E. B. Buynak, J. E. Whitman, and M. R. Hilleman: Live, Attenuated Mumps Virus Vaccine, New Engl. J. Med., 276:245, 1967.

Witte, J. J., and A. W. Karchmer: Surveillance of Mumps in the United States as Background for Use of Vaccine, U.S. Public Health Reports, 83:95, 1968.

Utz, J. P., V. N. Houk, and D. W. Alling: Studies of Mumps: IV. Viruria and Abnormal Renal Function, New Engl. J. Med., 270:1283, 1964.

232 CYTOMEGALIC INCLUSION DISEASE (Salivary Gland Virus Disease)

Walter H. Sheldon

DEFINITION. Cytomegalic inclusion disease (CID) is a viral infection which may be latent or active and often reflects age-related as well as congenital or acquired changes in host resistance. This disorder at one time was regarded as an affliction of babies, but is being encountered with increasing frequency in adults, generally as a complication of severe chronic debilitating disease. Recently, a self-limited infectious mononucleosis-like syndrome attributed to CID has been described in previously healthy persons. In this form, hepatitis may dominate the clinical picture.

ETIOLOGY. Present knowledge of the infection evolved from viral isolation and serologic techniques which are more sensitive than the morphologic demonstration of the distinctive nuclear inclusions first reported in 1904. Cytomegalovirus (CMV) was isolated in tissue culture by M. G. Smith in 1956. It is included in the *Herpes virus* family, produces striking acidophilic or amphophilic intranuclear (10 to 15 mμ) and inconspicuous basophilic cytoplasmic (2 to 4 mμ) inclusions. Electron-microscopic studies reveal that the intranuclear inclusions consist of proliferating viral particles in deoxyribonucleic acid matrix, while the cytoplasmic inclusions consist of lysosomes. The inclusions occur in all types of normal and neoplastic cells including white blood cells. The agent is sensitive to temperature and other environmental changes, but sorbitol or neutral glycerin preserves specimens for storage or shipment. Several antigenically heterogenous strains have been isolated which are species-specific for man and grow in human fibroblast cultures. CMV produces neutralizing and complement-fixing antibodies. Because human strains share a common complement-fixing antigen, the complement fixation test is generally used for serologic diagnosis. Antigenically distinct, species-specific CMV occur in mice and guinea pigs. The intranuclear inclusions of CMV have been seen in tissues of many mammals.

EPIDEMIOLOGY. The infection is worldwide and more prevalent where hygiene is poor. It may be congenital or acquired, latent or clinically apparent, and occurs in localized and disseminated form. In this country autopsy data show that infection is frequent in infancy (localized 10 to 12 percent, disseminated 1 to 2 percent) and is rare though increasing in adults. Serologic data indicate that antibody, which is relatively infrequent in early childhood, is present in about 15 percent of the population at age fifteen and in about 80 percent at age thirty-five. Antibody is found in about 50 percent of women of childbearing age, and elevated titers have been noted in pregnancy. The virus persists in the host for a long time, perhaps indefinitely, and is excreted in saliva and urine. Viral excretion in the presence of antibody often continues for months even in latent infection. Spread of the agent appears to require close and prolonged contact, which may explain the clustering of cases in families, schools, and hospitals. The importance of adult carriers is uncertain. The virus is also transmitted by transfusions. Transplacental transmission accounts for prenatal infection commonly followed by disease at birth or shortly thereafter. Newborns may also be infected by an apparently healthy contact who excretes the virus. Later in life inapparent infection appears to be common, and CID may result from either activated latent or newly acquired infection.

PATHOGENESIS AND PATHOLOGY. Localized or systemic CID is frequently associated with prolonged impaired host resistance. Latent and active infection occurs in benign and malignant disorders of the hematopoietic and lymphocytic-reticular tissues (various anemias, leukemias, lymphomas), other chronic debilitating diseases (renal failure, mucoviscidosis, malnutrition), and often after immunosuppressive measures employed for organ transplantation. It is a complication of many therapeutic measures, such as corticosteroids, antibiotics, antimetabolites, cytotoxins, and irradiation. The common denominator is a primary or acquired immunologic deficiency of immunoglobulin formation and/or cellular immunity. Serologic and some clinical data suggest that pregnancy might activate latent infection. Various forms of CID, generally with mild clinical manifestations, are being described with increasing frequency in apparently normal persons of all ages. This apparent increase in frequency may be due to improved hygiene, with less neonatal infection and an increase in the number of susceptible older persons, prolonged survival of patients with impaired host resistance, and to better diagnostic methods. The pathogenesis of the infection in infancy remains uncertain. Factors similar to those suggested in *Pneumocystis carinii* infection may be operative (Chap. 245), although prematurity and debilitation are not a frequent part of the clinical setting in which CID occurs. CID, however, may induce stillbirth or prematurity.

Enlarged cells, 25 to 40 M in diameter, with distinctive inclusions are the morphologic hallmark of the infection. They are easily seen with hematoxylin-eosin or Papanicolaou stains and are similar in all forms and sites of infection. It has been suggested that the large inclusions begin with the formation of small, sometimes multiple, pleomorphic Feulgen-positive intranuclear inclusions. Intact infected cells are not accompanied by inflammation, which occurs only after cell death. In adults the localized form most commonly consists of interstitial mononuclear cell pneumonitis or areas of gastrointestinal ulcerations. Other less frequent sites are the nasal mucosa, salivary gland, liver, and adrenal gland. Hepatitis even in the absence of the distinctive inclusions has been attributed to CID on serologic grounds. In the disseminated form nearly every tissue and organ have been affected, including the lung, alimentary canal, adrenal, liver, spleen, lymph nodes, pancreas, kidney, thyroid, and myocardium. In infancy the localized form is largely confined to the salivary glands, hence the original designation of salivary gland virus disease. In disseminated disease the more common sites are the salivary glands, kidney, liver, lung, pancreas, gastrointestinal tract, thyroid, adrenal, and brain.

Various other, sometimes multiple infections are associated with CMV infection. Bacterial infections are most common, but *P. carinii* pneumonia is frequent, and candidiasis, aspergillosis, and nocardiosis, various forms of herpes, as well as toxoplasmosis have been seen.

CLINICAL MANIFESTATIONS. In most adults CMV infection appears to be latent and becomes clinically apparent only in persons with chronic debilitating disease in whom host responses are impaired. The clinical manifestations may be masked by the underlying disorder, are non-specific, and vary according to the principal organ involved. The disease presents most commonly as acute pneumonia, but chronic lung disease, intestinal obstruction, malabsorption, colitis, and chronic hepatitis have been described. Rare instances of histologically proven CID manifested by either pneumonia or colitis without demonstrated underlying disease have been reported. Hepatitis and cirrhosis in infants and, on serologic grounds, chronic liver disease in normal adults have been attributed to the virus.

An *infectious mononucleosis-like syndrome* is also being ascribed to CMV infection on the basis of rising antibody titers and virus isolation. This illness was first noted after open-heart surgery where it seemed to be related primarily to transfusions with unrefrigerated blood, but has been described also in previously healthy persons. The patient is febrile and may complain of headache, back pain, or abdominal discomfort. The spleen and/or liver may be enlarged, and sometimes there is a transient maculopapular rash. Mild cervical and axillary lymph node enlargement occurs, but tonsillitis is absent. Absolute and relative lymphocytosis with atypical lymphocytes are always present. The heterophil antibody test is negative. Liver function tests are frequently abnormal. In a few instances, hepatitis with jaundice and hemolytic episodes is the presenting feature.

CMV infection is suspected as the cause of chronic cough and of an influenza-like illness in pregnancy because of the frequency with which these women subsequently deliver babies with prenatally acquired CID. If this finding is confirmed, it would be of considerable importance because surviving infants have had various grave oculocerebral abnormalities and mental retardation. Inapparent maternal infection during early gestation also has been implicated in other congenital defects. In infancy the clinical features of CID are quite constant and consist of hepatitis, hemolytic anemia, thrombocytopenia, interstitial pneumonia, and meningoencephalitis. In infants and older children with increased susceptibility to infection, a relationship between acquired hemolytic anemia and CMV infection with recurrent lymphadenitis has been described.

In adults the course of disseminated CID is generally fatal and the diagnosis is made at autopsy. The disease is often mild and self-limited when it presents as hepatitis, an infectious mononucleosis-like illness, or as a respiratory disorder. The evidence of a causal relationship of these manifestations to CMV infection is, however, not conclusive.

DIAGNOSIS. To establish the diagnosis, rising antibody titers are most useful. The virus may be isolated from tissue, blood, urine, or other body fluids, and the inclusions are sometimes demonstrated in biopsy specimens or in cell concentrates of fresh urine. While these findings are strongly suggestive of CID in the appropriate clinical setting, they do not exclude the possibility that CID may represent only coexisting latent infection. Chest roentgenograms may show interstitial pneumonitis or small nodular densities. The white blood cell count reveals no changes, with the exception of many atypical lymphocytes in the infectious mononucleosis-like syndrome. Other laboratory tests will reflect the underlying disease and the various sites of involvement but show no distinctive findings.

TREATMENT. There is no specific therapy. Beneficial effects have been attributed to the administration of interferon and particularly to the antiviral agent, floxuridine, given in combination with prednisone. The underlying disorder of which systemic CID in adults is frequently a complication should be treated vigorously.

REFERENCES

Hanshaw, J. B.: Congenital and Acquired Cytomegalovirus Infection, Pediat. Clin. N. Am., 13:181, 1966.

Klemola, E., L. Kääriäinen, R. von Essen, K. Haltia, A. Koivuniemi, and C.-H. von Bonsdorf: Further Studies on Cytomegalovirus Mononucleosis in Previously Healthy Individuals, Acta Med. Scand., 182:311, 1967.

Smith, D. R.: A Syndrome Resembling Infectious Mononucleosis after Open-heart Surgery, Brit. Med. J. 1:945, 1964.

Toghill, P. J., M. E. Bailey, R. Williams, R. Zeegen, and R. Bown: Cytomegalovirus Hepatitis in the Adult, Lancet, 1:1351, 1967.

Zuelzer, W. W., C. S. Stulberg, R. H. Page, J. Teruya, and A. J. Brough: Etiology and Pathogenesis of Acquired Hemolytic Anemia, Transfusion, 6:438, 1966.

233 YELLOW FEVER
Jay P. Sanford

DEFINITION. Yellow fever is an acute infectious disease of short duration and variable severity which is caused by a group B arbovirus, and is followed by lifelong immunity. The classical triad of symptoms, jaundice, hemorrhages, and intense albuminuria, is present only in severe infections, which are now known to comprise only a small proportion of cases.

PREVALENCE. Yellow fever remains the most dramatically serious arbovirus disease of the Tropics. For more than 200 years, after the first identifiable outbreak occurred in Yucatan in 1648, it was one of the great plagues of the world. As late as 1905, New Orleans and other southern United States ports experienced at least 5,000 cases and 1,000 deaths. Because of the existence of the sylvatic form of the disease, protective measures must be maintained against human disease, as demonstrated by recent outbreaks in Trinidad in 1954, Central America in 1948 to 1957, the Congo in 1958, and the Sudan and Ethiopia in 1959 to 1962. In 1965 an explosive epidemic erupted in Senegal.

EPIDEMIOLOGY. Human infection results from two basically different cycles of virus transmission, urban and sylvatic. The urban cycle is man-mosquito-man, *Aëdes aegypti*-transmitted yellow fever. After a 2-week extrinsic incubation period, mosquitoes can initiate infection. Sylvan yellow fever differs in various ecologic situations. In the rain forests of South and Central America, species of treetop *Haemogogus* or *Sabethes* mosquitoes maintain transmission in wild primates. Once infected, the mosquito vector remains infectious for life, and may serve as a reservoir as well as a vector. The incidence of overt disease and death in monkeys varies with the species involved. When man comes in proximity to the forest canopy mosquitoes, sporadic cases or focal outbreaks can occur. In East Africa, the mosquito-primate cycle is maintained by the forest canopy mosquito *Aëdes africanus,* which seldom feeds on man. The peridomestic mosquito *Aëdes simpsoni* feeds upon primates entering the village gardens and can then in turn transmit the virus to man. If yellow fever were reintroduced into urban areas, the urban cycle could be reinitiated with the potential for epidemic disease. Why yellow fever has never invaded Asia, despite the widespread distribution of man-biting *Aëdes aegypti* mosquitoes, has never been satisfactorily explained.

PATHOLOGY. Because of the abrupt onset and rapid course of the infection, the pathologic changes are acute. The lesions are predominantly visceral. The diagnosis of yellow fever in the experimental animal can be suspected by the presence of acidophilic degeneration in the Kupffer cells of the liver within 24 hr after inoculation. Necrobiosis and acidophilic necrosis of the parenchymal cells of the liver with the formation of *Councilman bodies* occur in a characteristically discontinuous fashion in the midzones of the liver lobules. In the kidney, the virus produces fatty changes, necrobiosis, and necrosis of the tubular epithelium. Multiple minute hemorrhages occur in the gastrointestinal tract. In the brain, the dominant lesion consists of perivascular hemorrhage, which is most frequently found in the subthalamic and periventricular region at the level of the mamillary bodies.

CLINICAL MANIFESTATIONS. The incubation period is 3 to 6 days. In accidental laboratory- or hospital-acquired infections longer incubation periods (10 to 13 days) have been reported. In *mild yellow fever* the only symptoms are the abrupt onset of fever and headache, which may last only 1 or 2 days. Additional symptoms include nausea, epistaxis, relative bradycardia (Faget's sign), and slight albuminuria. The mild illness lasts only 2 to 3 days and is like influenza. *Moderately severe* and *malignant* attacks of yellow fever are characterized by three distinct clinical periods: the period of infection, the period of remission, and the period of intoxication. Prodromal symptoms are usually absent. The onset is characteristically sudden, with headache, dizziness, and temperature elevations to 104°F without a relative bradycardia. Small children may have febrile convulsions. The headache is followed quickly by pains in the neck, back, and legs. Often there is nausea with vomiting and retching. Examination reveals a flushed face and injection of the conjunctivas. The congested eyes persist until the third day. The tongue becomes characteristic, with bright red margins and tip and a white furred center. Faget's sign appears by the second day. Epistaxis and gingival bleeding are common. On the third day of illness, the fever may fall by crisis, and the patient enters convalescence or, in the malignant form, copious hemorrhages, anuria, or delirium may occur. The stage of remission lasts from several hours to several days. In the third stage, the classic symptoms appear: the fever rises again but the pulse remains slow (Faget's sign). Jaundice becomes detectable about the third day; however, jaundice is often not a prominent symptom, even in fatal illnesses. Increased epistaxis, melena, and uterine hemorrhages are common, but gross hematuria is rare. Of the classical signs, "black vomit" is more characteristic than jaundice. It usually does not occur before the fourth day and is often associated with a fatal outcome. Albuminuria, which rarely develops before the third day, occurs in 90 percent and may be very intense (3.0 to 20.0 Gm albumin per liter). In spite of massive albuminuria, edema or ascites has not been encountered. In malignant infections, coma frequently occurs 2 or 3 days before death. Shortly before death, which usually occurs between the fourth and sixth days, the patient becomes delirious and wildly agitated. While the duration of fever in the third stage is usually 5 to 7 days, the period of intoxication is the most variable and may last up to 2 weeks. Clinical yellow fever is relatively free from complications; for some reason suppurative parotitis is the most striking. Clinical relapses do not occur.

LABORATORY FINDINGS. Early in the disease, progressive leukopenia may occur. By the fifth day, total leukocyte counts of 1,500 to 2,500 cells per cu mm are often found; the decrease is due mostly to a decrease in neutrophiles. Total leukocyte counts return to normal by the tenth day, and there may be a marked terminal leukocytosis in fatal cases. Hemoglobin values remain normal except terminally, when hemoconcentration may occur. Platelet counts are usually normal. Sophisticated coagulation studies have been performed only in rhesus monkeys experimentally infected with yellow fever. Within 72 hr after viral inoculation and prior to apparent clinical illness, a coagulation defect was observed. This was characterized by a prolonged one-stage prothrombin time and a prolonged partial thromboplastin time reflecting measured deficiencies in factors II, V, VII, VIII, IX, X, and XI. Both the euglobin lysis time and thrombin time were prolonged, suggesting a depression of plasminogen activation and accumulation of fibrinogen degradation products. At this time platelet counts and chemical measurements of fibrinogen were normal. During the subsequent 48 hr, these coagulation defects worsened as the monkeys developed clinical illness, and terminally, depression of platelet counts and fibrinogen levels occasionally were observed. The disturbances in coagulation occurred during the stage of viremia and existed before hepatic necrosis was visible in liver biopsy specimens. These data suggest that the hemorrhagic manifestations are primarily caused by a consumptive coagulopathy rather than by hepatic failure. Also, in experimental infections in primates, modest increases in total bilirubin, alkaline phosphatase, and marked increases in serum glutamic-oxalacetic transaminase occur. Electrocardiograms may show T-wave changes. Cerebrospinal fluid is normal.

DIAGNOSIS. There are three established procedures for the laboratory diagnosis of yellow fever: (1) Isolation of the virus from blood. This must be done early, preferably during the first 3 days. Caution must be exercised to avoid autoinoculation. (2) Diagnosis can also be based on the development of neutralizing antibody. (3) Diagnosis can also be reasonably based on the demonstration of the typical, although not completely specific, histopathologic lesions on liver biopsy.

TREATMENT. The management has been symptomatic and supportive. Current management should be based upon assessment and correction of the circulatory abnormalities. If evidence of disseminated intravascular coagulation is present, administration of heparin should be considered. Close attention to fluid and electrolyte balance is essential.

PROGNOSIS. The overall fatality rate in yellow fever is between 5 and 10 percent in clinical cases, and may be less because many infections are very mild or inapparent.

PREVENTION. Prophylaxis consists of vaccination and the eradication of A. aegypti mosquitoes. Two strains of attenuated yellow fever virus are available for the preparation of vaccines: the French neurotropic and the 17D strain. The vaccine prepared from the 17D strain consists of frozen, dried extract of infected chick embryos sealed in ampuls. For use, the virus is reconstituted by the addition of sterile physiologic saline solution. One subcutaneous injection of 0.5 ml will produce immunity in man. In rural areas, mass vaccination is the only effective protection against jungle yellow fever. The use of DDT spray on the walls of houses is effective in controlling mosquitoes, but presently no method is available for eradicating jungle yellow fever.

REFERENCES

Dennis, L. H., B. E. Reisberg, D. Crozier, and M. E. Conrad: The Original Hemorrhagic Fever: Yellow Fever, Blood, 30:858, 1967.

Kerr, J. A.: Clinical Aspects and Diagnosis of Yellow Fever, p. 389 in "Yellow Fever," G. K. Strode (Ed.), New York, McGraw-Hill Book Company, 1951.

Kirk, R.: An Epidemic of Yellow Fever in the Nuba Mountains, Anglo-Egyptian Sudan, Ann. Trop. Med. Parasitol., 35:67, 1941.

Lebrun, A. J.: Jungle Yellow Fever and Its Control in Gemena, Belgian Congo, Am. J. Trop. Med. Hyg., 12:398, 1963.

Work, T. H.: Virus Diseases in the Tropics, p. 1 in "A Manual of Tropical Medicine," 4th ed., G. W. Hunter, W. W. Frye, and J. C. Schwartzwelder (Eds.), Philadelphia, W. B. Saunders Company, 1966.

234 DENGUE FEVER
Jay P. Sanford

DEFINITION. Dengue is one of the arbovirus infections characterized by malaise, headache, generalized myalgia, lymphadenopathy, and rash. It is endemic over large areas of the tropics and subtropics. From 1963 to 1964 epidemic dengue occurred in the Caribbean, and a number of travelers returned to the United States with clinical illness. In these areas a high proportion of infections are inapparent or represent undifferentiated febrile illnesses. It is now recognized that the dengue syndrome can be caused by other arboviruses, hence the exact etiology of some of the earlier epidemics is uncertain.

ETIOLOGY. There are four distinct serogroups of dengue viruses, types 1, 2, 3, and 4, all of which are Group B arboviruses. The existence of at least two further antigenic types has been suggested. They are transmitted solely by mosquitoes of the genus *Aëdes*.

EPIDEMIOLOGY. So far as is known, dengue infections in nature involve only man and Aëdes mosquitoes. Attempts have been made to implicate lower vertebrates, especially monkeys, as reservoir sylvatic hosts, but the data are inconclusive. *Aëdes aegypti* is the most important worldwide vector species. This species, as well as the less common vector species, bite man readily or even preferentially, breed in small collections of water such as cisterns and backyard litter, and are peridomestic in nature. They fly during the day. Man appears to be uniformly susceptible, and susceptibility is not influenced by age, sex, or race. The disappearance of dengue from an area may be the result either of elimination of the vector or of exhaustion of the susceptible population. During outbreaks, attack rates may be very high: in Louisiana in 1922 the attack rate was estimated to be 1,740 per 100,000 (1.74 percent).

PATHOLOGY. The skin lesions in nonfatal uncomplicated disease produced in volunteers have been studied by biopsy. The chief abnormality occurred in small blood vessels and consisted of endothelial swelling, perivascular edema, and infiltration with mononuclear cells. Since the disease is self-limited, other studies have not been done.

CLINICAL MANIFESTATIONS. Dengue viruses frequently produce inapparent infections in man. When symptoms develop, three broad clinical patterns may be encountered: classical dengue, hemorrhagic fever (Chap. 235), and a mild atypical form. Classical dengue (break-bone fever) occurs primarily in nonimmune individuals, specifically nonindigenous adults and children. The usual incubation period is 5 to 8 days. Prodromal symptoms such as mild conjunctivitis or coryza may occur, followed in hours by the abrupt onset of a severe splitting headache, retroorbital pain, backache, especially in the lumbar area, and leg and joint pains. The headache is aggravated by movement. At least three-fourths of patients have ocular soreness with pain on moving the eyes. A few have mild photophobia. While true rigors are common during the course, they are usually not present at the onset (14 percent in one series). Additional symptoms include insomnia, anorexia with a loss of taste or bitter taste, and weakness. Mild transient rhinopharyngitis occurs in as many as one-quarter of individuals. Epistaxis has been observed. Examination reveals scleral injection (90 percent), tenderness upon pressure on the ocular globe, and nontender posterior cervical, epitrochlear, and inguinal lymphadenopathy. Over one-half of patients have an enanthem characterized initially by pinpoint-sized vesicles over the posterior half of the soft palate. The tongue is often coated. Skin rashes varying from diffuse flushing to scarlatiniform and morbilliform are frequently present over the thorax and inner aspects of the arms. These are transient and fade, only to be followed by a more apparent maculopapular rash which appears on the trunk on the third to the fifth day and spreads peripherally. The rash may be pruritic and generally terminates with desquamation. Extreme bradycardia is not observed. Within 2 to 3 days after the onset, the temperature may decrease to nearly normal and other symptoms disappear. The remission typically lasts 2 days and is followed by return of fever and the other symptoms, although they are generally less severe than during the initial phase. This "saddleback" diphasic febrile course is considered characteristic, but often is not encountered. The febrile illness usually lasts 5 to 6 days and terminates by crisis. Complaints of fatigue for several weeks after infection are common.

In addition to this "classical" syndrome, an atypically mild illness may occur. Symptoms include fever, anorexia, headache, and myalgia. On examination, evanescent rashes may be seen, but lymphadenopathy is usually absent. The course is usually less than 72 hr in duration.

At the onset both in classical and in mild dengue, the leukocyte counts may be low or normal; however, by the third to the fifth day, leukopenia, usually with counts of less than 5,000 per cu mm, and neutropenia are usually seen. Occasionally albuminuria of moderate degree occurs.

DIAGNOSIS. Virus isolation in tissue culture of serum obtained during the first days of illness is definitive. Diagnosis can be made by serologic tests employing paired sera for hemagglutination inhibition tests and complement fixation tests. Specific serologic diagnosis is complicated by cross-reactions with other group B arbovirus antibodies such as those following immunization with yellow fever vaccine.

TREATMENT. The treatment is entirely symptomatic.

PROGNOSIS. Mortality is nil.

PREVENTION. Attenuated vaccines are undergoing experimental evaluation but are not available. The hypothesis of "second infections" being responsible for the dengue hemorrhagic fever syndrome raises further questions about a program of active immunization. Control depends upon mosquito abatement.

REFERENCES

Clarke, D. H., and J. Casals: Arboviruses; Group B, p. 606 in "Viral and Rickettsial Infections of Man," 4th ed., F. L. Horsfall, Jr. and I. Tamm (Eds.), Philadelphia, J. B. Lippincott Company, 1965.

Diasio, J. S., and F. M. Richardson: Clinical Observations on Dengue Fever, Mil. Surg., 94:365, 1944.

Sabin, A. B.: Research on Dengue During World War II, Am. J. Trop. Med. Hyg., 1:30, 1952.

235 EPIDEMIC HEMORRHAGIC FEVER

Sheldon E. Greisman

DEFINITION. Epidemic hemorrhagic fever is the prototype of the viral hemorrhagic fevers, a group of illnesses characterized by an acute onset, thrombocytopenia, and widespread vascular injury with impaired vasomotor tone, enhanced capillary permeability, and a hemorrhagic diathesis. Included within this group is a variety of other distinct entities caused by viruses with no antigenic interrelationships and varying with respect to the specific clinical syndrome and pathologic findings. Certain of these entities and some important distinguishing features are outlined in Table 235-1.

HISTORY, ETIOLOGY, AND EPIDEMIOLOGY. Epidemic hemorrhagic fever was first recognized in Manchuria and Siberia by the Japanese and Russians about 3 decades ago. During the Korean War, the disease occurred among United Nations troops and was extensively investigated. It now is known to be widespread in European Russia and Scandinavia, and to extend westward as far as Hungary and Czechoslovakia.

Russian and Japanese workers have reported transmission of epidemic hemorrhagic fever to human subjects by intravenous or intramuscular injection of urine or blood taken from patients during the first 5 days of disease. Oral and intranasal routes of inoculation were ineffective. Preincubation of the acute phase with convalescent phase serum prevented transmission. The causative agent passed through filters which retained microbiologic agents larger than viruses. Neither these workers nor the Americans who investigated the Korean form were able to establish the agent in a laboratory host or in tissue culture.

Two seasonal peaks of incidence are characteristic of epidemic hemorrhagic fever, but sporadic cases occur throughout the year. Most of the 1,000 patients who were seen annually in Korea from 1951 to 1953 became ill between mid-April and early July or during October and November. The disease in Korea was limited to military personnel in rural areas north of Seoul. After the armistice, civilians of all ages contracted the disease upon returning to neglected farms in this area. In Europe, the disease affects civilians working in rural and forested areas. At least a thousand cases are reported annually in European Russia alone.

The majority of cases in Korea were isolated and widely spaced in time and place. In the small outbreaks, (1) there was no person-to-person spread of infection, (2) food and water were unimportant in epidemiology, and (3) infection followed exposure in a sharply localized area of abandoned farmland or scrub-covered terrain. It was assumed that trombiculid mites served as the vector for the agent of epidemic hemorrhagic fever and that small wild rodents provided the reservoir.

Table 235-1 indicates that epidemic hemorrhagic fever is distinct from Crimean and mid-Asian hemorrhagic fevers, which extend from the Balkans eastward across the southern U.S.S.R. These diseases do not demonstrate the renal changes typical of epidemic hemorrhagic fever, and the etiologic agents, which differ from that of epidemic hemorrhagic fever but which may be related to each other, are transmitted to man by *Hyalomma* ticks during the spring-summer season. Two other hemorrhagic fevers, also related to each other but distinct from those already mentioned, are Omsk hemorrhagic fever, which occurs in

Table 235-1. VIRAL HEMORRHAGIC FEVERS

Entity	Viral agent	Major age group infected	Vector	Renal injury	Characteristic leukocyte count	Mortality, %
Epidemic hemorrhagic fever	Not infective for animals or tissue culture	All ages	Mite (presumed)	++++	Leukocytosis	3–15
Crimean hemorrhagic fever Mid-Asian hemorrhagic fever	Not well characterized	Adults	Tick Person-to-person (minor)	±	Leukopenia	3–6 30–38
Omsk hemorrhagic fever Kyasanur Forest disease (India)	Related antigenically to Russian spring-summer encephalitis group viruses	Adults	Tick	++	Leukopenia	0.5–3 4–10
Philippine hemorrhagic fever Thailand hemorrhagic fever Malaysia hemorrhagic fever Calcutta hemorrhagic fever North and South Vietnam hemorrhagic fever Cambodian hemorrhagic fever	Dengue (usually types 1 to 4) or Chikungunya (less common)	Infants and small children	Mosquito	±	Leukopenia	1–23
Argentinian hemorrhagic fever Bolivian hemorrhagic fever	Junin Machupo (related antigenically to Junin)	Adults	Mite (presumed) Contamination of food and water by excreta of reservoir host, *Calomys callosus* (presumed) Person-to-person (minor)	++	Leukopenia	23 5–30
Yellow fever	Yellow fever virus	All ages	Mosquito	++	Leukopenia	5

western Siberia, and Kyasanur Forest disease, which is seen in central India. Both are caused by members of the Russian spring-summer group of viruses and are transmitted to man by *Dermacentor* ticks, which also serve as vectors in the natural cycle involving wild animals. Since 1950, febrile diseases with hemorrhagic manifestations have been described in the Philippines, Thailand, Malaysia, India, North and South Vietnam, and Cambodia. These are mosquito-borne infections caused by members of the dengue group of viruses. Concomitantly, viral diseases with a hemorrhagic diathesis have appeared in Argentina (initial recognized epidemic 1953) and in Bolivia (initial recognized epidemic 1959). The etiologic agents are related antigenically to each other and to the Tacaribe virus isolated from bats in Trinidad. The virus of Bolivian hemorrhagic fever has been isolated from the urine and feces of the rodent *Calomys callosus,* and although the major method of dissemination to man is uncertain, contamination of food and water has been suspected. Direct person-to-person spread of infection may also occur. In contrast, mites are the presumed vector of Argentinian hemorrhagic fever. Finally, a long-recognized viral illness with a hemorrhagic diathesis, yellow fever, occurs in large areas of South America and Africa but is unrelated to any of the above illnesses.

MANIFESTATIONS. Following an incubation period of about 2 weeks (extremes of 9 to 36 days), epidemic hemorrhagic fever begins abruptly, with frontal headache, chills, high fever, anorexia, and backache. Physical findings during the first several days of fever and prostration are limited to conjunctival injection and a cutaneous flush, especially about the face and neck. About the third day, petechiae appear on the palate, conjunctivas, axillary folds, and cutaneous areas subjected to mild trauma. Increased capillary permeability becomes clinically evident about the fourth day with the rapid appearance of pathognomonic severe proteinuria and edema of the conjunctivas and periorbital tissue. Edema in the lumbar gutters and mesentery, seen at autopsy, may contribute to the back and abdominal pain.

Fever subsides about the fifth day, but the course usually progresses through additional phases: hypotensive, oliguric, diuretic, and convalescent. Manifestations of increased capillary permeability, among them a rising hematocrit, progress during the hypotensive phase but abate rapidly when the oliguric phase develops, with its associated rising blood urea nitrogen and creatinine levels. With the onset of diuresis (usually from 3 to 6 liters daily) on about the tenth day, symptoms and abnormal physiologic findings generally disappear rapidly. However, renal tubular function is restored slowly, and normal concentrating capacity usually does not return until the fourth to sixth week of convalescence. Body weight, which may decrease as much as 30 lb during acute illness, is also restored slowly. Central-nervous-system symptoms are not specific and when present, in 10 to 15 percent of confirmed cases, are usually due to hemorrhage, uremia, and/or edema. This contrasts with Argentinian and Bolivian hemorrhagic fevers, where distinctive neurologic symptoms are frequent, and 50 percent of patients with Bolivian hemorrhagic fever have intention tremors of the tongue and hands.

PATHOPHYSIOLOGY. Injury to the smaller segments of the vascular system, resulting in reduced vasomotor tone, increased permeability, and increased fragility, are the basic derangements of epidemic hemorrhagic fever. The vascular injury is characteristically more intense in certain organs than in others, and selected, rather than uniform, vascular damage accounts for the extensive retroperitoneal edema in the absence of concomitant anasarca or pulmonary edema. Several mechanisms for the vascular injury have been considered: (1) direct viral invasion of vessel walls, (2) autonomic nervous system dysfunction, (3) hypersensitivity (this mechanism is probably involved in dengue hemorrhagic fevers), (4) thrombocytopenia. Their interrelationships and relative importance are not established.

The mechanisms responsible for the thrombocytopenia during the viral hemorrhagic fevers have received particular attention. Unlike the dengue hemorrhagic fevers, depressed megakaryocytopoiesis does not contribute to the thrombocytopenia of epidemic hemorrhagic fever; indeed, megakaryocytic hyperplasia is seen. Rather, the thrombocytopenia has been linked to disseminated intravascular coagulation with associated multiple defects in the first and second stages of coagulation, hypofibrinogenemia, and accumulation of fibrinogen degradation products. This coagulopathy has been suggested as the common denominator in the hemorrhagic diathesis of the viral hemorrhagic fevers.

The decrease in cardiac output, which constitutes the basis for the hypotensive phase of epidemic hemorrhagic fever, is attributable to decreased effective circulating blood volume because of capillary leakage of plasma and dilatation of capillary and venular beds. Impaired ability to compensate by elevating peripheral resistance inten-

sifies the hypotension. In hypotensive patients with high hematocrits, tachycardia, and cold extremities, administration of concentrated human albumin is helpful. Hypotensive subjects with normal or slightly elevated hematocrits, minimal tachycardia, and warm extremities have the least increases in peripheral vascular resistance, and although treatment with vasopressor agents restores arterial blood pressure toward normal, there is no proof that these drugs reduce mortality.

During the oliguric phase, the elevated hematocrit decreases rapidly; capillary permeability is repaired, and there is resorption of the interstitial fluid lost during the hypotensive phase. Approximately 20 percent of patients develop arterial blood pressures exceeding 140/90, which results from an increased cardiac output and/or increased peripheral resistance, but the mechanisms underlying these hemodynamic alterations are uncertain. Pulmonary edema is an important cause of death at this time. Phlebotomy may be lifesaving when pulmonary edema develops in hypertensive subjects, but is of little benefit in subjects with normotension. The acute renal failure and subsequent recovery during the oliguric and diuretic phases clinically resemble those seen following exposure to a variety of other severe injurious stimuli to the kidney (Chap. 300).

LABORATORY FINDINGS AND PATHOLOGY. Clinical laboratory data in epidemic hemorrhagic fever other than those already mentioned are (1) leukopenia during the initial 2 days of illness followed by leukocytosis of 10,000 to 50,000 per cu mm, with many immature granulocytes by the end of the first week, and (2) disturbances of electrolyte balance. The characteristic lesions at autopsy are found in the kidney, right atrium, and anterior pituitary gland. Grossly, the renal cortex appears pale; the pyramids appear intensely congested. Hemorrhagic lesions can be seen in the right atrial wall. The anterior pituitary appears intensely congested. During the hypotensive phase, gelatinous edema is found in the retroperitoneal tissues and mesentery; during the late oliguric phase, these tissues are usually dry. Inflammatory lesions of small vessels and thrombosis are conspicuously lacking, but intense capillary congestion is characteristic. Indeed, most of the areas which appear grossly hemorrhagic represent sites of extreme capillary dilatation. Varying degrees of necrosis occur in the anterior pituitary.

DIFFERENTIAL DIAGNOSIS. Epidemic hemorrhagic fever may be confused with leptospirosis, the typhus fevers, hemorrhagic smallpox, meningococcemia, idiopathic thrombocytopenic purpura, leukemia, hemorrhagic dengue, or even influenza. The diagnosis must be made on epidemiologic and clinical grounds because viral isolation techniques and serologic tests available for confirmation of many of the other hemorrhagic fevers are lacking. A history of exposure in an endemic area, particularly during a seasonal epidemic, and the appearance of marked proteinuria about the fourth day of fever, associated with a rising leukocyte count and thrombocytopenia, are virtually diagnostic.

TREATMENT AND PREVENTION. The treatment of epidemic hemorrhagic fever is entirely supportive; antibiotics, cortisone, antihistamines, and convalescent serum have been tried with no success. Treatment begins with early diagnosis and prompt but gentle transfer to a hospital with adequate facilities. During the febrile phase, complete bed rest, mild sedation, fluid balance with strict avoidance of overhydration, and an adequate but light diet are important. If the evidence that disseminated intravascular coagulation constitutes a common denominator of viral hemorrhagic fevers is substantiated, anticoagulants may prove an important therapeutic adjuvant. Once diuresis is established, attention must be paid to adequate replacement of fluid and electrolytes.

Vaccines are available for dengue, yellow fever, and Omsk hemorrhagic fever and are being developed for Argentinian and Bolivian hemorrhagic fevers, but failure to isolate the virus of epidemic hemorrhagic fever precludes vaccine prophylaxis. Prevention is based on avoidance of trombiculid mites, presumed vectors of the disease. These measures are (1) use of insect repellents for impregnation of clothes (benzyl benzoate) and application to exposed skin surfaces (dimethyl phthalate), (2) clearing of all vegetation from camp sites (bulldozing) and treatment of the area with residual insecticides such as lindane, (3) rodent control in and about camps by means of rodenticides. This method resulted in dramatic reductions in Bolivian hemorrhagic fever.

PROGNOSIS. Epidemic hemorrhagic fever varies greatly in severity. It may be so mild as to make diagnosis difficult; indeed, many suspected cases are not confirmed because the patients fail to develop typical renal manifestations. About 20 percent of patients with confirmed cases become critically ill. The following factors contribute to severity and influence the prognosis unfavorably: delayed initiation of medical care, rough transportation to the medical facility, prolonged high fever, severe dehydration with ketoacidosis, early excessive fluid replacement, prolonged or recurrent hypotension, persistent hemoconcentration, anuria, and progressive severe electrolyte disturbances. The fatality rate in cases among American soldiers in Korea was between 5 and 7 percent. Of these, deaths were approximately equally distributed through the hypotensive, oliguric, and diuretic phases. Complete recovery is the rule once the convalescent phase is reached.

REFERENCES

Dennis, L. H., M. B. Garvey, N. M. Tauraso, and M. E. Conrad: Disseminated Intravascular Coagulation: A Pathogenesis for Argentinian Hemorrhagic Fever, Clin. Res., 16:330, 1968.

Entwisle, G., and E. Hale: Hemodynamic Alterations in Hemorrhagic Fever, Circulation, 15:414, 1957.

Greisman, S. E.: Capillary Observations in Patients with Hemorrhagic Fever and Other Infectious Illnesses, J. Clin. Invest., 36:1688, 1957.

Johnson, K. M., S. B. Halstead, and S. N. Cohen: Hemorrhagic Fevers of Southeast Asia and South America: A Comparative Appraisal, Progr. Med. Virol., 9:105, 1967.

Smorodintsev, A. A., L. I. Kazbintsev, and V. G. Chudakov:
"Virus Hemorrhagic Fevers" (Trans. from Russian), Washington, D.C., The National Science Foundation, 1964.

Symposium on Epidemic Hemorrhagic Fever: Earle, D. P. (Ed.), Am. J. Med., 16:617, 1954.

236 COLORADO TICK FEVER
Jay P. Sanford

DEFINITION. Colorado tick fever is the only tick-transmitted virus disease of man that is recognized in the Western Hemisphere. While "mountain fever" had been described ever since the advent of immigrants to the Rocky Mountain region, Becker in 1930 differentiated it from mild Rocky Mountain spotted fever, established the clinical picture of disease, and renamed it Colorado tick fever.

ETIOLOGY. The causative agent in Colorado tick fever is an ungrouped arbovirus which has been isolated from patients with the syndrome.

PREVALENCE. The disease has been contracted only in Colorado, Idaho, Nevada, Wyoming, Montana, Utah and the eastern portions of Oregon, Washington, and California. However, the virus of Colorado tick fever has been reported to have been isolated from the dog tick, *Dermacentor variabilis*, obtained from Long Island. This observation has not been confirmed, but suggests the possibility that Colorado tick fever may occur over a wider geographic area. The actual prevalence is difficult to assess, but it is relatively common. Mild and clinically inapparent forms of the disease occur, but its frequency has never been determined. The number of cases of Colorado tick fever reported in Colorado is 20 times greater than that of Rocky Mountain spotted fever.

EPIDEMIOLOGY. Colorado tick fever is transmitted to man by the adult hard-shelled wood tick, *Dermacentor andersoni*. The virus has been found in as many as 14 percent of this species of ticks collected in endemic areas. Transovarial transmission of the virus in the tick has been established. Illness occurs primarily in the spring and summer months, with a predilection for April and May at lower altitudes and June and July at higher altitudes. Virus has been obtained from both the blood and the spinal fluid of patients during the acute illness.

CLINICAL MANIFESTATIONS. The incubation period is usually 3 to 6 days, and in most cases a history of tick bite can be obtained. Persons affected usually are those whose occupational or recreational activities bring them in contact with ticks. The disease may occur at any age. The clinical picture is characterized by the sudden onset of severe aching of the muscles of the back and legs, chilliness without true rigors, a rapid increase in temperature, which usually reaches 102 to 104°F, headache with pain on ocular movement, retroorbital pain, and photophobia. Occasionally nausea and vomiting occur. The physical findings are not specific. Tachycardia in proportion to the temperature, flushed facies, and variable conjunctival injection may be present. Occasionally the spleen is palpable. A rash is usually not present, but on occasion a petechial rash involving primarily the arms and legs or maculopapular rash over the entire body may occur. Rarely, punched-out ulcers may form at the site of tick bite. The fever with the associated symptoms lasts about 2 days, then abruptly lyses to normal or subnormal, leaving the patient very weak. After an afebrile period of about 2 days, the temperature recurs, may be higher than in the first phase, and may last as long as 3 days. Over 90 percent of patients show this saddleback pattern of temperature. Rarely there may be three febrile phases. The febrile episode may be followed by a period of weakness of several weeks' duration.

Evidence of central-nervous-system involvement has been recorded in a few patients. The findings are those of either an aseptic meningitis with stiffness of the neck or encephalitis with clouding of the sensorium, delirium and coma.

LABORATORY FINDINGS. The most important laboratory feature is moderate to marked leukopenia. On the first day of illness, the total leukocyte count may be at normal levels, but usually by the fifth or sixth day there has been a decrease to 2,000 to 3,000 per cu mm. Characteristically there is a proportionate decrease in lymphocytes and granulocytes. A moderate "left shift" in the neutrophilic series is usually apparent. Toxic changes in neutrophiles are often conspicuous and "virocyte" types of lymphocytes are frequently observed. Bone marrow examination reveals "maturation arrest" in the granulocytic series. Erythrocyte values remain normal. Thrombocytopenia has been recorded in an isolated case report. The blood picture returns to normal within a week after the fever subsides.

DIAGNOSIS. The diagnosis of Colorado tick fever is suspected on the basis of the epidemiologic history and clinical findings. The diagnosis can be established by the isolation of the virus from serum obtained during the febrile phase. Specific neutralizing or complement-fixing antibodies appear in the blood between the eighth and fourteenth days of illness. Because neutralizing antibodies persist for many years, demonstration of a rise in titer is required.

TREATMENT. Treatment is entirely symptomatic.

PROGNOSIS. The prognosis is excellent.

PREVENTION. No patients have been reported as having the disease twice. Active immunity with an attenuated virus has been produced but the immunization itself frequently produced mild disease. Prevention of Colorado tick fever is best carried out by avoiding contact with the wood tick.

REFERENCES

Becker, F. E.: Tick-borne Infections in Colorado, Colo. Med., 27:36, 1930.

Ecklund, C. M., G. M. Kohls, and J. M. Brennan: Distribution of Colorado Tick Fever and Virus-carrying Ticks, J.A.M.A., 157:335, 1955.

Florio, L., M. O. Stewart, and E. R. Mugroge: The Etiology of Colorado Tick Fever, J. Exp. Med., 83:1, 1946.

Lloyd, L. W.: Colorado Tick Fever, Med. Clinics N. Am., March, 1951.

Silver, H. K., G. Meiklejohn, and C. H. Kempe: Colorado Tick Fever, Am. J. Dis. Child., 101:30, 1961.

237 PHLEBOTOMUS FEVER
Jay P. Sanford

DEFINITION. Phlebotomus (sandfly, pappataci, or 3-day) fever is an acute, relatively mild, self-limited arbovirus infection which is characterized by malaise, headaches, and generalized myalgia.

ETIOLOGY. The disease is caused by at least two immunologically distinct ungrouped arboviruses, the Sicilian and Naples strains, but there may be additional immunologically distinct strains. The viruses have been adapted to white mice, but there is no evidence of an animal reservoir in nature.

PREVALENCE. The disease occurs throughout the Mediterranean basin, the Balkans, the Near and Middle East, the eastern part of Africa, the Soviet republics of Central Asia, West Pakistan, and possibly certain parts of southern China. In highly endemic areas, native populations acquire the disease at an early age and with repeated exposure develop and maintain high levels of immunity. The apparent absence of phlebotomus fever in indigenous adult populations residing in areas where sandflies are abundant can present a deceptive picture of the actual risk to susceptibles.

EPIDEMIOLOGY. The disease occurs during the hot, dry seasons (summer or autumn months) and is transmitted to humans by the bites of infected sandflies (*Phlebotomus papatasi*). *Phlebotomus papatasi* is a small fly which can penetrate ordinary house screens. Only the female bites and usually does so during the night. In persons who are not sensitive there is neither pain nor local irritation after the bite, hence only about 1 percent of patients will remember having been bitten. Approximately 7 days after feeding on an infected individual, the insect acquires the capacity to transmit infection. The sandflies continue to be infectious for their life span. Transovarial transmission of the virus to the next generation of insects has been demonstrated and offers the best explanation for the mechanism of over-winter survival of the virus. In man, the incubation period may be as short as 3 days. Viremia is present for at least 24 hr before and after the onset of fever, but is not detectable for more than 2 days after the onset of illness.

CLINICAL MANIFESTATIONS. The onset of symptoms is abrupt in over 90 percent of patients, with the temperature rapidly rising to its highest point, which may vary from 100 to 105°F. Headache is nearly always present, and is often accompanied by pain on moving the eyes and by retroorbital pain. Myalgia is common and may be localized to the chest, resembling pleurodynia, or to the abdomen. Other symptoms which occur (usually in less than 20 percent of patients) include vomiting, photophobia, giddiness, neck stiffness, alteration or loss of taste, and arthralgia. Physical signs include conjunctival injection in approximately one-third of patients. Small vesicles may be seen on the palate, and macular or urticarial rashes occur. The spleen is rarely palpable, and lymphadenopathy is absent. The pulse rate may be elevated in proportion to the temperature on the first day; thereafter bradycardia is often present. The fever persists 3 days in most patients, with defervescence in a staggered descent. Giddiness, weakness, and feelings of depression are frequently encountered during convalescence. Second attacks 2 to 12 weeks after the first occur in 15 percent of cases.

In common with other arbovirus infections, phlebotomus fever may be associated with aspetic meningitis. In one series, 12 percent of patients had symptoms and signs sufficient to warrant a lumbar puncture. Findings in these patients included pleocytosis, with an average cell count of 90 per cu mm and a predominance of either polymorphonuclear or mononuclear leukocytes. Spinal fluid protein concentration ranged from 20 to 130 mg per 100 ml. In another series mild papilledema was observed in a few patients with severe illness.

LABORATORY FINDINGS. The changes in leukocyte count constitute the only positive laboratory findings. Total leukocyte counts of less than 5,000 per cu mm are observed in 90 percent of patients if daily counts are done during the febrile period and convalescence. The leukopenia may not appear until the last day of fever or even after defervescence. The differential leukocyte count will reveal an absolute decrease in lymphocytes on the first day, accompanied by an increase in nonsegmented neutrophiles. During the second or third day, the number of lymphocytes begins to return to normal and may constitute 40 to 65 percent. At the same time, the number of segmented neutrophiles decreases, and immature cells increase sharply until they outnumber the segmented forms. The differential count usually returns to normal within 5 to 8 days after defervescence. Erythrocyte values remain normal, and urinalyses are usually normal.

DIAGNOSIS. In the absence of a specific serologic test, the diagnosis must be made on clinical and epidemiologic grounds.

TREATMENT. The disease is self-limited, and no specific therapy is available. Symptomatic care including bed rest, adequate fluid intake and analgesia with aspirin is recommended. Convalescence may require a week or longer.

PROGNOSIS. No fatalities are recorded among the tens of thousands of cases.

REFERENCES

Fleming, J., J. R. Bignall, and A. N. Blades: Sandfly Fever, Review of 664 Cases, Lancet, I: 443, 1947.

Sabin, A. B., C. B. Philip, and J. R. Paul: Phlebotomus (Papataci or Sandfly) Fever; Disease of Military Importance; Summary of Existing Knowledge and Preliminary Report of Original Observations, J.A.M.A., 125:603, 693, 1944.

238 WEST NILE FEVER
Jay P. Sanford

DEFINITION. West Nile virus is distributed from South Africa to southeastern India, but has been shown as a cause of significant disease only in the Near East, where it can produce a clinical picture closely resembling dengue.

ETIOLOGY. West Nile virus is a Group B arbovirus with pathogenicity for common laboratory animals. The virus multiplies and causes cytopathic effects in a variety of cells in tissue culture.

PREVALENCE. In 1940 the virus was isolated from the blood of a febrile patient. Subsequent serologic surveys demonstrated neutralizing antibodies against the virus to be widely prevalent in the native populations of Uganda, Kenya, the Congo, and the Sudan. However, the clinical manifestations were unknown until the virus was isolated from the blood of a child during an epidemic of febrile disease in Israel in 1951. Outbreaks of disease involving several hundred patients occurred in Israel in 1950 to 1952. In one outbreak, over 60 percent of the population developed overt disease.

EPIDEMIOLOGY. The disease is highly endemic in Egypt but goes largely unrecognized. Presumably the adult population is for the most part immune, and the infection in childhood is an undifferentiated mild febrile illness. The infection occurs in the summer both in Israel and in Egypt. The transmission cycle in Egypt is believed to be bird to mosquito to bird, with *Culex univittatus* as the principal vector. Although man and a variety of other vertebrates are infected by the virus, their involvement is believed to be tangential. In Israel, the most probable vectors are *Culex molestus* and *C. univittatus*.

CLINICAL MANIFESTATIONS. Most of the patients in Israel have been young adults, with neither sex predominating. The onset is usually abrupt and without prodromal symptoms. The temperature quickly rises to 101 to 104°F, with chills occurring in one-third of patients. Symptoms include drowsiness, severe frontal headache, ocular pain, and pain in the back. A small number of patients have anorexia, nausea, and dryness of the throat. Cough is uncommon (8 percent). Signs observed include flushing of the face, conjunctival injection, and coating of the tongue. The prominent finding is general enlargement of lymph nodes, which are of moderate size but are not hard and are only slightly tender. Occipital, axillary, and inguinal nodes are usually involved. The spleen and liver are slightly enlarged in a small proportion of patients. In one-half of the patients a rash may appear from the second to the fifth day of illness and persist for several hours or until defervescence. The rash occurs predominantly over the trunk and consists of pale roseolar maculopapular lesions. The illness is self-limited and lasts 3 to 5 days in 80 percent of patients.

In a few patients, transitory meningeal involvement may be encountered. Spinal fluid examinations may reveal a pleocytosis and some increase in protein concentration.

Leukopenia occurs in the majority of patients, and total leukocyte counts are lower than 4,000 per cu mm in one-third. Differential counts vary from a moderate shift to the left to a slight lymphocytosis.

Convalescence is often prolonged, lasting 1 to 2 weeks, with prominent symptoms of fatigue. Enlargement of lymph nodes subsides over several months. Only rarely have complications, sequelae, or fatalities been seen in natural infections, although in one outbreak in a group of elderly patients a high proportion of patients developed meningoencephalitis, and four fatalities ensued.

DIAGNOSIS. Accurate diagnosis rests on virus isolation, which can be accomplished because viremia persists for as long as 6 days, or the demonstration of a rising specific antibody titer.

TREATMENT. The treatment is symptomatic.

REFERENCES

Clarke, D. H., and J. Casals: Arboviruses: Group B, p. 606 in "Viral and Rickettsial Infections of Man," 4th ed., F. L. Horsfall, Jr., and I. Tamm (Eds.), Philadelphia, J. B. Lippincott Company, 1965.

Marberg, K., N. Goldblum, V. V. Sterk, W. Jasinska-Klingberg, and M. A. Klingberg: The Natural History of West Nile Fever. I. Clinical Observations During an Epidemic in Israel, Am. J. Hyg., 64:259, 1956.

Taylor, R. M., T. H. Work, H. S. Hurlbut, and F. Rizk: A Study of the Ecology of West Nile Virus in Egypt, Am. J. Trop. Med. Hyg., 5:579, 1956.

239 OTHER VIRAL FEVERS

Jay P. Sanford

Most viral infections in man are either asymptomatic or present as undifferentiated grippelike illnesses characterized by fever, malaise, headaches, and generalized myalgia. The similarities in clinical features between infections caused by viruses as dissimilar as the myxoviruses, e.g., influenza, rubella; the enteroviruses, e.g., poliovirus, Coxsackie virus, ECHO virus; some of the herpes viruses, e.g., cytomegalovirus; and the arboviruses usually preclude an etiologic diagnosis on the basis of clinical manifestations without ancillary information regarding epidemiologic features and serologic findings. The purpose of this chapter is to direct attention to the ever-expanding list of viruses, with particular attention to the arboviruses, which produce febrile disease in man. Because the number of agents is large, mention will be made of agents which have been best documented, have demonstrated unusual features, or seem to be of greatest potential significance.

ARBOVIRUSES

Arboviruses are distributed widely throughout the world and are of importance in both temperate and tropical zones. Representative viruses have been isolated in almost every geographic area outside of the polar regions. The survival of arboviruses in nature depends upon a complex cycle between the arthropod and vertebrate. The arthropod becomes generally infected, is infectious for life, and therefore serves as a reservoir as well as a vector.

Arbovirus infection of vertebrates is usually asymptomatic. The viremia which develops stimulates an immune response which sharply limits the duration of the viremia. In arbovirus infections other than urban yellow fever and dengue, infection of man represents an incidental occurrence which is tangential to the basic maintenance cycle. Hence, the isolation of virus from arthropod vectors or the detection of infection in the natural vertebrate host may provide a means for the early detection and enable the control of epizootic infection before significant spread to man occurs.

As determined by serologic evidence of host responses, at least 75 immunologically distinct arboviruses are capable of infecting man, while somewhat fewer have been incriminated as causing clinical disease. The spectrum of clinical illness produced by the arboviruses is varied both in predominant features and in severity. Five broad, often overlapping, and somewhat arbitrary clinical syndromes can be delineated (Table 239-1). Many of the more common of these infections have been considered in detail elsewhere: yellow fever (Chap. 233), dengue (Chap. 234), phlebotomus fever (Chap. 237), Colorado tick fever (Chap. 236), West Nile fever (Chap. 238), the epidemic hemorrhagic fevers (Chaps. 235), and the viral encephalitides (Chap. 218).

ARBOVIRUS INFECTIONS CHARACTERIZED PREDOMINANTLY BY MALAISE, HEADACHES, AND GENERALIZED MYALGIA

RIFT VALLEY FEVER. Rift Valley fever is an acute disease principally of sheep and cattle and first described in man during an investigation of an extensive epizotic of hepatitis in sheep in the Rift Valley in East Africa. The virus of Rift Valley fever is ungrouped and has no immunologic relationship with other arboviruses. During the extensive epizootic in sheep in 1930, workers associated with the investigations contracted a severe but limited febrile disease. A similar syndrome was common among the herders of infected flocks. More than 200 cases of human disease were originally recognized.

The infection is widespread in Africa, occurring in Kenya, Uganda, Anglo-Egyptian Sudan, French Equatorial Africa, and the Union of South Africa. Virus has been found in several species of mosquitoes: *Eretmapodites chrysogaster, Aëdes caballus, Aëdes circumluteolus,* and *Culex theileri.* Antibodies to Rift Valley fever have been found in wild field rats in Uganda. Man appears to be incidentally infected during the course of an epizootic. Although man presumably can be infected by arthropods, many human infections occur as a result of handling infected animal tissues. In addition, laboratory-acquired infections have been common, which suggests a respiratory route.

The incubation period is usually 3 to 6 days. The onset

Table 239-1. SUMMARY OF CLINICAL, VIROLOGIC, AND EPIDEMIOLOGIC FEATURES
OF ARBOVIRUSES ASSOCIATED WITH DISEASE IN MAN

Syndrome	Virus	Serologic group	Vector	Known geographic range of infection
Fever with malaise, headaches, generalized myalgia	Mayaro	A	Mosquito	Trinidad, Colombia, Brazil
	Mucambo	A	Mosquito	Brazil
	Uruma	A		Lowland Forest, Bolivia
	Kunjin	B	Mosquito	Northern Australia
	Spondweni	B	Mosquito	South Africa, Mozambique, Nigeria
	United States bat salivary gland	B	?	California, Texas, Sonora in Southwest North America
	Wesselsbron	B	Mosquito	South Africa, Bechuanaland
	Yellow fever	B	Mosquito	Africa, Central and South America
	Zika	B	Mosquito	Uganda, Nigeria
	Apeu	C	Mosquito	Brazil
	Caraparu	C	Mosquito	Brazil, Panama, Trinidad
	Itaqui	C	Mosquito	Brazil
	Madrid	C	?	Panama
	Marituba	C	Mosquito(?)	Brazil
	Murutucu	C	Mosquito(?)	Brazil
	Oriboca	C	Mosquito	Brazil
	Ossa	C	?	Panama
	Calovo	Bunyamwera	Mosquito	Czechoslovakia
	Germiston	Bunyamwera	Mosquito	South Africa, Angola
	Ilesha	Bunyamwera	Mosquito(?)	Nigeria
	Guaroa	Bunyamwera	Mosquito	Colombia, Brazil
	Tahyna	California	Mosquito	Czechoslovakia, Yugoslavia
	Catu	Guama	Mosquito	Brazil, Trinidad
	Guama	Guama	Mosquito	Brazil, Trinidad
	Oropouche	Simbu	Mosquito	Brazil, Trinidad
	Bwamba	Bwamba	Mosquito	Uganda
	Phlebotomus, Naples	Phlebotomus	Sandfly	Italy, Egypt, Iran, West Pakistan
	Phlebotomus, Sicilian	Phlebotomus	Sandfly	Italy, Egypt, Iran, Pakistan, Yugoslavia
	Chagres	Phlebotomus	?	Panama
	Candiru	Phlebotomus	?	Brazil
	Vesicular stomatitis	VSV	Sandfly, mosquito(?)	United States, Mexico, Panama, Venezuela, Colombia, Ecuador, Peru
	Colorado tick fever	Ungrouped	Hard tick	Western United States
	Nairobi sheep disease	Ungrouped	Hard tick	Kenya, Congo
	Rift Valley fever	Ungrouped	Mosquito	Africa
	Quaranfil	Ungrouped	Soft tick	Egypt, South Africa
	Piry	Ungrouped	?	Brazil
Fever with malaise, headaches, myalgia, *arthralgia*, and *rash*	Chikungunya	A	Mosquito	South, East, West, Central Africa, India, Thailand, Vietnam, Malaya
	Mayaro	A	Mosquito	Brazil, Trinidad
	O'nyong-nyong	A	Mosquito	East Africa, Senegal
	Sindbis	A	Mosquito	South and East Africa, Egypt, Israel, India, Malaya, Philippines, Australia
	Bunyamwera	Bunyamwera	Mosquito	South, East, West Africa
	Changuinola	Changuinola	Phlebotomus	Panama
Fever with malaise, headaches, myalgia, *rash*, and *lymphadenopathy*	Dengue 1	B	Mosquito	Hawaii, Oceana, New Guinea, Japan, Malaysia, Thailand, India
	Dengue 2	B	Mosquito	Circumglobal

Table 239-1. SUMMARY OF CLINICAL, VIROLOGIC, AND EPIDEMIOLOGIC FEATURES
OF ARBOVIRUSES ASSOCIATED WITH DISEASE IN MAN (*Continued*)

Syndrome	Virus	Serologic group	Vector	Known geographic range of infection
Fever with malaise, headaches, myalgia, *rash* and *lymphadenopathy* (continued)	Dengue 3	B	Mosquito	Caribbean, Oceana, Philippines, Thailand
	Dengue 4	B	Mosquito	Philippines, Thailand, India
	West Nile	B	Mosquito	South and West Africa, Rhone Delta, Near East, Israel, India, Malaysia, Borneo
Fever with headache, myalgia, prostration, and *hemorrhagic* signs	Chikungunya	A	Mosquito	Thailand, Malaysia, India, Vietnam
	Dengue 1	B	Mosquito	Thailand, India
	Dengue 2	B	Mosquito	Philippines, Vietnam, Thailand, Malaysia, India
	Dengue 3	B	Mosquito	Philippines, Thailand
	Dengue 4	B	Mosquito	Philippines, Thailand
	Kyasanur Forest disease	B	Tick	India
	Omsk hemorrhagic fever	B	Tick	Western Siberia, USSR
	Yellow fever	B	Mosquito	Africa, Central and South America
	Junin (Argentinian hemorrhagic fever)	Tacaribe	Rodent, mite(?)	Argentina
	Machupo (Bolivian hemorrhagic fever)	Tacaribe	Rodent, mite(?)	Eastern Bolivia
	Central Asian hemorrhagic fever	Ungrouped	Tick(?)	Central Asia, USSR
	Crimean type hemorrhagic fever	Ungrouped	Tick	Southern USSR
	Far Eastern or Korean hemorrhagic fever (hemorrhagic nephrosonephritis)	Ungrouped	Rodent, mite(?)	USSR, Manchuria, China, Korea
Fever with *central nervous system* involvement (meningitis to encephalitis)	See table in Chap. 218.			

is usually abrupt, with malaise, chilly sensation or rigors, headache, retroorbital pain, and generalized aching and backache. The temperature rises rapidly to 101 to 104°F. Later complaints include anorexia, loss of taste, epigastric pain, and photophobia. Examination is usually unremarkable except for flushing of the face and conjunctival injection. The temperature curve is often saddleback in type, with an initial elevation lasting 2 to 3 days, followed by a remission and second febrile period. Convalescence is usually rapid. Complications are rare; jaundice has not been seen in man. Macular exudates with decreased vision have been reported. One of the most characteristic findings is the initial normal total leukocyte count followed by leukopenia with a decrease in neutrophiles associated with an increase in band forms. The diagnosis is made by isolating the virus from the blood by inoculation of mice. In humans, viremia is present during the first 3 days. Neutralizing antibodies have been demonstrated as early as 4 days after onset. There is no specific treatment. The prognosis in human

infections is good. Only one fatality has been recorded, and in this instance death was not due directly to the infection.

MAYARO VIRUS. Mayaro virus was first isolated from man in Trinidad in 1954. Outbreaks involving a number of persons subsequently have occurred in Brazil and Bolivia. The virus has been isolated from a wild mosquito, *Mansonia venezuelensis*, and can be maintained serially in *Aëdes aegypti* and *Anopheles quadrimaculatus*. The mechanism of spread has not been determined, but the presence of viremia favors a biting arthropod vector. The predominance of illness and greater incidence of immunity in males suggests a forest infection. Symptoms include fever of several days' duration, which may be marked during the first 1 to 2 days. Systemic complaints include severe frontal headache, epigastric pain, backache, nausea, photophobia, and vertigo. Signs have included conjunctival injection, mild icterus in a few patients, and arthritis in at least one patient. The leukocyte count is in the range of 5,000 to 8,000 per cu mm. The illness in Bolivia was more severe, and several fatalities were reported.

BAT SALIVARY GLAND VIRUS. During the course of a survey for rabies infection in bats, an agent was obtained from the salivary glands of Mexican free-tailed bats in Texas. The virus is related to the St. Louis encephalitis complex of viruses (Group B). It is not known how the virus is maintained in nature. Five laboratory-acquired human infections have been recorded. The illnesses were characterized by fever associated with headache, myalgia, and a mild nonproductive cough. In two patients, there was evidence of central-nervous-system involvement with encephalitis and aseptic meningitis. One patient had oophoritis and two developed orchitis. By the sixth to seventh day of illness, leukopenia in the 2,000 to 3,000 per cu mm range was observed in two individuals.

ZIKA VIRUS. Zika virus was first isolated from a captive rhesus monkey in Uganda and subsequently from wild mosquitoes. Based upon serologic surveys, it is known to infect man in Uganda and Nigeria. During investigation in eastern Nigeria of an outbreak of jaundice that was suspected of being yellow fever, physicians isolated Zika virus from one patient and noted that two others had a rise in neutralizing antibodies. The symptoms in these patients included fever, arthralgia, and headache with retroorbital pain. Jaundice was present in one, and bile was demonstrated in the urine of another. Albuminuria was noted in one patient. Prothrombin times were normal. The clinical syndrome appears to simulate mild yellow fever.

BUNYAMWERA GROUP. Representative viruses of this group are found in all inhabited continents except Australia. Only four viruses of the group, Bunyamwera itself, Germiston, Ilesha, and Guaroa, have been associated with clinical disease. Based upon serologic surveys, there is evidence of a high prevalence of inapparent infection in some areas. The clinical patterns of infection due to Germiston, Ilesha, and Guaroa viruses seem similar, while infection due to Bunyamwera virus is often associated with arthralgia and may be associated with a rash. The mild clinical illness is characterized by low grade fever, headache, and myalgia which last several days, and it may be followed by weakness during convalescence.

VESICULAR STOMATITIS VIRUS. This virus disease of animals which chiefly affects cattle, horses, and swine appears in man as an acute self-limited infection with signs and symptoms quite similar to those of influenza. Two distinct serotypes, New Jersey and Indiana, have been recognized. Most of the outbreaks, especially in North America, have been due to the New Jersey serotype. Although most commonly occurring as a laboratory infection in man, this infection is transmissible under natural conditions. In one report, three-fourths of the laboratory personnel handling experimentally infected animals or manipulating the viruses developed neutralizing antibodies. In nature, the virus has been isolated from phlebotomus sandflies collected in a tropical rain forest in Panama and from a pool of *Aëdes spp.* (prob-

ably *dorsalis*) mosquitoes during an epizootic in New Mexico. In the areas of Panama which was involved, 17 to 35 percent of the population had neutralizing antibodies against VSV. Of the laboratory workers with serologic evidence of infection, approximately one-half reported clinical symptoms. In the majority of cases the incubation period has been 2 to 6 days, although symptoms have developed within 30 hr of accidental inoculation. The onset usually is sudden, with chills, fever, profuse diaphoresis, and generalized myalgia including pain on ocular movement. One-third to one-half of patients have sore throats, and 10 percent have coryza. Physical signs include a temperature of 102 to 104°F in severe cases; fever is absent in mild cases. Conjunctivitis is noted in 20 percent, and in some patients (10 percent), small raised vesicles may be present on the buccal mucosa. Submaxillary and cervical lymphadenitis is seen in approximately one-third of patients. A diphasic course is noted in approximately 10 percent of patients. Treatment is symptomatic.

ARBOVIRUS INFECTIONS CHARACTERIZED BY FEVER, MALAISE, ARTHRALGIA, AND RASH

CHIKUNGUNYA. In 1952 an epidemic of a disease similar to dengue occurred in Tanganyika, an area in which dengue had never been observed. The disease was given the name chikungunya ("that which bends up") from the local description of the sudden onset of distinctive joint pains. A Group A arbovirus was isolated in 1956 both from serum of patients ill with the disease and from a pool of *Aëdes aegypti* mosquitoes.

Chikungunya virus is responsible for a denguelike illness in South Africa, India, and Southeast Asia, as well as a rather mild form of hemorrhagic fever in Asiatic children (Chap. 235). Outbreaks have been associated with high attack rates, with as many as 80 percent of inhabitants in some settlements becoming ill. It is not known definitely what vertebrates and arthropods are involved in the wild transmission cycle. Because the virus has been isolated from *Aëdes africanus* and antibodies against the virus can be detected in chimpanzees, these may play a role in the natural cycle in Africa.

After an incubation period estimated at no less than 8 days, the onset is typically abrupt, with a rapid rise in temperature to 102 to 105°F, often associated with a rigor and headache. Pain in large joints occurs early, incapacitating some individuals within a few minutes of onset. The pain is frequently severe enough to prevent sleep. The arthralgia is often associated with objective arthritis. Sites of involvement include knees, ankles, shoulders, wrists, or proximal interphalangeal joints. Myalgia, especially backache, and malaise occur frequently. In 60 to 80 percent of patients a maculopapular eruption, which may appear at any time during the febrile course, is noted on the trunk or on the extensor surfaces of the extremities. Mild lymphadenopathy predominantly in the axillary or inguinal areas may be evident. Pharyngitis and conjunctival suffusion may be observed in a few patients. Elevated temperatures continue for 1 to 6 days, and in some patients an afebrile interval of 1 to 3 days is followed by a secondary rise in temperature. The joint pains sometimes continue after the temperature has returned to normal. In a few individuals, joint pains have persisted for up to 4 months. Hematocrit values remain normal. Total leukocyte counts may be less than 5,000 per cu mm in some patients, while in others they remain normal. Urinalyses are normal. There is no specific antiviral treatment. Anti-inflammatory agents such as aspirin or indomethacin have been utilized. No second attacks have been recognized, and in the absence of the hemorrhagic fever syndrome, no deaths have been described.

O'NYONG-NYONG. O'nyong-nyong fever was first noted as an epidemic illness characterized by joint pains, rash, and lymphadenopathy in the northern province of Uganda in 1959. The agent is a Group A arbovirus which shows close antigenic relationships with chikungunya and Semliki Forest viruses. The original outbreak was associated with an explosive epidemic which spread to Tanzania and other areas in East Africa. By 1961, 2 million cases were recorded. In some areas, 81 percent of the population had either clinical disease or inapparent infection. Local outbreaks extended over the entire year. All age groups were affected. The most likely vector is *Anopheles funestus*. The clinical features are similar to those of chikungunya virus infection.

SINDBIS VIRUS. Sindbis virus infection in man rarely presents as a clinical disease. Of five cases from Uganda, one patient gave a history of joint pain. In the only well-studied clinical illness, a South African woman had arthritis as a prominent finding. Two days after a headache she noted swelling in her hands and feet. Soon thereafter she developed a confluent macular rash, followed by vesicle formation. The small joints of the hands and feet were swollen at the time of examination. Slight swelling of the fingers was present at 10 weeks, although she had otherwise recovered.

OTHER ARBOVIRUSES

Epidemics of polyarthritis associated with rashes have been observed in Australia since 1928. The clinical and epidemiologic features of each outbreak were quite uniform, and therefore, the name *epidemic polyarthritis* was applied. More recently, a presumed etiologic agent (designated as Ross River virus) has been isolated. The clinical features include development of a rash on the cheeks and the forehead which occasionally spreads to the trunk and lasts 2 to 10 days. Mild joint pain occurs in two-thirds of patients. Temperature elevations are rarely recorded, but a few patients give a history of feverishness.

In addition, Mayaro and Bunyamwera viruses have been associated with the syndrome of rash and arthralgia. These have been discussed under their more common manifestations, the dengue syndromes.

ENCEPHALOMYOCARDITIS VIRUSES

The encephalomyocarditis viruses, Columbia S-K, MM, Mengo, EMC, are a group of small RNA viruses which are immunologically indistinguishable from each other. Rodents, in particular certain species of wild rats, constitute the major reservoir for EMC viruses. Strains also have been isolated from primates, swine, and other rodents from many parts of the world. Strains of Mengo virus have been isolated from mosquitoes (*Taeniorhynchus fuscopennatus*) in Uganda, but the epidemiologic evidence does not suggest that EMC viruses are arboviruses. The prevalence of neutralizing antibodies in surveys of healthy individuals in the United States, Germany, Sweden, and Mexico ranges up to 7 percent.

Human infections vary from inapparent to mild febrile illness to severe encephalomyelitis. Study of an outbreak of aseptic meningitis characterized by chills, fever, headache, stiff neck, and cerebrospinal fluid pleocytosis of 50 to 500 cells per cu mm which involved a group of 44 U.S. Army personnel in the Philippine Islands revealed that during convalescence 39 percent of the individuals had high titers of specific neutralizing antibodies. In this outbreak fever lasted 2 to 3 days and all patients recovered promptly without sequelae. Sporadic EMC virus isolates have been made from adults and children with illnesses diagnosed as paralytic poliomyelitis, the Guillain-Barre syndrome, and severe meningoencephalitis. Myocarditis has not been a feature of EMC virus infection in man. Nothing is known of the pathologic findings in man. The diagnosis of human EMC virus infection depends upon isolation of the virus from blood, cerebrospinal fluid, or stool or the demonstration of a rising titer of specific antibodies during convalescence. Treatment is symptomatic and supportive.

REFERENCES

Arboviruses

Anderson, S. G., and F. L. French: An Epidemic Exanthem Associated with Polyarthritis in the Murray Valley, 1956, Med. J. Aust., 2:113, 1957.

Casals, J., and D. H. Clarke: Arboviruses; Group A, p. 583 in "Viral and Rickettsial Infections of Man," 4th ed., F. L. Horsfall, Jr., and I. Tamm (Eds.), Philadelphia, J. B. Lippincott Company, 1965.

——, and ——: Arboviruses Other Than Groups A and B, p. 659 in "Viral and Rickettsial Infections of Man," 4th ed., F. L. Horsfall, Jr., and I. Tamm (Eds.), Philadelphia, J. B. Lippincott Company, 1965.

Clarke, D. H., and J. Casals: Arboviruses; Group B, p. 606 in "Viral and Rickettsial Infections of Man," 4th ed., F. L. Horsfall, Jr., and I. Tamm (Eds.), Philadelphia, J. B. Lippincott Company, 1965.

Daubney, R., J. R. Hudson, and P. C. Garnham: Enzootic Hepatitis or Rift Valley Fever, J. Pathol. Bacteriol., 34: 545, 1931.

Deller, J. J., Jr., and P. K. Russell: Chikungunya Disease, Am. J. Trop. Med. Hyg., 17:107, 1968.

Doherty, R. L., B. M. Gorman, R. H. Whitehead, and J. G. Carley: Studies of Epidemic Polyarthritis: The Significance of Three Group A Arboviruses Isolated from Mosquitoes in Queensland, Australas. Ann. Med., 13:322, 1964.

Fields, B. N., and K. Hawkins: Human Infection with the

Virus of Vesicular Stomatitis During an Epizootic, New Engl. J. Med., 277:989, 1967.

Malherbe, H., M. Strickland-Chomley, and A. L. Jackson: Sindbis Virus Infection in Man. Report of a Case with Recovery of Virus From Skin Lesions, S. Afr. Med. J., 37:547, 1963.

Patterson, W. C., L. O. Mott, and E. W. Jenney: A Study of Vesicular Stomatitis in Man, J. Am. Vet. Med. Ass., 133:57, 1958.

Robinson, M. C.: An Epidemic of Virus Disease in Southern Province, Tanganyika Territory, in 1952–53. I. Clinical Features, Trans. Roy. Soc. Trop. Med. Hyg., 49:28, 1955.

Schrire, L.: Macular Changes in Rift Valley Fever, S. Afr. Med. J., 25:926, 1951.

Shore, H.: O'nyong-nyong Fever: An Epidemic Virus Disease in East Africa. III. Some Clinical and Epidemiological Observations in the Northern Province of Uganda, Trans. Roy. Soc. Trop. Med. Hyg., 55:361, 1961.

Smithburn, K. C., A. F. Mahaffy, A. J. Haddow, S. F. Kitchen, and J. F. Smith: Rift Valley Fever, J. Immunol., 62:213, 1949.

Sudia, W. D., Fields, B. N., and Calisher, C. H.: Isolation of Vesicular Stomatitis Virus (Indiana Strain) and Other Viruses From Mosquitoes in New Mexico, 1965, Am. J. Epidemiol., 86:598, 1967.

Sulkin, S. E., K. F. Burns, D. F. Shelton, and C. Wallis: Bat Salivary Gland Virus: Infections of Man and Monkey, Texas Rept. Biol. Med., 20:113, 1962.

WHO Technical Report 219, Report of a Study Group: "Arthropod-Borne Viruses," Geneva, 1961.

Work, T. H.: Virus Diseases in the Tropics, p. 1 in "A Manual of Tropical Medicine," 4th ed., G. W. Hunter, W. W. Frye, and J. C. Schwartzwelder (Eds.), Philadelphia, W. B. Saunders Company, 1966.

Encephalomyocarditis Viruses

Gajdusek, D. C.: Encephalomyocarditis Infection in Childhood, Pediatrics, 16:902, 1955.

Smadel, J. E., and J. Warren: The Virus of Encephalomyocarditis and Its Apparent Causation of Disease in Man, J. Clin. Invest., 26:1197, 1947.

Warren, J.: Encephalomyocarditis Viruses, p. 562 in "Viral and Rickettsial Infections of Man," 4th ed., F. L. Horsfall, Jr., and I. Tamm (Eds.), Philadelphia, J. B. Lippincott Company, 1965.

Section 21

Diseases Caused by Protozoa

240 AMEBIASIS

James J. Plorde, Harry A. Feldman, and Ivan L. Bennett, Jr.

DEFINITION. Amebiasis is an infection of the large intestine produced by *Endamoeba histolytica*. It is an asymptomatic carrier state in most individuals, but disease ranging from chronic, mild diarrhea to fulminant dysentery is frequently produced. Among extraintestinal complications, the commonest is hepatic abscess, which may rupture into peritoneum, pleura, lung, or pericardium.

ETIOLOGY. There are at least six different species of ameba that parasitize the mouth and intestine of man. Of these, *E. histolytica* is the only one that causes disease and *E. coli* is the species with which it is most likely to be confused in examination of stools.

Endamoeba histolytica exists in two forms: the motile trophozoite and the nonmotile cyst. The trophozoite is the parasitic form and dwells in the wall and lumen of the colon, divides by binary fission, grows best under anaerobic conditions, and requires the presence of either bacteria or tissue substrates to satisfy its nutritional requirements. When diarrhea occurs, the trophozoites are passed unchanged in the liquid stool, where they can be distinguished by their rapid motility, ingestion of erythrocytes, and the sparsity of vacuoles and ingested bacteria within them. In the absence of diarrhea, the trophozoites encyst before leaving the gut. The cysts are highly resistant to environmental changes and are responsible for transmission of the disease. The cysts of *E. histolytica* can be distinguished from those of *E. coli* by their thin wall and their two thick chromated bodies.

Endamoeba histolytica strains have been classified into large and small races, depending upon whether they form cysts measuring more or less than 10 μ in diameter. While it is possible that small strains (sometimes called *E. hartmanni*) are somewhat less likely to produce symptoms than are the large strains, cyst size is apparently unstable and the often-heard statement that small strains are nonpathogenic for man is not justified.

Endamoeba histolytica occurs normally in the intestines of a few dogs, monkeys, and rats; these animals, rabbits, and kittens can also be infected experimentally. Amebas can be cultivated in artificial media, a procedure that is occasionally useful in diagnosis. With rare exceptions, the presence of bacteria in the culture medium is a prerequisite to multiplication of the protozoa.

EPIDEMIOLOGY. Because trophozoites die rapidly after leaving the intestine, patients with amebic dysentery are unimportant in transmission of the disease; asymptomatic cyst passers are the source of new infections.

Amebic infection is worldwide, although both symptomatic and subclinical infection are more frequent in tropical areas. Figures obtained from local and admittedly incomplete surveys indicate that the average incidence of asymptomatic carriers is 10 percent in Europe and the United States, 16 percent in Asia, and 17 percent in Africa. Cyst passers are more frequent among children and the inmates of institutions.

Cases of amebic dysentery are usually sporadic but epidemics, usually water-borne, have occurred. Outbreaks of amebiasis are never explosive, as are those produced by pathogenic intestinal bacteria, and may not be recognized for several weeks. The cysts are often transmitted by vegetables in countries where human excreta is used as fertilizer.

Symptomatic amebiasis is unusual below the age of ten years in temperate climates, and both intestinal and hepatic lesions predominate in adult males to an extent that is not readily explainable on the basis of different rates of exposure to infection.

PATHOGENESIS AND ANATOMIC CHANGES. After ingestion, cysts pass through the stomach unchanged. In the ileum, the cyst wall disintegrates and, eventually, eight trophozoites result. These immature amebas pass to the colon, where they attack the mucosa. Mucosal lesions too tiny to be detected probably occur in all infections. The sites of involvement in order of frequency are cecum and ascending colon, rectum, sigmoid, appendix, and terminal ileum.

The factors responsible for the development of ulceration extensive enough to cause symptoms in some individuals are not understood. The size of the inoculum and the virulence of the infecting organism are both important. The virulence seems to differ among strains, and there are some studies which suggest that it is increased with rapid passage from person to person. These factors alone, however, are insufficient to explain the occurrence of disease in only a small percentage of subjects exposed naturally to the same strain or in a minority of volunteers fed cysts from a single source. Certain experimental findings suggest strongly that the bacterial flora of the intestine may be a major determinant of the extent of amebic disease. The symbiosis between bacteria and amebas in artificial media has been mentioned. When 200 strains were cultured and tested for virulence in rabbits, disease was produced by only 4 percent grown without bacteria, by 35 percent grown with a single bacterial species, and by 85 percent grown with a mixed culture of several different bacteria. Germ-free animals cannot be infected with *E. histolytica* but become susceptible if the intestine is first allowed to acquire a normal complement of bacteria.

Amebic ulceration of the intestinal wall is characteristic. A small mucosal defect overlies a larger, burrowing area of necrosis in the submucosa and muscularis, producing a bottle-shaped lesion. There is little acute inflammatory response to the damage, and, in contrast to the picture in bacillary dysentery, the mucosa between ulcers is normal, without hyperemia. In the cecum and elsewhere, chronic infection leads to the formation of large masses of granulation tissue or "amebomas." Amebas can enter the portal circulation and lodge in venules; liquefaction necrosis of liver tissue leads to the formation of an abscess cavity. Rarely, embolization results in lung, brain or splenic abscess.

Because trophozoites in histologic sections of liver or intestine are usually seen lying free in small spaces, it has been said that *E. histolytica* destroys tissue through the elaboration of a "cytolytic ferment." Not only is there no evidence whatsoever that such a substance exists, but the histologic appearance is simply a shrinkage artifact of fixation.

CHRONIC AMEBIC DYSENTERY. Most patients with this commonest type of amebic disease cannot date the onset of illness accurately. There is intermittent diarrhea consisting of one to four foul-smelling stools daily, sometimes containing mucus and blood, alternating with periods of relative normality for months or years. Vague abdominal cramping, weight loss, and mild fever are frequent. In such cases of "walking dysentery" the only findings are wasting, occasional tender hepatomegaly (not indicative of hepatic abscess), and slight pain when the cecum and ascending colon are palpated. Sigmoidoscopy sometimes reveals typical ulcerations with normal intervening mucosa, or mucosal defects may be demonstrated radiologically in the right colon. Specific diagnosis depends upon finding the organisms in the feces.

ACUTE AMEBIC DYSENTERY. This type of amebiasis is unusual but was observed in several patients during the large epidemic in a Chicago hotel in 1933 when massive contamination of the water supply occurred through defective plumbing; it is more likely to be seen sporadically in tropical areas. The onset is abrupt, with high fever (104 to 105°F), severe abdominal cramps, and profuse, bloody diarrhea with tenesmus. There is diffuse abdominal tenderness, often so severe that peritonitis is suspected. Hepatomegaly is very frequent, and sigmoidoscopy almost always demonstrates extensive rectosigmoid ulceration. Trophozoites are numerous in stools and in material obtained directly from the ulcers.

AMEBOMA (AMEBIC GRANULOMA). Chronic infection can lead to the production of large masses of granulation tissue in the colon. When the entire circumference of the intestine is involved, there may be partial obstruction and a tender, sausage-shaped mass is often palpable. This lesion is most frequent in the cecum, where a palpable mass and radiologic demonstration of a ragged encroachment upon the lumen can lead to a mistaken diagnosis of adenocarcinoma. A history of diarrhea with blood and mucus may be elicited, but this is compatible with the diagnosis of cancer. The importance of searching for amebas in the feces of any patient with these findings is very great because surgical intervention in untreated ameboma can lead to peritonitis or perforation, pericecal abscess, and sinus formation with drainage of feculent material through the abdominal wall. In addition to cancer, these lesions are likely to be confused with tuberculosis or actinomycosis.

In the tropics, amebic ulceration of the appendix is responsible for a significant proportion of cases of appendicitis. Again, operative intervention is contraindicated before specific treatment. The majority of deaths among tourists infected during the 1933 Chicago epidemic were a direct result of laparotomy carried out for symptoms of appendicitis. The operations were performed in many different towns and cities after patients had returned home and before the significance of exposure in Chicago had been widely appreciated.

HEPATIC AMEBIASIS. The parasites usually reach the liver through the portal vein; rarely, they may traverse the lymphatic vessels. It has been believed for a long time that amebas which lodged in the liver could produce a diffuse hepatitis. Careful postmortem and biopsy studies indicate that the syndrome of tender hepatomegaly, right upper quadrant pain, fever, and leukocytosis in patients with amebic colitis is not a result of the presence of amebas in hepatic tissues, is accompanied by nonspecific periportal inflammation, and is rarely, if ever, a prelude to hepatic abscess. It is evident, then, that these manifestations are best regarded as an accompaniment of colitis and do not merit a separate diagnosis of "diffuse amebic hepatitis."

Hepatic abscess may develop insidiously, with fever, sweats, weight loss, and no local signs other than painless or slightly tender hepatomegaly. In other patients, there is abrupt onset, with chills, fever to 105°F, nausea, vomiting, severe upper abdominal pain, and polymorphonuclear leukocytosis. Initially, cholecystitis, perforated ulcer, or acute pancreatitis may be suspected.

Almost invariably, amebic abscess is localized in the posterior portion of the right lobe of the liver, because this lobe receives most of the blood draining the right colon through the "streaming" effect in portal vein flow. This location is responsible for several features that aid in diagnosis. *Point tenderness* in the posterolateral portion of a lower right intercostal space is frequent even in the absence of diffuse liver pain. Most abscesses enlarge upward, producing a bulge in the diaphragmatic dome, obliteration of the costophrenic gutter, small hydrothorax, basilar atelectasis, and pain referred to the right shoulder. Radiologically, unruptured abscesses do not show a fluid level, and calcification of the liver parenchyma is very rare. Isotope liver scan is invaluable in confirming both the presence and location of a liver abscess.

Needle puncture results in the withdrawal of "pus" which consists of liquefied, necrotic liver, the classic "chocolate syrup" or "anchovy paste" exudate; the pus contains no polymorphonuclear leukocytes (barring secondary bacterial infection) and, usually, no amebas. The parasites are localized in the cyst wall and may be demonstrated at times by a Vim-Silverman needle biopsy of the cyst wall following aspiration of the abscess.

Hepatic abscess complicates asymptomatic infection of the colon more often than symptomatic intestinal disease, another factor making recognition difficult. Trophozoites or cysts are demonstrable in the feces of only about one-eighth of patients with abscess, and fewer

than one-half can recall significant diarrheal illness.

PLEUROPULMONARY AMEBIASIS. The right pleural cavity and lung are involved by direct extension from the liver in 10 to 20 percent of patients with liver abscess. Rarely, amebic lung abscess has resulted from embolization rather than direct extension.

Manifestations are those of massive pleural effusion; aspiration of chocolate fluid is diagnostic, or if the lung parenchyma is involved and perforation into a bronchus occurs, patients expectorate large amounts of the typical exudate, some patients even commenting that the sputum "tastes like liver." Cough, pleural pain, fever, and leukocytosis are the rule, and secondary bacterial infection is frequent.

OTHER EXTRAINTESTINAL LESIONS. Rupture of liver abscess into the *pericardium* has occurred; these patients are often thought initially to have tuberculous pericarditis. *Peritonitis* is a result of perforation of colonic ulcer or rupture of liver abscess. Painful ulcers of the genitalia, perianal skin, or abdominal wall (draining sinuses), vaginitis, urethritis, and prostatitis are unusual complications resulting from extension of intestinal disease. Metastatic brain abscess is rare and an etiologic diagnosis is seldom made clinically. Splenic abscess has been reported but is very unusual.

DIAGNOSIS. The diagnosis of intestinal amebiasis depends upon identification of the organism in the stool or tissues. Formed stools are examined in saline and iodine mounts for amebic cysts; concentration methods will double the yield. Liquid stools must be examined immediately (or kept at body temperature until examination) in saline solution and using a warm stage if motile trophozoites are to be detected. Fixation of specimens in polyvinyl alcohol or merthiolate-iodine-formalin will preserve amebas for later identification. Careful examination of 4 to 6 stool specimens may be required for diagnosis.

Sigmoidoscopy is of value in symptomatic cases. The mucosal lesions should be aspirated and the material examined for trophozoites. Stained sections of biopsy material obtained from such lesions also will frequently reveal trophozoites.

The diagnosis of extraintestinal amebiasis is difficult. The parasite usually cannot be recovered from stool or tissue. Serologic tests employing purified antigens are positive in nearly all patients with proved amebic liver abscess, and in the majority of those with acute amebic dysentery. However, false positive results make these tests of more value in excluding the diagnosis rather than in confirming it. Cultivation of amebas from feces or pus is possible but is not practical in most laboratories. A most important diagnostic procedure in suspected liver abscess is a therapeutic trial of antiamebic drugs. The response is often dramatic within 3 days. In the event that demonstrating parasites is difficult, a therapeutic trial should be instituted without hesitation.

TREATMENT. Treatment should be aimed at relief of symptoms, replacement of fluid, electrolyte, and blood losses, and eradication of the organism. Eradication is confirmed by healing of lesions and by disappearance of either cysts or trophozoites from the stool. Amebicidal agents may act directly on the trophozoite or indirectly by destroying the intestinal bacteria upon which it is dependent for growth. The direct-acting amebicides can be divided further into those that act systemically and those that are active only within the lumen of the bowel by direct contact with the organisms. The large number of agents available indicates the lack of a single ideal drug. While most patients are eventually cured, initial improvement in chronic cases is frequently followed by relapse. In treatment, often a combination of drugs may be necessary to achieve cure.

The available drugs fall into several different groups. *Arsenicals:* Milibis (0.5 Gm three times daily for 1 week) is the least toxic of these preparations. It is effective only against intestinal trophozoites. *Halogenated hydroxyquinolines:* Diodoquin (0.65 Gm three times daily for 21 days) is used most frequently. Like Milibis it is a contact amebicide active only within the gut. *Antibiotics:* Oxytetracycline (Terramycin) is the most effective when given in dosage of 2.0 Gm daily for 10 days. Paromomycin (Humatin) given in a single dose (4.0 Gm or 1.0 Gm three times daily for 10 days) is also used. Both are effective only in intestinal amebiasis. *Aminoquinolines:* Chloroquine diphosphate (Aralen) is a systemic amebicide which is useful in hepatic disease because of its high concentration in the liver (0.5 Gm twice daily for 2 days and 0.5 Gm once daily for 12 to 19 days). *Alkaloids:* Emetine is a relatively toxic derivative of ipecac. When given intramuscularly (65 mg daily for no more than 10 days), it is highly effective in destroying trophozoites in tissue but does not affect these organisms in the gut. Dehydroemetine is apparently less toxic. This drug must also be given intramuscularly in dosage of 80 mg daily for no more than 10 days. Oral emetine preparations are effective against intestinal organisms but are not available in the United States. *Metronidazole* (Flagyl) taken orally in dosage of 800 mg three times daily for 10 days is unique because it is active against both intestinal and extraintestinal trophozoites. A related drug, niradazole (Ambulhar) is also effective but more toxic.

In asymptomatic or mildly symptomatic patients, Milibis and Diodoquin administered sequentially give good results. Paromomycin is also effective. Stools should be examined monthly for a year to detect relapse. If relapse occurs, retreatment should consist of a combination of Diodoquin and Terramycin. Chloroquine can be added for its potentiating effect on Terramycin as well as its ability to eradicate subclinical hepatic infection.

Treatment of acute dysentery involves control of symptoms as well as eradication of the organism. A number of regimens can be used:

1. Emetine or dehydroemetine given intramuscularly will control the acute attack. Because these drugs are toxic and cannot eliminate intestinal trophozoites, therapy with these drugs should be discontinued as soon as symptoms abate and a course of intestinal amebicides should be instituted. Terramycin or a combination of Diodoquin and Milibis is satisfactory. Usually emetine or dehydroemetine need be given for only 3 to 4 days to control the attack and are also effective in treating subclinical hepatic infection.

Emetine is quite toxic and produces abdominal pain, tremor, weakness, electrocardiographic abnormalities, and orthostatic hypotension. Dehydroemetine is less toxic, but neither drug should be given for more than 10 days and the dosage should not exceed 65 mg for emetine or 80 mg for dehydroemetine or 1 mg/Kg for either drug. Neither drug should be used in patients with renal, cardiac, or muscle disease, during pregnancy, or in children, unless all other drugs fail.

2. Terramycin will bring an acute attack under control although not as rapidly as emetine. It has the additional advantage of terminating the intestinal infection. A course of chloroquine should be given with Terramycin to eradicate subclinical hepatic infection.

3. Metronidazole. This agent controls symptoms, destroys intestinal trophozoites, and eradicates hepatic infection. If more extensive experience confirms the initial results, this agent could become the drug of choice in amebic dysentery.

4. If hepatic abscess is suspected, chloroquine is the drug of choice. It is effective, nontoxic, and produces symptomatic relief in 48 to 72 hr. Even large abscesses subside, but relapse is relatively frequent. If aspiration or a dramatic response to chloroquine prove that a hepatic abscess is of amebic etiology, emetine or dehydroemetine should be given for 10 days also to prevent relapse. Drainage of an amebic abscess usually is not necessary and should be performed only if there is localized swelling over the liver, marked elevation of the diaphragm, severe localized liver tenderness, and failure to respond to systemic amebicides. Adequate drainage can usually be accomplished by needle alone and surgical drainage is rarely necessary. The greatest hazard in needling an abscess is secondary bacterial infection.

Contact amebicides must be given in combination with emetine and chloroquine, to eradicate any intestinal trophozoites that might lead to relapse.

Amebiasis in locations other than the intestine and liver should be treated like hepatic amebiasis.

PROGNOSIS. Complete cure of intestinal amebiasis occurs in 75 to 95 percent of cases with repeated courses of therapy. The relapse rate is as high as 35 percent after a single course. The fatality rate is less than 5 percent.

Hepatic and pulmonary amebiasis are still attended by appreciable mortality, but no reliable figures are available.

PREVENTION. For the individual, avoidance of contaminated food and water, scalding of vegetables, and the use of iodine-releasing tablets in drinking water (chlorine, in the form of Halazone, is ineffective) are important measures. Globaline tablets, containing tetraglycine hydroperiodide, are convenient and effective.

Improvements in general sanitation and the detection of cyst passers and their removal from food-handling duties are general measures in prophylaxis, but such segregation of carriers is rarely practiced.

INFECTIONS DUE TO *HARTMANNELLA*

The free-living amebae which commonly inhabit soil and water and are usually considered to be nonpathogenic for man are called *Hartmannella* or *Acanthamoeba*. Several species have been described under the generic name *Hartmannella*, a term which will be used pending further clarification of their taxonomy. These amebae have been grown in monkey kidney and other tissue cultures, and some animals, including primates, experience both fatal and nonfatal infections when inoculated with species of *Hartmannella*. More importantly, a number of human cases of fatal meningitis have been caused by *Hartmannella* species. Three fatal cases occurred in boys following their swimming in two small, warm, Florida lakes. Similar organisms were cultured from the lakes. Seven fatal cases of meningoencephalitis occurred in July 1951, 1952, and 1966 in the vicinity of Richmond, Virginia. Each patient had been swimming in nearby lakes. A diagnosis of purulent meningitis was usually made, and the spinal fluids had leukocyte counts ranging from 870 to 21,450, mostly granulocytes. Protein was elevated and glucose was diminished. No bacteria were demonstrated either on smear or culture. Treatment with various antibiotics and sulfonamides was to no avail. The final diagnoses were made from the microscopic examination of the brains. Within a 4-year period, 16 fatal cases of amebic meningoencephalitis were identified in northern Bohemia. The age range was from eight to twenty-five years, and no patients responded to treatment with antibiotics and sulfonamides. All patients had been swimming in an indoor pool with chlorinated water maintained at 24°C. The average incubation period was about 7 days. The clinical courses of these and other cases have lasted from 1 to 8 days. The histologic examination often suggests that infection of the brain was by way of the nose.

Several new "viruses" have been demonstrated to be *Hartmannella* species. Wang and Feldman reported the isolation of 54 strains (three species) of *Hartmannella* in tissue cultures inoculated with pharyngeal swabs that had been obtained from members of a population of "normal" families which is under continuous surveillance for respiratory infections. Most isolates were obtained from young children, often less than one year of age. Several families had multiple isolations. No evident relationship could be established between the presence of amebae and clinical disease.

The treatment of human cases of amebic meningoencephalitis with antibiotics and sulfonamides has been unsuccessful. Emetine was not very effective against the free-living amoebae in vitro, but carbarsone, a pentavalent arsenical seemed to affect them adversely. A clinical trial with this drug may be warranted should an infection of this type be recognized or suspected.

It is not possible at this time to define the spectrum of human illness which may be caused by *Hartmannella*

but it is very likely that these organisms will increase in importance.

REFERENCES

Amebiasis

Belding, D. L., and H. W. Brown: "Basic Clinical Parasitology," New York, Appleton-Century-Crofts, Inc., 1964.

Kessel, J. F., W. P. Lewis, C. M. Pasquel, and J. A. Turner: Indirect Hemagglutination and Complement Fixation Tests in Amebiasis, Am. J. Trop. Med. Hyg., 14:540, 1965.

Lamont, N. McE., and N. R. Pooler: Hepatic Amoebiasis, Quart. J. Med., 27:389, 1958.

Powell, S. J., A. J. Wilmot, and R. Elsdon-Dew: Further Trials of Metronidazole in Amebic Dysentery and Amebic Liver Abscess., Ann. Trop. Med. Parasit., 61:511, 1967.

Powell, S. J., A. J. Wilmot, I. Macleod, and R. Elsdon-Dew: A Comparative Trial of Dehydroemetine, Emetine Hydrochloride, and Chloroquin in the Treatment of Amebic Liver Abscess., Ann. Trop. Med. Parasit., 59:496, 1965.

Wilmot, A. J.: "Clinical Amoebiasis," Philadelphia, F. A. Davis Company, 1962.

Hartmannella

Butt, C. G.: Primary Amebic Meningoencephalitis, New Engl. J. Med., 274:1473, 1966.

Callicott, J. H., Jr.: Amebic Meningoencephalitis Due to Free-living Amebas of the Hartmannella (Acanthamoeba)-Naegleria Group, Am. J. Clin. Path., 49:84, 1968.

Cerva, L., and K. Novak: Amoebic Meningoencephalitis: Sixteen Fatalities, Science, 160:92, 1968.

Culbertson, C. G.: Pathogenic Acanthamoeba (Hartmannella), Am. J. Clin. Path., 35:195, 1961.

Wang, S. S., and H. A. Feldman: Isolation of Hartmannella Species from Human Throats, New Engl. J. Med., 277:174, 1967.

241 MALARIA
James J. Plorde and Ivan L. Bennett, Jr.

DEFINITION. Malaria is a protozoan disease transmitted to man by the bite of *Anopheles* mosquitoes. It remains the major infectious disease problem in the world. The increasing import of malaria into the United States by travelers and military personnel has caused a resurgence of interest in this disease. Malaria is characterized by rigors, fever, splenomegaly, anemia, and a chronic, relapsing course.

ETIOLOGY. The causative organisms are protozoa of the genus *Plasmodium*. The four species known to infect man do not produce disease in lower animals, although many species affecting animals and birds are known. *Plasmodium vivax* causes tertian malaria; *P. malariae* causes quartan malaria; *P. falciparum* causes malignant tertian (estivoautumnal) malaria; *P. ovale* causes ovale tertian malaria, a relatively rare and mild illness.

Man is the intermediate and the mosquito the definitive host. In man, after a stage of exoerythrocytic development in the liver, the parasites reproduce asexually in circulating erythrocytes. They first appear in the red cells as *ring forms;* after several divisions, daughter cells (*merozoites*) fill the corpuscle, which ruptures and releases them (sporulation) to parasitize additional erythrocytes. With repetition of this cycle, some of the red cells become filled with sexual forms (*gametocytes*); these do not induce cell lysis and are unable to undergo further development unless ingested by an appropriate mosquito during a blood meal. In the stomach of the mosquito fertilization occurs, and the resulting *ookinete* encysts on the outer surface of the stomach and releases myriads of *sporozoites.* These migrate to the salivary glands and, if inoculated into a human subject, lead to repetition of asexual multiplication. There is variation in this cycle among different species, and several intermediate stages occur.

The asexual cycle in the erythrocyte requires 36 to 48 hr for *P. falciparum,* 48 hr for *P. vivax* and *P. ovale,* and 72 hr for *P. malariae.* The periodicity of febrile paroxysms in infections by the different species coincides with the cyclic discharge of merozoites. The incubation period between bite of an infected mosquito and onset of symptoms is 10 to 14 days in vivax and falciparum malaria and 18 days to 6 weeks in quartan infections. There is good evidence for the existence of several strains of each species of human malarial *Plasmodium,* and greater virulence of some strains is suggested by the consistent severity of the clinical illnesses which they produce.

EPIDEMIOLOGY. Malaria survives only in areas where the mosquito and the infected human populations remain above a *critical density* for each. These critical densities are interdependent, but either may fluctuate in a given area. Control measures are directed toward reducing both populations to levels that are too low for the infection to survive. Important procedures include drainage or filling of breeding areas, use of residual insecticide sprays (this has largely replaced the use of oil or other antilarval measures), screening, use of skin repellents, effective treatment of cases, and large-scale suppressive drug programs in some human populations.

An active international cooperative program aimed at the eradication of malaria has resulted in a significant decline in the incidence of the disease since 1945. In over three-quarters of the original malarial areas of the world, the disease has been eradicated or active eradication programs have been instituted. The presence of mobile populations, outdoor biting mosquitoes, and high levels of disease transmission make successful eradication in the remaining areas less certain. Furthermore, the emergence of insecticide-resistant mosquitoes and drug-resistant parasites as well as a variety of administrative problems have produced serious setbacks to several previously successful eradication programs. The demonstration of naturally occurring simian malaria in man has raised the question of an animal reservoir of the disease. Although this may not prove to be a major problem, the global eradication of malaria remains today a distant goal.

PATHOGENESIS AND PATHOLOGY. The invasion, alteration, and destruction of red cells by malaria parasites, systemic and local circulatory changes, and immune phenomena are probably all important in the pathophysiology of malaria. Malaria species differ significantly in their ability to invade red cells. *Plasmodium vivax* and *P. ovale* attack only immature erythrocytes and *P. malariae,* only senescent ones. During infection with these species, therefore, no more than 1 or 2 percent of cells are involved at any one time. *Plasmodium falciparum* invades red cells regardless of age and may cause extremely high levels of parasitemia. Only the presence of certain abnormal hemoglobins, notably S, is capable of limiting parasitemia produced by the species. Whether the same protective effect is exerted in hemoglobin C, thalassemia, and G-6-PD deficiency awaits confirmation.

Once parasitized, the cells may be destroyed at the time of sporulation or phagocytosed in the liver or spleen. In the spleen the parasites are also removed from some cells, and the intact erythrocytes are returned into the circulation. However, anemia usually develops, and in the case of falciparum malaria, may be severe. This species also induces physical changes in parasitized cells resulting in intravascular agglutination and sludging.

Although paroxysms of fever coincide with sporulation and the destruction of red cells, the cause of the fever remains obscure and may be related to release of an endogenous pyrogen from injured cells.

The circulatory changes in malaria are characterized by vasoconstriction during the "cold" stage followed by vasodilation during the "hot" stage. In falciparum malaria vasodilation in the skin is accompanied by hypotension, decreased central venous pressure, increased radioiodinated serum albumin space, and increased excretion of aldosterone, suggesting a decrease in effective circulating blood volume due to enhanced vascular permeability and/or capacitance. On the other hand, there may be localized vasospasm, obstruction of capillaries with agglutinated red cells, and intravascular coagulation which may compromise perfusion to vital organs such as the kidney, brain, liver, and lung.

Normal as well as parasitized red cells are destroyed in malaria. This phenomenon occurs in all forms but is most profound during blackwater fever. Hypersplenism results in erythrophagocytosis but there is also evidence that immune mechanisms may be operative in excess red cell destruction and renal disease. Host gamma and beta-1C-globulin deposits have been noted along the glomerular capillary basement membrane of patients with the nephrosis of quartan malaria.

Negroes seem to be peculiarly resistant to *P. vivax* infection; the mechanism for this is unknown.

Immunity in malaria is mediated by species specific IgG and IgM antibodies which appear early in malaria infection in response to the erythrocytic phase of parasitemia. These antibodies have an antiplasmodial effect. The relative rarity of malaria in young infants has been attributed to transplacental passage of IgG antibodies. While immunity in malaria has been thought to be strain specific, different strains appear to share common antigens. Furthermore, there appear to be antigenic changes in the parasites during chronic simian malaria which may provide an explanation for the relapsing course of malarial infection.

MANIFESTATIONS. General. There is some variation in malaria produced by the different plasmodia, but in all, chills, fever, headache, muscle pains, splenomegaly, and anemia are common. Herpes labialis is frequent and usually appears after the infection is well established. Hepatomegaly, mild icterus, and edema are often observed, especially in estivoautumnal infections. Urticaria is common in patients with chronic malaria.

The hall mark of the disease is the malarial *paroxysm*, which recurs regularly in all but falciparum infections. The typical paroxysm begins with a rigor that lasts 20 to 60 min—the "cold stage"—followed by a "hot stage" of 3 to 8 hr with temperature of 104 to 107°F. The "wet stage" consists of defervescence with profuse diaphoresis and leaves the patient exhausted.

First attacks are often severe, but repeated episodes become milder, although debilitation may be progressive. In untreated cases, the attacks may persist for weeks. The paroxysms eventually become more irregular and less frequent and finally cease, corresponding with the disappearance of parasites from the blood and marking the end of the primary attack. Relapses occur when exoerythrocytic parasites persisting in the liver reinvade the bloodstream.

Tertian Malaria (P. vivax or P. ovale). This infection is rarely fatal, although relapses are common, and it is the most difficult to cure. A prodrome of myalgia, headache, chilliness, and low-grade fever for 48 to 72 hr heralds the onset of the acute illness. Initially, the fever may be irregular because the maturation cycle of the parasite is not synchronized. Synchronization usually occurs toward the end of the first week, and typical paroxysms then occur on alternate days. The spleen becomes palpable at the end of the second week. Infections with *P. ovale* tend to be milder, and primary attacks shorter than those caused by *P. vivax*.

Quartan Malaria (P. malariae). Paroxysms occur every third day and tend to be regular. The disease is usually more disabling than tertian but responds well to treatment. Edema, albuminuria, and hematuria (*not* hemoglobinuria), a clinical state similar to acute hemorrhagic nephritis, occasionally appear during the course. This complication should not be confused with *blackwater fever*. Chronic *P. malariae* infection may be associated with nephrosis, which is poorly understood.

Estivoautumnal Malaria (P. falciparum). Because of an asynchronous cycle of multiplication, the onset may be insidious and fever continuous, remittent or irregular. Typical paroxysms occur in a minority of patients. Splenomegaly occurs rapidly and mental confusion, postural hypotension, edema and gastrointestinal symptoms are common. If the acute attack is treated rapidly, the disease is usually mild and recovery uneventful. If left untreated anemia becomes severe, and the decreased effective circulating blood volume results in capillary blockage that can give rise to serious complications. This feature of *P. falci-*

parum infections accounts for the protean manifestations of estivoautumnal malaria, and the high morbidity and mortality associated with it. Depending upon the organ system involved, several so-called *pernicious syndromes* are seen. *Cerebral malaria* can lead to hemiplegia, convulsions, delirium, hyperpyrexia, coma, and rapid death. When the *pulmonary* circulation is involved, there may be cough and blood-streaked sputum, leading to confusion with many other diseases of the lung. The splanchnic capillaries can be obstructed, with consequent vomiting, abdominal pain, diarrhea, or melena. Such patients are sometimes thought to have bacillary dysentery or cholera. Fever in these disorders may be low or absent. Indeed, in patients with predominantly gastrointestinal manifestations, there are usually cold clammy skin, hypotension, profound weakness, and repeated syncopal attacks, so-called *algid malaria*. Tender hepatomegaly, with or without jaundice, and acute renal failure are common. The pernicious syndromes should be anticipated if more than 5 per cent of red cells are parasitized.

Blackwater Fever. This is a disorder that occurs in association with malaria, particularly and perhaps only with *P. falciparum* infections. The usual attack begins with a rigor and fever followed by massive intravascular hemolysis, icterus, hemoglobinuria, collapse, and often acute renal failure and uremia. The pathologic findings in the kidney are necrosis of tubules and occasionally hemoglobin casts. The mortality is 20 to 30 percent, and survivors are very likely to experience hemolytic episodes with subsequent malarial infections.

Although blackwater fever is often classified as one of the "pernicious" complications of estivoautumnal malaria, its etiology is obscure. In many patients, parasitemia is absent at the time hemolysis occurs. Because blackwater fever has usually occurred in patients with chronic falciparum infections who were treated with quinine, it was suggested that the hemolysis results from an autoimmune reaction to the red cells that have been altered by the drug or parasite or both. However, blackwater fever can occur in patients not given drugs. The institution of an appropriate regimen for acute renal failure (Chap. 300) will reduce the fatality rate considerably.

Complications. In addition to the several complications already mentioned, others deserve comment. Rupture of the spleen is relatively rare, but malaria is by far the commonest cause of spontaneous rupture and predisposes to traumatic rupture of this organ.

Chronic malaria or repeated infection in an endemic area leads to anemia, debility, and cachexia. Secondary bacterial infection is often the immediate cause of death. Bacillary dysentery, cholera, and pyogenic pneumonia are common. Tuberculous foci often extend in malarial patients, and miliary tuberculosis is occasionally observed.

LABORATORY FINDINGS. The blood leukocyte count is low or normal. The erythrocyte sedimentation rate is elevated. Plasmodia are demonstrable in smears of peripheral blood from the vast majority of patients with symptomatic malaria. When the disease is suspected, appropriately stained blood films should be examined diligently. For the inexperienced examiner, a thin smear of fingertip blood on a clean glass slide should be stained with Wright, Giemsa, or Hastings stain. Parasitized erythrocytes are most frequent at the edges of a smear; extracellular parasites are not found. Thick smears should be thoroughly dried and stained with diluted Giemsa or Field stain. This method has the advantage of concentrating the parasites, but artefacts are numerous, and correct interpretation of these preparations requires much experience.

The morphology of the four species of plasmodia that infect man is specific enough to allow identification in blood smears. The parasitized red cells in *P. vivax* infections are enlarged, pale, and may contain diffuse bright red dots (Schaffner's dots), and the parasite presents in a wide variety of shapes and sizes; in *P. ovale* infections, the red cells containing parasites are oval but otherwise resemble those in *P. vivax*; in *P. malariae* the red cells are of normal size and do not contain dots. The parasites often present in "band" forms and the merozoites are arranged in a rosette around central pigment; in *P. falciparum* infections the rings are very small, may contain two rather than one chromatin dot, and often are found lying flat against the margin of the cell. Only the ring stages of the asexual forms are found in the peripheral smear, and there may be more than one ring in a single red cell. The gametocytes are distinctively large and banana-shaped.

There is no advantage over blood of material obtained by splenic or sternal puncture. The administration of epinephrine with the idea of dislodging parasites by producing contraction of the spleen has been advocated, but results are irregular. Serologic tests are used primarily for epidemiologic rather than diagnostic purposes.

DIAGNOSIS. The most important diagnostic test is the search for parasites in peripheral blood. Because the intensity of parasitemia varies greatly from hour to hour, particularly in *P. falciparum* infections, blood smears should be examined repeatedly and at frequent intervals. History of residence in an endemic area, previous attacks of malaria, typical malarial paroxysms, or some artificial exposure (blood transfusion, narcotic injections in an addict) should suggest the disease. Splenomegaly is an almost invariable finding during the second week of illness. Leukocytosis is *not* a feature of malaria.

While final cure of malaria may be difficult, particularly in *P. vivax* infections, almost all cases will respond symptomatically to quinine or one of the newer antimalarial drugs, and failure of response to a therapeutic trial argues strongly against the diagnosis.

TREATMENT. The use of appropriate chemotherapy can suppress symptoms in individuals exposed in endemic areas or cure malarial infection completely. The emergence of drug-resistent falciparum malaria in Brazil, Colombia, Venezuela, and Southeast Asia, however, necessitates the use of drug combinations in the treatment of this infection.

Treatment of Acute Attack. Treatment of an acute attack can be accomplished with chloroquine for all types of malaria except drug-resistant falciparum infection. Administration of 0.6 Gm of chloroquine base (four tablets) followed by 0.3 Gm 6 hr later and then 0.3 Gm daily for 2 days usually produces complete subsidence of symptoms and destruction of the erythrocytic forms of the parasite. If vomiting is present, chloroquine hydrochloride should be given intramuscularly in dosage of 0.2 to 0.3 Gm of base every 6 hr. Oral therapy should be resumed as soon as possible.

If the patient has contracted malaria in an area known to harbor drug-resistant *P. falciparum,* he should be treated with a combination of quinine, pyrimethamine, and one of the sulfonamides or sulfones. *Quinine sulfate,* 0.6 Gm orally three times a day, should be given for 14 days. If nausea and vomiting preclude oral therapy, quinine dihydrochloride diluted in saline or glucose can be given very slowly intravenously. The dose may be repeated every 6 hr, but oral therapy should be instituted as soon as possible. In the presence of renal failure, the dose of quinine should be limited to 0.6 Gm a day, and the drug should not be given if acute massive hemolysis occurs. An overdose of quinine produces cinchonism of which tinnitus is an early manifestation. The drug may also cause mild hemolysis, allergic purpura, and drug fever. Pyrimethamine should be given orally in dosage of 25 mg three times daily for 3 days. This is an antifolate agent and may cause megaloblastic anemia. Sulfisoxazole, 2.0 Gm initially and then 0.5 Gm every 6 hr for 5 days should be given concurrently with the other 2 drugs. Pyrimethamine with a sulfonamide may be as effective as the three-drug regimen but acts more slowly.

Patients should be followed for 1 month to detect recrudescence of the infection, and if there is evidence of recurrence, retreatment with pyrimethamine and a sulfonamide should be instituted.

Radical Cure. *Plasmodium vivax, P. ovale,* and *P. malariae* all persist in the liver in the exocrythrocytic stage and in this form are not affected by drugs used in the treatment of the acute attack. Unless destroyed, they will eventually reinvade the bloodstream. Primaquine base 15 mg by mouth daily for 14 days will effect a radical cure in most cases. If relapse occurs after primaquine therapy, a second course of the drug should be given. This agent may cause hemolysis in patients with G-6-PD deficiency, but in the dosage recommended hemolysis is rare and usually mild.

Treatment of Complications. This includes careful attention to fluid and electrolyte balance, prevention of fluid overload in patients with oliguria, and early diagnosis and treatment of renal failure. In severe hemolysis large doses of steroids may be helpful in combating hemolysis. Transfusions should be given in severe hemolysis, care being taken to match the patient's cells and plasma with that of the donor. Dexamethasone has been helpful in management of cerebral edema.

Suppressive Therapy. Although it is not possible to prevent infection with chemotherapeutic agents, it is possible to suppress symptoms while residing in an endemic area by the administration of chloroquine base in dosage of 300 mg weekly (2 tablets Aralen). If the medication is continued for 1 month after leaving the area, sensitive strains of *P. falciparum* will be eradicated. *Plasmodium ovale, P. malariae,* and *P. vivax* will produce clinical manifestations some weeks or months after chloroquine is discontinued because of their persistence outside red cells. This can be circumvented by administration of primaquine after chloroquine is discontinued. Chloroquine is not effective in suppressing drug-resistant *P. falciparum.*

REFERENCES

Blount, R. E.: Management of Chloroquine-Resistant Falciparum Malaria, A.M.A. Arch. Intern. Med., 119:557, 1967.

Conrad, M. E.: Pathophysiology of Malaria: Hematologic Observations in Human and Animal Studies, Ann. Int. Med., 70:134, 1969.

Dukes, D. C., B. J. Sealey, and J. I. Forbes: Oliguric Renal Failure in Blackwater Fever, Am. J. Med., 45:899, 1968.

Hunter, G. W., W. W. Frye, and J. C. Swartzwelder: "A Manual of Tropical Medicine," 4th ed., Philadelphia, W. B. Saunders Company, 1966.

Maegrath, B. G.: The Physiologic Approach to the Problems of Malaria, Brit. Med. Bull., 8:28, 1951.

Malloy, J. P., M. H. Brooks, and K. G. Barry: Pathophysiology of Acute Falciparum Malaria, Am. J. Med., 43:745, 1967.

Neva, F. A.: Malaria—Recent Progress and Problems, New Engl. J. Med., 277:1241, 1967.

Russell, P. F., L. S. West, R. D. Manwell, and G. MacDonald: "Practical Malariology," 2d ed., Fairlawn, N.J., Oxford University Press, 1963.

242 LEISHMANIASIS

James J. Plorde and
Ivan L. Bennett, Jr.

DEFINITION. Leishmaniasis designates three separate disorders of man that are produced by protozoa of the genus *Leishmania.* All are transmitted by the bite of sandflies (*Phlebotomus*).

ETIOLOGY AND PATHOGENESIS. There is confusion over speciation of *Leishmania.* These organisms appear morphologically identical and must be differentiated by serologic techniques which are not entirely satisfactory. There are antigenic differences among various strains of *Leishmania* species, but the significance of these differences is not known. Four species are generally recognized: *L. donovani, L. tropica, L. mexicana,* and *L. brasiliensis.* Two others, *L. peruviana* and *L. pifanoi,* are thought to be variations of *L. brasiliensis.*

Leishmania donovani is the cause of kala-azar, the visceral form of leishmaniasis (dumdum fever, tropical splenomegaly, Burdwan fever, Sirkari disease, *Ponos, Mard el Bicha*).

Leishmania tropica causes Old World cutaneous leishmaniasis or oriental sore, also known as Delhi boil, Bagdad boil, Aleppo button, and Salek and Pendeh sore.

Leishmania mexicana produces a cutaneous leishmania-

sis known as forest yaws, bay sore, and *chiclero ulcer. Leishmania brasiliensis* is the cause of American mucocutaneous leishmaniasis also known as *espundia. Leishmania brasiliensis* (var.) *peruviana* produces *uta,* another type of cutaneous leishmaniasis, and *Leishmaniasis tegumentaria diffusa* is caused by *L. brasiliensis* (var.) *pifanoi.*

In the sandfly, the parasites assume the flagellated leptomonas form, but in man, the organisms lose their flagella, enter mononuclear phagocytes, and multiply as small, rounded leishmanial forms 2 to 3 μ in diameter, the pathognomonic "Leishman-Donovan bodies."

In man continued intracellular multiplication of the parasite leads to rupture of the affected phagocyte and invasion of other cells, resulting in extensive histiocytic proliferation which is followed by infiltration with plasma cells and lymphocytes. The course of the disease from this point is apparently determined by the host's immunologic reaction, which is poorly understood. In cutaneous leishmaniasis the secondary cellular infiltration is associated with a reduction in the number of parasites, the development of a delayed skin (leishmanin) reaction, and spontaneous cure. In the mucocutaneous form, the spontaneous disappearance of the primary lesion may be followed by destructive metastatic mucocutaneous lesions at some later date. An interesting exception to the general pattern in cutaneous disease is *leishmaniasis tegumentaria diffusa* in which there is no infiltration of lymphocytes and plasma cells, the leishmanin reaction is negative, and the skin lesions become chronic, progressive and disseminated. In visceral leishmaniasis, the cellular changes are similar to those seen in cutaneous disease. However, the skin test remains negative, and the parasites spread to reticuloendothelial cells throughout the body. This spread is associated with development of marked hyperglobulinemia. Circulating antibodies which are rarely seen in cutaneous forms of the disease are detectable but do not seem to have a protective function. A positive skin test develops in the visceral form after successful treatment.

KALA-AZAR

DISTRIBUTION AND EPIDEMIOLOGY. Kala-azar occurs in China, Russia, India, Egypt, Sudan, East Africa, several Mediterranean countries, including Greece, Crete, and Malta, and a few areas of South and Central America. Although the manifestations of the disease throughout this area, which touches all continents but Australia, are basically similar, certain definite peculiarities in its behavior justify classification of visceral leishmaniasis into at least three main types. These differences are attributed to variations in the strains of *L. donovani* in a given area and, perhaps more important, to the length of time that the disease has been endemic in a population. It is believed that kala-azar (and also infection by *L. tropica*) is introduced into a new area from animal reservoirs and that this "primitive" or zoonotic infection is likely to result in many cases of acute, rapidly fatal illness among the population coming into contact with the parasites for the first time. After generations, kala-azar becomes endemic, the disease assumes a more chronic form, and the main or only reservoir of infection, especially in urban areas, is man.

Mediterranean, or *infantile*, *kala-azar* is primarily a disease of children under the age of two years and has its reservoir in dogs, jackals, and foxes. Adults are by no means spared, but the preceding sentence describes the predominant pattern of the disorder as it occurs in the Mediterranean area, China, Russia, and Latin America.

Indian kala-azar shows no special predilection for infants and has never been found in dogs or other animals in India, indicating that the human reservoir is responsible for perpetuation of the disease.

Sudanese, or *Egyptian*, *kala-azar* shows no predilection for children, is endemic in gerbils and other rodents in many areas, and is more resistant to therapy with antimony compounds than that found in the rest of the world.

MANIFESTATIONS. The incubation period varies from 10 days to 1 year but is usually about 3 months. No lesion appears at the site of the infecting bite in most cases, but a primary "chancre" which heals with scarring before the onset of systemic symptoms is commonly noted in the African disease. The organisms multiply extensively in the macrophages of spleen, liver, bone marrow, and lymph nodes, accounting for many of the manifestations of the disease. Organisms may be found in the blood for several months before the onset of symptoms.

Fever, which is characterized at times by two daily spikes, may be abrupt or gradual in onset. It persists for 1 to 6 weeks and then disappears only to reappear at irregular intervals during the course of the illness. Although prostration is absent even during periods of high fever, there is progressive weakness, pallor, weight loss, and tachycardia. Gastrointestinal disturbances are frequent in Indian cases. Physical findings include enormous splenomegaly, lymphadenopathy, hepatomegaly, and often, edema, which tends to conceal the extent of the wasting. The proliferation of parasite-loaded histiocytes in the bone marrow and in the enlarged spleen make anemia the rule, and thrombocytopenia with gingival and other mucosal bleeding is common. The peripheral leukocyte count is low (usually less than 4,000 per cu mm); in children, granulocytosis with cancrum oris (noma) and secondary pulmonary or intestinal infections contribute to the high mortality.

Hyperglobulinemia is universally present. Proteinuria and hematuria are frequent in the course of kala-azar, and symptoms of heart failure can occur terminally; uremia due to renal amyloidosis may complicate chronic cases.

DIAGNOSIS. The diagnosis is made by finding leishmania in stained preparations of blood (often possible in Indian but rarely so in Sudanese kala-azar), bone marrow, lymph nodes, or material obtained by hepatic or splenic puncture. The last is the best source of organisms, but the spleen should be needled only by an expert. The organisms will grow out as flagellated forms in simple media containing blood incubated at 28°C.

A complement fixation test using an antigen from *Mycobacterium phlei* gives positive results in 95 percent of patients with kala-azar, but tuberculosis gives positive test results also. Fluorescent antibody and indirect hemagglutination tests with leishmanial antigens are more specific but are not generally available. The leishmanin skin test is negative during active kala-azar but becomes positive several months after successful treatment of the disease.

TREATMENT. Rest, good diet, transfusions, and treatment of complicating infections, of which tuberculosis, bacterial pneumonia, amebiasis, and bacillary dysentery are the more important, must supplement or precede specific therapy. Pentavalent antimony compounds are highly effective against the parasites. Neostibosan, as a 25 percent solution, can be given intravenously or intramuscularly on alternate days. A total of 3 to 4 Gm in 10 injections is needed. Urea stibamine is popular in India. Solustibosan, neostam, and Pentostam are effective antimony compounds that come as permanently stable solutions in ampuls for injection.

More than 90 percent of cases respond promptly to antimony, except in Africa, where the cure rate is as low as 70 percent. Resistant cases should be treated with 2 percent pentamidine (two courses of 5 to 10 intravenous or intramuscular injections each of 2 to 4 mg per kg on alternate days) or with the more effective hydroxystilbamidine given intravenously as 10 daily injections of a fresh solution in dosage of 0.25 Gm daily. The course may have to be repeated in African Kala-azar. Amphotericin B has been effective in some cases.

POST-KALA-AZAR DERMAL LEISHMANIASIS. Patients treated successfully with antimony compounds for kala-azar may later develop cutaneous lesions called "leishmanoids," in which *Leishmania* are demonstrable. These are rare in Mediterranean or Chinese kala-azar. They occur after a latent period of 1 to 2 years in as many as 10 percent of Indian cases, and in 30 percent of Sudanese cases, they occur almost immediately after systemic symptoms subside. The lesions range from patchy areas of depigmentation to erythematous papules and confluent nodules which may involve the ears and mucous membranes and have been mistaken for leprosy.

Antimony will cure these dermal leishmanoids, but the response is slow.

PROGNOSIS AND CONTROL. The mortality in untreated kala-azar is 95 percent in adults and 80 percent in children. This has been greatly reduced by treatment with antimony and the aromatic diamidines.

The treatment of the disease in man, the elimination of diseased dogs, and the use of DDT residual sprays against sandflies are the important preventive measures. Incidence of the disease has diminished greatly in many areas where DDT has been used to eradicate malaria—an unexpected added benefit of this program. When the vectors are exophilic, control is difficult. Attempts at vaccination with avirulent strains of *L. donovani* have been unsuccessful.

AMERICAN CUTANEOUS LEISHMANIASIS

These diseases occur in every country of Central and South America except Chile. In some areas, 10 to 20 percent of the population are infected. There are four varieties of American cutaneous leishmaniasis. All begin with a local lesion at the site of the infecting sandfly bite after an incubation period of from 10 days to 3 months.

Chiclero ulcer, which is found in Mexico, Panama, British Honduras, and Brazil is a zoonosis caused by *L. mexicana.* The disease occurs naturally in several arboreal rodents. It is occasionally transmitted to men entering forests to harvest chicle. The disease is characterized by lesions on the ear which are chronic, show little ulceration, and lead to deformities through scarring. The leishmanin skin test is positive. Spontaneous healing is the rule, and parasites are never numerous in the lesions. Mucosal ulceration does not occur. Successful treatment with both metranidazole and cycloguanil pamoate (which may also be useful as a chemoprophylactic agent) has been reported.

Uta, which occurs in cooler climates and at altitudes of more than 2,000 ft, consists of single or multiple skin ulcers in which parasites are readily demonstrable. Spontaneous healing within 3 months to a year is the rule, and mucosal spread is unusual. The etiologic agent is *L. brasiliensis* (var.) *peruviana,* and the reservoir is the domestic dog. With widespread use of insecticides in Peru, the disease has almost disappeared.

In tropical Latin America, *L. brasiliensis* causes the better-known and more serious *espundia.* The epidemiology of the lesion is poorly defined. The initial skin lesion enlarges progressively, and secondary bacterial infection is frequent. The disease may spread by direct extension or by lymphatics to the mucosal surfaces of the mouth and nose where, after the primary lesion has healed, painful, destructive, and mutilating erosions scar and distort the involved structures. Fever, anemia, and weight loss accompany these mucosal complications. Destruction of the nasal septum produces a characteristic deformity called *tapir nose* or *camel nose.* The hard palate may be destroyed, and largyngeal erosion can lead to aphonia. In Negroes, the lesion is often hypertrophic, and large polypoid masses deform the lips and cheeks, perhaps representing a type of keloid reaction. This can be mistaken for South American blastomycosis (Chap. 186). Secondary bacterial infection, inanition, and respiratory obstruction lead to death.

The diagnosis is made by finding the organisms in scrapings or by culture. The leishmanin skin test is specific and highly useful. Treatment consists of antibiotics for bacterial infections and antimonials, preferably sodium antimony tartrate, which is given intravenously as 1 or 2 percent solution, the dose being increased on al-

ternate days from 0.04 Gm initially to a maximum of 0.28 Gm, until a total of 2.2 Gm has been given. Pentavalent antimonials and Amphotericin B have also been used with some success in this disease.

The early lesions respond well, but even with repeated courses of antimony, the mucosal complications of the espundia type heal slowly; in advanced cases, the prognosis is very poor.

Leishmaniasis tegumentaria diffusa is caused by *L. brasiliensis* (var.) *pifanoi.* This remarkable disease is characterized by massive dissemination of skin lesions without visceral involvement. The clinical picture often bears a striking resemblance to lepromatous leprosy (Chap. 175). The diagnosis is not difficult because the lesion contains large numbers of organisms. In contrast to all other types of cutaneous leishmaniasis, the leishmanin skin test is negative. A similar disease caused by *L. tropica* has been described in Ethiopia. The disease is progressive and very refractory to treatment. Glucantime, amphotericin B, and pentamidine have been used to reduce remissions but cure is rare.

OLD WORLD CUTANEOUS LEISHMANIASIS: ORIENTAL SORE

This, the least serious form of human leishmaniasis, consists of localized cutaneous ulceration which heals spontaneously and is endemic in the European countries bordering the eastern Mediterranean, in North Africa, Asia Minor, Southwest Asia, and India. Two major strains of the causative organism, *L. tropica,* produce similar but distinctive clinical syndromes. Homologous immunity after recovery from infection by either strain is solid and lifelong. Infection with *L. tropica* (var.) *major* protects against *L. tropica* (var.) *minor,* but the opposite is not the case. The rural or moist type, caused by (var.) *major,* has its reservoir in gerbils and other small rodents; the ulcers usually appear on the extremities 2 to 6 weeks after the bite of the sandfly and are accompanied by regional lymphadenopathy in a majority of cases. Spontaneous healing occurs within 3 to 6 months, leaving a depigmented, pitted scar.

The incubation period in the *urban,* or *dry,* type ranges from 2 months to more than a year. The lesion is usually facial and begins as a pruritic, purplish nodule (the "Aleppo button"), which slowly enlarges and finally breaks down after 3 or 4 months. Healing of the indolent, granulomatous ulcer may require a year or more; lymphatic involvement is uncommon. Man is the only known reservoir of infection.

The typical oriental sore is a sharply punched-out, ragged ulcer about 1 in. in diameter, surrounded by an erythematous rim. Satellite lesions which fuse with the original are not rare. The center of the granulating base of the ulcer frequently contains a hard excrescence called the *Montpellier sign* or the *rake* beneath which the parasites are most likely to be found when scrapings are examined.

The wet and dry types occur together in Asia Minor;

indeed, it is not rare to find simultaneous infections in the same patient. In Africa, Southeastern Europe, and India, only the dry type is prevalent.

Diagnosis is usually made on clinical grounds and is confirmed by finding the parasites, which occur both intra- and extracellularly. Pyogenic infection makes direct visualization difficult, but *L. tropica* can be cultured in Novy-MacNeal-Nicolle medium at room temperature, and a skin test using *L. tropica* antigen becomes positive in the vast majority of patients with the disease.

Treatment should include vigorous measures for bacterial infection, such as hot soaks and appropriate systemic antibiotics. Local infiltration with a 2 percent solution of berberine sulfate weekly for 3 weeks is very effective in early lesions, but nothing seems to speed the subsidence of established ulcers except control of secondary infection. Systemic antimonials may be required where ulceration is extensive or multiple. In endemic areas the custom is to withhold treatment directed against the parasite until the initial nodule ulcerates, to assure the development of immunity against reinfection.

Prevention consists of use of insect repellents on exposed parts of the body, residual DDT sprays, and fine-mesh screening for dwellings. The lesions should be covered to prevent infection of vectors and, of course, contact with the lesion or its discharges should be avoided.

In Asia Minor, a relapsing form known as *leishmaniasis recidiva* is common. Nodules appear at the periphery of the scarred area and mimic lupus vulgaris so closely that errors in diagnosis are very frequent.

REFERENCES

Adler, S.: Immunology of Leishmaniasis, Israel J. Med. Sci., 1:9, 1965.

Convit, J., and F. Kerdel-Vegas: Disseminated Cutaneous Leishmaniasis, Arch. Dermatol., 91:439, 1965.

Faust, E. C., and P. F. Russell: "Clinical Parasitology," Philadelphia, Lea & Febiger, 1964.

Hunter, G. W., W. W. Frye, and J. C. Swartzwelder: "A Manual of Tropical Medicine," 4th ed., Philadelphia, W. B. Saunders Company, 1966.

Lainson, R., and J. Strangeways-Dixon: The Epidemiology of Dermal Leishmaniasis in British Honduras, Trans. Roy. Soc. Trop. Med. Hyg., 58:316, 1964.

243 TRYPANOSOMIASIS

James J. Plorde and Ivan L. Bennett, Jr.

DEFINITION. Trypanosomiasis designates infection produced by protozoans of the genus *Trypanosoma*. These organisms are responsible for numerous diseases in animals and for three separate disorders in man, Gambian or mid-African sleeping sickness, Rhodesian or East African sleeping sickness, and Chagas' disease in Central and South America.

ETIOLOGY. Trypanosomes are fusiform organisms, recognized by an undulating membrane which extends along the length of the cell and terminates in an anterior flagellum. The morphologic characteristics of many species are so nearly identical that they are distinguishable only by their pathogenicity for certain animals, differences in biochemical requirements, and ability to multiply in insects.

Most species are transmitted to vertebrate hosts by insects and undergo a part of their life cycle in the vector, but direct transmission between warm-blooded hosts is the rule for others. *Trypanosoma gambiense*, the cause of mid-African sleeping sickness, is transmitted to man by riverine tsetse flies (*Glossina*), and *T. rhodesiense* (East African) by woodland tsetse flies. *Trypanosoma cruzi*, the agent of Chagas' disease, is carried by reduviid ("assassin" or "kissing") bugs, primarily those of the genera *Triatoma*, *Panstrongylus*, and *Rhodnius*. Transmission of the trypanosomes of sleeping sickness occurs by what is referred to as the "anterior station;" after multiplication in the intestine of the tsetse fly, the parasites migrate to the salivary glands and are discharged when a host is bitten. The agent of Chagas' disease, however, multiplies only in the gut of the vector and is discharged in the feces, infection of man occurring through contamination of the bite wound; this is transmission by the "posterior station."

Trypanosomiasis in animals is a great economic problem in many parts of the world. Indeed, it is said that an area of approximately 4 million square miles in Africa is now essentially unpopulated because of the impossibility of keeping domestic animals in these areas where tsetse flies are infected with *T. brucei*, the cause of *nagana*, a fatal disease of cattle and horses. Among the more important trypanosomal diseases of animals are *dourine* in horses and donkeys, caused by *T. equiperdum*, which is transmitted by sexual intercourse and is worldwide; *souma*, caused by *T. vivax* in horses and cattle (Africa); *surra*, caused by *T. evansi* in horses, cattle, and dogs (Asia, Australia, Madagascar); *mal de caderas*, caused by *T. equinum* in horses and cattle (South America); and *murina de caderas*, caused by *T. hippicum* in horses and mules (Central America). The epidemiology of each of the three trypanosomiases of man is discussed separately below.

GAMBIAN SLEEPING SICKNESS. This disease occurs in tropical west and central Africa, especially along the Congo River and its tributaries. Though swine and goats are suspected of harboring *T. gambiense*, man is the only known reservoir. The vectors are the palpalis group of tsetse flies that live near water, and the highest incidence of the disease is in young men, a result of increased exposure to the flies. Less than 5 percent of flies are infected, even in the most notorious endemic foci.

The disease in man has customarily been described as proceeding through several classic "stages" interspersed with periods of remission or quiescence. Actually, there is tremendous variation in the severity, symptoms, duration, and outcome of the disease, all apparently dependent upon the resistance of the host, and the many so-called types or stages of trypanosomiasis are better understood in these terms than on the basis of duration of infection alone.

The *incubation period* is usually about 2 weeks but rarely may be as long as 3 years. The infecting bite, especially in Europeans, may show an erythematous nodule with a pale halo, the *trypanosomal chancre,* which subsides gradually. The parasites multiply locally, enter lymphatics, and appear in the blood about 3 weeks after the bite of the tsetse fly. In the usual case, the patient experiences bouts of fever for months. The temperature can exceed 106°F, and during these episodes, rashes of various types are common. These may be generalized, pruritic papular eruptions or erythema nodosum. In Caucasians, a characteristic circinate erythema resembling erythema marginatum is frequent. Transient firm areas of subcutaneous edema localized to the hands, feet, or periorbital tissue may appear. Severe headache and tachycardia accompany fever and, as the illness progresses, weight loss and progressive debilitation ensue. Tender lymphadenopathy, with gradual induration of the nodes, and splenomegaly are almost invariably present. The lymph nodes of the posterior cervical triangles are especially prominent; this is referred to as *Winterbottom's sign.* Insomnia, inability to concentrate, paresthesias, and formication are frequent, and most patients demonstrate a peculiar delayed sensation to pain combined with deep, aching hyperesthesia that can be elicited by a light blow with any hard object, known as *Kerandel's sign.* The illness can terminate spontaneously after weeks or months or can drag on intermittently for years. Death is often from intercurrent infection, of which bacillary and amebic dysentery, malaria, and bacterial (often pneumococcal) pneumonia are the most important.

Eventually, the parasites enter the central nervous system, usually about 1 year after the onset of illness, although it may occur much earlier or may be delayed for as long as 8 years. Cerebral trypanosomiasis can be explosive, causing repeated convulsions or deep coma and death within a few days. Most patients show gradual progression to the classic picture of *sleeping sickness.* Although spontaneous recovery is not rare in early trypanosomiasis, untreated *sleeping sickness* is almost invariably fatal within 4 to 8 months. The patient develops a vacant expression, the eyelids droop, the lower lip hangs loosely, and it becomes more and more difficult to gain his attention or prod him to any activity. Patients will eat when offered food, but they never ask for it or engage in spontaneous conversation, and speech gradually becomes blurred and indistinct. Tremors of the hands and tongue, choreiform movements, seizures with transient paralysis, loss of sphincter control, ophthalmoplegia, extensor plantar responses, and finally death in coma, status epilepticus, or from hyperpyrexia follow inexorably.

The overall mortality of Gambian trypanosomiasis is 25 to 50 percent; with chemotherapy, this can be reduced to 5 or 10 percent.

Anemia and *hyperglobulinemia* are invariably present, and spontaneous clumping of erythrocytes in blood specimens is grossly evident in many cases. The sedimentation rate is rapid, and peripheral monocytosis is frequent.

The *cerebrospinal fluid* shows mononuclear pleocytosis and increased protein content in sleeping sickness. The colloidal gold curve is tabetic. The protein content is a better index of severity of disease and therapeutic response than is the number of cells.

Fever, lymphadenopathy, Winterbottom's and Kerandel's signs, splenomegaly, and anemia in a resident of an endemic area make the clinical diagnosis relatively easy. *Irregular fever, lymphadenopathy, and especially circinate erythema in any Caucasian who has resided in Africa within 7 years should arouse suspicion of trypanosomiasis.* Although malaria, kala-azar, Hodgkin's disease, and leprosy are sometimes confused with early trypanosomiasis, the proper diagnosis usually becomes evident within a short time.

The definitive diagnosis depends upon finding the trypanosomes in the blood, aspirate of lymph node, or cerebrospinal fluid. These should be examined first in wet mounts; actively motile organisms are seen easily under high power. For final identification thin and thick blood films should be stained with Wright's or Giemsa stain. If the blood smears are negative, citrated blood should be centrifuged at 1000 rpm for 10 min and the supernatant (including the leukocytes) recentrifuged at 2000 rpm for 15 min and the sediment examined. Cerebrospinal fluid should be centrifuged at 2,000 rpm for 15 min before examination. If these methods are negative, rats or guinea pigs may be inoculated and examined after several weeks. A severalfold increase of IgM globulins is of some confirmatory value. Complement fixation and indirect fluorescent antibody tests are used in endemic areas.

Antrypol (Bayer 205, suramin) is the most effective agent before central-nervous-system involvement has occurred. The initial dose should be limited to 1.0 ml because of possible idiosyncrasy to the drug. If red cells, casts, or protein appear in the urine, therapy should be discontinued; otherwise, 10 injections at intervals of 4 to 7 days should be given, each dose consisting of 10 ml of a fresh 10 percent solution. Pentamidine given in water either intramuscularly or intravenously on alternate days for 8 to 10 injections is effective in early disease. The dose is 2 to 4 mg per kg for each injection. When the agent is given too rapidly by the intravenous route, it may cause hypotension.

Lumbar puncture should always be performed in patients who are about to undergo therapy for trypanosomiasis. If the central nervous system is involved, agents that will penetrate the blood-brain barrier must be used; for this purpose, the most effective agent is tryparsamide given intravenously as a fresh 20 percent solution in water once weekly for 8 to 15 weeks. The initial dose should consist of 1 Gm, and subsequent doses should be 2 Gm weekly. A course of injections may be repeated after a rest of 1 month. Arsenical hepatitis or dermatitis, abdominal cramps, and most important, optic atrophy may result from tryparsamide; ocular symptoms make cessation of the drug mandatory. *Antrypol* or *pen-*

tamidine should be used in conjunction with tryparsamide. *Mel B* (*Arsobal*) an arsenical derivative of BAL, is effective both in early and late cases. It can be given intravenously in dosage of 3.6 mg per kg daily for 4 days and should be followed by 4 more daily injections after an interval of 1 week. Recovery rates as high as 50 percent have followed intensive therapy in sleeping sickness.

Prevention includes use of repellents and protective clothing (gloves, head nets) in endemic areas and chemoprophylaxis with 1.0 Gm of *Antrypol* every 2 months or pentamidine 3 mg per kg every 6 months for each member of the population. Elimination of the vector is presently a hopeless undertaking in many areas. Indeed it has been easier to move whole villages out of infested areas than to eradicate tsetse flies.

RHODESIAN SLEEPING SICKNESS. This disease is found in tropical east Africa where the etiologic agent, *T. rhodesiense*, is transmitted by woodland tsetse flies. Antelopes are known reservoirs, and other wild animals are also suspected of harboring the parasite. A recent epidemic of Rhodesian sleeping sickness in Kenya was transmitted by a peridomestic tsetse which is the normal vector of Gambian disease. More than 60 percent of human infections occur in adult males. Rhodesian trypanosomiasis is a more acute and severe disease than the Gambian form, usually terminating fatally within a year. Fever is higher, emaciation more rapid, and lymphatic involvement is less evident. Death from intercurrent infection, myocarditis, or "toxemia" usually occurs before there is appreciable central-nervous-system involvement; although lethargy and somnolence are seen, the typical sleeping sickness syndrome is rare.

Rhodesian trypanosomiasis is more resistant to treatment than the Gambian disease. *Antrypol* is effective only if given within 3 weeks of the onset of symptoms; *Mel B* can be used in cases discovered too late for treatment with Antrypol; and *tryparsamide* should be given immediately if there is any evidence of neurologic disease. No drug is really effective in advanced cases.

Prevention is complicated because of the much greater problems of eradicating woodland tsetse flies than the riverine and the need to shift populations into noninfected areas. Although chronic human cases are relatively rare, the existence of animal reservoirs makes it impossible to prevent continuing infection of the vectors. Chemoprophylaxis is the same as for the Gambian disease. Individual protection with repellents, netting, etc., is, of course, important.

The disease is almost invariably fatal if untreated. Intensive treatment results in cure of about 50 percent of early cases, but this falls to 15 percent in advanced disease.

CHAGAS' DISEASE (American Trypanosomiasis). This infection occurs from Argentina and Chile to southern Mexico, where it is a major and perhaps the primary cause of heart disease in the rural areas. The etiologic agent, *T. cruzi,* has been found in "assassin" and "kissing" bugs along our southern boundaries, but very few authenticated cases are known in which the disease was acquired in the United States. Both domestic and wild animals, especially the opossum and armadillo, may serve as reservoirs for the infection in these reduviid bugs. Infection in man usually begins with acute systemic symptoms and then becomes chronic, resembling kala-azar more than the sleeping sickness of Africa. The parasites multiply intracellularly in a leishmania form, morphologically indistinguishable from the Leishman-Donovan bodies of kala-azar, but they assume the trypanosomal form in the bloodstream.

The vector attacks man at night, usually biting the face at a mucocutaneous junction (hence the name *kissing bug*), most frequently the lip or outer canthus of the eye. An erythematous nodule, the *chagoma* appears within a few days at the initial site where the parasites have gained entrance from the infected feces of the vector. Secondary nodules are sometimes seen along draining lymphatics. *After an incubation period* of 2 weeks, there is the onset of *fever* (coincident with the appearance of parasitemia, which lasts for 30 to 60 days), and a morbilliform or urticarial *skin eruption,* which subsides after a few days. Painless *unilateral palpebral edema and conjunctivitis,* known as *Romaña's sign,* may occur during the first febrile week. The parasites spread systemically, showing a predilection for histiocytes, skeletal muscle, heart muscle, and the central nervous system, resulting in generalized lymphadenopathy and hepatosplenomegaly. Myositis may be attended by extensive gelatinous edema (pseudomyxedema) of the face and trunk, and the differentiation of Chagas' disease from cretinism and endemic goiter is sometimes surprisingly difficult. When meningoencephalitis complicates the acute illness in children, the mortality is 40 percent. An extensive acute myocarditis is sometimes accompanied by pericardial effusion and can result in heart failure. The duration of this acute stage is variable. When meningoencephalitis or severe heart disease is present, the disease may end fatally in a few days or weeks. More often it resolves slowly during a several week period. Moreover, the process usually becomes chronic and slowly progressive resulting in a number of late manifestations. Most patients presenting with these late manifestations, however, deny a history of acute illness suggesting that subclinical infections often progress to chronic disease. Chronic *neurologic* manifestations including convulsions, paresis, intention tremor, and personality disorders have been reported but have been poorly documented. Better established is the role of *T. cruzi* in the genesis of *megaesophagus* and *megacolon.* The parasite evokes inflammatory changes in and around the ganglionic nerve cells resulting in dilatation and malfunction of these organs. The most important late manifestation is *heart disease,* which may affect as many as 10 percent of the rural population in endemic areas. Symptoms and signs range from arrhythmias and heart block to chronic congestive heart failure. Sudden cardiac arrest is reportedly common. At autopsy, the hearts of patients with Chagas' disease may show a peculiar herniation of the endocardium through the apical muscle bundles. There is debate whether the heart disease is caused by an inflammatory destruction of the myocardium or by a loss of ganglion cells depriving the heart of parasympathetic innervation. Both factors may be operative.

Trypanosoma cruzi is easily grown in blood broth incubated at 28°C. The technique of *xenodiagnosis* is often used in endemic areas; a laboratory-reared vector, known to be parasite-free, is allowed to feed on suspected cases, and 2 weeks later, the insect's intestinal contents are examined for parasites. Confusion sometimes arises from the finding of trypanosomes in blood. Many children in Venezuela and other South American countries are infected with a harmless species, *T. rangeli*, which produces no symptoms but may be present in the blood for many months. Utilizing both culture and xenodiagnosis repeatedly, organisms can be recovered from most acute cases and from up to 40 percent of chronic ones. Biopsy of an involved lymph node or calf muscle may reveal the organism during the initial illness when the parasites cannot be recovered from the blood. The Machado-Guerreiro test (a complement fixation reaction) is most helpful in the diagnosis of chronic cases and in survey work. Fluorescent antibody and hemagglutination inhibition tests have been introduced which may be useful.

There is *no specific treatment* for Chagas' disease. Prevention consists of using residual insecticide sprays—of which benzene hexachloride (BHC) is the most effective—on the walls of houses, the main habitat of the vectors. Reinfestation, however, may occur within a year or two of spraying.

REFERENCES

Ashcroft, M. T.: A Critical Review of the Epidemiology of Human Trypanosomiasis in Africa, Trop. Dis. Bull., 56: 1073, 1959.

Brown, H. W., and D. L. Belding.: "Basic Clinical Parsitology," 2d ed., New York, Appleton-Century-Crofts, Inc., 1964.

Duggan, A. J.: An Appraisal of the Clinical Problems of Gambian Sleeping Sickness, J. Trop. Med. Hyg., 67:268, 1959.

Hunter, G. W., W. W. Frye, and J. C. Swartzwelder: "A Manual of Tropical Medicine," 4th ed., Philadelphia, W. B. Saunders Company, 1966.

The Etiology of Chagas' Myocarditis, Lancet, 1:1150, 1965.

244 TOXOPLASMOSIS
Harry A. Feldman

DEFINITION. Toxoplasmosis is caused by *Toxoplasma gondii*, an obligate intracellular parasite which is widely distributed among mammals and birds. It is usually, but not definitely, classified as a protozoon. In man it produces either acquired (usually asymptomatic) or congenital (generally symptomatic) infections.

HISTORY. First demonstrated in 1908 by Nicolle and Manceaux in a North African rodent, the gondii, and in the same year by Splendore in Brazil, toxoplasma were proved to cause human disease in 1939 when Wolfe, Cowen, and Paige reported that several neonatal cases of fatal encephalomyelitis had resulted from congenital infections with this parasite. A few cases of acquired infection were reported subsequently, but the parasite excited interest primarily as the cause of an uncommon congenital disease. That it did more became evident following the almost simultaneous descriptions of dye, complement fixation, and skin tests; subsequently, other serologic procedures were introduced. Their application has demonstrated that toxoplasma frequently infect man and animals and that human congenital toxoplasmosis is only one aspect of its disease spectrum.

ETIOLOGY. *Toxoplasma gondii* is considered to be a protozoon, but its taxonomic classification has not been settled. All strains are antigenically similar and of the same species. The organism measures about 3 by 6 μ and may appear crescentic, oval, or round. It divides by endodyogeny and is best stained with either Wright's or Giemsa stains. Toxoplasma are unique in that they may infect any mammalian or avian cell, except nonnucleated erythrocytes. They can be maintained in mice or tissue culture or embryonated eggs but do not multiply except in the presence of living cells. Under special conditions they can be frozen and stored, but ordinary freezing kills them. Live parasites persist in cysts which can be found in any tissue, but especially, in muscle and the central nervous system.

EPIDEMIOLOGY. Serologic surveys indicate that toxoplasma infections are worldwide in distribution. With the dye test, the most sensitive indicator of antibody, it has been demonstrated that approximately 33 percent of the inhabitants of several American cities and Haiti, 63 percent of Hondurans, and 70 percent of Tahitian natives had positive tests. In contrast, 1 percent of the inhabitants of several islands off of the northern coast of Australia, 4 percent of Navajo Indians, and 11 percent of a sample of Icelanders had positive reactions. Among American military recruits, marked differences were found in the prevalence of antibodies among those originating from different areas of the United States. East Coast recruits were 20 percent positive, but only 3 and 8 percent, respectively, from the Mountain and Pacific Coast regions reacted similarly. Overall, 14 percent of the American recruits were positive in comparison with 51 and 56 percent, respectively, of Colombian and Brazilian recruits.

Two longitudinal studies of seroconversions in American families are especially informative. In the one, conducted in Cleveland, it was found that during the 10-year observation period that only four individuals who had no hemagglutinating antibodies at the start acquired them subsequently. Among a group of Syracuse families, in a 4-year period, three had seroconversions, or 1 in 2392 person-months of observation. In neither study was it possible to identify an associated clinical illness.

In animal surveys, cats, goats, guinea pigs, sheep, swine, and to a lesser extent, rabbits and pigeons often have had positive tests. It is clear from these data that toxoplasma infections are frequent in man and animals, but that there is considerable variation in their prevalence from place to place and in different species.

The pathways whereby man and animals acquire parasites generally are unknown. Human-to-human transfer seems not to occur except from mother to fetus. It has long been known that animals can acquire infections by cannibalizing other infected animals. This information may be applicable to man, since Desmonts has shown that children without antibodies acquire them following the ingestion of undercooked mutton and beef. No clinical illnesses were noted. This does not explain the route by which herbivores acquire toxoplasma. Human infections are contracted in any season and with equal frequency by the two sexes.

Recent reports that *Toxocara cati* excretes toxoplasma-infected eggs following the ingestion of toxoplasma by nematode infested cats led to the conclusion that an additional transmission system existed. Subsequently it was shown that toxocara does not participate in this chain and that the cat excretes a new resistant, infectious cyst form of toxoplasma. Whether such cysts occur in other species and their relation to the pathogenesis of toxoplasmosis remains to be determined.

CLINICAL MANIFESTATIONS. Congenital Toxoplasmosis. Congenitally infected infants may be born prematurely or at term and stillborn or alive with active disease, which can be expressed by chorioretinitis, convulsions, fever, icterus, hepatomegaly, rash, splenomegaly, and xanthochromic spinal fluid in various combinations. The newborn infant may have none of these signs, but subsequently, hydrocephaly or microcephaly, chorioretinitis, psychomotor retardation, cerebral calcifications, and convulsions may appear, either singly or in combination. A fatality rate of 11 percent was noted in one series of 141 cases of congenital toxoplasmosis. The most common residuals in congenitally affected children are chorioretinitis, cerebral calcifications, psychomotor retardation, hydro- or microcephaly, and convulsions. Any or all of these may follow other congenital infections, especially those due to cytomegalic virus (Chap. 232). The mothers of congenitally damaged offspring ordinarily are unaware of having had any specific illnesses during the pregnancy and should be advised that future pregnancies can be undertaken with confidence because a repetition will not occur. This complication only occurs in a female who happens to be pregnant when she has an asymptomatic parasitemia with her initial toxoplasma infection.

Acquired Toxoplasmosis. Although the clinical features show great variability in proved cases of acquired toxoplasmosis, certain manifestations are suggestive of this disease. Maculopapular rashes often appear soon after the clinical onset of the illness and tend to disappear in 3 to 4 days. Lymphadenopathy is common and may be so prominent as to suggest primary lymphatic disease. Encephalitis may be present alone or in combination with other manifestations. Myalgias, arthralgias, myocarditis, and pneumonitis also have been noted. Siim described a syndrome which resembles infectious mononucleosis in that lymphadenopathy and lymphocytosis with atypical lymphocytes are present, but the heterophile reactions are negative. Parasites have been demonstrated in lymph nodes removed from such patients, some of whom were afebrile.

Toxoplasma have been isolated from several cases of posterior granulomatous uveitis, presumably the result of acquired infections. The proportion of such cases which is caused by toxoplasma has not been established. In contrast to congenital chorioretinitis, which is usually bilateral, the acquired form seems to be unilateral.

The incubation period, recovery and mortality rates, average duration of illness, and the residual defects resulting from acquired toxoplasmosis are unknown. Cerebral calcifications are not found in postnatally acquired infections.

LABORATORY DIAGNOSIS. A specific diagnosis may be made by serologic methods, by demonstrating the organism in smears, or by their cultivation in mice. Toxoplasma can be identified in cerebrospinal fluid sediments with Wright's or Giemsa stains, or occasionally, in biopsied lymph node or muscle. Laboratory-reared mice are best for isolation trials from fresh spinal fluid sediment (when acute central-nervous-systems signs are present) or suspensions of tissue.

Serum antibodies can be detected with the dye, complement fixation, hemagglutination, or immunofluorescence tests. The results are most helpful when they are negative or when a rising titer is demonstrated. Dye test antibodies appear early and persist for many years. Complement-fixing antibodies are slower to develop and disappear more rapidly. A high dye test titer (1:256 or more) and a negative complement fixation reaction in the same serum suggest either very recently acquired infection or the serologic residual of a previous one. Hemagglutinating antibodies seem to parallel dye test antibodies, but on occasion the results of the two tests are quite divergent.

Antibodies of the IgM class have been demonstrated by immunofluorescence and suggest a recent, active infection. This reaction should be especially useful in helping to differentiate between passively transferred antibodies and congenital infection in newborns.

Skin test antigens prepared from mouse peritoneal fluid or embryonated eggs have been used and yield reactions of the delayed type. Although still popular in some parts of the world, their use is not recommended.

TREATMENT. There is evidence from the treatment of experimental infections that a combination of sulfonamide and 5-p-chlorophenyl-2,4-diamino-6-ethylpyrimidine (Daraprim) is more effective than sulfonamide alone. Combinations of sulfadiazine or triple sulfonamides and Daraprim have been reported to yield excellent results in some cases of uveitis but have not affected others at all. Information on the effectiveness of this regimen in systemic toxoplasmosis is inadequate, but it does appear to control acute symptoms without eradicating encysted organisms. This drug combination is not specific for toxoplasmosis, and the patient's response does not prove the diagnosis. The sulfonamide should be administered in dosage of 2 to 4 Gm daily along with 50 mg

Daraprim daily in adults. Since Daraprim is an antifolic agent, leukocyte counts should be determined at least twice weekly. The dose of Daraprim probably should be halved after 2 weeks, and 1 month of treatment certainly constitutes an adequate trial. The leukopenia and thrombocytopenia which may result from Daraprim administration can be corrected by simultaneous administration of Leucovorin calcium and yeast cakes without interfering with the antitoxoplasmic effect of the drug.

REFERENCES

Feldman, H. A.: Medical Progress, Toxoplasmosis, New Engl. J. Med., 279:1370 and 1431, 1968.

Maumenee, A. E., and A. M. Silverstein: "Immunopathology of Uveitis," Baltimore, The Williams & Wilkins Company, 1964.

——: "Toxoplasmosis," Baltimore, The Williams & Wilkins Company, 1962.

Siim, J. Chr.: "Human Toxoplasmosis," Baltimore, The Williams & Wilkins Company, 1960.

245 PNEUMOCYSTIS CARINII PNEUMONIA (Pneumocystosis, Interstitial Plasma Cell Pneumonia)

Walter H. Sheldon

DEFINITION. *Pneumocystis carinii* (P.c.) pneumonia is an infection that becomes apparent clinically in patients with impaired host defenses. The disorder originally observed in premature or debilitated infants is being reported with increasing frequency in adults with either primary or secondary immunologic deficiency states, and instead of being a clinical curiosity, the disease is likely to become a common complication of transplantation surgery, tumor chemotherapy, and other states of increased host susceptibility. Pulmonary insufficiency is the cardinal clinical manifestation.

ETIOLOGY. *Pneumocystis carinii* first was seen by Chagas in 1909 and regarded as a form of *Trypanosoma cruzi* but was recognized as a different parasite by M. and Mme Delanoë, who in 1914 gave it the present name. The agent has not been cultured, and its taxonomic position remains uncertain; some consider it a protozoon, others regard it as a fungus. The consistent presence of P.c. in the pulmonary lesions of patients with the disease is the primary evidence for the causative role of the agent. Similar findings in laboratory animals with experimentally induced disease and serologic studies in man support the etiologic role of pneumocystis. The organism is best seen in smears as a minute oval or crescentic structure measuring 2 to 4 μ with a single nucleuslike body or as a cyst ranging from 5 to 10 μ and containing 2 to 8 bodies. Electron microscopic studies reveal a complex structure with organelles and suggest the capacity for protein synthesis and oxidative metabolism. Many

dyes, but *not* hematoxylin-eosin, stain the agent, which is also readily seen with phase microscopy and has been demonstrated with fluorescent antibody techniques. Silver impregnation methods are most useful for survey of preparations, and the structural detail is best observed with the Giemsa stain. The organism in patients everywhere is morphologically similar to that in animals but species-specific serologic differences may exist.

EPIDEMIOLOGY. In the absence of in vitro culture techniques and of readily applicable serologic tests, the incidence of P.c. infection is uncertain and epidemiologic data are based on indirect evidence. Morphologic observations supported by some serologic findings indicate that latent infection is not rare in man and is frequent in many animals including those commonly used in the laboratory. In man the disease is worldwide, and isolated cases occur in all age groups and in epidemics in nurseries. Retrospective study of autopsy files has uncovered typical instances of the infection antedating the description of the entity shortly after World War II. Clinical observations such as the reduction of nursery epidemics by isolation measures, the clustering of cases in families, and the apparently sequential occurrence in hospital room mates suggest that the disease is contagious and acquired by inhalation from patients with clinically apparent infection, asymptomatic carriers, and perhaps also from infected rodents. The incubation period is 1 to 2 months. Rare instances of P.c. pneumonia acquired in utero, probably by transplacental transmission, have been reported.

PATHOGENESIS. Clinical and experimental observations indicate that P.c. is of low virulence and slow to proliferate. It is possible that the presence of another living agent is needed for it to multiply. The frequent occurrence of progressive P.c. pneumonia in patients of all ages with primary or secondary immunologic deficiency states emphasizes the essential role of lowered host resistance in progressive infection. The disease has been encountered as a complication of neoplasia, particularly malignancies of the lymphocyte-reticular tissues, various anemias, cyclic neutropenia, collagen-vascular and autoimmune diseases, and renal failure. The common denominator in most patients has been their prolonged survival while treated with one or several agents such as corticosteroids, antimetabolites, cytotoxic substances, antibiotics, ionizing radiation, and colloidal gold. When some of these substances are administered to mice, rats, or rabbits, P.c. pneumonia will be produced or latent infection will be transformed into progressive disease. Suitable conditions for the proliferation of P.c. appear to occur in man and may be produced in animals not only by massive depression of the immune system but also by deficits which are thought to affect primarily only one aspect of the immune response such as antibody formation or cellular immunity. Fatal P.c. pneumonia, however, has also been reported in a few children and adults without demonstrated underlying disease. In some of these instances, exposure to massive doses of the infectious agent has been postulated.

The pathogenesis remains uncertain in the largest group of patients, in whom the disease was first described in Europe under the name of *interstitial plasma cell pneumonia*. These are premature or debilitated newborns in whom P.c. pneumonia occurs chiefly as epidemic outbreaks in nurseries with a peak incidence at the age of three to four months. Because this peak coincides with the period of physiologic hypoimmunoglobulinemia in the newborn, a relative or as yet unrecognized immunologic deficit has been suspected but remains unproven. However, in the absence of a correlation between the infection and immunoglobulin abnormalities a deficiency of cellular host defenses has been considered. Some evidence suggests that the mononuclear cell phase of inflammation in normal full-term infants is quantitatively less and morphologically different from that of healthy adults. A physiologic immaturity of the lymphocyte-mononuclear cell system which is involved in the cellular immune response, combined with age-related under-developed and incomplete immunoglobulin synthesis might in the presence of appropriate amounts of the infectious agent permit the development of P.c. pneumonia, particularly in the premature. Increased host susceptibility has also been attributed to chronic lung injury subsequent to presumably unrelated respiratory infections and to previous antimicrobial therapy which in animals activates latent P.c. infection.

Many other, often multiple infections occur in patients of all ages with P.c. pneumonia. Most common are acute and chronic bacterial infections, including tuberculosis and leprosy. Localized and disseminated cytomegalic inclusion disease is particularly frequent. Other concurrent infections are measles, vaccinia, candidiasis, aspergillosis, histoplasmosis, nocardiosis, cryptococcosis, and trypanosomiasis cruzi.

PATHOLOGIC FINDINGS. Gross findings in widespread disease show massively consolidated lungs without pleuritis. The process may be focal and confined to the central and dorsal lung areas. Histologically the alveoli are distended by a virtually typical, foamy material teeming with organisms. Hyaline membranes may be present. The sparse cellular response consists of mononuclear cells and occasionally giant cells. Alveolar septal infiltration by plasma cells, a prominent feature in many cases, is absent in others. Septal fibrosis is generally slight. These changes appear to be reversible. Granuloma formation, focal fibrosis, and calcification have been noted. Fragments of the alveolar contents in bronchi may account for dissemination throughout the lung. In latent infection the lesions are minute and generally few, foamy intraalveolar material is lacking, organisms are scant, and mononuclear cells are sparse. The infection is confined to the lung, but in a few instances organisms have been seen in regional lymph nodes. Systemic dissemination of the infection with focal lesions in distant sites is rare.

CLINICAL MANIFESTATIONS. Generally, the onset is insidious. The fully developed clinical picture is characterized by extreme dyspnea and tachypnea with respiratory rates up to and over 80 per min. Flaring of the nostrils, sternal retraction, and pronounced use of the auxiliary respiratory muscles are present. The face is covered with perspiration, and the patient is anxious, cyanotic, and pale. Sometimes there is a dry cough which, together with the cyanosis, is made worse by any movement. When present, fever is slight. Pulmonary physical findings are scanty, which contrasts with the sometimes grave clinical state of the patient and the extensive lung involvement seen roentgenologically. Roentgenographic abnormalities may precede symptoms by months and usually consist of soft infiltrates, spreading from the hilum to the base and later to the entire lung but often sparing the upper lobes. Pleural effusions do not occur. Emphysema may be present. Laboratory studies reveal no consistent alterations of the white blood cell count, serum proteins, or any other parameters. Pulmonary function tests show primarily a diffusion defect. Complications include pneumothorax from a ruptured emphysematous bleb and rib fractures attributed to forced respiratory movements. Often the disease progresses relentlessly and death occurs by asphyxia or cardiac failure after 6 to 10 weeks.

DIAGNOSIS. The diagnosis depends on the morphologic demonstration of the agent. Material for histologic study may be obtained by aspiration of coughed-up hypopharyngeal and tracheal secretions, tracheal lavage, or by open or needle biopsy of the lung. Although successful in some hands, examination of secretions has, in general, yielded poor results. However, this procedure may become most useful if the recently reported staining of the organism by specific fluorescent antibody is confirmed and can be applied routinely. Because of possible subsequent pneumothorax and bleeding, needle biopsy involves considerable risk and open lung biopsy seems safer. A complement fixation test widely used in Europe is not available in this country, where it may not even be applicable because of possible serologic differences in the organism.

COURSE. In the absence of a simple diagnostic test, morbidity and mortality figures are uncertain. Beyond doubt, P.c. infection is not rare at any age, and P.c. pneumonia is likely to become more frequent. When associated with significant predisposing disorders, the prognosis is grave. An overall mortality of 40 to 50 percent has been suggested. Remissions and spontaneous cures (reported as 20 to 50 percent in some large series) occur, making claims of therapeutic success hard to evaluate.

TREATMENT. Recent clinical and experimental observations report distinctly encouraging results for treatment with pentamidine isothionate in dosage of 4 mg per kg body weight given in a single intramuscular injection for 12 to 14 days. In desperately ill patients the drug has been given intravenously. Combined treatment with pyrimethamine, 25 mg per day, and sulfadiazine, 1 to 4 Gm per day, both given orally, may also have beneficial effect. Megaloblastic anemia has been an occasional side effect but is correctable with folinic acid without apparently affecting the efficacy of the antiprotozoan drugs. Antibiotics, commercial immunoglobulin, and convalescent serum have had no success. Symptomatic treatment with oxygen and digitalis may be indicated.

REFERENCES

Ivády, G., L. Páldy, M. Koltay, G. Tóth, and Z. Kovács: Pneumocystis Carinii Pneumonia, Lancet, 1:616, 1967.

Ruskin, J., and J. S. Remington: The Compromised Host and Infection. I. Pneumocystis carinii Pneumonia, J.A.M.A., 202:1070, 1967.

Sheldon, W. H.: Pulmonary Pneumocystis Carinii Infection, J. Pediat., 61:780, 1962.

246 MINOR PROTOZOAN DISEASES

James J. Plorde and Ivan L. Bennett, Jr.

TRICHOMONIASIS

Of the many members of the genus *Trichomonas,* three are parasites of man: *T. hominis* in the intestine, *T. tenax* in the oral cavity, and *T. vaginalis,* the only one capable of producing disease, in the vagina and urethra. All three possess four anterior flagella, and their morphology is quite similar; *T. vaginalis* is the largest, however, and confusion in diagnosis is rare because of the anatomic specificity of their habitats.

Trichomonas vaginalis, despite some question about its role as a primary pathogen, is associated with persistent vaginitis in about 20 percent of parasitized women. Manifestations include itching, burning, and profuse, creamy, yellow, frothy leukorrhea. Examination shows inflammation ranging from mild hyperemia of the vaginal vault to extensive erosion, petechial hemorrhages, and perineal intertrigo.

The diagnosis is made by examining a fresh unstained drop of the discharge, which will be found to contain numerous motile trichomonads. The organisms are often present in urine. In males, a mild, usually asymptomatic urethritis is produced. The importance of the disease in males has to do with the transmission of infection by sexual contact, although the disease is also spread by toilet articles, fomites, etc.

Trichomoniasis is sometimes responsible for confusing changes in the cytologic pattern of exfoliated vaginal cells. However, ordinary Papanicolaou preparations are not well suited to establishing the diagnosis of this infection, and when it is suspected, fresh material should be looked at immediately.

Treatment consists of attention to personal hygiene and the local application of an appropriate compound. Floraquin and acetarsone have been used as insufflated powders or suppositories with success. Systemic therapy with metronidazole (Flagyl) has been quite effective. A dose of 1 Gm daily for 10 days will eliminate most infections in women. Infected sexual partners should be treated concurrently to prevent reinfection. Otherwise, infection in males seldom requires therapy. Tetracyclines are said to be effective but favor the development of vaginal moniliasis.

GIARDIASIS (Lambliasis)

Giardia lamblia is a pear-shaped, multiflagellar, protozoan parasite of the human duodenum. It possesses two large nuclei which give the organism the appearance of a face with two large eyes when viewed under the microscope. The parasite is capable of invading the intestinal mucosa. The response to infestation is highly variable and seems related at least in part to host factors. Children are three times more likely to be parasitized than adults and probably have more prominent clinical manifestations. Gastrectomy or decreased gastric acidity in adults may increase their susceptibility. Giardiasis also has been reported frequently in patients with immunoglobulin deficiencies.

Most often the infection is asymptomatic, but in some patients nausea, flatulence, epigastric pain, and distension occur. Sometimes patients have watery diarrhea and lose weight. These symptoms are more common in children and are usually self-limited. Rarely, fulminating and extensive duodenal ulceration have been described. Radiographically, asymptomatic carriers may show irritability of the duodenal bulb. Chronic giardiasis may lead to malabsorption, the pathogenesis of which is poorly understood. Mechanical blockage of microvilli by the parasites, competition between the organisms and host for nutrients, altered motility, and mucosal invasion have been suggested as possible mechanisms. Jejunal biopsy of patients infested with giardia sometimes shows flattening of the microvilli and an inflammatory infiltrate. Both malabsorption and the jejunal lesions have been reversed with specific treatment.

The diagnosis is made by finding the parasites in duodenal washings, jejunal biopsies, or diarrheal stools. Cyst forms are often passed; they contain two to four nuclei and are readily identified when stained with iodine.

Treatment consists of the administration of 0.1 Gm Atabrine hydrochloride three times daily for 3 days, a regimen which eliminates the organisms in 90 percent of the cases. Metronidazole (Flagyl) 250 mg twice daily for 5 to 7 days has also been effective. Treatment is necessary only in symptomatic cases. The frequency of infestation in children bears out transmission by the fecal-oral route, and reinfection will occur unless appropriate measures are taken.

COCCIDIOSIS

This is a relatively unusual disease characterized by fever, abdominal pain, and diarrhea, which results from ingestion of the oocysts or spores of *Isospora belli* or *I. hominis.* Volunteers develop symptoms about 1 week after ingestion, and the disease subsides spontaneously after 1 to 4 weeks. Infection is much more common in children and is worldwide in distribution, especially in tropical areas. The diagnosis is made by finding oocysts of the organisms in zinc sulfate concentrates of feces.

Isospora species occur in many lower animals, but only the dog is suspected of playing any part as a reservoir of the species that are pathogenic for man.

Diagnosis can be confused if oocysts of other members of the order Coccidia are ingested in fish or meat and appear in the feces without undergoing any change in the intestinal tract.

No treatment other than symptomatic is needed as the infection is self-limited.

BALANTIDIASIS

Balantidium coli, the largest protozoon of man, inhabits the large intestine. In addition to producing an asymptomatic carrier state, it elicits disease ranging from mild recurrent diarrhea to fulminant ulceration with perforation and death. In many respects the disease is similar to amebiasis in its range of manifestations, exclusive of spread to the liver.

The illness has been reproduced by feeding the organism to volunteers. The diagnosis is made by finding the parasites in the stool, but repeated examinations may be required because shedding of balantidium is intermittent. The disease is more likely to occur in tropical areas, but at least 60 cases have been reported in the United States. Swine are frequent carriers of *B. coli,* but there is great doubt about their role in the spread of the disease to man.

The tetracyclines in ordinary doses are highly effective in treatment, as is Diodoquin in a dosage of 0.65 Gm three times daily for 3 weeks.

REFERENCES

General

Brown, H. W., and D. L. Belding: "Basic Clinical Parasitology," New York, Appleton-Century-Crofts, Inc., 1964.

Balantidiasis

Shookhoff, H. B.: *Balantidium coli* Infection with Special Reference to Treatment, Am. J. Trop. Med., 34:442, 1951.

Swartzwelder, J. C.: Balantidiasis, Am. J. Dig. Dis., 17:173, 1950.

Coccidiosis

Matsubayashi, H., and F. Nozawa: Experimental Infection of *Isospora hominis* in Man, Am. J. Trop. Med., 28:633, 1948.

Smitskamp, H., and E. Oey-Muller: Geographical Distribution and Clinical Significance of Human Coccidiosis, Trop. Geog. Med., 18:133, 1966.

Giardiasis

Brandborg, L. L., C. B. Tankersley, S. Gottlieb, M. Baranick, and V. E. Sartor: Histological Demonstration of Mucosal Invasion by *Giardia Lamblia* in Man, Gastroenterol., 52: 143, 1967.

Hoskins, L. C., S. J. Winawer, S. A. Broitman, L. S. Gottlieb, and N. Zamcheck, Clinical Giardiasis and Intestinal Malabsorption, Gastroenterol., 53:265, 1967.

Rendtorff, R. C.: Experimental Transmission of Human Intestinal Protozoan Parasites; *Giardia lamblia* Cysts Given in Capsules, Am. J. Hyg., 59:209, 1954.

Yardley, J. H., J. Takano, and T. R. Hendrix: Epithelial and Other Mucosal Lesions of the Jejunum in Giardiasis: Jejunal Biopsy Studies, Bull. Johns Hopkins Hosp., 115: 389, 1964.

Trichomoniasis

Kotcher, E., C. A. Frick, and L. O. Giesel: The Effect of Metranidazole on Vaginal Microbiology and Maternal and Neonatal Hematology, Am. J. Obstet. Gynecol., 88: 184, 1964.

Section 22

Diseases Caused by Worms

INTRODUCTION

Ivan L. Bennett, Jr.

Human diseases produced by worms, or, more properly, *helminths,* are truly global in their occurrence. In the Arctic and in most temperate countries, these parasites are a source of annoyance and discomfort but, generally speaking, they are not major health hazards. For climatic, socioeconomic, ethnic, and other environmental reasons, however, serious helminthic disorders are highly prevalent in many tropical areas. The devastating effects of such diseases as hookworm, echinococcosis, filariasis, and schistosomiasis in terms of disability, economic loss, and lagging of progress in developing countries are almost inestimable.

It is abundantly clear that the eventual control and eradication of helminthic diseases will require preventive measures on a massive scale, including broad public health measures, improvement of sanitation, water supply, and transportation, changes in agricultural methods, abolition of long-held customs of diet and daily living, and even a modification in religious practices. Though these aspects are mentioned in the chapters which follow, the main emphasis in this section is on the recognition and treatment of these diseases as they occur in the individual patient.

CLASSIFICATION. The worms of importance in human disease include the flukes (class Trematoda) and the tapeworms (class Cestoda) of the phylum Platyhelminthes (flatworms); class Nematoda of the phylum Nemathelminthes (roundworms); and class Hirudinea (leeches) of the phylum Annelida (segmented worms).

Medical helminthology is only a small fraction of the study of parasites, and a textbook of medicine cannot hope to include definitive information concerning morphologic variation and the details of identification of parasites, which, in the last analysis, depends upon special skill and long experience. References to more complete treatises are appended at the end of each chapter.

LIFE CYCLES AND THE HOST. Most helminths (as is true of other parasites) have developed life cycles involving one or more vertebrate or invertebrate hosts. The life cycle of some parasites is so complicated that it is difficult to see how they persist; indeed, for some species which produce disease in man (sparganosis), the complete life cycle is still unknown.

Lower animals harboring parasites which infect man are called *reservoir* hosts. The parasite reaches maturity in the *final* or *definitive* host. In the *intermediate* host (of which there may be more than one), the parasite passes through a larval stage. Man may develop disease as an *intermediate* or as a *definitive* host; sometimes he is a substitute or incidental host for parasites which ordinarily affect lower animals.

Programs of prevention and control depend on the discovery of those stages in the life cycle of a parasite which are vulnerable to attack by chemicals, environmental alterations, or elimination of a necessary host.

TRAVEL. Large migrations in the past have introduced helminthic diseases into new localities, examples being the spread of the fish tapeworm from Northern Europe to the United States, and the introduction of filariasis, hookworm (*Necator*), and dracunculosis (Guinea worm) into the New World by the importation of slaves from Africa.

Rapid transportation, greater travel by tourists, and increased military and civilian service in foreign countries now allow for exposure of many individuals all over the world to parasitic diseases which may not be manifested until their return to nonendemic areas and may, therefore, pose great problems in diagnosis. "Exotic" tropical diseases are now of more than academic interest to the practitioner. Furthermore, the firm commitment of the United States and other Western nations to render help to developing countries carries with it a need for special emphasis on the principal medical and health problems in all areas of the world.

MANIFESTATIONS OF HELMINTHIC DISEASE. The symptoms and signs elicited by helminths are largely dependent on the tissues and organs involved, the production of chemical or mechanical injury by the parasite, and the development of hypersensitivity of the host to components of the parasite. Systemic symptoms such as fever, weight loss, or anemia, gastrointestinal dysfunction, a variety of cutaneous and systemic manifestations of allergy, and evidence of central-nervous-system disease are common to many of these disorders and will be detailed in the chapters to follow. Treatment often causes an exacerbation of allergic manifestations, and caution in initiating therapy is mandatory in many of these diseases.

DIAGNOSIS. Clinical diagnosis of parasitic disease in an endemic area is sometimes accurate, but even the most experienced physician must seek laboratory confirmation in view of the many overlapping syndromes which these diseases can create.

In nonendemic areas, a physician must be alert to the possibility of parasitic disease in individuals who may have been exposed in a foreign country. Once the possibility of helminthic disease is recognized, the physician must have knowledge of the proper specimens—feces, urine, blood, sputum, biopsy, etc.—to obtain or examination and must have available the services of a competent laboratory for diagnosis.

REFERENCES

Brown, H. W., and D. L. Belding: "Basic Clinical Parasitology," New York, Appleton-Century-Crofts, Inc., 1964.

Faust, E. C., and P. F. Russell: "Craig and Faust's Clinical Parasitology," 7th ed., Philadelphia, Lea & Febiger, 1964.

Hunter, G. W., III, W. W. Frye, and J. C. Swartzwelder: "A Manual of Tropical Medicine," 3d ed., Philadelphia, W. B. Saunders Company, 1960.

Lenczner, M., and T. Owen: "The Impact of Tropical and Parasitic Diseases in a Non-endemic Area, Can. Med. Assoc. J., 82:805, 1960.

Manson-Bahr, P.: "Manson's Tropical Diseases," 15th ed., London, Cassell and Co., Ltd., 1960.

Markell, E. K., and M. Voge: "Medical Parasitology," 2d ed., Philadelphia, W. B. Saunders Company, 1965.

Soulsby, E. J. L.: Immunity to Helminths—Recent Advances, Vet. Record, 72:322, 1960.

Stoll, N. R.: The Worms—Can We Vaccinate against Them? Am. J. Trop. Med. Hyg., 10:293, 1961.

Weller, T. H.: Tropical Medicine Today, New Engl. J. Med., 264:911, 1961.

247 TRICHINOSIS
Ivan L. Bennett, Jr., and Robert G. Petersdorf

DEFINITION. Trichinosis is caused by the intestinal nematode *Trichinella spiralis*. The disease is characterized by diarrhea during the development of the adults in the intestine and by myositis, fever, prostration, periorbital edema, and, occasionally, evidence of myocarditis or encephalitis during the stage of larval migration and invasion.

ETIOLOGY. Trichinosis in man is contracted by ingestion of meat containing the encysted larvae of *T. spiralis*. The meat is almost always pork, although a number of infections from bear meat have been observed, particularly in Northern Canada and Alaska. There are no intermediate hosts, and both the adult and larval stages develop in the same host. Infection has been produced or observed in the bear, wild boar, wolf, coyote, fox, muskrat, horse, cow, dog, cat, rabbit, guinea pig, mouse, and marine mammals, in addition to the rat and the pig. Man is particularly susceptible; most fowl are resistant. Among pigs, infection is contracted following feeding of uncooked pork scraps, less often by eating infected rats. The incidence of infection in pigs has been reduced by laws requiring that garbage be cooked thoroughly before being fed. Rats also feed on uncooked pork scraps and, in addition, maintain a high incidence of infection by their cannibalism.

Soon after ingestion, the larvae are liberated from their cysts by gastric digestion and migrate into the intestinal mucosa, where copulation takes place. The male dies, and within a week, the viviparous female is discharging larvae ($100 \times 6\ \mu$), which enter vascular channels and are distributed throughout the body. Larviposition continues for about 4 to 6 weeks. The larvae enter skeletal muscle and encyst. The muscles of the diaphragm, tongue, and eye, the deltoid, pectoral, and intercostal muscles are most often affected. Larvae carried to sites other than skeletal muscles do not encyst but disintegrate. The life cycle can be carried further only if a new host ingests the encysted larvae.

EPIDEMIOLOGY. Trichinosis is common in Europe and North America and uncommon in other parts of the world, including the Tropics. In the United States, the incidence of infection (as detected by finding calcified cysts at autopsy) has declined from 15.9 to 4.5 percent. This decline in incidence has been due to (1) a decrease of trichinosis in pigs, (2) a decrease in use of pork as compared with beef, (3) better techniques for deep-freezing pork, and (4) better education, which has led to more thorough cooking of pork products.

PATHOLOGY. The most striking lesions are in the skeletal muscles, where there is a severe myositis with basophilic granular degeneration of the invaded muscle fiber. Adjacent fibers exhibit hyaline or hydropic degeneration, and the focus becomes infiltrated with neutrophilic and eosinophilic leukocytes, some lymphocytes, and mononuclear macrophages. Hyperemia, edema, and hemorrhages are constant features.

Larvae do not encyst in cardiac muscle, but an intense myocarditis has been observed in fatal cases.

In cases of central-nervous-system involvement, there may be granulomatous nodules, and vasculitis involving small arterioles and capillaries of the brain and meninges. Encystment of larvae in the brain is unusual.

CLINICAL MANIFESTATIONS. The first symptoms usually appear within 1 to 2 days after ingestion of the uncooked or undercooked meat montaining encysted larvae. At that time diarrhea, abdominal pain, nausea, and sometimes prostration and fever develop. The next stage, that of muscular invasion, begins about the end of the first week and may last as long as 6 weeks. During this period, patients have fever, edema of the eyelids, conjunctivitis and subconjunctival hemorrhages, muscle pain and tenderness, and often severe weakness. There may be a maculopapular rash which lasts for several days and

subungual "splinter hemorrhages." Central-nervous-system involvement may be evident as polyneuritis, poliomyelitis, myasthenia, meningitis, encephalitis, focal or diffuse pareses, delirium, psychosis, and coma. Despite the severity of central-nervous-system involvement in some patients, the CSF (cerebrospinal fluid) remains normal.

Myocarditis is characterized by persistent tachycardia or development of congestive heart failure. There may be marked electrocardiographic alterations, including T-wave changes and conduction abnormalities.

LABORATORY FINDINGS. The most constant finding, and one of significance early in the course of the disease, is the eosinophilic leukocytosis (over 500 eosinophilic leukocytes per cu mm) which generally appears before the end of the second week. In cases of moderate severity, the proportion of eosinophilic leukocytes ranges between 15 and 50 percent. In severe cases, particularly terminally, the eosinophilic leukocytosis may disappear entirely.

The skin test to larval antigen becomes positive early in the third week of infection, with a wheal of 5 mm or more appearing within 30 min. The usual positive response is an immediate reaction, but early in the infection (before the seventeenth day) the response may be of the delayed type. The antigens vary in their sensitivity, and care must be taken to employ a potent preparation.

There is a variety of serologic tests for trichinosis, including the precipitin reaction, the bentonite flocculation test, the complement fixation test, and the indirect fluorescent antibody test. The last of these is probably the most accurate. These serologic tests all become positive by about the third week of the disease and may remain positive for several years. The serologic tests are most valuable if they are negative initially and then turn positive or if there is a change in titer.

Muscle biopsy remains the most useful site for demonstration of larvae or cysts. Myositis is a significant finding even in the absence of larvae or cysts.

In severe trichinosis there may be marked hypoalbuminemia, probably because of protein leakage from damaged capillaries. During the fourth, fifth, and sixth weeks of the disease, concomitant with a rise in antibody, diffuse hypergammaglobulinemia occurs. There may be moderate rises in SGOT (serum glutamic oxaloacetic transaminase), probably related to myositis, and the sedimentation rate is characteristically slow.

DIFFERENTIAL DIAGNOSIS. Trichinosis must be differentiated from diseases which are characterized by eosinophilia (such as Hodgkin's disease, eosinophilic leukemia, and periarteritis nodosa) and from entities which are characterized by myopathy, such as dermatomyositis. When the central nervous system is involved, the diagnosis may be very difficult.

TREATMENT. Thiabendazole, in dosage of 50 mg/kg/day for 5 to 7 days, has resulted in dramatic improvement in a number of patients with trichinosis. Within 48 hr of receiving this drug the patient has usually experienced subjective improvement, relief of muscle pain and tenderness, and lysis of fever. The drug has been associated with nausea, vomiting, abdominal discomfort, dermatitis, and drug fever, but despite these drawbacks it appears promising. It has not been uniformly larvicidal.

Patients with "allergic" manifestations of trichinosis, including angioedema and urticaria as well as central-nervous-system involvement, should be treated with ACTH and/or prednisone in dosage of 60 mg per day. Response to steroids usually has been prompt, particularly in central-nervous-system trichinosis. Not all focal lesions have resolved, however.

Other measures should be directed at relief of pain and maintenance of adequate caloric and fluid intake.

PROGNOSIS. The prognosis in trichinosis has improved markedly, and even when the central nervous system is involved, the mortality rate has fallen to under 10 percent. The overall mortality rate is probably less than 5 percent.

PREVENTION. The responsibility for control rests with the consumer. Adequate cooking of pork involves heating all portions of the meat to 55°C. Freezing procedures to kill the larvae require a temperature of −15°C for 20 days or −18°C for 24 hr. Proper smoking and pickling will also destroy the larvae. Important in control is the cooking of garbage fed to hogs. There is no practical method of inspection which will detect trichinous pork.

REFERENCES

Dalessio, D. J., and H. G. Wolff: *Trichinella spiralis* Infection of the Central Nervous System, Arch. Neurol., 4:407, 1961.

Gould, S. E.: "Trichinosis," Springfield, Ill., Charles C Thomas, Publisher, 1945.

Hall, W. J., III, and W. R. McCabe: Trichinosis. Report of a Small Outbreak with Observations of Thiabendazole Therapy, Arch. Intern. Med., 119:65, 1967.

Kagan, I. G.: Trichinosis: A Review of Biologic, Serologic and Immunologic Aspects, J. Infect. Dis., 107:65, 1960.

Kean, B. H., and D. W. Hoskins: Treatment of Trichinosis with Thiabendazole. A Preliminary Report, J.A.M.A., 190:116, 1964.

Most, H.: Trichinellosis in the United States, J.A.M.A., 193: 871, 1965.

Rachón, K., J. Januszkiewicz, and H. Wehr: Serum Proteins in Human Trichinosis, Am. J. Med., 44:937, 1968.

Sulzer, A. J., and E. S. Chisholm: Camparison of the IFA and Other Tests for *Trichinella spiralis* Antibodies, Public Health Report U.S., 81:729, 1966.

Wilson, R.: Bear Meat Trichinosis, Ann. Intern. Med., 65:965, 1967.

248 OTHER INTESTINAL NEMATODES

James J. Plorde, Ivan L. Bennett, Jr., and Robert G. Petersdorf

HOOKWORM DISEASE

Hookworm disease is a symptomatic infection caused by *Ancylostoma duodenale* or *Necator americanus*. Assymptomatic infection may be termed simply *hookworm infection,* and the individual with such infection is called a carrier.

ETIOLOGY. *Ancylostoma duodenale,* also known as the "Old World" hookworm, possesses four prominent hooklike teeth in its adult stage. The adults are about 1 cm long and inhabit the upper part of the small intestine of man, where they attach to the mucosa by means of the mouth parts and suck blood. Each adult extracts 0.15 ml blood daily. The adults migrate within the small intestine, and each site of attachment persists temporarily as a bleeding point. Following fertilization, the female liberates eggs which measure about $40 \times 60 \mu$ and are usually in the two- to four-celled stage when discharged in the feces.

Necator americanus, the "New World" hookworm, has a buccal capsule containing dorsal and ventral plates rather than teeth. It is slightly smaller and causes much less blood loss than *A. duodenale.*

The life cycles of both hookworms are similar. Development to the filariform or infective stage occurs outside the body. The larvae then penetrate the skin to enter vessels which carry them to the lungs. The larvae leave the alveolar capillaries, enter the alveoli, ascend the respiratory tree, enter the pharynx, and are swallowed. They reach the intestine about 1 week after penetration of the skin, and mature within 3 to 5 weeks. Adults have been known to survive in the human intestine for as long as 15 years.

EPIDEMIOLOGY. Conditions conducive to the development of the hookworm egg into infective filariform larvae are found in tropical and semitropical regions in which rainfall is plentiful. Hookworm infection occurs where there is opportunity for contact of the skin with contaminated soil. The disease may also be acquired by oral ingestion, but this is of little importance.

The white race is probably more susceptible to symptomatic infection than the Negro, but this is rarely of clinical significance. Probably because of greater exposure, males show a higher incidence of infection than females.

Repeated infections of hookworm in dogs results in immunity and elimination of the parasite. It seems probable that a similar phenomenon occurs in human infections. When the possibility of reinfection is eliminated, the majority of worms is eliminated spontaneously within 1 or 2 years.

In general, *Ancylostoma* presents a greater public health hazard than *N. americanus,* the species which is most prevalent in the Southern United States, because it is more persistent in the environment, more harmful to the host, and less amenable to treatment.

PATHOGENESIS AND CLINICAL MANIFESTATIONS. During the invasion of the exposed skin by the larvae, there are erythema and edema, with severe pruritus. These manifestations are more marked in *N. americanus* infection than in *A. duodenale* infection. The lesions are most common about the feet, particularly between the toes, and have been termed "ground itch."

During migration through the lungs, cough and, in

severe infections, fever are common. The pulmonary symptoms were particularly troublesome to soldiers engaged in close combat in the Asiatic campaign in World War II. Usually, however, pulmonary involvement does not give rise to clinical symptoms.

Various gastrointestinal symptoms, ranging from vague epigastric distress and picca to typical ulcer pain, have been reported in association with hookworm infection. Roentgenographic studies may reveal nonspecific changes such as excessive peristalsis and "puddling," particularly in the proximal jejunum. However, gross and microscopic examination of the bowel itself reveals conspicuously little damage. Previous reports of absorptive abnormalities in hookworm infection have not been supported.

The major clinical manifestations of hookworm disease clearly are those of iron-deficiency anemia consequent to chronic intestinal blood loss. Whether anemia develops and how severe it becomes depend on the balance between iron lost in the gut and iron absorbed from the diet. In many endemic areas, dietary iron is largely of vegetable origin and is absorbed poorly. General dietary deficiency also may lower resistance to parasitic infections. The severity of the disease and the prognosis depend on such factors as the age of the patient, the magnitude of the worm burden, the duration of the disease, and diet. Young children often have extreme anemia, with cardiac insufficiency and anasarca. Those who survive to puberty show retarded physical, mental, and sexual development. Milder degrees of the disease, as seen in older children and adults, are characterized by lassitude, dyspnea, palpitation, tachycardia, constipation, and pallor of the skin and mucous membranes. Poor diet influences the course of hookworm disease unfavorably.

Asymptomatic infections outnumber symptomatic infections, considering all age groups, twenty to forty times in endemic areas. The worm burden is small in asymptomatic infections, and the carrier state is probably indicative of some degree of acquired host resistance.

LABORATORY FINDINGS. In symptomatic infection, hookworm eggs are usually numerous enough to be detected by microscopic examination of a direct fecal smear. Abdominal and pulmonary symptoms appear before eggs are discharged, although a presumptive diagnosis may be made on the basis of the clinical history and the eosinophilic leukocytosis.

The feces seldom contain gross blood in hookworm disease, although tests for occult blood are usually positive. *Trichostrongylus* eggs are larger and in a later stage of maturation when observed in a fresh fecal specimen than are those of *Necator* or *Ancylostoma*.

Generally, the leukocyte count is normal or slightly elevated, and the percentage of eosinophils is increased to 15 or 30 percent. However, in some early cases, leukocytosis may be marked, with an eosinophilia as high as 70 or 80 percent. In general, the more severe the anemia, the less the eosinophilia. The anemia is characteristically hypochromic and microcytic.

DIFFERENTIAL DIAGNOSIS. Since hookworm disease oc-

curs in areas in which beriberi and malaria are also more common, these diseases must be differentiated from hookworm disease, or their coexistence must be established.

TREATMENT. Specific therapy for the infection and that directed toward improvement of nutrition and the anemia should be considered simultaneously. In the usual case, anthelmintics may be administered immediately, followed by iron therapy and a high protein diet. A number of satisfactory antihelmintic agents are available, but the drug of choice is tetrachlorethylene (TCE). In most instances a single dose of this agent will decrease the worm load substantially. Complete cure may require several courses of treatment but is not necessary in endemic areas; the aim of therapy is reduction of the worm load to an asymptomatic level. Tetrachlorethylene is administered as a single 5-ml oral dose mixed in a glass of water. Children should receive 0.10 ml per kg (to a maximum of 5 ml) by the same route. The night before treatment, the patient is permitted a light, fat-free meal. The following morning, breakfast is omitted and the drug is administered. No food is permitted for 4 hr and no alcohol for 24 hr. Purgation following administration of the drug is no longer recommended. Treatment can be repeated in a week if complete cure is desired and has not been accomplished. The drug is inexpensive, nontoxic, and ideal for mass therapy. If ascariasis is also present, it should be treated first with piperazine citrate (see Ascariasis below).

Biphenium hydroxynaphthoate (Alcopar) is also a drug of low toxicity which is said to be more effective than TCE against *A. duodenale* but possibly less effective against *N. americanus*. In mixed infections with Ascaris it can be used alone because it is active against both types of parasite. A single dose of 5 Gm biphenium hydroxynaphthoate is dispersed in water and ingested in the morning on an empty stomach. No food is permitted for 2 hr, and no purgation is recommended. The dose for children is the same as for adults. In *N. americanus* infections, treatment should be repeated on three consecutive days. Another drug which has been introduced for treatment of hookworm infections is thiabendazole (Mintezal). This is a broad-spectrum drug which is effective against ascaris, trichuris, and strongyloides as well as hookworm. The dose is 25 mg per kg twice a day for 2 or 3 days. Twenty-five percent of patients treated with this agent develop nausea and vomiting.

The anemia requires iron replacement.

When anemia is severe and there is malnutrition with anasarca, blood transfusions and a high protein diet should be given before drug treatment is begun. Blood should be given in an amount sufficient to raise the hemoglobin level to 10 Gm per 100 ml. In advanced cases it may be necessary to delay drug treatment for 2 to 3 weeks.

PROGNOSIS. Generally, the immediate prognosis is good. When opportunity for reinfection persists and nutrition cannot be maintained, a state of chronic debility develops. Maturation of children is impaired, and intercurrent disease is a serious problem in adults.

PREVENTION. Many of the measures required are obvious but difficult to apply on a large scale. Even if facilities for proper disposal of feces are provided, it is no simple matter to educate the population in their use. Soil pollution must be eliminated, and until this is accomplished, avoidance of direct skin contact with the soil (by wearing shoes) is mandatory. Periodic mass treatment of the population has been used in some hookworm control programs.

CREEPING ERUPTION
(Cutaneous Larva Migrans)

DEFINITION. Creeping eruption is an infection of the skin in man caused by the larvae of the dog and cat hookworm, *Ancylostoma brasiliense.* The other dog hookworms, *A. caninum* and *Uncinaria stenocephala,* and the horse botfly, *Gasterophilus,* in their larval stage may produce a similar cutaneous infection.

ETIOLOGY. *Ancylostoma brasiliense* reaches adulthood regularly only in the dog and cat. The larvae emerging from eggs discharged in the feces develop to the filariform stage and then are capable of penetrating the skin. In man, the larvae usually remain in the skin and migrate, producing an irregular erythematous tunnel visible on the skin surface.

EPIDEMIOLOGY AND DISTRIBUTION. Transmission to man requires environmental temperature and humidity appropriate for development of the egg to the infective filariform larva stage. Beaches and other moist, sandy areas are hazardous, because animals choose such areas for defecation, and the *A. brasiliense* eggs develop well in such soil.

PATHOGENESIS AND CLINICAL MANIFESTATIONS. The site of penetration of the skin by the larva becomes apparent in a few hours. The migration of the larva in the skin is accompanied by severe itching. Scratching may lead to bacterial infection. In the course of 1 week, the initial red papule develops into an irregular, erythematous, linear lesion which may attain a length of 15 to 20 cm.

Wright and Gold have observed Loeffler's syndrome in 26 of 52 cases of creeping eruption. Transient, migratory pulmonary infiltrations associated with an increased number of eosinophils in the blood and sputum were interpreted as an allergic reaction to the helminthic infection.

LABORATORY FINDINGS. Eosinophils occur in the lesion, but eosinophilic leukocytosis is slight, except when Loeffler's syndrome appears. The percentage of eosinophils in the blood may then rise to 50 percent, and in the sputum to 90 percent.

TREATMENT. Thiabendazole is the drug of choice; it should be given orally in the dosage suggested for hookworm, or it may be applied topically as a 10 percent aqueous suspension. Topical administration avoids systemic toxicity. Carbon dioxide snow or ethyl chloride applied to the advancing portion of the lesion is effective and practical, when there are only a few lesions. Superficial bacterial infections are improved by the application of wet dressings and elevation of the extremity. For intense itching, oral antihistaminics may be of aid.

PROGNOSIS. Untreated infections last several months. Treatment, which is usually sought because of severe pruritus, is usually successful.

PREVENTION. Dogs and cats should be prevented from contaminating recreation areas.

STRONGYLOIDIASIS

DEFINITION. Strongyloidiasis is an intestinal infection of man and other mammals, caused by *Strongyloides stercoralis.*

ETIOLOGY. The adult female resides in the mucosa of the upper part of the small intestine and lays eggs which develop into rhabditiform larvae which are excreted in the feces. Further larval development may take one of several courses: (1) In a suitable external environment, the indirect, or sexual, cycle occurs. (2) Under less-suitable external circumstances, the rhabditiform larvae develop into the infective filariform stage (direct, or asexual, cycle). (3) Development to the infective stage is thought to take place in the large intestine, the filariform larvae then entering the body through the intestinal wall or the perianal skin. This type of "autoinfection" may explain the long persistence (20 to 30 years) of strongyloidiasis in patients who have left endemic areas and also may account for the extremely heavy worm loads in some individuals.

The migration of the filariform larvae of *S. stercoralis* after entering the skin, the oral mucosa, or the intestinal mucosa resembles that of hookworm larvae. In the intestine the females burrow into the mucosa, from which site embryonated eggs are discharged.

EPIDEMIOLOGY AND DISTRIBUTION. The usual mode of infection is the penetration of the skin by larvae. Some infections may result from ingestion of contaminated food and drink, and some are believed to be transmitted by contact. This disease is endemic in the Tropics, although sporadic cases appear in temperate countries.

PATHOGENESIS AND CLINICAL MANIFESTATIONS. The initial cutaneous penetration of the filariform larvae usually produces no symptoms. Cough, dyspnea, and gross hemoptysis occasionally may accompany migration through the lungs. Roentgenograms may show pulmonary infiltration at this time.

Epigastric pain and tenderness, nausea, flatulence, vomiting, and diarrhea alternating with constipation may be observed during the intestinal phase. Transitory skin eruptions characterized by blotchy erythema, serpiginous lesions, and urticaria may recur at irregular intervals and apparently are related to episodes of acute infection. As with hookworm infection, many asymptomatic infections occur, and most symptomatic infections occasion only vague abdominal complaints.

In massive infection, there may be serious complications. These are particularly likely to occur during treatment with corticosteroids. Presumably these drugs facilitate the transformation of rhabditiform larvae to the infective filariform stage within the lumen of the intestine, resulting in autoinfection. A severe form of ulcerative colitis, accompanied by intestinal perforation and peritonitis, has been encountered. In one fatal case, pulmonary hemorrhage and edema were observed and larvae were found in the myocardium, lungs, trachea, liver, gallbladder, and intestine.

LABORATORY FINDINGS. Although clinical findings may be suggestive, the definitive diagnosis can be made only in the laboratory. Fresh fecal specimens should be examined to avoid confusion with hookworm infection; generally, fresh specimens contain *larvae* in strongyloidiasis infections, while in hookworm infection they contain *eggs*. If pulmonary involvement is present, the sputum should be examined for larvae. Microscopic examination of the duodenal washings may also establish the diagnosis.

Eosinophilic leukocytosis is common, except in very severe cases. When eosinophilia occurs in association with peptic ulcer symptoms strongyloidiasis should be suspected.

TREATMENT. Dithiazanine no longer can be recommended because it has caused fatal intoxication in several cases. The drug of choice is thiabendazole, which should be given orally in dosage of 25 mg per kg twice a day for 2 or 3 days. Light-headedness, nausea, and vomiting are common accompaniments of therapy with this agent. Hypersensitivity reactions may occur but usually respond to treatment with antihistamines.

PROGNOSIS. In the usual case, the prognosis is good. Since the occurrence of hyperinfection is unpredictable, every effort should be made to eradicate the infection in each case. In severe cases with hyperinfection, the prognosis is poor.

PREVENTION. In general, the measures are those for the control of hookworm infection. In addition, it is well to remember that infection may be contracted by ingestion of contaminated food (especially uncooked vegetables) or of contaminated drinking water and by contact.

ASCARIASIS

DEFINITION. Ascariasis is an infection of man caused by *Ascaris lumbricoides* and characterized by an early pulmonary phase related to larval migration and a later, prolonged intestinal phase. It is estimated that 25 percent of the world's population is infested with this nematode.

ETIOLOGY. The adult ascarids are large (20 to 40 cm in length) and cylindric, with blunt ends. The eggs are elliptic (30 to 40 μ $\times$ 50 to 60 μ) and have an irregular, dense outer shell and a regular, translucent inner shell. Under proper conditions of warmth and moisture the ovum develops to the infective larval stage in about 4 to 5 weeks. When the egg is ingested at this stage, the larva is liberated in the small intestine. It migrates through the wall and ultimately reaches the lungs. After about 10 days in the pulmonary capillaries and alveoli, the larvae pass in turn to the bronchioles, bronchi, trachea, and epiglottis, are swallowed, and develop into male and female adults in the small intestine. The adult has a life span of 6 to 18 months.

EPIDEMIOLOGY AND DISTRIBUTION. Infection follows the ingestion of the embryonated egg contained in contaminated food, or, more commonly, the introduction of the eggs into the mouth by the hands after contact with contaminated soil. Since the eggs are resistant to desiccation and wide variations in temperature, the disease is worldwide.

PATHOGENESIS AND CLINICAL MANIFESTATIONS. Because of the extensive migration of which both the larvae and adults are capable, clinical manifestations may be unusually diverse. In heavy infections, severe bronchopneumonia, occasionally fatal in children, may occur during the migration of the larvae through the lungs. Adult worms may cause no symptoms if the infection is light and may be detected accidentally when an adult worm is vomited or passed in the stool. Heavier infections may cause abdominal pain, and occasionally a bolus of worms may result in partial or complete intestinal obstruction in the ileocecal area. Obstruction often follows febrile illnesses which stimulate the worms to increased motility. Rarely an adult ascarid will migrate into the appendix, bile ducts, or pancreatic ducts, causing obstruction of these organs.

LABORATORY FINDINGS. The diagnosis is usually made by finding the ova in the feces. The intact ova are characteristic and not easily confused with those of other helminths.

Symptomatic infection, especially during the phase of larval migration through the lungs, is usually accompanied by fever and eosinophilic leukocytosis.

TREATMENT. Only symptomatic treatment can be used during the period of pulmonary involvement by the migrating larvae. For removal of the adult worms from the intestines, piperazine citrate, as a flavored syrup administered in a single dose after breakfast on two successive days, will cure the majority of cases. The dose of piperazine is 150 mg per kg, with a maximum of 3 Gm. No particular dietary regulation is necessary. The drug must be administered with caution to patients with renal insufficiency, because impaired elimination may produce neurotoxic signs. In intestinal obstruction, nasogastric suction should be initiated. After vomiting is controlled, piperazine should be given through the nasogastric tube every 12 to 24 hr in dosage of 65 mg per kg (maximum 1.0 Gm) for six doses. Surgery usually is not required.

While piperazine citrate is the treatment of choice, thiabendazole (see Strongyloidiasis, above) or biphenium hydroxynaphthoate (see Hookworm Disease, above) may be used. When both ascariasis and trichuriasis are present, treatment with thiabendazole is effective. When both ascariasis and infection with *A. duodenale* are present, treatment with biphenium hydroxynaphthoate is recommended.

PROGNOSIS. The prognosis in intestinal infection is generally good. When acute or chronic obstruction of ducts or hollow viscera has occurred, the immediate prognosis is determined by the promptness of diagnosis and treatment.

PREVENTION. Ascariasis is primarily a household infection of rural areas. All infections should be treated, personal hygiene stressed, and adequate toilet facilities provided.

VISCERAL LARVA MIGRANS

This is a clinical syndrome usually, but not exclusively, seen in children. Hepatosplenomegaly, skin rash, and recurrent pneumonitis with wheezing respiratory distress are frequent. There is often a history of dirt eating and contact with dogs or cats. Ocular involvement, which may be mistaken for retinoblastoma, and convulsions may also be observed.

Leukocytosis with eosinophilia to high levels (over 60 percent) and hypergammaglobulinemia are common. Anti-IgG factors have been reported in the serum of children with this syndrome. The eosinophils are unusual in that they are large and have vacuolated cytoplasm containing granules which vary in size and are present in smaller than normal numbers.

This syndrome, with various degrees of clinical severity, follows the ingestion of the infective eggs of nematodes whose life cycle is not completed in man. It is caused most often by nematodes whose life cycle is completed in the dog (*Toxocara canis*) or in the cat (*Toxocara cati*). Larvae of the *Toxocara* become widely disseminated in the body and incite a granulomatous reaction. Lesions are prominent in the liver, lungs, skeletal muscle, and brain. Larvae with eosinophilic leukocytic and granulomatous reactions have been noted in liver biopsies.

The clinical diagnosis may be made on the basis of the findings described. A hemagglutination test employing ascaris and toxocara antigens has been demonstrated by Jung and Pacheco to be a valuable aid in the laboratory diagnosis of visceral larva migrans. This is another variety of helminthic infection capable of causing Loeffler's syndrome. When the respiratory difficulty is pronounced, administration of ACTH or adrenocortical steroids is helpful. A small number of cases has been treated successfully with thiabendazole in dosage of 25 mg per kg twice daily for 1 to 4 weeks.

Control measures are directed toward preventing ingestion of the toxocara eggs. Removal or repeated treatment of infected cats and dogs must be considered, as well as modifying the diet to reduce the temptation to ingest contaminated materials.

ENTEROBIASIS

DEFINITION. Enterobiasis (pinworm, seatworm, or threadworm infection; oxyuriasis) is an intestinal infection of man caused by *Enterobius vermicularis* and characterized by perianal pruritus.

ETIOLOGY. The female averages 10 mm in length, the male 3 mm. The eggs are deposited by the female on the perineal skin, the migration generally occurring at night. Each egg contains an embryo which, within a few hours, develops into the infective larva. After the egg has been ingested, the larva is released in the small intestine and, in less than 1 month from the time of ingestion, newly developed gravid females are again discharging eggs. They are planoconvex and measure approximately 20 × 50 μ. The shell is clear and doubly contoured.

EPIDEMIOLOGY AND DISTRIBUTION. The eggs usually reach the host by way of contaminated hands, food, or drink, although airborne transmission is possible. They are relatively resistant to desiccation, and transmission within family and children's groups occurs readily. Enterobiasis is found in all climates and is probably the most common helminthic infection of man. Its low incidence in some tropical areas, however, defies explanation.

CLINICAL MANIFESTATIONS. The most common symptom is pruritus ani, which is most troublesome at night, being related to the migration of the gravid female worms. Scratching may lead to perineal eczema or pyogenic infection.

LABORATORY FINDINGS. Examination for ova of material obtained from the perineal skin by means of a cellophane or Scotch tape swab is the preferable method for the detection of enterobiasis. Searching for ova in the feces is rarely helpful. Scrapings from under the nails may reveal ova. The diagnosis is sometimes made by finding adult worms in feces following a laxative or an enema. Eosinophilic leukocytosis is not a typical finding.

TREATMENT. All infected individuals in a family or communal group should be treated simultaneously. Drug treatment must be combined with such measures as (1) providing a sleeping garment which prevents contamination of the fingers with ova from the perianal region, (2) instituting a morning shower, (3) lukewarm water enemas, and (4) local antipruritic ointments. It is relatively easy to reduce the worm burden and to make the infection asymptomatic, but eradication or cure is very difficult.

Pyrvinium pamoate (Povan) is the drug of choice. A single dose of 5 mg per kg is given orally, in tablet or liquid form. This compound turns the stool red and may stain bedclothes or undergarments. An acceptable alternative is piperazine citrate, which is highly effective when prescribed in a single course of 7 days. It is given in syrup each day before breakfast, with a total daily dose of 250 mg for children weighing up to 15 lb, 500 mg for those weighing between 16 and 30 lb, 1 Gm for those between 31 and 60 lb, and 2 Gm for those over 60 lb (Brown). When renal insufficiency is present, piperazine should be given in smaller dosage to avoid neurotoxicity.

PROGNOSIS. The prognosis with reference to the duration of infection is good, particularly when the other measures mentioned are carried out in addition to drug treatment.

PREVENTION. Methods of preventing autoinfection and dissemination within a group involving children are extremely difficult to enforce. Personal environmental hygiene should be stressed, and anthelmintic and symptomatic treatment of pruritus ani should be instituted. To control infection within a group, simultaneous treatment of all cases is mandatory.

TRICHURIASIS

DEFINITION. Trichuriasis (whipworm infection, trichocephaliasis) is an intestinal infection of man caused by *Trichuris trichiura* and is characterized by invasion of the colonic mucosa by the adult trichuris.

ETIOLOGY. The adult whipworms possess a threadlike anterior two-thirds and a stouter posterior third, giving them a whiplike structure. The eggs are characteristically barrel-shaped, brown, and translucent, with knoblike extremities.

EPIDEMIOLOGY. The mode of spread resembles that of ascariasis, the eggs generally being introduced into the mouth by contaminated fingers.

PATHOGENESIS AND CLINICAL MANIFESTATIONS. Symptomatic infection generally requires the presence of large numbers of adult whipworms and may be correlated in part with the degree of mucosal involvement. Heavy infections usually occur only in children and may be accompanied by nausea, abdominal pain, diarrhea, dysentery, and rectal prolapse.

LABORATORY FINDINGS. In symptomatic infection, large numbers of eggs are present in the feces and there may be eosinophilic leukocytosis and anemia.

TREATMENT. Thiabendazole, 25 mg per kg twice daily for 2 or 3 days, is effective, although less so in trichuriasis than in hookworm infection and strongyloidiasis. A 5-day course of pyrvinium pamoate or a 7-day course of piperazine citrate is also acceptable therapy (see Enterobiasis).

PROGNOSIS. Whipworm infection, unless characterized by severe diarrhea, blood loss, and systemic reaction, usually responds well to treatment. Serious infections may require supportive treatment as well as chemotherapy.

PREVENTION. Measures recommended for ascariasis apply also to trichuriasis.

TRICHOSTRONGYLIASIS

DEFINITION. Trichostrongyliasis is an intestinal infection of man and other mammalian hosts, including sheep, goats, and cattle.

ETIOLOGY. Almost a dozen species of *Trichostrongylus* are known to have infected man. Few human infections have been reported in the United States. In view of the high frequency of animal infections here, the low incidence of human infections is difficult to understand. The possibility exists that some such infections are mistaken for hookworm infection.

The ova resemble those of the hookworm but are larger and, when observed in a fresh fecal specimen, show a more advanced stage of segmentation (16- to 32-celled stage).

PATHOGENESIS. Infection is acquired by ingestion of the larvae, rather than by their penetration of the skin. The adult maintains residence in the intestine for long periods. Sandground, who infected himself, observed infection to last more than 8 years.

MANIFESTATIONS. Diarrhea is observed occasionally when infection is massive, but most infections are asymptomatic. The parasite owes its importance primarily to the resemblance of its ova to those of the hookworms. Moreover, because the trichostrongylidae do not respond to anthelmintics effective in hookworm infection, it may be assumed incorrectly that one is dealing with refractory hookworm infection.

LABORATORY DIAGNOSIS. The diagnosis depends on the finding of the ova in the feces. Since they are few, they are usually found only when a concentration method is used. In symptomatic infections, there may be leukocytosis with marked eosinophilia (e.g., 80 percent).

TREATMENT. These infections do not respond to tetrachlorethylene. Thiabendazole, 25 mg per kg twice daily for 2 or 3 days, or piperazine citrate as used against enterobiasis is effective in symptomatic infections.

PREVENTION. Contamination of the hands is to be avoided, as well as food grown in contaminated soil.

ANGIOSTRONGYLIASIS

The rat lungworm, *Angiostrongylus cantonensis*, is the etiologic agent of a fatal form of eosinophilic meningitis which has been reported from Tahiti, Hawaii, Vietnam, and Thailand. Living *angiostrongylus* has also been removed from the eye of patients without central-nervous-system involvement. Freshwater snails serve as the intermediate hosts of *A. cantonensis*, and man acquires the infection by ingestion of raw snails.

The nematode produces extensive tissue damage by moving through the brain when alive, and provokes a marked inflammatory reaction when dead. The inflammation is characterized by (1) dilatation of almost all blood vessels, particularly the veins, in the subarachnoid space; (2) marked eosinophilic infiltration of the meninges and brain substance, probably related to the presence of dead parasites, and (3) granuloma formation around dead parasites and the necrotic debris which ensheathes the worm. Charcot-Leyden crystals within macrophages are prominent.

Clinically, eosinophilic meningoencephalitis is indistinguishable from other meningitides. The cerebrospinal fluid contains several hundred cells per cubic millimeter, mostly eosinophils, and the cerebrospinal fluid protein level is elevated. There may not be an eosinophilia in the peripheral blood.

Although most of the reports of this disease deal with fatal cases, it is likely that nonfatal infections occur. There is no effective treatment. The best preventive approach is to warn the populace in endemic areas against eating raw snails.

INTESTINAL CAPILLARIASIS

Intestinal capillariasis is an infection of man caused by the roundworm *Capillaria philippinensis*. This species of capillaria was first discovered in 1963 from a fatal human infection occurring in the Philippines. The infection results in severe illness with a high mortality rate. Clinical studies have shown a severe protein-losing enteropathy and malabsorption of fats and sugars. This species of capillaria is the first of its genus found to infect the human intestine and the first to infect man in epidemic proportions. Of the more than 250 known species of capillaria which parasitize most classes of vertebrates, only three have been shown to infect man, and these have accounted for 16 sporadic cases reported in various parts of the world.

Capillaria are nematodes of the family Trichuroidea, and are closely related to comembers Trichuris and Trichinella. Adult *C. philippinensis* are small, measuring 2 to 4 mm in length. The peanut-shaped eggs have flattened bipolar plugs and an average size of 42×20 μ. The adults inhabit the mucosa of the small intestine, especially the jejunum. Adults, larval forms, and eggs are found in the stool.

The infection has been found only in persons residing in the Ilocano ethnic region in Northwest Luzon, Philippines. Since 1966 the disease has occurred in epidemic form and more than 1,000 cases and 100 deaths have been reported. Males are infected more frequently than females, perhaps because of occupational exposure. Prior to the discovery of an effective chemotherapeutic agent, the mortality rate in untreated cases was about 30 percent. With chemotherapy, the case fatality rate has been reduced to 6 percent.

The mode of transmission and life cycle of the parasite are not established. The presence of many adult worms, larviparous females, embryonated eggs, and all larval stages in human intestinal contents suggests that autoinfection may be part of the life cycle; this would allow for direct transmission by the fecal-oral route. In addition, indirect evidence indicates that man-to-man transmission occurs. The mechanism by which man originally became infected remains obscure. Because the Ilocano people of the region eat many animal foods raw or semi-cooked, numerous species of local fauna have been examined for capillaria, but without success. Experimental transmission studies in which embryonated eggs have been fed laboratory animals, including primates, have failed to result in infection.

Adult worms in large numbers invade the small-intestinal mucosa and cause a severe protein-losing enteropathy and malabsorption. Autopsy studies have failed to show extraintestinal spread of the parasite. Initial symptoms of intestinal "gurgling" (borborygmi) and recurrent vague abdominal pain are followed, usually within 2 to 3 weeks, by a voluminous watery diarrhea. Other findings, consistent with the basic pathophysiologic process, are anorexia, vomiting, weight loss, muscle wasting and weakness, hyporeflexia, and edema. Abdominal tenderness and distension may occur. The period between onset of symptoms and death is usually 2 to 3 months. Subclinical infection has not been noted.

The diagnosis is made by finding ova in the stool. *Capillaria philippinensis* ova must be differentiated from those of *Trichuris trichiura*, which are similar. Care

must be taken that capillaria are not overlooked in patients with *Trichuris* infections because in the endemic area most patients with capillariasis have coexistent *Trichuris* infection.

Administration of thiabendazole, combined with fluid and electrolyte replacement, leads to dramatic improvement. Thiabendazole therapy must be given over a prolonged period to prevent relapse. A divided dose of 25 mg per kg body weight per day is given for 1 month. On this schedule ova disappear from the stool within 2 weeks. Stools should be examined biweekly for 2 months following cessation of treatment.

REFERENCES

Beaver, P. C.: Larva Migrans, Exp. Parasitol., 5:587, 1956.

Beck, J. W., D. Saavedra, G. J. Antell, and H. Tejeiro: The Treatment of Pinworm Infections in Humans (Enterobiasis) with Pyrvinium Chloride and Pyrvinium Pamoate, Am. J. Trop. Med., 8:349, 1959.

Brown, H. W., K. Chan, and K. L. Hussey: Treatment of Enterobiasis and Ascariasis with Piperazine, J.A.M.A., 161:515, 1956.

Chitwood, M. B., C. Velasquez, and N. G. Salazar: *Capillaria philippinensis* N. (Nematoda: Trichinellida) from the Intestine of Man in the Philippines, J. Parasitol., 54:368, 1968.

Davis, C. M., and R. M. Israel: Treatment of Creeping Eruption with Topical Thiabendazole, Arch. Dermatol. 97: 325, 1968.

Duguid, I. M.: Features of Ocular Infestation by Toxocara, Brit. J. Ophthalmol., 45:789, 1961.

Franz, K. H., W. J. Schneider, and M. H. Pohlman: Clinical Trials with Thiabendazole against Intestinal Nematodes Infecting Humans, Am. J. Trop. Med., 14:383, 1965.

Gelpi, A. P., and A. Mustafa: Ascaris Pneumonia, Am. J. Med., 44:377, 1968.

Getz, L.: Massive Infection with *Trichuris trichiura* in Children, Am. J. Dis. Child., 70:19, 1945.

Heiner, D. C., and S. V. Kevy: Visceral Larva Migrans: Report of the Syndrome in Three Siblings, New Engl. J. Med., 254:629, 1956.

Hsieh, H.-C., H. W. Brown, M. Fite, L.-P. Chow, C.-S. Cheng, and C.-C. Hsu: The Treatment of Hookworm, *Ascaris* and *Trichuris* Infections with Biphenium Hydroxynaphthoate, Am. J. Trop. Med. Hyg., 9:185, 1960.

Jung, R. C., and G. Pacheco: Use of a Hemagglutination Test in Visceral Larva Migrans, Am. J. Trop. Med. Hyg., 9: 185, 1960.

Karpinski, F. E., E. A. Everts-Suarez, and W. G. Sawitz: Larval Granulomatosis (Visceral Larva Migrans), A.M.A. J. Dis. Child., 92:34, 1956.

Markell, E. K.: Pseudohookworm Infection—Trichostrongyliasis. Treatment with Thiabendazole, New Engl. J. Med., 278:831, 1968.

Nelson, J. D., T. H. McConnell, and D. V. Moore: Thiabendazole Therapy of Visceral Larva Migrans: A Case Report, Am. J. Trop. Med. Hyg., 15:930, 1966.

Ochsner, A., E. G. DeBakey, and J. L. Dixon: Complications of Ascariasis Requiring Surgical Treatment, A.M.A. J. Dis. Child., 77:389, 1949.

Roche, M., and M. Layrisse: The Nature and Causes of

Hookworm Anemia, Am. J. Trop. Med. Hyg., 15:1029, 1966.

Stemmerman, G. N.: Strongyloidiasis in Migrants. Pathological and Clinical Considerations, Gastroenterology, 53:59, 1967.

Swartzwelder, J. C.: Clinical *Trichocephalus trichuris* Infection, Am. J. Trop. Med., 19:473, 1939.

Tangchai, P., S. W. Nye, and P. C. Beaver: Eosinophilic Meningoencephalitis Caused by Angiostrongyliasis in Thailand, Am. J. Trop. Med. Hyg., 16:454, 1967.

Whalen, G. E., E. B. Rosenberg, G. T. Strickland, R. A. Gutman, J. H. Cross, R. H. Watten, C. Uylangco, and J. J. Dizon: Intestinal Capillariasis, Lancet, I:13, 1969.

Wright, D. O., and E. M. Gold: Loeffler's Syndrome Associated with Creeping Eruption, Arch. Intern. Med., 78·303, 1946.

249   FILARIASIS

*James J. Plorde and
Ivan L. Bennett, Jr.*

DEFINITION. Filariasis is a group of disorders produced by infection with nematodes of the superfamily Filarioidea. These worms invade the subcutaneous tissues and lymphatics of man, producing reactions ranging from acute inflammation to chronic scarring. The clinical pictures produced by various species in this group are more or less specific. The term *filariasis* is commonly used to designate the disease produced by *Wuchereria bancrofti* or *Brugia malayi*, the organisms responsible for elephantiasis. The disorders associated with infection by *Loa loa* or *Onchocerca volvulus* are usually referred to as *loiasis* and *onchocerciasis*.

FILARIASIS (Bancroftian and Malayan)

ETIOLOGY AND EPIDEMIOLOGY. The threadlike adult worms live coiled together in the lymphatics of man. The male *W. bancrofti* measures 35 mm and the female 80 to 100 mm. The *B. malayi* adults are about one-half as long. Gravid females release microfilariae in large numbers into the lymphatics. These embryos, which are sheathed, measure approximately 200 to 300 μ. They eventually reach the peripheral blood, where further development depends on their ingestion by a proper mosquito vector. Species of *Culex, Aëdes,* and *Anopheles* transmit Bancroftian filariasis; *Mansonia* and *Anopheles* serve as vectors in Malayan disease. After further development in the vector, larvae migrate to the mouthparts and, if inoculated into a human host, reach maturity in about a year. In the absence of reinfection, man harbors microfilariae for 5 to 10 years, the reproductive life of the adult worms. In most *W. bancrofti* and *B. malayi* infections, the microfilariae are found in the blood in greatest numbers between 9 P.M. and 2 A.M. During the day, apparently in response to changes in oxygen tension, they accumulate in the pulmonary vessels and disappear from the peripheral blood. However, in some endemic areas this nocturnal periodicity is not seen and may actually be replaced with a diurnal periodicity in which the peak occurs in the early evenings (subperiodic form). Periodicity is of epidemiologic significance because it determines which species of mosquito serves as the vector. Furthermore, several nonperiodic forms of *B. malayi* have been found in animals, suggesting the possibility that this disease has an animal reservoir.

Wuchereria bancrofti infection is endemic between latitudes 41°N and 30°S. Distribution is irregular, and there are many peculiar "skip areas" in this geographic pattern, presumably because the endemic disease can be maintained only where human infection and mosquitoes are prevalent. *Brugia malayi* infection is much more restricted in its distribution and occurs in India, Ceylon, Burma, Thailand, Vietnam, China, South Korea, Japan, Malaysia, Indonesia, Borneo, and New Guinea. There were approximately 15,000 *W. bancrofti* infections among American military personnel in World War II.

A small endemic focus of *W. bancrofti* once existed near Charleston, S.C., but no new cases have been observed in several years.

PATHOGENESIS. Pathologic changes are caused primarily by the presence of the adult worm in the lymphatics and may be divided into inflammatory and obstructive. The inflammatory response, most marked around dead or dying worms, consists of infiltration with lymphocytes, plasma cells, and eosinophils. This is followed by a granulomatous reaction which may lead to lymphatic obstruction. There are hyperplasia of lymphatic endothelium, acute lymphangitis, and thrombosis. Repetition of this process over a period of years leads to permanent lymphatic obstruction. The tissues become edematous, thickened, and fibrotic. Dilated lymphatics may rupture into surrounding tissue. Elephantiasis is actually a relatively unusual complication of filarial infections. If repeated reinfections do not occur, the disease is self-limited.

MANIFESTATIONS. Symptoms may occur within 3 months of infection, but ordinarily the incubation period is 8 to 12 months. The clinical findings closely reflect the pathologic changes, with inflammation early in the disease followed by obstruction later. Inflammatory filariasis consists of a series of brief febrile attacks occurring over a period of weeks. Fever is usually low grade but may reach 104°F and be accompanied by chills and sweats. Other symptoms include headache, nausea and vomiting, photophobia, and muscle pain. If the involved lymphatics lie close to the surface, the local symptoms dominate the clinical picture. Lymphangitis is very common, involving the legs more frequently than the arms. It often begins as a tender spot in the region of the malleoli or femoral area and spreads centrifugally. The involved vessels are palpably tender and painful. The overlying skin is red and swollen. When abdominal lymphatics are involved, the picture may simulate that of an acute condition of the abdomen. In Bancroftian filariasis the vessels of the spermatic cord and testes may be involved, resulting in painful orchitis, epididymitis, or funiculitis. Lymphadenitis almost always accompanies and may sometimes precede lymphangitis. The inguinal, femoral, and epitrochelar nodes are involved. Abscesses which may form about involved lymphatics and lymph nodes may discharge to the surface, resulting in persistently draining sinus tracts. The acute manifestations last only a few days and then subside spontaneously, only to recur at irregular intervals over a period of weeks or months. Recovery finally ensues. With repeated infections, slowly progressive lymphatic obstruction may develop in areas where the inflammatory reactions have occurred previously. Edema, ascites, lymph scrotum-hydrocele, pleural effusion, or joint effusion may appear as a result of interference with lymphatic drainage. Lymphadenopathy persists. The lymphatic vessels become palpably enlarged as tense elastic masses beneath the skin, especially in the femoral, inguinal, and scrotal areas. They may rupture and form draining sinuses. Internal rupture of lymphatics may give rise to chylous ascites or chyluria. In a small percentage of cases elephantiasis develops. This complication is rare below the age of twenty even in natives of heavily infested areas. The chronic obstructive phase of the disease often is punctuated by acute inflammatory episodes.

DIAGNOSIS. A history of exposure, the long incubation period, the occurrence of typical inflammatory episodes, and the finding of regional lymphadenopathy, thickening of the spermatic cord, or swelling of an extremity should suggest the diagnosis. There is usually eosinophilia during acute episodes. Lymphangiography may reveal dilated afferent and small efferent lymphatics. The definitive diagnosis depends on demonstration of the parasite. Although adult worms can be demonstrated in biopsied lymph nodes, biopsy is not recommended because it may interfere further with lymphatic drainage. Microfilariae are found in the blood during intermediate stages but not early or late in the disease. As in malaria, they are demonstrated best in thick smears. Concentration methods may be used if the parasite is not found in thick smears. Microfilariae are motile and sometimes may be seen in wet mounts. Because the appearance of microfilariae in peripheral blood is periodic, it is essential to obtain blood at appropriate times. Microfilariae may also be found in lymphatic fluid, hydrocele fluid, ascites, and pleural fluid. Complement fixation and skin tests are available and, although not completely reliable, are helpful when microfilariae cannot be demonstrated.

TREATMENT. Diethylcarbamazine (Hetrazan) rapidly eliminates microfilariae from the blood. It probably also kills or injures adult worms, impairing their ability to reproduce, and clears microfilariae permanently from the bloodstream of many patients. The drug is given in dosage of 2 mg per kg three times a day for 3 or 4 weeks. Treatment with this agent is often followed by allergic reactions to the dying parasite. These reactions may be quite severe, especially in Malayan filariasis. They can be controlled with aspirin, antihistamines, or steroid hormones. In heavy infections, it may be desirable to begin treatment with antihistamines before administration of Hetrazan.

Antimony compounds have no place in the treatment of filariasis.

Reassurance of the patient is very important in this disease. Vaccines and antiserums are valueless. Pressure bandages and surgery sometimes benefit elephantiasis. The prognosis for life is excellent, particularly if infected individuals leave endemic areas or otherwise avoid reinfections. Disease control is accomplished by combining mass treatment with mosquito control measures.

ONCHOCERCIASIS ("RIVER BLINDNESS")

This infection is produced by *Onchocerca volvulus* and is transmitted by flies of the genus *Simulium*, which breed along fast-moving streams. The disease is widespread in southern Mexico and Guatemala and is common in Central Africa. It is estimated that at least 20 million individuals are infected and that about 5 percent of these are blind as a result of the disease. Onchocerciasis is characterized by subcutaneous nodules, a pruritic skin rash, and ocular lesions. Adult worms are found coiled together in the fibrous subcutaneous nodules. In South America the nodules are found most frequently over the head; in Africa they occur primarily over the trunk. The gravid female worms release unsheathed microfilariae which are actively motile and which migrate in the skin, subcutaneous tissue, and eye until they die or are ingested by a feeding simulium fly. The pathologic changes occur as a result of a hypersensitivity reaction to dead or dying microfilariae. The skin lesions may appear as an erysipelas-like reaction over the face or a pruritic papular rash over one extremity. In chronic cases, lichenification and depigmentation may be present. The most serious complication of onchocerciasis are eye lesions, which are usually found in patients who have been heavily infected for a prolonged period of time. A punctate keratitis and iridocyclitis may eventually lead to blindness.

The parasites may be eliminated by excision of nodules on the head and neck, a procedure which is useful in preventing ocular complications, or by chemotherapy. Hetrazan kills the microfilariae but has little effect on the adult worm. Rapid destruction of microfilariae may cause severe allergic reactions which may result in severe ocular damage if the eye is involved. Adrenal steroids are useful in minimizing these allergic reactions. Suramin is effective in killing the adult worms but is nephrotoxic and must be used with care. The prognosis is favorable unless ocular invasion occurs or the number of nodules exceeds 50.

LOIASIS

This form of filariasis is produced by *Loa loa* and is prevalent in West and Central Africa. The infection is transmitted by flies of the genus *Chrysops*. Localized areas of allergic inflammation in the subcutaneous tissues known as *Calabar swellings* are the hallmark of the disease, although infestation may be completely asymptomatic. The adult worms are sometimes visible beneath the conjunctiva, and *Loa loa* is often called the *eye worm.* Diagnosis can be made by finding the adult worm or by demonstrating microfilariae in contents of Calabar swellings or in blood smears. Treatment is symptomatic, and the prognosis is good. An association between loiasis and endomyocardial fibrosis has been reported.

REFERENCES

Adams, A. R. D., and B. G. Maegrath: "Clinical Tropical Medicine," 4th ed., Philadelphia, F. A. Davis Company., 1966.

Cahill, K. M., and R. L. Kaiser: Lymphangiography in Bancroftian Filariasis, Trans. Roy. Soc. Trop. Med. Hyg., 58:356, 1964.

Choyce, D. P.: Onchocerciasis: Ophthalmic Aspects, Trans. Roy. Soc. Trop. Med. Hyg., 60:720, 1966.

Hawking, F.: The 24-hour Periodicity of Microfilariae: Biological Mechanisms Responsible for Its Production and Control, Proc. Roy. Soc., London, Ser. B, 169:59, 1967.

Hunter, G. W., W. W. Frye, and J. C. Swartzwelder: "A Manual of Tropical Medicine," 4th ed., Philadelphia, W. B. Saunders Company, 1966.

McGregor, I. A., and H. M. Gilles: Further Studies on the Control of Bancroftian Filariasis in West Africa by Means of Diethylcarbamazine, Ann. Trop. Med. Parasitol., 54:415, 1960.

Manson-Bahr, P.: The Story of *Filaria bancrofti,* a Critical Review, J. Trop. Med. Hyg., 62:53, 85, 106, 138, 100, 1959.

Ive, F. A., A. J. P. Willis, A. C. Ikeme, and I. F. Brockington: Endomyocardial Fibrosis and Filariasis, Quart. J. Med., 36:495, 1967.

Woodruff, A. W., O. P. Choyce, F. Muci-Mendoza, M. Hills, and L. E. Pettit: Onchocerciasis in Guatemala, Trans. Roy. Soc. Trop. Med. Hyg., 60:707, 1966.

World Health Organization Tech. Rep., ser. 359, 1967. (WHO Expert Committee on Filariasis—Wuchereria and Brugia infections—2d report.)

250 SCHISTOSOMIASIS (Bilharziasis)

James J. Plorde and
Ivan L. Bennett, Jr.

DEFINITION. Schistosomiasis (bilharziasis) designates a group of diseases produced by three closely related species of digenetic trematodes, or blood flukes, belonging to the family Schistosomatidae—*Schistosoma mansoni, S. haematobium,* and *S. japonicum.* These flukes inhabit the circulatory system of man and animals living in tropical and subtropical countries. The organs and tissues most frequently affected are the colon, urinary bladder, liver, lungs, and central nervous system.

ETIOLOGY AND LIFE CYCLE. The adult worms which grow and mature within the portal venous system of the liver measure 1 to 2 cm in length. The male has a central trough, the gynecophoral canal, that enfolds the longer slender female during most of its life. After copulation the male carries the female against the flow of portal blood to the small mesenteric vessels. *Schistosoma japonicum* ascends the superior mesenteric vein and S. *mansoni,* the inferior mesenteric vein. Both eventually reach the submucosal vessels of the small intestine; S. *japonicum* ends up in the ascending colon and S. *mansoni,* in the descending colon and rectum. *Schistosoma haematobium* finds its way through the hemorrhoidal anastomoses to the systemic capillaries of the bladder and other pelvic organs. When they can travel no further, the female deposits her eggs one by one, slowly retreating down the vessel in front of them. As the egg matures, it secretes a lytic substance which destroys the surrounding tissue. If the egg lies close to the mucosal surface, it ruptures into the lumen of the gut (or bladder in the case of S. *haematobium*) and is carried to the outside in the urine or feces. On reaching fresh water, the eggs quickly hatch, liberating ciliated *miracidia.* These miracidia have a life span of 8 hr in which to search out and penetrate the specific snail host which is appropriate to its species. Within the snail the miracidia are transformed into thousands of infective larvae called *cercariae.* When cercariae are released 1 to 2 months after the original penetration of the snail, they swim around vigorously and if they contact human skin within 2 days, they penetrate it and become *schistosomulae.* Within 24 hr the schistosomulae work their way into the peripheral venules and are carried to the right side of the heart and then to the pulmonary capillaries. After some delay, they enter the systemic circulation. Those parasites that survive the passage through the mesenteric capillary bed finally reach the portal venous system, where they mature into adult flukes in 4 to 10 weeks.

EPIDEMIOLOGY AND CONTROL. Schistosomiasis is possibly the most important of the helminthic diseases because of its worldwide distribution and the extensive pathologic changes produced by the parasites. It is believed that about 150 million persons are affected by this condition. Control measures have been relatively ineffective.

The continuing presence of schistosomiasis depends on the disposal of human excrement into fresh water, the presence of suitable snail hosts, and the exposure of persons to water infested with cercarias. Promiscuous defecation, latrine drainage, and unsanitary sewage disposal are the more important sources of pollution of streams and rivers. The disease is contracted by persons washing clothes, bathing, wading, or working in contaminated water. Schistosomiasis is more frequently encountered in rural than in urban communities.

Of these three disease-producing blood flukes of man, S. *mansoni* is the most common in the Western Hemisphere. It was brought to the Caribbean area and South America by African slaves. In South America it is present in Venezuela, Dutch Guiana, and Brazil. In Africa, it occurs in the Nile Delta, Sudan, Zanzibar, Madagascar, and Central Africa.

Schistosoma japonicum affects the agricultural population in Japan, China, the Philippines, and Thailand. Men are more frequently infected than women. An important source of infection in the Orient is the use of human excreta as a fertilizer in vegetable gardens.

Schistosoma haematobium is distributed widely throughout the African continent and, to a much less extent, is found in Spain, Portugal, Cyprus, and Greece. In Africa, it is highly prevalent among the agricultural population of the Nile Valley.

The best attack on schistosomiasis is preventive. Public health measures, including proper disposal of human excrement, provision of pure water supplies, and anthelmintic therapy, should be carried out in endemic areas. The effectiveness of these measures is diminished if there are significant animal reservoirs of the disease, as in S. *japonicum* and possibly in S. *mansoni* infections. Extermination of the mollusk intermediate host by chemical agents in areas where the infestation rate is high is an extremely costly undertaking. Available molluscicides include copper sulfate, pentachlorophenate, and niclosamide (Bayluside). This drug appears to be the most effective, but the selection of an agent is determined in large part by the nature of the habitat.

SCHISTOSOMIASIS MANSONI
(Intestinal Bilharziasis, Schistosomal Dysentery)

ETIOLOGY. *Schistosoma mansoni* is distinguished from the two other major species by the structure of its eggs and the adult flukes. The eggs are bluntly oval, have a lateral spine, and measure about 140 by about 60 μ. They are passed in feces and, rarely, in the urine. The intermediate snail hosts belong to the genera *Australorbis* or *Tropicorbis* in America and *Biomphalaria* in Africa. Man is thought to be the principal host, but baboons in Kenya have been found to be infected naturally. It is not known as yet whether they constitute an important reservoir of the disease independent of man.

PATHOLOGY AND PATHOGENESIS. Schistosomiasis mansoni is divisible into three stages: (1) an early stage of migration, during which the schistosomulae are carried by the blood to the liver and mature into adult parasites within intrahepatic portal veins; (2) an intermediate stage, during which ova are accumulating in various viscera; and (3) a late stage, characterized by scarring and fibrosis.

The greatest damage to man is caused by the eggs or their secretions. Reactions may take the form of a hypersensitivity reaction, intravascular obstruction, granuloma formation and eventual fibrosis. However, the secretions, metabolic products, and toxins of the adult worms are believed by some investigators to play an important role. As long as they are living, the adult parasites apparently produce no reaction, but when they die numerous eosinophils gather about them.

Eggs that are passed into the lumen of the bowel cause little tissue damage, but if retained, they elicit an eosinophilic and mononuclear cell infiltration. This is followed by granuloma or pseudotubercle formation. Healing occurs by formation of fibrous tissue and calcification.

In the bowel, congestion of the colonic mucosa, punctate hemorrhages, and thickening of the wall due to edema and fibrosis of the submucosa are the main findings; in Egypt, pedunculated or sessile polyps were commonly found in the rectum, but this is now unusual. Ova transported from the colon by venous blood are retained in the hepatic portal spaces, where they may produce an endophlebitis. Pseudotubercles form around them, accompanied by eosinophils. The organ is enlarged during the intermediate stage but later contracts as a characteristic periportal fibrosis develops. The larger portal veins are surrounded by collars of fibrous tissue, resulting in a severe presinusoidal form of portal hypertension which frequently leads to marked splenic enlargement. With the development of portocaval anastomoses, some eggs are carried past the liver to the vessels of the lung, where they may produce an inflammatory endarteritis with deposition of hyaline, granuloma formation, and obstruction of pulmonary arterioles. There may be interstitial fibrosis and destruction of pulmonary capillaries. On roentgenogram the granulomas may resemble miliary tuberculosis. In time cor pulmonale may develop. Occasionally ova are carried to the spinal cord through anastomotic venous channels. The resulting inflammatory reaction may lead to various neurologic manifestations.

MANIFESTATIONS. The finding of schistosome ova in the stools of apparently healthy individuals is a relatively frequent occurrence in endemic areas. Because the parasites do not multiply within the human host, symptomatic disease is dependent on the continued exposure to infection.

Itching and urticaria, sometimes with fever, are common but not invariable after exposure. Anorexia, headache, generalized aches and pains, and diarrhea accompanied by abdominal discomfort soon follow and last 1 to 2 weeks. These symptoms occur after invasion of the parasite and during the periods of migration of the larvae. From 30 to 70 days following exposure, when the schistosomulae have become adult males and females and oviposition has occurred, more severe symptoms may appear. These apparently are caused by an allergic response to the growing antigenic mass of ova and adult parasites and consist of high fever, chills, cough, urticaria, abdominal pain, diarrhea, and occasionally melena. Physical examination shows lymphadenopathy, an enlarged tender liver, and fine scattered rales. Sigmoidoscopy reveals an inflamed, engorged mucosa with small areas of ulceration and hemorrhage. The peripheral blood shows an eosinophilic leukocytosis. Ova may not be present in the stool initially but usually appear within a few weeks. The clinical picture in severe infections resembles that of typhoid except for the eosinophilia. This acute illness may last as long as 3 months and subsides gradually. When the initial infection is not severe or when anthelmintic treatment is given, the patient may recover rapidly.

Deposition of eggs continues during the life of the female worm (which may be as long as 30 years) and recurrence of these acute symptoms is common.

The late clinical manifestations are related to granuloma formation, vascular obstruction, and fibrosis elicited by ova in the tissues. Abdominal pain, diarrhea with or without blood, intestinal obstruction, and rectal prolapse reflect the pathologic changes in the colon. The periportal fibrosis in the liver and resulting portal hypertension cause splenomegaly, anemia, leukopenia, and thrombocytopenia. Massive hematemesis from ruptured gastroesophageal varices is a common cause of death. The liver is enlarged, but hepatocellular function usually is well preserved, and spider nevi, gynecomastia, jaundice, and ascites are uncommon.

In some patients, particularly adolescents in whom irreversible vascular changes have occurred in the lungs, pulmonary hypertension associated with chronic cor pulmonale dominates the clinical picture. Deposition of eggs in the spinal cord may result in transverse myelitis.

DIAGNOSIS AND LABORATORY FINDINGS. Diagnosis depends on finding the ova in the stools or the rectal mucosa. By the use of methods for stool concentration, a greater number of eggs is picked up from a given specimen, and a larger number of cases may be detected.

By means of a Jackson's laryngoscopic forceps 35 cm long, a piece of mucosa 2 to 3 mm in diameter can readily be obtained through a proctoscope. When this unstained tissue is compressed between two glass slides, the ova can be recognized easily under the low-powered lens of a microscope. It is believed by many investigators that rectal biopsy is the most reliable method of diagnosis; a very small piece of tissue may contain up to several hundred ova. In many cases in which repeated stool examinations have been negative, rectal biopsy has shown living or dead ova. Occasionally, however, stools contain ova when biopsy is negative.

An intradermal test is available and may be helpful in diagnosis. It is quite sensitive except in children and becomes positive about 2 months after infection. It is not species-specific, however, and 25 percent of patients with a history of "swimmers' itch" also react to the antigen. Because it remains positive despite cure, it is valuable in epidemiologic surveys.

The complement fixation test is the most reliable serologic test available. It becomes positive early in the course of infection, often before eggs can be recovered. Like the intradermal test, it is not species-specific. A cercarial slide flocculation test may provide a simple reliable tool for serologic surveys. Positive serologic or skin tests should lead to a vigorous search for eggs by concentration methods or rectal biopsy, but positive tests are not themselves an indication for treatment.

TREATMENT. Certain trivalent antimony compounds are effective against *S. mansoni*. These are tartar emetic (antimony potassium tartrate), stibophen (Fuadin), and antimony dimercaptosuccinate (Astiban). *Tartar emetic* remains the most effective agent available but is also the most toxic. Antimony sodium tartrate is less toxic than the potassium salt and is the form generally used. It is administered intravenously as a freshly prepared 0.5 percent solution. The drug must be given slowly. Extravasation into surrounding tissue leads to painful necrosis. The initial dose is 0.04 Gm; subsequent doses are given on alternate days and gradually increased to a maximum of 0.12 Gm by the fifth dose. A total of 1.8 to 2.2 Gm should be given. The patient should be hospitalized during treatment and should remain at bed rest for a few hours after each injection. Temporary ECG changes are common during therapy; they consist primarily of repolarization abnormalities which disappear a few days after the drug is discontinued. However, arrhythmias, collapse, and sudden death have been reported. Antimonials also may cause hepatitis, acute nephritis, hemolytic anemia, and thrombocytopenic purpura. Any of these complications calls for immediate discontinuation of therapy. Nausea and joint pains can usually be controlled by decreasing the individual dose or increasing the intervals between doses. Heart, renal, or liver disease constitutes a contraindication to therapy with this group of agents.

Fuadin contains 6.3 percent trivalent antimony and is less toxic, but also less effective, than tartar emetic. If the drug can be given intramuscularly, then daily injections of 1.5, 3.5, and 5 ml are given for the first 3 days. 5.0 ml is then given every other day until a total of 100 ml of a 6.3 percent solution has been given. Pain at the site of administration is common.

Astiban appears to be as effective as tartar emetic but is much less toxic. It is given by intramuscular injection as a 10 percent solution for five doses, for a total of 35 to 50 mg per kg (maximum 2.0 Gm). Toxic side effects are mitigated if injections are given at weekly intervals.

Ambilhar (Niradazole) can be taken orally in dosage of 25 mg per kg every day for 5 to 7 days, and may be as effective as Astiban. Although ECG changes occur with this drug also, they are lesss common than with antimonial therapy. However, there has been a high incidence of neurologic abnormalities, and as many as 80 percent of patients receiving the drug show eletroencephalographic changes. Psychotic episodes or convulsions, which disappear when the drug is discontinued, have also been reported. This drug is not available in the United States.

Success of treatment is judged by the disappearance of eggs from the stool, reduction in eosinophils, and alleviation of symptoms. Patients should be examined monthly for 12 months to detect relapses. If living eggs are found, retreatment is indicated. In the late stages of the disease, therapeutic measures are palliative, since the patient is suffering from fibrosis of the liver, portal hypertension, or hypersplenism. The indications for surgical procedures are the same as for the other forms of portal hypertension.

PROGNOSIS. The prognosis is good when the symptoms are mainly secondary to colitis, but when the liver, spleen, and lungs are involved, the prognosis is poor.

SCHISTOSOMIASIS JAPONICA
(Eastern Schistosomiasis, Katayama Disease)

ETIOLOGY. The oval eggs are shorter, wider, and smaller than those of the other two species, measuring about 90 × 70 μ. Mature eggs have a minute hook, or spine, laterally situated and smaller than that of S. mansoni. The ova are passed in the feces only. The life cycle is similar to that of S. mansoni, but various species of Oncomelania snails are utilized as intermediate hosts. Schistosoma japonicum lives in the inferior mesenteric venules but frequently migrates into the venules draining the large intestine and oviposits there. Water buffalo, horses, cattle, pigs, dogs, and cats as well as man may harbor the parasite, and some of these species serve as important reservoirs.

PATHOLOGY. Schistosoma japonicum resembles the mansoni type, but because of the much greater number of ova deposited by the female worms in the former disease, the manifestations are frequently more severe. Fibrosis of the liver develops earlier, and the duration of the disease is shorter—death often ensuing in 2 to 5 years. In advanced cases the gross postmortem findings are emaciation and pallor; a large or contracted liver with periportal fibrosis; splenomegaly, with fibrosis of pulp; ascites; fibrotic nodules over the colonic peritoneum; fibrous thickening and rigidity of the colon, with small polyps projecting from the mucosa; and thickening and fibrosis of the omentum. Microscopically, the tissue changes are similar to those of schistosomiasis mansoni. Eggs are more frequently found in ectopic locations, especially the central nervous system, than is the case with S. mansoni.

MANIFESTATIONS. Following penetration of cercarias through the skin, allergic manifestations such as urticaria, itching, localized dermatitis, cough, and angioneurotic edema accompanied by fever and diarrhea may appear. From 4 to 6 weeks after exposure, gastrointestinal symptoms are evident, a result of ulcerations produced in the intestinal walls by the large number of eggs. Bloody mucoid stools, or periods of bloody diarrhea accompanied by abdominal pain, may be present. If untreated, symptoms may last for several months. The liver enlarges and becomes tender, and splenomegaly develops.

As the disease progresses, signs of portal obstruction, such as engorgement of superficial abdominal veins, ascites, etc., appear. Some individuals present marked splenomegaly, a small contracted liver, profound anemia, leukopenia, and thrombocytopenia associated with severe malnutrition and hypoproteinemia. The majority of individuals suffering from schistosomiasis japonica die of cirrhosis and cachexia, massive hemorrhage from rupture of esophageal varices, or intercurrent infections.

Central-nervous-system lesions occur more frequently in the brain than in the spinal cord and appear clinically as an expanding tumor.

DIAGNOSIS AND LABORATORY FINDINGS. The characteristic ova must be found in the stools in order to establish the diagnosis. In established cases, ova are more difficult to demonstrate in the stools or in rectal biopsy; the intradermal and complement fixation tests are valuable in these instances.

TREATMENT. In general, S. japonicum infections are more difficult to treat, and relapses are more frequent. The drug of choice is sodium antimony tartrate; a total dose of 2.2 Gm should be given in the manner outlined for S. mansoni. If a lesion is present in the brain, prompt treatment may forestall the need for surgical intervention. Astiban may be used as an alternative drug. Portacaval shunt may be necessary to control bleeding from esophageal varices.

PROGNOSIS. If the condition is not treated early, prognosis is poor in the majority of cases encountered in endemic communities.

SCHISTOSOMIASIS HAEMATOBIA
(Genitourinary Schistosomiasis, Endemic Hematuria)

ETIOLOGY AND LIFE CYCLE. The eggs are compact, elongated spindles, dilated in the middle and measuring about 140 by about 50 μ. At one pole they present a short terminal spine. The ova are passed in the urine, and occasionally in the feces. The life cycle is similar to that of S. mansoni. The adult worms live in the hemorrhoidal plexus of veins, some going to the rectum for oviposition but most of them passing on to the vesical plexus. The intermediate hosts are snails of the genera Bulimus, Physopsis, and Ferrissia.

PATHOLOGY. In the urinary bladder, large numbers of ova are deposited in the submucosa and give rise to dense infiltration with eosinophils, lymphocytes, and plasma cells. These foci, or "pseudoabscesses," apparently represent an allergic reaction to the eggs. The trigone is involved at first, but soon the entire mucosa is thickened and ulcerated. In chronic infections, the other coats become scarred and the muscularis hypertrophies. Pedunculated papillomas often develop at the trigone and about the urethral orifices. The bladder capacity becomes greatly reduced as the organ loses its contractility. Lesions occur in the distal third of the ureters in many cases, causing obstruction and hydronephrosis. Bacterial pyelonephritis may occur. In about 10 percent of cases, calculi develop in the bladder, renal pelvis, or ureters. Fistulas between the urogenital tract and intestines may develop. The prostate and seminal vesicles may be affected, and lymph blockage may produce an elephantoid condition of the genitalia. The cervix and vagina can be infected by extension from the bladder. Carcinoma of the bladder is a frequent late complication in Egypt but not in other areas. Because the ova are deposited in the vesical plexus, ectopic eggs are carried to the lungs rather than to the liver, resulting in the early appearance of pulmonary hypertension and cor pulmonale.

MANIFESTATIONS. Painful micturition, frequency, and hematuria are the leading symptoms. Secondary bacterial infection of the urinary tract is frequent, and repeated hemorrhages from the bladder produce severe anemia. Salmonellosis, including the carrier state and bacteremia, is frequently associated with S. *haematobium* infection.

DIAGNOSIS AND LABORATORY FINDINGS. As in the other types of schistosomiasis, diagnosis is made by finding the characteristic ova in the urinary sediment, in tissues obtained from vesical mucosa, or, less frequently, in the stools.

TREATMENT. Chemotherapy is effective early in the disease but is contraindicated when urinary obstruction and infection have supervened. The drugs are the same as those recommended for S. *mansoni*. Surgery may be required for abscesses, fistulas, strictures, papillomas, and various other complications involving the bladder. Chemotherapy is indicated for secondary bacterial infections of the urinary tract. The criteria of cure are the absence of ova in the urine and bladder wall and the disappearance of ulcerative granulomatous lesions, as revealed by cystoscopic examination.

PROGNOSIS. Provided treatment is started without further delay, prognosis is good in recent infection, fair when damage to the bladder and urinary infection have already occurred. Prognosis is very poor in chronic, late infections. After age forty-five, the mortality rate increases fourfold. The frequent coexistence of infection with S. *mansoni* aggravates prognosis and the clinical picture.

SCHISTOSOME DERMATITIS

DEFINITION AND GEOGRAPHIC DISTRIBUTIONS. Certain nonhuman schistosome cercarias may penetrate the skin of man and cause a dermatitis. This condition is known as *schistosome dermatitis*, or "swimmer's itch," and is common in many parts of the world. The condition apparently does not develop after a single contact with cercarias, but it ensues following multiple exposures. Definitive hosts of some of the schistosomes producing dermatitis are the muskrat and migratory birds. Again, snails are intermediate hosts.

Schistosome dermatitis has been reported from the freshwater areas of north central United States, Canada, Oregon, Central America, Western Europe (particularly Switzerland), and the Far East.

A seawater dermatitis believed to be produced by nonhuman schistosome cercarias has been reported in New York, Rhode Island, California, Hawaii, and Florida.

PATHOGENESIS AND CLINICAL MANIFESTATIONS. Because the dermatitis develops only after multiple exposures, the condition is believed to represent an allergic reaction, the nonhuman cercarias being the sensitizing agents. Exposed individuals show positive intradermal reaction when tested with cercarial antigen.

TREATMENT. Local application of antipruritic lotions such as calamine with menthol or phenol is used to allay itching and thereby reduce the likelihood of secondary infection. Local treatment with antihistaminic drugs will relieve the pruritus.

PREVENTION. Immediate drying of the skin after swimming has been recommended as a prophylactic measure. This will not completely prevent lesions, since some penetration occurs during immersion. Dimethyl phthalate cream has been reported as an effective cercarial repellent.

In some areas, control has been effected by destruction of snails. Copper sulfate and copper carbonate have been used for this purpose. Treatment of shallow waters where snails are abundant has been moderately effective.

REFERENCES

Amaury, C.: Hemodynamic Studies of Portal Hypertension in Schistosomiasis Am. J. Med., 44:547, 1968.

Cheever, A. W., and Z. A. Andrade: Pathologic Lesions Associated with *Schistosoma mansoni* Infection in Man, Trans. Roy. Soc. Trop. Med. Hyg., 61:626, 1967.

Chemotherapy of Bilharziasis. Report of a WHO Scientific Group, World Health Organ. Tech. Rep. Ser., no. 317, 1966.

Davis, A.: Field Trials of Ambilhar in the Treatment of Urinary Bilharziasis in School Children, Bull. World Health Organ. 35:827, 1966.

Diaz-Rivera, R., F. Ramos-Morales, F. Koppisch, M. R. Garcia Palmieri, A. A. Cintron-Rivera, E. J. Marchand, O. Gonzalez, and M. W. Torregrosa: Acute Manson's Schistosomiasis, Am. J. Med., 21:918, 1956.

El-Din Hathout, S., Y. Abd El-Ghaffar, and A. Y. Awny: Salmonellosis Complicating Schistosomiasis in Egypt. A New Clinical Appreciation, Am. J. Trop. Med. Hyg., 16:462, 1967.

Epidemiology and Control of Schistosomiasis. Report of a WHO Expert Committee, World Health Organ. Tech. Rep. Ser., no. 372, 1967.

Garcia-Palmieri, M. R., and R. A. Marcial-Rojas: The Protean Manifestations of Schistosomiasis Mansoni. A Clinical Pathologic Correlation, Ann. Intern. Med., 57:763, 1962.

Kagan, I. G., and J. Pellegrino: A Critical Review of Immunologic Methods for the Diagnosis of Bilharziasis, Bull. World Health Organ., 25:611, 1961.

——, D. W. Rairigh, and R. L. Kaiser: A Clinical, Parasitologic and Immunologic Study of Schistosomiasis in 103 Puerto Rican Males Residing in the United States, Ann. Intern. Med., 56:457, 1962.

Marcial-Rojas, R. A., and R. E. Fial: Neurologic Complications of Schistosomiasis. Review of the Literature and Report of Two Cases of Transverse Myelitis Due to S. *mansoni*, Ann. Intern. Med., 59:215, 1963.

Orris, L., and F. C. Combes: Clam Digger's Dermatitis: Schistosome Dermatitis from Sea Water, A.M.A. Arch. Dermatol. Syphilol., 66:367, 1952.

Powell, S. J.: Natural History of Urinary Tract Bilharziasis in Durban, S. African Med. J., 41:991, 1967.

Zaki, M. H., S. DeRamos, H. B. Shookhoff, and M. Sterman: Further Trials with Astiban in *Schistosomiasis mansoni*:

The Effect of Increased Dosage, Am. J. Trop. Med. Hyg., 15:725, 1966.

251 OTHER TREMATODES OR FLUKES
James J. Plorde and
Ivan L. Bennett, Jr.

PARAGONIMIASIS

Paragonimiasis (endemic hemoptysis) is an infection of the lung caused by the trematode, *Paragonimus westermani*. The dog, cat, pig, rat, and wild carnivores are definitive hosts for the parasite, in addition to man. The infection is acquired by ingestion of cysts in the second intermediate host, a crab or crayfish. The metacercariae excyst in the duodenum, burrow through the intestinal wall into the peritoneal cavity, and migrate through the diaphragm and into the lung, where they become encapsulated. The pulmonary lesions are cysts with fibrous walls measuring up to 1 cm in diameter. Small fibrous nodules representing reaction around deposited eggs also occur. Eggs appear in the feces when sputum from pulmonary lesions is swallowed. In heavy infections, lesions are also found in the liver, mesentery, skeletal muscle, and brain, and cases are often classified as pulmonary, abdominal, or cerebral. In the pulmonary type, the clinical picture is one of chronic bronchitis or bronchiectasis with production of brownish sputum and hemoptysis. A poorly resolving pulmonary infiltrate, lung abscess, or pleural effusion may be present in heavy infections. Abdominal pain and dysentery characterize the abdominal type. Various types of paralysis and epilepsy are observed with cerebral involvement. Eosinophilia is a constant finding. In attempting to establish the diagnosis, eggs should be sought in the sputum and feces. Complement fixation and skin tests may be helpful.

Bithionol is the drug of choice. From 30 to 40 mg per kg in divided doses should be given every other day for a total of 10 to 15 treatment days. The symptoms disappear rapidly, and most infiltrates resolve within 3 months. Side effects are minor and consist of nausea, vomiting, and urticaria. Emetine and chloroquine are less satisfactory. Prevention of superinfection by the same parasite is important, because the disease is self-limiting.

Paragonimiasis has probably the widest geographic distribution of any of the diseases produced by the hermaphroditic trematodes. It is endemic in many parts of the Far East and has been reported from parts of Africa and northern South America.

The most practical control measure is the adequate cooking of all shellfish before it is eaten.

CLONORCHIASIS

DEFINITION. Clonorchiasis is caused by *Clonorchis sinensis* and is characterized by hepatic lesions produced by the adult worms in the biliary passages.

ETIOLOGY. *Clonorchis sinensis*, the most important liver fluke of man, measures about 15 × 5 mm. Infection is a result of ingestion of raw fish containing the larval clonorchis. Many mammals can serve as definitive hosts (dog, cat, pig, badger, guinea pig, and others). The encysted larva is released and migrates from the duodenum into the biliary tract, where it develops into the adult form. Judging from studies on individuals who have left the Far East, the major endemic area, the adult clonorchis is capable of living as long as 25 years.

CLINICAL MANIFESTATIONS. Most infections are asymptomatic. Although there are proliferations of the biliary epithelium, thickening and dilatation of the bile ducts, chronic pericholangitis, and atrophy of the parenchyma, the usual manifestations of cirrhosis are rare. Attacks of suppurative cholangitis following biliary obstruction with dead flukes have been reported. The adult worms may infest the pancreatic ducts, where they can cause squamous metaplasia and periductal fibrosis.

LABORATORY DIAGNOSIS. The diagnosis usually depends on the demonstration of the eggs in the feces or the duodenal contents. An antigen extracted from adult worms can be used in a complement fixation test for the detection of the host's antibody response. Skin tests are also useful.

TREATMENT. No consistently effective treatment is known, but some success has been noted with gentian violet and chloroquine diphosphate. Gentian violet is given orally in enteric-coated tablets in dosage of 60 mg three times a day with meals for 30 days. Chloroquine is prescribed in a dose of 0.25 Gm twice daily for 28 days. Infections which do not respond to this dosage should be treated for an additional 2- to 3-week period Good results have been claimed with hexachloroparaxylol (Hetol) but more experience with this drug is needed before it can be recommended for general use.

PREVENTION. Thorough cooking of freshwater fish will prevent infection.

OPISTHORCHIASIS

Opisthorchiasis is caused by *Opisthorchis felineus* or *O. viverini* and is characterized by hepatic lesions produced by adult worms in the larger bile ducts. The life cycle resembles that of *C. sinensis*, with lesions and clinical manifestations like those produced by *C. sinensis*. The geographic distribution differs in that it is endemic in Eastern and Central Europe and in Siberia and occurs in some parts of Asia. The diagnosis usually is based on the finding of the eggs in the feces or duodenal contents. Treatment as recommended for clonorchiasis may be used. Infection can be prevented by eating only well-cooked fish.

FASCIOLIASIS

Fascioliasis is caused by the hermaphroditic leaf-shaped fluke *Fasciola hepatica*, which inhabits the bile ducts of the definitive host. When fully matured, the adult measures about 3×1 cm and discharges large operculate eggs 140×70 mm.

Fascioliasis produces so-called "liver rot" in sheep, the principal definitive host. The disease is most common in sheep- and cattle-raising countries but has been reported from many parts of the world. In North America it occurs in the Southern and Western United States, Central America, and in the Caribbean Islands.

Infection is contracted by ingestion of the encysted form of the fluke attached to edible aquatic plants such as watercress. The larvae excyst in the duodenum, migrate through the intestinal wall, pass into the peritoneal cavity, penetrate the liver capsule, and finally reach the bile ducts, where they mature.

Early clinical manifestations are related to the migration of the larval form to and within the liver. Epigastric pain, fever, diarrhea, jaundice, urticaria, pruritus, arthralgia, and eosinophilia may be observed during this stage. Fibrosis of the liver similar to that found in clonorchiasis appears only after prolonged residence of many adult worms in the bile ducts. A pharyngeal form of the disease, called "halzoun," can result from eating infected raw liver, the young adults attaching themselves to the pharyngeal mucosa, occasionally interfering with respiration.

The diagnosis usually is based on the finding of the eggs in the feces or in the duodenal contents. It is difficult to distinguish the eggs from those of *Fasciolopsis buski.* Complement fixation, hemagglutination, and precipitin tests have been reported to be helpful. A skin test is also available.

Treatment is unsatisfactory. Emetine hydrochloride in dosage of 30 mg per day intramuscularly for 18 days may be helpful and at times curative. The drug should not be given to patients with chronic cardiac or renal disease or to children.

To prevent infection, aquatic plants such as watercress should not be eaten, vegetables grown in fields irrigated with polluted water should be boiled, and safe drinking water should be provided.

FASCIOLOPSIASIS

Fasciolopsiasis is caused by the large intestinal fluke *Fasciolopsis buski,* which inhabits the upper part of the intestine of its definitive host. The principal definitive host is the pig. In parts of China, India, and other areas in the Far East, infection of man is contracted following ingestion, or peeling with the teeth, of water chestnuts and other edible aquatic plants. The large adults attach themselves to the intestinal mucosa, and these sites may later ulcerate. Diarrhea and abdominal pain appear early. Later, if heavy infection continues, asthenia with ascites and anasarca occurs. Diagnosis is based upon the history and the finding of eggs in the feces. The eggs resemble those of *Fasciola hepatica.* The prognosis in untreated heavy infections, especially in children, is poor. Hexylresorcinol is the preferred therapeutic agent and can be expected to cure or markedly reduce the worm burden in the majority of cases. The drug should be given in a single dose with a glass of water on an empty stomach. The pills must be swallowed intact to prevent burning of the oropharynx. No food should be taken for 4 hr, and a saline purge should be administered 24 hr after treatment. The dose for adults is 1.0 Gm. The most practicable control measure is the brief immersion of all edible aquatic plants in boiling water.

REFERENCES

Chan, P. H., and T. B. Teoh: The Pathology of *Clonorchis sinensis* Infestation of the Pancreas, J. Pathol. Bacteriol., 93:185, 1967.

Edelman, M. H., and C. L. Springarn: Clonorchiasis in the United States, J.A.M.A., 140:1147, 1949.

Hunter, G. W., W. W. Frye, and J. C. Swartzwelder: "A Manual of Tropical Medicine," 4th ed., Philadelphia, W. B. Saunders Company, 1966.

Koenigstein, R. P.: Observations on the Epidemiology of Infections with *Clonorchis sinensis,* Trans. Roy. Soc. Trop. Med. Hyg., 42:503, 1949.

McFadzean, A. J. S., and R. T. T. Yeung: Hypoglycemia in Suppurative Pancholangitis Due to *Clonorchis sinensis,* Trans. Roy. Soc. Trop. Med. Hyg., 59:179, 1965.

Neghme, A., and M. Ossandon: Ectopic and Hepatic Human Fascioliasis, Am. J. Trop. Med., 23:545, 1943.

Ross, J. A., W. E. Kershae, and A. L. Kurowski: The Radiological Diagnosis of Paragonimiasis with Report of a Case, Brit. J. Radiol., 25:579, 1952.

Sadun, E. H., and A. A. Buck: Paragonimiasis in South Korea —Immunodiagnostic, Epidemiologic, Clinical, Roentgenologic and Therapeutic Studies, Am. J. Trop. Med. Hyg., 9:562, 1960.

Tillman, A. J. B., and H. S. Phillips: Pulmonary Paragonimiasis, Am. J. Med., 5:167, 1948.

Yokogawa, M., M. Iwasaki, N. Shigeyasu, H. Hirose, T. Okura, and M. Tsuji: Chemotherapy of Paragonimiasis with Bithionol, Am. J. Trop. Med. Hyg., 12:859, 1963.

252 CESTODES, OR TAPEWORMS

James J. Plorde and
Ivan L. Bennett, Jr.

TAENIASIS SAGINATA

DEFINITION. *Taenia saginata,* the beef tapeworm, is a hermaphroditic cestode which inhabits the intestinal tract of man, its only definitive host.

ETIOLOGY AND PATHOGENESIS. In its adult stage, *T. saginata* measures 5 to 10 m in length and possesses about 1,000 proglottids. The gravid proglottid measures about 5×20 mm and possesses 15 to 30 lateral uterine branches, thus distinguishing it from *Taenia solium,* which has 8 to 12. The head, or scolex, measures 1 to 2 mm in diameter and possesses prominent suckers but no hooks. The eggs are ovid, 30×40 μ, and are indistinguishable from those of *T. solium.* When the eggs are ingested by cattle, the embryo is released in the intestine, invades the intestinal wall, and is carried by vascular channels to striated muscle in the hind limbs, diaphragm, and tongue, the common sites for formation of the cysticercus stage (*Cysticercus bovis*). *Cysticercus bovis* measures about 5×10 mm and consists of a scolex held in a cystlike structure. After ingestion of the cyst in raw or undercooked beef by man, it requires about 2 months for the adult worm to develop in the intestine.

DISTRIBUTION. Taeniasis saginata occurs in all countries in which it is the custom to eat raw or undercooked beef. It has been estimated that there are about 20 million infected individuals in the U.S.S.R., and in the world's population almost 40 million. Beef tapeworm is not very common in the United States, but it is the most prevalent infection of this type in the Northern states.

CLINICAL MANIFESTATIONS. In probably the majority of cases the disease is asymptomatic. Epigastric discomfort, diarrhea, hunger sensations, weight loss, irritability, nausea, and rarely an increase in appetite have been reported in association with *T. saginata* infections.

Movements of the worm are sometimes apparent to the host. Rarely, segments become impacted in the vermiform appendix, with development of appendicitis.

LABORATORY FINDINGS. The diagnosis is usually made by the finding of proglottids in the feces. If it is believed that proglottids have been passed, but none is available for examination, the perianal region should be examined as for pinworm infection, using the Scotch tape swab. By this method 85 to 95 percent of infections may be detected, whereas by stool examination only 50 to 75 percent can be recognized. When the scolex is obtained, it may be examined for suckers and the absence of rostellum and hooks, to identify it as *T. saginata*. The above study is necessary, since the ova observed in the feces cannot be distinguished from those of *T. solium*. A slight eosinophilia may accompany this infection.

TREATMENT. Experience with Atabrine has shown it to be a highly efficacious agent. The evening before the Atabrine is to be administered, the patient takes 30 Gm sodium or magnesium sulfate in a glass of water. The following morning, while still fasting, he takes 1.0 Gm Atabrine as 2 tablets of 0.1 Gm each at 5-min intervals. Nausea, vomiting, and abdominal pain are quite common. Then 2 hr later a second dose of sodium or magnesium sulfate is taken. When successful, such treatment will remove the entire worm, which will be found to be stained yellow. If the scolex has not been removed, the tapeworm will regenerate after 2 or 3 months. A newer and highly effective taenicide is niclosamide (Yomesan), which digests the scolex and immature segments of the worm. This drug can be given without preparation or purge in two 1-Gm doses 1 hr apart. Few side effects have been reported.

PREVENTION. The only practical means of preventing infection is the thorough cooking of beef. Temperatures as low as 71°C for as little as 5 min will destroy *C. bovis*. Refrigeration and salting for prolonged periods also destroy the cysticercus. Adequate meat inspection and proper disposal of human excreta will also aid in control.

TAENIASIS SOLIUM

DEFINITION. *Taenia solium*, the pork tapeworm, usually manifests itself as a parasite of man by inhabiting the intestinal lumen. Man is the only definitive host and under some circumstances may act also as the intermediate host harboring the larval stage, *Cysticercus cellulosae*. The usual intermediate host is the hog.

DISTRIBUTION. Taeniasis solium is worldwide but is most common in the U.S.S.R., Asia, and Africa.

ETIOLOGY AND PATHOGENESIS. The hermaphroditic adult tapeworm measures about 3 m in length and possesses a globular scolex containing a rostellum with about two dozen hooklets. There are seldom more than 1,000 proglottids. The gravid proglottid measures about 6×12 mm and contains a uterus with 8 to 12 lateral branchings. The eggs resemble those of *T. saginata*. When ova are ingested by the hog, the embryo is released from the egg, penetrates the intestinal wall, and is carried by vascular channels to all parts of the body. Localization with development to the encysted larval stage, *C. cellulosae* ("bladder worm"), occurs predominantly in striated muscle of the tongue, neck, and trunk. The cysticerci are ovoid, gray-white, opalescent structures about 1 cm in diameter. Man becomes infected following ingestion of undercooked pork containing cysticerci. The scolex is freed and attaches itself to the intestinal mucosa, and development to the adult stage begins at this time.

CLINICAL MANIFESTATIONS. Clinical manifestations resemble those associated with *T. saginata*. The clinical picture is entirely different when man serves as the intermediate host. This form of the disease can occur after ingestion of the eggs or the return of gravid segments to the stomach by reverse peristalsis. The released embryos bore into the intestinal wall and are distributed by vascular channels to various parts of the body. Cysticerci develop in the subcutaneous tissues, in muscles, in viscera, and—of most significance—in the eye and brain. Only a moderate tissue reaction occurs while the scolex is viable. The dead larva, however, behaves as a foreign body and provokes a marked tissue response. Symptoms are related to active larval encystment only in heavy infections. Muscular pains, weakness, and slight fever may be observed. The involvement in the brain may be in the form of a meningoencephalitis when the cysticerci are widely distributed. However, epilepsy, brain tumor, encephalitis, and other types of neurologic disorder may be simulated. Degenerated cysticerci ultimately calcify.

Infection with the adult worm can be detected by finding eggs in perianal scrapings or in the feces. However, to differentiate *T. solium* from *T. saginata* infection, proglottids or the scolex must be examined. Cystercercosis should be suspected in an individual who has lived in a hyperendemic area and who develops neurologic findings. Biopsy of subcutaneous nodules may lead to the identification of typical encysted larvae. Roentgenograms of the soft tissues also often reveal calcified cysticerci. Group-specific serologic tests may aid in the diagnosis. The prognosis is in large part determined by the stage and location of the parasite. Surgery may be necessary in cerebral and ocular cysticercosis.

TREATMENT. For removal of the worm in the adult stage, see Taeniasis Saginata, above. It is well to administer an antiemetic before giving Atabrine, to prevent reverse peristalsis, with return of the eggs to the stomach and release of the embryos. Because Yomesan does not destroy the eggs, treatment with this drug should be followed with a purge to prevent autoinfection.

PREVENTION. The simplest and most effective preventive measure is the thorough cooking of pork. Treatment of recognized cases will reduce the hazard of larval stage development as well as the spread of the infection.

HYMENOLEPIASIS NANA

DEFINITION. Hymenolepiasis nana is an intestinal infection of man caused by *Hymenolepis nana,* the dwarf tapeworm.

ETIOLOGY. The life cycle is unique in that both the larval and adult phases occur in the same host. Man, mice, and rats readily contract infection upon ingestion of the eggs. The adult measures about 2 cm in length and may possess more than 100 proglottids.

DISTRIBUTION. Dwarf tapeworm infection has been reported in temperate and tropical regions around the globe. It is the most common tapeworm found in the United States, most of the infections occurring in the Southern states.

CLINICAL MANIFESTATIONS. This tapeworm infection is characterized by the presence of many adult worms in the host's intestine. When infection is massive, diarrhea and abdominal pain occur.

TREATMENT. Atabrine, as prescribed for taeniasis saginata, is moderately effective. Because various stages of the helminth are present simultaneously, it is necessary to repeat the course of Atabrine at least once, after an interval of 2 weeks. Yomesan, as given for taeniasis, is often effective. It should be followed by a purge to prevent autoinfection.

PREVENTION. This is a difficult problem, similar to that encountered in enterobiasis. Only a single host is involved, and the eggs are immediately infective. Personal hygiene should be stressed. The contamination of food by rats and mice should be prevented.

DIPHYLLOBOTHRIASIS LATUM

DEFINITION. *Diphyllobothrium latum,* the fish tapeworm or broad tapeworm, produces a disease in its definitive hosts, including man, characterized by the presence of the adult worm in the intestinal lumen.

ETIOLOGY. The adult worm may be as long as 5 to 10 m and possess between 3,000 and 4,000 proglottids.

PATHOGENESIS. Ingestion of infected raw fish results in infection by the so-called *pleroceroid larva* or *Sparganum,* for which the fish is the intermediate host. The larva matures in the intestine and after 3 weeks is an adult, capable of discharging eggs. The adults of *D. latum* have been known to survive for 5 to 10 years.

DISTRIBUTION. The infection is common in the Baltic and Scandinavian countries, Switzerland, Italy, Russia, Japan, Chile, and Central Africa. It also occurs in the north central United States, south central Canada, and Florida.

CLINICAL MANIFESTATIONS. Most infections are asymptomatic or produce slight transient abdominal discomfort. Rarely, there may be severe cramping abdominal pain, vomiting, weakness, and loss of weight.

Tapeworm *anemia,* with erythrocyte counts ranging from half a million to 2 million, has many features in common with Addisonian pernicious anemia, including central-nervous-system involvement. Patients with the tapeworm produce intrinsic factor but do not respond when given extrinsic factor and normal gastric juice (intrinsic factor) as long as the infection persists. The location of the worm in the intestine is important, anemia occurring only when the tapeworm is in the proximal small intestine. Large amounts of vitamin B_{12} have been demonstrated in the tapeworm, presumably absorbed from the host's intestine. *Taenia saginata,* which does not produce pernicious tapeworm anemia, contains about 2 percent as much vitamin B_{12} as *D. latum.* The appearance of anemia is certainly related to vitamin B_{12} absorption and possibly also to decreased production of intrinsic factor or inadequate extrinsic factor. It is apparent that the tapeworm and the host compete for vitamin B_{12}.

TREATMENT. Atabrine as prescribed for taeniasis saginata will cure most infections. Yomesan is probably also effective. In the presence of severe macrocytic anemia, parenteral vitamin B_{12} should be given.

PREVENTION. The only practical control measure is the thorough cooking of all freshwater fish. To reduce contamination of waterways, dogs and cats should not be fed raw freshwater fish.

SPARGANOSIS

The *Sparganum,* or plerocercoid larva, of *Diphyllobothrium mansoni* will develop in man following ingestion (usually in drinking water) of a *Cyclops* bearing the procercoid larva. Sparganosis also follows ingestion of infected frogs or application of infected fresh frog flesh as a poultice. The frog tissues contain the Sparganum, which is capable of invading human tissues. The dog and cat are definitive hosts for *D. mansoni.* The location of the larvae determines the prognosis of the infection in man. Surgery and local injection of ethyl alcohol with epinephrine-free procaine to kill the worms is the preferred method of treatment. Novarsenobenzol given intravenously is also said to be effective.

ECHINOCOCCIASIS

DEFINITION. Echinococciasis may be caused by the larval stage of *Echinococcus granulosus* or *E. multilocularis.* These species of echinococcus are distinct morphologically and biologically. In man, *E. granulosus* produces cystic, expanding lesions, involving the liver and lungs primarily, whereas the lesions of *E. multilocularis* are destructive because of their invasive character.

ETIOLOGY. *Echinococcus granulosus* infection in man, cattle, sheep, horses, and hogs, the principal intermediate hosts, is contracted by ingestion of the eggs present in the feces of the dog, the principal definitive host. Following ingestion, the embryos escape from the eggs, penetrate the intestinal mucosa, and enter venous and lymphatic channels. Some soon arrive in the liver and may form hydatid cysts there, and those entering the lymphatics are carried ultimately to the lungs. There is no exogenous budding from the wall of the cyst, only endogenous. Transmission to the definitive host occurs following ingestion of the hydatid cysts which contain scolices. An adult worm may develop from each scolex in the intestine of the dog, wolf, coyote, and other of the *Canidae*. The adult is small, measuring about 5 mm in length, and consists of no more than five or six segments. *Echinococcus multilocularis* infection is manifested by the same type of invasive larval-produced lesion as is observed in the natural intermediate host for this stage, the microtine rodents. The adult, or tapeworm, stage is found in the dog and fox.

DISTRIBUTION. Echinococciasis caused by *E. granulosus* has its highest incidence in sheep- and cattle-raising countries, particularly in North and South Africa, Australia, Central Europe, and South America. In Iceland, a high incidence of infection in man and the dog has been markedly reduced by control measures. In the Southern, Western, and Southwestern areas of the United States, the infection is established, and a small number of cases is reported each year. *Echinococcus multilocularis* has been identified in Eurasia, Alaska, and the Kuriles and adjacent islands.

PATHOGENESIS AND CLINICAL MANIFESTATIONS. Two principal types of lesion develop in the intermediate host: the unilocular type of *E. granulosus* and the alveolar type of *E. multilocularis*. The former is more common, grows slowly, and consists of an external laminated cuticula and an inner germinal layer. Fluid fills and distends the cyst. Daughter cysts and brood capsules develop from the germinal layer, representing endogenous development. "Hydatid sand" found in the cyst consists of scolices liberated from ruptured brood capsules. Exogenous development results from evagination of the cyst wall and ultimately produces the multilocular or alveolar type of lesion. Metastatic lesions occur when growth extends into vessels.

Symptoms produced depend on the size attained by the cystic lesion and the amount of tissue destroyed. Unilocular lesions may become barren following resolution of secondary bacterial infection. Rupture into the peritoneal or pleural cavities may produce an anaphylactoid reaction, which occasionally is fatal. The unilocular type of hepatic lesion progresses slowly and is most amenable to surgical treatment. The alveolar type progresses more rapidly, with metastatic lesions developing in the bones, brain, and other sites. Pathologic fractures occur, and cerebral involvement may be manifested by epilepsy.

DIAGNOSIS AND TREATMENT. Clinical manifestations seldom are characteristic enough to suggest the diagnosis, but roentgenographic appearance of the lesion, especially when calcification is present, is often helpful. Eosinophilia is suggestive, although seldom present. Inquiry should be made concerning residence in an endemic area, and skin tests (Casoni's or substitute antigen) and serologic tests performed, before exploration is considered. Of the various serologic tests, the indirect hemagglutination test seems the most sensitive. It is positive in three-quarters or more of patients with liver cysts and in one-third to one-half of patients with lung disease. The latex agglutination and bentonite flocculation tests are simpler but not as reliable. Nearly 90 percent of patients with echinococciasis will have either a positive skin test or a positive indirect hemagglutination reaction. Exploration may be required as both a diagnostic and a therapeutic measure. Because of serious reactions to the leakage of cyst fluid into the tissues and body cavities, aspiration should be attempted only during exploration. Aspirated cyst fluid should be examined carefully for scolices, hooklets, and laminated cyst wall. The size of the lesion will determine whether excision or marsupialization is the procedure of choice. Surgical treatment offers the only hope of cure. The contents of the cyst should be sterilized with 10 ml of 10 percent Formalin before an attempt to drain or excise the lesion is made.

PREVENTION. In prevention, (1) contact with infected dogs should be avoided, particularly fecal contamination of the hands and food; (2) infected carcasses and offal should be burned or buried, in order to prevent access of dogs to material containing scolices; and (3) dogs should be treated if found to be infected. The reduction of the incidence of echinococciasis in Iceland is an example of the efficacy of control measures.

REFERENCES

Bakir, F.: Serious Complications of Hydatid Cyst of the Lung, Am. Rev. Resp. Dis., 96:483, 1967.

Beaver, P. C., and W. A. Sodeman: Treatment of *Hymenolepiasis nana* Infection with Atabrine, J. Trop. Med. Hyg., 55:97, 1952.

Bonne, C.: Researches on Sparganosis in the Netherlands East Indies, Am. J. Trop. Med., 22:643, 1942.

Corkum, K. C.: Sparganosis in Some Vertebrates of Louisiana and Observations in a Human Infection, J. Parasitol., 52:444, 1966.

Dixon, H. B. F., and D. W. Smithers: Epilepsy in Cysticercosis, Quart. J. Med., 3:603, 1934.

Dungal, N.: Echinococcosis in Iceland, Am. J. Med. Sci., 212:12, 1946.

Halawani, A., et al.: Treatment of Tapeworms with Atabrine, J. Roy. Egypt. Med. Assoc., 31:956, 1948.

Hunter, G. W., W. W. Frye, and J. C. Swartzwelder: "A Manual of Tropical Medicine," 4th ed., Philadelphia, W. B. Saunders Company, 1966.

Hutchinson, W. F., and M. W. Bryan: Studies on the Hydatid Worm *Echinococcus granulosus*: I and II, Am. J. Trop. Med. Hyg., 9:606, 612, 1960.

Kagan, I. G., J. J. Osimani, J. C. Varela, and P. S. Allain: Evaluation of Intradermal and Serologic Tests for the Diagnosis of Hydatid Disease, Am. J. Trop. Med. Hyg., 15:172, 1966.

Mueller, J. F., E. P. Hart, and W. P. Walsh: Human Sparganosis in the United States, J. Parasitol., 49:294, 1963.

Newman, C. M., and B. S. Aron: Roentgen Diagnosis of Tapeworm Infestation, J. Mt. Sinai Hosp., 28:91, 1961.

Obrador, S.: Clinical Aspects of Cerebral Cysticercosis, Arch. Neurol. Psychiat., 59:457, 1948.

Powell, S. J., E. M. Proctor, A. J. Wilmott, and I. N. MacLeod: Cysticercosis and Epilepsy in Africans, Ann. Trop. Med. Parasitol., 60:152, 1966.

Rausch, R.: Studies on the Helminth Fauna of Alaska: XXX. The Occurrence of *Echinococcus multilocularis* Leuckart, 1863, on the Mainland of Alaska, Am. J. Trop. Med. Hyg., 5:1086, 1956.

Von Bonsdorff, B., W. Nyberg, and R. Grasbeck: Vitamin B_{12} Deficiency in Carriers of the Fish Tapeworm, *Diphyllobothrium latum*, Acta Haematol., 24:15, 1960.

253 HIRUDINIASIS

Ivan L. Bennett, Jr.

DEFINITION AND ETIOLOGY. Human hirudiniasis results from the attachment of *Hirudinea* or leeches to the skin or, rarely, to internal mucosal surfaces. Leeches are found in lakes, ponds, and tropical forests and vary in size from a few millimeters to several centimeters in length. They attach themselves firmly to a host and suck blood. Because their salivary secretion contains an anticoagulant, the puncture wounds at the attachment site may continue to bleed freely after the dislodgment of the parasite.

Land leeches are found on bushes in tropical areas of Asia and South America, and man is infected by contact with the foliage. Attachment of aquatic species occurs during swimming or wading in infested waters. Rarely, young leeches may be ingested in drinking water, an event that can lead to serious illness.

MANIFESTATIONS. *External* hirudiniasis is painless and is called to the victim's attention by finding the parasites or the bleeding puncture wounds left when the engorged leeches detach. With heavy infestations, significant amounts of blood may be lost.

Internal or *atrial* hirudiniasis results from the attachment of small leeches to the mucosa of the upper part of the respiratory tract, larynx, trachea, or esophagus. Infestation of the vagina, bladder, or urethra has occurred in swimmers. As the leeches engorge and grow, they produce symptoms of obstruction, often with bleeding. Pharyngeal blockage is referred to as "halzoun." Hoarseness, cough, nasal obstruction, dysphagia, nausea, and dysuria are frequent, as are hemoptysis, hematemesis, melena, and hematuria. Anemia may be severe, and death has occurred from obstruction of the epiglottis.

TREATMENT. Leeches must be removed with care to avoid leaving mouth parts in the wound. Application of a lighted cigarette or vinegar will help with complete removal. Skin wounds should be cleaned and covered; secondary infection is the only complication.

Removal of leeches from the genitourinary tract is facilitated by irrigation. In the respiratory tract, endoscopy and removal are necessary with the use of topical anesthesia.

PREVENTION. Use of chemical repellents on skin and clothing and boiling of water are the only measures needed to avoid hirudiniasis.

REFERENCES

Chin, T. H.: Further Note on Leech Infestation of Man, J. Parasitol., 35:215, 1949.

Masterson, E. W. G.: Hirudinea as a Human Parasite in Palestine, Parasitology, 1:182, 1908.

Walton, B. C., R. Traub, and H. D. Newson: Efficacy of Clothing Impregnants M-2065 and M-2066 against Terrestrial Leeches in North Borneo, Am. J. Trop. Med., 5:190, 1956.

Section 23

Diseases of Uncertain Etiology

254 SARCOIDOSIS

Carol J. Johns

DEFINITION. A definition adopted by the 1960 International Conference of Sarcoidosis states:

Sarcoidosis is a systemic, granulomatous disease of undetermined etiology and pathogenesis. Mediastinal and peripheral lymph nodes, lungs, liver, spleen, skin, eyes, phalangeal bones, and parotid glands are most often involved but other organs or tissues may be affected. The Kveim reaction is frequently positive, and tuberculin type hypersensitivities are frequently depressed. Other important laboratory findings are hypercalcuria and increased serum globulin. The characteristic histologic appearance of epithelioid tubercles with little or no necrosis is not pathognomonic and tuberculosis, fungal infection, beryllium disease and local sarcoid tissue reactions must be excluded. The diagnosis should be regarded as established for clinical purposes in patients who have consistent clinical features together with biopsy evidence of epithelioid tubercles or a positive Kveim test.

There is no basis for altering this definition. Manifestations vary from incidental radiologic findings without associated symptoms to severe incapacity and death. The course may be one of complete spontaneous remission with no evidence of residual disease, of persistent abnormalities with little or no disability, or of progressive deterioration and death.

ETIOLOGY. The cause of sarcoidosis remains unknown. Originally, it was thought to be a special form of tuberculosis in which the atypical features were explained by some unusual reactivity of the host or some alteration in the tubercle bacillus. This hypothesis continues to have adherents, chiefly because of the occurrence of tuberculosis before, during, or following clinical sarcoidosis and the occasional identification of mycobacteria from "sarcoid" tissue. Also, mycobacteriophages in the absence of phage-neutralizing antibodies in some sarcoid patients have been observed. Lysogenic mutants then might be produced, but may be unrecognizable as the etiologic agent.

A second hypothesis is that one or several as yet unidentified specific inciting agents are responsible for the tissue reaction and clinical picture. These have included viruses, atypical mycobacteria, fungi, and pine pollen, but no definite relationship has been established. Support for the single agent hypothesis is found in the findings of comparable clinical disease and positive Kveim reactions when a single splenic suspension was used.

A third hypothesis favors a particular state of host reactivity to one or more agents. Altered host reactivity could be a result of genetic susceptibility as well as unidentified factors of hypersensitivity. This idea is in accord with the familial aggregations of sarcoidosis, observed immunologic abnormalities, and the occurrence in sarcoidosis of manifestations common to hypersensitivity diseases such as erythema nodosum, uveitis, arthritis, arteritis, and thyroiditis. Siltzbach has suggested that mycobacteria or other agents might act as an immunologic sensitizer in a manner analogous to Freund's adjuvant, with the later development of a granulomatous reaction.

EPIDEMIOLOGY. Sarcoidosis has been observed in virtually every country in which it has been sought. Prevalence rates are largely determined by rates of disease recognition; therefore, figures collected in different parts of the world cannot be compared. Negroes are ten times more commonly affected than Caucasians in the United States, and the incidence in females is usually double that in males. An increased incidence in relation to pregnancy and lactation has been noted, especially in patients with erythema nodosum. The disease is most frequent in the third and fourth decades of life, but the range begins in childhood, particularly around ado-

lescence, and extends to the sixth and seventh decade. Sarcoidosis has been observed in siblings and in parent and child but not in husband and wife. There is no evidence for patient-to-patient transmission.

PATHOLOGY. The granulomatous inflammatory changes of sarcoidosis may occur in almost any organ. The hard tubercles are generally sharply demarcated from surrounding tissues but may coalesce. Some central fibrinoid necrosis may occur, but caseation is usually absent, and inflammatory reaction is minimal. Giant cells containing laminated calcific Schaumann bodies or stellate "asteroid" bodies are frequent, but neither of these inclusions is found solely in sarcoidosis.

Similar histologic changes can be seen in tuberculosis, fungus infections, leprosy, tertiary syphilis, beryllium disease, "farmer's lung," foreign body reactions, lymphomas, and lymph nodes draining malignant tumors. The histologic picture in sarcoid is not specific for that disease alone, and the above-mentioned possibilities cannot be excluded in the absence of other data.

Adrenal steroids apparently cause a prompt reduction in the nonspecific cellular inflammatory reaction of an acute or subacute process and hasten involution and resorption of the "sarcoid" tubercles. It is not known whether these hormones prevent or lessen scarring.

Autopsy material on patients with long-standing sarcoidosis may reveal widespread tubercles in many organs, a few scattered tubercles or focal hyaline scarring, or rarely, no residual changes. Histologic changes have been described in cases where there has been no previous clinical suspicion of sarcoidosis.

MANIFESTATIONS. Clinical manifestations of sarcoidosis generally depend on the activity, degree, and site of tissue involvment. Impairment of function is caused both by active granulomatous disease and by secondary fibrosis.

Constitutional Symptoms. In some instances the presenting features are those of nonspecific constitutional manifestations, with fever, weight loss, fatigue, weakness, and malaise. *Fever* is generally slight and of incidental importance. However, the initial picture may be that of "fever of unknown origin" without localizing signs or symptoms, and daily temperature elevation to over 101°F may persist for months. This type of disease is often accompanied by active granulomatous changes and an inflammatory reaction in the liver. Fever in association with *erythema nodosum* is another form in which sarcoidosis may become evident. This syndrome includes transient tender erythematous subcutaneous nodules over the pretibial areas, arthralgias, and pulmonary hilar adenopathy on x-ray. Hepatic tubercles and a positive Kveim reaction are frequent. This syndrome has been regarded as an early manifestation of sarcoidosis and noted frequently in young women in Scandinavia and Great Britain. It is also observed in the United States, may be overlooked easily, and has a favorable prognosis.

Another common mode of presentation is that of asymptomatic *lymphadenopathy*, particularly involving the mediastinal and hilar nodes. Vague substernal chest discomfort may be the only complaint. Readily palpable peripheral nodes which are discrete, firm, and nontender often attract attention. There may be generalized lymphadenopathy or involvement may be localized to the cervical, axillary, and femoral nodes. Usually, the changes are symmetric, and the epitrochlear nodes are palpable.

Lungs. Pulmonary involvement is the most common and, perhaps, the most important manifestation of sarcoidosis. Serious parenchymal changes with or without hilar adenopathy are evident on x-ray in about 50 percent of all patients. Varying and impressive degrees of dyspnea and cough are noted. A discrepancy in which the radiologic changes exceed the symptoms and signs is a diagnostic clue in early sarcoidosis. In some patients, usually Caucasian, striking radiologic changes may be associated with no symptoms and ventilatory and diffusion measurements are normal. In others, often Negroes, pathologic and physiologic abnormalities may be present when the x-ray shows only hilar adenopathy without parenchymal lesions. There may be progression from mild exertional dyspnea to severe incapacity and cyanosis at rest. This results from extensive interstitial changes which impair oxygenation by destruction of effective diffusing surface. Compensatory hyperventilation is often noted. Symptoms are less severe or lacking altogether if the process chiefly involves the lymphatics in the interlobular septums. Large rounded intrapulmonary masses which may resemble metastatic tumor are probably a result of primary involvement of lymphoid tissue or localized infiltrates producing minimal physiologic disturbance and minimal symptoms despite their dramatic x-ray appearance. Pleural effusions are unusual and should lead to the suspicion that other disease is present.

Cough may be severe and incapacitating and may occur in paroxysms which can even lead to vomiting. Sputum is scanty; occasional blood streaking results from the strain of coughing or endobronchial granulomas. Wheezing is occasionally produced by localized bronchial lesions with stenosis. Physical findings are variable and nonspecific. Respiratory excursion may be restricted, crackling rales may be heard diffusely or at the lung bases, and P_2 may be accentuated or split if pulmonary hypertension exists.

Bronchoscopy generally reveals normal mucosa, although in a few cases it shows granulomatous inflammatory changes. Granulomas may be demonstrated occasionally in grossly normal appearing mucosa.

The course of pulmonary sarcoid may be one of complete and spontaneous resolution of symptoms and radiologic changes, or there may be residual impairment of pulmonary function.

In some patients sarcoidosis is a chronic progressive disease, and pulmonary insufficiency and cor pulmonale occur as late features. Bronchiolostenosis resulting from peribronchial fibrosis and mucosal changes may result in localized emphysema, giving rise to cystic changes, usually in the upper lung fields. With superimposed bacterial infection a bronchiectasis-like picture results. Large cavitary or bullous lesions are rare but can lead to large and repeated hemoptyses, which are occasionally fatal. Such lesions may also form the locus for an aspergilloma with which hemoptyses or disseminated aspergillus infection are hazards. Steroids and frequent use of antibiotics probably predispose to aspergillosis. Surgical management is rarely feasible because of the diffuse and restrictive nature of the disease. Spontaneous pneumothorax is an occasional complication of lung involvement.

Eyes. Acute granulomatous uveitis may be the initial manifestation of sarcoidosis. Ocular disease may progress to severe visual impairment and blindness with corneal and lenticular opacities and secondary glaucoma. A careful slit-lamp examination is worthwhile in all patients with sarcoid to detect early evidence of anterior uveitis. Lacrimal gland enlargement, conjunctival infiltrations, and keratoconjunctivitis sicca of the type seen in Sjogren's syndrome (Chap. 386) are common. Exophthalmos has been observed, as have retinal lesions with vasculitis producing papillitis and periphlebitis.

Skin. Lesions occur in about 30 percent of patients and vary from extensive erythematous, infiltrated, and raised lesions to small nondescript plaques and papules. Increased or decreased pigmentation is frequently noted. Sarcoid changes often occur at sites of old scars or recent injury. Subcutaneous nodular infiltrations occur, and in rare instances calcification of such lesions has been observed. Alopecia occurs if the scalp is affected. Erythema nodosum lesions in early sarcoidosis usually present a histologic picture of a nonspecific vasculitis.

Liver. Clinical manifestations of hepatic sarcoidosis are present in only about 20 percent of cases. Nevertheless, hepatic tubercles can be found by biopsy in about 75 percent and provide one of the most useful means of obtaining histologic confirmation of the diagnosis. Asymptomatic hepatomegaly is frequent. Severe jaundice is unusual, but mild increase in bilirubin and striking elevation of serum alkaline phosphatase level are seen frequently. Intense pruritus may be the presenting manifestation. The spectrum of hepatic sarcoid includes the incidental tubercle, tubercles with surrounding nonspecific inflammatory reaction, chronic active granulomatous hepatitis, postnecrotic cirrhosis with or without portal hypertension, and portal hypertension without significant cirrhosis. Esophageal varices have been demonstrated in patients with portal hypertension, and shunt procedures occasionally have been required. Response to steroids has been disappointing in severe hepatic sarcoid. In some patients the granulomatous disease is limited to the liver, spleen, and abdominal nodes without other clinical or radiographic evidence of sarcoidosis.

Spleen. Mild splenomegaly occurs in 20 to 30 percent of cases, but enlargement may be striking. Sarcoidosis can lead to "hypersplenism," with anemia, leukopenia, and thrombocytopenia. This condition may persist for 10 to 20 years without undue complications, although splenectomy will result in hematologic improvement. Response to steroids has been observed also.

Kidneys. Impaired renal function may occur secondary to hypercalcemia and hypercalcuria, hyperuricemia, and less commonly, because of direct granulomatous involvement. Nephrocalcinosis and renal calculi are common.

Heart. Effects are usually secondary to lung disease, with pulmonary hypertension and cor pulmonale. Primary myocardial sarcoidosis is most commonly manifested by conduction disturbances and paroxysmal arrhythmias.

Salivary Glands. Asymptomatic enlargement of the parotid, sublingual, and submaxillary glands occurs in about 6 percent of cases. Spontaneous regression commonly occurs. A syndrome of fever, uveitis, and lacrimal and salivary gland enlargement is known as uveoparotid fever, or Heerfordt's syndrome. Facial nerve palsies may be associated with parotid disease.

Muscle. Sarcoid granulomas occur in muscles far more frequently than is clinically indicated by pain and weakness. In a few cases symptoms may be severe and incapacitating. Muscle biopsy is likely to be positive in such patients and also in those with polyarthralgias.

Joints. Arthralgias may occur independently as an early prominent feature but are more common in association with erythema nodosum. Chronic migratory arthritis may respond to colchicine. Sarcoid tubercles have been observed in biopsies of synovium. Transient knee effusions are occasionally noted. Chronic periarticular swelling and tenderness may be associated with bony changes in the fingers and toes and skin lesions.

Bones. Asymptomatic, punched-out lesions in the distal phalanges of the hands and feet are visible in roentgenograms in about 10 percent of cases. Associated overlying skin changes are common. Radiolucent skull lesions have been noted in a few patients. "Routine" hand x-rays are not likely to be abnormal in the absence of overlying skin changes.

Nervous System. Neurologic manifestations are variable. Cranial and peripheral nerves may be affected by direct involvement of the nerve sheaths or roots. Facial nerve palsies, which may be bilateral and sequential, are the commonest neurologic finding and may undergo full remission. A granulomatous basilar meningitis can affect the cranial nerves and produce pleocytosis and elevation of the spinal fluid protein. Pituitary involvement produces diabetes insipidus. Involvement of the choroid plexuses may obstruct the ventricles. Cortical changes can result in convulsive seizures.

Other Tissues. Rarely involvement of the tonsils and laryngeal, buccal, and nasal mucosa (often with associated sinusitis) has been encountered. Mucosal lesions are usually associated with cutaneous sarcoid. Sarcoid lesions have been found in thyroid, parathyroid, and pancreatic tissues, and gastric granulomas have resulted in bleeding and perforation. Sarcoid involving the adrenal, cervix, uterus, epididymis, or testis is very unusual.

LABORATORY FINDINGS. Mild anemia, leukopenia, eosinophilia, and elevated sedimentation rate are common in active disease. Thrombocytopenia is unusual but may be severe.

Delayed Skin Reactions. Tuberculin anergy is noted in about two-thirds of patients. Associated generalized cutaneous anergy to other commonly occurring antigens such as *Candida albicans, Trichophyton,* and mumps virus has been noted. This depression of delayed skin reactivity is considered to be an important feature of sarcoidosis, but it varies with the duration and activity of the disease.

Chemical Studies. Hypergammaglobulinemia and reduction of serum albumin are common. Hypercalcuria results from increased intestinal absorption of calcium, which is apparently related to increased sensitivity to vitamin D. Serum uric acid level may be elevated even in the absence of renal insufficiency. Elevation of serum alkaline phosphatase level is attributable to intrahepatic tubercles rather than to bone lesions and may reach levels of 60 to 80 Bodansky units, or more than 100 King-Armstrong units.

Roentgenographic Studies. Approximately 90 percent of patients will eventually show intrathoracic disease on chest x-ray. Bilateral hilar adenopathy, often with associated right paratracheal adenopathy, is a common feature. Unilateral hilar adenopathy is unusual and should initiate a search for other diseases. Patients may be grouped according to apparent severity and chronicity of the radiologic picture as follows: group I—hilar adenopathy with no parenchymal changes; group II—hilar adenopathy and diffuse parenchymal changes; group III —diffuse parenchymal changes without hilar adenopathy; group IV—chronic parenchymal changes of more than 2 years' duration with pulmonary fibrosis. The pulmonary changes are generally symmetrical, and may present a diffuse ground-glass appearance, fine reticular or miliary lesions, large nodular lesions, or multiple large confluent infiltrates resembling metastatic tumors. Fine diffuse interstitial fibrosis may be present. Pulmonary fibrosis may produce contraction and distortion, and extensive cystic and bullous lesions are common in the late stages. Bony changes in the phalanges and skull may occur.

Pulmonary Function Tests. These tests commonly demonstrate restriction, decreased compliance, and loss of effective diffusing surface. Vital capacity is reduced. Measurements of oxygen- and carbon monoxide–diffusing capacity are frequently reduced even in the absence of demonstrable radiologic changes or clinical symptoms. Measurements of vital capacity and diffusing capacity may serve as indicators of progression of disease. In diffuse disease, arterial blood studies reveal with exercise a reduced P_{O_2} because of perfusion of poorly ventilated areas of the lung. The arterial P_{CO_2} is commonly below normal because of contemporary hyperventilation. Because ventilatory obstruction occurs only occasionally, and then in severe, late stages of pulmonary fibrosis, carbon dioxide retention with elevation of arterial P_{CO_2} is a late and unusual feature. Significant impairment of pulmonary function frequently remains even after radiologic clearing. Following steroid therapy or a spontaneous remission, the vital capacity tends to return toward normal, but may remain somewhat reduced. The diffusing capacity may improve significantly but usually stabilizes well below normal despite complete remission of all symptoms. Improvement in diffusing capacity is less frequent than is that of the vital capacity. Deterioration of pulmonary function may occur gradually without significant radiologic detriment.

DIAGNOSIS. The diagnosis of sarcoidosis depends on

consistent clinical features together with histologic evidence of epithelioid tubercles from tissue biopsy or from a positive Kveim reaction. To exclude local sarcoid tissue reaction, as in nodes draining a malignant tumor, evidence of involvement of more than one site is desirable. Careful search for tubercle bacilli, fungi, and foreign bodies must be made in all histologic sections. A positive Kveim reaction is perhaps the most specific feature and helps to exclude other granulomatous processes. Tissue biopsy for histologic diagnosis is most readily and easily obtained from superficial or palpable lesions in skin, lymph nodes, conjunctiva, and nasal, buccal, and bronchial mucosa. Almost any palpable lymph node is likely to be positive. Epitrochlear and supraclavicular nodes will verify the diagnosis in a high percentage of cases. Liver biopsies reveal granulomas in 70 to 80 percent of cases even without clinical evidence of impaired hepatic function. Biopsy of the gastrocnemius muscle frequently reveals granulomatous changes in patients with arthralgias and erythema nodosum. In the absence of palpable peripheral lymph nodes or dermal lesions, biopsy of liver, deeper lymph nodes (as with mediastinoscopy), or muscle is in order. Lung biopsy is generally reserved for patients in whom other diagnostic maneuvers have not been successful or in whom the exclusion of other diseases is urgent.

Kveim Reaction. In 50 to 80 percent of patients with sarcoidosis, the intracutaneous injection of a heat-sterilized suspension of human sarcoid tissues (spleen or lymph nodes) produces a papulonodular lesion with epithelioid tubercles. The nodule must be biopsied in 4 to 6 weeks to confirm the histologic picture of sarcoid. Each batch of test material should be assayed in patients of known reactivity. When this type of standardized material is used, a positive reaction provides strong support for the diagnosis of sarcoidosis. Tests in patients with a variety of granulomatous and collagen vascular diseases have revealed only 2 to 5 percent false positives, but many false negatives are encountered in patients later shown to have sarcoidosis. The reaction is less likely to be positive in long-standing inactive disease, in the absence of lymph node involvement, and during steroid therapy. The Kveim test is particularly likely to be positive in the presence of significant lymphadenopathy of recent onset, in association with erythema nodosum, and when sarcoid skin lesions are present. The nature of the Kveim reaction is not understood.

PROGNOSIS. Sarcoidosis is frequently asymptomatic and often undergoes complete spontaneous remission with subsequent normal life expectancy. There may be impressive clearing of radiologic lesions, especially when the disease seems limited to the thorax. Following a spontaneous remission, recurrence is most unusual. Such remissions are most frequent in the syndrome of erythema nodosum and hilar adenopathy. This "benign" form is more common in Caucasians than in Negroes, where chronic progressive disease is more frequently encountered. Systemic manifestations which include skin, bone, eyes, salivary glands, and hepatosplenomegaly herald a less favorable prognosis. Sarcoidosis is directly responsible for death in only 10 percent of recognized cases. Death is usually related to pulmonary insufficiency and cor pulmonale.

The influence of steroids on the prognosis is not clear. Some patients remain in remission after steroids, but the disease commonly recurs as the dose is reduced, even when therapy has been continued for 2 or more years. It is thought that steroids prevent the progression of disease, but healing may occur with hyaline scarring. Steroids clearly cannot reverse a fibrotic process. Early steroid therapy offers more hope than that initiated after 1 to 2 years of disease.

TREATMENT. Relatively asymptomatic patients require no treatment. *Adrenal steroids* are the recommended agents to suppress the active inflammatory reaction and provide symptomatic improvement. Indications for treatment are (1) active ocular disease; (2) progressive pulmonary involvement; (3) persistent hypercalcemia or hypercalcuria; (4) central-nervous-system involvement with significant functional impairment; (5) persistent systemic evidence of illness such as fever and weight loss; and (6) involvement of a vital organ.

Steroids are most frequently required for symptomatic lung disease. Even relatively asymptomatic lung disease should be treated if there is no evidence of spontaneous regression in 6 months, or if there is progression in 3 months. Asymptomatic hilar adenopathy without evidence of parenchymal disease does not require therapy.

Prednisone is administered in initial divided daily doses of 40 mg, with 2-week periods on daily doses of 40, 30, and 25 mg, and then, maintenance doses of 20 to 10 mg. Symptomatic improvement occurs in 1 to 2 weeks, and the disease regresses over a period of several months. Therapy probably should be continued for a minimum of 6 months, with periodic attempts thereafter to reduce dosage or eliminate the drug. Objective criteria such as x-rays and measurements of pulmonary function are important. Some patients will remain in remission after 6 to 18 months of treatment. Maintenance therapy for many years has proved necessary in many patients in whom relapses recur at a dose below 15 mg. Tapering of the dose must be done slowly, with decrements of 2.5 mg no oftener than at 2- to 4-week intervals if long-term treatment has been used. Lifelong therapy may be required. Careful documentation and observation during tapering is essential in planning treatment. The efficacy of alternate day dosage is not well established, but this regimen can be used for maintenance therapy. It is probably not advisable for initial management. Endocrine side effects with weight gain of 20 to 50 lb have been observed in some women, and diabetes has appeared in some patients. Increased susceptibility to bacterial and fungus infection has been of some concern but is not a major problem. Local steroid therapy has been effective in ocular sarcoid with anterior uveitis or iritis, although there is the risk of glaucoma. Intradermal steroids have been used with some success for disfiguring cutaneous lesions.

Oxyphenbutasone also has been observed to produce radiologic remission comparable to that of steroids in a small series of relatively asymptomatic patients. There is less experience with this drug than with steroids.

Chloroquine (Aralen) in doses of 250 to 500 mg daily has been observed to induce improvement in skin lesions over periods of several weeks, but relapse is the rule when the drug is withdrawn. Remission may be maintained with as little as 125 mg daily. Hypercalcemia has also appeared to respond to chloroquine. Other beneficial effects of chloroquine in sarcoidosis have been less certain and slower, although temporary radiologic remissions of lung disease have been noted after 4 months of chloroquine sulfate in 400- to 600- mg daily doses.

Colchicine has been thought to provide symptomatic improvement in chronic arthritis associated with sarcoidosis.

Oxygen therapy is indicated and efficacious in severe lung disease if there is arterial desaturation. It can be safely administered because carbon dioxide retention is unlikely.

Antituberculous therapy is ineffective in sarcoidosis. However, prophylactic isoniazid is sometimes recommended for Negro patients with extensive pulmonary disease, in areas with high risks of exposure to tuberculosis, and for patients who are tuberculin positive.

COMPLICATIONS. The complications are related to the effects of severe and progressive disease in various organs, the side effects of therapy, and superimposed infection. An increased incidence of tuberculosis in association with sarcoidosis has been recognized. Superimposed fungus infections seem to be increasing. Aspergillosis with "fungus balls" developing in cysts has occurred. Candidiasis and cryptococcosis in association with sarcoidosis have also been noted. It is highly probable that long-term steroid and antimicrobial therapy predispose to these fungus infections.

REFERENCES

"Bibliography on Sarcoidosis, 1878–1963," National Library of Medicine, U.S. Dept. Health, Education, and Welfare, 1964.

Cummings, M. M., and J. F. Hammarsten: Sarcoidosis, Ann. Rev. Med., 13:19–40, 1962.

Longcope, W. T., and D. G. Freiman: A Study of Sarcoidosis: Based on a Combined Investigation of 160 Cases Including 30 Autopsies from The Johns Hopkins Hospital and Massachusetts General Hospital, Medicine, 31:1–132, 1952.

Mayock, R. L., P. Bertrand, C. E. Morrison, and J. H. Scott: Manifestations of Sarcoidosis: Analysis of 145 Patients, with a Review of 9 Series Selected from the Literature, Am. J. Med., 35:67–89, 1963.

Proceedings of the International Conference on Sarcoidosis, June 1–3, 1960, Am. Rev. Resp. Dis., 84(part 2):1–183, 1961.

Proceedings of the Third International Conference on Sarcoidosis, Sept. 11–14, 1963, Acta Med. Scand., 176(suppl. 425):1–310, 1964.

Reisner, D.: Observations on the Course and Prognosis of Sarcoidosis, with Special Consideration of its Intra-

thoracic Manifestations, Am. Rev. Resp. Dis. 96:361–80, 1967.

La Sarcoidose, Rapports de la IVᵉ Conférence Internationale Paris, 12–15 Septembre, 1966, J. Turiaf, and J. Chabot (Eds.), Paris, Masson et Cie, 1967.

Smellie, H., and C. Hoyle: The Natural History of Pulmonary Sarcoidosis, Quart. J. Med., 29:539–558, 1960.

255 INFECTIOUS MONONUCLEOSIS
M. M. Wintrobe

DEFINITION. This disorder of unknown cause is usually benign and probably of infectious origin. It is characterized by irregular fever, sore throat, lymphadenopathy, and enlargement of the spleen, as well as by an absolute lymphocytosis made up of cells of a peculiar type. High concentrations of antibodies against sheep erythrocytes are demonstrable in the blood serum.

HISTORY. Since the designation "infectious mononucleosis" was first proposed by Sprunt and Evans in 1920, an ever-increasing number of cases has been observed and reported, especially since 1935. This is at least in part because of better recognition of the disease. Prior to 1920 a few sporadic cases had been observed. The relationship of epidemics in children and in adults described under the title of "glandular fever" to infectious mononucleosis is in doubt because in most instances appropriate serologic techniques were not used, and when they were, the results were indefinite and irregular.

ETIOLOGY AND PATHOGENESIS. This is a disease of young people, including children, which has now been observed practically throughout the world. In the United States, infectious mononucleosis has been less frequent in Negroes than in white persons. It is relatively common in interns, medical students, and nurses, but many cases among other persons undoubtedly pass unnoticed. The mild or nonspecific character of many of the symptoms may be responsible, or the fact that appropriate blood examinations have not been made. With increasing frequency, sporadic cases have been observed wherever young people live together, as in boarding schools, colleges, and military groups. Infectious mononucleosis is quite uncommon over the age of forty but has been encountered occasionally.

The cause is unknown, although it is generally believed that the disease is infectious in nature.

Patients with infectious mononucleosis have been shown to develop high antibody titers to a herpes-type virus. This agent, which has been called the EB virus, originally was found in cell lines derived from burkitt lymphomas. These observations strongly support the possibility that EB or a closely related virus is the etiologic agent of infectious mononucleosis.

PATHOLOGY. The outstanding features are the diffuse distribution of the tissue lesions and the involvement of the lymphoid tissue. In the latter the gross findings are observed. Histologically, widespread focal lesions are found, consisting of perivascular aggregates of normal and abnormal lymphocytes. Hyperplasia of nasopharyngeal lymphoid tissue is constant. Lymph node reactions range from a predominantly follicular hyperplasia to a blurred pattern due to proliferation of lymphocytic and reticuloendothelial elements in the medullary cords which may resemble the findings in malignant lymphoma.

CLINICAL PICTURE. In the absence of a demonstrable etiologic agent, some have assumed that the clinical manifestations of infectious mononucleosis are protean and have been willing to include under this diagnosis many cases of otherwise unexplained, self-limited febrile disorders with clinical and hematologic features somewhat resembling those of infectious mononucleosis, especially when occurring in young persons. This does not seem to be justified. For the present, at least, it would seem better to restrict the diagnosis to cases in which the lymphocytes constitute more than 50 percent of the leukocytes, "atypical" lymphocytes are present, and both these features have been present for a period of at least 10 days. In addition, the titer of heterophil antibodies, after guinea pig absorption, should be at least 1:56. The clinical picture of the disorder, so defined, is quite consistent.

Three clinical stages can be identified, namely, (1) a prodromal period of 3 to 6 days, characterized by nonspecific features similar to those of other infections and during which diagnosis may be difficult; (2) a mid-stage of 4 to 20 days during which the full-blown disease presents itself; and (3) the stage of convalescence.

The incubation period is uncertain and may be as long as 4 to 7 weeks. The onset is gradual, but ultimately bilateral *lymph node enlargement* develops in practically all cases. The cervical glands are always affected, the axillary and inguinal frequently but not invariably. Involvement of the posterior cervical nodes is of value in differentiation from other forms of pharyngitis. The glands are affected singly or in groups. Local heat, redness, and marked tenderness of the glands are conspicuously absent. The *spleen* is enlarged in at least 50 percent of cases.

The most common *syndrome* is the *pharyngeal* (80 percent of cases). Pharyngeal inflammation varies in intensity, but hyperplasia of pharyngeal lymphoid tissue is almost always present. The palatal arch and uvula often have a gelatinous appearance, but significant edema of the uvula is unusual. In some cases the throat presents the typical picture of follicular tonsillitis or that of Vincent's angina or of diphtheria. Stomatitis may be present.

The *fever* is of no characteristic type. It may be transient in degree, but in one-sixth to one-third of cases the temperature reaches a peak of 103 to 104°F; it is only occasionally higher. The temperature may rise in a remittent manner in the course of 4 to 8 days. A secondary rise after an initial drop to normal may accompany the onset of glandular swelling or sore throat.

A *typhoidal syndrome,* with fever, malaise, and headache predominating, is seen in 12 percent of cases. The headache may be so severe as to suggest meningitis. Gastrointestinal symptoms are rare.

In about 8 percent of cases *icterus* occurs and the picture of hepatitis is found. In the majority of cases, however, hepatitis without jaundice is present, as judged by liver function tests. The hepatic disease is usually mild.

Edema of the eyelids has been described in a third of the cases and a palatal enanthem in almost as many. The latter consists of 5 to 20 pinhead-sized red spots, usually at the junction of the soft and hard palates, which appear in crops, darken in about 48 hr, and disappear after 3 or 4 days. Cutaneous lesions are unusual except for faint erythema or, rarely, a maculopapular eruption. Petechial hemorrhages and purpura are encountered sometimes, and other hemorrhagic manifestations, such as epistaxis, may occur.

Other manifestations are rare. These include abdominal pain of a type to suggest acute appendicitis, possibly due to swelling of mesenteric nodes; cardiac and pulmonary manifestations, such as tachycardia, cyanosis, signs of pericarditis, transient T wave changes, and enlargement of mediastinal lymph nodes or pulmonary parenchymal changes; and a variety of neurologic manifestations. The last include headache, blurring of vision, even convulsions, stupor, coma, bradycardia, stiff neck, the Guillain-Barré syndrome, and encephalitis.

Convalescence is sometimes slow and may be associated with marked prostration. Recrudescences are very common. Relapse has occurred in about 6 percent of cases. Recovery is the rule, but death has been observed in a few instances from such complications as rupture of the spleen, respiratory paralysis in association with nervous system involvement, pneumonia, edema of the glottis, and hemorrhage from a deep tonsillar ulceration.

BLOOD PICTURE. The leukocyte count is usually increased but, in the first week especially, there may be leukopenia due to granulocytopenia. The leukocytosis is usually moderate (10,000 to 15,000 cells per cu mm), but it may sometimes be very marked. It is due to an increase in number of lymphocytes, and these, in the main, are of a peculiar type: their nucleus may be oval, kidney-shaped, or slightly lobulated, and the cytoplasm often is somewhat basophilic and may be vacuolated or foamy in appearance. The nuclear chromatin is usually coarse and irregular, and nucleoli are rarely seen. These cells make up 60 percent or more of all the leukocytes.

The characteristic changes in the leukocytes may appear as early as the second day of illness or as late as the twelfth day. They attain a peak by the seventh to tenth day and persist usually for 1 to 2 months.

Anemia is extremely rare, but several instances of hemolytic anemia complicating infectious mononucleosis have been reported. Thrombocytopenia is rare, but in a few cases the clinical picture resembled that of idiopathic thrombocytopenic purpura. The bone marrow reveals a slight myeloid hyperplasia and immaturity; there may be an increase in number of lymphocytes.

The serum characteristically contains agglutinins against sheep red cells in high titer (heterophil antibodies, Paul-Bunnell test). This has been observed, in different series and according to the diagnostic criteria of the authors, in 60 to 100 percent of cases. The Paul-Bunnell test is actually nonspecific. Anti-sheep agglutinins are present in titers up to 1:28 in most normal persons and occasionally even in a titer of 1:56. In various infections a titer of 1:112 and occasionally of 1:224 may be seen. Persons receiving injections of horse serum and horse immune serum may develop titers as high as any seen in infectious mononucleosis. For these reasons it is generally considered that in the presence of clinical and hematologic findings suggestive of infectious mononucleosis, only a titer of 1:224 or higher can be interpreted as confirming the diagnosis. When there is doubt, a differential test is required. This is based on the observation that heterophil antibodies in normal serum, in horse serum sensitization, and in a variety of infections can be absorbed completely by guinea pig kidney. On the other hand, anti-sheep agglutinins in infectious mononucleosis are never completely removed by treating the serum with guinea pig kidney although they are, as a rule, completely removed by beef red cells. The differential test is carried out by absorbing a portion of the patient's serum with guinea pig kidney and another portion with beef red cells. After this the absorbed specimens are tested for sheep red cell agglutination.

Horse agglutinins have been found to be as specific but more sensitive than sheep agglutinins, and horse erythrocytes are now used in preference to sheep erythrocytes in the differential test. Formalinized horse red cells serve as the immunologic indicator in the very simple and highly specific "mono" test.

In infectious mononucleosis, highest heterophil antibody titers are found usually during the second and third weeks of illness and, as a rule, positive reactions last 4 to 8 weeks. The titer bears no relation to the severity of the disease or the degree of lymphocytosis.

A 100 percent increase in IgM globulins and a 50 percent increase in IgG accompanies the increase in heterophil antibodies and a linear relation between IgM levels and heterophil antibody titers has been observed. It is postulated that the agent causing infectious mononucleosis shares antigenic determinants with the heterophil antigen on sheep cells. Additional serum protein alterations which may occur in this disease include the appearance of the cold agglutinating antibody anti-i, and transiently positive serologic tests for syphilis and for rheumatoid factors.

Renal function is rarely impaired, but albumin and red cells may be found in the *urine*. The *cerebrospinal fluid* pressure may be moderately elevated, and pleocytosis due to lymphocytes may be found.

DIAGNOSIS. Glandular enlargement, sore throat, fever, the characteristic cells in the blood, and an increased titer of heterophil antibodies are a combination of findings which makes recognition of infectious mononucleosis easy in most instances. Some investigators have been willing to define infectious mononucleosis quite broadly. However, it seems reasonable to require a minimum of 20 percent lymphocytes of the characteristic type at the time of the fever peak and a positive heterophil antibody reaction. In the absence of a positive heterophil antibody test, it is difficult to maintain the diagnosis. The paradox of a positive heterophil antibody test unaccompanied by characteristic clinical and hematologic features of infectious mononucleosis can be explained by persistence of antibodies from an earlier unrecognized attack and, in rare instances, by a resurgence of heterophil antibodies with another illness.

The above criteria should help to differentiate infectious mononucleosis from other infectious disorders. It may be added that certain symptoms are so unusual in infectious mononucleosis that their presence militates against the diagnosis; namely, nasal discharge or congestion, paroxysmal harassing cough, sputum, chest pain, joint pains, painful or extremely tender lymph nodes, watery diarrhea, and hematuria or dysuria.

Lymphocytosis, relative or absolute, may be encountered regularly or occasionally in a number of the diseases with which infectious mononucleosis may be confused on clinical grounds. Marked leukocytosis (40,000 cells per cu mm or even higher), chiefly due to the presence of small lymphocytes of normal appearance, characterizes a benign disorder, *acute infectious lymphocytosis*, which has been observed chiefly in children and is accompanied by only mild constitutional manifestations and no lymphadenopathy, splenomegaly, or positive heterophil agglutination reactions.

The clinical picture may be like that of serum sickness, a condition in which lymphocytes quite similar to those seen in infectious mononucleosis may be found and a positive heterophil antibody test may be obtained. The differential test is required to distinguish between the antibody reactions in infectious mononucleosis and the rise in titer produced by horse serum.

It is not rare for infectious mononucleosis to be confused with acute leukemia. Differentiation depends on the demonstration of very immature leukocytes ("blasts") in the blood or the bone marrow and the presence of anemia and thrombocytopenia, both of which are rare in infectious mononucleosis. The heterophil antibody test will be negative.

Following open-heart surgery a syndrome characterized by daily remittent fever, splenomegaly, less often adenopathy and a rubelliform rash, together with "infectious mononucleosis" cells in the blood has been observed in 3 to 11 percent of cases. The heterophil antibody test is negative. This picture also has been described following blood transfusion and in a few otherwise normal adults. The disorder is attributed to cytomegalic virus infection (Chap. 232).

TREATMENT. There is no specific therapy. Sodium perborate mouth washes are recommended since Vincent's infection is frequently associated with infectious mononucleosis. Many agents have been advocated, such as arsenicals, penicillin, the tetracyclines, and chloroquine, but such claims are difficult to evaluate. As a rule, without treatment, the irregular fever persists for 1 to 3 weeks, and subjective symptoms disappear in 2 to 4 weeks. *Relapses* are not uncommon and may be late, but recurrences are very rare. The positive heterophil antibody reaction may persist for as long as 5 or 6 months. In instances of more than average severity, adrenocorticosteroid therapy will give symptomatic relief and shorten the febrile period, but such treatment, if used, should be continued for only 5 to 10 days.

REFERENCES

Hoagland, R. J.: Infectious Mononucleosis, New York, Grune & Stratton, Inc., 1967.

Klemola, E., et al.: Further Studies on Cytomegalovirus Mononucleosis in Previously Healthy Individuals, Acta Med. Scand., 182:311, 1967.

Niederman, J. C., R. W. McCollum, G. Henle, and W. Henle: Infectious Mononucleosis, J.A.M.A., 203:205, 1968.

Wintrobe, M. M.: "Clinical Hematology," 6th ed., Philadelphia, Lea & Febiger, 1967.

256 FAMILIAL MEDITERRANEAN FEVER (Familial Paroxysmal Polyserositis)

Sheldon M. Wolff

DEFINITION. Familial Mediterranean fever (FMF) is an inherited disorder of unknown etiology, characterized by recurrent episodes of fever, peritonitis, and/or pleuritis. Arthritis, skin lesions, and amyloidosis are seen in some patients.

HISTORY. Although the first report of FMF was by Janeway and Mosenthal in 1908, it was not until the report of five cases by Siegal in 1945 that attention was focused on FMF as a distinct entity. Subsequently, some authors have not applied strict clinical criteria, however, and many patients with other diseases have been reported as having FMF. The detailed and extensive descriptions by Heller and Sohar have clarified many of the clinical aspects of FMF.

TERMINOLOGY. The variety of names given to FMF has led to confusion concerning its clinical features. None of the names, including *FMF*, is completely satisfactory, but FMF has received the widest acceptance. Such terms as *periodic disease, periodic peritonitis, la maladie periodique,* etc. are inaccurate because the disease often is not cyclical. *Benign paroxysmal peritonitis* is inappropriate because many of the patients have involvement of serosal surfaces other than the peritoneum, and some die of amyloidosis. *Familial paroxysmal polyserositis* is an acceptable alternative for the term *FMF*.

ETHNOLOGY AND GENETICS. FMF occurs predominantly in patients of non-Ashkenazic (Sephardic) Jewish, Armenian, and Arabic ancestry. However, the disease is not restricted to these groups, and has been seen in patients of Italian, Ashkenazic Jewish, and Irish descent as well as others.

The best studies of the genetics of FMF have been done in Israel, where relatively homogeneous population groups exist. In Israel, the disease appears to be inherited as an autosomal recessive. Nevertheless, a large number of patients give no family history of the disease. Con-

sanguinity among the parents of FMF patients is as high as 20 percent, a figure which may be an underestimate because most patients came from very inbred ethnic groups. Approximately 60 percent of patients are male.

ETIOLOGY. Although numerous pathogenetic mechanisms have been suggested, the etiology of FMF is unknown. Fever and inflammation are such prominent signs that frequent attempts have been made to implicate infectious agents and/or their products. It has been suggested that FMF is a form of brucellosis or tuberculosis. Suffice it to say that extensive studies utilizing modern microbiologic and serologic techniques have failed to implicate these or any other specific infectious agents.

It has been reported that FMF is due to an allergy to milk or to hypersensitivity to tuberculoprotein, but such a hypersensitive state has not been substantiated. There is no firm evidence favoring an autoimmune etiology.

Reimann has suggested that FMF, like many other recurring illnesses ("periodic diseases"), may be a pathologic exaggeration of normal periodic temperature rhythmicity. However, extensive studies of temperature and other circadian rhythms in FMF patients have failed to demonstrate alterations from normal.

Because many FMF patients note that certain emotional or environmental changes may have profound effects on the frequency with which episodes of their disease occur, a psychosomatic basis has been suggested for the illness. There is no question that most patients eventually have transient or even permanent psychologic alterations, which probably reflect their reaction to a chronic recurring illness that is forever threatening their social, economic, and personal well-being, but there is no evidence for a functional etiology for FMF.

The demonstration that FMF is inherited as an autosomal recessive disorder has led to the thesis that it is another inborn error of metabolism. In view of initial optimistic reports that restriction of dietary fat ameliorates the course of FMF, it was thought that the disorder might be one of altered lipid metabolism. Despite extensive studies, no such error has been found. Reported instances of excessive urinary excretion of porphyrins in FMF are probably examples of true porphyria and not FMF.

Bondy and his colleagues reported that blood levels of unconjugated etiocholanolone were elevated during fever in 13 patients, 6 of whom had FMF. Subsequent studies, however, showed only inconstant correlation between levels of etiocholanolone and fever. The possible role of etiocholanolone and other steroids in FMF will be discussed below.

PATHOLOGY. Despite the striking clinical manifestations during an acute attack of FMF, no specific pathologic alterations have been found. Most FMF patients undergo at least one laparotomy, and only acute peritoneal inflammation in which the exudate contains a predominance of polymorphonuclear leukocytes is present. A disproportionately large number of male patients develops gallbladder disease with and without cholelithiasis, but extensive histopathologic examination has failed to reveal any specific pathologic changes. Pleural and joint inflammation are also nonspecific.

In the amyloidosis which accompanies FMF, amyloid is deposited in the intima and media of the arterioles, the subendothelial region of venules, the glomeruli, and the spleen. Aside from their vessels, the heart and liver are uninvolved.

MANIFESTATIONS. In the majority of patients, the symptoms of FMF begin between the ages of five and fifteen, although attacks sometime commence during infancy, and onset has occurred as late as age thirty-eight. The duration and frequency of attacks vary greatly in the same patient, and there is no set rhythm or periodicity to their occurrence. The usual acute episode lasts 24 to 48 hr, but some may be prolonged for 7 to 10 days. The attacks range in frequency from twice weekly to once a year, but 2 to 4 weeks is the commonest interval. Spontaneous remissions lasting up to 4 years have been seen. In the majority of cases, pregnancy is associated with an absence of acute episodes, and many patients note less frequent attacks in the summer than in the winter. There tends to be a decrease in the severity and frequency of the attacks with age or with development of amyloidosis.

Fever. Fever is a cardinal manifestation of FMF and is present during most but not all attacks. Rarely, fever may be present without serositis. The temperature rise may be preceded by a chill, and will peak in 12 to 24 hr. Defervescence is often accompanied by diaphoresis. The fever ranges from 38.5 to 40°C but is quite variable.

Abdominal Pain. Abdominal pain occurs in more than 95 percent of patients, and may vary in severity in the same patient. Minor premonitory discomfort may precede an acute episode by 24 to 48 hr. The pain usually starts in one quadrant and then spreads to involve the whole abdomen. The initial site is usually very tender. Tenderness may remain localized with referred pain in other areas, and there may be radiation to the back. There may be splinting of the chest and pain in one or both shoulders, typical of diaphragmatic irritation. Nausea and vomiting sometimes occur. The abdomen is usually distended, and may become rigid with decreased or absent bowel sounds. On x ray, the wall of the small intestine may appear edematous, transit of barium is slowed, and fluid levels may be seen. Because the manifestations of an acute abdominal attack can simulate those of a perforated viscus so closely, patients should be advised to have an elective appendectomy between attacks so that acute appendicitis will not obfuscate the picture at a later date. An abdominal operation may precipitate an acute attack of FMF which may be confused with other postoperative complications.

Chest Pain. Most patients with abdominal attacks have referred chest pain at one time or another, and 75 percent also develop acute pleuritic pain with or without abdominal symptoms. In 30 percent, the attacks of pleuritis precede the onset of abdominal attacks by varying periods of time and a small number of patients never develops abdominal attacks. Chest pain is usually unilateral and is associated with diminished breath sounds, a friction rub, or a transient pleural effusion.

Joint Pain. In Israel, 75 percent of patients report at least one episode of acute arthritis. Arthritis can be distinct from abdominal or pleural attacks, can be acute or, rarely, chronic, and may involve one or several joints. Effusions are common and the large joints are involved most frequently. Radiologic findings are nonspecific. Despite careful search, frank arthritis rarely has been seen in the United States. Some patients have a history of rheumatic fever–like illness in childhood, but in a large series of patients, including 20 from the Middle East, acute arthritis was not observed. Mild arthralgia is common during acute attacks but is nonspecific and can be seen in many febrile illnesses, including experimentally induced hyperthermia.

Skin Manifestations. Skin involvement is reported by 25 to 35 percent of patients. These lesions consist of painful, erythematous areas of swelling from 5 to 20 cm in diameter, usually located on the lower legs, the medial malleolus, or the dorsum of the foot. They may occur without abdominal or pleural pain and subside within 24 to 48 hr.

Other Signs and Symptoms. Involvement of other serosal membranes has been reported, but pericarditis is rare, and it is probable that descriptions of recurrent meningitis have been diseases other than FMF. Hematuria, splenomegaly, and small white dots called "colloid bodies" in the ocular fundus are among the findings of questionable significance. Rarely migrainelike headaches accompany acute abdominal attacks, and some patients have become somewhat irrational or show extreme emotional lability during attacks. Whether these are primary manifestations of FMF or secondary effects of pain and fever is not known.

Complications. The most serious complication of FMF in the United States is drug addiction or habituation, and obviously efforts should be made to avoid use of narcotics. Depression and lack of motivation are common, and patients with FMF require considerable encouragement and support. A striking number of patients in one American series have developed gallbladder disease.

Another major complication of FMF is *amyloidosis*. Some investigators believe that few patients in Israel escape this complication and that it is an expression of the same gene that is responsible for the other manifestations of FMF. If the attacks occur first, as they do in over 90 percent of the patients, the patients are classified as being of phenotype I. Amyloidosis also occurs in siblings of FMF patients or precedes the abdominal attacks (phenotype II). The infiltration by amyloid involves the kidneys, and death is often attributable to renal failure.

Amyloidosis has been reported in Israel and North Africa, but despite careful search, there has been only one reported instance of amyloidosis complicating FMF in the United States, and that occurred in a young man of Dutch ancestry. These findings are even more striking because there are probably as many known FMF patients in the United States (400 to 500 patients) as in Israel (470 patients). These differences are unexplained and suggest that environmental or nutritional, as well as genetic, factors may play a role in the development of amyloidosis in FMF (Chap. 114).

LABORATORY FINDINGS. There is no specific diagnostic test. Polymorphonuclear leukocytosis ranging from 15,000 to 30,000 is almost invariable during acute attacks. The erythrocyte sedimentation rate is elevated during attacks but returns to normal between attacks. Plasma fibrinogen, serum haptoglobin, ceruloplasmin, and C-reactive protein increase during the episodes. Plasma lipids are normal, and there are no consistent abnormalities of hepatic or renal function. When amyloidosis is present, laboratory findings are typical of a nephrotic syndrome followed by renal insufficiency. Electrocardiographic and electroencephalographic changes are inconstant and nonspecific.

DIAGNOSIS. When the typical acute attacks of FMF occur in an individual of appropriate ethnic background who has a family history of FMF, the diagnosis is easy. On the other hand, if the disease has not been present in the family and the patient resides in a community where FMF is rare, the diagnosis can be very difficult.

Most patients with undiagnosed FMF have had one or more abdominal operations with no relief of symptoms. When a patient is seen for the first time, a variety of other febrile illnesses must be excluded by appropriate study or observation. These include acute appendicitis, acute pancreatitis, porphyria, cholecystitis, intestinal obstruction, and other major abdominal catastrophes.

Some of the inherited forms of the hyperlipidemias (Chap. 113) may mimic the clinical picture of FMF, but measurement of serum cholesterol and triglycerides will eliminate them from consideration. The patient with FMF is not immune to the other diseases, and when an attack differs from the usual pattern or is more prolonged, consideration should be given to other diagnostic possibilities. The pleural form of the disease is sometimes difficult to differentiate from acute pulmonary infection or infarction, but the rapid disappearance of signs and symptoms resolves the problem. The joint manifestations may be more prolonged than other forms of FMF, and differentiation from septic arthritis, gout, and acute rheumatoid disease may be necessary. The erythema is sometimes difficult to differentiate from superficial thrombophlebitis or cellulitis.

Whether or not the patient is of the appropriate ethnic group, the most difficult diagnostic problem in FMF is the patient who presents with fever alone. In this situation, an extensive diagnostic work-up for fever of unknown origin may be required. Fortunately, such patients are rare and all eventually develop serosal involvement. Until specific diagnostic tests for FMF are available, patients with recurrent fever but without signs of inflammation of one of the serosal membranes should not be categorized as having FMF.

PROGNOSIS. The prognosis of the patient with FMF varies greatly according to the country in which he lives. In the United States, the prognosis for long life is excellent. Despite the severity of the symptoms during some acute attacks, most patients are remarkably free of any debilitation during the intervals between attacks. With encouragement and an understanding of their disease, most FMF patients lead fairly normal lives. The greatest hazard to patients is prolonged periods of hospitalization due to erroneous diagnoses or failure to understand the disease. The liberal and injudicious use of narcotics for analgesia in these patients can lead to major psychologic and health problems. Establishment of a reasonable doctor-patient relationship and education of the patient will avoid this hazard. In the United States, the prognosis of patients with FMF does not seem to be different from that of patients with other chronic nonfatal illnesses. Death usually results from causes unrelated to the underlying disease.

The complication of amyloidosis in Israel, parts of North Africa, Turkey, and other parts of the Middle East, makes the prognosis quite different from that in America. Approximately 25 percent of FMF patients in Israel are known to have amyloidosis, and this complication usually leads to death. Because a majority of patients under observation in Israel are under forty years of age, it has been suggested that fatal amyloidosis may eventually occur in nearly all patients. This would explain the rarity of older patients in that area.

TREATMENT. Many forms of therapy have been tried in FMF, but no specific or uniformly effective therapeutic agent or regimen has been found. Antibiotics, hormones, antipyretic and anti-inflammatory agents, immunotherapy, psychotherapy, elimination diets, and many other agents and programs have been attempted. Chloroquine and phenylbutazone have been reported to be successful in treating FMF, but other investigators have failed to substantiate these findings. Adrenal cortical steroids have been used extensively to suppress some of the signs of inflammation, but attacks recur upon steroid withdrawal. In fact, some patients have noted increased numbers of attacks while taking corticosteroids. Symptomatic therapy and support are all that can be offered to FMF patients. Narcotics should be avoided whenever possible.

ETIOCHOLANOLONE AND THE PYROGENIC STEROIDS

In 1957, Kappas et al. reported that certain 5 β-H, C-19 steroids of endogenous human origin would induce inflammation and fever when administered to human volunteers. Etiocholanolone was the prototype of this group of hormone metabolites. Shortly thereafter, Bondy and his colleagues reported high levels of plasma unconjugated etiocholanolone in association with fever in two patients. Since that time, much has been written about the possible role of these steroids in the pathogenesis of certain recurrent fevers of unexplained etiology, including FMF. It is for this reason that special mention should be made of these compounds.

There is no question that many C-19, C-21, C-24 steroids with a 5-β-H configuration are potent inducers of fever, inflammation, granulocytosis, and other biologic effects when they are administered to man. Despite these observations, there is considerable doubt that these compounds play a role in human disease. Investigators have been hampered by the lack of a sensitive and reproducible method for detection of minute concentrations in biologic fluids. Nevertheless, the potential importance of compounds such as etiocholanolone in human febrile disease should not be disregarded until such techniques are at hand. When precise methodology is available, some of these endogenous human products may turn out to be important not only in the pathogenesis of FMF but in other conditions of unknown etiology which are characterized by fever and inflammation. In the light of available data, however, none of these steroids has been shown to cause human disease or its symptoms; to assign a pathogenetic role to them at this time leads to confusion and tends to impede the search for the etiology of these diseases.

REFERENCES

Bondy, P. K., G. L. Cohn, and P. B. Gregory: Etiocholanolone Fever, Medicine, 44:249, 1965.

Ehrenfeld, E. N., M. Eliakim, and M. Rachmilewitz: Recurrent Polyserositis (Familial Mediterranean Fever; Periodic Disease). A Report of Fifty-five Cases, Am. J. Med., 31:107, 1961.

Heller, H., E. Sohar, and L. Sherf: Familial Mediterranean Fever, Arch. Intern. Med., 102:50, 1958.

Kappas, A., and R. H. Palmer: Thermogenic Properties of Steroids, in "Methods in Hormone Research," vol. 4, R. I. Dorfman (Ed.), New York, Academic Press, Inc., 1965.

Reimann, H. A.: "Periodic Diseases," Philadelphia, F. A. Davis Company, 1963.

Siegal, S.: Familial Paroxysmal Polyserositis. Analysis of Fifty Cases, Am. J. Med., 36:893, 1964.

Sohar, E., J. Gafni, M. Pras, and H. Heller: Familial Mediterranean Fever, Am. J. Med., 43:227, 1967.

Wolff, S. M., H. R. Kimball, S. Perry, R. Root, and A. Kappas: The Biological Properties of Etiocholanolone, Ann. Intern. Med. 67:1268, 1967.

257 MIDLINE GRANULOMA
Lawrence E. Shulman

DEFINITION. This peculiar condition, also known as *lethal midline granuloma* or *granuloma gangraenescens*, is characterized by progressive destruction of the soft tissues and bony structures of the face, terminating almost invariably in death after several months or a few years of illness. It occurs mostly in young adults and the middle-aged, and is more common in men. The first case was described by McBride in 1897, and since then more than 200 cases have been reported, mostly in the otolaryngologic literature.

ETIOLOGY AND PATHOLOGY. Not only is the cause of midline granuloma unknown, but the category of disease in which it belongs is uncertain. There is disagreement as to whether it is primarily (1) vascular or allergic, (2) neoplastic, or (3) infectious. Only a few complete autopsy studies have been reported. In half of them, lesions have been found in skin, lungs, and mesenteric lymph nodes as well as the face.

Histologically, the lesions of midline granuloma vary from case to case and also from one area to another in the individual case. The most common finding in the facial lesion is chronic inflammation. In the face and elsewhere there are focal areas of necrosis and necrotic small blood vessels, often containing granular thrombi, suggesting that the process is primarily vascular. The vascular lesions, however, differ from those of polyarteritis nodosa because inflammatory cells are absent. Some areas contain large numbers of cells of varying sizes with large, pale, multilobulated nuclei, simulating Hodgkin's disease and mycosis fungoides. In other areas, hyperchromatic nuclei and numerous mitotic figures resemble those seen in undifferentiated tumors.

CLINICAL FEATURES. Midline granuloma begins with a prodromal period of months to years of nasal obstruction and discharge, at first mucoid and later purulent. During this time, the patient is usually thought to have allergic rhinitis or sinusitis. Progressive inflammation and ulceration follow. The first ulcerations are found in the nasal septum, the mucosa or skin of the alae nasi, or the center of the palate. The lesions invade underlying cartilage and bone, giving rise to septal or palatal perforations. The process spreads by local extension to involve the rest of the nose, paranasal sinuses, eyes, mouth, pharynx, and larynx. Eventually, the structures of the midface are totally destroyed by erosion. Gradually, the functions of sight, speech, and ventilation are impaired or lost. The end result is the formation of a large cavity, founded above by the frontal bone and superior aspect of the orbits and below by the mandible, which is never affected.

During periods of activity, and especially preterminally, the patient becomes febrile. Usually the fever does not respond to chemotherapy appropriate for the secondary bacterial infection which is almost always present. Moreover, even in the presence of obvious pyogenic infection, the patient often fails to develop leukocytosis and during the later stages may become chronically leukopenic. Another curious feature is the absence of cervical lymphadenopathy during periods of active inflammation and progression of the disease. A few patients show red, raised, indurated areas on the skin of the legs and abdomen, resembling those of erythema nodosum clinically and histologically. There is no anemia, and the bone marrow and serum proteins are normal. Microbiologic investigations have consistently failed to detect a specific virus, bacterium, or fungus.

The course of the disease varies greatly; some cases last for more than a decade with long periods of quiescence, and others are fulminant, ending fatally after a few months. Death usually results from meningitis, pneumonia, inanition, or massive hemorrhage. Rarely, the disease may be nonfatal.

DIAGNOSIS. During the early phases of midline granuloma it is important to rule out several specific nasal and facial conditons, many of which are treatable. These include leprosy, syphilis, yaws (gangosa), tuberculosis (lupus vulgaris), glanders, leishmaniasis, blastomycosis, and coccidioidomycosis; chromate poisoning; lupus erythematosus; and also lymphomas, mycosis fungoides, and other malignant tumors. Midline granuloma is differentiated from Wegener's granulomatosis by absence of generalized arteritis and glomerulonephritis. Early in the disease, the differential diagnosis between these two may be difficult. Noma is readily distinguished by its being largely restricted to children and involving the cheeks and mouth but not the nose.

TREATMENT. No effective therapy for midline granuloma has been found. The disease progresses despite administration of antibiotics or adrenocortical steroids. A few early reports of benefit following radiotherapy have not been substantiated by further experience. Recent encouraging reports of benefit from immunosuppressive agents, often with concomitant corticosteroids, require confirmation. Radical surgical excision is no more effective than conservative debridement. Various prostheses designed to maintain the integrity of the normal facial passages are helpful both functionally and cosmetically.

REFERENCES

Edgerton, M. T., and J. D. Desprez: Lethal Midline Granuloma of the Face, Brit. J. Plast. Surg., 9:200, 1956.

James, A. E., Jr.: Malignant Lymphoma as Cause of Midline Granuloma, A.M.A. Arch. Inter. Med., 115:200, 1965.

Pardo-Castello, V., F. L. Blanco, and R. Rivera del Sol: Granuloma Crangraenescens, Southern Med. J., 46:149, 1953.

Spear, G. S., and W. G. Walker, Jr.; Lethal Midline Granuloma (Granuloma Grangraenescens) at Autopsy, Bull. Johns Hopkins Hosp., 99:313, 1956.

Index

Index

Boldface page numbers refer to the principal discussion of a subject. Under a general category the subentries for specific conditions may refer to the principal discussion only, and more information will be found under the name of the condition. See muscle diseases and muscular dystrophy.

Friedländer bacilli (*see Klebsiella pneumoniae*)
Friedreich's ataxia, **1724**, 1832
heart disease in, 1234
Frigidity, 280
Froehlich's syndrome, 434
brain tumor and, 1782
Frommel-Chiari syndrome, 431, **565**
Frontal lobe ataxia, gait, 134
Frostbite, 701
"Frozen shoulder," 1954
Fructosuria, 541
FSH (*see* Follicle-stimulating hormone)
FTA (*see* Fluorescent treponemal antibody test)
Fuadin (stibophen) for schistosomiasis, 1059
Fugues, hysterical, 1866–1867
Fungizone (*see* Amphotericin B)
Fungous infections, **906–921**
pathogenesis, 906
skin, 1987–1990
tuberculosis confused with, 879
Funnel chest (pectus excavatum), 1301
FUO (*see* Fever, of unknown origin)
Furadantin (*see* Nitrofurantoin)
Furosemide for heart disease, 1141
Furuncles (boils), 780
Fusospirochetal infections, 847–848

Gaisbock's syndrome, 1642
Gait, **131–134**
athetotic, 133
in beriberi, 406–407
cerebellar, 125, 132
in cerebellar ataxia, 132, 133, 1829
in cerebral palsy, 1842–1843
choreic, 133
drunken, 133–134
dystonic, 133
examination of, 131, 1690
festinating, 132–133, 1826
in Friedreich's ataxia, 1724
frontal lobe ataxia, 134
in Huntington's chorea, 1821
hysterical, 134, 1867
in kuru, 983
labyrinthine function and, 131
in muscular dystrophy, 133, 1906
in Parkinson's disease, 1826
senile, 134
spastic (hemiplegic and paraplegic), 132
staggering, 133–134
steppage (drop-foot, equine), 133
in tabes dorsalis, 891
in vertigo, 129
waddling, 133
Galactorrhea, 431
Galactosemia, 580, **628–629**, 1848
liver disorders, 1563
Galactosylceramidoses, 636–637
Galactosylsulfatidosis, 636–637
Gallbladder disorders, **1565–1574**
cancer, 1567, 1574
cholecystitis: acute, 1567, 1570
chronic, 1567, 1570–1571

Gallbladder disorders:
cholecystitis: infections, 802, 1574
congenital abnormalities, 1574
gallstones (*see* Gallstones)
hydrops, 1572
pain, 46–47, 1566
polyps, 1574
postcholecystectomy syndrome, 1572–1573
radiologic diagnosis, 1567–1569
rupture, 1574
symptoms, 1566–1567
Gallop:
in aortic stenosis, 1193
in heart failure, 1136
presystolic (atrial), 1083, 1084
protodiastolic, 1084
Gallstones (cholelithiasis), 1569–1570
in anemia, 1616
biliary colic and, 1566, 1569–1571
ileus, 1571–1572
pancreatitis and, 1578–1579, 1584
radiologic studies, 1567–1569
treatment, 1570, 1572
after vagotomy, 1458
Gambian sleeping sickness, 1037–1039
Gamma aminobutyric acid (GABA), 169
Gamma-globulins, **351–356**
disorders of, 354–355
γA, 352
congenital absence of, 351
γG, 348, 352–353
in virus diseases, 942
γM, 942
impaired cellular immunity and, 349–350
properties, 352
structure, 348, 352–354
in treatment of chickenpox, 994
of immunologic deficiency diseases, 350–351
of measles, 986, 987
of pertussis, 824
of rubella, 988
(*See also* Agammaglobulinemia; Hypogammaglobulinemia; Immunoglobulins)
Gamma rays, 714
Gamstorp's disease (adynamia episodica hereditaria), 1914
Ganglioneuroma, mediastinal, 1347
Ganglionic blocking agents, 1258–1262
(*See also* Adrenergic blocking agents)
Ganglions:
basal (*see* Basal ganglions)
dorsal root, pain in extremities and, 80
geniculate, 1716
Ganglioside lipoidosis (*see* Tay-Sachs disease)
Gangliosidoses, 636
generalized, 1823
(*See also* Amaurotic familial idiocy)
Gangosa, 899
Gangrene:
anaerobic streptococcus and, 794
of feet, 1270

Gangrene:
of feet: in diabetes, 537–538
gas (*see* Gas gangrene)
heat application as cause, 80
in typhus, 933
in vascular disease, 1267, 1269, 1270
Ganser's syndrome, 1867
Gantrisin (sulfisoxazole), 740, 741
Garamycin (*see* Gentamicin)
Gardner's syndrome, 1995
Gargoylism (Hunter-Hurler syndrome), 1823
dwarfism in, 1839
genetics, 19
Gas (gases):
blood, measurement, 1283
intestinal, 242, 248
Gas exchange in respiration, 1279–1280
Gas gangrene (clostridial myositis), 861–862
diagnosis, 863
treatment, 863–864
Gas inhalation:
lung disorders, 1322–1323
poisoning, 649, 661
Gasoline poisoning, 659
Gastrectomy:
anemia after, 1458, 1597
complications, 1457–1458
malabsorption syndrome, 1458, 1476–1477
postgastrectomy syndrome (dumping syndrome), 1457–1458
Gastric juice (*see* Gastric secretion)
Gastric lavage, 645, 678, 683
contraindications, 649, 651
Gastric mucosa:
prolapse, 1466
Gastric resection for peptic ulcer, 1450
Gastric retention, 1465–1466
Gastric retention, 1465–1466
Gastric secretion:
control, 1443
diagnostic studies, 1435
mechanism, 1442–1443
in peptic ulcer, 1445, 1451
Gastric ulcer, 1450–1452
(*See also* Peptic ulcer)
Gastric varices, bleeding from, 252
Gastritis, **1463–1465**
acute, 1463
antral, 1465
benign giant hypertrophic, 1464
chronic, 1463–1464
corrosive, 1464
emphysematous, 1464–1465
hemorrhage from, 252, 1463
phlegmonous, 1464
postoperative, 1457
specific, 1464–1465
treatment, 1464
vomiting in, 246, 1463
Gastroenteritis:
appendicitis confused with, 1497
Escherichia coli infection, 803
salmonella, 817–818
viral, 249, **966**
Gastroileal reflex, 247
Gastrointestinal disorders, **1433–1518**
in Addison's disease, 507